Fig. A1-3 Verruca vulgaris. The skin lesions are firm, skin-colored papules 1 to 10 mm or rarely larger, with a hyperkeratotic surface and with vegetations. There are often characteristic ''red dots'' (thrombosing capillary loops) seen with a hand lens (see Chap. 196).

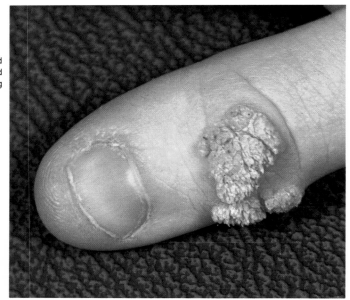

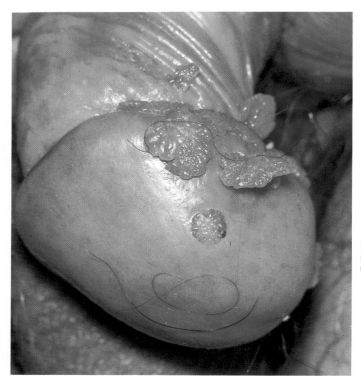

Fig. A1-4 Condylomata acuminata. The skin lesions are skin-colored, pinhead, soft papules or cauliflower-like masses that are filiform or sessile (especially on the penis) (see Chaps. 196 and 200).

Fig. A1-5 Psoriasis vulgaris. The skin lesions are papules and plaques with marked silvery-white scaling, sharply marginated, and/or pustules. Erythroderma is a rare form of psoriasis (see Chap. 42).

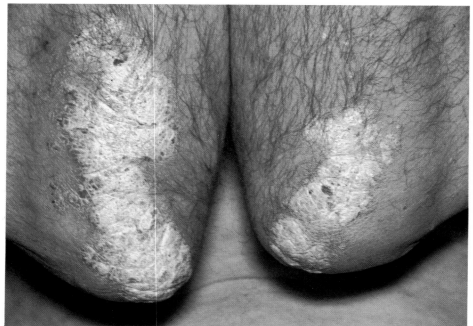

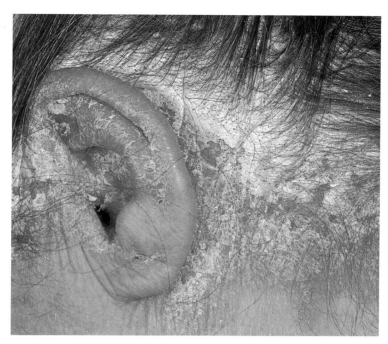

Fig. A1-6 Psoriasis of the scalp. The plaques often have thick, adherent, very white scales; fissures and exudation are common, especially behind the ears. There is usually little or no hair loss despite marked skin involvement. Lichenification is often superimposed on the basic psoriatic lesion (see Chap. 42).

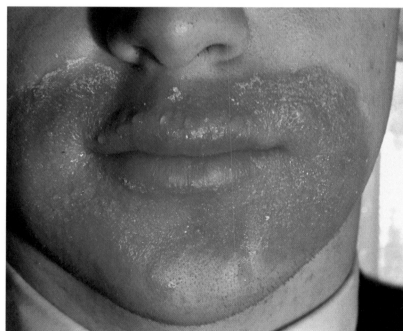

Fig. A1-7 Contact eczematous dermatitis. The skin lesions in acute contact dermatitis consist of irregular, poorly outlined patches of erythema and edema on which are superimposed closely spaced, nonumbilicated vesicles, punctate erosions exuding serum, and crusts (see Chap. 117).

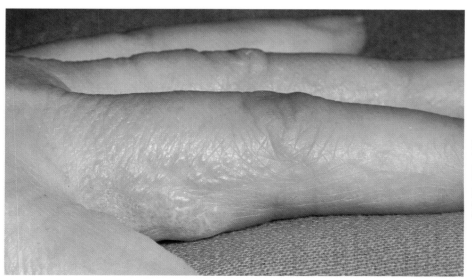

Fig A1-8 Pompholyx (dyshidrotic eczema). The skin lesions are vesicles, usually small (1.0 mm), deep-seated, and appearing like "tapioca" in clusters. Occasionally bullae are present, especially on the feet. Later there is scaling, lichenification, painful fissures, and erosions (see Chap. 116).

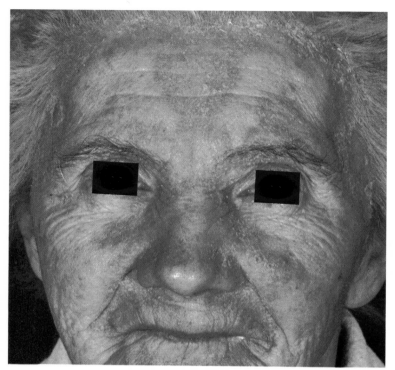

Fig. A1-9   Seborrheic dermatitis. The skin lesions consist of white or yellowish-red, often greasy, scaling macules and papules of varying size, rather sharply marginated. ''Sticky'' crusts and fissures are common when the external ear and scalp are involved (weeping) (see Chap. 84).

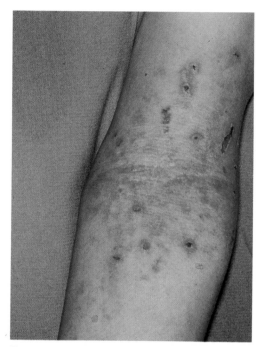

Fig. A1-10   Atopic eczematous dermatitis. The skin lesions include papular and lichenified plaques, excoriations, erosions, dry and wet crusts, and cracks (fissures) (see Chap. 119).

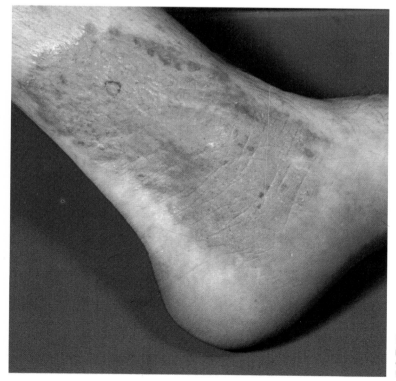

Fig. A1-11   Localized lichenification (lichen simplex). The skin lesion is a solid plaque of lichenification; scaling is minimal except in nuchal lichen simplex (see Chap. 119).

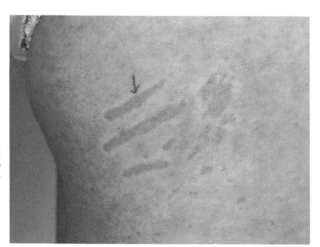

Fig. A1-12 Urticaria. The skin lesions in cholinergic urticaria consist of small (1 to 2 mm) papules (wheals). In common urticaria there are small papules (1.0 cm) to large edematous plaques (8.0 cm). In angioedema, skin-colored enlargement of a portion of the face (eyelids, lips, tongue) or extremity may occur (see Chap. 105).

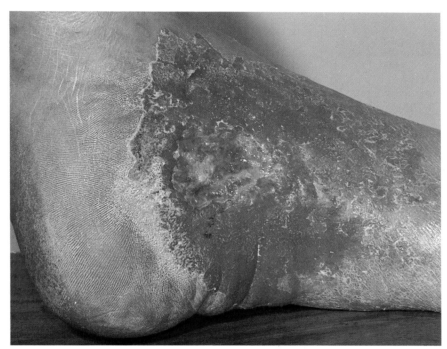

Fig. A1-13 Stasis dermatitis and ulcer. The skin lesions comprise multiple, irregularly demarcated shallow ulcerations with a yellow base surrounded by an erythematous oozing area (see Chap. 171).

Fig. A1-14 Tinea pedis is a superficial infection caused by dermatophytes (fungi). It is characterized by scaling, maceration, fissures, vesicles or bullae, and erosions. The fissures can be an important portal of entry for streptococci (see Chap. 181).

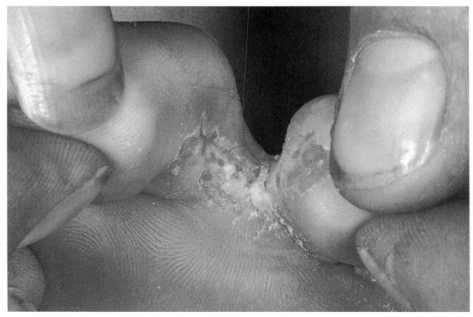

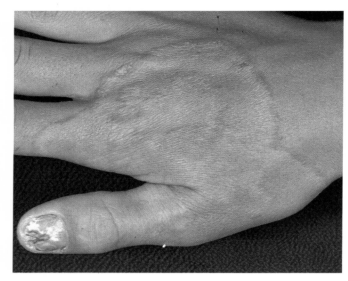

Fig. A1-15 **Tinea manus** on the dorsum of the hand. A large area is less tanned than the surrounding skin and is bordered by a narrow erythematous, slightly indurated, delicate scaling zone. The margin is quite sharp and somewhat polycyclic (see Chap. 181).

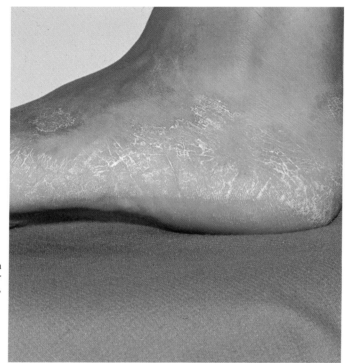

Fig. A1-16 **Tinea pedis.** The soles, sides of the feet, and the heels show a faint pink color, and are covered with fine silvery-white scales. The upper border of these areas is irregular. Some of the nails are yellowish, thickened, and cracked (see Chap. 181).

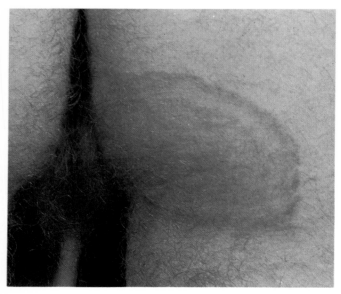

Fig. A1-17 **Tinea cruris.** The skin lesions are plaques with scaling sharp margins with occasional pustules and central clearing (see Chap. 181).

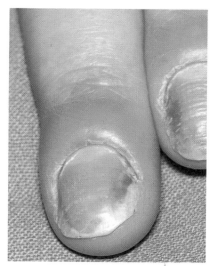

Fig. A1-18 Onychia and paronychia from *Candida albicans.* Redness and swelling of the nail folds. The eponychia are absent. The sides of the nails are yellowish gray and show distal onycholysis and an irregular surface. Paronychia is often erroneously regarded as a pyogenic infection and treated with antibiotics (see Chap. 181).

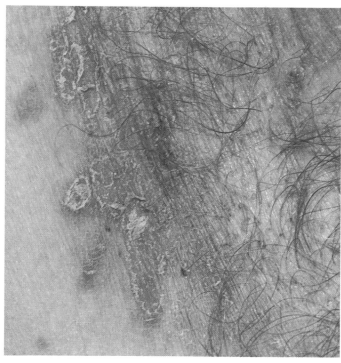

Fig. A1-19 Candidiasis (intertriginous). In the right groin, a nonindurated, fairly sharp but irregularly demarcated erythematous area with easily detachable cigarette-paper-like scaling that follows the borders of the lesion, occasionally circular, resulting in a scaling collar. Outside the main lesion are some smaller similar lesions (satellites) (see Chap. 181).

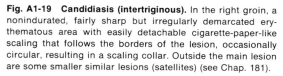

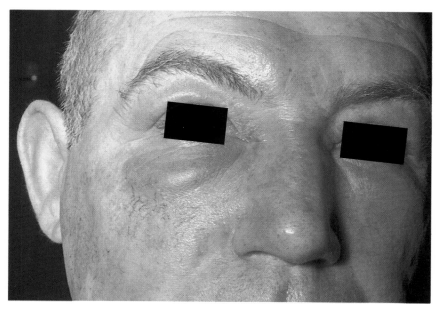

Fig. A1-20 Erysipelas. The skin lesion is usually a bright red plaque, enlarging peripherally with an advancing, elevated, sharp margin. On palpation there is an indurated lesion with "peau d'orange" appearance; warm and tender to touch (see Chap. 176).

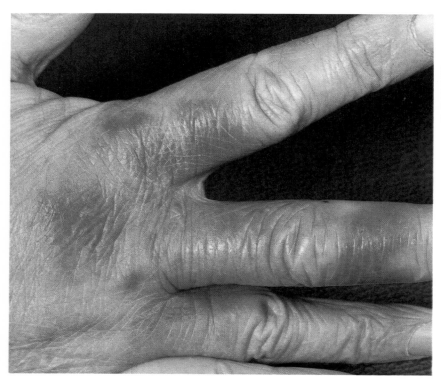

Fig. A1-21 Erysipeloid. Dusky red, sharply demarcated, slightly infiltrated macules, 1 to 3 cm in diameter, irregularly disseminated over the backs of the fingers. Vesicles rarely occur. The lesions are not hot or tender (see Chap. 176).

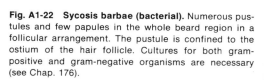

Fig. A1-22 Sycosis barbae (bacterial). Numerous pustules and few papules in the whole beard region in a follicular arrangement. The pustule is confined to the ostium of the hair follicle. Cultures for both gram-positive and gram-negative organisms are necessary (see Chap. 176).

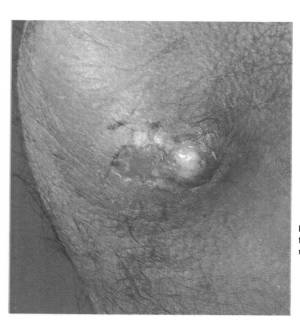

Fig. A1-23 Furuncle. The skin lesion is a tender, hard nodule which may become fluctuant and rupture, forming an ulcer. There is an erythematous halo surrounding the nodule. Furuncles are exquisitely tender and painful (see Chap. 176).

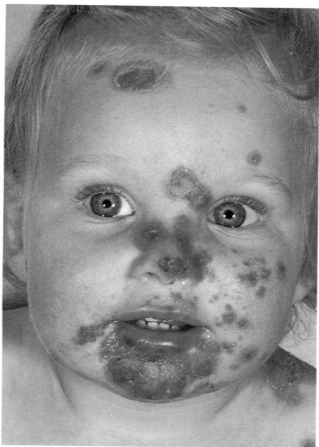

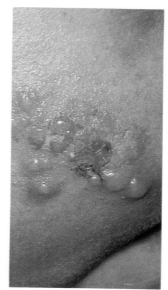

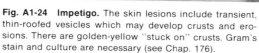

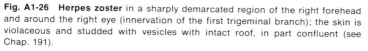

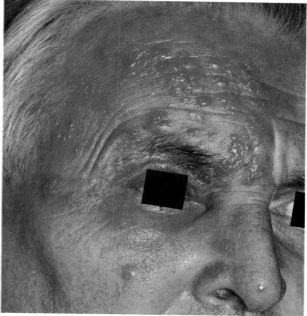

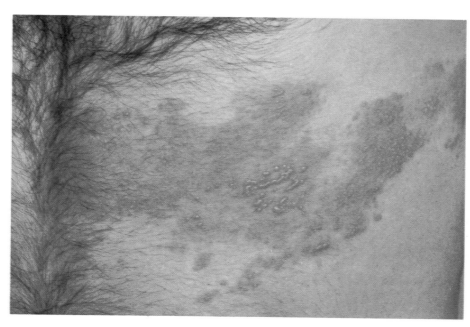

Fig. A1-25 **Herpes simplex** is an acute vesicular eruption of the skin and mucous membrane caused by *Herpesvirus hominis*. Recurrences are common and can be precipitated by fever, sunlight, and other nonspecific events. Note the grouped vesicles and bullae on the erythematous base. The lesion may be linear and be confused with herpes zoster infection. Cultures are sometimes necessary to identify herpes simplex (see Chap. 190).

Fig. A1-24 **Impetigo.** The skin lesions include transient, thin-roofed vesicles which may develop crusts and erosions. There are golden-yellow "stuck on" crusts. Gram's stain and culture are necessary (see Chap. 176).

Fig. A1-26 **Herpes zoster** in a sharply demarcated region of the right forehead and around the right eye (innervation of the first trigeminal branch); the skin is violaceous and studded with vesicles with intact roof, in part confluent (see Chap. 191).

Fig. A1-27 **Herpes zoster.** Illustrated in the region of the ninth and tenth ribs is a patchy red area comprised of clusters of vesicles. Localization of herpes zoster to the thoracic area occurs in 50 percent of the patients (see Chap. 191).

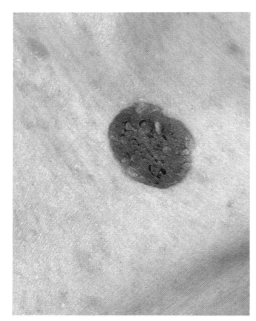

Fig. A1-28 Seborrheic keratosis appears in middle life and may be on the exposed or unexposed areas but is especially common on the trunk. The lesions are irregularly round or oval, flattopped papules or plaques that seem "stuck" on the skin. The margins are sharp, and the surface is often warty or consists of multiple tiny projections (vegetation). In fair-skinned persons, the lesions are light brown at first but, enlarging, become more heavily pigmented and may be confused with malignant melanoma.

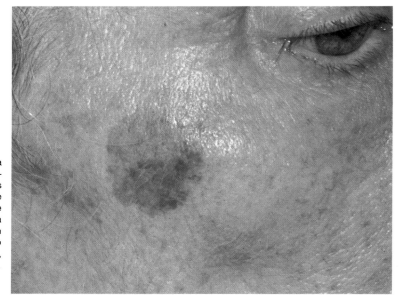

Fig. A1-29 Solar lentigo occurs as a single macule or as a group of isolated, sharply circumscribed macules on the exposed areas, especially on the dorsal surfaces of the hands and arms and on the forehead and cheeks. The macules are usually light yellowish brown, but may be dark brown; the color is somewhat variegated rather than uniform as it is in a café au lait macule. Rarely, dark brown areas develop in these lesions, and then the condition is called *lentigo maligna*, which may slowly develop, over a period of years, into a melanoma (lentigo maligna melanoma) (see Chap. 81).

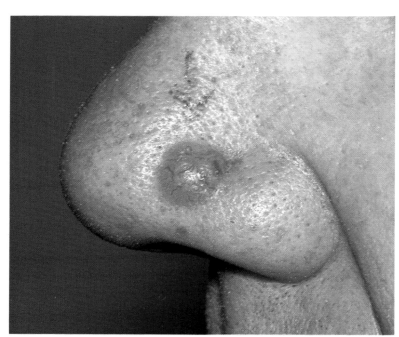

Fig. A1-30 Basal cell carcinoma. The skin lesion is a papule or nodule which is translucent, pearly, and shiny. An ulcer (often covered with a crust) may occur in the center of the nodule. There is usually telangiectasia. The lesion is hard, not firm (see Chap. 76).

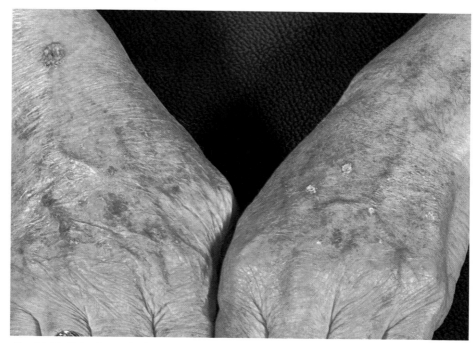

Fig. A1-31 Solar keratosis. The skin lesion consists of an adherent, hyperkeratotic scale, which is removed with difficulty and pain. There may be nodular lesions. A rough, coarse sandpaper-like "feel" is evident in most lesions (see Chap. 74).

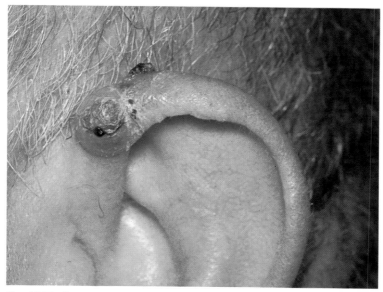

Fig. A1-32 Squamous cell carcinoma. The skin lesion is an indurated papule, plaque, or hard nodule with an adherent, keratotic scale, often eroded, crusted, and ulcerated (see Chap. 75).

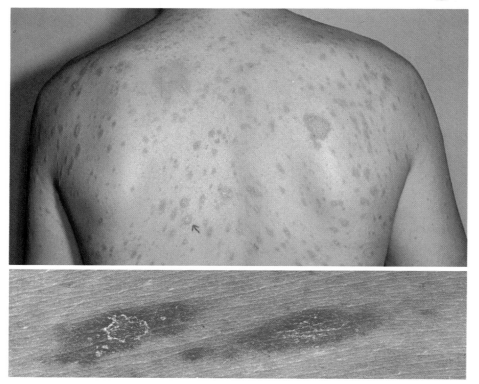

Fig. A1-33 Pityriasis rosea. The first skin lesion is often a single herald plaque, 2 to 5 cm in diameter, bright red, with a fine scale. There is an exanthem with fine-scaling macules and very slightly raised papules with a highly characteristic marginal collarette, as illustrated in the lower picture (see Chap. 85).

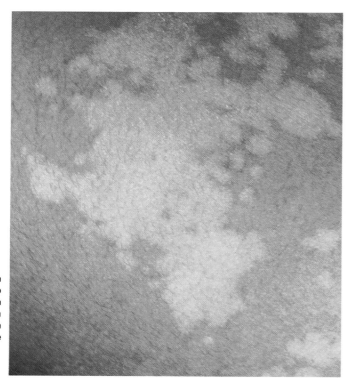

Fig. A1-34 Tinea (pityriasis) versicolor is a relatively common disorder occurring primarily on the trunk and appearing in two forms, as scattered, 3- to 5-mm, very slightly scaling, brown macules, or as whitish macules that may be confused with vitiligo. The fungal spores and hyphae can be demonstrated on direct examination of the scales using potassium hydroxide (see Chaps. 79 and 181).

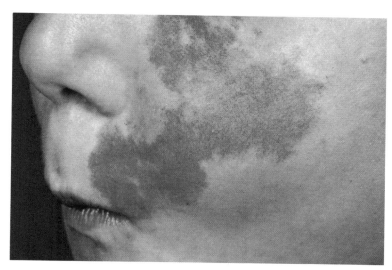

Fig. A1-35 Capillary hemangioma, port-wine stain, nevus flammeus. These vascular hamartomas are irregularly shaped, red or violaceous macules that are present at birth and never disappear; the pigmentation reflects permanent dilatation of capillaries in the dermis (see Chap. 95).

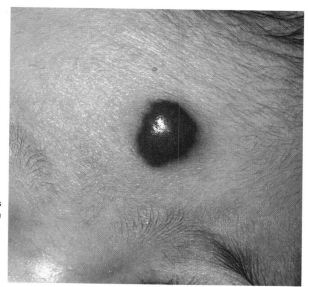

Fig. A1-36 Strawberry nevus (angiomatous nevus). An angiomatous nevus is a soft, bright red, vascular nodule that develops at birth or soon after birth and disappears spontaneously by the fifth year (see Chap. 95).

CUTANEOUS MANIFESTATIONS OF DISEASES IN OTHER ORGAN SYSTEMS

Klaus Wolff and Thomas B. Fitzpatrick

Each of the following disorders is an example of either multisystem disease with skin manifestations or of serious disorders involving the skin that can be potentially fatal. The skin lesions serve as signals indicating disease that may hold serious implications for the patient. They are as important and as specific as the discovery of palpable lymph nodes or an abnormal CT scan.

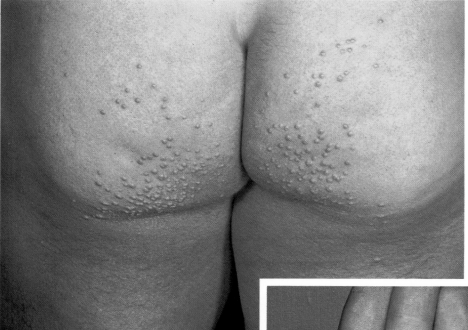

a

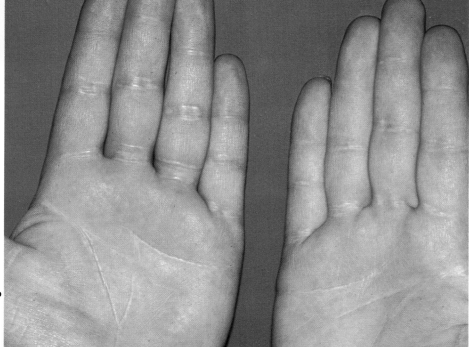

b

Fig. A2-1 **(a) Xanthomata papuloeruptiva in type IV hyperlipoproteinemia and diabetes.** There are disseminated, discrete, yellow papules, 1 to 3 mm in diameter, on the buttocks. The yellow papules are often surrounded by a red halo. **(b) Xanthomata striata palmaria in type III hyperlipoproteinemia.** The creases of the palms are yellow. The palmar creases of the metacarpophalangeal and interphalangeal joints show elevated yellow streaks.

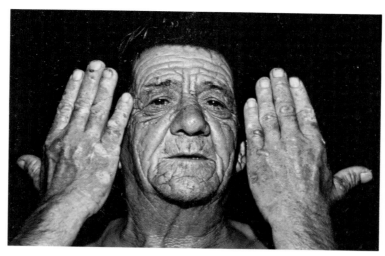

Fig. A2-2   Porphyria cutanea tarda. Violaceous suffusion in the periorbital skin is evident. There are bullae, erosions and pink atrophic scars at sites of previous bullae on the dorsa of the hands.

Fig. A2-3   Necrobiosis lipoidica. The lesion often begins as a small, dusky red, elevated nodule with a sharp border. It slowly enlarges, becomes flattened and eventually depressed as the dermis becomes atrophic. The color becomes brownish yellow except for the border, which may remain reddened. Delicate vessels can be seen through the atrophic epidermis.

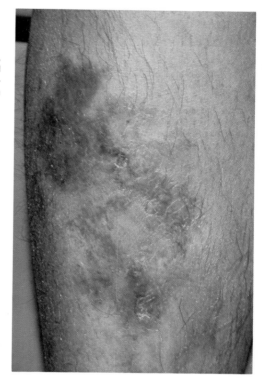

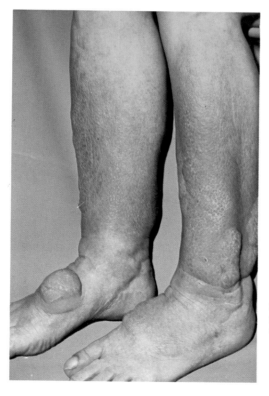

Fig. A2-4   Pretibial myxedema. This illustration exhibits bilateral, asymptomatic, raised, firm nodules that are pink, flesh colored, or purplish brown. The overlying epidermis is smooth but can become verrucous.

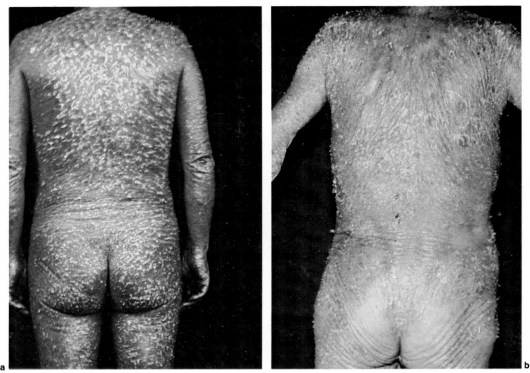

a   b

Fig. A2-12   (a) Exfoliative erythroderma (psoriasis). There is uniform redness, infiltration, thickening of the skin, and massive desquamation. The diagnosis in this patient was established by the patient's previous history of typical psoriasis. **(b) Exfoliative erythroderma (cutaneous T-cell lymphoma).** As in psoriasis, there is generalized redness, thickening of the skin, and desquamation. Generalized lymphadenopathy, circulating abnormal T cells, and skin histopathology showing T-cell lymphoma established the diagnosis of Sézary's syndrome.

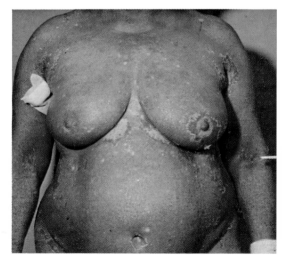

a

Fig. A2-13   (a) Exfoliative erythroderma (pityriasis rubra pilaris). Generalized redness and thickening of skin here results from the coalescence of minute, slightly scaling papules. Sparing of small, well-defined areas of normal skin (at the border of which individual papules can still be discerned), diffuse hyperkeratosis of the palms and soles, pronounced scaling of the scalp, and the histopathology established the diagnosis. **(b) Exfoliative erythroderma (drug-induced).** Diffuse redness of skin and focal scaling result from the confluence of a macular rash. The history of sulfonamide medication five days prior to the onset of the rash and of a similar eruption following sulfonamides at a previous occasion, involvement of the mucous membranes, and the histopathology established the diagnosis.

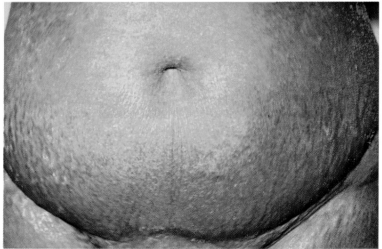

b

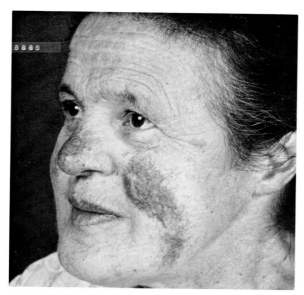

Fig. A2-14 Sarcoidosis. Purple infiltrated plaques on the face.

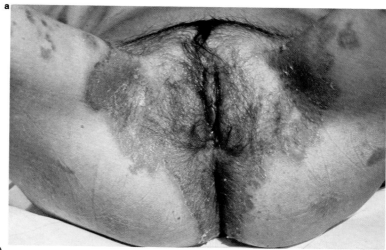

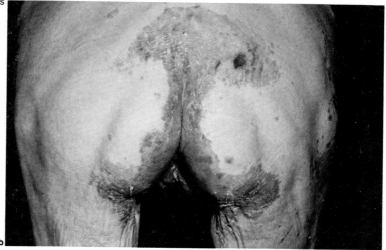

Fig. A2-15 Glucagonoma (a) and **acquired zinc deficiency (b).** Circinate and gyrate areas of blistering, erosion, and maceration. The eruption is often mistaken for psoriasis or mucocutaneous moniliasis.

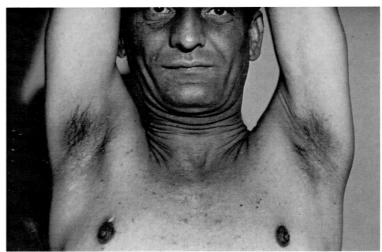

Fig. A2-16 Acanthosis nigricans (malignant form).
Confluent, hyperpigmented, velvety, hyperkeratotic
plaques involving the axillae.

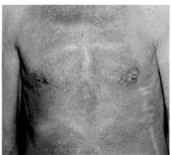

Fig. A2-17 Carcinoid showing the effect of stroking. In contrast to the
flushing that occurs in other disorders, the flush in carcinoid is typically a
panorama of colors, ranging from bizarre pinkish orange to bright red to
violaceous to blanching white. The flush (which lasts only a few minutes)
spreads from the face to the neck, shoulders, chest, and arms.

DIFFERENTIAL DIAGNOSIS OF RASHES IN THE ACUTELY ILL FEBRILE PATIENT AND IN LIFE-THREATENING DISEASES

Thomas B. Fitzpatrick and
Richard A. Johnson

The sudden appearance of a rash and fever is frightening for the patient. Medical advice is immediately sought and often in the emergency units of hospitals; about 10 percent of all patients seeking emergency medical care have a dermatologic problem.

The diagnosis of an acute rash with a fever is a clinical challenge. Rarely in clinical practice do physicians have to "lean" on their eyes as much as when confronted by an acutely ill patient with fever and a skin eruption. If a diagnosis is not established promptly in certain patients (e.g., those having septicemia), life-saving treatment may be delayed unnecessarily.

The cutaneous findings alone may be diagnostic before confirmatory laboratory data are available. As in the problems of the acute abdomen, the results of some laboratory tests, such as microbiologic cultures, and serologic titers, may be available only after days to weeks. On the basis of a differential diagnosis, appropriate therapy—whether antibiotics, corticosteroids, or treatment of symptoms—may be started. Furthermore, prompt diagnosis and isolation of the patient with a contagious disease prevents spread to other persons, which may have serious consequences. For example, varicella in adults can rarely be fatal. Contagious diseases presenting with rash and fever as the major findings include *viral infections* (varicella, vaccinia, variola, herpes simplex, measles, rubella, enterovirus and adenovirus infections), *bacterial infections* (streptococcal, staphylococcal, meningococcal), and *secondary syphilis*.

The physical diagnosis of skin eruptions is a discipline based on accurate observation, with precise identification of the type of skin lesion being essential (see Chap. 4). The physician must not only identify and classify the *type* of skin lesion but look for additional morphologic clues such as: the *configuration* (annular? iris?) of the individual lesion; the *arrangement* of the lesions (zosteriform? linear?); the *distribution pattern* (exposed areas? centripetal or centrifugal? mucous membranes?). In the differential diagnosis of exanthems it is important to determine by history the *site* of the rash, *first appearance* (the rash of Rocky Mountain spotted fever characteristically appears first on the wrists and ankles), and the *temporal evolution* of the rash (measles spreads from head to toes in a period of 3 days while the rash of rubella spreads from head to toes in 1 day and has largely disappeared in 3 days).

Although there is some overlap, the differential diagnostic possibilities may be grouped into three main categories according to the type of lesion (see Table A3-1).

Table A3-1   Rash and fever in the acutely ill patient: diagnosis according to type of lesion

Diseases	Macules or papules	Vesicles, bullae, or pustules	Purpuric macules, papules, or vesicles
Drug hypersensitivity	x	x	x
Systemic lupus erythematosus	x	x	x
Dermatomyositis	x		
Serum sickness (manifested only as wheals)	x		
Urticaria, acute (viral hepatitis)	x		
Allergic vasculitis (manifested as urticaria)	x		x
Hypereosinophilic syndrome	x		x
Erythema marginatum	x		
Erythema multiforme	x	x	
Acquired immune deficiency syndrome	x		x
Toxic epidermal necrolysis	x	x	
Staphylococcal scalded-skin syndrome	x	x	
Staphylococcal toxic shock syndrome	x	x	
Kawasaki disease (mucocutaneous lymph node syndrome)	x		

Table A3-1   Rash and fever in the acutely ill patient: diagnosis according to type of lesion (continued)

Diseases	Macules or papules	Vesicles, bullae, or pustules	Purpuric macules, papules, or vesicles
Scarlet fever	x		
Erysipelas	x	x	x
Erythema infectiosum (fifth disease)	x		
Measles (rubeola)	x		
German measles (rubella)	x		
Enterovirus infections (echo, Coxsackie)	x	x	x
Adenovirus infections	x		
Pityriasis rosea	x		
Chickenpox (varicella)	x	x	
Generalized herpes zoster		x	
Disseminated herpes simplex		x	
Eczema herpeticum		x	
Eczema vaccinatum		x	
Rickettsial diseases:			
Eastern hemisphere spotted fever	x		
Rickettsialpox		x	
Rocky Mountain spotted fever	x	x	x
Typhus, louse-borne ("epidemic")	x		x
Typhus, murine (endemic)	x		
Typhoid fever	x		
Secondary syphilis	x		
Lyme disease (erythema chronicum migrans)	x		
Bacteremias:			
Gonococcemia			x
Meningococcemia	x	x	x
Due to *Pseudomonas aeruginosa*		x	x
Staphylococcal		x	x
Bacterial endocarditis	x	x	x

Laboratory tests available for quick diagnosis

The physician should make use of the following laboratory tests immediately or within 8 h:

1. *Direct smear from the base of a vesicle.* This procedure, known as the *Tzanck test*, is performed by unroofing an intact vesicle, gently scraping the base with a curved scalpel blade, and smearing the contents on a slide. After air drying, the smear is stained with Wright's or Giemsa's stain and examined for multinucleated giant cells (Fig. 4-19). These altered epidermal cells are present in the herpes simplex-herpes zoster-varicella group but are not present in the vaccinia-variola group of viruses.
2. *Gram's stain of aspirates or scraping.* Organisms can be seen in the lesions of typhoid and in acute meningococcemia, and rarely in the skin lesions of gonococcemia.
3. *Dark-field examination.* In the skin lesions of secondary syphilis, repeated examination of papules may show *Treponema pallidum*. This is not reliable in mucous membrane as nonpathogenic organisms

are almost impossible to differentiate from *T. pallidum*.
4. *Biopsy of the skin lesions.* A 3- to 4-mm trephine under local anesthesia is used. In many laboratories this can be processed within 8 h if necessary. A diagnosis can be made in instances of Rocky Mountain spotted fever, systemic lupus erythematosus, erythema multiforme bullosum, toxic epidermal necrolysis, herpes zoster, allergic vasculitis, and some bacteremias.
5. *Blood and urine examinations.* Blood culture, rapid serologic test for syphilis, and LE preparation require 24 h. Examination of urine sediment may reveal red cell casts in allergic vasculitis.

We wish to express our appreciation to M. Fisher, M.D., D. S. Feingold, M.D., T. C. Peebles, M.D., A. N. Weinberg. M.D., N. Fiumara, M.D., and E. S. Murray, M.D., of Boston for their valuable assistance in the preparation of this section and for some of the photographs. We are indebted also to E. G. L. Bywaters, M.B., F.R.C.P., of London and to the National Communicable Disease Center, Atlanta, Georgia, for some of the photographs.

Fig. A3-1 Drug hypersensitivities may be manifested by all three categories of lesions. The main characteristics that differentiate them from other eruptions include: **(1)** a sudden onset; **(2)** a symmetrical, frequently generalized distribution; and **(3)** the bright red color shown here (so characteristic in hue that it is called "drug red"). The lesions occurring in drug reactions are always erythematous and may be only macular, papular (shown here), or urticarial (wheals) (see Chap. 115).

The most common type of drug eruption is urticaria, followed by the exanthematous eruptions, which resemble viral exanthems (measles-like or morbilliform) or scarlet fever (scarlatiniform). Seen less frequently are erythema multiforme, eczematous eruptions, toxic epidermal necrolysis, and drug-induced systemic lupus erythematosus. Infectious mononucleosis also alters reactivity to ampicillin. In series of patients with sore throats who have received ampicillin for presumed streptococcal pharyngitis or tonsillitis, 85 to 100 percent have been reported to have an exanthematous drug eruption. Although rashes do occur with infectious mononucleosis, the frequency without ampicillin is low (3 percent).

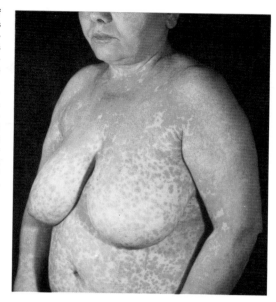

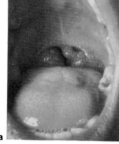

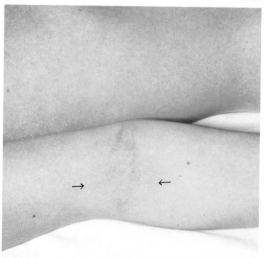

b   a

c

Fig. A3-2 Scarlet fever (scarlatina) is a streptococcal infection with high temperature and a painful tonsillopharyngitis **(a)** with lymphadenopathy or wound sepsis followed by the appearance of a diffuse erythematous rash. The rash is most often produced by the erythrogenic exotoxin elaborated by some strains of group A streptococci. Strains of *S. aureus* can also synthesize an erythrogenic exotoxin and produce a scarlatiniform exanthem. The rash usually appears on the neck first and then rapidly spreads to the trunk and then to the extremities. This total involvement of the body is complete in about 36 h. This diffuse, bright red rash consists of numerous punctate, papular lesions at the site of hair follicles that feel like rough sandpaper. On the face, there are usually no discrete lesions, but there is a marked flushing of the cheeks and forehead that contrasts sharply with the characteristic circumoral pallor. The rash is accentuated in the body folds and the antecubital fossae; the eruption in these locations may become petechial (Pastia's sign) **(b)**. There are often also purpuric macules on the palate **(c)** and uvula. On the tongue, which is usually coated, there are enlarged red fungiform papillae that are found in the first 24 h after the appearance of the rash (this condition is called the "strawberry tongue"). A striking sheetlike desquamation occurs, especially on the palms and soles, as the eruption fades. There is a polymorphonuclear leukocytosis. The diagnosis can be confirmed by throat or wound culture or by a rise in antistreptolysin O titer (see Chap. 176).

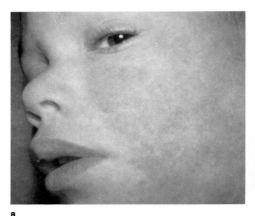

a

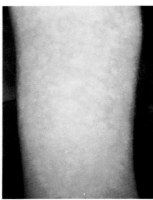

b

Fig. A3-3 Erythema infectiosum (fifth disease) has, as its characteristic feature, a "slapped-face" appearance **(a)** that results from a confluent erythema and edema of the cheeks and occurs with absent or mild prodrome (headache, nausea, musculoskeletal pain); later, an erythematous macular, papular, or urticarial eruption appears on the trunk and extremities. The central clearing of the papular lesions results in a striking rosette and lacelike formation **(b).**

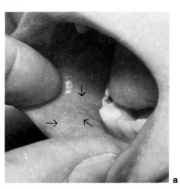

a

Fig. A3-4 Measles (rubeola; morbilli) has a characteristic prodrome of 3 to 4 days that consists of coryza, a striking palpebral conjunctivitis with photophobia, and a "barking" cough. The first lesions appear on the soft palate as blotchy erythema, but the most pathognomonic lesions of the prodrome, if present, are the Koplik spots **(a),** which appear as tiny white lesions surrounded by an erythematous ring ("grains of sand"). Koplik's spots precede the onset of the generalized rash by 1 to 2 days, remain for 2 to 3 days, and are usually heavily clustered on the buccal mucosa opposite the second molars. The purplish red rash on the body appears first behind the ears and over the forehead and then spreads slowly to involve the entire body by the third day: the eruption extends downward over the neck and shoulders and trunk and then distally over the upper and lower extremities; the spread of this rash over the central parts of the trunk **(b)** first is in contrast with that of German measles, which spreads rapidly to involve the entire body in 1 day. The measles rash remains in its original site while it spreads to the extremities, in contrast with the rash in rubella, which disappears from each site as it spreads. The erythematous macular and papular lesions, which were discrete **(c),** become confluent on the face and upper part of the neck, whereas they may remain discrete on the legs. As the rash disappears, it becomes brownish yellow, owing to capillary hemorrhages (see Chap. 186).

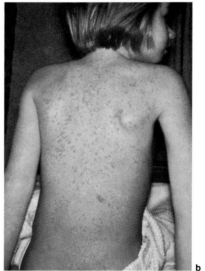

b

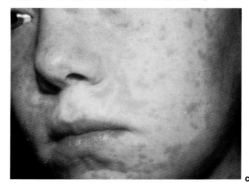

c

Fig. A3-5 German measles (rubella) is characterized by a usually mild prodrome consisting of fever and generalized lymphadenopathy with typical, but not pathognomonic, involvement of the suboccipital, postauricular, and cervical nodes. One to 7 days after the appearance of the lymphadenopathy, the rash appears, involves the entire body within 1 day, and *lasts only 2 to 3 days.* The exanthem begins on the hairline and face as shown here and spreads rapidly to involve the neck, trunk, and extremities, usually within 1 day of onset in contrast with measles, which spreads more slowly. Typical rubella lesions begin as quite discrete macules, but rapidly become rose-pink papules. The rash consists of a generalized eruption of discrete lesions on the first day, fades on the face and becomes confluent on the trunk on the second day, and usually disappears by the third day. In contrast with the rash of measles, the rash of rubella disappears from each site as it spreads and is not associated with desquamation. Synovitis (manifested as arthralgia) of fingers, wrists, knees, and ankles occurs in 40 percent of female adults (see Chap. 185).

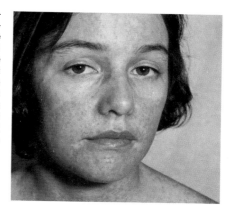

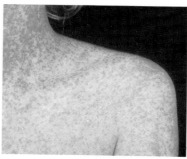

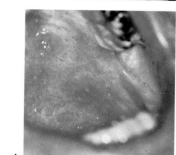

a

b

Fig. A3-6 Enterovirus (Coxsackie A and B, and echo) and adenovirus infections may cause bilaterally symmetrical urticarial eruptions, as well as macular, papular **(a)**, and vesicular eruptions. Purpuric macules resembling those found in meningococcemia may be seen. There may be a vesicular exanthem, especially on the palate **(b)**.

The exanthematous eruption in the febrile patient poses a diagnostic problem. Both viral and drug eruptions appear relatively abruptly, that is, within 24 h. Both types appear symmetrically and centripetally, which suggests a systemic cause rather than a topical or local cause. Concomitant findings such as an exanthem, coryza, pharyngitis, or gastroenteritis are often helpful in distinguishing between viral and drug eruptions. However, often the patient with such a condition has taken a medication such as penicillin, which makes the distinction difficult. Peripheral eosinophilia occurs with drug eruptions and is useful evidence when detected in a differential white blood cell count.

Hand-foot-and-mouth disease is manifested by vesicles, bullae, and pustules, often linear **(c)**, on an erythematous base. They are often painful and are usually found on the fingers and toes **(d)**. There may be an associated vesicular exanthem **(b)**. The causative agent is usually Coxsackie virus A16, although rarely it may be A5 (see Chap. 188).

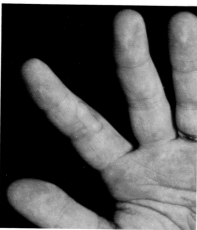

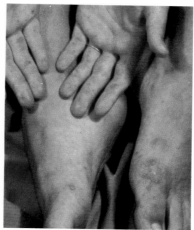

c   d

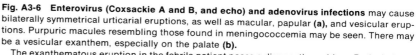

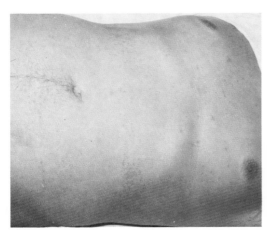

Fig. A3-7 Typhoid fever is manifested in the skin by the appearance, 7 to 10 days after the onset of a high temperature, of the characteristic "rose spots." The lesions occur in 75 percent of patients. These lesions are 1- to 3-mm pink *papules* that blanch on pressure. There are few lesions, usually only 10 to 20, located on the upper part of the abdomen, lower part of the chest, or middle of the back. In the untreated patient, the rose spots usually become brownish as they subside, and they disappear in 3 to 4 days, but other new crops may emerge over the 2 to 3 weeks. Bacteria can sometimes be demonstrated with Gram's stain in preparations from the papules (see Chap. 177).

Fig. A3-8 Secondary syphilis is manifested by generalized, symmetrical copper-colored **(a)** scaling or nonscaling macules and papules of the skin and characteristic desquamative papules of the palms and soles **(b).** Additional findings include annular lesions around facial orifices, mucous patches (small erosions) in the mouth **(c),** moth-eaten alopecia, moist anogenital papules (condylomata lata), iritis. Lymphadenopathy is present in 70 percent of patients, and most often occurs in cervical, occipital, and epitrochlear nodes. A dark-field examination of skin lesions can confirm the diagnosis immediately. Fever is present in only 14 percent of patients, but a sore throat is present in 50 percent of patients (see Chap. 201).

a

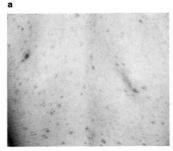

b

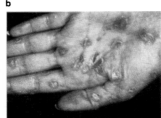

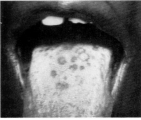

c

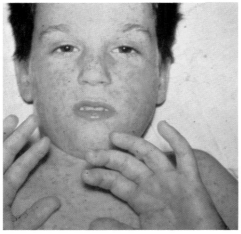

Fig. A3-9 Rocky Mountain spotted fever, secondary to a tick bite, is manifested by a rash that appears on the second to the fourth day of the illness (fever, chills, severe frontal headache, myalgia, and arthralgia). *The eruption first appears on the wrists, ankles, and forearms* as pink macules. After 6 to 18 h, the eruption characteristically (and somewhat uniquely among the acute infections with fever) includes involvement of the palms and soles early in the course of the eruption; of the few acute conditions that involve the palms and soles (drug reactions, secondary syphilis, erythema multiforme), Rocky Mountain spotted fever is by far the most serious because it is a treatable disease, with an overall mortality rate in untreated cases of 20 percent and of 50 percent in older persons. After involving the palms and soles, the eruption extends centrally to the rest of the arms, the thighs, trunk, and face. The eruption, in its early stages, is erythematous and macular, and only after 2 to 4 days does the rash become papular and more deeply red and then purpuric as seen here. It should be repeatedly stressed, however, that early diagnosis may save the patient's life. The most important clues to the diagnosis of Rocky Mountain spotted fever are **(1)** the spreading of the rash to the palms and soles in an acutely ill patient with a fever and **(2)** the history of exposure in an endemic area (Rocky Mountain area and the Atlantic coastal states from Massachusetts to Florida). Skin biopsy with results available in 8 h establishes the diagnosis, as the organism can often be demonstrated in the endothellal cells of the blood vessels of the dermis (see Chap. 183).

Fig. A3-10 Erythema multiforme (bullosum) develops suddenly in a symmetrical distribution favoring the extensor surfaces and distal parts of the extremities including the dorsa of the hands and feet. The palms and soles are characteristically involved, even if the dorsal surfaces are not. Oral lesions often occur and include erosions of the cheeks, gums, and tongue, and swelling and crusting of the lips. Early lesions may resemble urticarial wheals but unlike urticarial lesions which fade in several hours, the papules may remain for days. Shown here is the characteristic target (iris) lesion, which consists of a clear red area as a periphery surrounding a pale zone and a central livid area that may contain a bulla or a tiny vesicle; target lesions may not be seen in the early phases of the disease (see Chap. 53).

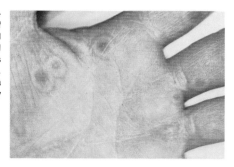

Fig. A3-11 Erythema marginatum, seen in 10 percent of patients, mostly children, with rheumatic fever, is characterized by a rapidly spreading, ringed eruption, sometimes with raised margins, and sometimes macular. The lesion may start as a small erythematous macule or papule and spreads peripherally, leaving a pale, or sometimes pigmented, inactive center. The outstanding characteristic of the eruption is its rapid spread, which may be 2 to 10 mm in 12 h. The ringed eruptions (shown) usually occur on the trunk and on the extremities and may involve the proximal areas of the hands or even the face. Although the advancing periphery is usually circular initially, it may later become either polycyclic or irregular (geographic). The rash may precede, but usually follows, the joint involvement. Erythema marginatum is usually associated with carditis, but may occasionally occur alone (see Chap. 157).

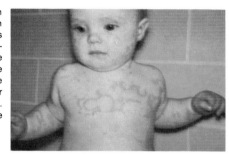

a
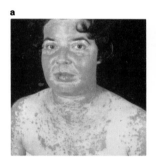

b
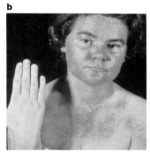

Fig. A3-12 Systemic lupus erythematosus is manifested in 40 percent of patients by bright, erythematous, scaling macules, papules, and plaques, usually on the light-exposed areas of the face ("butterfly") and body **(a);** the plaques consist of telangiectasia, and may contain follicular plugs. There may also be periungual atrophy and telangiectasia **(c).** The results of skin biopsy and immunofluorescence can be obtained within 8 h (see Chap. 152 and Figs. A2-8 and A2-9).

Dermatomyositis is manifested by a periorbital heliotrope hue **(b)** and periungual atrophy and telangiectasia **(c);** there may also be erythematous telangiectatic plaques with scaling over the bony prominences of the extremities **(b).** There is usually an associated weakness of the proximal muscle groups of the upper and lower extremities, making it difficult or impossible for the patient to arise from a supine position (see Chap. 153 and Fig. A2-5).

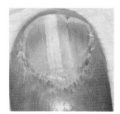

c

Fig. A3-13 "Serum sickness" is manifested first by erythema and intense pruritus and may appear initially and most intensely at the site at which the serum or drug was administered. The urticarial lesions (wheals) may become annular, polycyclic (as here), or even have the shape of the target lesions of erythema multiforme. Fever is present from the onset. Arthralgia and arthritis are common and are usually migratory and involve the distal large joints. Lymphadenopathy is common and frequently precedes the skin eruption (see Chap. 105).

Acute urticaria occurs during the early stages of infectious hepatitis and infectious mononucleosis. In viral hepatitis the rash and pruritus appear before jaundice develops. In both viral hepatitis and infectious mononucleosis urticarial lesions are the most frequent rash but morbilliform and erythema multiforme-type lesions also occur. Diagnosis is made by the heterophil test or by detection of the hepatitis-associated antigen.

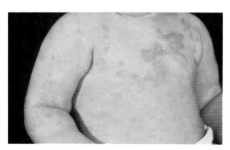

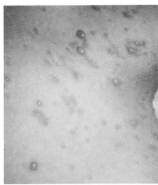

a

Fig. A3-14 Varicella is characterized by centripetally distributed, superficial lesions that develop rapidly from the macular stage to the crusting stage. All these stages of development **(a)** are present in the acute phase of the disease. Varicella appears in successive crops over a period of 3 to 5 days. There are more lesions over the thorax and proximal extremities than there are over the neck, face, and distal extremities. The most characteristic lesion is a tiny vesicle, occasionally umbilicated **(b),** on an erythematous base **(a),** which has been described as a "dewdrop on a rose petal." When material from early lesions is treated with Giemsa's or Wright's stain, it is usually possible to demonstrate multinucleated giant cells, and this finding distinguishes varicella and herpes zoster from variola and vaccinia, in which no giant cells are present. A chest x-ray should be obtained in adolescents and young adults to detect asymptomatic pneumonitis (see Chap. 191).

Generalized herpes zoster is manifested by lesions in a dermatomal distribution and, in addition, widely scattered, few or many, vesicles and pustules in different stages of development, as in varicella. Umbilication of the lesions is often present. Some patients with generalized herpes zoster may have impaired immune mechanism due either to lymphoma or leukemia or immunosuppressive therapy. Disseminated infection with herpes simplex virus is the only other cause of a generalized vesiculopustular eruption with multinucleated giant cells (Tzanck test) (see Chap. 191).

Disseminated vaccinia occurs following vaccination and is manifested by a generalized vesicular eruption that heals without scarring. Umbilicated pustules are almost always present. Vaccinia virus may be transmitted to the abnormal skin of other persons. This condition is called *eczema vaccinatum.* Vaccinia virus may also be transmitted to patients who have pemphigus, dermatitis herpetiformis, or multiple skin injuries (abrasions or heat burns) (see Chap. 192).

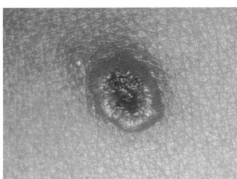

b

Fig. A3-15 Eczema herpeticum is characterized by fever and the sudden development of vesicles in eczematous areas. These vesicles occur singly at first, but may later occur in small herpetiform groupings as seen here, and are the result of accidental herpes virus exposure in patients with atopic dermatitis. Eczema herpeticum usually occurs as a manifestation of a primary infection in patients with atopic dermatitis. Recurrent herpes simplex may also occur in atopic dermatitis following the initial primary infection (see Chap. 190).

Disseminated herpes simplex is characterized by a generalized distribution of grouped vesicles; these groupings may be confluent in many areas. Umbilicated lesions are usually present. Material from early lesions in both eczema herpeticum and disseminated herpes simplex reveals multinucleated giant cells in Giemsa-stained or Wright-stained preparations. The specific diagnosis is made by culture of the virus from the skin lesions. The term *Kaposi's varicelliform eruption* is applied to both eczema vaccinatum and eczema herpeticum.

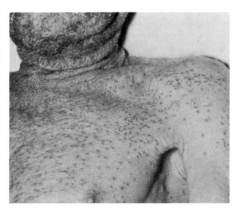

Fig. A3-16 Toxic epidermal necrolysis is characterized by epidermal necrosis of varying depth and extent. In newborns and infants the disease *scalded-skin syndrome* (see Chap. 55) is caused by an exotoxin produced by *S. aureus,* phage type 71. The staphylococcus may colonize the nose, conjunctivae, or umbilical stump without causing clinically apparent infection, but may elaborate an exotoxin that is carried hematogenously to the skin. In the newborn and infant the toxin causes necrosis of the upper half of the viable epidermis.

Patients are brought for emergency evaluation because of the sudden occurrence of irritability, possibly mild fever, and tender skin. On examination in the early stage, erythema and tenderness are noted in the flexural areas of skin in the neck, axillae, antecubital fossae, and inguinal folds. The epidermis may shear off if a frictional force is applied to it (Nikolsky's sign). Within 1 to 2 days, all the skin may appear erythematous. Bullae do not occur.

In the adult, staphylococcal exotoxin is rarely a factor in toxic epidermal necrolysis. Drugs are common etiologic agents. In some cases the cause is undetermined. The drugs most frequently implicated are the hydantoins, barbiturates, sulfonamides, thiazide diuretics, oral hypoglycemic agents, and phenylbutazone. The reaction may occur within a few days of initiation of a new drug or it may occur after the same drug has been taken for many years. Within 24 to 48 h the entire epidermis, as well as the mucosa of the conjunctivae, nose, and oropharynx, may become necrotic. The epidermis shears off when the patient moves or is examined (as illustrated here). Skin usually shows necrosis of the epidermis to the basal layer, which creates the clinical impression of a second-degree thermal burn. Extracellular fluid does not usually accumulate beneath the epidermis as bullae since there is little vascular damage. Initially the patient may be remarkably alert but in pain after stripping of the epidermis, or may be obtunded.

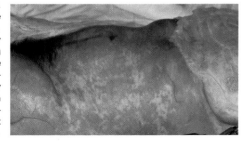

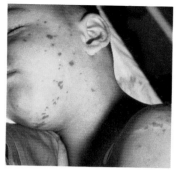

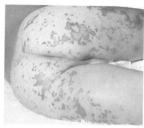

Fig. A3-17 **Meningococcemia** in its *acute* form is characterized by polymorphous lesions, but petechiae are predominant. The petechiae are somewhat irregular with a smudged appearance and may have a slightly raised, pale-grayish vesicular or pustular center. Occasionally, on careful examination, it is possible to demonstrate gram-negative diplococci obtained from the center of these lesions. The lesions are located mainly on the extremities or trunk in a random asymmetrical pattern. A progressive increase in the number of petechiae may be followed by a coalescence of lesions to form gross ecchymotic areas; the skin may become gangrenous in these areas of extensive involvement, making the condition indistinguishable from purpura fulminans. *Chronic meningococcemia* is manifested by various types of lesions that come and go in crops with the fluctuations in the fever. They vary in size from 1 to 20 mm and consist of **(1)** purpuric papular lesions, which are the most common (called palpable purpura) **(a)**; **(2)** slightly indurated and tender erythema nodosum-like lesions, mainly on the lower extremities; **(3)** petechiae with vesicular or pustular centers; **(4)** tiny purpuric papules with an areola of paler erythema; **(5)** purpuric macules with gunmetal-gray infarcted centers **(b)**. It is not usually possible to demonstrate bacteria in the lesions of chronic meningococcemia (see Chap. 177).

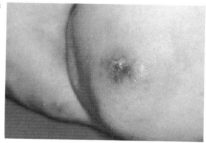

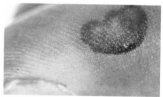

Fig. A3-18 **Gonococcemia,** which occurs most often in young females, is manifested by purpuric macules, purpuric papules, purpuric vesicles **(a and b),** purpuric bullae, or purpuric infarcts **(b),** and also pustules which may be surrounded by a narrow rim of purpura. Migratory polyarthritis and tenosynovitis are usually present. The lesions are so few in number they can be counted, are often painful, and occur predominantly around the joints **(a)** (see Chap. 205).

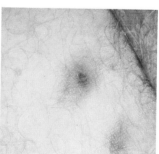

Fig. A3-19 **Pseudomonas septicemia** occurs usually in hospitalized individuals who have other underlying medical problems. Often these patients are infants, or those adults who are receiving immunosuppressive agents or antibiotics. The patients usually have a toxic febrile illness, and, although the lesions are slightly painful, the patients are usually too sick to complain about them. The skin lesions are some of the most characteristic features of *Pseudomonas* septicemia, and consist of four types: **(1)** vesicles and bullae, which occur singly and in clusters and frequently, as they evolve, become hemorrhagic like those shown here; **(2)** necrotic ulcerations (ecthyma gangrenosum), which are round, indurated, and painless with a central black or grayish black eschar and a surrounding erythema and are almost always located in the anogenital area or axillae; **(3)** gangrenous cellulitis, which has a more sharply demarcated, superficial, painless, necrotic area that may resemble a decubitus ulcer; and **(4)** macular and papular lesions that are small, oval, and painless, located primarily over the trunk, and resemble the "rose spots" of typhoid fever (see Chap. 177).

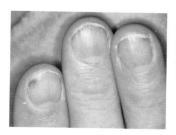

Fig. A3-20 **Subacute bacterial endocarditis,** caused by streptococcus viridans and group D streptococci, is manifested by painful urticaria-like nodules in the pulp of the fingers and toes (Osler's nodes), purpuric macules of the acral areas (Janeway's lesions), and subungual splinter hemorrhages as shown here (see Chap. 176). Splinter hemorrhages are frequently seen in trichinosis and in 10 percent of hospitalized medical patients. Petechiae may also occur in crops on the skin or on the mucosae of the conjunctiva or palate.

Fig. A3-21 "Allergic" vasculitis is characterized by *symmetrical* red papules ("palpable purpura"), usually on the lower extremities. The purpuric lesions frequently develop into bullae and infarcts, and may be associated with arthralgia, abdominal pain, melena, and neuropathy. Red cell casts may be present in the urine sediment. Biopsy of the purpuric papules shows a necrotizing angiitis involving the venules of the dermal vascular plexus (see Chap. 107).

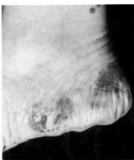
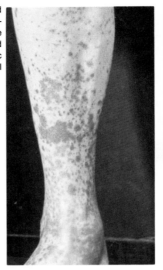

OCULOCUTANEOUS DISEASES

David D. Donaldson

On first thought one might assume that a discussion of the eye in reference to dermatologic disorders would primarily involve the lid as the specific cutaneous tissue. Nothing could be less true. Not only the lids but a surprising number of the structures of the eye, both external and internal, are affected by systemic diseases characteristically associated with the skin. These parallel findings provide useful and often highly significant information for research and diagnosis. This discussion does not include oculocutaneous lesions of the lid, as they are typically so similar in nature to lesions occurring in other areas that they are of no special interest here. A number of objective findings in the eye are highly characteristic, if not pathognomonic, of systemic diseases. The internal structures of the eye, such as the iris, lens, and retina, as well as the external portions of the eye, the conjunctiva and cornea, provide unique opportunities to study the relationship of ocular to dermatologic disorders. Important diagnostic criteria for the physician are seen in oculocutaneous disorders, such as ochronosis, which is characterized by the typical scleral and corneal pigmentation, or pseudoxanthoma elasticum, in which the classic angioid streaks in the fundus can be observed. Frequently, these ocular changes are easily discernible without special equipment. Therefore, it is evident that a familiarity with the eye manifestations of oculocutaneous disorders substantially increases the physician's ability in the field of clinical diagnosis. It is hoped that this section will illustrate some of the more common and significant oculocutaneous disorders, so that the reader can become aware of these findings. (See Table A4-1.)

Table A4-1   Oculocutaneous disorders

Eye changes in disorders primarily affecting the skin and mucous membrane:
   Nevus of Ota (oculodermal melanocytosis) (Fig. A4-1)
   Rosacea (Fig. A4-2)
   Hemangiomas (Fig. A4-3)
   Erythema multiforme (Fig. A4-4)
   Behçet's syndrome (Fig. A4-5)
   Benign mucosal pemphigoid (Fig. A4-6)
   Atopic dermatitis (Fig. A4-7)
Cutaneous and eye lesions in nutritional, metabolic, and heritable disorders:
   Vitamin A deficiency (Fig. A4-8)
   Alkaptonuria (Fig. A4-9)
   Pseudoxanthoma elasticum (Fig. A4-10)
   Tuberous sclerosis (Fig. A4-11)
Ocular manifestations of diseases involving the skin and multiple organ systems
   Vogt-Koyanagi-Harada syndrome (Fig. A4-12)
   Ataxia-telangiectasia (Fig. A4-13)
   Lupus erythematosus (Fig. A4-14)
   Dermatomyositis (Fig. A4-15)
   Sjögren's syndrome (Fig. A4-16)
   Sarcoidosis (Fig. A4-17)
Disorders due to microbial agents with skin and eye manifestations
   Tuberculosis (Fig. A4-18)
   Herpes simplex (Fig. A4-19)
   Herpes zoster (Fig. A4-20)
   Vaccinia (Fig. A4-21)
   Varicella (Fig. A4-22)
   Molluscum contagiosum (Fig. A4-23)
   Syphilis (Fig. 4-24)
   Gonococcal infection (Fig. A4-25)

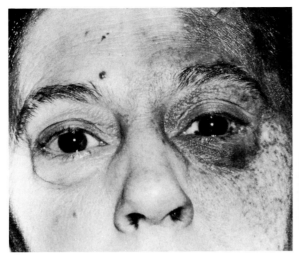

Fig. A4-1 **Congenital melanosis oculi** is a condition in which there is unilateral excessive melanin pigmentation of the uvea and episclera. If the pigmentation involves the lids or skin of the face, then the condition is usually known as the nevus of Ota or oculodermal melanocytosis **(a).** The condition is sometimes hereditary. The most prominent ocular findings are patchy episcleral pigmentation, usually bluish in color, and a darker iris on the involved side **(b).** Funduscopy shows that the fundus of the involved side is also darker. A very small number of patients with this condition develop malignant melanoma of the choroid or pigmentary glaucoma (Fig. A8-30).

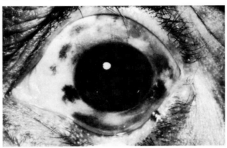

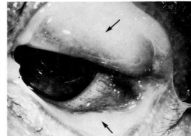

Fig. A4-2 **Rosacea** often presents with a chronic blepharoconjunctivitis. The more rare but more serious marginal ulceration of the cornea may lead to considerable loss of vision. Typically, there is a scleritis and peripheral keratitis with vascularization and loss of corneal stroma (arrows). Complications include vascularization involving the pupillary region, secondary iritis, and perforation of the cornea. The course is chronic and recurrences are common.

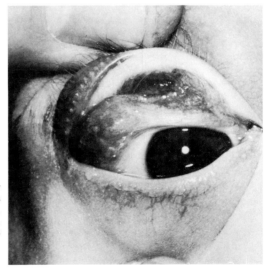

Fig. A4-3 **Hemangiomas** may involve the eyelids or the conjunctiva. The capillary type may be part of the Sturge–Weber syndrome in which an entire half of the face is involved. Hemangioma may be serious in that, if the lid and conjunctiva are involved, the child may not be able to open the eye, and an amblyopia (from disuse) may result. As elsewhere in the body, spontaneous regression is usually seen within the first 5 years of life.

Fig. A4-4 **Erythema multiforme** has ocular manifestations of a catarrhal, purulent, or pseudomembranous conjunctivitis. The pseudomembranous form (arrows) **(a)** is the most common, and usually results in permanent scarring, symblepharon formation, and keratitis sicca. The late sequelae include complete keratinization of the conjunctiva and cornea and severe loss of vision **(b).**

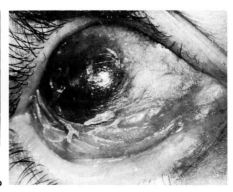

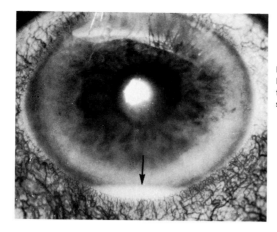

Fig. A4-5 Behçet's syndrome has the ocular findings of recurrent uveitis with hypopyon and retinal vasculitis. The uveitis is bilateral and both anterior and posterior and occurs in crises at intervals of several months. The hypopyon (arrow) is sterile and present throughout the acute phase of the anterior uveitis.

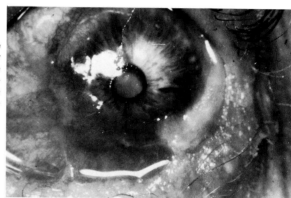

Fig. A4-6 Benign mucosal pemphigold is a slowly progressive disease which primarily affects the mucous membranes of the eyes. Over many years, there is symblepharon formation and scarring of the lids to the globe. Later there is keratinization of the conjunctiva and the cornea, ultimately giving an appearance of the eyes indistinguishable from the late stages of erythema multiforme. Topical corticosteroids may delay the progression of the disease process.

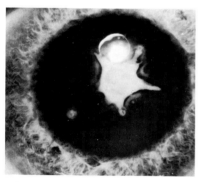

Fig. A4-7 Cataracts in chronic atopic eczema may develop in patients between the ages of 15 and 30. The typical opacity of the lens lies just beneath the anterior lens capsule and consists of a central dense plaque or "shield" with fingerlike projections toward the periphery. These cataracts are usually bilateral. There is a high incidence of retinal detachment in patients with these atopic cataracts.

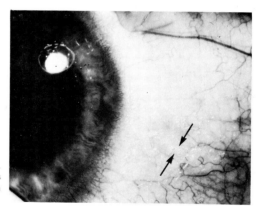

Fig. A4-8 Xerosis of the conjunctiva in vitamin A deficiency is characterized by a roughened, granular conjunctival surface and a thick, pearly, foamy exudate. This exudate, which is always in the interpalpebral region, can be wiped away and is known as a Bitot's spot (arrows). In severe prolonged vitamin A deficiency, corneal ulceration and keratomalacia may develop.

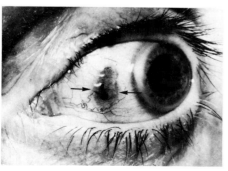

Fig. A4-9 Ochronosis (alkaptonuria) has pathognomonic ocular signs. The first sign to appear is that of grayish black scleral pigmentation anterior to the tendon insertions of the horizontal recti muscles (arrows). At times pigmentation of the elastic tissue in a pinguecula may be stained a dark brown or black and usually has the configuration of small, dark rings. In advanced cases of ochronosis, Bowman's membrane, adjacent to the limbus, may have areas of black pigmentation (Fig. A8-41).

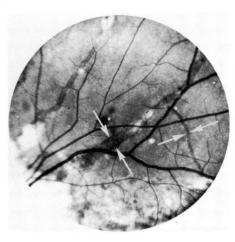

Fig. A4-10 Pseudoxanthoma elasticum usually produces the typical fundus findings of angioid streaks. These red, brown, or gray streaks (arrows) radiate from the disk and resemble vessels. However, they have irregular margins, vary considerably in width, and are sometimes concentric with the disk. Macular degeneration (seen at the bottom of the photograph) due to recurrent hemorrhages is a common late finding and is associated with marked reduction in vision.

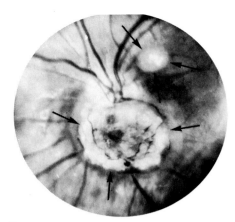

Fig. A4-11 Tuberous sclerosis frequently has eye findings which are characterized by whitish, refractile tumor masses (arrows) in the fundus, often having a mulberrylike appearance. When these are on the optic nerve head they may be confused with hyaline bodies (drusen) of the nerve head. However, when multiple or not on the nerve head, they are almost pathognomonic of tuberous sclerosis. Occasionally portions of these tumors become pinched off and float free in the vitreous. The vision may be affected depending on the location of the lesion.

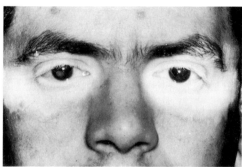

a

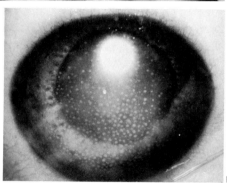

b

Fig. A4-12 Vogt–Koyanagi–Harada syndrome is characterized by an exudative iridocyclitis and choroiditis associated with a patchy depigmentation of the skin and hair about the eyes (a). Frequently there is tinnitus and deafness, and there may be a pleocytosis of the cerebrospinal fluid. The disease typically occurs in young men and the only known treatment is symptomatic. The syndrome frequently runs a long course with recurrent attacks of iridocyclitis with multiple keratic precipitates of the cornea (b), and may progress to total blindness in both eyes.

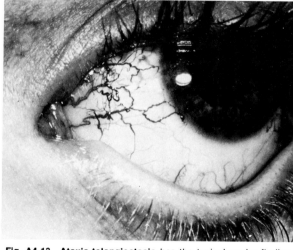

Fig. A4-13 Ataxia-telangiectasia has the typical ocular finding of telangiectatic vessels in the inner and outer canthal regions. These are usually bilateral and symmetrical and give the initial impression of a low-grade conjunctivitis. These patients also exhibit a defect in executing voluntary ocular movements and in maintaining full excursions of the eyes.

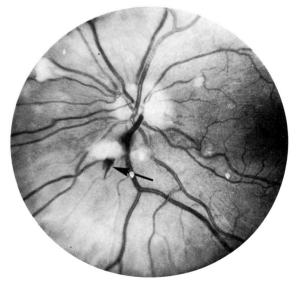

Fig. A4-14 Ocular findings in systemic lupus erythematosus are usually confined to the fundus. These consist of fluffy white exudates called cytoid bodies which are usually superficial in the retina. Superficial retinal hemorrhages (arrow) and circumpapillary edema may be present.

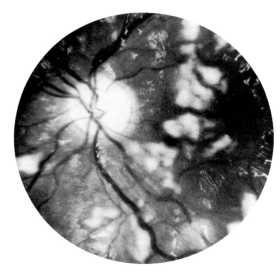

Fig. A4-15 Dermatomyositis produces superficial large white exudates, flame-shaped hemorrhages, and dilated veins in the ocular fundus. The vision may not be affected by this retinal pathology; however, retinal findings usually parallel the severity of the generalized disease process.

Fig. A4-16 Sjögren's syndrome is often associated with rheumatoid arthritis and is believed to be a systemic disease manifested by decreased lacrimal and salivary secretions. The ocular signs and symptoms are photophobia, dry eyes, sensation of foreign body in the eyes, and a mucoid, thick secretion on the conjunctiva and cornea (arrow). Shredding of the conjunctival and corneal epithelium is visible with a slit lamp and with special supravital stains used in the eye, such as rose bengal. The test for deficiency of tear formation (Schirmer test) is always positive. The treatment consists of the use of artificial tears such as polyvinyl alcohol. In advanced cases, occlusion of the lacrimal puncta may be necessary.

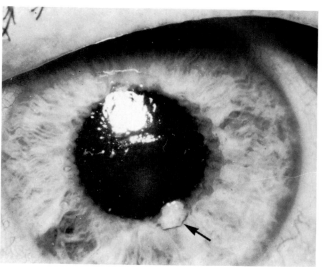

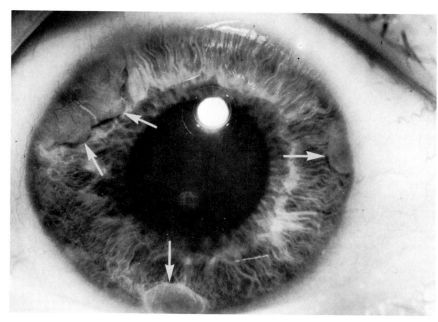

Fig. A4-17 Sarcoidosis (Boeck's sarcoid) produces a bilateral anterior uveitis with the typical granulomatous "mutton-fat" type of keratic precipitates. Almost pathognomonic are fleshy, vascularized nodules of tissue on the iris, if they are present (arrows). The uveitis may resolve spontaneously, or, occasionally, may lead to permanent loss of vision and even phthisis bulbi. Treatment of the uveitis is usually successful with both systemically administered and topical corticosteroids. Other pathology in the eye associated with sarcoidosis is white perivenous infiltrates in the retina and deposition of calcium in Bowman's membrane (band keratopathy) secondary to the hypercalcemia of this condition.

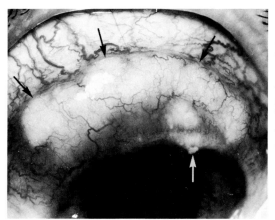

Fig. A4-18 **Tuberculoma** is one form of ocular involvement with the tubercle bacillus. This presents as yellow or gray subconjunctival nodules which may invade the cornea (arrows). Other forms of conjunctival involvement include: the ulcerative type in which there are one or more ulcers; the hypertrophic papillary type characterized by outgrowths of flattened granulation tissue; and the polypoid type showing a pedunculated fibroma of the tarsal conjunctiva. The tubercle bacillus may affect the uveal tract, causing "mutton-fat" keratic precipitates in the anterior segment and a recurrent chorioretinitis in the posterior segment. The treatment of ocular tuberculosis is the same as that used for the systemic disease.

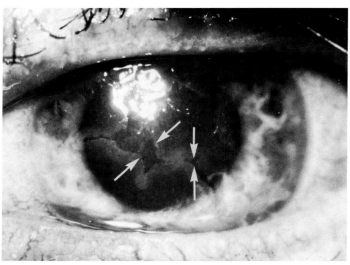

Fig. A4-19 **Herpes simplex infections** may involve the lids, conjunctiva, and cornea, the latter being the most serious, because severe loss of vision may occur. The typical lesion of the cornea is the well-known dendritic ulcer, which primarily affects the epithelium but may later extend into the corneal stroma. Dendritic ulcers of the cornea (arrows) are occasionally seen in herpes zoster infections but are characteristic of involvement of the cornea by herpes simplex. Topical idoxuridine arrests the development of the virus, while corticosteroid medications usually enhance its invasion into the cornea.

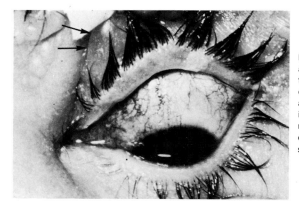

Fig. A4-20 **Herpes zoster** involvement of the eye is usually associated with a unilateral involvement of the ophthalmic division of the trigeminal nerve, typically with vesicular lesions of the lids (arrows). The typical lesion of the cornea involves the periphery with vascularization and ulceration. Occasionally, dendritic ulcers are seen which are indistinguishable from those found in herpes simplex keratitis. The most serious complication is a uveitis which may be intense and prolonged, producing many keratic precipitates and secondary glaucoma. Permanent loss of vision and even phthisis bulbi can result. The uveitis is usually treated with topical corticosteroids and atropine.

Fig. A4-21 **Vaccinia** of the eyes is usually the result of a secondary inoculation either from the patient's own recent vaccination or from that of another person. The lesions of the eyelids are identical to those elsewhere on the body and produce marked swelling. About one-third of the patients with lid involvement also have a corneal ulcer, which may lead to perforation of the globe. The lid lesions frequently heal with considerable scarring and permanent loss of lashes.

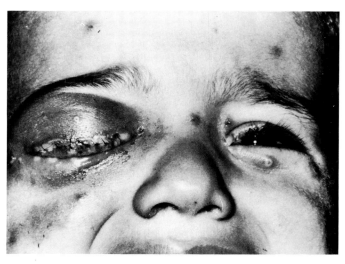

Fig. A4-22 Varicella (chickenpox) occasionally involves the lids, conjunctiva, or cornea, resulting in an excavated ulcer. Superficial corneal involvement (arrows) usually has a rapid course, healing with little cicatrization. The rare interstitial or deep type causes more swelling and has a longer course with considerable residual scarring.

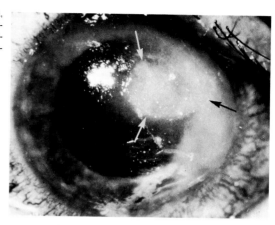

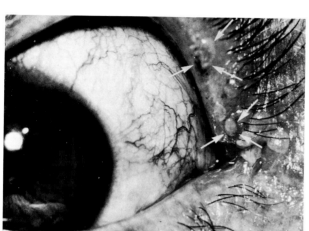

Fig. A4-23 Molluscum contagiosum of the lids (arrows) even of insignificant size, may produce a follicular or papillary conjunctivitis which will respond only to the elimination of the molluscum contagiosum lesion. Occasionally, a superficial punctate keratitis is found, associated with molluscum contagiosum.

Fig. A4-24 Congenital syphilis may present with only a positive serology and an interstitial keratitis. The onset of luetic keratitis appears between the sixth and twelfth year but may be much later in life. It is almost always bilateral but it usually does not develop in both eyes simultaneously. The first ocular manifestations of interstitial keratitis are ciliary injection, photophobia, and lacrimation. Later, iritis, corneal edema, and vascularization gradually develop, with intense photophobia as a major symptom. As the blood vessels invade the cornea, the edematous stroma slowly clears, the central region clearing last. The final result is usually a relatively clear cornea containing many ghost vessels which are the residual of the old vascular channels and which remain throughout life.

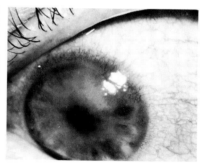

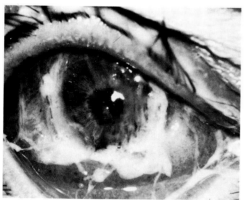

Fig. A4-25 Gonococcal conjunctivitis typically produces an acute purulent reaction without involvement of the cornea in the adult. However, the infant eye may become infected during the birth process. Gonococci can penetrate the intact neonatal corneal epithelium, leading ultimately to severe corneal ulceration and permanent loss of vision. Topical and systemic penicillin is the preferred treatment.

Fig. A4-26 Corticosteroid cataracts as typically seen in the posterior subcapsular region of the lens. The opacities are granular and densest in the axial portion of the lens (arrows). They are seen in patients who have been on long-term corticosteroid therapy systemically (and sometimes topically) for treatment of various chronic conditions, as was the case with this patient with pemphigus vulgaris. They are usually bilateral and may require cataract extraction if they become sufficiently dense to interfere with vision and if the patient's general condition is not too serious.

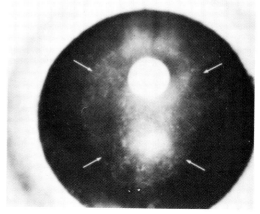

CLINICAL RECOGNITION OF PRIMARY MALIGNANT MELANOMA AND OF ITS PRECURSORS

Thomas B. Fitzpatrick, Martin C. Mihm, Jr., Arthur J. Sober, and Arthur R. Rhodes

Melanoma, the curable of the serious cancers

Until about 20 years ago, the dismal prognosis—the dreaded advance of "black cancer"—dominated the physician's attitude toward melanoma. Extensive studies of melanoma patients over the past two decades have laid the groundwork for a complete reversal of this negative situation. The results of these studies, based on the correlation of clinical and microscopic findings, have sharply altered our concepts of melanoma and its precursor lesions such as the dysplastic nevus; defined the histopathologic nature of the disease, especially the growth patterns; provided a method for estimating prognosis by measurement of the depth of the lesion, and, most important, established simple diagnostic criteria for detecting early-stage tumors and precursor lesions by visual inspection, using only the naked eye.

Given the irreversible character of advanced melanoma, their rising incidence presents a special challenge to physicians: how to distinguish early surgically curable melanoma from the many common benign pigmented lesions that are seen in everyday practice.

Failure to make this distinction can have serious consequences. In the absence of treatment, melanoma may lie dormant for an indefinite period; but once in motion, it may progress rapidly, with devastating destructiveness.

Unlike most cancers, metastatic melanoma shows no significant response to any of the various antineoplastic therapeutic modalities—surgical, chemical, radiologic, immunologic—that are used in the management of neoplastic disease. The inexorable progress of advanced melanoma is generally rapid and lethal.

The unique aspect of primary melanoma of the skin among all the potentially fatal malignant tumors (breast, stomach, uterus, lung, colon) is its easy access, not only for gross examination with the naked eye, but for histologic study—a biopsy is easily obtained and decisive. This easy accessibility is especially important in primary melanoma because curability is directly related to the size and depth of invasion of the tumor—a growth that in the most common type, the superficial spreading melanoma, fortunately proceeds relatively slowly over a period of a few years. This provides a "grace" period in which early tumors can be detected.

The task, therefore, is to define the clinical criteria of early lesions and this has been done over the past two decades. Early melanoma is usually easy to spot with the naked eye. Moreover, as stated previously, the prognosis of melanoma is related to the depth of invasion into the skin—early "thin" primary melanoma has a 95 to 100 percent survival rate while "thick" lesions have a dismal prognosis and there is no successful treatment for metastatic melanoma. Thus, primary melanoma of the skin is a potentially fatal skin cancer affecting persons in middle life (and increasingly young adults) that can be cured if detected early and surgically removed.

Failure to recognize malignant melanoma in its early stages may be largely attributed to the inadequacy of traditional diagnostic criteria, according to which physicians were taught to suspect only pigmented lesions that exhibited recent growth, darkening, bleeding, or ulceration. While recent enlargement and changes in color are diagnostic features of early melanoma (occurring in 70 percent of early lesions), bleeding and ulceration typify a late stage of the disease, when the melanoma has already invaded the skin deeply and the prognosis is poor.

In the vast majority of cases, early melanoma can be easily recognized by three physical characteristics—coloration, contour, and size—of the lesion. Although the same characteristics are sometimes present in other types of lesions (e.g., seborrheic keratoses, pyogenic granulomas, and pigmented basal cell epitheliomas), the likelihood of false-positive diagnoses is minimized once the clinician becomes familiar with the typical features of primary cutaneous melanoma. Moreover, since biopsy should be considered mandatory for all suspected lesions, the risks of making a false-positive diagnosis are negligible when compared with the potential consequences of a false-negative or a missed diagnosis of melanoma.

Clinical signs

The three positive clinical signs suggesting melanoma in a pigmented lesion are, in order of importance, variegated color, irregular border, and size.

1. *Variegated color.* Displayed in a disorderly, haphazard pigment pattern, this is a frequent characteristic of malignant melanoma, especially the superficial spreading type. The colors indicative of malignancy are shades of red, white, and blue. Blue, the most ominous color, is produced by the Tyndall effect of light scattering from brown melanin pigment deep within the dermis. White, gray, and pink shades indicate focal areas of partial regression, which occurs spontaneously in some cases. Some malignant melanomas, particularly the nodular type, are not diversified but are uniform in color—usually bluish black, bluish gray, or bluish red. Any marked change in the color of a lesion is another warning sign of melanoma.

2. *Irregular border.* Often marked by an angular indentation or notch, this is the second most helpful sign in the diagnosis of malignant melanoma, especially the superficial spreading and the lentigo maligna types.

3. *Size.* An increase in size is typical of early melanomas, especially when it occurs rapidly enough to be of concern to the patient.

Visual inspection can be significantly enhanced by two simple tools that no physician should be without: a penlight for viewing lesions with oblique lighting and a 7× magnifying lens for observing details that are otherwise overlooked, especially the presence of subtle gray or blue colors.

The precursor lesion: dysplastic melanocytic nevus

While early diagnosis of primary melanoma is the key to prevention of metastatic disease, the emphasis now in the 1980s is on the recognition of individuals at in-

creased risk for development of melanoma: a family history of melanoma and/or the presence of one or more precursor lesions. The known precursor lesions of melanoma are lentigo maligna, congenital melanocytic nevi, certain types of acral and mucosal pigmented lesions, and the most significant of all the precursors, the dysplastic melanocytic nevus. The dysplastic melanocytic nevus is an atypical-appearing variant of melanocytic nevi and consists of intraepidermal melanocytic dysplasia. Intraepidermal melanocytic dysplasia is to cutaneous melanoma what actinic (solar) keratosis is to squamous cell carcinoma, namely, a proliferation of variable atypical intraepidermal melanocytes that are morphologically intermediate between normal and malignant. Dysplastic melanocytic nevi represent both a marker for individuals at increased risk for developing melanoma, as well as histogenic precursors of melanoma.

All physicians are in a unique position to prevent melanoma by recognizing, amid a large variety of pigmented lesions, an early melanoma by the variegation of color (especially a gray color). Now, however, he or she can recognize the dysplastic nevi that have the same features as early melanoma: variegation of color (dysplastic nevi never have gray or blue hues) and irregular borders (although not quite as marked as most primary melanomas). It is useful to recall that the most common presentation of cutaneous melanoma is a changing mole, an atypical-appearing mole, or a mole "marching out of step" with the other lesions in an individual.

A comparison of the clinical features of early superficial spreading melanoma with some premalignant and benign melanocytic lesions is presented in Table A5-1.

Table A5-1 Clinical features of early superficial spreading melanoma compared with some premalignant and benign melanocytic lesions (in white adults)

	Type of lesion	Size	Color	Border	Shape
Superficial spreading melanoma (early)	Plaque (rarely macular)	5–15 mm or larger	Variegated, disorderly pattern with admixture of dark brown, black, blue, gray-white, pink, red	Usually irregular, may have a notch	Round, oval, arciform, or very irregular contour
Dysplastic melanocytic nevus	Macule, usually with slightly raised areas	5–10 mm or larger	Variegated, disorderly color pattern: pink, tan, brown, dark brown	Usually irregular, poorly circumscribed	Round, oval, or irregularly angulated contour
Lentigo maligna	Macule	5–30 mm or larger			
Congenital nevocytic nevus (small)	Plaque	10 mm*	Uniform orderly pattern: tan to dark brown	Regular, discrete	Round or oval
Common acquired melanocytic nevus	Macule (small) papule nodule	≤ 10 mm	Orderly color pattern: pink, flesh, tan, brown	Regular, discrete	Round or oval

*May be smaller but then virtually indistinguishable from the common acquired melanocytic nevus.

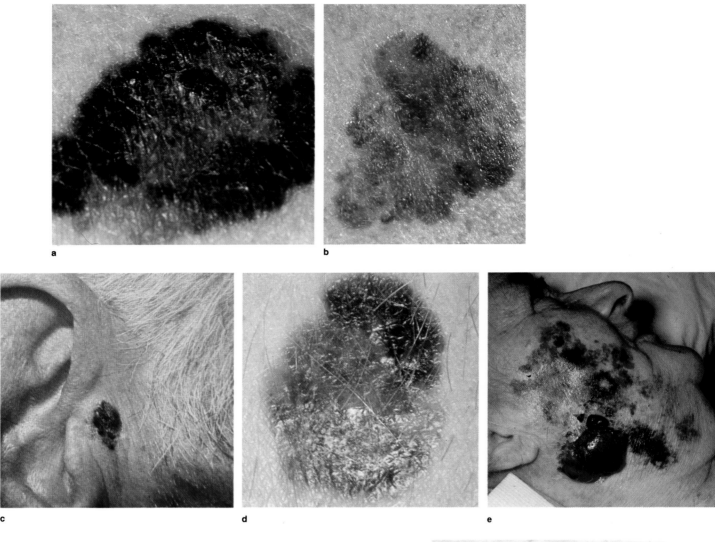

a

b

c

d

e

f

Fig. A5-1 Malignant melanoma. On close inspection melanomas shown above are characterized by irregular surface **(a)**, irregular border and notching **(b)**, and nodularity **(c)**. Also shown are a reniform melanoma **(d)**, an extensive lentigo maligna on face of patient **(e)** and a regressive melanoma characterized by grayish color infiltrated with pink areas **(f)**. *(From Hospital Practice, January 1982, with permission.)*

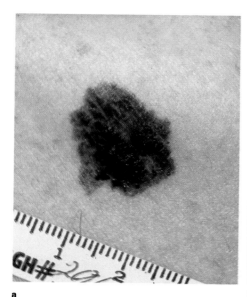
a

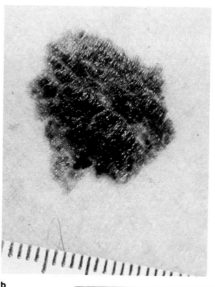
b

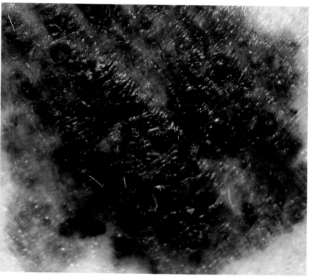
c

Fig. A5-2 Superficial spreading melanoma. Photographs illustrate the importance of close examination of cutaneous lesions. **(a)** One sees the lesion as it would appear to an examiner standing far enough from the patient to include a substantial portion of the body in his or her visual field. Note the notch at 6:30 o'clock. **(b)** Close-up view, still with the naked eye, in which pigmentation becomes more obvious. **(c)** Under a hand-held lens (7×), bluish coloration and irregular surface typical of melanoma becomes obvious. *(From Hospital Practice, January 1982, with permission.)*

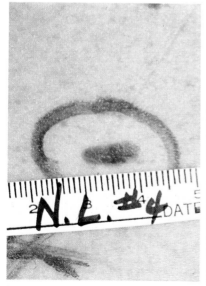
a

Fig. A5-3 Dysplastic nevi. Precursor lesions with high probability of evolving into melanomas. **(a)** Dysplastic nevi on the back. **(b)** Close-up of circled lesion in **(a)** shows suspicious pigmentation. **(c)** A dysplastic nevus. *(From Hospital Practice, January 1982, with permission.)*

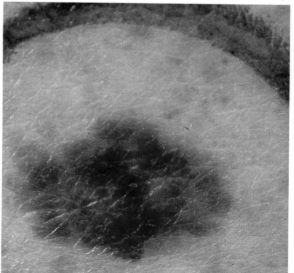
b

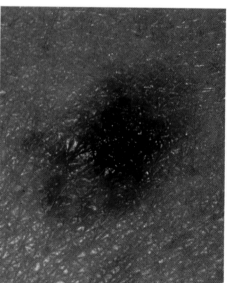
c

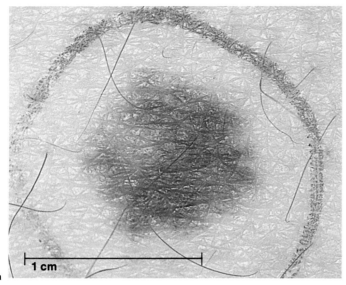

a

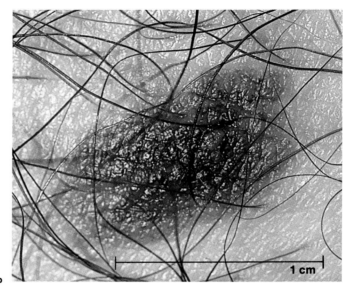

b

Fig. A5-4 Dysplastic melanocytic nevi. (a) Round, essentially macular lesions in which the slightly elevated area is present at 12:00 o'clock. The elevation is detectable only by oblique lighting. Note striking variegation of color with tan, brown, and pink areas. **(b)** This lesion is more obviously elevated in the central portion. Note "pebbly" surface. Both lesions have indistinct and irregular borders. *(From Dermatologic Capsule & Comment 7(4):4, 1985, with permission.)*

Fig. A5-5 Malignant melanoma—dysplastic nevus syndrome. This 28-year-old woman gave a history of a rapidly growing (3 to 6 months), asymptomatic lesion on her right scapular area. Her mother had melanoma and both mother and siblings had many dark "moles." Diagnosis: **(1)** Superficial spreading melanoma, level IV, 4.75 mm. **(2)** Regional nodes—of 32 removed, 1 was positive. **(3)** Dysplastic nevus syndrome with family history of melanoma. Note primary lesion and many dark "moles" on back **(a)** and dysplastic nevi on untanned areas under the bathing suit straps **(b)**. *(From Dermatologic Capsule & Comment 6(4):3, 1984, with permission.)*

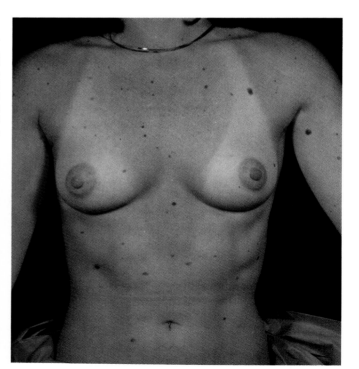

b

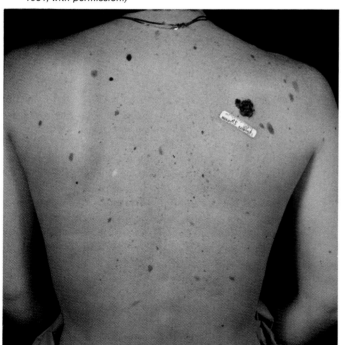

a

TROPICAL DERMATOLOGY

Gunnar Lomholt

Tropical dermatology is presumably best defined as dermatology in tropical areas. Most of the "usual" skin diseases are seen in the tropics but the clinical manifestations often differ from those encountered in more moderate climates and in individuals from a different ethnic and environmental background. In addition, there are a number of "exotic" diseases usually not seen in so-called developed countries. These diseases mirror the poverty and the bad living conditions of the people living in the tropics. Undernourishment coupled with other environmental factors such as heat, humidity, and parasites including insects, helminths, and fungi determine the spectrum of diseases. The main problems are malnutrition, tuberculosis, and leprosy.

It is not intended here to give a complete review of all conditions seen in the tropics as most of these are described in detail in other chapters of the book. Instead, the present account, which is based on the author's own experience in Uganda, attempts to emphasize the special aspects of dermatology in tropical climates and regions and to illustrate some of the more common and important conditions. This is particularly true for leprosy, which is the main "dermatologic" disease in the tropical world with approximately 12 to 18 million persons suffering from it.

General statements regarding skin diseases in tropical areas are often based on experience from one area, and this is particularly true for the African continent. Without doubt there are great differences between East and West Africa and between the northern and southern parts. The genetic background of the population is different and so are climatic and other environmental factors. For instance, psoriasis is very uncommon in West Africa, but in East Africa it is a common disease, presumably with a prevalence more or less equal to that in the Mediterranean area. The occurrence of diseases depends also, for example, on the living conditions for vectors. The sand fly is the vector for leishmaniasis. This insect does not occur in Uganda and leishmaniasis is therefore practically absent from this country in contrast to the Sudan and Ethiopia. One usually does not look for a disease which is "known not to exist" in the particular area. Partly because of this, loa loa was never diagnosed in Uganda; however, one day when microfilariae were unexpectedly found in the peripheral blood of a patient we became alerted. In the course of a few months we detected no less than 20 cases previously diagnosed as Quincke's edema and urticaria.

Skin infestations are common. Scabies is often extensive with severe secondary infection. In contrast to the usual procedure, we generally gave antiscabies treatment at once, even to patients with quite severe infections, because our expeience was that many patients did not come for the specific treatment when they had improved. Pediculosis corporis and capitis are other common infestations. Tungiasis usually is treated by the patients themselves by removing the sand flea (*Tunga penetrans*) with a needle. In some cases the lesions might be mistaken for plantar warts or corns.

Skin infections are extremely common in tropical areas, especially among children. Papular urticaria leads to repeated attacks of impetigo and ecthyma, owing to constant scratching and infection. Perhaps these severe skin infections are responsible for some of the many cases of glomerulonephritis of unknown origin seen among small children. The staphylococcal scalded-skin syndrome is also seen.

The frequency of tinea is very high; among school children in Kampala we found a prevalence between 4 and 8 percent. Tinea versicolor affects a high proportion of all people living in tropical areas. The deep fungus infections are some of the most impressive diseases in the tropics but of various importance to different areas. The treatment is difficult and often unsatisfactory.

Onchocerciasis is a common disease not only in South America but also in Africa, occurring in a broad belt around the equator. We found suramin to be an extremely toxic therapeutic agent for our patients and had to abandon this as a routine. One reason is presumably that most patients had anemia caused by the widespread infection with hookworms.

Miliaria is very common in equatorial Africa, especially in small children, and sweat gland abscesses are seen in children with malnutrition. On the other hand, allergic contact dermatitis was impressively uncommon in our clinic in contrast to nummular eczematous dermatitis. Ulcers were seen frequently, some phagedenic (so-called tropical ulcers), others caused by *Mycobacterium ulcerans* (Buruli ulcers). Leg ulcers are seen also in patients with sickle cell anemia, whereas the usually venous ulcers of the legs are nearly unknown. For unknown reasons varicose veins are extremely uncommon even in women with many children.

Several of the common skin diseases have special features in African blacks living in the tropical regions of this continent. Lichen planus is much more common than in the United States, quite often producing lesions on the face; atrophic annular lesions are encountered frequently and achromic lesions may be seen; on the other hand, buccal lesions are rare but the lips are often affected. Extensive, widespread lesions are commonly seen even in children. Seborrheic dermatitis is common in East Africa and most cases of exfoliative dermatitis are caused by this condition. The affected areas are often hypopigmented with a follicular keratosis. Lichen spinulosus is often found in African children. Children with the clinical features of lichen scrofulosorum are regularly seen without any evidence of tuberculosis.

The incidence of bullous conditions was high in our clinic. Of the pemphigus group, pemphigus foliaceus, usually starting as pemphigus erythematosus, is the most frequently diagnosed and, like fogo selvagem, can also be seen in children. Impressive in the author's experience, was the great number of cases of dermatitis herpetiformis encountered, especially in children in whom the disease often presented as extensive bullous eruptions. Generalized exudative erythema multiforme and idiopathic or drug-induced forms of toxic epidermal necrolysis were regularly seen. A very common condition is fixed drug eruption usually caused by phenolphthalein; long-standing melanosis following skin eruptions is very common.

Basal cell carcinoma is extremely rare among Africans in contrast to Europeans and Indians. Squamous cell carcinoma is, however, quite common, for instance in chronic ulcers, patients with xeroderma pigmentosum, and in albinos. Burkitt's lymphoma and Kaposi's sarcoma are common conditions in East Africa.

Venereal diseases are a great public health problem all over the world but especially in developing countries. In our clinic, 19,000 cases of gonorrhea, 2,000 cases of early contagious syphilis, and 1,000 cases of chancroid were diagnosed in 1972. These figures presumably account for only one-third of the cases in Kampala.

All clinical manifestations of syphilis were seen. Characteristic were the annular lesions of the face and the extensive eruptions of condylomata lata. Syphilis serology may present difficulties because of many false-positive reagin reactions, in our clinic about 50 percent. In addition, we also found a rather high number of false-negative reagin reactions in secondary syphilis. Late cutaneous manifestations of syphilis were rare in contrast to cardiovascular syphilis, and general paralysis and tabes dorsalis are nearly unknown. Many cases of early congenital syphilis are not diagnosed. Only 40 cases were seen in our clinic in 1972. The most impressive feature was the very extensive involvement of the long bones. We did not diagnose a single case of late congenital syphilis.

Leprosy

The infection with *Mycobacterium leprae* presents a spectrum of clinical manifestations depending upon the host's resistance. Generally accepted is the Ridley-Jopling classification based on clinical, bacteriologic, histologic and immunologic features of leprosy: TT, BT, BB, BL, and LL.

Leprosy is, however, not only a skin disease. In the tuberculoid end of the spectrum the nerves are involved and lepromatous leprosy is a universal infection affecting many organs. The nerves involved in leprosy are the subcutaneous nerves and superficial nerve trunks. The most important are: the ulnar, facial, external popliteal, posterior tibial, supraorbital, median, and trigeminus nerves. Both motor and sensory nerve fibers are affected.

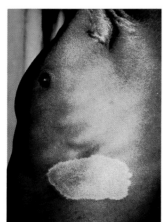

Fig. A6-1 TT leprosy. A person with high resistance but not full resistance develops the TT type of leprosy. The patient is able to restrict the infection to a single, well-defined lesion. This lesion is anesthetic and hypopigmented; in the African it is the typical color of copper. *M. leprae* not demonstrable; the lepromin test is positive.

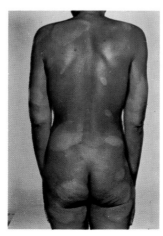

Fig. A6-2 BT leprosy. With less resistance the patient develops several lesions. This is the most common form of leprosy in Africa.

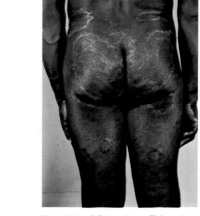

Fig. A6-3 BB leprosy. This represents the middle of the spectrum, midborderline leprosy. The lesions are often annular. *M. leprae* moderate in skin lesions.

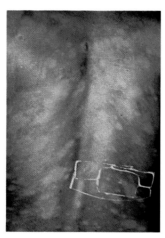

Fig. A6-4 LL leprosy. The diffuse form of lepromatous leprosy. An abundance of *M. leprae* everywhere in the skin; lepromin test negative.

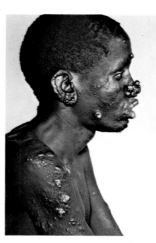

Fig. A6-5 LL leprosy. An advanced, late, nodular type of lepromatous leprosy.

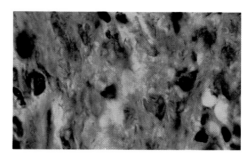

Fig. A6-6 M. leprae from a patient with lepromatous leprosy. Ziehl–Neelsen staining.

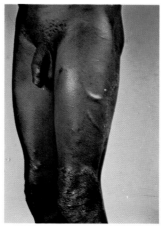

Fig. A6-7 Thickening of subcutaneous nerves in a patient with tuberculoid leprosy.

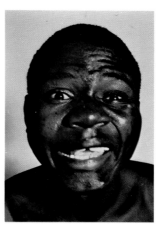

Fig. A6-8 Facial paralysis in tuberculoid leprosy.

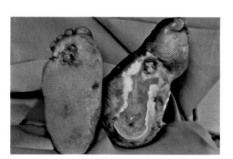

Fig. A6-9 Severe trophic ulcers caused by anesthesia of the feet.

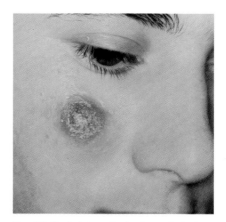

Fig. A6-10 Leishmaniasis. An early lesion. Leishmaniasis is so varied in its clinical manifestations that it might mimic a boil, lupus vulgaris, syphilis, and leprosy in all its forms: tuberculoid, borderline, and lepromatous.

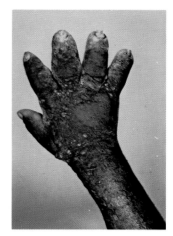

Fig. A6-11 Kaposi's sarcoma. Nodular lesions with severe lymphedema of the hand. Kaposi's sarcoma is common in equatorial Africa. Most cases in adults are of nodular type.

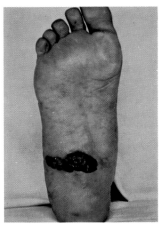

Fig. A6-12 Melanoma. Most cases of melanoma in African blacks occur on the soles. The reason is presumably that many tribes have pigmented nevi in the soles which have considerable junctional activity; possibly, chronic traumatization by walking barefoot plays a pathogenic role.

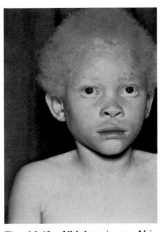

Fig. A6-13 Albinism in an African child. This child has nystagmus and solar keratoses. These patients develop extensive squamous cell carcinomas at an early age. Only a few survive to the age of 25.

Fig. A6-14 Pellagra is a common disease in East Africa. The staple diet of this area consists of banana and maize, which are poor in B vitamins and protein. One of the typical skin manifestations is a photodermatitis localized to the V of the neck. The beneficial effect of niacin or B-complex products is usually dramatic.

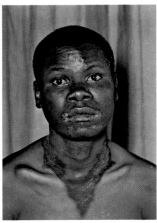

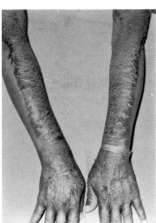

Fig. A6-15 Photodermatitis localized to the dorsa of the hands and forearms. A typical skin manifestation of **pellagra.**

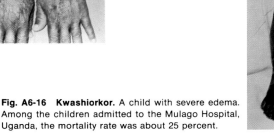

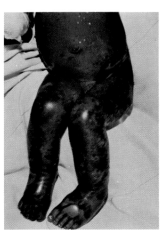

Fig. A6-17 Malnutrition is a milder form of kwashiorkor caused by undernourishment and often also malabsorption. The children have red hair, moon face, and "cracked skin."

Fig. A6-16 Kwashiorkor. A child with severe edema. Among the children admitted to the Mulago Hospital, Uganda, the mortality rate was about 25 percent.

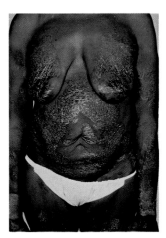

Fig. A6-18 Erythrasma. Extensive eruptions are often seen in Africa. This patient had had the disease for more than 20 years. Treatment with tetracyclines for 14 days cleared the lesions completely.

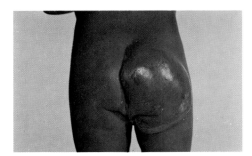

Fig. A6-19 Subcutaneous phycomycosis. The clinical features are often diagnostic: an extensive, subcutaneous, hard infiltration involves fat and muscles; the border is lobulated. Usually one can press one's fingertips beneath the border of the well-defined tumor.

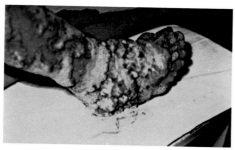

Fig. A6-20 Chromoblastomycosis. Extensive verrucous lesions on the lower extremity.

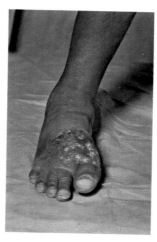

Fig. A6-21 Madura foot (mycetoma). The color and size of the grains in the discharge are helpful in classifying the causing agent.

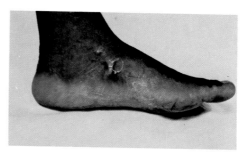

Fig. A6-22 African histoplasmosis caused by *Histoplasma duboisii.* Some patients have molluscum contagiosum-like papular lesions in the face.

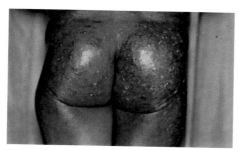
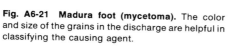

Fig. A6-23 Onchocerciasis. Severe lichenification on the buttocks with papular lesions caused by microfilariae. Nodular lesions with adult worms are not seen. They are mainly localized over bony prominences of the hips, ribs, knees, and elbows.

Fig. A6-24 Guinea worm (dracunculosis). The worm is seen on the medial side of the foot.

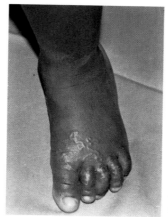

Fig. A6-25 Larva migrans (creeping eruption). This eruption was effectively treated by freezing with ethyl chloride, a simple treatment widely used in epidemic areas.

PEDIATRIC DERMATOLOGY

Ferdinando Gianotti and
Ruggero Caputo

Infants and children represent approximately one-sixth of the world population. At one time or another, they are all subject to cutaneous disorders, a fact that by itself underlines the importance of pediatric dermatology. The significance of this particular subspecialty also becomes evident if one takes into account that it encompasses: (1) diseases specific for the pediatric age group; (2) the large number of exanthematous conditions, most of which are infectious in nature and preferentially occur in children; (3) common skin conditions which, in the child, present in a different way than in the adult; and (4) many genetic disorders, already evident in the newborn or infant.

As in the adult, cutaneous signs and symptoms in the child allow the early recognition of diseases in other organ systems. Most infectious diseases can be identified through their cutaneous lesions; histiocytosis X can be diagnosed in the skin when visceral lesions are not yet detectable and the same is true for acrodermatitis enteropathica and some immunologic disorders. The importance of recognizing and treating such severe diseases before irreversible damage has occurred need not be stressed.

Inflammatory conditions of infancy

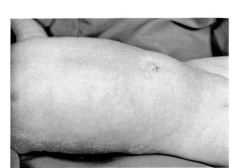

Fig. A7-1 Erythema toxicum neonatorum. This common eruption, which initially is papuloerythematous and subsequently micropustular and is usually confined to the trunk, may be present at birth or appears within the first 2 days of life. The micropustules are sterile and rich in eosinophils. The eruption subsides spontaneously within 10 days and its etiology is unknown.

a

b

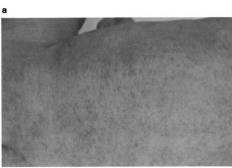

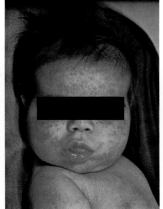

c

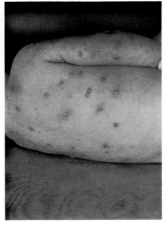

Fig. A7-2 Eosinophilic papulovesicular dermatitis of infancy. Papuloerythematous **(a)** and occasionally vesiculopustular eruptions **(b)** also occur in children over 2 months of age. The lesions are disseminate, showing a predilection for the head and trunk, and are rich in eosinophils. In older babies they may be less numerous **(c)** and papular, and are accompanied by pronounced eosinophilia of the peripheral blood. These eruptions do not itch, they recur over several months, and are not due to insect bites or scabies from which they have to be differentiated.

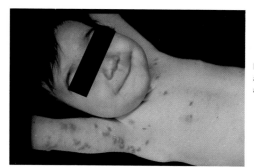

Fig. A7-3 Nodular lesions due to scabies. Nodular granulomas due to scabies are also rich in eosinophils and occur during the first years of life. The most common sites are the axillae, penis, and scrotum, where they persist for long periods of time.

b

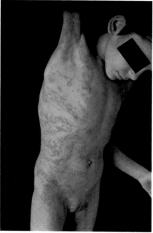

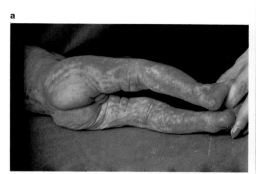

a

Fig. A7-4 Incontinentia pigmenti. Full-blown incontinentia pigmenti presents as a congenital bullous condition. It is only rarely familial and almost always occurs in females. It usually develops during the first days of life and manifests as an erythematous and subsequently bullous eruption, distributed along Blaschko's lines on the limbs and the trunk, while the head is usually spared. The lesions are rich in eosinophils; in the bullous stage there is pronounced blood eosinophilia (up to 60 percent). After one or more months, the bullous stage is followed by a papuloverrucous stage **(a)** and, finally, by the pigmentary stage **(b)**; the latter is characteristic for the disease and lasts from 2 to 10 or more years. Some cases present with the pigmentary stage at birth, the earlier stages having presumably taken place during intrauterine life. In many cases there may be other, associated anomalies of the skin (atrophic and cicatricial alopecia, nail dystrophy, impairment of sweating) and of the teeth, eyes, heart, and the nervous system.

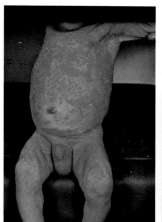

Fig. A7-5 Seborrheic dermatitis. This erythematous dermatitis is associated with greasy parakeratotic scaling and is thus commonly known as "milk crust." It appears during the first few weeks of life, usually starting on the scalp and the retroauricular folds, where it may lead to the development of a cap of yellowish scales or to transient alopecia. The condition subsequently spreads to involve the inguinal **(a)**, axillary, intergluteal, and nuchal folds, where lesions become erosive, oozing, and exhibit deep fissures. On the trunk, lesions spread by peripheral growth and are covered with dry scales, while the face is erythematous with prominent scaling of the eyebrows and nasolabial folds **(b)**. There is no itching. The condition is often accompanied by gastrointestinal disturbances and thrush is sometimes present.

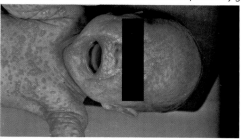

Superinfection of skin lesions by *Candida albicans* is heralded by superficial micropustules; eczematization may occur either as a consequence of inadequate treatment, or as an early manifestation of atopic dermatitis and is characterized by the appearance of vesicles or exudative papules on the cheeks. Generalized seborrheic dermatitis evolves into Leiner's disease (see Fig. A7-12).

Seborrheic dermatitis usually persists for a few weeks and rarely recurs. Its pathogenesis is unknown. Milk, by breast- or bottle-feeding, is not responsible for the disorder and it is therefore totally unnecessary to discontinue its administration.

a   b

Fig. A7-6 Dermatitis of the diaper area. Persistent occlusion of the diaper area by waterproof pants often leads to erythematous and infiltrated lesions in this region. Common sites are the skin of the pubis, external genitalia, intergluteal folds, and thighs but, in contrast to intertrigo, the bottoms of the folds usually remain unaffected *(diaper dermatitis)*. In long-lasting diaper dermatitis, isolated or grouped, eroded or even ulcerated papules appear, probably owing to chronic infections. This is termed *syphiloid dermatitis of Sevestre–Jacquet* **(a)**; it responds to topical treatment with erythromycin. Diffusely erythematous diaper dermatitis may exhibit psoriasiform scaling, and psoriasiform lesions may spread to involve the trunk, limbs, and scalp *(psoriasiform diaper dermatitis)* **(b)**. The authors believe that in most cases this is a peculiar expression of seborrheic dermatitis; however, in some cases it does represent early psoriasis. Differential diagnosis is difficult even by histology. While the former heals definitively, psoriasis will sooner or later recur.

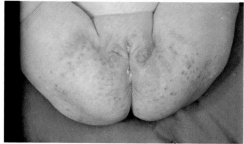

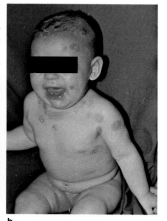

a   b

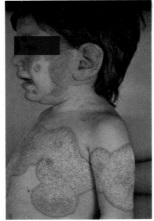

Fig. A7-7 Candidiasis. *Candida albicans* infections have become increasingly common, possibly as a consequence of treatments with antibiotics and corticosteroids. Most newborn babies soon become carriers of *Candida* and develop sensitivity to candidine. Stomatitis caused by *Candida* is extremely frequent and is characterized by white plaques of the oral mucosa which can be wiped off easily. In addition, babies may exhibit pelèche, cheilitis, lingua nigra, perioral pustular and squamous or crusted lesions, and extensive intertrigo and psoriasiform or pustular plaques which expand peripherally and may occasionally spread to involve the entire skin. Vulvovaginitis, perianal dermatitis, paronychia, and onychomycosis may develop. Symmetrical vesicular eruptions, termed *monilids,* are believed to represent a reaction of the sensitized host to the yeast or its products. Immunodeficient children or children with hypoparathyroidism may exhibit verrucose, papular-crusted, or hyperkeratotic lesions (granulomatous candidiasis) seen here; this condition can become generalized and involve internal organs.

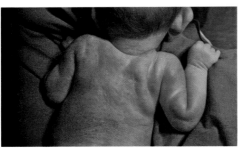

Fig. A7-8 Subcutaneous fat necrosis. This condition occurs shortly after birth and presents as reddish, firm, subcutaneous nodules and plaques of variable size; the cheeks, back, arms, buttocks, and thighs may be affected. These indurations are nonpitting and are well defined; after weeks or months they soften and resolve spontaneously without residual atrophy. Histologically there is fat necrosis and an inflammatory reaction with giant cells. Triglyceride crystals, visible in frozen sections, are present in lipocytes and giant cells; in routine paraffin sections their sites appear as needle-shaped clefts. Calcium deposits may be observed. These lesions occur in healthy infants born at term, the pathogenesis is not known and trauma is not involved.

In premature and debilitated newborns, *sclerema neonatorum* may develop during the first days of life. In this condition there is a diffuse and rapidly spreading hardening of the subcutaneous fat of large areas of symmetrical distribution. The entire skin may be involved and appear uniformly thickened, hardened, and cold. The joints often become immobile and there may be lesions in the visceral fat. The persistence of sclerema beyond 2 weeks is usually fatal.

Histologically there are wide fibrous bands within the subcutis; needlelike clefts, previously occupied by triglyceride crystals, are apparent in fat cells but, in contrast to subcutaneous fat necrosis, there is no fat necrosis or inflammation or giant cells, and calcium is not deposited.

Cold panniculitis may develop in infants, particularly on the face and legs. One or two days after exposure to cold, red, indurated plaques or nodules appear in the subcutaneous tissue with the overlying skin firmly bound to these lesions; they subside spontaneously within a short time. Histologically, one finds perivascular lymphohistiocytic infiltrates and lipid cysts derived from ruptured fat cells.

Erythrodermas of infancy

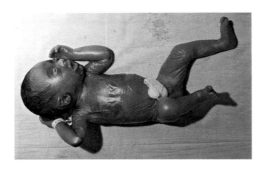

Fig. A7-9 Collodion baby. At birth, babies with X-linked and lamellar ichthyosis and with ichthyosiform erythroderma may occasionally be enveloped by a "collodion" membrane. After shedding of the membrane, collodion babies may exhibit a normal skin and some authorities therefore believe that the membrane is a persistent periderm coming off at a late stage. Usually, however, there is either a gradual transition to X-linked ichthyosis, in which case the characteristic corneal opacities are present, or to lamellar ichthyosis or ichthyosiform erythroderma; in this case ectropion and eclabion develop.

Fig. A7-10 Erythrodermic psoriasis. This is really a congenital form of psoriasis, but it may also develop in early infancy. Grossly and histologically, it resembles ichthyosiform erythroderma with marked shedding of large, micaceous scales. Some normal skin areas may be present but only the development of typical psoriatic patches or lesions of pustular psoriasis during childhood allow an unequivocal diagnosis.

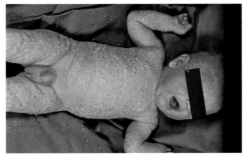

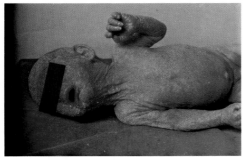

Fig. A7-11 Ichthyosiform erythroderma. This is a more severe condition characterized by a dry, scaly mantle encasing erythrodermic skin; there is ectropion, and eclabion may cause feeding problems. Bullae are never present. Generalized erythroderma persists throughout childhood and beyond, but it may become less marked with age.

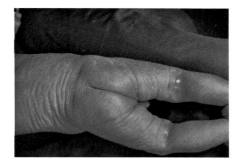

Fig. A7-12   Leiner's disease. Erythrodermic seborrheic dermatitis (Leiner's disease) occurs between the second and sixth month of life. It develops rapidly and combines erythroderma, edema, greasy scaling, and shiny, oozing erosions. Gastrointestinal disturbances may occur and dehydration, disturbances of the electrolyte balance, and hypoproteinemia may develop. Reactive lymphadenitis may occasionally be present. These infants are prone to acquire gram-negative and *Candida* infections and apparently have a defect in the function of the fifth component of complement (C5). The prognosis is usually good; correction of the electrolyte balance and the administration of fresh plasma may become necessary in patients with severe enteropathy.

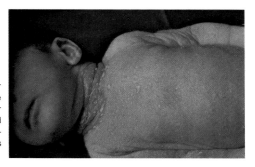

Fig. A7-13   Ritter's disease. Ritter's disease (dermatitis exfoliative neonatorum) or the *staphylococcal scalded-skin syndrome* is caused by an exotoxin of certain phage group 2 staphylococci either following bullous (staphylococcal) impetigo or other staphylococcal infections at distant sites. Flaccid bullae arise on reddened skin and where the epithelium is not yet detached, it can be easily dislodged by rubbing (positive Nikolsky's sign). This is due to a subgranular acantholytic process. The mortality is low if antibiotic therapy is quickly instituted.

Generalized bullous conditions

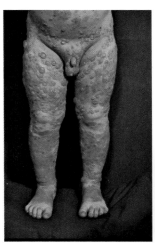

Fig. A7-14   Dermatitis herpetiformis. Dermatitis herpetiformis of childhood usually appears between the second and sixth years of age. It is a polymorphous skin eruption, consisting of figurate erythemas, urticarial lesions, and isolated or grouped vesicles and blisters **(a).** Lesions may be generalized or involve only specific regions, particularly the lower abdomen, and the intergluteal and perioral regions. Successive eruptions continue for months and years. Itching is often present. General health remains undisturbed even after years of disease but some of these children have a gluten-sensitive enteropathy. Granular deposits of IgA are characteristically found by immunofluorescence at the tips of the dermal papillae of perilesional or uninvolved skin. In many cases, the disease presents only with a few discrete papular or vesicular lesions. Oral administration of 10 to 20 drops of 50% potassium iodide is usually followed by a bullous eruption **(b and c),** which can be used as a diagnostic test. *Chronic bullous dermatosis of childhood* and *bullous pemphigoid* are clinically similar to the bullous forms of dermatitis herpetiformis but the former exhibits linear IgA and the latter IgG and C3 at the dermal-epidermal junction.

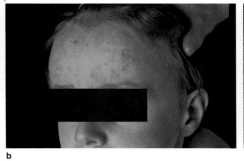

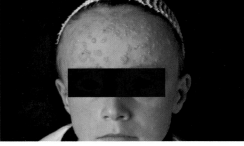

b   c

Fig. A7-15   Epidermolysis bullosa, recessive. Autosomal recessive epidermolysis bullosa can be subclassified as follows.
   Junctional epidermolysis bullosa (epidermolysis bullosa letalis). Large blisters and extensive shedding of the epidermis **(a),** often affecting the whole skin except for palms and soles, can be present from birth. Lesions show little tendency to heal, there is no scarring, and many of these children die during the first months of life.
   Dystrophic epidermolysis bullosa (dystrophica). In this disease, blisters are continuously formed leading to cicatricial atrophy so that, over several years' time, there is loss of nails, and fingers and toes undergo pseudofusion with mittenlike epidermal encasements **(b).** Severe oral and esophageal involvement can be observed. Teeth are dystrophic. There is retardation of growth and development and death may occur early in life.
   The blisters of recessive epidermolysis bullosa are always formed at the dermal-epidermal junction. In the junctional form, the plane of cleavage lies between the plasma membrane of basal cells and the basal lamina. In the scarring form the dermal-epidermal separation takes place just beneath the basal lamina, due to the congenital absence of anchoring fibrils (dermolytic epidermolysis bullosa).

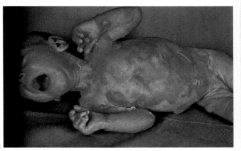

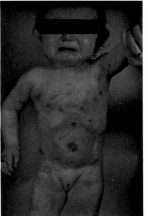

a   b

Papular conditions

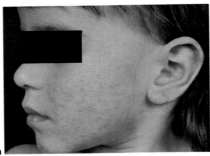

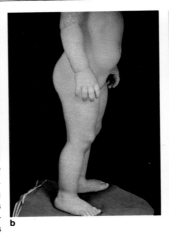

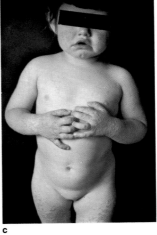

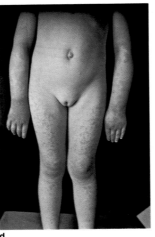

Fig. A7-16 Acrodermatitis. *Papular acrodermatitis of childhood (PAC)* (formerly Gianotti–Crosti syndrome) is a fairly common infectious disease which is characterized by nonrelapsing, nonitching papular lesions usually on the face **(a)**, buttocks, and limbs **(b)**; it is not very contagious and lasts for 20 to 25 days. Associated symptoms are **(1)** an enlargement of inguinal and axillary lymph nodes due to a reactive reticulohistiocytic lymphadenitis, and **(2)** an acute hepatitis, which is usually anicteric, lasts for at least 2 months but may progress to chronic aggressive hepatitis and is always associated with hepatitis B antigen (HBsAg, any subtype). The authors consider PAC a clinical condition due to primary infection with HB virus, acquired via the oral route or through mucous membranes. HBAg carriers are often found among the family members of a child with PAC.

In childhood, there are also other types of papular or papulovesicular eruptions, preferentially localized on acral regions. They may or may not itch, they may be purpuric or nonpurpuric, and the lesions may be disseminate **(c)** or coalesce to larger patches **(d)**; they are associated with reactive lymphadenitis. These eruptions may accompany or follow other diseases (such as infectious mononucleosis) or have an unknown cause. The latter should be classified as *papulovesicular acrolocated syndrome* until their pathogenesis is clarified.

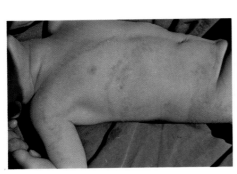

Fig. A7-17 Lichen striatus. While lichen planus is quite rare in children but does exhibit typical papular or verrucous lesions and lichen nitidus shows the same lesions and localizations as in adults, lichen striatus is fairly common in children between 2 and 6 years of age. The condition has a rapid onset and presents with red or yellowish or brown and white papules which are aligned along the so-called Blaschko lines. The striae may be verrucous and do not itch; they may be single or multiple and are always unilateral. The eruption spontaneously subsides after a few months. Its etiology and pathogenesis are unknown.

Fig. A7-18 Pityriasis lichenoides. This disorder occurs mainly in childhood. Histologically there is lymphocytic vasculitis; and clinically several forms, differing in severity and localization, can be distinguished. Erythematous papules, often covered with a thin scale adhering to the center, are symmetrically disseminated over the entire skin or are more rarely confined to the limbs and buttocks or occur almost exclusively on the trunk. The condition is rather uncommon in the infant but when it occurs the manifestations may be severe. Individual lesions last several weeks and often lead to transient leukoderma. The course is unpredictable but the general health is not impaired.

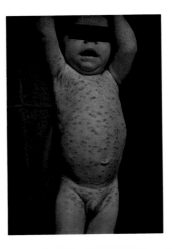

Mesenchymal disorders and metabolic diseases

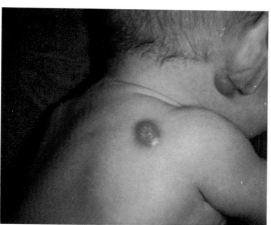

Fig. A7-19 Juvenile xanthogranuloma. This is a self-healing, eruptive, histiocytic granuloma which is not due to or accompanied by disorders of lipid or glucose metabolism. The onset is usually in early infancy, although lesions may occasionally be present at birth. Typical lesions are firm, erythematous or brownish nodules measuring 2 to 30 mm in diameter, which become xanthomatous after a few weeks or months. Nodules are solitary or may occur as multiple, small lesions disseminated all over the body.

When large nodules are present they may be a sign of visceral involvement (lungs, bones, testes, pericardium); specific ocular lesions, mainly affecting the uvea, may appear during infancy. They may cause hemorrhage of the anterior chamber and glaucoma. Visceral xanthogranulomas, like skin lesions, heal spontaneously within a few years. It is fairly common to find café au lait spots, typical of von Recklinghausen's neurofibromatosis, accompanied by small, multiple xanthogranulomas in children.

Histologically, the xanthogranulomas initially consist almost exclusively of monomorphous histiocytes; subsequently, their cytoplasm becomes foamy, with the appearance of multinucleate giant cells (Touton and foreign-body) and inflammatory cells. Lipids are confined to the cytoplasm of histiocytic cells and there are no extracellular lipid deposits.

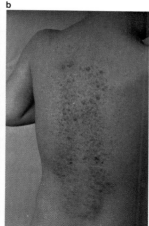

Fig. A7-20 Papular histiocytosis of the head. The main clinical feature of this self-healing histiocytosis is the appearance of yellowish and brownish papules about 2 to 3 mm in diameter on the upper part of the face as shown here; lesions subsequently spread over the whole head, involving also the backs of the ears and the neck and they may also occur on the arms and chest. In the latter region they always remain flat. The lesions persist for several years after which they flatten; atrophic macules result. The health and development of these children is unimpaired and there is no visceral involvement. Histologically, early lesions consist of histiocytes and a few lymphocytes; lipids are absent. In older lesions there are more lymphocytes and occasional cells contain lipids. The histiocytes are rich in peculiar wormlike particles, as revealed by electron microscopy, but there is no similarity to xanthogranuloma, to the xanthomatoses, or to histiocytosis X.

Fig. A7-21 Mastocytosis (urticaria pigmentosa). This papular condition is due to the accumulation of mast cells within the skin. Rubbing of lesions leads to mast cell degranulation, histamine release, and urtication. Skin manifestations may be present at birth but usually appear between the third and ninth month of life and last until puberty. Systemic involvement is rare in children and the prognosis is good.

Well-known manifestations of mastocytosis are (1) solitary or multiple macular or papular lesions of a yellowish to brown color and (2) yellow to brown nodular lesions. There is also a rare diffuse form which may present as (1) urticaria-like mastocytosis (a) in which the skin color is normal or slightly yellow; massive urtication is frequent and the condition is thus confused with urticaria; blister formation may occur; or (2) pachyerythrodermic mastocytosis (b) in which massive infiltration by mast cells results in a marked thickening and erythrodermic appearance of the entire skin and pruritus is severe.

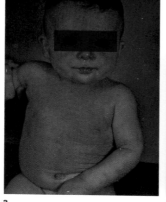

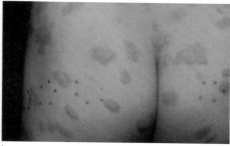

a

b

Fig. A7-22 Histiocytosis X. Histiocytosis X includes Letterer–Siwe disease (LS), Hand–Schüller–Christian disease (HSC) and eosinophilic granuloma (EG). These conditions are due to a proliferation of histiocytes which characteristically contain Langerhans granules. The evolution and course of histiocytosis X varies with the clinical form: it is rapid and disseminated in LS, disseminated but chronic in HSC, localized and chronic in EG. These three syndromes are thus different expressions of the same disorder as demonstrated by transitions from one form to the other, either spontaneously or after treatment. In children, the cutaneous manifestations of disseminated histiocytosis X develop early and in a typical fashion so that they often represent the only detectable signs of this disease.

A close relationship between age of onset and severity of the disease has been demonstrated: the earlier the onset, the more organs are involved, the quicker the course, and the higher the chance of death. The organs most commonly involved are the skin and the bones, but whereas skin lesions are indicative of severe disease, bone lesions are a more benign sign.

In LS lesions are characteristically localized on the chest, abdomen, and scalp (a). They represent pink to reddish papules, 1 to 2 mm in diameter topped by yellowish scales and crusts. Intralesional purpura, subungual petechiae, and ulcerations of mucous membranes are indicative of severe disease.

In HSC skin lesions appear in one-third of the cases. In the eruptive stage they resemble those of LS while in the chronic stage they are either sparse and discrete or grouped in the mediothoracic and dorsal regions (b) or on the scalp.

In the child, EG only rarely causes skin or mucosal lesions. The former are often found in the genital region.

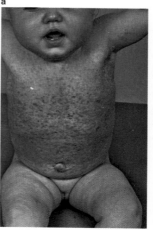

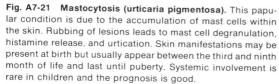

a

b

DISORDERS OF MELANIN PIGMENTATION

Thomas B. Fitzpatrick

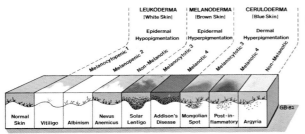

Fig. A8-1 Clinicopathologic classification of pigmentary disorders.

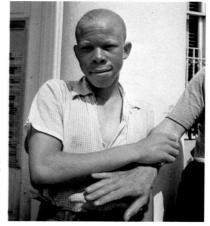

Fig. A8-2 **Oculocutaneous albinism** in a 17-year-old black from Nassau. The albinotic skin of this boy, although darker than normal tanned Caucasian skin, is markedly lighter than the normal skin of his heavily pigmented siblings. This albino also has nystagmus, iris translucence, and reduction of visual acuity, as well as a dilution of skin color.

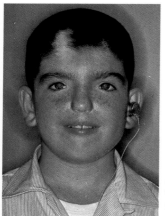

Fig. A8-3 **Waardenburg's syndrome** in a 15-year-old boy. The white forelock is hardly visible. (It often disappears entirely.) The patient has lateral displacement of the medial canthi and uses a hearing aid.

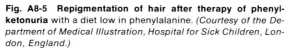

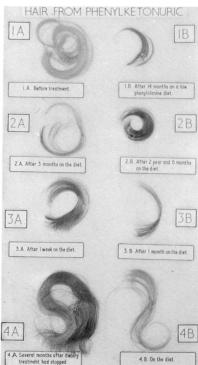

Fig. A8-5 **Repigmentation of hair after therapy of phenylketonuria** with a diet low in phenylalanine. *(Courtesy of the Department of Medical Illustration, Hospital for Sick Children, London, England.)*

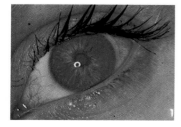

Fig. A8-4 **Iris translucence in oculocutaneous albinism.** The light from the strobe appears as pink areas in the iris. Iris translucence is easily detected by placing a point source of light on the sclera and pointing the light toward the optic disk. (The eyelashes have been artificially darkened.)

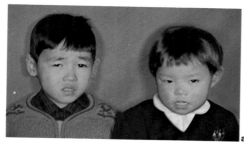

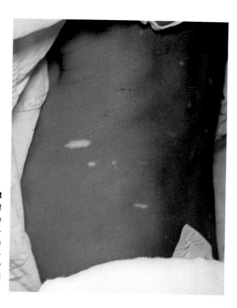

Fig. A8-6 Dilution of hair color in phenylketonuria.
(a) The Japanese child on the right has phenyl-ketonuria and characteristically lighter hair (i.e., brown). **(b)** The hair samples show this contrast in color even more strikingly.

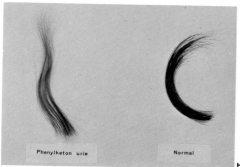

Phenylketon urie   Normal

Fig. A8-7 Hypomelanotic macules in a black infant with tuberous sclerosis. The most typical shapes of hypomelanosis are visible on the trunk: lance-ovate ("ash leaf") and polygonal ("thumb-print"). The lesions are not totally white, as in vitiligo. In persons with white skin it is necessary to use a Wood's lamp to detect the white macules. The use of Wood's lamp is now a standard practice in the examination of infants and children with mental retardation or with seizures.

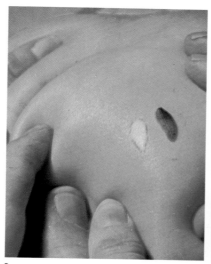

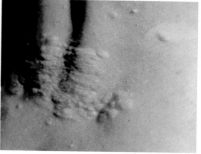

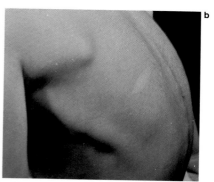

Fig. A8-8 "Ash-leaf" hypomelanotic macules in tuberous sclerosis. (a) Typical lesion with a mountain-ash leaflet placed alongside. **(b)** Typical lance-ovate lesion on the trunk of a severely retarded child. This white macule could easily be overlooked without examination by Wood's lamp. **(c)** At the upper right, a typical ash-leaf spot, and, at the left, a large fibrous plaque, or "shagreen" patch; this patch is a characteristic skin lesion of tuberous sclerosis but is not nearly so frequently present as are the hypomelanotic macules, which are present at birth and persist throughout life. Facial angio-fibromas appear only after 2 years and are much less frequently present.

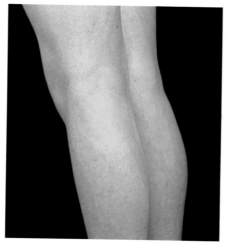

Fig. A8-9 Nevus depigmentosus in a white child. The long linear streaks of hypomelanosis occur in a bizarre, almost artificial, configuration. These lesions may be overlooked in white untanned skin and are easily identified with Wood's lamp.

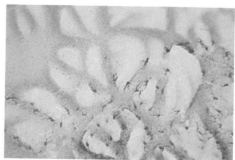

Fig. A8-10 Epidermis, whole mount, separated from the dermis by trypsin digestion, and incubated in dopa solution. The thin slice of skin was taken from a **vitiligo** patient and included a normally pigmented area and a vitiligo area. ×10. *(Courtesy of G. Szabó, Ph.D.)*

At the upper left, the **vitiligo** area shows an absence of dopa-positive melanocytes, and at the lower right, the normal skin shows normal dopa-positive melanocytes.

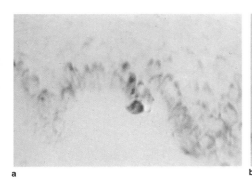

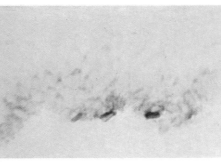

a

b

Fig. A8-11 Skin from a black infant with tuberous sclerosis. ×100. **(a)** A control specimen from the normally pigmented skin which shows an intense dopa reaction. **(b)** A specimen from the hypomelanotic area adjacent to the control skin which shows smaller melanocytes and marked reduction of the dopa reaction.

Fig. A8-12 Idiopathic guttate hypomelanosis. (a) Lesions on the leg of a black. **(b)** Close-up of lesions in which the characteristic sharp margins of the hypomelanosis are evident.

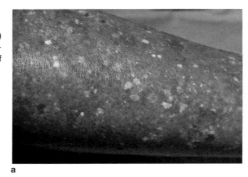

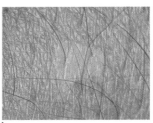

b

a

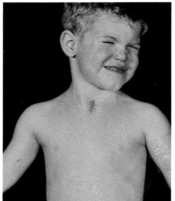

Fig. A8-13 Chédiak–Higashi syndrome. (a) Dilution of skin color and photophobia in a 9-year-old boy. **(b)** Giant cytoplasmic particles in the leukocytes.

 This rare, fatal disorder of childhood exhibits features of oculocutaneous albinism (nystagmus, iris translucency) but the hair color is often a striking metallic gray. *(Courtesy of O. C. Stegmaier, M.D.)*

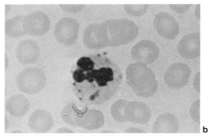

a

b

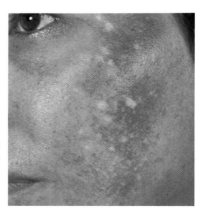

Fig. A8-14 Hypomelanosis following topical application of monobenzyl ether of hydroquinone for treatment of melasma, which is still present. The hypomelanosis is usually irreversible even with psoralen photochemotherapy.

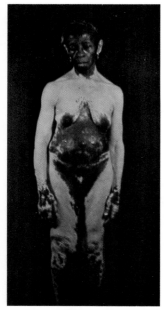

Fig. A8-15 Vitiligo. Striking contrast of normal black pigmentation and vitiliginous areas. Vitiligo in blacks and in East Indians is a medical tragedy because of the striking disfigurement.

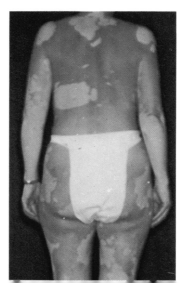

Fig. A8-16 Addison's disease with vitiligo-like hypomelanosis.

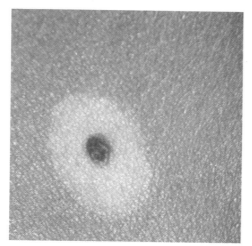

Fig. A8-17 Halo nevus. The pigmented melanocytic lesion may disappear spontaneously and the white macule completely repigment.

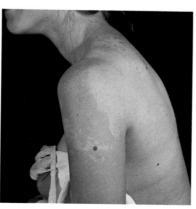

Fig. A8-18 Tinea (pityriasis) versicolor with vitiligo-like hypomelanosis. The hypomelanosis may persist for months after virtual disappearance of the fungal infection. The hypopigmented areas mimic vitiligo. Careful search with Wood's lamp will usually detect remaining foci of fluorescent, scaling areas in which the organisms can be demonstrated.

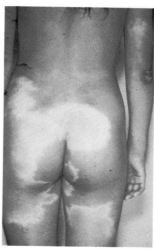

Fig. A8-19 Tuberculoid leprosy with vitiligo-like hypomelanosis. In India, vitiligo is often confused with leprosy, and vitiligo is called "white leprosy." The white macules of leprosy, however, have a loss of tactile sensation, a decreased thermal sensation, and reduced or absent sweating. *(Courtesy of U.S. Public Health Service Hospital, Carville, Louisiana.)*

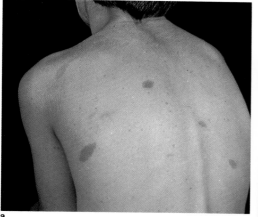

a

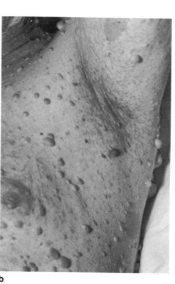

b

Fig. A8-20 Café au lait hypermelanotic macules in neurofibromatosis. (a) Typical occurrence of the macules on the trunk. **(b)** Axillary frecklelike pigmentation that is almost pathognomonic of neurofibromatosis.

Fig. A8-21 Melanotic macules in Albright's syndrome. These macules are indistinguishable from the café au lait macules in neurofibromatosis (see Chap. 79).

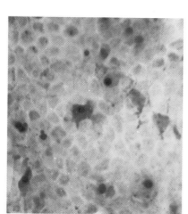

Fig. A8-22 Epidermal whole mount of a café au lait macule in neurofibromatosis. Large pigment granules can be seen in the melanocytes and in the malpighian cells. Dopa; ×64. In electron micrography these large pigment granules are a special type of large spherical organelle called the *melanin macroglobule* (see Chap. 79).

Fig. A8-23 Peutz–Jeghers syndrome. (a) Macules on the buccal mucosae that are blue or blue-black and are pathognomonic. **(b)** Punctate dark brown macules that typically occur on the lips, around the mouth, and on the fingers. The pigmented macules may disappear on the lips but not on the buccal mucosa.

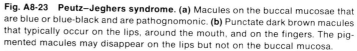

a

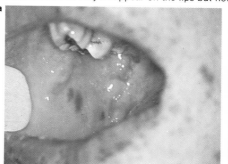

b

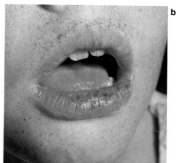

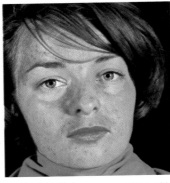

Fig. A8-24 Melasma associated with ingestion of progestational agents.

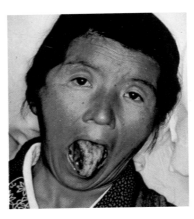

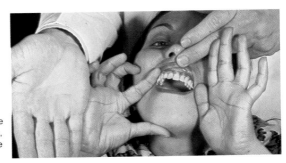

Fig. A8-25 Diffuse brown hypermelanosis of the skin and slate gray or blue pigmentation of the mucous membrane in Addison's disease.

Fig. A8-26 Addisonian type pigmentation of the mucous membrane and palmar creases occurs normally in Asiatics, blacks, Amerindians, and in some whites. Illustrated here is increased pigmentation of the gums and palmar creases in a 35-year-old Gypsy woman.

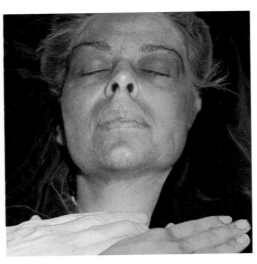

Fig. A8-27 Diffuse brown hypermelanosis, in a patient with a functioning chromophobe adenoma, that followed bilateral adrenalectomy for adrenocortical hyperplasia. The hypermelanosis disappears following treatment of the tumor.

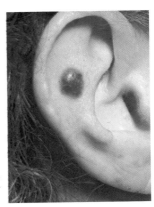

Fig. A8-28 Blue nevus (dermal melanocytoma) that has been present on the ear since birth. Blue nevus can mimic nodular malignant melanoma, and all blue papules or nodules should be excised or biopsied for histologic confirmation of the clinical diagnosis.

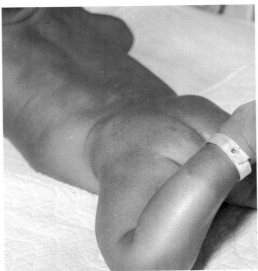

Fig. A8-29 Dermal melanocytosis (Mongolian spots) in a black infant. These lesions almost always virtually disappear in childhood.

Fig. A8-30 Oculodermal melanocytosis (nevus fuscocaerulius ophthalmomaxillaris of Ota) in a black. This pigmentation is not usually congenital, but develops at puberty and does not disappear. Both epidermal and dermal pigmentation may occur.

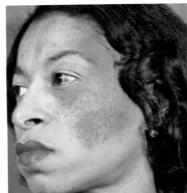

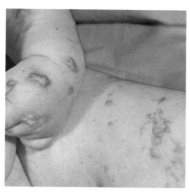

Fig. A8-31 Incontinentia pigmenti, showing bizarre, macular hyperpigmentation and vesicular and papular lesions. This pigmentation is dermal and therefore does not increase in intensity when viewed with Wood's lamp.

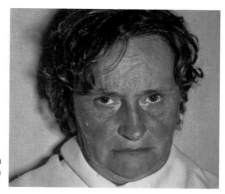

Fig. A8-32 Purple pigmentation in a schizophrenic patient after prolonged high dosage of chlorpromazine.

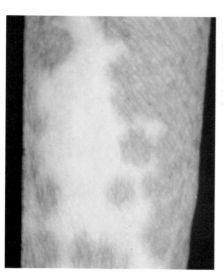

Fig. A8-33 Hypomelanosis in pinta. The late or dyschromic phase of pinta is characterized by deep blue or slate gray pigmentation. Later, vitiligo-like hypomelanosis occurs, especially over bony prominences.

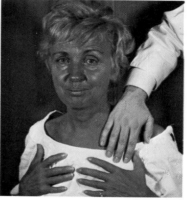

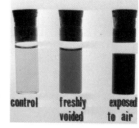

control   freshly voided   exposed to air

Fig. A8-34 Slate gray dermal pigmentation with metastatic melanoma and melanogenuria. (a) Diffuse blue argyria-like hypermelanosis. This patient died 1 month after this photograph was taken, illustrating that this bizarre argyria-like blue pigmentation is a terminal complication. **(b)** Dark urine from a patient with melanogenuria, compared with normal urine.

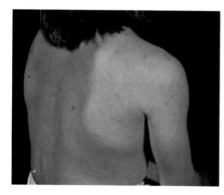

Fig. A8-35 Erythema dyschromicum perstans. There are randomly distributed, faintly blue macules on the trunk. All of the patients with this disease seen in the past 25 years at the Department of Dermatology, Harvard Medical School, present with blue or slate gray macules *without* presence of inflammation or a previous history of an erythematous, raised border, as in the original description by Ramirez of San Salvador (see Chap. 79).

Fig. A8-36 Melasma treated with hydroquinone, 2%, in a washable base. **(a)** The patient before therapy. **(b)** The patient after 2 months of therapy. The lesions can still be seen with Wood's lamp after the hyperpigmentation is no longer detectable in visible light.

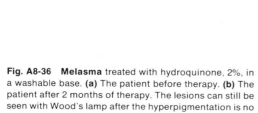

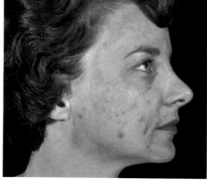

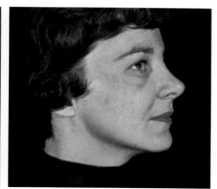

a   b

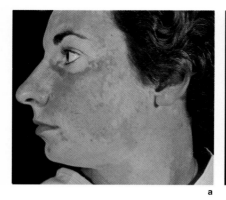
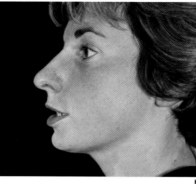

a

b

Fig. A8-37 Depigmentation of the normal skin color with topical application of 20% monobenzyl ether of hydroquinone (MBH) in a patient with generalized vitiligo. **(a)** Normally pigmented skin to which the applications were made. **(b)** The permanent loss of skin color after treatment. Although spotty, recurrences may occur in the summer; these recurrences respond to further treatment with MBH. This patient has remained virtually free of pigment for 10 years.

In vitiligo of late middle life involving more than 70 percent of the skin surface, use of MBH is a very effective method of treatment (see Chap. 79).

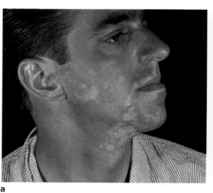
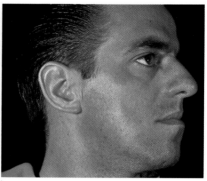

Fig. A8-38 Treatment of vitiligo with orally administered trioxsalen. (a) The patient before therapy. **(b)** The patient after treatment with trioxsalen, 40 mg daily, with daily exposure to the sun for the 5 months of May through September. Such a rapid, complete repigmentation is infrequent. Most patients using either trioxsalen or methoxsalen with sunlight or long-wave photochemotherapy require over 100 exposures to achieve cosmetically satisfactory repigmentation (see Chap. 79).

a

b

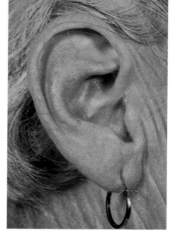

Fig. A8-39 Ochronotic discoloration seen through the thin area of skin overlying the pigmented cartilage of the ear. *(Courtesy of Dr. Brian R. Entwisle, Melbourne, Australia.)*

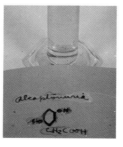

Fig. A8-40 The glass cylinder in the background contains urine from a patient with alkaptonuria. The urine itself was used to write on the photographic paper, then alkali was added. The homogentisic acid in the urine acted as a photographic developer.

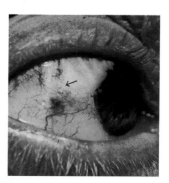

Fig. A8-41 Ochronotic scleral pigmentation.

DERMATOLOGY IN GENERAL MEDICINE

EDITORS

Thomas B. Fitzpatrick, M.D., Ph.D.
Edward Wigglesworth Professor of Dermatology
Chairman, Department of Dermatology
Harvard Medical School
Chief, Dermatology Service
Massachusetts General Hospital, Boston

Arthur Z. Eisen, M.D.
Winifred A. and Emma R. Showman Professor of Medicine
Head, Division of Dermatology
Washington University School of Medicine
Dermatologist-in-Chief
Barnes Hospital, St. Louis

Klaus Wolff, M.D.
Professor and Chairman, Department of Dermatology I
University of Vienna Medical School
Chief, Dermatology Service I
General Hospital of Vienna, Vienna

Irwin M. Freedberg, M.D.
George Miller MacKee Professor and Chairman
Department of Dermatology
New York University
School of Medicine, New York

K. Frank Austen, M.D.
Theodore B. Bayles Professor of Medicine
Harvard Medical School
Chairman, Department of Rheumatology and Immunology
Brigham and Women's Hospital, Boston

DERMATOLOGY IN GENERAL MEDICINE

Textbook and Atlas

Third Edition

McGRAW-HILL BOOK COMPANY • NEW YORK • ST. LOUIS • SAN FRANCISCO • AUCKLAND • BOGOTÁ
HAMBURG • JOHANNESBURG • LISBON • LONDON • MADRID • MEXICO • MILAN • MONTREAL • NEW DELHI
PANAMA • PARIS • SAN JUAN • SÃO PAULO • SINGAPORE • SYDNEY • TOKYO • TORONTO

NOTICE

Medicine is an ever-changing science. As new research and
clinical experience broaden our knowledge, changes in treatment and drug therapy are required. The editors and the publisher of this work have made every effort to ensure that the
drug dosage schedules herein are accurate and in accord with
the standards accepted at the time of publication. Readers are
advised, however, to check the product information sheet
included in the package of each drug they plan to administer to
be certain that changes have not been made in the recommended dose or in the contraindications for administration.
This recommendation is of particular importance in regard to
new or infrequently used drugs.

DERMATOLOGY IN GENERAL MEDICINE

Copyright © 1987, 1979, 1971 by McGraw-Hill, Inc. All rights
reserved. Printed in the United States of America. No part of
this publication may be reproduced, stored in a retrieval system, or transmitted, in any form or by any means, electronic,
mechanical, photocopying, recording, or otherwise, without
the prior written permission of the publisher.

1234567890 DOWDOW 89876

This book was set in Times Roman by Ruttle, Shaw &
Wetherill, Inc. The editors were J. Dereck Jeffers, Eileen
Scott, and Julia White; the cover was designed by Edward
R. Schultheis; the production supervisor was Ave McCracken.
R. R. Donnelley & Sons Company was printer and binder.

Library of Congress Cataloging in Publication Data
Main entry under title:

Dermatology in general medicine.

   Includes bibliographies and index.
   1. Dermatology. 2. Cutaneous manifestations of general
diseases. I. Fitzpatrick, Thomas B. [DNLM: 1. Skin diseases. 2. Skin
Manifestations.   WR 100 D4383]
RL71.D46   1987   616.5   86-10633
ISBN 0-07-079689-0 (set)
ISBN 0-07-021205-8 (v. 1)
ISBN 0-07-021206 (v. 2)

Preface

The Third Edition of *Dermatology in General Medicine* is a major revision with 60 additional chapters and 120 new contributors. Through this edition we are attempting to keep pace with new developments in dermatology: aging of the skin; pathophysiology of pruritus; physiology and pharmacology of the skin including cutaneous circulation, hormone receptors, and metabolism of drugs; chemical and viral carcinogenesis; dermatopathology; therapeutics including topical and systemic therapy, especially recently introduced modalities such as PUVA photochemotherapy, retinoids, cytotoxic agents, antiviral agents, and pharmacokinetics in relation to topical therapy; benign and dysplastic melanocytic nevi; cutaneous aspects of cardiopulmonary diseases, cutaneous manifestations of immunodeficiency disorders.

Some of the chapters and sections in this edition are, in fact, monographs with detailed documentation, some chapters have been completely rewritten by new authors, and others have been extensively revised and updated. The discussion on photomedicine has now been expanded to ten chapters.

Special features are an Atlas of Common Skin Disorders with 36 new color plates, a new color Atlas of Cutaneous Manifestations of Multisystem Disease with detailed legends, and a new color Atlas of Clinical Recognition of Primary Melanoma and its Precursors.

The new edition again presents comprehensive discussions of the basic sciences as they relate to the skin and its pathophysiology, and we have included those disorders limited to the skin such as psoriasis and eczema and a major consideration of the cutaneous manifestations of diseases in other organ systems.

Although the book is aimed primarily at the dermatologist, it should also be valuable for medical students, general internists and medical specialists (gastroenterologists, rheumatologists, endocrinologists, and infectious disease physicians), primary care physicians, pediatricians, neurologists, pathologists, surgeons, psychiatrists, and dentists.

The editors are deeply grateful to Patricia K. Novak who has assiduously assembled all three editions of this textbook.

We wish also to acknowledge the cooperation of those persons at the McGraw-Hill Book Company with whom we worked—J. Dereck Jeffers, Eileen Scott, Julia White, Edward R. Schultheis, and Ave McCracken

Thomas B. Fitzpatrick
Arthur Z. Eisen
Klaus Wolff
Irwin M. Freedberg
K. Frank Austen

Contents

PART FIVE

Section 26

DISORDERS DUE TO MICROBIAL AGENTS

Bacterial Diseases with Cutaneous Involvement

Section 27

Fungal Diseases with Cutaneous Involvement

Section 28

Rickettsial and Viral Diseases with Cutaneous Involvement

Section 29

Sexually Transmitted Diseases

Section 30   Animal Bites, Infestations, and Insect Bites and Stings

Section 31   Skin Manifestations of Immunosuppression

PART SIX   THERAPEUTICS

Section 32   Topical Modalities

Section 33   Systemic Therapy

PART SEVEN   PEDIATRIC DERMATOLOGY

Section 34   Pediatric Dermatology

PART EIGHT   DERMATOLOGIC ATLAS

ATLAS

List of Contributors

A. Bernard Ackerman, M.D. Professor of Dermatology and Pathology, and Director, Dermatopathology, New York University School of Medicine, New York

Raymond D. Adams, M.A., M.D., M.A. (Hon.), D.Sc. (Hon.), M.D. (Hon.) Bullard Professor of Neuropathy (Emeritus), Harvard Medical School; Senior Neurologist, Massachusetts General Hospital; Director (Emeritus), E. K. Shriver Center, Boston.

Oscar M. Alvarez, Ph.D. Scientist, Bioderm Medical Inc., Princeton.

Arthur J. Ammann, M.D. Adjunct Professor of Pediatrics and Pediatric Immunology/Rheumatology, School of Medicine, University of California, San Francisco.

Warren A. Andiman, M.D. Associate Professor, Pediatrics and Epidemiology and Public Health, Yale University School of Medicine, New Haven.

Elliot J. Androphy, M.D. Medical Staff Fellow, Dermatology Branch and Laboratory of Cellular Oncology, National Cancer Institute, National Institutes of Health, Bethesda.

Howell O. Archard, D.D.S. Associate Professor of Dentistry, School of Dental Medicine, State University of New York at Stony Brook, Stony Brook.

Kenneth A. Arndt, M.D. Professor of Dermatology, Harvard Medical School; Dermatologist-in-Chief, Beth Israel Hospital, Boston.

Frank C. Arnett, Jr., M.D. Professor of Internal Medicine, The University of Texas Health Science Center at Houston, Houston.

Dalal Assaad, M.D., F.R.C.P.(C) Consultant Dermatologist and Dermatopathologist, Sunnybrook Medical Centre; Assistant Professor, University of Toronto, Toronto.

K. Frank Austen, M.D. Theodore B. Bayles Professor of Medicine, Harvard Medical School; Chairman, Department of Rheumatology and Immunology, Brigham and Women's Hospital, Boston.

Howard P. Baden, M.D. Professor of Dermatology, Harvard Medical School; Dermatologist, Massachusetts General Hospital, Boston.

Ann Sullivan Baker, M.D. Assistant Professor of Medicine, Harvard Medical School; Associate Physician, Infectious Disease Unit, Massachusetts General Hospital, Boston.

Eugene A. Bauer, M.D. Professor of Medicine, Division of Dermatology, Department of Medicine, Washington University School of Medicine, St. Louis.

Jeffrey D. Bernhard, M.D. Assistant Professor of Medicine; Director, Division of Dermatology; Director of Phototherapy Center, Department of Medicine, University of Massachusetts Medical Center, Worcester.

Arthur P. Bertolino, M.D., Ph.D. Assistant Professor of Dermatology, New York University School of Medicine, New York.

David R. Bickers, M.D. Professor and Chairman, Department of Dermatology, Case Western Reserve University; Director, Dermatology Services, University Hospitals and Veterans Administration Medical Center, Cleveland.

Alf Björnberg, M.D. Associate Professor of Dermatology, Department of Dermatology, University of Lund, Lund.

Claudine Blanchet-Bardon, M.D. Director, Pre-Natal Diagnosis Unit, Department of Dermatology, Hôpital Saint-Louis, Paris.

Irvin H. Blank, Ch.E., M.Sc., Ph.D. Associate Biochemist, Massachusetts General Hospital; formerly Assistant Professor of Dermatology, Harvard Medical School, Boston.

Edward E. Bondi, M.D. Associate Professor of Dermatology, University of Pennsylvania School of Medicine, Philadelphia.

Conrado C. Bondoc, M.D. Assistant Professor of Surgery, Harvard Medical School; Associate Visiting Surgeon, Massachusetts General Hospital and Shriners Burns Institute, Boston.

Martine Bouclier, Ph.D. Senior Biochemist and Pharmacologist, Department of Experimental Pharmacology and Toxicology, Centre International de Recherches Dermatologiques, Valbonne.

H. Bryan Brewer, Jr., M.D. Chief, Molecular Disease Branch, National Heart, Lung, and Blood Institute, National Institutes of Health, Bethesda.

Robert A. Briggaman, M.D. Professor of Dermatology, Department of Dermatology, University of North Carolina School of Medicine, Chapel Hill.

Michael B. Brodin, M.D. Assistant Clinical Professor of Dermatology, New York University School of Medicine, New York.

Stanley G. Browne, C.M.G., O.B.E., M.D., F.R.C.P., F.R.C.S., D.T.M. Ex-Secretary, The International Leprosy Association, Sutton, England.

Philip A. Brunell, M.D. Professor and Division Head, Infectious Diseases, Department of Pediatrics, The University of Texas Health Science Center, San Antonio.

Walter H. C. Burgdorf, M.D. Professor and Chairman, Department of Dermatology, The University of New Mexico, Albuquerque.

Robert E. Burgeson, Ph.D. Associate Research Director, Portland Research Unit, Shriners Hospital for Crippled Children, Portland, Oregon.

John F. Burke, M.D. Helen Andrus Benedict Professor of Surgery, Harvard Medical School; Chief of Trauma Services, Massachusetts General Hospital, Boston.

Eric G. L. Bywaters, C.B.E., M.B., B.S. (London), M.D. (Liège Hon.), F.R.C.P. (London), F.A.C.P., F.A.C.P. & S. of Canada Emeritus Professor of Rheumatology, Department of Medicine, Royal Postgraduate Medical School, University of London, London.

Gary W. Cage, M.D. Assistant Clinical Professor of Medicine (Dermatology), Georgetown University; Consultant, Dermatology Branch, National Cancer Institute, National Institutes of Health, Bethesda.

Evan Calkins, M.D. Professor of Medicine; Head, Division of Geriatrics and Gerontology, Department of Medicine, State University of New York at Buffalo; Head, Section on Gerontology, Buffalo Veterans Administration Medical Center, Buffalo.

Ruggero Caputo, M.D. Professor of Dermatology, 1° Dermatologic Clinic, University of Milan, Milan.

D. Martin Carter, M.D., Ph.D. Professor and Senior Physician, Laboratory for Investigative Dermatology, The Rockefeller University, New York.

Enno Christophers, M.D. Professor and Chairman, Department of Dermatology, University of Kiel, Kiel.

Jay D. Coffman, M.D. Professor of Medicine, Boston University School of Medicine; Chief, Peripheral Vascular Section, University Hospital, Boston.

Marcus A. Conant, M.D. Clinical Professor of Dermatology, University of California Medical Center, San Francisco.

Louis Z. Cooper, M.D. Professor of Pediatrics, College of Physicians and Surgeons of Columbia University; Director of Pediatrics, St. Luke's/Roosevelt Hospital Center, New York.

Thomas W. Cooper, M.D. Adjunct Assistant Professor of Clinical Medicine (Dermatology), Dartmouth Medical School, Hanover.

Allen C. Crocker, M.D. Senior Associate in Medicine and Director, Developmental Evaluation Clinic, The Children's Hospital; Associate Professor of Pediatrics, Harvard Medical School; Lecturer in Maternal and Child Health, Harvard School of Public Health, Boston.

Clyde S. Crumpacker, M.D. Associate Professor of Medicine, Harvard Medical School; Infectious Disease Unit, Beth Israel Hospital, Boston.

Mark V. Dahl, M.D. Associate Professor of Dermatology, University of Minnesota Medical School, Minneapolis.

Sven-Erik Dahlén, M.D., Ph.D. Assistant Professor of Physiology, Department of Physiology, and the National Institute of Environmental Medicine, Karolinska Institute, Stockholm.

Farrington Daniels, Jr., M.D., M.P.H. Professor Emeritus of Medicine and Public Health, Cornell University Medical College, New York; Visiting Emeritus Professor, Department of Medicine, The University of Wisconsin, Madison.

Michel Demarchez, Ph.D. Biologist, Department of Cell Biology, Centre International de Recherches Dermatologiques, Valbonne.

Robert J. Desnick, Ph.D., M.D. Arthur J. and Nellie Z. Cohen Professor of Pediatrics and Genetics, and Chief, Division of Medical Genetics, Mount Sinai School of Medicine, New York.

Kevin M. Diette, M.D. Assistant Clinical Professor of Dermatology, Yale University School of Medicine, New Haven.

John J. DiGiovanna, M.D. Senior Staff Fellow, Dermatology Branch, National Cancer Institute, National Institutes of Health, Bethesda.

David D. Donaldson, M.D. Clinical Associate Professor of Ophthalmology, University of South Florida, Tampa; Lecturer, Harvard Medical School; Surgeon Emeritus, Massachusetts Eye and Ear Infirmary, Boston.

Donald T. Downing, Ph.D. Professor, Department of Dermatology, University of Iowa College of Medicine, Iowa City.

William H. Eaglstein, M.D. Professor and Chairman, Department of Dermatology, University of Pittsburgh School of Medicine, Pittsburgh.

J. John Ebling, D.Sc., Ph.D., C.Biol., F.I.Biol. Emeritus Professor of Zoology, The University of Sheffield; Independent Research Worker, Academic Division of Medicine (Sub-Department of Dermatology), Royal Hallamshire Hospital, Sheffield.

Richard L. Edelson, M.D. Professor and Chairman, Department of Dermatology, Yale University School of Medicine, New Haven.

Edward A. Edwards, M.D. Chief, Rehabilitation Medicine Service, Boston Veterans Administration Outpatient Clinic; Surgeon Emeritus, Peter Bent Brigham Hospital; Clinical Professor Emeritus of Anatomy, Harvard Medical School, Boston.

Arthur Z. Eisen, M.D. Winifred A. and Emma R. Showman Professor of Dermatology and Professor of Medicine; Head, Division of Dermatology, Washington University School of Medicine; Dermatologist-in-Chief, Barnes Hospital, St. Louis.

Peter M. Elias, M.D. Chief, Dermatology Service, Veterans Administration Medical Center, San Francisco, and Clinical Professor of Dermatology, University of California School of Medicine, San Francisco.

Edward A. Emmett, M.B., B.S., M.S., F.R.A.C.P. Professor and Director, Division of Occupational Medicine, The Johns Hopkins Medical Institutions, Baltimore.

Edgar G. Engleman, M.D. Associate Professor of Pathology and Medicine, Stanford University School of Medicine, Stanford.

Ervin H. Epstein, Jr., M.D. Clinical Professor and Research Dermatologist, Department of Dermatology, University of California, San Francisco.

William L. Epstein, M.D. Professor, Department of Dermatology, University of California, San Francisco.

Fuad S. Farah, M.D. Professor of Medicine and Chief, Dermatology Section, State University of New York Upstate Medical Center, Syracuse.

Evan R. Farmer, M.D. Associate Professor of Dermatology, Johns Hopkins University School of Medicine; Director, Division of Dermatopathology and Oral Pathology, The Johns Hopkins Medical Institutions, Baltimore.

David S. Feingold, M.D. Professor and Chairman, Department of Dermatology, Tufts University School of Medicine and New England Medical Center Hospital, Boston.

Donna Felsenstein, M.D. Instructor in Medicine, Harvard Medical School; Assistant in Medicine, Massachusetts General Hospital, Boston.

Jessica Fewkes, M.D. Instructor, Harvard Medical School, Assistant Dermatologist, Massachusetts General Hospital, Boston.

George H. Findlay, D.Sc., M.D., F.R.S.(S.Afr) Professor and Head, Department of Dermatology, Faculty of Medicine, The University of Pretoria, Pretoria.

Thomas B. Fitzpatrick, M.D., Ph.D. Edward Wigglesworth Professor of Dermatology and Chairman, Department of Dermatology, Harvard Medical School; Chief, Dermatology Service, Massachusetts General Hospital, Boston.

Raul Fleischmajer, M.D. Professor and Chairman, Department of Dermatology, Mount Sinai School of Medicine, The Mount Sinai Hospital, New York.

P. Donald Forbes, Ph.D. Associate Director, Center for Photobiology, Temple University School of Medicine, Philadelphia.

Andrew G. Franks, Jr., M.D., F.A.C.P. Assistant Clinical Professor of Dermatology, New York University School of Medicine; Assistant Clinical Professor of Medicine (Rheumatology), New York Medical College; Chief of Dermatology, Cabrini Medical Center; Associate Rheumatologist, Lenox Hill Hospital, New York.

Donald S. Fredrickson, M.D., M.D. (Hon.), D.Sc. (Hon.) President, Howard Hughes Medical Institute, Bethesda.

Irwin M. Freedberg, M.D. George Miller MacKee Professor and Chairman, Department of Dermatology, New York University School of Medicine, New York.

Norbert Freinkel, M.D. C. F. Kettering Professor of Medicine; Director, Center for Endocrinology, Metabolism and Nutrition; Director Endocrine-Metabolic Clinics, Northwestern University Medical School, Chicago.

Ruth K. Freinkel, M.D. Professor of Dermatology and Cell Biology-Anatomy, Northwestern University Medical School, Chicago.

Peter O. Fritsch, M.D. Professor and Chairman, Department of Dermatology, University of Innsbruck, Innsbruck.

Lynn From, M.D., F.R.C.P.(C) Pathologist-in-Chief, Women's College Hospital; Associate Professor, University of Toronto, Toronto.

Vincent A. Fulginiti, M.D. Professor and Head, Department of Pediatrics; Vice Dean, College of Medicine, The University of Arizona Health Sciences Center, Tucson.

Kenneth H. Fye, M.D., F.A.C.P. Rheumatologist, Greenbrae, California.

Richard W. Gange, M.D. Assistant Professor of Dermatology, Harvard Medical School; Assistant in Dermatology, Massachusetts General Hospital, Boston.

Joseph Gazith, Ph.D. Senior Biochemist, Department of Pharmacological Biochemistry, Centre International de Recherches Dermatologiques, Valbonne.

Raif S. Geha, M.D. Chief, Division of Allergy, Department of Medicine, The Children's Hospital; Associate Professor, Harvard Medical School, Boston.

Stephen E. Gellis, M.D. Assistant Professor of Dermatology and Pediatrics, Tufts Medical School; Dermatologist, New England Medical Center, Boston.

Sydney S. Gellis, M.D. Professor of Pediatrics and Chairman (Emeritus), Tufts University School of Medicine, Boston.

Feroze N. Ghadially, M.B., B.S. (Bom), M.B., B.S. (Lond), M.D. Ph.D., D.Sc.(Lond), Hon. D.Sc.(Guelph), F.R.C.Path., F.R.C.P.(C), F.R.S.A. Izaak Walton Killam Laureate of the Canada Council; W. S. Lindsay Professor of the College of Medicine, and Professor of Pathology, University of Saskatchewan, Saskatoon.

Fernando Gianotti, M.D. Professor of Dermatology, University of Milan, Milan.

Irma Gigli, M.D. Professor of Medicine and Chief, Division of Dermatology, University of California, San Diego.

Barbara A. Gilchrest, M.D. Professor and Chairman, Department of Dermatology, Boston University School of Medicine; Chief, Cutaneous Gerontology Laboratory, USDA Human Nutrition Center on Aging, Tufts University, Boston.

James N. Gilliam, M.D. Professor and Chairman, Department of Dermatology, Professor of Internal Medicine, Southwestern Medical School, Dallas.

Lowell A. Goldsmith, M.D. James H. Sterner Professor of Dermatology and Chief, Dermatology Unit, the University of Rochester Medical Center, Rochester.

Robert W. Goltz, M.B., M.D. Professor and Head Emeritus, Department of Dermatology, University of Minnesota Medical School, Minneapolis; Adjunct Professor of Medicine, University of California, San Diego.

Ernesto Gonzalez, M.D. Assistant Professor of Dermatology, Harvard Medical School; Director, Dermatology Ambulatory Services, Massachusetts General Hospital, Boston.

J. Blake Goslen, M.D. Assistant Professor, Department of Internal Medicine (Dermatology), Washington University School of Medicine, St. Louis.

Richard D. Granstein, M.D. Assistant Professor of Dermatology, Harvard Medical School; Assistant in Dermatology, Massachusetts General Hospital, Boston.

Seymour J. Gray, M.D., Ph.D. Formerly Associate Clinical Professor of Medicine, Harvard Medical School, Boston.

Malcolm W. Greaves, M.D., Ph.D. Professor and Chairman of Dermatology, Institute of Dermatology, University of London; Consultant Dermatologist, St. James Hospital for Diseases of the Skin; Hon. Senior Lecturer, Department of Pharmacology, University College, London.

Franz Greiter, Ph.D. Professor, Technical University, Vienna.

F. Carl Grumet, M.D. Associate Professor of Pathology and Director, Transfusion Service, Stanford University School of Medicine, Stanford.

Ken Hashimoto, M.D. Professor and Chairman, Department of Dermatology and Syphilology, Wayne State University School of Medicine, Detroit.

Harley A. Haynes, M.D. Associate Professor of Dermatology, Harvard Medical School; Director, Dermatology Division, Brigham and Women's Hospital; Chief, Dermatology, West Roxbury Veterans Administration Hospital, Boston.

Vincent J. Hearing, Ph.D. Laboratory of Cell Biology, National Cancer Institute, National Institutes of Health, Bethesda.

Peter J. Heenan, M.B., F.R.C.Path., F.R.C.P.A. Sir Charles Gairdner Hospital and University of Western Australia, Nedlands.

Martin S. Hirsch, M.D. Associate Professor of Medicine, Harvard Medical School; Associate Physician, Massachusetts General Hospital, Boston.

Karen A. Holbrook, Ph.D. Professor of Biological Structure, Adjunct Professor of Medicine (Dermatology), Associate Dean for Scientific Affairs, University of Washington School of Medicine, Seattle.

Karl Holubar, M.D. Professor and Chairman, Department of Dermatology, Hadassah University Hospital, Hebrew University, Jerusalem.

Herbert Hönigsmann, M.D. Professor of Dermatology, Department of Dermatology I, University of Vienna Medical School, Vienna.

Antoinette F. Hood, M.D. Associate Professor, Department of Dermatology, Johns Hopkins University School of Medicine, Baltimore.

Yoshiaki Hori, M.D., Ph.D. Professor and Chairman, Department of Dermatology, Yamanashi Medical College, Yamanashi, Japan.

Harry J. Hurley, Jr., M.D., D.Sc.(Med.) Clinical Professor of Dermatology, University of Pennsylvania School of Medicine; Attending Dermatologist, Hospital of the University of Pennsylvania, Philadelphia, and Mercy Catholic Medical Center, Darby.

D. Geraint James, M.A., M.D., F.R.C.P. Dean and Physician, Royal Northern Hospital; Consultant Ophthalmic Physician, St. Thomas' Hospital; Consulting Physician to the Royal Navy, London.

Kowichi Jimbow, M.D. Associate Professor, Department of Dermatology, Sapporo Medical College, Sapporo.

Richard A. Johnson, M.D.C.M. Clinical Instructor in Dermatology, Harvard Medical School; Clinical Associate in Dermatology, Massachusetts General Hospital, Boston.

Robert E. Jordon, M.D. Professor and Chairman, Department of Dermatology, The University of Texas Medical School, Houston.

Ben Z. Katz, M.D. Postdoctoral Fellow, Pediatric Infectious Diseases, Yale University School of Medicine, New Haven.

Stephen I. Katz, M.D., Ph.D. Chief, Dermatology Branch, National Cancer Institute, National Institutes of Health, Bethesda.

Helmut Kerl, M.D. Professor of Dermatology, Department of Dermatology, University of Graz, Graz, Austria.

Rebecca E. I. Kerr, M.B., Ch.B., F.R.C.P. Consultant in Dermatology, Stobhill General Hospital; Honorary Clinical Lecturer, The University of Glasgow, Glasgow.

Abdul-Ghani Kibbi, M.D. Research Fellow in Dermatology, Department of Pathology, Massachusetts General Hospital, Harvard Medical School, Boston.

Lloyd E. King, Jr., M.D., Ph.D. Professor of Medicine, Vanderbilt University; Chief of Dermatology, Vanderbilt University and Veterans Administration Medical Centers, Nashville.

Albert M. Kligman, M.D., Ph.D. Professor of Dermatology, Duhring Laboratories, Department of Dermatology, University of Pennsylvania School of Medicine, Philadelphia.

Lorraine H. Kligman, Ph.D. Assistant Research Professor, Department of Dermatology, University of Pennsylvania School of Medicine, Philadelphia.

George S. Kobayashi, Ph.D. Professor, Departments of Internal Medicine and of Microbiology and Immunology, Washington University School of Medicine, St. Louis.

Irene E. Kochevar, Ph.D. Principal Associate, Department of Dermatology, Harvard Medical School, Massachusetts General Hospital, Boston.

Kenneth H. Kraemer, M.D., Research Scientist, Laboratory of Molecular Carcinogenesis, National Cancer Institute, National Institutes of Health, Bethesda.

Stephen M. Krane, M.D., M.A.(Hon.) Professor of Medicine, Harvard Medical School; Chief, Arthritis Unit, Massachusetts General Hospital, Boston.

Eric W. Kraus, M.D. Lieutenant Colonel, United States Army, Medical Corps, Staff Dermatologist, Brooke Army Medical Center, Fort Sam Houston; Associate Clinical Professor, University of Texas Health Sciences Center, San Antonio.

Gerald G. Krueger, M.D. Professor of Medicine and Head, Division of Dermatology, Department of Internal Medicine, University of Utah School of Medicine, Salt Lake City.

W. Clark Lambert, M.D., Ph.D. Associate Professor of Pathology and Director, Division of Dermatopathology, and Associate Professor of Medicine and Vice Chairman, Division of Dermatology, UMDNJ-New Jersey Medical School, Newark.

Thomas J. Lawley, M.D. Senior Investigator, Dermatology Branch, National Institutes of Health, Bethesda.

Gerald S. Lazarus, M.D. Milton B. Hartzell Professor and Chairman, Department of Dermatology, University of Pennsylvania School of Medicine, Philadelphia.

Ullin W. Leavell, Jr., M.D. Professor of Medicine (Dermatology), University of Kentucky Medical Center, Lexington.

Donald Y. M. Leung, M.D., Ph.D. Assistant Professor of Pediatrics, Harvard Medical School; Assistant in Medicine, Department of Medicine, The Children's Hospital, Boston.

Walter F. Lever, M.D. Professor Emeritus of Dermatology, Tufts University School of Medicine, Boston.

Robert A. Lewis, M.D. Associate Professor of Medicine, Harvard Medical School, Boston; Director of Basic Research, Syntex Corporation, Palo Alto.

David L. Livingston, M.D. Professor of Medicine, Harvard Medical School; Physician, Brigham and Women's Hospital; Chief, Laboratory of Neoplastic Disease Mechanisms, Dana-Farber Cancer Institute, Boston.

Gunnar Lomholt, M.D., M.D.h.c. Tutor in Dermatology and Venereology, Lilongwe School of Health Sciences, and Head, Department of Dermatology, Kamuzu Central Hospital, Malawi; formerly Senior Lecturer in Dermatology, Venereology, and Leprology, Makere University, Uganda; formerly Professor of Dermatology, Tromsoe University, Norway; formerly Head, Department of Dermatology, Helsingborg, Sweden.

Douglas R. Lowy, M.D. Chief, Laboratory of Cellular Oncology, National Cancer Institute, National Institutes of Health, Bethesda.

Anton F. H. Luger, M.D. Professor of Dermatology. Head, Ludwig Boltzmann Institute for Venereal Diseases, Krankenhaus Lainz; Vienna.

Marvin A. Lutzner, M.D. Medical Director, U.S. Public Health Service (Ret.), National Cancer Institute, National Institutes of Health, Bethesda.

Frederick D. Malkinson, M.D., D.M.D. The Clark W. Finnerud, M.D. Professor and Chairman, Department of Dermatology, Rush-Presbyterian-St. Luke's Medical Center, Chicago.

Janet M. Marks, M.A., D.M., F.R.C.P. Senior Lecturer in Dermatology, The University of Newcastle upon Tyne; Honorary Consultant Dermatologist, Newcastle upon Tyne Hospitals, Newcastle upon Tyne.

Victor A. McKusick, M.D., F.A.C.P., F.R.C.P.(Lond), D.Sc. (Hon.) University Professor of Medical Genetics, Johns Hopkins University School of Medicine, Baltimore.

Donald S. McLaren, M.D., Ph.D., D.T.M.&H., F.R.C.P. Reader in Medicine, Department of Medicine, University Medical School, Edinburgh.

David I. McLean, M.D., F.R.C.P. (C) Assistant Professor, Division of Dermatology, Department of Medicine, University of British Columbia; Chairman, Skin Tumor Group, Cancer Control Agency of British Columbia, Vancouver.

Richard H. Meade, III, M.D. Internist, Arlington, Massachusetts.

Paula V. Mendenhall, Pharm.D. Manager, Pharmaceutical Technical Services, Syntex (U.S.A.) Inc., Palo Alto.

Martin C. Mihm, Jr., M.D. Professor of Pathology, Harvard Medical School; Chief, Dermatopathology, Massachusetts General Hospital and Harvard Medical School, Boston.

Lawrence M. Miller, M.D. Assistant Clinical Professor of Medicine, Harvard Medical School; Associate Physician, Massachusetts General Hospital, Boston.

John A. Mills, M.D. Associate Professor of Medicine, Harvard Medical School; Physician, Massachusetts General Hospital, Boston.

Frederic E. Mohs, M.D. Emeritus Professor of Surgery, University of Wisconsin School of Medicine; Emeritus Director of Chemosurgery Clinic, University Hospital and Clinics, Madison.

David B. Mosher, M.D. Clinical Instructor in Dermatology, Harvard Medical School; Clinical Associate, Massachusetts General Hospital, Boston.

Theodore Nadelson, M.D. Chief, Psychiatry Service, Veterans Administration Medical Center; Clinical Professor of Psychiatry, Tufts University School of Medicine, Boston.

Kenneth H. Neldner, M.D. Professor and Chairman, Department of Dermatology, Texas Tech University Health Sciences Center, Lubbock.

Thomas P. Nigra, B.S., M.D. Chairman, Department of Dermatology, The Washington Hospital Center; Clinical Professor of Dermatology, George Washington University Medical Center; Vice Chairman, Dermatology, Children's Hospital, National Medical Center, Washington, D.C.

Jean-Paul Ortonne, M.D. Professor of Dermatology, Nice University School of Medicine; Chief, Department of Dermatology, Hôpital Pasteur, Nice.

Michael N. Oxman, M.D. Professor of Medicine and Pathology, University of California, San Diego; Chief, Infectious Diseases and Clinical Virology Sections, Veterans Administration Medical Center, San Diego.

John A. Parrish, M.D. Director, Wellman Research Laboratory, Massachusetts General Hospital; Professor of Dermatology, Harvard Medical School; Professor, Division of Health Sciences and Technology, Massachusetts Institute of Technology, Boston.

Robert H. Parrott, M.D. Director Emeritus, Children's Hospital National Medical Center; Professor, Department of Child Health and Development, George Washington University School of Medicine and Health Sciences, Washington, D.C.

Steven M. Passman, M.D. Clinical Assistant Professor of Internal Medicine and of Pediatrics, University of Kansas School of Medicine, Wichita.

Madhu A. Pathak, B.Sc. (Hon.), M.S. (Tech.), M.S., Ph.D. Senior Associate in Dermatology, Harvard Medical School, Massachusetts General Hospital, Boston.

Jennifer A. K. Patterson, M.D. Assistant Professor, Department of Dermatology, New York University School of Medicine, Director, Inpatient and Consultative Services and Associate Attending Physician, Department of Dermatology, Bellvue Hospital Center, New York.

Barry S. Paul, M.D. Clinical Instructor in Dermatology, Harvard Medical School; Clinical Associate in Dermatology, Massachusetts General Hospital; Associate Dermatologist, Beth Israel Hospital, Boston.

Gary L. Peck, M.D. Senior Investigator, Dermatology Branch, National Cancer Institute, National Institutes of Health, Bethesda.

Stephanie H. Pincus, M.D. Associate Professor, Tufts University School of Medicine; Vice Chairman, Department of Dermatology, New England Medical Center, Boston.

Sheldon R. Pinnell, M.D. Professor of Medicine and Chief, Division of Dermatology, Duke University Medical Center, Durham.

Gerd Plewig, M.D. Professor and Chairman, Department of Dermatology, University of Düsseldorf; Direktor, Universitätshautklinik, Düsseldorf.

Machiel K. Polano, M.D. Emeritus Professor and Chairman, Department of Dermatology, University Hospital, Leiden.

Maria Ponec, Ph.D. Department of Dermatology, University Hospital, Leiden.

Thomas T. Provost, M.D. The Noxell Professor and Chairman, Department of Dermatology, The Johns Hopkins Medical Institutions, Baltimore.

Michel Pruniéras, M.D. Professor Agréré de Dermatologie, Directeur de Recherche, à l'Institut National de la Santé et de la Recherche Médicale, Paris.

Walter C. Quevedo, Jr., Ph.D. Professor of Biology, Division of Biology and Medicine, Brown University, Providence.

Christopher J. Quirk, M.B., B.S., F.A.C.D. Department of Dermatology, Fremantle Hospital, Fremantle, Western Australia.

Rhonda E. Rand, M.D. Dermatologist, Beverly Hills.

Riley S. Rees, M.D. Associate Professor of Plastic Surgery, Vanderbilt University, Nashville.

Uwe Reichert, Ph.D. Professor, Centre International de Recherches Dermatologiques, Valbonne.

Arthur R. Rhodes, M.D., M.P.H. Chief, Division of Dermatology, Department of Medicine, The Children's Hospital; Assistant Professor of Dermatology, Harvard Medical School, Boston.

David Robertshaw, D.V.M., Ph.D. Professor and Head, Department of Physiology and Biophysics, College of Veterinary Medicine and Biomedical Sciences, Colorado State University, Fort Collins, Colorado.

Paul L. Romain, M.D. Assistant Professor of Medicine, Tufts University School of Medicine; Assistant Physician, Division of Rheumatology/Immunology, Department of Medicine, New England Medical Center, Boston.

Hans Rorsman, M.D. Professor and Chairman, Department of Dermatology, University of Lund, Lund.

Fred S. Rosen, M.D. James L. Gamble Professor of Pediatrics, Harvard Medical School; Chief, Immunology Division, The Children's Hospital, Boston.

Richard B. Rothenberg, M.D., M.P.H. Assistant Director for Science, Division of Chronic Disease Control, Centers for Disease Control, Atlanta.

Naomi F. Rothfield, M.D. Professor of Medicine and Chief, Division of Rheumatic Diseases, The University of Connecticut Health Center, Farmington.

John W. Rowe, M.D. Associate Professor of Medicine, Harvard Medical School; Chief, Gerontology Division, Department of Medicine, Beth Israel Hospital, Boston.

Andrew H. Rudolph, M.D. Clinical Professor of Dermatology, Baylor College of Medicine, Houston.

Imrich Sarkany, F.R.C.P. Consultant Physician for Diseases of the Skin, The Royal Free Hospital, London.

Kenzo Sato, M.D., Ph.D. Associate Professor of Dermatology, The University of Iowa Hospitals and Clinics, Iowa City.

Hans Schaefer, Ph.D. Professor of Biochemistry and Director, Centre International de Recherches Dermatologiques, Valbonne.

William Schaffner, M.D. Professor and Chairman, Department of Preventive Medicine and Chief, Division of Infectious Diseases, Department of Medicine, Vanderbilt University School of Medicine, Nashville.

Wolfgang Shalla, M.D. Head, Department of Pharmacokinetics and Clinical Pharmacology, Centre International de Recherches Dermatologiques, Valbonne.

Robert J. Scheuplein, Ph.D. Deputy Director for Toxicological Sciences, Food and Drug Administration; Center for Food Safety and Applied Nutrition, Washington, D.C.

Stuart F. Schlossman, M.D. Professor of Medicine, Harvard Medical School; Chief, Division of Tumor Immunology, Dana-Farber Cancer Institute, Boston.

Robert A. Schwartz, M.D., M.P.H., F.A.C.P. Associate Professor and Chairman, Division of Dermatology, UMDNJ New Jersey Medical School; Chief, Dermatology Service, UMDNJ University Hospital, Newark.

J. Edwin Seegmiller, M.D. Professor of Medicine and Head, Division of Arthritis; Director, Institute for Research on Aging, University of California San Diego, La Jolla.

Philippe Sengel, Dr. ès Sciences Laboratoire de Zoologie et Biologie Animale, Université Scientifique, Technologique et Médicale de Grenoble, Grenoble.

H. Jean Shadomy, M.A., Ph.D. Professor of Microbiology and Immunology, Medicine, Pathology and Biology, Virginia Commonwealth University-Medical College of Virginia, Richmond.

Braham Shroot, B.Sc., Ph.D. Deputy Director, Department of Biochemistry, Centre International de Recherches Dermatologiques, Valbonne.

Sam Shuster, M.B., Ph.D., F.R.C.P. Professor and Head, Dermatology Department, University of Newcastle upon Tyne; Consultant Dermatologist, Newcastle Health Authority, Newcastle upon Tyne.

Harry Shwachman, B.S., M.D. Professor Emeritus of Pediatrics, Harvard Medical School; Chief (Emeritus), Clinical Nutrition Division, The Children's Hospital, Boston.

Jeremiah E. Silbert, M.D. Director, Connective Tissue Research Laboratory, Veterans Administration Outpatient Clinic, Boston; Professor of Medicine, Harvard Medical School, Boston.

Arthur J. Sober, M.D. Associate Professor of Dermatology, Harvard Medical School; Associate Dermatologist, Massachusetts General Hospital, Boston.

Richard D. Sontheimer, M.D. Associate Professor of Dermatology and Internal Medicine, Southwestern Medical School, Dallas.

Nicholas A. Soter, M.D. Professor of Dermatology, New York University School of Medicine; Attending Physician, University Hospital, Bellevue Hospital, and Manhattan Veterans Administration Hospital, New York.

Richard F. Spark, M.D. Associate Clinical Professor of Medicine, Harvard Medical School; Associate Physician, Beth Israel Hospital, Boston.

Timothy J. Stafford, Ph.D., M.D. Associate Professor of Anaesthesiology, University of Massachusetts Medical Center, Worcester.

Robert S. Stern, M.D. Associate Professor of Dermatology, Harvard Medical School; Dermatologist, Beth Israel Hospital, Boston.

Mary Ellen Stewart, Ph.D. Associate Research Scientist, Department of Dermatology, University of Iowa College of Medicine, Iowa City.

Georg Stingl, M.D. Professor of Dermatology, Department of Dermatology I, University of Vienna Medical School, Vienna.

Howard L. Stoll, Jr., M.D. Clinical Associate Professor of Dermatology, State University of New York at Buffalo; Chief, Department of Dermatology, Roswell Park Memorial Institute, Buffalo.

John S. Strauss, M.D. Professor and Head, Department of Dermatology, University of Iowa College of Medicine, Iowa City.

George P. Stricklin, M.D., Ph.D. Division of Dermatology, Veterans Administration Medical Center and University of Tennessee, Memphis.

Dick Suurmond, M.D. Professor and Chairman, Department of Dermatology, University Hospital, Leiden.

Gunnar Swanbeck, M.D. Professor and Chairman, Department of Dermatology, University of Gothenberg, Göteborg.

Morton N. Swartz, M.D., F.A.C.P. Professor of Medicine, Harvard Medical School; Chief, Infectious Disease Unit, Massachusetts General Hospital, Boston.

Charles C. Sweeley, Ph.D. Professor of Biochemistry, Michigan State University, East Lansing.

George Szabó, Ph.D. Senior Associate in Oral Biology and Pathophysiology (Anatomy), Harvard School of Dental Medicine; Lecturer on Dermatology, Harvard Medical School; Associate Biologist, Massachusetts General Hospital, Boston.

Allister Taggart, M.D., M.R.C.P. Consultant Physician and Senior Lecturer, Department of Therapeutics and Pharmacology, The Queen's University of Belfast, Belfast.

Norman Talal, M.D. Professor of Medicine and Microbiology and Head, Division of Clinical Immunology, The University of Texas Health Science Center at San Antonio; Chief, Section of Clinical Immunology, Audie Murphy Memorial Veterans Hospital, San Antonio.

Oon Tian Tan, M.D. Assistant Professor of Dermatology, Department of Dermatology, Boston University School of Medicine, Boston.

Gert Tappeiner, M.D. Associate Professor, Department of Dermatology I, University of Vienna Medical School, Vienna.

Francisco A. Tausk, M.D. Assistant Researcher, Division of Dermatology, University of California, San Diego.

John Thomson, M.D., F.R.C.P., D.Obst., R.C.O.G. Consultant in Dermatology, The Royal Infirmary; Honorary Clinical Lecturer, The University of Glasgow, Glasgow.

John P. Tindall, M.D., M.P.H. Deputy Commander, USAF Academy Hospital, Colorado Springs; Formerly Professor of Dermatology, Duke University Medical Center, Durham.

Jouni Uitto, M.D., Ph.D. Professor of Medicine, University of California at Los Angeles; Associate Chief and Director of Research, Division of Dermatology, Harbor-UCLA Medical Center, Torrance.

Frederick Urbach, M.D., F.A.C.P. Professor and Acting Chairman, Department of Dermatology, and Director, Center for Photobiology, Temple University School of Medicine, Philadelphia.

John P. Utz, M.S., M.D. Professor of Medicine, Georgetown University School of Medicine, Washington, D.C.

Christopher F. H. Vickers, M.D., F.R.C.P. Professor of Dermatology, University of Liverpool, Royal Liverpool Hospital, and Alder Hey Children's Hospital, Liverpool.

Jan Waldenström, M.D., D.Sc.h.c., F.A.C.P., F.R.C.P. Professor Emeritus of Internal Medicine, University of Lund, Malmö General Hospital, Malmö.

Elaine Waldo, M.D. Associate Professor of Clinical Pathology, New York University Medical Center, New York.

Stephen I. Wasserman, M.D. Professor of Medicine, UCSD School of Medicine; Director, Division of Allergy, Department of Medicine, UCSD Medical Center, San Diego.

Arnold N. Weinberg, M.D. Professor of Medicine, Harvard Medical School; Physician, Infectious Disease Unit, Massachusetts General Hospital, Boston.

Gerald D. Weinstein, M.D. Chairman and Professor, Department of Dermatology, University of California, Irvine.

Howard G. Welgus, M.D. Assistant Professor of Medicine, Division of Dermatology, Washington University School of Medicine; Chief, Division of Dermatology, The Jewish Hospital of St. Louis, St. Louis.

Peter F. Weller, M.D. Assistant Professor of Medicine, Harvard Medical School; Assistant Physician, Beth Israel Hospital, Boston.

William L. Weston, M.D. Professor and Chairman, Department of Dermatology, and Professor of Pediatrics, University of Colorado Medical Center, Denver.

Michael W. Wick, M.D., Ph.D. Associate Professor of Dermatology, Harvard Medical School; Chief, Skin Cancer Clinic, Dana-Farber Cancer Institute; Dermatologist, New England Deaconess Hospital, Boston.

Bruce U. Wintroub, M.D. Chairman, Department of Dermatology, University of California School of Medicine, San Francisco.

Arthur Wiskemann, M.D. Professor of Dermatology and Chief, Section of Dermatologic Radiology, Hamburg University Hospital, Hamburg.

Klaus Wolff, M.D. Professor and Chairman, Department of Dermatology I, University of Vienna Medical School; Chief, Dermatology Service I, General Hospital of Vienna, Vienna.

Sheldon M. Wolff, M.D. Physician-in-Chief, New England Medical Center; Endicott Professor and Chairman, Department of Medicine, Tufts University School of Medicine, Boston.

Elisabeth C. Wolff-Schreiner, M.D. Associate Professor of Dermatology, Department of Dermatology I, University of Vienna Medical School, Vienna.

David T. Woodley, M.D. Associate Professor, Department of Dermatology, University of North Carolina, Chapel Hill.

Verna Wright, M.D., F.R.C.P. Professor of Rheumatology, Rheumatism Research Unit, University Department of Medicine, General Infirmary, Leeds.

Stuart H. Yuspa, M.D. Chief, Laboratory of Cellular Carcinogenesis and Tumor Promotion, Division of Cancer Etiology, National Cancer Institute, National Institutes of Health, Bethesda.

Nardo Zaias, M.D. Dermatologist and Dermatopathologist; Senior Attending Physician, Mount Sinai Medical Center, Miami Beach.

John L. Ziegler, M.D. Associate Chief of Staff/Education, Veterans Administration Medical Center, San Francisco; Professor of Medicine, University of California, San Francisco.

Dorothea Zucker-Franklin, M.D. Professor of Medicine, New York University School of Medicine, New York.

The color photographs herein were done by H. Korff and J.v.d. Walle of the Audiovisual Service of the Medical Faculty in Leiden. The Netherlands, and are from the collection of the Department of Dermatology, University Medical Centre, Leiden. The color plates were prepared in the lithographic institute Sturm of Basel, Switzerland, on appointment by CIBA-GEIGY, Basel. The superb co-operation of CIBA-GEIGY is gratefully acknowledged.

PART FOUR

DERMATOLOGY AND INTERNAL MEDICINE

Section 24

Cutaneous lesions in nutritional, metabolic, and heritable disorders

CHAPTER 136

CUTANEOUS CHANGES IN NUTRITIONAL DISORDERS

Donald S. McLaren

The scope of disordered nutrition is wide, relating not only to possible deficiency of a wide variety of nutrients, but also to an excess of some, and arising secondarily from failure of utilization as well as from a primary dietary imbalance. Although disease states such as pellagra, scurvy, and kwashiorkor have skin lesions prominent among their symptomatology, it is important to appreciate that they, like all nutritional disorders, are generalized conditions affecting many systems. Furthermore, an inadequate diet tends to lead to multiple deficiencies. The accessibility of the skin and its appendages and mucous membranes to examination makes them especially valuable in clinical diagnosis.

Proteins and energy

Experimental starvation in adults

The most thorough study of the effects of inanition on the skin of human volunteers was made as part of the monumental Minnesota experiment [1]. The skin of the subjects, after 23 weeks on a diet providing only 1570 kcal, was thinner than normal, dry, inelastic, pallid, and grayish in color. It was cold and "dead" to the touch with a tendency to cyanosis in cold weather. All these signs were very suggestive of those commonly seen in old age. Less regular in occurrence was the rough gooseflesh appearance similar to the follicular hyperkeratosis associated by some with vitamin A deficiency (see "Vitamin A Deficiency" below). A patchy, dirty brownish pigmentation situated anywhere on the body, but most commonly on the face, was found to some degree but never sufficiently marked to resemble pellagra. The hair was dry, dull, and "staring," with a tendency to cease growing and to fall out very easily, very

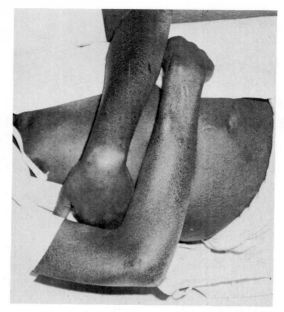

Fig. 136-1   A fine mosaic-like fissuring of the skin on the extensor aspects of the forearms and the abdomen in an African patient.

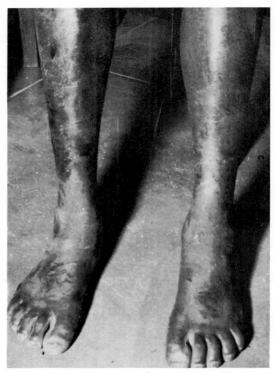

Fig. 136-2   Patchy hyperpigmented changes of the skin on the shins and dorsa of the feet in a symptom-free African subject.

much as described in protein-energy malnutrition in children (see "Kwashiorkor" below).

Privation starvation in adults

In times of famine and war many abnormal appearances of the skin have been described, in addition to the obvious loss of subcutaneous fat. Some of these changes may be attributed to starvation, but others are undoubtedly more closely related to the breakdown of sanitary and medical facilities at such times. Pallor of the skin is often more than can be explained by anemia, and the skin is abnormally cold as a result of vasoconstriction. In victims of famine and prisoners of war, the skin has frequently been described as dry, rough, scaly, thin, and inelastic—resembling the skin of old age. A similar appearance is found in anorexia nervosa and, indeed, in any prolonged wasting disease, whatever the cause. In undernourished, dark-skinned people, fine mosaiclike fissuring of the skin (Fig. 136-1) is extremely common, as are burnished, hyperpigmented lesions over the shins and dorsa of the feet (Fig. 136-2). These appearances are probably related to repeated minor trauma in individuals with chronic marginal undernutrition.

Follicular hyperkeratosis and folliculosis have been reputed to be associated with undernutrition. The former is recognized clinically as small, hard, elevated nodules around the hair follicles, giving the skin a "nutmeg grater" texture. The follicles may be filled with keratotic plugs. Exactly what is meant by *folliculosis* in nutrition survey reports is far from clear. It usually seems to mean a relative prominence of the hair follicle due to thinning of the epidermal, dermal, and subcutaneous layers of the skin; it is also called *follicular pouting* and *permanent gooseflesh*. The clinical status of these appearances is in dispute (see "Vitamin A Deficiency" below).

Pigmentary changes in the skin are characteristic of semistarvation. Their color is usually brownish, darker than ordinary suntan, and they usually manifest around the mouth and eyes and on the malar prominences. Less commonly the hands, arms, and trunk are involved. The changes are not like those seen in pellagra.

Changes in the hair have also been reported to occur frequently in semistarvation. It is thin, grows slowly, falls out prematurely, and rapidly becomes gray. The nails grow slowly and may be fissured. Some have reported a pronounced development of downy hair (lanugo) all over the body, especially on the face and nape of the neck in children, as well as in patients with anorexia nervosa.

Starvation in children (marasmus) (Fig. A6-17)

Total inanition in the child, with intake of all nutrients affected but in particular proteins and energy, soon leads to suppression of growth, negative nitrogen balance due to catabolism of tissue protein for energy, and the state of *marasmus* (Greek, "wasting"). This is one form of what is now termed *protein-energy malnutrition* of early childhood (see also "Kwashiorkor" below). It is widely prevalent throughout the developing regions of the world and is to a large extent responsible for the high mortality in infancy and early childhood. The disturbed nutrition is usually secondary to weaning problems resulting from ignorance, poor hygiene, and economic and cultural factors.

In contrast to kwashiorkor, there is classically no clinical edema or dermatosis in marasmus. As in the undernourished adult, the skin is dry, wrinkled, and loose, due to marked loss of subcutaneous fat. The "monkey

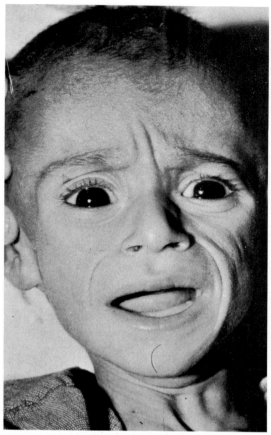

Fig. 136-3 "Monkey facies" in a marasmic Arab child with wrinkled skin and loss of subcutaneous fat.

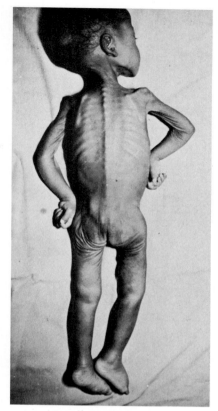

Fig. 136-4   The general appearance in marasmus.

facies'' with loss of the buccal fat pads is characteristic (Figs. 136-3 and 136-4). There is some evidence to suggest that pitting edema is seen only if the subcutaneous fat is largely preserved, as in kwashiorkor.

Kwashiorkor (Fig. A6-16)

This form of protein-energy malnutrition results from a diet quantitatively and qualitatively poor in protein with an adequate and often excessive intake of energy from starch or sugar. Characteristically, the weanling child is affected; in additon to the dermatosis and hair changes to be described below, there are typically retarded growth, hypoalbuminemia, edema, moon face, fatty liver, and psychomotor change. Much less commonly, a similar clinical picture has been reported in school-age children and young adults, and several cases are on record following extensive intestinal surgical treatment resulting in a secondary type of protein malnutrition.

The skin lesions are not invariably present in kwashiorkor, but when present they are diagnostic and characteristic. They are more frequent and severe in dark-skinned races; the basic change is depigmentation. The first sign is circumoral pallor; pallor is also marked on the legs. The skin is stretched with edema, and the pallor may be due as much to thinning and distension of the skin as to actual loss of pigment. Localized losses of pigment may follow abrasions, wounds, ulceration, etc.

The characteristic dermatosis in white-skinned infants starts with erythema. At first the skin blanches on pressure, but this is rapidly followed by small, dusky, purple patches which do not blanch. On dark skins, purple areas darken within a few hours of appearing. They have a burnished surface and feel almost waxy to the touch. They have an absolutely sharp edge and appear raised above the surrounding skin, as if small particles of enamel paint had been applied. They are most common in areas subject to pressure, especially if combined with moisture resulting from sweat or any other secretions or discharge. The diaper area is affected early, but so also are the trochanters, knees, ankles, elbows, and areas of pressure on the trunk. The dermatosis seldom appears on areas exposed to sunlight, and, in contrast to pellagra, it spares the feet and dorsa of the hands.

Whereas in mild cases patients show only a superficial desquamation, in severe cases there are large areas of erosion in which much skin is lost. This characteristic dermatosis was given the descriptive names of "enamel paint," "flaky paint," and "crazy paving" dermatosis (Figs. 136-5 and 136-6).

Advanced cases may also show linear fissuring in the flexures, around the pinna, on the back of the knee, in front of the elbow, in the axilla, between the toes, at the edge of the foreskin, and in the center of the lips. All these lesions appear to be caused by intermittent tension, and those occurring at the corners of the mouth should be distinguished from the angular stomatitis of riboflavin deficiency, in which there is usually a heaped-up, sodden appearance (Fig. 136-7, see also Fig. 136-14).

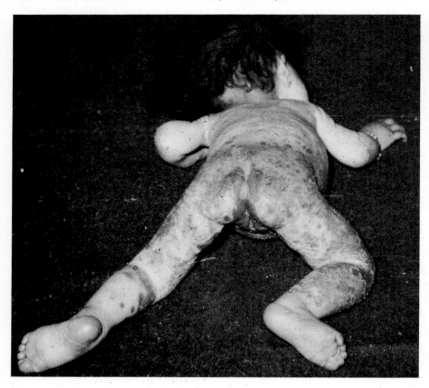

Fig. 136-5 Severe "enamel paint" dermatosis of kwashiorkor in a fair-skinned Arab child. (Courtesy of Dr. E. Shirajian, Luzmila Hospital, Amman, Jordan.)

One of the milder skin changes in kwashiorkor, and the most commonly observed sign involving the skin in fair-skinned children, is a dry, fine desquamation with cracking along the natural lines to give "mosaic skin" or "cracked skin." The shins, outer sides of the thighs, and back of the trunk are areas most commonly affected. In fair Arab children the changes are especially prone to affect the forehead with some hyperpigmentation (Fig. 136-8).

Occasionally on the dorsum of the foot, on the buttocks, or on sites not obviously related to pressure, a large bulla may form and break, leaving a shallow depression.

In advanced kwashiorkor the skin is very easily damaged. Bony points on the pelvis and over the elbows and knees are easily rubbed raw. Special care has to be taken in nursing these cases, most especially if metabolic experiments are being carried out that necessitate keeping the child on a special bed for continuous collection of stools and urine.

True pellagrous skin changes can occur in children with evidence of kwashiorkor. This is especially apt to arise when children are weaned onto a diet containing much maize flour, as in South and Central Africa. It is also possible that the dermatosis of kwashiorkor is related to deficiency of B vitamins, as well as to protein or amino acid malnutrition.

The nails are often thin and soft in kwashiorkor, and this may be particularly obvious when healthy new nails start to grow, forming a mass at the nail base that is completely separated from the old nail.

The hair in kwashiorkor shows depigmentation, is sparse, is thin in texture, and comes out easily. None of these changes is specific to kwashiorkor; in malnourished Arab children they are seen about as frequently accompanying marasmus. Kwashiorkor may be diagnosed without the presence of hair changes, although this is rather unusual. Normally black hair becomes brown or reddish,

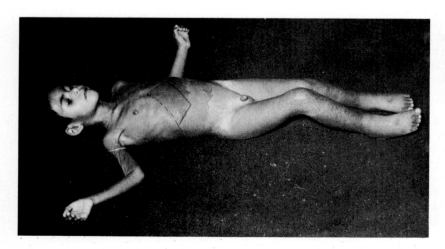

Fig. 136-6 Marasmic kwashiorkor in adolescent Arab boy, showing typical hyperpigmentation, edema of lower extremities, wasting of trunk and upper limbs, hepatomegaly, and hypogonadism. (Courtesy of Dr. E. Shirajian, Luzmila Hospital, Amman, Jordan.)

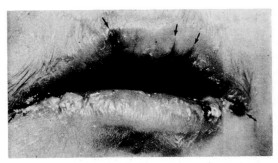

Fig. 136-7   Fissuring of lips in child with kwashiorkor (compare with riboflavin deficiency in Fig. 136-14).

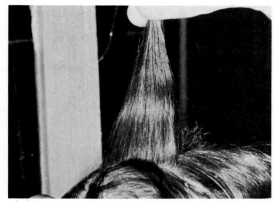

Fig. 136-9   The flag sign in a Salvadoran child with kwashiorkor.

and brown hair turns blond. Somehow the idea has spread that kwashiorkor means "red boy," red referring to the hair change. The word *kwashiorkor,* however (taken from the Ga language of Ghana), means, "the sickness of the weanling," an apt description of the pathogenesis of the condition. There are many causes of bleaching of the hair other than malnutrition—such as sunlight, ultraviolet radiation, and oxidizing agents—and care must be exercised in interpretation. Especially striking is the flag sign (*signe de la bandera*) affecting long and normally dark hair in which the hair grown during periods of inadequate nutrition is pale, so that alternating bands of dark and pale hair can be seen along a single strand, recording alternating periods of adequate and inadequate nutrition (Fig. 136-9).

The other changes undergone by the hair are more constant and more reliable than the alterations in color described above. The growth of hair is sparse and it comes out easily. There may be recession from the temporal regions and loss from the back of the head, probably due to pressure when the child lies down. Loss of hair may be extreme in advanced cases. The texture of the hair becomes softer and finer than normal for a child of that age and culture. It tends to be unruly and to resemble the "staring" coat of some animals described in nutritional deficiency. The eyelashes may undergo the same change, having a "broomstick" appearance.

In health, most of the scalp hairs are in the anagen or active growth phase and few in the telogen or resting phase. In early protein-energy malnutrition this is reversed

and analysis of the hair cycle has been advocated as a diagnostic procedure.

Cancrum oris (noma, necrotizing ulcerative gingivitis)

The cause of this destructive lesion (Fig. 136-10), usually involving the face in the region of the mouth, is not clear. Malnutrition in the form of kwashiorkor or marasmus is almost always present, but it is sometimes difficult to decide whether the nutritional deficiency is primary or secondary. Likewise the role played by the constantly present Vincent's organisms is obscure.

Infants and preschool children are most commonly affected. Cancrum oris is reported not infrequently from all parts of Africa, Southeast Asia, and tropical America. It used to occur in white children following measles, typhus, or typhoid fever but is now very rare.

Most cases probably start as an area of ulcerative gingivitis with a tender, firm swelling of the upper gum and underlying bone and some swelling of the overlying part of the face. Very soon the teeth loosen, and inflammation spreads into the underlying bone with osteitis and a sequestrum. The cheek usually ulcerates, producing a cavity

Fig. 136-10   Massive destruction of face due to noma in a Tanzanian child.

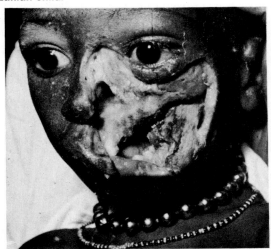

Fig. 136-8   Scaly hyperpigmented dermatosis of forehead of Arab child with kwashiorkor. (Courtesy of Dr. E. Shirajian, Luzmila Hospital, Amman, Jordan.)

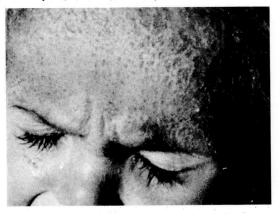

leading directly into the mouth. Occasionally the process originates in the nose, vulva, or elsewhere.

Without treatment there is rapid progress of the disease, frequently leading to death. The introduction of antibiotics (penicillin, erythromycin, or tetracycline) has revolutionized the treatment of these cases, although massive residual defects continue to present almost insuperable plastic surgery problems, particularly in relation to the relatively primitive facilities usually available. A full diet is of great value, especially one rich in protein, high in energy, and providing all vitamins. Feeding difficulties necessarily create problems in achieving adequate nutrition.

Tropical ulcer (tropical sloughing phagedena)

This chronic condition, affecting chiefly the lower limbs above the malleoli, shares with cancrum oris the frequent background of general malnutrition of the patient and the occurrence of Vincent's organisms in the lesions. However, adults rather than children are usually affected. It is especially prevalent in hot and humid weather, among workers on plantations, and among troops in the tropics. The relationship to poor nutrition is not invariable, but a good diet, rest, and antibiotics give good results.

The disease starts with the formation of a larger or smaller blister with serosanguinolent contents. When the bulla ruptures, an ash-gray moist slough is exposed. The sloughing process extends rapidly, until the skin and subcutaneous fascia over quite a large area may be converted into a yellowish, moist, foul-smelling ulcer. In extensive cases, muscles, tendons, nerves, vessels, and even the periosteum may have shared in the gangrenous process. Even after healing, deformity may ensue from ankylosis, and a contracting cicatrix may strangulate a vital part, necessitating amputation. Smaller healed tropical ulcers leave behind tissue-paper-like scars with pigmented edges. These are prone to break down.

Obesity

Skin disorders tend to be common in the obese. Excessive fat folds lead to intertrigo from friction between skin surfaces and to maceration of the skin from accumulated moisture in the folds. Infection frequently supervenes, particularly with staphylococci, dermatophytes, and yeast. The obese become overheated easily and sweat more profusely because of the thick layers of subcutaneous fat; areas of inflammation and skin rashes are thus exaggerated. Many obese patients have either a diabetic tendency or frank diabetes with all the accompanying dermatoses. It is important in all these circumstances that due attention be paid during treatment to measures aimed at correction of the underlying obesity; otherwise local treatment of the skin lesions will remain purely palliative.

Vitamins

Vitamin A (retinol)

This fat-soluble vitamin is found only in the animal kingdom. Many plants contain one or more of the several provitamin carotenoids of which beta-carotene is the most active. Vitamin A, as the aldehyde (retinal), has a well-known role in night vision, and the earliest clinical manifestation of vitamin A deficiency is impairment of dark adaptation. In animals, deficiency of vitamin A has been shown to have profound effects, including cessation of growth, death, congenital malformations, and severe damage, especially to epithelial tissues. In both humans and animals, severe deficiency produces destructive eye lesions affecting the conjunctiva (xerosis conjunctivae, Bitot's spots) and cornea (xerosis corneae and keratomalacia) (see Fig. A4-8). Recent work implicates vitamin A as a factor influencing lability of lysosome membranes, glycosaminoglycan metabolism, and cell-mediated immunity.

Vitamin A deficiency. There is general agreement that severely malnourished patients with the pathognomonic ocular lesions of vitamin A deficiency, namely, xerosis of the conjunctiva and cornea and keratomalacia, may also show changes in the skin attributable to the same cause. The skin over large areas of the body is dry, wrinkled, and covered with fine scales. These changes were described in China more than 30 years ago, together with deep, excavating lesions, which were termed *dermomalacia*. Marked changes of this type are quite uncommon, even in children with bilateral keratomalacia (Fig. 136-11).

Histologically, those skin lesions that can confidently be attributed to vitamin A deficiency represent primary hyperkeratinization and hyperplasia of the epidermis, including the lining of the hair follicles and sebaceous glands. Most characteristically in the conjunctiva and cornea, vitamin A deficiency causes metaplasia, but in the skin there

Fig. 136-11 Advanced keratomalacia due to vitamin A deficiency (serum vitamin A 2 μg/dL; normal: 20 to 50 μg) in a 5-month-old Arab child.

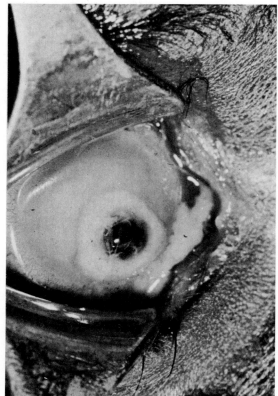

is an accentuation of a process of progressive keratinization normally inherent here.

In infants and very young children, before the pilosebaceous follicle has fully matured, simple xerosis, or xeroderma, is usually the characteristic feature. The stratum corneum is usually several times its normal thickness, and there is blockage of sweat ducts and hyperkeratinization of the follicle lining.

Adults, especially those who have exhibited the advanced ocular manifestations, have shown grosser changes. The stratum corneum forms a broad network or even horny plates, with abundant desquamation of fine scales. The stratum lucidum and stratum granulosum remain unchanged. The basal layers are unaltered except for increased melanin deposition. Sebaceous glands are reduced in number, sweat gland ducts are occluded by keratinous material, and although the glands are normal in appearance, they are probably hypofunctional. Except for perifollicular infiltration, the dermis is normal. It is significant that the follicular reaction is minimal in those cases with marked hyperkeratosis and pathognomonic eye lesions; this is in contrast to the pronounced reaction in the very common follicular hyperkeratosis usually unaccompanied by generalized hyperkeratosis or eye changes.

It is the follicular eruption (Fig. 136-12), termed *follicular hyperkeratosis* by Frazier and Hu [2], that has proved to be so controversial. It is interesting to note that Pillat, the ophthalmologist, made no reference to this, although he was working in the same hospital and the 14 cases that Frazier and Hu reported were drawn from a group of 209 soldiers with ocular lesions seen by Pillat. The follicular changes were described as occurring on a background of a generally dry and rough skin. Spinous papules appeared at the tips of the hair follicles. First affected were the anterolateral aspects of the thighs and the posterolateral parts of the upper forearms. The eruptions slowly spread to the extensor surface of upper and lower limbs, the shoulders, the lower part of the abdomen, and, to a lesser extent, the chest, back, and buttocks. Each papule had a keratotic plug at its apex, projecting as a hard spinous process. The eruption was usually abundant and symmetrical. With a generally good diet and cod liver oil (up to 30 mL daily) the skin lesions improved slowly, but even after 2 months the skin had not regained its normal appearance.

Subsequently, under the name of *phrynoderma*, or "toad skin," such follicular changes, frequently of a much milder nature and more limited distribution, have been attributed to nutritional deficiency. Not only deficiency of vitamin A, but deficiency of linoleic acid or vitamins of the B complex have all been implicated.

The evidence from deprivation experiments in humans does not support the contention that follicular hyperkeratosis can be associated specifically with vitamin A deficiency. In the Sheffield experiment [3] 20 men and 3 women received a diet deficient in vitamin A and carotene for periods ranging from 6½ to 25 months. With regard to the minimal skin changes observed, it was concluded that the enlargement and hyperkeratosis of the hair follicles that occurred among both the supplemented and the deprived group fluctuated in both extent and size of the eruption independently of the state of vitamin A nutrition.

In view of the lack of proof of nutritional deficiency as the cause of hyperfollicular keratosis, it is especially im-

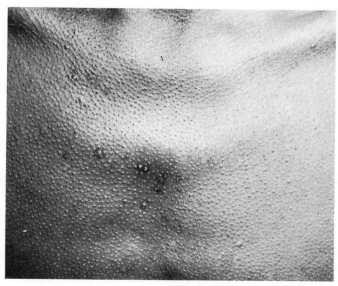

Fig. 136-12 Follicular hyperkeratosis of the chest in an East African adult male. (The appearance is typical, but there is no conclusive evidence of the precise cause.)

portant to explore the possibility of other diagnoses. The distribution of the lesions and infrequency of pustulation should rule out acne vulgaris; the rarity of the eruption in postpuberal females and in adolescent children seems incompatible with keratosis pilaris, and the relatively rare Darier's disease may be excluded by the absence of familial tendency and the demonstration of dyskeratotic changes in the skin specimen.

Massive oral vitamin A therapy has been advocated for many skin conditions of unknown cause, including some mentioned above, that pose problems of differential diagnosis. Other conditions include pityriasis rubra pilaris (Devergie's disease), keratosis palmaris et plantaris, ichthyosis, and pachyonychia. In none of these conditions has a deficiency of vitamin A been demonstrated. In the past, very large doses (ranging from 75,000 to 400,000 units of vitamin A daily), many times the normal requirement, have been given for prolonged periods, resulting in chronic toxicity [see "Vitamin A Toxicity (Hypervitaminosis A)" below].

In recent years retinoic acid has been used in the treatment of several skin diseases. Tretinoin (as 0.05% solution, 0.025%, and 0.01% gel, or 0.1% and 0.05% cream) has become a frequently used modality in the treatment and prevention of comedonal and inflammatory acne of all grades [4]. Derivatives of vitamin A are being used orally for severe cystic acne (see Chap. 67) with striking results and for diseases of keratinization.

Vitamin A toxicity (hypervitaminosis A). The skin is frequently involved in both acute and chronic forms. Desquamation over large areas of the body, accompanied by severe headache and vomiting, has occurred in arctic explorers after a single meal of the liver of polar bear, bearded seal, or their sledge dogs previously fed on the livers of these animals. Chronic poisoning results from injudicious therapeutic use of the vitamin. The bizarre symptomatology includes coarsening of the skin with pruritus and loss of hair. In patients with this process diagnosis of brain tumor, psychoneurosis, generalized infectious arthritis, Addison's disease, hepatitis, and dermatomyositis may be made before the true nature of the process is determined.

Both acute and chronic manifestations of hypervitaminosis A must be watched for in young children; increasing numbers of such cases are being reported in the literature. Central nervous system and bone changes are especially common, but pruritus and desquamation are not infrequent.

Withdrawal of vitamin A brings about gradual improvement over several weeks, and, in spite of the alarming manifestations of vitamin A poisoning, no fatalities have been reported.

Carotenoderma. The time taken to produce clinically appreciable pigmentation depends to some extent on dietary consumption of carotenoids. In one instance 1.8 kg of carrots were consumed weekly for 7 months. Children develop carotenoderma more readily than adults. An infant developed the skin pigmentation after only 2 months on the breast milk of its carotenemic mother, while another born pigmented to such a mother remained yellow until weaned. Appropriate laboratory tests, including determination of total serum carotenoids (usual range for healthy adults: 40 to 150 μg/dL), will differentiate hypercarotenosis from hemolytic anemia, pernicious anemia, obstructive jaundice, etc. It is especially likely to occur during wartime with rationing of meat, butter, and cheese, and increased consumption of fresh vegetables. It is endemic in parts of the world (e.g., West Africa) where red palm oil is used for cooking.

Excess carotene is in part excreted in sweat and reabsorbed by the horny layer of the skin. Deposition occurs first and predominantly in the nasolabial folds and over the forehead, where sebaceous glands abound, and on the palms and the soles where the horny layer of the skin is thickest. It is found to a lesser degree on the upper eyelids, inner canthi, ears, and anterior folds of the axillae, and over areas subject to pressure, e.g., the elbows, knees, and malleoli. This uneven distribution helps to distinguish carotenoderma from jaundice.

Carotenoderma is usually not noticeable until the serum level is 3 or 4 times normal. The color of the skin is canary yellow, ochre, or golden. It never has the bronze, orange, saffron, or green tint of jaundice. Mucous membranes, including the sclerae, are not stained by carotene. Subconjunctival or submucosal fat, if present, may be stained and lead to confusion. Other points of differentiation from jaundice are that hypercarotenosis does not cause itching and does not significantly change the color of urine or stools. It has to be borne in mind that some carotene is present in all normal skin. Carotenoderma is said to develop more readily in those who sweat profusely. As far as is known, hypercarotenosis in all its forms appears to be harmless. If of dietary origin, it slowly disappears when the intake is reduced to normal levels.

In diabetes mellitus there is frequently a raised serum carotene level, but carotenoderma develops in only about 10 percent of cases. In this disease it is probably due to a high dietary consumption, but there may possibly be impaired conversion of carotene to vitamin A. Some patients with hypothyroidism also have carotenoderma, and this

may be related to the known function of thyroid hormone in facilitating carotene conversion. Hypercarotenemia has been consistently reported in anorexia nervosa. It occasionally amounts to carotenoderma and is of obscure origin.

Vitamins of the B complex

Niacin (pellagra) (Figs. A6-14 and A6-15). The amide of niacin is an important constituent of coenzyme I (oxidized form of nicotinamide-adenine dinucleotide, NAD) and coenzyme II (reduced form of nicotinamide-adenine dinucleotide, NADP) which either donate or accept hydrogen ions in vital oxidation-reduction reactions. The essential amino acid, tryptophan, can be converted in the body to niacin, about 60 mg of tryptophan being the dietary equivalent of 1 mg of niacin. The cause of pellagra is still not entirely clear. It may arise on a diet deficient in niacin or tryptophan, or more commonly both, and amino acid imbalance also may play a part. In practice, a predominantly maize diet is usually implicated. Besides the dermatosis, there are important gastrointestinal and nervous system changes.

The dermatosis is usually preceded by prodromal symptoms, especially of the digestive system. The changes are characteristic and pathognomonic, and their distribution is determined especially by exposure to the sun and by local pressure. The diagnosis of pellagra is difficult in the absence of the dermatosis. It begins as an erythema on the dorsa of the hands, with pruritus and burning. It is characteristically symmetrical. There is slight edema of the skin. In some patients, several days after the onset of the erythema, blisters appear; these run together to form bullae and then break. In others, dry brown scales form. On the face, the scales are thicker and larger and, here, frequently become pustular.

In the second stage the dermatosis becomes hard, rough, cracked, blackish, and brittle. The epidermis of the fingers thickens, and the articular folds disappear. Painful fissures develop in the palms and on the digits. The skin may look like that of the goose; hence the term *goose skin*. When the deficiency state is far advanced, the skin becomes progressively harder, drier, more cracked, and covered with scales and blackish crusts that are due to hemorrhages.

The usual sites are the face, neck, and dorsal surfaces of the hands, arms, and feet. The changes rarely are seen elsewhere. The dorsa of the hands are the most frequent site; here the lesions may extend up the arm to form the "glove," or "gauntlet," of pellagra. The symmetry and clear line of demarcation from normal skin are especially striking. On the feet the lesions usually do not rise proximal to the malleoli, which are included; the heels remain free. Distally the eruption ends at the toes or on the backs of the great toes. The front and back of the leg may be involved to form a "boot."

On the face the symmetry of the lesions is striking. They tend to spread from the sides to the rest of the nose, to the forehead, cheeks, chin, lips, and, more rarely, eyelids and ears. The "butterfly" appearance common to lupus erythematosus is frequent. On the forehead there is always a narrow border of normal skin between the erythema and the hair. The face is often only slightly affected. The facial

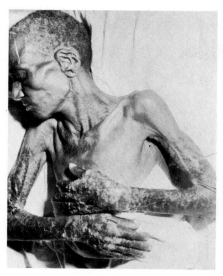

Fig. 136-13 Elderly East African female in the acute phase of pellagrous dermatosis. Note the Casal necklace, only very early involvement of the face, and exudative crusted lesions of the hands and arms.

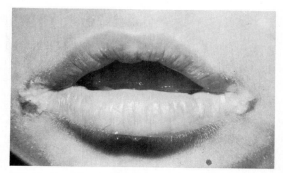

Fig. 136-14 Angular stomatitis with maceration in an Arab child. Riboflavin excretion in the urine was diminished.

lesions never appear independently of lesions on the hands and elsewhere.

Casal's "necklace" extends as a fairly broad band, or collar, entirely around the neck (Fig. 136-13). If the band is incomplete, the lesions are striking in their symmetry. The upper border reaches somewhat below the hairline to the larynx anteriorly. The lower border begins under the vertebra prominens and extends to the edge of the manubrium. In many instances the necklace has an anterior continuation, or broad "cravat," extending from the manubrium over the sternum to the level of the nipples, ending in a point or square. Men, women, and children have the necklace, and it is always accompanied by the characteristic dermatitis elsewhere.

Other sites occasionally affected are the shoulders, elbows, forearms, and knees. The so-called pellagrous vulvitis, vaginitis, and lesions of the perianal region and scrotum are dealt with as part of the "oro-oculo-genital" syndrome [see "Riboflavin (Oro-oculo-genital Syndrome)" below].

Healing usually takes place centrifugally with the line of demarcation remaining actively inflamed after the center of the lesion has desquamated. Specific therapy consists of the oral administration of 100 to 300 mg of niacinamide daily in divided doses. The amide is preferable since it does not precipitate the vasomotor disturbances resulting from administration of niacin in large doses. A similar dose is given subcutaneously where diarrhea or a noncooperative patient makes oral administration ineffective or difficult. Multivitamins (especially other vitamins of the B complex) and a high-quality protein diet (100 to 150 g per day) should be given.

Riboflavin (oro-oculo-genital syndrome). This vitamin has coenzyme function in the chain of reversible oxidation-reduction reactions on which tissue respiration depends. A variety of lesions has been produced by experimental

deficiency in animals, but in humans the changes appear to be rather trivial, occurring mainly in the skin and mucous membranes.

For many years a syndrome resembling pellagra but without the typical dermatosis had been known, going by the rather confusing name of *pellagra sine pellagra*. Sebrell and Butler [5] studied a group of patients on a diet low in riboflavin and nicotinic acid and showed that the manifestations of pellagra sine pellagra were due to riboflavin deficiency. The changes produced in this way commenced with pallor of the mucosa in the angles of the mouth. This was soon followed by maceration and superficial linear fissures (Fig. 136-14). These fissures remained moist and became crusted. The skin of the nasolabial folds, on the alae nasi, in the vestibule of the nose, and sometimes on the ears and at the inner and outer canthi of the eyelids became rather greasy and scaly (Figs. 136-15 and 136-16). Many other human experiments have subsequently been carried out, and it is now clear that these signs do develop in subjects subsisting for long periods (1 to 2 years) on diets very low in riboflavin (less than about 0.55 mg per day) and are not influenced by low dietary levels of nicotinic acid or tryptophan.

In addition to these changes (angular stomatitis, nasolabial seborrhea, or shark skin, and angular blepharitis), other alterations of the skin and mucous membranes also have been associated with human riboflavin deficiency, but it needs to be emphasized that none is pathognomonic. These changes include (1) soggy, white, angular lesions of the mouth, usually termed *perlèche* (French, *perlècher*, "to lick thoroughly with the tongue"), often associated with moniliasis; (2) involvement of the vermilion border of the lips including vertical fissuring, usually termed *cheilosis* (Greek, *cheilos*, "lip"); (3) a glossitis in which the tongue frequently has a magenta color; (4) corneal vascularization; and (5) lesions of the scrotum and vulva.

The dermatosis affecting the genital area has frequently been reported to be the earliest manifestation of riboflavin deficiency and also one of the most common. It may begin either as a patchy redness associated with scaling of the superficial epithelium or as a fine powdery desquamation without any color change. In chronic cases lichenification is a feature, and far-advanced lesions are raw and extend up the shaft of the penis or onto the inner aspects of the thighs. The response to treatment (5 mg of riboflavin daily) is usually quite dramatic.

Sideropenic anemia with epithelial lesions (Plummer-

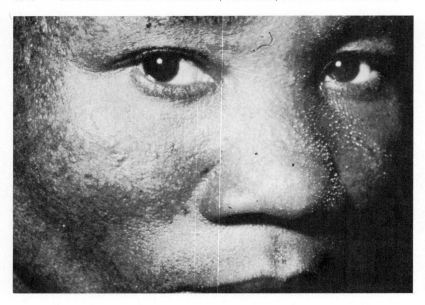

Fig. 136-15 Early nasolabial seborrhea in an African boy.

Vinson syndrome), which has a little-understood relationship to postcricoid carcinoma, may be accompanied by evidence of riboflavin deficiency.

Pyridoxine (vitamin B_6). Pyridoxine acts mainly as a coenzyme in the decarboxylation and transamination of a number of amino acids. It also plays a part in the enzymes concerned with the conversion of linoleic to arachidonic acid and in adrenocortical function. There are a few reports in the literature of response of both microcytic hypochromic and megaloblastic types of anemia to pyridoxine therapy. In pyridoxine dependency, in which there is no deficiency of the coenzyme form of the vitamin but a defect in the apoenzyme protein, reversal of the clinical and biochemical changes is obtained only with massive doses of pyridoxine. One form of dependency is familial xanthurenic aciduria with urticaria as the main feature.

Adults living on a pyridoxine-deficient diet for up to 2 months remained symptom-free. However, Vilter and his associates [6] described symptoms of pyridoxine deficiency after prolonged administration of an antimetabolite, desoxypyridoxine. These included seborrhea-like changes around the eyes, nose, and mouth, and cheilosis. No response occurred to thiamin, riboflavin, and niacinamide but the process cleared completely with pyridoxine. During the test period there was increased excretion of xanthurenic acid.

Drugs that may impair pyridoxine metabolism include isoniazid, hydralazine, DL-penicillamine, and oral contraceptives.

Vitamin B_{12} (cobalamin). This vitamin, together with folic acid, is involved in the synthesis of deoxyribonucleic acid (DNA). There are several reports of symmetrical hyperpigmentation of the extremities over the palms and dorsal aspects of the hands and around the wrists and forearms, and also involving the lower limbs with a similar distribution in patients with vitamin B_{12} deficiency. In one case epidermal cells in areas of pigmentation had abnormally large nuclei. Lesions have responded to treatment.

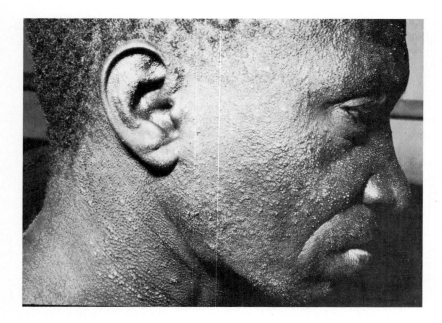

Fig. 136-16 Marked "shark skin" in an African. Riboflavin deficiency was suspected as the cause in both this case and that in Fig. 136-15.

Biotin. This substance is a growth factor for yeast and also the curative factor for raw egg-white injury which results from avidin antagonism of biotin. A generalized exfoliative dermatitis results in animals deficient in biotin.

A similar, milder condition has been produced experimentally in human volunteers fed a diet with minimal biotin and containing large amounts of raw egg white. A prompt response occurred with 75 to 300 µg biotin per day. Several patients receiving prolonged total parenteral nutrition without added biotin have developed scaling eczematoid lesions of the arms, legs, and feet, nasal and genital excoriations, cheilosis, waxy pallor of the face, alopecia, lethargy, and hypotonia, all of which responded to added biotin [7].

Pantothenic acid. This is a component of coenzyme A and is involved in the process of acetylation. No deficiency symptoms have been reported in humans; experiments feeding metabolic antagonists have not produced deficiency states that could be rapidly reversed by giving pantothenic acid alone. Further investigation has failed to confirm that it is of any value in the "burning feet" syndrome.

Vitamin C (scurvy)

In the deficiency state, collagen formation is impaired as a result of failure in hydroxylation of protocollagen, proline, and lysine. Clinically, changes have been described in bones, mucous membranes (Fig. 136-17), skin, and blood.

In human deprivation experiments [8,9], the first changes noted were enlargement and keratosis of the hair follicles chiefly on the outer aspect of the upper arm. The follicles became plugged by horny material in which the hair was coiled or looped, the so-called swan neck deformity. The number of enlarged follicles increased over ensuing weeks and months; the main areas affected were the upper arms, back, buttocks, backs of thighs, calves, and shins. A few weeks later the enlarged follicles turned red, due to congestion and proliferation of blood vessels around the hair follicles. The color deepened to dark purple over another week or two when the follicles became hemorrhagic; there was no bleaching on compression. Follicles on the legs showed the greatest tendency to become hemorrhagic. If acne had been present in a mild form at the start of the experiment, the lesions increased in size and became hemorrhagic.

Gum changes were most marked in those volunteers who showed evidence of gingivitis and periodontal disease at the start of the experiment. The earliest signs (after about 6 months of deprivation) were reddening, swelling, and tiny hemorrhages in the tips of the interdental papillae. Grosser changes observed in a few subjects consisted of a purplish, swollen, and spongy appearance of the gums, part of the tissue becoming necrotic with some bleeding. Aphthous ulcers, tenderness and pain, nontypical hemorrhages into the gums, and small extravasations without swelling in places other than the interdental papillae were all observed just as frequently in the supplemented as in the nonsupplemented group, and were therefore not related to diet. Gum changes are not present in edentulous patients.

During the later stages of experimental deficiency, scars, where experimental wounds had been excised, became red

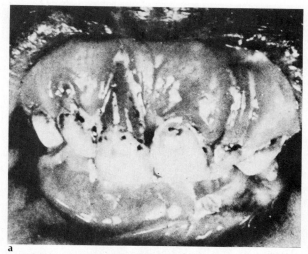

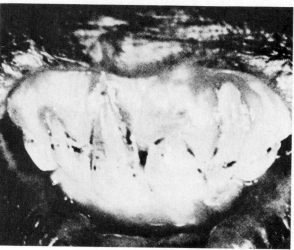

Fig. 136-17 Scorbutic gum changes in an adult who also has gum infection and poor dental hygiene. (a) On admission; note the characteristic gum redness and "hypertrophy." (b) After therapy with vitamin C. *(Courtesy of Dr. Charles S. Davidson.)*

and livid as a result of hemorrhages into the scar tissue and surrounding skin. New wounds made at the stage of pronounced scurvy failed to heal at the normal rate. Scorbutic patients respond dramatically to the administration of vitamin C. Infants should receive 150 to 300 mg of vitamin C daily by mouth, in divided doses, for 10 days, followed by 150 mg daily for a month. Thereafter a daily intake of 30 to 60 mg should be ensured in the form of fresh citrus fruits and juices. Adults should receive up to 800 mg daily in divided doses, for 1 week, and half this amount daily until complete recovery.

Vitamin K

Vitamin K is necessary for the synthesis of calcium-binding prothrombin by the liver. The hypoprothrombinemia of vitamin K deficiency may cause bleeding to occur almost anywhere in the body including the skin. Ecchymoses may appear, associated with mild trauma, and massive hemorrhage may occur beneath the skin within muscles, partic-

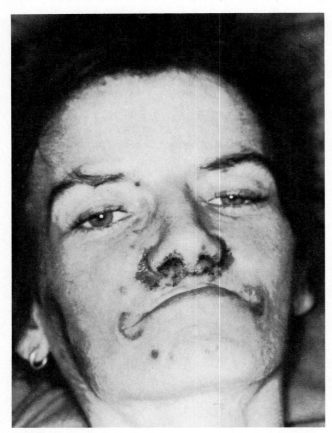

Fig. 136-18 Dermatosis of zinc deficiency in a patient with alcoholic cirrhosis. (Courtesy of Dr. A. Ilchyshyn.)

ularly of the extremities. In hemorrhagic disease of the newborn, areas of predilection are the umbilicus, skin, nose and mouth, intestine, and cerebrum. Differentiation has to be made from scurvy, hemophilia, and thrombocytopenia, but the clinical features are different, as are results of tests of clot time, plasma prothrombin, bleeding time, and capillary fragility.

Intramuscular phytonadione (vitamin K_1) is curative, 10 mg in adults, 2 mg in young children, and 1 mg in the newborn who should receive it routinely.

Essential fatty acids

On a fat-free diet rats fail to thrive and they develop skin lesions. Certain polyunsaturated fatty acids (linoleic, linolenic, and arachidonic) are curative. Arachidonic acid is synthesized in the body from linoleic acid, which is an essential dietary nutrient. The deficiency state has been produced in a variety of animal species. Growth failure and a dry, scaly skin have resulted in young children fed a diet very low in polyunsaturated fat.

Any natural diet readily supplies the 1 to 2 percent of total energy required in the form of essential fatty acids. Prolonged total parenteral nutrition, with concentrated glucose as the sole energy source, has resulted in deficiency, evidenced first by an abnormal plasma fatty acid pattern (a ratio of 20:3 ω 9 to 20:4 of 0.4 or over is diagnostic) and later by skin changes similar to those produced in experimental animals. These changes can be prevented by the

now standard practice of infusing at least 500 ml of 10% fat emulsion twice a week [10].

Essential elements

Iron

Chronic iron deficiency causes spoon-shaped deformity (koilonychia) of fingernails and toenails. Iron overload results in bronzing of the skin (see ''Hemochromatosis'' in Chap. 69) and is a major causative factor in porphyria cutanea tarda (see Chap. 143).

Zinc

Acrodermatitis enteropathica is an autosomal recessive condition due to impaired absorption of zinc (see Chap. 137). Deficiency has frequently been reported in patients receiving prolonged total parenteral nutrition [11] when zinc is not added to the nutrients. Clinical signs have included eczematous lesions of the face, mouth, and genitalia (Fig. 136-18).

Copper

Menkes' kinky hair syndrome is an X-linked recessive disorder caused by defective copper absorption (see Chap. 65). Infants on an exclusively milk diet or prolonged total parenteral nutrition have developed a copper-responsive syndrome consisting of anemia, bone changes, psychomotor retardation, and depigmentation of hair and skin with distended blood vessels due to defective elastin formation [12].

Selenium

One infant on prolonged total parenteral nutrition developed a white appearance of the fingernail beds reversed by selenium [13].

References

1. Keys A et al: *The Biology of Human Starvation*, 2 vols. Minneapolis, Univ of Minnesota Press, 1950
2. Frazier CN, Hu CK: Cutaneous lesions associated with deficiency in vitamin A in man. *Arch Intern Med* **48:**507, 1931
3. Hume EM, Krebs HA (Comps): *Vitamin A Requirements of Human Adults: Experimental Study of Vitamin A Deprivation in Man. Report of Vitamin A Subcommittee of Accessory Food Factors Committee.* Medical Research Council Special Report Series, no 264. London, Her Majesty's Stationery Office, 1949
4. Olsen TG: Therapy of acne. *Med Clin North Am* **66:**851, 1982
5. Sebrell WH, Butler RE: Riboflavin deficiency in man: preliminary note. *Public Health Rep* **53:**2282, 1938
6. Vilter RW et al: Effect of vitamin B_6 deficiency induced by desoxypyridoxine in human beings. *J Lab Clin Med* **42:**335, 1953
7. Innis SM, Allardyce DB: Possible biotin deficiency in adults receiving long-term parenteral nutrition. *Am J Clin Nutr* **37:**185, 1983
8. Bartley W et al: *Vitamin C Requirements of Human Adults. Report by Vitamin C Subcommittee of Accessory Food Factors Committee and A. E. Barnes, and Others.* Medical Re-

search Council Special Report Series, no 280. London, Her Majesty's Stationery Office, 1953

9. Hodges RE et al: Clinical manifestations of ascorbic acid deficiency in man. *Am J Clin Nutr* **24**:432, 1971

10. Fleming CR et al: Essential fatty acid deficiency in adults receiving total parenteral nutrition. *Am J Clin Nutr* **29**:976, 1976

11. Younoszai HD: Clinical zinc deficiency in total parenteral nutrition: zinc supplementation. *Journal of Parenteral and Enteral Nutrition* **7**:72, 1983

12. Bennani-Smires C et al: Infantile nutritional copper deficiency *Am J Dis Child* **134**:1156, 1980

13. Kien CL, Ganther HE: Manifestations of chronic selenium deficiency in a child receiving total parenteral nutrition. *Am J Clin Nutr* **37**:319, 1983

CHAPTER 137

ACRODERMATITIS ENTEROPATHICA AND OTHER ZINC-DEFICIENCY DISORDERS

Kenneth H. Neldner

Acrodermatitis enteropathica

Definition

Acrodermatitis enteropathica (AE) is a rare inherited disorder, transmitted as an autosomal recessive trait. Prior to the discovery by Moynahan and Barnes [1] in 1973 that the disorder was caused by an inability to absorb sufficient zinc from the diet, the disease was usually fatal in infancy or early childhood. It is now rapidly and dramatically cured by simple dietary supplementation with zinc salts.

The clinical syndrome is characterized by a basic triad of acral dermatitis, alopecia, and diarrhea. The distribution of the rash (face, hands, feet, anogenital area) has become recognized as a virtually pathognomonic cutaneous marker for zinc deficiency, whether secondary to AE or any of the numerous recently recognized nonhereditary causes for zinc deficiency.

Historical aspects

Acrodermatitis enteropathica was originally described by Danbolt and Closs [2] in 1943. In 1953 Dillaha et al [3] reported some therapeutic success with oral diiodohydroxyquin which was effective in controlling many aspects of AE, at least to a degree that would allow the children to survive but with varying degrees of morbidity. While studying a patient with AE and associated lactose intolerance in 1973, Moynahan and Barnes [1] made the observation during various dietary manipulations that alterations in zinc concentrations affected the well-being of the patient, leading to the discovery that AE was a disease of zinc deficiency.

Epidemiology

Acrodermatitis enteropathica has worldwide distribution with no apparent predilection for race or sex. Because of the early interest in the disease throughout Europe, particularly northern Europe, there are seemingly larger numbers of cases reported from these geographic areas.

The present ease of diagnosis and treatment of AE has now relegated it to the status of a relatively minor and insignificant disease. It remains, however, one of the more intriguing disorders known to medical science because seldom in human physiology have so many physical (and emotional) signs and symptoms been attributable to a deficiency of one single element, all of which are dramatically reversed by simple dietary supplementation with zinc. The opportunities for research appear endless, yet the disease is seldom studied, perhaps due in part to the fact that it is now so easily treated that cases are seldom referred to academic centers.

Etiology

After AE was discovered to be a disorder of zinc deficiency, the one missing link in its pathogenesis was to determine the mechanism by which zinc is absorbed from the diet, a process that is not totally lacking in AE because the patients can absorb a small amount of zinc from an average diet and a simple increase in dietary zinc will rapidly raise plasma levels to normal and cure the disease. The fact that zinc in human milk is much more biologically available to infants with AE than that from bovine milk, with essentially equal zinc concentration, has led to much interest in comparing the two milks in an effort to find a specific ligand involved in basic transport mechanisms for zinc, in addition to a possible species-specific zinc-binding ligand (ZBL) for humans that might be abnormal in AE. Thus far the search has shown the process to be complex and controversial. Those studies representing major lines of investigation are presented in brief overview.

Eckert et al [4] found the zinc in human milk to be associated with a low-M_r ligand ($\sim 10,000$) and the zinc of bovine milk was contained in higher-M_r fractions. Hurley

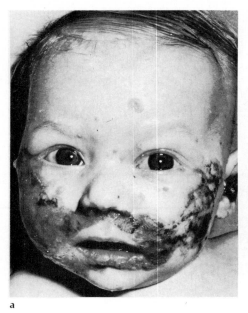
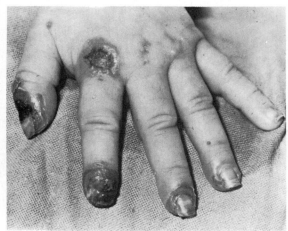

a   b

Fig. 137-1 Acrodermatitis enteropathica. Erosive and crusted lesions. (a) On the face. (b) On the hands and paronychial area.

et al [5] and Casey et al [6] have found a similarly sized low-M_r zinc ligand in human duodenal-pancreatic secretions, adding to the impression that the size of the ZBL was critical. Casey and coworkers [7] also found that the low-M_r ligand of duodenal-pancreatic secretions of patients with AE contained much less zinc than similar secretions from normal controls, suggesting that the ZBL in the duodenum of patients with AE was in some way less efficient.

More recently Cousins and Smith [8] found only 10 percent of the zinc in fat-free human milk to be associated with a low-M_r ZBL of <2000. But when additional zinc was added in vitro almost all of it became associated with this low-M_r fraction, suggesting that the overall concentration of zinc in milk determined how much of it appeared in which fraction. They also postulated that the difference in total protein of human milk (5.3 mg/ml) compared to bovine milk (29.0 mg/ml) also influenced the bioavailability of zinc in some unknown way.

Lönnerdal et al [9] and Menard and Cousins [10] found intestinal zinc to be complexed with citrate (M_r600 to 650) which they believe to be a major intestinal ZBL. However Oestreicher and Cousins [11] have reported that the addition of citrate to milk does not enhance absorption of zinc in the rat.

To further complicate the picture, other ZBLs have been reported to exist. Song [12] has proposed that prostaglandin E_2 has a role in zinc absorption from the gut. Evans and Johnson [13] have shown that picolinic acid, present in milk and duodenal contents, has a high affinity for zinc, but Rebello et al [14] found the intestinal concentration of picolinic acid to be so low that a significant role in zinc absorption is highly questionable.

Other factors such as the overall state of total-body zinc nutriture of the host will influence zinc absorption, i.e., the zinc-depleted individual will absorb zinc much more avidly than one in a zinc adequate or excess state. Complex and poorly understood interactions with other trace elements, particularly copper, lead, iron, and cadmium, are known to alter absorption [15]. Once zinc is absorbed by the intestinal villous brush border, another complex series of homeostatic events regulates the transport of zinc into the circulation and then on to the liver and kidneys where a final poorly understood surveillance system operates to regulate how much zinc will be preserved and how much excreted. These mechanisms appear to function normally in AE. The defect therefore lies somewhere in the early stages of zinc nutriture where the chemical form and the structure in which dietary zinc is presented to the intestinal mucosal brush border is in some way deficient or aberrant.

Clinical manifestations

The acute syndrome of AE usually begins within days to a few weeks after birth in infants bottle-fed with bovine milk or soon after weaning from the breast in older infants. Acral dermatitis begins slowly with dry, scaly, eczematous plaques on the face, scalp, and anogenital areas (Figs. 137-1 and 137-2). Perlèche is a common early sign. All lesions become progressively worse as vesicobullous, pustular, and erosive lesions develop. Superficial oral aphthous-like lesions may appear. The hands and feet are soon involved, commonly with paronychia and a brightly erythematous dermatitis of the palmar and finger creases plus annular lesions with collarette scaling. As the dermatitis worsens, secondary infections with bacteria and *Candida albicans* are common aggravating factors. Alopecia gradually worsens with time. Diarrhea is the most variable and may be only intermittent or totally absent. If diarrhea is severe and persistent, the clinical course will be further complicated by the loss of fluids, electrolytes, and other nutrients.

Within a few weeks, failure of growth becomes apparent.

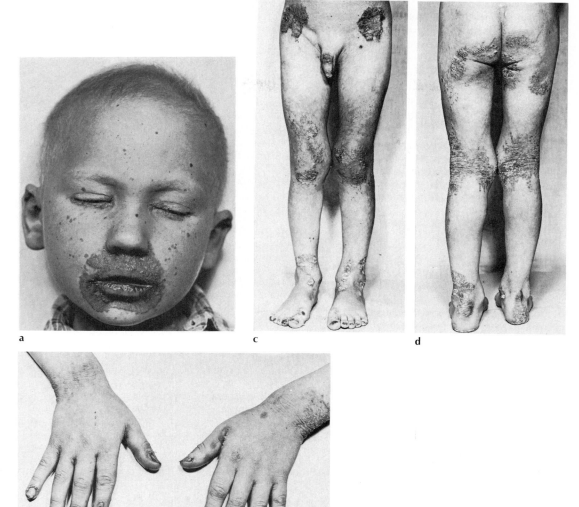

Fig. 137-2   Acrodermatitis enteropathica. Characteristic lesions (a) on the face, (b) on the hands, (c) on the anterior aspect of the lower extremities, (d) on the posterior aspect of the lower extremities.

Emotional and mental disturbances are common manifestations of zinc deficiency although difficult to evaluate. They are often best appreciated at the time when zinc supplementation is instituted resulting in rather rapid improvement in mood, disposition, and irritability within 24 to 48 h.

Photophobia develops gradually and is believed to be due to the fact that retinal binding protein is known to require zinc for its function. Other manifestations include anorexia, hypogeusia, hyosmia, hypogonadism, anemia, and impaired wound healing. The presence and severity of these findings will depend on the depth and duration of zinc deficiency.

Prior to the use of zinc in AE, fertility was low in those who reached reproductive age and congenital malformations were common, particularly those involving the central nervous system. Rat dams placed on severe zinc restriction for as short a period as four or five days prior to mating had litters with increased fetal resorption and more pups born with congenital anomalies than their zinc-adequate controls [16].

Biochemistry of zinc metabolism

Even though zinc was known to be required for normal growth and development in the rat since 1934, it was not established as an essential human nutrient by the National Research Council until 1974 when a recommended dietary allowance (RDA) was set at 15 mg per day.

The adult body contains 2 to 3 g of zinc, which is about half the iron content and some 10 to 20 times more than other trace elements such as copper, magnesium, and nickel. The zinc cation exists almost totally in the Zn^{++} oxidation state and does not readily undergo further oxidation or reduction, providing a stability which is believed to be significant in zinc biochemistry such as hydrolysis and transfer or addition to double bonds.

The average diet in the United States provides approximately 12 to 15 mg of elemental zinc per day. Body stores and homeostatic mechanisms combine to insure adequate supplies during times of reduced intake; however, during periods of dietary deprivation, the body will soon fall into a negative metabolic balance. In the rat, a negative balance develops within a few days after being fed a zinc-deficient diet, causing a rapid reduction in DNA synthesis [17]. Normally, about 30 percent of the daily intake is absorbed, although this figure is variable. Specific mechanisms of absorption have been discussed under "Etiology." The intravascular transport of zinc is primarily as a loosely bound complex with albumin (60 to 70 percent) and lesser amounts more tightly bound to alpha$_2$-macroglobulin (10 to 20 percent), transferrin (1 to 5 percent), amino acid chelates (5 to 10 percent), and IgG ($<$1 percent).

All body tissues contain zinc. Muscle, bone, and the prostate gland have the richest stores. In the skin, zinc is concentrated in the epidermis which contains up to five to six times greater concentration compared to the dermis [18,19]. Zinc also concentrates in hair, but changes in zinc nutriture of the host will be reflected in hair zinc concentration only after prolonged periods of deprivation (or excess), so its quantitation is unreliable for assessment of short-term or recent events.

The principal biochemical function of zinc is through its incorporation into a wide range of enzymes. Since zinc was discovered in 1940 to be present in carbonic anhydrase, the list of zinc metalloenzymes has grown to over 200 if those from nonhuman species are included [20]. All six classes of enzymes contain zinc metalloenzymes, the largest number being found in the hydrolases (Class III). There are two basic types of zinc-activated enzymes; one is a metal-enzyme complex that readily dissociates but requires the presence of zinc for continued activity, and the other in which zinc is firmly bound to the active site and will not dissociate during isolation of the enzyme.

Zinc deficiency also has significant adverse effects on the immune system. In both AE and an animal model of AE (Danish Black Pied Friesian breed of cattle) [21], thymic atrophy is one consequence of the disorder. As a result, thymocytes and cellular immune functions, particularly a wide range of T-cell functions, are depressed. This aspect of zinc deficiency has been reviewed by Good et al [21]. Neutrophils, peripheral blood monocytes, tissue macrophages, and mast cells also require optimal concentrations of zinc for normal function [22].

Recent reviews of the biochemistry and physiology of zinc metabolism have been written by Prasad [23] and Forbes [24].

Acquired (conditioned) zinc deficiency

In recent years a number of acquired (conditioned) zinc deficiency states have been described. Any disorder causing malabsorption, abnormal excretion, general catabolism, or certain iatrogenically induced drug or nutritional factors may deplete the body stores of zinc through various mechanisms.

A list of potential causes for acquired zinc deficiency and their basic mechanisms is presented in Table 137-1. The most common are those involving medical diseases of the gastrointestinal tract such as chronic mucosal disease with diarrhea (Fig. 137-3) or steatorrhea, pancreatic insuf-

Table 137-1   Acquired (conditioned) zinc deficiencies

Disorder	Etiology
Gastrointestinal:	
Mucosal diseases	Diarrhea
Malabsorption syndromes	Diarrhea
Pancreatic disorders	Reduced zinc ligands
Cirrhosis	Increased urinary loss
Postgastrectomy syndrome	Diarrhea
Blind loop syndromes	Diarrhea
Dietary factors:	
High dietary phytate	Chelation
Alcoholism	Increased urinary loss
Total parenteral nutrition	Lack of zinc supplementation
Trauma:	
Burns	Exudation, catabolism
Postsurgical procedure	Catabolism, anorexia
Malignancy:	
All types	Catabolism, anorexia
Renal disorders:	
Renal tubular disease	Failure to resorb zinc
Nephrotic syndrome	Proteinuria
Dialysis	Loss of zinc in dialyzate
Infection:	
Parasitic	Chronic blood loss
Bacterial, viral	Redistribution, urinary loss
Miscellaneous:	
Antimetabolite drug therapy	Catabolism
Chelation drug therapy	Chelation-urinary loss
Diabetes mellitus	Urinary loss
Hemolytic anemias	Urinary loss of erythrocyte zinc
Collagen-vascular diseases	Catabolism
Pregnancy	Increased fetal requirements

ficiency and cirrhosis, or surgically induced conditions such as postsurgical gastrectomy or bowel resection with blind-loop syndromes. If patients with any of these conditions become so ill as to require total parenteral nutrition (TPN), zinc deficiency almost always develops within four to six weeks unless adequate supplementation is provided in the TPN solutions [25].

When the deficiency reaches a critical level, a broad range of clinical manifestations begins to appear. The earliest of these will often be subtle and unrecognized as being related to zinc metabolism. Systemic manifestations such as hypogeusia, hyposmia, anorexia, and minor mental disturbances are common early findings. The skin may show early seborrheic dermatitis-like changes (see Fig. A2-15b) along with perlèche. As the zinc deficit deepens, the skin reaction becomes a good marker, showing an acral dermatitis that mimics AE in all respects. Diffuse alopecia follows but diarrhea may be variable. Emotional disturbances often become more marked, with depression, mental lethargy, and general irritability most prominent. Progressive anorexia may accelerate the total process by further reducing dietary intake of all nutrients.

The possibility of low-grade chronic zinc deficiency is of interest and may be much more common than presently recognized. Prasad et al [26] studied members of rural Egyptian and Iranian communities and found chronic zinc

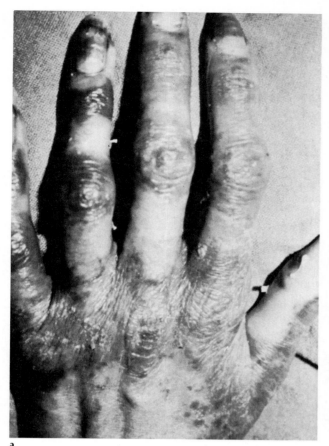

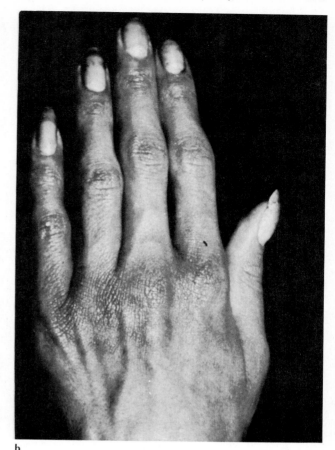

a

b

Fig. 137-3 (a) Hand of a 25-year-old woman with severe acquired zinc deficiency secondary to prolonged nausea, vomiting, diarrhea, and weight loss. She was also on total parenteral nutrition for two weeks prior to this photograph. Plasma zinc concentration was 25 μg/dL. (b) Same patient after 10 days of oral zinc supplementation and no topical therapy.

deficiency secondary to diets high in zinc-binding phytates and low in zinc-containing meats and sea foods. Major overt manifestations were dwarfism, hypogonadism, dry rashes, and anemia, which in most instances responded to zinc supplementation. Because of the known concentration of zinc in the epidermis and therefore a presumed involvement in epidermal physiology, the possibility of chronic low-grade zinc deficiency producing heretofore unrecognized skin reactions seems worthy of future consideration. The known suppressing effect of zinc deficiency on immune mechanisms also creates the potential for more generalized systemic disorders of immunosuppression that may also have a cutaneous component.

Laboratory diagnosis of zinc deficiency

The laboratory verification of zinc deficiency is the same as for hereditary deficiency (AE) or any of the acquired forms. Plasma or serum zinc levels are currently the easiest, best, and most commonly used method for assessing zinc status. It is, however, well recognized that blood levels fluctuate rapidly following infection, injury, burns, or any sudden stressful stimuli, resulting in redistribution of zinc from the blood to other sites. Blood levels during such events may, therefore, not give a true presentation of total

zinc nutriture. Normal plasma levels are 70 to 110 μg/dL. (Serum levels are 80 to 120 μ/dL.) Urinary zinc excretion is highly variable under normal circumstances but does gradually decrease as zinc deficiency progresses. The normal urinary excretion ranges from 200 to 500 μg/24 h. Hair zinc concentration is commonly measured but again reflects only the long-term zinc status. Its use and interpretation will therefore depend upon the clinical situation and type of information desired. Serum alkaline phosphatase activity is a moderately sensitive indicator of zinc status, although not a particularly early marker of deficiency. Another zinc metalloenzyme that is relatively easily measured is erythrocyte carbonic anhydrase activity, but it is known to be a poor indicator of zinc deficiency. Its activity remains near normal until profound and prolonged deficiency exists. Leukocyte zinc has been shown to be quite sensitive to early minor changes in total-body zinc nutriture but has the disadvantage of being a difficult and expensive assay [27].

It should also be emphasized that specimen collections and laboratory technique are important. Contamination with environmental zinc in collecting tubes or containers plus laboratory contamination in the handling and transfer of specimens and in the preparation of laboratory chemicals and solutions is a constant threat. Spurious laboratory results will, therefore, almost always be on the side of higher than actual values which may lead to a missed diagnosis of impending or borderline zinc deficiency.

Treatment of zinc deficiency

The treatment of zinc deficiency is essentially that of dietary or intravenous supplementation with zinc salts, no matter what the etiology. In most instances, dietary supplementation with two to three times the RDA in doses of 30 to 55 mg of elemental Zn^{++} daily will be adequate to restore a normal zinc status within days to a few weeks, depending on the degree of depletion. In all circumstances, a rapid clinical response will occur with dramatic reversal of many manifestations within hours to days [28]. Severe infected and erosive skin lesions will heal within one to two weeks without additional topical therapy. Diarrhea, if present, often stops within 24 h. Rapid improvement in mental disturbances is usually detectable within 24 to 48 h. In children, a surge of total-body and hair growth can be detected within three to four weeks after commencing zinc therapy.

Any of the zinc compounds available appear to work well (zinc sulfate, zinc acetate, zinc gluconate, zinc chloride, amino acid chelates). However, $ZnSO_4$ has been recommended more for oral supplementation and $ZnCl_2$ for intravenous use. Dosage prescribed must be based on the amount of elemental zinc present in the preparation, which varies from one compound to another. For example, a standard capsule of 220 mg of $ZnSO_4 \cdot 7\ H_2O$ contains approximately 55 mg Zn^{++} which is an adequate daily dose for most deficient individuals.

High, pharmacologic doses of oral zinc have been recommended by some investigators for the therapy of sickle cell anemia, acne, delayed wound healing, and leg ulcers. All of these conditions will improve with zinc therapy if a preceding zinc deficiency existed. However, it is generally believed that proof is lacking for a pharmacologic effect over and above that of restoration of a normal zinc nutritional status. Furthermore, the threat of zinc toxicity must be guarded against if prolonged high doses are ingested.

Zinc toxicity

Most heavy metals, including zinc, become toxic if taken to excess. Moderate overdose is eliminated through homeostatic mechanisms involving decreased absorption and/or increased urinary and biliary excretions. However, plasma levels of 150 to 300 μg/dL (normal, 70 to 110 μg/dL) are easily achieved by persons ingesting zinc supplements of 50 to 100 mg Zn^{++} daily. Such doses usually produce no immediately apparent adverse effects although the long-term safety of such a dose is unknown.

$ZnSO_4$ is listed in the *U.S. Pharmacopeia* as an emetic. Not surprisingly its most common adverse effect is stomach irritation with nausea, vomiting, and mild gastric hemorrhage.

Acute and fatal zinc toxicity has been reported following large accidental oral and intravenous overdose [29]. Chronic toxicity among zinc smelter workers is known as "metal fume fever" which causes fever, chills, gastroenteritis, and pulmonary symptoms [30]. Rats and mice fed moderate overdose for long periods have shown reduced growth rates, anemia, declining rates of reproduction, hypertrophy of the adrenal cortex, and pancreatic islets [31]. The finding that moderate to high (160 mg Zn^{++} daily) overdose was atherogenic in humans was reported by Hooper et al [32], but it has been found more recently that lower doses of zinc have no effect on high-density lipoprotein cholesterol [33].

A reciprocal interaction with copper is well recognized [34]. Patients receiving prolonged oral zinc supplementation are prone to develop hypocupremia as a consequence of long-standing hyperzincemia. One adverse effect of hypocupremia is a refractory microcytic anemia that will not respond to iron therapy until the serum copper level is normalized [35]. Neutropenia and hypoceruloplasminemia also occur with hypocupremia.

It is recommended that patients on long-term zinc therapy should be monitored periodically with the following tests: plasma zinc concentrations taken as a fasting A.M. specimen to regulate dosage, complete hemogram with erythrocyte indices, leukocyte differential count, serum copper level, and a stool examination for occult blood.

References

1. Moynahan EJ, Barnes PM: Zinc deficiency and a synthetic diet for lactose intolerance. *Lancet* **1:**676, 1973
2. Danbolt N, Closs K: Acrodermatitis enteropathica. *Acta Derm Venereol (Stockh)* **23:**127, 1943
3. Dillaha CJ et al: Acrodermatitis enteropathica: review of the literature and a report of a case successfully treated with Diodiquin. *JAMA* **152:**509, 1953
4. Eckert CD et al: Zinc binding: a difference between human and bovine milk. *Science* **195:**789, 1977
5. Hurley LS et al: Zinc binding ligands in milk and intestine: a role in neonatal nutrition. *Proc Natl Acad Sci USA* **74:**3547, 1977
6. Casey CE et al: Zinc binding in human duodenal secretions. *Lancet* **2:**423, 1978
7. Casey CE et al: Zinc binding in human duodenal secretions. *J Pediatr* **95:**1008, 1979
8. Cousins RJ, Smith KT: Zinc-binding properties of bovine and human milk in vitro: influence of changes in zinc content. *Am J Clin Nutr* **33:**1083, 1980
9. Lönnerdal B et al: Isolation of a low molecular weight zinc binding ligand from human milk. *J Inorg Biochem* **12:**71, 1980
10. Menard MD, Cousins RJ : Effect of citrate, glutathione and picolinate on zinc transport by brush border membrane vesicles from rat intestine. *J Nutr* **113:**1653, 1983
11. Oestreicher P, Cousins RJ: Influence of intraluminal constituents on zinc absorption by isolated, vascularly profused rat intestine. *J Nutr* **112:**1978, 1982
12. Song MK: Evidence for an important role of prostaglandin E_2 and F_2 in the regulation of zinc transport in the rat. *J Nutr* **109:**2152, 1979
13. Evans GW, Johnson PE: Characterization and quantitation of a zinc binding ligand from human milk. *Pediatr Res* **14:**870, 1980
14. Rebello T et al: Picolinic acid in milk, pancreatic juice and intestine: inadequate for role in zinc absorption. *Am J Clin Nutr* **35:**1, 1982
15. Solomons NW: Competitive mineral-mineral interaction in the intestine: implications for zinc absorption in humans, in *Nutritional Bioavailability of Zinc*, edited by GE Inglett. Washington, DC, ACS Symposium Series, 1983, p 247
16. Hurley LS, Baly DL: The effects of zinc deficiency during pregnancy, in *Clinical, Biochemical and Nutritional Aspects*

of Trace Elements, edited by AS Prasad. New York, Alan R Liss, 1982, p 145

17. Prasad AS, Oberleas D: Thymidine kinase activity and incorporation of thymidine into DNA in zinc deficient tissues. *J Lab Clin Med* **83**:634, 1974

18. Michaëlsson G et al: Zinc in epidermis and dermis of normal subjects. *Acta Derm Venereol (Stockh)* **60**:295, 1980

19. Molokhia M, Portnoy B: Neutron activation analysis of trace elements in skin: III. Zinc in normal skin. *Br J Dermatol* **81**:759, 1969

20. Vallee BL, Galdes A: The metallobiochemistry of zinc enzymes. *Adv Enzymol* **56**:284, 1984

21. Good RA et al: Zinc and immunity, in *Clinical, Biochemical and Nutritional Aspects of Trace Elements,* edited by AS Prasad. New York, Alan R Liss, 1982, p 189

22. Beisel WR: The role of zinc in neutrophil function, in *Clinical, Biochemical and Nutritional Aspects of Trace Elements,* edited by AS Prasad. New York, Alan R Liss, 1982, p 203

23. Prasad AS: Clinical biochemistry and nutritional spectrum of zinc deficiency in human subjects: an update. *Nutr Rev* **41**:197, 1983

24. Forbes RM: Use of laboratory animals to define physiological functions and bioavailability of zinc. *Fed Proc* **43**:2835, 1984

25. Wolman SL et al: Zinc and total parenteral nutrition: requirements and metabolic effects. *Gastroenterology* **73**:458, 1979

26. Prasad AS et al: Zinc metabolism in patients with a syndrome of iron deficiency anemia, hypogonadism and dwarfism. *J Lab Clin Med* **61**:537, 1963

27. Prasad AS et al: Experimental zinc deficiency in humans. *An Intern Med* **89**:483, 1978

28. Neldner KH, Hambridge KM: Zinc therapy of acrodermatitis enteropathica. *N Engl J Med* **292**:879, 1975

29. Brocks A et al: Acute intravenous zinc poisoning. *Br Med J* **28**:1390, 1977

30. Papp JP: Metal fume fever. *Postgrad Med* **43**:160, 1968

31. Aughey E et al: The effect of oral zinc supplementation in the mouse. *J Comp Pathol* **87**:1, 1977

32. Hooper PL et al: Zinc lowers high-density lipoprotein-cholesterol levels. *JAMA* **244**:1960, 1980

33. Crounse SF et al: Zinc ingestion and lipoprotein values in sedentary and endurance trained men. *JAMA* **252**:785, 1984

34. Kirchgessner M et al: Interactions of essential metals in human physiology, in *Clinical, Biochemical and Nutritional Aspects of Trace Elements,* edited by AS Prasad. New York, Alan R Liss, 1982, p 477

35. Solomons NW et al: Studies on the bioavailability of zinc in humans: mechanism of the intestinal interaction of non heme iron and zinc. *J Nutr* **113**:337, 1983

CHAPTER 138

GENETICS IN RELATION TO THE SKIN

Lowell A. Goldsmith and Victor A. McKusick

Understanding genetic principles and methods is essential to understanding the basis and the treatment of many skin diseases. In common skin disorders, such as atopic dermatitis and psoriasis, genetic factors play a significant role, but the genetics are often complex and environmental factors are very significant. In contrast, many relatively rare disorders are the result primarily of a single mutant gene. Although individually rare, these conditions, in the aggregate, represent an important body of disease. In Table 138-1 are listed the relative incidences of some of the more common genetic diseases determined by a single gene locus. In Table 138-2, for comparison, are data on some of the rarer genetic diseases.

When the mutant gene in a single dose (or heterozygous state) results in the particular clinical phenotype, the condition is said to be dominant; when the mutant gene must be present in double dose (or homozygous state) to produce abnormality, the resulting disorder is said to be recessive. When the mutant gene is on the X chromosome, the condition produced thereby is called sex-linked, or more precisely X-linked. X-linked conditions may also be dominant or recessive depending on whether the heterozygous female does or does not show the phenotype. When the mutant gene is on one of the 22 pairs of autosomes (non-sex chromosomes) the disorder is referred to as autosomal. Although means are not yet available for curing

genetic disease in terms of repairing the defect in the gene, many hereditary disorders are now amenable to satisfactory treatment aimed at averting the deleterious effects of the genes. Examples in the skin include zinc supplementation to treat acrodermatitis enteropathica, a low-tyrosine, low-phenylalanine diet to treat tyrosinemia II (Richner-Hanhart syndrome), or the administration of oral beta-carotene for erythropoietic protoporphyria.

Pedigree patterns

An understanding of the characteristic pedigree patterns of rare, simple inherited ("Mendelizing") disorders is essential to counseling prospective parents on the risk of having affected children. As stated above, the three main patterns of inheritance are autosomal dominant, autosomal recessive, and X-linked recessive.

Autosomal dominant

Apart from the recipients of new mutations, persons affected with rare autosomal dominant disorders have one affected parent and the condition is transmitted from generation to generation. Both males and females are affected in approximately equal numbers and both males and females can transmit the disorder. On the average, when an

Table 138-1 Frequency of genetic skin diseases

Variegate porphyria (South Africa)	1:330
Hemochromatosis	1:400
Cystic fibrosis	1:2000
X-linked ichthyosis	1:6000 males
Phenylketonuria (classical)	1:11,000
Oculocutaneous albinism (tyrosinase positive)	{ 1:37,000 white { 1:15,000 black
Oculocutaneous albinism (tyrosinase negative)	{ 1:39,000 white { 1:28,000 black
Fabry's disease	1:40,000
Ehlers-Danlos (all types)	1:50,000
Argininosuccinate lyase deficiency	1:70,000
Variegate porphyria (Finland)	1:75,000
Menkes' disease	1:100,000
Xeroderma pigmentosum	1:250,000
Prolidase deficiency	1:600,000

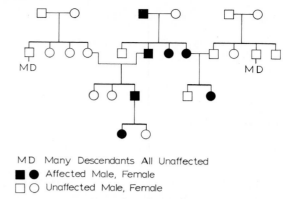

MD Many Descendants All Unaffected
■ ● Affected Male, Female
□ ○ Unaffected Male, Female

Fig. 138-1 Idealized autosomal dominant pedigree pattern. The condition is transmitted from generation to generation by affected males or females to males or females.

affected person is married to an unaffected person, half the children will have the condition. In Fig. 138-1, an idealized autosomal dominant pedigree pattern is illustrated and in Fig. 138-2, an actual pedigree of a kindred with monilethrix. It must be emphasized that the expected 50:50 ratio will probably be found only when many pedigrees or an exceptionally extensive, single pedigree are available for analysis.

Autosomal recessive

Typically, rare autosomal recessive disorders occur in brothers and sisters, both of whose parents are unaffected. The parents are related to each other more often than the average, and the rarer the condition, the more likely the parental consanguinity. Provided that affected individuals do not marry a relative, their children are unlikely to manifest the condition. An idealized pedigree is shown in Fig. 138-3, and Fig. 138-4 illustrates a kindred with epidermolysis bullosa letalis. Both parents of all the individuals marked as affected could be traced back to one common ancestral couple, one of whom was presumably heterozygous for the mutant gene. This family belonged to the Old Order Amish, where exact pedigree data are available for many generations. This is an example of inbreeding. Inbreeding per se does not alter the frequency of genes in a population. What it does is to increase homozygosity and therefore undesirable recessive traits. If a person who is homozygous for a particular recessive gene, and therefore affected, does not reproduce because of the grave nature of the hereditary ailment, inbreeding may actually lead to a decline of the frequency of the gene in the given population. Consanguinity plays little part in rare X-linked recessive and autosomal dominant disorders.

X-linked recessive

These conditions occur almost exclusively in males, but the gene is transmitted by carrier females, who have the gene only in a single dose (heterozygous state). An affected male cannot transmit the disorder to any of his sons, who are all normal, but all his daughters are carriers (obligatory heterozygotes). Occasionally, some females show clinical abnormalities as evidence of the carrier state, and this phenomenon can be explained by the Lyon hypothesis.

Dr. Mary Lyon suggested that early in embryogenesis one X chromosome in each cell of the normal XX female becomes genetically inactive; that which one is inactive is a random matter; and that once it had been "decided" whether the X chromosome from the female's mother or that from her father will be the active one in a given cell, all descendants of that cell "abide by the decision." Thus, the adult female is a mosaic of two classes of cells, those with the paternal X as the active one and those with the maternal X as the active one. The inactive X chromosome forms the Barr body, or sex chromatin.

The Lyon hypothesis provides an explanation for an intermediate level of gene effect in the heterozygous female and for its rather wide variability. By chance alone, rare individuals may have all cells of a particular type with the mutant X chromosome as the inactive one, in which case no abnormality will be detectable by even the most sensitive methods. However, in many X-linked conditions, such as anhidrotic ectodermal dysplasia, some carrier females demonstrate abnormal features, suggesting that the mutant X chromosome is active in some cell lines. Indeed, patchy abnormalities, such as the Lyon principle would predict, have been observed in females heterozygous for this gene. An idealized pedigree of X-linked inheritance is given in Fig. 138-5 and an example of a family with X-linked ichthyosis in Fig. 138-6. Since the short arm of the X chromosome is not completely inactivated, loci on the short arm of the X chromosome such as that for X-linked ichthyosis and the Xg^a blood group do not undergo complete inactivation.

In X-linked dominant inheritance both males and females

Table 138-2 Rare genetic skin diseases

	No. of cases reported
Tyrosinemia II (Richner-Hanhart syndrome)	26
Farber's lipogranulomatosis (ceramidase deficiency)	27
α-Fucosidosis	30–60
Hartnup disease	60
Congenital erythropoietic porphyria	60–80
Refsum's disease	100

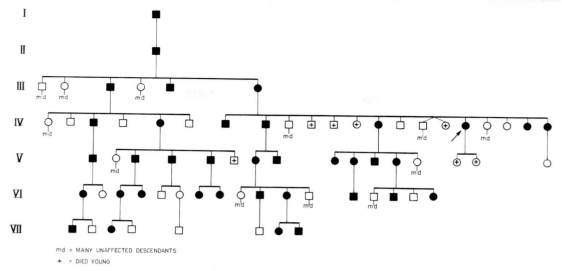

Fig. 138-2   Monilethrix. Although the degree of alopecia was highly variable, all affected persons had an affected parent. *(From McKusick VA: Medical Genetics 1961–63: An Annotated Review. Oxford, Pergamon, 1966.)*

are affected, and the pedigree patterns may superficially resemble those of autosomal dominant inheritance. There is, however, one important difference. An affected male transmits the disorder to all of his daughters and to none of his sons. X-linked dominant inheritance, lethal in males, has been postulated for one variety of incontinentia pigmenti. This explains pedigrees where more than one member of the family is affected and the condition is seen only in females. Affected males may appear as spontaneous abortions or die so early that pregnancy would not be recognized. A half-chromatid mutation model in which the gamete has one normal and one mutant cell was proposed to explain incontinentia pigmenti, but this model has been refuted on the basis of a mother and a son with incontinentia pigmenti. This is the only male with the disease with an affected mother; the other six males who are reported

are sporadic cases. An idealized pedigree is given in Fig. 138-7. Incontinentia pigmenti is probably an example of genetic and clinical heterogeneity, but hypotheses on the mode of inheritance must always explain the fact that all but a few affected persons are female. X-linked dominant inheritance with lethality in hemizygous affected males has also been proposed to explain the pedigree of focal dermal hypoplasia.

The term *sex-linked* is used if an autosomal disorder is confined to one sex. Such conditions may be seen either in males or females, and a definite mode of inheritance is not implied by the use of this term. When only males or only females in a given family are affected with a condition, this may be an example of sex limitation but it is more likely the result of chance. Sex linkage, better called X linkage, results in a specific pedigree pattern, as described above. True sex-limited conditions, that is, disorders which have manifestations in one sex only, are rare. *Sex-influenced* is the term used when an autosomal trait occurs more often, although not exclusively, in one sex.

A second possible type of sex-linked transmission is that observed with genes carried on the Y chromosome. Since this chromosome determines the maleness of an individual, and must be inherited from the father, all the sons and none of the daughters of the affected person will manifest the disorder. The most famous supposed example of this mode of inheritance, the porcupine men (epidermolytic hyperkeratosis), has not been substantiated by recent research. There is some evidence that hairy ears (Fig. 138-8), a trait more frequent in some areas of India than elsewhere, may be transmitted in this way. An illustrative pedigree is given in Fig. 138-9.

Mutation

The gene responsible for many simply inherited disorders originated by mutation in a recent past or more remotely past generation. Most simply inherited disorders are the

Fig. 138-3   **Idealized autosomal recessive pedigree pattern. The parents are unaffected and consanguinity is common.**

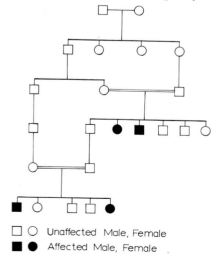

☐ ◯ Unaffected Male, Female
■ ● Affected Male, Female

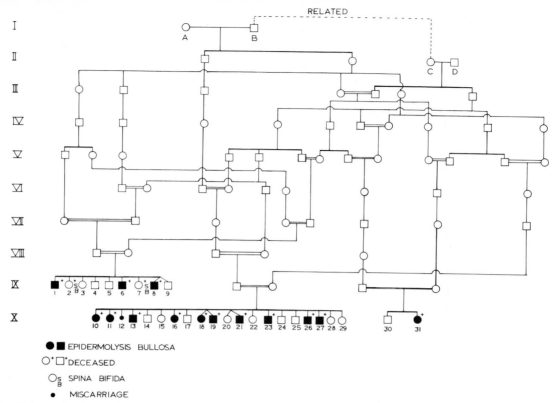

Fig. 138-4 Epidermolysis bullosa letalis. A pedigree from the Old Order Amish showing considerable consanguinity.

result of point mutation, i.e., a change in the sequence of purine-pyrimidine bases in the DNA molecule. This change is at a level far below that which can be detected by the available methods of chromosome study and the karyotype is normal in patients with straightforward dominant, recessive, or X-linked disorders. In the case of autosomal dominant conditions and X-linked conditions, the new mu-

tation may have occurred in the germ cell, egg, or sperm which participated in the origin of the specific person under observation. If such was the case, then that person will present a sporadic case, and no family history of the disorder will be obtained. In the case of many disorders, it is probably valid to assume genetic equilibrium; the loss of genes from the population, due to failure of the affected individuals to have as many children as the population as a whole, is balanced by the addition of new mutant genes through the process of mutation. The proportion of all cases observed that are new mutants, as opposed to familial cases, will be higher the lower the fertility of affected persons. For instance, probably about 15 percent of cases of the Marfan syndrome are new mutants. In X-linked recessive conditions such as Duchenne's muscular dystrophy or agammaglobulinemia, in which the affected males do not survive to have children, it can be shown that one-third of the cases are new mutants, and two-thirds have a carrier mother and are therefore inherited. In epidermolytic hyperkeratosis, new mutations are common.

Thus, sporadic cases of hereditary disease may represent new dominant or X-linked mutants. Another frequent mechanism for sporadic cases is the chance occurrence of only one case of a recessive disorder in the family. Human families are small and a family may have only one child affected by a given recessive disorder. In fact, it can be calculated that of all two-child families with one child affected by a given recessive disorder, the other child will be normal in 86 percent of instances; in three-child families only one child will be affected in 73 percent of instances, and so on.

Fig. 138-5 Idealized X-linked recessive pedigree pattern. Only males are affected and the gene is transmitted by carrier females.

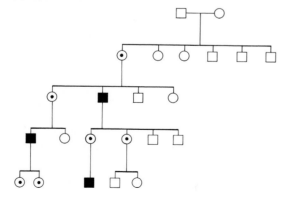

☐○ Unaffected Male, Non-carrier Female
■ Affected Male
⊙ Carrier Female

Fig. 138-6 X-linked ichthyosis. No evidence of ichthyosis in the heterozygous females.

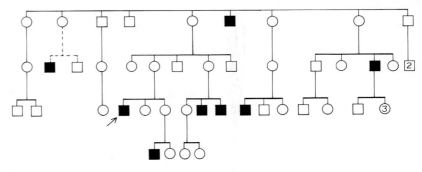

■ Affected Male

For the sporadic cases of most autosomal dominant disorders studied from this point of view, it has been possible to demonstrate a paternal age effect. For example, the average age of fathers of sporadic cases of achondroplastic dwarfism is about 7 years greater than the average. Maternal age per se is probably not a factor although a "maternal age effect" is well known in certain chromosomal aberrations, notably Down's syndrome.

Variability of genetic diseases

The physician must deal with the marked variability in the expression of abnormal genotypes. This is especially a problem when deciding whether a new mutation has occurred and whether manifestations of a deleterious gene are present in a carrier of that gene who may be asymptomatic and essentially normal. In those cases in which specific quantitative biochemical tests are available, the presence of an abnormal gene, even in a completely asymptomatic carrier, can be determined.

Several terms are used to deal with the question of variability; their usage is often confused and a brief discussion of these terms is in order.

Penetrance is the ability to detect any manifestation of an abnormal genotype. If the phenotypic manifestations of a genotype are not discernible, the gene would be nonpenetrant. Penetrance is an operational term depending on

how well one can analyze for evidence of the abnormal genotype. If one could determine detailed DNA sequences, an abnormal genotype could always be detected. If a trait is not penetrant, its expressivity must be none.

Expressivity defines the degree of expression (severity) of a trait. It is a designation of the qualitative and quantitative manifestations of a specific genotype, and is the variability in phenotype produced by a given genotype.

Pleiotropy refers to the multiple phenotypic effects due to the primary actions of an abnormal genotype. Single autosomal genes such as those for Gardner's syndrome, pachyonychia congenita, neurofibromatosis, or the X-linked gene for Menkes' disease cause multiple phenotypic effects in several organ systems. The expressivity or even the penetrance of these traits may differ in individuals in the same family or between families. The elucidation of the basic defects in these diseases will allow one to understand the multiple manifestations of an abnormal genotype. In most cases, pleiotropy is not due to the close linkage of several genes on a chromosome.

Heterogeneity. Many genetic diseases, e.g., albinism, epidermolysis bullosa, ichthyosis, Ehlers-Danlos syndrome, and cutis laxa, are really groups of diseases: within

Fig. 138-8 Hairy ear rims in a male.

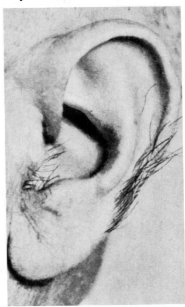

Fig. 138-7 Idealized pedigree pattern of X-linked dominant trait lethal in the male.

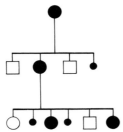

● ○ Affected and Unaffected Female

□ Unaffected Male

● Abortion

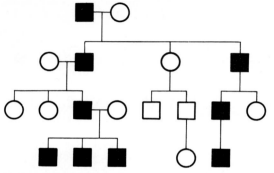

Fig. 138-9 Idealized Y-linked pedigree pattern. All the sons of an affected male must be affected.

each group biochemical and genetic analysis shows multiple forms of the diseases, which can be distinguished. The recognition of heterogeneity requires certainty of diagnosis when genetic counseling is contemplated.

Another source of variability is the fact that two conditions may have clinical features in common. For instance, patients with Darier's disease may show lesions of acrokeratosis verruciformis. There are several possible explanations for this finding. First, there is a single gene with variable expression in different patients. Second, there are two separate genes, and an affected individual may by chance have both conditions. Third, there may be three genes, one for Darier's disease, one for acrokeratosis verruciformis, and a third which has manifestations of both disorders. Such a problem can generally be resolved only by detailed pedigree studies of many kindreds, and it may be very important to do this. For instance, some patients with multiple epidermal and sebaceous cysts have polyps

in the bowel which undergo malignant change, but it is not known whether all patients with numerous wens are at risk.

Three other terms are useful when discussing some genetic diseases, but they often lead to confusion: phenocopy, congenital, and linkage.

Phenocopy. Environmental (nongenetic) causes may mimic inherited diseases. The vascular lesions of the CRST form of systemic sclerosis mimic very closely the telangiectatic lesions of Rendu-Weber-Osler disease. The recognition of phenocopies is of importance when considering prognosis and counseling for an individual condition.

Congenital. The words *congenital* ("present at birth") and *familial* do not necessarily imply that a condition is genetically determined.

Linkage. Linkage is the occurrence of two loci on one chromosome, sufficiently close together that something less than completely independent assortment takes place. Examples of linkage in dermatology are (1) the gene for the nail-patella syndrome and those for the ABO blood group system are on the same autosome, so that the nail-patella syndrome tends to occur in members of a given blood type in a family, and (2) the gene for the Xg blood group and X-linked ichthyosis are each inherited on the X chromosome and therefore the ichthyosis is associated with a given Xg group in a family. Because of the phenomenon of crossing over, by which even closely linked genes become separated after the passage of generations, genetic linkage produces no permanent association of traits in the population. Linkage of traits is now of extreme importance since chromosome mapping is highly advanced and many traits have been linked to the HLA region of chromosome 6 and to other discrete chromosomal regions. Gene mapping with banding patterns can demonstrate karyotypic

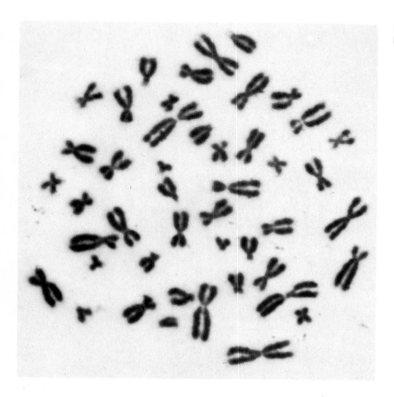

Fig. 138-10 Chromosomes of a single human white blood cell in the metaphase stage of mitosis.

markers of a genetic trait. Gene mapping using restriction endonucleases to digest the DNA can demonstrate structural markers at the level of the DNA that can be closely linked with abnormal genotypes.

Chromosomes and chromosomal disorders

Genes are arranged and organized in supramolecular groups, the chromosomes. Techniques for the culture of cells and analysis of their chromosomes allowed the definition of the chromosomal basis of several diseases. Recent techniques with the use of fluorescent dyes and special staining techniques (banding) have increased the resolution of the cytogenetic techniques possible with the light microscope. Besides a large number of congenital diseases diagnosable by chromosomal analysis, acquired diseases such as chronic myelogenous leukemia, some patients with T-cell lymphoma (mycosis fungoides), and retinoblastoma also have characteristic chromosomal alterations.

In clinical practice, lymphocytes are stimulated to divide by phytohemagglutinin and their chromosomes are then studied (Fig. 138-10). The chromosomes of a single such cell are examined with light microscopy at a magnification of about 1800×, and the 46 chromosomes are arranged in what is known as a karyotype (Fig. 138-11a and b). The autosomes occur in 22 pairs; the sex chromosomes are X and Y in the male, two X's in the female. Note that each of the 46 chromosomes consists, at this state of cell division (metaphase), of two chromatids attached at what is called the centromere. Each chromatid is destined to form the particular chromosome in one of the two daughter cells.

Recently, many genetic diseases have been mapped to particular chromosomes and portions of chromosomes (Fig. 138-12). Abnormalities of chromosome number include: trisomy (three of a particular chromosome rather than two), monosomy (absence of an autosome), deletion of a long or a short arm of a chromosome, and the presence of an additional portion of a chromosome (often because of translocation).

Since multiple genes will be lost or increased due to a chromosomal aberration, the disorders associated with chromosomes often are serious (or even lethal) and may involve malformations of many organ systems.

In certain of the chromosomal disorders the skin manifestations of the disease are prominent. The prominent skin manifestations are grouped in Table 138-3. The complete phenotypes of many of these syndromes are discussed in other sections of the book.

Several disorders with prominent skin manifestations have evidence of chromosomal instability which is detectable by karyotypic analysis of the cultured cells (Table 138-4). Detailed descriptions of these disorders can be found elsewhere in the text. Malignancies of various types are increased in these diseases. In ataxia-telangiectasia and Fanconi's anemia there is evidence that heterozygotes have an increased incidence of cancer.

Genetic counseling

Genetic counseling is an integral part of the practice of medicine and usually requires the services of a specialist in medical genetics. Once the diagnosis is established be-

yond doubt and the mode of inheritance is known, there is no reason why any dermatologist should not be able to advise patients correctly and sympathetically. The familiarity with the disease in question allows the dermatologist to discuss the disease, its various manifestations, and its degree of variability with authority.

The aims of counseling include an explanation of the nature of the defect, the mathematics of the risk of recurrence, and the detailed knowledge of what recurrence would entail. Counseling, besides being preventive medicine, often allows the relief of parental guilt and can allay rather than increase anxiety. For example, it may not be clear to the person that he or she cannot transmit the given disorder. The nonaffected brother of a patient with Fabry's disease, or with X-linked ichthyosis, need not worry about his male children, but he may not know that. The adult normal son of a patient with epidermolytic hyperkeratosis (a condition inherited as a dominant) will also not transmit the condition to his children. A patient with the recessively inherited form of pseudoxanthoma elasticum (PXE), which leads to serious visual impairment and vascular disease, will have children all of whom are normal, provided that he or she does not marry a person who is heterozygous for the PXE gene. In many congenital malformations such as congenital heart disease and harelip-cleft palate, and in disorders such as epilepsy, the risk is of the order of a few percent, but the patient often has an exaggerated impression of the risk in future pregnancies.

Genetic counseling must be based on a familiarity with genetic principles and on a familiarity with the usual behavior of hereditary and congenital abnormalities, not only in terms of mode of inheritance, but also in terms of range of severity, social consequences of the disorder, and the availability of therapy. As in other clinical prognostication, a sense of proportion and a quality of compassion are valuable if not essential.

Special problems that arise during counseling include the fact that the parents and patients often have a limited knowledge of biology, genetics, and probability. It must be remembered that the burden imposed by a disease rather than the strict mathematical risk of recurrence often will determine the decision about reproduction. It must be remembered that if a couple has three children with a given recessive disorder, then the chance of a fourth being affected is still 1:4. "Chance has no memory," and even if the couple has 10 children the chance with each succeeding pregnancy is still the same, 1:4. Similarly, with autosomal dominant conditions, with one parent affected, the chance of each child having the same condition is 50 percent.

The prevailing philosophy is that in giving genetic counseling, one states the risk in as precise mathematical terms as possible (with ancillary information on the range of severity that can be expected, the prospects for treatment, and so on) and leaves the decision as to the course of action to the prospective parents.

Prognosis and counseling in those conditions in which the genetics is still unclear is more difficult. In those circumstances one must use empirical data which suggest, for example, that if both parents have psoriasis, the probability is 60 to 75 percent that a child will have psoriasis; if one parent and a child of that union have psoriasis, then the chance is approximately 30 percent that another child

(Text continued on page 1631.)

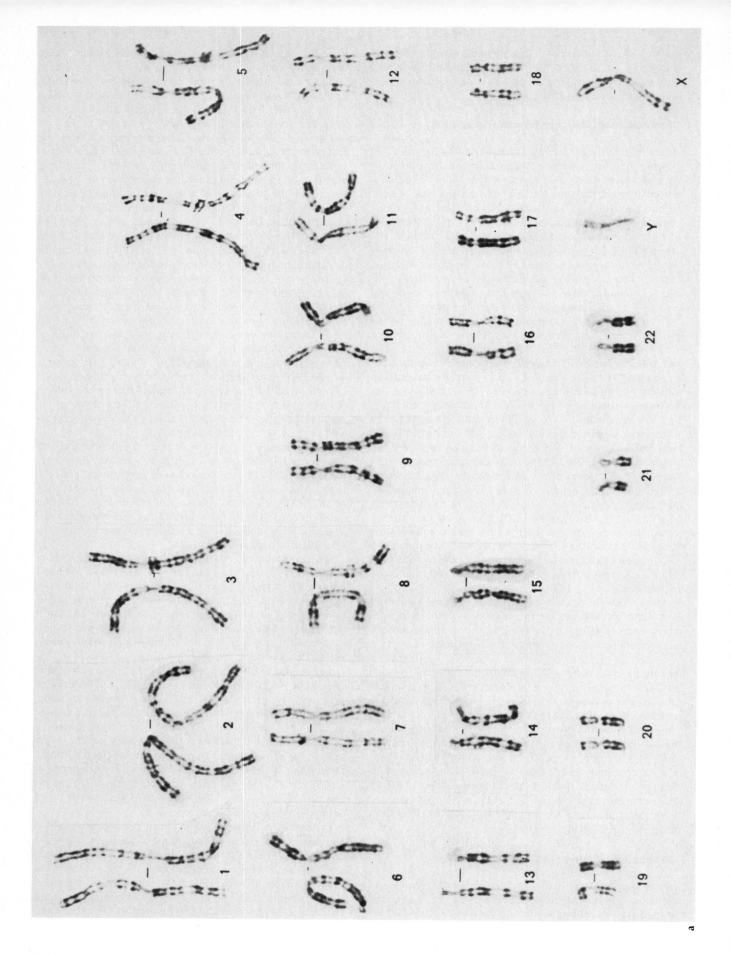

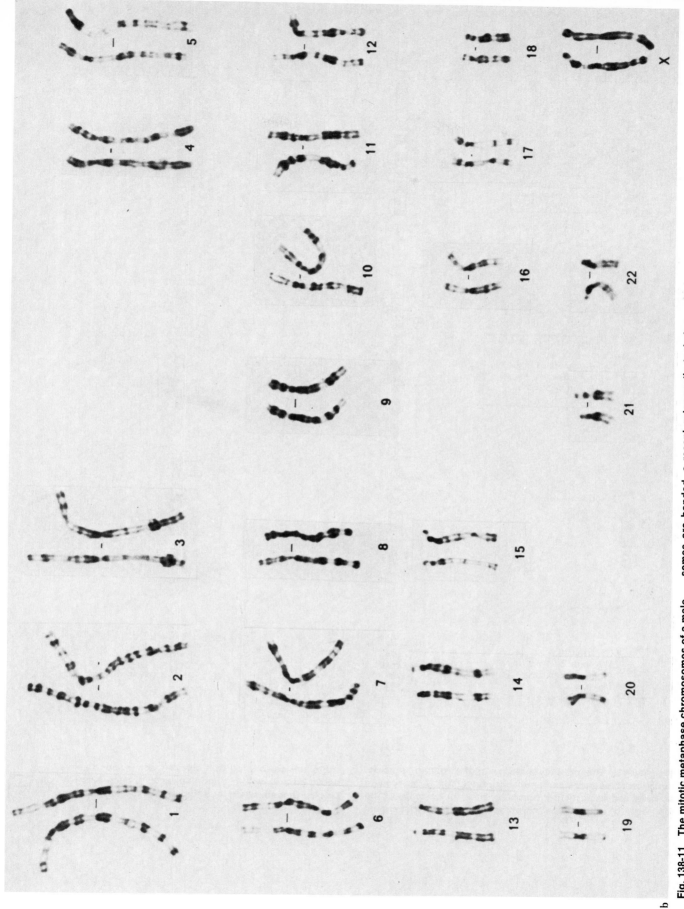

Fig. 138-11 The mitotic metaphase chromosomes of a male (a) and female (b) arranged in a karyotype. The chromo- somes are banded, a recent cytogenetic technique which has increased the resolution of the human karyotype.

b

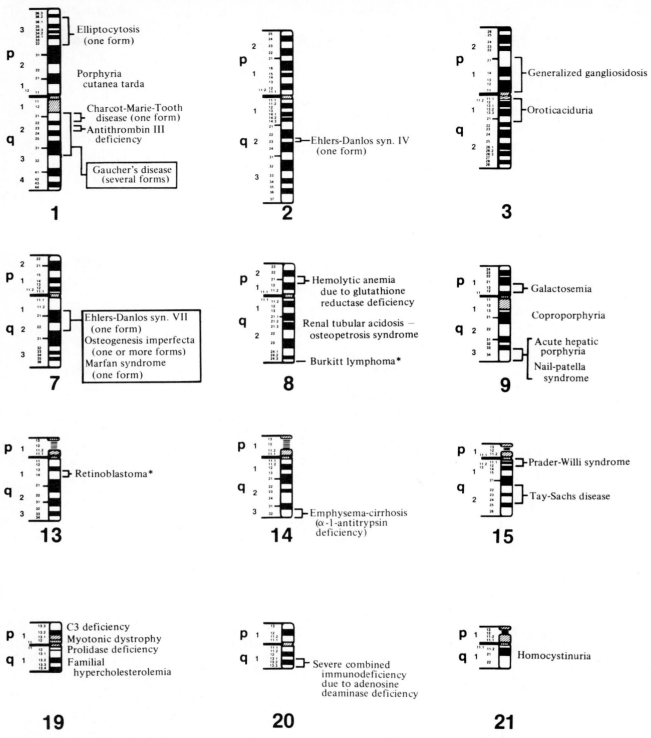

Fig. 138-12 The morbid anatomy of the human genome. Location of diseases on human chromosomes. Diseases can be localized to particular bands, or the short arm (p) or the long arm (q) of individual chromosomes. Many biochemical traits, not associated with disease, are mapped as well. □ : allelic disorders; [ ] : "nondisease"; * : neoplasm with specific chromosomal change and/or relation to oncogene.

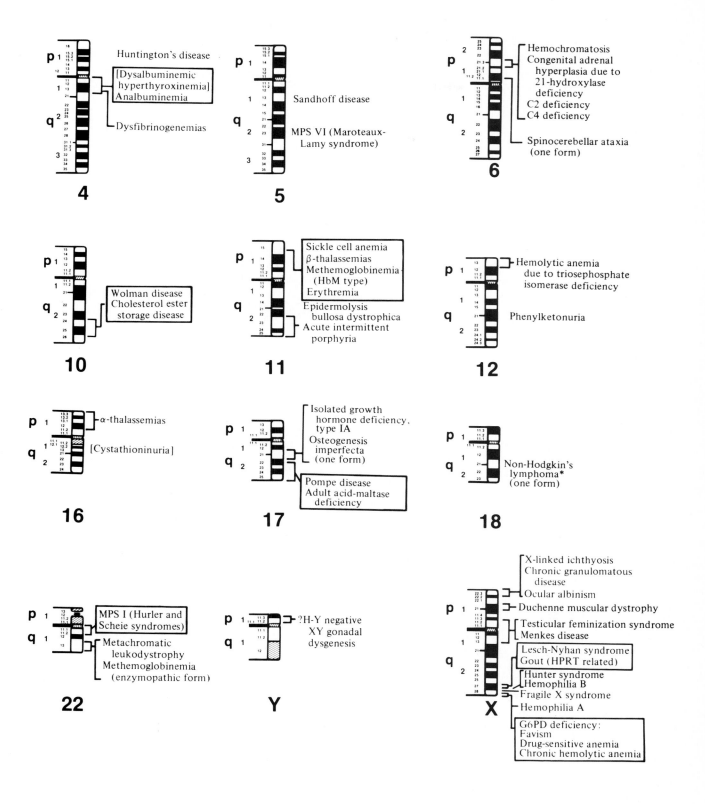

Table 138-3 Skin manifestations associated with chromosomal defects

Disease	Defect	Skin manifestations
Turner's syndrome	XO [deficiency of one X chromosome or presence of an abnormal X chromosome, XX$_I$ (iso-X)]	Congenital and persistent lymphedema Hypoplastic nails Increased number of nevi Redundant skin on neck Low posterior hair line Increased aging of skin
Klinefelter's syndrome	XXY (XXY mosaics, XXXY, XXYY)	Thirteen percent with leg ulcers
XYY	Extra Y chromosome	Cystic acne Varicose veins and ulceration
4p—	Deletion of the short arm of chromosome 4	Central scalp defects
Trisomy 8	Extra autosome	Short nails No patella (Important to distinguish trisomy 8 from the nail-patella syndrome)
Inversion 9	Pericentric inversion of chromosome 9	Inversion of 9, usually harmless polymorphism Features of anhidrotic ectodermal dysplasia in obligate females with inversion; obligate females without inversion. One family.
Trisomy 10	Extra autosome	Congenital scalp defect
Trisomy 13	Trisomy 13 (D group) Extra autosome	Scalp defects (parietal-occipital) Low posterior hairline Redundant skin on neck Nails narrow and hyperconvex Scrotal-type skin extending to tip of penis
Ring 13	Deletion of portions of 13 associated with ring formation	Epicanthal fold Alopecia and (?) scalp defect Symmetrical hypopigmentation (arciform)
Ring 14	Ring of chromosome 14	Epicanthal folds Café au lait macules (some linear) Redundant neck skin Multiple depigmented macules Seizure (myotonic) (Need to consider in differential diagnosis of tuberous sclerosis)
Ring 17	Ring of chromosome 17	Multiple café au lait macules
18p—	Deletion of the short chromosome 18	Congenital alopecia
Trisomy 18	Extra autosome (E group)	Redundant skin on posterior neck Hypoplastic nails
Down's syndrome	Trisomy 21 (as an additional autosome or due to a translocation)	Elastosis perforans serpiginosa Vasculature instability (acrocyanosis, cutis marmorata) Premature wrinkling of the skin Frequent syringomas Frequent alopecia areata Hyperkeratotic palms, skin, and ichthyosis-like changes Fissured and furrowed skin (xerosis)
Monosomy 21 (mosaic)		EEC syndrome (ectrodactyly, ectodermal dysplasia, cleft lip and palate) Sparse scalp hair

Table 138-4   Genetic diseases with skin manifestations, neoplasia, and chromosomal instability

Disease	Chromosomal abnormalities	Associated neoplastic diseases
Ataxia-telangiectasia	↑ Chromosome breaks	Lymphosarcoma; lymphocytic leukemia
Bloom's syndrome	↑ Chromosome breaks ↑ Chromosome rearrangements ↑ Sister chromatid exchanges Decreased rate of DNA replication ↑ Quadriradial configuration	Gastric adenocarcinoma Leukemia Lymphosarcoma Sigmoid adenocarcinoma Squamous cell carcinoma (oral, esophagus)
Dyskeratosis congenita	↑ Sister chromatid exchanges Normal breaks	Squamous cell carcinoma (tongue, oral, esophagus, nasopharynx, cervix, skin) Mucinous carcinoma (rectum) Adenocarcinoma (rectum)
Fanconi's aplastic anemia	↑ Breaks ↑ Chromatid exchanges Endoreduplication	Squamous cell carcinoma (anus, vulva, oral)
Gardner's syndrome	↑ Tetraploidy in skin fibroblasts	Adenocarcinoma (colon, rectum)
Werner's syndrome	↑ Rearrangements (variegated translocation mosaicism)	Fibrosarcoma, meningioma, leiomyosarcoma

will have psoriasis; and if the union of two normal parents has produced a child with psoriasis, the probability is 15 to 20 percent for another child with psoriasis.

Prenatal diagnosis

The ability to determine fetal sex from amniotic fluid cells makes it possible to predict the likelihood of many diseases with dermatologic manifestations (Table 138-5). In Goltz's syndrome and incontinentia pigmenti, one-half of the female fetuses will be affected with serious, nontreatable manifestations and abortion should be considered. In the other diseases in Table 138-5, one-half of male fetuses will be affected with serious, currently nontreatable diseases. In those disorders in which biochemical testing is possible,

a 100 percent accurate diagnosis can be made of an affected male fetus. The diagnosis of metabolic diseases with skin manifestations, including xeroderma pigmentosum, hypercholesterolemia, Hurler's syndrome, and Niemann-Pick disease, has been made using biochemical analysis of amniotic fluid cells. The chromosomal disorders with skin manifestations can be diagnosed by analyzing the karyotype of the amniotic fluid cells.

Fetoscopy, the direct visualization of the fetus, will allow the dermatologist to visualize the fetal skin in utero and to further extend the list of diseases diagnosable before birth. The harlequin fetus, forms of epidermolysis bullosa, albinism, and the Sjögren-Larsson syndrome have been detected by fetoscopy, skin biopsy, and study of the involved skin.

Some dermatologic disorders where the pattern of inheritance has been established are listed in Tables 138-6 and 138-7. They are separated into groups on the basis of their major phenotypic features. Representative X-linked diseases are listed in the counseling and prenatal diagnosis portion of this chapter. For a guide to the literature on the genetics and nosology of the genetic disorders of the skin, see McKusick's *Mendelian Inheritance in Man: Catalogs of Autosomal Dominant, Autosomal Recessive, and X-Linked Phenotypes.*

In summary, for a large number of conditions seen in dermatologic practice, exact information is available for their mode of inheritance, and the basic principles of genetic counseling have been established. With some common disorders such as atopic eczema and psoriasis, the inheritance has, however, not been established beyond doubt, and the etiology is probably multifactorial. In these circumstances counseling is necessarily more indefinite, but the chance of an affected person having affected children, or of unaffected parents with one affected child having other children with the disorder, should not be exaggerated and is less than in single gene conditions.

Table 138-5   Candidates for prenatal sex determination in X-linked diseases

Sex determination alone necessary (no current biochemical marker):
  Albinism with deafness
  Anhidrotic ectodermal dysplasia
  Dyskeratosis congenita
  Goltz's syndrome
  Incontinentia pigmenti
  Wiskott-Aldrich syndrome
Sex determination and/or special biochemical studies:
  Fabry's disease
  Hunter's syndrome (mucopolysaccharidosis II)
  Lesch-Nyhan syndrome
  Menkes' disease
  X-linked ichthyosis with steroid sulfatase deficiency*

* Since the skin manifestations of this disease are readily treatable, this may not be necessary; however, diagnosis may be necessary to suitably treat the mother during labor, which is often complicated.

Table 138-6   Autosomal dominant skin diseases (classified according to major skin phenotypic features

Blistering:
  Epidermolysis bullosa (Cockayne)
  Epidermolysis bullosa dystrophica
  Epidermolysis bullosa simplex
  Pemphigus, benign familial (Hailey-Hailey)
Connective tissue abnormalities:
  Cutis laxa
  Ehlers-Danlos syndrome
  Familial pachydermoperiostosis
  Hereditary sclerosing poikiloderma
  Lipoatrophic diabetes
  Marfan's syndrome
  Multiple benign ring-shaped skin creases
  Pseudoxanthoma elasticum
  Sclerotylosis
Gastrointestinal and skin:
  Gardner's syndrome
  Keratoderma with esophageal cancer
  Peutz-Jeghers syndrome
Hair abnormalities:
  Congenital scalp defect
  Distichiasis and lymphedema
  Hidrotic epidermal dysplasia
  Hypertrichosis universalis
  Marie-Unna hair dystrophy
  Milia and decreased hair density
  Monilethrix
  Pili annulati
  Trichorhinophalangeal syndrome
  Wooly hair
Hyperkeratosis:
  Acrokeratosis verruciformis (Hopf)
  Bullous ichthyosiform erythroderma
  Darier's disease
  Erythrokeratoderma variabilis
  Hidrotic ectodermal dysplasia
  Howel-Evans syndrome (with esophageal cancer)
  Ichthyosis hystrix gravior
  Ichthyosis vulgaris (ichthyosis simplex)
  Keratoderma palmaris et plantaris, diffuse, linear, punctate
  Naegli's syndrome
  Pachyonychia congenita
Hyperpigmentation:
  Familial lichen amyloidosis
  Familial progressive hyperpigmentation
  Leopard syndrome (progressive lentiginosis)
  Lipoatrophic diabetes
  Naegli's syndrome
  Peutz-Jeghers syndrome
Hypopigmentation:
  Albinism
  Albinism and deafness
  Incontinentia pigmenti achromians
Blistering:
  Acrodermatitis enteropathica
  Congenital erythropoietic porphyria
  Epidermolysis bullosa dystrophica
  Epidermolysis bullosa letalis
  Tyrosinemia II

Piebaldism
Tuberous sclerosis
Waardenburg's syndrome
Light sensitivity:
  Albinism
  Erythropoietic protoporphyria
  Piebaldism
  Porphyria, variegate (South African)
Nail plate and nail bed defects:
  Anonychia ectrodactyly
  Epidermolysis bullosa dystrophica
  Hereditary koilonychia
  Hidrotic ectodermal dystrophica
  Leukonychia totalis
  Nail-patella syndrome
  Pachyonychia congenita
  Pachyonychia congenita with steatocystoma multiplex
  Tuberous sclerosis
Tumors (benign or malignant):
  Basal cell nevus syndrome
  Bushke-Oldendorff syndrome (osteopoikilosis with connective tissue nevus)
  Cowden's syndrome (multiple hamartoma syndrome)
  Epitheliomas, hereditary benign cystic (Brooke-Fordyce)
  Gardner's syndrome
  Malignant melanoma
  Multiple cylindromas (Ancell-Spiegler)
  Multiple leiomyomata
  Multiple lipomatosis
  Neurofibromatosis (von Recklinghausen's)
  Steatocystoma multiplex (multiple sebaceous cysts) with pachyonychia congenita
  Tuberous sclerosis
Urticaria and edema:
  Cold hypersensitivity
  Cold hypersensitivity with paramyotonia
  Familial angioedema
  Familial localized heat urticaria
  Lymphedema and distichiasis
  Lymphedema, hereditary (I or Nonne-Milroy type)
  Lymphedema, hereditary (II or Neige type)
  Periodic fever
  Urticaria, deafness, and amyloidosis
Vascular skin lesions:
  Blue rubber bleb nevus syndrome
  Glomus tumors
  Hereditary hemorrhagic telangiectasia (Rendu-Weber-Osler)
  Maffuci's syndrome
Keratoderma palmaris et plantaris with periodontopathia (Papillon-Lefèvre syndrome)
Mal de Meleda
Refsum's syndrome
Sjögren-Larsson syndrome

Table 138-7   Autosomal recessive skin diseases (classified according to major skin features)

Connective tissue abnormalities:	Tyrosinemia II (Richner-Hanhart syndrome)
Alkaptonuria	Hyperpigmentation:
Cockayne's syndrome	Fanconi's syndrome
Conradi's disease	Gaucher's disease
Cutis laxa	Niemann-Pick disease
Ehlers-Danlos syndrome	Wilson's disease
Homocystinuria	Hypopigmentation:
Lipoid proteinosis	Albinism
Mucopolysaccharidoses	Chédiak-Higashi syndrome
Progeria	Light sensitivity:
Pseudoxanthoma elasticum	Albinism
Seip-Lawrence syndrome	Aspartylglycoaminuria
Werner's syndrome	Cockayne's syndrome
Hair abnormalities:	Congenital erythropoietic porphyria
Argininosuccinic aciduria	Hartnup's disease
Biotin-responsive carboxylase	Phenylketonuria
deficiency	Xeroderma pigmentosum
Cartilage-hair hypoplasia	Multiple skin papules:
Chédiak-Higashi disease	Epidermodysplasia verruciformis
Cornelia de Lange syndrome	Farber's lipogranulomatosis
Hallermann-Streiff syndrome	Hunter's syndrome
Homocystinuria	Juvenile fibromatosis
Marinesco-Sjögren syndrome	Lipoid proteinosis
Low-sulfur hair syndrome	Pseudoxanthoma elasticum
Phenylketonuria	Skin ulcers:
Vitamin D-resistant rickets (type II) with	Prolidase deficiency
alopecia	Werner's syndrome
Werner's (premature graying)	Tumors:
Hyperkeratosis:	Xeroderma pigmentosum
Conradi's disease	Vascular skin lesions:
Harlequin fetus	Ataxia-telangiectasia
Ichthyosiform erythroderma (nonbullous)	Bloom's syndrome
Ichthyosis, lamellar, of the newborn	Fucosidosis type II
Keratoderma palmaris et plantaris with	Rothmund-Thomson syndrome
corneal dystrophy	Sialidosis, juvenile type II

Bibliography

Alper JC: Principles of genetics as related to the chromosome disorders and congenital malformations with reference to prenatal diagnosis and genetic counseling. *J Am Acad Dermatol* **4**:379, 1981

Bergsma D (ed): *Birth Defects Compendium*, 2d ed. New York, Alan R Liss, 1979

Der Kaloustian VM, Kurban AK: *Genetic Diseases of the Skin.* Springer-Verlag, 1979

Goldsmith LA: Principles of genetics as applied to dermatologic diseases. *J Am Acad Dermatol* **4**:255, 1981

Hecht F et al: Incontinentia pigmenti: occurrence in Arizona Indians and evidence against the half-chromadic mutation model, *Dysmorphology*, Part B of *Annual Review of Birth Defects, 1981*, edited by WL Nyhan, KL Jones. New York, Alan R Liss,

1982, p 89

McKusick VA: *Mendelian Inheritance in Man: Catalogs of Autosomal Dominant, Autosomal Recessive, and X-Linked Phenotypes,* 5th ed. Baltimore, Johns Hopkins Press, 1978

McKusick VA: *Mendelian Inheritance in Man: Catalogs of Autosomal Dominant, Autosomal Recessive, and X-Linked Phenotypes,* 5th ed. Baltimore, Johns Hopkins Press, 1978

Montagna W et al (eds): Proceedings of the XIII Annual Symposium on the Biology of Skin. *J Invest Dermatol* **60**:339, 1973

Nyhan WL, Sakati NO: *Genetic and Malformation Syndromes in Clinical Medicine.* Chicago, Year Book, 1976

Roberts JAF: *An Introduction to Medical Genetics,* 5th ed. London, Oxford Univ Press, 1970

Stanbury JB et al (eds): *The Metabolic Basis of Inherited Disease,* 5th ed. New York, McGraw-Hill, 1983

CUTANEOUS CHANGES IN ERRORS OF AMINO ACID METABOLISM: TYROSINEMIA II, PHENYLKETONURIA, AND ARGININOSUCCINIC ACIDURIA

Lowell A. Goldsmith

This chapter emphasizes skin disorders in which an abnormality of amino acid metabolism causes specific cutaneous syndromes. The general aspects of amino acid metabolism are reviewed elsewhere [1–3].

Tyrosinemia II

Definition

Tyrosinemia type II (Richner-Hanhart syndrome) is a distinctive clinical syndrome involving the eyes, skin, and frequently the central nervous system. Tyrosine is elevated because of a deficiency of hepatic tyrosine aminotransferase.

General features of the patients

Fewer than 30 patients with this clinical syndrome have been reported [4], all with tyrosinemia, phenolicaciduria, and inflammatory skin and eye lesions. Both sexes are affected equally; the disease is worldwide in distribution. There is frequent consanguinity [4], which is strongly suggestive of autosomal recessive inheritance.

Dermatologic features. Patients have hyperkeratotic skin lesions limited to the palms and soles [5–8]. Lesions usually begin during the first year of life; in one patient, the first lesions were at age 6 [9]. The skin lesions are painful, nonpruritic, and are frequently associated with hyperhidrosis (Fig. 139-1). The pain has been intense enough to cause patients to crawl rather than apply pressure to the lesions. Bullous lesions rapidly progress to erosions; these then become crusted and hyperkeratotic. Lesions are frequently linear. The fingertips and hypothenar eminences are frequently involved. One patient had hyperkeratotic subungual lesions; one was possibly hyperpigmented.

Ophthalmologic features. Eye lesions occur weeks to months before the skin lesions. Eye symptoms start as early as 2 weeks of age and as late as 8 years. Tearing, redness, pain, and photophobia are early signs; late signs include corneal clouding and central or paracentral opacities which initially are intraepithelial and progress to superficial or deep dendritic ulcers in some patients (Fig. 139-2). Neovascularization is prominent. Chronic results of the eye disease include scarring, nystagmus, and exodeviation. One patient had a persistent conjunctival plaque

[9]. Topical therapy is ineffective, and herpes simplex and bacterial cultures are consistently negative.

Neurologic features. Mental retardation of varying degrees is reported, as is normal mental development.

Other organ system involvement. Renal and hepatic function tests have been uniformly normal. One of the patients [10] had multiple congenital anomalies, including microcephaly, cleft lip and palate, inguinal hernias, talipes equinovarus, and the absence of one kidney.

Laboratory findings

Amino acid abnormalities. The blood and urine tyrosine levels of the affected patients are markedly elevated. Other amino acids have not been increased. Urinary tyrosine metabolites are elevated; these include p-hydroxyphenylpyruvic acid, p-hydroxyphenyllactic acid, p-hydroxyphenylacetic acid, tyrosine, and N-acetyltyrosine (Fig. 139-3). All of the metabolic effects are consequences of the deficiency of hepatic tyrosine aminotransferase.

Tyrosine aminotransferase (TAT) is a pyridoxal phosphate-dependent cytoplasmic enzyme which transaminates tyrosine-forming p-hydroxyphenylpyruvate (PHPPA). The liver is the richest source of TAT; this specific TAT is not present in skin. The liver biopsy shows little or no soluble TAT, although there is normal or slightly increased mitochondrial tyrosine (aspartate) transaminase activity [8,11]. In mitochondria, aspartate aminotransferase utilizes tyrosine as a substrate and is responsible for the production of increased amounts of PHPPA from the increased amounts of tyrosine available in tyrosinemia II. Since mitochondria do not have PHPPA oxidase activity, PHPPA and its metabolic products increase and appear in the urine [11]. This creates the unusual situation in which metabolites are increased both proximally and distally to the defective enzyme (Fig. 139-4).

Histopathology. Routine histopathology which shows hyperkeratosis, parakeratosis, and acanthosis is not diagnostic. In one patient, the biopsy was interpreted as showing epidermolytic hyperkeratosis [5]; however, review of the published biopsy does not support that specific diagnosis.

In one patient, the palmar papules showed parakeratosis with homogeneous, refractile, eosinophilic inclusions 2 to 3 μm in diameter in the stratum corneum and stratum

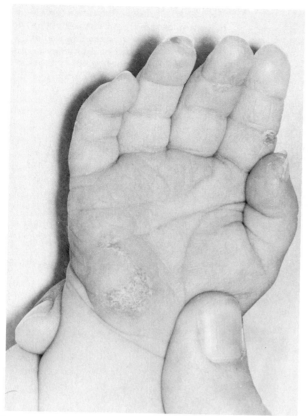

Fig. 139-1 Hyperkeratotic and erosive lesions in patient with tyrosinemia II.

spinosum [9]. Electron microscopy in one case suggested that the 2- to 3-μm inclusions were lipid-like granules. Discrete 100-Å filaments and myelin-like figures were intermixed with lipid-like droplets [9]. These electron microscopic results were interpreted as showing possible lysosomal activation. Extensive electron microscopic studies in three patients showed increases in tonofibrils and keratohyalin and very tightly packed microtubular and microfibrillar masses [12].

The conjunctival plaques of one patient showed eosinophilic inclusions in the superficial epithelial cells and a plasma cell infiltrate. Electron microscopy [13] revealed aggregated clumps of chromatin, and increased numbers of fibrils, forming bundles. The superficial epithelial cells contained membrane-bound, alcian blue-positive inclusion bodies 0.5 to 1.0 μm in diameter. Endothelial cells of the vessels contained similar inclusions and whorled membranous substances. In fibroblasts, dark bodies consisting of fine, needlelike crystals were found. A second conjunctival biopsy, 2 years after the initial biopsy, revealed no infiltration, but persistence of the inclusions in the epithelium and fibrocytes was seen [13].

Pathophysiology of the skin and eye lesions in tyrosinemia II. Rats fed a 12 percent protein diet with 0.5 to 2.0 percent tyrosine developed a syndrome resembling tyrosinemia II with weight loss, a shortened life, keratitis, conjunctivitis, alopecia, chelitis, and inflammatory toe changes [14]. The high tyrosine syndrome in rats was ameliorated by increasing the protein content of the diet or adding threonine [15]

or thiouracil. Inducers of tyrosine aminotransferase, e.g., glucagon, phenobarbital, corticosteroids, and steroids devoid of glucocorticoid activity (e.g., pregnenolone-16 α-carbonitrile or progesterone), prevented the syndrome [16].

The affected animals had photophobia, corneal erosions, exudate, and panblepharitis. Microscopically [17], the initial lesion was epithelial edema associated with disorganization of the basal cells and polymorphonuclear leukocyte (PMNL) infiltration. The PMNL invaded the epithelium stroma and the anterior chamber. After 1 week, the cornea was opaque, thickened, and vascularized. By 2 to 3 weeks, the cornea was ulcerated.

The eyes contained birefringent crystals limited to the areas of corneal damage. The crystals were long (10 to 25 μm), slender (0.5 to 1.1 μm), and appeared to be membrane-bound; the crystals passed from cell to cell and penetrated nuclei. Multinucleate cells, vacuoles, autophagic vacuoles, and multivesicular bodies were present, which suggested lysosomal activation by the tyrosine crystals.

In unpublished studies, skin lesions in the rats were limited to the bottoms of the feet and the nail beds. The histologic changes were limited to the volar surfaces of the feet and the nail beds. Initially, there was dyskeratosis followed by local areas of intense PMNL infiltration, erosions, crusting, and hyperkeratosis. Subcorneal collections of PMNL were seen first focally and then diffusely. By days 5 to 7 there were extravasated erythrocytes, basal cell vesiculation, subepidermal vesiculation, and necrotic epidermis. Biopsies of the tail and back epidermis, even after epidermal cell division was stimulated, showed no evidence of inflammation.

There are ranch mink and dogs with the clinical metabolic features of tyrosinemia [18,19] as well. The reason for the localization of the lesions to the eyes and volar skin in human, mink, and canine tyrosinemia II and in experimental tyrosinemia is unknown. Studies of the rat cornea showed that inflammation was limited to the location of crystal deposition [20], suggesting the importance of tyrosine crystals as a factor in the initiation of inflammation. Electron microscopic studies of both human and rat tissues showed evidence of lysosomal activation and cytoskeletal disorganization.

In vitro studies showed that tyrosine crystals can cause release of lysosomal enzymes [21]. The model of tyrosine crystals as lysosome labilizers is unique in that the tyrosine crystals are not phagocytosed into the cell but form within the cell and possibly within lysosomes. Within the cells, the initially soluble tyrosine, either because of changes in pH, ionic strength, carrier proteins, or other protective factors, crystallizes and then interacts with lysosomes and other membrane-bound structures. It is hypothesized that by this mechanism tyrosine crystals induce lysosomal rupture with the subsequent release of proteolytic enzymes and chemotactic factors, which in turn initiate PMNL infiltration and grossly visible inflammation.

Treatment

With a low-tyrosine, low-phenylalanine diet (Mead Johnson), there is a rapid decrease in tyrosine to normal levels (Fig. 139-5). Skin and eye lesions resolved within days [7] in all individuals treated with the diet. Normal growth and

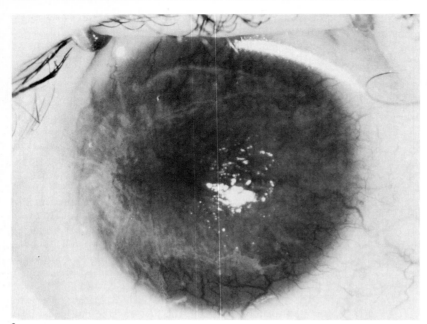

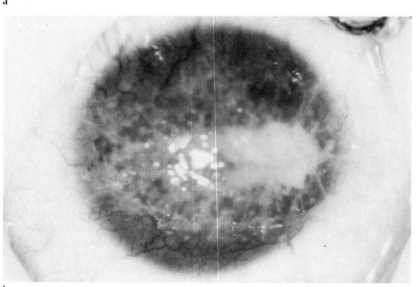

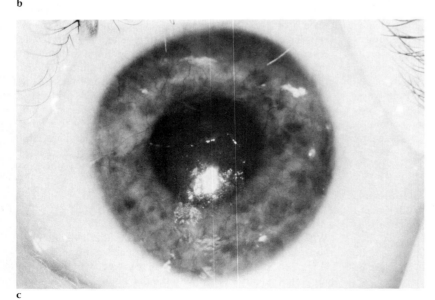

Fig. 139-2 Corneal changes in tyrosinemia II. Cornea before treatment, left eye (a) corneal opacity and neovascularization are prominent. The right eye (b) has even more extensive involvement. After 6 weeks of therapy there is marked clearing of the lesions (c).

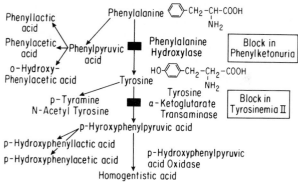

Fig. 139-3 Metabolic scheme of phenylalanine, tyrosine, and their derivatives.

development took place in a patient when kept on the diet for 30 months starting at the age of 14 months. In this patient, 6 weeks after diet therapy was begun, the corneas were much clearer and less injected (Fig. 139-2c) and the patient had vision sufficient to follow colored objects during play. At age 6 years, examination showed only remnants of vessels and vision was normal except for myopia. Other patients have had slower resolution of symptoms. A 55-year-old man with tyrosinemia II had diffuse plantar hyperkeratosis (Fig. 139-6) which responded to a low-tyrosine, low-phenylalanine diet [8].

Two adults have responded objectively to an aromatic retinoid (Ro 10-9359) (1.0 mg/kg per day). Interestingly, there was resolution without decreases in plasma tyrosine [22]. In none of the patients studied has there been response to cortisone acetate, ascorbic acid, pyridoxine, or folic acid, which are cofactors or known inducers of TAT and PHPPA oxidase.

Prenatal diagnosis and heterozygote determination have not yet been possible.

Since the consequences of tyrosinemia II are serious,

Fig. 139-4 Tyrosine metabolism in normal subjects and in tyrosinemia II. The hepatic metabolism is depicted with the normal metabolic pathways in bold arrows. The pathway in disease is in broken arrows.

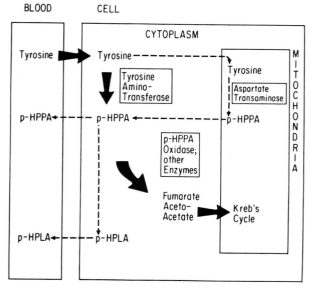

and a safe treatment is available, a patient presenting with any atypical bullous or hyperkeratotic disease on the palms and soles in the first months of life should be screened for tyrosine and its metabolites; simple screening tests (nitrosonaphthol in the presence of nitric acid and sodium nitrite) are available in most hospital laboratories [1]. Amino acid analysis by ion-exchange chromatography is necessary to confirm the diagnosis and follow the response to diet therapy.

Differential diagnosis

Clinical disorders of tyrosine metabolism. The disorders of tyrosine metabolism have a bewildering set of names. Tyrosinemia II (Richner-Hanhart syndrome) is distinct from all the others; none of the others has any skin manifestations. These diseases are more completely reviewed elsewhere [4].

Neonatal tyrosinemia is a common transient condition with decreased amounts of PHPPA oxidase apoenzyme and a relative deficiency of ascorbic acid contributing to the tyrosinemia, tyrosinuria, and increased excretion of tyrosine metabolites. Treatment is with ascorbic acid supplementation and a low-protein diet.

Hereditary tyrosinemia (tyrosinosis, tyrosinemia type I) is an autosomal, recessively inherited, severe liver and renal disease. In the first 6 months of life, there are fever, edema, vomiting, a peculiar odor, hematuria, diarrhea, jaundice, hepatosplenomegaly, and the Fanconi syndrome. The basic biochemical defect is presumed to be fumarylacetoacetate deficiency with resulting increases in succinylacetone. Tyrosinemia, tyrosinuria, increased plasma PHPPA, hypermethioninemia, increased δ-amino levulinic acid, increased catecholamines, and the renal findings of the Fanconi syndrome are present. Succinylacetone inhibits δ-amino levulinic acid dehydratase and probably other enzymes, leading to the multiplicity of metabolic defects.

Some other patients with disorders of tyrosine metabolism have had similar metabolic profiles to those seen in tyrosinemia II, but have not had the complete clinical syndrome [4].

Classical Richner-Hanhart syndrome. The Richner-Hanhart syndrome classically consists of keratosis palmoplantaris, persistent dendritic lesions of the cornea with unaffected corneal sensitivity, photophobia, tearing, frequent profound mental retardation, and autosomal recessive inheritance. In a review [23] of the classical syndrome, 14 cases from 10 families are discussed. All had corneal disease, 12 had keratosis palmoplantaris, and 8 were retarded. Consanguinity was common. Although none of the 14 patients had the extensive eye lesions of the patient in Fig. 139-2, it is suspected most of these patients had tyrosinemia II.

An autosomal dominantly inherited syndrome of volar keratosis and keratitis which is clinically similar to tyrosinemia was described in one family by Zmegac and Sarajlic [24]. The involvement was more extensive than the classical Richner-Hanhart syndrome and was similar to the patients with tyrosinemia II. The keratitis of the Spanglang-Tappeiner syndrome [25], which is associated with palmar and plantar keratosis, appears to be related to lipid infiltration of the cornea.

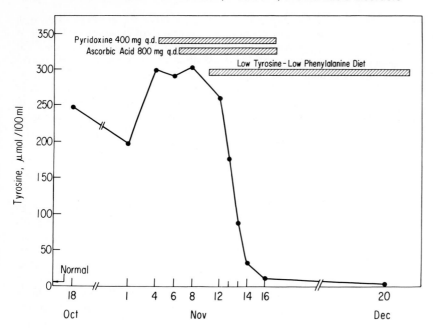

Fig. 139-5 The response of elevated plasma tyrosine to a low-tyrosine, low-phenylalanine diet and failure of response to various cofactors in a patient with tyrosinemia II.

Phenylketonuria

Definition

Phenylketonuria (PKU) is an autosomal, recessively inherited disease due to a deficiency of hepatic phenylalanine hydroxylase or cofactors for the phenylalanine hydroxylating system. The increased levels of phenylalanine are associated with mental retardation, seizures, decreased pigmentation of the skin, hair, and eyes, and eczematous dermatitis.

Clinical features

This common metabolic defect occurs in 1 of 10,000 births and can be detected by screening procedures in neonatal life. One percent of institutionalized retarded patients have PKU. Mental retardation, athetosis, restlessness, increased tendon reflexes and muscle tone, hyperkinesis, tremors, and seizures accompany the untreated disease. The general features of the disease, its biochemistry, heterozygote detection, and treatment are reviewed elsewhere [26].

Patients with phenylketonuria have an increased incidence of eczematous dermatitis, pigment dilution of hair and skin color, and occasionally sclerodermatous skin changes. Other changes reported include a decreased number of pigmented nevi, and an increased incidence of keratosis pilaris [27]. Skin phenylalanine levels are higher in PKU skin than in normal skin [28].

Atopic dermatitis has been found to be increased in studies by Fleisher and Zeligman [29] and Braun-Falco and Geissler [27]. In the former study, atopic dermatitis was present in 3 of 23 patients, while in the latter, it was present in 15 of 25 patients. A potential mechanism suggested for the increased incidence of atopic disease is an increased tendency to vasoconstriction in PKU [30]. Dramatic clearing of eczema with a low-phenylalanine diet has been reported in some patients. It is possible that an inborn tendency to eczematous dermatitis has been nonspecifically

triggered in these patients, although normal patients with eczema have no abnormality of phenylalanine metabolism detectable after a phenylalanine load [31]. Patients with PKU often have a lighter hair and eye color than their siblings [32]. The color changes may be especially striking in the rare black or Japanese patient with PKU whose eye or hair color may be very different from that of other members of the ethnic group (Fig. A8-6). With a low-phenylalanine diet, or with aging alone, hair color darkens. When tyrosine is added to the diet of patients with PKU, hair darkens; if tyrosine is removed, the hair will lighten and banded hair is produced (Fig. A8-5). The increased levels of phenylalanine and its oxidation products (phenylpyruvic acid, *o*-hydroxyphenylacetic acid, phenylacetic acid) inhibit the enzyme, tyrosinase, and therefore reduce melanization [33] (Fig. 139-3).

The sclerodermatous changes in PKU are very striking and have been reviewed by Jablonska and Stachow [34]. Nine patients with PKU have had the onset of indurated areas of skin, most prominent on the thighs and associated with contractures, during the first year of life. Acral areas of the body were least affected in contradistinction to systemic sclerosis. Biopsy showed increased fibroblasts and histiocytes, and atrophy of skin appendages. The elastic fibers were scanty and fragmented and were thus different from those found in true scleroderma. With dietary control the sclerodermatous lesions cleared. The lesions may be due to alterations in tryptophan metabolism which occur in patients with phenylketonuria; tryptophan absorption is decreased in the presence of high blood levels of phenylalanine [35]. In experimental phenylketonuria, there is an abnormal tubulin due to decreased posttranslational addition of tyrosine to tubulin α-chains [36]. This may explain some of the tissue effects in PKU.

Diagnosis

Phenylalanine can be quantitated by ion exchange chromatography. Increased levels of its metabolites in the urine are detected by a screening test in which $FeCl_3$ forms a

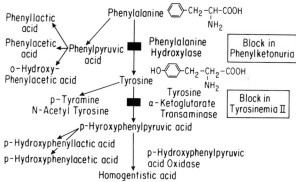

Fig. 139-3 Metabolic scheme of phenylalanine, tyrosine, and their derivatives.

development took place in a patient when kept on the diet for 30 months starting at the age of 14 months. In this patient, 6 weeks after diet therapy was begun, the corneas were much clearer and less injected (Fig. 139-2c) and the patient had vision sufficient to follow colored objects during play. At age 6 years, examination showed only remnants of vessels and vision was normal except for myopia. Other patients have had slower resolution of symptoms. A 55-year-old man with tyrosinemia II had diffuse plantar hyperkeratosis (Fig. 139-6) which responded to a low-tyrosine, low-phenylalanine diet [8].

Two adults have responded objectively to an aromatic retinoid (Ro 10-9359) (1.0 mg/kg per day). Interestingly, there was resolution without decreases in plasma tyrosine [22]. In none of the patients studied has there been response to cortisone acetate, ascorbic acid, pyridoxine, or folic acid, which are cofactors or known inducers of TAT and PHPPA oxidase.

Prenatal diagnosis and heterozygote determination have not yet been possible.

Since the consequences of tyrosinemia II are serious,

Fig. 139-4 Tyrosine metabolism in normal subjects and in tyrosinemia II. The hepatic metabolism is depicted with the normal metabolic pathways in bold arrows. The pathway in disease is in broken arrows.

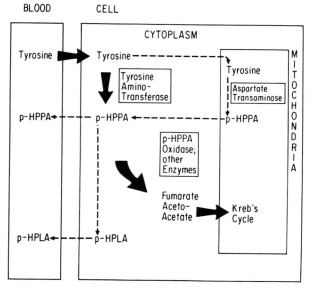

and a safe treatment is available, a patient presenting with any atypical bullous or hyperkeratotic disease on the palms and soles in the first months of life should be screened for tyrosine and its metabolites; simple screening tests (nitrosonaphthol in the presence of nitric acid and sodium nitrite) are available in most hospital laboratories [1]. Amino acid analysis by ion-exchange chromatography is necessary to confirm the diagnosis and follow the response to diet therapy.

Differential diagnosis

Clinical disorders of tyrosine metabolism. The disorders of tyrosine metabolism have a bewildering set of names. Tyrosinemia II (Richner-Hanhart syndrome) is distinct from all the others; none of the others has any skin manifestations. These diseases are more completely reviewed elsewhere [4].

Neonatal tyrosinemia is a common transient condition with decreased amounts of PHPPA oxidase apoenzyme and a relative deficiency of ascorbic acid contributing to the tyrosinemia, tyrosinuria, and increased excretion of tyrosine metabolites. Treatment is with ascorbic acid supplementation and a low-protein diet.

Hereditary tyrosinemia (tyrosinosis, tyrosinemia type I) is an autosomal, recessively inherited, severe liver and renal disease. In the first 6 months of life, there are fever, edema, vomiting, a peculiar odor, hematuria, diarrhea, jaundice, hepatosplenomegaly, and the Fanconi syndrome. The basic biochemical defect is presumed to be fumarylacetoacetate deficiency with resulting increases in succinylacetone. Tyrosinemia, tyrosinuria, increased plasma PHPPA, hypermethioninemia, increased δ-amino levulinic acid, increased catecholamines, and the renal findings of the Fanconi syndrome are present. Succinylacetone inhibits δ-amino levulinic acid dehydratase and probably other enzymes, leading to the multiplicity of metabolic defects.

Some other patients with disorders of tyrosine metabolism have had similar metabolic profiles to those seen in tyrosinemia II, but have not had the complete clinical syndrome [4].

Classical Richner-Hanhart syndrome. The Richner-Hanhart syndrome classically consists of keratosis palmoplantaris, persistent dendritic lesions of the cornea with unaffected corneal sensitivity, photophobia, tearing, frequent profound mental retardation, and autosomal recessive inheritance. In a review [23] of the classical syndrome, 14 cases from 10 families are discussed. All had corneal disease, 12 had keratosis palmoplantaris, and 8 were retarded. Consanguinity was common. Although none of the 14 patients had the extensive eye lesions of the patient in Fig. 139-2, it is suspected most of these patients had tyrosinemia II.

An autosomal dominantly inherited syndrome of volar keratosis and keratitis which is clinically similar to tyrosinemia was described in one family by Zmegac and Sarajlic [24]. The involvement was more extensive than the classical Richner-Hanhart syndrome and was similar to the patients with tyrosinemia II. The keratitis of the Spanglang-Tappeiner syndrome [25], which is associated with palmar and plantar keratosis, appears to be related to lipid infiltration of the cornea.

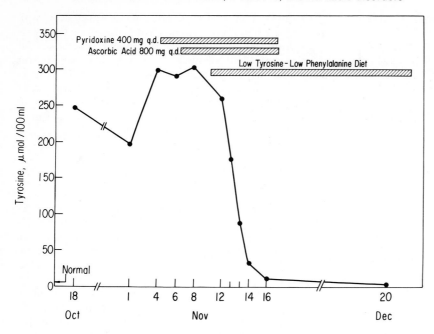

Fig. 139-5 The response of elevated plasma tyrosine to a low-tyrosine, low-phenylalanine diet and failure of response to various cofactors in a patient with tyrosinemia II.

Phenylketonuria

Definition

Phenylketonuria (PKU) is an autosomal, recessively inherited disease due to a deficiency of hepatic phenylalanine hydroxylase or cofactors for the phenylalanine hydroxylating system. The increased levels of phenylalanine are associated with mental retardation, seizures, decreased pigmentation of the skin, hair, and eyes, and eczematous dermatitis.

Clinical features

This common metabolic defect occurs in 1 of 10,000 births and can be detected by screening procedures in neonatal life. One percent of institutionalized retarded patients have PKU. Mental retardation, athetosis, restlessness, increased tendon reflexes and muscle tone, hyperkinesis, tremors, and seizures accompany the untreated disease. The general features of the disease, its biochemistry, heterozygote detection, and treatment are reviewed elsewhere [26].

Patients with phenylketonuria have an increased incidence of eczematous dermatitis, pigment dilution of hair and skin color, and occasionally sclerodermatous skin changes. Other changes reported include a decreased number of pigmented nevi, and an increased incidence of keratosis pilaris [27]. Skin phenylalanine levels are higher in PKU skin than in normal skin [28].

Atopic dermatitis has been found to be increased in studies by Fleisher and Zeligman [29] and Braun-Falco and Geissler [27]. In the former study, atopic dermatitis was present in 3 of 23 patients, while in the latter, it was present in 15 of 25 patients. A potential mechanism suggested for the increased incidence of atopic disease is an increased tendency to vasoconstriction in PKU [30]. Dramatic clearing of eczema with a low-phenylalanine diet has been reported in some patients. It is possible that an inborn tendency to eczematous dermatitis has been nonspecifically triggered in these patients, although normal patients with eczema have no abnormality of phenylalanine metabolism detectable after a phenylalanine load [31]. Patients with PKU often have a lighter hair and eye color than their siblings [32]. The color changes may be especially striking in the rare black or Japanese patient with PKU whose eye or hair color may be very different from that of other members of the ethnic group (Fig. A8-6). With a low-phenylalanine diet, or with aging alone, hair color darkens. When tyrosine is added to the diet of patients with PKU, hair darkens; if tyrosine is removed, the hair will lighten and banded hair is produced (Fig. A8-5). The increased levels of phenylalanine and its oxidation products (phenylpyruvic acid, *o*-hydroxyphenylacetic acid, phenylacetic acid) inhibit the enzyme, tyrosinase, and therefore reduce melanization [33] (Fig. 139-3).

The sclerodermatous changes in PKU are very striking and have been reviewed by Jablonska and Stachow [34]. Nine patients with PKU have had the onset of indurated areas of skin, most prominent on the thighs and associated with contractures, during the first year of life. Acral areas of the body were least affected in contradistinction to systemic sclerosis. Biopsy showed increased fibroblasts and histiocytes, and atrophy of skin appendages. The elastic fibers were scanty and fragmented and were thus different from those found in true scleroderma. With dietary control the sclerodermatous lesions cleared. The lesions may be due to alterations in tryptophan metabolism which occur in patients with phenylketonuria; tryptophan absorption is decreased in the presence of high blood levels of phenylalanine [35]. In experimental phenylketonuria, there is an abnormal tubulin due to decreased posttranslational addition of tyrosine to tubulin α-chains [36]. This may explain some of the tissue effects in PKU.

Diagnosis

Phenylalanine can be quantitated by ion exchange chromatography. Increased levels of its metabolites in the urine are detected by a screening test in which $FeCl_3$ forms a

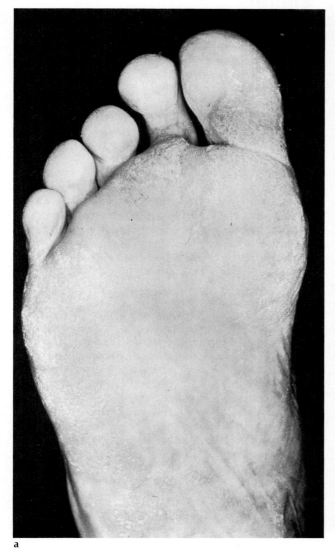
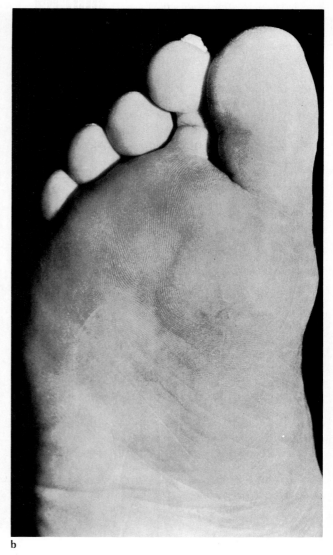

a

b

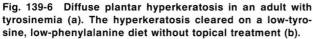

Fig. 139-6 Diffuse plantar hyperkeratosis in an adult with tyrosinemia (a). The hyperkeratosis cleared on a low-tyrosine, low-phenylalanine diet without topical treatment (b).

bluish green (olive-green) color in the presence of phenylpyruvic acid. The chemical determination distinguishes PKU from the various forms of oculocutaneous albinism and Chédiak-Higashi disease, which are also associated with pigment dilution.

Treatment

A low-phenylalanine diet results in increased pigmentation, and often clearing of the eczema. Over-rigorous control of diet can lead to protein deficiency and an eczematous dermatitis.

Argininosuccinic aciduria

Definition and clinical features

Argininosuccinic aciduria (ASA) is characterized by hepatomegaly, mental retardation, seizures, episodic lethargy and ataxia, autosomal recessive inheritance, and friable,

brittle hair with the morphology of trichorrhexis nodosa. The deficiency of an essential enzyme in the urea cycle, argininosuccinase (argininosuccinate lyase), causes an increase in blood ammonia, and citrullinemia. Argininosuccinate is increased in the blood and spinal fluid and is excreted in large amounts (2 to 9 g per day) in the urine.

The detailed clinical and biochemical features of the disease and the principles of therapy have been reviewed [37]. The disease presents in the neonatal period as failure to thrive and ammonia intoxication, or in the second year of life with psychomotor retardation, seizures, and ataxia.

Hair defects

Clinical and morphologic. About half of the reported patients have had abnormally friable hair with visible trichorrhexis nodosa; the other half have grossly normal hair [37,38]. Brushing and combing accentuate breaking (i.e., "brittle" hair) [38]. No definite correlation can be made between liver ASAase level, argininosuccinic acid levels, arginine levels, and the degree of hair abnormalities; some patients with severe ASA have had seemingly normal hair. Some patients' hair has improved with diet [39], or without specific therapy [40]. One patient of Hartlage et al [41], had trichorrhexis nodosa at birth and improvement in her hair with the addition of increased amounts of arginine to the diet. Eyelashes, eyebrows, and general body hair [38] as well as the nails [42] may be involved.

There is variation in diameter within the same hair, and torsion, grooving, and irregular contours of the intrafollicular portions of growing hairs [38]. With polarizing microscopy, there is no uniform cortical or medullary structure and no correlation of the lesion to polarized or nonpolarized regions [38]. Stains of the hair with acridine orange and subsequent fluorescent microscopy show red fluorescence instead of the green fluorescence seen in ordinary, mechanically induced trichorrhexis nodosa [42].

Molecular nature of hair defect. During stress-strain testing in air, ASA hair broke prematurely at the end of the Hookean portion of the stress-strain curve [43], and Young's modulus of elasticity was less than 50 percent of normal. In two patients [44], there was no argininosuccinic acid in the hair, and the only abnormality in amino acid content was a decreased serine level. In another patient [43] the amino acid content was normal except for a cystine value one-half that of normal.

The basic nature of the hair defect is unknown. Are the brittle hair and the trichorrhexis nodosa a consequence of the deficiency of a product from the urea cycle, e.g., arginine, or is the hair defect related to an excess of one of the products which is increased due to argininosuccinate lyase deficiency? The administration of argininosuccinic acid to adult rats did not cause any specific effects, although there are no data on whether the argininosuccinic acid was absorbed from the gut [40].

Increasing the arginine in the diet aids hair growth and structure in this disease, suggesting that the decrease in arginine may be related to the defective hair. Since the urea cycle is depressed in ASA, the arginine required for protein synthesis would come predominantly from dietary sources. Hair protein is rich in arginine (up to 10 percent of the amino acid residues are arginine) and, furthermore, the citrulline present in certain specialized proteins in the medulla and internal root sheath is derived from arginine [45]. Increased ammonia levels also might inhibit ϵ-(γ-glutamyl)lysine bond formation which is important for stabilization of the internal root sheath and medulla. The fumarate derived from ASA is important for the Krebs tricarboxylic acid cycle and this cycle might be altered in ASA with consequent abnormalities of hair metabolism and growth.

Other disorders of the urea cycle [37]

In citrullinemia, a rare recessive disease due to the absence of argininosuccinic acid synthetase, there are somatic and mental retardation and increased levels of blood, urine, and cerebral spinal fluid citrulline, low to normal values of plasma arginine, and increased blood ammonia [37]. Hair from a patient with citrullinemia [46] was lightly pigmented, grew only to a length of 6 cm, and showed irregular areas of dystrophy and interruption of the cuticle. The

hair of an adult with the syndrome was said to be normal. More clinical details on the hair of these and similar patients and further studies of their hair would be of interest.

In lysinuric protein intolerance, which is due to defective transport, the skin may be hyperelastic, joints hypermobile, and the hair sparse and brittle [37]. One-half of the patients have been from Finland. Mice with deficiency in the X-linked urea cycle enzyme, ornithine carbamyl transferase, have sparse hair, but hair defects are not described in humans with the mutation.

Diagnosis

Retardation, ammonia intolerance, and abnormal hair will suggest the syndrome. The diagnosis is confirmed by high-voltage electrophoresis or ion-exchange chromatography of the urine, blood, or spinal fluid. Only a tiny percentage of the cases of trichorrhexis nodosa and brittle hair are due to argininosuccinic aciduria.

Microargininosuccinic aciduria

In true argininosuccinic aciduria, urinary ASA ranges between 2 and 9 g per day. In contradistinction, there have been instances of normal individuals excreting a few milligrams of argininosuccinic acid a day and some of these patients have had monilethrix [47,48], trichorrhexis nodosa [49], or pili torti [48]. In some of these cases ASA was not correctly identified [49], or it may have had dietary sources. In any case, it is difficult to make a cause-and-effect relationship between these trivial levels of argininosuccinic acid and the associated hair defects.

References

1. Scriver CR et al: *Amino Acid Metabolism and Its Disorders.* Philadelphia, WB Saunders, 1973
2. Nyhan WL: *Heritable Disorders of Amino Acid Metabolism: Patterns of Clinical Expression and Genetic Variation.* New York, John Wiley & Sons, 1974
3. Stanbury JB et al (eds): *The Metabolic Basis of Inherited Disease,* 5th ed. New York, McGraw-Hill, 1983
4. Goldsmith LA: Tyrosinemia and related disorders, in *Metabolic Basis of Inherited Disease,* 5th ed, edited by JB Stanbury et al. New York, McGraw-Hill, 1983, p 287
5. Zaleski WA et al: Skin lesions in tyrosinosis: response to dietary treatment. *Br J Dermatol* **88**:335, 1973
6. Billson FA, Danks DM: Corneal and skin change in tyrosinemia. *Aust J Ophthalmol* **3**:112, 1975
7. Goldsmith LA, Reed J: Tyrosine-induced eye and skin lesions. A treatable genetic disease. *JAMA* **236**:382, 1976
8. Goldsmith LA et al: Hepatic enzymes of tyrosine metabolism in tyrosinemia II. *J Invest Dermatol* **83**:530, 1979
9. Goldsmith LA et al: Tyrosinemia with plantar and palmar keratosis and keratitis. *J Pediatr* **83**:798, 1973
10. Burns RP: Soluble tyrosine aminotransferase deficiency: an unusual cause of corneal ulcers. *Am J Ophthalmol* **73**:400, 1972
11. Fellman JH et al: Soluble and mitochondrial forms of tyrosine aminotransferase. Relationship to human tyrosinemia. *Biochemistry* **8**:615, 1969
12. Bohnert A, Anton-Lamprecht I: Richner-Hanhart's syndrome: ultrastructural abnormalities of epidermal keratinization indicating a causal relationship to high intracellular tyrosine levels. *J Invest Dermatol* **79**:68, 1982

13. Bienfang DC et al: The Richner-Hanhart syndrome. Report of a case with associated tyrosinemia. *Arch Ophthalmol* **94:**1133, 1976

14. Schweizer W: Studies on the effect of L-tyrosine on the white rat. *J Physiol (Lond)* **106:**167, 1947

15. Alam SQ et al: Effect of threonine on the toxicity of excess tyrosine and cataract formation in the rat. *J Nutr* **89:**90, 1966

16. Selye H: Steroids influencing the toxicity of L-tyrosine. *J Nutr* **101:**515, 1971

17. Beard ME et al: Histopathology of keratopathy in the tyrosine-fed rat. *Invest Ophthalmol* **13:**1037, 1974

18. Goldsmith LA et al: Tyrosine aminotransferase deficiency in mink *(Mustela vison)*: a model for human tyrosinemia II. *Biochem Genet* **19:**687, 1981

19. Jezyk PF et al: Screening for inborn errors of metabolism in dogs and cats, in *Animal Models of Inherited Metabolic Diseases,* edited by RJ Desnick. New York, Alan R Liss, 1982, p 93

20. Gipson IK et al: Crystals in corneal epithelial lesions of tyrosine fed rats. *Invest Ophthalmol* **14:**937, 1975

21. Goldsmith LA: Hemolysis and lysosomal activation by solid-state tyrosine. *Biochem Biophys Res Commun* **64:**558, 1975

22. Hunziker N et al: Richner-Hanhart syndrome (RHS)–tyrosinemia type II and oral aromatic retinoid (Ro 10-9359). Report of two cases, in *Retinoids. Advances in Basic Research and Therapy,* edited by CE Orfanos et al. New York, Springer-Verlag, 1981, p 453

23. Franceschetti AT et al: Die Cornea beim Richner-Hanhart Syndrom. *Berl Dtsch Ophthalmol Ges* **71:**109, 1971

24. Zmegac ZJ, Sarajlic MV: A rare form of an inheritable palmar and plantar keratosis. *Dermatologica* **130:**40, 1964

25. Geeraets WJ: *Ocular Syndromes.* Philadelphia, Lea & Febiger, 1976

26. Tourian A, Sidbury JB: Phenylketonuria and hyperphenylalaninemia, in *The Metabolic Basis of Inherited Disease,* 5th ed, edited by JB Stanbury et al. New York, McGraw-Hill, 1983, p 270

27. Braun-Falco O, Geissler H: Skin phenomena in phenylketonuria. *Med Welt* **37:**1941, 1964

28. Fisch RO et al: Studies of phenylketonuria with dermatitis. *J Am Acad Dermatol* **4:**284, 1981

29. Fleisher TL, Zeligman I: Cutaneous findings in phenylketonuria. *Arch Dermatol* **81:**898, 1960

30. Solomon LM, Desai K: Phenylketonuria. *Cutis* **4:**1233, 1968

31. Vickers CFH: Eczema and phenylketonuria. *Trans St Johns Hosp Dermatol Soc* **50:**56, 1964

32. Berg JM, Stern J: Iris color in phenylketonuria. *Ann Human Genet* **22:**370, 1958

33. Miyamoto M, Fitzpatrick TB: Competitive inhibition of mammalian tyrosinase by phenylalanine and in relationship to hair pigmentation in phenylketonuria. *Nature* **179:**199, 1957

34. Jablonska S, Stachow A: Scleroderma-like lesions in phenylketonuria (PKU), in *Scleroderma and Pseudoscleroderma,* 2d ed, edited by S Jablonska. Warsaw, Polish Medical Publishers, 1975, p 489

35. Yarbro MT, Anderson JA: Tryptophan metabolism in phenylketonuria. *J Pediatr* **68:**895, 1966

36. Rodriguex JA, Borisy GG: Experimental phenylketonuria: replacement of carboxyl terminal tyrosine by phenylalanine in infant rat brain tubulin. *Science* **206:**463, 1979

37. Walser M: Urea cycle disorders and other hereditary hyperammonemic syndromes, in *The Metabolic Basis of Inherited Disease,* 5th ed, edited by JB Stanbury et al. New York, McGraw-Hill, 1983, p 402

38. Rauschkolb EW et al: Hair fragility—an important clue to aminoacidopathy in mental retardation. *Cutis* **4:**1315, 1968

39. Coryell ME et al: A familial study of a human enzyme defect, argininosuccinic aciduria. *Biochem Biophys Res Commun* **14:**307, 1964

40. Westall RG: Treatment of argininosuccinic aciduria. *Am J Dis Child* **113:**160, 1967

41. Hartlage RL et al: Argininosuccinic aciduria: perinatal diagnosis and early dietary management. *J Pediatr* **85:**86, 1974

42. Levin B et al: Argininosuccinic aciduria. An inborn error of amino acid metabolism. *Arch Dis Child* **36:**622, 1961

43. Potter JL et al: Argininosuccinic-aciduria—the hair abnormality. *Am J Dis Child* **127:**724, 1974

44. Van Sande M: Hair amino acids: normal values and results in metabolic errors. *Arch Dis Child* **45:**678, 1970

45. Rogers GE, Harding HWJ: Molecular mechanisms in the formation of hair, in *Biology and Disease of the Hair,* edited by T Kobori, W Montagna. Baltimore, University Park Press, 1976, p 411

46. Porter PS: The genetics of human hair growth. *Birth Defects* **12:**69, 1971

47. Grosfeld JCM et al: Argininosuccinic aciduria in monilethrix. *Lancet* **2:**789, 1964

48. Winther A, Bundgaard L: Argininosuccinic aciduria in hereditary hair diseases. *Acta Derm Venereol (Stockh)* **48:**567, 1968

49. Efron ML, Hoefnagel D: Argininosuccinic acid in monilethrix. *Lancet* **1:**321, 1966

CHAPTER 140

CUTANEOUS CHANGES IN ERRORS OF AMINO ACID METABOLISM: ALKAPTONURIA

Lowell A. Goldsmith

Definition

Alkaptonuria is a rare autosomal recessive disorder caused by the inherited deficiency of homogentisic acid oxidase, the sole catabolic enzyme for homogentisic acid (HGA). Excessive HGA is excreted in the urine, which often turns dark, and HGA accumulates in connective tissues including the skin.

Historical aspects [1]

In 1859 Boedeker originally used the term *alcapton* to denote a urinary substance with great avidity for oxygen at an alkaline pH; later he spelled the word alkapton. In 1866 Virchow saw the diffuse bluish black pigmentary changes of connective tissue, in a presumably alkaptonuric individual, and called the condition *ochronosis* because of the ochre (yellow) hue seen microscopically. The prediction of Garrod, set forth in 1908, that alkaptonuria was caused by a specific enzyme deficiency was fully confirmed 50 years later when La Du and associates demonstrated the absence of hepatic HGA oxidase in an alkaptonuric patient.

Epidemiology

Alkaptonuria is inherited as an autosomal recessive trait; those pedigrees that support a dominant mode of transmission and contain a high degree of consanguinity, when subjected to careful scrutiny, are called "pseudodominants." Alkaptonuria in the total population is quite rare (1:250,000), but clusters of high incidence are found in certain groups with significant inbreeding, e.g., in Slovakia and the Dominican Republic. In Slovakian newborns the incidence is 1:25,000 [2]. Disease distribution is worldwide and there is an approximately equal incidence in both sexes.

Etiology and pathogenesis [3]

The biochemical pathway by which phenylalanine and tyrosine normally undergo oxidative degradation to acetoacetic acid is shown in Fig. 140-1. HGA (2,5-dihydroxyphenylacetic acid), the last molecule in the sequence to contain an intact aromatic ring, is cleaved to maleylacetoacetic acid. The enzyme catalyzing ring cleavage, HGA oxidase, is normally present in the soluble fraction of liver and kidney cells, but not other tissues. It is highly specific for HGA. Atmospheric oxygen, ferrous ion, and sulfhydryl groups are required for enzymatic function. Quinones inhibit the enzyme. HGA oxidase activity is totally absent in both liver and kidney tissue from alkaptonuric subjects. Whether there is inactive enzymatic protein is unknown as is the detailed molecular pathobiology of the disease. In patients with alkaptonuria, HGA either undergoes renal excretion or is transformed to ochronotic pigment within connective tissue. HGA may not be present in the first days of life due to the absence of enzymatic activity of other enzymes in the pathway of tyrosine catabolism.

Infusion studies have shown that the renal clearance of HGA is extremely high (up to 400 to 500 mL/min) in both normal and alkaptonuric subjects, indicating active tubular secretion of HGA [3]. It is important to determine the possible inhibitors of this secretion, since drugs which may inhibit this secretion may be an important factor in ochronosis. This explains the observation that in alkaptonuria, with relatively low fasting plasma concentrations of HGA (in the range of 3 mg/dL), excretion may be up to 4 to 8 g per day. Once excreted, HGA (which is itself colorless in solution) gradually oxidizes to dark products. Oxidation occurs gradually when the urine is exposed to air, but can be markedly hastened by alkalinization. Urinary pH is the major variable causing the darkening of the urine and some patients with acidic urine may *never* have spontaneously black urine. Urinary HGA varies at least 10-fold in concentration. A diet high in protein or tyrosine increases the amount of HGA excreted in disease.

The precise manner by which HGA accumulation in tissues leads to ochronosis is only partially understood. A presumed HGA polymer has never been characterized. When HGA is injected into guinea pigs it has a high predilection to localize in skin and cartilage; benzoquinoneacetic acid (BQA), the highly reactive quinone of HGA, binds irreversibly to connective tissue. Homogentisic acid polyphenol oxidase, a copper-containing enzyme, in human, guinea pig, and rabbit skin and cartilage, catalyzes the oxidation of HGA into ochronotic pigment. In the presence of increased HGA this enzyme may form BQA which can then be polymerized by the same polyphenol oxidase [4].

The demonstration of experimental ochronosis by prolonged feeding of high tyrosine diets to rats [5] may be of particular value in delineating the precise interaction between HGA and its products and connective tissue. In this animal model, joint capsules, sternum, and trachea were affected and there was increased nonsulfated acid mucopolysaccharides and decreased sulfated mucopolysaccharides. HGA and BQA were in the subcutaneous tissue.

**Fig. 140-1   Metabolic pathway of phenyla-
lanine and tyrosine degradation.**

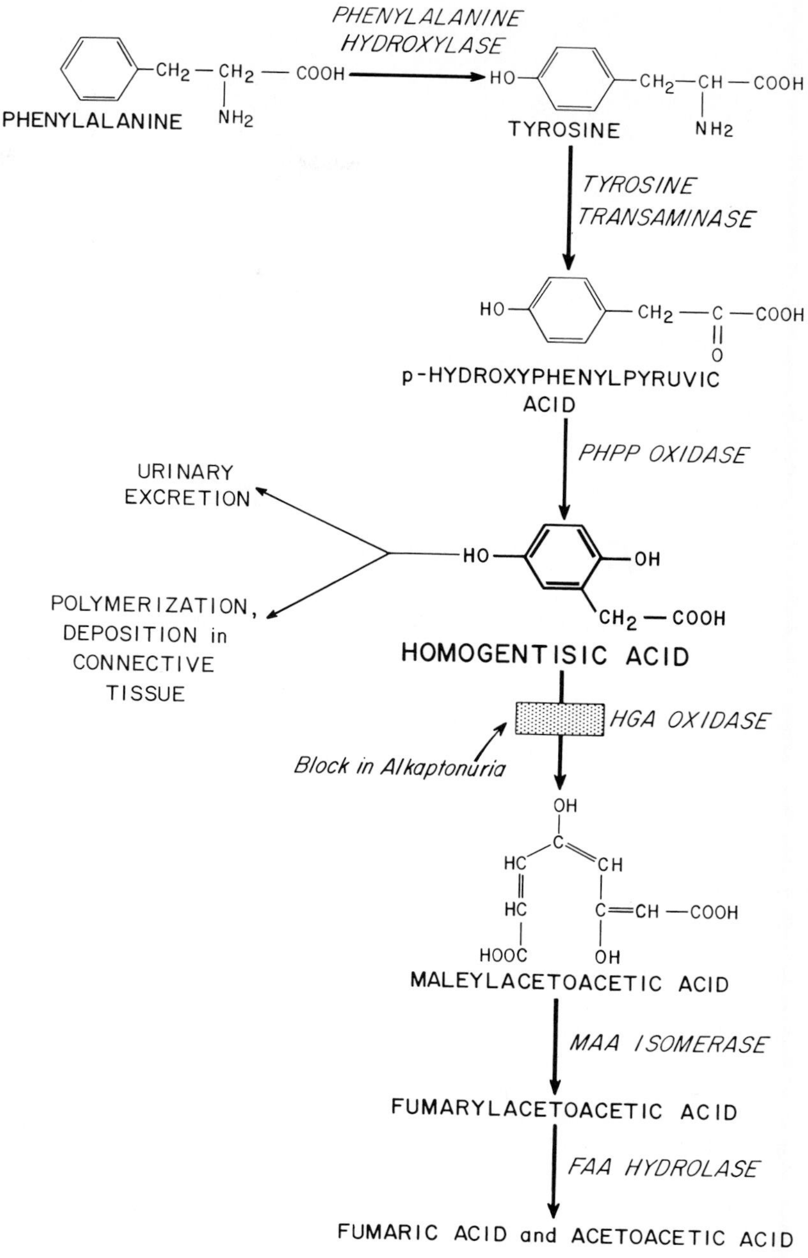

Alkaptonuria also has been produced in experimental animals by L-phenylalanine feeding, diets deficient in sulfur
amino acids or tryptophan and the iron chelator α,α'-di-
pyridyl. In patients with tyrosinemia II (see Chap. 139)
there is no evidence of increased HGA or of dermal pigmentation.

Homogentisic acid inhibits the enzyme lysyl hydroxylase
in chick embryo calvaria [6], suggesting that a reduction
of the structural integrity of collagen consequent to deficient hydroxylysine-derived cross-linkages may be responsible for cartilaginous degeneration in alkaptonuria. The
plasma level of HGA, approximately 0.1 mM, would cause
30 percent inhibition of lysyl hydroxylase. Milch has
shown that autooxidized polymers of HGA combine with
collagen chains to form significant cross-linking in vitro
[7].

Clinical manifestations [1,2]

Although many classic descriptions of the clinical presentation of alkaptonuria cite dark urine as the initial manifestation, this is not always the case. The urine is most apt
to discolor rapidly at a pH above 7.0 and when reducing
substances such as ascorbic acid, which normally protect
HGA from oxidation, are not present in sufficient quantity.

An early diagnosis of alkaptonuria is frequently made
when: (1) it is specifically sought because of familial history; (2) discoloration of diapers occurs after cleansing in
(alkaline) soap; (3) the urinary pH favors the polymerization of HGA; or (4) testing for urinary glucose with Benedict's solution yields an orange precipitate (indicating a
reducing substance) accompanied by a dark supernatant.
A positive Benedict's reaction and a negative glucose anal-

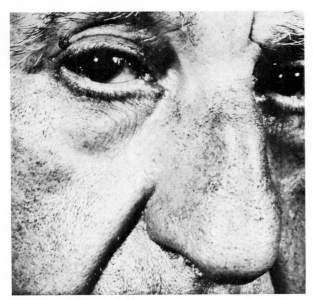

Fig. 140-2 Punctate, blue dermal pigmentation in alkaptonuric ochronosis in a butterfly distribution on the nose and cheeks.

ysis with a glucose oxidase test reagent strongly suggest the diagnosis.

Although the diagnosis of alkaptonuria may be made during childhood, individuals rarely develop pathologically significant changes in connective tissue until they reach their third or fourth decade. If coincidental renal disease prevents effective HGA excretion, the development of ochronosis may be accelerated.

Dark brown or black cerumen may be present in the first decade even in those less than 5 years of age [2]. Axillary skin pigmentation (greenish blue, blue, greenish yellow, or brown) may be present late in the first decade and may be accompanied by underwear staining. The pigmentation is in the pattern of glandular orifices. Changes in the ear cartilage usually do not occur until late in the third decade. In addition to pigmentation, calcification leads to irregularly thickened pinnae.

The visible changes that occur with the passage of time are due primarily to the formation of ochronotic pigment granules in the dermis and sweat follicles, and, most importantly, to the transmission of ochronotic discoloration through thin areas of skin overlying pigmented cartilage and tendon. The latter type, which is fairly uniform in ochronosis, is most apparent at the nose tip, ear (Fig. A8-39), costochondral junctions, and extensor tendons of the hands. Intrinsic pigmentation of the skin is typically less prominent, but may occur in a butterfly pattern on the nose and cheeks (Fig. 140-2). Rarely, bluish gray fingernails [1] and intensely dark nevi have been reported.

A grayish blue tinge overlying ear cartilage occurs relatively early in the course of ochronosis. Later in the disease, structural changes result in loss of transillumination, stiffening, and eventual calcification of the pinnae. Black cerumen is frequently present. The tympanic membrane may be blue. Tinnitus and variable degrees of deafness have been ascribed to ochronotic degeneration of the tympanic membrane and underlying ossicles. Laryngeal and tracheal cartilage become heavily pigmented but do not cause symptoms.

Ochronotic pigment sometimes accumulates in the outer ocular tissues: sclerae (Figs. A4-9 and A8-41), corneas, conjunctivae, and tarsal plates. Scleral discoloration is generally restricted to that portion of the globe exposed by the palpebral fissure. The scleral pigmentation is usually triangular in shape with the base of the triangle facing the cornea at the site of recti muscle insertion [3]. Tiny ''oil droplets'' of ochronotic pigment appear at the inner and outer poles of the corneas in advanced ochronosis.

Insidious progression of ochronotic arthropathy, which generally begins in the third and fourth decades in males and about 10 years later in females, is the most disabling manifestation of alkaptonuria. The disease is more severe in males. Bouts of acute inflammation may occur. Hip, knee, and shoulder limitation are early signs. Lumbar pain, lordosis, kyphosis, and sciatica are common. Roentgenograms show a characteristic appearance of early calcification of the intervertebral disc and, later, narrowing of the intervertebral spaces with eventual disc collapse and progressive loss of height (Fig. 140-3). In addition to the spine, ochronotic arthropathy typically involves larger joints, such as the shoulders, knees, and hips. The hands and feet are generally spared. Pseudogout has been reported to coexist with ochronosis [8].

There is some suggestion of an increased incidence of cardiovascular disease in ochronosis but accelerated arteriosclerosis has not been clearly documented. At postmortem examination, pigmentation is commonly observed in the heart valves, annuli, and in arteriosclerotic plaques. A case of aortic valve stenosis has been attributed to the deposition of ochronotic pigment [9].

Prostatic symptoms in older males frequently are due to the formation of soft pigmented calculi in the alkaline secretions of the ducts and sinuses of that gland. Porous black renal stones containing calcium, phosphate, and oxalate have also been reported in patients with alkaptonuria.

Laboratory findings

Aside from the excretion of homogentisic acid, alkaptonuric patients show no abnormalities discernible on routine clinical laboratory tests. Normal individuals do not excrete HGA; therefore, darkening of the urine upon addition of sodium hydroxide is presumptive evidence of alkaptonuria.

Other tests based on the reducing properties of HGA include the black reaction after treatment with $FeCl_3$, and blackening of photographic emulsion paper upon application of a drop of alkaptonuric urine followed by a drop of sodium hydroxide (Fig. A8-40). A screening test with sodium hydroxide-impregnated filter paper is sensitive and useful for field studies [2]. Specific identification and quantitation of urinary (as well as blood) HGA can be achieved by the use of a direct spectrophotometric method employing HGA oxidase.

With the development of ochronotic arthropathy, x-rays of the spine show characteristic disc calcification which rarely occurs in other forms of spondylitis. Periostitis, ligamental calcification, and sacroiliac sclerosis are not features of ochronotic spondylitis.

Pathology

Yellow to light brown (ochre) pigment granules, which gave the original designation of ochronosis, are present as free bodies and in dermal macrophages [10]. Irregular masses may be over 100 μm in diameter. The pigment is not bleached by 10% H_2O_2 after 72 h [10].

Electron microscopic studies show smaller-sized homogeneous bodies fusing to form larger non-membrane-bound structures [10]. Although the original pigment is brown, scattering of light from it makes involved skin appear blue.

The tendency of connective tissue and, in particular, cartilage to gradually darken over the years constitutes the cardinal pathologic finding in alkaptonuria. Intervertebral discs are pigmented ("jet black") and darken when examined. Articular cartilage, when heavily pigmented, displays the degenerative changes of fibrillation, fissuring, fragmentation, and erosion to bare bone [11].

Diagnosis and differential diagnosis

The diagnosis of alkaptonuria may be made on the basis of typical urinary discoloration or may await the onset of ochronosis in adulthood. Inasmuch as the disease behaves in a quite stereotypical manner with few confusing variants in its mode of presentation, it has been concluded that the diagnosis need only to be thought of to be made. Other causes of dark urine—melaninuria, porphyria, myoglobinuria, bilirubinuria, hematuria, etc.—ought not to be confused with alkaptonuria. An ochronotic-like pigmentation of skin and cartilage has been iatrogenically produced by quinacrine administration over a period of months. Pigmentation due to antimalarial treatment is usually much more pronounced on mucosal surfaces and will fluoresce with a Wood's lamp.

Ochronotic pigmentation has also resulted from chronic application of carbolic acid to cutaneous ulcers, a form of therapy rarely used today. In a patient described by Osler and Garrod [12] the blue color was present on the sclera, the conchar concavity of the antihelix, and extensor tendons of the hands. The pigment on the eyes and ears regressed during hospitalization and upon discontinuation of carbolic acid. The light-related distribution of pigmentation was noted by the authors.

It is possible that the *reversible* ochronotic pigment caused by prolonged carbolic acid treatment is due to the HGA polyphenol oxidase polymerizing the carbolic acid to a HGA polymer-*like* substance which differs from the polymer found in the genetic disease by its reversibility.

Exogenous ochronosis has been reported in a number of South Africans who used strong hydroquinone bleaching creams for a prolonged period [13]. An occupationally induced blue-black dermal pigment resembling ochronosis has been described in a tiler who handled glues, varnishes, dyes, diluents, and stain removers [14]. Ochronotic arthropathy does not occur in these iatrogenic forms of hyperpigmentation.

Treatment

It is disappointing that despite advances in our biochemical understanding of alkaptonuria and the disposition of accumulated HGA to form ochronotic pigment in connective tissue, this information has yet to be translated into a successful therapeutic program for managing the disease. The treatment of ochronotic arthropathy centers about the

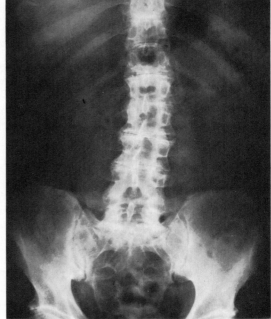

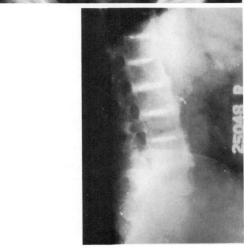

Fig. 140-3 Roentgenographic findings in ochronosis. (a) Calcification of the intervertebral discs and disc collapse. (b) Marked intervertebral disc calcification.

proper balance of rest, physiotherapy, and analgesia. Prosthetic joint replacement is apt to be of considerable benefit for patients with advanced degenerative joint changes.

Course and prognosis

The ultimate course in adults with alkaptonuria is that of increasing pigmentation and skeletal incapacity. Little can be done to interrupt this progression; however, the disease is not incompatible with a normal life span, and the oldest patient on record lived to 99 years of age.

Acknowledgment

The author is indebted to the earlier version of this chapter, in the first and second editions of this book, which was written by Dr. Stephen E. Goldfinger.

References

1. O'Brien WM et al: Biochemical, pathologic and clinical aspects of alcaptonuria, ochronosis and ochronotic arthropathy. *Am J Med* **34**:813, 1963
2. Sřseň S: Alkaptonuria. *Johns Hopkins Med J* **145**:217, 1979
3. La Du BN: Alcaptonuria, in *The Metabolic Basis of Inherited Disease,* 3d ed, edited by JB Stanbury et al. New York, McGraw-Hill, 1972 p 308
4. Zannoni VG et al: Oxidation of homogentisic acid to ochronotic pigment in connective tissue. *Biochim Biophys Acta* **177**:94, 1969
5. Blivaiss BB et al: Experimental ochronosis: induction in rats by long-term feeding with L-tyrosine. *Arch Pathol* **82**:45, 1966
6. Murray JC et al: *In vitro* inhibition of chick embryo lysyl hydroxylase by homogentisic acid. A proposed connective tissue defect in alkaptonuria. *J Clin Invest* **59**:1071, 1977
7. Milch RA: Studies of alcaptonuria: mechanisms of swelling of homogentisic acid-collagen preparations. *Arthritis Rheum* **4**:253, 1961
8. Rynes RI et al: Pseudogout in ochronosis. *Arthritis Rheum* **18**:21, 1975
9. Gould L et al: Cardiac manifestations of ochronosis. *J Thorac Cardiovasc Surg* **72**:788, 1976
10. Attwood HD et al: A histological, histochemical and ultrastructural study of dermal ochronosis. *Pathology* **3**:115, 1971
11. O'Brien WM et al: Studies on the pathogenesis of ochronotic arthropathy. *Arthritis Rheum* **4**:137, 1961
12. Reid E et al: On ochronosis: the clinical features, the urine. *Q J Med* **1**:199, 1908
13. Findlay GH et al: Exogenous ochronosis and pigmented colloid milium from hydroquinone bleaching creams. *Br J Dermatol* **93**:613, 1975
14. Dupré A et al: Idiopathic pigmentation of the hands: professional exogenous ochronosis? New entity? *Arch Dermatol Res* **266**:1, 1979

CHAPTER 141

DISORDERS OF GAMMA GLOBULINS

AGAMMAGLOBULINEMIAS

Fred S. Rosen

Definition

The agammaglobulinemias are a group of diseases characterized by very low serum concentrations of gamma globulin, impairment of antibody formation, and undue susceptibility to infection. Agammaglobulinemia has multiple etiologies; a classification is given in Table 141-1.

Etiology and pathogenesis

The agammaglobulinemias may be divided into two major groups on the basis of their pathogenic mechanisms. In the first group, the deficiency is due to a greatly diminished rate of gamma globulin synthesis. There is an absence or very marked diminution in the number of plasma cells in the lymphoid tissue of these individuals. B lymphocytes are absent from the blood or are abnormal and fail to mature sufficiently to secrete antibody.

In the second group, hypogammaglobulinemia, which is accompanied by hypoalbuminemia, is due to increased catabolism of gamma globulin as a result of gastrointestinal loss, exudation from the skin, or proteinuria. The lymphoid tissue of patients with this type of process is normal. Despite low serum concentrations of gamma globulin, such individuals remain immunologically competent and exhibit less susceptibility to infection.

General clinical manifestations

In general, the outstanding clinical manifestation of the antibody deficiency syndrome is recurrent severe infection due to the common pyogenic bacteria—*Diplococcus pneu-* *moniae, Hemophilus influenzae, Staphylococcus aureus* (see Fig. 141-1), and *Streptococcus pyogenes*. Infections most frequently involve the skin (see below), the middle ear, the conjunctiva, the respiratory tract, and the meninges. On physical examination, particularly of children, very small tonsils and adenoids are noted.

Chronic nonsuppurative arthritis is a common complication of agammaglobulinemia, particularly in patients with the congenital type. Persistent diarrhea with a sprue-like syndrome is frequently seen in adults. Hypersplenism also occurs in some adults with acquired agammaglobulinemia. Hematologic abnormalities such as recurrent neutropenia, hemolytic anemia, and thrombocytopenia may occur in any of these patients.

Laboratory findings

Accurate diagnosis of the various agammaglobulinemic syndromes requires the application of several immunochemical measurements which are not always readily available. Paper electrophoresis, which is very useful in the diagnosis and follow-up of hypergammaglobulinemic states, provides only crude quantitation in the low ranges of gamma globulin concentration. Serum from an individual suspected to have agammaglobulinemia should optimally be examined by immunoelectrophoresis and other immunochemical procedures so that the various immune globulins (IgG, IgA, IgM) can be quantitated.

Failure of a patient to respond to any one of a number of antigens can be determined more rapidly. Absence of the isohemagglutinins or failure to respond to diphtheria or tetanus toxoid or the H and O antigens of typhoid vaccine are useful for this purpose.

Delayed-hypersensitivity testing differentiates patients with T-cell defect. Transcobalamine II deficiency is associated with megaloblastic anemia and the failure of B-cell

Table 141-1 Agammaglobulinemias: a classification of syndromes

Type	Sex	Age of onset	Etiology	Pathology of lymphoid tissue
Agammaglobulinemia:				
Transient	Both	4–8 months	Delayed maturation	Immature lymphoid follicles; few plasma cells; normal B cells; deficient helper T cells
Congenital	Males	5 months or older	X-linked recessive	No plasma cells or follicles; no B cells
Acquired				
Secondary	Both	Any age	Lymphoreticular malignant	Neoplasia
Primary	Both	Any age	Idiopathic	Abiotrophy or hypertrophy of follicles; very few plasma cells; abnormal B cells
Selective immunoglobulin deficiency (dysgammaglobulinemia)	Both	Any age	X-linked recessive or idiopathic	Normal or absent follicles; abnormal B cells
Hypogammaglobulinemia, secondary to:				
Nephrotic syndrome	Both	Any age	Unknown	None
Exudative enteropathy	Both	Any age	Gastrointestinal inflammatory disease or lymphangiectasia	None
Exudative skin lesions	Both	Any age	Severe eczema, burns, pemphigus, exfoliative dermatitis	None
Severe combined immuno-deficiency:				
With generalized hematopoietic hypoplasia	Both	1–2 days	Autosomal recessive; hypoplasia of thymic epithelium; no Hassall's corpuscles	Absence of lymphocytes and myelocytes
Autosomal recessive	Both	2–8 months	Same as above	Absence of T lymphocytes
X-linked	Males	2–14 months	X-linked recessive; hypoplasia of thymic epithelium; no Hassall's corpuscles	Few B lymphocytes; no T lymphocytes
Thymic aplasia	Both	1 week	Congenital	Complete absence of thymus and parathyroids

maturation. A properly prepared *Monilia* antigen almost universally elicits a delayed-sensitivity response in individuals over 6 to 7 months of age. Infants with T-cell defects do not respond. Some patients with Boeck's sarcoid, Hodgkin's disease, chronic lymphatic leukemia, and intestinal lymphangioectasia may also be unresponsive to delayed-hypersensitivity antigens. Dinitrochlorobenzene (DNCB) may be used to induce skin-contact type of delayed hypersensitivity by direct application to the skin. Applied as a patch test in a dilution of 1:100 10 days after the vesicant dose, DNCB will induce a delayed sensitivity response in over 90 percent of normal and agammaglobulinemic individuals.

T and B lymphocytes can readily be enumerated in the blood by most medical center laboratories. Profound T-cell deficiency can result from genetic deficiency of the enzymes adenosine deaminase or purine nucleoside phosphorylase.

Dermatologic aspects

Transient, congenital, sporadic, and acquired agammaglobulinemias

One of the most common primary manifestations is recurrent and severe furunculosis, usually caused by *Staphylococcus aureus* (Fig. 141-1). Severe cicatrization of the skin may result from repeated episodes of pyoderma.

A dermatomyositis-like syndrome has been observed,

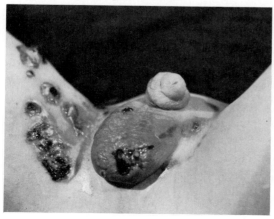

Fig. 141-1 Pyoderma due to *Staphylococcus aureus* in a boy with congenital agammaglobulinemia.

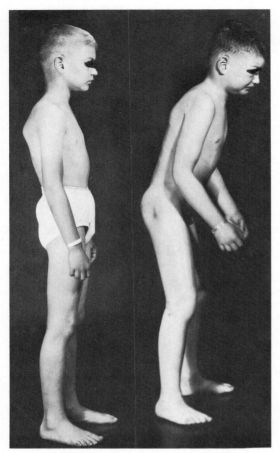

Fig. 141-2   Dermatomyositis-like disease in a boy with congenital agammaglobulinemia at the onset of symptoms (left) and 1 year later (right).

later in the course of the disease, in several children with agammaglobulinemia (Fig. 141-2). The skin over extensor surfaces of the joints develops the typical violaceous lesions of dermatomyositis. There is brawny, almost ligneous edema, and induration of the subcutaneous tissues occurs.

This complication has been fatal after a period of months. It is due to infection with echo virus, an organism that can be recovered from cerebrospinal fluid.

Drug eruptions, poison ivy, angioedema, and eczema occur frequently in patients with agammaglobulinemia. Cutaneous and visceral granulomas of unknown cause frequently complicate acquired agammaglobulinemia in adults (Fig. 141-3), and the late development of infiltration of the skin as part of generalized lymphomatous disease has been observed.

The course of the viral exanthems is usually normal in children with agammaglobulinemia. Extensive manifestations of verruca vulgaris have been noted in a few cases of dysgammaglobulinemia (usually absence of IgA or IgG with elevated γM-globulins) (Fig. 141-4). Vitiligo in association with pernicious anemia is common with acquired agammaglobulinemia.

Almost all patients with dysgammaglobulinemia and several with agammaglobulinemia have recurrent neutropenia accompanied by indolent aphthous ulcers in the mouth. Rarely, a pathogenic organism is isolated from these ulcers.

Secondary hypogammaglobulinemia

As mentioned above, patients who have secondary hypogammaglobulinemia are immunologically competent despite their low serum gamma globulin concentration. Infection occurs less frequently in patients with this problem, but recurrent pneumococcal peritonitis, bacteremia, and a rather diffuse erysipelas-like, tender cellulitis of the edematous skin are often seen in the nephrotic syndrome. This may be the result of the very low concentration of gamma globulins in the extracellular fluid due to the combination of low serum levels and dilution by the massive edema.

Thymic aplasia and severe combined immunodeficiency

Besides pyoderma, a frequent early manifestation of agammaglobulinemia, infants with failure of thymic embryogenesis manifest other dermatologic complications. Exten-

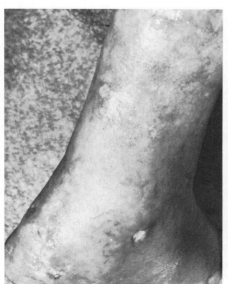

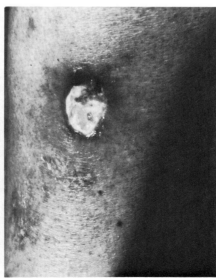

Fig. 141-3   Ulcers and scarring on the legs of a man with acquired agammaglobulinemia. Both caseating and noncaseating granulomas were found in the skin and viscera. (Case Records of MGH #61963. N Engl J Med 268:204, 1963.)

a   b

Fig. 141-4 Extensive infection with verruca vulgaris in a boy with congenital dysgammaglobulinemia type I.

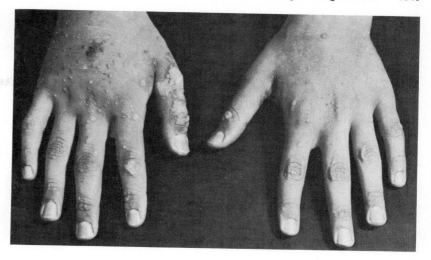

sive cutaneous and oral moniliasis, persisting beyond the neonatal period, is the most common presenting complaint in these infants (Fig. 141-5). A persistent morbilliform rash is suggestive of chronic graft-versus-host disease or measles infection that cannot be terminated. When vaccinated, these infants developed fatal progressive vaccinia gangrenosa. Hemorrhagic varicella has also been seen. No therapy has been of any avail in these complications.

In contrast to patients with agammaglobulinemia who have normal or near normal first and second set graft rejection, infants with no T cells accept homografts and manifest no signs of rejection macroscopically or microscopically.

Miscellaneous conditions

The *Wiskott-Aldrich syndrome* is characterized by severe eczematous dermatitis and thrombocytopenic purpura. These male infants (the disease is transmitted as an X-linked recessive) have recurrent pyogenic infections and bloody diarrhea. Isohemagglutinins are absent from their blood, IgM is usually decreased, and IgA is often markedly increased in the serum. The disease has been corrected with bone marrow transplants. Splenectomy is sometimes advised to control thrombocytopenia. Prophylactic antibiotics must be maintained postoperatively.

Hereditary ataxia-telangiectasia is inherited as an autosomal recessive trait. These children develop ocular (see Fig. A4-13) and cutaneous telangiectases, particularly about the collar area and in the creases of the arms. The disease is also manifested by progressive cerebellar degeneration and sinobronchopulmonary infections. Delayed-hypersensitivity reactions are blunted. In 70 to 80 percent of cases, the serum IgA is absent whereas the other immunoglobulins are normal. In both the Wiskott-Aldrich syndrome and hereditary ataxia-telangiectasia, there is a marked tendency toward development of lymphoreticular malignancies.

Fig. 141-5 Oral moniliasis in an infant with X-linked thymic epithelial hypoplasia.

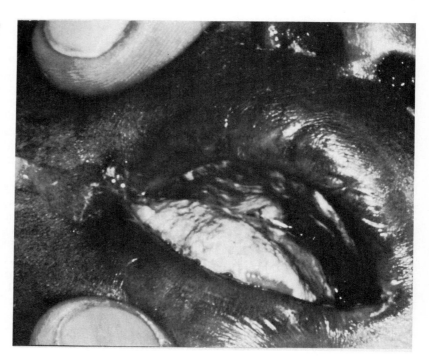

Chronic granulomatous disease usually afflicts males and is transmitted as an X-linked characteristic. Affected male infants develop chronic, suppurative microabscesses first of the skin and lymph nodes and ultimately of all the viscera, prior to death (Fig. 141-6). Lymph nodes, liver, and spleen are enlarged, and the serum contains markedly elevated concentrations of all immunoglobulins. The defect resides in the polymorphonuclear leukocytes which are morphologically normal but functionally deficient. In the usual form, these leukocytes are capable of phagocytosis, but incapable of subsequent intracellular killing of the bacteria—a metabolic defect which is manifested by an inability to operate the hexose monophosphate shunt during phagocytosis and to oxidize NADH and NADPH. This biochemical defect can be readily demonstrated by the failure of the leukocytes to reduce nitroblue tetrazolium dye from the colorless to the deep blue state during phagocytosis.

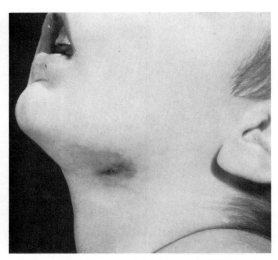

Fig. 141-6 **Scars from chronic cervical adenitis in a boy with chronic granulomatous disease.**

Treatment

Acute infections require intensive antimicrobial chemotherapy in all cases. Gamma globulin replacement therapy is a successful prophylactic measure only in the agammaglobulinemias. It is of no avail in halting or preventing the fatal complications of the various thymic disorders. Since secondary hypogammaglobulinemias are due to abnormal loss or destruction of gamma globulin, exogenous gamma globulin is rapidly catabolized after injection into these patients.

The aim of gamma globulin replacement therapy is to keep the gamma globulin level above 150 mg/dL. Since the serum of the newly diagnosed patient usually contains less than 100 mg/dL, a loading dose of 1.2 to 1.8 mg/kg is given followed by a maintenance dose of 0.6/kg at monthly intervals. At the present time, these large doses must be given intramuscularly, but efforts are now being directed toward preparation of a gamma globulin derivative safe for intravenous use.

Bone marrow transplants have corrected T-cell deficiency.

Bibliography

Rosen FS et al: Primary immunodeficiency diseases. Report prepared for the WHO by a Scientific Group on Immuno-deficiency. *Clin Immunol Immunopathol* **28**:450, 1983

DYSPROTEINEMIAS

Jan Waldenström

Definition

The definition of the word *dysproteinemia* may seem difficult at first. A great number of different diseases lead to changes in the plasma proteins that must be regarded as purely symptomatic: increases in fibrinogen and haptoglobin and decrease in albumin are common symptoms of many acute clinical conditions. These changes are not included in the group that we call dysproteinemia. Regarding the gamma globulin fraction that includes the so-called

immunoglobulins, it is clear that both acute and especially chronic infections might cause changes. In some chronic infections, for instance lymphopathia venereum (Nicholas-Favre), there may be very marked chronic increases in gamma globulin. It is well known that this disease may have several cutaneous manifestations. By definition such conditions are not included among the dysproteinemias and will not be treated here.

On the whole it may be said that chronic increase in gamma globulin not caused by infections may be of two types. One is characterized by the development of a narrow band and the other by a broad increase in the whole gamma fraction, often stretching into the beta globulins. I call the first type monoclonal, as we have reason to believe that it is caused by increase in one special individual gamma globulin molecule produced by the descendants of one gamma globulin-forming cell delivering its product in increased quantities. Together they may be imagined as a special clone or cell line.

Space does not permit a discussion of the many arguments in favor of the hypothesis that the protein contained in the narrow band is homogeneous. At all events the designation monoclonal seems handy and is probably correct. Nobody could deny that the broad fraction must contain the product of many proliferating clones and therefore be polyclonal. From the work with electrophoresis, ultracentrifugation, and immunoelectrophoresis, we know that the normal gamma fraction is not homogeneous. There are molecules with different molecular weight, different carbohydrate content, and different immunologic characteristics. Regarding molecular weight there are two distinct types, "normal" gamma globulin with a molecular weight of 150,000 and the so-called gamma macroglobulin with a molecular weight of 1,000,000. This is often expressed as the sedimentation constant (S = Svedberg unit) in the ultracentrifuge. The first-named group (7 S) constitutes the bulk of the entire gamma globulin and is immunologically characterized as IgG. Another smaller group is called IgA (7 S or 10 to 11 S), whereas the macroglobulin is designated as IgM (19 to 20 S) [1]. Monoclonal globulins are seen chiefly in myeloma and in macroglobulinemia: IgG and IgA in the first-named disease, IgM in the last. There also are

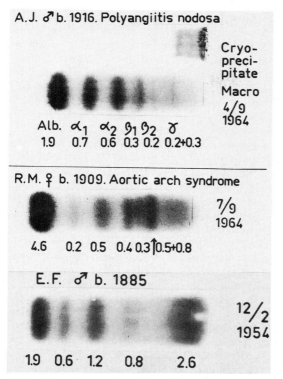

A. J. ♂ b. 1916. Polyangiitis nodosa

Cryo-preci-pitate
Macro
4/9
1964

| Alb. | α₁ | α₂ | β₁ | β₂ | γ |
| 1.9 | 0.7 | 0.6 | 0.3 | 0.2 | 0.2+0.3 |

R. M. ♀ b. 1909. Aortic arch syndrome

7/9
1964

4.6   0.2   0.5   0.4 0.3|0.5+0.8

E. F. ♂ b. 1885

12/2
1954

1.9   0.6   1.2   0.8   2.6

Fig. 141-7   The pictures show the difference between monoclonal and polyclonal increase in gamma globulin. The upper picture (A. J.) shows electrophoresis from a serum where all the cryoprecipitate has disappeared before electrophoresis; it has been redissolved in the upper part of this diagram. The picture E. F. comes from a patient with hyperglobulinemic purpura and a polyclonal broad increase in gamma globulin.

numerous persons who have monoclonal globulins of any one among the three types without having or developing any symptoms of disease. Such conditions have been described by the author with the designation benign monoclonal gammopathy [2].

Polyclonal gammaglobulinemia

Polyclonal hypergammaglobulinemia is found in many conditions, which are sometimes interpreted as being autoimmune. It contains members of all three groups, IgG, IgA, and IgM (see Fig. 141-7). It is also common to see with this several serologic reactions in high titers, such as false-positive Wassermann, rheumatoid factors, antinuclear factors, thyroid and other organ antibodies, LE cell factors, etc. This shows that there is a large diversity in the synthesis of gamma globulin molecules.

Purpura hyperglobulinemica

Purpura hyperglobulinemica is one syndrome where cutaneous lesions together with polyclonal hypergammaglobulinemia may be the only symptom of disease. This is what is called *purpura hyperglobulinemica* here. It is usual that these persons have extremely high polyclonal gamma globulin values with well-preserved serum albumin. This probably indicates the presence of large immune complexes

with little influence on colloid osmotic pressure. In many cases there is overlapping with other clinical syndromes, such as sarcoidosis and chronic sialoadenitis (Sjögren). The author has a number of patients in whom no other signs of disease will be found than an extremely chronic but relapsing orthostatic purpura, leaving scattered pigmentations on the lower legs and extreme hyperglobulinemia. The fact that the gamma globulin pattern is polyclonal, such as we see it in the autoimmune diseases, might induce us to regard this as an example of autoimmunity, just as chronic thyroiditis, chronic sialoadenitis, and chronic hepatitis with polyclonal gamma globulin is now regarded as indicating autoimmunity [2].

Capra and Kunkel et al have carefully studied the reason why the rheumatoid factor is often strongly positive. Ultracentrifugation of serum and plasma showed large amounts of complexes with sedimentation coefficients of between 7 and 19 S. They probably represent IgG–anti-IgG complexes and are not identical with the common rheumatoid factor that is an IgM [3]. This fact has also been stressed by Kyle et al who found that the rheumatoid factor activity was still present after treatment of the serum with mercaptoethanol. This indicates that the factor is not an IgM. Among the 24 patients studied by Kyle et al only one had a negative rheumatoid factor activity [4]. Capra and Kunkel investigated latex fixation in the sera from 16 persons and found high titers in all. It seems convincing that immune complex formation is a basic process in the development of the purpura.

In our own material from Sweden I have seen more than 20 female patients and only 3 males. The diagnosis should therefore be made with special critique in men. The patients are usually middle-aged or elderly, but one of our patients had had purpura and unexplained maximal ESR since the age of 9 [2]. The purpura begins insidiously, always on the lower legs. It appears in crops, usually after special strain (dancing the whole night in one of my first patients). Some patients maintain that carrying heavy things with arms stretched may produce spots on the arms. The Rumpel-Leede test is positive. Sometimes there are somewhat bigger spots and even slightly elevated papules. Itching is usually absent or very slight, but tingling and burning may cause considerable discomfort. The patient's complaints are mostly connected with cosmetic problems in this age of nylon. It should be remembered that the purpura is located only in the skin, and bleedings in internal organs have never been seen. A great many such cases have been described from different countries. Some authors have adopted the expression purpura hyperglobulinemia. This is a linguistic misnomer since -ica denotes the adjective [5].

Therapy is difficult. Recently, a patient with typical hyperglobulinemic purpura was found to have a thymoma. After this was removed the purpura disappeared and did not recur during a considerable observation time. In other patients treated with thioguanine results seem to have been excellent, but it may be questioned whether such toxic substances should be used in the treatment of a comparatively benign disease. The author and many others have tried steroids without much influence on the purpura. We have not regarded such treatment as indicated. In my follow-up of patients, some of whom were first seen as early as 1943, I have seen only one woman who had become free of symptoms when I saw her 30 years later. Spontaneous remission must be very rare (see also [4]).

We observed for many years a patient who had only the typical purpura but belonged to a family in which two sisters had SLE with marked hypergammaglobulinemia and another sister had only the latter abnormality together with chronic unexplained maximal elevation of the ESR. She was still alive 25 years later and in good condition. After treatment with phenylbutazone our patient with purpura developed a typical attack of SLE and later died from this disease [6]. Such and other similar observations make us believe that purpura hyperglobulinemica is related to the collagen or autoimmune conditions. It is characteristic that these patients do not have chronic arthritis; rheumatic purpura with acute attacks is something different. Also Henoch-Schönlein's purpura has a different clinical picture that is not seen in purpura hyperglobulinemica, such as colicky pain, intestinal bleeding, and acute arthritis, even if transitions may be found.

Monoclonal hyperglobulinemia

In this group, myeloma is without any doubt the most common and therefore the most important malady. It is usually maintained that plasmocytoma initially does not occur in the skin. From studies in the literature and from my own large experience with this disease I can subscribe to this statement. Patients are seen, however, where myeloma in late stages may infiltrate the skin and cause bluish, multiple, nodular lesions. It is possible that in some of these patients reticular cells are proliferating. Bulging skeletal tumors from the skull do not belong to the skin.

Recently a new group of myeloma patients has been described from Japan. Characteristically, they have low M components. Many show osteosclerosis with or without polyneuropathy. A few male patients have shown gynecomastia. Many patients have had pigmentations and localized hypertrichosis [7–9].

One complication that is not too uncommon in myeloma is so-called atypical amyloidosis. Its connection with myeloma cannot be treated here, but it is equally certain that the two diseases may occur together and that they may sometimes be entirely separate. An intriguing dermatologic symptom in atypical or primary amyloidosis is the fact that small petechial bleedings occur in certain areas of the body and may be quasidiagnostic. This is true of the periocular and perianal bleedings, and I have suspected atypical amyloidosis several times from this symptom [9]. These patients have had typical monoclonal globulin changes, and at least one of them also had clinical myeloma. Very rare instances of amyloidosis in the skin in myeloma patients have been published, one by Mandema [10] with pictures.

Another rare cutaneous lesion that seems to belong to the monoclonal dysproteinemias is so-called lichen myxoedematosus or papular mucinosis. This disease is characterized by whitish lichenoid macules which tend to form plaques and occur symmetrically. They are follicular and often distributed in rows; sometimes the skin is thickened. The characteristic histologic picture is explained by the fact that many cells stain positively with alcian blue, indicating that they contain acid mucopolysaccharides. The prognosis seems good, with survival for many years. Osserman and Takatsuki [11] think the deposits in the skin

found on histologic examination consist of the pathologic gamma globulin. A myeloma patient with the same skin lesion has been reported by Perry et al [12]. No convincing signs of myeloma were found in the eight patients mentioned by James et al [13] nor in other patients where a myeloma-like protein was discovered. Nor has papular mucinosis been discovered as a symptom in myeloma. Plasmocytosis of the bone marrow was noted by some authors, however. All patients had IgG bands of narrow type on paper electrophoresis. The globulin was extremely basic. James et al [13] determined the light chain type of 8 proteins; they were all lambda type. In view of the fact that only one-third of monoclonal proteins seen in myeloma are lambda, this type of light chain must be highly prevalent in papular mucinosis M components. In this connection it should be remembered that Harboe and Lind [14] found 100 consecutive anti-I cold agglutinins to be kappa type macroglobulins. Osserman and Takatsuki [11] published two instances of this disease, in which a monoclonal increase in gamma globulins of the IgG type was noted. The marrow showed a plasmocytic proliferation.

A group of German dermatologists [15] have published a paper on pyodermia ulcerosa serpiginosa (dermatitis ulcerosa) "occurring in multiple myeloma." Six patients had chronic deep ulcerations in the skin of the lower legs and were severely incapacitated. Four sera contained monoclonal globulin, all of which were of IgA type. In three patients no myeloma was found, but the fourth was regarded as a probable instance of this disease. Similar, as yet unpublished, observations are known to me. We have observed in Malmö a male patient with long-lasting (13 years) deep ulcerations of unknown cause on the legs, high ESR, proteinuria, and massive hypertension. He had a very marked monoclonal globulin band, IgG 5.2 g/dL, and we regarded the diagnosis of myeloma as fairly certain in spite of the fact that his skeletal roentgenogram was negative and his bone marrow plasma cell count was only 7.2 percent. The patient died at home and there was only partial postmortem that was not sufficient to exclude myeloma. In this patient an IgG globulin was present. Among our patients with clear-cut myeloma we have never seen any such ulcers. They must be rare.

In 1978 we published a report of a patient with pyoderma gangrenosum and a monoclonal IgA globulin. The diagnosis of myeloma was never definitely established, but was regarded as possible. The patient was therefore treated with Melphalan. Her general condition improved, but in the meantime a carcinoma of the colon had been removed. After Melphalan treatment her bilateral ulcerations healed. When she died of myocardial infarction, the postmortem showed no signs of myeloma and no ulcerations.

An interesting dermatologic finding has recently been published [16].

Cryoglobulinemia

We do not know the exact role of the myeloma globulins in the development of cutaneous symptoms except when cryoglobulins are present. It had long been known that some globulins precipitate in the cold, but the occurrence of clinical symptoms that could be connected with such intravascular precipitations was realized by Flemberg [17] and by Lerner and Watson [18] in the United States. The

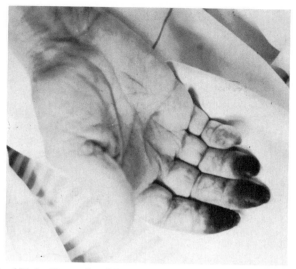

Fig. 141-8 Necrosis of fingertips in a patient with cryoglobulin precipitating at 25°C.

latter authors coined the expression cryoglobulin, and this has since been widely used (see Fig. 141-8). There are three types of abnormal behavior in the cold that are connected with the presence of cryoglobulins: (1) very strong gradual increase in viscosity with decreasing temperature until a gel is formed; (2) stratification of the serum with an upper limpid zone and a lower gel that contains most of the globulin; and (3) precipitation of solid globulin, sometimes in the form of crystals. It is possible that some of the gels are exceptionally caused by such precipitates because they are thixotropic and disappear on violent shaking with the precipitation of needle-like crystals. One of the first Swedish cases with myeloma and purpura belonged to this group. It is interesting to note that cryoglobulins may be either IgG or IgM (macroglobulin). One of my first three patients with macroglobulinemia had a cryoglobulin that formed gels but did not cause any clinical symptoms. As a matter of fact I have never seen cold purpura in this disease.

It should be realized that some cryoglobulins are at the same time euglobulins, i.e., they are precipitated on dilution with water (Sia water test). We have also seen a patient whose macrocryoglobulin had the activity of a cold agglutinin. (For pictures and case history see Ref. 2, page 77.) These interrelations make it difficult to judge the mechanism of the skin symptoms. On the whole it may be said that some patients with cryoglobulins develop a cold urticaria on cooling the skin locally [19].

In typical cryoglobulinemic purpura you would expect to see purpuric spots. This was found in seven cases of essential cryoglobulinemia and cold urticaria quoted by James et al [13]. In many instances the urticaria has probably not been noted. In some patients with cryoglobulins larger ecchymoses are seen, sometimes leading to gangrene of the skin. In other patients with this type of globulin, necrosis of fingertips is observed. One of our cases had large ulcers on the legs and developed gangrene of the fingertips. Both radiologic and anatomic investigations revealed signs of "arteritis" in this patient. We do not know whether the arteritic process causes cryoglobulins or vice versa. There are still many problems that await solution in this group of maladies. Livedo reticularis in amplissima forma was present in one of our patients with cryoglobulins (see [20]).

The commonly accepted theory is that protein "plugs" cause ischemia with secondary bleeding or even necrosis. The work of James et al on degranulation of mast cells may throw new light on some of these problems. I have seen the autopsy of one patient with severe myeloma whom we had treated with Melphalan very successfully for nearly 7 years. He had a massive, noncrystallizing 7-S IgG cryoglobulin but never any skin symptoms.

One interesting finding in these cold syndromes is acrocyanosis—what is in the United States commonly called the Raynaud's syndrome. It has long been known that female patients especially may develop white fingers that then turn blue in the cold. In severe cases we may see gangrene, and the patient who was just mentioned had had acrocyanosis before her fingertips became necrotic. The relationship of this finding to cold-precipitating proteins is not clear. We know the syndrome is not rare in SLE and similar autoimmune conditions commonly accompanied by polyclonal increase in gamma globulins and sometimes by cryoglobulinemia. We have observed this latter symptom in several of our cases but have never been convinced about its pathogenic importance. On the other hand, I have seen several patients with very severe acrocyanotic episodes in the cold without any demonstrable disturbances of serum globulins; however, local cooling of the skin in these patients may cause urticaria [20].

Very rarely, patients with cryoglobulinemia have had quite serious symptoms with necrosis of the distal parts of their fingers (see Fig. 141-8). These cold syndromes deserve a thorough study since they may shed light on the eternal question of how cooling causes disease. It has usually been maintained that "purpura" develops in patients with cryoglobulins. I have seen some patients where it would be more appropriate to talk about ecchymoses.

Acrocyanosis is sometimes seen in another type of dysproteinemia. These patients develop a reddish blue color of their fingers and often also of nose and ears in the cold. If one hand is put into cold water and the other is kept in water of 37°C, after cooling very remarkable differences are noticed, as the latter regains normal color rapidly. The differential diagnosis of the various conditions with acrocyanosis is a subject that should deserve special treatment. The type we are talking of here is present in patients with high titers of cold agglutinins. These antibodies generally agglutinate red corpuscles from all persons except those who have a very rare, genetically determined, special blood group. Cold agglutinins also cause clumping of red cells from various animals in the cold. The so-called cold agglutinin disease is usually present together with chronic hemolytic anemia but it is remarkable that hemolysis may occur independent of unusual cooling, whereas the acrocyanosis is always caused by low temperatures.

We have been able to observe a patient who had cold agglutinin disease with cold hemoglobinuria. When he lived indoors there were no signs of hyperhemolysis, he had no anemia, no anhaptoglobinemia, and a normal endogenous CO production. After 30 min in a cold room ($+4$°C) his haptoglobin disappeared and the urine contained hemoglobin, but there was no measurable anemia, even when the serum iron rose from 56 γ/dL to 106 in 2 h. Both his fingers and his toes became dark blue in the cold. He had a macroglobulin cold agglutinin of β mobility. Table 4 in [2] shows the seemingly haphazard combination of symptoms in 6 patients with high cold agglutinins in our hospital.

Investigations have shown that the cold agglutinin is a macroglobulin (IgM). In many patients it occurs in such great quantities that the picture of a monoclonal globulin increase is seen. By adsorption experiments with red cells in the cold it has been possible to remove the macroglobulin from some sera. It may then be eluted by bringing the red cells to 37°C.

It is common to find that cold agglutinin disease is a special entity that does not seem to be connected with any other clinical picture such as lymphoma, except in rare cases. The macroglobulin increase could therefore be regarded as idiopathic and I have called all these conditions, where a monoclonal globulin is present at the same levels during many years without decreasing or increasing, essential monoclonal hyperglobulinemia [13]. By *essential* I mean that no primary disease can be found and that the increase in monoclonal globulin is the central symptom. If by chance this globulin behaves like a cryoglobulin or like a cold agglutinin, the characteristic clinical picture may arise. The large majority of these globulins do not have any pathologic effects, except when the macroglobulins rise to very high concentration, when the blood becomes highly viscous. We have also been able to find rare instances of myeloma, and some "essential" increase in IgG globulin, in which the globulin has shown antistreptolysin or antistaphylolysin activities. Such cases are very rare and the presence of the globulin does not give any clinical symptoms, but the cases illustrate that many different types of gamma globulin-producing cells may proliferate and release their product.

During recent years, observations have been published in which patients with monoclonal gamma globulins have had signs of generalized arteritis, sometimes of the nodosa type (see Fig. 141-7). In such cases it is not rare to find plasma cell infiltrates around the vessels, especially on the legs. Sometimes sores may develop. It is very hard to decide whether these patients have the gamma globulin disturbance from the beginning, this leading to "arteritis," or whether the arteritic process causes proliferation of a plasma cell clone [2]. For the time being it seems best to refrain from such speculations and simply state the facts.

References

1. Waldenström J: Abnormal proteins in myeloma. *Adv Intern Med* **5**:398, 1952

2. Waldenström J: *Monoclonal and Polyclonal Hypergammaglobulinemia: Clinical and Biological Significance.* London, Cambridge Univ Press, 1968

3. Capra JD, Kunkel HG: Hypergammaglobulinemic purpura. Studies on the unusual anti-gamma-globulins characteristic of the sera of these patients. *Medicine (Baltimore)* **50**:125, 1971

4. Kyle RA et al: Benign hypergammaglobulinemic purpura of Waldenström. *Medicine (Baltimore)* **50**:113, 1971

5. Waldenström J: Three new cases of purpura hyperglobulinemica. A study in long-lasting benign increase in serum globulin. *Acta Med Scand [Suppl]* **226**:931, 1952

6. Leonhardt T: Family studies in systemic lupus erythematosus. *Acta Med Scand [Suppl]* **416**:1, 1964

7. Takatsuki K, Sanada I: Plasma cell dyscrasia with polyneuropathy and endocrine disorders: clinical and laboratory features of 109 reported cases. *Jpn J Clin Oncol* **13**:543, 1983

8. Waldenström JG et al: Osteosclerotic "plasmocytoma" with polyneuropathy, hypertrichosis and diabetes. *Acta Med Scand* **203**:297, 1978

9. Hällén J, Rudin R: Peri-collagenous amyloidosis. *Acta Med Scand* **179**:483, 1966

10. Mandema E: Over het multipel myeloom, het solitaire plasmocytoom en de macroglobulinaemie. Thesis, Groningen, Dijkstra's Drukkerij NV, 1956

11. Osserman EF, Takatsuki K: Considerations regarding the pathogenesis of the plasmacytic dyscrasias. *Series Haematologica* **4**:28, 1965

12. Perry HO et al: Further observations on lichen myxedematosus. *Ann Intern Med* **53**:955, 1960

13. James K et al: Studies on a unique diagnostic serum globulin in papular mucinosis (lichen myxedematosus). *Clin Exp Immunol* **2**:153, 1967

14. Harboe M, Lind K: Light chain types of transiently occurring cold haemagglutinins. *Scand J Haematol* **3**:269, 1966

15. Röckl H et al: Über das Vorkommen von Paraproteinämie bei Pyodermia ulcerosa serpiginosa (Pyoderma gangraenosum-Dermatitis ulcerosa). *Hautarzt* **15**:165, 1964

16. Möller H et al: Pyoderma gangraenosum (dermatitis ulcerosa) and monoclonal (IgA) globulin healed after Melphalan treatment. *Acta Med Scand* **203**:293, 1978

17. Flemberg T: Några fall med patologiskt förändrad blodaggvita. *Nord Med* **37**:330, 1948

18. Lerner AB, Watson CJ: Studies of cryoglobulins; unusual purpura associated with presence of high concentration of cryoglobulin (cold precipitable serum globulin). *Am J Med Sci* **214**:410, 1947

19. Waldenström JG, Raiend Ü: Plasmapheresis and cold sensitivity of immunoglobulin molecules. I. A study of hyperviscosity, cryoglobulinemia, euglobulinemia and macroglobulinemia vera. II. A study of macroglobulinemia polyclonalis spuria and immune complex disease. *Acta Med Scand* **216**:449, 1984

20. Waldenström J: Studies on conditions associated with disturbed gamma globulin formation (gammapathies). *Harvey Lect* **56**:211, 1961

AMYLOIDOSIS OF THE SKIN

Evan Calkins

Definition and classification of amyloidosis

Characterized, easily identified, and, to some extent, defined by its unique affinity to Congo red and certain other dyes [1], amyloid has provided a fertile ground for studies by clinicians and pathologists over the course of approximately 100 years [2–4]. Although it was thought initially that amyloid was a degradation product of cellulose, it is now recognized that the term refers to a group of proteinaceous deposits which appear hyaline and slightly eosinophilic on hematoxylin and eosin stain, yet have a high affinity for certain dyes, notably Congo red [1]. When one examines Congo red-stained tissue slices, 8 μm in thickness, under polarized light, amyloid exhibits a characteristic birefringence, which is apple green. An even more striking, though less specific, optical effect is achieved following staining with fluorescent dyes (thioflavine S & T) and ultraviolet examination [5]. Through use of these staining techniques, one can identify minute traces of amyloid in histologic specimens. This point must be kept in mind when, as a clinician, one hears that traces of amyloid are present in a given tissue. Amyloid, in trace amounts, will be found in many tissues, especially those from older patients. Deposits of this sort can be identified in one organ or another in 90 percent of all persons dying at age 90 or older [6]. Thus, the disease *amyloidosis* is not defined merely by the presence of amyloid on histologic examination; instead, the material must be present in a sufficient amount and location so as to induce symptoms or, possibly, death.

Approximately 25 years ago it was first observed that amyloid is not, in fact, amorphous or hyaline in nature but is composed, to a considerable degree, of fibrils with distinctive ultrastructural characteristics [7,8]. X-ray diffraction analysis of fibrils demonstrated, in each instance studied, that they exhibited a secondary chemical configuration of a cross-beta antiparallel beta-pleated sheet [9]. This is one of the three major conformations exhibited by mammalian proteins [10], the others being alpha helices and random coils.

The presence, in amyloid deposits, of fibrils with identical or nearly identical ultrastructural characteristics suggested, initially, that amyloid is a uniform substance, occurring as an end result of a variety of pathologic processes. Subsequently, immunochemical and amino acid sequence studies showed that amyloid fibrils from individual patients are, in many instances, quite different [11], exhibiting homologies with a variety of normal body proteins. These include immunoglobulin light chains [12], a variety of polypeptide hormones [13] (including insulin [14] and calcitonin [15]), prealbumin [16], and a normal serum protein (SAA) [17,18] which exhibits many of the charac-

teristics of an acute phase reactant [19]. The fact that all of these proteins studied to date, with which amyloid fibrils exhibit homology, have been shown to exhibit the secondary chemical structure of the beta-pleated sheet, provides added support to their role as precursor proteins in the process of amyloidogenesis. The precise means by which these precursors are transformed into the amyloid fibrils and the factors influencing this process are not yet fully understood (see further discussion at the end of this chapter).

A classification of these putative amyloid precursors and of the related amyloid substances is outlined in Tables 142-1 and 142-2 [20,21].

The amyloid syndromes which have been studied, classified, and reclassified over the past 100 years are now beginning to emerge with clearer definition [22]. Amyloidosis accompanying multiple myeloma or occurring spontaneously in association with defects in immunoglobulin metabolism, previously known as "primary" amyloidosis, is now referred to as amyloid AL (referring to light chains). Persons with this form of amyloidosis usually develop cardiac involvement, frequently with heart block, angina-like pain, and congestive heart failure. Approximately half of these individuals develop renal involvement, with massive proteinuria and renal failure, and many of them manifest macroglossia and skin manifestations (to be discussed below). Although some patients may survive for periods of 10 or more years, the mean duration of life after onset of symptoms is more often short, averaging, in one study, two years [22].

Amyloid AA, formerly known as secondary amyloid, occurs in association with prolonged inflammatory diseases such as tuberculosis, regional ileitis, or severe decubiti. Patients primarily exhibit renal involvement, with nephrotic syndrome and ultimately renal failure. The skin is usually asymptomatic and normal in appearance. In some instances, remission will occur following eradication of the inflammatory disease. More often, death ensues. In one study [22], survival averaged four to five years from initial recognition of the amyloid process.

Several forms of amyloid occur in association with aging. ASc refers to amyloid accumulation in the heart. At least two distinctive clinical and histologic patterns have been defined [23], one of which is occasionally associated with intractable congestive failure [22]. The course of illness of these patients is usually prolonged, with a mean duration in one study of 15 years [22]. Other forms of amyloidosis, occurring in advanced age, include the accumulation of amyloid in the meningeal vessels, or in the cerebral cortex in the form of senile plaques. These lesions are present in high concentration in many patients with senile dementia of the Alzheimer type [24].

Table 142-1   Amyloidosis, an evolving classification (1984)

"Clinical type" of amyloidosis	Putative precursor	Designation
I. Systemic		
A. Immunoglobulin related		
Primary sporadic accompanying multiple myeloma	Immunoglobulin light chain	AL
B. "Secondary"	SAA (an acute phase reactant)	AA
C. Heredofamilial		
Accompanying familial Mediterranean fever neuropathy (see below)	SAA	AA
II. Localized		
A. Immunoglobulin related		
(Skin, bladder, ureter, larynx, trachea, breast, etc.)	Immunoglobulin light chain	AL
B. Localized "secondary"		
Skin, GI tract, etc.	To be determined	
C. Epidermal origin		
Lichen amyloidosis (may be familial)	?Keratin or related protein	
Macular amyloidosis (may be familial)	To be determined	
D. Peripheral neuropathy (may also be present under I.A. above)		
Portuguese type	Prealbumin	AFp
Japanese type	Prealbumin	AFj
Indian type	Prealbumin	
E. Endocrine origin		
Thyroid	Precalcitonin	AEt
Pancreas	?Proinsulin	
III. Senile		
A. Cardiovascular		
Aortic	To be determined	
Isolated atrial	To be determined	
"Senile cardiac amyloid"	Similar or identical to prealbumin	ASc_1
B. Brain		
Senile plaques	To be determined	ASb_1
Meninges	To be determined	ASb_2
C. Other		

Note: This table depicts how dermatologic amyloid may be viewed in the context of the classification system currently being developed by investigators concerned with the *general* problem of amyloidosis. The third column, presently incomplete, reflects the extent to which there is general agreement, at present.

Amyloidosis of the skin

In the context outlined above, amyloidosis of the skin represents an area of tissue involvement, by the amyloid process, comparable to many other tissues cited. As with the upper respiratory tract and genitourinary tract [25], amyloid may accumulate in the skin as the sole tissue involved. Trace accumulations of this sort may occur in association with other dermatologic lesions. These localized traces are asymptomatic. They are not accompanied by widespread organ system involvement and they do not present any harm to the patient.

Primary localized cutaneous amyloidosis (PLCA)

Derived from epidermal cells. *Lichen amyloidosis* is by far the most common form of amyloidosis associated with the skin [26–28]. Although this condition is rare among Europeans and North Americans, it is commonly encountered in South Americans and Asians, especially Chinese and Malaysians [29], in whom it may exhibit a striking familial presentation. In one report [30] 19 cases were described in a family of 56 persons, spanning four generations. In this and other reports of familial amyloidosis [31] the condition is transmitted as a Mendelian autosomal dominant trait, with variable penetrance.

Occurring in persons of all ages, the condition initially presents with intense pruritus, characteristically on the anterior aspect of the shins, accompanied by discrete small papules 1 to 3 mm in diameter (Fig. 142-1) These range in color from that of normal skin to yellowish brown or gray. Later, these coalesce to form firm, nontender, discrete hyperkeratotic plaques. The lesions gradually spread to involve the calves, thighs, ankles, dorsa of feet, and oc-

Table 142-2 Classification of amyloidosis of the skin

I. Primary localized cutaneous amyloidosis
  A. Derived from epidermal cells
    1. Lichen amyloidosis
    2. Macular amyloidosis
  B. Nodular or tumefaction amyloidosis
II. Secondary localized cutaneous amyloidosis
III. Amyloidosis of the skin associated with systemic amyloidosis
  A. Immunoglobulin related (AL)
    1. Primary systemic amyloidosis
    2. Amyloidosis accompanying multiple myeloma
  B. Other forms
    1. Amyloidosis AA
    2. Familial amyloidosis
    3. Senile amyloidosis
IV. Systemic amyloidosis AA associated with dermatologic conditions

Note: This classification is designed to assist in categorizing presently available clinical literature. The terms "primary" and "secondary" refer, here, to the absence or presence, respectively, of a recognizable etiologically related condition.

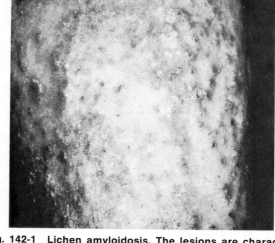

Fig. 142-1 Lichen amyloidosis. The lesions are characteristically very pruritic and some excoriations may be seen.

casionally the anterior aspect of the forearms and abdominal or chest wall. Although the pruritus lessens with time, the lesions may remain for years.

On histologic examination the lesions exhibit marked hyperkeratosis of the epidermis, with papillomatosis and downward proliferation of the rete ridges. The amyloid, identified on electron microscopy by its characteristic fibrillar appearance, is seen in close association with the fibroblasts in the dermal papillae. Amyloid fibrils may, sometimes, be seen within the cytoplasm of the fibroblasts. The amyloid accumulations are usually separated from the epidermis by a thin layer of collagen. The epidermis itself may be thinned or, alternatively, the keratin layer may be compact and locally thickened. In sharp distinction from amyloid accompanying *systemic* amyloidosis, the deeper dermis, subcutaneous tissues, and small blood vessels are uninvolved by the amyloid process.

Systemic pathology, in patients with lichen amyloidosis, has shown no consistent abnormalities. Recent evidence suggests that, in this condition, the fibrils may be derived from a degradation product of keratin (see subsequent discussion).

Macular amyloidosis, less common than lichen amyloidosis, is characterized by grayish brown macules (Fig. 142-2). In some patients these coalesce to form a wavy linear pattern, described as a ripple-like appearance [32]. In others, they aggregate to form poorly delineated, hyperpigmented plaques. These lesions occur in a symmetrical distribution over the shins, thighs, arms, breasts, upper back, and buttocks. They are moderately pruritic.

On pathologic examination, the changes appear identical to those of lichen amyloidosis, except that there is no epidermal hyperplasia. It has been suggested that macular amyloidosis is a form of lichen amyloidosis. Macular amyloidosis may, in time, evolve into lichen amyloidosis and the term *biphasic amyloidosis* has been proposed to describe the condition of patients who, at one time or another, exhibit both of these forms of primary cutaneous amyloidosis [33,34]. Several investigators have identified

instances of localized cutaneous amyloidosis manifested by poikiloderma-like changes, and proposed that this be regarded, along with lichenoid and macular amyloidosis, as a third form of primary localized cutaneous amyloidosis [35]. Although, like lichen amyloidosis, macular amyloidosis is almost always localized to the skin, one investigator [36] has described a patient in whom amyloid infiltration was also present in the larynx and nasopharynx.

Nodular or tumefaction amyloidosis. The clinical appearance and histology of nodular or tumefaction amyloid, when localized to the skin, is identical with that occurring when nodular or tumefaction amyloid is part of systemic amyloidosis [37–39]. It is characterized by single or multiple nodules occurring on the face, extremities, trunk, or genital area. The nodules range in size from that of a pinhead to several centimeters in diameter. They are slightly raised, firm, and white, pink, or yellowish brown in color. They are not tender or pruritic. Histologic examination shows amyloid infiltration of the subcutaneous tissue and dermis and, in some instances, the walls of blood vessels (Fig. 142-3).

Occasionally the deposits may become very large in size. Amyloid tumors have been described in the abdominal wall, inguinal region, extremities, breast, and scalp. While these lesions may occur as a reflection of multisystem involvement in systemic immunoglobulin-related amyloidosis (AL), they may represent the sole area of clinical involvement in this entity. Kyle and Bayrd [37] have noted, in their series of 236 cases of systemic amyloidosis AL, all of whom exhibited abnormal immunoglobulins in serum or urine, that the amyloid deposits were localized to a single tissue in 9 percent of the instances. In addition to skin, other tissues in which localized amyloid accumulation occurred included the urinary bladder, renal pelvis, ureter and urethra, orbit, breast, stomach, bowel, mesentery, palate, and larynx [37]. Nodular or tumefaction amyloid may also occur in the absence of any demonstrable evidence of a generalized defect in immunoglobulin metabolism.

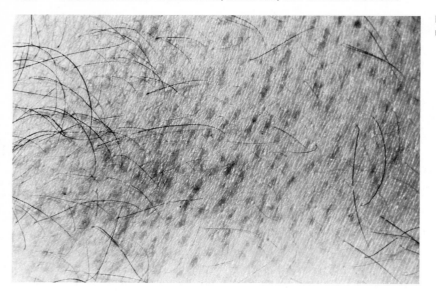

Fig. 142-2 Grayish brown macules occurring in "macular" amyloidosis.

Secondary localized cutaneous amyloidosis

Traces of amyloid not infrequently occur in the immediate vicinity of other dermatologic lesions [40,41]. Malak and Smith [41] underscored this association in a study of 640 consecutive skin biopsies submitted to a dermatopathology laboratory. Amyloid, as evidenced by positive staining with thioflavine T and Congo red stains, was present in 17 instances. Nine of these occurred in the 88 patients with basal cell epitheliomas, 2 in the 22 cases of squamous cell epithelioma, 1 in the 42 cases of seborrheic keratosis, 1 in 16 cases of fibroma, and 1 in 11 cases of severe actinic keratosis. The authors correctly emphasized the need to differentiate a *specific* association between the localized secondary amyloidosis and the other dermatologic entity, and the coincidental occurrence of the nonamyloid dermatosis and lichen amyloidosis. Malak and Smith [41] compared this lesion to the localized amyloidosis that may be noted in tumors in other tissues, such as uterine polyps, lymphomas, and mediastinal sarcomas. The amyloid, in these instances, is an incidental finding, unaccompanied by specific clinical manifestations. The nature and source of the amyloid fibers in these conditions have not yet been defined.

Amyloidosis of the skin associated with systemic amyloidosis

Immunoglobulin related (AL). Dermatologic involvement is present in one-third to one-half of patients with systemic amyloidosis (AL), whether or not associated with multiple myeloma [42–44]. In many of these instances this is an early and, possibly, the first clinical manifestation of the systemic process. Because of this fact, and the characteristic nature of the lesions, amyloidosis of the skin provides an important clue to the correct diagnosis in some patients with multisystem disease, the nature of which otherwise appears obscure.

In our experience and that of Kyle [44] the most common dermatologic manifestation of amyloid AL is purpura. While this may be localized to the folds of the skin in the inguinal area, neck, or around the ears or eyes (Fig. 142-4), it may also occur on the broad surfaces of the back (Fig. 142-5), chest, face, abdomen, or extremities. The purpuric lesions are variable in size. They may be very small, resembling petechiae, or may extend to 1 cm or more in diameter. In the latter instances the borders are usually very irregular. They are not painful, rarely itch, and usually fade over the course of several weeks or months. Deep purpura of the eyelids is especially characteristic of amyloidosis (Fig. 142-6). Kyle has pointed out that periorbital purpura may become more pronounced after proctoscopy, vomiting, coughing, or the Valsalva maneuver [44]. In some patients, in whom the purpura is not evident spontaneously, it can be elucidated by drawing a dull object, such as a key, across the skin with moderate pressure. The purpura is due, primarily, to the amyloid infiltration of the very small blood vessels, leading them to become friable or "leaky." In some cases the purpura may also reflect a deficiency of clotting factor X or IX, which may accompany amyloidosis AL [45,46].

Next in frequency, or in some series [43] in even greater frequency, are papules. These range in size from that of the head of a pin to two or three times that size. The

Fig. 142-3 Amyloidosis. Amyloid is frequently deposited about and within the walls of small blood vessels. ×100. (Micrograph by Wallace H. Clark, Jr., M.D.)

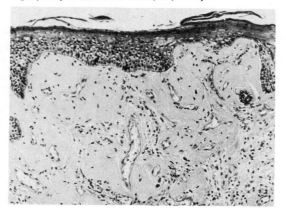

Fig. 142-4 Hemorrhagic papules on the eyelid in amyloidosis AL.

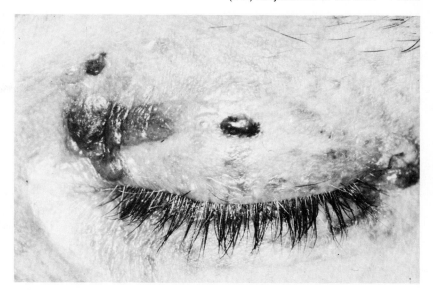

papules are flattopped, slightly raised, smooth, waxy, nontender, and nonpruritic (Fig. 142-7). Although they may be deep red in color, reflecting a hemorrhagic component, they are more often of a pale hue, either white or light yellow. Not infrequently the deposits are larger, forming nodules which are usually discrete. Especially apt to occur on the face, eyelids, or scalp, the papules or nodules may also occur on the tongue (Fig. 142-8) or on a flat surface such as a palm. Amyloid nodules, resembling condylomata lata, have been described on the labia and perianal skin [47].

At times the nodules may coalesce to form a scleroderma-like picture. This may involve the face, neck, and hands, including fingertips. When located adjacent to joints or tendons (of the fingers, for example), the lesions and the tightening of the skin associated with them may impair joint motion, resulting in flexion deformities [48]. The nod-

ules, like the papules, frequently become purpuric, often secondary to relatively minor trauma. Occasionally, if large, they may become ulcerated.

In some cases, amyloidosis AL may result in alopecia. While this process may occasionally be complete, it is usually patchy and confined to the scalp [42] (Fig. 142-9). In rare cases bullous eruptions have been seen on the extremities, trunk, or oral mucosa [49–51].

Fig. 142-6 Purpura of the eyelids, which is very characteristic of systemic amyloidosis AL.

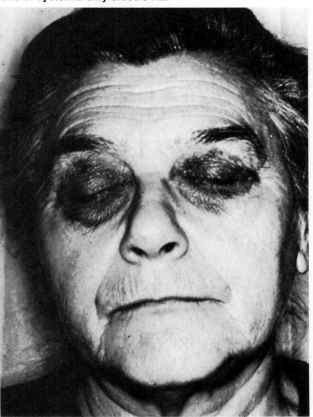

Fig. 142-5 Irregularly shaped purpuric lesions in amyloidosis AL.

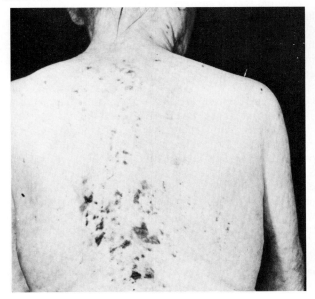

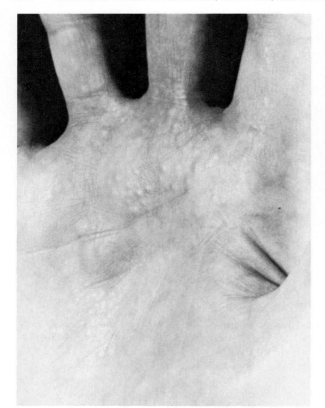

Fig. 142-7 Discrete papules occurring on the palm in amyloidosis AL.

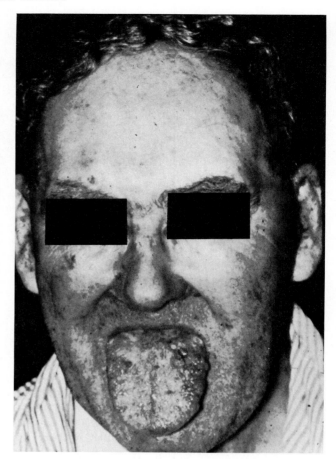

Fig. 142-8 Papules and nodules on the tongue in systemic amyloidosis AL.

Histologic examination of the skin reveals the epidermis to be uninvolved. The amyloid infiltration is confined to the dermis (Fig. 142-3). Amyloid, with its apple-green bi-refringence when viewed under polarized light, can be distinguished from collagen bundles, identified by bright white birefringence. In identifying the presence of amyloid on histologic examination it is important to request the pathologist to cut sections 6 to 8 μm in thickness. The reason is that the staining characteristics of amyloid are lost when thinner sections are used.

Specific areas of involvement were catalogued in the excellent study by Rubinow and Cohen [43]. Amyloid was most consistently noted in the walls of the arteries, venules, and capillaries in the dermis and subcutaneous tissue. In some instances, vascular walls were extensively infiltrated. Sweat glands and the extravascular tissues of the dermis were frequently involved. The presence of amyloid in the subcutaneous fat was evidenced by the appearance of characteristic amyloid rings around individual fat cells. In some instances, amyloid accumulated adjacent to the hair follicles and, occasionally, within the hair shaft itself. In the report by Rubinow and Cohen [43], the authors noted histologic changes of the sort described above in 11 of 27 patients without clinical evidence of skin involvement and in 5 of 7 biopsies of clinically uninvolved skin in patients who did exhibit skin involvement.

In addition to changes in the skin itself, patients with systemic amyloidosis may also exhibit abnormalities that reflect involvement of tissues beneath the dermis. An example is carpal tunnel syndrome, frequently seen in pa-

tients with amyloid accompanying multiple myeloma [52,53]. This is characterized by numbness and tingling of the fingertips, especially the thumb, second and third fingers, often occurring at night, and by weakness, especially in apposition of thumb and little finger. This entity is frequently accompanied by visible or palpable swelling at the wrist, and by slight swelling of the hand.

Amyloid may occasionally infiltrate the skeletal musculature, producing a sense of firmness to the overlying skin. Conversely, in occasional patients, the pulp of the fingertips will become flaccid and seemingly ''empty,'' due, one presumes, to amyloid infiltration of the very small peripheral vessels (Fig. 142-10).

The physician who, on the basis of these manifestations, becomes suspicious that the patient may have amyloidosis, should look for other clinical evidence of this disease, such as an enlarged, stiffened tongue (Fig. 142-11), albuminuria, partial heart block, evidence of multiple myeloma, or the presence of immunoglobulin light chains in blood or urine. Screening for the latter is done by obtaining serum protein electrophoresis and immunoelectrophoresis, and electrophoresis and immunoelectrophoresis of a urine specimen which has been concentrated prior to analysis [54]. Referral to an internist for further examination is recommended.

Other forms of amyloid (AA, AF, and AS). Dermatologic involvement of the skin in ''secondary'' amyloidosis (AA) is analogous to amyloid involvement of the heart [22] in

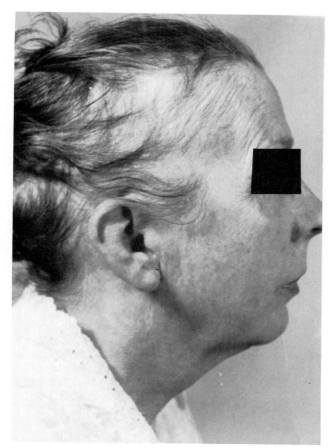

Fig. 142-9 Patchy alopecia in a patient with amyloid AL.

this form of systemic disease. In both organs, while the changes are evident histologically in all or nearly all cases, they are rarely if ever associated with clinical manifestations. While dermatologic features, such as purpuric nodules or plaques have been reported in an occasional patient with amyloidosis accompanying prolonged inflammatory disease [55], it is now recognized that the mere association of systemic amyloidosis and an inflammatory disease does not yield proof that the relationship is more than coincidental [22]. The use of the potassium permanganate staining technique [56,57] provides a simple, inexpensive means of differentiating amyloid AA from amyloid AL or AS in parenchymal tissues in these forms of systemic amyloidosis.

Based upon earlier studies [58], indicating that amyloid deposits occur in subcutaneous fat in most cases of secondary amyloidosis (AA), Westermark and Stenkvist have performed multiple, fine-needle biopsies of subcutaneous fat in patients with amyloidosis and have stained air-dried smears of the aspirated material with alkaline Congo red [59]. Positive results by this procedure were corroborated on rectal biopsy or autopsy in all of the nine patients studied (eight of whom had amyloidosis AA).

Senile amyloidosis (amyloid AS) has not, as yet, been shown to be accompanied by histologic or clinical involvement of the skin. Certain dermatologic changes may, however, be seen in association with familial forms of amyloidosis (amyloid AP). These may be secondary to underlying neuropathy. An example is the anhidrosis and muscle atro-

phy which accompanies severe cases of primary familial amyloidosis of Andrade (AFp) [16,60]. This syndrome, endemic in a small region of Portugal north of Porto, is also frequently seen in persons of Brazilian ancestry. Similarly, patients with one of the rare familial neuropathic forms of amyloidosis may exhibit atrophy of the skin of the extremities secondary to marked peripheral neuropathy.

Amyloidosis AA associated with inflammatory processes of the skin

As pointed out by Brownstein and Helwig [61], "Several forms of cutaneous amyloidosis are recognized, but it is not generally appreciated that certain dermatoses may be *complicated* by systemic amyloidosis." In a review of 100 autopsy cases of systemic amyloidosis AA conducted at the Armed Forces Institute of Pathology, these authors identified eight patients in whom the amyloidosis was preceded by severe chronic dermatoses. Case reports were presented for six of these, with the following diagnoses: stasis dermatitis and recurrent ulcers over 25 years, markedly ulcerated basal cell carcinoma, hidradenitis suppurativa, generalized psoriasis and psoriatic arthritis, dystrophic epidermolysis bullosa, and advanced lepromatous leprosy. Mendel et al [62] reported seven cases of renal amyloidosis in 150 consecutively examined drug addicts who had received serial intravenous or, in one instance, subcutaneous injections. Twenty-three of these patients had localized chronic skin infections; over one-fourth of these had renal amyloidosis. Similar observations have been reported by others [63,64]. Other dermatologic conditions that have been reported in association with secondary amyloidosis (AA) include chronically infected burns, epidermolysis bullosa acquisita, dermatomyositis, hidradenitis suppurativa, and X-linked anhidrotic ectodermal dysplasia [28].

Pathogenesis of amyloidosis of the skin

Studies referred to earlier in this chapter make it quite clear that amyloid fibrils are formed from precursor proteins or polypeptides which exhibit the cross-beta antiparallel beta-pleated sheet conformation and, under appropriate stimulus, become linked together to form amyloid fibrils. The process by which this linkage takes place and the factors that control it are not clearly understood. In vitro studies [65] have indicated that amyloid fibrils can be formed through a process of degradation of serum protein A by the action of macrophages. Whether this mechanism is operative in other forms of amyloidosis is not known.

Although there has long been a debate as to whether amyloidogenesis takes place in situ or whether the precursors circulate and are deposited in locations far from their site of formation, it is now generally accepted that either pattern may be at work in different forms of amyloidosis. For example, it seems reasonable to assume that amyloid accumulation surrounding medullary carcinoma of the thyroid is formed through transformation of prethyrocalcitonin, synthesized by the thyroid gland. On the other hand, in amyloidosis AL, the precursor immunoglobulins are, presumably, synthesized by plasma cells, primarily in the bone marrow, and transformed into amyloid fibrils at the

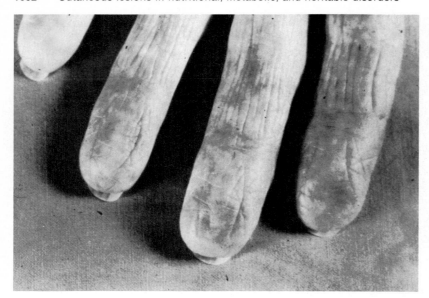

Fig. 142-10 Flaccid fingertips that look "empty" related to amyloid infiltration of small peripheral vessels.

sites of deposition in blood vessel walls and tissue parenchyma.

Over the past two or three years, application of sensitive immunohistologic techniques has provided increased understanding of the nature of the amyloid fibrils in the various forms of amyloidosis involving the skin. These studies have provided added grounds for a clear differentiation of the lichenoid and macular forms of primary localized cutaneous amyloidosis from the nodular or tumefaction forms. In the latter entities, it is now accepted that the amyloid fibrils are comprised primarily of immunoglobulin light chains. Although some immunofluorescence studies have demonstrated that immunoglobulins, kappa and lambda light chains, and complement are present in the deposits of macular and papular amyloid [66,67], there is now a general consensus that the fibrils themselves are not composed of immunoglobulins but, instead, absorb these substances in a nonspecific fashion [68,69]. Evidence also suggests that, in these forms of amyloidosis, the fibrils are composed neither of amyloid protein AA nor, in all likelihood, of prealbumin [70]. The fact that, in lichen amyloidosis, amyloid in the skin exhibits the so-called resistant reaction to potassium permanganate [56,57] does not prove or even suggest that this form of amyloid is of the AA type, as proposed by Maeda et al [71]. Amyloid AA characteristically exhibits the "sensitive" response to potassium permanganate, while lichen amyloid shares with amyloid AL and AS the property of "resistance." Immunohistologic studies have shown that neither lichenoid nor macular amyloid contains amyloid AA, AL, ASc, or AEt [72,73]. While the nature of the fibrils in lichen amyloid has not been elucidated, clearly the best evidence suggests that they have a close relationship with keratin-like material derived from tonofilaments of epidermal cells [74–77]. Striking similarities have been observed between keratin and amyloid [78]. There are, however, distinct differences between colloid, which is also derived from necrotic keratinocytes, and amyloid. For example, colloid does not evidence the Congo red birefringence that is characteristic of amyloid. These differences suggest that in lichen amy-

loidosis the keratin material must be modified in some way. In this regard it should be noted that one of the characteristics this form of amyloid shares with most others is the presence, in small concentration, of a substance known as P-component, which is homologous with a normal serum protein referred to as SAP (serum amyloid P-component). So consistent is the presence of P-component in lichen amyloidosis that Breathnach et al [69] have utilized an indirect immunofluorescence method, using specific fluorescence with anti-SAP, to identify these deposits.

In short, these histochemical and immunochemical studies provide clear grounds for supporting the clinical differentiation between papular and macular PLCA and nodular and tumefaction forms. While the latter entities appear to represent one form of immunoglobulin-derived amyloid (AL), the precise nature and source of origin of the fibrilloprotein in the former still requires further study.

Recent studies by an Israeli group [79,80] have established an in vitro model for studying factors influencing solubilization of amyloid fibrils AA.

Although these observations have not been corroborated by others, they add further impetus to the need to study more actively the process of amyloid resorption. It seems likely that amyloid is a dynamic substance that is constantly being deposited and resorbed. The defect in amyloidosis may represent an alteration in the balance between these control factors.

The therapeutic implications of this observation are very exciting. In the preliminary studies of Kedar et al [80] three agents (ascorbic acid, sodium citrate, and EDTA) were found to neutralize the effect of the inhibitor protein, thus restoring the amyloid degrading activity of the amyloidotic serum to normal. Although ascorbic acid has been tried as a therapeutic agent in amyloidosis with only equivocal results, the observation of Kedar et al may provide an important aid in the development of improved treatment of amyloidosis through the availability of a much more rapid means of assessing the effectiveness of therapeutic agents.

Recent studies have led to an increasing awareness of

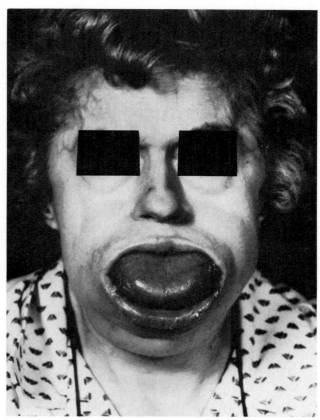

Fig. 142-11   Enlarged, stiffened tongue characteristic of systemic amyloidosis AL.

the biologic importance of SAA, the serum protein homologous with amyloid protein AA in the acute phase response which occurs following serious injury or infection. Changes that accompany this response include an increase of approximately 50 percent in the concentration of ceruloplasmin and C3, a twofold increase in the concentration of alpha$_1$-acid glycoprotein, fibrinogen, and several other substances, and an increase of several hundredfold or more in C-reactive protein and SAA [81,82].

SAA is synthesized by the liver [83]. Its rate of synthesis depends on a stimulating substance, similar if not identical with interleukin 1 [84,85]. This term refers to a soluble monokyne synthesized by macrophages in response to inflammatory or antigenic stimulation. Many individuals experience, at various periods, marked increases in concentration of SAA; few, however, develop amyloidosis. The factors that determine the formation of amyloid AA, presumably from the precursor protein SAA, are not fully understood. Kesilevsky and Boudreau [85] have recently obtained data, using a mouse model of experimental amyloidosis, which suggests that an amyloid enhancing factor (AEF), which can be extracted from spleens of preamyloidotic mice, may alter the acute phase response so that amyloid fibrils will be deposited in the spleen [86]. The interrelationship of the precursors, mediators, and enhancers of amyloid deposition has recently been reviewed [87].

Amyloid P-component referred to earlier, is present in all or nearly all amyloid deposits in quantities amounting to 10 to 15 percent of isolated amyloid fibril weight [87,88]. The role of this component is not yet understood. The

serum protein with which it is homologous, SAP, has a number of similarities to C-reactive protein. Both exhibit an almost identical pentameric structure on electron microscopy. Both exhibit calcium-dependent ligand binding capacity and extensive homology of amino acid sequence. The two are not identical, however. The P-component has been shown to be a normal constituent of human glomerular basement membrane and of elastic fiber microfibrils. It acts as an acute phase reactant in the mouse, but not in other species. The fact that this component appears to be present in all forms of amyloid, without regard to the specific chemical nature or presumptive precursor of the amyloid fibril, suggests that it may play an important role in the genesis of this group of tissue deposits.

In summary, therefore, there has been a rapid expansion of our knowledge concerning the nature of the amyloid fibril in the various forms of amyloidosis, in the identity of the putative precursor compounds, and in the biologic factors and forces involved. We still lack information, however, concerning the precise mechanism by which amyloid fibrils are formed from the precursor proteins, and how this process can be prevented or reversed.

Therapy of amyloidosis

With regard to therapy of systemic amyloidosis, it has been shown that colchicine treatment of patients with familial Mediterranean fever prevents amyloid deposition [89–92]. Colchicine has also been shown to inhibit the deposit of amyloid AA in the mouse model [93]. In the accelerated model of mouse amyloidosis, it has been shown to slow the rate of amyloid deposition if given early in the induction period [94]. This effect is accompanied by a temporary decrease in SAA concentration. The effectiveness of this agent in various forms of human amyloidosis (including amyloidosis accompanying familial Mediterranean fever, once established) [92] has been much less encouraging.

Dimethyl sulfoxide (DMSO) has also been shown to be effective in the treatment of experimental amyloidosis [95]. In the accelerated mouse model, DMSO is most effective when given during the period of rapid amyloid deposition, early in the course of the condition [94]. In the mouse, DMSO treatment has a more profound inhibiting effect on amyloidogenesis than does colchicine, and its administration is accompanied by a more significant and prolonged decrease in the serum concentration of SAA [95]. DMSO was shown to be effective in a small group of patients with amyloidosis AA secondary to rheumatoid arthritis [96] but its value in the treatment of amyloid AL has so far proved disappointing [97]. In addition, the sickening odor experienced by patients receiving this medication has inhibited its extensive use. Localized treatment of patients with amyloid infiltration of the skin would seem to represent a logical area for clinical study, but we are not aware of reports concerning this avenue of treatment.

Treatment of patients with amyloidosis AL with melphalan and prednisone, in the regimen that has proved effective in multiple myeloma, appears eminently logical. Unfortunately, while this treatment is effective for myeloma, its inconsistent effectiveness in inducing remissions of amyloid, as balanced against its toxicity, tempers its widespread use in amyloidosis except when associated with myeloma [98,99].

For most patients, therefore, careful, thoughtful, symptomatic therapy, explanation of the nature of the disease, and the use of agents such as ascorbic acid and colchicine which are, at least, relatively harmless provide the best approach to treatment. It seems likely that the rapid expansion of our knowledge concerning the nature and pathogenesis of this group of diseases will soon lead to more effective therapy.

References

1. Puchtler H, Sweat F: Congo red as a stain for fluorescence microscopy of amyloid. *J Histochem Cytochem* **13**:693, 1965
2. Franklin EC: Amyloid and amyloidosis of the skin. *J Invest Dermatol* **67**:451, 1976
3. Kyle RA: Amyloidosis. Part 1. *Int J Dermatol* **19**:537, 1980
4. Cohen AS: An update of clinical, pathologic and biochemical aspects of amyloidosis. *Int J Dermatol* **20**:515, 1981
5. Vassar PS, Culling CFA: Fluorescent stains with special reference to amyloid and connective tissues. *Arch Pathol* **68**:487, 1959
6. Wright JR et al: Relationship of amyloid to aging: review of the literature and systematic study of 83 patients derived from a general hospital population. *Medicine (Baltimore)* **48**:39, 1969
7. Cohen AS, Calkins E: Electronmicroscopic observation on a fibrous component in amyloid of diverse origins. *Nature* **183**:1202, 1959
8. Shirahama T, Cohen AS: High resolution electron microscopic analysis of the amyloid fibril. *J Cell Biol* **33**:679, 1967
9. Glenner GG: Amyloid deposits and amyloidosis: the beta fibrilloses. *N Engl J Med* **302**:1283, 1333, 1980
10. Pauling L, Corey RB: Configuration of polypeptide chains with favored orientation around single bonds: two new pleated sheets. *Proc Natl Acad Sci USA* **37**:729, 1951
11. Benditt EP, Eriksen N: Chemical classes of amyloid substance. *Am J Pathol* **65**:231, 1971
12. Glenner GG et al: Amyloid fibril proteins: proof of homology with immunoglobulin light chains by sequence analysis. *Science* **172**:1150, 1971
13. Westermark P et al: Amyloid in polypeptide hormone-producing tumors. *Lab Invest* **37**:212, 1977
14. Westermark P: Amyloid of human islets of Langerhans. II. Electron microscopic analysis of isolated amyloid. *Virchows Arch [Pathol Anat]* **373**:161, 1977
15. Tashjian AH et al: Human calcitonin, immunologic assay, cytologic localization and studies on medullary thyroid carcinoma. *Am J Med* **56**:840, 1974
16. Costa PP et al: Amyloid fibrilprotein related to prealbumin in familial amyloidotic polyneuropathy. *Proc Natl Acad Sci USA* **75**:4499, 1978
17. Levin M et al: The amino acid sequence of a major nonimmunoglobulin component of some amyloid fibrils. *J Clin Invest* **51**:2773, 1972
18. Sipe JD et al: Amyloid fibril protein AA: purification and properties of the antigenically related serum component as determined by solid phase radioimmunoassay. *J Immunol* **16**:1151, 1976
19. Stearman RS et al: Regulation of synthesis of amyloid A-related protein, in *C-Reactive Protein and the Plasma Protein Response to Tissue Injury,* edited by I Kushner et al. New York, Annals of the New York Academy of Sciences, 1982, p 106
20. Benditt EP et al: Guidelines for nomenclature, in *Amyloid and Amyloidosis,* edited by GG Glenner et al. Amsterdam/Oxford/Princeton, Excerpta Medica, 1980
21. Cohen AS, Wegelius O: Classification of amyloid 1979–80. *Arthritis Rheum* **23**:644, 1980
22. Wright JR, Calkins E: Clinical-pathologic differentiation of common amyloid syndromes. *Medicine (Baltimore)* **60**:429, 1981
23. Cornwell GG et al: Frequency and distribution of senile cardiovascular amyloid. *Am J Med* **75**:618, 1983
24. Glenner GG: Current knowledge of amyloid deposits as applied to senile plaques and congophilic angiopathy, in *Alzheimer's Disease: Senile Dementia and Related Disorders,* edited by R Katzman et al. New York, Raven Press, 1978, p 493
25. Fujihara S, Glenner GG: Primary localized amyloidosis of the genitourinary tract: immunohistochemical study on 11 cases. *Lab Invest* **44**:55, 1981
26. Brownstein MY, Helwig EB: The cutaneous amyloidoses. I. Localized forms. *Arch Dermatol* **102**:8, 1971
27. Hashimoto K, Yoong OLL: Lichen amyloidosis. Some new findings. *Arch Dermatol* **104**:648, 1971
28. Kyle RA: Amyloidosis. Part 3. *Int J Dermatol* **20**:75, 1981
29. Wong CK: Lichen amyloidosis; a relatively common skin disorder in Taiwan. *Arch Dermatol* **110**:438, 1974
30. Rajagopalan K, Tay CH: Familial lichen amyloidosis: report of 19 cases in 4 generations of a Chinese family in Malaysia. *Br J Dermatol* **87**:123, 1972
31. Vasily DB et al: Familial primary cutaneous amyloidosis. *Arch Dermatol* **114**:1173, 1978
32. Brownstein MH, Hashimoto K: Macular amyloidosis. *Arch Dermatol* **106**:50, 1972
33. Brownstein MH et al: Biphasic amyloidosis; link between macular and lichenoid forms. *Br J Dermatol* **88**:25, 1973
34. Bedi TR, Data BN: Diffuse biphasic primary cutaneous amyloidosis. *Dermatologica* **158**:433, 1979
35. Ogino A, Tanaka S: Poikiloderma-like cutaneous amyloidosis. *Dermatologica* **155**:301, 1977
36. Gottschalk L: Macular amyloidosis with localized amyloid of the upper air passages. *Arch Dermatol* **111**:1017, 1975
37. Kyle RA, Bayrd ED: Amyloidosis: review of 236 cases. *Medicine (Baltimore)* **54**:271, 1975
38. Chapel TA: Nodular primary localized cutaneous amyloidosis. *Arch Dermatol* **113**:1248, 1977
39. Ratz JL, Bailen PL: Cutaneous amyloidosis; a case report of the tumefaction variant and a review of the spectrum of clinical presentations. *J Am Acad Dermatol* **4**:21, 1981
40. Tsuti T et al: Secondary localized cutaneous amyloidosis in solar elastosis. *Br J Dermatol* **106**:469, 1982
41. Malak JA, Smith EW: Secondary localized cutaneous amyloidosis. *Arch Dermatol* **86**:125, 1962
42. Brownstein MH, Helwig EB: The cutaneous amyloidoses. II. Systemic forms. *Arch Dermatol* **103**:20, 1971
43. Rubinow A, Cohen AS: Skin involvement in generalized amyloidosis: a study of clinically involved and uninvolved skin in 50 patients with primary and secondary amyloidosis. *Ann Intern Med* **88**:781, 1978
44. Kyle RA: Amyloidosis. Part 2. *Int J Dermatol* **120**:20, 1981
45. Furie AB et al: Mechanism of factor X deficiency in systemic amyloidosis. *N Engl J Med* **304**:827, 1981
46. Greipp PR et al: Factor X deficiency in amyloidosis: a critical review. *Am J Hematol* **11**:443, 1981
47. Goltz RW: Systematized amyloidosis: a review of the skin and mucous membrane lesions and a report of two cases. *Medicine (Baltimore)* **31**:381, 1952
48. Gordon DA et al: Amyloid arthritis simulating rheumatoid disease in five patients with multiple myeloma. *Am J Med* **55**:142, 1973
49. Holden CA et al: Trauma induced bullae: the presenting feature of systemic amyloidosis associated with plasma cell dyscrasia. *Br J Dermatol* **107**:701, 1982
50. Northover JMA et al: Bullous lesions of the skin and mucous membranes in primary amyloidosis. *Postgrad Med J* **48**:351, 1972

51. Chow C et al: Bullous amyloidosis. *Arch Dermatol* 95:622, 1967

52. Lambird PA, Hartmann WH: Hereditary amyloidosis, the flexor retinaculum and the carpal tunnel syndrome. *Am J Clin Pathol* 52:714, 1969

53. Bashan FO: Amyloidosis and the carpal tunnel syndrome. *Am J Clin Pathol* 61:711, 1974

54. Calkins E, Wright JR: Amyloidosis, in *Principles of Immunologic Diagnosis in Medicine,* edited by F Milgrom et al. Philadelphia, Lea & Febiger, 1981, p 341

55. Michelson HE, Lynch FW: Systemic amyloidosis of the skin and muscles. *Arch Dermatol Syphilol* 29:805, 1934

56. Wright JR et al: Potassium permanganate reaction to amyloidosis: a histologic method to assist in differentiating forms of this disease. *Lab Invest* 36:274, 1977

57. van Rijswijk MH, van Heuden CWGJ: The potassium permanganate method: a reliable method for differentiating amyloid AA from other forms of amyloid in routine laboratory practice. *Am J Pathol* 97:43, 1979

58. Westermark P: Occurrence of amyloid deposits in the skin in secondary systemic amyloidosis. *Acta Pathol Microbiol Scand [A]* 80:718, 1972

59. Westermark P, Stenkvist B: A new method for the diagnosis of systemic amyloidosis. *Arch Intern Med* 132:522, 1973

60. Andrade C: Peculiar form of peripheral neuropathy; familial atypical generalized amyloidosis with special involvement of peripheral nerves. *Brain* 75:408, 1952

61. Brownstein MH, Helwig EB: Systemic amyloidosis complicating dermatoses. *Arch Dermatol* 102:1, 1970

62. Mendel S et al: AA protein-related renal amyloidosis in drug addicts. *Am J Pathol* 112:195, 1983

63. Jacob H et al: Amyloid secondary to drug abuse and chronic skin suppuration. *Arch Intern Med* 138:1150, 1978

64. Scholes J et al: Amyloidosis in chronic heroin addicts with the nephrotic syndrome. *Ann Intern Med* 91:26, 1979

65. Lavie G et al: Degradation of serum amyloid A protein by surface associated enzymes of human blood monocytes. *J Exp Med* 148:1020, 1978

66. MacDonald DM et al: Immunofluorescence studies in primary localized cutaneous amyloidosis. *Br J Dermatol* 96:635, 1977

67. MacDonald DM et al: Localized cutaneous amyloidosis; a clinical review of 100 cases including immunofluorescence studies, in *Amyloid and Amyloidosis,* edited by GG Glenner et al. Amsterdam/Oxford/Princeton, Excerpta Medica, 1980, p 239

68. Danno K, Imamura S: Deposition of complement C1q in primary localized cutaneous amyloidosis. *Br J Dermatol* 107:129, 1982

69. Breathnach SM et al: Immunohistochemical deposition of amyloid P component in skin of normal subjects and patients with cutaneous amyloidosis. *Br J Dermatol* 105:115, 1981

70. Breathnach SM et al: Primary localized cutaneous amyloidosis: dermal amyloid deposits do not bind antibodies to amyloid A protein, prealbumin or fibronectin. *Br J Dermatol* 107:453, 1982

71. Maeda H et al: Epidermal origin of the amyloid in localized cutaneous amyloidosis. *Br J Dermatol* 106:345, 1982

72. Cornwell GG III et al: Senile cardiac amyloid evidence that fibrils contain a protein immunologically related to prealbumin. *Immunology* 44:447, 1981

73. Norén P et al: Immunofluorescence and histochemical studies of localized cutaneous amyloidosis. *Br J Dermatol* 108:277, 1983

74. Hashimoto K, Kumakiri M: Colloid-amyloid bodies in PUVA treated psoriatic patients. *J Invest Dermatol* 72:70, 1979

75. Kumakiri M, Hashimoto K: Histogenesis of primary localized cutaneous amyloidosis: sequential change of epidermal keratinocytes to amyloid via filamentous degradation. *J Invest Dermatol* 73:150, 1979

76. Masu S et al: Amyloid in localized cutaneous amyloidosis: immunofluorescence studies with anti-keratin antiserum especially concerning the difference between systemic and localized cutaneous amyloidosis. *Acta Derm Venereol (Stockh)* 61:381, 1981

77. Kobayashi H, Hashimoto K: Antigenic identity of amyloid in localized cutaneous amyloidosis with keratin (abstr). *J Invest Dermatol* 76:320, 1981

78. Gueft B: The analogy of amyloid and keratin as suggested by x-ray, amino acid, and ultrastructural analysis. *Mt Sinai J Med (NY)* 39:91, 1972

79. Kedar I et al: Demonstration of amyloid degrading activity in normal human serum. *Proc Soc Exp Biol Med* 145:343, 1974

80. Kedar I et al: Degradation of amyloid by a serum component and inhibition of degradation: a dynamic concept of amyloid deposition. *J Lab Clin Med* 99:693, 1982

81. Kushner I: The phenomenon of the acute phase response, in *C-Reactive Protein and the Plasma Protein Response to Tissue Injury,* edited by I Kushner et al. New York, Annals of the New York Academy of Sciences, 1982, p 39

82. Benson MD: *In vitro* synthesis of the acute phase reactant SAA by hepatocytes, in *C-Reactive Protein and the Plasma Protein Response to Tissue Injury,* edited by I Kushner et al. New York, Annals of the New York Academy of Sciences, 1982, p 116

83. Sipe JD et al: The role of interleukin 1 in acute phase serum amyloid A (SAA) and serum amyloid P (SAP) biosynthesis, in *C-Reactive Protein and the Plasma Protein Response to Tissue Injury,* edited by I Kushner et al. New York, Annals of the New York Academy of Sciences, 1982, p 137

84. Vogel SN, Sipe JD: The role of macrophages in the acute phase SAA response to endotoxin. *Surv Immunol Res* 1:235, 1982

85. Kesilevsky R, Boudreau L: Kinetics of amyloid deposition. I. The effects of amyloid-enhancing factor and splenectomy. *Lab Invest* 48:53, 1983

86. Cohen AS et al: Editorial: Amyloid proteins, precursors, mediator, and enhancer. *Lab Invest* 48:1, 1983

87. Skinner M et al: Studies in amyloid protein AP, in *Amyloid and Amyloidogenesis,* edited by GG Glenner et al. Amsterdam/Oxford/Princeton, Excerpta Medica, 1980, p 384

88. Peppys MB et al: Biology of serum amyloid P component, in *C-Reactive Protein and the Plasma Protein Response to Tissue Injury,* edited by I Kushner et al. New York, Annals of the New York Academy of Sciences, 1982, p 286

89. Dyck RF et al: Amyloid P component in a constituent of normal human glomerular basement membrane. *J Exp Med* 152:1162, 1980

90. Zemer D et al: A controlled trial of colchicine in preventing attacks of familial Mediterranean fever. *N Engl J Med* 291:932, 1974

91. Dinarello CA et al: Colchicine therapy for familial Mediterranean fever. A double-blind study. *N Engl J Med* 291:934, 1974

92. Zemer D et al: Daily prophylactic colchicine in familial Mediterranean fever, in *Amyloid and Amyloidosis,* edited by GG Glenner et al. Amsterdam/Oxford/Princeton, Excerpta Medica, 1980, p 580

93. Shirahama T, Cohen AS: Blockage of amyloid induction by colchicine in an animal model. *J Exp Med* 140:1102, 1974

94. Kesilevsky R et al: Kinetics of amyloid deposition. II. The effect of DMSO and colchicine therapy. *Lab Invest* 48:60, 1983

95. Kedar I et al: Treatment of experimental murine amyloidosis with dimethyl sulfoxide. *Eur J Clin Invest* 7:149, 1977

96. van Rijswijk MH et al: Successful treatment with DMSO of

human amyloidosis secondary to rheumatoid arthritis, in *Amyloid and Amyloidosis,* edited by GG Glenner et al. Amsterdam/Oxford/Princeton, Excerpta Medica, 1980, p 570

97. Osserman EF et al: Further studies of therapy of amyloidosis with DMSO, in *Amyloid and Amyloidosis,* edited by GG Glenner et al. Amsterdam/Oxford/Princeton, Excerpta Medica, 1980, p 563

98. Kyle RA, Greipp PR: Primary systemic amyloidosis: comparison of melphalan and prednisone versus placebo. *Blood* **54:**818, 1978

99. Korkery J et al: Resolution of amyloidosis and plasma cell dyscrasia with combination therapy. *Lancet* **2:**425, 1978

CHAPTER 143

THE PORPHYRIAS

David R. Bickers and Madhu A. Pathak

The porphyrias are among the most intriguing diseases of humans. Widely variable, even bizarre in their clinical manifestations, these disorders of porphyrin or porphyrin precursor metabolism result from aberrations in the control of the porphyrin-heme biosynthetic pathway. Heme, the end product of the pathway, is a tetrapyrrole, protoporphyrin (PROTO), chelated with ferrous iron. Because of its special ability to bind and release oxygen, heme functions in numerous metabolic pathways of living organisms. Heme is the prosthetic group for a number of proteins including hemoglobin, myoglobin, catalases, peroxidases, cytochromes P-450 and P-448 and a_3, etc.; without this iron-chelated tetrapyrrole, most essential biochemical pathways in the body could not function. Chlorophyll, a magnesium-chelated porphyrin, is another important tetrapyrrole, which is critical for photosynthesis, the specialized energy-storing system found in plants in which the conversion of light energy into stabilized chemical energy is achieved with a sequence of oxidation-reduction reactions. The corrin ring, a cobalt-chelated tetrapyrrole, is a major constituent of vitamin B_{12}, the lack of which results in pernicious anemia. Porphyrins, therefore, are ubiquitous and essential biochemical constituents of living beings. The biologic importance of the porphyrins and their iron complexes in metabolism lies in their capacity to act as mediators of oxidation reactions and either as oxidative components in the metabolism of steroids, drugs, and environmental chemicals or as a means of exchanging gases such as oxygen and carbon dioxide between the environment and the tissues of the body.

Daily synthesis of porphyrins and heme in humans occurs in amounts sufficient to provide for the body's metabolic requirements. The control of heme synthesis is so precise that, under normal circumstances, microgram quantities or less of pathway intermediates are present in plasma, red blood cells (RBC), urine, and stool (see Table 143-1).

Porphyria results from either inherited or acquired abnormalities in heme synthesis causing excessive accumulation of heme pathway intermediates in the body. Each type of human porphyria appears to be characterized by deficient activity of specific enzymes, as shown in Table 143-2. The different porphyrias arising from such derangements of normal heme synthesis manifest patterns of accumulation and excretion of specific porphyrins and/or their precursors [1,2]. In general, the major porphyrin or porphyrin precursor excreted in a given porphyria is the substrate for the defective enzyme. The different porphyrias arising from such derangements of normal heme synthesis are also characterized by accumulation and excretion of specific porphyrins and/or their precursors (Table 143-3). These intermediates, when present in excess amounts, exert toxic effects that are likely responsible for the expression of clinical porphyria.

The porphyrias are of particular dermatologic interest because several of them have distinct cutaneous manifestations that may permit diagnosis from clinical signs alone. Furthermore, simple laboratory procedures, easily performed in a physician's office, can confirm a clinically suspected diagnosis in many instances and can also help to initiate appropriate therapeutic measures for the amelioration of the biochemical derangements and the clinical symptoms of these diseases.

Historical aspects

One of the first known reported cases of cutaneous porphyria was that of Schultz [3], who described a 33-year-old man with marked cutaneous photosensitivity and splenomegaly which he called pemphigus leprosus, a bullous disease. The urine was red. Spectroscopic studies by Schultz and subsequently by Baumstark [4] identified abnormal urinary pigments which were named urorubrohematin and urofuscohematin. This abnormal pigment was most likely uroporphyrin (URO) and this patient probably had porphyria, but of what type is disputed [5]. Anderson [6] reported two brothers with a scarring photosensitivity which he called hydroa aestivale. Beginning in childhood, this disease was said to be associated with "hematoporphyrin" in the urine. He implied that the abnormal urinary pigment was related to the skin disease.

Detailed studies by Günther early in this century led to the first classification of the porphyrias [7]. Günther felt that the dark pigment in the urine of patients with porphyria was the synthetic porphyrin, hematoporphyrin, but subsequent studies by Fischer proved that this pigment was a natural porphyrin which he named URO since it was isolated from the urine of a patient with congenital porphyria

Table 143-1   Normal values of porphyrins and porphyrin precursors in humans

Porphyrins or precursors	Urine (μg/24 h)	RBC (μg/100 mL packed cells)	Plasma (μg/100 mL)	Feces (μg/g dry wt)
δ-Aminolevulinic acid (ALA)	4000	–	–	–
Porphobilinogen (PBG)	1500	–	–	–
Uroporphyrin (URO)	40	0–2.0	0–2	10–50
Coproporphyrin (COPRO)	280	0–2.0	0–1	10–50
Protoporphyrin (PROTO)	Absent	90	0–2	0–20
X-porphyrin	Absent	Absent	Absent	Trace
Isocoproporphyrin (ISOCOPRO)	Absent	Absent	Absent	
	(nmol/day)	(nmol/dL)	(nmol/dL)	(nmol/g dry weight)
δ-Aminolevulinic acid (ALA)	4.6×10^4	–	–	–
Porphobilinogen (PBG)	8.8×10^3	–	–	–
Uroporphyrin (URO)	40		–	24
Coproporphyrin (COPRO)	280		–	46
Protoporphyrin (PROTO)	0	285	0.5	134

[8]. The detailed study of Mathias Petry, the celebrated but unfortunate patient with congenital erythropoietic porphyria (EP), added greatly to modern knowledge of porphyria and of the cutaneous photosensitivity associated with it [9,10]. This is an excellent example of the interaction of basic science and clinical medicine leading to important new knowledge about the metabolic basis of a human disease.

Other types of porphyria known as acute intermittent porphyria (AIP) and porphyria cutanea tarda (PCT) were first defined in Sweden by Waldenström in 1937 [11]. Subsequently, Brunsting [12], Waldenström [13], and Schmid [14] further characterized PCT in various human populations and showed that environmental factors such as drugs and chemicals could influence the clinical expression of this disease. Barnes [15], Dean [16], and Dean and Barnes [17] described a type of porphyria characterized by cutaneous manifestations identical to those of PCT and acute attacks identical to those of AIP. Known as variegate porphyria (VP), this disease occurs most frequently in South African whites.

In the past several years it has become apparent that VP

occurs in other areas of the world, including the United States, much more commonly than previously appreciated [18–22].

Another porphyria of bone marrow origin, erythropoietic protoporphyria (EPP) was described in 1961 by Magnus et al in England [23] and an extremely rare disorder, erythropoietic coproporphyria, was identified in Germany by Heilmeyer and Clotten in 1964 [24]. In 1955 Berger and Goldberg in Scotland first described hereditary coproporphyria (HCP) [25]. Finally, the most recently identified disorder known as hepatoerythropoietic porphyria (HEP) was described in 1969 by Pinõl-Aguadé [26].

Porphyrin-heme biosynthesis

Most mammalian cells, including those in the epidermis and dermis, can synthesize the heme required for formation of essential heme-proteins; however, the major sites of heme synthesis in the body are the bone marrow and the liver.

Heme is the prosthetic group for a number of hemoproteins, including hemoglobin, myoglobin, mitochondrial cy-

Table 143-2   Enzyme activities in various porphyrias

Enzyme	Tissue	Postulated enzymatic defect
δ-Aminolevulinic acid synthase (ALAS)	Liver, kidney, fibroblasts, lymphocytes	Increased activity in AIP, HCP, and VP
δ-Aminolevulinic acid dehydrase (ALAD)	Erythrocytes, liver, kidney	Decreased in lead intoxication
Porphobilinogen deaminase (PBGD)	Erythrocytes, liver, fibroblasts, lymphocytes, amnion cells	Decreased in AIP
Uroporphyrinogen-III cosynthase (UROCOSYN-III)	Erythrocytes, fibroblasts	Decreased in EP
Uroporphyrinogen decarboxylase (UROGEND)	Erythrocytes, liver	Decreased in PCT and HEP
Coproporphyrinogen oxidase (COPROGENO)	Fibroblasts, lymphocytes, liver	Decreased in HCP
Protoporphyrinogen oxidase (PROTOGENO)	Liver, fibroblasts	Decreased in VP
Ferrochelatase	Bone marrow, fibroblasts	Decreased in EPP, in lead poisoning, and ? in VP

Table 143-3 Biochemical features of the porphyrias

Type of porphyria	Blood				Stool			Urine				
	RBC URO	RBC COPRO	RBC PROTO	Plasma	URO	COPRO	PROTO	Color	ALA	PBG	URO	COPRO
Erythropoietic:												
Erythropoietic porphyria (EP)	++++	+++	+++	↑ URO & COPRO	+	+++ *	+	Pink to red	N	N	++++ *	++ *
Erythropoietic protoporphyria (EPP)	N	N to +	++++	↑ PROTO	N	++	++ to ++++	N	N	N	N	N
Hepatic:												
Acute intermittent porphyria (AIP)												
Latent	N	N	N	N	N to +	N to +	N to +	Red to purple	+ to +++	+ to +++	N	N to +
Acute	N	N	N	N	N to +	N to +	N to +	Red to purple	++ to ++++	++ to ++++	+++	++
Porphyria variegata (VP)												
Latent	N	N	N	?N	N	+++	++++	N	N	N	N	N
Acute	N	N	N	?N	++	++	+++	Pink to red	++ to +++	++ to +++	+++	+++
Porphyria cutanea tarda (PCT)	N	N	N	↑ URO	++	+++	+ ISOCOPRO	Pink to red	N	N	++++	++
Hereditary copro-porphyria (HCP)												
Latent	N	N	N	?N	++	++++	N to +	N	N to +	N to +	N	N
Acute	N	N	N	?N	+	+++	N to +	Red	++ to N	++ to N	++	++++
Hepatoerythro-poietic porphyria (HEP)	N	+/−	+++	↑ URO ↑ PROTO	N	ISOCOPRO COPRO	N	Pink to red			+++	ISOCOPRO

N = normal, + = above normal, + + = moderately increased, + + + and + + + + = greatly increased; URO = uroporphyrin, COPRO = coproporphyrin, PROTO = protoporphyrin, and ISOCOPRO = isocoproporphyrin. Findings of major diagnostic importance are boxed.
* Type 1 isomers

tochromes, microsomal cytochromes (including cytochrome P-450), catalase, peroxidase, tryptophan pyrrolase, and prostaglandin endoperoxide synthase. The two body organs that produce the vast majority of heme in humans are the liver and the bone marrow. Approximately 85 percent of heme synthesis occurs in bone marrow where it is utilized for the production of hemoglobin. Most remaining heme synthesis occurs in the liver for making cytochrome P-450, catalase, and various mitochondrial cytochromes. Heme is a critical cellular constituent essential for a variety of metabolic processes primarily because of its unique ability to take up and release oxygen and to facilitate oxygen transport. Heme synthesis is regulated by the interplay of a number of factors and is directly dependent upon its concentration within cells and upon the requirements of the cell for production of the various hemoproteins described above. Many of these have rapid turnover times (minutes to hours) thereby necessitating continuously high rates of hepatic heme synthesis (e.g., cytochrome P-450, an important membrane-bound enzyme in the liver involved in the detoxification and metabolism of drugs, has a half-life of 90 to 180 min) [1]. This regulation (and indeed the ability to synthesize heme at all) is dependent upon a series of eight intracellular enzymes whose sequential catalytic activity culminates in heme synthesis. Abnormal control of heme synthesis may result from partial defects in enzymes of the pathway and this may occur as the result of inherited and/or environmental factors. One result of such abnormal control is the accumulation in the body of one or more heme pathway intermediates such as the porphyrins or their precursors which are associated with the clinical disorders that are collectively referred to as the porphyrias. Studies by Schmid and coworkers first clearly proved that the porphyrias reflect derangements in heme synthesis in the liver or the bone marrow [27]. While a diagnosis of porphyria can often be made from a careful history and physical examination, the definitive diagnosis rests upon measurements of porphyrin and/or porphyrin excretion or the activity of one or another of the enzymes in the heme pathway (Table 143-3). Each porphyria demonstrates a unique pattern of porphyrin or porphyrin precursor accumulation in blood, urine, and/or feces. To fully comprehend the meaning as well as the importance of these measurements, it is necessary to have a clear understanding of current concepts regarding the regulation of heme synthesis. The steps involved in the biosynthesis of porphyrins and heme are outlined in Figs. 143-1 and 143-2 and have recently been summarized with extensive references to the details of the individual steps [28–30].

Delta-aminolevulinic acid synthase (ALAS) (Fig. 143-2a)

Heme synthesis begins in the mitochondrion of the cell where succinate and glycine are conjugated to form the aminoketone delta-aminolevulinic acid (ALA). ALAS is the mitochondrial enzyme that catalyzes the formation of ALA. ALAS has the lowest catalytic activity (30 to 50 nm ALA formed/g liver) of any of the other enzymes in the heme pathway. Furthermore, it has a very short half-life (1 to 3 h) compared to other mitochondrial enzymes which generally have half-lives on the order of 3 to 5 days [28]. ALAS is synthesized on ribosomes in the cytosol in an aggregated form consisting of a dimer of two identical, catalytically active subunits of molecular weight 51,000 linked to two catalytically inactive subunits of molecular weights of 79,000 and 120,000 [31]. This is transported into the mitochondrion where the small, catalytically active subunits are released and can produce ALA from glycine and succinate [32].

The major significance of this enzyme is its regulatory role in controlling the rate of heme synthesis in the liver. The putative pool of hepatocellular free heme is thought to regulate heme synthesis by directly influencing the ac-

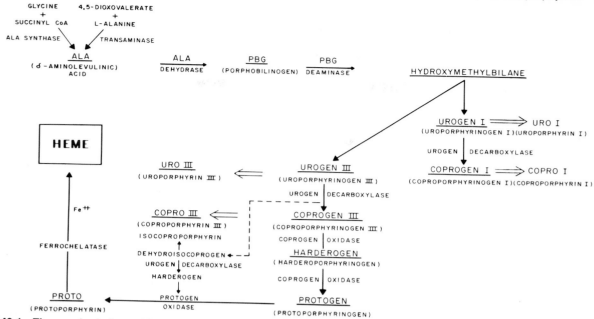

Fig. 143-1 The porphyrin-heme biosynthetic pathway.

tivity of mitochondrial ALAS in two ways: (1) by inhibiting ALAS activity or (2) by controlling its rate of synthesis. ALAS activity is increased in the liver of patients with those hepatic porphyrias in which acute attacks characterized by a neurologic-visceral symptom complex occur. This increase in ALAS is a major marker for AIP, VP, and HCP. It is also an inducible enzyme, and factors that lead to further increases in activity of ALAS are accompanied by exacerbation of the clinical manifestations of these types of porphyria. Conversely, factors that reduce ALAS activity are often useful therapeutically in those porphyrias characterized by elevated activity of the enzyme. The importance of ALAS for the regulation of heme synthesis will be discussed later in the chapter.

It should be pointed out that there is some evidence to suggest that a second mitochondrial enzyme in mammalian liver known as L-alanine-4,5-dioxovalerate (DOVA) aminotransferase can catalyze a transamination between L-alanine and DOVA, yielding ALA (Fig. 143-2a) and pyruvate [33]. The importance of this reaction for production of tetrapyrroles in certain plants is well known but its role in human heme synthesis remains to be defined.

Delta-aminolevulinic acid dehydrase (ALAD)

In the next reaction two molecules of ALA are combined to form the monopyrrole porphobilinogen (PBG) (Fig. 143-2a). Known as delta-aminolevulinic acid dehydrase (ALAD), this enzyme is present in the cytoplasm of the cell. ALAD activity is 50 to 100 times that of ALAS so that virtually all of the ALA synthesized is converted to PBG [28]. ALAD is a sulfhydryl-dependent enzyme which requires zinc for catalytic activity and is very sensitive to heavy metals such as lead. Decreased ALAD activity in the RBC is an excellent indicator and a most sensitive test for detecting lead poisoning [34]. Experimental studies indicate that iron-loading in rats results in a marked decrease

in hepatic ALAD activity [35]. Several patients with neurologic signs and symptoms similar to those occurring in the acute hepatic porphyrias have been reported to have reduced ALAD activity without any evidence of lead intoxication [36]. The etiology of the reduced ALAD activity in these patients is currently unexplained. In addition, patients with one form of hereditary tyrosinemia produce increased amounts of succinylacetone, a close structural analog of ALA, and a potent competitive inhibitor of ALAD activity [37]. These individuals are also said to suffer acute attacks similar to those observed in the acute hepatic porphyrias [38].

Porphobilinogen deaminase (PBGD)

This is the third enzyme in the pathway which in the past was known as uroporphyrinogen synthetase. It combines four molecules of the monopyrrole PBG to form the linear tetrapyrrole, hydroxymethylbilane (Fig. 143-2b) which cyclizes spontaneously to form the initial porphyrinogen or tetrapyrrole known as uroporphyrinogen I (UROGEN I) (Fig. 143-2c). Depending on the manner in which the PBG molecules are arranged, several different isomers of the tetrapyrroles are possible. The sole difference between type I and type III porphyrinogens is that one of the four pyrrole rings is "flipped over." Only two of them (labeled I and III) are known to occur in the mammalian heme synthetic pathway. The enzyme has been purified from human RBC and shown to have a molecular weight of approximately 40,000 and a pH maximum of 8.2 [39]. Except for ALAS, PBGD is present in the lowest concentration of any enzyme in the heme pathway. This suggests that factors (genetic or acquired) that influence PBGD activity may have important regulatory influences on the rate of heme synthesis. Consequently if excessive PBG is formed because of increased ALAS activity, as is often seen in the acute hepatic porphyrias, there may be only partial conversion of this monopyrrole to UROGEN I. These factors account for the elevated urinary PBG characteristic of attacks of the acute hepatic porphyrias. PBGD activity is known to be reduced by about 50 percent in the tissue of patients with AIP and is currently thought to be the primary enzymatic abnormality in this autosomal dominant disorder [40,41].

ALA and PBG, the two aliphatic nonporphyrin precursors of heme, are excreted primarily in the urine and normally this amounts to less than 4000 and 1500 μg of each, respectively, per 24 h (Table 143-1). However, in some types of porphyria (AIP and VP) there may be a 10- to 100-fold increase in urinary excretion of ALA and PBG which can be detected using relatively simple diagnostic tests. For example, PBG reacts with Ehrlich's reagent which contains p-dimethylaminobenzaldehyde in hydrochloric acid to give a positive red-color reaction (Watson-Schwartz test) during attacks of AIP and VP [42]. This cherry-red chromogen is water-soluble and cannot be extracted in chloroform or butanol when PBG is elevated.

Uroporphyrinogen III cosynthase (UROCOSYN III)

By simple inversion of one PBG molecule during synthesis of UROGEN I, the III isomer is formed (Fig. 143-2d). This apparently minor structural alteration is of considerable

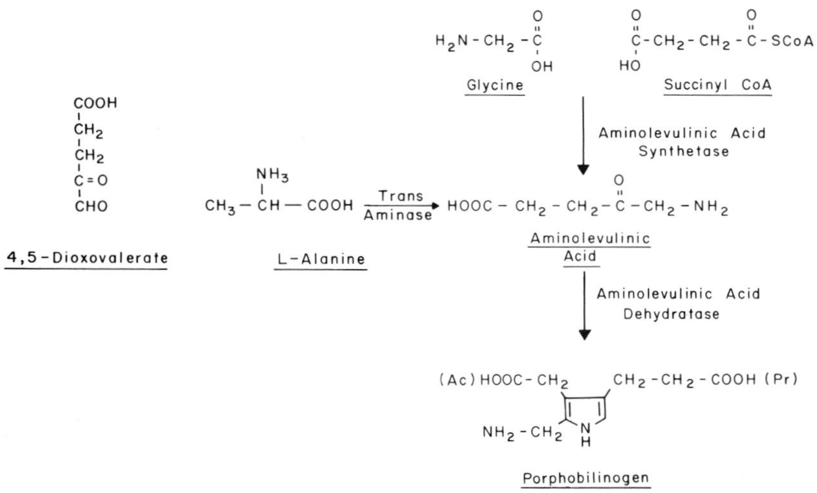

Fig. 143-2 (a and b).

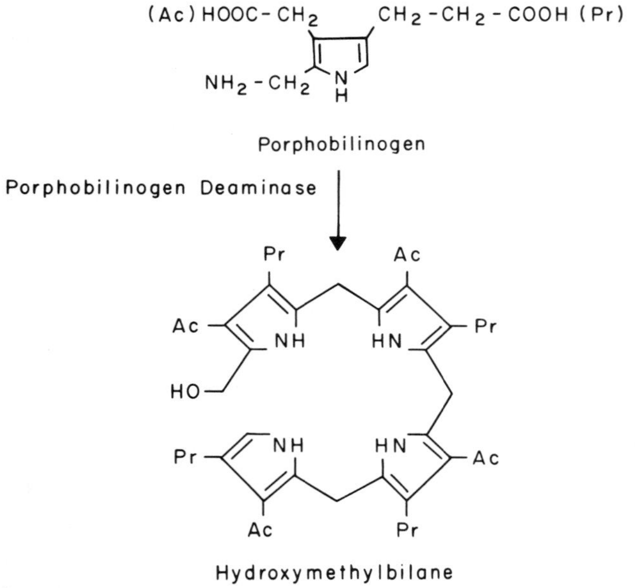

Fig. 143-2 (a) Delta-aminolevulinic acid can be formed in two separate ways. Two molecules of aminolevulinic acid are then combined to form the monopyrrole porphobilinogen. (b) Four molecules of porphobilinogen are converted to a linear tetrapyrrole, hydroxymethylbilane, which can cyclize spontaneously to form uroporphyrinogen. (c) Hydroxymethylbilane forms uroporphyrinogen I. The four acetyl groups of uroporphyrinogen I are sequentially decarboxylated by uroporphyrinogen decarboxylase to form coproporphyrogen I. (d) Hydroxymethylbilane can form uroporphyrinogen I or be converted to uroporphyrinogen III by the enzyme uroporphyrinogen III cosynthase. In this reaction one of the monopyrrole rings is "flipped over." (e) The acetyl groups of uroporphyrinogen III are sequentially decarboxylated by uroporphyrinogen decarboxylase to form 5-carboxylporphyrinogen. (f) 5-Carboxylporphyrinogen either can undergo decarboxylation of its last acetyl group by uroporphyrinogen decarboxylase to form coproporphyrinogen I or III or can undergo oxidative decarboxylation of one propionyl group by coproporphyrinogen oxidase to form dehydroisocoproporphyrinogen. (g) Coproporphyrinogen III is converted to harderoporphyrinogen and to protoporphyrinogen by the enzyme coproporphyrinogen oxidase which oxidatively decarboxylates each of the propionyl groups. (h) The final acetyl group of dehydroisocoproporphyrinogen can undergo decarboxylation by uroporphyrinogen decarboxylase to form harderoporphyrinogen. (i) Dehydroisocoproporphyrinogen can undergo hydration to form isocoproporphyrinogen which can spontaneously oxidize to form isocoproporphyrin. (j) Protoporphyrinogen is converted to protoporphyrin IX by protoporphyrinogen oxidase. Protoporphyrin IX is converted to heme by ferrochelatase which catalyzes the insertion of ferrous iron into the molecule.

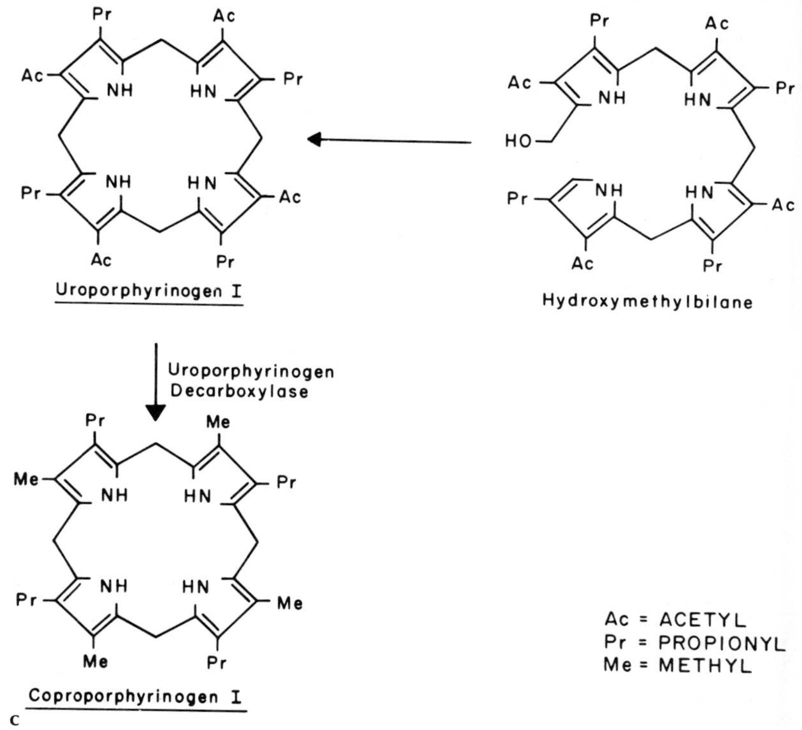

Uroporphyrinogen I

Hydroxymethylbilane

Uroporphyrinogen
Decarboxylase

Coproporphyrinogen I

c

Ac = ACETYL
Pr = PROPIONYL
Me = METHYL

Hydroxymethylbilane

Uroporphyrinogen III
Cosynthetase

Uroporphyrinogen III

Uroporphyrinogen
Decarboxylase

5 Carboxylporphyrinogen

Ac = ACETYL
Pr = PROPIONYL
Me = METHYL

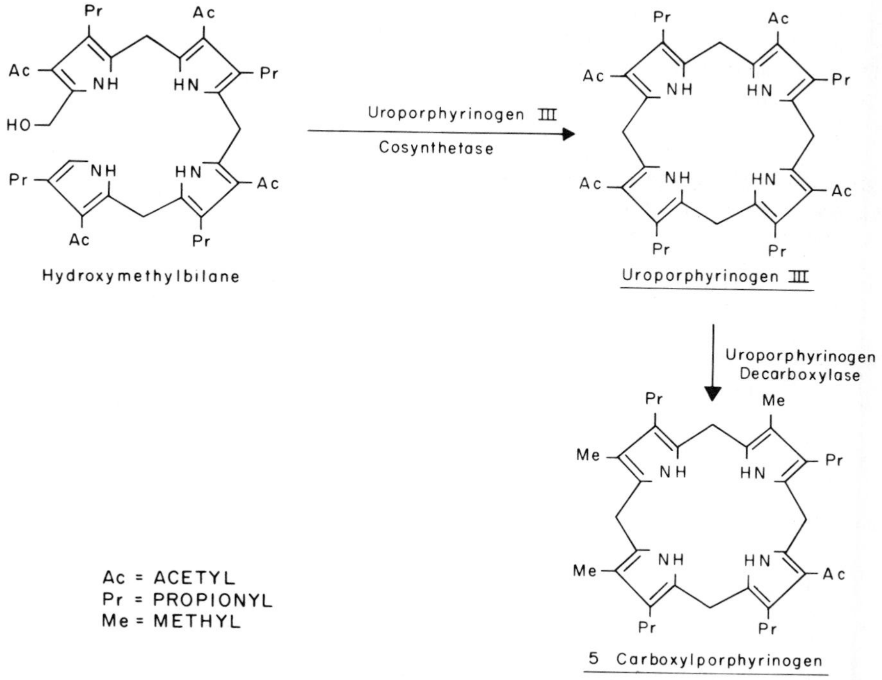

d

Fig. 143-2 (c and d).

Uroporphyrinogen III

↓ Uroporphyrinogen Decarboxylase

5 Carboxylporphyrinogen

Ac = ACETYL
Pr = PROPIONYL
Me = METHYL

e

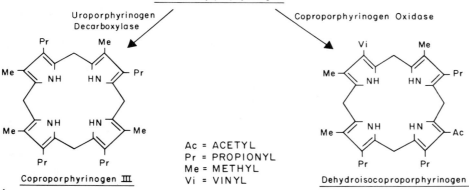

5 Carboxylporphyrinogen

Uroporphyrinogen Decarboxylase

Coproporphyrinogen Oxidase

Coproporphyrinogen III

Ac = ACETYL
Pr = PROPIONYL
Me = METHYL
Vi = VINYL

Dehydroisocoproporphyrinogen

f

Fig. 143-2 (e and f).

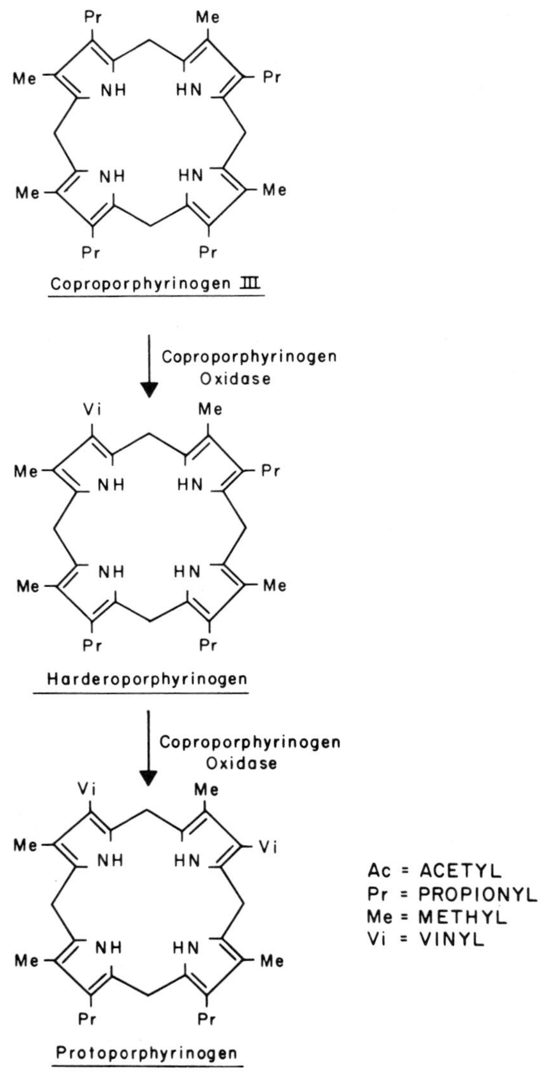

Coproporphyrinogen III

↓ Coproporphyrinogen Oxidase

Harderoporphyrinogen

↓ Coproporphyrinogen Oxidase

Protoporphyrinogen

Ac = ACETYL
Pr = PROPIONYL
Me = METHYL
Vi = VINYL

g

Fig. 143-2 (g).

biologic importance since only the III isomer can proceed to the formation of heme. Heme is a type III porphyrin and no type I heme has been identified in nature, thus making production of the I isomer an essentially "dead end" pathway. The formation of UROGEN III is catalyzed by the cytoplasmic enzyme UROCOSYN III, which is closely linked to PBGD. This enzyme is thermolabile, exhibits maximum catalytic activity at pH 7.8, and is inhibited by heavy metals such as zinc, cadmium, and copper [43]. In most tissues UROCOSYN III is present in considerable excess as compared to PBGD, thus assuring maximum conversion of the I to the III isomer. The only difference between the I and III isomers of each of the porphyrinogens is the reversal of the side chains on the "D" ring of the tetrapyrrole molecule. The importance of UROCOSYN III is amply illustrated by the disease EP (Günther's disease), an autosomal recessive disorder in which the enzyme is deficient and there is a major increase in RBC URO I and COPRO I and in the urinary excretion of UROGEN I and URO I [44].

Uroporphyrinogen decarboxylase (UROGEND)

UROGEN I and III each contain eight carboxyl groups as side chains, four of which are acetate (-CH$_2$COOH) and four of which are propionate (-CH$_2$-CH$_2$-COOH) moieties (Fig. 143-2c and d). The soluble enzyme UROGEND catalyzes the sequential decarboxylation of the four acetate groups to methyl groups (Fig. 143-2c to e). Decarboxylation first occurs on ring D, then the enzyme turns around to decarboxylate rings A, B, and C. This converts the original 8-carboxyl porphyrinogen (UROGEN I or III) first to 7-carboxyl, then to 6-carboxyl, and 5-carboxyl porphyrinogen. The 5-carboxyl porphyrinogen can then undergo decarboxylation of its last acetyl group to form the 4-carboxyl porphyrinogen which is known as coproporphyrinogen (COPROGEN I or III) (Fig. 143-2c and f). As discussed above, COPROGEN I cannot be further metabolized to heme. Mauzerall and Granick first showed that UROGEN III is decarboxylated twice as rapidly as UROGEN I by UROGEND [45]. This has recently been confirmed in studies with the purified enzyme prepared from human erythrocytes [46]. The purified human enzyme has a molecular weight of 46,000 and its activity is inhibited by metals such as copper and mercury [46].

UROGEND activity is reduced in patients with PCT and HEP [47–51]. Hepatic UROGEND activity is also inhibited by certain chlorinated hydrocarbons (e.g., hexachlorobenzene and chlorinated phenols [52–53]. High concentrations of hepatic iron have long been suspected of inhibiting liver UROGEND [54] activity in PCT but recent studies with the purified human erythrocyte enzyme have failed to verify this concept [46].

Coproporphyrinogen oxidase (COPROGENO)

COPROGEN III has four carboxyl groups, each of which is part of a propionate side chain. COPROGENO, a mitochondrial enzyme of molecular weight 72,000, catalyzes the sequential oxidative decarboxylation of two of the propionate groups, forming first 3-carboxyl porphyrinogen or harderoporphyrinogen (HARDEROGEN) and then 2-carboxylporphyrinogen or protoporphyrinogen (PROTOGEN) [55] (Fig. 143-2g). The activity of this enzyme is reduced in patients with HCP [56]. It should be recalled that COPROGEN I is not a substrate for COPROGENO and thus I isomers are not further metabolized.

Modification of the normal heme synthesis pathway has been discovered in PCT. No additional enzymes or enzymatic reactions are involved but there is a reversal in the sequence of action of the enzymes UROGEND and CO-PROGENO [28]. As shown in Fig. 143-2f, UROGEND normally acts on 5-carboxylporphyrinogen to decarboxylate the final remaining acetate group, forming a tetracarboxyl porphyrinogen known as COPROGEN III. This is subsequently converted to protoporphyrinogen by CO-PROGENO (Fig. 143-2g). However, in PCT where URO-GEND is deficient, COPROGENO may first oxidatively decarboxylate a propionate group on 5-carboxylporphyrinogen to form dehydroisocoproporphyrinogen (Fig. 143-2f). The acetyl group on dehydroisocoproporphyrinogen can be decarboxylated by UROGEND to form HARDEROGEN, resulting in diversion back into the nor-

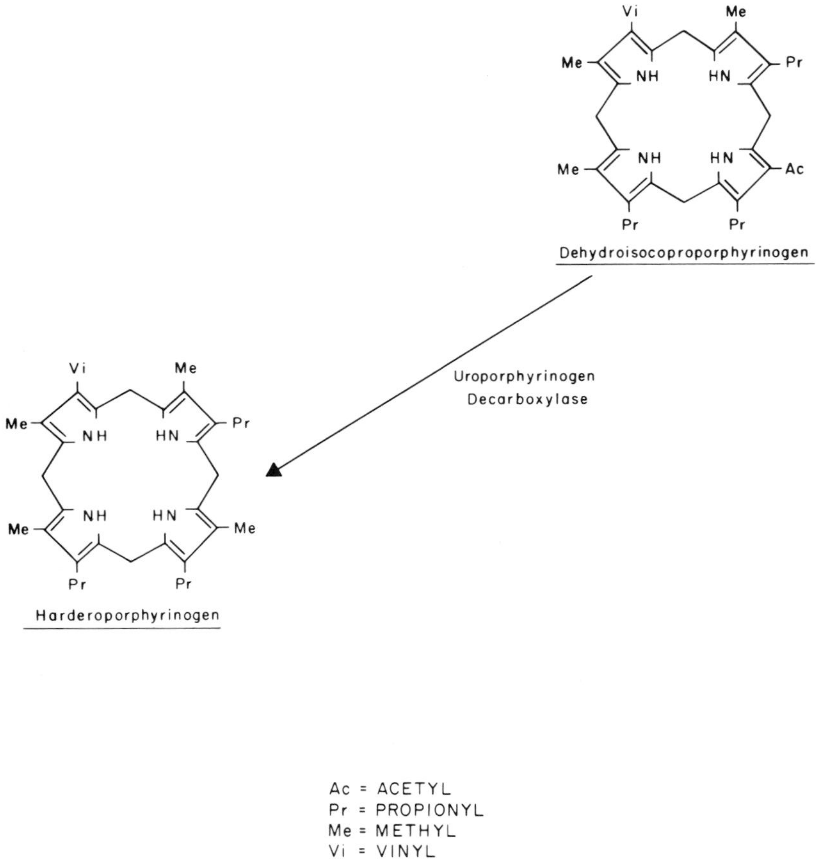

Dehydroisocoproporphyrinogen

Uroporphyrinogen
Decarboxylase

Harderoporphyrinogen

Ac = ACETYL
Pr = PROPIONYL
Me = METHYL
Vi = VINYL

h

Fig. 143-2 (h).

mal heme synthesis pathway (Fig. 143-2h). Alternatively, dehydroisocoproporphyrinogen can undergo hydration to isocoproporphyrinogen (Fig. 143-2i). These steps rarely, if ever, occur during the normal process of heme synthesis but become important in certain of the porphyrias such as PCT where they provide one explanation for the increased isocoproporphyrin (ISOCOPRO) characteristically found in the feces of patients with this disease [57].

Protoporphyrinogen oxidase (PROTOGENO)

The oxidation of PROTOGEN to PROTO is catalyzed by the mitochondrial enzyme protoporphyrinogen oxidase (PROTOGENO) (Fig. 143-2j). This reaction can also occur nonenzymatically but the enzyme appears to be necessary for heme synthesis to proceed at a normal rate [58]. There is experimental evidence to indicate that PROTOGENO activity is reduced in patients with VP [59].

Ferrochelatase

The final step in the formation of heme, the incorporation of ferrous iron (Fe^{+2}) into PROTO is catalyzed by the mitochondrial enzyme ferrochelatase. As will be discussed below, there is some evidence that this enzyme may be rate-limiting for bone marrow heme synthesis [60]. Ferrochelatase activity has been shown to be reduced in fibroblasts and hepatocytes of patients with EPP [61–64]. Qualitative as well as quantitative differences in ferrochelatase

activity are present in EPP patients as compared to normals. This has led to the suggestion that in patients with this disease there may be a variant form of ferrochelatase rather than simply reduced activity of the normal enzyme [65].

The end product, ferrous-PROTO or heme, diffuses out of the mitochondrion into the cytoplasm where it is available to function as a prosthetic group by combining with appropriate apoproteins.

It is important to emphasize that porphyrinogens (reduced porphyrins) are the true intermediates in heme synthesis. The irreversibly oxidized porphyrins, with the exception of PROTO, do not function as substrates for the enzymes of the pathway. Thus, porphyrins are actually heme pathway by-products, which are of special interest to dermatologists because of their unique photosensitizing properties.

Regulation of heme synthesis

Evidence that ALAS is the rate-limiting enzyme for heme synthesis in the liver was first provided in a classic study by Granick and Urata [66]. They showed that following administration of the drug 3,5-dicarbethoxy-1,4-dihydrocollidine (DDC) to guinea pigs, hepatic ALAS activity was increased whereas no induction effect on any other heme pathway enzyme could be demonstrated. This was the first evidence that control of heme synthesis could be depen-

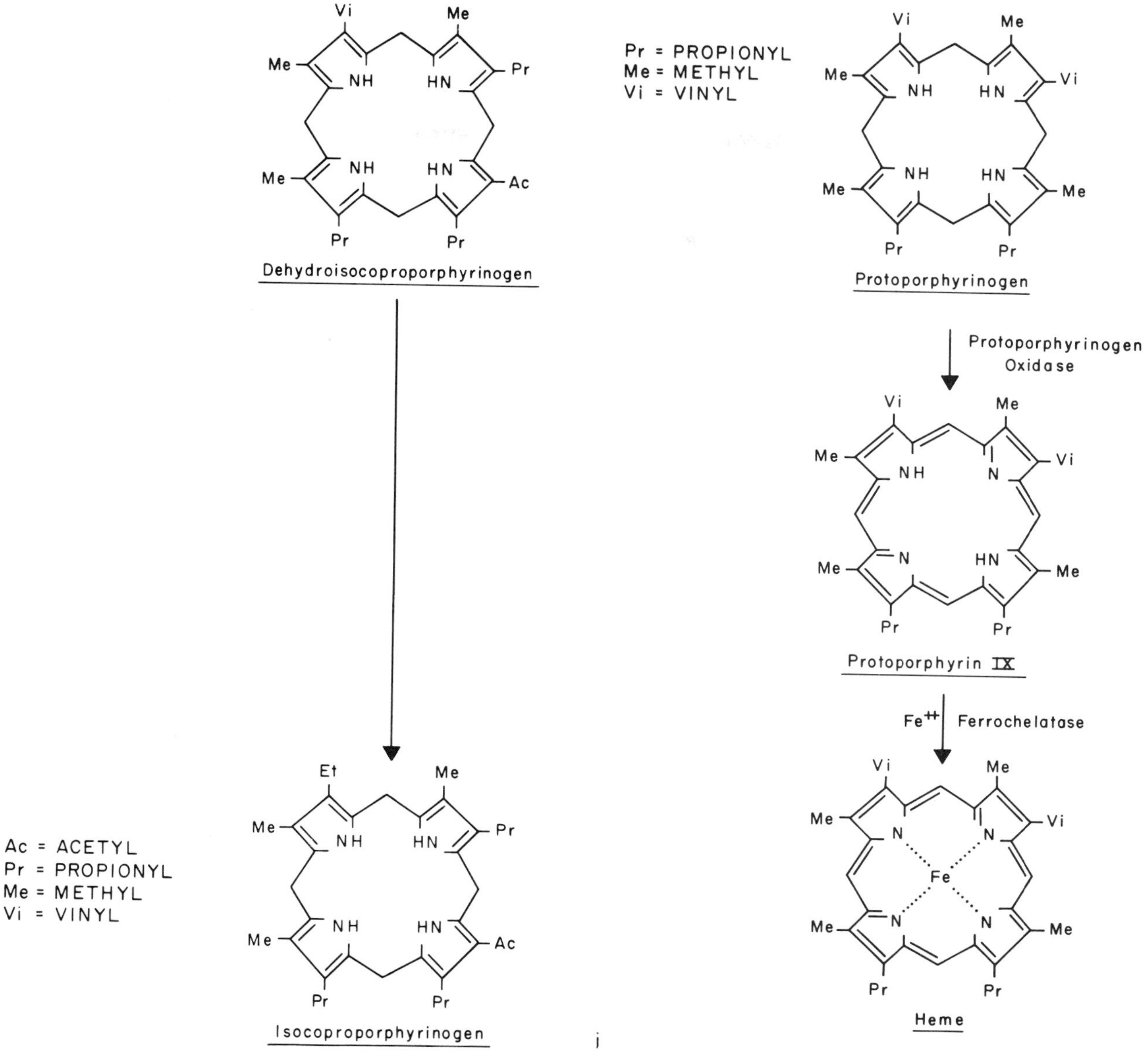

Dehydroisocoproporphyrinogen

Pr = PROPIONYL
Me = METHYL
Vi = VINYL

Protoporphyrinogen

Protoporphyrinogen Oxidase

Protoporphyrin IX

Fe++ | Ferrochelatase

Heme

Ac = ACETYL
Pr = PROPIONYL
Me = METHYL
Vi = VINYL

Isocoproporphyrinogen

Fig. 143-2 (i and j).

dent upon changes in ALAS activity in the cell and that environmental agents could directly affect this enzyme.

Subsequent studies by Marver et al [67] showed that other drugs such as allylisopropylacetamide (AIA) had similar induction effects on ALAS in rat liver. The demonstration that selected environmental agents could enhance the activity of hepatic ALAS coupled with the known excessive urinary excretion of ALA and PBG in AIP, led to the finding that ALAS activity is increased in the liver of patients with this disease [68–70].

Granick [71] has proposed a model for the control of heme synthesis based on studies of genetic regulation in bacteria [72]. There are at least two general mechanisms whereby the activity of rate-limiting enzymes such as ALAS could be controlled. One is by end-product inhibition and the other by end-product repression. Heme could alter the activity of ALAS by directly inhibiting the enzyme. This has been demonstrated in the bacterium *Rhodopseudomonas spheroides* [73]. However, there is cur-

rently no evidence that the levels of heme required for this direct inhibitory effect can be achieved in mammalian cells in vivo [74].

End-product repression of ALAS by heme has been demonstrated in chick embryo liver at concentrations that can be achieved in vivo [75]. Theoretically, heme could repress ALAS at either the transcriptional (messenger RNA) or the translational (ribosomal RNA) level and evidence for both has been published [76–77].

Granick's hypothetical mechanism for repression of ALAS by heme is shown in Fig. 143-3. Heme, the end product, functions as a corepressor and binds to a putative aporepressor protein. The complete repressor molecule can block the structural gene coding for ALAS, thereby decreasing the rate of synthesis of the enzyme which in turn results in lower heme levels in the cell. As heme levels diminish, the corepressor will not occupy all available aporepressor binding sites so that the repressor does not function. This derepression leads to enhanced synthesis of

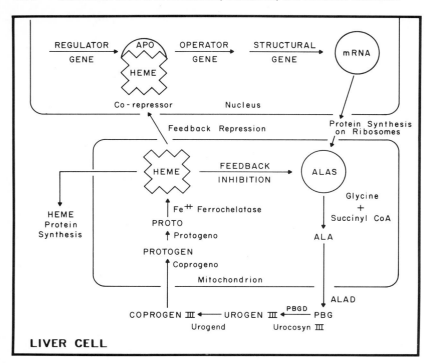

Fig. 143-3 Heme is capable of regulating its synthesis by either directly inhibiting or repressing the synthesis of its rate-limiting enzyme, ALAS. The repression may result from the binding of heme to an aporepressor protein which, when combined, becomes a functional unit.

ALAS until heme levels rise sufficiently to again form the complete repressor molecule. Any biochemical event that leads to decreased heme levels in the cell can theoretically result in induction of ALAS. For example, administration of a drug such as AIA to rats causes rapid depletion of cytochrome P-450 and heme in liver microsomes and suggests that reduced heme levels lead to the enhanced hepatic ALAS activity evoked by the drug [78]. In other studies, it has been shown that DDC, also an ALAS inducer, inhibits ferrochelatase activity which could also result in decreased heme levels in the cell, in turn leading to loss of feedback repression of the synthesis of ALAS [79]. However, DDC is a much more potent inhibitor of ferrochelatase than of ALAS and no temporal relationship can be shown between the two effects in chick embryo liver [80].

On the other hand, heme can induce the catalytic activity

of and be destroyed by the microsomal heme-catabolizing enzyme, heme oxygenase, in the cell [81]. It seems likely that an unbound or free fraction of heme within the cell, the level of which is dependent upon its concomitant synthesis and degradation, as well as its binding to apoproteins, could well be the critical determinant for regulation of the synthesis of ALAS (Fig. 143-4). While such a fraction has not been proved to exist it is reasonable to speculate that heme can regulate its own production by controlling ALAS activity. Finally, metabolically or chemically generated intermediates such as lipid peroxides may cause liver damage and concomitant heme destruction in the hepatocyte [82,83].

From the preceding discussion, it can be seen that one factor that could influence intracellular heme levels is the concentration and turnover rate of hepatic cytosolic mitochondrial and microsomal cytochromes (e.g., P-450). Ac-

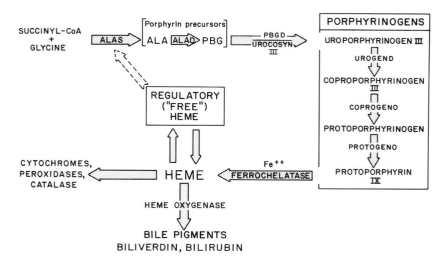

Fig. 143-4 A regulatory pool of "free" heme unbound to apoproteins may be the critical determinant controlling its synthesis.

celerated turnover rates of their apoprotein moieties result in increased demand for heme, thereby diminishing the free heme pool and enhancing synthesis of ALAS. In patients with acute hepatic porphyria, this increase in ALAS activity and the metabolic products generated as a consequence of the increased catalytic activity may well be the direct cause of the clinical manifestations.

The barbiturates have long been known to precipitate attacks in patients with acute hepatic porphyria. These drugs are also known to cause enhanced synthesis of apo-cytochrome P-450, which creates a demand for heme to produce the functional holocytochrome [84,85]. Conversely, there is evidence that a high carbohydrate diet, which has been used therapeutically for attacks of the acute hepatic porphyrias [86], may reduce P-450 turnover rates in cultured hepatocytes, thereby diminishing the utilization of heme [87]. While the explanations for this effect remain unsatisfactory, it would explain the beneficial effect of "glucose loading" which is observed clinically in these patients. Similarly, this could explain exacerbation of acute hepatic porphyria in patients following starvation [88,89].

Inhibition of the activity of other enzymes in the heme pathway could also result in reduced intracellular heme concentration, thereby enhancing ALAS activity. For example, griseofulvin, similar to DDC, is a potent inhibitor of ferrochelatase, and blocks the conversion of PROTO to heme. This could explain the observed ability of this medication to induce acute attacks in some patients with acute hepatic porphyria [88]. Similarly, certain sulfonamides have been shown to inhibit PBGD and may exacerbate acute hepatic porphyria in this fashion [90].

Since ALAS activity can be inhibited and its synthesis repressed by increased levels of intracellular heme, administration of exogenous heme might be expected to inhibit induction of the enzyme. Indeed, infusions of hematin, an oxidized form of heme, have been utilized with considerable success in the management of attacks of the acute hepatic porphyrias [91–93] (see "Acute Intermittent Porphyria" and "Variegate Porphyria" below).

In bone marrow there is some experimental evidence that ferrochelatase rather than ALAS is the rate-limiting step for heme synthesis [94]. Consequently, factors that decisively influence the clinical course of acute hepatic porphyria are generally without effect in patients with porphyrias of bone marrow origin. For example, griseofulvin-mediated inhibition of ferrochelatase has not been associated with a clinical worsening of EPP in humans. In mice, this inhibitory effect of the drug occurs predominantly in the liver [95] and it is possible that it may exert a similar effect in humans. Indeed, Rimington and coworkers showed that individuals treated with griseofulvin may have elevated fecal porphyrin excretion though they do not have clinically manifested porphyria [96].

Like ALAS, ferrochelatase activity appears to be influenced by numerous factors. Its activity can be augmented by elevated levels of the reduced form of glutathione and by fatty acids, whereas lead and other heavy metals can inhibit it [97].

It is important to recall that the body's daily demand for heme production is rather high since hemoglobin and the hepatic heme-proteins must be continuously regenerated. This is due to the obligate breakdown of heme into the linear tetrapyrroles, biliverdin and bilirubin. Thus 50 to 60 mg of heme are produced by the body each day whereas only a few hundred micrograms of porphyrins are excreted. This represents 2 percent or less of the heme that is produced. In the porphyrias, excretion of porphyrins and porphyrin precursors increases enormously because of inherited and/or environmentally induced changes in the activity of enzymes in the heme pathway (Table 143-2). How these porphyrins are excreted (i.e., in urine or feces) depends upon their solubility in water. The distribution of porphyrins between urinary and biliary routes of excretion is related to their solubility properties. URO, with 8-carboxyl groups, is water-soluble and therefore is predominantly excreted in the urine, while the most insoluble (hydrophobic) PROTO, is exclusively excreted in the bile. Isomers of COPRO follow a mixed route, with preferential excretion of the Type I isomer in the bile and Type III in the urine. From the preceding discussion it should be clear that the early intermediates (ALA, PBG, UROGEN) are very polar and are therefore quite water-soluble. As a result, they are excreted primarily in the urine. These factors are of great importance in the selection of appropriate specimens for diagnostic tests. For instance, in a patient suspected of having EPP or VP, the increased PROTO excretion will be overlooked if only the urine is tested and not the feces.

Drug-induced porphyria

Drug exacerbation of human porphyria has been known for nearly a century, since Stokvis [98] first reported two women who had acute abdominal pain and excreted dark red urine following the ingestion of the sedative sulfonal. He suggested that the red urinary pigment in these patients was related to hematoporphyrin. Duesberg [99] reported fatal porphyria in a patient treated with large amounts of Sedormid in which symptoms of acute porphyria appeared. Subsequent studies of sizable numbers of patients with AIP in Sweden, Great Britain, South Africa, and the United States have all emphasized the relationship of ingestion of barbiturates to acute attacks of porphyria [100–102]. However, some patients with unquestioned hereditary porphyria may receive the barbiturates or other potent inducing drugs at times without incident only to have an acute attack result at another time. It is now clear that other drugs in addition to Sedormid will cause porphyria in the absence of any identifiable genetic predisposition, producing a biochemical and clinical disturbance similar to that of other human porphyrias (e.g., hexachlorobenzene (HCB) and PCT in Turkey). Drugs that have been incriminated in the precipitation of acute attacks of porphyria include anticonvulsants, barbiturate and nonbarbiturate sedatives, griseofulvin, and sex steroid hormones, to name but a few (see Table 143-4).

Ingestion of some drugs may be associated with increased excretion of porphyrins or porphyrin precursors in some normal individuals, e.g., griseofulvin and oral contraceptives [79,103]. Drugs thus may have stimulatory effects on the heme pathway in humans without inducing any clinical evidence of porphyria.

A wide variety of drugs and chemicals has been observed to evoke typical porphyria in diverse groups of individuals. There was one "epidemic" of more than 3000 cases of chemically induced porphyria in Turkey following the oral

Table 143-4   Drugs potentially hazardous in patients with the acute porphyrias

Amphetamines
Analgesics:
  Aminopyrine, antipyrine, amidopyrine, dichloralphenazone, diclophenac, phenylbutazone, fentanyl
Anaesthetics:
  Althesine, barbiturates (Pentothal), enflurane, halothane, methoxyflurane
Anticonvulsants:
  Carbamazepine, diphenylhydantoin, ethosuximide, mephenytoin, methsuximide, phensuximide, primidone, trimethadione,
    valproate
Antihypertensives:
  Clonidine, hydralazine, methyldopa, pargyline, phenoxybenzamine, spironolactone
Antimicrobial agents:
  Chloramphenicol, griseofulvin, pyrazinamide, novobiocin, sulfonamides
Barbiturates
Chloroquine
Dapsone
Diethylpropion
Dramamine
Ergot preparations
Ethchlorvynol
Ethyl alcohol
Furosemide
Hormones:
  Estrogens, progesterones
Hyoscine-N-butylbromide
Imipramine
Nikethamide
Nonbarbiturate hypnotics:
  Chlormethazone, glutethimide, meprobamate, methylprylon, sulphonal, trional
Pentazocine
Pyrazinamide
Sedormid
Sulfonylureas:
  Tolbutamide, chlorpropamide
Theophylline
Tranquilizers:
  Chlordiazepoxide, clonazepam, diazepam, oxazepam, flurazepam

ingestion of the fungicide HCB [104]. This was one of the first known instances in which exposure of a population of diverse genetic backgrounds to a chemical substance resulted in human porphyria. Industrial workers exposed to chlorinated phenols have developed PCT [105]. Interestingly, follow-up evaluation of these same workers several years later revealed no clinical porphyria, probably due to the introduction of stringent safety measures to minimize clinical exposure [106]. Lynch et al [107] also showed that

exposure to chlorinated phenols, inadvertently produced by mixing commonly available household cleansers, resulted in typical PCT in a woman working as a janitor. How chlorinated phenols induce PCT is not clear, but experimental evidence suggests that these compounds or metabolites of these compounds can inhibit hepatic URO-GEND activity [108].

Alcohol and estrogens are also known to be associated with PCT [12,109]. However, only a minority of individuals

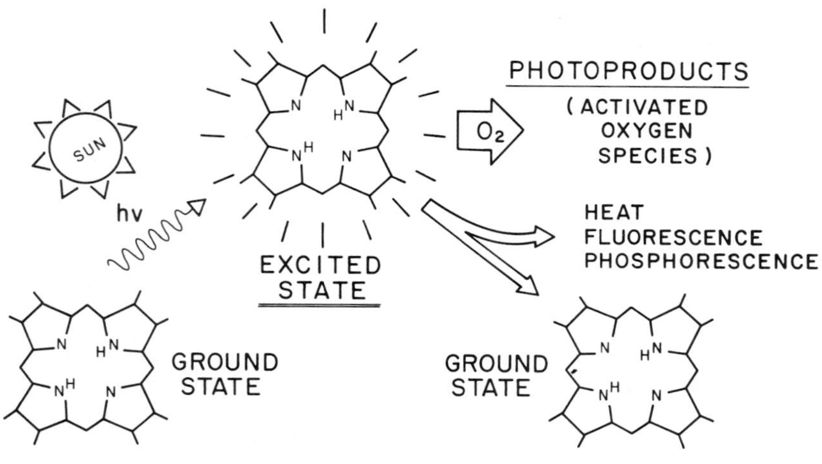

Fig. 143-5 Photoexcited porphyrins release energy in a variety of ways when returning to their ground state and these may contribute to damaging reactions in biologic systems.

exposed to alcohol and estrogens develop clinically manifest porphyria. This suggests that there is a specific genetic susceptibility to PCT which is precipitated by exposure to alcohol or estrogens in some individuals [110–112]. Latent cases of PCT have been observed in the relatives of affected individuals [113].

Possible mechanisms of porphyrin-induced photosensitivity

Increased cutaneous photosensitivity to visible light is commonly seen in patients with several different porphyrias (EP, EPP, PCT, VP, HCP, and HEP) in whom plasma and tissue porphyrins are increased. Patients with lead intoxication (PbI) and patients with AIP, however, do not manifest any increased sensitivity to light—the former (PbI) because the increased PROTO is zinc-chelated and trapped within the RBC and cannot diffuse into the tissues; and the latter (AIP) because only nonphotosensitizing porphyrin precursors are present in substantially increased amounts. The cutaneous photosensitivity may range from simple acute burning, itching, and swelling during the course of sun exposure to chronic edema, erythema, vesicle or bulla formation, lichenification, and scarring reactions. Many of the changes, both acute and chronic, in the light-exposed skin of patients with cutaneous porphyria can be related to the interaction of light with excess circulating porphyrins present in cutaneous tissue.

The first experimental evidence for the photosensitizing property of porphyrins in human skin was provided by the heroic self-experiment of Meyer-Betz [114]. After injecting himself intravenously with 200 mg of hematoporphyrin and exposing his skin to sunlight, he observed marked erythema and edema in light-exposed body areas. With the increasing use of hematoporphyrin derivative (HPD) as a substance for the early diagnosis and treatment of human malignancy, this phenomenon of cutaneous photosensitivity is reported to be occurring with increasing frequency [115-117].

Porphyrins such as URO, COPRO, and PROTO absorb light intensely in the 400 ± 10 nm range, the so-called Soret band. Absorption of this radiant energy in the visible spectrum causes porphyrins to become photoactivated and thus biologically reactive. When porphyrins absorb light energy, orbital electrons in the molecule are raised from their normal ground state energy levels to higher "excited state" energy levels in which the molecule is more reactive. One such state of porphyrin is referred to as the triplet state, a metastable excited or reactive state of relatively long life.

The energy-rich photoexcited porphyrins may produce toxic effects by evoking changes in cell membranes, nucleic acids, structural proteins, or enzymes in an energy transfer type of reaction. Then, as the excited triplet state porphyrin returns to its normal ground state, it releases energy in the form of light (fluorescence/phosphorescence), heat, or by transfer of its energy to the cell constituents (Fig. 143-5). Porphyrin-photosensitized damage to biologic systems (cell membrane or DNA damage) appears to be mediated by the triplet state of porphyrins. The long-lived triplet sensitizer state of a porphyrin permits it to undergo primary reactions with molecules in its immediate vicinity. The majority of porphyrin-sensitized photoreactions in bi-

ology involve, in fact, sensitized photooxidation processes. It has been recently demonstrated, however, that the porphyrin molecule can also transfer its absorbed energy to oxygen molecules, thereby creating "excited oxygen" states [118–121]. Various forms of excited oxygen capable of causing tissue damage are known to exist, including singlet oxygen ($^1O_2$), superoxide anion ($O_{\bar{2}}$), or superoxide radical ($HO_{\bar{2}}$). Photoexcited porphyrins (URO, COPRO, PROTO, etc.) commonly generate $^1O_2$ and rarely $O_{\bar{2}}$. In some cases the sensitized porphyrin reacts with oxygen to yield hydrogen peroxide or with water to form hydroxyl radicals. Those processes in which activated oxygen species play a role are referred to as photodynamic reactions [122].

The photosensitizing action of porphyrins may thus be characterized as an oxygen-dependent, sensitized photooxidation reaction. In this photooxidation reaction there is a transfer of excitation energy from the triplet state of the porphyrin molecule to molecular oxygen, resulting in the generation of singlet oxygen as shown schematically below:

$$P_O \text{--------} {}^1P$$
$$^1P \text{--------} {}^3P$$
$$^3P + {}^3O_2 \text{--------} P_O + {}^1O_2$$
$$^1O_2 + A \text{--------} AO_2 \text{ or } AOX$$

In this reaction P_0, ^1P, and ^3P represent the ground state, the singlet excited state, and the triplet excited state of the porphyrin, respectively. $^3O_2$ represents the stable triplet ground state of oxygen and $^1O_2$ represents the excited and reactive form of singlet oxygen that combines with the biologic acceptor molecule A to give a peroxide AO_2 or the fully oxidized form of the substrate AOX. The biologic substrates that seem to be most susceptible are lipids in cellular membranes and organelles or nuclear DNA.

While these concepts regarding excited porphyrins and oxygen are valid in simple systems, their applicability to complex tissues such as the skin remains to be verified. Several hypotheses have been advanced regarding the mechanism of porphyrin-induced photosensitivity. One hypothesis involves the transfer of energy from excited species of oxygen to water or to lipids, creating hydrogen and/or lipid peroxides [123]. These peroxides, in turn could produce oxidative damage to lipid-rich cellular membranes (Fig. 143-6). Evidence for this type of reaction has come from the demonstration of porphyrin-UV-induced crosslinkage of proteins within RBC membranes [124–126] and destruction of fibroblast membrane sulfhydryl groups [127]. If such damage occurs in plasma membranes in cells in or adjacent to the skin, it could result in tissue destruction and possibly explain the photosensitivity seen in the cutaneous porphyrias. Goldstein and Harber showed that photoexcitation of PROTO-enriched RBC resulted in the formation of hydrogen peroxide and lipid peroxides, each of which would be highly destructive to lipid-rich membranous structures [128]. There is evidence in RBC of peroxidation of cholesterol groups in the cell membrane resulting in hemolysis following exposure to UV radiation and PROTO [129].

Other membrane-bound cellular structures could also be targets for this type of damage. Allison et al have suggested that porphyrins and light can initiate free radical reactions and that lysosomal membranes might be attacked in this

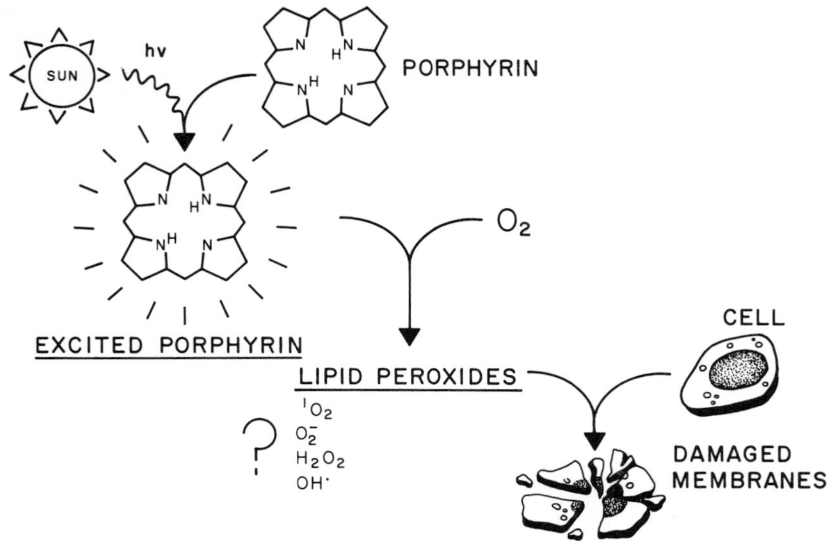

Fig. 143-6 Lipid peroxide formation in membranes may be a major common pathway for cellular damage by porphyrin photosensitization.

manner, resulting in leakage of proteases with subsequent cellular damage [130]. While there is indirect histochemical evidence for lysosomal enzyme release in sun-exposed skin of patients with porphyria, in vitro studies have shown that it followed rather than preceded cell damage [131,132]. If confirmed, this would suggest that lysosomal damage may be the result rather than the cause of porphyrin photosensitization.

Other studies have suggested that mitochondria are targets for this type of membrane attack. Ultrastructural studies of lymphoma cells treated with hematoporphyrin and UV radiation revealed that mitochondrial damage occurred first, followed by damage to the endoplasmic reticulum and finally to the nucleus [133].

It is also clear that porphyrins and 400-nm light can damage hepatic and epidermal microsomal cytochrome P-450 in vitro, a pathologic process mediated by singlet oxygen [121,134]. Thus, microsomal membranes are another potential target for cell damage due to porphyrin photosensitization.

While these reports have focused primarily on alteration of cell membranes as the target for porphyrin photosensitization, other investigators have proposed that changes in DNA may also be important in its pathogenesis [135]. DNA exposed to visible light and hematoporphyrin manifests selective degradation of the guanine moiety [136]. Such DNA damage could lead to subsequent abnormalities in protein synthesis, resulting in extensive cellular damage.

In still other investigations, porphyrin photosensitization has been studied in cultured human fibroblasts [137]. These cells were shown to have substantially reduced viability following treatment with PROTO and light. There was no evidence of release of lysosomal enzymes, again suggesting that damage to this organelle may not be a primary event in porphyrin photosensitization. Pyknotic nuclei, vacuolated cytoplasm, and surface blebs were observed in these fibroblasts treated with PROTO and light, indicating that extensive cell damage had occurred. Furthermore, denaturation of intracellular proteins was also shown to occur in the photosensitized cells.

A newer concept regarding the pathogenesis of cutaneous photosensitivity in porphyria has focused on the possible role of complement-derived mediators of inflammation in the production of skin lesions in vivo. Activation of the complement cascade in serum of patients with EPP and PCT exposed to UV radiation in vitro was shown to occur [138,139]. Furthermore, complement components have been detected in the fluid of suction blisters induced in the skin of patients with EPP. Increased amounts of C5a, a potent chemotactic substance, are present in both serum and blister fluid. These data have led Lim and Gigli to propose a role for complement activation by porphyrin and light in the pathogenesis of the skin photosensitivity seen in the cutaneous porphyrias [140].

Fluorescent microscopy of snap-frozen sections of skin biopsies obtained from patients with cutaneous porphyria has revealed reddish-pink fluorescence indicative of porphyrins in both the epidermis and dermis. This fluorescence is present in the epidermis around hair roots (in the juxtacapillary spaces of the papillary bodies) and in the reticular dermis [141; Pathak, unpublished observations]. The sparse red fluorescence is low in intensity, often unstable, and difficult to photograph.

Several investigators have studied the relation between the absorption spectrum of porphyrins and the photocutaneous responses in the skin of porphyric patients [142–145]. The published action spectra of these investigators are in close agreement with the absorption spectra of the porphyrins (see Fig. 143-7). Peak skin reactivity is around 400 nm with a lesser response between 500 to 650 nm. It should be noted that skin responses to the sunburn spectrum (290 to 320 nm) and minimal erythema dose (MED) values are normal in patients with PCT, EPP, or VP (unpublished observation).

While the photochemical reactions that evoke skin lesions in vivo remain poorly understood, the oxidative hypothesis involving the formation of peroxide, free-radicals, or singlet oxygen is strengthened by in vitro and in vivo studies showing the photoprotective effect of β-carotene, a known quencher of both singlet oxygen and free radicals [146–150].

As will be discussed below, the patterns of cutaneous photosensitivity in the porphyrias vary considerably. This variation is likely due to the differing aqueous and lipid

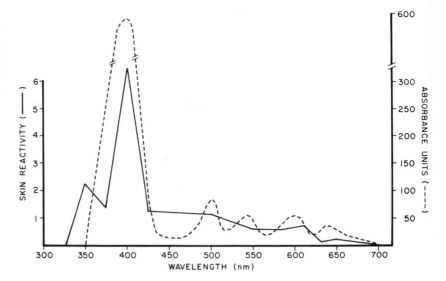

Fig. 143-7 Action spectrum for skin photosensitivity in a patient with erythropoietic protoporphyria. The ordinate scale represents skin reactivity for whealing (arbitrary units). The broken line represents absorption bands on a typical photosensitizing porphyrin. *(Adapted from Magnus [162].)*

solubilities of the various porphyrins. Thus PROTO accumulates primarily in lipophilic environments such as membranes whereas water-soluble URO accumulates in hydrophilic structures. These differences in lipid and water solubility could result in variable cellular localization of the particular porphyrin, which might account for the contrasting signs and symptoms of cutaneous photosensitivity observed in patients with EPP and PCT. Experimental studies have shown that the lipid solubility of porphyrins can dramatically alter their phototoxic effects in membrane models [151].

Classification of the porphyrias

Although each porphyria is biochemically unique since it is the consequence of an enzyme abnormality in heme synthesis, an acceptable and accurate classification of the porphyrias will be feasible only when specific genetic defects for each disease have been precisely defined. At present most classifications are based on the abnormal porphyrin patterns found either in tissues or in the urine or feces of patients with these disorders. This concept, however, has limitations because, in some porphyrias, the biochemical patterns of porphyrin excretion can overlap.

The porphyrias have been classified by Günther [7,152], Waldenström [11,13], Watson et al [153], and Schmid et al [27]. The classification used here (Table 143-5) is an extension of that originally proposed by Watson et al [153], Schmid [27], and more recently by Magnus [154].

Erythropoietic porphyria (EP) (Table 143-6)

Historical aspects

This disease was originally named hematoporphyria congenita by Günther in 1911 and the first published case of porphyria was probably of this type [3]. Several reports in the 1920s described this disorder in detail [155–157].

Perhaps the most careful studies ever performed in a patient with any type of porphyria were those conducted by Günther between 1911 and 1936 on a patient named Mathias Petry. Günther's studies were complemented bio-chemically by Hans Fischer. Fundamental studies concerning the chemical nature of the excessive porphyrin produced in this patient revealed that this was a new type of porphyrin which Fischer named URO since it was in highest concentration in the urine [8]. This was the first definite evidence that the type of porphyrin observed in excess in human porphyria was not hematoporphyrin. A recent excellent review of EP has been published by Ippen and Fuchs [158].

Etiology

Basically, EP consists of a genetic disturbance in porphyrin metabolism which primarily involves the hematopoietic system. The etiology of EP remains unknown although most clinical evidence suggests that EP is due to an enzyme defect, presumably of UROCOSYN III, inherited as an autosomal recessive trait. Romeo and Levin [44] suggest that there is a deficiency of erythrocyte UROCOSYN III in bone marrow hemolysates of EP patients. In further studies these workers also showed evidence for decreased UROCOSYN III activity in latent cases of EP [159]. However, these findings are disputed by Miyagi et al [160], who suggest that the fault lies in a mutation causing increased ALAS or PBGD activity rather than decreased UROCOSYN III. The picture is further clouded by the report of Kushner et al [161] who demonstrated diminished activity of UROGEND in one patient with congenital erythropoietic porphyria and dyserythropoiesis.

Table 143-5 Classification of human porphyrias

Tissue origin	Type
Erythropoietic	Erythropoietic porphyria (EP)
	Erythropoietic protoporphyria (EPP)
	Erythropoietic coproporphyria (ECP)
Hepatic	Acute intermittent porphyria (AIP)
	Variegate porphyria (VP)
	Hereditary coproporphyria (HCP)
	Porphyria cutanea tarda (PCT)
Hepatic/	Harderoporphyria
erythropoietic?	Hepatoerythropoietic porphyria (HEP)

Table 143-6   Erythropoietic porphyria

Synonyms	Günther's disease
	Congenital photosensitive porphyria
	Erythropoietic uroporphyria
Inheritance	Autosomal recessive
Age of onset	Usually infancy or first decade
Incidence	Very rare (less than 100 reported cases)
Photosensitivity	Marked, early in childhood
Skin reactions	Early: Vesicles, bullae, erosions, hypertrichosis of lanugo hair, and in the brows and eyelashes, hypermelanosis, skin sensitivity to trauma
	Late: Scarring with atrophy, mutilating deformities of hands, ears, face and nose, cicatrizing alopecia, sclerodermoid changes
Clinical findings	Hemolytic anemia, erythrodontia, splenomegaly, skin photosensitivity, pink-red urine, fluorescent red blood cells and normoblasts, scleral ulceration of the eyes
Biochemical defects	Excretory: mainly elevated URO I and COPRO I in urine and feces
	Enzymatic: UROCOSYN III deficiency
	? Increased PBGD activity
	? Decreased UROGEND in some cases

Epidemiology

EP has been observed to occur in countries around the world and it is among the rarest of the cutaneous porphyrias. Nearly all cases begin in childhood [162] and only a few in adult life [163,164]. It is of considerable interest that congenital EP occurs in a number of mammals including swine, cattle, and cats [165–167], and these animal models have greatly aided research in this disease.

Clinical manifestations

The disease usually presents itself in the first few months of life with moderate to severe cutaneous photosensitivity associated with pinkish red urine which stains the diaper. The infant may scream during sun exposure. In some cases, clinical signs and symptoms of EP are evident immediately after birth while in others these may be delayed for months or even years [158,168].

The dramatic skin changes are the result of severe cutaneous photosensitivity. EP causes the most mutilating skin lesions of any of the porphyrias. The photosensitivity is apparently due to the excessive URO I and COPRO I in RBC, plasma, and skin.

The skin manifestations include vesicles and bullae, which may contain pink fluorescent fluid, become secondarily infected, heal slowly, and after repetitive episodes, scar. This may lead to loss of acral tissue such as the tips of the ears, the nose, and fingers (Fig. 143-8). In association with these destructive changes there may develop a peculiar kind of hirsutism, the hair often being quite long and dark, even with a lanugo-like texture. This is particularly evident in light-exposed body areas such as the face, neck, and extremities. The scalp may develop a cicatrizing alo-

pecia. Other chronic findings include eye changes (photophobia, keratoconjunctivitis, ectropion, symblepharon) and irregular hyper- and hypopigmentation of the skin. Increased fragility of the skin is often seen. Erythrodontia (red-stained teeth) is a common finding in both deciduous and permanent teeth. Occasionally the diagnosis of EP is made from the deep mahogany color of the first teeth. Under a Wood's lamp the teeth exhibit a reddish pink fluorescence characteristic of porphyrins. The urine also fluoresces reddish pink.

In addition to cutaneous lesions, there is often hemolytic anemia and splenomegaly [169]. Many bone marrow normoblasts fluoresce intensely red. The erythrocyte lifespan is usually shorter than normal (36 vs. 120 days). Whether the hemolytic anemia is due to "photohemolysis" of circulating porphyrin-laden erythrocytes or to an associated intracorpuscular red cell defect is unresolved [170,171].

Laboratory findings

The pink to burgundy red color of the urine from excess URO I is often visible on inspection. Marrow normoblasts exhibit relatively stable fluorescence and contain markedly elevated URO I, COPRO I, and PROTO. Urinary excretion of ALA and PBG is normal. COPRO I may be present in large amounts in the feces. Typical biochemical findings of EP are summarized in Tables 143-3 and 143-6. At autopsy, the most striking finding in these patients is the reddish brown discoloration of the skeleton and the teeth, and when examined with Wood's lamp they exhibit intense red fluorescence.

Histopathology

The bullous lesion of EP is subepidermal with varying degrees of inflammation, usually slight. Thickening of collagen bundles may be seen in areas of scarring. Connective tissue fibrosis is often seen. Perivascular deposits of porphyrin can be found when the unstained sections of skin or liver are viewed with a fluorescence microscope.

Differential diagnosis

The diagnosis of EP can usually be made from the pattern of severe photosensitivity associated with red fluorescent urine and erythrodontia. Distinguishing EP from other congenital types of photodermatosis is relatively simple since only patients with xeroderma pigmentosum exhibit such extensive mutilation of the sun-exposed skin which is often accompanied by pigmentary change and cutaneous neoplasia. In epidermolysis bullosa, the mutilating skin changes may resemble those of EP, but determination of urinary and RBC porphyrins differentiates the two conditions. Hemolytic anemia rarely occurs in epidermolysis bullosa. Furthermore, skin lesions in EP occur on light-exposed body areas whereas the lesions of epidermolysis bullosa are more often seen in areas of repeated trauma. Other bullous diseases, including hydroa vacciniforme and pemphigoid, and other photosensitizing porphyrias such as EPP and PCT present distinctive cutaneous syndromes in most instances. Patients with hepatic porphyrias such as PCT and VP can be differentiated from EP by the normal PROTO content of their erythrocytes. The cutaneous man-

Fig. 143-8 Congenital erythropoietic porphyria (Günther's disease) shows severe scarring, damage of the ear and nose cartilage, hair loss, and discolored teeth. *(Courtesy of Drs. A. Wiskemann and J. Kimmig, University Skin Clinic, Hamburg.)*

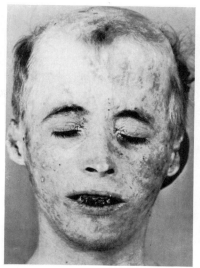 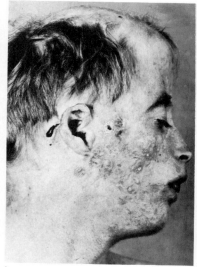

a   b

ifestations of HEP may be strikingly similar to those in EP and measurement or RBC PROTO or RBC UROCOSYN III and UROGEND activity may be decisive.

Treatment

The treatment of EP is difficult and unsatisfactory at present. It is essentially preventive and symptomatic, including avoidance of sun exposure, surveillance of the anemia, and treatment of recurrent skin infection. Protection from sunlight is absolutely essential and this alone may be of substantial benefit. Topical sunscreens are relatively little used since the only ones effective at wavelengths greater than 400 nm are those containing light-opaque substances such as zinc oxide or titanium dioxide which are cosmetically unsatisfactory to patients and messy to use. The efficacy of oral administration of β-carotene (120 to 180 mg daily) in EP is not proved although there are reports that it may improve light tolerance (D. J. Cripps, personal communication). Splenectomy has been performed in several patients because of intractable hemolytic anemia and has occasionally resulted in marked improvement both in the anemia and in cutaneous photosensitivity [5,170]. Unfortunately, this desirable therapeutic effect has not occurred in all cases. Suppression of erythropoiesis by transfusion of packed erythrocytes causes a marked decrease in porphyrin production and excretion with concomitant decrease in erythropoiesis, erythropoietin production, and plasma iron turnover [172]. Watson and Bossenmaier [173] gave intravenous hematin to one patient with EP and were able to produce an apparent feedback repression of porphyrin biosynthesis, followed by a decline of porphyrin levels in urine, plasma, and erythrocytes. This interesting finding requires further evaluation.

Erythropoietic protoporphyria (EPP) (Table 143-7)

Historical aspects

Although the disorder was first reported by Kosenow and Treibs [174] and Langhof et al [175], it was first clearly

defined and named by Magnus et al [23] who described their patient in detail in 1961 and showed a relationship between the protoporphyrinemia and the photosensitivity in the Soret band. This disease escaped detection for many years for at least two reasons: (1) objective clinical signs of skin photosensitivity associated with EPP are much milder than those of EP and (2) excessive porphyrins are almost never found in the urine of patients with EPP due to the virtual insolubility of PROTO in water. The entity

Table 143-7   Erythropoietic protoporphyria

Synonym	Erythrohepatic protoporphyria
Inheritance	Autosomal dominant
Age of onset	Early childhood
Photosensitivity	Mild to severe
Skin reactions	Acute: Edematous plaques, erythema, urticaria (occasional), purpura, rare bullae on the nose and hands
	Chronic: Shallow waxy scars over nose and dorsa of hands; "aged" knuckles; skin thickening of exposed areas; erosions, crusts, and diffuse infiltration and wrinkling of the face
Clinical findings	Pruritus, burning, and stinging of skin often during the first few minutes of sun exposure; erythema and edema; waxy thickening of the knuckles and nose with fine linear scarring
	Cholelithiasis, terminal hepatic failure in a small percentage of patients
Biochemical defects	Excretory: Normal porphyrins in urine; elevated PROTO in feces; RBC and plasma have increased PROTO
	Enzymatic: Ferrochelatase deficiency as manifest in RBC, skin fibroblasts, liver, and bone marrow

became established only after porphyrins were measured in RBC and feces [23].

The first patient reported by Magnus et al [23] was a 35-year-old male who had suffered from solar urticaria since the age of 8. His urinary porphyrins were normal but RBC and fecal PROTO were elevated and there was intense, transient red fluorescence of bone marrow normoblasts. Using a monochromator, Magnus et al were able to produce an abnormal cutaneous response of erythema, edema, and whealing in the skin of the patient following exposure to 400 nm radiation. No such reactions occurred in skin of normal individuals similarly irradiated.

Etiology

The specific enzyme defect in EPP is believed to occur at the step where PROTO is converted to heme by ferrochelatase. Several studies have demonstrated deficient ferrochelatase activity in RBC and cultured skin fibroblasts of patients and unaffected carriers of EPP [61–64]. Further studies have shown that the activity of ferrochelatase in cultured skin fibroblasts of EPP patients is only 10 to 25 percent of normal [176]. The markedly reduced catalytic activity is associated with increased affinity for the porphyrin substrate. Mitogen-stimulated lymphocytes have also been used to demonstrate the enzyme defect in EPP [177]. It is of interest that this disease occurs in cattle but in that species there is autosomal recessive inheritance of the enzyme defect [178].

Epidemiology

The inheritance of EPP has autosomal dominant features [179–185]. The sex incidence appears equal in most series. The infrequency in parents and children of affected families is consistent with a partial recessive factor [186]; evidently the mode of inheritance is complex. Cutaneous photosensitivity begins in childhood in the majority of patients (average age of onset, 4.3 years) [182].

Although the exact incidence of EPP is unknown, it has been reported with increasing frequency since 1961, indicating that it is one of the more common types of porphyria. Since the cutaneous photosensitivity may be mild and nondisfiguring, especially in patients living in less sunny areas, there are undoubtedly large numbers of unreported patients. Studies from one laboratory performing diagnostic tests for RBC porphyrins in patients with suspected cutaneous photosensitivity indicated that 8 percent of such samples demonstrate elevated RBC PROTO levels diagnostic of EPP. The disease has been reported from many countries around the world, including the United Kingdom, Holland, Denmark, and the United States in particular [187–189]. Possibly no ethnic group is spared and cases have now been reported in both Hispanic and black Americans [184,189].

Clinical manifestations

The disease begins early in life and is characterized by cutaneous photosensitivity and by elevated PROTO in RBC, feces, and plasma but there is no excess porphyrin excretion in the urine except when hepatic failure occurs as a terminal event. Photosensitivity usually begins in childhood and occurs on sun-exposed areas such as the

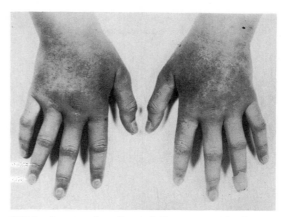

Fig. 143-9 A case of erythropoietic protoporphyria showing swelling and purpura on dorsa of hands resulting from exposure to solar radiation. *(Courtesy of Dr. E. Gasser-Wolff; Helv Paediatr Acta 20:598, 1965.)*

nose, cheeks, and dorsal aspects of the hands. The acute episodes of cutaneous photosensitivity include a burning, stinging (smarting), and itching in light-exposed skin, particularly the face and hands. Photosensitivity often occurs early in the spring and diminishes in the winter. The skin lesions may be erythematous, edematous, or urticarial; their severity may seem inconsistent with that of the subjective symptoms. The acute symptoms or lesions often develop during sun exposure or immediately thereafter. When placed in direct sunlight, infants may cry; older children and adults will often complain, within 5 to 10 min, of a burning sensation or pruritus. This may be followed in several hours by an increase in symptoms and diffuse swelling of the light-exposed skin (Fig. 143-9). Some patients may notice erythema with or without edema. Rarely, patients may exhibit urticaria or purpura. Sun exposure through window glass, e.g., an automobile window or even light-weight clothing will elicit the symptoms. Depending upon the duration and intensity of sun exposure, discomfort may persist from hours to days. Bullae are rare but purpura in fair-skinned individuals who inadvertently overexpose their face either in summer or on snow-covered mountains in winter has frequently been observed. The skin lesions may resolve slowly leaving small, atrophic, waxy scars (Fig. 143-10). These are most often seen on the dorsa of the hands, the nose, around the eyes, and on the pinnae. There may be some pursing of perioral skin (pseudorhagades). The skin of the knuckles and fingers, particularly over the metacarpophalangeal and interphalangeal joints, often appears thickened, wrinkled, and waxy, suggesting a premature aging (so-called old knuckles in a child). This subtle change, once recognized, is pathognomonic, particularly in children. Superficial scarring on the bridge of the nose and small, circular, shallow scars may be seen on the face and on the back of the neck. Vesicular or bullous lesions rarely occur in EPP in temperate climates although they have occurred in patients exposed to tropical sunlight. The course of EPP is evidently prolonged. The porphyrin abnormality remains throughout life, although some patients seem to be less symptomatic later in life.

Controversy exists concerning the tissue origin of the excessive PROTO in the plasma, the RBC, or the feces of

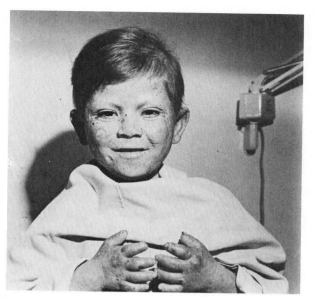

Fig. 143-10 A case of erythropoietic protoporphyria showing atrophic waxy scars, mutilations, and crusted lesions on face and hands. The hands also show severe edema. The mutilating skin lesions are the result of severe photosensitivity due to excessive protoporphyrin. *(Courtesy of Dr. A. Kurban, American University of Beirut.)*

patients with EPP. Studies from several laboratories have shown either that RBC PROTO levels alone are sufficient to explain the increased levels of PROTO [190–192] or that hepatic PROTO production must contribute to the excessively high levels of circulating PROTO [193–195]. Experimental studies have shown that the increased erythrocyte PROTO burden can be derived from both erythroid and hepatic sources [196].

The data of Piomelli et al [192] indicate that during the process of maturation of reticulocytes into adult erythrocytes, excessive PROTO leaks from the RBC into the plasma and subsequently is cleared by the liver. These findings suggest that most of the PROTO in liver and feces originates from the bone marrow. It is important to note that, in EPP, PROTO is unchelated by metals such as zinc. This metal-free PROTO can readily diffuse out of the RBC in the circulation. Thus, younger RBC contain elevated PROTO and as these cells mature, the PROTO levels diminish. This, perhaps, explains why, in EPP, not all RBC fluoresce [197]. Approximately 5 to 30 percent of RBC exhibit characteristic fluorescence when examined under a fluorescent microscope.

Associated findings are few in most patients with EPP. There is no erythrodontia, and hemolytic anemia is decidedly uncommon although about 11 percent of patients with EPP have a mild anemia of unknown cause [150]. No hypertrichosis, milia, sclerodermoid change, or hyperpigmentation occurs in EPP. Hemolytic anemia with cirrhosis and hypersplenism has been reported, and in at least one patient the degree of hemolysis, the porphyrin excretion, and the cutaneous photosensitivity all decreased following splenectomy [198].

Gallstones have been reported in some patients with EPP at a relatively early age, e.g., where 12 percent of patients had cholelithiasis, of whom three underwent cholecystec-

tomy [199]. Careful study of all gallstones obtained at surgery from two EPP patients showed that they contained large amounts of PROTO [199; Pathak and Bickers, unpublished observations].

Light microscopy of liver biopsies has revealed slight portal and periportal fibrosis and deposition of brown pigment which may occlude bile canaliculi and ducts and is also present in hepatocytes, in Kupffer cells, and in periportal macrophages. The pigment is birefringent on polarization microscopy [200–201]. Hepatocytes may also contain cytoplasmic or mitochondrial inclusions which at the ultrastructural level appear as needlelike crystals probably due to precipitated PROTO [202,203] (Fig. 143-11).

Terminal hepatic failure has been reported in about 20 patients with EPP [204–210]. These individuals ranged from 11 to 58 years of age; all were jaundiced, had hepatic cirrhosis, and died in hepatic coma or as a consequence of portal hypertension. The mechanism of this type of hepatic failure remains unexplained. Experimental studies have shown that perfusion of rat liver with PROTO induces a dose-dependent cholestasis that could contribute to the hepatotoxic effect of PROTO [211]. The hepatic pathology could be secondary to the accumulation of PROTO leaked from RBC that is incompletely cleared by the liver. In most cases, the development of jaundice has usually presaged rapid hepatic failure with coma and death. Awareness of this serious complication of EPP should be kept in mind by dermatologists as well as gastroenterologists.

Laboratory findings

The diagnosis of EPP is made by detecting elevated levels of free PROTO in the RBC and/or feces (see Tables 143-3 and 143-7). In addition, there may be increased plasma PROTO, increased fecal COPRO, and occasionally slightly increased RBC COPRO. In the individual patient with EPP, the excessive PROTO may be found in one or more of these compartments. In incomplete expression of EPP, only the fecal PROTO may be elevated [212]. Examination of a blood smear under a fluorescent microscope equipped with a mercury lamp or tungsten-iodide lamp emitting 400-nm radiation and a dark-field condensor reveals red-fluorescing RBC (5 to 30 percent). This fluorescence is often transient, quite light-sensitive, and the procedure should be carried out in subdued light or preferably in the dark [213]. Poh-Fitzpatrick et al [213] have devised a rapid quantitative microfluorometric assay for free erythrocyte PROTO which is useful as a screening test for suspected EPP. Finger-prick samples of blood collected on filter paper are used for this test. In one series of 32 patients with EPP, the RBC PROTO levels ranged from 131 to 1617 µg per dL of RBC (normal less than 90 µg per dL of RBC) [182].

The characteristic action spectrum of skin reactivity to light in the 400-nm range is the main evidence that porphyrins present in skin are responsible for the abnormal cutaneous photosensitivity reaction (see Fig. 143-7). The photosensitizing activity of porphyrins is most probably related to the light absorption and emission characteristics of these tetrapyrroles. In EPP, elevated plasma and RBC PROTO in metal-free form presumably can diffuse into vessel walls, endothelial cells, pericytes, or even into the extracellular fluid that bathes the dermis and perhaps even

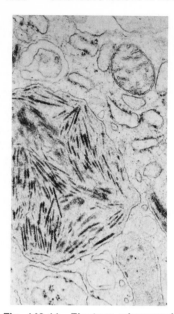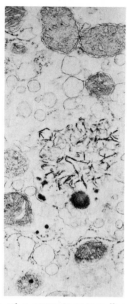

Fig. 143-11   Electron micrographs of a percutaneous liver biopsy specimen obtained from a patient with erythropoietic protoporphyria. Numerous rod-shaped crystals and electron-dense clumps of pigment are seen in the hepatocytes and Kupffer cells. When viewed under the microscope, these dense clumps of pigment exhibit an orange-red fluorescence and striking birefringence. *(Courtesy of Drs. K. Wolff and H. Hönigsmann, University of Vienna.)*

the epidermis as well. The mechanism whereby PROTO evokes damaging cutaneous responses is not clear. There is some evidence to suggest that unchelated (metal-free) PROTO may be responsible for the skin photosensitivity reactions. Evidence for this has come from studies designed to explain the perplexing observation that in lead poisoning and in iron-deficiency anemia, conditions in which RBC PROTO levels are similar to those found in EPP, cutaneous photosensitivity does not occur. Studies by Piomelli et al [192] and Lamola et al [214] suggest that in these nonphotosensitizing disorders the excessive PROTO is probably chelated with zinc and bound to globin chains in the RBC. This renders it incapable of diffusing into the plasma and then into cutaneous tissue, and explains why plasma PROTO is not elevated in these non-photosensitizing disorders. In EPP, however, the majority of the excessive PROTO is probably unchelated or free. Free PROTO can diffuse out of the RBC and is detectable in the plasma of patients with EPP who manifest cutaneous photosensitivity [171]. In one study a patient with sidero-blastic anemia had marked increases in free PROTO both in the RBC and in the plasma but had no cutaneous photosensitivity [215]. Since ferrochelatase activity was normal in this patient, it is possible that the excessive free PROTO was readily converted to heme in the skin, thereby precluding cutaneous accumulation of PROTO and associated photosensitivity. It has also been suggested that the absence of hemolytic anemia in EPP is due to the unique capacity of PROTO to move out of the RBC and to bind to albumin in the plasma [216]. The porphyrin does not remain within the lipid-rich red cell membrane sufficiently long for light exposure to cause damage and serum albumin

has a potent inhibitory effect on photohemolysis in EPP [217].

Histopathology

Specific findings are limited to sun-exposed skin. The epidermis may show mild acanthosis and hyperkeratosis, but the major changes are seen in the dermis. There is often marked eosinophilic homogenization and thickening of vessels in the papillary dermis due to the accumulation of an amorphous, homogeneous, slightly basophilic substance (hyaline-like) in and around the vessel walls [182]. The perivascular deposits of concentric eosinophilic layers of hyaline-like material stains strongly positive with periodic acid-Schiff (PAS) and is diastase positive (see Fig. 143-12). Histochemical studies suggest that this material may be a neutral glycoprotein with smaller amounts of acid muco-polysaccharide and lipids [218]. The histologic findings are apparently similar to those of lipoid proteinosis (hyalinosis cutis et mucosae) in which hyaline material may be seen not only in a perivascular distribution but also around sweat glands and nerves [219]. Electron microscopic studies in EPP show that the amorphous material consists of a multilayered, partially fragmented basement membrane and finely fibrillar material of moderate density which permeates and surrounds the vessel walls [220]. Other studies have shown that type IV collagen and laminin as well as amyloid P and fibronectin are deposited in the walls of dermal blood vessels [221,222].

Differential diagnosis

EPP must be differentiated from other causes of photosensitivity, primarily hydroa aestivale, polymorphous light eruption (PMLE), idiopathic solar urticaria, lipoid proteinosis, and other types of porphyria. Contact dermatitis and angioneurotic edema should also be considered. In PMLE, the lesions are characteristically papules, plaques, and papulovesicles. A family history of photosensitivity is less common. Burning and smarting of the skin during or soon after sun exposure is unusual in PMLE whereas it is a common occurrence in EPP. Skin biopsy with PAS staining may also be helpful in differentiating between PMLE and EPP. Idiopathic solar urticaria is not associated with elevated RBC or fecal PROTO. Contact dermatitis may involve non-light-exposed areas such as the skin folds and the submental areas. Patch testing with a suspected allergen and negative porphyrin values help to differentiate this condition. The lesions of angioneurotic edema may occur anywhere on the body including the mucous membranes. Because discomfort is often disproportionate to visible lesions, EPP has been confused with psychoneurosis or even malingering. This problem in differential diagnosis is readily solved by porphyrin determinations. ECP, an extremely rare condition, should also be considered in the differential diagnosis [24]. Clinically it resembles EPP and could only be diagnosed by chromatographic study of RBC porphyrins. The rare genodermatosis, lipoid proteinosis, may be confused with EPP due to a superficially similar histologic appearance of increased PAS-positive material in the upper dermis. In EPP, the PAS-positive material is usually limited to sun-exposed skin; in lipoid proteinosis, however, this material may be seen in any skin area. Idiopathic solar

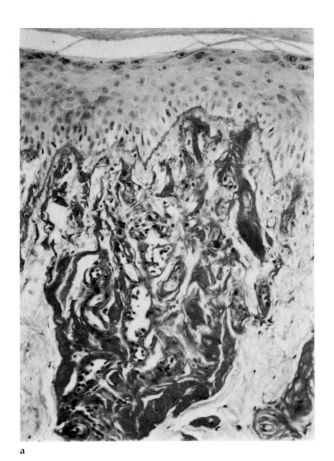

a

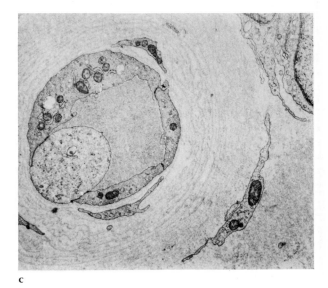

c

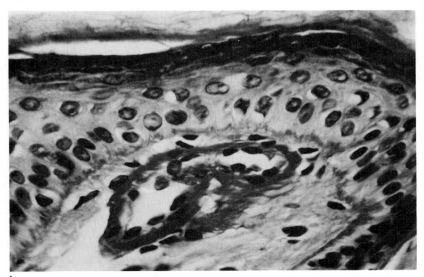

b

Fig. 143-12 (a) A biopsy of light-exposed skin from a patient with erythropoietic protoporphyria. There is marked thickening of the blood vessel walls of the upper dermis. The capillaries in the upper dermis are surrounded by a hyaline-like material. (b) Periodic acid-Schiff (PAS) stain of biopsy from light-exposed skin from a patient with erythropoietic protoporphyria, showing PAS-positive carbohydrate protein complex with lipid also present. These histologic features were not unlike those found in lipoid proteinosis. (c) Electron micrograph of biopsy of chronically exposed skin from a patient with erythropoietic protoporphyria. Multiple concentric basal laminae surrounding dermal blood vessels and finely fibrillar material admixed with amorphous masses within perivascular tissue are shown. *(Courtesy of Drs. K. Wolff and H. Hönigsmann, University of Vienna.)*

urticaria can be differentiated by measurement of PROTO levels in RBC and feces.

Treatment

The treatment of EPP has been aided by the introduction of beta carotene (Solatene). Formerly, the only treatment consisted of measures to protect the skin against UV and visible radiation. Topical sunscreens, antimalarial drugs, cholestyramine, and vitamins E and C have all been suggested but have not been shown to be effective [182]. As reported by Mathews-Roth et al [149,150,223], beta carotene (60 to 180 mg per day p.o.) has been found helpful in preventing or ameliorating the skin photosensitivity of EPP. Eighty-four percent of 133 patients claimed to triple their tolerance to sunlight after an adequate course of beta carotene exceeding two months. The therapeutic effectiveness of the drug has been confirmed by several groups of investigators [224–228]. These results are, however, based on limited controlled laboratory testing and uncontrolled clinical impressions; the one attempt at a controlled trial of short duration failed to confirm the therapeutic effectiveness of beta carotene [229]. Serum carotene levels should be maintained at a minimum of 600 μg per dL. In adult patients, this can usually be achieved by oral administration of 3 to 6 30-mg capsules per day which will produce serum carotene levels of 600 to 800 μg per dL after 4 to 6 weeks of therapy. Children under 12 years of age may receive 30 to 90 mg daily. Maximum effectiveness may not occur until 1 to 3 months after initiating therapy. The drug is remarkably well tolerated at these doses and there are no known toxic systemic effects of beta carotene. The drug in recommended doses has not caused any bone marrow abnormality or any aberrations of hepatic or renal function. Occasionally diarrhea occurs in a small number of patients. Orange or rusty discoloration of stools is common and is not an indication for discontinuing treatment. The only side effect of note is the visible yellowing of the skin that occurs as a result of carotenoderma. Topical application of beta carotene in cream form (1 to 5%) to light-exposed skin areas of EPP patients is totally ineffective; the photolability of carotenoid pigments results in rapid destruction of the applied beta carotene (Pathak, unpublished observations). The mechanism of the photoprotective effect of beta carotene is not precisely known. It does not appear to function as a protective filter to screen out potentially harmful solar radiation (380 to 550 nm). It does, however, appear to be capable of quenching excited singlet oxygen and of trapping free radicals formed by the interaction of light with PROTO. In vitro studies using various porphyrins have verified the production of $^1O_2$ and its quenching by beta carotene [230]. It should be remembered that beta carotene has no effect on the metabolism of porphyrins or on the biochemical abnormality of EPP. Patients with adequate blood levels of the drug may still become photosensitive following sun exposure. In many geographic regions it is often possible to discontinue the drug until spring.

Management of the hepatic failure remains unsatisfactory. Some clinical and biochemical improvement has been observed with the use of the anionic binding resin cholestyramine and the antioxidant vitamin E [203,210]. However, well-controlled studies are needed to verify their ther-apeutic efficacy in EPP. Hematin infusions have been used to temporarily decrease the production of heme and are associated with a decrease in fecal and plasma PROTO in some patients [196,231]. The efficacy of this approach remains poorly defined. The use of RBC exchanges with autologous washed cells has also been explored for its ability to induce clinical and biochemical remission of EPP. Bechtel et al showed that transfusion therapy in one patient with EPP resulted in a marked decrease in photosensitivity associated with a decline in free erythrocyte PROTO levels [232].

Erythropoietic coproporphyria (ECP)

There are only three known cases of this entity that have been published. Heilmeyer and Clotten have described the disorder in some detail [24]. Elevated PROTO and COPRO were found in the RBC of one patient. More recently Topi et al described two brothers with cutaneous photosensitivity similar to that of EPP with elevated RBC PROTO and COPRO III in each [233]. Very little is known about this disease.

Porphyria cutanea tarda (PCT) (Table 143-8)

Historical aspects

Porphyria cutanea tarda was originally classified by Günther as hematoporphyria chronica. He described it as a syndrome of skin lesions and darkly colored urine occurring later in life than either congenital or acute porphyria [7]. It was said not to be associated with acute attacks of abdominal pain or neurologic dysfunction. Waldenström [11,13] first named the disease PCT and observed that Swedish patients with acute attacks of porphyria (AIP) never developed cutaneous porphyria. He suggested that these two disorders were completely distinct, PCT being primarily acquired and AIP familial.

Following Waldenström's description of PCT in 1937, scattered case reports appeared in the literature. Early experience with this disorder in the United States was carefully described by Brunsting and his coworkers at the Mayo Clinic [12,234,235]. Shortly thereafter, patients with a comparable clinical picture were described in South Africa [236–238]. Finally, and even more confusing, it became clear that there were a small number of patients in the United States and a larger number in South Africa who manifested both the cutaneous changes of PCT as well as intermittent attacks of AIP. In South Africa, this was called VP, whereas initially in the United States it was known as mixed porphyria [101,239]. There is general agreement now on the use of the term VP to describe this disorder in the United States [18–22].

Etiology

Complete understanding of the etiology of PCT has been hampered by clinical evidence suggesting that there are several distinct forms of the disease. Thus many patients who in retrospect clearly had VP were often initially classified as PCT if the cutaneous manifestations of their disease predominated [240]. The additional knowledge that exposure to toxic environmental chemicals such as HCB

Table 143-8 Porphyria cutanea tarda

Synonyms	Symptomatic porphyria; acquired hepatic porphyria; chemical porphyria
Inheritance	Unclear; autosomal dominant in some patients
Age of onset	Usually in third or fourth decade; rare before puberty
Photosensitivity	Moderate to severe
Skin reactions	Vesicular, bullous and ulcerative lesions, primarily on light-exposed skin; increased skin fragility to mechanical trauma; hyperpigmentation and sclerodermoid plaques; scarring alopecia; milia on fingers and hands; hypertrichosis and periorbital violaceous suffusion
Clinical findings	Diabetes mellitus in about 25 percent of patients; rare hepatic tumor; increased liver iron stores; increased serum iron
Biochemical defects	Excretory: Increased urinary URO (I > III) and 7-carboxyl porphyrins (III > 1); increased ISOCOPRO in urine and feces
	Enzymatic: Deficiency of UROGEND in liver and RBC of some patients and their families
Differential diagnosis	"Pseudo-PCT": Drugs (sulfonamides, nalidixic acid, furosemide, tetracyline), hemodialysis, epidermolysis bullosa acquisita
	Porphyria variegata (VP): An autosomal dominant, potentially fatal disease following ingestion of barbiturates and sulfonamides, has identical skin lesions to PCT. High stool PROTO is distinctive for VP. Also VP patients have acute attacks, usually precipitated by drugs and characterized by acute abdominal pain, and elevated levels of PBG can be detected in the urine by the Watson-Schwartz test.

or chlorinated phenols induced a PCT-like syndrome, despite no clear evidence of genetic susceptibility, also made classification of PCT difficult. However, Kushner et al [47] and Benedetto et al [111] have suggested that in some patients with PCT there is a specific inherited deficiency of UROGEND and the defect is inherited as an autosomal dominant trait. Deficient activity of the enzyme was observed in the liver and RBC of patients with the disease and clinically unaffected family members, suggesting that PCT may be due to a genetically transmitted defect. The demonstrable UROGEND deficiency in both sexes and in members of four successive generations of a single family suggests that this is an autosomal dominant disorder [111]. Elder et al [241] have confirmed the enzyme deficiency in the liver of patients with sporadic (nonfamilial) PCT, but found normal activity in RBC and in cultured skin fibroblasts, a finding confirmed by others [112]. From these studies it was concluded that inheritance of deficient UROGEND in RBC and liver is an uncommon cause of PCT

and that in the more common nonfamilial PCT the enzyme is deficient only in the liver, which could be explained either by a gene defect restricted to the liver or by exposure to chemicals which selectively inhibit the hepatic but not the RBC enzyme.

Most classifications of PCT separate the disorder into at least two broad categories: (1) PCT-symptomatic or sporadic, (2) PCT-hereditary (Table 143-8). Symptomatic or sporadic PCT is assumed to be an acquired abnormality due to the effects of environmentally encountered substances (Table 143-9). Such exposure may provoke porphyria only in selected individuals ingesting alcohol and estrogens or in practically all exposed individuals (HCB). The term PCT-hereditary has been used to describe those patients who had other family members with the same disease. It is unclear whether some of the early studies in which patients were reported as having hereditary PCT actually had VP, an autosomal dominant disorder. This remains an unsolved problem. Studies by Watson et al in the United States [242] and by Day et al in South Africa [243] have shown that PCT and VP may occur in different members of the same family, so-called dual porphyria.

Alcohol. Ethanol has been shown to induce hepatic ALAS in patients with PCT [244]. Erythrocyte UROGEND activity is diminished in healthy subjects following acute ethanol ingestion and in chronic alcoholics [245,246]. It should be emphasized that ethanol in addition to its ability to enhance ALAS activity can also inhibit the activity of other enzymes in the heme pathway, including ferrochelatase and ALAD. Chronic alcoholism leads to suppression of erythropoiesis [247] and increased absorption of dietary iron, although whether the increased iron absorption of alcoholism is related to the characteristic hepatic siderosis of PCT is unknown. A recent study showing that hepatic ALAS is increased in cirrhotic liver of individuals without porphyria raises questions concerning the relevance of alcohol effects on ALAS in the clinical expression of PCT [248].

Estrogens. The widespread use of estrogens as contraceptive agents or as hormone supplements in females and as adjunctive hormonal therapy in males with prostatic carcinoma has been associated with an increasing number of cases of PCT [109,249–251]. The mechanism of the estrogen effect on the expression of PCT is not established. Levere [252] has shown that diethylstilbesterol, an estrogen, induces hepatic ALAS. This alone, however, would not explain the distinctive porphyrin excretion pattern found in PCT.

Hexachlorobenzene (HCB). This fungicide caused an "epidemic" of a PCT-like syndrome in southeastern Turkey in the 1950s [14,104,253]. It was added as a preservative to wheat intended for planting but, because of a famine, sev-

Table 143-9 Drugs and chemicals associated with the clinical expression of porphyria cutanea tarda

Ethyl alcohol	Iron
Estrogenic hormones	Tetrachlorodibenzo-*p*-dioxin
Hexachlorobenzene	Polychlorinated biphenyls
Chlorinated phenols	

eral thousand individuals of diverse ethnic origin, mostly children, ingested the seed wheat and subsequently developed typical PCT. The porphyrin excretion pattern and the cutaneous syndrome in these patients was similar to that seen in PCT evoked by ethanol or estrogens. The outbreak of PCT in Turkey caused by ingestion of HCB indicated that the disease can be acquired in nongenetically predisposed individuals.

Twenty-five years after onset, the most common clinical findings in these HCB-poisoned individuals were those of chronic porphyria including sclerodermoid scarring (84 percent), hyperpigmentation (78 percent), hirsutism (49 percent), and increased skin fragility (38 percent) [254,255]. A painless arthritis was seen in two out of three affected individuals and a variety of neurologic signs and symptoms were seen in the majority. Stool and urine URO remained elevated in many patients.

Experimental studies have shown that the chronic administration of HCB to experimental animals produces excessive porphyrin accumulation in the liver in a pattern quite similar to that seen in PCT in humans [256,257]. These data are consistent with the hypothesis that chlorinated hydrocarbons such as HCB or their metabolites inhibit hepatic UROGEND, leading to excessive hepatic storage of URO and other acetate substituted porphyrins [52]. It is of interest that experimental studies have shown that HCB can inactivate UROGEND by abolishing catalytic activity without changing the amount of immunoreactive enzyme protein [258]. Chemical porphyria, similar to PCT, is caused by other chlorinated hydrocarbons such as the polychlorinated biphenyls and 2,3,7,8-tetrachlorodibenzo-*p*-dioxin (TCDD), a by-product in the synthesis of the herbicide 2,4,5-trichlorophenoxyacetic acid [259,260].

Tetrachlorodibenzo-*p*-dioxin (TCDD). TCDD is known to be one of the most toxic environmental pollutant chemicals yet identified. Among its numerous toxic effects are chloracne, liver damage, and hepatic porphyria in experimental animals and perhaps also in humans [261–264]. It has been shown that the hepatic porphyrinogenic effect of TCDD can be abolished in mice by first depleting the animals of iron [54,265]. Furthermore, it is known that highly inbred mouse strains vary in their susceptibility to induction of hepatic porphyria by TCDD, indicating that the porphyrogenic effect of this hydrocarbon is modulated by as yet undefined genetic factors [266].

Iron. Hepatic iron overload accompanies clinical PCT in practically all cases [267] and elevation of plasma iron is found in one-third to one-half of patients [249]. Stainable iron can be seen both in Kupffer cells and in hepatocytes. Lundvall [268] has pointed out that histochemical staining for iron may not provide an accurate assessment of total hepatic iron stores. In PCT, the quantity of iron that can be mobilized by phlebotomy indicates that total iron stores are approximately twice normal [269,270]. Detailed ferrokinetic studies in patients with PCT have been normal [271]. The long remissions that follow repeated phlebotomy and the apparent ineffectiveness of this treatment if supplemental iron is administered concomitantly suggest that iron plays a role in the excessive hepatic porphyrin production of PCT [267]. PCT is particularly common where alcoholism and iron overload occur together.

The role of iron in the pathogenesis of PCT is undoubt-

edly a complex one and several hypotheses have been proposed to explain it. It was thought by some that iron is capable of directly inhibiting UROGEND [272] and that iron may have a permissive effect on the inhibitory effect of chlorinated phenols on hepatic UROGEND in chick embryo liver [54]. When added as ferrous iron to crude liver homogenates, there is accumulation of URO and 7-carboxylporphyrin [272,273]. Furthermore, it has been shown that the porphyrinogenic effect of TCDD can be largely abolished by concomitant iron depletion [265]. However, studies with purified UROGEND prepared from human erythrocytes have shown that the purified enzyme is not inhibited by Fe^{++} or Fe^{+++} suggesting that the role of this metal in the pathogenesis of PCT may not involve direct inhibition of the enzyme [46]. To add further confusion, some workers have suggested that iron can activate UROGEND [274] whereas others have shown no effect by the metal on the enzyme [275]. Acute iron loading of rats causes a 70 to 80 percent decrease in the activity of ALAD which in turn can diminish hepatic heme synthesis and increase ALAS activity [34]. Chronic iron overload can produce peroxidative damage to lipid-rich mitochondrial and microsomal membranes in the liver of experimental animals but the relation of this toxic effect to changes in hepatic heme synthesis has not been clearly defined [83,276].

Iron can also enhance the induction response of hepatic ALAS to drugs [277]. This iron-augmented increase in ALAS activity could lead to enhanced porphyrinogenesis, though this alone would not explain the porphyrin excretion pattern seen in PCT. Finally, Kushner et al have shown that addition of ferrous iron to liver in vitro causes a marked increase in porphyrin synthesis and inhibits URO-COSYN III activity [278]. This latter effect would explain the URO isomer I excess characteristic of PCT. The multiple effects of iron on heme synthesis have been nicely summarized [279–281].

The sclerodermoid changes that are seen primarily in the skin of patients with PCT, HEP, and EP include indurated hypopigmented plaques and scarring which can occur in both light-exposed and light-protected skin sites. Experimental studies have shown that URO I, the major excess porphyrin in these disorders, when added to human fibroblasts in vitro, causes a specific increase in collagen synthesis. This occurs in both the presence and the absence of 400-nm radiation, indicating that porphyrins have biologic effects independent of their photosensitizing properties [282].

From these known effects of alcohol, estrogens, chlorinated hydrocarbons, and iron on the heme pathway it is clear that each of these could contribute to the excessive hepatic porphyrinogenesis characteristic of PCT. The clinical expression of PCT is therefore dependent upon the interaction of a number of factors both genetic and environmental. However, it is important to note that the ingestion of drugs usually associated with inducing acute attacks of AIP, VP, or HCP (see Table 143-4) does not appear to lead to exacerbations of PCT.

Epidemiology

PCT occurs throughout the world [283–285]. The disease most often begins in middle-aged individuals but occasion-

Fig. 143-13 **A case of porphyria cutanea tarda showing bullae and depigmented scars.** *(Courtesy of Dr. L. Eales, Groote Schurr Hospital, Capetown).*

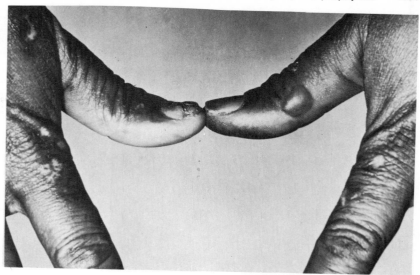

ally occurs in prepuberal children [286]. Prior to the widespread use of oral contraceptives PCT developed predominantly in males. Thus, in the past, a typical patient with PCT might have been described as a middle-aged male in good general health who regularly consumed significant amounts of alcohol. Brunsting's experience at the Mayo Clinic illustrates this clearly [12]: of 34 patients, 26 were male and more than 90 percent consumed moderate to heavy amounts of alcohol.

In contrast, experience with 40 patients over the past decade indicates that the sex incidence is now approximately equal [249]: in this series 21 patients were male and 19 were female. The earlier sex difference probably reflected a higher incidence of male alcoholism. PCT is frequently seen in young women below the age of 30 [287,288]. The rising incidence of PCT in females is probably due to the widespread ingestion of estrogens in oral contraceptives or in hormone supplements [289]. It should be noted that males treated with estrogens, for example as adjunctive therapy for carcinoma of the prostate, have also developed PCT [109,250].

Clinical manifestations

Vesicles and bullae occur predominantly in areas subject to repeated trauma (see Figs. 143-13 to 143-16). There is an increased susceptibility to minor mechanical trauma and the patient often notices a gradual increase in skin fragility, usually on the dorsa of the hands, but occasionally on the feet as well (Fig. 143-15). Inadvertent minor trauma to the hand results in shearing away of the skin, leaving multiple indolent, red to purple erosions that heal only slowly (Fig. 143-16). The traumatized skin becomes crusted and, as the lesions resolve, areas of scarring may ensue. Numerous small milia can develop, particularly on the fingers and hands. These are pearly white to yellow, spherical, subepidermal inclusions, 1 to 5 mm in diameter, and characteristically are present in each of the hepatic porphyrias with cutaneous photosensitivity (PCT and VP) (Figs. 143-14 and 143-16). *Patients are often unaware that sunlight plays a role in producing their lesions since the acute photosensitivity so characteristic of the erythropoietic porphyrias is rare in PCT.* However, most patients do recognize that

Fig. 143-14 **A case of porphyria cutanea tarda showing bullae and erosions on the hands.** *(Courtesy of Drs. A. Wiskemann and J. Kimmig, University Skin Clinic, Hamburg.)*

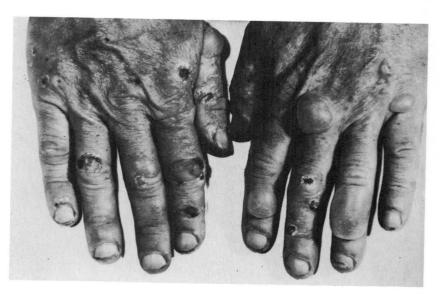

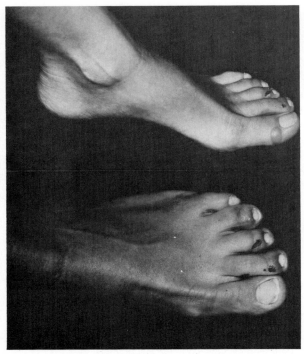

Fig. 143-15 A bullous eruption with erosions on the feet in a patient with porphyria cutanea tarda.

mental changes in light exposure. It is of interest that variations in environmental light exposure can affect hepatic ALAS activity [292,293].

Other skin changes that are seen in PCT include hyperpigmentation and hypopigmentation that may be mottled, resembling chloasma or melasma (Fig. 143-17). There may be an associated purplish red ("heliotrope") suffusion of the central part of the face, particularly involving the periorbital areas, which may bear a striking resemblance to the plethora seen in polycythemia rubra vera (see Fig. A2-2). This is not seen in the porphyrias of bone marrow origin.

Hypertrichosis (nonvirilizing) is a useful diagnostic sign that often brings the female patient to the dermatologist (Fig. 143-18). The hair may vary in texture between fine and coarse and in color between light and dark. These hairs are particularly prominent along the temples and the cheeks but may occasionally involve the trunk and extremities in severe cases. Such hair may continue to grow and to darken and thicken, particularly on the cheeks and on the forehead between the eyes and at the hairline of the scalp. Males may complain that shaving is more difficult and that the growth pattern of their beard has changed. Hypertrichosis may be the presenting symptom in women with PCT. A particularly severe form of hypertrichosis may occur in younger children with PCT. Thus, in the reports of HCB poisoning in Turkey, some of the children were described as "monkey-like" because of marked hypertrichosis [104]. The mechanism of this phenomenon is unknown; androgen levels are reported to be normal. The hypertrichosis of PCT usually improves slowly following appropriate treatment. Sclerodermoid plaques may develop on both light-exposed and on the less-covered body areas. These are usually scattered, waxy yellow to white, indurated plaques that closely resemble, both clinically and histopathologically, morphea or scleroderma and are often seen in light-exposed areas. As discussed above, URO I stimulates collagen synthesis in human skin fibroblasts [282]. In a few patients, calcification has developed in these

their skin condition worsens in the spring and summer and seems to improve in the fall and winter. It is of interest that porphyrin excretion in PCT appears to increase in summer months and to decrease in winter months [290]. Whether increased duration of sun exposure and photocatalyzed oxidation of porphyrin precursors account for this seasonal variation in porphyrin excretion and clinical expression of the disease remains unknown. However, the work of Jones et al [291] suggests there is a circadian activity of porphyrin metabolism susceptible to environ-

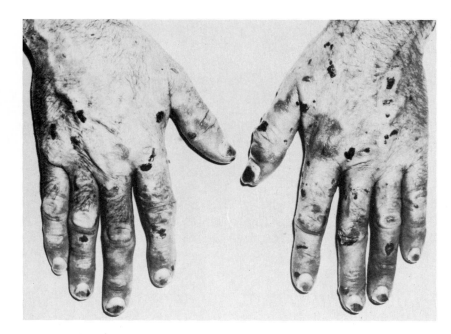

Fig. 143-16 A case of porphyria cutanea tarda showing bullae and erosions on the hands. Several areas show hypopigmented scarring. (Courtesy of Drs. H. Wallace and G. Wells, St. Thomas Hospital, London.)

Fig. 143-17 Porphyria cutanea tarda, which exhibits marked "wrinkling" of the face and depigmented scars on the dorsa of the hands.

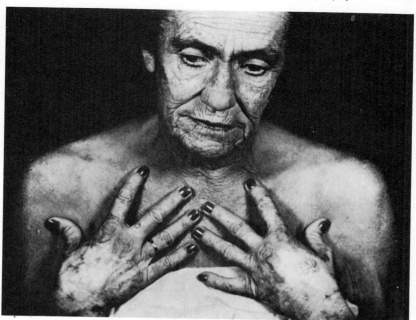

sclerodermoid plaques, necessitating excision and grafting of skin.

PCT-like syndromes are occasionally seen in association with other conditions including hepatic tumors [294–298], hepatitis [299,300], and lupus erythematosus [301,302]. Subepidermal bullous dermatoses mimicking PCT clinically and histologically have been described (see "Pseudoporphyria" below). A number of cases have occurred in patients with renal failure undergoing hemodialysis [303–309]. Associations with sarcoidosis [310] and Sjögren's syndrome [311] have also been reported.

Laboratory findings

Virtually all patients with PCT have excessive total body iron stores manifest as increased serum iron and/or hepatocellular iron. Occasionally there is mild erythrocytosis. A diabetic glucose tolerance test occurs in 25 percent of patients and cryoglobulinemia has been detected occasionally [312].

Patients with PCT excrete increased amounts of porphyrins in the urine which may exhibit characteristic pink-red fluorescence when examined with a Wood's lamp. The porphyrin excretion pattern of PCT has three main features: (1) increased urinary excretion of URO and of other acetate-substituted porphyrins, (2) a distinctive pattern of excretion of isomer series I and III porphyrins, and (3) increased excretion of fecal and urinary ISOCOPRO [313–319]. PCT patients excrete greatly increased amounts of urinary 8-carboxyl URO and also prophyrins with 7-, 6-, and 5-carboxyl groups; 4-carboxyl porphyrin (COPRO) is also increased but to a lesser extent than URO and rarely surpasses 600 μg/24 h (see Table 143-3). In PCT, the hepatic UROGEND deficiency results in the accumulation of dehydroisocoproporphyrinogen (Fig. 143-2b). ISOCOPRO is derived from this moiety which in turn is derived from 5-carboxylporphyrinogen III (Figs. 143-1 and 143-2i). The enzyme COPROGENO can utilize this as a substrate to form dehydroisocoproporphyrinogen.

The 8-carboxyl URO and 7-carboxyl porphyrins are the predominant urinary porphyrins in PCT (greater than 90 percent of total porphyrins). The urinary porphyrin excretion pattern is a mixture of type I and type III isomers. URO is about 60 percent type I isomer and 40 percent type III; 7- and 6-carboxyl porphyrins are greater than 90 percent type III and less than 10 percent type I isomer; 5- and 4-carboxyl porphyrins are about 50 percent each isomer. This distinctive isomer pattern is found consistently in patients with PCT [320,321].

In general, only trace amounts of URO are present in the stools of normal individuals. There is some fecal porphyrin excretion in PCT. This consists primarily of ISOCOPRO (type III), 7-carboxyl porphyrin, and lesser amounts of URO and COPRO.

In summary, the characteristic excretion pattern of PCT is as follows: in urine there is elevated URO (I isomer 60 to 70 percent) and 7-carboxyl porphyrin (III isomer greater than 90 percent) and lesser elevations of 6-, 5-, and 4-carboxyl prophyrins. Two ISOCOPROS have also been identified in the urine of PCT patients [314]. ISOCOPRO (COPRO with one acetate side group) is found in large amounts in the feces [313].

The ratio of URO to COPRO in the urine is often helpful in differentiating PCT and VP. Thus, in PCT, the URO:COPRO ratio is usually greater than 3:1, whereas in VP the ratio is less than 1:1. Occasionally, 24-h urine porphyrins will be normal or only slightly increased in a patient with the cutaneous findings of PCT. This should alert the physician to evaluate stool porphyrins since these are elevated in patients with VP (see "Variegate Porphyria" below).

The constellation of clinical and laboratory findings including examination of the urine with a readily available Wood's lamp often suffices to make the diagnosis of PCT [57]. Suspected PCT can frequently be confirmed by acidifying a random urine sample with a few drops of 10% hydrochloric acid or acetic acid and looking for orange-red fluorescence. The sensitivity of the screening test can be

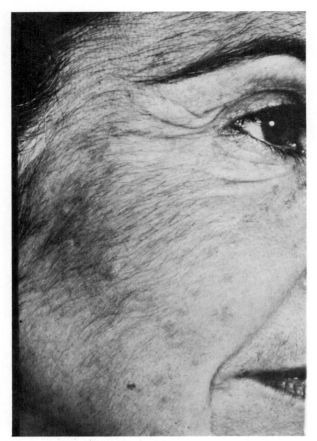

Fig. 143-18 Facial hypertrichosis in a female patient with porphyria cutanea tarda who received estrogen therapy. Thick black hair growth is seen on the cheeks and in the periorbital region. This growth of hair often extends to the forehead. (Reproduced with permission of Yearbook of Dermatology, Chicago, Year Book, 1975, and Professor L. C. Harber.)

enhanced by addition of talc to the urine, shaking, centrifuging, and examining the talc pellet for fluorescence. If in doubt, this test can be modified as follows [57,322,323]. To 5 ml of urine (freshly voided or 24-h specimen), add 5 to 10 drops (0.5 ml) glacial acetic acid and 2.5 ml ethyl acetate. Shake and allow to settle. Examine the upper aqueous layer with a Wood's lamp for characteristic red-pink porphyrin fluorescence.

It should be emphasized that patients who appear clinically to have PCT may have a negative fluorescent screening test for porphyrins and only slightly elevated total 24-h urine porphyrins. In such patients, it is absolutely essential to perform quantitative 24-h urine URO and COPRO determinations and stool PROTO determinations which almost always permit delineation of PCT from VP.

Histopathology

The characteristic histopathologic finding in PCT is a subepidermal bulla (Figs. 143-19 and 143-20). Bullae characteristically show a corrugated, undulating base that has been termed festooned [324]. There is little or no inflammatory infiltrate. PAS stain reveals a mild degree of thickening of the papillary vessel wall, not nearly so marked as

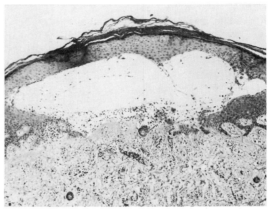

Fig. 143-19 Porphyria cutanea tarda: subepidermal vesiculation in an early lesion. The subepidermal vesiculation of porphyria may occur with only a sparse, inflammatory cell infiltrate. ×40. (Courtesy of Dr. W. H. Clark, Jr., University of Pennsylvania.)

that seen in patients with EPP. Reticulin staining demonstrates slight proliferation of reticulin fibers along the basement membrane [325]. Deposition of complement components and of immunoglobulins has been demonstrated. IgG deposition at the dermal-epidermal junction and in and around vessel walls is present in affected skin of patients with PCT [326]. These changes are most apparent in sun-exposed areas of patients with active disease and high urinary porphyrin excretion and decrease substantially in patients after appropriate treatment. It is also possible that the deposition of immunoglobulins and complement is a nonspecific result of injury to the cutaneous tissue. The locus of damage to the upper dermal vessels and the dermal-epidermal junction suggests that damage to these areas

Fig. 143-20 Porphyria cutanea tarda: subepidermal vesiculation in a late lesion. There is virtually no inflammatory response, but the form of the dermal papillae is partially preserved. ×100. (Courtesy of Dr. W. H. Clark, Jr., University of Pennsylvania.)

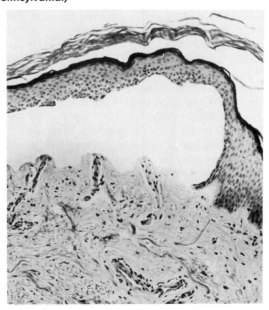

evoked by porphyrin photosensitivity may be responsible for the unique skin fragility seen in PCT. Several studies have shown increased porphyrin concentrations in the skin of patients with PCT [327–329]. With rare exception, blisters have not been induced by phototesting [142]; however, Magnus et al [143,330] and Rimington et al [145], using a monochromator, have been able to produce both erythema and delayed edema in the skin of patients with PCT. Runge and Watson [141] and Pathak (unpublished observations) have also produced erythema and edema of light-exposed skin by preexposure to infrared radiation followed by exposure to 400-nm radiation in PCT patients.

Differential diagnosis

Other dermatoses that can be confused with PCT include VP, HEP, hydroa aestivale, hydroa vacciniforme, scleroderma, pellagra, neurotic excoriations, PMLE, and bullous erosive conditions such as pemphigus vulgaris, pemphigoid, epidermolysis bullosa, bullous dermatosis of hemodialysis, and dermatitis herpetiformis. Each of these can readily be differentiated on histopathologic grounds, by immunofluorescence tests, or by appropriate porphyrin studies. Careful evaluation of urine, stool, and plasma porphyrins will almost always permit confirmation of the diagnosis of PCT. It should be emphasized that patients with PCT are not prone to the acute life-threatening attacks characteristic of AIP and VP. A very limited number of drugs and chemicals, particularly alcohol, estrogens, and selected halogenated hydrocarbons seem capable of evoking the disease (Table 143-9). Drugs such as barbiturates, which are contraindicated in AIP, have been administered to PCT patients without untoward effect. Drugs such as nalidixic acid, furosemide, and the tetracyclines may rarely produce clinical signs closely resembling PCT (see "Pseudoporphyria" below). VP has skin lesions identical to PCT, but elevated fecal PROTO and the urinary porphyrin excretion pattern can usually differentiate this disease.

Treatment

Initially, a careful history should be taken in an effort to identify an environmental toxin, e.g., alcohol, estrogen, or chlorinated hydrocarbon, that may have triggered the disease. These should be strictly avoided if possible; often this alone can lead to gradual improvement in the disease [331]. However, in most patients with PCT more aggressive treatment is usually necessary and this currently consists of either repeated phlebotomy [331–336] or orally administered chloroquine [337–341] or a combination of both [342,343]. Other forms of treatment that have been advocated include administration of iron chelators [344,345], metabolic alkalinization of the urine [346,347], and oral administration of cholestyramine [348]. In this chapter only phlebotomy and chloroquine will be discussed since these are most effective in the treatment of PCT.

Phlebotomy. Phlebotomy is the treatment of choice for PCT. Numerous reports have emphasized the safety and efficacy of this form of therapy [331–336] which was introduced by Ippen in 1961. Phlebotomy is apparently effective because it depletes the excessive hepatic iron stores characteristic of PCT [267,268,273,331]. Biochemical remission

of PCT has occurred in patients treated with phlebotomy who had iron overload as well as in patients with quantitatively normal iron stores. Replenishment of iron following phlebotomy-induced remission of PCT may result in biochemical and clinical exacerbation of the disease [267,273]. Abstinence from the porphyrinogenic agent alone, especially alcohol, may induce a clinical and biochemical remission although this may take months to years [11,331].

There are several interesting hypotheses concerning the mechanism whereby phlebotomy-induced depletion of excess iron leads to improvement in PCT and these include the following.

1. *Iron effect on ALAS.* Iron can enhance the induction response of ALAS to drugs [277] and the hepatic porphyrinogenic response to HCB in experimental animals [256]. Depletion of iron could render ALAS less inducible and thereby diminish hepatic prophyrinogenesis.
2. *Iron depletion effects on other heme pathway enzymes.* The studies of Kushner et al showing that ferrous iron inhibits UROGEND [272] and increases the rate of hepatic porphyrin synthesis from ALA or PBG [278] suggest that removal of iron can allow UROGEND activity to return to normal and/or reduce excessive porphyrinogenesis. Iron depletion can also reverse the decreases in ALAD and increases in ALAS induced by iron loading [276].
3. *Iron effects on hepatic lipid peroxidation.* Iron depletion could reverse this response by the liver to iron overload [83].

Phlebotomy can easily be carried out in the dermatologist's office. In most reported series the total amount of blood removed has varied widely, ranging usually from 1,500 to 12,000 mL [267,268,331,333,336]. It is most convenient to use plastic blood-drawing bags available in any blood bank. Approximately 500 mL of blood is removed at weekly or biweekly intervals until the hemoglobin decreases to 10 to 11 g per dL or until the serum iron drops to 50 to 60 μg per dL. Patients are strongly encouraged to discontinue or decrease exposure to porphyrinogenic agents since this usually hastens clinical and biochemical remission.

It is particularly important to reassure the patient that clinical improvement may not become apparent for variable intervals after beginning the phlebotomies. Porphyrin excretion continues to fall long after phlebotomies are discontinued. Ramsay et al [331] have shown that in more than 90 percent of patients treated with regular phlebotomy, urinary URO excretion reached normal levels (less than 100 μg per 24 h) after 5 to 12 months. Blistering is the first sign to disappear, followed by improvement in skin fragility, and in hypertrichosis over a period of 3 to 18 months. Even sclerodermoid changes can resolve slowly although this may take several years [331,336]. There is little or no published information on follow-up of treatment for longer than about 5 years, but most relapsed patients have again responded to a second or third series of phlebotomies [336]. The length of remission induced by phlebotomy varies widely but, in the authors' experience, has ranged from 6 months to more than 8 years [349]. Follow-up studies show that at least 5 to 10 percent of patients will relapse within one year.

Phlebotomy is a safe, effective, and relatively simple form of therapy with minimum associated morbidity. A few patients may complain of mild to moderate fatigue and weakness during the treatment period but this usually resolves as the hemoglobin returns to normal. In the authors' experience, phlebotomy is the treatment of choice for PCT.

Chloroquine. The antimalarial aminoquinolines, chloroquine (Aralen) and hydroxychloroquine (Plaquenil), have also been recommended for treating PCT [350]. Linden et al [351] reported that five days following oral administration of chloroquine a 48-year-old man developed acute abdominal pain and dark red urine. It was felt that chloroquine had caused an attack of acute porphyria. In some patients with lupus erythematosus, chloroquine treatment has inadvertently unmasked latent PCT. In 1957, London [352] first suggested that chloroquine was useful in treating PCT. One patient had no toxic reaction to the drug (500 mg daily for several months) and the cutaneous signs of the disease cleared within a year. Vogler et al [337] and Kowertz [338] recommended the use of chloroquine in doses of 500 mg daily for 8 days. Kowertz feels that the associated hepatotoxic response seen in PCT patients treated with chloroquine is a necessary and acceptable risk, since prolonged remissions of PCT usually ensue after such treatment. Liver function tests usually reveal marked hepatocellular dysfunction with large increases in serum SGOT, SGPT, and bilirubin. These usually return to normal levels over a period of several weeks. The clinical and biochemical remission of PCT obtained with chloroquine appears to be identical in all respects to that evoked by phlebotomy. However, it has been reported that rapid relapse occurred in several patients treated with hydroxychloroquine [353]. There is a marked increase in urinary URO excretion in patients receiving this drug. This effect of chloroquine does not occur as a result of the hepatotoxic response per se, but seems to be due to removal of porphyrins from the liver as a complex with the drug [354].

The mechanism of chloroquine action in PCT is not completely clear. Scholnick et al [354] have shown that chloroquine binds to hepatocellular porphyrins, making them more water soluble. The water-soluble chloroquine–porphyrin complex then diffuses rapidly from the hepatocyte and is excreted. Taljaard et al [350], however, feel that chloroquine binds to iron in the hepatocyte and the bound iron is then excreted. This has been confirmed in selected patients [353].

The concept of using low-dose chloroquine therapy to reduce the severity of the hepatoxtoxic effect in PCT was first suggested by Saltzer et al [355]. Remission of PCT was obtained in a single patient who received 50 mg of chloroquine twice weekly for 7 months. Taljaard et al [350] extended these studies and reported good results in seven of eight PCT patients treated with chloroquine sulfate (330 mg base) twice weekly for several months. Kordac et al [340] have reported the successful use of low-dose chloroquine (125 mg twice weekly for 8 to 18 months) in 112 patients with PCT. Complete clinical and biochemical remission occurred in all patients. Furthermore, 73 of these patients remained in remission for more than 4 years.

Chloroquine therapy appears to have a place in the management of PCT. There are selected patients who are not good candidates for phlebotomy, i.e., those with anemia. The authors suggest the following regimen for chloroquine administration in PCT. After obtaining baseline urinary porphyrin values and liver function tests, a single "test dose" of chloroquine base of 125 mg is administered. Liver function tests are repeated in one week and if there are no abnormalities the drug is then administered in doses of 125 mg twice weekly. Liver function tests and urinary porphyrins are monitored bimonthly and the medication continued until urinary URO is less than 100 μg per 24 h. This usually requires 6 to 12 months of treatment. Studies comparing the therapeutic efficacy of phlebotomy with that of low-dose chloroquine have shown each to be superior [356,357].

In one study, Swanbeck and Wennersten [342] suggest that the combination of phlebotomy and high-dose chloroquine treatment may reduce the severity of the hepatotoxic response to chloroquine and also induce remission of the disease. Patients are treated with a series of one to four phlebotomies prior to starting high-dose chloroquine (250 mg daily for 7 days). The procedure is repeated when signs of biochemical or clinical relapse occur. Relapse occurred in 43 percent of patients treated with this regimen with symptom-free periods of 1 to 2.5 years thereafter [343].

It should be emphasized that despite the tendency of the antimalarials to evoke hepatotoxic responses in patients with PCT, there is no evidence to suggest that the changes in hepatocellular pathology characteristic of PCT worsen as a result of treatment with these drugs [358].

Acute intermittent porphyria (AIP) (Table 143-10)

Historical aspects

The disease has been known since the late nineteenth century when Stokvis [98] first reported the case of a woman who ingested the drug sulfonal and then became acutely ill, excreted dark red urine, and died. Barker and Estes first suggested the familial nature of the disease when they reported recurrent episodes of abdominal pain, muscle weakness, and neurologic dysfunction in an 18-year-old female [359]. Two sisters were said to be similarly affected.

The first detailed clinical description of AIP was that of Waldenström [11] who described a total of 179 cases in Sweden. Of these, 103 were said to have acute porphyria characterized by periodic attacks of abdominal pain with constipation, nervous and mental symptoms, and paralysis. This was accompanied by increased urinary excretion of PBG. Several excellent reviews have summarized the clinical and biochemical features of AIP [13,28,29, 100,102,360].

Concepts concerning the etiology of AIP have undergone change as new biochemical knowledge has accumulated. Because of the characteristic pattern of excessive urinary excretion of ALA and PBG, it was first thought that AIP was an "overproduction" disease, manifested by increased levels of the enzyme ALAS. The studies of Granick and Urata [66] had shown that ALAS is the rate-limiting enzyme for the heme pathway and that the enzyme is inducible by drugs (see Table 143-4 and "Drug-Induced Porphyria" above). This observation suggested that the excessive ALA and PBG excretion seen in AIP could be explained by enhanced activity of ALAS. Several groups then showed that hepatic ALAS activity was indeed increased in AIP [68–70,361]. It was proposed that an op-

Table 143-10 Acute intermittent porphyria

Synonym	Swedish porphyria
Inheritance	Autosomal dominant
Age of onset	10 to 40; extremely rare prior to puberty
Incidence	1.5:100,000; more common in Scandinavia
Photosensitivity	None
Skin reactions	None
Clinical findings	Acute attacks with a neurologic–visceral symptom complex; this includes abdominal pain, constipation, and muscle weakness occasionally leading to paralysis and death; bizarre, neurotic or psychotic behavior; acute attacks often precipitated by drugs
Biochemical defects	Excretory: Elevated ALA and PBG in the urine during and between attacks
	Enzymatic: PBGD deficiency in liver, RBC, lymphocytes, and skin fibroblasts; increased hepatic ALAS; decreased hepatic steroid 5-α reductase

erator constitutive gene defect in AIP was responsible for this increased ALAS activity [68]. It is now clear that the enzyme PBGD, which converts PBG to UROGEN I, is deficient in the liver [69], cultured skin fibroblasts [362], organ-cultured skin [363], and cultured lymphocytes [364] of affected individuals and latent carriers of the disease. This helps to explain the excessive ALA and PBG excretion of AIP. PBGD activity in AIP is approximately 50 percent of that in unaffected normals, consistent with an autosomal dominant mode of inheritance. The decreased PBGD may lead to a partial block in heme synthesis which in turn leads to derepression of ALAS as discussed previously (see "Regulation of Heme Synthesis" above).

A most important concept is that, although AIP appears to be inherited as an autosomal dominant trait, many latent carriers of the PBGD defect never suffer an acute attack of porphyria. The gene defect alone seems to be inconsequential unless the individual is exposed to precipitating factors, among which are drugs (see Table 143-4) [28,365,366]. Other precipitating factors besides drugs include steroid hormones and their metabolites [367], starvation [368], and infections [102].

Steroid hormones and their metabolites are known to be potent inducers of ALAS in chick embryo liver [369]. There is good clinical evidence that aberrations in sex steroid hormone metabolism could play a role in precipitating AIP. Thus, the absence of attacks prior to puberty, the female predominance, the repeated association of attacks with specific phases of the menstrual cycle, the exacerbations seen during pregnancy or in patients who receive hormone therapy, all suggest that sex steroids participate in the clinical expression of AIP. A number of C19 and C21 steroid hormones are potent inducers of ALAS in chick embryo liver [369]. Initially, it was thought that only 5β steroid metabolites had such induction effects. Other studies, however, indicate that both 5α and 5β metabolites can induce hepatic ALAS [370,371]. Kappas et al [367] have suggested that AIP patients have a defect in sex

hormone biotransformation such that liver microsomal 5α-reductase activity is decreased. Furthermore, these workers have demonstrated that while patients with expressed and latent AIP are homogeneous insofar as diminished erythrocyte PBGD is concerned, impairment of 5α-reduction of steroid hormones occurred only in patients with a history of acute attacks [372]. How the hormone biotransformation anomaly may trigger an attack of porphyria is unknown, although it is of interest that administration of barbiturates to normal subjects can alter steroid hormone biotransformation in a pattern similar to that seen in patients with clinically expressed AIP [373]. Thus, one possible triggering mechanism of acute porphyria by drugs could relate to associated changes in sex steroid hormone metabolism.

Epidemiology

AIP is an autosomal dominant disease which is rarely, if ever, manifest before puberty. Most published series emphasize the female predominance of affected patients ranging from ratios of 1.5:1 to 2.0:1 [11,28,100]. The incidence in the human population is approximately 1.5:100,000 in most areas of the world. However, in Scandinavia, particularly Lapland, Waldenström [11] has shown that the incidence is much higher (1:1000).

Clinical manifestations (see Table 143-10)

All of the clinical signs and symptoms of AIP may be related to the autonomic nervous system [5]. These include autonomic neuropathy (abdominal pain, constipation, vomiting and hypertension, peripheral neuropathy, weakness, and paresis anywhere in the body), bulbar paresis (respiratory failure), and hypothalamic dysfunction (inappropriate antidiuretic hormone [ADH] secretion). The acute attack is characterized by abdominal pain, neurologic and psychiatric symptoms and is often precipitated by ingestion of drugs such as those listed in Table 143-4.

There are no cutaneous lesions related to photosensitivity in AIP. This is logical since the abnormal excretion pattern of the disease consists mostly of the porphyrin precursors ALA and PBG, which are not photosensitizers. Thus, little if any excessive photosensitizing porphyrins accumulate in these patients [374].

Abdominal pain occurs in 80 to 90 percent of patients during an acute attack. (Between attacks patients are often completely symptom-free.) The pain may be diffuse or localized and is often intermittent and spastic. Vomiting and constipation are frequently associated. Mild fever and leukocytosis may occur, making differential diagnosis extremely difficult. This is one reason many patients with AIP have undergone repeated exploratory laparotomies before the diagnosis was finally established.

Peripheral neuropathy is a major part of the clinical syndrome in many patients. This may vary from localized pain and weakness to complete generalized flaccid paralysis. Patients may succumb to the disease, usually due to respiratory failure, or may improve slowly though residual muscle weakness may persist for extended periods in some cases.

Other findings in AIP include profound hyponatremia which may be due to several factors, including gastrointestinal sodium loss, renal sodium loss, imprudent fluid therapy, or to inappropriate ADH secretion [375]. Evidence for the latter is based on the observed damage to cells in the supraoptic nuclei of the hypothalamus in autopsy specimens from patients with AIP [376,377].

Individual patients may demonstrate striking differences in the severity and frequency of attacks. Thus, one patient may have a single mild attack with no further difficulty whereas others may have repeated attacks culminating in irreversible muscle weakness, paralysis, and death. The factors responsible for these differences are unknown.

Laboratory findings

The primary biochemical abnormality in AIP, the PBGD deficiency, causes excessive urinary excretion of ALA and PBG. Urinary porphyrins may also be elevated [37] (Table 143-3). Urinary excretion of ALA and PBG as high as 100 mg per 24 h may occur during an acute attack. During clinical remission of the disease, urinary excretion of ALA and PBG usually remains somewhat elevated. This is in contrast to patients with VP who often exhibit normal urinary excretion of ALA and PBG between acute attacks.

Two rapid screening tests are available to test freshly voided urine for increased PBG. The first is simply to expose the urine to bright sunlight for several hours. Darkening to a deep red color suggests that PBG is present but does not prove it. (Porphobilin, another dark pigment, can also be photocatalytically formed in urine.) The second rapid screening test known as the Hoesch test is also a simple procedure for detecting the excessive urinary PBG [378]. To 2 ml of Ehrlich's reagent (3 g of *p*-dimethylaminobenzaldehyde dissolved in 125 mL of acetic acid and 24 mL of perchloric acid) add 2 drops of fresh urine. A uniform cherry-red color of the sample indicates a positive reaction [379]. This test is based upon the formation of a chromogen by PBG and Ehrlich's aldehyde reagent that produces a red pigment with strong absorbance at 552 nm. The well-known Watson-Schwartz test is based on this same principle although a number of refinements have helped to enhance its accuracy [5,27]. In patients with suspected porphyria, quantitative measurement of urinary ALA and PBG is best done using column chromatography with ion-exchange resins.

In addition to measuring urinary ALA and PBG, it is now possible to directly measure PBGD activity in patients with suspected AIP. Using RBC lysates or mitogen-stimulated lymphocytes, it has been shown that PBGD activity is decreased approximately 50 percent in both affected and in latent individuals with AIP [41,364]. Hypercholesterolemia [380,381] and elevated serum protein-bound iodine (PBI) [382] are occasionally seen without evidence of thyroid disease in patients with AIP.

Histopathology

Histopathologic findings of skin are unremarkable.

Differential diagnosis

The clinical manifestations of AIP are so variable and resemble so many different types of systemic disease that Waldenström has used the term ''little imitator'' to de-

scribe it [11,13]. Several excellent reviews have summarized the differential clinical features of AIP [28,29,100,102].

Treatment

Unfortunately, there is still no specific treatment for AIP. Avoidance of precipitating factors such as drugs (Table 143-4), sex steroid hormones, starvation, etc., are important preventive measures.

For the patient in an acute attack with pain, muscle weakness, and paralysis, skilled nursing in an intensive care setting may be critical to survival, particularly for patients in respiratory distress. It is generally agreed that most drugs should be avoided if at all possible. However, the phenothiazines are often useful in allaying apprehension and may even have some beneficial effect on the associated autonomic dysfunction. Opiates are useful for analgesia. Fluids should be administered cautiously because of the hyponatremia associated with inappropriate ADH secretion that can occur.

The two forms of treatment that are currently recommended include: (1) glucose loading and (2) hematin infusions. Glucose loading evolved as a form of treatment for AIP because of the knowledge that prior feeding of carbohydrate could diminish the induction of hepatic ALAS by porphyrogenic drugs in rat liver [383]. Felsher and Redeker [88] showed that high carbohydrate intake reduced urinary ALA and PBG excretion in AIP. This is thought to be due to a glucose effect which reduces the inducibility of hepatic ALAS. This form of treatment has been used extensively and appears to be helpful in many cases [28,268]. Large amounts of glucose (up to 500 g per day) may be required.

The second type of therapy for AIP is that of hematin (ferric PROTO hydroxide) infusions [93,383–387]. Hematin therapy is based on the hypothetical concept that the end product, heme, can inhibit or repress ALAS by a feedback mechanism leading to decreased formation of ALA and PBG by the liver and reduction in plasma and urinary ALA and PBG. Hematin is a structural analog of heme in which the iron is in the Fe^{+++} form. The general experience with hematin has been that biochemical improvement is more predictable than abatement of the clinical signs and symptoms. Hematin infusions (4 mg/kg intravenously in 500 mL of saline once or twice daily) have resulted, after 48 to 72 h, in a marked decrease in ALA and PBG excretion in the urine and in diminished leukocyte ALAS activity [93]. Clinical manifestations, particularly abdominal pain and neuropathy, have shown improvement in some cases. It should be emphasized that hematin is not innocuous. Transient renal insufficiency and a coagulopathy have been reported in selected patients [388,389].

Variegate porphyria (VP) (Table 143-11)

Historical aspects

Previously known as mixed porphyria, this disease has been a source of much confusion in the classification of porphyria. In 1957, Waldenström revised his original 1937 classification of the porphyrias and described two different types of PCT: (1) PCT symptomatica, (2) PCT hereditaria

Table 143-11   Variegate porphyria

Synonyms	Mixed porphyria; South African porphyria; protocoproporphyria hereditaria
Inheritance	Autosomal dominant
Age of onset	Usually between ages 15 to 30
Incidence	Common in South Africa; relatively rare elsewhere
Photosensitivity	Similar to PCT
Skin lesions	Similar to PCT
Clinical findings	Acute attacks similar to AIP; history of acute episodes of abdominal pain, nausea, vomiting, behavioral disturbances, paralysis and seizures. Drugs, particularly barbiturates, hydantoin, griseofulvin, sulfonamides; hormone preparations containing estrogens and progestins; ethanol; infection; acute illness; and starvation provoke acute attacks
Biochemical defects	Excretory: Increased PROTO, COPRO, and X-porphyrin in feces; increased ALA and PBG in urine during acute attacks; normal between attacks Enzymatic: Decreased PROTOGENO in fibroblasts; some evidence for decreased ferrochelatase; increased hepatic ALAS

(protocoproporphyria) [13]. PCT symptomatica was said to be the typical PCT with onset of cutaneous lesions in middle age or later, occurring predominantly in males who ingested moderate to heavy quantities of ethanol. PCT hereditaria was said to occur in individuals at a much younger age (15 to 30 years). Large amounts of PROTO and COPRO were excreted in the stool and these patients had acute attacks indistinguishable from those of AIP. Waldenström suggested that this disease be named protocoproporphyria to separate it from PCT in which fecal porphyrins were usually elevated to a lesser extent.

Barnes [15,390] had described a similar disorder in South Africa. However, not being a physician, he found it difficult to pursue detailed clinical studies. Soon thereafter Geoffrey Dean went to South Africa and in collaboration with Barnes began a careful evaluation of families affected with this type of porphyria [16,391]. Because it presents in a variety of forms, Dean and Barnes proposed the name porphyria variegata to describe the porphyria commonly seen in the South African white population. The entire adventure has been summarized in a fascinating book [101]. These patients had intermittent attacks typical of AIP usually following ingestion of barbiturates or sulfonamides. These attacks, predominantly affecting females, were identical to those described in Waldenström's patients with AIP, and most, if not all, such acute attacks could be avoided by eliminating exposure to inducing drugs. It is of interest that one report has shown that a weight-reduction diet triggered an attack of VP [87]. Furthermore, Dean was able to obtain detailed histories and family trees from the patients and subsequently saw numerous family members, predominantly males, with a clinical picture practically identical to that of PCT, hence the name VP.

Etiology

The cause of VP, like that of AIP, has not been defined though the excretory differences suggest that each must be due to separate genetic traits. Dowdle et al [361] have shown that hepatic ALAS is elevated in the liver of VP patients just as in AIP. This is a nonspecific finding since it occurs in each of the acute hepatic porphyrias. Becker et al [64] have suggested that RBC ferrochelatase activity is decreased approximately 50 percent in patients with VP. This could explain the fecal excretion patterns but does not account for the skin photosensitivity resembling PCT. Other studies suggest that decreased PROTOGENO activity is the primary enzyme defect in VP [58,392].

Epidemiology

This form of porphyria is quite common among the white and colored South Africans because of the "founder" effect. A high proportion of the present population is descended from a pair of early settlers who emigrated to South Africa from Holland in 1688. The disease is inherited as an autosomal dominant trait, and the incidence in South Africa is rather high, approximately 1:300 individuals in the white population.

In comparing the cutaneous manifestations of PCT and VP, it seems they are probably indistinguishable. It is of interest that among the black peoples of South Africa, typical PCT without associated acute attacks also occurs [236]. There is apparently no family history, and porphyrin excretion patterns are as for PCT, not VP. Excessive intake of home-brewed spirits (Kaffir beer) and dietary overload of iron from cooking vessels are considered important factors in the development of the disease. Thus, VP of the descendants of the Dutch immigrants of South Africa is quite distinct from the PCT seen in the native blacks. Finally, Dean has pointed out that the so-called Cape coloured, who are descendants of white European and Indian immigrants who intermarried with black natives, may have VP and PCT in the same family [101]. VP has been identified in all areas of the world. Our recent findings of five families in New England suggest that VP may be more prevalent than previously appreciated [22].

Clinical manifestations

The clinical manifestations of VP include those of AIP and PCT, either or both of which may occur in the same individual [393]. In general, females have more frequent acute attacks typical of AIP and males have the cutaneous lesions of PCT. One major difference between VP and PCT is that the skin reactions usually develop at an earlier age (second and third decades) as compared to PCT (fourth and fifth decades). The clinical features of VP are: (1) positive personal or family history of chronic skin involvement with or without attacks of abdominal pain, constipation, vomiting, muscle weakness, and neuropsychiatric manifestations of stupor and coma, and (2) photocutaneous lesions associated with minor mechanical trauma. The skin lesions of VP are indistinguishable from those of PCT.

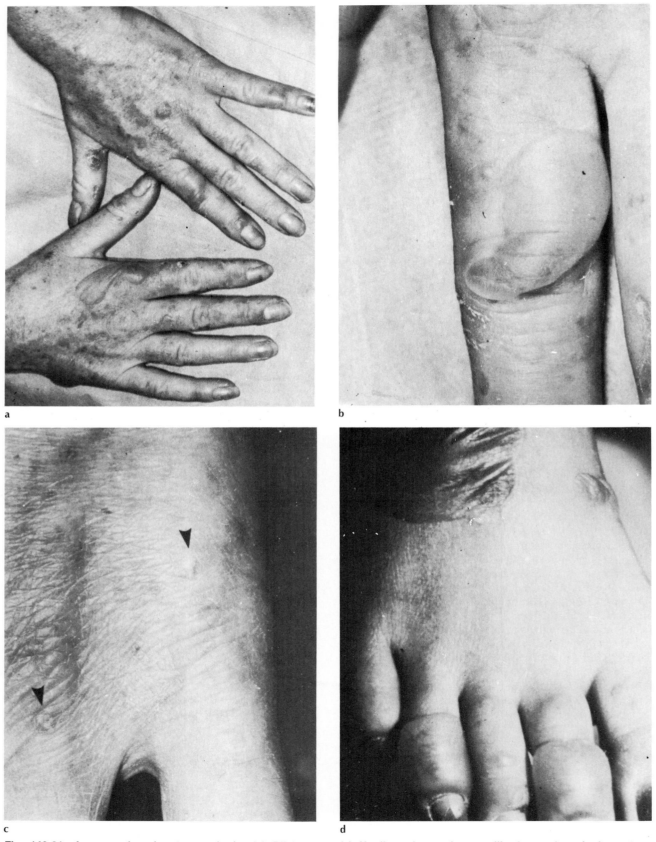

Fig. 143-21 A case of variegate porphyria. (a) Blisters, crusted erosions, and pigmentary changes over the dorsa of the hands and fingers. (b) Close-up view of index finger shows an intact blister with milia and pigmentary changes. (c) Healing phase shows milia (arrows) and pigmentary changes. (d) Large bullae of dorsum of foot and toes. *Note:* Patients with porphyria cutanea tarda have indistinguishable cutaneous findings.

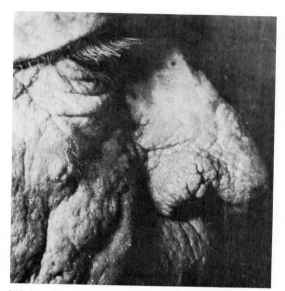

Fig. 143-22 A case of variegate porphyria showing a peculiar leathery thickening of skin of the face of a patient chronically exposed to strong sunlight. A similar appearance has been noted in South African patients with erythropoietic protoporphyria. *(Courtesy of Drs. G. H. Findlay, F. P. Scott, and D. J. Cripps; Br J Dermatol 78:69, 1966.)*

These include bullae, erosions, or ulcers following minor trauma of light-exposed skin (Fig. 143-21). Blisters are often blood-tinged, heal slowly, and form milia with some scarring. Occasionally the patient gives a history of acute sun sensitivity occurring during or soon after a period of exposure. This may include burning, erythema, and edema. In its chronic state the skin changes include crusting, depigmented scarring, and hypertrichosis [394] (Fig. 143-22). The skin manifestations in no way correlate with the acute attacks in most patients.

Laboratory findings

Urinary ALA and PBG are elevated during acute attacks of VP (when the Watson-Schwartz test may be positive) but characteristically fall to normal levels between attacks (see Table 143-3), whereas in AIP patients, the urinary ALA and PBG are elevated, both during and between attacks. Another distinguishing feature of the two disorders is the stool porphyrin excretion. Asymptomatic patients with VP have marked elevations of stool PROTO and CO-PRO between attacks [22,57]. These may fluctuate somewhat during acute systemic attacks but the feces will always contain markedly elevated levels of both these porphyrins. In AIP, fecal porphyrins are not elevated between attacks and usually increase only slightly during an acute attack of the disease. Rimington et al [395] have suggested that a markedly hydrophilic ether-insoluble porphyrin-peptide conjugate is present in the stools of patients with VP. The name X-porphyrin was given to this peculiar porphyrin since it could only be extracted from stool with a mixture of urea and the detergent, Triton-X. Elder et al [396] have questioned the usefulness of measuring the X-porphyrin in differentiating VP from other types of hepatic porphyria. In these studies, X-porphyrin was detected in

the stools of patients with active PCT and the levels overlapped considerably with those found in patients with VP.

Eales et al [397] have suggested that certain patterns of fecal and urinary porphyrin excretion may help in distinguishing VP from PCT, e.g., urinary URO is only moderately elevated in VP and is usually less than COPRO. This is in marked contrast to active PCT where the reverse pattern is seen, viz. urinary URO is much higher than COPRO. Again in VP, fecal porphyrins exceed 500 μg/g dry weight in 92 percent of patients, whereas in PCT this amount of stool porphyrin is excreted by only 1 percent of patients. Furthermore, the ratio of stool PROTO to CO-PRO in VP usually exceeds 1.5:1 whereas in PCT the ratio is almost always less than 1:1 due to the increased ISO-COPRO content characteristic of this disease. It is of interest that stool porphyrin excretion patterns consistent with both VP and PCT have been found in different members of single families [242,243]. One patient with VP had large elevations of stool PROTO and COPRO with normal ISOCOPRO, whereas a brother had markedly elevated urinary URO, mildly elevated stool PROTO and COPRO (ratio 1:6), and a large amount of fecal ISOCOPRO, all consistent with PCT. Watson et al [242] suggested that this might be due to a double heterozygosity of VP and PCT analogous to that seen in hemoglobin sickle cell disease. This interesting finding awaits confirmation and clarification.

Poh-Fitzpatrick has shown that saline-diluted plasma specimens from patients with VP have characteristic fluorescence emission spectra that can be used to differentiate this disease from other forms of acute porphyria, PCT, EPP, and lead poisoning (Table 143-12) [398].

Histopathology

The skin lesions of VP are subepidermal bullae indistinguishable from those of PCT.

Differential diagnosis

The differential diagnosis of VP should be considered from two perspectives. Acute attacks of abdominal pain and neurologic signs and symptoms are identical to those described for AIP. Fecal PROTO and COPRO determinations and plasma fluorescence spectra are decisive in making the diagnosis [57]. The skin lesions of VP are identical to those of PCT and, as such, the differential diagnosis includes the bullous diseases as well as other photosensitivity disorders. In VP, the stool PROTO and COPRO are usually markedly elevated and urinary COPRO exceeds URO. In

Table 143-12 Fluorescence characteristics of native porphyrin-protein complexes of plasma diluted with 1:10 phosphate-buffered solution

Type	Excitation (nm)	Emission (nm)
Erythropoietic porphyria (EP)	398	619
Erythropoietic protoporphyria (EPP)	409	634
Porphyria cutanea tarda (PCT)	398	619
Variegate porphyria (VP)	405	626
Acute intermittent porphyria (AIP)	398	619
Hereditary coproporphyria (HCP)	398	619

HCP there may be identical acute attacks but markedly elevated fecal COPRO III is diagnostic for this disease. The presence of skin lesions rules out AIP.

Treatment

Preventive treatment of VP is identical to that described in AIP, viz. avoidance of inducing drugs (see Table 143-4). Patients should, insofar as possible, avoid medications in general, and suspicious drugs in particular. Glucose loading and hematin infusions have also been used with ill-defined success. Treatment of cutaneous lesions similar to that of PCT has been tried, but neither phlebotomy nor the anti-malarials have proved effective [399,400]. Beta-carotene may occasionally be helpful [22].

Hereditary coproporphyria (HCP) (Table 143-13)

Historical aspects

This rare disorder was first described by Watson et al [401] in two completely asymptomatic individuals who excreted large amounts of COPRO III in the feces and to a lesser extent in the urine. The condition was named HCP by Berger and Goldberg [25], who described similar findings in a 10-year-old Swiss boy and three relatives. These individuals were also completely asymptomatic.

In 1967 Goldberg et al [402] reported 10 cases of HCP and reviewed 20 more in the literature. They found that HCP was associated with acute attacks similar in many ways to those seen in AIP and VP although severe neurologic sequelae seemed to occur less often. In addition, most acute attacks of HCP seemed to be precipitated by ingestion of drugs. During acute attacks urinary ALA and PBG are elevated just as in AIP and VP; however, a marked elevation of fecal COPRO is diagnostic of HCP.

Cutaneous photosensitivity has been reported in some patients though the pattern has not been consistent. Many of these patients have developed acute photosensitivity in conjunction with evidence of hepatocellular dysfunction and jaundice. Brodie et al [403] reviewed the known cases of HCP and found that 20 percent had suffered cutaneous photosensitivity reactions of an unspecified type and 35 percent acute attacks similar to those of AIP or VP.

Etiology

The etiology of HCP is unknown. Recent evidence suggests that there is a deficiency in COPROGENO activity. This has been demonstrated in cultured skin fibroblasts, in RBC, and in leukocytes of affected individuals [404–405]. Enzyme activity is approximately 50 percent of that of normals or patients with other forms of porphyria. Hepatic ALAS is reported to be elevated in this disease [406].

Epidemiology

The disease appears to occur worldwide and, like AIP, to have a female preponderance and probably to have an autosomal dominant transmittance.

The recently defined porphyria known as harderoporphyria appears to be a variant of HCP in which COPRO-GENO activity is 10 percent of control values [407]. Ki-

Table 143-13 Hereditary coproporphyria

Synonym	Idiopathic coproporphyria
Inheritance	Autosomal dominant
Age of onset	Any age
Incidence	Rare
Photosensitivity	Occurs infrequently
Skin reactions	Usually blistering
Biochemical defects	Excretory: Marked elevation of fecal and urinary COPRO III during and between attacks
	Enzymatic: COPROGENO deficiency in lymphocytes and fibroblasts; increased hepatic ALAS

netic properties of the enzyme were abnormal with a Michaelis constant 15- to 20-fold higher than normal values when using COPROGEN or HARDEROGEN as substrates. V_{max} was half the normal value. This disease has been identified in three siblings and it is speculated that these patients may be homozygous for a gene that causes HCP in some families.

Clinical manifestations

The acute attacks are similar to those of AIP. Cutaneous photosensitivity is relatively uncommon but has been reported in one patient by Hunter et al [408]. A 17-year-old female developed jaundice and the sudden onset of a "blistering eruption" on sun-exposed areas. This appears to have resembled PCT. Between attacks the only abnormality is the extremely high level of fecal COPRO III. In general, it appears that this disorder is not associated with acute attacks as severe as those of AIP or VP.

Laboratory findings

Markedly elevated fecal COPRO, more than 90 percent of which is the III isomer, is present at all times in these patients. In addition, the feces also contain increased amounts of hepta-, hexa-, and pentacarboxylic porphyrins. Urinary COPRO III is also raised as are ALA and PBG during attacks. The latter usually fall to near normal levels in remission.

Histopathology

No histology has yet been reported.

Differential diagnosis

Acute attacks are similar to those of AIP. The differential diagnosis rests on stool porphyrin determinations and measurement of COPROGENO in fibroblasts or leukocytes. The skin lesions are said to resemble PCT although no definitive evidence for this has been reported.

Treatment

Avoidance of inducing drugs, glucose-loading, and hematin infusions may be helpful.

Hepatoerythropoietic porphyria (HEP) (Table 143-14)

Historical aspects

In 1969 Pinōl-Aguadé et al in Spain first reported the occurrence of a new and biochemically unclassifiable type of porphyria [26]. Since that time at least eight additional cases of a similar nature have been reported [51,408–411].

Etiology

The cause of HEP is unknown but the available evidence indicates that it may be inherited as an autosomal recessive trait. The primary enzyme defect that has been identified is a profound decrease in UROGEND activity [50]. Measurement of the enzyme in hemolyzed whole blood or skin fibroblasts from three unrelated patients with the disease showed that it was 7 to 8 percent of normal levels. The father of one HEP patient was heterozygous for the same enzyme defect, suggesting that patients with HEP are homozygous for the gene that causes PCT. There is no evidence, as yet, to show that clinical expression of HEP is related to exposure to environmental drugs or chemicals as is true for PCT.

Epidemiology

All of the cases that have been reported thus far have come from Europe and the disease appears to be inherited in some instances as an autosomal recessive.

Clinical manifestations

This disease is usually manifest before 2 years of age with dark urine being the most frequently observed sign. Marked cutaneous photosensitivity including blistering, burning, and pruritus occurs usually during the first summer of life. The photosensitivity seems to diminish with age and is followed by hypertrichosis, hyperpigmentation, and scleroderma-like scarring similar to that seen in Gün-

ther's disease. Ocular manifestations include ectropion associated with cutaneous sclerosis and scleromalacia perforans. Splenomegaly has occurred in a small percentage of affected individuals, particularly after the age of 10, and hemolytic anemia has been documented as well. In some patients liver function tests have been abnormal but serum iron and iron binding are normal.

In summary, the clinical manifestations of HEP are strikingly similar to those of Günther's disease while the biochemical abnormalities are suggestive of a severe form of PCT mixed with EPP [50].

Laboratory findings

Elevated urinary URO (I, III), elevated fecal COPRO and ISOCOPRO, and elevated RBC PROTO have been observed in all patients. These findings suggest that there is abnormal porphyrin synthesis in both the liver and the bone marrow.

Histopathology

PAS-positive material in and around dermal capillaries has been observed [412].

Differential diagnosis

The clinical differential diagnosis is essentially that of Günther's disease and the two diseases are so similar that laboratory studies are necessary to identify HEP. Unlike Günther's disease in which increased RBC URO is a characteristic finding, in HEP there is elevated RBC PROTO. The urinary porphyrin pattern is similar to that found in PCT with high URO (URO:COPRO ratio greater than 5:1).

Treatment

There is no known treatment aside from careful photoprotection.

Pseudoporphyria

The term *pseudoporphyria* can be utilized to describe a number of acquired cutaneous disorders involving traumatized skin sites that are characterized by the development of increased skin fragility and blistering which evolves through crusting and heals leaving milia with scarring. This occurs in selected patients undergoing hemodialysis and may or may not be associated with abnormal porphyrin metabolism [303–309].

In addition, patients receiving drugs such as nalidixic acid, furosemide, and the tetracyclines may occasionally exhibit similar findings [412–416]. Careful assessment of blood, plasma, urine, and feces reveals completely normal porphyrin levels in such patients. The pathogenesis of these reactions is likely a direct phototoxic response although this is somewhat controversial. In most cases the cutaneous changes have improved slowly after discontinuation of the drug. In the case of tetracycline, the light microscopic immunofluorescence and electron microscope changes in the skin were shown to be identical to those seen in PCT and VP [416]. A similar eruption has been described in diabetes mellitus [322,417,418].

Table 143-14 Hepatoerythropoietic porphyria

Synonym	Hepatoerythrocytic porphyria
Inheritance	?
Age of onset	Early infancy, before age 2
Incidence	Extremely rare
Photosensitivity	Marked
Skin reactions	Early: Vesicles, bullae, erosions
	Late: Hypertrichosis, scleroderma-like scarring, hyperpigmentation, mutilating scarring deformities of acral areas such as hands, ears, face and nose; cicatrizing alopecia
Clinical findings	Moderate normochromic anemia; ? hemolytic anemia; erythrodontia
Biochemical defects	Excretory: Elevated URO (I–III) and 7-carboxyl porphyrin (III) in urine; elevated URO, COPRO, and ISO-COPRO in feces; elevated PROTO in RBC
	Enzymatic: Markedly decreased RBC UROGEND

Table 143-15 Procedures for evaluation of patients with various porphyrias

Erythropoietic porphyria

Detailed family history
Examine urine: pink-red color and fluorescence
Examine teeth with Wood's lamp for erythrodontia
Examine photosensitivity of skin and eyes (photophobia),
   keratoconjunctivitis, and hypertrichosis
Quantitative RBC, stool, and urine porphyrin (24-h
   specimens) for URO-1 and COPRO-1
Thin-layer chromatography of extracted porphyrins
Complete blood count including reticulocytes
Measure RBC PBGD and UROCOSYN III activity

Erythropoietic protoporphyria

Detailed family history
Skin biopsy from light-exposed area; perform PAS stain
Quantitative RBC and stool PROTO
Liver function tests
Measure RBC ferrochelatase activity
Determine spectral sensitivity of skin in Soret band (400–
   420 nm)

Porphyria cutanea tarda

Detailed history of drug and/or chemical exposure
Detailed family history
Skin biopsy of intact vesicle/bulla; perform PAS stain
Check random urine for fluorescence with Wood's lamp
Quantitative urine and stool URO, COPRO, ISOCOPRO
   (24-h specimens)
Thin-layer chromatography of extracted porphyrins
Complete blood count including reticulocytes, serum iron
   and total iron binding capacity, liver function tests,
   glucose tolerance test, liver scan
Liver biopsy, check for fluorescence, perform iron stains
Measure hepatic and RBC UROGEND activity

Acute intermittent porphyria

Detailed history of drug and/or chemical exposure
Detailed family history
Watson-Schwartz or Hoesch test on urine
Quantitative urine ALA and PBG (24-h specimens)
Liver function tests, glucose tolerance test, serum
   cholesterol, serum and urine osmolality
Measure RBC PBGD activity

Variegate porphyria

Detailed family history
Skin biopsy of intact vesicle/bulla
Quantitative stool and urine uro-, copro-, and
   protoporphyrin, and X-porphyrins (24-h specimens)
Thin-layer chromatography of extracted porphyrins
Quantitative urine ALA and PBG (24-h specimens)
Measure RBC PROTOGENO activity

Hereditary coproporphyria

Detailed family history
Quantitative urine and stool for COPRO
Thin-layer chromatography of extracted porphyrins
Liver function tests
Measure RBC COPROGENO activity

Hepatoerythropoietic porphyria

Detailed family history
Quantitative URO and COPRO in urine and stool
Quantitative PROTO in RBC
Measure RBC UROGEND activity

Procedures for evaluation of various porphyrias

In Table 143-15 are listed procedures for evaluation of patients with various porphyrias [57].

Qualitative screening tests for determining porphyrins (office methods) [57,419]

Reagents

(a) Amyl alcohol; (b) ethyl acetate:glacial acetic acid (4:1 v/v mixture); (c) diethylether; (d) amyl alcohol:glacial acetic acid:diethyl mixture (1:1:1 v/v) made fresh; (e) hydrochloric acid 1.5 N or 10%; (f) Ehrlich's reagent containing reagent grade 0.7 g p-dimethylaminobenzaldehyde plus 150 ml concentrated hydrochloric acid to 100 ml water and stored in amber-colored bottle; (g) sodium acetate, saturated solution; (h) chloroform; (i) N butanol; and (j) pH test paper with pH range 4 to 5.

Apparatus

Wood's lamp emitting UVA radiation (320 to 400 nm) or fluorescent black light tube lamp; and test tubes, glass rods, and medicine droppers.

Urinary screening tests for porphyrins

Urine containing excess porphyrins may show rusty color in daylight or ordinary room light. When viewed under Wood's lamp or black light tubes, it may show red or pink fluorescence. Normal urine shows bluish white or greenish blue fluorescence. The addition of 3 to 4 drops of 1.5 N HCl or glacial acetic acid helps in intensifying the pink-red fluorescence color characteristic of porphyrins. If in doubt, this test can be modified as follows: to 5 ml of urine (freshly voided or 24-h specimen), 5 to 10 drops (0.5 ml) of glacial acetic and 2.5 ml of ethyl acetate are added. One can substitute amyl alcohol for ethyl acetate. The mixture is shaken well and allowed to settle. The upper layer is examined under Wood's lamp. Pink or red fluorescence indicates excess porphyrins.

This test is usually positive in all porphyrias except in patients with EPP, in which the urinary porphyrins are always in the normal range. A distinction must be made between porphyrinurias and porphyrias. The former is a symptom of an acute febrile state, lead or arsenic poisoning, pernicious anemia, cirrhosis, malignancies, etc., wherein the excretion of coproporphyrin (COPRO) may be elevated. Porphyrias, on the other hand, result from either inherited or acquired abnormalities in heme synthesis causing excessive accumulation and excretion of porphyrin pathway intermediates.

Urinary porphobilinogen (PBG) test

PBG in urine is evaluated by the well-known Watson-Schwartz test [42]. In a large test tube, 2.5 mL of Ehrlich's reagent and 2.5 ml urine are mixed. Five milliliters of saturated solution of sodium acetate is added, and the pH is checked and adjusted between 4 to 5. If no color develops, the test is negative. If a red color develops, 5 ml chloroform or butanol is added. This helps to differentiate the color formed with PBG from urobilinogen or indole. PBG-positive color cannot be extracted in $CHCl_3$ or butanol. A cherry-red color remaining in the aqueous phase, therefore, indicates that the PBG test is positive.

This test may be positive in urine of patients with a AIP, VP, and occasionally, in HCP.

The Hoesch test [378] is comparable to the Watson-Schwartz test in its sensitivity and reliability; moreover, false-positive reactions secondary to urobilinogen are not encountered. For suspected cases of AIP and VP, 2 to 3 ml of modified Ehrlich's reagent [20 g p-dimethylamino-benzaldehyde diluted to 1000 mL with HCl (6 mol/liter)] is pipetted in a test tube. Two or three drops of fresh urine specimen is added. Instantaneous cherry-red color present, initially at the top of the solution (miniscus) and subsequently throughout the tube on brief agitation, indicates a positive test for PBG.

Screening test for fecal porphyrin [57,322,419]

This is a valuable test and is often positive in EP, EPP, VP, and HCP. In rare instances, patients with PCT may give a weakly positive reaction.

When viewed with Wood's lamp, a stool specimen containing abnormally high levels of porphyrins may fluoresce red when it is thinly smeared on a filter paper or on the flat surface of a glass slide; however, it is best to examine the fluorescence by extracting the stool porphyrins into an acidified organic solvent. In a test tube, a small lump of stool (pea size) is mixed with 4 ml of the solvent mixture containing amyl alcohol, glacial acetic acid, and ether reagent. The mixture is shaken well and allowed to settle. The supernatant is transferred to another tube with the aid of a pipette. Two milliliters of 1.5 N HCl is added and mixed vigorously. The HCl layer is examined for red or pink fluorescence under Wood's lamp.

Eales et al [397] have also described a modified version of this screening test for the detection of abnormal levels of fecal porphyrin. In a centrifuge tube, a small lump of feces (pea size) is mixed with 1 ml of glacial acetic acid and stirred with a glass rod. The suspension is mixed thoroughly with 5 to 7 ml of ether and centrifuged. The supernatant is decanted and 1 ml of 1.5 N HCl is added. After thorough shaking the aqueous phase and ether phase are allowed to separate. A positive test is indicated by red fluorescence in the acid phase. The porphyrins derived from dietary chlorophyll generally remain in the ether phase. The test is quite sensitive, and all positive tests should be followed by quantitative measurements of porphyrins.

Screening tests for porphyrins in blood [57,322,419]

Blood should be collected in a tube containing anticoagulants (heparin or EDTA) and kept in the dark, preferably wrapped with either aluminum foil or paper. Protoporphyrin (PROTO) is usually stable for 5 to 7 days at 5°C or lower. Excess PROTO may be detected by a simple office procedure based on solvent partition or by fluorescence microscopy of RBC. Rimington and Cripps [420] developed a simple extraction procedure using 0.1 to 0.2 ml blood in a test tube, adding 2.5 ml of ether:acetic acid (5:1 v/v) with thorough shaking. The dark brown RBC are allowed to

sediment, and the supernatant is pipetted to another tube in which 0.5 ml of 3 M HCl is added to extract the porphyrins. The aqueous HCl phase is examined for orange-red fluorescence with Wood's lamp or fluorescent black light emitting UVA radiation.

Examination of a patient's blood smear made on a glass slide is one of the most reliable and rapid methods for diagnosing patients with EP, EPP, and lead intoxication with the aid of a fluorescence microscope equipped with a 100-W tungsten-iodine or xenon-arc lamp, dark-field condenser, and appropriate glass filters transmitting 400 nm radiation. Excess porphyrins in RBC can be visualized by detecting the fluorocytes with intense orange-red fluorescence [419,420]. Two slides are usually prepared: (a) a thin smear with 2 drops of whole blood spread uniformly over two-thirds of the area of the slide; and (b) a saline diluted smear (1 drop blood plus 2 drops of saline) under a transparent coverslip. The slides are examined with the aid of a dark-field condenser and nonfluorescent oil immersion. The blue-violet radiation (360 to 420 nm) that excites porphyrin to fluoresce is allowed to impinge on RBC, and the cells are focused through a dark-field condenser covered with a thin oil film. The red fluorescence due to PROTO or URO and COPRO can be seen through a yellow-orange filter interposed between the objective of the microscope and the eyes of the observer.

RBC from patients with EPP exhibit rather bright red, transient fluorescence which is stable for about 45 to 60 s. Patients with EP exhibit similar fluorescence which is, however, more stable than the fluorescence emitted by EPP cells. The RBC fluorescence of EP patients lasts for at least 3 min or longer. Xenon and mercury-arc lamps appear to be more intense than the tungsten-iodide lamp and quickly photodegrade PROTO in RBC. A heat absorption filter (Schott BG-38) and blue or violet light-transmitting filter (Schott BG-12) should be placed in the light beam before it reaches and photoactivates the RBC porphyrins to fluoresce. Positive tests are indicated by the presence of 5 to 30 percent fluorocytes in blood of patients with EPP. Patients with EP exhibit 30 to 50 percent fluorescent erythrocytes. Fluorescence of cell nuclei may be seen in many circulating immature erythroid cells in EP, but not in EPP or lead intoxication. The fluorescence in RBC of patients with lead intoxication is very evanescent and lasts but a few seconds.

Added in Proof

Studies on the effect of heme on hepatic ALAS indicate that heme can inhibit synthesis of the enzyme and that this effect may be based upon diminished peptide chain elongation [421]. Furthermore, heme was shown to inhibit translocation of ALAS from cytosol into the mitochondrion which could provide a regulatory control mechanism for heme synthesis in liver cells [422]. It is of interest that insulin and glucose have also been shown to inhibit translocation of ALAS from the cytosol into the mitochondrial matrix and this effect may relate to the ability of these two substances to increase the free heme pool [423].

Recent studies on other enzymes in the heme pathway indicate that cell-free translation of UROD can be achieved in a reticulocyte lysate under the direction of messenger RNAs isolated from human fetal liver and human reticulocytes [424]. Human liver ferrochelatase was shown to have high zinc-chelatase activity with endogenous zinc and this affinity of the enzyme for zinc lowers the actual determination of ferrochelatase activity with iron as substrate [425]. The role of human ferrochelatase in zinc-PROTO synthesis suggests that in patients with iron deficiency anemia and lead poisoning a deficiency of available iron leads to the increase in zinc-PROTO that characterizes these disorders. Furthermore, in EPP, where defective ferrochelatase activity occurs, PROTO rather than zinc-PROTO preferentially accumulates.

Further verification of the functional importance of an intracellular regulatory heme pool has come from studies with tin-PROTO, a powerful competitive inhibitor of heme oxygenase which degrades heme into bile pigments [426]. It has been proposed that the degree of heme saturation of the heme-protein tryptophan pyrrolase may serve as a useful index of the regulatory heme fraction in liver cells. Administration of tin-PROTO to animals causes near-total heme saturation of the enzyme suggesting that by inhibiting heme degradation by heme oxygenase, the intracellular level of this moiety rises, thereby increasing heme saturation of tryptophan pyrrolase.

Additional studies on the regulatory control of heme synthesis in erythrocytes undergoing differentiation indicate that the addition of dimethylsulfoxide to mouse Friend virus-transformed erythroleukemia cells leads to increased ALAD activity as a result of de novo synthesis of the enzyme [427]. Addition of succinylacetone, a potent inhibitor of ALAD, to these cells in vitro caused a major increase in ALAS activity [428]. Since inhibition of ALAD results in diminished heme production, these results suggest that heme may exert negative control on its own synthesis in the differentiating erythroid system by an effect on ALAS.

Newer studies on the mechanism of cutaneous photosensitization by porphyrins verified that in vivo irradiation of the skin of patients with PCT and EPP was associated with activation of the complement system as assessed by diminution of the hemolytic titers of the third and fifth components of complement and by the generation of increased chemotactic activity for polymorphonuclear leukocytes [429]. Similar findings were obtained in irradiated sera from rats rendered porphyric by orally administered hexachlorobenzene [430]. In further studies in experimental animals, it was shown that H_1 and H_2 histamine antagonists can suppress the tissue injury evoked by porphyrin photosensitization [431].

A new hypothesis regarding the inheritance pattern of EPP has been proposed. A study of patients, sibs, and children led to the conclusion that EPP may be inherited as an autosomal recessive disease in a 3-allele system [432].

Experimental studies have suggested that cholic acid administration to animals can enhance PROTO transport into bile, thereby reducing hepatic PROTO deposition and leading to improvement in associated abnormalities of liver morphology. This suggests the possibility that bile salts may be of some therapeutic benefit in patients with EPP with developing hepatic failure. Another therapeutic approach that has been employed in EPP is the combination of erythrocyte exchange and plasmapheresis [433,434].

Further confirmation of iron overload as an etiologic factor in PCT has come from studies showing elevated serum ferritin in the majority of patients in one series [435]. More recent studies on the role of iron in inhibiting hepatic UROD have suggested a dual inhibitory effect of the metal on this enzyme [436]. This could relate either to direct interaction of Fe^{2+} or Zn^{2+} with essential sulfhydryl groups of the enzyme or to the generation of free radicals in the presence of oxygen and an electron donor such as cysteine. These could either cause oxidative injury to the enzyme or oxidize the porphyrinogen substrates to non-metabolizable porphyrins.

Newer studies on UROD activity in familial PCT using a direct and noncompetitive enzyme immunoassay revealed that in familial PCT immunoreactive protein was decreased (51 percent) to the same extent as catalytic activity (48 percent) [437]. Furthermore, it was shown that in two cases of HEP there was severe UROD deficiency and that patients with this disease are homozygous cases of familial PCT.

Follow-up studies on individuals in Turkey poisoned with hexachlorobenzene in the 1950s revealed persistence of neurologic, dermatologic, and orthopedic abnormalities [438]. Cutaneous stigmata include: severe residual scarring (85 percent), pinched facies (42 percent), hirsutism (47 percent), and hyperpigmentation.

Confirmation of the therapeutic efficacy of nothing other than avoidance of hepatic toxins in PCT has appeared [439]. The effectiveness of low-dose oral chloroquine (125 mg twice weekly) was also reaffirmed in patients treated for a mean of 14.9 months during which all went into clinical and biochemical remission [440]. Relapses did occur in four patients requiring further therapy. In another study, hydroxychloroquine (200 mg twice weekly) was also found to be effective in PCT [441]. The mechanism of action of chloroquine remains controversial, but one study suggests that the drug may diminish hepatic ALAS activity [442].

In Scandinavia, concomitant existence of hepatocellular carcinoma and AIP were reported in 11 patients [443]. The antiepileptic drug carbamazepine was shown to induce a nonhereditary form of acute hepatic porphyria and the drug was also shown to have a direct suppressive effect on UROS in a group of epileptic patients receiving it [444].

Cyclical attacks of AIP premenstrually in one patient were shown to be prevented with a long-acting agonist of luteinizing hormone-releasing hormone [445].

The growing awarness of VP has been emphasized by a study of a kindred in Ireland in which eight members had clinical and biochemical evidence of this disease [446]. Similarly HCP has been studied carefully in a large English family where 27 affected individuals were identified [447]. Symptomatic illness was almost always elicited by the ingestion of drugs.

Finally, an effort has been made to classify the various types of pseudoporphyria into those related to drugs such as tetracycline, nalidixic acid and furosemide and those associated with chronic renal failure and hemodialysis [448].

References

1. Elder GH: Enzymatic defects in porphyria: an overview. *Semin Liver Dis* **2**:87, 1982
2. del C Batelle AM: Porphyrins and porphyrias: etiopatho-

genesis, clinics, and treatment. *Int J Biochem* **12**:671, 1980

3. Schultz JH: *Ein Fall von Pemphigus leprosus complicirt durch Lepra visceralis.* Greifswald, Kunike, 1874
4. Baumstark F: Zwei pathologische Hamfarbstoffe. *Arch Dtsch Ges Physiol* **9**:568, 1874
5. Taddeini L, Watson CJ: The clinical porphyrias. *Semin Hematol* **5**:335, 1968
6. Anderson TM: Hydroa aestivale in two brothers, complicated with the presence of haematoporphyrin in the urine. *Br J Dermatol* **10**:1, 1898
7. Günther J: Die Hamatoporphyrie. *Dtsch Arch Klin Med* **105**:89, 1911
8. Fischer H: Uber das Urinporphyrin. *Z Physiol Chem* **95**:34, 1915
9. Fischer H et al: Zur Kenntnis der naturlichen Porphyrine: Chemische Befund bei einem Fall von Porphyrinurie (Petry). *Z Physiol Chem* **150**:44, 1925
10. Borst M. Konigsdorffer H Jr: *Untersuchungen über Porphyrie mit besonderer Berucksichtigung der Porphyria congenita.* Stuttgart, Hirzel, 1929
11. Waldenström J: Studien über Porphyrie. *Acta Med Scand [Suppl]* **82**:1, 1937
12. Brunsting LA: Observations on porphyria cutanea tarda. *Arch Dermatol Syphilol.* **70**:551, 1954
13. Waldenström J: The porphyrias as inborn errors of metabolism. *Am J Med* **22**:758, 1957
14. Schmid R: Cutaneous porphyria in Turkey. *N Engl J Med* **263**:397, 1960
15. Barnes HD: A note on porphyrinuria with a resumé of eleven South African cases. *Clin Proc* **4**:269, 1945
16. Dean G: Porphyria. *Br Med J* **2**:1291, 1953
17. Dean G, Barnes HD: Porphyria in Sweden and South Africa. *S Afr Med J* **33**:246, 1959
18. Fromke VL et al: Porphyria variegata. Study of a large kindred in the United States. *Am J Med* **65**:80, 1978
19. Mustajoki P: Variegate porphyria. *Ann Intern Med* **89**:238, 1978
20. Corey TJ et al: Variegate porphyria: clinical and laboratory features. *J Am Acad Dermatol* **2**:36, 1980
21. Mustajoki P: Variegate porphyria: twelve years experience in Finland. *Q J Med* **49**:191, 1980
22. Muhlbauer JE et al: Variegate porphyria in New England. *JAMA* **247**:3095, 1982
23. Magnus IA et al: Erythropoietic protoporphyria: a new porphyria syndrome with solar urticaria due to protoporphyrinaemia. *Lancet* **2**:448, 1961
24. Heilmeyer L, Clotten R: Congenital erythropoietic coproporphyria. *German Med Monthly* **9**:353, 1964
25. Berger H, Goldberg A: Hereditary coproporphyria. *Br Med J* **2**:85, 1955
26. Pinōl-Aguadé J et al: A case of biochemically unclassifiable hepatic porphyria. *Br J Dermatol* **81**:270, 1969
27. Schmid R et al: Porphyrin content of bone marrow and liver in the various forms of porphyria. *Arch Intern Med* **93**:167, 1954
28. Kappas A et al: The porphyrias, in *The Metabolic Basis of Inherited Disease,* 5th ed, edited by JB Stanbury et al. New York, McGraw-Hill, 1983, p 1301
29. Tschudy DP, Lamon JM: Porphyrin metabolism and the porphyrias, in *Duncan's Diseases of Metabolism,* 8th ed, edited by PK Bondy, CE Rosenberg. Philadelphia, WB Saunders, 1980, p 939
30. Doss MO: Hepatic porphyrias: pathobiochemical, diagnostic and therapeutic implications. *Prog Liver Dis* **7**:573, 1982
31. Nakakuki M et al: Purification and some properties of δ-aminolevulinate synthase from the rat liver cytosol fraction and immunochemical identity of the cytosolic enzyme and the mitochondrial enzyme. *J Biol Chem* **255**:1738, 1980
32. Ohashi A, Sinohara H: Incorporation of δ-aminolevulinate synthase of rat liver into the mitochondrion *in vitro. Biochem Biophys Res Commun* **84**:76, 1978
33. Morton KA et al: Biosynthesis of delta-aminolevulinic acid and heme from 4,5-dioxovalerate in the rat. *J Clin Invest* **71**:1744, 1983
34. Granick JL et al: Studies in lead poisoning. II. Correlations between the ratio of activated and inactivated δ-aminolevulinate dehydratase of whole blood and the blood lead level. *Biochem Med* **8**:149, 1973
35. Bonkowsky HL et al: Iron and the liver: acute effects of iron-loading on hepatic heme synthesis of rats. *J Clin Invest* **71**:1175, 1983
36. Doss MR et al: New type of hepatic porphyria with porphobilinogen synthase defect and intermittent acute clinical manifestation. *Klin Wochenschr* **57**:1123, 1977
37. Sassa S, Kappas A: Herediatry tyrosinemia and the heme biosynthesis pathway. Profound inhibition of δ-aminolevulinic acid dehydratase by succinylacetone. *J Clin Invest* **71**:625, 1983
38. Strife CF et al: Tyrosinemia with acute intermittent porphyria: aminolevulinic acid dehydratase deficiency related to elevated urinary aminolevulinic acid levels. *J Pediatr* **90**:400, 1977
39. Anderson PM, Desnick RJ: Purification and properties of uroporphyrinogen I synthase from human erythrocytes. Identification of stable enzyme-substrate intermediates. *J Biol Chem* **255**:1993, 1980
40. Strand LJ et al: Heme biosynthesis in intermittent acute porphyria: decreased hepatic conversion of porphobilinogen to porphyrins and increased delta-aminolevulinic acid synthetase activity. *Proc Natl Acad Sci USA* **67**:1315, 1970
41. Meyer UA et al: Intermittent acute porphyria: demonstration of a genetic defect in porphobilinogen metabolism. *N Engl J Med* **286**:1277, 1972
42. Watson CJ, Schwartz S: A simple test for urinary porphobilinogen. *Proc Soc Exp Biol Med* **47**:393, 1941
43. Clement RP et al: Rat hepatic uroporphyrinogen III cosynthase: purification, properties and inhibition of metal ions. *Arch Biochem Biophys* **214**:657, 1982
44. Romeo G, Levin EY: Uroporphyrinogen III cosynthetase in human congenital erythropoietic porphyria. *Proc Natl Acad Sci* **63**:856, 1969
45. Mauzerall D, Granick S: Porphyrin biosynthesis in erythrocytes. III. Uroporphyrinogen and its decarboxylase. *J Biol Chem* **232**:1141, 1958
46. deVerneuil H et al: Purification and properties of uroporphyrinogen decarboxylase from human erythrocytes. A single enzyme catalyzing the four sequential decarboxylations of uroporphyrinogens I and III. *J Biol Chem* **258**:2454, 1983
47. Kushner JP et al: An inherited enzymatic defect in porphyria cutanea tarda: decreased uroporphyrinogen decarboxylase activity. *J Clin Invest* **58**:1089, 1976
48. Elder GH et al: Decreased activity of hepatic uroporphyrinogen decarboxylase in sporadic porphyria cutanea tarda. *N Engl J Med* **299**:274, 1978
49. Felsher BF et al: Red-cell uroporphyrinogen decarboxylase activity in porphyria cutanea tarda and other forms of porphyria. *N Engl J Med* **299**:1095, 1978
50. Felsher BF et al: Decreased hepatic uroporphyrinogen decarboxylase activity in porphyria cutanea tarda. *N Engl J Med* **306**:766, 1982
51. Elder GH et al: Hepatoerythropoietic porphyria. A new uroporphyrinogen decarboxylase defect on homozygous porphyria cutanea tarda. *Lancet* **1**:916, 1981
52. Sinclair PR, Granick S: Uroporphyrin induced by chlorinated hydrocarbons (lindane, polychlorinated biphenyls, tetrachlorodibenzo-p-dioxin): requirements for endogenous iron, protein synthesis and drug metabolizing activity. *Biochem Biophys Res Commun* **61**:124, 1974

53. Goldstein JA et al: Effects of pentachlorophenol on hepatic drug-metabolizing enzymes and porphyria related to contamination with chlorinated dibenzo-p-dioxins and dibenzofurans. *Biochem Pharmacol* **26**:1549, 1977

54. Jones KG et al: The role of iron in the toxicity of 2,3,7,8-tetrachlorodibenzo(p)dioxin (TCDD). *Toxicol Appl Pharmacol* **61**:74, 1981

55. Yoshinaga T, Sano S: Coproporphyrinogen oxidase. I. Purication, properties and activation by phospholipids. *J Biol Chem* **255**:4722, 1980

56. Brodie MJ et al: Hereditary coproporphyria. *Q J Med* **46**:229, 1977

57. Pathak MA, West JD: Porphyrias: office procedures and laboratory tests for diagnosis of porphyrin abnormalities. *Acta Derm Venereol [Suppl] (Stockh)* **100**:91, 1982

58. Poulson R: The enzymic conversion of protoporphyrinogen IX to protoporphyrin IX in mammalian mitochondria. *J Biol Chem* **251**:3730, 1976

59. Brenner DA, Bloomer JR: The enzymatic defect in variegate porphyria. Studies with human cultured skin fibroblasts. *N Engl J Med* **302**:765, 1980

60. Rutherford T et al: Heme biosynthesis in Friend erythroleukemia cells: control by ferrochelatase. *Proc Natl Acad Sci USA* **76**:833, 1979

61. Bonkowsky HL et al: Heme synthetase activity in human protoporphyria: demonstration of the defect in liver and cultured skin fibroblasts. *J Clin Invest* **56**:1149, 1975

62. de Goeij AFPN et al: Decreased haem synthetase activity in blood cells of patients with erythropoietic protoporphyria. *Eur J Clin Invest* **5**:397, 1975

63. Bloomer JR et al: Inheritance in protoporphyria. *Lancet* **2**:226, 1976

64. Becker DM et al: Reduced ferrochelatase activity: a defect common to porphyria variegata and protoporphyria. *Br J Haematol* **36**:171, 1977

65. Kramer S, Viljoen JD: Erythropoietic protoporphyria: evidence that it is due to a variant ferrochelatase. *Int J Biochem* **12**:925, 1980

66. Granick S, Urata G: Increase in activity of delta-aminolevulinic acid synthetase in liver mitochondria induced by feeding of 3,5-dicarbethoxyl-1,4-dihydrocollidine. *J Biol Chem* **238**:821, 1963

67. Marver HS et al: Delta-aminolevulinic acid synthetase. II. Induction in rat liver. *J Biol Chem* **241**:4323, 1966

68. Tschudy DP et al: Acute intermittent porphyria: the first "overproduction disease" localized to a specific enzyme. *Proc Natl Acad Sci USA* **53**:841, 1965

69. Nakao K et al: Activity of amino-laevulinic acid synthetase in normal and porphyric human livers. *Nature* **210**:838, 1966

70. Sweeney VP et al: Acute intermittent porphyria: increased ALA-synthetase activity during an acute attack. *Brain* **93**:369, 1970

71. Granick S: The induction in vitro of the synthesis of delta-aminolevulinic synthetase in chemical porphyria: a response to certain drugs, sex hormones, and foreign chemicals. *J Biol Chem* **241**:1359, 1966

72. Jacob F, Monod J: On the regulation of gene activity: cellular regulatory mechanisms. *Cold Spring Harbor Symp Quant Biol* **26**:193, 1961

73. Lascelles J: The synthesis of enzymes concerned in bacteriochlorophyll formation in growing cultures of *Rhodopseudomonas spheroides*. *J Gen Microbiol* **23**:487, 1960

74. Sinclair PR, Granick S: Heme control of the synthesis of delta-aminolevulinic acid synthetase in cultured chick embryo liver cells. *Ann NY Acad Sci* **244**:509, 1975

75. Sassa S, Granick S: Induction of delta-aminolevulinic acid synthetase, in chick embryo liver cell in culture. *Proc Natl Acad Sci USA* **67**:517, 1970

76. Strand LJ et al: The induction of delta-aminolevulinic acid synthetase in cultured liver cells. The effects of end product and inhibitors of heme synthesis. *J Biol Chem* **247**:2820, 1972

77. Whiting MJ: Synthesis of delta-aminolaevulinate synthetase by isolated liver polyribosomes. *Biochem J* **158**:391, 1976

78. DeMatteis F: Rapid loss of cytochrome P-450 and heme caused in the liver microsomes by the porphyrogenic agent 2-allyl-2-isopropyl-acetamide. *FEBS Lett* **6**:343, 1970

79. DeMatteis F, Gibbs AH: Stimulation of the pathway of porphyrin synthesis in the liver of rats and mice by griseofulvin, 3,5-diethoxcarbonyl-1,4-dihydrocollidine and related drugs: evidence for two basically different mechanisms. *Biochem J* **146**:285, 1975

80. Rifkind AB: Maintenance of microsomal hemoprotein concentrations following inhibition of ferrochelatase activity by 3,5-diethoxycarbonyl-1,4-dihydrocollidine in chick embryo liver. *J Biol Chem* **254**:4636, 1979

81. Yoshinaga T et al: Purification and properties of bovine spleen heme oxygenase amino acid composition and sites of action of inhibitors of heme oxidation. *J Biol Chem* **257**:7778, 1982

82. DeMatteis F, Sparks RG: Iron-dependent loss of liver cytochrome P-450 haem in vivo and in vitro. *FEBS Lett* **29**:141, 1973

83. Bacon BR et al: Hepatic lipid peroxidation in vivo in rats with chronic iron overload. *J Clin Invest* **71**:429, 1983

84. Rajamanickam C et al: On the sequence of reactions leading to cytochrome P-450 synthesis: effect of drugs. *J Biol Chem* **250**:2305, 1975

85. Correia MA et al: Incorporation of exogenous heme into hepatic cytochrome P-450 *in vivo*. *J Biol Chem* **254**:15, 1979

86. Tschudy DP et al: Acute intermittent porphyria: clinical and selected research aspects. *Ann Intern Med* **83**:851, 1975

87. Giger U, Meyer UA: Induction of delta-aminolevulinate synthase and cytochrome P-450 hemoproteins in hepatocyte culture. Effect of glucose and hormones. *J Biol Chem* **256**:11182, 1981

88. Felsher BF, Redeker AG: Acute intermittent porphyria: effect of diet and griseofulvin. *Medicine (Baltimore)* **46**:217, 1967

89. Quiroz-Kendall E et al: Acute variegate porphyria following a Scarsdale Gourmet Diet. *J Am Acad Dermatol* **8**:46, 1983

90. Rifkind AB: Drug-induced exacerbations of porphyria. *Primary Care* **3**:665, 1976

91. Dhar GJ et al: Effects of hematin in hepatic porphyria. *Ann Intern Med* **83**:20, 1975

92. Watson CJ et al: Use of hematin in the acute attack of the "inducible" hepatic porphyrias. *Adv Intern Med* **233**:265, 1978

93. McColl KEL et al: Treatment with haematin in acute hepatic porphyria. *Q J Med* **198**:161, 1981

94. Canepa ET et al: Properties of the cobaltochelatase and the ferrochelatase. *Enzyme* **26**:288, 1981

95. Poh-Fitzpatrick MB, Lamola AA: Comparative study of protoporphyrins in erythropoietic protoporphyria and griseofulvin-induced murine protoporphyria. *J Clin Invest* **60**:380, 1977

96. Rimington C et al: Griseofulvin administration and porphyrin metabolism. *Lancet* **2**:318, 1963

97. Taketani S, Tokunaga R: Rat liver ferrochelatase: purification, properties and stimulation by fatty acids. *J Biol Chem* **256**:12748, 1981

98. Stokvis BJ: Over twee zeldzame kleurstotten in urine van zicken. *Ned Tijdschr Geneeskd* **25**:409, 1889

99. Duesberg G: Toxische Porphyrie: *Munch Med Wochenschr* **79**:1821, 1932

100. Goldberg A: Acute intermittent porphyria: study of 50 cases. *Q J Med* **28**:183, 1959

101. Dean G: *The Porphyrias*. Philadelphia, Lippincott, 1963

102. Stein JA, Tschudy DP: Acute intermittent porphyria: a clin-

ical and biochemical study of 46 patients. *Medicine (Baltimore)* 49:1, 1970

103. Koskelo P et al: Urinary excretion of porphyrin precursors and coproporphyrin in healthy females on oral contraceptive. *Br Med J* 1:652, 1966

104. Cam C, Nigogosyan G: Acquired toxic porphyria cutanea tarda due to hexachlorobenzene. *JAMA* 183:88, 1963

105. Bleiberg J et al: Industrially acquired porphyria. *Arch Dermatol* 89:793, 1964

106. Poland AP et al: A health survey of workers in a 2,4-D and a 2,4,5-T plant. *Arch Environ Health* 22:316, 1971

107. Lynch RE et al: Porphyria cutanea tarda associated with disinfectant misuse. *Arch Intern Med* 135:549, 1975

108. Elder GH et al: The effect of the porphyrinogenic compound, hexachlorobenzene, on the activity of hepatic uroporphyrinogen decarboxylase in the rat. *Clin Sci Mol Med* 51:71, 1976

109. Roenigk HH Jr, Gottlob NE: Estrogen-induced porphyria cutanea tarda. *Arch Dermatol* 102:260, 1970

110. Dehlin O et al: Porphyria cutanea tarda—a genetic disease? *Acta Med Scand* 194:265, 1973

111. Benedetto AV et al: Porphyria cutanea tarda in three generations of a single family. *N Engl J Med* 298:358, 1978

112. de Verneuil H et al: Familial and sporadic porphyria cutanea. Two different diseases. *Hum Genet* 44:145, 1978

113. Elder GH et al: Identification of two types of porphyria cutanea tarda by measurement of erythrocyte uroporphyrinogen decarboxylase. *Clin Sci* 58:477, 1980

114. Meyer-Betz F: Untersuchungen uber die biologische (photodynamische) Wirkung des Hamatoporphyrins und andere derivate des Blut und Gallenfarbstoffes. *Dtsch Arch Klin Med* 112:476, 1913

115. Lipson RL et al: The use of a derivative of hematoporphyrin in tumor detection. *J Natl Cancer Inst* 26:1, 1961

116. Zalar GL et al: Induction of drug photosensitization in man after parenteral exposure to hematoporphyrin. *Arch Dermatol* 113:1392, 1977

117. Leroy D et al: Photosensitization complications after intramuscular injections of hematoporphyrin. *Ann Dermatol Venereol* 108:95, 1981

118. Bodaness RS, Chan PC: Singlet oxygen as a mediator in the hematoporphyrin-catalyzed photooxidation of NADPH to NADP$^+$ in deuterium oxide. *J Biol Chem* 252:8554, 1977

119. Cauzzo G et al: The effects of chemical structure on the photosensitizing efficiencies of porphyrins. *Photochem Photobiol* 25:389, 1977

120. Kessel D, Rossi E: Determinants of porphyrin-induced photo-oxidation characterized by fluorescence and absorption spectra. *Photochem Photobiol* 35:37, 1982

121. Bickers DR et al: Hematoporphyrin photosensitization of epidermal microsomes results in destruction of cytochrome P-450 and in decreased monooxygenase activities and heme content. *Biochem Biophys Res Commun* 108:1032, 1982

122. Blum HF: *Photodynamic Action and Diseases Caused by Light.* Princeton, Reinhold, 1941

123. Hochstein P, Ernster L: Microsomal peroxidation of lipids and its possible role in cellular injury, in *CIBA Foundation Symposium on Cellular Injury,* edited by AVS De Reuck, J Snight. Boston, Little, Brown, 1964, p 123

124. Dubbelman TMAR et al: Photodynamic effects of protoporphyrin on red blood cell deformability. *Biochem Biophys Res Commun* 77:811, 1977

125. Dubbelman TMAR et al: Protoporphyrin sensitized photodynamic modification of proteins in isolated human red blood cell membranes. *Photochem Photobiol* 28:197, 1978

126. Girotti AW: Protoporphyrin-sensitized photodamage in isolated membranes of human erythrocytes. *Biochemistry* 18:4403, 1979

127. Schothorst AA et al: Photochemical damage to skin fibro-

blasts caused by protoporphyrin and violet light. *Arch Dermatol Res* 268:31, 1980

128. Goldstein BD, Harber LC: Erythropoietic protoporphyria: lipid peroxidation and red cell membrane damage associated with photohemolysis. *J Clin Invest* 51:892, 1972

129. Lamola AA et al: Cholesterol hydroperoxide formation in red cell membranes and photohemolysis in erythropoietic protoporphyria. *Science* 179:1131, 1973

130. Allison AC et al: Role of lysosomes and of cell membranes in photosensitization. *Nature* 209:874, 1966

131. Sandberg S: Protoporphyrin-induced photodamage to mitochondria and lysosomes from rat liver. *Clin Chim Acta* 111:55, 1981

132. Sandberg S, Romslo I: Phototoxicity of protoporphyrin as related to its subcellular localization in mice livers after short-term feeding with griseofulvin. *Biochem J* 198:67, 1981

133. Coppola A et al: Ultrastructural changes in lymphoma cells treated with hematoporphyrin and light. *Am J Pathol* 99:175, 1980

134. Dixit R et al: Destruction of cytochrome P-450 by reactive oxygen species generated during photosensitization of hematoporphyrin derivative. *Photochem Photobiol* 37:173, 1983

135. Gutter B et al: The photodynamic modification of DNA by hematoporphyrin. *Biochim Biophys Acta* 475:307, 1977

136. Canti G et al: Hematoporphyrin-treated murine lymphocytes: in vitro inhibition of DNA synthesis and light-mediated inactivation of cells responsible for GVHR. *Photochem Photobiol* 34:589, 1981

137. Wakulchik SD et al: Photolysis of protoporphyrin-treated human fibroblasts *in vitro.* Studies on the mechanism. *J Lab Clin Med* 96:158, 1980

138. Gigli I et al: Erythropoietic protoporphyria: photoactivation of the complement system. *J Clin Invest* 66:517, 1980

139. Lim HW et al: Generation of chemotactic activity in serum from patients with erythropoietic protoporphyria and porphyria cutanea tarda. *N Engl J Med* 304:212, 1981

140. Lim HW, Gigli I: Role of complement in porphyrin-induced photosensitivity. *J Invest Dermatol* 76:4, 1981

141. Runge W, Watson CJ: Experimental production of skin lesions in human cutaneous porphyria. *Proc Soc Exp Biol Med* 109:809, 1962

142. Wiskemann A, Wulf K: Zur Lichtprovokastion der Porphyrin-Dermatosen. *Arch Klin Exp Dermatol* 209:454, 1959

143. Magnus IA et al: The action spectrum for skin lesions in porphyria cutanea tarda. *Lancet* 1:912, 1959

144. Gordon W: The detection of photosensitivity in porphyria using filtered sunlight. *S Afr J Lab Clin Med* 9:245, 1963

145. Rimington C et al: Porphyria and photosensitivity. *Q J Med* 36:29, 1967

146. Mathews MM: Protective effect of beta-carotene against lethal photosensitization by hematoporphyrin. *Nature* 203:1092, 1964

147. Fujimori E, Tavla N: Light-induced electron transfer between chlorophyll and hydroquinone and the effect of oxygen and beta-carotene. *Photochem Photobiol* 5:877, 1966

148. Foote CS, Denny RW: Chemistry of singlet oxygen. VII. Quenching by beta-carotene. *J Am Chem Soc* 90:6233, 1968

149. Mathews-Roth MM et al: Beta-carotene as a photoprotective agent in erythropoietic protoporphyria. *N Engl J Med* 282:1231, 1970

150. Mathews-Roth MM et al: Beta-carotene as an oral photoprotective agent in erythropoietic protoporphyria. *JAMA* 228:1004, 1974

151. Emiliani C, Delmelle M: The lipid solubility of porphyrins modulates their phototoxicity in membrane models. *Photochem Photobiol* 37:487, 1983

152. Günther H: Die Bedeutung der Hamatoporphyrine in Physiologie und Pathologie. *Ergeb Allerg Pathol* 20:608, 1922

153. Watson CJ et al: The manifestations of the different forms of porphyria in relation to chemical findings. *Trans Assoc Am Physicians* **64**:345, 1951

154. Magnus IA: *Dermatological Photobiology*. London, Blackwell, 1976

155. Mackey L, Garrod AE: A further contribution to the study of congenital porphyrinuria (haematoporphyria congenita). *Q J Med* **19**:357, 1925

156. Ashby HT: Haematoporphyria congenita (congenital porphyrinuria): its association with hydroa vacciniforme and pigmentation of the teeth. *Q J Med* **19**:375, 1925

157. Gray AMH: Haematoporphyria congenita with hydroa vacciniforme and hirsuties. *Q J Med* **19**:381, 1925

158. Ippen H, Fuchs T: Congenital porphyria, *Clin Haematol* **9**:323, 1980

159. Romeo G et al: Uroporphyrinogen III cosynthetase activity in an asymptomatic carrier of congenital erythropoietic porphyria. *Biochem Genet* **4**:719, 1970

160. Miyagi K et al: The activities of uroporphyrinogen synthetase and cosynthetase in congenital erythropoietic porphyria (CEP). *Am J Hematol* **1**:3, 1976

161. Kushner JP et al: Congenital erythropoietic porphyria, diminished activity of uroporphyrinogen decarboxylase and dyserythropoiesis. *Blood* **59**:725, 1982

162. Magnus IA: The cutaneous porphyrias. *Semin Hematol* **5**:380, 1968

163. Kramer S et al: The anemia of erythropoietic porphyria with the first description of the disease in an elderly patient. *Br J Haematol* **11**:666, 1965

164. Pain RW et al: Erythropoietic uroporphyria of Günther first presenting at 58 years with positive family studies. *Br Med J* **2**:621, 1975

165. Clare NT, Stevens EH: Congenital porphyria in pigs. *Nature* **153**:252, 1944

166. Watson CJ et al: Some studies of the comparative biology of human and bovine erythropoietic porphyria. *Arch Intern Med* **103**:436, 1959

167. Giddens WE et al: Feline congenital erythropoietic porphyria associated with severe anemia and renal disease. *Am J Pathol* **80**:367, 1975

168. Nordmann Y, Deybach JC: Congenital erythropoietic porphyria. *Semin Liver Dis* **2**:154, 1982

169. Haining RG et al: Congenital erythropoietic porphyria. I. Case report, special studies and therapy. *Am J Med* **43**:624, 1968

170. Rosenthal IM et al: Effect of splenectomy on porphyria erythropoietica. *Pediatrics* **15**:663, 1955

171. Poh-Fitzpatrick MB: Erythropoietic porphyrias: current mechanistic, diagnostic and therapeutic considerations. *Semin Hematol* **14**:211, 1977

172. Haining RG et al: Congenital erythropoietic porphyria. II. The effects of induced polycythemia. *Blood* **36**:297, 1970

173. Watson CJ, Bossenmaier I: Repression by hematin of porphyrin biosynthesis in erythrocyte precursors in congenital erythropoietic porphyria. *Proc Natl Acad Sci USA* **71**:278, 1974

174. Kosenow W, Treibs A. Lichtüberemfindlichkeit und Porphyrinamie. *Z Kinderheilkd* **73**:82, 1953

175. Langhof H et al: Untersuchungen zur familiären protoporphyrinamischen Lichturticaria. *Arch Klin Exp Dermatol* **212**:506, 1961

176. Bloomer JR: Characterization of deficient heme synthase activity in protoporphyria with cultured skin fibroblasts. *J Clin Invest* **65**:321, 1980

177. Sassa S et al: Studies in porphyria. Functional evidence for a partial deficiency of ferrochelatase activity in mitogen-stimulated lymphocytes from patients with erythropoietic protoporphyria. *J Clin Invest* **69**:809, 1982

178. Bloomer JR et al: Bovine protoporphyria: documentation of autosomal recessive inheritance and comparison with the human disease through measurement of heme synthase activity. *Am J Hum Genet* **34**:322, 1982

179. Bloomer JR et al: Inheritance in protoporphyria. *Lancet* **2**:226, 1976

180. Haeger-Aronsen B, Krook G: Erythropoietic protoporphyria: a study of known cases in Sweden. *Acta Med Scand* **179**:48, 1966

181. Reed WB et al: Erythropoietic protoporphyria: a clinical and genetic study. *JAMA* **214**:1064, 1970

182. DeLeo VA et al: Erythropoietic protoporphyria. *Am J Med* **60**:8, 1976

183. DeGoeif AFPM: Biochemical aspects of erythropoietic protoporphyria. *Dermatologica* **163**:232, 1981

184. Poh-Fitzpatrick MB: Erythropoietic protoporphyria. *Int J Dermatol* **17**:359, 1978

185. Kansky A, Bercu M: Erythropoietic protoporphyria in Slovenia. Epidemiologic study. *Dermatologica* **163**:232, 1981

186. Went LN et al: In, *Proceedings of the XIV International Congress of Dermatology,* series no. 289, edited by F Flarer, S Serri. Amsterdam, Excerpta Medica, 1972, p 401

187. Bhutani LK et al: Erythropoietic protoporphyria: first report in an Indian. *Br Med J* **2**:741, 1972

188. Schmidt H et al: Erythropoietic protoporphyria: a clinical study based on 29 cases in 14 families. *Arch Dermatol* **110**:58, 1974

189. Bovenmayer DA: First report of EPP cases in the American Negro. *Cutis* **18**:227, 1976

190. Cripps DJ, McEachen WN: Hepatic and erythropoietic protoporphyria. *Arch Pathol* **91**:497, 1971

191. Schwartz S et al: Erythropoietic defects in protoporphyria: a study of factors involved in labeling of porphyrins and bile pigments from ALA-^{3}H and glycine-^{14}C. *J Lab Clin Med* **78**:411, 1971

192. Piomelli S et al: Erythropoietic protoporphyria and lead intoxication: the molecular basis for difference in cutaneous photosensitivity. I. Different rates of disappearance of protoporphyrin from the erythrocytes, both in vivo and in vitro. *J Clin Invest* **56**:1519, 1975

193. Gray CH et al: Isotope studies on a case of erythropoietic protoporphyria. *Clin Sci* **26**:7, 1964

194. Scholnick P et al: Erythropoietic protoporphyria: evidence for multiple sites of excess protoporphyrin formation. *J Clin Invest* **50**:203, 1971

195. Nicholson DC et al: Isotopic studies of the erythropoietic and hepatic components of congenital porphyria and "erythropoietic" protoporphyria. *Clin Sci* **44**:135, 1973

196. Lamon JM et al: Hepatic protoporphyrin production in human protoporphyria. *Gastroenterology* **79**:115, 1980

197. Kaplowitz N et al: Isolation of erythrocytes with normal protoporphyrin levels in erythropoietic protoporphyria. *N Engl J Med* **278**:1077, 1968

198. Porter FS, Lowe BA: Congenital erythropoietic protoporphyria. I. Case reports, clinical studies and porphyria analyses in two brothers. *Blood* **22**:521, 1963

199. Cripps DJ, Scheuer PJ: Hepatobiliary changes in erythropoietic protoporphyria. *Arch Pathol* **80**:500, 1965

200. Klatskin G, Bloomer JR: Birefringence of hepatic pigment deposits in erythropoietic protoporphyria: specificity and sensitivity of polarization microscopy in the identification of hepatic protoporphyrin deposits. *Gastroenterology* **67**:295, 1974

201. Bloomer JR et al: Hepatic disease in erythropoietic protoporphyria. *Am J Med* **58**:869, 1975

202. Cripps DJ et al: Erythropoietic protoporphyria: juvenile protoporphyrin hepatopathy cirrhosis and death. *Pediatrics* **91**:744, 1977

203. Bloomer JR: Pathogenesis and therapy of liver disease in protoporphyria. *Yale J Biol Med* **52**:39, 1979

204. Barnes HD et al: Erythropoietic protoporphyria hepatitis. *J Clin Pathol* **21:**157, 1968

205. Scott AJ et al: Erythropoietic protoporphyria with features of a sideroblastic anemia terminating in liver failure. *Am J Med* **54:**251, 1973

206. Nicholson DC, Zawirska B: Porphyrin production in terminal erythropoietic protoporphyria, in *Porphyrins in Human Diseases. First International Porphyrin Meeting, Freiburg,* edited by M Doss, P Nawrocki. Basel, Karger, 1976, p 137

207. Cripps DJ, Goldfarb SS: Erythropoietic protoporphyria: hepatic cirrhosis. *Br J Dermatol* **98:**349, 1978

208. Wells MM et al: Erythropoietic protoporphyria with hepatic cirrhosis. *Arch Dermatol* **116:**429, 1980

209. Macdonald DM et al: The histopathology and ultrastructure of liver disease in erythropoietic protoporphyria. *Br J Dermatol* **104:**7, 1981

210. Romslo I et al: Erythropoietic protoporphyria terminating in liver failure. *Arch Dermatol* **118:**668, 1982

211. Avner DL et al: Protoporphyrin-induced cholestasis in the isolated in situ perfused rat liver. *J Clin Invest* **67:**385, 1981

212. Poh-Fitzpatrick MB, DeLeo VA: Rates of plasma porphyrin disappearance in fluorescent vs. red incandescent light exposure. *J Invest Dermatol* **69:**510, 1977

213. Poh-Fitzpatrick MB et al: Rapid quantitative assay for erythrocyte porphyrins. *Arch Dermatol* **110:**225, 1974

214. Lamola AA et al: Erythropoietic protoporphyria and Pb intoxication: the molecular basis for difference in cutaneous photosensitivity. II. Different binding of erythrocyte protoporphyrin to hemoglobin. *J Clin Invest* **56:**1528, 1975

215. Romslo I et al: Sideroblastic anemia with markedly increased free erythrocyte protoporphyrin without dermal photosensitivity. *Blood* **59:**628, 1982

216. Sandberg S, Brun A: Light-induced protoporphyrin release from erythrocytes in erythropoietic protoporphyria. *J Clin Invest* **70:**693, 1982

217. Joenje H et al: Inhibitory effect of palsma on photohemolysis in erythropoietic protoporphyria. *Dermatologica* **163:**285, 1981

218. Peterka EA et al: Erythropoietic protoporphyria. II. Histological and histochemical studies of cutaneous lesions. *Arch Dermatol* **92:**357, 1965

219. Cripps DJ et al: Four cases of erythropoietic protoporphyria presenting as light-sensitive lipoid proteinosis. *Proc R Soc Med* **57:**1095, 1964

220. Ryan EA, Madill GT: Electron microscopy of the skin in erythropoietic protoporphyria. *Br J Dermatol* **80:**561, 1968

221. Wick G et al: Immunofluorescence demonstration of type IV collagen and a noncollagenous glycoprotein in thickened vascular basal membranes in protoporphyria. *J Invest Dermatol* **73:**335, 1979

222. Breathnach SM et al: Immunohistochemical studies of amyloid P component and fibronectin in erythropoietic protoporphyria. *Br J Dermatol* **108:**267, 1983

223. Mathews-Roth MM et al: Beta-carotene therapy for erythropoietic protoporphyria and other diseases. *Arch Dermatol* **113:**1229, 1977

224. Baart de la Faille H et al: Beta-carotene as a treatment for photosensitivity due to erythropoietic protoporphyria. *Dermatologica* **145:**389, 1972

225. Krook G, Haeger-Aronsen B: Erythrohepatic protoporphyria and its treatment with beta-carotene. *Acta Derm Venereol (Stockh)* **54:**39, 1974

226. Gschnait F, Wolff K: Die erythropoietische Protoporphyrie. *Hautarzt* **25:**72, 1974

227. Thomas K et al: Beta-carotene in erythropoietic protoporphyria: 5 years' experience. *Dermatologica* **159:**82, 1979

228. Krook G, Haeger-Aronsen B: Beta-carotene in the treatment of erythropoietic protoporphyria. A short review. *Acta Derm Venereol [Suppl] (Stockh)* **100:**125, 1982

229. Corbett NF et al: The long term treatment with beta-carotene in erythropoietic protoporphyria: a controlled trial. *Br J Dermatol* **97:**653, 1977

230. Joshi PC, Pathak MA: Production of singlet oxygen and superoxide radicals by psoralens and their biological significance. *Biochem Biophys Res Commun* **112:**638, 1983

231. Bloomer JR, Pierach CA: Effect of hematin administration to patients with protoporphyria and liver disease. *Hepatology* **2:**817, 1982

232. Bechtel MA et al: Transfusion therapy in a patient with erythropoietic protoporphyria. *Arch Dermatol* **47:**99, 1981

233. Topi G et al: Coproporphirie erithropoetique congenitales observée chez un frère et une soeur. *Ann Dermatol Venereol* **104:**68, 1977

234. Brunsting LA, Mason HC: Porphyria with epidermolysis bullosa: report of a case of the tardive congenital type with demonstration of latent porphyria in a sister of the patient. *JAMA* **132:**509, 1946

235. Brunsting LA, Mason HL: Porphyria with cutaneous manifestations. *Arch Dermatol Syphilol* **60:**66, 1949

236. Eales L: Cutaneous porphyria: observations on 111 cases in three racial groups. *S Afr J Lab Clin Med* **6:**63, 1960

237. Lamont NM et al: Porphyria in the African. *Q J Med* **30:**373, 1961

238. Eales L: Porphyria as seen in Cape Towne: a survey of 250 patients and some recent studies. *S Afr J Lab Clin Med* **9:**151, 1963

239. Watson CJ: The problem of porphyria: some facts and questions. *N Engl J Med* **263:**1205, 1960

240. Holti G et al: Investigation of porphyria cutanea tarda. *Q J Med* **27:**1, 1958

241. Elder GH et al: Decreased activity of hepatic uroporphyrinogen decarboxylase in sporadic porphyria cutanea tarda. *N Engl J Med* **299:**274, 1978

242. Watson CJ et al: Porphyria variegata and porphyria cutanea tarda in siblings: chemical and genetic aspects. *Proc Natl Acad Sci USA* **72:**5126, 1975

243. Day RS et al: Coexistent variegate porphyria and porphyria cutanea tarda. *N Engl J Med* **307:**36, 1982

244. Shaley BC et al: Effect of ethanol on liver and aminolaevulinate synthetase activity and urinary porphyrin excretion in symptomatic porphyria. *Br J Haematol* **17:**389, 1969

245. McColl KEL et al: Acute ethanol ingestion and haem biosynthesis in healthy subjects. *Eur J Clin Invest* **10:**107, 1980

246. McColl KEL et al: Abnormal haem biosynthesis in chronic alcoholics. *Eur J Clin Invest* **11:**461, 1981

247. Hourihane DO, Weir DG: Suppression of erythropoiesis by alcohol. *Br Med J* **1:**86, 1970

248. Kodama T et al: Changes in aminolevulinate synthase and aminolevulinate dehydratase activity and cirrhotic liver. *Gastroenterology* **84:**236, 1983

249. Grossman ME et al: Porphyria cutanea tarda. Clinical features and laboratory findings in 40 patients. *Am J Med* **67:**277, 1979

250. Harber LC, Bickers DR: The porphyrias: basic science aspects, clinical diagnosis and management, in *Yearbook of Dermatology,* edited by F Malkinson, R Pearson. Chicago, Year Book, 1975, p 9

251. Taylor JS, Roenigk HH Jr: Estrogen-induced porphyria cutanea tarda, in *Porphyrins in Human Disease,* edited by M Doss, P Marocki. Basel, Karger, 1976, p 328

252. Levere RD: Stilbesterol-induced porphyria: increased hepatic delta-aminolevulinic acid synthetase. *Blood* **28:**569, 1966

253. Ochner RK, Schmid R: Acquired porphyria in man and rat due to hexachlorobenzene intoxication. *Nature* **189:**499, 1961

254. Peters HA: Hexachlorobenzene poisoning in Turkey. *Fed Proc* **35:**2400, 1976

255. Cripps DJ et al: Porphyria turcica. Twenty years after hexachlorobenzene intoxication. *Arch Dermatol* **116**:46, 1980

256. Stonard MD: Experimental hepatic porphyria induced by hexachlorobenzene as a model for human symptomatic porphyria. *Br J Haematol* **27**:617, 1974

257. Courtney KD: Hexachlorobenzene (HCB): a review. *Environ Res* **20**:225, 1979

258. Elder GH, Sheppard DM: Immunoreactive uroporphyrinogen decarboxylase is unchanged in porphyria caused by TCDD and hexachlorobenzene. *Biochem Biophys Res Commun* **109**:113, 1982

259. Goldstein JA et al: Effects of pentachlorophenol on hepatic drug-metabolizing enzymes and porphyria related to contamination with chlorinated dibenzo-*p*-dioxins and dibenzofurans. *Biochem Pharmacol* **26**:1549, 1977

260. Poland AP, Glover E: 2,3,7,8-Tetrachlorodibenzo-*p*-dioxin: a potent inducer of delta-aminolevulinic acid synthetase. *Science* **179**:476, 1973

261. Goldstein JA et al: Hepatic porphyria induced by 2,3,7,8-tetrachlorodibenzo(p)dioxin in the mouse. *Res Commun Chem Pathol Pharmacol* **6**:919, 1973

262. May G: Chloracne from the accidental production of tetrachlorodibenzodioxin. *Br J Ind Med* **30**:276, 1973

263. Schwetz BA et al: Toxicology of chlorinated dibenzo-(p)dioxins. *Environ Health Perspect* **5**:87, 1973

264. Strik JJTWA: Porphyrinogenic action of polyhalogenated aromatic compounds, with special reference to porphyria and environmental impact, in *Diagnosis and Therapy of Porphyrias and Lead Intoxication,* edited by M Doss. Berlin/Heidelberg, Springer-Verlag, 1978, p 151

265. Sweeney GD et al: Iron deficiency prevents liver toxicity of 2,3,7,8-tetrachlorodibenzo-*p*-dioxin. *Science* **204**:332, 1979

266. Jones KG, Sweeney GD: Dependence of the porphyrogenic effect of 2,3,7,8-tetrachlorodibenzo(p)dioxin upon inheritance of aryl hydrocarbon hydroxylase responsiveness. *Toxicol Appl Pharmacol* **53**:42, 1980

267. Lundvall O: The effect of replenishment of iron stores after phlebotomy therapy in porphyria cutanea tarda. *Acta Med Scand* **189**:51, 1971

268. Lundvall O: The effect of phlebotomy therapy in porphyria cutanea tarda: its relation to the phlebotomy-induced reduction of iron stores. *Acta Med Scand* **189**:33, 1971

269. Epstein JH, Pinski JB: Porphyria cutanea tarda: association with abnormal iron metabolism. *Arch Dermatol* **92**:362, 1965

270. Turnbull A: Iron metabolism in the porphyrias. *Br J Dermatol* **84**:380, 1971

271. Turnbull A et al: Iron metabolism in porphyria cutanea tarda and in erythropoietic protoporphyria. *Q J Med* **42**:341, 1973

272. Kushner JP et al: The role of iron in the pathogenesis of porphyria cutanea tarda. II. Inhibition of uroporphyrinogen decarboxylase. *J Clin Invest* **56**:661, 1975

273. Felsher BF et al: Iron and hepatic uroporphyrin synthesis: relations in porphyria cutanea tarda. *JAMA* **226**:663, 1973

274. Blekkenhorst GH et al: Iron and porphyria cutanea tarda: activation of uroporphyrinogen decarboxylase by ferrous iron. *S Afr Med J* **56**:918, 1979

275. Woods JS et al: Studies on the action of porphyrinogenic trace metals on the activity of hepatic uroporphyrinogen decarboxylase. *Biochem Biophys Res Commun* **103**:264, 1981

276. Bonkowsky HL et al: Iron and the liver. Acute and long-term effects of iron-loading on hepatic haem metabolism. *Biochem J* **196**:57, 1981

277. Stein JA et al: Delta-aminolevulinic acid synthetase. III. Synergistic effect of chelated iron on induction. *J Biol Chem* **245**:2213, 1970

278. Kushner JP et al: The role of iron in the pathogenesis of porphyria cutanea tarda: an in vitro model. *J Clin Invest* **51**:3044, 1972

279. DeMatteis F, Stonard J: Experimental porphyrias as models for human hepatic porphyrias. *Semin Hematol* **14**:187, 1977

280. Felsher BF, Kushner JP: Hepatic siderosis and porphyria cutanea tarda: relation of iron excess to the metabolic defect. *Semin Hematol* **14**:243, 1977

281. Elder GH: Haem synthesis and breakdown, in *Iron in Biochemistry and Medicine II,* edited by A Jacobs, M Worwood. London/New York, Academic Press, 1980, p 245

282. Varigos G et al: Uroporphyrin I stimulation of collagen biosynthesis in human skin fibroblasts. A unique dark effect of porphyrin. *J Clin Invest* **69**:129, 1982

283. Waldenström J: Geography and genetics of the porphyrias. *Acta Derm Venereol [Suppl] (Stockh)* **100**:43, 1982

284. Pimstone NR: Porphyria cutanea tarda. *Semin Liver Dis* **2**:125, 1982

285. DiPadova C et al: Effects of phlebotomy on urinary porphyrin pattern and liver histology in patients with porphyria cutanea tarda. *Am J Med Sci* **285**:2, 1983

286. Welland FH, Carlsen RA: Porphyria cutanea tarda in an 8 year-old boy. *Arch Dermatol* **99**:451, 1969

287. Enriquez de Salamanca R et al: Patterns of porphyrin-excretion in female estrogen-induced porphyria cutanea tarda. *Arch Dermatol Res* **274**:179, 1982

288. Gilchrest B et al: Porphyria cutanea tarda in young women. *Arch Dermatol* **111**:263, 1975

289. Becker FT: Porphyria cutanea tarda induced by estrogens. *Arch Dermatol* **92**:252, 1965

290. Burnett JW, Pathak MA: Effect of light upon porphyrin metabolism of rats. *Arch Dermatol* **89**:257, 1964

291. Jones K et al: Environmental lighting and porphyrin metabolism in rat, in *Porphyrins in Human Diseases. First International Porphyrin Meeting, Freiburg,* edited by M Doss, P Nawrocki. Basel, Karger, 1976, p 385

292. Magnus IA et al: The effect of environmental lighting on porphyrin metabolism in the rat. *Nature* **250**:504, 1974

293. Bickers DR et al: The effect of environmental light exposure on drug-induced porphyria in the rat. *Photochem Photobiol* **24**:551, 1976

294. Tio TH et al: Acquired porphyria from a liver tumor. *Clin Sci* **16**:517, 1957

295. Waddington RT: A case of primary liver tumor associated with porphyria. *Br J Surg* **59**:653, 1972

296. Keczkes K, Barker DJ: Malignant hepatoma associated with acquired hepatic cutaneous porphyria. *Arch Dermatol* **112**:78, 1976

297. Grossman M, Bickers DR: Porphyria cutanea tarda and hepatic tumor. *Cutis* **21**:782, 1978

298. Solis JA et al: Association of porphyria cutanea tarda and primary liver cancer. *J Dermatol (Tokyo)* **9**:131, 1982

299. Burnett JW et al: Haemophilia, hepatitis and porphyria. *Br J Dermatol* **97**:353, 1977

300. Uthemann H et al: Serologische Hepatitis-B-Marker bei Porphyrie cutanea tarda: *Dtsch Med Worchenschr* **105**:1718, 1980

301. Cram DL et al: Lupus erythematosus and porphyria. *Arch Dermatol* **103**:779, 1973

302. Clemmensen O, Thomsen K: Porphyria cutanea tarda and systemic lupus erythematosus. *Arch Dermatol* **118**:160, 1982

303. Korting GW: Porphyria-cutanea tarda-artige Hautveranderungen bei Langzeit hamodialysepatienten. *Dermatologica* **150**:58, 1975

304. Poh-Fitzpatrick MB et al: Porphyria cutanea tarda in two patients treated with hemodialysis for chronic renal failure. *N Engl J Med* **299**:292, 1978

305. Day RS, Eales L: Porphyrins in chronic renal failure. *Nephron* **26**:90, 1980

306. Poh-Fitzpatrick MB et al: Porphyria cutanea tarda associated with chronic renal disease and hemodialysis. *Arch Dermatol* **116**:191, 1980

307. Day RS et al: Porphyrias and the kidney. *Nephron* **28**:261, 1981

308. Disler P et al: Treatment of hemodialysis-related porphyria cutanea tarda with plasma exchange. *Am J Med* **72**:989, 1982

309. Hanno R, Callen JP: Porphyria cutanea tarda as a cause of bullous dermatosis of hemodialysis. A case report and review of the literature. *Cutis* **28**:261, 1981

310. Mann RJ, Harman RR: Porphyria cutanea tarda and sarcoidosis. *Clin Exp Dermatol* **7**:619, 1982

311. Ramasamy R, Kubik MM: Porphyria cutanea tarda in association with Sjögren's syndrome. *Practitioner* **226**:1297, 1982

312. Biro I et al: Cryoglobulinemia and porphyria hepatica chronica (porphyria cutanea tarda). *Acta Derm Venereol (Stockh)* **44**:226, 1964

313. Elder GH: Porphyrin metabolism in porphyria cutanea tarda. *Semin Hematol* **14**:227, 1977

314. Smith SG: Porphyrins found in urine of patient with symptomatic porphyria. *Biochem Soc Trans* **5**:1472, 1977

315. Perrot H et al: Urinary porphyrin excretion in various types of porphyria. Thin-layer chromatographic study. *Dermatologica* **161**:167, 1980

316. With TK et al: Comparison of the porphyrin patterns in patients with porphyria cutanea tarda in Czechoslovakia and Denmark. *Int J Biochem* **13**:769, 1981

317. Hill RH Jr et al: Development and utilization of a procedure for measuring urinary porphyrins by high-performance liquid chromatography. *J Chromatogr* **232**:251, 1982

318. Jackson AH et al: High-pressure liquid chromatographic analysis of tetracarboxylic porphyrins in hepatic porphyrias. *Biochem J* **207**:599, 1982

319. Nonaka S et al: Urinary porphyrin analyses in patients with porphyria cutanea tarda. *J Dermatol (Tokyo)* **9**:397, 1982

320. Perrot H et al: Faecal porphyrin excretion in various types of porphyria. Thin layer chromatographic study. *Arch Dermatol Res* **263**:67, 1978

321. Smith SG et al: A comparison of porphyrin excretion patterns from hepatoerythropoietic porphyria (HEP) and porphyria cutanea tarda (PCT), in *Proceedings of the XVI International Congress of Dermatology*, edited by A Kukita, M Seiji. Tokyo, Univ of Tokyo Press, 1982, p 264

322. Cripps DJ, Peters HA: Fluorescing erythrocytes and porphyrin screening tests on urine, blood and stool. *Arch Dermatol* **96**:712, 1967

323. Harber LC, Bickers DR: Laboratory tests for the diagnosis of porphyrias, in *Photosensitivity Diseases: Principles of Diagnosis and Treatment*. Philadelphia, WB Saunders, 1981, p 346

324. Bolgert N et al: La porphyrie cutanée de l'adulte: étude de neuf cas et description. *Sem Hop Paris* **29**:1587, 1953

325. Cormane RH et al: Histopathology of the skin in acquired and hereditary porphyria cutanea tarda. *Br J Dermatol* **85**:531, 1971

326. Epstein JH et al: Cutaneous changes in the porphyrias. *Arch Dermatol* **107**:689, 1973

327. Pathak MA, Burnett JW: The porphyrin content of skin. *J Invest Dermatol* **43**:119, 1964

328. Pathak MA, Burnett JW: The intracellular localization of porphyrins. *J Invest Dermatol* **43**:421, 1964

329. Molina L et al: Skin porphyrin assay in porphyria. *Clin Chim Acta* **83**:55, 1978

330. Magnus IA: Action spectroscopy of the skin in porphyria. *Acta Derm Venereol [Suppl] (Stockh)* **100**:47, 1982

331. Ramsay CA et al: The treatment of porphyria cutanea tarda by venesection. *Q J Med* **43**:1, 1974

332. Ippen H: Allgemeinsymptome der spaten Hautporphyrie (Porphyria cutanea tarda) als Hisweise fur deren Behandlung. *Dtsch Med Wochenschr* **86**:127, 1961

333. Epstein JH, Redeker AG: Porphyria cutanea tarda: a study of the effect of phlebotomy. *N Engl J Med* **279**:1301, 1968

334. Lundvall O, Weinfeld A: Studies of the clinical and metabolic effects of phlebotomy treatment in porphyria cutanea tarda. *Acta Med Scand* **184**:191, 1968

335. Ippen H: Treatment of porphyria cutanea tarda by phlebotomy. *Semin Hematol* **14**:253, 1977

336. Lundvall O: Phlebotomy treatment of porphyria cutanea tarda. *Acta Derm Venereol [Suppl] (Stockh)* **100**:107, 1982

337. Vogler WR et al: Biochemical effects of chloroquine therapy in porphyria cutanea tarda. *Am J Med* **49**:316, 1970

338. Kowertz MJ: The therapeutic effect of chloroquine. *JAMA* **223**:515, 1973

339. Kordac V, Semradova M: Treatment of porphyria cutanea tarda with chloroquine. *Br J Dermatol* **90**:95, 1974

340. Kordac V et al: Chloroquine in the treatment of porphyria cutanea tarda. *N Engl J Med* **296**:949, 1977

341. Tsega E et al: Chloroquine in the treatment of porphyria cutanea tarda. *Trans R Soc Trop Med Hyg* **75**:401, 1981

342. Swanbeck G, Wennersten G: Treatment of porphyria cutanea tarda with chloroquine and phlebotomy. *Br J Dermatol* **97**:77, 1977

343. Wennersten G, Ros AM: Chloroquine in treatment of porphyria cutanea tarda. Long-term efficacy of combined phlebotomy and high-dose chloroquine therapy. *Acta Derm Venereol [Suppl] (Stockh)* **100**:119, 1982

344. Donald GF et al: Current concepts of cutaneous porphyria and its treatment with particular reference to the use of sodium calcium edetate. *Br J Dermatol* **82**:70, 1970

345. Thivolet J et al: Traitement des porphyries cutanées tardines par les chelateurs du fer (EDTA Desferral). *Lyon Med* **218**:225, 1967

346. Bourke E et al: Effect of urinary pH on excretion of porphyrins. *Lancet* **1**:1394, 1966

347. Wiegand SE et al: Metabolic alkalinization in porphyria cutanea tarda. *Arch Dermatol* **100**:544, 1969

348. Stathers GM: Porphyrin-binding effect of cholestyramine. *Lancet* **2**:780, 1966

349. Harber LC, Bickers DR: The porphyrias, in *Photosensitivity Diseases: Principles of Diagnosis and Treatment*. Philadelphia, WB Saunders, 1981, p 189

350. Taljaard JJF et al: Studies on low-dose chloroquine therapy and the action of chloroquine in symptomatic porphyria. *Br J Dermatol* **87**:261, 1972

351. Linden IH et al: Development of porphyria during chloroquine therapy for chronic discoid lupus erythematosus. *Calif Med* **81**:235, 1954

352. London ID: Porphyria cutanea tarda: report of a case successfully treated with chloroquine. *Arch Dermatol* **75**:801, 1957

353. Malkinson FD, Levitt L: Hydroxychloroquine treatment of porphyria cutanea tarda. *Arch Dermatol* **116**:1147, 1980

354. Scholnick PL et al: The molecular basis of the action of chloroquine in porphyria cutanea tarda. *J Invest Dermatol* **61**:226, 1973

355. Saltzer EI et al: Porphyria cutanea tarda: remission following chloroquine administration without adverse effects. *Arch Dermatol* **98**:496, 1968

356. Malina L, Chlumsky J: A comparative study of the results of phlebotomy therapy and low-dose chloroquine treatment in porphyria cutanea tarda. *Acta Derm Venereol (Stockh)* **61**:346, 1981

357. Cainelli T et al: Hydroxychloroquine versus phlebotomy in the treatment of porphyria cutanea tarda. *Br J Dermatol* **108**:593, 1983

358. Chlumska A et al: Liver changes in porphyria cutanea tarda patients treated with chloroquine. *Br J Dermatol* **102**:261, 1980

359. Barker LF, Estes WF: Family hematoporphyrinuria and its association with chronic gastroduodenal dilatation, peculiar fits and acute polyneuritis. *JAMA* **59**:718, 1912

360. Bonkowsky HL, Schady WL: Neurologic manifestations of acute porphyria. *Semin Liver Dis* **2**:108, 1982

361. Dowdle EB et al: Delta-aminolevulinic acid synthetase activity in normal and porphyric human liver. *S Afr Med J* **41**:1093, 1967

362. Sassa S et al: Effect of lead and genetic factors on heme biosynthesis in human red cells. *Ann NY Acad Sci* **244**:419, 1975

363. Bickers DR et al: Studies in porphyria. VI. Biosynthesis of porphyrins in mammalian skin and in the skin of porphyric patients. *J Invest Dermatol* **68**:5, 1977

364. Sassa S et al: Studies in porphyria. VII. Induction of uroporphyrinogen-I synthetase and expression of the gene defect of acute intermittent porphyria in mitogen-stimulated human lymphocytes. *J Clin Invest* **61**:499, 1978

365. DeMatteis F: Disturbances of liver porphyrin metabolism caused by drugs. *Pharmacol Rev* **19**:523, 1967

366. McColl KEL, Moore MR: The acute porphyrias—an example of pharmacogenetic disease. *Scott Med J* **26**:32, 1981

367. Kappas A et al: A defect of steroid hormone metabolism in acute intermittent porphyria. *Fed Proc* **31**:1293, 1972

368. Welland FH et al: Factors affecting the excretion of porphyrin precursors by patients with acute intermittent porphyria. I. The effect of diet. *Metabolism* **13**:232, 1964

369. Granick S, Kappas A: Steroid induction of porphyrin synthesis in liver cell culture: structural basis and possible physiological role in the control of heme formation. *J Biol Chem* **242**:4587, 1967

370. Edwards AM, Elliott WH: Induction of delta-aminolevulinic acid synthetase in isolated rat liver cells by steroids. *J Biol Chem* **250**:2750, 1975

371. Stephens JK et al: Porphyrin induction: equivalent effect of $5\alpha H$ and $5\beta H$ steroids in chick embryo liver cells. *Science* **197**:659, 1977

372. Anderson KE et al: Studies in porphyria. VIII. Relationship of the 5α-reductive metabolism of steroid hormones to clinical expression of the genetic effect in acute intermittent porphyria. *Am J Med* **66**:644, 1979

373. Kappas A et al: Induction of a deficiency of steroid Δ^4-5-α-reductase activity in liver by a porphyrinogenic drug. *J Clin Invest* **59**:159, 1977

374. Wetterberg L et al: Why is the patient with acute intermittent porphyria not light sensitive? *Acta Derm Venereol [Suppl] (Stockh)* **100**:73, 1982

375. Perlroth MG et al: Acute intermittent porphyria: new morphologic and biochemical findings. *Am J Med* **41**:149, 1966

376. Stein JA et al: Abnormal iron and water metabolism in acute intermittent porphyria with new morphologic findings. *Am J Med* **53**:784, 1972

377. Doss M et al: Biochemical course in acute intermittent porphyria, in *Porphyrins in Human Diseases. First International Porphyrin Meeting, Freiburg*, edited by M Doss, P Nawrocki. Basel, Karger, 1976, p 206

378. Hoesch K: Uber die Auswertung der Urobilinogenurie und die "umgekehrte" Urobilinogenurie. *Dtsch Med Wochenschr* **72**:704, 1947

379. Tiepermann RV, Doss M: Simple diagnostic test for urinary porphobilinogen and porphyrins, in *Porphyrins in Human Diseases. First International Porphyrin Meeting, Freiburg*, edited by M Doss, P Nawrocki, Basel, Karger, 1976 p 249

380. Taddeini L et al: Hypercholesterolemia in experimental and human hepatic porphyria. *Metabolism* **13**:691, 1964

381. Lees RS et al: Hyperbeta-lipoproteinemia in acute intermittent porphyria. *N Engl J Med* **282**:432, 1970

382. Hellman ES et al: Elevation of the serum protein-bound iodine in acute intermittent porphyria. *J Clin Endocrinol* **23**:1185, 1963

383. Tschudy DP et al: The effect of carbohydrate feeding on the induction of delta-aminolevulinic acid synthetase. *Metabolism* **13**:396, 1964

384. Bonkowsky HL et al: Repression of the overproduction of porphyrin precursors in acute intermittent porphyria by intravenous infusions of hematin. *Proc Natl Acad Sci USA* **68**:2725, 1971

385. Watson CJ et al: Postulated deficiency of hepatic heme and repair by hematin infusions in the inducible hepatic porphyrias. *Proc Natl Acad Sci USA* **74**:2118, 1977

386. Watson CJ: Hematin and porphyria. *N Engl J Med* **293**:605, 1979

387. Pierach CA: Hematin therapy for the porphyric attack. *Semin Liver Dis* **2**:125, 1982

388. Dhar GJ et al: Transitory renal failure following rapid administration of a relatively large amount of hematin in a patient with acute intermittent porphyria in remission. *Acta Med Scand* **203**:437, 1978

389. Glueck R et al: Hematin: unique effects on hemostasis. *Blood* **61**:243, 1983

390. Barnes HD: Further South African cases of porphyrinuria. *S Afr J Clin Sci* **2**:117, 1951

391. Dean G, Barnes HD: The inheritance of porphyria. *Br Med J* **2**:89, 1955

392. Deyback JC et al: The inherited enzymatic defect in porphyria variegata. *Hum Genet* **58**:425, 1981

393. Dean G: Porphyria variegata. *Acta Derm Venereol [Suppl] (Stockh)* **100**:81, 1982

394. Dean G: Porphyria turcica. *Arch Dermatol* **117**:318, 1981

395. Rimington C et al: The excretion of porphyrin-peptide conjugates in porphyria variegata. *Clin Sci* **35**:211, 1968

396. Elder GH et al: Faecal "X" porphyrin in the hepatic porphyrias. *Enzyme* **17**:29, 1974

397. Eales L et al: The place of screening tests and quantitative investigations in the diagnosis of the porphyrias, with particular reference to variegate and symptomatic porphyria. *S Afr Med J* **40**:63, 1966

398. Poh-Fitzpatrick MB: A plasma porphyrin fluorescence marker for variegate porphyria. *Arch Dermatol* **116**:543, 1980

399. Cramers M, Jepsen LV: Porphyria variegata: failure of chloroquine treatment. *Acta Derm Venereol (Stockh)* **60**:89, 1980

400. Perrot H et al: La porphyrie variegata (à propos de 4 cas). *Lyon Med* **235**:905, 1976

401. Watson CJ et al: Studies of coproporphyrin. III. Idiopathic coproporphyrinuria. A hitherto unrecognized form characterized by lack of symptoms in spite of the excretion of large amounts of coproporphyrin. *J Clin Invest* **28**:465, 1949

402. Goldberg A et al: Hereditary coproporphyria. *Lancet* **1**:632, 1967

403. Brodie NJ et al: Hereditary coproporphyria. *Q J Med* **46**:229, 1977

404. Grandchamp B, Nordmann Y: Decreased lymphocyte and coproporphyrinogen-free oxidase activity in hereditary coproporphyria. *Biochem Biophys Res Commun* **74**:1089, 1977

405. Elder GH et al: The primary enzyme defect in hereditary coproporphyria. *Lancet* **2**:1217, 1976

406. McIntyre N et al: Hepatic delta-aminolevulinic acid synthetase in an attack of hereditary coproporphyria and during remission. *Lancet* **1**:560, 1971

407. Nordmann Y et al: Harderoporphyria: a variant hereditary coproporphyria. *J Clin Invest* **72**:1139, 1983

408. Hunter JAA et al: Hereditary coproporphyria: photosensitivity jaundice and neuropsychiatric manifestations associated with pregnancy. *Br J Dermatol* **84**:301, 1971

409. Pinõl-Aguadé J et al: Hepato-erythrocytic porphyria: a new type of porphyria. *Ann Dermatol Syphiligr (Paris)* **102**:129, 1975

410. Czarnecki DB: Hepatoerythropoietic porphyria. *Arch Dermatol* **116**:307, 1980

411. Lim HW, Poh-Fitzpatrick MB: Hepatoerythropoietic por-

phyria: a variant of childhood-onset porphyria cutanea tarda. *J Am Acad Dermatol* **11**:1103, 1984

412. Birkett DA et al: Phototoxic bullous eruptions due to nalidixic acid. *Br J Dermatol* **81**:342, 1969

413. Luscombe HA: Photosensitivity reaction to nalidixic acid. *Arch Dermatol* **101**:122, 1970

414. Burry JN, Lawrence JR: Phototoxic blisters from high furosemide dosage. *Br J Dermatol* **94**:495, 1976

415. Zugerman C, LaVoo EJ: Erythema multiforme caused by oral furosemide. *Arch Dermatol* **116**:518, 1980

416. Epstein JH et al: Porphyria-like cutaneous changes induced by tetracycline hydrochloride photosensitization. *Arch Dermatol* **112**:661, 1976

417. Rocca FP, Pereya E: Phlyctenar lesions in the feet of diabetic patients. *Diabetes* **12**:220, 1963

418. Bernstein JE et al: Bullous eruption of diabetes mellitus. *Arch Dermatol* **115**:324, 1979

419. Poh-Fitzpatrick MB: Laboratory testing in the porphyrias. *Int J Dermatol* **18**:453, 1979

420. Rimington C, Cripps DJ: Biochemical and fluorescence-microscopy screening tests for erythropoietic protoporphyria. *Lancet* **1**:624, 1965

421. Yamamoto M et al: Translational inhibition by heme of the synthesis of hepatic δ-aminolevulinate synthase in a cell-free system. *Biochem Biophys Res Commun* **115**:225, 1983

422. Hyashi N et al: Inhibition by hemin of in vitro translocation of chicken liver δ-aminolevulinate synthase into mitochondria. *Biochem Biophys Res Commun* **115**:700, 1985

423. DeLoskey RJ, Beattie DS: The effects of insulin and glucose on the induction and intracellular translocation of δ-aminolevulinic acid synthase. *Arch Biochem Biophys* **233**:64, 1984

424. Grandchamp B et al: Cell-free translation of human uroporphyrinogen decarboxylase m RNAs. *Biochem Biophys Res Commun* **118**:378, 1984

425. Camadro J-M et al: Kinetic studies of human liver ferrochelatase. Role of endogenous metals. *J Biol Chem* **259**:5678, 1984

426. Kappas A et al: SN-protoporphyrin rapidly and markedly enhances the heme saturation of hepatic tryptophan pyrrolase. Evidence that this synthetic metalloporphyrin increased the functional content of heme in the liver. *J Clin Invest* **75**:302, 1985

427. Chang CS, Sassa S: Induction of δ-aminolevulinic acid dehydratase in mouse Friend virus-transformed erythroleukemia cells during erythroid differentiation. *Blood* **64**:64, 1984

428. Beaumont C et al: Effects of succinylacetone on dimethylsulfoxide-mediated induction of heme pathway enzymes in mouse Friend-virus-transformed erythroleukemia cells. *Exp Cell Res* **154**:474, 1984

429. Lim HW et al: Activation of the complement system in patients with porphyrias after irradiation *in vivo. J Clin Invest* **74**:1976, 1984

430. Torinuki W et al: Activation of the alternative complement pathway by 405nm light in serum from porphyric rat. *Acta Derm Venereol (Stockh)* **64**:367, 1984

431. Lim HW et al: Delayed phase of hematoporphyrin-induced phototoxicity: modulation by complement, leukocytes and antihistamines. *J Invest Dermatol* **84**:114, 1985

432. Went LN, Klasen EC: Genetic aspects of erythropoietic protoporphyria. *Ann Hum Genet* **48**:105, 1984

433. Lefkowitch JH et al: Cholic acid amelioration of light and electron microscopic hepatic lesions in experimental protoporphyria. *Hepatology* **3**:399, 1983

434. Spiva DA, Lewis CE: Erythropoietic protoporphyria: therapeutic response to combined erythrocyte exchange and plasmapheresis. *Photodermatology* **1**:211, 1984

435. Disler PB et al: Serum ferritin levels in patients with porphyria cutanea tarda. *Dermatologica* **168**:16, 1984

436. Mukerji SK et al: Dual mechanism of inhibition of rat liver uroporphyrinogen decarboxylase activity by ferrous iron: its potential role in the genesis of porphyria cutanea tarda. *Gastroenterology* **87**:1248, 1984

437. de Verneuil H et al: Enzymatic and immunological studies of uroporphyrinogen decarboxylase in familial porphyria cutanea tarda and hepatoerythropoietic porphyria. *Am J Hum Genet* **36**:613, 1984

438. Cripps DJ et al: Porphyria turcica due to hexachlorobenzene: a 20 to 30 year follow-up study on 204 patients. *Br J Dermatol* **111**:413, 1984

439. Topi GC et al: Recovery from porphyria cutanea tarda with no specific therapy other than avoidance of hepatic toxins. *Br J Dermatol* **111**:75, 1984

440. Ashton RE et al: Low-dose oral chloroquine in the treatment of porphyria cutanea tarda. *Br J Dermatol* **111**:609, 1984

441. Marchesi L et al: A comparative trial of desferrioxamine and hydroxychloroquine for treatment of porphyria cutanea tarda in alcoholic patients. *Photodermatology* **1**:286, 1984

442. Goerz G et al: Influence of chloroquine on the porphyrin metabolism. *Arch Dermatol Res* **277**:114, 1985

443. Lithner F, Wetterberg L: Hepatocellular carcinoma in patients with acute intermittent porphyria. *Acta Med Scand* **215**:271, 1984

444. Laiwak AACY et al: Carbamazepine-induced non-hereditary acute porphyria. *Lancet* **1**:790, 1983

445. Anderson KE et al: Prevention of cyclical attacks of acute intermittent porphyria with a long-acting agonist of luteinizing hormone-releasing hormone. *N Engl J Med* **331**:643, 1984

446. McGrath H et al: An Irish family with variegate porphyria. *Clin Exp Dermatol* **9**:583, 1984

447. Andrews J et al: Hereditary coproporphyria: incidence in a large English family. *J Med Genet* **21**:341, 1984

448. Harber LC, Bickers DR: Porphyria and pseudoporphyria. *J Invest Dermatol* **82**:207, 1984

CHAPTER 144

SKIN MANIFESTATIONS OF GOUT

J. Edwin Seegmiller

Gouty arthritis presents clinically as a severe, recurrent monoarticular arthritis of sudden onset occurring predominantly in males during mature years. The patients frequently have a family history of the same disease. Hyperuricemia precedes development of clinical gout by many years and leads to deposition of crystals of monosodium urate in and about the joints from the supersaturated concentration present in serum [1–3]. The acute attack represents an inflammatory response directed toward the crystals undergoing phagocytosis by polymorphonuclear leukocytes in the same way as would invading microorganisms. Large aggregates of these same crystals form the characteristic tophi found in the subcutaneous tissue overlying joints, tendons, or cartilage, particularly of the ear. If untreated, the tophi will show progressive enlargement, and when they are near the surface of the skin they exhibit a characteristic mottled salmon-pink color and can intermittently drain a clear, amber fluid containing white flecks of monosodium urate crystals. When viewed microscopically, these crystals are needle shaped and negatively birefringent under cross-polarizing filters. The same deposits frequently are found in the kidney and are associated with progressive renal damage, while precipitation of free uric acid in the urinary tract can result in formation of renal calculi in a significant portion of gouty patients. Asymptomatic hyperuricemia, sometimes associated with renal calculi, is also found in many relatives of gouty patients who may never develop symptoms of the disease.

Hyperuricemia and gout are found associated with a wide range of other diseases. These include psoriasis [4], proliferative disorders of the hematopoietic system, primary or secondary renal damage, hypertension, obesity, myocardial infarction, hyper- or hypoparathyroidism, and myxedema. Hyperuricemia and gout can result from thiazides and other diuretics and can be a late effect of lead poisoning. In addition, hyperuricemia accompanies Down's syndrome (mongolism), type I glycogen storage disease (with absence of glucose 6-phosphatase), hereditary nephritis, pituitrin-resistant diabetes insipidus, and an X-linked neurologic disorder with compulsive automutilation described by Lesch and Nyhan [2]. The latter is caused by a severe genetic deficiency of the enzyme hypoxanthine-guanine phosphoribosyltransferase. Another X-linked form of gout which is, in some families, associated with deafness results from a threefold increase in phosphoribosylpyrophosphate synthetase activity [5,6].

Clinical features of the arthritis are the same regardless of the cause of the hyperuricemia. In some instances the acute attack of gouty arthritis has been the presenting symptom of the underlying disease. In recent years a start has been made in identifying genetic deficiencies of specific enzymes of purine metabolsim associated with purine overproduction in gouty arthritis [7].

Historical aspects

Gout has been on the forefront in the historical development of many medical concepts. The unusual clinical features permitted it to be distinguished from other ailments by Hippocrates at a very early stage in medical history and the specific treatment of the acute attack with the drug colchicine was introduced in the fifth century. Sydenham's description in 1563 of his own personal experience with the disease remains a classic of descriptive medicine. The early interest of the chemists in the disease, and, more recently, the biochemists, has resulted in substantial advances in our scientific understanding of gout throughout the years. Scheele in 1776 first isolated uric acid from a urinary concretion and some 20 years later Wallaston isolated the same substance from a gouty tophus which he reportedly removed from his own ear. The demonstration of hyperuricemia in gout by Garrod in 1848 provided the first use of an abnormality in a chemical component of serum as an aid to the diagnosis of a metabolic disease. It also provided the first application of chemical principles to the understanding of the pathology of the disease [1].

No disease has enjoyed a more royal patronage than gout. The list of gouty personages of fame is astonishingly long and through their vicissitudes, gout has changed the course of history. A less admirable image has been the popular association of gout with luxurious living and excessive indulgence in natural appetites, giving rise to the moralistic view that gout is nature's retribution for intemperate living and quite impossible to treat medically. This view is being dispelled to some extent by the identification of both specific hereditary and environmental factors that can contribute to the development of hyperuricemia and gout. Furthermore the introduction of new drugs and the more effective use of colchicine have now minimized the disability and deformity heretofore produced by this ancient malady [8].

Epidemiology

Gouty arthritis accounts for 5 percent of the patients seen with arthritis at major clinics. It has been found in all races but appears in unusually high incidence among Filipinos who have migrated to the United States or Hawaii and certain people of the South Pacific islands where it is frequently associated with obesity. Gout is primarily a disease of males (95 percent of cases) and usually appears between the third and sixth decades of life. When it does appear in women it is usually after the menopause. The fact that the mean serum urate of women is lower than that of men by about 1mg/dL until after the menopause provides the most reasonable explanation for this sex difference in incidence of the disease. The frequency of hyperuricemia and gout

Fig. 144-1   A possible mechanism of acute gouty arthritis. *(From Seegmiller JE, Howell RR: Arthritis Rheum 5:616, 1962. Reproduced with permission of the publisher.)*

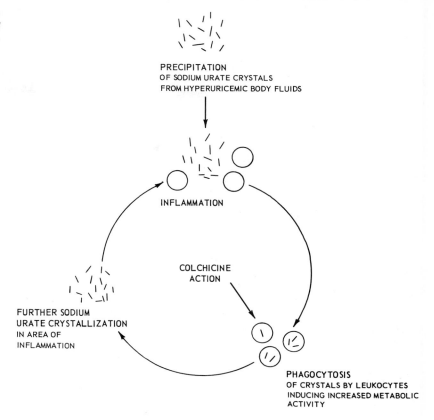

PRECIPITATION
OF SODIUM URATE CRYSTALS
FROM HYPERURICEMIC BODY FLUIDS

INFLAMMATION

COLCHICINE
ACTION

FURTHER SODIUM
URATE CRYSTALLIZATION
IN AREA OF
INFLAMMATION

PHAGOCYTOSIS
OF CRYSTALS BY LEUKOCYTES
INDUCING INCREASED METABOLIC
ACTIVITY

is increasing in the more affluent countries of the world. A low but statistically significant, positive correlation between serum urate concentration and intelligence as well as academic and professional achievement has been reported.

Etiology and pathogenesis

The principal clinical features of gouty arthritis can be related to the limited solubility of uric acid and its monosodium salt in body fluids. The crystals of monosodium urate monohydrate deposited in and about the joints can produce an inflammatory reaction. A vicious cycle of inflammatory reactions leading to more crystal deposition and additional inflammatory reaction directed toward such crystals has been proposed to account for the acute attack of gouty arthritis (Fig. 144-1). Colchicine presumably interrupts the cycle through a metabolic effect on leukocytes. At the more acid pH of the urinary tract, crystals of free uric acid are precipitated and give rise to kidney stones in 20 to 40 percent of gouty patients.

The demonstration by Simkin [9] that urate moves from a traumatic effusion of a joint at a rate roughly half that of water, provides a mechanism for concentrating urate transiently within the joint cavity, particularly if the joint had been previously injured. The possibility of such an injury in the form of preexisting osteoarthritis setting the stage for a traumatic effusion of the first metatarsophalangeal joint by reason of the high weight-bearing stresses to which it is subject in normal walking, provides an ingenious explanation for the predilection for gouty arthritis to attack the first metatarsophalangeal joint. Presumably the onset of the attack during the early morning hours reflects crystal formation during the partial resolution of the traumatic effusion which would attend the elevation of the feet to the horizontal position during nocturnal slumber.

The hyperuricemia of gout results from a variety of biochemical and physiologic abnormalities as shown in Fig. 144-2. In some patients the diminished renal excretion of uric acid accounts for the hyperuricemia, while in others an excessive production of uric acid from increased purine biosynthesis is found either as a primary metabolic abnormality or secondary to the turnover of tissue nucleic acids in a myeloproliferative disease. In still other gouty patients both excessive synthesis of uric acid and decreased renal excretion of uric acid are found. Patients with gout are therefore a very heterogeneous group; a variety of specific underlying disorders of physiology or metabolism rather than a uniform defect in a single enzyme accounts for their hyperuricemia.

As noted above, several types of specific enzyme defects have been identified among patients with severe gout, associated with purine overproduction. Two of these are X-linked disorders. One is a deficiency in an enzyme of purine metabolism, hypoxanthine-guanine phosphoribosyltransferase (HPRT), and is associated with the most severe degree of excessive production of uric acid yet found and with a wide range of clinical expression [10]. Patients with virtually complete deficiency of HPRT show a severe and incapacitating neurologic disease often classed as cerebral palsy, consisting of choreoathetosis, spasticity, and some degree of mental retardation with a dramatic, compulsive self-mutilation (the Lesch-Nyhan syndrome). Other patients with as little as 1 percent of normal HPRT activity in the erythrocytes have no neurologic disease and present with a high incidence of uric acid renal calculi and severe

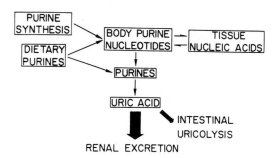

NORMAL

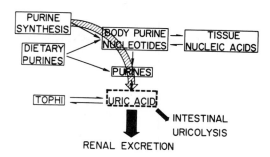

PRIMARY GOUT
With overproduction of uric acid

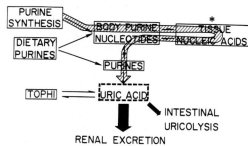

SECONDARY GOUT
Associated with myeloproliferative disease

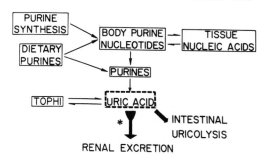

PRIMARY GOUT
With diminished renal excretion of uric acid

Fig. 144-2   Origin and disposition of uric acid in normal man and causes of hyperuricemia in gout. *(From Seegmiller JE et al: N Engl J Med 268:712, 764, 821, 1963. Reproduced with permission of the publisher.)*

gouty arthritis in adolescence or early adult life. Patients in families having lesser amounts of HPRT enzyme manifest, in addition, a variety of mild neurologic disorders.

The second X-linked disorder associated with gout and overproduction of purine consists of a high specific activity (2 to 3 times normal) of the enzyme phosphoribosylpyrophosphate synthetase. Two families have been found in whom this enzyme defect is associated with deafness [5,6]. Cells of patients with both of these disorders show a high intracellular concentration of the substrate for the presumed rate-limiting reaction of purine synthesis, phosphoribosylpyrophosphate.

Severe gouty arthritis is also a major clinical problem of patients with type I glycogen storage disease (glucose 6-phosphatase deficiency) who live to adult life. They show not only a renal retention of uric acid associated with a profound lactic acidemia and ketonemia but also an excessive rate of purine synthesis. Some evidence has been presented in support of the view that the overproduction of purines results from an intermittent glucogen-mediated increase in glycogen breakdown which induces a secondary depletion of ATP and inorganic phosphate within the cells, thus leading to an excessive rate of purine synthesis. Both the lactic acidemia and excessive rate of purine synthesis can be alleviated by continuous feedings by a nasal gastric tube, suggesting that they are a direct consequence in these patients of hypoglycemia [11].

Not all patients with essential hyperuricemia develop gout, but the chance of developing gouty arthritis seems to be increased by the degree of hyperuricemia and the duration of exposure to hyperuricemia.

Clinical manifestations

History

Acute gout. A typical patient with gout is an adult male, usually in his thirties or forties, who gives a history of the sudden onset over a few hours of an excruciating, throbbing pain, usually in a single peripheral joint, frequently the first metatarsophalangeal joint which appears warm, red, and so exquisitely tender that even the touch of a bedsheet is intolerable to the patient. The patient is incapacitated and unable to use the limb. Frequently the overlying warmth and redness is interpreted as a cellulitis from an infectious process or as a sprain developing after minimal trauma. If undiagnosed and untreated, the acute attack will gradually subside over a period of days to weeks with complete recovery of normal function lasting months to years.

Tophaceous gout. If untreated, the natural history is one of recurrent acute attacks in different joints over the years at progressively more frequent intervals. Eventually full re-

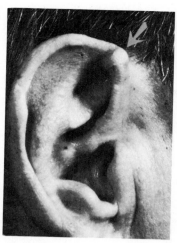

Fig. 144-3   Nonpainful nodule of the ear: tophaceous gout. *(From Kingery FAJ:* JAMA 2:137, 1966.)

covery between attacks does not occur, thereby merging into the stage of chronic tophaceous gout. At this stage the cumulative tophaceous deposits erode into bone and cartilage, causing structural damage that is only partially reversible. Impairment of renal function by the disease can lead to a progressive decrease in ability to excrete uric acid, thereby accelerating the pathologic process.

Cutaneous findings

The area involved by the acute attack shows the classical signs of an acute inflammatory process consisting of warmth, tenderness, swelling, as well as varying degrees of redness. As the acute attack diminishes, the involved area often assumes a violaceous hue and the skin may show desquamation.

The tophaceous deposit is a highly specific lesion of gout which should not be confused with the deposits of xanthoma tuberosum, rheumatoid nodules, or Darwinian tubercles of the ear. Subcutaneous lesions have a characteristic salmon-pink color and are seen most commonly on the helix of the ear (Fig. 144-3), over the bursa of the

Fig. 144-4   Tophaceous gout.

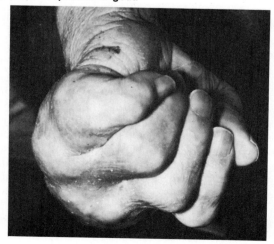

elbow, and about the digits of the hands and feet (Fig. 144-4). When very large, they usually drain a chalky white material consisting of crystals of monosodium urate (Fig. 144-5). In gout associated with psoriasis, the excessive uric acid synthesis is a consequence of the more rapid turnover of nucleic acid associated with proliferation of the epidermal cells and is diminished when the proliferation process is brought under control [4].

Other physical findings

A fever and systemic symptoms not infrequently accompany the acute attack. Although the acute attack of gout does not produce permanent joint damage, the bony erosions from tophaceous deposits are readily demonstrable by x-ray as characteristic punched-out lesions in subchondral areas of bone of peripheral joints, most commonly the first metatarsophalangeal joint. Gout patients have a high incidence of renal calculi that may produce symptoms. The physical findings characteristic of any one of the variety of underlying diseases associated with hyperuricemia listed above may also be found.

Laboratory findings

Hyperuricemia (a serum urate above 7.0 mg/dL) is found in virtually all gouty patients, although an occasional patient may show a serum urate value in the high normal range, particularly during the acute attack. As methodology has improved, the number of instances of gouty arthritis with normal serum urate has diminished. Leukocytosis and an increased sedimentation rate accompany the generalized inflammatory reaction. In advanced stages of renal damage the serum creatinine is first elevated, followed by an increase in uric acid content. Laboratory tests also may show evidence of polycythemia, hemolytic anemia, other hematologic disorders, abnormalities of calcium metabolism, or hypothyroidism among gouty patients.

Pathology

The characteristic lesion of gout is the deposit of crystals of needle-shaped monosodium urate and the accompanying inflammatory reaction of the surrounding tissue. However, tissue deposits of urate crystals almost invariably are dissolved away during formalin fixation and aqueous staining routinely used in preparation of histologic specimens. Fixation in absolute ethanol or freezing is required for preservation of crystals in histologic materials. Crystals are brilliantly anisotropic when viewed microscopically with polarized light, and in the staining technique of DeGalantha the urate crystals appear brownish black. Deposits of elongated urate crystals in the interstices of the renal pyramids are seen in many of the patients with long-standing gout. These deposits are accompanied by evidence of chronic pyelonephritis which does not need to be bacterial in origin. A high incidence of arteriolar nephrosclerosis and chronic glomerulonephritis also has been found.

Diagnosis and differential diagnosis

In most patients the clinical features of the acute attack are sufficiently characteristic to permit a presumptive di-

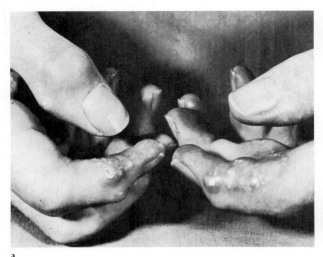
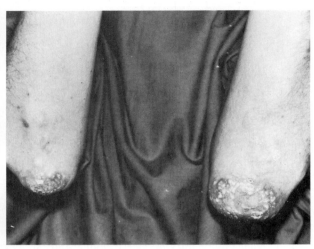

a   b

Fig. 144-5   Tophaceous gout. Chalky white material is present within lesions on the fingers (a) and elbows (b).

agnosis if the possibility of gout is but considered. The subsequent demonstration of hyperuricemia and the clinical response of the arthritis to colchicine within 24 to 48 h of treatment provides confirmation of the diagnosis. A positive diagnosis can be established by demonstration of urate crystals in the material removed with a needle or expressed from a subcutaneous tophus or in fluid aspirated from a synovial effusion. Monosodium urate crystals have a needle-like shape and are intensely birefringent, so are readily detected through polarizing filters attached to an ordinary light microscope. The acute attack of gout is often confused with severe cellulitis or septic arthritis; however, regional lymphadenopathy is seldom seen in acute gout and a septic process is often surrounded by doughlike, pitting edema. Synovial fluid examination and culture provide a definitive answer. Biopsy of the subcutaneous nodule with fixation in alcohol provides histologic distinction between the gouty tophus and the rheumatoid nodule of rheumatoid arthritis. Chondrocalcinosis (pseudogout) also shows birefringent crystals (calcium pyrophosphate) in the synovial fluid but the calcium deposited in the knee or wrist joint serves to distinguish it from gout by x-ray. Other types of arthritis to be considered include osteoarthritis, Reiter's syndrome, and palindromic rheumatism.

Treatment

Acute gouty arthritis

The affected joints should be kept at complete rest. A narcotic is often required for analgesia. As early as possible in the attack, one of the drugs discussed below should be administered to control the inflammation. Treatment with drugs that lower serum urate should not be started until the acute attack is well under control because of their tendency to cause an exacerbation of the acute attack.

Colchicine (0.5 mg) is given hourly until relief is obtained or until nausea, vomiting, or diarrhea occur, at which time the drug is discontinued. Because of its specific effect on acute gouty arthritis, colchicine remains the drug of choice for the presenting attack, particularly if the diagnosis is in doubt. It is helpful in aborting an incipient attack and less effective if given late in the course of an attack. Administration of 2.0 mg diluted in 20 ml of saline by the intravenous route is very effective, particularly for a patient with peptic ulcer or before or after surgery since this route avoids the gastrointestinal side effects that often accompany oral colchicine. No more than 5 mg in divided doses should be given by the intravenous route over a 48-h period and even this dose should be given only to patients with normal renal function.

Adrenocorticotropic hormone (ACTH) in long-acting repository gel form at a dosage of 50 to 100 units administered intramuscularly provides effective control of even very severe attacks. Colchicine (0.5 mg, 2 to 3 times daily) should be given concurrently to prevent a "rebound" attack.

Alternative methods of terminating the acute attack of gouty arthritis include phenylbutazone or oxyphenbutazone given orally at a dose of 0.4 g followed by 0.1 to 0.2 g at 4 and 8 h, and by 0.1 g four times daily for the second and third day. The drug is then stopped.

Indomethacin at a dose of 50 mg three times daily for 2 to 3 days is also effective but sometimes produces the side effect of headache. Other newer anti-inflammatory drugs have also been found to be effective in terminating acute attacks of gouty arthritis.

Preventive therapy

Colchicine, 0.5 mg taken 2 to 4 times daily depending on tolerance to gastrointestinal side effects, is very effective in preventing acute attacks. However, it does nothing to prevent the more serious joint destruction by tophaceous deposits. This aspect of the disease, as well as the progressive renal damage, presumably can be arrested by lowering the serum urate concentration to the normal range (below 7.0 mg/dL) by the use of one of a number of drugs. The serum urate should be determined every few weeks as a guide to the proper dose of medication during the period when therapy is initiated. Prophylactic daily colchicine is especially important during the initiation and the first 3 to 4 months of therapy with drugs used to lower the serum urate content in order to suppress the tendency of gout patients to develop acute attacks during this time. Patients should always be warned that they are at greater risk for developing an acute attack during this period and should be advised to take an extra tablet of colchicine at the appearance of the very first symptom suggestive of an impending acute attack.

Since therapy with a drug for lowering the serum urate is a commitment to lifelong medication, the proper drug for each particular patient's need should be selected. This can be determined most readily by assessing the 24-h urinary excretion of uric acid while the patient is maintained on a diet virtually free of purine compounds. For this purpose meat, fish, fowl, the high-purine vegetables (peas, beans, and other leguminous plants), as well as all fermented or alcohol-containing beverages, and caffeine-containing drinks are eliminated from the diet for a 6-day period. Twenty-four-hour urines are then collected over the last 3 days of the diet, each in a separate bottle containing 3 ml of toluene as preservative, and the urine is stored at room temperature until analysis to minimize the deposition of crystalline uric acid that tends to occur at lower temperatures. Uricosuric drugs, as well as drugs that cause urate retention such as salicylate and most antihypertensive drugs except the spironolactones are also eliminated during the evaluation period on the diet. The drug acetaminophen (Tylenol) should be used in place of aspirin or other salicylate-containing medication by all gout patients for mild analgesia.

The purine-free diet and urine collection are most conveniently instituted immediately after the patient presents with his acute attack of gout. At this time he is well motivated to follow a diet virtually free of purines. In addition, time must be allowed for resolving the acute attack of gout before instituting any therapy with uricosuric drugs, otherwise the acute attack may not be as promptly resolved.

The 24-h urines are analyzed for uric acid and creatinine; the latter compound provides an index of complete 24-h collection. Excretion of quantities of uric acid greater than 600 mg for 24 h is indicative of purine overproduction and is indication for beginning the xanthine oxidase inhibitor allopurinol (Zyloprim) which blocks uric acid production by specifically reducing purine overproduction. Other indications for allopurinol are a uric acid/creatinine ratio of the morning urine above 0.7, a history of renal calculi composed of uric acid, or the presence of impaired renal function.

Allopurinol has a prolonged therapeutic action and is available in 0.1- and 0.3-g tablets. The usual dosage is 0.1 to 0.4 g daily and is particularly useful for patients resistant or intolerant to uricosuric drugs. In addition, it is specifically indicated for patients who are producing excessive quantities of uric acid in the 24-h urine as stated above. Other indications for use of allopurinol are the presence of renal dysfunction or a history of frequent uric acid calculi of the urinary tract. It is effective in preventing uric acid stone formation as well as dissolving calculi already formed. It can be used in combination with uricosuric drugs, if necessary, but such combined therapy is seldom required.

Excretion of quantities of uric acid less than 600 mg per 24 h in the absence of evidence of renal impairment indicates a normal production of uric acid and a probable specifically diminished renal clearance of uric acid as the basis for hyperuricemia. Therefore, a uricosuric drug provides the specific correction to normalize this aberration of renal physiology.

Probenecid acts to increase the renal excretion of uric acid. It is begun at a low dose of 0.25 g twice daily and gradually increased over a week's time to the usual maintenance dose of 0.5 g 2 to 3 times daily. It may be increased to as high as 3.0 g daily if necessary to produce a normal serum urate concentration.

Sulfinpyrazone provides a much greater uricosuric action and is often required in the presence of renal impairment. It is begun at a dose of 50 mg twice daily and increased over a week to 0.1 g 3 to 4 times daily. Up to 0.8 g per day can be administered if necessary.

Adjuncts to treatment

A high fluid intake of at least 3 L per day will be of value in preventing uric acid precipitation in the urinary tract. Since low-calorie diets can exacerbate hyperuricemia and provoke acute attacks of gout, any weight reduction is best deferred until the serum urate concentration has been brought under control and the disease is quiescent. Avoidance of high-purine foods may be helpful until the serum urate has been brought under control, then a regular diet is advised.

Prognosis

As a result of improvement in therapy over the past three decades almost all patients with gouty arthritis can now look forward to a full and productive life without serious disability from their arthritis or uric acid stones of the urinary tract. This can be achieved by early diagnosis, continuous medical supervision, and institution of a preventive program of management which includes assessment of serum urate concentration taken before the morning medications at 6-month intervals with appropriate adjustment of drug dosage to assure the maintenance of serum urate concentrations well within the normal range of less than 7.0 mg/dL.

References

1. Garrod AB: *The Nature and Treatment of Gout and Rheumatic Gout.* London, Walton and Maberly, 1859
2. Seegmiller JE: Diseases of purine and pyrimidine metabolism, in *Metabolic Control and Disease,* 8th ed, edited by PK Bondy, LE Rosenberg. Philadelphia, WB Saunders, 1980, p 777
3. Wyngaarden JB, Kelley WN: *Gout and Hyperuricemia.* New York, Grune & Stratton, 1976
4. Eisen AZ, Seegmiller JE: Uric acid metabolism in psoriasis. *J Clin Invest* **40**:1486, 1961
5. Becker MA et al: Variant human phosphoribosylpyrophosphate synthetase altered in regulatory and catalytic functions. *J Clin Invest* **65**:109, 1980
6. Simmonds HA et al: Evidence of a new syndrome involving hereditary uric acid overproduction, neurological complications and deafness. *Adv Exp Med Biol* **165** (**pt A**):97, 1984
7. Seegmiller JE: Disorders of purine and pyrimidine metabolism, in *The Principles and Practice of Medical Genetics,*

edited by A Emery, D Rimoin. New York, Churchill Livingstone, 1984, p 97

8. Talbott JR, Yu T-F: *Gout and Uric Acid Metabolism.* New York, Stratton Intercontinental Medical Book Corp, 1976
9. Simkin PA: The pathogenesis of podagra. *Ann Intern Med* **86:**230, 1977
10. Seegmiller JE: Inherited deficiency of hypoxanthine-guanine phosphoribosyltransferase in X-linked uric aciduria (the Lesch-Nyhan syndrome and its variants), in *Advances in Human Genetics,* edited by H Harris, K Hirschhorn. New York, Plenum Press, 1976, vol 6, p 75
11. Greene HL et al: ATP depletion. A possible role in hyperuricemia in glycogen storage disease Type I. *J Clin Invest* **62:**321, 1978

CHAPTER 145

DYSLIPOPROTEINEMIAS AND XANTHOMATOSES

H. Bryan Brewer, Jr. and Donald S. Fredrickson

Transport in extracellular fluids of large quantities of poorly soluble lipids is an important metabolic requirement. Plasma lipids are transported by lipoproteins, collections of particles composed of several lipids (including cholesterol, triglycerides, and phospholipids) and proteins called apolipoproteins. Abnormalities of lipid transport often appear clinically as abnormal plasma concentrations of cholesterol or triglycerides (dyslipidemia). Such abnormalities are best understood by their translation into dyslipoproteinemias and by quantitating the concentrations and composition of the plasma lipoproteins in which lipids are transported. A frequent clinical expression of dyslipoproteinemia is deposits of lipoprotein components in skin, subcutaneous tissues, and tendons called *xanthomas.* Frequently, dermatologists are the first physicians called upon to interpret such lesions. The diseases represented are diverse, numerous, and of considerable importance because of their relationship to vascular disease.

Knowledge of the plasma lipoproteins is growing steadily. The minimum required for proper understanding of the basis for dyslipidemia, dyslipoproteinemia, and xanthomatosis is presented in this chapter. Normal values for plasma concentrations of cholesterol and triglycerides are given in Table 145-1.

Classification of lipoproteins

In clinical medicine as well as in biomedical research the lipoproteins are usually classified on the basis of their electrophoretic mobility and hydrated density. Plasma lipoproteins are separated by electrophoresis into those that remain at the origin or migrate into the β (β lipoproteins), α_2 (pre-β lipoproteins), or α_1 (alpha lipoproteins) globulin zones. Five major classes of lipoproteins are separable by ultracentrifugation: chylomicrons, very low density lipoproteins (VLDL), intermediate density lipoproteins (IDL), low density lipoproteins (LDL), and high density lipoproteins (HDL). The lipoproteins which remain at the origin on electrophoresis are synonymous with chylomicrons, those of pre-β mobility with VLDL, β with LDL, and α lipoproteins with HDL.

Apolipoproteins

Thirteen major human plasma apolipoproteins have been identified and characterized (Table 145-2). The major apolipoprotein associated with LDL is apoB, and the two principal apolipoproteins of HDL are apoA-I and apoA-II. In addition to serving as structural constituents of the lipoproteins, the functions of the apolipoproteins include: (1) participating as a cofactor or activator of enzymes involved in lipoprotein-lipid metabolism; (2) interacting with a specific receptor site on cells and thereby directing lipoprotein catabolism; and (3) facilitating exchange of lipids (cholesteryl esters, triglycerides, and phospholipids) between lipoprotein particles. The well-established functions of the different apolipoproteins are summarized in Table 145-3.

The apolipoprotein B cascades

A conceptual overview of the known features of lipoprotein metabolism is schematically shown in Fig. 145-1. The metabolic relationships of the principal lipoprotein classes containing apoB may be considered to consist of two major "cascades." The *first apoB cascade* involves the stepwise metabolism of chylomicrons secreted by the intestine. The major function of these triglyceride-rich lipoproteins is to transport dietary lipids from the intestine to the liver. The chylomicrons secreted by the intestine contain a form of apoB synthesized by the intestine designated as apoB-48. Shortly after secretion, the triglyceride-rich chylomicrons rapidly acquire other apolipoproteins, particularly apoC-II and apoE transferred from HDL. ApoC-II is a cofactor required for optimal activity of lipoprotein lipase (Table 145-3), an enzyme attached to the capillary endothelium which catalyzes the hydrolysis of triglycerides to free fatty acids and monoglycerides. After entering the plasma, the triglycerides on chylomicrons rapidly undergo hydrolysis and the chylomicrons are sequentially reduced to "remnants" first having the density of VLDL and then of IDL. The chylomicron remnants are then removed from the plasma by binding to receptors having an affinity for apoE.

Table 145-1 Normal plasma lipid and lipoprotein levels

Age	Cholesterol		Triglycerides		VLDL		LDL		HDL	
					Male					
0–19	155	(120–195)	65	(55–115)	10	(1–20)	95	(65–130)	50	(35–70)
20–29	170	(125–225)	100	(45–185)	15	(2–30)	110	(70–155)	45	(30–65)
30–39	200	(145–265)	130	(50–285)	25	(4–50)	130	(80–190)	45	(30–65)
40–49	210	(155–270)	150	(55–300)	25	(5–55)	140	(95–195)	45	(30–65)
50–59	215	(155–275)	145	(60–290)	25	(5–55)	145	(90–200)	45	(30–70)
60+	215	(160–280)	135	(65–245)	20	(2–40)	145	(90–200)	50	(30–75)
					Female					
0–19	160	(125–205)	70	(35–125)	10	(2–15)	100	(65–140)	50	(35–70)
20–29	175	(125–235)	90	(40–165)	15	(2–30)	110	(65–160)	55	(35–80)
30–39	185	(135–240)	90	(40–185)	15	(2–30)	115	(75–165)	55	(35–80)
40–49	200	(150–265)	105	(45–210)	15	(3–40)	130	(80–180)	60	(35–90)
50–59	225	(165–290)	125	(55–250)	20	(2–45)	75	(90–205)	60	(40–90)
60+	230	(170–290)	130	(60–270)	15	(1–45)	150	(95–220)	65	(35–95)

Values are adopted from Lipid Research Clinics Study and expressed as mg/dL. Values are mean with 5 and 95 percentile limits in parentheses; VLDL, LDL, and HDL values are expressed in terms of cholesterol content (Lipid Research Clinics Population Studies Data Book, vol I. DHHS, NIH Publication No. 80-1527, 1980).

The remnants are then taken up by endocytosis and their constitutents catabolized by the hepatocyte (Fig. 145-1).

The *second apoB cascade* involves hydrolysis of triglyceride-rich VLDL secreted by the liver. These lipoprotein particles contain apoB-100, a larger molecular weight form of apoB secreted from the liver. The triglycerides on VLDL also undergo hydrolysis by lipoprotein lipase and are serially converted to lipoproteins with the density of IDL and, finally, LDL. During the conversion of IDL to LDL, apoC-II and apoE dissociate from IDL and reassociate with HDL. The resulting LDL contain almost exclusively apoB-100 (Fig. 145-1). A second lipolytic enzyme, hepatic lipase, appears to be involved in the conversion of IDL to LDL; this enzyme may function both as a triglyceryl hydrolase and as a phospholipase. LDL containing apoB-100 interact with receptors on the plasma membrane of cells in the liver, adrenal, and peripheral cells (e.g., smooth muscle cells and fibroblasts). This receptor has a high affinity for apolipoproteins B and E. Following interaction with LDL the receptor and lipoproteins undergo endocytosis and the components of LDL are catabolized (Fig. 145-1).

High density lipoproteins

HDL arise in plasma by several pathways including direct synthesis and secretion by the intestine and liver. The HDL particles in plasma also acquire lipids and apolipoproteins arising from the catabolism of triglyceride-rich apoB containing lipoproteins. It is thought that HDL function partly as a "reservoir" for apolipoproteins (e.g., apoC-II and apoE) during lipoprotein metabolism. HDL may also interact with specific receptors to initiate the transport of excess cholesterol from cells back to the liver. This still hypothetical process is often termed *reverse cholesterol transport*. It is proposed to begin with the removal from cells of cholesterol largely as the unesterified sterol, which is then esterified in the plasma by the enzyme lecithin cholesteryl acyltransferase (LCAT). The cholesteryl esters are transferred to the core of the lipoprotein particles and exchange between different lipoprotein particles (e.g., HDL and VLDL). The esterification of cholesterol in plasma, the exchange of cholesteryl esters between lipoproteins, and the HDL-facilitated movement of intracellular cholesterol into plasma are considered to be important

Table 145-2 Major human plasma apolipoproteins

Apolipoprotein	Major density class	Approximate molecular weight	Major site of synthesis in humans
A-I	HDL	28,000	Liver-intestine
A-II	HDL	18,000	Liver-intestine
A-IV	Chylomicrons	45,000	Intestine
B-100	VLDL-IDL-LDL	375,000	Liver
B-48	Chylomicrons-VLDL-IDL	180,000	Intestine
C-I	Chylomicrons-VLDL-HDL	6,500	Liver
C-II	Chylomicrons-VLDL-HDL	10,000	Liver
C-III$_{0-2}$	Chylomicrons-VLDL-HDL	10,000	Liver
D	HDL	20,000	?
E$_{2-4}$	Chylomicrons-VLDL-HDL	40,000	Liver
F	HDL	30,000	?
G	VHDL	75,000	?
H	Chylomicrons	45,000	?

Table 145-3 Physiologic functions of human plasma apolipoproteins

Physiologic function	Apolipoprotein
Cofactor for enzyme	
Lipoprotein lipase	apoC-II
Lecithin cholesterol acyltransferase (LCAT)	apoA-I
Ligand on lipoprotein particle for interaction with receptor site on cells	
Chylomicron remnant	apoE
LDL	apoB-100
HDL	apoA-I and apoE
Structural protein on lipoprotein particle	
Intestinal chylomicron	apoB-48
Hepatogenous VLDL	apoB-100
HDL	apoA-I

elements in cholesterol metabolism and related to the development of atherosclerosis.

Dyslipoproteinemia

Specific defects in lipoprotein metabolism usually involve either abnormal increases (hyperlipoproteinemia) or decreases (hypolipoproteinemia) in concentrations of specific classes of plasma lipoproteins. Sometimes abnormal plasma lipoproteins are also present. Some dyslipoproteinemias may be associated with distinct clinical syndromes. History, physical examination, and laboratory evaluation all contribute to establishing the diagnosis.

Lipoprotein patterns

Separation of the syndromes associated with *hyperlipoproteinemia* is often assisted by initial separation of the lipo-

Fig. 145-1 Schematic overview of human lipoprotein metabolism. The metabolism of the principal lipoprotein classes containing apoB may be conceptualized as consisting of two major cascades. (A) The *first apoB cascade* involves chylomicrons containing apoB-48 secreted by the intestine. The triglycerides on the chylomicrons undergo lipolysis by the enzyme lipoprotein lipase and chylomicron remnants are formed with densities initially of VLDL and finally of IDL. (B) The *second apoB cascade* involves triglyceride-rich VLDL containing apoB-100 secreted by the liver. The triglycerides on VLDL are hydrolyzed and VLDL undergoes serial conver-

sion to IDL and then LDL. During metabolism some of the VLDL remnants are taken up by the liver. Shortly after secretion, triglyceride-rich particles from both the liver and intestine acquire apoC-II and apoE from HDL. ApoC-II is a cofactor for lipoprotein lipase, and apoE facilitates the receptor-mediated endocytosis and catabolism of remnants by the liver. ApoB-100, the predominant apolipoprotein on LDL, interacts with a high-affinity receptor on peripheral cells and hepatocytes, culminating in LDL endocytosis and catabolism of LDL. (See text for further details.)

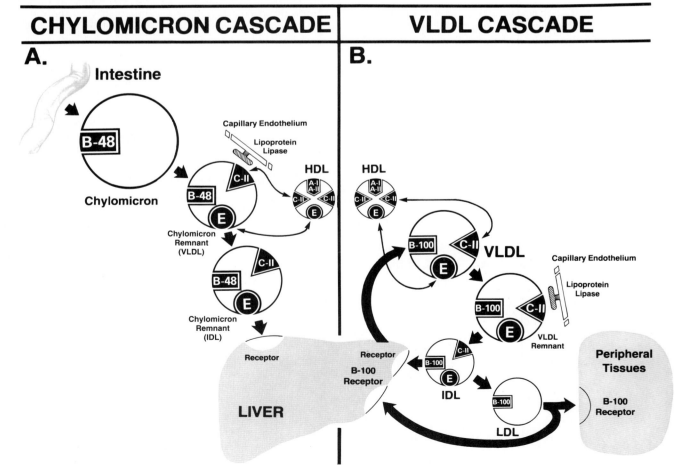

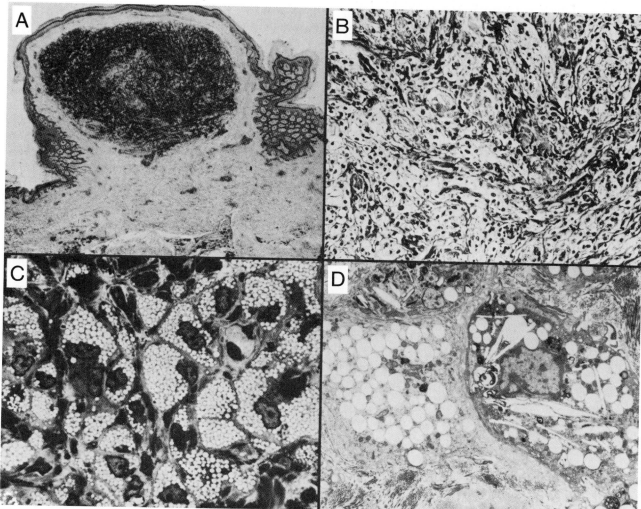

Fig. 145-2 Histologic features of tuberous and tendon xanthomas. (A) Cross section of xanthomas in the Achilles tendon from a patient with familial hypercholesterolemia. A frozen section was stained with oil red O. A tuberous xanthoma containing foam cells and extracellular lipid (dark mass) is shown overlying a tendon xanthoma (×25). (B) Light micrograph of a tuberous xanthoma containing numerous foam cells interspersed in fibrous tissue (×200). (C) High magnification (×600) of the xanthoma illustrated in (B) showing extensive vacuolation due to lipid accumulation in foam cells. (D) Electron micrograph of a tendon xanthoma (B and C) demonstrating the presence of lipid droplets, cholesterol crystals, and electron-dense inclusions in foam cells (×5000).

protein pattern into one of the general lipoprotein phenotypes (types I to V). *Hypolipoproteinemia* also is separable into syndromes expressed as reductions in HDL or in apoB-containing lipoproteins (i.e., chylomicrons, VLDL, IDL, and LDL). Sometimes concentrations of both are affected. Initial classification helps to sharpen differential diagnosis including separation of primary (genetic) defects from dyslipoproteinemias *secondary* to other disorders, to anticipate the clinical course including complications, and to select the most effective therapy. Consideration of lipoproteins, rather than lipids, also provides a more flexible framework for adjusting to the rapidly expanding knowledge about these disorders.

Xanthomas

The skin is a particularly valuable index for the diagnosis of dyslipoproteinemias and for following the effects of treatment. Different xanthomas frequently represent the hallmarks of particular syndromes. Xanthoma (Greek: *xanthoas*, "yellow," + -*oma*, "tumor," - perhaps from *onkona*, "swelling") are lipid deposits in skin and subcutaneous tissues. Historically, xanthomas were recognized before dyslipidemias, and descriptive terms including *xanthoma diabeticorum, xanthoma tendinosum* or *xanthoma tuberosum multiplex* were once used nosologically.

Xanthomas associated with the dyslipoproteinemias are frequently classified as eruptive, tuberous, planar, or tendinous. The principal microscopic feature of all xanthomas is lipid-laden macrophages or foam cells surrounded by collagen-rich stroma, connective tissue cells, and blood vessels (Fig. 145-2). In most xanthomas the major lipid stored is cholesteryl ester, although the transient eruptive xanthomas early contain primarily triglycerides. The majority of the excess lipid is intracellular although tendon xanthomas frequently contain extracellular clumps of cholesterol crystals which react strongly with lipid stains. In unstained frozen sections, the foam cells contain nonfluorescent, birefringent lipid droplets and a few autofluorescent, nonbirefringent cytoplasmic granules. By electron microscopy the lipid appears as droplets, crystals, concentric lamellar bodies, and ceroid-like material (Fig. 145-2D). The foam cells stain intensely with Sudan, oil red O, the Schultz stain for cholesterol, and faintly with Baker hematoxylin or periodic acid-Schiff stains.

The dermatologist may find it particularly useful to use xanthomas for orientation to syndromes of hyperlipoproteinemia. We, therefore, use eruptive, planar, and tendinous xanthomas as rubrics to delineate the dyslipoproteinemias.

Hyperlipoproteinemias

Severe chylomicronemia with or without eruptive xanthomas (lipoprotein lipase deficiency, apoC-II deficiency, type I hyperlipoproteinemia, or type V hyperlipoproteinemia)

Clinical syndrome. Plasma triglyceride concentrations are labile depending primarily upon the time relationship of sampling to the intake of fat. In general, fasting plasma concentrations over 300 mg/dL are abnormal (Table 145-1). Chylomicrons are normally seen in plasma only a few hours after one has eaten a fatty meal. At plasma concentrations of triglycerides exceeding 1500 mg/dL, there is usually a distinct accumulation of chylomicrons. These are visible as a distinct creamy layer on top of plasma left overnight in a refrigerator at 4°C. If the infranatant is cloudy, significant elevations of VLDL (or IDL) concentration(s) are also present.

Above triglyceride concentrations of 1500 to 2000 mg/dL, a frequent symptom complex or *chylomicronemia syndrome* often appears. The clinical manifestations of the chylomicronemia syndrome are eruptive xanthomas, lipemia retinalis, and sometimes pancreatitis. Additional symptoms may include dry eyes and dry mouth, numbness or tingling in the extremities, abdominal pains of uncertain origin, depression, memory loss, and emotional lability. The majority of the symptoms are ameliorated with the reduction in plasma triglycerides. A history of prior exploratory surgery because of abdominal pain is not unusual, and patients may ultimately develop chronic pancreatitis.

Over the years two general categories of patients with severe chylomicronemia have been identified. In one, the elevated triglycerides appear primarily in chylomicrons (type I hyperlipoproteinemia, exogenous hypertriglyceridemia). In the other, the triglyceride elevations represent both chylomicrons and VLDL (type V hyperlipoproteinemia, mixed exogenous and endogenous hypertriglyceridemia). Actually, patients with either the type I or type V lipoproteinemia have elevations of both apoB-48 and apoB-100 in the triglyceride-rich lipoproteins. Thus, triglyceride-rich lipoproteins synthesized by both the liver and intestine accumulate in plasma in all severely hypertriglyceridemic patients.

The type of defect in patients with severe hypertriglyceridemia is suggested by the age of onset of the chylomicronemia syndrome. Patients with signs and symptoms

before puberty nearly always have genetic defects in triglyceride metabolism involving lipoprotein lipase activity (Table 145-3, Fig. 145-3). A primary deficiency of lipoprotein lipase activity results in defective lipolysis of chylomicrons and hepatogeneous VLDL with accumulation of very large triglyceride-rich lipoprotein particles in plasma, the classic type I phenotype (Fig. 145-3). Recently, a deficiency of apoC-II has also been recognized as a cause of severe hypertriglyceridemia and the type I phenotype. These patients have a severe reduction in lipoprotein lipase activity secondary to an absence of normal amounts of the apoC-II cofactor. The clinical manifestations of apoC-II also appear before puberty; however, the signs and symptoms tend to be less dramatic than in familial lipoprotein lipase deficiency.

The molecular defect(s) in patients who develop severe hypertriglyceridemia in the fourth and fifth decades are incompletely understood. These patients have no detectable abnormality in lipoprotein lipase or apoC-II. Yet they have elevated concentrations of plasma chylomicrons as well as VLDL and are classified as having type V hyperlipoproteinemia. The diagnosis must be pursued to separate primary or familial forms of type V from secondary hypertriglyceridemia due to uncontrolled diabetes and other diseases. The differentiation of whether the hyperlipidemia is secondary to chronic pancreatitis or vice versa may sometimes be academic with respect to the clinical care of the patient.

A number of other patients have dyslipoproteinemias that are characterized by mild hypertriglyceridemia with plasma triglycerides of 300 to 500 mg/dL. These patients have a type IV lipoprotein pattern (elevations of plasma VLDL without chylomicrons). Two other inheritable disorders, *familial hypertriglyceridemia* and *combined hyperlipidemia* (multiple lipoprotein phenotypes), have been identified as subgroups within this cadre of hypertriglyceridemic patients. The majority of patients with the type IV phenotype are asymptomatic and have few physical manifestations of hyperlipidemia. Patients with combined hyperlipidemia may have tendon xanthomas and an increased incidence of premature cardiovascular disease (see below). Occasionally, mildly affected patients with familial hypertriglyceridemia or combined hyperlipidemia may develop the chylomicronemia syndrome secondary to the additive effect of environmental factors (alcohol, obesity), separate diseases (hypothyroidism, diabetes), or medications (estrogens).

Physical examination. The characteristic xanthoma accompanying the chylomicronemia syndrome is the eruptive xanthoma (Fig. 145-4A). These are usually asymptomatic, discrete papules 5 to 6 mm in size, with a yellow center and red halo. During resolution the inflammatory character of the lesions resolves and the papules become waxy yellow in appearance. These xanthomas result from the phagocytosis of triglyceride-rich lipoproteins by macrophages in the skin. Eruptive xanthomas may suddenly appear in showers and they disappear with the decline of the acute transient elevations in plasma triglycerides. Sometimes the xanthomas persist if the triglycerides remain elevated (Fig. 145-4C and D). Eruptive xanthomas have a predilection to form on pressure points on the extensor surfaces of the elbows, back, buttocks (Fig. A2-1a), and knees. Frequently,

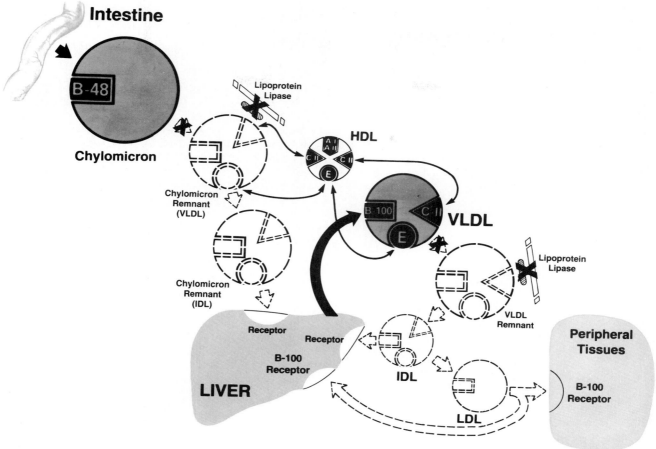

Fig. 145-3 Schematic view of the block in lipoprotein metabolism in patients with the chylomicronemia syndrome and the type I phenotype. Molecular defects underlying this syndrome include primarily a deficiency of lipoprotein lipase activity and a deficiency of the cofactor for lipoprotein lipase, apoC-II.

eruptive xanthomas are missed on physical examination unless great care has been taken to search for the lesions.

Occasionally, eruptive xanthomas may become confluent and associated with tuberous xanthomas. These hybrid lesions have been termed *tuboeruptive xanthomas* and are typical of patients with type III hyperlipoproteinemia (see below).

Lipemia retinalis can be detected in the fundus of the eye when triglyceride levels reach 3000 to 4000 mg/dL (Fig. 145-4B). The retinal arterioles and venules appear pale pink due to light scattering of the large chylomicron particles. Vision is not reduced and there are no clinical sequelae of lipemia retinalis.

Hepatosplenomegaly associated with abdominal pain and tenderness is a frequent physical manifestation of the hyperchylomicronemia syndrome. The hepatosplenomegaly is secondary to lipid accumulation in the parenchymal and reticuloendothelial tissues. Acute right and left upper quadrant pain may develop with rapid elevations in plasma triglycerides, often mimicking an acute abdominal emergency. With reduction in plasma triglycerides, hepatosplenomegaly may decrease and the symptoms abate. Abdominal pain in patients with the chylomicronemia syndrome is frequently due to acute pancreatitis which can have a fatal outcome. Chronic pancreatitis is a frequent and important sequela of the syndrome. The evaluation of abdominal pain in the patient with hyperchylomicronemia is often a test of the clinical acumen of the physician.

Neuropsychiatric symptoms are frequently present in patients with severe elevations in plasma triglycerides, especially with primary type V hyperlipoproteinemia. The symptoms are often bizarre, follow no neurologic patterns, and include paresthesias, dysthesias, acute memory loss, personality changes, depression, and mild dementia. Physical findings are not consistent with any specific neurologic syndrome. The severity of the symptoms appears to be correlated with the elevation of the plasma triglycerides.

Therapy. Patients with severe chylomicronemia with or without VLDL elevations respond to dietary restriction of fats. Selected patients with type V hyperlipoproteinemia may require drug therapy with norethindrone acetate, nicotinic acid, or lopid. The hyperlipoproteinemia in patients whose clinical course is complicated by an additional disease (e.g., diabetes, hypothyroidism) can be markedly improved by treatment of the acquired disease.

Defective removal of lipoprotein remnants with or without planar and tuboeruptive xanthomas (type III hyperlipoproteinemia, apoE absence, defective apoE, apoE₂ phenotype or dysbetalipoproteinemia)

Clinical syndrome. Patients with delayed removal of lipoprotein remnants often develop hyperlipidemia and clinical symptomatology in the fourth and fifth decades. This dyslipoproteinemia has been designated as *type III hyperli-*

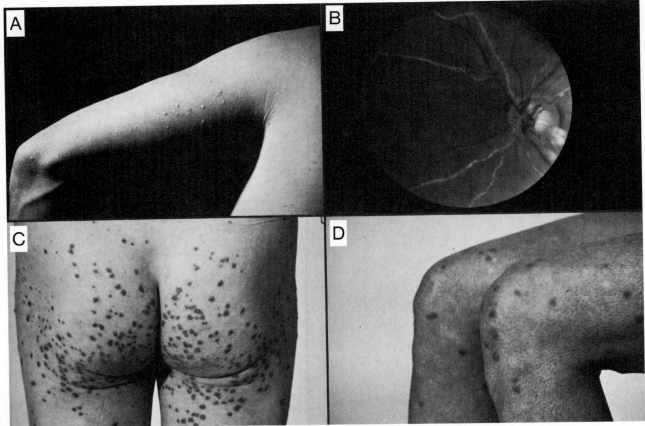

Fig. 145-4   Clinical manifestations of the chylomicronemia syndrome include eruptive xanthomas (A) and lipemia retinalis (B), both of which may be evanescent. Persistent, pain- **ful, erythematous eruptive xanthomas may occasionally be observed in patients with type V hyperlipoproteinemia (C and D).**

poproteinemia. Type III hyperlipoproteinemia is of particular importance due to the increased incidence of premature cardiovascular disease. Untreated patients with type III hyperlipoproteinemia have virtually pathognomonic planar xanthomas on the palmar creases of their hands and tuberous xanthomas on the elbows, knees, and buttocks. Plasma concentrations of both triglycerides and cholesterol are elevated (frequently about equally), and the principal elevation of the plasma lipoproteins involves IDL. These lipoproteins are cholesterol-rich, migrate as an extra beta band on high-resolution agarose gel electrophoresis of plasma, and migrate in the beta position on lipoprotein electrophoresis following separation by ultracentrifugation of the plasma lipoproteins at a density less than 1.006 g/mL. These beta migrating lipoproteins have been designated as floating beta lipoproteins. An additional important diagnostic feature of this dyslipoproteinemia is a VLDL-cholesterol to plasma triglyceride ratio greater than 0.3. In normal subjects this ratio is less than 0.3.

Apolipoprotein E. A key role in the metabolism and cellular uptake of triglyceride-rich lipoproteins is played by apoE. Population and structural analyses have indicated that apoE is controlled at a single genetic locus with an unusual degree of polymorphism. There are three common alleles in the general population which have been designated E^2, E^3, and E^4. The three E apolipoproteins encoded by these three alleles are separable by isoelectrofocusing and are

codified as $apoE_2$, $apoE_3$, and $apoE_4$. Six major apoE phenotypes are present in the population including homozygotes for apolipoprotein E_2, E_3, and E_4 as well as heterozygotes for apolipoproteins $E_{2/3}$, $E_{2/4}$, and $E_{3/4}$. Differences in the apoE isoproteins have been shown to be due to one or two amino acid substitutions involving cysteine and arginine interchanges in the amino acid sequences. $ApoE_2$ contains two cysteine residues, $apoE_3$, a cysteine and arginine, and $apoE_4$, two arginine residues.

Epidemiologic studies have established the frequency of the E alleles and lipoprotein profiles in the general and hyperlipidemic population. The predominant E isoprotein in the normolipidemic population is $apoE_3$. An increased frequency of the E^2 allele ($apoE_2$ phenotype) or E^0 allele ($apoE$ absence) has been observed in patients with type III hyperlipoproteinemia. In early adult life, nearly all subjects with the $apoE_{2/2}$ phenotype are normolipidemic and in fact may be hypolipidemic. Subjects with the $apoE_{2/2}$ phenotype and no hyperlipidemia are categorized as normolipidemic E^2 homozygotes or subjects with dysbetalipoproteinemia. They also have an elevated synthesis and plasma level of apoE.

In the fourth and fifth decades, some subjects either lacking apoE (E^0) or with the $apoE_{2/2}$ phenotype develop hyperlipidemia and have a lipoprotein pattern characteristic of type III. Genetic and kindred studies in hyperlipidemic subjects have suggested that the $apoE_{2/2}$ phenotype per se is a permissive defect and that an additional factor

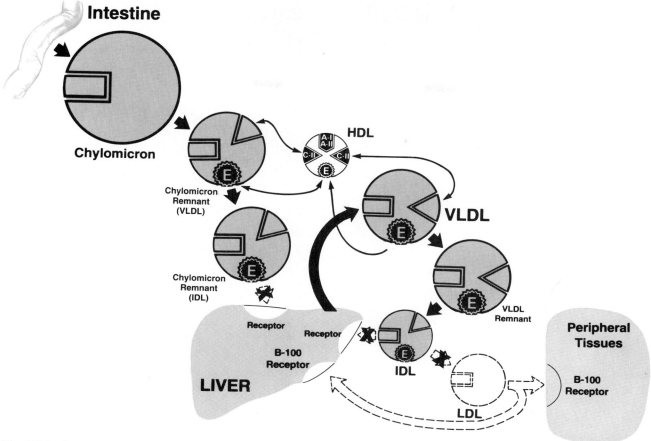

Fig. 145-5 Schematic model of the defect in lipoprotein metabolism in patients with type III hyperlipoproteinemia. The block is characterized by a defect in removal of remnants of both the chylomicron and hepatogenous VLDL cascades due to a defect in the apoE-mediated uptake of lipoprotein remnants. These patients may be missing apoE (E^0 allele) or more commonly have an abnormal apoE ($apoE_2$, E^2 allele) resulting in the accumulation of lipoproteins and hyperlipidemia.

(e.g., obesity or separate dyslipoproteinemia) is required for the patient to become hyperlipidemic and develop type III hyperlipoproteinemia.

The lipoproteins that accumulate in type III hyperlipoproteinemia contain both apoB-48 and apoB-100, indicating that there is defective metabolism of lipoproteins of both intestinal (chylomicron) and liver (VLDL) origin (Fig. 145-5). The delay in catabolism of these lipoproteins is due to the absence of apoE or the presence of $apoE_2$ which results in defective binding to the hepatic apoE receptor. Remnants, therefore, persist in the circulation for an abnormally long time and are susceptible to uptake by macrophages. Lipid accumulations in these cells underlie the development of xanthomas and unusual lipid deposits such as those observed in the atrial endothelium. Presumably, this is also the basis for an increased incidence of coronary and peripheral arterial disease in patients with type III hyperlipoproteinemia.

Physical findings. One of the fascinating features of type III hyperlipoproteinemia is the appearance of planar xanthomas (xanthoma striata palmaris) that are nearly pathognomonic of this disorder (Fig. 145-6A). These xanthomas are frequently accompanied by tuberous lesions over the elbows, knees, and buttocks (Fig. 145-6B and D). Occasionally, the patients may also develop Achilles tendon

xanthomas, which are characteristic of patients with hypercholesterolemia, and an elevation of plasma LDL (see below). These xanthomas contain foam cells filled with cholesteryl esters.

Other physical findings in patients with type III hyperlipoproteinemia relate to the increased frequency of atherosclerosis observed in these patients and include evidence of both cardiac as well as peripheral vascular disease. Peripheral vascular disease is particularly frequent in this dyslipoproteinemia. The atherosclerotic lesions in patients with type III hyperlipoproteinemia are similar to those observed in the absence of hyperlipidemia and in other hyperlipidemic phenotypes.

Therapy. Before the institution of therapy for type III hyperlipoproteinemia, aggravating factors should be excluded, including diabetes mellitus or other diseases that mimic or exaggerate the abnormal lipoprotein patterns (systemic lupus erythematosus, paraproteinemias, and especially hypothyroidism). Modification of diet and caloric restriction, if appropriate, are very effective in lowering plasma lipids in patients with the uncomplicated phenotype. Additional lowering may be achieved by drug therapy with clofibrate, nicotinic acid, or lopid. Alcohol intake should be sharply limited since it often exaggerates the hyperlipidemia. Effective control of type III hyperlipopro-

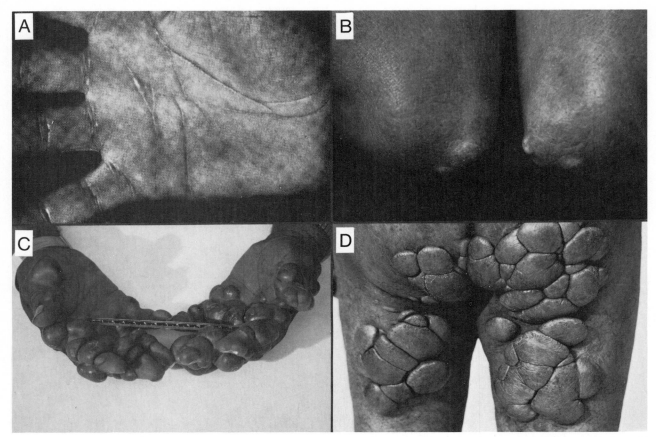

Fig. 145-6   Palmar (A) and tuberous (B) xanthomas characteristic of patients with a defect in the removal of remnant lipoproteins and the type III phenotype. Extensive tuberous xanthomas (C and D) observed in an occasional patient with type III hyperlipoproteinemia.

teinemia with diet and/or drug therapy leads to rapid resolution of xanthomas.

Elevated LDL levels with or without tendon xanthomas (defective LDL receptor, familial hypercholesterolemia, familial combined hyperlipidemia, type II hyperlipoproteinemia)

Clinical syndrome. The important manifestations of hypercholesterolemia associated with an increased level of plasma LDL include arcus juvenilis, tendon xanthomas, and premature coronary artery disease. The dyslipoproteinemia characterized by an increased plasma LDL is type II hyperlipoproteinemia (type IIa is characterized by an increase in LDL, and type IIb with an increase in both LDL and VLDL).

Type II hyperlipoproteinemia is a generic term which may result from a number of different causes. These include at least three different genetically determined diseases: familial hypercholesterolemia (FH), familial combined hyperlipidemia (FCH), and polygenic hypercholesterolemia (PH).

Familial hypercholesterolemia. One of the most important dyslipoproteinemias, FH, is a relatively common codominant disease with a gene frequency of approximately 1:500 in the general population. Heterozygotes for FH have el-

evated plasma cholesterol and LDL levels from birth. As an adult the patient's plasma cholesterols are usually in the 300 to 400 mg/dL range. Clinical manifestations typically do not develop until the third and fourth decades. At this time xanthomas appear, most characteristically in the Achilles tendons and extensor tendons of the hands; occasionally in tendons about the knee and elbow. Arcus juvenilis and xanthelasma may also be present in FH patients. The most significant clinical manifestation of heterozygous FH is the tendency to develop coronary artery disease several decades earlier than other 30- to 60-year-old males. Premature occurrence of coronary artery disease also occurs in female heterozygotes but lags about 10 years behind male heterozygotes.

Homozygotes for FH have markedly elevated cholesterol and LDL at birth, and during the first few years of life plasma cholesterol levels range from 700 to 1200 mg/dL. In the early years, a unique yellowish planar xanthoma may develop in the interdigital webs of the hands and at pressure points or sites of trauma, particularly over the knees, elbows, and buttocks. Large xanthomas, particularly in the Achilles tendons, but also over the elbows, ankles, and hands, as well as arcus juvenilis, and xanthelasma are characteristic of homozygous FH. Of paramount clinical importance in homozygous patients is the very early development of severe coronary artery disease; myocardial infarction can occur in the first and second decades

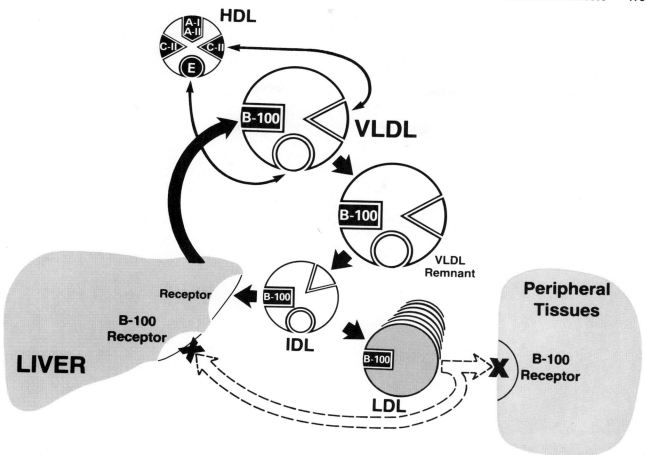

Fig. 145-7 Schematic view of the defect in lipoprotein metabolism characterized by tendon xanthomas and hyperbetalipoproteinemia observed in patients with familial hypercholesterolemia and the type II phenotype. The molecular defect in familial hypercholesterolemia is a defect in the LDL receptor process on both liver and peripheral cells.

of life and life expectancy rarely extends beyond the third decade.

The molecular defect in FH is now well understood and has been extensively studied in fibroblast cells and the liver. Circulating LDL normally binds to a high-affinity receptor on cellular membranes initiating a receptor-mediated endocytosis (Fig. 145-1). In FH, one of numerous primary defects in the structure and function of the LDL receptor process results in defective cellular uptake of LDL (Fig. 145-7). The resulting deficiency of LDL uptake results in a marked increase in circulating plasma LDL and a reduction in the uptake of LDL by high-affinity processes. The steady-state level of LDL is far above the level of normal subjects.

Patients with homozygous FH were initially subdivided into receptor "negative" or "defective" depending on the residual capacity of the cellular receptor system. Recent studies have indicated that there are several mutant alleles at the LDL receptor locus which result in varying defects in the synthesis and function of the LDL receptor. The degree of residual receptor function is correlated with clinical onset of symptoms, severity of disease, and response to treatment. Patients with the most severe deficiencies of receptor function are symptomatic at an earlier age, develop more virulent cardiovascular disease, and are more resistant to therapy. The spectrum of clinical disease in patients with heterozygous FH is broad, in keeping with

the considerable polymorphism underlying the changes in the receptor gene.

Familial combined hyperlipidemia. One of the most common monogenetic disorders in humans is FCH. The gene frequency assuming a single defect has been estimated to be as high as 1:300. The clinical manifestations of FCH generally appear in the fourth and fifth decades. The characteristic feature of FCH is paradoxically the variability of the plasma lipoprotein phenotype in the proband and the affected relatives. The most frequent lipoprotein patterns observed are types IIa, IIb, and IV. The molecular defect in FCH is unknown, and the diagnosis is presumptive and established only by analysis of the pattern of dyslipoproteinemia in the propositus and family members. No homozygotes for FCH have been identified, although a number of genetic compounds, i.e., one gene for FCH and the other for some other form of hyperlipoproteinemia, have been suspected. Available data suggest that at least a subset of patients with FCH have increased synthesis of LDL and an increased ratio of apoB-100 to cholesterol in plasma LDL. A receptor-mediated defect in LDL catabolism such as that present in FH has not been shown.

The majority of patients with FCH have no xanthomas, although tendon xanthomas, arcus juvenilis, and xanthelasma may be observed. The most frequent as well as significant clinical manifestation of FCH is the develop-

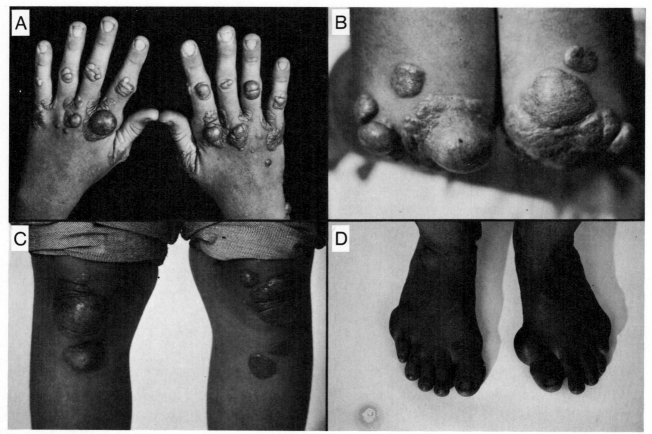

Fig. 145-8   Characteristic tuberous and tendon xanthomas observed in a patient with homozygous familial hypercholesterolemia.

ment of premature cardiovascular disease which is very similar in severity and clinical course to that observed in heterozygotes for FH.

Type II hyperlipoproteinemia may also occur as one or more disorders having polygenic inheritance. Whatever the molecular defect(s), these patients have variable clinical manifestations with respect to degree of hypercholesterolemia and severity of premature cardiovascular disease.

Physical examination. Heterozygotes as well as homozygotes for FH have tendon xanthomas located in the Achilles tendons and the tendons of the dorsa of the hands (Figs. 145-8 and 145-9). In homozygotes, the characteristic and usually earliest physical manifestation of hypercholesterolemia is the appearance of planar xanthomas in the webs of the hands and on the elbows, knees, and buttocks (Fig. 145-8). These xanthomas do not appear in the heterozygous adult with FH. Xanthelasmas often accompany type II hyperlipoproteinemia; however, these lesions are not diagnostic of hyperlipoproteinemia (Fig. 145-9).

Histologically, tendon xanthomas contain macrophages so laden with lipid droplets that they form foam cells which are interspersed among the fibrous stroma. The cytoplasmic lipid droplets predominantly contain cholesteryl esters, which are birefringent and positive for the oil red O stain. Arcus juvenilis, a grayish white ring in the cornea, is due to the accumulation of lipid droplets (Fig. 145-8A). Superficially, the arcus appears to extend not quite to the

limbus, leaving a clear margin of iris. By slit lamp examination, however, the lipid droplets extend diagonally through the entire thickness of the cornea. Arcus in children is practically always a sign of hyperbetalipoproteinemia. In older subjects its diagnostic value gradually diminishes with age. In blacks, arcus is commonly observed without hyperlipidemia.

Therapy. The treatment of adults with type II hyperlipoproteinemia begins with a low-fat, low-cholesterol diet (less than 300 mg/day) with a polyunsaturated:saturated fat ratio of 1.0:1.5. Patients who require additional therapy to reduce their plasma cholesterol levels below 250 mg/dL can be treated with a single drug or a combination of drugs that decreases synthesis (niacin) and increases the catabolism (cholestyramine/cholestipol) of lipoproteins. FCH and FH heterozygotes often require therapy with both niacin and cholestyramine which frequently lowers cholesterol levels by as much as 50 percent. Other drugs such as mevinolin which decrease cholesterol synthesis are still experimental but show great potential as therapeutic agents in patients with hypercholesterolemia, particularly in combination with bile acid binding resins.

Treatment of patients with homozygous FH must be aggressive due to the malignant nature of the premature cardiovascular disease. A low-fat, low-cholesterol diet with a polyunsaturated:saturated fat ratio of 1.0:1.5 and combination drug therapy (e.g., cholestyramine and niacin)

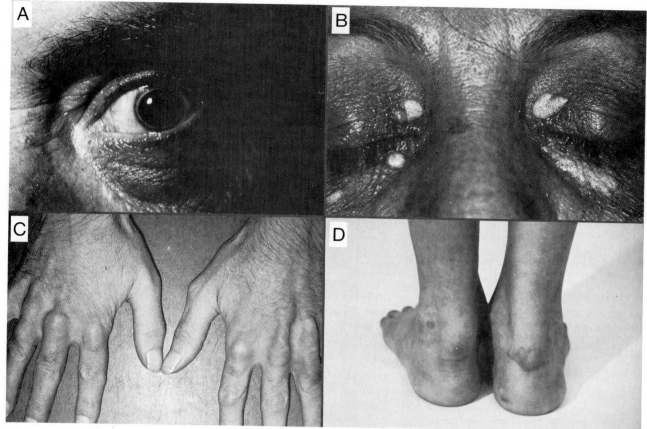

Fig. 145-9 Clinical manifestations of hyperbetalipoprotein-emia in a patient with heterozygous familial hypercholester-olemia. Arcus juvenilis (A), xanthelasma (B), tendon xantho- **mas in the extensor tendons of the hand (C), and Achilles tendons (D) are characteristic of this disease.**

should be actively pursued. If significant lowering of plasma cholesterol (at least to below 500 mg/dL) is not achieved, additional therapeutic intervention should be considered in FH homozygotes. Effective in limited series of patients have been portacaval shunt (lowering plasma cholesterol concentrations by approximately 35 percent) and bimonthly plasma exchanges. As the molecular defects in patients with the type II phenotype and hypercholester-olemia continue to be elucidated, including finer detail of LDL receptor defects (FH) and FCH, drug therapy will become more selective and one will be required to individ-ualize therapy to maximize effective reduction of plasma cholesterol.

Other sterol-storage diseases associated with tendon xanthomas

Cerebrotendinous xanthomatosis (CTX). CLINICAL SYN-DROME. CTX is a rare autosomal recessive disease char-acterized by the accumulation of cholestanol (5,6-dihy-droxycholesterol) in plasma lipoproteins and tissues. The cardinal manifestations of CTX include xanthomas, cata-racts, severe neurologic deficiencies, mental retardation, dementia, and cardiovascular disease. The xanthomas may be widespread and most commonly occur in tendons, brain, and lungs.

The onset of the clinical manifestations of CTX are fre-quently insidious and variable in presentation. They may

not become clearly manifested until the teen years. Initial symptoms may be related to xanthomas, neurologic dys-function with dementia, and ataxia or cataracts. A young person presenting with tendon xanthomas, cataracts, and normal plasma lipids should raise the suspicion of CTX. Neurologic dysfunction, often devastating in the late stages of the disease, may initially be only a minor manifestation of the disease. Premature atherosclerotic cardiovascular disease may occur in patients with CTX.

The diagnosis of CTX is established by quantitation of cholestanol in plasma or tissues. The bile characteristically contains an increase in biliary cholestanol, decreased chen-odeoxycholic acid, and a marked elevation in glucuronide-conjugated bile alcohols. Plasma VLDL and LDL concen-trations are usually normal. The concentrations of plasma HDL may be low and the composition is abnormal with increased triglycerides and reduced cholesteryl esters. The protein to cholesteryl ester ratio is also increased and there is a relative increase in the ratio of the concentrations of apoA-I to apoA-II. The clinical and biochemical signifi-cance of the low HDL in the pathogenesis of the premature cardiovascular disease in CTX has not been definitively established.

Cholestanol in CTX appears to be derived almost exclu-sively from cholesterol. Cholestanol, like cholesterol, ex-ists both in the free as well as the fatty acyl ester form. Cholestanol and cholesteryl esters are transported on plasma lipoproteins, primarily LDL.

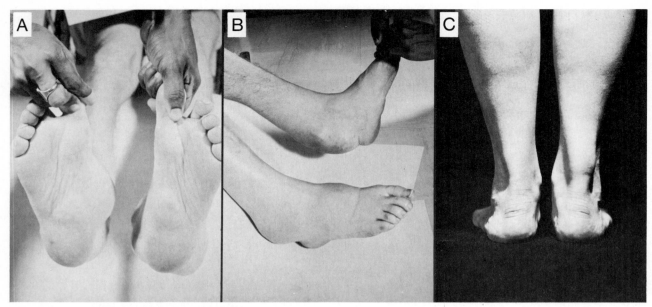

Fig. 145-10 Tendon xanthomas observed in patients with cerebrotendinous xanthomatosis. *(Courtesy of Dr. Gerald Salen, Veterans Administration Hospital Center, East Orange, New Jersey.)*

The clinical features of CTX reflect the tissue accumulation of sterols including cholestanol. In the final stages of the disease the neurologic deterioration may be severe. Death usually occurs between the fourth and sixth decades and usually results from severe neurologic deficiencies with pseudobulbar paralysis or acute myocardial infarction.

The biochemical defect in CTX has been proposed to be a reduction in the activity of one of the hepatic enzymes involved in the biosynthesis of bile acids. The block in biosynthesis of bile acids results in a marked deficiency of biliary cholic and chenodeoxycholic acid, and the secretion into the bile of increased levels of cholestanol and glucuronide C_{27} bile alcohols. The increased tissue deposits of cholesteryl and cholestanol esters may signify an increased hepatic synthesis of cholesterol and cholestanol due to a lack of bile acids in the enterohepatic circulation and loss of normal feedback control of sterol biosynthesis.

PHYSICAL EXAMINATION. The major clinical findings in patients with CTX are tendon xanthomas, cataracts, and neurologic deficiencies. By the second and third decades large tendon xanthomas are characteristically present in the Achilles tendons, extensor tendons of the hand, and tibial tuberosities (Fig. 145-10). These xanthomas are indistinguishable in gross or histologic appearance from the lesions present in patients with hypercholesterolemia and hyperbetalipoproteinemia. The major lipids deposited are cholesteryl esters. The presence of a significant cholestanol content provides a definitive diagnosis of CTX. Xanthomas also occur at unique sites including the cerebellum, forebrain, lung, and bone, which are never involved in familial hypercholesterolemia.

Zonular cortical lens cataracts are also a well-documented feature of CTX. The devastating neurologic involvement may include dementia, mental retardation, spasticity, ataxia, tremors, muscular atrophy, and pseudobulbar paralysis. The neurologic symptoms are correlated anatomically with lipid accumulation and demyelination.

THERAPY. Recently, patients with CTX have been treated with chenodeoxycholic acid, which inhibits biosynthesis of abnormal bile acids and results in a reduction of plasma cholestanol concentrations. The effect of such treatment on the relentless progression of the clinical manifestations of CTX is as yet uncertain.

Sitosterolemia. CLINICAL SYNDROME. Sitosterolemia is a rare autosomal recessive disease characterized by an accumulation in plasma and tissue of plant sterols including sitosterol, campesterol, and stigmasterol. Increased plasma concentrations of plant sterols are frequently accompanied by an increase in cholesterol levels and hyperapobetalipoproteinemia.

The clinical manifestations begin in childhood or the first and second decades of life. Tendon xanthomas are common, yet the plasma cholesterol may be normal instead of elevated. A child with tendon xanthoma without hypercholesterolemia requires consideration of sitosterolemia, and the disease should be considered in young patients with tendon xanthomas and hypercholesterolemia. LDL receptor function is normal, and occasionally some of these patients have been classified as "pseudofamilial hypercholesterolemia."

The definitive diagnosis of sitosterolemia may be made by the determination of increased plasma levels of plant sterols (upper limit of normal 0.5 percent total plasma sterols), which are transported primarily within LDL. The plant sterol content of xanthomas is greater than 10 percent; however, the predominant sterol present in xanthomas remains cholesterol. The fecal bile acid pattern is unusual in that it contains deoxycholic and lithocholic acids. There is also an increase in fecal bile alcohols.

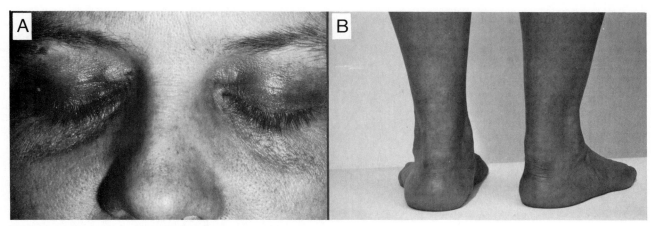

Fig. 145-11 Clinical features of sitosterolemia include xan-thelasma (A) and Achilles tendon xanthomas (B). The tendon xanthomas in sitosterolemia are indistinguishable from those present in familial hypercholesterolemia (Fig. 145-9).

The molecular defect in sitosterolemia is as yet unknown. Metabolic studies have revealed that there is an increased absorption of all sterols including cholesterol, plant and shellfish sterols. The defect appears to be the loss of the ability of the cell to differentiate among the sterols of different sources. In addition, there appears to be a defect in the hepatic excretion of the plant and shellfish sterols resulting in delayed clearance of the absorbed sterols. Cholesterol and plant sterols accumulate in tendon as well as subcutaneous xanthomas and accelerated atherosclerosis is not uncommon.

PHYSICAL EXAMINATION. The principal manifestations of sitosterolemia are tendon as well as subcutaneous xanthomas, xanthelasma, and premature cardiovascular disease (Fig. 145-11). Hemolytic anemia and arcus juvenilis may also be present. Signs of cardiovascular disease may be present depending on the age of the patient. Cataracts are not present.

THERAPY. The usual therapy of sitosterolemia with xanthomatosis is a diet restricted in plant sterols, which is opposite to the diet prescribed for patients with hypercholesterolemia and elevated plasma LDL. Vegetable fats including vegetable oils, shortenings, and margarines as well as plant foods such as nuts, seeds, chocolate, and olives are eliminated. In addition to diet therapy, cholestyramine and neomycin have been reported to reduce plasma and sterol accumulation. No definitive long-term studies are currently available to establish whether diet and/or drug therapy will decrease the risk of the development of premature cardiovascular disease in these patients.

Hypolipoproteinemias

The dyslipoproteinemias characterized by abnormally low concentrations of plasma lipoproteins involve primarily HDL or all apoB-containing lipoproteins (i.e., chylomicrons, VLDL, IDL, and LDL).

HDL deficiency

Tangier disease. CLINICAL SYNDROME. Tangier disease is an inheritable disorder characterized clinically by orange tonsils, cloudy corneas, hepatosplenomegaly, lymphadenopathy, and intermittent peripheral neuropathy.

The diagnosis of Tangier disease should be suspected when the plasma cholesterol is below 120 mg/dL and the triglycerides slightly elevated or normal. Marked deficiencies of HDL, apoA-I, and apoA-II (less than 2 to 5 percent of normal) are characteristic of Tangier disease.

The onset of the clinical manifestations of Tangier disease is insidious and reflects the tissue accumulation of cholesteryl esters. The most important sites of deposition, the pharyngeal tonsils, can provide the diagnosis of Tangier disease at a glance but usually these have been removed long before the physician sees the patient. Enlargement of the liver and spleen is modest, if present, and due to lipid accumulation in the reticuloendothelial system. Hypersplenism is rare. The removal of the spleen, however, may lead to hyperplasia of the reticuloendothelial cells in the omentum and other areas of the body. Transient and recurrent peripheral neuropathy appears to be due to an accumulation of lipid within the nerve sheaths. Neurologic symptoms including motor weakness, paresthesias, and dysesthesias may occur and wax and wane. The clinical course of patients with Tangier disease is extremely variable, and the diagnosis may not be established until the third or fourth decade. Premature cardiovascular disease is not a prominent feature.

The catabolism of the plasma HDL in Tangier disease is aberrant, the lipoproteins leaving the plasma at a rate far faster than normal. Evidence has been presented recently that this could be due to abnormal handling of Tangier HDL by macrophages. Normally HDL appear to be shunted through macrophages and emerge to be carried away in the plasma, while Tangier HDL may be abnormally diverted to lysosomes where they are destroyed. The abnormal signal to the macrophages could be a posttranslational change in the apoA-I in Tangier disease, for the structural gene directing synthesis of apoA-I is isomorphic in normals and patients with Tangier disease.

PHYSICAL EXAMINATION. The unique clinical feature of Tangier disease is lobulated, bright orange-yellow tonsils (Fig. 145-12A). If the tonsils have been removed, pharyngeal tags of orange-yellow tissue may sometimes be ob-

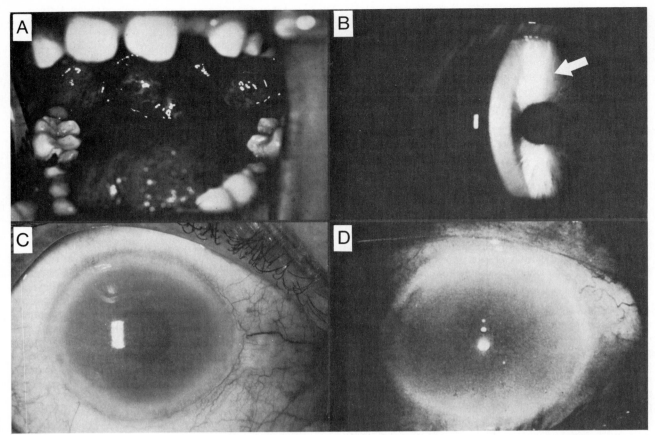

Fig. 145-12 Clinical manifestations of patients with HDL deficiency. Orange-yellow tonsils (A) are pathognomonic for Tangier disease. A varying degree of corneal opacification is characteristic of patients with HDL deficiency. Corneal opacification (arrow) is mild in Tangier disease and requires slit lamp examination (B); however, significant opacification is observed in lecithin cholesteryl acyltransferase deficiency (LCAT deficiency) (C). Severe corneal opacification is the hallmark of patients with fish eye disease (D). *(Courtesy of Professor L. Carlson, Karolinska Institute, Stockholm, Sweden.)*

served. The rectal mucosa has a similar appearance, and storage of cholesteryl esters in foam cells in the rectal mucosa may establish the diagnosis.

Asymptomatic corneal infiltrates, requiring slit lamp examination for identification, are frequently present (Fig. 145-12B). Mild hepatosplenomegaly and lymphadenopathy may be observed. The transient neuropathy may be detected by decreased deep tendon reflexes and sensory-motor abnormalities.

THERAPY. There is no specific therapy for Tangier disease.

Familial lecithin: cholesteryl acyltransferase (LCAT) deficiency. CLINICAL SYNDROME. LCAT deficiency is a rare autosomal recessive disease in which deficiency of the plasma enzyme leads to dyslipoproteinemia and lipid deposition in the cornea, kidney, and cardiovascular system. The resulting damage to the kidney and heart reduces life expectancy.

The onset of clinical manifestations in patients homozygous for LCAT deficiency usually begins in childhood with the development of corneal opacities. During the next two decades anemia appears and then ensues the more ominous development of renal failure with proteinuria and premature cardiovascular disease.

The deficiency of LCAT results in increased plasma levels of unesterified cholesterol as well as lecithin, and a reduction in cholesteryl esters and lysolecithin. Plasma triglyceride concentrations are frequently elevated, and total cholesterol reduced. Plasma lipoproteins have an abnormal lipid composition and vesicular lipoproteins are present in LDL. LDL and HDL are particularly rich in triglycerides, and discoidal particles containing predominately apoE or apoA-I and apoA-II are present within HDL.

The deficiency of LCAT enzymic activity has important implications for plasma transport of cholesterol and cholesteryl esters. The ability of HDL to function in reverse cholesterol transport (reviewed above) is compromised, since free cholesterol derived from peripheral cells is normally esterified by LCAT and transferred to the hydrophobic core of the lipoprotein particle or exchanged into chylomicrons, VLDL, or LDL. Changes in cellular membranes (e.g., red cell membranes) and the vascular wall also result from the abnormality in cholesterol transport and esterification. The abnormalities in red blood cell membranes lead to hemolysis, and accumulation of lipids in the kidney results in renal deficiency and the development of cardiovascular disease.

PHYSICAL EXAMINATION. Corneal opacities are a characteristic clinical feature of LCAT deficiency (Fig. 145-12C). These are due to punctate stromal deposits, resembling those present in Tangier disease. No characteristic xanthomas are present in patients with LCAT deficiency. Signs of renal failure and atherosclerotic changes in major arteries due to premature cardiovascular disease usually occur during the later stages of the disease.

THERAPY. No definitive therapy is currently available for patients with LCAT deficiency. Renal transplant should be considered; however, the underlying enzyme defect presents a significant hazard to the graft.

Deficiency of ApoA-I and ApoC-III. A rare familial disease has been recognized in two separate kindreds in which there is a deficiency of both apolipoproteins A-I and C-III. Homozygotes lack apoA-I and apoC-III, have a virtual absence of HDL, and suffer severe premature cardiovascular disease. Plasma levels of apoA-I and apoC-III in heterozygotes are approximately 50 percent of normal levels. In the first reported kindred the female propositus had mild corneal opacifications in addition to premature coronary artery disease. Plasma VLDL and LDL concentrations were normal, and there were no xanthomas.

In the second kindred, two young women had yellowish planar xanthomas on the face and trunk, and corneal opacities in addition to extensive atherosclerosis. Plasma concentrations of VLDL and HDL were reduced and LDL was normal.

The deficiency of plasma apoA-I and apoC-III in both kindreds is likely due to a defect in expression of the apoA-I and apoC-III genes, both of which have been localized to human chromosome 11. The resulting severe deficiency of HDL is presumably responsible for the severe premature cardiovascular disease observed in these kindreds.

Fish eye disease. This rare disorder has been reported in two Swedish kindreds and is characterized clinically by severe corneal opacities (Fig. 145-12D), elevated plasma triglycerides, HDL levels reduced to 10 percent of normal, and atherosclerosis late in life. No xanthomas or lipid accumulation in parenchymal or reticuloendothelial tissue have been reported and the molecular defect in fish eye disease is unknown.

Deficiency of apoB-containing lipoproteins

Abetalipoproteinemia. CLINICAL SYNDROME. Abetalipoproteinemia is an autosomal recessive disease characterized in homozygotes by the absence of all lipoproteins containing both apolipoproteins B-48 and B-100. These include chylomicrons, VLDL, IDL, and LDL. The plasma concentrations of both triglycerides and cholesterol are thus extremely low (below 50 mg/dL). HDL are the only plasma lipoproteins and their composition is abnormal with increased proportions of free to esterified cholesterol and sphingomyelin to phosphatidylcholine. The heterozygotes for classical abetalipoproteinemia (see "Familial Hypobetalipoproteinemia" below) have no known clinical or biochemical abnormalities.

The clinical manifestations of abetalipoproteinemia include steatorrhea, retinitis pigmentosa, hemolytic anemia, and severe neurologic impairment. The first signs to appear are often related to malabsorption of fat during the first years of life. Radiographic findings are not diagnostic. Biopsy of the small intestine reveals a snow-white mucosa with unblunted, well-formed villi containing lipid-laden mucosal cells. These mucosal findings are characteristic and distinguish abetalipoproteinemia from celiac disease. Of clinical importance is the severe malabsorption of fat-soluble vitamins particularly A and E. Visual symptoms often present as night blindness due to vitamin A deficiency. During the course of the disease nystagmus becomes a common sign, and retinal degeneration may result in decreased visual acuity.

Acanthocytes with altered cholesterol and phospholipid composition appear and lead to episodes of hemolysis and anemia.

The most disabling manifestations of abetalipoproteinemia are neurologic dysfunctions including loss of motor as well as sensory function and ability to walk. The neurologic defects have been presumed to be due to a profound deficiency of vitamin E. During the late stages of the disease these symptoms may be severe. Death usually occurs in the fourth or fifth decade and may be related to cardiac arrhythmias.

The molecular defect in abetalipoproteinemia is unknown. Neither apolipoproteins B-48 or B-100 are present in plasma and no apoB immunoreactivity is detectable in the intestinal mucosa by immunofluorescence techniques. It is therefore probable that apoB-containing lipoproteins are not synthesized by the liver or intestinal cells. The inability to synthesize and secrete chylomicrons by the intestine results in malabsorption and deficiency of fat-soluble vitamins. The absence of hepatic production of VLDL severely diminishes the transport of endogeneous triglycerides and abolishes the transport of cholesterol to peripheral cells via the LDL receptor pathway.

PHYSICAL EXAMINATION. Decreased visual acuity, retinitis pigmentosa, and nystagmus are prominent physical findings (Fig. 145-13). Neurologic deficiencies may be severe with marked dysarthria, ataxia, loss of deep tendon reflexes, and decreased sensory discrimination. Cardiac arrhythmias may be detected.

THERAPY. Reduction in dietary fat may reduce diarrhea and fat malabsorption. Medium-chain triglycerides which are absorbed directly into the portal system can be used to supplement the fat-restricted diet. Large doses of water-soluble vitamins A and E may retard both retinal and central nervous system degeneration. Current studies with high-dose vitamin supplementation suggest that ocular as well as neurologic disease may be stabilized or prevented if such treatment is initiated at an early age.

Familial hypobetalipoproteinemia. CLINICAL SYNDROME. Familial hypobetalipoproteinemia is a rare autosomal disease which, like classical abetalipoproteinemia, is characterized in the homozygote by the absences of apoB-48 and apoB-100 containing lipoproteins in plasma. There are two major differences between these two clinical syndromes. First, the clinical manifestations of homozygous hypobetalipoproteinemia are milder than abetalipoproteinemia. Second, the heterozygous carrier state of familial hypobetalipoproteinemia is detectable by reduced concentrations of plasma LDL. In the homozygote, malabsorption of fat-soluble vitamins and lipid-laden columnar epithelial

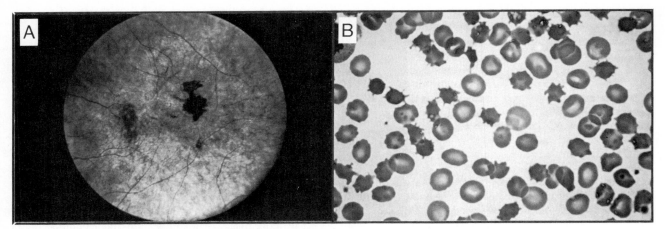

Fig. 145-13 Abetalipoproteinemia is characterized clinically by atypical retinitis pigmentosa (A) and acanthocytosis (B).

cells are present on intestinal biopsy. Acanthocytes are present in peripheral blood; however, hemolytic anemia is less frequent than in abetalipoproteinemia. Ocular manifestations include night blindness and the development of progressive retinal degeneration. Of particular importance in the clinical course of the disease in hypobetalipoproteinemia is the sparing of the neuromuscular system. The majority of the patients have minimal ataxia, cerebellar signs, and motor-sensory dysfunction. The reported cases have no difficulty in walking, which is in marked contrast to the severe neurologic dysfunctions observed in abetalipoproteinemia.

The biochemical basis of familial hypobetalipoproteinemia, like abetalipoproteinemia, appears to be a lack of biosynthesis of apoB, leading to a reduction in the formation of chylomicrons and hepatogenous VLDL. The molecular defect(s) in familial hypobetalipoproteinemia could include abnormalities at a number of sites in the intracellular assembly and transport of triglyceride-rich lipoproteins.

THERAPY. No therapy is required for heterozygotes. Homozygous patients with low plasma concentrations of fat-soluble vitamins should receive supplementation of large doses of vitamins A and E. The effect of high-dose therapy of vitamins A and E on the clinical progression of the disease has not been definitively ascertained.

Normotriglyceridemic abetalipoproteinemia. This rare disorder was discovered in a preadolescent female with plasma concentrations of cholesterol and triglycerides of 25 mg/dL and 30 mg/dL, respectively. Triglyceride-rich lipoproteins were present within VLDL; however, LDL were absent. Absorption of dietary fat was normal and plasma triglycerides increased after a fat meal. HDL levels were low and, in contrast to abetalipoproteinemia, the major HDL subfraction was HDL_3 and not HDL_2.

Clinically, the patient was obese, retarded, and had mild ataxia. There was no evidence of retinitis pigmentosa, and only a few acanthocytes were present in the peripheral smear. Vitamin A levels were normal; however, plasma vitamin E was undetectable.

The biochemical defect in normotriglyceridemic abetalipoproteinemia is the absence of apoB-100 containing lipoproteins in plasma. ApoB-48 containing lipoproteins from the intestine are present which is consistent with the ability of the patient to transport dietary lipid. Intestinal biopsy after a fat load was normal. The unique defect in this patient appears to be the lack of biosynthesis or processing of apoB-100 containing lipoproteins in the liver. These results support the concept that apolipoproteins B-48 and B-100 are under separate genetic control. Treatment of this patient has involved vitamin E supplementation with apparent improvement in her ataxia.

Bibliography

Brewer HB et al: Type III hyperlipoproteinemia: diagnosis, molecular defects, pathology, and treatment. *Ann Intern Med* **98:**623, 1983

Lippel K (ed): *Proceedings of the Workshop on Apolipoprotein Quantification.* DHHS NIH Publication No. 83-1266, 1983

Scanu AM, Landsberger FR (eds): Lipoprotein structure. *Ann NY Acad Sci* **348:**1, 1980

Stanbury JB et al (eds): *The Metabolic Basis of Inherited Disease,* 5th ed. Chap 29, Familial lipoprotein deficiency: abetalipoproteinemias, hypobetalipoproteinemias, and Tangier disease; Chap 30, Familial lipoprotein lipase deficiency and related disorders of chylomicron metabolism; Chap 31, Familial lecithin: cholesterol acyltransferase deficiency; Chap 32, Familial type 3 hyperlipoproteinemia (dysbetalipoproteinemia); familial hypercholesterolemia; Chap 34, Familial disease with storage of sterols other than cholesterol: cerebrotendinous xanthomatosis. New York, McGraw-Hill, 1983

CHAPTER 146

FABRY'S DISEASE: α-GALACTOSIDASE A DEFICIENCY (ANGIOKERATOMA CORPORIS DIFFUSUM UNIVERSALE)

Robert J. Desnick and Charles C. Sweeley

Fabry's disease, an inborn error of glycosphingolipid metabolism, results from the defective activity of the lysosomal enzyme, α-galactosidase A. The enzymatic defect, transmitted by an X-linked recessive gene, leads to the progressive deposition of neutral glycosphingolipids with terminal α-galactosyl moieties in most visceral tissues and fluids of the body (Fig. 146-1). The predominant glycosphingolipid accumulated in this disorder is globotriaosylceramide. The birefringent deposits are primarily found in the lysosomes of the vascular endothelium; progressive endothelial glycosphingolipid accumulation results in ischemia and infarction and leads to the major clinical manifestations of the disease. The glycosphingolipids also accumulate in perithelial and smooth muscle cells of the cardiovascular-renal system, and to a lesser extent in reticuloendothelial, myocardial, and connective tissue cells of the cornea, kidney, and other tissues, and in ganglion and perineural cells of the autonomic nervous system.

Clinically, hemizygous males have a characteristic skin lesion which led to the descriptive name of *angiokeratoma corporis diffusum universale*. They also have acroparesthesias, episodic crises of excruciating pain, corneal and lenticular opacities, hypohidrosis, and cardiac and renal dysfunction. Death usually occurs in adult life from renal, cardiac, and/or cerebral complications of their vascular disease. Heterozygous females are usually asymptomatic and are most likely to show the corneal opacities.

Historical aspects

In 1898, two dermatologists, Anderson [1] in England and Fabry [2] in Germany, independently described the first patients with angiokeratoma corporis diffusum. Anderson designated his case as one of angiokeratoma. His original patient was a 39-year-old male who had proteinuria, finger deformities, varicose veins, and lymphedema. Because of the proteinuria, Anderson suspected that the disease was a generalized disorder and astutely suggested that abnormal vessels might be present in the kidneys as well as in the skin. He also correctly noted that "the vascular lesion was not a new formation, as implied by the suffix 'oma', but an ectasia of cutaneous capillaries" [1]. Fabry originally made the diagnosis of purpura nodularis in a 13-year-old male whom he followed over the next 30 years (Fig. 146-2). He documented the presence of albuminuria, further described the cutaneous lesions, noting the presence of small-vessel aneurysms [3], and subsequently classified

his case to be one of *angiokeratoma corporis diffusum*, a designation that has persisted.

Several individuals made early contributions to the clinical description of the disease. Steiner and Voerner [4] and Gunther [5] described a hemizygous male with anhidrosis and intermittent acroparesthesias that were aggravated by hot or cold weather. Examination of a skin biopsy showed atrophy of the sweat glands and aneurysmal dilatation of the capillaries. Weicksel [6] first described the characteristic corneal opacities and the vascular abnormalities in the retina and conjunctiva. In 1947, Pompen and coworkers [7] reported the first postmortem findings in two affected brothers who died from renal failure. The most significant observation was the presence of abnormal vacuoles in blood vessels throughout their bodies. From these findings, they suggested that the disease was a generalized storage disorder. Subsequently, Scriba definitively established the lipid nature of the storage material [8] and Hornbostel and Scriba were the first to confirm the diagnosis histologically in a living patient by demonstrating the refractile lipid deposits in vessels of a skin biopsy specimen [9]. Although the familial occurrence of the disease was recognized earlier [10], it was not until 1965 that Opitz et al [11] documented the X-linked recessive inheritance of the disorder by pedigree analysis.

In 1963, Sweeley and Klionsky [12] isolated and characterized two neutral glycosphingolipids—globotriaosylceramide (Gal-Gal-Glc-Cer) and galabiosylceramide (Gal-Gal-Cer)—from the kidney of a Fabry hemizygote obtained at autopsy. On the basis of these findings, they classified Fabry's disease as a sphingolipidosis. Subsequent chemical analyses of various Fabry tissues and fluids [13–16] have demonstrated the marked accumulation of Gal-Gal-Glc-Cer, and to a lesser extent, Gal-Gal-Cer. In addition, the accumulation of blood group B substances, glycosphingolipids with terminal α-galactosyl moieties, have been reported in affected individuals with B or AB blood types [17].

In 1967, Brady et al [18] demonstrated that the enzymatic defect was in ceramide trihexosidase, a lysosomal galactosyl hydrolase required for the catabolism of Gal-Gal-Glc-Cer (Fig. 146-1). Kint [19], using synthetic substrates, characterized the defective enzymatic activity as an α-galactosyl hydrolase (designated α-galactosidase A). Shortly thereafter, several laboratories independently demonstrated that the accumulated glycosphingolipid substrates, including blood group B substances, all had α-

Trihexosyl Ceramide

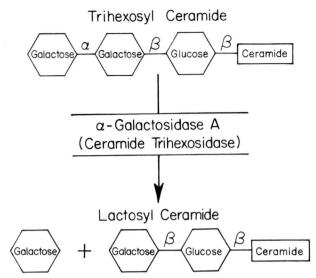

Fig. 146-1 The metabolic defect in Fabry's disease. Defective α-galactosidase A activity results in the accumulation of its major glycosphingolipid substrate, trihexosyl ceramide, which is also termed globotriaosylceramide.

linked terminal galactosyl residues. The elucidation of the specific enzymatic defect permitted the enzymatic diagnosis of affected hemizygous males, identification of heterozygous carrier females [20,21] and the prenatal diagnosis of hemizygous fetuses [22,23]. In addition, pilot trials of α-galactosidase A replacement have been reported [24–26]. The recent molecular cloning of a cDNA encoding the structural gene for human α-galactosidase A [27] should

Fig. 146-2 Distribution of angiokeratoma in the 30-year-old patient originally described by Dr. J. Fabry [2].

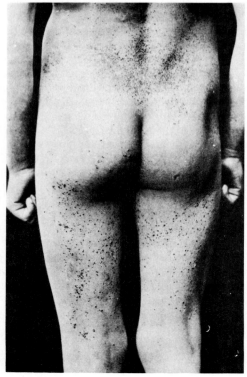

Table 146-1 Major clinical manifestations in hemizygotes with Fabry's disease

Vascular glycolipid deposition	Manifestation
Skin	Angiokeratoma
Peripheral nerves	Excruciating pain; acroparesthesias
Heart	Ischemia and infarctions
Brain	TIA and strokes
Kidney	Renal failure
Average age at death	41 years

facilitate characterization of the disease mutations, improve diagnosis especially of heterozygous carriers, and stimulate efforts to treat the disease.

Various designations have been used to identify this disorder. In keeping with the terminology applied to other lipidoses, and for the benefit of information retrieval, it would seem advisable to retain the commonly used eponym and to append the specific enzymatic defect. Thus, an appropriate designation is *Fabry's disease: α-galactosidase A deficiency.* Comprehensive reviews on the clinical, pathologic, biochemical, and genetic aspects of the disease are available [28–31].

Clinical manifestations

The hemizygote

The clinical manifestations of Fabry's disease predominantly result from the progressive deposition of Gal-Gal-Glc-Cer in the vascular endothelium (Table 146-1). Onset of the disease usually occurs during childhood or adolescence. Early manifestations include periodic crises of severe pain in the extremities (acroparesthesias), the appearance of vascular cutaneous lesions (angiokeratoma), hypohidrosis, and characteristic corneal and lenticular opacities.

Pain. The single most debilitating symptom of Fabry's disease is the pain, of which two types have been described: episodic crises and constant discomfort [10,32]. The painful crises most often begin in childhood or early adolescence and signal clinical onset of the disease. Lasting from minutes to several days, these "Fabry crises" consist of agonizing, burning pain initially in the palms and soles. Often the pain will radiate to the proximal extremities and other parts of the body. Attacks of abdominal or flank pain may simulate appendicitis or renal colic. The painful crises are usually triggered by exercise, fatigue, emotional stress, or rapid changes in temperature and humidity. With increasing age, the periodic crises usually decrease in frequency and severity; however, in some patients, they may occur more frequently and the pain can be so excruciating that the patient may contemplate suicide. Because the pain usually is associated with a low-grade fever and an elevated erythrocyte sedimentation rate, these symptoms frequently have led to the misdiagnosis of rheumatic fever, neurosis, or erythromelalgia [32].

In addition to these intermittent crises, most patients complain of a nagging, constant discomfort in their hands and feet characterized by burning, tingling paresthesias

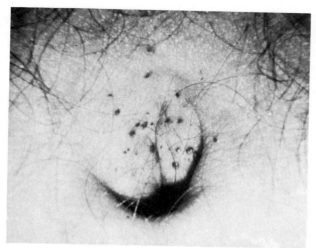

Fig. 146-3 Clusters of dark red angiokeratomas in the umbilical area of a hemizygote with Fabry's disease.

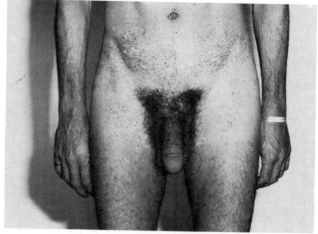

Fig. 146-4 Typical "swim suit" distribution of the angiokeratoma in a 28-year-old hemizygote with Fabry's disease.

[32]. These acroparesthesias may occur daily, usually during late afternoon, and may represent an attenuated form of the excruciating episodic crises. Although pain is a hallmark of the disease, it should be noted that about 10 to 20 percent of older patients deny a history of Fabry crises or acroparesthesias.

Skin lesions. Angiectases may be one of the earliest manifestations and may lead to diagnosis in childhood. There is a progressive increase in the number and size of these cutaneous vascular lesions with age. Classically, the angiokeratomata develop slowly as clusters of individual, punctuate, dark red to blue-black angiectases in the superficial layers of the skin (Fig. 146-3). The lesions may be flat or slightly raised and do not blanch with pressure. There is a slight hyperkeratosis notable in larger lesions. The clusters of lesions are most dense between the umbilicus and the knees and have a tendency toward bilateral symmetry (Fig. 146-4). The hips, back, thighs, buttocks, penis, and scrotum are most commonly involved, but there is a wide variation in the pattern of distribution and density of the lesions. Involvement of the oral mucosa and conjunctiva is common and other mucosal areas also may be involved. Variants without the characteristic skin lesions have been reported [33–36]. Although the angiectases may not be detected readily in some patients, careful examination of the skin, especially the scrotum and umbilicus, may reveal the presence of isolated lesions. In addition to these vascular lesions, anhidrosis, or more commonly hypohidrosis, is an early and almost constant finding.

Cardiac, cerebral, and renal vascular manifestations. With increasing age, the major morbid symptoms of the disease result from the progressive infiltration of glycosphingolipid in the vascular system. Cardiac disease occurs in most hemizygous males; common clinical manifestations include anginal chest pain, myocardial ischemia and infarction, congestive heart failure, and cardiac enlargement [37,38]. These findings may be accentuated by systemic hypertension related to vascular involvement of renal parenchymal vessels. Mitral insufficiency is the most frequent valvular lesion. Involvement of the myocardium and possibly the

conduction system results in electrocardiographic abnormalities which may show left ventricular hypertrophy, ST segment changes, and T wave inversion; other abnormalities including arrhythmias and an abbreviated PR interval have been reported [39]. Electrocardiographic patterns consistent with myocardial infarction have been seen. However, several cases with electrocardiographic changes indicating infarction had no evidence of myocardial necrosis at postmortem examination; the ECG changes were probably related to glycosphingolipid deposition in the myocardium [38]. Echocardiographic studies reveal an increased incidence of mitral valve prolapse and an increased thickness of the interventricular septum and the left ventricular posterior wall, particularly in adult hemizygous males [40,41]. In addition, hypertrophic obstructive cardiomegaly has been reported [42].

Cerebrovascular manifestations result primarily from multifocal small-vessel involvement and may include thromboses, basilar artery ischemia and aneurysm, seizures, hemiplegia, hemianesthesia, aphasia, labyrinthine disorders, or frank cerebral hemorrhage. Personality changes and psychotic behavior may become manifest with increasing age. A transient state of disorientation and confusion may occur in association with electrolyte imbalance secondary to renal disease. Severe neurologic signs may be present without evidence of major thrombosis or hypertension and are due presumably to multifocal small-vessel occlusive disease.

Progressive glycosphingolipid deposition in the kidney results in proteinuria and other signs of renal impairment, with gradual deterioration of renal function and development of azotemia in middle age. During childhood and adolescence, protein, casts, red cells, and desquamated kidney and urinary tract cells may appear in the urine. Birefringent lipid globules with characteristic "Maltese crosses" can be observed free in the urine and within desquamated urinary sediment cells by polarization microscopy (Fig. 146-5). With age, progressive renal impairment is evidenced by significant proteinuria, isosthenuria (specific gravities of 1.008 to 1.012), and alterations of other renal tubular functions including tubular reabsorption, secretion, and excretion [43]. Polyuria and a syn-

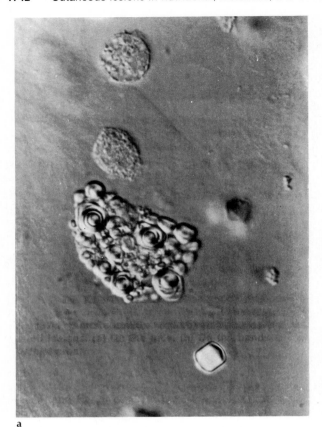

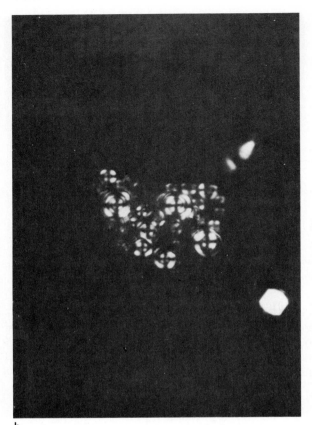

Fig. 146-5 **Photomicrographs of the urinary sediment from a heterozygote showing lipid accumulation by interference-microscopy (a) and polarization light microscopy (b). Note** **that Maltese crosses are observed under polarization. ×1000.**

drome similar to vasopressin-resistant diabetes insipidus occasionally develop. Gradual deterioration of renal function and the development of azotemia usually occur in the third to fourth decades of life, although the renal failure has been reported in the second decade. Death most often results from uremia unless chronic hemodialysis or renal transplantation is undertaken. The mean age at death of 94 hemizygous males who were not treated for uremia was 41 years [44], but occasionally an affected individual has survived into his sixties.

Ocular features. Ocular involvement is most prominent in the cornea, lens, conjunctiva, and retina [45–47]. A characteristic corneal opacity, observed only by slit-lamp microscopy, is found in males with the disease and in most heterozygous females (Fig. 146-6). The earliest lesion is a diffuse haziness in the subepithelial layer. In more advanced cases, the opacities appear as whorled streaks extending from a central vortex to the periphery of the cornea. Typically, the whorl-like opacities are inferior and cream-colored; however, they range from white to golden brown and may be very faint. An identical familial corneal dystrophy, termed *cornea verticillata,* was described by Gruber in 1946 [48]; subsequent investigation of these patients revealed that they were hemizygotes and heterozygotes for Fabry's disease [47]. An indistinguishable, drug-induced phenocopy of the Fabry corneal dystrophy occurs in patients on long-term chloroquine or amiodarone ther-

apy (see "Genetics"). Interestingly, a report has suggested that the corneal lesions regress in patients who wear contact lenses [49].

Two specific types of lenticular changes have been described. A granular anterior capsular or subcapsular deposit has been observed in about one-third of hemizygous males, but rarely in heterozygous females. Typically, these lenticular opacities are bilateral and inferior in position. They frequently appear in a "propeller-like" distribution, i.e., wedge-shaped with their bases near the lenticular equator and aligned radially with the apices toward the center of the anterior capsule. A second, and possibly unique, lenticular opacity has been observed in both hemizygous and heterozygous individuals [45,46]. It may be the first ocular manifestation to appear. The opacity is posterior, linear, and appears as a whitish, almost translucent, spokelike deposit of fine granular material on or near the posterior lens capsule. These lines usually radiate from the central part of the posterior cortex. This unusual opacity has been termed the "Fabry cataract" [45] and is best seen by retroillumination.

Conjunctival and retinal vascular lesions are common and represent part of the diffuse systemic vascular involvement. These vascular lesions occur early in life in normotensive individuals and are characterized by mild to marked tortuosity of the conjunctival and retinal vessels. There is an aneurysmal dilatation of thin-walled venules as well as angulation and segmental, sausagelike dilatation

Fig. 146-6 Corneal opacity in a heterozygote observed by slit-lamp microscopy. The corneal involvement results from subepithelial glycosphingolipid deposition.

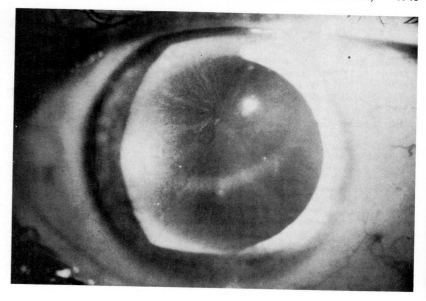

of veins typically seen on the inferior bulbar conjunctiva. As the disease progresses, retinal changes associated with the development of hypertension and uremia may be superimposed. Vision is not impaired by the vascular lesions in the conjunctiva and retina or by the corneal dystrophy. However, acute visual loss has occurred in hemizygotes as a result of unilateral total central retinal artery occlusion [45].

Other ocular findings have included lid edema in the absence of renal insufficiency, myelinated nerve fibers radiating from the optic disc, mild optic atrophy, papilledema, peripapillary edema, nystagmus, and internuclear ophthalmoplegia [45–47].

Other clinical features. Because of the widespread visceral distribution of the glycosphingolipid deposits, signs and symptoms of this disorder arise in many other organs and systems. Several patients have had chronic bronchitis, wheezing respiration, or dyspnea with alveolar capillary block. Pulmonary function studies in older hemizygotes may show significant airflow obstruction, reduced diffusing capacity, and a reduction in the $V_{max_{25}}$ values. Roentgenographic studies may reveal hyperinflation and/or bullous disease. Smokers have greater airflow obstruction than expected from smoking alone. In general, hemizygotes do not manifest significant clinical or functional pulmonary involvement on a primary basis [50]. Presumably the reported findings of pneumothorax, pleural effusions, and pulmonary edema were secondary to primary cardiac, vascular, and/or renal insufficiency. However, primary pulmonary involvement has been reported in the absence of cardiac or renal disease [51].

Lymphedema of the legs may be present in adulthood without hypoproteinemia, varices, or any clinically manifest vascular disease. This symptom presumably reflects the progressive glycosphingolipid deposition in the lymphatic vessels and lymph nodes. Many patients have varicose leg veins and hemorrhoids. Priapism also has been reported.

Episodic diarrhea and, to a lesser extent, nausea, vomiting, and flank pain, are the most common gastrointestinal complaints [52]; these symptoms may be related to deposition of glycosphingolipid in intestinal small vessels and in the autonomic ganglia of the bowel [53]. Perforation of the small bowel has been described. Although intestinal malabsorption has been reported, it is not a recognized feature of the disease. Radiologic studies reveal thickened, edematous folds and mild dilatation of the small bowel, a granular-appearing ileum, and the loss of haustral markings throughout the colon, particularly in the distal segments [52]. The symptomatology and pathophysiology of the gastrointestinal involvement have been reviewed [52–54].

Anemia is probably due to decreased red blood cell survival. A decreased serum iron concentration, normal red blood cell fragility, and an elevated reticulocyte count have been reported [28]. Lipid-laden, foamy-appearing macrophages are present in the bone marrow. The spleen is not enlarged.

Many patients have evidence of musculoskeletal involvement. A characteristic permanent deformity arises from changes in the distal interphalangeal joint of the fingers, causing limited extension of the terminal joints [10]. Avascular necrosis of the head of the femur or talus, multiple small infarct-like opacities in the femoral heads, and involvement of the metacarpals, metatarsals, and temporal mandibular joint have been described.

Many hemizygous males appear to have retarded growth or delayed puberty and sparse, fine facial and body hair. In some kindreds, an acromegalic-like appearance has been reported. Affected individuals may complain of fatigue and weakness and may be incapacitated for prolonged periods of time.

The heterozygote

The clinical course and prognosis of heterozygotes and hemizygotes differ significantly. Heterozygotes experience little difficulty in adult life when hemizygous males already have severe renal and/or cardiac involvement. Although most biochemically documented heterozygotes are asymptomatic throughout a normal lifespan, with increasing age, many manifest minor symptoms of the disease (Table

Table 146-2 Clinical manifestations in heterozygotes for Fabry's disease

Manifestation	Estimated incidence*	Remarks
Corneal dystrophy	~ 80%	Useful for heterozygote identification
Angiokeratoma	~ 30%	Single or isolated lesions
Acroparesthesias	< 10%	Infrequent; hands and feet; RLQ
Hypohidrosis	< 1%	Rare variants†
Cardiac involvement	< 1%	Rare variants†
CNS involvement	< 1%	Rare variants†
Renal failure	< 1%	Rare variants†

* Based on review of over 122 heterozygous females, 1 to 85 years old, evaluated at our Center.
† Rare variants with 0 to 5 percent α-galactosidase A activity.

146-2). Some heterozygotes will develop cardiac involvement with advanced age [55]. However, a few heterozygotes have been reported in whom the expression was comparable to that observed in severely affected hemizygous males [37,56]. In contrast, obligate heterozygotes (daughters of affected hemizygous males) without clinical or biochemical evidence of the disease have also been described [57], further documenting the extensive variability of the heterozygote expression in this disease. Of more than 150 heterozygotes reported in the literature, corneal involvement is the most frequent and often the singular manifestation [45]; frequently the corneal dystrophy is more prominent than in affected males in the same family. However, biochemically documented and/or obligate heterozygous females without corneal opacities have been described [10,46,57].

The skin lesions are much less prominent in affected females than in males; often they are not clinically manifest. The lesions may occur in the characteristic distribution; isolated lesions may occasionally be seen on the breasts, lips, and trunk. The lesions have been detected in heterozygotes during childhood. Skin biopsies of clinically uninvolved skin from obligate heterozygotes obtained in the first decade of life contain deposits of glycosphingolipid in the vascular endothelial and muscularis cells.

Other manifestations may include intermittent pain in the extremities, edema (particularly of the ankles), vascular lesions in the conjunctiva and retina, and cardiovascular changes such as hypertension, electrocardiographic abnormalities, and left ventricular hypertrophy [10,34,44]. Basilar artery aneurysms also have been reported. Urologic symptoms in heterozygotes include hyposthenuria, the occurrence of erythrocytes, leukocytes, and granular and hyaline casts in the urinary sediment, proteinuria, and other signs of renal impairment. Mucosal lesions, hypohidrosis, and diarrhea have been recorded less frequently. Heterozygotes may develop arthritis in the distal interphalangeal joints of the fingers.

Pathology

Morphologically, Fabry's disease is characterized by widespread tissue deposits of crystalline glycosphingolipid which show birefringence with typical Maltese crosses under polarization microscopy (Fig. 146-5). The glycosphingolipid is deposited in all areas of the body, occurring predominantly in the lysosomes of endothelial, perithelial, and smooth-muscle cells of blood vessels (Fig. 146-7) and, to a lesser degree, in histiocytic and reticular cells of connective tissue. Lipid deposits are also prominent in epithelial cells of the cornea and glomeruli and tubules of the kidney, in muscle fibers of the heart, and in ganglion cells of the autonomic system.

Pathology of the skin

The skin lesions are telangiectases or small superficial angiomas (Fig. 146-8). After a silent period, cumulative vascular damage leads eventually to clinically apparent and progressive angiectases. This sequence is suggested by the biopsy finding of lipid deposits in areas of clinically normal skin [58,59] or in patients with no skin lesions [60], and by recognition of patients who have visceral lesions but whose skin lesions either were of minimal consequence or were

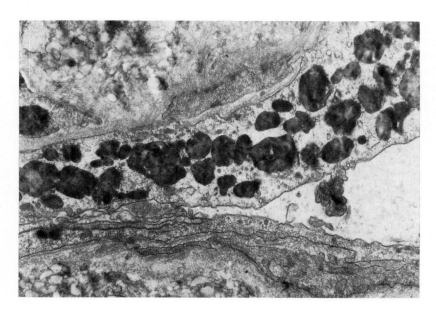

Fig. 146-7 Electron micrograph of a section of an arteriole from the jejunum of a hemizygote showing the marked accumulation of concentric lamellar inclusions in the lysosomes of the vascular endothelium. The progressive lysosomal deposition of the glycosphingolipid substrate leads to the narrowing and eventual occlusion of the vascular lumen. × 25,000 *(Courtesy of Dr. J. G. White, University of Minnesota.)*

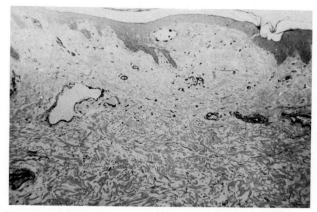

Fig. 146-8 Telangiectatic vessels in the dermis that are typical of the changes seen in the skin.

delayed. The pathologic involvement was observed in the vascular endothelium and perithelium of clinically normal skin from a 1-year-old hemizygote [59].

Capillaries, venules, and arterioles contain pathologic lipid storage in the endothelium, perithelium, and smooth muscle (Fig. 146-7). There is marked dilatation of the capillaries of the dermal papillae. Deeper vessels show less dilatation and aneurysm formation. Lipid stores have been noted in arrectores pilorum muscles, sweat gland epithelium, and perineural cells [58–62]. Similar findings have been observed in gingival tissues. Atrophic or scarce sweat and sebaceous glands have been reported.

The fully developed classic lesions are usually located in the upper dermis, where they may produce elevation, flattening, or hypertrophy of the epithelium. The larger lesions may have a slight to moderate hyperkeratosis, hence the term *angiokeratoma*. As in all forms of angiokeratomas, the hypertrophy and hyperkeratosis may be secondary to pressure on the epithelium by the underlying dilated vessel.

Fig. 146-9 Photomicrograph of glomerulus and renal tubules from a 35-year-old hemizygote. The epithelial cells of the parietal and visceral layers of Bowman's capsule show multiple vacuoles from which the stored glycosphingolipids were extracted during fixation and staining. Zenker's fixation, paraffin embedding, hematoxylin and eosin. × 225.

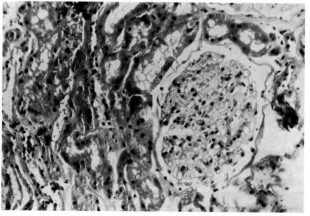

Pathology of the kidney

The earliest lesions are due to the accumulation of glycosphingolipid in endothelial and epithelial cells of the glomerulus and of Bowman's space and in the epithelium of the loops of Henle and of distal tubules (Fig. 146-9). In later stages and, to a lesser degree, proximal tubules, interstitial histiocytes and fibrocytes may show lipid accumulation. Lipid-laden distal tubular epithelial cells desquamate and may be detected in the urinary sediment (Fig. 146-5).

Concurrently, renal blood vessels are involved progressively and often extensively. An early finding is the presence of arterial fibrinoid deposits which may result from the necrosis of severely involved muscular cells. Other histologic changes in the kidney are the sequelae of nonspecific, end-stage renal disease with evidence of severe arteriolar sclerosis, glomerular atrophy and fibrosis, pseudotubular proliferation of residual glomerular epithelium, tubular atrophy, and diffuse interstitial fibrosis. Renal size increases during the third decade of life followed by a decrease in the fourth and fifth decades. The renal involvement has been the subject of comprehensive reviews [43,61,63].

Pathology of the nervous system

Vascular involvement also is prominent in the nervous system [64–71] and presumably accounts for the observation of minor EEG and EMG abnormalities in these patients. In addition, vascular ischemia and lipid deposition in the perineurium may cause the peripheral nerve conduction abnormalities of slowed conduction velocities and distal latency, respectively. In both heterozygotes and hemizygotes, glycosphingolipid deposition in nervous tissue appears to be limited to perineural sheath cells of peripheral nerves, neurons of the peripheral and central autonomic nervous system, and certain primary neurons of somatic afferent pathways [8,65–69,72]. Lipid deposition was observed in Schwann cells by some, but not by other investigators [68,69]. Qualitative [65–68] and quantitative [67] studies of peripheral sensory neurons in sural nerves and spinal ganglia have shown preferential loss of small myelinated and unmyelinated fibers as well as small cell bodies of spinal ganglia [67,73].

Brain stem centers that are involved include the nuclei gracilis and cuneatus, the dorsal autonomic vagal nuclei, salivary nuclei, nucleus ambiguus, thalamus, reticular substance, mesencephalic nucleus of the fifth nerve, and the substantia nigra [67,68]. Hemisphere involvement has been noted in the amygdaloid, hypothalamic, and hippocampal nuclei. Recent studies have revealed abnormal lipid deposits in the fifth and sixth cortical layers of the inferior temporal gyrus, the Edinger-Westphal nucleus, the parasympathetic cell column, and the midline nucleus [68]. Lipid storage in neuronal cells of the anterior and posterior lobes of the pituitary has been described. Detailed reviews of the neurologic findings are available [68,72].

Pathology of the eye

Histologically, abnormal glycosphingolipid deposits are found in endothelial, perivascular, and smooth-muscle cells of all ocular and orbital vessels, in smooth muscle of the iris and ciliary body, in perineural cells, and in connective tissue of the lens and cornea [74,75]. Inclusions have been localized in the epithelium of the conjunctiva, cornea, and lens, and, by electron microscopy, in the basal layer of conjunctival epithelial cells as well as in the surface epithelium. There may be hyperplasia and edema of corneal epithelial cells. Bowman's membrane appears normal and no deposits are observed in the stroma or endothelium by light or electron microscopy. It has been suggested that the whorl-like corneal dystrophic pattern may result from the formation of a series of subepithelial ridges or from the reduplication of the basement membrane [74,75].

Pathology of the heart

The progressive deposition of glycosphingolipid in myocardial cells and valvular fibroblasts appears to be a primary cause of cardiac disease in hemizygotes and some heterozygotes [16,37,38]. Gross cardiomegaly involving all chambers has been observed. Most commonly, the left atrium and ventricle are enlarged and the ventricular walls and septum are markedly thickened; right atrial and ventricular dilatation and enlargement are variable findings. Within the myocardial cells, there is extensive glycosphingolipid deposition around the nucleus and between myofibrils. The vessels show marked hypertrophy of the endothelial cells and smooth-muscle cells secondary to lipid deposition.

Mitral and tricuspid valves have numerous lipid-laden cells embedded in fibrous tissue [16]. The most common valvular defect is thickening and interchordal hooding of the leaflets of the mitral valve, with normal chordae tendineae and either normal or thickened and shortened papillary muscles. The tricuspid valve may be similarly involved; the aortic and pulmonary valves are usually normal. Clinical and pathologic features of cardiac involvement in both hemizygotes and heterozygotes have been reviewed [16,37,38].

Histochemistry and ultrastructure

The accumulated glycosphingolipids are birefringent and show a Maltese cross configuration in polarized light (Fig. 146-5). They can be stained in frozen sections with lipid-soluble dyes, and may be removed from tissues by the process of dehydration and embedding in paraffin. If lipid-solubilizing procedures are used, empty vacuoles are observed by light microscopy. Most of the lipid crystals are retained through alcohol dehydration, but are lost on exposure to xylene or pyridine. Exposure of formalin-fixed tissue to 3% potassium chromate for one week helps to preserve the lipid; improved fixation of the lipid deposits can be achieved with 1% calcium formol. A comparison of various fixation and embedding techniques to preserve the storage material has been reported [76]. A modified PAS stain specific for neutral glycosphingolipids [77], and a positive test for sphingosine [78] have served to confirm the chemical identification of the accumulated glycosphingolipids. Peroxidase- or fluorescent-labeled *Bandeiraea simplicifolia* lectin, which is specific for α-D-galactosyl residues, and anti-globotriaosylceramide antibodies also have been used to selectively stain the glycosphingolipid substrates [76,79,80].

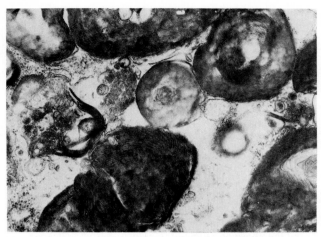

Fig. 146-10 Electron photomicrograph of a section of the mitral valve from a hemizygote with Fabry's disease, showing the concentric lamellar inclusions in lysosomes of fibrocytes. × 65,000. *(Courtesy of Dr. H. L. Sharp.)*

The ultrastructural characteristics of the lesions and of the lipid inclusions in various tissues from hemizygous males have been described extensively (e.g., [81–83]). At high resolution, a typical pattern of concentric or lamellar inclusions with alternating light- and dark-staining bands is observed (Fig. 146-10). The periodicity of these bands has been reported variably as 40 to 50 Å, 50 to 60 Å, 60 to 65 Å, or as great as 98 Å. The electron-dense component is 20 to 30 Å in thickness. These inclusions have coarser periods of 150 to 200 Å.

The metabolic defect in Fabry's disease

The enzymatic defect

The primary metabolic defect in Fabry's disease is the defective activity of the lysosomal enzyme, α-galactosidase A [18,19], in the tissues and fluids of affected individuals. The deficient activity in hemizygotes and heterozygotes has been demonstrated with the radiolabeled natural substrate, globotriaosylceramide [18], and with synthetic chromogenic or fluorogenic substrates (e.g., [19–21]). Studies with the synthetic substrates have revealed that affected hemizygotes have residual α-galactosidase activity which is approximately 10 to 25 percent of that observed in material from normal subjects. The residual activity was determined to be due to the presence of another enzyme, α-N-acetylgalactosaminidase (previously designated α-galactosidase B) on the basis of physical, kinetic, and immunologic properties [20,21,84–88].

The inability to detect α-galactosidase A activity in affected hemizygotes is consistent with the accumulation of glycosphingolipid substrates with terminal α-galactosyl moieties. The intermediate levels of α-galactosidase A activity in most heterozygous females are associated with a less severe accumulation of globotriaosylceramide and galabiosylceramide in plasma, urinary sediment, and cultured skin fibroblasts, as shown in Table 146-3. In addition, the observed transmission of the defective α-galactosidase A activity in families with Fabry's disease is consistent with

Table 146-3 Mean concentration of globotriaosylceramide and galabiosylceramide in various sources from normal individuals and hemizygotes and heterozygotes with Fabry's disease

Glycosphingolipid/source	Normal	Heterozygotes	Hemizygotes
Globotriaosylceramide:			
Plasma	2.1*	4.5	7.6
Urinary sediment	26*	405	1570
Cultured fibroblasts	660*	1260	2430
Galabiosylceramide:			
Plasma	n.d.†	n.d.	n.d.
Urinary sediment	trace	183	247
Cultured fibroblasts	n.d.	n.d.	n.d.

* Concentrations expressed as nmol/mL plasma, nmol/24 h urine, nmol/g dry weight cultured fibroblasts.
† n.d. = not detectable.
Sources: Vance et al [13], Desnick et al [14], Dawson et al [89].

the inheritance of a mutant gene for this catalytic gene product on the X chromosome (see "Genetics").

α-Galactosidase A isolated from normal tissues and fluids is a relatively heat-labile glycoprotein that catalyzes the hydrolysis of substrates possessing α-galactosidic residues, including various synthetic water-soluble substrates and naturally occurring glycosphingolipids and glycoproteins. Maximal activity of α-galactosidase A is obtained at about pH 4.5 with 4-methylumbelliferyl-α-galactoside. The Michaelis constant (K_m) of the reaction with this substrate is about 2.5 mM [20,86,90–92]. The highest specific activities obtained to date were reported with human liver [91], spleen, and placenta [90]. In addition, a heat-stable glycoprotein activator has been identified which enhances α-galactosidase activity in vitro [93]. The M_r of native α-galactosidase A from human tissues is approximately 101,000 [90–92,94]. Polyacrylamide gel electrophoresis in the presence of sodium dodecyl sulfate (SDS) has consistently shown a diffuse band of subunits with M_r of about 49,000 [27,90–92,95], indicating that the enzyme probably has a homodimeric structure. Biosynthetic studies have shown that the enzyme is synthesized as a precursor ($M_r \cong 58,000$) which is processed to a mature enzyme ($M_r \cong 49,000$) in cultured Chang liver cells [95].

α-Galactosidase A is a glycoprotein containing one or more asparagine-linked complex oligosaccharide chains. Multiple forms are observed upon isoelectric focusing of purified preparations from plasma and various tissues. The isoelectric points of the tissue forms of α-galactosidase A range from 4.4 to as high as 5.1 [90], whereas the plasma form has a pI of 4.2 [92]. The plasma and tissue forms of the enzyme are converted by neuraminidase to a single form with a sharp isoelectric focusing band of higher pI, suggesting that the heterogeneity is the result of variations in the amount of sialic acid on the carbohydrate chain. It has been suggested that the plasma form may contain 10 to 12 sialic acid residues, whereas the placental form of α-galactosidase A has only 1 or 2 residues [90]. This property is of considerable importance in connection with the circulatory half-life of enzyme administered intravenously to patients with Fabry's disease [26], and may also be a factor determining which organs acquire enzyme activity after infusion.

The more heat-stable form of α-galactosidase activity in human tissues, called α-galactosidase B, has been purified to apparent homogeneity from human liver and placenta [94,96]. Kinetic studies of α-galactosidase B indicate that it probably functions in vivo as an α-N-acetylgalactosaminidase rather than as an α-galactosidase [87,88, 94,96]. Based on biochemical and immunologic studies [86,94,97], it has been concluded that α-galactosidase B is probably identical to the α-N-acetylgalactosaminidases isolated independently from various sources by monitoring activity with *p*-nitrophenyl-α-N-acetylgalactosaminide [98].

The nature of accumulated glycosphingolipids

The deficient activity of α-galactosidase A in patients with Fabry's disease leads to the progressive accumulation of glycosphingolipids with terminal α-galactosyl residues in the lysosomes of most non-neural tissues and in body fluids. These substances are structurally and metabolically members of a family of glycosphingolipids that are widely distributed in human tissues as normal constituents of plasma membranes and possibly of subcellular membranes as well. The lipoidal moiety of glycosphingolipids is a hydrophobic structure called *ceramide,* which consists of a mixture of 4-sphingenine long-chain aliphatic amines joined in amide linkages with various fatty acids. Carbohydrate groups are attached by a glycosidic linkage between the reducing end of the carbohydrate and the terminal hydroxyl group of the ceramide.

$$\text{Carbohydrate} \cdots \text{O—CH}_2\text{CHCHC}=\text{C(CH}_2)_{12}\text{CH}_3$$

Ceramide

The glycosphingolipids involved in Fabry's disease are of the type called neutral glycosphingolipids, as contrasted with the gangliosides, which contain one or more acidic sialic acid groups, and the sulfoglycosphingolipids, which contain a sulfate monoester group on the carbohydrate moiety.

In living organisms, the glycosphingolipids are localized in the membranes of cells and in transport complexes such as lipoproteins. During their synthesis, and when ex-

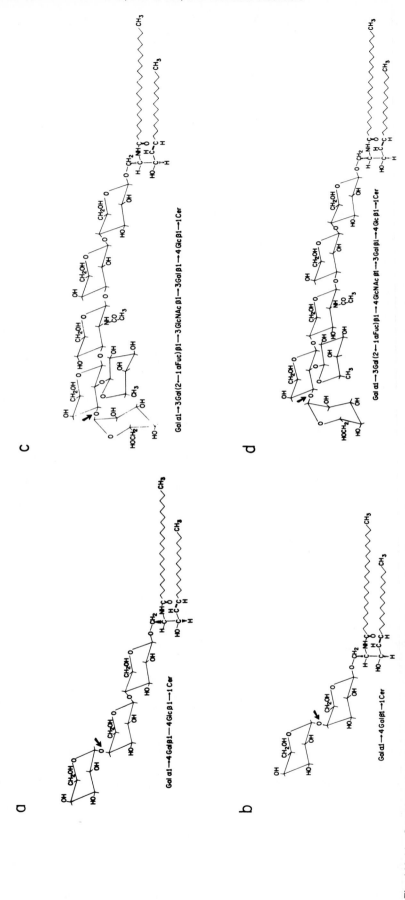

Fig. 146-11   Complete chemical structures of the neutral glycosphingolipids that accumulate in Fabry's disease. (a) Globotriaosylceramide, Gal-Gal-Glc-Cer, the major accumulated substrate. (b) Galabiosylceramide, Gal-Gal-Cer. (c and d) The blood group B antigenic glycosphingolipids which accumulate in blood group B and AB patients. The arrows indicate the α-galactosyl bonds which are normally cleaved by α-galactosidase A.

changed from one membrane to another, they may be attached to cytosolic exchange proteins [99]. Glycosphingolipids of the plasma membrane are believed to be associated primarily with the outer half of the bilayer in such a way that the carbohydrate residues extend from the surface of the cell into the extracellular environment.

In Fabry's disease there is widespread accumulation of the glycosphingolipid, globotriaosylceramide [Gal($\alpha1\rightarrow4$) Gal($\beta1\rightarrow4$)Glc($\beta1\rightarrow1'$)Cer], particularly in the lysosomes of vascular endothelial cells as well as in epithelial and perithelial cells of most organs. Chemical analyses have shown that the accumulated glycosphingolipid isolated from tissues of patients with Fabry's disease is identical with that of normal tissues. The positions of glycosidic linkages, the anomeric configurations of these linkages, and the fatty acid compositions of globotriaosylceramide from normal and Fabry tissue have been rigorously established [28]. The complete structure of this glycosphingolipid, shown in Fig. 146-11a, has been chemically synthesized [100]. It is notable that globotriaosylceramide is a cell-specific marker for Burkitt's lymphoma [101].

A second neutral glycosphingolipid, galabiosylceramide [Gal($\alpha1\rightarrow4$)Gal($\beta1\rightarrow1'$)Cer], also occurs in abnormally high concentrations in the kidneys, pancreas, and urinary sediment of patients with Fabry's disease [12,14,15]. Some of this glycosphingolipid may also occur abnormally in other tissues as well, such as lung and the right-sided heart structures [16]. The chemical structure of the carbohydrate moiety of galabiosylceramide obtained from Fabry kidney has been established [28]. The complete structure is shown in Fig. 146-11b.

Other accumulated glycosphingolipids were identified in patients who had blood group B activity. Certain tissues from such patients contained abnormal quantities of two neutral glycosphingolipids that inhibit blood group B-specific hemagglutination, (IV^2-α-fucosyl-IV^3-α-galactosyl-lactotetraosylceramide and IV^2-α-fucosyl-IV^3-α-galactosyl-neolactotetraosylceramide) [17]. These substances have been shown to occur on the membranes of human erythrocytes which express the blood group B antigens [17]. The structures of the glycosphingolipids from Fabry tissues were established by biochemical, enzymatic, and immunologic properties to be identical to the H$_1$ and H$_2$ glycosphingolipids of human erythrocytes [17]. The complete structures of these blood group B-active glycosphingolipids are shown in Fig. 146-11c and d.

Abnormal distribution in tissues

The distribution of glycosphingolipids in the organs and tissues of patients with Fabry's disease has been investigated (e.g., [12,15]). Increased concentrations of globotriaosylceramide were found in all sources analyzed except erythrocytes [13,15], which indicates that most tissues are involved in the catabolism of these glycosphingolipids. In one affected male, the magnitude of glycosphingolipid accumulation was 30- to 300-fold higher than normal levels [15]. The greatest levels were observed in kidney, lymph nodes, vessels, prostate, and autonomic ganglia. In addition, the accumulation of galabiosylceramide has been reported to occur only in the kidney, pancreas, heart, lungs, and urinary sediment [12,14–16]. Table 146-3 indicates the average levels of the globotriaosylceramide and galabiosyl-

ceramide in plasma, urinary sediment, and cultured skin fibroblasts from hemizygotes, heterozygotes, and normal subjects. The two blood group B-active neutral glycosphingolipids have only been found accumulated in Fabry patients who have blood group B specificity [17].

Pathophysiology

The pattern of glycosphingolipid deposition in Fabry's disease, particularly its predilection for vascular endothelial and smooth-muscle cells, is uniquely different from that seen in other glycosphingolipidoses [102]. However, the origin of the accumulated glycosphingolipid substrates has not been fully clarified. Certainly there is a significant contribution from the endogenous synthesis and subsequent lysosomal accumulation of terminal α-galactosyl containing glycosphingolipids following autophagy of cellular membranous material containing these lipid substrates. Endogenous metabolism presumably is the major source of substrate accumulation in avascular sites such as cornea and in neural cells which presumably are protected from the increased circulating levels of Gal-Gal-Glc-Cer by the blood-brain barrier. In addition, the turnover of Gal-Gal-Glc-Cer, and particularly its precursor, globotetraosylceramide (globoside) which are present in higher concentrations in normal renal tissue than in any other tissue, are presumably responsible for the endogenous renal deposition of the Fabry substrate.

The unique cellular and tissue distribution of accumulated Gal-Gal-Glc-Cer, particularly in the vascular endothelium (Fig. 146-7) and smooth muscle, suggests that a significant intracellular contribution may be derived by the endocytosis or diffusion of Gal-Gal-Glc-Cer from the circulation where the concentration is three- to tenfold higher than that of normal individuals. In Fabry hemizygotes and normal individuals, the circulating Gal-Gal-Glc-Cer is primarily transported in the low-density (LDL) and high-density (HDL) lipoprotein fractions [28,103–105]. In plasma from hemizygotes, the accumulated Gal-Gal-Glc-Cer is distributed in the LDL and HDL fractions in proportions similar to those in normal plasma, approximately 60 and 30 percent, respectively. The finding that little, if any, substrate deposition occurs in Fabry hepatocytes (in contrast to the accumulation in Kupffer cells [76,106]) supports the contention that Gal-Gal-Glc-Cer synthesized by the hepatocyte is associated with lipoprotein and secreted as a complex [107]. In support of this concept is the fact that patients with hypercholesterolemia have proportional plasma elevations of both LDL and neutral glycosphingolipids including Gal-Gal-Glc-Cer [103]. The circulating Gal-Gal-Glc-Cer then presumably gains access to vascular endothelial and smooth-muscle cells throughout the body by the high-affinity lipoprotein receptor-mediated uptake pathway [108–110]. Deposits in other tissues also may be derived to a lesser extent from receptor-independent diffusion or by nonabsorptive endocytosis of globoside- or Gal-Gal-Glc-Cer-lipoprotein complexes from the plasma. Since lysosomes in all cells are deficient in the α-galactosidase A activity needed to degrade the accumulated glycosphingolipids, they accumulate within extended multivesicular bodies or, in more advanced stages, as free intracytoplasmic masses which may lead to cellular dysfunction or degeneration.

In addition to hepatocyte biosynthesis, glycosphingolipids are synthesized in the bone marrow where they become incorporated into the membranes of the formed blood elements [13,111,112]. It has been postulated that erythrocyte globoside (Gal-Nac-Gal-Gal-Glc-Cer), the predominant glycosphingolipid of erythrocytes and the catabolic precursor of Gal-Gal-Glc-Cer (Fig. 146-11), may be another major metabolic source of the circulating pathogenic lipid. Globoside is presumably released into the circulation from senescent erythrocytes [111] and is subsequently catabolized (presumably in the spleen) to Gal-Gal-Glc-Cer. In Fabry's disease, the Gal-Gal-Glc-Cer cannot be metabolized and may be partly released into the circulation where it can be incorporated into both HDL and LDL fractions [107], and/or rapidly cleared by the liver as has been shown for intravenously administered neutral glycosphingolipids [113]. Thus, the turnover of erythrocyte and other membrane glycosphingolipids may contribute significantly to the substrate load in Fabry's disease. In addition, a minor amount of Gal-Gal-Glc-Cer may be "excreted" into the circulation from the secondary lysosomes of various cell types throughout the body. Since the glycosphingolipid cannot be catabolized in the circulation, it would slowly accumulate at a rate reflecting the turnover of various cells, the contribution from exocytosis, lipoprotein uptake, and/or diffusion.

The metabolism of at least two other compounds is also abnormal, as demonstrated by the accumulation of galabiosylceramide, Gal-Gal-Cer, and the blood group B antigenic substances. Hemizygous and heterozygous individuals who are blood group type B or AB appear to be more severely affected, presumably due to the additional accumulation of B-specific glycosphingolipids [30]. Thus, the total amount of glycosphingolipid stored in a given tissue depends on time, the rate of accumulation from intracellular and circulatory sources, the possibilities for excretion, the individual's ABO blood type, and the presence or absence of residual α-galactosidase A activity (see "Genetic Variants").

The pattern of glycosphingolipid accumulation, predominantly in the cardiovascular-renal system, best correlates pathophysiologically with the major clinical manifestations of the disease as selectively described below.

Pathophysiology of the vasculature

Narrowing, dilatation, motor unresponsiveness, and instability of blood vessels are major features of the altered physiology in Fabry's disease. The swollen vascular endothelial cells, often accompanied by endothelial proliferation, encroach upon the lumen (Fig. 146-7) causing a focal increase of intraluminal pressure, dilatation, and angiectases as well as peripheral ischemia or frank infarction [114]. Such changes are frequently the precursors of thromboses and infarcts of the brain and other tissues. Muscle and peripheral nerve ischemia may contribute to the pain or fatigue [70,115].

There may be progressive aneurysmal dilatation of the weakened vascular wall. This process is apparent in the progressive dilatation and microaneurysm formation of the retinal and conjunctival vessels and in the transition from normality to telangiectasia and frank angiokeratoma in the skin.

Observed alterations of vasomotor control may reflect either the vascular lesions themselves or the extensive glycosphingolipid deposits in autonomic ganglia and perineural sheath cells (e.g., [71,116,117]). Both hemizygotes and heterozygotes with Fabry's disease demonstrate an impaired ability for vasoconstriction, and the more severely involved hemizygotes show, in addition, an inability to vasodilate. Such a combined vascular and neural lesion may also explain the clinically observed temperature intolerance.

Pathophysiology of the nervous system

The involvement of peripheral and central autonomic nerve cells may be responsible for the paresthesias, pain, hypohidrosis, such gastrointestinal symptoms as nausea and diarrhea, and a variety of vague neurologic signs and symptoms. Fukuhara et al [115] found marked degeneration of the secretory cells and myoepithelial cells of sweat glands by electron microscopy and proposed that the hypohidrosis was due to local lipid deposition rather than autonomic nervous system involvement. The episodic fevers may be related to lesions of the hypothalamus [72]. The observations of a selective decrease in the number of unmyelinated and small myelinated fibers in peripheral nerves [65,68,69,73,116,118,119] have led to the suggestion that the selective damage to these fibers may account for the pain production and hypohidrosis in this disorder. Studies of autonomic function revealed sympathetic and parasympathetic dysfunction, particularly in distal cutaneous responses [71,116]. Alternatively, it has been suggested that the lipid deposition in the vasa nervorum may lead to the acroparesthesias rather than involvement of the autonomic nervous system [115,116,118].

Pathophysiology of the kidney

The observed disorders in renal function have their basis in lesions of the nephron and of the renal vasculature, and possibly in disorders of the posterior pituitary and hypothalamus. Early glycosphingolipid deposits antedate clinical signs and symptoms. During this early period, the lesions of the renal vasculature are less prominent than those of the nephron, and renal architecture is maintained. The observed mild proteinuria may be explained by alteration of the glomerular epithelial cells and their foot processes [63] or by increased desquamation of lipid-laden tubular epithelial cells [79].

Loss of renal concentrating ability with polyuria and polydypsia may occur well in advance of a significant decrease in glomerular filtration or evidence of renal failure [43]. The defect in concentrating ability may be due to decreased water permeability of the distal tubules and collecting ducts secondary to lipid deposition. The diabetes insipidus-like syndrome, which is not related to faulty electrolyte transfer in distal tubules, may result from tubular insensitivity to antidiuretic hormone or to combined dysfunction of the renal tubular cells and lesions of the glycosphingolipid-laden supraoptic nucleus, and antidiuretic center of the hypothalamus. The later and more severe renal changes are the result of vascular lesions and of hypertension.

Pathophysiology of the heart

The progressive deposition of glycosphingolipids in the myocardial cells, the valvular fibroblasts, and the coronary vessels is the primary cause of cardiac disease in hemizygotes and some heterozygotes [16,37,38]. The frequent findings of left ventricular hypertrophy and mitral insufficiency are presumably related to the fact that the left ventricular myocardium and the mitral valve are the sites of the most marked lipid deposition in the heart [16]. The abnormally short PR interval and the finding of cardiomyopathy on EKG may be related to lipid deposition in the myocardium and/or conduction system [39]. The marked deposition of Gal-Gal-Glc-Cer in the coronary arteries leads to myocardial ischemia and frank infarction [16,37,38].

Other involvement

Pulmonary symptoms have been attributed to involvement of lung vasculature or bronchial and mucous gland epithelium [50]. The airflow obstruction may be due to the loss of elastic recoil secondary to lipid deposition in lung parenchyma. The lymphedema presumably results from lymphatic obstruction or venous insufficiency secondary to lipid-laden endothelial cells.

Reports of growth retardation, delayed puberty, abnormal beard, or impaired fertility associated with a decrease of gonadotropins, may correlate with observations of testicular atrophy [120] or with glycosphingolipid storage in anterior and posterior lobes of the pituitary gland [76] or in the interstitial cells of the testis. No explanations have been offered for the frequently observed acromegalic-like appearance.

Genetics

Mode of inheritance

Fabry's disease is transmitted by an X-linked recessive gene which normally encodes the gene product, α-galactosidase A. Somatic cell hybridization studies of human–hamster hybrid fibroblasts have localized the α-galactosidase A structural gene to a narrow region on the long arm of the X-chromosome, Xq21-q22 [121,222]. The gene for human α-galactosidase B (α-N-acetylgalactosaminidase) has been assigned to chromosome 22 by somatic cell hybridization techniques [123], further distinguishing α-galactosidases A and B at the genic level. The evidence for the X-linked recessive inheritance of this disease has been reviewed in detail [28].

The frequency of Fabry's disease has not been determined; the disease is rare and it is estimated that the incidence is about 1:40,000. Of the over 400 described cases of hemizygous males, most are white; however, black, Latin American, Egyptian, and Oriental cases have been observed.

The Fabry gene is highly penetrant in the hemizygote. Clinical onset is variable, occurring usually during childhood, but may be delayed until the second or third decade. Both intrafamilial and interfamilial variations in the clinical expression have been reported, the intrafamilial being less than the interfamilial variation.

Expressivity in the heterozygote is variable. Approximately 30 percent of the heterozygotes have a few, isolated skin lesions, a smaller percentage have the characteristic intermittent pain in the extremities, and about 80 percent have whorl-like corneal dystrophy. Proven heterozygotes may be completely asymptomatic throughout a normal life span. Obligate heterozygotes without any clinical manifestations and with normal levels of leukocyte α-galactosidase and urinary sediment glycosphingolipids have been reported [57,124]. In contrast, complete clinical and biochemical expression of the disease, as severe as in affected hemizygotes, has been documented in several heterozygotes [37,124]. The markedly variable expression of the Fabry gene in heterozygous females is anticipated for X-linked enzymatic deficiencies by the random X-inactivation hypothesis [125]. At the cellular level, this hypothesis predicts that heterozygotes for X-linked enzymatic defects will have two populations of cells, one clone with mutant and the other with normal enzymatic activity. Two such populations have been cloned from individual cultured skin fibroblasts from obligate heterozygotes, one with normal and the other with defective α-galactosidase A activities [126]. Ultrastructural examination of renal tissue from heterozygotes also demonstrated two populations of glomerular, interstitial, and vascular cells: one normal, the other in which glycosphingolipid deposition was observed.

Genetic variants

Although most affected hemizygotes present with the typical clinical features and disease progression, rare variants have been described with milder disease manifestations [35,127–129]. In contrast to the typical patients who have nondetectable α-galactosidase A activity, biochemical investigation of these variants has revealed the presence of residual α-galactosidase A activity. The occurrence of the residual activity in the variants is consistent with less substrate accumulation and attenuation or absence of the characteristic clinical manifestations.

In 1971, Clarke et al [35] described a 38-year-old Italian male who presented with proteinuria and hypercholesterolemia; biopsied renal tissue revealed the typical histologic and ultrastructural abnormalities of Fabry's disease. There was no history of acroparesthesias and no angiokeratoma or corneal opacities were observed. Urinary sediment glycosphingolipid analyses demonstrated levels of Gal-Gal-Glc-Cer in the heterozygote range and low levels of Gal-Gal-Cer [35]. This patient died at age 49 years after a second myocardial infarction. His total α-galactosidase activities (A and B) in cultured skin fibroblasts and leukocytes were about 30 percent of normal. Subsequently, the residual α-galactosidase A in cultured fibroblasts was partially purified and shown to have kinetic and thermostability properties similar to normal α-galactosidase A. About 20 percent of normal α-galactosidase A activity was detected in fibroblasts, but the amount of cross-reactive immunologic material (CRIM) was not quantitated [130].

More recently, we evaluated a 42-year-old male with severe rheumatoid arthritis and proteinuria, who was referred following renal biopsy which revealed ultrastructural findings consistent with Fabry's disease [127]. He denied a history of acroparesthesias or hypohidrosis. No angiokeratoma, corneal or lenticular opacities, or cardiac manifestations were found. Creatinine clearance and concentrating ability were normal. Levels of α-galactosidase A activity were about 1 percent of normal in plasma and urine, confirming the diagnosis. Specific immunoprecipitation with monospecific anti-α-galactosidase A antibodies demonstrated residual A activity in granulocytes, lymphocytes, platelets, liver, and cultured fibroblasts ranging from 9 to 37 percent of normal levels. The immunoprecipitated residual α-galactosidase A activity from fibroblasts had the same kinetic and physical properties as the immunoprecipitated enzyme from normal fibroblasts. However, compared to the normal enzyme, the residual fibroblast α-galactosidase A was more thermolabile at pH 4.6 and 50°C, and significantly more pH unstable at pH 7.4 and 37°C; this is consistent with the extremely low enzyme level in plasma and urine. Interestingly, the levels of Gal-Gal-Glc-Cer in plasma and urinary sediment were in the low heterozygote ranges. No lysosomal inclusions were observed in hepatocytes or Kupffer cells in biopsied liver. Rocket immunoelectrophoresis studies demonstrated that the level of α-galactosidase A activity corresponded to the amount of enzyme protein. These findings are consistent with a stability mutation, resulting in an enzyme with normal kinetics. In this variant, it appears that 10 to 40 percent of normal intracellular activity is sufficient to prevent the majority of the clinical manifestations of the disease. In addition, the finding of only 1 percent of enzymatic activity in the plasma and low levels of plasma Gal-Gal-Glc-Cer suggests that circulating enzyme is not required to catabolize the plasma substrate.

Several other variants also have been reported. Bach et al [128] described a 51-year-old asymptomatic male who had 10 percent of normal α-galactosidase A activity and normal levels of globotriaosylceramide in his urinary sediment. Further enzymatic studies revealed that the residual enzymatic activity had a K_m value which was fourfold higher than normal and an increased stability. Kobayashi et al [129] studied a 26-year-old Japanese variant who had a history of acroparesthesias, but no angiokeratomas, keratopathy, or hypohidrosis. Although the level of α-galactosidase A activity in this patient was typical of classical hemizygotes, loading studies indicated that his cultured skin fibroblasts were able to hydrolyze some of the exogenously supplied substrate.

Genetic nature of the enzymatic defect

Several different mutations involving the α-galactosidase A structural gene have been presumptively identified by biochemical and immunologic techniques, although the number of unrelated hemizygotes studied to date is small. These include the atypical variants with residual α-galactosidase A activity (described in the preceding section), classical hemizygotes with no detectable activity and very low, but detectable levels of enzyme protein, and classical hemizygotes with no detectable α-galactosidase A activity or enzyme protein. Efforts in our laboratory have been directed to determine the presence of CRIM to normal α-galactosidase A in classical hemizygotes with Fabry's disease. Using a monospecific rabbit antibody to homogeneous placental α-galactosidase A (which does not cross-react with α-galactosidase B), the presence of CRIM was evaluated by rocket immunoelectrophoresis in tissues from

six unrelated Fabry hemizygotes, who had no detectable α-galactosidase A activity. To date, tissues from four hemizygotes were CRIM-negative; however, CRIM corresponding to about 1 to 5 percent of normal enzyme protein levels was detected in the tissues of two other unrelated hemizygotes. Other investigators have detected only CRIM-negative mutations [131,132]. These findings support the presence of heterogeneity in the structural gene mutations responsible for this disease.

Presumably, variants with residual activity and classical hemizygotes with immunologically detectable, but nonfunctional enzyme protein result from point mutations in the α-galactosidase A structural gene. The classical hemizygotes with no detectable enzymatic activity or enzyme protein may result from (1) point mutations which alter the enzyme conformation, rendering it markedly unstable and subject to rapid degradation, (2) point mutations which cause premature termination of transcription or translation or mRNA processing defects, or (3) partial or complete gene deletions, analogous to those recently identified in the β-thalassemias [133]. The recent cloning of a cDNA for human α-galactosidase A [27] should permit the elucidation of the molecular defects underlying the enzyme deficiency in unrelated families as well as provide the means for carrier identification by gene analysis.

Phenocopies

A phenocopy is a phenotypic mimic or simulation of a specific genetic trait. Since a phenocopy is usually the result of environmental factors, it is not inherited. There are two such phenocopies for Fabry's disease, one that mimics the characteristic corneal opacity and another that causes renal functional and ultrastructural changes resembling those in hemizygotes. Since the diagnosis of Fabry's disease is often suspected from an eye examination or renal evaluation for proteinuria, these phenocopies have significant diagnostic import.

The whorl-like keratopathy of Fabry's disease is readily distinguishable from the corneal opacities of other lysosomal storage diseases, but is clinically and ultrastructurally identical to the corneal dystrophy associated with long-term chloroquine therapy [134,135]. Chloroquine has been shown to concentrate rapidly in lysosomes, increase the intralysosomal pH, decrease the activity of specific lysosomal hydrolases, alter the rate of proteolysis, and cause the formation of lysosomal inclusions. Based on these findings, it has been proposed that the chloroquine-induced keratopathy results from the pH inactivation of lysosomal α-galactosidase A and the subsequent accumulation of Gal-Gal-Glc-Cer [135]. In support of this concept is the finding that corneal α-galactosidase A is more sensitive to increasing pH in vitro than other lysosomal hydrolases [136]. Similar studies have shown that chloroquine inactivated the α-galactosidase A activity in cultured human skin fibroblasts [137]. These findings demonstrate the likely mechanism responsible for the phenocopy and represent the first biochemical elucidation of a human phenocopy. More recently, amiodarone has been shown to cause a phenocopy of the Fabry keratopathy; although presumed to act like chloroquine, the mechanism underlying the amiodarone-induced pathology has not been characterized [138].

Another tissue-specific phenocopy of Fabry's disease

occurs in individuals who are environmentally exposed to silica dust. The pulmonary complications of silicolipoproteinosis have been described, but the renal manifestations of proteinuria and lipiduria have received little attention. Ultrastructural examination of renal tissue from these individuals has revealed the typical electron-dense lamellar inclusions in the lysosomes of glomerular epithelial and endothelial cells and proximal and distal tubular cells observed in Fabry's disease [139]. The levels of α-galactosidase A and urinary sediment glycosphingolipids were normal in one such patient [139]. Although the mechanism responsible for the silica-induced phenocopy is unknown, the finding of such lesions in biopsied renal tissue should include silicosis as well as Fabry's disease in the differential diagnosis.

Genetic counseling

Genetic counseling should be available to all families in which the diagnosis of Fabry's disease is made. Inheritance of the Fabry gene from hemizygotes and heterozygotes should be considered, since both genotypes transmit the gene. All sons of hemizygous males will be unaffected, but all daughters will be obligate carriers of the gene. On the average, half the sons of heterozygous females will have the disease and half the daughters will be carriers. All possible carriers among close female relatives should be examined clinically and biochemically for heterozygote identification. Fabry's disease has been detected antenatally from cultured fetal cells and amniotic fluid obtained by amniocentesis as well as from chorionic villus samples (see "Prenatal Diagnosis").

Diagnosis

Clinical evaluation

The clinical diagnosis in hemizygous males is most readily made from the history and by observation of the characteristic skin lesions and corneal dystrophy. The most common childhood symptom before appearance of the cutaneous lesions is recurrent fever in association with pain of the hands and feet. The disorder has been often misdiagnosed as rheumatic fever, neurosis, erythromelalgia, or collagen vascular disease. Differential diagnosis of the cutaneous lesions must exclude the angiokeratoma of Fordyce [140,141], angiokeratoma of Mibelli [142], and angiokeratoma circumscriptum [143,144], none of which has the typical histologic or ultrastructural pathology of the Fabry lesion (Fig. 146-8). The angiokeratomata of Fordyce are similar in appearance to those of Fabry's disease, but are limited to the scrotum, and usually appear after age 30. The angiokeratomata of Mibelli are warty lesions on the extensor surfaces of extremities in young adults which are associated with chilblains. Angiokeratomata circumscriptum or neviformus can occur anywhere on the body, are clinically and histologically similar to those of Fordyce, and are not associated with chilblains.

Angiokeratomata reportedly similar to or indistinguishable from the clinical appearance and distribution of the cutaneous lesions in Fabry's disease have been described in patients with other lysosomal storage diseases, including fucosidosis [145], sialidosis (α-neuraminidase deficiency with or without β-galactosidase deficiency) [146], adult-type β-galactosidase deficiency [147], aspartylglucosaminuria [148], and a recently reported lysosomal disorder which presents with mental retardation and some features of the mucopolysaccharidoses [149]. Ultrastructural examination of these lesions reveals lysosomal substrate deposition which differs in the fine structural appearance of the respective storage material. In addition, patients with classical-appearing angiokeratoma, but no other clinical symptoms or morphologic evidence of lysosomal storage have been described [150,151]; these patients have had normal levels of α-galactosidase A and other lysosomal hydrolase activities. Clinical and pathologic details of the differential diagnosis of the skin lesions are available in reviews [58,152–154].

Presumptive diagnosis of hemizygotes can be made by a careful ophthalmologic examination, demonstration of the birefringent inclusions in the urinary sediment, or by skin or bone marrow biopsy. The observation of the characteristic corneal dystrophy observed by slit-lamp examination should aid in the diagnosis. Biopsied skin will reveal the characteristic refractile lipid inclusions (Maltese crosses) in blood vessels [59]. Lipid-containing macrophages may also be observed in bone marrow aspirates. Women suspected of being heterozygous carriers of the Fabry gene should be carefully examined for evidence of the characteristic corneal opacity by slit-lamp microscopy and for isolated skin lesions, particularly on the breasts, back, trunk, and posterolateral thighs. Detection may also be accomplished by the histologic finding of lipid-laden cells in biopsied skin, tissues, or in the urinary sediment.

Biochemical confirmation

All suspect hemizygotes should be confirmed biochemically by the demonstration of deficient α-galactosidase A activities in plasma or serum, leukocytes, tears, biopsied tissues, or cultured skin fibroblasts (e.g., [20,21,84,85, 155,156]). Alternatively, multiprocedural glycosphingolipid analyses can be accomplished to demonstrate the increased levels of Gal-Gal-Glc-Cer in urinary sediment, plasma, or cultured skin fibroblasts [13,14,89] (Table 146-3).

Suspect heterozygotes should be biochemically identified by their intermediate levels of α-galactosidase A activity in the above sources (Fig. 146-12). If borderline normal values of α-galactosidase A activity are obtained, then the enzyme levels should be determined in a series of single hair roots, which are presumably derived from single cells and should express either normal or hemizygous levels of activity [157–159]. The genotypic diagnosis also may be made by the demonstration of increased concentrations of Gal-Gal-Glc-Cer and Gal-Gal-Cer in urinary sediment. Further documentation of heterozygosity, if necessary, can be accomplished by cloning cultured skin fibroblasts followed by the demonstration of two cell populations, normal and deficient, for α-galactosidase A activity [80,126].

Prenatal diagnosis

Prenatal diagnosis of Fabry's disease can be accomplished by the assay of α-galactosidase A activity in chorionic villi obtained at 9 to 10 weeks of pregnancy or in cultured amniotic cells obtained by amniocentesis at approximately 15 weeks of pregnancy [22,23,160,161]. The prenatal diagnosis of an affected hemizygous male fetus minimally

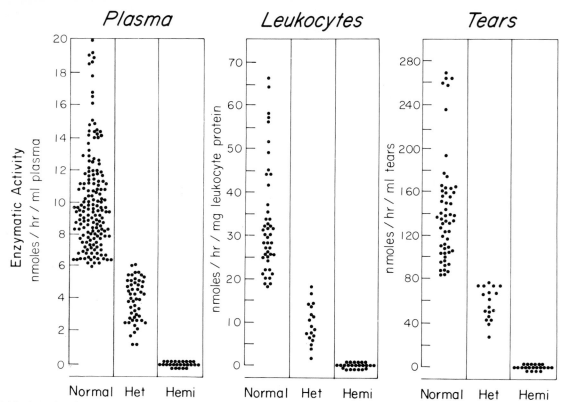

Fig. 146-12 Levels of α-galactosidase A activity in plasma (or serum), isolated leukocytes, and tears from normal individuals and heterozygotes (Het) and hemizygotes (Hemi) with Fabry's disease.

requires the demonstration of deficient α-galactosidase A activity and an XY karyotype.

Biochemical and ultrastructural studies of tissues from fetuses with Fabry's disease have been reported [22,160,161]. Consistent with the prenatal diagnosis, the α-galactosidase A activity was defective in all tissues studied; increased concentrations of globotriaosylceramide were found in all tissues analyzed with the exception of neural tissues [160]. Histologic and light microscopic examination of various tissues were unremarkable, but ultrastructural examination revealed electron-dense concentric lamellar inclusions in the lysosomes of vascular endothelium, renal tubules, and epithelial and endothelial cells of renal glomeruli [160,161].

Treatment

Medical management

In Fabry's disease the chronicity of the clinical events causes severe debilitation and incapacity that extends over years. The single most debilitating and morbid aspect of Fabry's disease is the excruciating pain. The pathophysiologic events that cause the incapacitating episodes of pain or the chronic burning acroparesthesias have not been clarified. Numerous drugs have been tried for the relief of these agonizing pains [10]. The α-adrenergic blocking agent, phenoxybenzamine, which increases peripheral vas-

cular flow, has been administered for pain relief; although this drug provided relief in a hemizygote on several occasions, priapism and epistasis were early complications in two other hemizygotes [162]. With the exception of centrally acting narcotic analgesics, which have been only partially effective, conventional analgesic agents have not been successful. However, prophylactic administration of low maintenance dosages of diphenylhydantoin have been found to provide relief from the periodic crises of excruciating pain and constant discomfort in hemizygotes and heterozygotes [32]. Lenoir et al [163] noted that carbamazepine also provided pain relief. The combination of diphenylhydantoin and carbamazepine significantly reduced the pain in an affected hemizygote [164]. Subsequent reports have further documented the effectiveness of diphenylhydantoin and/or carbamazepine in the prevention and amelioration of these debilitating pains [165].

Care of patients with regard to cardiac, pulmonary, and central nervous system manifestations remains nonspecific and symptomatic. Obstructive lung disease has been documented in older hemizygotes and heterozygotes, with more severe impairment in smokers; therefore, patients should be discouraged from smoking. Since renal insufficiency is the most frequent late complication in patients with this disease, chronic hemodialysis and/or renal transplantation have become life-saving procedures. In addition to treatment of the renal failure, kidney transplantation has been undertaken to determine whether the allograft could provide normal α-galactosidase A for substrate metabolism [56,166]. Hypothetically, the normal kidney might metabolize the accumulated substrate by uptake and catabolism within the allograft and/or by the release of the active enzyme into the circulation for uptake and metabolism in other tissues such as the vascular endothelium. Although biochemical and/or clinical improvement have been reported in several recipients (e.g. [56,166–170]), no biochemical effect could be demonstrated in other recipients [171–174]. Patients with successful engraftment who survived for more than ten years, have expired from cardiac disease complications [175,176]. Thus, the use of renal allografts to alter the rate of progressive substrate accumulation remains unclear and further studies are required to determine the long-term biochemical effects of this strategy. In view of these results, renal transplantation should be undertaken only in patients with clinically significant renal failure.

At present, the most practical and effective therapy is preventive. Screening of all suspect heterozygotes, genetic counseling, and prenatal diagnostic studies should be made available to all at-risk families (see "Genetics"). Family and vocational counseling should be provided, especially to families with affected children. Often, parents, teachers, and/or physicians misinterpret the excruciating pain experienced during childhood as psychosomatic, especially in the absence of any objective physical or laboratory findings. Since physical exertion, emotional stresses, and fatigue, as well as rapid changes in the environmental temperature and humidity can trigger these painful episodes, appropriate arrangements must be made with physical education teachers and other individuals to minimize or eliminate stressful activities. In addition, young hemizygotes should be allowed to pursue selected activities and be permitted to stop these activities at their own discretion. Within this perspective, reasonable occupational and vocational objectives should be pursued. Vocational counseling should discourage occupations that require significant manual dexterity, physical exertion, emotional stress, or exposure to rapid changes in temperature or humidity.

Enzyme replacement and substrate depletion strategies

Attempts to replace the defective α-galactosidase A activity with normal enzyme have been undertaken in vitro and in vivo. Studies using partially purified α-galactosidase A from fig [177] and human sources [177,179; D. L. Johnson and R. J. Desnick, unpublished results] supplied in the media of cultured skin fibroblasts from Fabry hemizygotes demonstrated the ability of the exogenous enzyme to gain access to and catabolize the accumulated substrate, Gal-Gal-Glc-Cer. These in vitro studies indicated the feasibility of enzyme replacement and in particular, demonstrated that low levels (~5 percent) of exogenous enzyme, particularly the high uptake form [178], were capable of effecting normalization of substrate metabolism.

Several in vivo exploratory studies of enzyme replacement have been undertaken to determine whether such endeavors can decrease the circulating accumulated substrate concentration. Normal plasma containing active enzyme has been administered to hemizygotes with Fabry's

disease [24]. Although active enzyme and decreased levels of Gal-Gal-Glc-Cer were demonstrated in the recipients' plasmas, the major limitation was the short half-life ($T_{1/2}$ ~ 95 min) of the infused enzymatic activity. Subsequently, Brady and coworkers [25] partially purified a tissue form of α-galactosidase A from human placenta and intravenously administered single doses to two patients (6,000 and 11,000 units, respectively). The exogenous activity was rapidly cleared from the recipients' circulation with half-lives of 10 and 12 min, respectively. The plasma substrate was decreased about 50 percent at 45 min with a return to the preinfusion level by 48 h. In addition, the administered activity was detected in percutaneously biopsied liver at 1 h [25].

More recently, a clinical trial of enzyme replacement was performed involving multiple injections of purified splenic and plasmic forms of α-galactosidase A into two brothers with Fabry's disease [26]. This trial confirmed the previously observed differences in clearance rates of enzyme from the circulation and demonstrated for the first time the differential substrate depletion and reaccumulation kinetics for enzyme purified from tissue vs. plasma sources [180]. The differential plasma clearance of these enzyme forms was presumably related to differences in the posttranslational modifications of these glycoproteins. The splenic form, which was rapidly cleared from the circulation ($T_{1/2} \cong 10$ min), contained few sialic acid residues. The plasma form, however, was highly sialylated and was retained in the circulation ($T_{1/2} \cong 70$ min) [26]. These results are in accordance with the Ashwell model for the prolonged retention of sialylated glycoproteins in the circulation and the rapid clearance of desialylated glycoproteins [181].

A marked difference in the clearance of circulating substrate was observed after the administration of these isozymes [26,180,182]. Administration of α-galactosidase A isolated from human spleen effected a rapid decrease in the plasma concentration of accumulated substrate. The level of the circulating substrate decreased to approximately 50 percent of the preinfusion values 15 min after injection followed by a rapid return to preinfusion levels by 2 to 3 h. In contrast, the administration of α-galactosidase A from human plasma resulted in a prolonged depletion of the circulating substrate. At 2 h after injection, the levels of Gal-Gal-Glc-Cer were decreased by 50 to 70 percent of the preinfusion values. Significantly, low levels were retained up to 12 to 24 h and the substrate levels slowly returned to preinfusion levels after 36 to 72 h. When the total amount of substrate cleared with time was calculated by integrating the mean concentrations of Gal-Gal-Glc-Cer, the plasma enzyme appeared to have cleared about 25 times more substrate over time than the splenic form. When two doses are administered on subsequent days, the plasma substrate level was reduced into normal range [180]. In addition, these clinical trials demonstrated that multiple doses of either partially purified enzyme, administered over a 117-day period, did not elicit an immune response in the recipients. Although these studies demonstrated the feasibility of enzyme therapy for Fabry's disease, the current limitation of this approach is the availability of the purified human enzyme. The recent cloning of a cDNA encoding α-galactosidase A [27] will facilitate efforts to use recombinant DNA techniques for the expression of large amounts of enzyme for future trials of replacement therapy and, perhaps, gene replacement.

Recently, fetal liver has been transplanted in three hemizygotes with Fabry's disease in an attempt to replace the deficient enzyme [183]. The rise and subsequent fall in the levels of serum α-fetoprotein evidenced the initial survival and subsequent maturation (or possible loss) of the fetal cells. Following transplantation, the α-galactosidase A levels in sera and leukocytes were unchanged and the substrate levels in urine and sera were slightly decreased. However, the recipients noted subjective clinical improvement (e.g., increased sweating, no acroparesthesias, slightly decreased angiokeratoma). The effectiveness of fetal liver transplantation must await the long-term evaluation of these recipients to document its efficacy.

Another approach that has been employed to deplete the accumulated circulating substrate is chronic plasmapheresis [184]. Three plasmaphereses, performed at two-day intervals, resulted in a 70 percent reduction of the level of circulating Gal-Gal-Glc-Cer to a value within the normal range. A total of 23 mg of substrate was removed. The plasma substrate levels slowly returned to preplasmapheresis levels in five days. Similar results have been observed with chronic plasmapheresis performed over a six-month period (D. F. Bishop and R. J. Desnick, unpublished data). The major question to be resolved is whether intervention by chronic plasmapheresis will deplete enough substrate, compared to that newly synthesized, so that the net result is decreased substrate deposition in the target sites of pathology, the vascular endothelium. Thus, further evaluation is required to determine the value of this strategy in Fabry's disease. Another therapeutic attempt to decrease the plasma substrate levels involved chronic phlebotomies which were performed in an attempt to remove senescent erythrocytes, a source of the accumulated glycosphingolipid [185]. However, following chronic blood depletion for almost six months, the levels of plasma Gal-Gal-Glc-Cer unexpectedly increased, indicating that this approach was not therapeutic.

Recent reviews of the various approaches for the treatment of enzyme deficiency diseases are available [186,187].

References

1. Anderson W: A case of angiokeratoma. *Br J Dermatol* **10**:113, 1898
2. Fabry J: Ein Beitrag zur Kenntnis der Purpura haemorrhagica nodularis (Purpura papulosa haemorrhagica Hebra). *Arch Derm Syph (Berlin)* **43**:187, 1898
3. Fabry J: Weiterer Beitrag zur Klinik des Angiokeratoma naeviforme (Naevus angiokeratosus). *Dermatol Wochenschr* **90**:339, 1930
4. Steiner L, Voerner H: Angiomatosis miliaris: eine ideiopathische Gefasserkrankung. *Dtsch Arch Klin Med* **96**:105, 1909
5. Gunther H: Anhidrosis und Diabetes insipidus. *Z Klin Med* **78**:53, 1913
6. Weicksel J: Angiomatosis, bzw. Angiokeratosis universalis (eine sehr seltene Haut- und Gafasskrankheit). *Dtsch Med Wochenschr* **51**:898, 1925
7. Pompen AWM et al: Angiokeratoma corporis diffusum (universale) Fabry, as a sign of an unknown internal disease: two autopsy reports. *Acta Med Scand* **128**:234, 1947
8. Scriba K: Zur Pathogenese des Angiokeratoma diffusum Fabry mit cardio-vasorenalem Symptomenkomplex. *Vehr Dtsch Ges Pathol* **34**:221, 1950
9. Hornbostel H, Scriba K: Zur Diagnostik des Angiokeratoma Fabry mit kardio-vasorenalem Symptomenkomplex als Phosphatidspeicherungskrankheit durch Probeexcision der Haut. *Klin Wochenschr* **31**:68, 1953
10. Wise D et al: Angiokeratoma corporis diffusum: a clinical study of eight affected families. *Q J Med* **31**:177, 1962
11. Opitz JM et al: The genetics of angiokeratoma corporis diffusum (Fabry's disease), and its linkage with Xg(a) locus. *Am J Hum Genet* **17**:325, 1965
12. Sweeley CC, Klionsky B: Fabry's disease: classification as a sphingolipidosis and partial characterization of a novel glycolipid. *J Biol Chem* **238**:3148, 1963
13. Vance DE et al: Concentrations of glycosyl ceramides in plasma and red cells in Fabry's disease: a glycolipid lipidosis. *J Lipid Res* **10**:188, 1969
14. Desnick RJ et al: Diagnosis of glycosphingolipidoses by urinary sediment analysis. *N Engl J Med* **284**:739, 1971
15. Schibanoff JM et al: Tissue distribution of glycosphingolipids in a case of Fabry's disease. *J Lipid Res* **10**:515, 1969
16. Desnick RJ et al: Cardiac valvular anomalies in Fabry's disease: clinical, morphologic and biochemical studies. *Circulation* **54**: 818, 1976
17. Wherret JR, Hakomori S: Characterization of a blood group B glycolipid, accumulating in the pancreas of a patient with Fabry's disease. *J Biol Chem* **218**:3046, 1973
18. Brady RO et al: Enzymatic defect in Fabry's disease: ceramide trihexosidase deficiency. *N Engl J Med* **276**:1163, 1967
19. Kint JA: Fabry's disease, α-galactosidase deficiency. *Science* **167**:1268, 1970
20. Desnick RJ et al: Enzymatic diagnosis of hemizygotes and heterozygotes. Fabry's disease. *J Lab Clin Med* **81**:157, 1973
21. Johnson DL et al: Fabry disease: diagnosis of hemizygotes and heterozygotes by α-galactosidase A activity in tears. *Clin Chim Acta* **63**:81, 1975
22. Brady RO et al: Fabry's disease: antenatal diagnosis. *Science* **172**:172, 1971
23. Desnick RJ, Sweeley CC: Prenatal detection of Fabry's disease, in *Antenatal Diagnosis,* edited by A Dorfman. Chicago, Univ of Chicago Press, 1971, p 185
24. Mapes CA et al: Enzyme replacement in Fabry's disease, an inborn error of metabolism. *Science* **169**:987, 1970
25. Brady RO et al: Replacement therapy for inherited enzyme deficiency: use of purified ceramidetrihexosidase in Fabry's disease. *N Engl J Med* **289**:9, 1973
26. Desnick RJ et al: Enzyme therapy XII: Enzyme therapy in Fabry's disease: differential enzyme and substrate clearance kinetics of plasma and splenic α-galactosidase isozymes. *Proc Natl Acad Sci USA* **76**:5326, 1979
27. Calhoun DH et al: Fabry disease: isolation of a cDNA clone encoding human α-galactosidase A. *Proc Natl Acad Sci USA* **82**:7364, 1985
28. Desnick RJ, Sweeley C: Fabry's disease: defective α-galactosidase A, in *Metabolic Basis of Inherited Disease,* 5th ed, edited by JB Stanbury et al. New York, McGraw-Hill, 1983, p 906
29. Kahlke W: Angiokeratoma corporis diffusum (Fabry's disease), in *Lipids and Lipidoses,* edited by G Schettler. Berlin, Springer, 1967, p 332
30. Kint JA, Carton D: Fabry's disease, in *Lysosomes and Storage Diseases,* edited by HG Hers, F Van Hoof. New York, Academic Press, 1973, p 347
31. Dean K, Sweeley C: Fabry disease, in *Practical Enzymology of the Sphingolipidoses,* edited by RH Glew, SP Peters. New York, Alan R Liss, 1977, p 173
32. Lockman LA et al: Relief of pain of Fabry's disease by diphenylhydantoin. *Neurology* **23**:871, 1973

33. Urbain G et al: Fabry's disease without skin lesions. *Lancet* **1**:1111, 1967

34. Wallace RD, Cooper WJ: Angiokeratoma corporis diffusum universale (Fabry). *Am J Med* **39**:656, 1965

35. Clarke JTR et al: Ceramide trihexosidosis (Fabry's disease) without skin lesions. *N Engl J Med* **284**:233, 1971

36. Ainsworth SK, Smith RM: A case study of Fabry's disease occurring in a black kindred without peripheral neuropathy or skin lesions. *Lab Invest* **38**:373, 1978

37. Ferrans VJ et al: The heart in Fabry's disease: a histochemical and electron microscopic study. *Am J Cardiol* **24**:95, 1969

38. Becker AE et al: Cardiac manifestations of Fabry's disease. Report of a case with mitral insufficiency and electrocardiographic evidence of myocardial infarction. *Am J Cardiol* **36**:829, 1975

39. Mehta J et al: Electrocardiographic and vectorcardiographic abnormalities in Fabry's disease. *Am Heart J* **93**:699, 1977

40. Bass JL et al: The M-mode echocardiogram in Fabry's disease. *Am Heart J* **100**:807, 1980

41. Goldman M et al: Echocardiographic abnormality and disease severity in Fabry disease. *Am J Cardiol,* in press

42. Colucci WS et al: Hypertrophic obstructive cardiomyopathy due to Fabry's disease. *N Engl J Med* **307**:926, 1982

43. Pabico RC et al: Renal pathologic lesions and functional alterations in a man with Fabry's disease. *Am J Med* **55**:415, 1973

44. Colombi A et al: Angiokeratoma corporis diffusum—Fabry's disease. *Helv Med Acta* **34**:67, 1967

45. Sher NA et al: The ocular manifestations in Fabry's disease. *Arch Ophthalmol* **97**:671, 1979

46. Spaeth GL, Frost P: Fabry's disease: its ocular manifestations. *Arch Ophthalmol* **74**:760, 1965

47. Franceschetti ATh: La cornea verticillata (Gruber) et ses relations avec la maladie de Fabry (angiokeratom corporis diffusum). *Ophthalmologica* **156**:232, 1968

48. Gruber H: Cornea verticillata. *Ophthalmologica* **111**:120, 1946

49. Terlinde R et al: Ruckbildung der cornea verticillata bei Morbus Fabry durch kontaktlinsen-erste beobachtungen. *Contactologia* **4**:20, 1982

50. Bartimmon EE Jr et al: Pulmonary involvement in Fabry's disease: a reappraisal. Follow up of a San Diego kindred and review of the literature. *Am J Med* **53**:755, 1972

51. Kariman K et al: Pulmonary involvement in Fabry's disease. *Am J Med* **64**:911, 1978

52. Rowe JW et al: Intestinal manifestations of Fabry's disease. *Ann Intern Med* **81**:628, 1974

53. Sheth KJ et al: Gastrointestinal structure and function in Fabry's disease. *Am J Gastroenterol* **76**:246, 1981

54. O'Brien BD et al: Pathophysiologic and ultrastructural basis for intestinal symptoms in Fabry's disease. *Gastroenterology* **82**:957, 1982

55. Broadbent JC et al: Fabry cardiomyopathy in the female confirmed by endomyocardial biopsy. *Mayo Clin Proc* **56**:623, 1981

56. Desnick RJ et al: Correction of enzymatic deficiencies by renal transplantation: Fabry's disease. *Surgery* **72**:203, 1972

57. Avila JL et al: Fabry's disease: normal α-galactosidase activity and urinary-sediment glycosphingolipid levels in two obligate heterozygotes. *Br J Dermatol* **89**:149, 1973

58. Sagebiel RW, Parker F: Cutaneous lesions of Fabry's disease: glycolipid lipidosis—light and electron microscopic findings. *J Invest Dermatol* **50**:208, 1968

59. Breathnach SM et al: Anderson-Fabry disease: characteristic ultrastructural features in cutaneous blood vessels in a 1 year old boy. *Br J Dermatol* **103**:81, 1980

60. Tarnowski WM, Hashimoto K: New light microscopic skin findings in Fabry's disease. *Acta Derm Venereol (Stockh)* **49**:386, 1969

61. Morel-Maroger L et al: Des rapports avec l'angiokeratose de Fabry et la cytodystrophie renale familiale. *Bull Soc Med Hop Paris* **117**:49, 1966

62. Hashimoto K et al: Angiokeratoma corporis diffusum (Fabry): histochemical and electron microscopic studies of the skin. *J Invest Dermatol* **44**:119, 1965

63. McNary W, Lowenstein LM: A morphological study of the renal lesion in angiokeratoma corporis diffusum universale (Fabry's disease). *J Urol* **93**:641, 1965

64. Grunnet ML, Spilsbury PR: The central nervous system in Fabry's disease. *Arch Neurol* **28**:231, 1973

65. Kocen RS, Thomas PK: Peripheral nerve involvement in Fabry's disease. *Arch Neurol* **22**:81, 1970

66. Kahn P: Anderson-Fabry disease: a histopathological study of three cases with observations on the mechanism of production of pain. *J Neurol Neurosurg Psychiatry* **36**:1053, 1973

67. Ohnishi A, Dyck PJ: Loss of small peripheral sensory neurons in Fabry disease. Histologic and morphometric evaluation of cutaneous nerves, spinal ganglia, and posterior columns. *Arch Neurol* **31**:120, 1974

68. Sung JH et al: Neuropathology of Fabry's disease. in *Proceedings of the VIIth International Congress of Neuropathology, Budapest, Hungary.* Excerpta Medico Series, 1974, p 267

69. Sung JH: Autonomic neurons affected by lipid storage in the spinal cord of Fabry's disease: distribution of autonomic neurons in the sacral cord. *J Neuropathol Exp Neurol* **38**:87, 1979

70. Cable WJ et al: Fabry disease: significance of ultrastructural localization of lipid inclusions in dermal nerves. *Neurology* **32**:347, 1982

71. Cable WJL et al: Fabry disease: impaired autonomic function. *Neurology* **32**:498, 1982

72. Rahman AN, Lindenberg R: The neuropathology of hereditary dystopic lipidosis. *Arch Neurol* **9**:373, 1963

73. Gemignani F et al: Pathological study of the sural nerve in Fabry's disease. *Eur Neurol* **23**:173, 1984

74. Witschel H, Mathyl J: Morphological elements of the specific ocular changes in morbus Fabry. *Klin Monatsbl Augenheilkd* **154**:599, 1969

75. Font RL, Fine BS: Ocular pathology in Fabry's disease. Histochemical and electron microscopic observations. *Am J Ophthalmol* **73**:419, 1972

76. Farragina T et al: Light and electron microscopic histochemistry of Fabry disease. *Am J Pathol* **103**:247, 1981

77. Lehner T, Adams CWM: Lipid histochemistry of Fabry's disease. *J Pathol Bacteriol* **95**:411, 1968

78. Van Mullem PJ, Ruiter M: Histochemical studies on lipid metabolism in so-called Fabry's disease (angiokeratoma corporis diffusum). *Arch Klin Exp Dermatol* **232**:148, 1968

79. Chatterjee S et al: Immunohistochemical localization of glycosphingolipid in urinary renal tubular cells in Fabry's disease. *Am J Clin Pathol* **82**:24, 1984

80. Robinson D, Khalfan HA: Fabry's disease. Identification of carrier status by fluorescent/electron binding. *Biochem Soc Transactions* **12**:1063, 1984

81. Van Mullem PJ, Ruiter M: Fine structure of the skin in angiokeratoma corporis diffusum (Fabry's disease). *J Pathol* **101**:221, 1970

82. Hashimoto K et al: Angiokeratoma corporis diffusum (Fabry disease). *Arch Dermatol* **112**:1416, 1976

83. Nakamura T et al: Angiokeratoma corporis diffusum (Fabry disease): ultrastructural studies of the skin. *Acta Derm Venereol (Stockh)* **61**:37, 1981

84. Beutler E, Kuhl W: Biochemical and electrophoretic studies

of α-galactosidase in normal man, in patients with Fabry's disease, and in Equidae. *Am J Hum Genet* **24**:237, 1972

85. Wood S, Nadler HL: Fabry's disease: absence of an α-galactosidase isozyme. *Am J Hum Genet* **24**:250, 1972

86. Beutler E, Kuhl W: Purification and properties of human α-galactosidases. *J Biol Chem* **247**:7195, 1972

87. Dean KJ et al: The identification of α-galactosidase B from human liver as an α-N-acetylgalactosaminidase. *Biochem Biophys Res Commun* **77**:1411, 1977

88. Schram AW et al: The identity of α-galactosidase B from human liver. *Biochim Biophys Acta* **482**:138, 1977

89. Dawson G et al: Glycosphingolipids in cultured human fibroblasts. II. Characterization and metabolism in fibroblasts from patients with inborn errors of glycosphingolipid and mucopolysaccharide metabolism. *J Biol Chem* **247**:5951, 1972

90. Bishop DF, Desnick RJ: Affinity purification of α-galactosidase A from human spleen, placenta and plasma with elimination of pyrogen contamination. *J Biol Chem* **256**:1307, 1981

91. Dean KJ, Sweeley CC: Studies on human liver α-galactosidases. I. Purification of α-galactosidase A and its enzymatic properties with glycolipid and oligosaccharide substrates. *J Biol Chem* **254**:9994, 1979

92. Bishop DF, Sweeley CC: Plasma α-galactosidase A. Properties and comparisons with tissue α-galactosidases. *Biochim Biophys Acta* **525**:339, 1978

93. Gartner S et al: Activator protein for the degradation of globotriaosylceramide by human a-galactosidase. *J Biol Chem* **258**:12378, 1983

94. Kusiak JW et al: Purification and properties of the two major isozymes of α-galactosidase from human placenta. *J Biol Chem* **253**:184, 1978

95. LeDonne NC et al: Biosynthesis of α-galactosidase A in cultured chang liver cells. *Arch Biochem Biophys* **224**:186, 1983

96. Dean K, Sweeley CC: Studies on human liver α-galactosidases. II. Purification and enzymatic properties of α-galactosidase B (α-N-acetylgalactosaminidase). *J Biol Chem* **254**:10001, 1979

97. Schram AW et al: Enzymological properties and immunological characterization of α-galactosidase isozymes from normal and Fabry human liver. *Biochim Biophys Acta* **482**:125, 1977

98. Sung S-SJ, Sweeley CC: Purification and partial characterization of porcine liver α-N-acetylgalactosaminidase. *J Biol Chem* **255**:6589, 1980

99. Crain RC, Zilversmit DB: Net transfer of phospholipid by the nonspecific phospholipid transfer proteins from bovine liver. *Biochim Biophys Acta* **620**:37, 1980

100. Shapiro D, Archer AJ: Total synthesis of ceramide trihexoside accumulating with Fabry's disease. *Chem Phys Lipids* **197**:206, 1978

101. Nudelman E et al: A glycolipid antigen associated with Burkitt lymphoma defined by a monoclonal antibody. *Science* **220**:509, 1983

102. Johnson DL, Desnick RJ: Molecular pathology of Fabry's disease: physical and kinetic properties of α-galactosidase A in cultured human endothelial cells. *Biochim Biophys Acta* **538**:195, 1978

103. Dawson G et al: Distribution of glycosphingolipids in the serum lipoproteins of normal human subjects and patients with hypo- and hyperlipidemias. *J Lipid Res* **17**:125, 1976

104. Clarke JTR et al: Neutral glycosphingolipids of serum lipoproteins in Fabry's disease. *Biochim Biophys Acta* **431**:317, 1976

105. Van den Bergh FAJTM, Tager JM: Localization of neutral glycosphingolipids in human plasma. *Biochim Biophys Acta* **441**:391, 1976

106. Meuweissen SGM et al: Ultrastructural and biochemical liver analyses in Fabry's disease. *Hepatology* **2**:263, 1982

107. Clarke JTR, Stoltz JM: Uptake of radiolabeled galactosyl-(α1 4)-galactosyl-(β 4)-glucosylceramide by human lipoproteins *in vitro*. *Biochim Biophys Acta* **441**:165, 1976

108. Stein O, Stein Y: High density lipoproteins reduce the uptake of low density lipoproteins by human endothelial cells in culture. *Biochim Biophys Acta* **431**:363, 1976

109. Goldstein JL, Brown MS: The low density lipoprotein pathway and its relation to atherosclerosis. *Annu Rev Biochem* **46**:897, 1977

110. Vlodavsky I et al: Role of contact inhibition in the regulation of receptor-mediated uptake of low density lipoprotein in cultured vascular endothelial cells. *Proc Natl Acad Sci USA* **75**:356, 1979

111. Dawson G, Sweeley CC: *In vivo* studies on glycosphingolipid metabolism in porcine blood. *J Biol Chem* **245**:410, 1970

112. Tao RVP: Biochemistry and metabolism of mammalian blood glycosphingolipids. Ph.D. Thesis, Michigan State University, 1973

113. Barkai A, DiCesare JL: Influence of sialic acid groups on the retention of glycosphingolipids in blood plasma. *Biochim Biophys Acta* **389**:287, 1975

114. Nakamura T et al: Angiokeratoma corporis diffusum (Fabry disease): ultrastructural studies of the skin. *Acta Derm Venereol (Stockh)* **61**:37, 1981

115. Fukuhara N et al: Fabry's disease on the mechanism of the peripheral nerve involvement. *Acta Neuropathol (Berl)* **33**:9, 1975

116. Dvorak AM et al: Diagnostic electron microscopy. II. Fabry's disease: use of biopsies from uninvolved skin. Acute and chronic changes involving the microvasculature and small unmyelinated nerves. *Pathol Annu* **16**:139, 1981

117. Seino Y et al: Peripheral hemodynamics in patients with Fabry's disease. *Am Heart J* **105**:783, 1983

118. Sheth KJ, Swick HM: Peripheral nerve conduction in Fabry disease. *Ann Neurol* **7**:319, 1980

119. Pelissier JF et al: Morphological and biochemical changes in muscle and peripheral nerve in Fabry's disease. *Muscle Nerve* **4**:381, 1981

120. Vogelberg KH et al: Lipoidchemische Untersuchungen beim Angiokeratoma corporis diffusum (Fabry-Syndrome). *Klin Wochenschr* **47**:916, 1969

121. Grzeschik K et al: X-linkage of human α-galactosidase. *Nature [New Biol]* **240**:48, 1972

122. Fox MF et al: Regional localization of α-galactosidase (GLA) to Xpter → q22, hexosaminidase B (HEXB) to 5q13 → qter, and arylsulfatase B (ARSB) to 5pter → q13. *Cytogenet Cell Genet* **38**:45, 1984

123. de Groot PG et al: Localization of a gene for human α-galactosidase A B (-N-acetyl-α-galactosaminidase) on chromosome 22. *Hum Genet* **44**:305, 1978

124. Rietra PJGM et al: The use of biochemical parameters for the detection of Fabry's disease. *J Mol Med* **1**:237, 1976

125. Lyon M: Gene action in the X-chromosome of the mouse (*Mus muscularus* L.). *Nature* **190**:372, 1961

126. Romeo G, Migeon BR: Genetic inactivation of the α-galactosidase locus in carriers of Fabry's disease. *Science* **170**:180, 1970

127. Bishop DF et al: Fabry disease: an asymptomatic hemizygote with significant residual α-galactosidase A activity (abstr). *Am J Hum Genet* **33**:71A, 1981

128. Bach G et al: Pseudodeficiency of α-galactosidase A. *Clin Genet* **21**:59, 1982

129. Kobayashi T et al: Fabry's disease with partially deficient hydrolysis of ceramide trihexoside. *J Neurol Sci* **67**:179, 1985

130. Romeo G et al: Residual activity of α-galactosidase A in Fabry's disease. *Biochem Genet* **13**:615, 1975

131. Beutler E, Kuhl W: Absence of cross-reactive antigen in Fabry disease. *N Engl J Med* **289:**694, 1973

132. Rietra PJGM et al: Investigation of the α-galactosidase deficiency in Fabry's disease using antibodies against the purified enzyme. *Eur J Biochem* **46:**89, 1974

133. Orkin SH, Kazazian HH Jr: The mutation and polymorphism of the human β-globin gene and its surrounding DNA. *Annu Rev Genet* **18:**131, 1984

134. Francois J, de Becker L: Les manifestations oculaires de l'intoxication chloroquine. *Ann Oculist* **198:**513, 1965

135. Desnick RJ et al: Fabry keratopathy: molecular pathology of the chloroquine-induced phenocopy. *Am J Hum Genet* **26:**26a, 1974

136. Whitley CB: Studies of heritable and induced lysosomopathies. Ph.D. Thesis, University of Minnesota, 1977

137. De Groot PG et al: Inactivation by chloroquine of α-galactosidase in cultured human skin fibroblasts. *Exp Cell Res* **136:**327, 1981

138. Whitley CB et al: Amiodarone phenocopy of Fabry's keratopathy. *JAMA* **249:**2177, 1983

139. Banks DE et al: Silicon nephropathy mimicking Fabry's disease. *Am J Nephr* **3:**279, 1983

140. Imperial R, Heliwig EB: Angiokeratoma of the scrotum (Fordyce type). *J Urol* **98:**379, 1967

141. Fordyce JA: Angiokeratoma of the scrotum. *J Cutan Genitourin Dis* **14:**81, 1896

142. Traub EF, Tolmach JA: Angiokeratoma. Comprehensive study of the literature and report of a case. *Arch Dermatol Syphilol* **24:**39, 1931

143. Dammert K: Angiokeratosis naeviformis—a form of naevus telangiectatieus lateralis (naevus flammeus). *Dermatologica* **130:**17, 1965

144. Goldman L et al: Thrombotic angiokeratoma circumscriptum simulating melanoma. *Arch Dermatol* **117:**138, 1981

145. Epinette WW et al: Angiokeratoma corporis diffusum with α-L-fucosidase deficiency. *Arch Dermatol* **107:**755, 1973

146. Miyatake T et al: Adult type neuronal storage disease with neuraminidase deficiency. *Ann Neurol* **6:**232, 1978

147. Wenger DA et al: Adult G_{M1} gangliosidosis: clinical and biochemical studies on two patients and comparison to other patients called variant or adult G_{M1} gangliosidosis. *Clin Genet* **17:**323, 1980

148. Gehler J et al: Clinical and biochemical delineation of aspartylglycosaminuria as observed in two members of an Italian family. *Helv Paediatr Acta* **36:**179, 1981

149. McCallum DI et al: Angiokeratoma corporis diffusum with features of a mucopolysaccharidosis. *J Med Genet* **17:**21, 1980

150. Holmes RC et al: Angiokeratoma corporis diffusum in a patient with normal enzyme activities. *J Am Acad Dermatol* **10:**384, 1984

151. Crovato F, Rebora A: Angiokeratoma corporis diffusum and normal enzyme activities. *J Am Acad Dermatol* **12:**885, 1985

152. Frost P et al: Fabry's disease: glycolipid lipidosis. Skin manifestations. *Arch Intern Med* **117:**440, 1966

153. Imperial R, Heliwig EB: Angiokeratoma: a clinicopathological study. *Arch Dermatol* **95:**166, 1967

154. Van Mullem PJ, Ruiter M: Electron microscopic study of the skin in angiokeratoma corporis diffusum. *Arch Klin Exp Dermatol* **226:**453, 1966

155. Ho MW et al: Fabry's disease: evidence for a physically altered α-galactosidase. *Am J Hum Genet* **24:**256, 1972

156. Mayes JS et al: Differential assay for lysosomal α-galactosidases in human tissues and its application to Fabry's disease. *Clin Chim Acta* **112:**247, 1981

157. Grimm T et al: Fabry's disease: heterozygote detection by hair root analysis. *Hum Genet* **32:**329, 1976

158. Spense MW et al: Heterozygote detection in angiokeratoma corporis diffusum (Anderson-Fabry disease). *J Med Genet* **14:**91, 1977

159. Vermorken AJM et al: Fabry's disease: biochemical and histochemical studies on hair roots for carrier detection. *Br J Dermatol* **98:**191, 1978

160. Desnick RJ et al: Prenatal diagnosis of glycosphingolipidoses: Sandhoff's and Fabry's diseases. *J Pediatr* **83:**149, 1973

161. Malouf M et al: Ultrastructural changes in antenatal Fabry's disease. *Am J Pathol* **82:**132, 1976

162. Funderburk SJ et al: Priaprism after phenoxybenzamine in a patient with Fabry's disease. *N Engl J Med* **290:**630, 1974

163. Lenoir G et al: La maladie de Fabry. Traitement du syndrome acrodyniforme par la carbamazepine. *Arch Fr Pediatr* **34:**704, 1977

164. Atzpodien W et al: Angiokeratoma corporis diffusum (Morbus Fabry). Biochemische diagnostik im Blutplasma. *Dtsch Med Wochenschr* **100:**423, 1975

165. Dupperrat B et al: Maladie de Fabry. Angiokeratomes presents a la naissance. Action de la diphenylhydantoine sur les crises douloureuses. *Ann Dermatol Syphiligr (Paris)* **102:**392, 1975

166. Philippart M et al: Reversal of an inborn sphingolipidosis (Fabry's disease) by kidney transplantation. *Ann Intern Med* **77:**195, 1972

167. Desnick RJ et al: Fabry disease: correction of the enzymatic deficiency by renal transplantation, in *Enzyme Therapy in Genetic Diseases,* edited by RJ Desnick et al. Baltimore, Williams & Wilkins, 1973, p 88

168. Jacky E: Fabrysche Erkrankung (Angiokeratoma corporis diffusum universale): gunstiger Verlauf nach Nierentransplantation. *Schweiz Med Wochenschr* **106:**703, 1976

169. Buhler FR et al: Kidney transplantation in Fabry's disease. *Br Med J* **3:**28, 1973

170. Clement M et al: Renal transplantation in Anderson-Fabry disease. *J R Soc Med* **75:**557, 1982

171. Clarke JTR et al: Enzyme replacement therapy by renal allotransplantation in Fabry's disease. *N Engl J Med* **287:**1215, 1972

172. Spense MW et al: Failure to correct the metabolic defect by renal allotransplantation in Fabry's disease. *Ann Intern Med* **84:**13, 1976

173. Grunfeld JP et al: Le transplantation renale chez les sujets atteints de maladie de Fabry. *Neuv Presse Med* **4:**2081, 1975

174. Van den Bergh FAJTM et al: Therapeutic implications of renal transplantation in a patient with Fabry's disease. *Acta Med Scand* **200:**249, 1976

175. Bannwart F: Morbus Fabry. Licht- und elektronenmikroskopischer Herzbefund 12 Jahre nach erfolgreicher Nierentransplantation. *Schweiz Med Wochenschr* **112:**1742, 1982

176. Kramer W et al: Progressive cardiac involvement by Fabry's disease despite successful renal allotransplantation. *Int J Cardiol* **7:**72, 1984

177. Dawson G et al: Correction of the enzymatic defect in cultured fibroblasts from patients with Fabry's disease: treatment with purified α-galactosidase from Ficin. *Pediatr Res* **7:**684, 1973

178. Mayes JS et al: Endocytosis of lysosomal alpha-galactosidase A by cultured fibroblasts from patients with Fabry disease. *Am J Hum Genet* **34:**602, 1982

179. Hasholt L, Sorensen SA: A microtechnique for quantitative measurements of acid hydrolyses in fibroblasts. Its application in diagnosis of Fabry disease and enzyme replacement studies. *Clin Chim Acta* **142:**257, 1984

180. Desnick RJ et al: Enzyme therapy XVII: metabolic and immunologic evaluation of α-galactosidase A replacement in Fabry disease, in *Enzyme Therapy in Genetic Diseases: 2,* edited by RJ Desnick. New York, Alan R Liss, 1980, p 393

181. Ashwell G, Morell AG: The role of surface carbohydrates in

the hepatic recognition and transport of circulating glycoproteins. *Adv Enzymol* **41**:99, 1974

182. Bishop DF et al: Enzyme therapy XX: further evidence for the differential *in vivo* fate of human splenic and plasma forms of α-galactosidase A in Fabry disease. Recovery of exogenous activity from hepatic tissue, in *Lysosomes and Lysosomal Storage Diseases,* edited by JW Callahan, JA Lowden. New York, Raven Press, 1981, p 381

183. Touraine JL et al: Maladie de Fabry: deux maladies ameliorées par la greffe de cullules de foie foetal. *Nouv Presse Med* **8**:1499, 1979

184. Pyeritz RE et al: Plasma exchange removes glycosphingolipid in Fabry disease. *Am J Med Genet* **7**:301, 1980

185. Beutler E et al: The effect of phlebotomy as a treatment of Fabry disease. *Biochem Med* **30**:363, 1983

186. Desnick RJ (ed): *Enzyme Therapy in Genetic Diseases:* 2. New York, Alan R Liss, 1980

187. Desnick RJ, Grabowski GA: Advances in the treatment of inherited metabolic diseases. *Adv Hum Genet* **11**:281, 1981

CHAPTER 147

LIPOID PROTEINOSIS

George H. Findlay

Lipoid proteinosis (hyalinosis cutis et mucosae, Urbach-Wiethe disease) is a disease with four main features: a unique interstitial tissue deposit, a distinctive genetic background, a characteristic pattern of lesions, and a regular sequence of evolution [1].

1. *Deposits*. The unique deposit occurring in connective tissues in lipoid proteinosis is a pale-staining material which appears hyaline in the light microscope. Absorbed in the hyaline material are droplets of a lipid mixture (neutral fat, cholesterol) with no distinctive constituents. It is not produced through any local or general disorder of lipid metabolism. The periodic acid-Schiff stain on the hyaline is positive, but there is no evidence favoring any one of the histochemically identifiable carbohydrates. Considering the hyaline to be a glycoprotein, the nondescript term *lipoid proteinosis* can be seen to apply to the condition.

Ultrastructurally the hyaline has a fibrogranular appearance. It is surrounded by areas having an entirely normal connective tissue structure. In the hyaline mass, true collagen fibrils may be embedded. There is no evidence that the hyaline is derived from elastin, anchoring fibrils, fibrin, amyloid, or metachromatic mucopolysaccharides. In the skin, concentric calcified granules may also be seen by electron microscopy. This tendency to calcify is a feature of the cerebral lesions.

Various cell constituents have been held responsible for producing the special hyaline material. Contributions to the hyaline may to some extent be forthcoming from certain fibroblasts, smooth muscle, myoepithelial and Schwann cells. However the sources having at present the greater claim as the main producers of hyaline are the vascular endothelial and perithelial cells, and the basal cells of the epidermis and its derivatives. These are characteristically the generators of basement membranes [2–6]. Both under the electron microscope and with indirect immunofluorescence the perivascular hyaline shows a marked increase in basal lamina constituents—type IV collagen and the noncollagenous glycoprotein, laminin, which forms the normal lamina lucida. The reduplicated basal lamina contains the fibrogranular (hyaline) material between its layers, shading off to pure hyaline deposits beyond, which yield a single band of noncollagenous glycoprotein, presumably laminin, on electrophoretic separation. The pericytes and associated endothelial cells are morphologically hyperactive. Some of these also contain myofibrils in the cytoplasm, and in various respects some may resemble myofibroblasts.

In the regions affected by these excessive hyaline deposits, the alterations are traceable to a variety of basal lamina-producing cell systems. This suggests that the fault lies in the regulation of basal laminae in that region. Theoretically there could be a deficient, inhibited, or difficult lysis of the laminar material, or a fault in the inhibitory feedback loop, with consequent overproduction of these components. Other structural glycoproteins may be added by fibroblasts to the ground-substance hyaline in areas beyond the basal laminae.

The sources and nature of the hyaline are now more clearly understood, but the reasons for its presence in excess are still speculative. A time is approaching when it should be possible to replace the vague names applied to the disease with some more accurate descriptive term for the pathologic process.

2. *Genetics* [7]. Lipoid proteinosis is inherited as a monogenetic autosomal recessive disorder of normal chromosome pattern. The mutation rate must be low, but in some geographically isolated regions where intermarriage is common, the gene frequency in the population may rise considerably. Otherwise, the disease is seen infrequently. Nevertheless, it occurs in all populations and on all continents throughout the world, with certain nests of high frequency in some special regions. The disease hinders the homozygote occupationally, socially, and in marriage. The heterozygote shows virtually no lesions, but may possibly be identifiable by minor signs, such as abnormalities in the formation or number of teeth. If the particular recessive gene controls a single enzyme defect, it is still not known where this defect lies.

3. *Evolution.* Mild changes must precede birth, causing lack of development of certain tooth germs, and at birth the infant has a veiled, hoarse cry. Although skin infections with scarring are considered to be an early sign in infancy and childhood, these signs already reflect a weakness at the dermal-epidermal junction which only develops its hyaline deposits rather later. Mucosal signs are already present at this stage as a rule.

The disease picture gradually establishes itself in the first few years of life. In adolescence the signs become more extensive but remain stable thereafter, with minor fluctuations.

Lipoid proteinosis does not regularly shorten life, but respiratory obstruction and the neurologic complications are likely to increase the risks of an early death.

4. *Distribution pattern of the lesions* [8]. The main localization of lipoid proteinosis is in the skin and mucosae of the "muzzle" region. The cerebral representation of the muzzle, the rhinencephalon, where taste, smell, and correlated reflexes are controlled, is also affected by the disease.

Besides the head, the skin surface is diffusely affected. Special exaggeration of the changes is seen at orifices, folds, commissures, pressure areas, transitional sites, and sites of injury or wear and tear. The buccal, pharyngeal, and laryngeal mucosae contain deposits as well, but below the level of the neck the mucosal deposits are insignificant.

In the brain, the territory of the anterior choroidal artery and the amygdaloid nucleus in the temporal lobe are mainly affected. In these areas the arteriocapillary walls are hyaline and calcified, while in the surrounding tissue calcification and ossification have been noted. In remoter regions of the brain, thrombosis, calcification, infarction, and demyelination have been observed [7]. The presence of these changes can be most regularly shown during life by CT scanning. Scanography shows the brain calcification better and more frequently, while the rest of this examination is likely to emphasize the degenerative and involutional changes elsewhere in the brain [9,10].

Histologically, the distribution of hyaline may be seen [11] in the arteriocapillary walls and the epithelial and adnexal basement membrane regions. Some obstruction and mild interference with blood flow, nerve function, sweating, and hair growth may result. Spread occurs into the dermis, submucosae, along muscles and nerves, etc. There is no phagocytosis or inflammatory response around the hyaline. Physiologic abnormalities in cultured fibroblasts from a patient have been noted. These affect the metabolic activity, hexuronic acid uptake, and the uptake and release of labeled sulfate [12].

Clinical features

Mucosae: The buccal and throat mucosae, from the lips inward to the vocal cords and beyond, stiffen from birth or within a few years. Nothing can be seen at first. What can be heard is increasing hoarseness from the inelastic vocal cords [13]. To appreciate the tense texture of the lips and buccal cavity, these areas must be thoroughly palpated with the examining fingers.

Early skin changes: The cheek skin of an affected white baby is waxy and translucent. In darker subjects, color

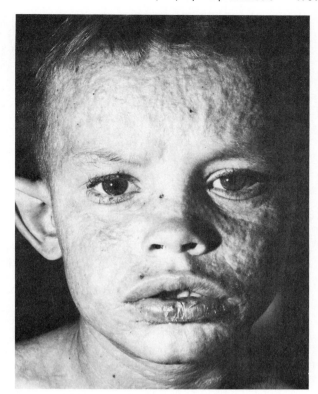

Fig. 147-1 Lipoid proteinosis in boy of 7 years. Eyelids, lips, and face infiltrated with hyaline. Scattered blood crusts and depressed scars.

changes are not obvious, and palpation with close inspection is needed.

Surface defects: The papillary layer of the dermis is readily damaged from early on. Papules, blisters, blood crusts, and mild dermatitis are present. The skin is easily scratched, injured, and infected, with ulceration, scabbing, and slow healing. Scars that result are depressed, linear, foveate, acneform, varioliform, ecthymatous, papulonecrotic, or with a shape determined by injury. Although worst on the face, these scars are widespread (Fig. 147-1).

Increase of infiltration: Hyaline deposits gradually become more clearly visible in the susceptible regions. They take on a papular, nodular, plaquelike, reticulate, or striate arrangement. Areas of movement, pressure, and exposure are more prominently affected (Fig. 147-2). The skin starts to remind one of the knobby surface of a citrus fruit such as a mandarin or a lime. The tongue is firm and tied down. A hoarse voice with inability to protrude the tongue may give the correct diagnosis within seconds. Eating and speech are laborious. The soft palate, epiglottic folds, and larynx become papular, thickened, and deformed.

Effect on larger ducts: The parotid duct, the lacrimal punctum, the airway through the larynx, and subglottic region may become stenosed and readily obstructed.

Prominent secondary signs: Papules may accumulate at the angles of the mouth. On the edges of the eyelids, such papules are famous for resembling a string of beads. Striae appear on flexural skin or on the sides of the neck. Indirect consequences of the disease include hypohidrosis, hypotrichosis, and poor nail growth. Fragility, itching, capillary proliferation, and regional hyperkeratosis are also seen.

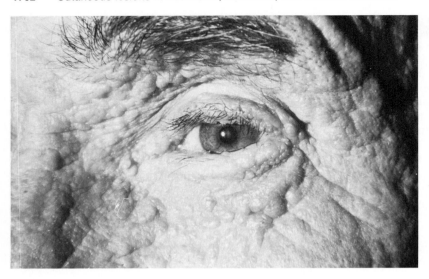

Fig. 147-2 Lipoid proteinosis in an adult. Characteristic papulation around the eye.

Neurologic manifestations: Temporal lobe type epilepsy is traceable to the specific vascular and degenerative changes, with calcification (Fig. 147-3) in the hippocampus. These changes form an integral part of lipoid proteinosis, and the calcification, when present radiologically, is pathognomonic (see also "Distribution pattern of the lesions" above, for pathology). These calcified nodules, however, need not be present in every case. Epileptic attacks develop in later childhood—major, minor, uncinate, akinetic, and psychomotor types (rage attacks). Intellectual impairment is variable. One of our patients was renowned for his witty repartee, but killed himself through an addiction to horse and motorcycle racing. Others have tended to be rather dull and stupid.

Interdisciplinary summary for cases of lipoid proteinosis

Neuropsychiatry: Epilepsy and abnormal behavior should be investigated and controlled.

Radiology: Hippocampal calcifications on either side of the sella turcica are seen. CT scans may be helpful. Deformities of the pharynx and larynx can be shown by contrast methods.

Ophthalmology: Marginal beading of the eyelids is the principal sign. Eyelash distortion and minor fundus changes such as drusen may occur.

Leprology: Hoarseness, hair loss, and skin infiltrates may be mistaken for leprosy.

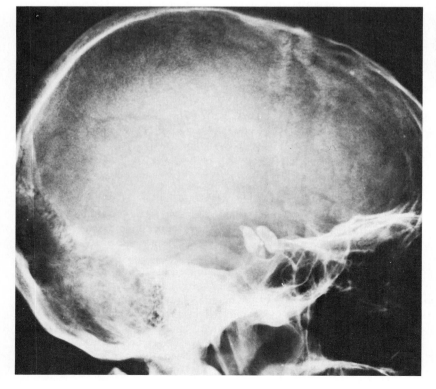

Fig. 147-3 Calcifications in the hippocampus, one bean-shaped focus lying on either side of the midline at the level of the sella turcica. This appearance is pathognomonic of lipoid proteinosis.

Surgery: Laryngeal and sublaryngeal stenosis and obstruction may require tracheostomy. The vocal cords may on occasion be stripped of nodules. Parotid ducts may need opening if occluded. Parotid abscesses unwisely drained may lead to fistulae. Planing operations may be considered for cosmetic improvement.

Pathology: Pathologists are expected to distinguish between hyaline appearances in biopsy material, as compared with colloid, elastosis, amyloid, and other types of hyaline.

Differential diagnosis

Erythropoietic protoporphyria produces similar deposits around the skin vessels, though only in sun-exposed sites. The mucosae are unaltered, causing confusion with lipoid proteinosis only where there is little hoarseness in the latter disease. Causalgic burning from sun exposure, with skin swelling and behavior disturbances, are characteristic of erythropoietic protoporphyria. These symptoms are relieved by sun protection and applications of ice. These cases were formerly regarded as "light sensitive lipoid proteinosis." This classification is obsolete, and raised erythrocyte protoporphyrin levels settle the diagnosis. Erythropoietic protoporphyria is also now more easily treatable.

Treatment

Only the complications of lipoid proteinosis are treatable: eczema, surface infection, epilepsy, respiratory and parotid obstruction, etc. Stripping of the vocal cords or planing of the skin is possible, but hyaline removed in this way is apt to re-form.

References

1. Hofer PA: Urbach-Wiethe disease. A review. *Acta Derm Venereol (Stockh)* **53 (suppl 71)**:1, 1973
2. Ishibashi A: Histogenesis of hyalinosis cutis et mucosae. *J Dermatol (Tokyo)* **5**:265, 1978
3. Dupré A et al: Étude ultrastructurale d'un cas de hyalinose cutanéo-mugueuse. *Ann Dermatol Venereol* **108**:1003, 1981
4. Fleischmajer R et al: Hyalinosis cutis et mucosae. A basal lamina disease (abstr). *J Invest Dermatol* **76**:314, 1981
5. Fleischmajer R et al: Ultrastructure and composition of connective tissue in hyalinosis cutis et mucosae skin. *J Invest Dermatol* **82**:252, 1984
6. Ishibashi A: Hyalinosis cutis et mucosae. *Dermatologica* **165**:7, 1982
7. Meenan FOC et al: Lipoid proteinosis: a clinical, pathological and genetic study. *Q J Med* **47**:549, 1978
8. Findlay GH: Studies in morphogenetic dermatology: the brain calcifications of lipoid proteinosis. *Trans St Johns Hosp Dermatol Soc* **60**:152, 1974
9. Boudouresques J, Boudouresques G: Maladie d'Urbach-Wiethe avec calcification temporales à la scanographie. *Nouv Presse Med* **8**:2483, 1979
10. Leonard JN et al: CT scan appearances in a patient with lipoid proteinosis. *Br J Radiol* **54**:1098, 1981
11. Hofer PA et al: A clinical and histopathological study of 27 cases of Urbach-Wiethe disease. *Acta Pathol Microbiol Scand [A]* **Suppl 245**:1, 1974
12. Bauer EA et al: Lipoid proteinosis: in vivo and in vitro evidence for a lysosomal storage disease. *J Invest Dermatol* **76**:119, 1981
13. Harper JI et al: Oropharyngeal and laryngeal lesions in lipoid proteinosis. *J Laryngol Otol* **97**:877, 1983

CHAPTER 148

SKIN AND SUBCUTANEOUS TISSUE: CALCIFICATION, OSSIFICATION, AND NEOPLASMS

CALCIFICATION AND OSSIFICATION OF THE SKIN AND SUBCUTANEOUS TISSUES

Lawrence M. Miller and Stephen M. Krane

Calcification and/or ossification of the skin or subcutaneous tissues occurs in a wide variety of unrelated disorders. In some conditions the deposition of the solid, inorganic mineral phase containing calcium and phosphate ions is not organized in the manner that characterizes bone as a tissue and is therefore termed *calcification.* In other conditions the mineral phase is deposited in well-formed bone and is termed *heterotopic ossification.* It has not been established that calcification must precede the formation of heterotopic bone. Moreover, when calcification of the

type described above does occur in the skin or subcutaneous tissues, it is usually not converted into true bone. The fundamental mechanisms responsible for the deposition of the mineral phase in these two forms are probably different.

The complex biologic process whereby inorganic ions are deposited as a solid phase in bone, tooth enamel, and dentine is not completely understood. Therefore, the process of pathologic mineralizaton of tissues that are normally not mineralized is even more obscure. The regulation of calcium metabolism, calcification, and bone formation have been completely presented elsewhere [1,2], but will be briefly reviewed here. Parathyroid hormone, vitamin D, and calcitonin are involved.

Normal mechanism of calcification and ossification

Calcium and phosphate ions (and/or complexes of these ions) may be viewed as existing in solution in the extracellular fluid in metastable equilibrium. Such solutions are capable of remaining stable indefinitely although under certain conditions new, even more stable (solid) phases can be formed. The formation of the solid inorganic mineral component of bone and other calcified tissues results from a physical change of state, that is, a phase transformation from ions in solution to the solid. In normally mineralized tissues this solid, inorganic phase is organized with respect to its organic matrix, resulting in a structural two-phase system. In bone and dentine the matrix consists largely of collagen; in enamel, the matrix consists of unique noncollagenous proteins. When calcification of the aorta occurs, the mineral phase appears to be related to the elastin fibers. Heavy metal ions, when linked to the polypeptide chains of elastin, have positions that may be occupied by inorganic orthophosphate ions to which calcium is then bound, as demonstrated by in vitro experiments. Reconstituted, purified collagen fibrils as well as demineralized collagen of bone and dentine are capable of inducing the formation (nucleation) of apatite crystals from solutions of calcium and phosphate ions in vitro which do not form the solid phase in the absence of collagen. Present evidence indicates that the phase transformation induced by collagen fibrils is facilitated by the manner in which the collagen macromolecules are packed in the native-type fibril as a result of (1) a specific steric relationship around constituent amino acids, (2) a distribution of electrostatic charges, or (3) the internal "space geometry" within the fibril.

Evidence that supports the important role of phosphorus in biologic mineralization has been obtained both from studies of disease and experiments in vitro. It has been suggested that phosphorus possesses a number of theoretical advantages over calcium in initiating or participating in the formation of crystal nuclei by organic matrices. Moreover, in in vitro experiments using isolated mitochrondria, it has been demonstrated that only in the presence of ATP and organic phosphates are the mitochondria capable of a significant concentration of calcium, allowing the solid phase to form. Massive increases in the amount of calcium in the presence of anions, other than phosphates, do not allow the mineral phase to form. Apatites are essentially phosphate salts, the structural characteristics of the apatite lattice being primarily determined by the organization of the phosphate groups in the unit cell of the crystal. The organic matrices of mineralized tissues all contain protein-bound organic phosphorus although the actual amounts vary depending on age and species. The organic matrices can be phosphorylated by protein phosphokinases with adenosine triphosphate as the phosphoryl donor. It has been proposed that such covalently bound phosphorus might be important in initiating the formation of crystal nuclei from solutions containing calcium and in organic phosphate ions or clusters of these ions. The effects of phosphate in stimulating bone "turnover" and

healing the bone diseases in adults with hypophosphatemic osteomalacia are striking, and are not explained simply on the basis of providing phosphate ions for crystal growth. The key role of phosphate in mineralization of normally calcified tissues may also be extended to situations of aberrant "calcification."

The initial fragments of the solid phase that are thus formed increase in size to clearly defined particles by the process of crystal growth. It is important to consider that the rate of nucleation of the new phase is strikingly dependent on the degree of metastability of the system, which among other factors is a function of the concentration of calcium and phosphate ions (or complexes of these ions) in solution. At very low concentrations of calcium and phosphate in solution, a new phase cannot be formed. At very high concentrations, probably never observed in biologic situations, spontaneous precipitation in the bulk of the solutions may occur.

Although collagen extracted from bone, as well as a portion of the collagen from skin, tendon, and fascia, are designated type I collagens with the same amino acid sequence, significant posttranslational modifications and mechanical differences exist, as well as differences in packing arrangements. Nonetheless, since collagen from sources other than bone is capable of initiating mineralization under specified conditions, mechanisms must normally be operative which prevent the calcification of these soft tissues or facilitate mineralization of the tissues normally unmineralized. There is evidence that tissue proteoglycans inhibit mineralization and that such substances are removed precisely at the mineralizing front in bone. Other inhibitors may be components of the extracellular fluid, such as inorganic pyrophosphate which is effective in inhibiting mineralization at very low concentrations. Alkaline phosphatase which is present in high concentration in the osteoblast has the ability to remove inorganic pyrophosphate and allow mineralization to proceed where it is biologically appropriate. The organic matrix in instances of pathologic ectopic calcification consists of proteins other than collagens, particularly acidic proteins [3]. Some of these proteins contain glutamic acid residues which are modified by the addition of an extra carboxyl group on the side chain (γ-carboxyglutamic acid). The γ-carboxyglutamic acid residues are formed through the action of vitamin K-dependent enzymes. These residues confer on the proteins additional calcium-binding properties which may also have a role in the initiation of calcification.

Under circumstances in which the aberrant mineralization occurs in the form of true heterotopic bone, the organization of the connective tissue cells that have undergone metaplasia into osteoblasts may result in conditions that are more favorable for mineralization. For example, this could result from (1) the formation of collagen with structural properties more closely resembling those of bone collagen, (2) changes in the proteoglycans, or (3) aberration in the local concentration of calcium and/or phosphate ions. Although metaplastic bone has been produced under a variety of experimental conditions, the underlying mechanisms still have not been clarified.

Whatever the underlying process that results in abnormal calcification of skin, the analysis of the mineral phase by x-ray diffraction has revealed the presence of hydroxyapatite. However, since the mineral phase in bone itself has now been shown to consist of so-called amorphous calcium–phosphate in addition to poorly crystalline apatite, it is probable that abnormal calcification also will show the existence of this amorphous calcium–phosphate phase as well. The mineral is amorphous in the sense that a coherent x-ray diffraction pattern is not obtained although short-range order is present as shown by infrared spectroscopy, and the mineral is well-defined chemically. It is probable that the abnormal skin calcifications are associated with collagen or elastin despite the difficulties in defining the organization of these deposits by conventional light microscopy. However, once the formation of the inorganic phase occurs in aberrant locations, crystal growth may then proceed to result in a disorganized mass of mineral having no resemblance to the highly organized, two-phase system of bones, and having the consistency of a semifluid, pastelike material.

Aberrant calcification of the skin

With this background, the abnormal calcification in the skin and subcutaneous tissues may be viewed as of three general types:

1. *Calcification without ossification in association with increased concentrations of calcium and/or inorganic phosphate ions in the extracellular fluid.* Under the circumstances in which skin and subcutaneous calcification is observed clinically, such as in hypervitaminosis D, the hypercalcemia is usually accompanied by some increase in levels of phosphate in the serum as well. Although the metastability of the extracellular fluid is increased, deposition of the mineral occurs more commonly in preferential locations, such as in areas surrounding large joints, suggesting that other factors may play a role in the localization of the calcification. In these clinical situations, calcification in the early stages also tends to be localized in such tissues as the cornea, gastric mucosa, renal parenchyma, and blood vessels. Local factors, such as alterations in pH with a tendency toward alkalosis, must therefore also be operative.

2. *Calcification without ossification in association with normal concentrations of calcium and inorganic phosphate ions in the extracellular fluid.* The term *dystrophic calcification* has been used to describe the situations in which this occurs, implying that the disturbance is a local one, ascribable either to the loss of normal inhibitors or to the creation of new conditions more favorable for calcification to proceed. Under these circumstances, neither the loss of a specific inhibitor nor the presence of calcification-inducing substances has yet been demonstrated. The calcinosis that may accompany scleroderma is an example of this type of abnormal calcification. Trauma of different types (physical, thermal) may predispose to calcification.

3. *True ossification* (heterotopic bone formation). Cutaneous or subcutaneous ossification may be seen, for example, in myositis ossificans or pseudohypoparathyroidism.

In Table 148-1 are listed various diseases associated with skin or subcutaneous calcification which may be grouped according to the general classification described above. The features of these categories are presented here.

Diseases associated with increased concentrations of calcium and/or inorganic phosphate ions in the extracellular fluid

It has been well established that hypercalcemia, regardless of cause, may lead to impaired renal function. The increase in metastability of the serum in any hypercalcemic state is ascribable, therefore, not only to the hypercalcemia per se, but also to the increase in the concentration of inorganic phosphate which results from the renal insufficiency.

The concept that the serum phosphorus level may be of critical importance in aberrant calcifications of this type is supported by the chemical data associated with renal failure. Under these circumstances the serum phosphorus is usually elevated because of the inability of the kidney to clear this ion. The serum calcium level is often low, presumably due to impaired intestinal absorption, which in turn may be ascribed to insufficient renal 1-hydroxylation of 25-hydroxycholecalciferol (the 1,25-dihydroxycholecalciferol is the active form of the hormone). The low level of ionized calcium in the serum is a stimulus to increase secretion of parathyroid hormone which results in resorption of both calcium and phosphorus as well as organic matrix components from bone. This sequence of events may then result in "secondary" parathyroid hyperplasia. The net effect of the increased secretion of parathyroid hormone is to further increase the level of serum phosphorus which is already elevated. Moreover, pyrophosphate metabolism may be abnormal in the uremic patient [4]. Skin and subcutaneous calcification may then occur. If the serum phosphorus level is lowered by dialysis or by binding of the ion in the lumen of the gastrointestinal tract with the use of aluminum hydroxide gel, the mass of the calci-

---

Table 148-1 Disorders associated with aberrant calcification and ossification of the skin and subcutaneous tissues

I. Calcification of the skin and/or subcutaneous tissues
   A. Diseases associated with increased concentrations of calcium and/or inorganic phosphate ions in the extracellular fluid
      1. Renal failure
      2. Milk-alkali syndrome
      3. Hyperparathyroidism
      4. Hypervitaminosis D
      5. Tumoral calcinosis*
      6. Other
   B. Diseases associated with normal concentrations of calcium and inorganic phosphate ions in the extracellular fluid
      1. Progressive systemic sclerosis (scleroderma)
      2. Polymyositis (including dermatomyositis)
      3. Miscellaneous disorders
         a. Skin trauma* (physical, thermal)
         b. Venous stasis*
         c. Ehlers–Danlos syndrome
         d. Parasitic infestations
         e. Werner's syndrome
II. Ossification of the skin and/or subcutaneous tissues
   A. Skin tumors
   B. Hypoparathyroidism, pseudohypoparathyroidism, and pseudopseudohypoparathyroidism
   C. Myositis ossificans
   D. Neurologic diseases

* Indicates that the disorder may not belong in this category, as explained in the text.

fications in the skin and subcutaneous tissues may then decrease or disappear. These calcifications are usually located around large joints and may be disabling by virtue of their size, which correlates best with the degree of hyperphosphatemia. These nodular depositions may appear following an episode of paraarticular inflammation but more often are small, multiple, and asymptomatic. Those that have been analyzed contain hydroxyapatite.

The calcifications that occur in patients with the milk-alkali syndrome share many clinical features with those seen in uremia. This syndrome, which is usually accompanied by some degree of renal failure, is attributable to the consumption of large quantities of calcium, usually in the form of milk, in addition to antacids. Hypercalcemia is a consistent feature. Other features of this syndrome are kidney stones containing calcium, calcification of the renal parenchyma, and metabolic alkalosis. The levels of serum phosphorus are usually elevated, presumably due to impaired renal function in the face of increased intake. When an absorbable antacid such as calcium carbonate is ingested, the chemical changes may be dramatic. In one reported case the serum calcium rose from 10 to 18 mg/dL over a 10-day period. There are no distinctive characteristics as to the size or distribution of the calcifications but, as in other forms of metastatic deposition, they tend to occur around large joints. Disappearance of the intracutaneous and subcutaneous lesions have been observed when the offending agents have been withdrawn. The differential diagnosis between the milk-alkali syndrome and primary hyperparathyroidism may be difficult. This is especially true when renal failure has supervened in the latter condition. The diagnosis of the milk-alkali syndrome can be made only when the serum calcium level returns to normal upon reduction of the excessive calcium intake.

It is of interest that calcification of the skin rarely occurs in uncomplicated primary hyperparathyroidism, despite the presence of hypercalcemia. The action of parathyroid hormone under these circumstances results in excessive renal losses of phosphorus via the kidney, leading to hypophosphatemia. While the degree of hypercalcemia in primary hyperparathyroidism may exceed that seen in the milk-alkali syndrome, metastatic skin calcification does not occur unless renal failure and associated hyperphosphatemia supervene. These clinical observations further support the central role of phosphorus in the genesis of metastatic ''calcification.''

Hypervitaminosis D, which usually results in some degree of renal failure, may also be accompanied by calcific subcutaneous masses. Formerly, when large doses of vitamin D were used in therapy of such diseases as rheumatoid arthritis, metastatic calcifications around joints were frequently reported; uncontrolled administration of vitamin D is currently not encountered very often. The normal adult requirement for this vitamin is approximately 100 IU (0.0025 mg) per day. Paraarticular calcific masses have developed when doses as low as 50,000 IU (1.25 mg) per day have been consumed over an extended period of time. Hypercalcemia and renal impairment have been observed as early as 12 days when the dose has exceeded 500,000 IU (12.5 mg) per day. The metastatic calcifications usually do not form unless some degree of hyperphosphatemia is also present. When aspirated, they contain the same type of pasty-white material that can be obtained

from metastatic deposits regardless of their cause. Administration of radioisotopes such as ^{47}Ca has demonstrated that rapid exchange of calcium ions takes place between the masses and the extracellular fluid. These masses usually have an alkaline milieu, with levels of pH as high as 8 having been reported.

Tumoral calcinosis clinically resembles this group of diseases in many respects. The masses of calcium are located around large joints and have the above characteristics. Reported cases have shown no other abnormalities other than minimal hyperphosphatemia in some instances. The abnormalities are limited to the skin and subcutaneous tissues, sparing all internal organs. Approximately 130 cases of this condition have been reported, many in nonwhites [5], with most cases in the younger age group and a 2:1 male predominance. Several familial occurrences have been noted, although not in successive generations, suggesting an autosomal recessive inheritance pattern in some instances. Formerly this entity had been included among the dystrophic calcifications, but this concept has been questioned in view of the observations of the hyperphosphatemia and the effect of induced phosphate deprivation on reducing or eliminating the calcific masses [6]. The most common areas of calcification are around the hips and elbows. Histologic examination has shown areas of edema, presumed to be the initial event, followed by ''degradation'' of collagen, which then mineralizes. In those cases that were extensively studied, other abnormalities included an increase in the urinary hydroxyproline excretion presumably reflecting collagen degradation, normal renal tubular reabsorption of phosphorus, and low levels of urinary calcium excretion. Treatment consists of reduction in calcium and phosphorus intake and using aluminum hydroxide gels to bind intestinal phosphorus and prevent its absorption. Urinary calcium excretion has risen using this therapy and the calcific masses have disappeared. Both calcium and phosphorus balances have become negative and the urinary hydroxyproline excretion decreased. No clinical or chemical osteomalacia developed, but bone biopsies have not been performed. The increase in urinary calcium and phosphorus excretion presumably reflects depletion from the tumoral masses. One case of massive osteolysis (phantom bone disease) has been reported as the cause of subsequent tumoral calcinosis, raising the issue of trauma as an etiologic factor in tumoral calcinosis [7].

Reports of the spontaneous occurrence of skin and subcutaneous calcification in destructive bone disease (metastatic neoplasia, multiple myeloma, leukemia, Paget's disease) are rare. In some instances of hypercalcemia associated with malignancies treated with large doses of phosphate, extensive metastatic calcification has been observed. Calcification of eccrine sweat ducts has been reported in a patient with pancreatitis and hypercalcemia [8].

Diseases associated with normal concentrations of calcium and inorganic phosphate in the extracellular fluid

Since the first clinical report of calcinosis in 1878, there have been numerous attempts to define this condition. In 1936 Rothstein and Welt [9] reviewed 39 cases. Polymyositis (with or without skin involvement) and progressive

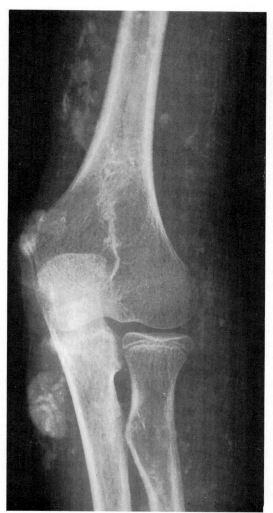

Fig. 148-1   Radiograph of an elbow from a 10-year-old girl with polymyositis.

systemic sclerosis were the most common disorders associated with the cutaneous calcification. When no specific disease entity could be established, muscle weakness suggestive of polymyositis was prevalent. Wheeler et al [10] reviewed the literature from 1938 to 1952 and described an additional 66 cases of "normocalcemic" calcinosis. In 51 of these the diagnosis of polymyositis or progressive systemic sclerosis was evident. Sufficient data were lacking in the remaining 15 cases to make a definitive diagnosis but the above-named conditions were also suspected. It was Wheeler's conclusion that so-called calcinosis circumscripta or calcinosis universalis was rarely a primary diagnosis, but rather was usually associated with progressive systemic sclerosis [11] or polymyositis. There remain, however, a number of instances in which no underlying myositis or scleroderma can be demonstrated. The calcifications that occur in patients with progressive systemic sclerosis tend to be small and localized to the hands, feet, knees, and hips, but larger deposits widely distributed have also been observed. They usually, but not always, occur in areas where the skin is already involved. Inflammation around these deposits may be observed and pasty material may extrude spontaneously with subsequent ulceration and

scarring. The course of the disease in patients with progressive systemic sclerosis does not appear to be modified by the occurrence of calcifications. A recent review of 45 patients with systemic sclerosis disclosed secondary hyperparathyroidism (elevated serum PTH, low ionized serum calcium, decreased urinary calcium and phosphate) in patients with calcinosis compared to those without it [12]. There is no effective therapy for the calcifications. Trials of phosphate depletion or the use of the diphosphonate, disodium etidronate as a potential calcification inhibitor have been unsuccessful.

Calcifications that occur in polymyositis and dermatomyositis may be found in the muscles, skin, tendons, and subcutaneous tissues (Fig. 148-1). They are usually more extensive and larger in size than those in progressive systemic sclerosis. The buttocks, thighs, arms, and trunk can be severely involved, and ulcerations as well as local inflammatory reactions are common (Fig. 148-2). The face and neck are rarely involved. Severe clinical complications of calcification occur almost exclusively in the juvenile form of the disease. Contractures of joints, muscle atrophy, and failure of a limb to develop are also noted. Wheeler et al [10] have stated that occasional spontaneous remissions with resolution of the calcific deposits may sometimes occur, although this has not been noted in the calcifications associated with progressive systemic sclerosis. There is no known abnormality of calcium or phosphorus metabolism in either of the above diseases.

It may be difficult on occasion to differentiate between progressive systemic sclerosis and polymyositis since there are overlapping features common to both diseases. Calcification of the skin has also been reported infrequently in localized scleroderma [13], systemic lupus erythematosus, and rheumatoid arthritis, but it is difficult to be sure that these cases do not represent mixed connective tissue disease, a disorder which may have features of both systemic lupus erythematosus and progressive systemic sclerosis. This may be of clinical significance since the mixed connective tissue disease syndrome often responds to corticosteroid therapy [14], whereas this mode of treatment has no value in progressive systemic sclerosis.

Miscellaneous disorders with calcification

There is abundant clinical evidence that skin injured by physical or thermal trauma [15] may eventually calcify. True bone formation may occur in laparotomy scars, primarily in midline incisions involving the linea alba. Since this structure is derived from the sternum, it has been suggested that the cells in the linea alba retain their capacity to form true bone. In one series, 86 of 88 cases occurred in males [16]. Reversible penile calcifications have been noted with the anticancer drug, bleomycin, and idiopathic penile calcification has also been reported [17,18].

Prolonged venous stasis of the lower extremity, which is accompanied by stasis dermatitis and recurrent ulceration, may be complicated by calcification or ossification. The mineral is found localized to subcutaneous tissues, sparing skin and muscles [19]. Radiographs often show a straight edge when seen in profile; periostitis is a common accompaniment. Laminograms may reveal the presence of calcification when plain films are not rewarding and CAT scans may also be helpful [20]. Biopsy material has shown

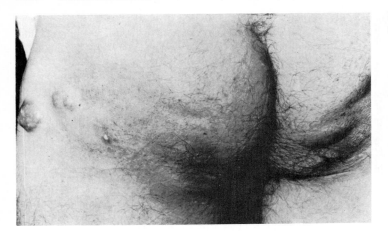

Fig. 148-2   Calcifications on the buttocks and hip in a patient with polymyositis.

true bone with typical marrow in a number of instances. The incidence of this complication in chronic venous stasis may be as high as 10 percent. The therapeutic value in removing these calcific deposits is still in doubt.

The *Ehlers–Danlos syndrome* and *pseudoxanthoma elasticum* are discussed in detail in Chap. 149. The subcutaneous calcifications that occur in the Ehlers–Danlos syndrome have a characteristic radiographic appearance. They are usually ovoid in shape (so-called spherules), with a dense outer shell surrounding a more diffuse and less dense central core. These spherules, which do not usually exceed 6 mm in the greatest dimension, most frequently occur in the lower extremities but may also occur in the arms. Histologically, the spherules are calcified necrotic fat or fibrocaseous material surrounded by dense fibrous tissue capsules which also may calcify; however, not all of the spherules calcify. In pseudoxanthoma elasticum [21] calcifications that are seen on roentgenograms are usually localized in the walls of blood vessels. However, extravascular subcutaneous calcifications also have been described. In affected patients a high calcium intake in adolescence has been correlated with clinical severity [22]. A number of larvae as well as the adult forms of several parasites may die and become calcified in the skin or subcutaneous tissues [23]. The larval form of the tapeworm *Taenia solium* appears radiographically as a calcific density several millimeters long and a few millimeters wide, oriented along the long axis of muscle fibers. When they are found in the skin, they have a more rounded appearance, with the perimeter of the calcification more dense than the central portion. The female guinea worm (*Dracunculus medinensis*) can measure up to 100 cm and is apparent radiographically in the subcutaneous tissues as a tubelike structure that does not follow the course of blood vessels. In loiasis, the adult worms live in the subcutaneous tissues and are most often found radiographically in the hands as thin, calcified threads measuring 3 to 6 cm in length. Their presence may result in an inflammatory response in the tendons of the hands. Echinococcus cysts (hydatid disease) may rarely be found in the proximal portion of the extremities. These calcified cysts are usually fragmented.

Werner's syndrome is characterized by premature senility, diabetes mellitus, hypogonadism, and a generalized mediosclerosis of arteries beginning in the third decade of life. Arterial calcification is located in the distal part of the lower extremities but subcutaneous calcifications, mostly in the soft tissues around the knees and ankles, have also been described.

Aberrant ossification of the skin and subcutaneous tissues

Skin tumors

Ossification has been observed in a variety of skin tumors including pyogenic granulomas, fibroxanthomas, nevi, basal cell carcinomas, pilomatrixomas, and chondroid syringomas [24–27]. When nevi or basal cell carcinomas ossify, they are almost always located on the face. The term *osteoma cutis* has been applied to the rare patient with acne vulgaris in whom the skin may exhibit loci of ossification as well as the above-mentioned tumors.

Hypoparathyroidism

Aberrant calcifications may occur in patients with hypoparathyroidism. However, this is not seen except in rare instances in the basal ganglia of patients whose disorder results from alteration or injury to the parathyroid glands in the course of thyroid or other neck surgery. It is, therefore, unlikely that the calcification of the skin or subcutaneous tissues that occurs in patients with hypoparathyroidism of other causes can be ascribed to the changes in the concentration of calcium and inorganic phosphate in the extracellular fluid. Hypocalcemia, usually accompanied by some degree of hyperphosphatemia, is the usual biochemical alteration.

In idiopathic hypoparathyroidism, the parathyroid glands are either absent or replaced by fat or fibrous tissue. The injection of standard doses of parathyroid hormone produces prompt phosphaturia and an increase in excretion of cAMP. These patients are usually of normal stature and intelligence but frequently have other associated disorders, such as adrenal insufficency, cutaneous candidiasis, steatorrhea, macrocytic anemia, and cirrhosis of the liver. When aberrant calcification does occur, it is usually intracranial, most often in the basal ganglia.

Pseudohypoparathyroidism is the term coined by Albright and his colleagues to distinguish a separate group of presumably hypoparathyroid patients [28]. The concentrations of calcium and phosphorus in the serum are the same as those in idiopathic and surgical hypoparathyroidism, but the clinical picture is distinctive. The typical patient is short, thickset, with a round face, and shortened metacarpal and/or metatarsal bones. Calcification of basal ganglia is also seen. In addition, in this disease approximately 60 percent of the patients have subcutaneous ossifications which may present as hard, nontender nodules. They are more common in the extremities and tend to localize around large joints, but may be found anywhere. All reported biopsies have revealed the presence of true bone. The administration of parathyroid extract fails to produce the expected phosphaturic or cAMP response. In the few cases in which neck surgery has been performed, parathyroid glands which appear normal or hyperplastic have been found. Serum levels of immunoreactive parathyroid hormone are elevated and the parathyroid glands have been shown to contain biologically active parathyroid hormone which cross-reacts immunologically with purified parathyroid hormone. These and other observations regarding the renal defect in the excretion of cAMP when parathyroid hormone is administered support Albright's hypothesis that this disorder is due to end-organ resistance of the hormone rather than to its absence.

Pseudopseudohypoparathyroidism is the term applied to the patient with normal concentrations of calcium and phosphate in the serum but with other clinical features similar to those of patients with pseudohypoparathyroidism, including subcutaneous ossifications. The presence of subcutaneous ossification in these individuals further supports the concept that the alterations in concentrations of calcium and phosphate in the extracellular fluid are not the cause of the subcutaneous lesions.

Myositis ossificans

Myositis ossificans refers to the formation of true bone in muscles. This condition may be divided into two groups. The more common form is secondary to muscle trauma in which the aberrant ossification is localized to the area of traumatic involvement. The second variety has been termed *myositis ossificans progressiva* and refers to a systemic disorder of unknown cause.

Traumatic myositis ossificans may occur in any muscle, but the most common sites are the flexors of the upper arm and the quadriceps femoris. A doughy mass is present a few hours following physical injury, and heterotopic ossification may be observed within a month. As bone is formed, the serum alkaline phosphatase may rise slightly, but the concentrations of calcium and phosphate in the serum remain normal. Ackerman [29] has pointed out the necessity of distinguishing this disease from various types of sarcoma in order to avoid mutilating surgery. So-called zone phenomena are present in the histology of traumatic myositis ossificans. The zones are comprised of a central undifferentiated area which may be difficult to distinguish from true sarcoma. This is surrounded by a zone of osteoid, which is, in turn, encapsulated by true bone. Such zone phenomena are not seen in sarcomas. Ectopic ossification is also seen as a complication of hip surgery but rarely produces functional deficit.

Myositis ossificans progressiva is usually recognized within the first few years of life. Diagnostic features are the progressive nature of the muscle ossification associated with several congenital abnormalities, the most common of which is microdactylia or adactylia of the thumbs and great toes. There have been reports of multiple affected members of the same family, suggesting an inherited basis for the disorder. The levels of calcium, phosphate, and alkaline phosphatase in the serum are usually normal.

Lutwak [30] studied one case of this disease extensively. He found the overall metabolism of calcium and phosphorus to be normal. Using radioactive calcium kinetic techniques, he demonstrated the turnover of calcium to be increased, reflecting the large amount of extraskeletal bone. The course of the disease was not affected by corticosteroids.

Neurologic disorders

Neurologic disorders may be associated with deposition of bone around large joints. Paraplegia, hemiplegia, and head injury are the most common causes. This complication always occurs below the level of the neurologic injury. The tissues around the joints become inflamed and ossification follows within a few weeks. There is usually a rise in the serum alkaline phosphatase, which heralds the metastatic ossification. Radiation therapy and surgery have not been of benefit [31]. In paraplegia, the problem is often belated. A similar process has been reported distal to the joint which had been immobilized by a thermal injury.

Approach to the patient

Calcification and/or ossification in and under the skin is detected clinically or radiographically and requires precise definition.

Attention to the etiology may have considerable therapeutic importance since the soft tissue calcifications of hypervitaminosis D, renal failure, and the milk-alkali syndrome, as well as tumoral calcinosis, can be made to diminish or disappear if appropriate measures are taken. The so-called dystrophic calcification associated with skin and muscle diseases (scleroderma and dermatomyositis) is less amenable to therapy.

References

1. Glimcher M: Composition, structure and organization of bone and other mineralized tissues and the mechanism of calcification, in *Handbook of Physiology,* vol VII, *Parathyroid Gland,* edited by RO Greep, EB Astwood. Washington, DC, American Physiological Society, 1976, p 25
2. Bronner F, Coburn JW (eds): *Disorders of Mineral Metabolism,* vol II, *Calcium Physiology.* New York, Academic Press, 1982, 568 pp
3. Lian JB et al: The presence of γ-carboxyglutamic acid in the proteins associated with ectopic calcification. *Biochem Biophys Res Commun* **73:**349, 1976
4. Alfrey A, Solomons CC: Bone pyrophosphate in uremia and its association with extraosseous calcification. *J Clin Invest* **57:**700, 1976
5. Veress B et al: Tumoral lipocalcinosis. *J Pathol* **119:**113, 1976
6. Mozaffarian G et al: Treatment of tumoral calcinosis with phosphorus deprivation. *Ann Intern Med* **77:**741, 1972
7. Frame B et al: Massive osteolysis and tumoral calcinosis. *Am J Med* **50:**408, 1971
8. Greenebaum E: Metastatic calcification in skin: exclusive involvement of eccrine sweat ducts. A case report. *Hum Pathol* **11:**287, 1980
9. Rothstein JL, Welt S: Calcinosis universalis and calcinosis circumscripta in infancy and in childhood: three cases of cal-

cinosis universalis, with a review of the literature. *Am J Dis Child* **52**:368, 1936

10. Wheeler CE et al: Soft tissue calcification with special reference to its occurrence in the "collagen diseases." *Ann Intern Med* **36**:1050, 1952
11. Rosenberg JN: Calcinosis in scleroderma. *Proc R Soc Med* **69**:264, 1976
12. Serup J, Hagdrup HK: Parathyroid hormone and calcium metabolism in generalized scleroderma. *Arch Dermatol Res* **276**:91, 1984
13. Hazen PG, Askari A: Localized scleroderma with cutaneous calcinosis. A distinctive variant. *Arch Dermatol* **115**:871, 1979
14. Sharpe GC: Mixed connective tissue disease. *Arthritis Rheum* **20**:S181, 1977
15. Hogan VM, Conway H: Calcification of burn scars. *Plast Reconstr Surg* **33**:559, 1964
16. Lehrman A et al: Heterotropic bone in laparotomy scars. *Am J Surg* **104**:591, 1962
17. Hutchinson IF et al: Idiopathic calcinosis cutis of the penis. *Br J Dermatol* **102**:341, 1980
18. Theuvenet WJ et al: Massive deformation of the scrotal wall by idiopathic calcinosis of the scrotum. *Plast Reconstr Surg* **74**:539, 1984
19. Beninson J, Morales A: Subcutaneous calcification in leg ulcers: three cases. *Arch Dermatol* **90**:314, 1964
20. Mahoney PD et al: Osteoma cutis: computed tomographic appearance. *J Comput Tomogr* **9**:61, 1985
21. Goodman RM et al: Pseudoxanthoma elasticum: a clinical and histopathological study. *Medicine (Baltimore)* **42**:297, 1963
22. Renie WA et al: Pseudoxanthoma elasticum: high calcium intake in early life correlates with severity. *Am J Med Genet* **19**:235, 1984
23. Gaylor BW, Brogdon BG: Soft tissue calcifications in the extremities in systemic disease. *Am J Med Sci* **249**:590, 1965
24. Fulton RA et al: Bone formation in a cutaneous pyogenic granuloma. *Br J Dermatol* **102**:351, 1980
25. Chen KT: Atypical fibroxanthoma of the skin with osteoid production. *Arch Dermatol* **116**:113, 1980
26. Tomsick RS, Menn H: Ossifying basal cell epithelioma. *Int J Dermatol* **21**:218, 1982
27. Roth SI et al: Cutaneous ossification: report of 120 cases and review of the literature. *Arch Pathol* **76**:44, 1963
28. Bronsky D et al: Idiopathic hypoparathyroidism and pseudohypoparathyroidism: case reports and review of the literature. *Medicine (Baltimore)* **37**:317, 1958
29. Ackerman LV: Extra-osseous localized non-neoplastic bone and cartilage formation (so-called myositis ossificans): clinical and pathological confusion with malignant neoplasms. *J Bone Joint Surg* **40A**:279, 1958
30. Lutwak I: Myositis ossificans progressiva: mineral, metabolic and radioactive calcium studies of the effects of hormones. *Am J Med* **37**:269, 1964
31. Rosen AJ: Ectopic calcification around joints of paralysed limbs in hemiplegia, diffuse brain damage, and other neurological diseases. *Ann Rheum Dis* **34**:499, 1975

NEOPLASMS OF SUBCUTANEOUS FAT

Elaine Waldo and A. Bernard Ackerman

There are two types of adipose tissue, so-called white and brown, in both of which large amounts of fat are contained in cytoplasmic vacuoles. White fat constitutes the bulk of human adipose tissue and is distributed subcutaneously throughout the body in a panniculus, whereas brown fat (best developed in hibernating animals) in hu-

mans is concentrated principally in the intrascapular region, neck, axillae, and retroperitoneum.

Neoplasms may arise from any of the mesodermal cells that are normally lodged in the subcutis, namely, lipocytes, fibroblasts, and endothelial cells. The classification of neoplasms of the subcutaneous fat that follows is based upon cellular composition (Table 148-2).

Benign Lipoblastoma and Lipoblastomatosis

The term *lipoblastomatosis* [1] describes an asymptomatic, nontender proliferation of immature fat cells that occurs in very young children. About 88 percent of such lesions appear before 3 years of age. This benign neoplasm is more common in boys and, in them, appears mainly on the extremities, particularly the lower ones. Histologically, the neoplasm resembles fetal fat and consists of lipoblasts that vary from small, univacuolated signet-ring forms to large, multivacuolated cells separated into lobules by highly vascularized connective tissue [1,2] (Fig. 148-3). A myxoid stroma is often the supporting structure. Electron microscopy also demonstrates the cellular spectrum of the tumor and supports the concept of its relationship to fetal white fat [3].

Two variants of the lesion have been described, namely, a more common, benign, circumscribed, noninfiltrating type, and a more aggressive, deeply situated, diffuse type that tends to recur upon attempted extirpation.

Although the term lipoblastomatosis has been used for both types, it is suggested [1] that the designation *benign lipoblastoma* be used for the circumscribed type and *benign lipoblastomatosis* for the diffuse type.

Hibernoma

Hibernoma is a solitary, circumscribed, benign neoplasm of brown lipoblasts aggregated into variably sized lobules of polyhedral cells that contain vacuoles in finely granular eosinophilic cytoplasms and central round or oval nuclei (Fig. 148-4). Septa divide the lobules of well-vascularized connective tissue [4].

Hibernomas show no predilection for sex or age. They most often occur in the interscapular region, but sometimes in the neck, axillae, and mediastinum.

Hibernoma resembles closely the brown adipose tissue that is normal in many hibernating animals. The cells are oval or polygonal and less than half the size (25 to 40 μm in diameter) of the cells of white fat (120 μm); their nuclei are round and situated centrally within the cells, and their

Table 148-2 Classification of tumors of the subcutaneous fat

Embryonic white lipoblasts: benign lipoblastoma and lipoblastomatosis
Embryonic brown lipoblasts: hibernoma
Mature white lipocytes: lipoma, adiposis dolorosa (Dercum's disease)
Mature white lipocytes and endothelial cells: angiolipoma (infiltrating and noninfiltrating)
Mature white lipocytes, fibrocytes, collagen: spindle cell lipoma, pleomorphic lipoma
Atypical white lipocytes: liposarcoma

Fig. 148-3 Lipoblastomatosis. Variously sized lipoblasts are arranged in a lobular configuration. ×85.

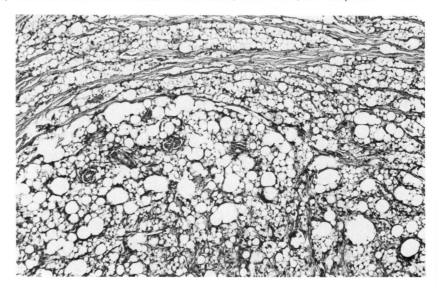

Fig. 148-4 Hibernoma. The subcutis has largely been replaced by cells with a central nucleus and numerous small vacuoles in a granular cytoplasm. These vacuolated cells have been likened to mulberries. ×220.

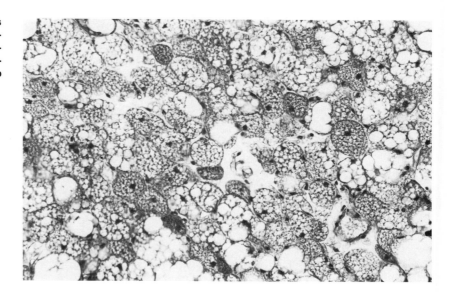

Fig. 148-5 Angiolipoma. The neoplasm is well circumscribed and consists of arterioles; venules; capillaries, some of which are thrombosed; and mature fat cells. × 85.

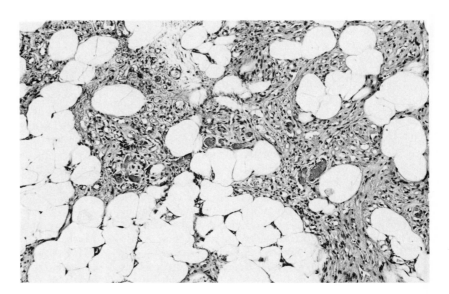

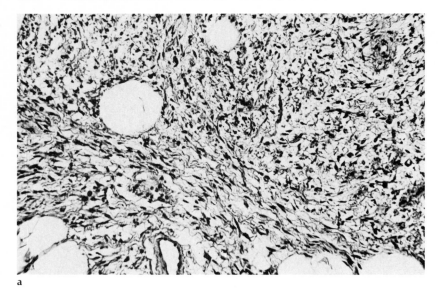

a

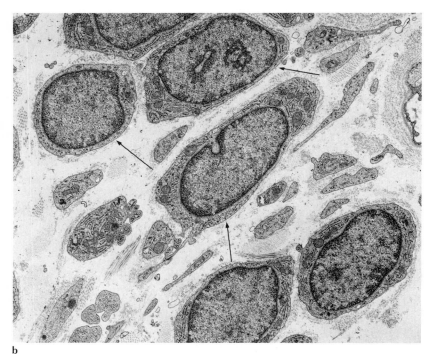

b

Fig. 148-6 Spindle cell lipoma. There are increased numbers of hyperchromatic spindle, fibroblast-like cells in a myxomatous stroma. Many of the fibroblast-like cells are surrounded by a discontinuous basal lamina (arrows). (a) ×170. (b) ×6,000.

cytoplasm is granular. The brown color results from the combination of abundant lipochrome and high vascularity.

Lipoma

A lipoma is a nonpainful, usually well-circumscribed, benign neoplasm of mature lipocytes. The lesions tend to be solitary, but some are multiple [5].

Lipomas may appear at any age, but particularly in the age group between 40 and 60. They are more common in women, but multiple tumors are more common in men. Their distribution may be widespread, but the majority occur in the subcutaneous tissue of the neck, back, arms, and shoulders. They may reach enormous sizes.

Microscopy shows lipomas to be composed of mature fat; lipomas do not usually have well-organized fibrous septa that divide fat lobules as does normal subcutaneous fat. Compression of the surrounding connective tissue by the gradually expanding lipoma often gives the impression of encapsulation [5]. Multiple, asymmetrical lipomas associated with pain are termed *lipoma dolorosa*. Liposarcomas tend to arise de novo and not in preexisting lipomas.

Adiposis dolorosa (Dercum's disease)

The four major clinical manifestations of Dercum's disease are (1) nodules of fat in the subcutis, (2) pain associated with the adiposity, (3) asthenia, and (4) psychic disturbances [6,7]. The painful fat nodules may be widespread, giving the impression of ordinary obesity, especially of the abdomen, thighs, buttocks, and arms. The cause of pain is unknown. Asthenia may be the presenting sign, and it may

Fig. 148-7 Pleomorphic lipoma. There are multinucleated giant cells many of which have a floret-like arrangement in association with dense bundles of mature collagen and variable sized fat cells. ×400.

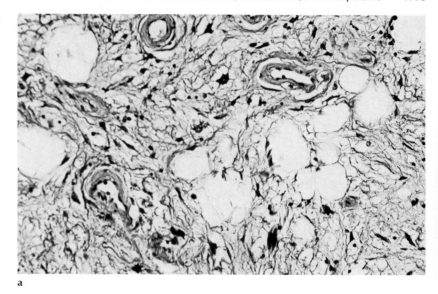

a

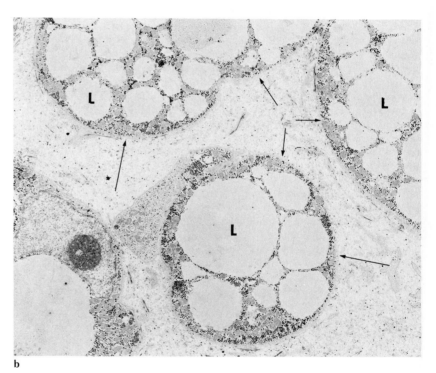

b

be so severe that the patients, who are most often older women, are incapacitated by it.

Histologic examination of the lesions shows only nodular connections of mature fat cells.

Angiolipoma

Howard and Helwig [8] defined *angiolipomas* as a painful mass usually occurring shortly after puberty and situated in the subcutaneous tissue, most often of the trunk or extremities. It is a well-circumscribed, benign neoploasm composed of mature fat cells and well-developed arterioles, venules, and capillaries, in which fibrin thrombi often form (Fig. 148-5). Angiolipomas require merely conservative surgical excision (enucleation) and usually do not recur.

A rare variant of angiolipoma extends into deeper structures like skeletal muscle and bone, and tends to recur unless widely excised. This type is also painful, occurs in young adults, and usually involves the lower extremities. The histologic appearance of infiltrating angiolipoma is similar to that of the noninfiltrating form [9,10].

Spindle cell lipoma

In 1975, Enzinger and Harvey [11] described a variant of lipoma that was often misinterpreted as liposarcoma and which they named *spindle cell lipoma*. This lesion is a single, slow-growing, superficially or deeply situated, painless nodule that grows to about 5 cm in diameter, occurs on the back, shoulders, or neck, and is most frequent in

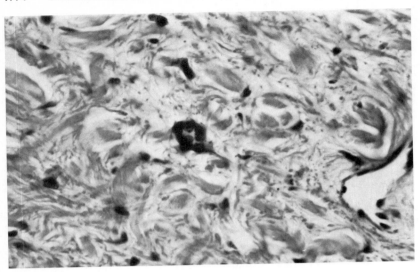

Fig. 148-8 Liposarcoma. Bizarre lipoblasts are present in highly vascularized myxomatous stroma (a). Rounded tumor cells with multiple, cytoplasmic, nonmembrane-bound lipid vacuoles (b) and surrounding basal lamina (arrows). (a) ×170. (b) ×4,000. *(Electron micrograph courtesy of Dr. J. C. Vuletin.)*

men (about 90 percent of cases) between 45 and 70 years of age.

Microscopy shows a well-circumscribed collection of mature fat cells separated or partly replaced by groups of small, slender spindle cells in a localized portion of an ordinary lipomatous neoplasm. In others, the spindle cells compose, or are distributed diffusely throughout, the entire lesion [11,12] (Fig. 148-6). In the latter case, the proliferating spindle cells and the collagen they make may obscure the essential lipomatous nature of the process. Usually, the spindle cells are oriented along bundles of collagen, sometimes they are arranged in a palisade.

In general, the spindle cells are remarkably uniform but, rarely, they show marked atypicality with nuclear pleomorphism and hyperchromasia. However, mitotic figures are hardly ever seen. Thick collagen bundles, a myxoid matrix, and an inconspicuous vascular pattern are other characteristics of this benign neoplasm.

Biologically, spindle cell lipomas, like others so far discussed, are wholly benign. Surgical excision is curative.

Pleomorphic lipoma

Recently a neoplasm that simulates a sclerosing or pleomorphic liposarcoma has been described [13]. It is usually a painless, circumscribed subcutaneous mass that occurs predominantly in men in their fifth to seventh decades and is situated in the shoulder or neck regions. Rarely does a pleomorphic lipoma measure more than 6 cm. Microscopically, it is composed of variably sized fat cells and bizarre pleomorphic multinucleated giant cells many of which have a floret-like arrangement of nuclei associated with dense bundles of mature collagen (Fig. 148-7).

This neoplasm is benign and most probably represents a pleomorphic variant of spindle cell lipoma.

Liposarcoma

In 1962, Enzinger and Winslow [14] wrote as follows: "Among mesenchymal neoplasms, liposarcomas are probably unsurpassed by their wide range in structure and behaviour. In fact, the variations are so striking that it seems more apt to regard them as groups of closely related neoplasms, rather than a well-defined single entity. Since liposarcomas may range from frankly malignant neoplasms to borderline cases of low-grade malignancy, careful histologic classification is mandatory for determining prognosis and selection of proper type of therapy." Their judgement obtains to this day for the degree of differentiation is the most reliable yardstick in the determination of clinical behavior [15].

Liposarcomas are malignant mesenchymal neoplasms composed of atypical adipose cells that most often occur in the large connective tissue zones between muscles of the lower extremities (especially the popliteal fossa and medial thigh), buttocks, and shoulders. They are deep-seated neoplasms affecting men between ages 50 and 55 years most frequently, and often presenting as palpable masses which sometimes may be astoundingly large, weighing in excess of 50 pounds. Liposarcomas in children are very rare [16].

Although liposarcomas in the shoulder, neck, and face region may arise in the subcutaneous fat, most liposarcomas do not have their origin in the subcutis, but in the deeper structures.

Several histologic classifications for liposarcomas have been proposed. One morphologic classification divides liposarcomas into four types, namely (1) myxoid (by far the most common), (2) round cell, (3) well-differentiated, and (4) pleomorphic. More than one pattern may be present in the same specimen. The neoplasms are composed of proliferating lipoblasts which, depending on the subtype, have different cytologic appearances ranging from stellate and spindle to bizarre, uniloculated, or multioculated. In addition to cytologic variation, there are marked differences in amount of lipid deposition, vascularity, mitotic activity, and in stroma, which range from myxoid to sclerotic [14]. Often a plexiform pattern of capillaries is seen (Fig. 148-8).

Findings by electron microscopy suggest that a continuum of stages of differentiation from fibroblast to mature lipocyte can be found in each of the neoplasm types [17]. However, one type of incompletely differentiated cell may predominate in the various types of liposarcoma.

The well-differentiated and myxoid liposarcomas have the best prognosis; the round-cell and pleomorphic types have the worst. The former infiltrate locally, tend to recur, but seldom metastasize. The latter metastasize to the lungs, liver, and bone marrow. Radical surgery is the treatment for the primary neoplasm; failure of complete ablation is ominous.

Neoplasms incidentally in the subcutis

Some neoplasms, benign or malignant, may extend into the subcutaneous fat from the dermis above (e.g., dermatofibrosarcoma protuberans) or from the fascia below (e.g., nodular fasciitis). Rarely, basal cell carcinomas and squamous cell carcinomas get that deep. Metastatically malignant neoplasms (e.g., malignant melanomas) may also be situated in the subcutaneous fat.

References

1. Velios F et al: Lipoblastomatosis: a tumor of fetal fat different from hibernoma. *Am J Pathol* **34:**1149, 1958
2. Chung EB, Enzinger FM: Benign lipoblastomatosis. *Cancer* **32:**482, 1973
3. Alba Greco M, Garcia RL, Vuletin JC: Benign lipoblastomatosis: ultrastructure and histogenesis. *Cancer* **45:**511, 1980
4. Sutherland JC et al: Hibernoma: a tumor of brown fat. *Cancer* **5:**364, 1952
5. Adam FE et al: *Lipomas*. Am J Cancer **16:**1104, 1932
6. Stout AP, Lattes R: *Atlas of Tumor Pathology: Tumors of the Soft Tissues,* 2d series, fascicle 1. Washington, DC, AFIP, 1966, p 52
7. Wohl MG, Pastor N: Adipositas dolorosa (Dercum's disease). *JAMA* **110:**1261, 1938
8. Howard WR, Helwig EG: Angiolipoma. *Arch Dermatol* **82:**924, 1960
9. Lin JJ, Lin F: Two entities in angiolipoma. *Cancer* **34:**720, 1974
10. Stimpson N: Infiltrating angiolipoma of skeletal muscle. *Br J Surg* **58:**464, 1971
11. Enzinger FM, Harvey DA: Spindle cell lipoma. *Cancer* **36:**1852, 1975
12. Angervall I et al: Spindle cell lipoma. *Acta Pathol Microbiol Scand [A]* **84:**477, 1976
13. Schmookler BM, Enzinger FM: Pleiomorphic lipoma: a benign tumor simulating liposarcoma. *Cancer* **47:**126, 1981
14. Enzinger FM, Winslow DJ: Liposarcoma. *Virchows Arch [Pathol Anat]* **335:**367, 1962
15. Enzinger FM, Weiss SW: *Soft Tissue Tumors*. St. Louis, CV Mosby, 1983, pp 248, 276
16. Kauffman SI, Stout AP: Lipoblastic tumors and children. *Cancer* **12:**912, 1959
17. Yao SF et al: Ultrastructure of benign and malignant adipose tissue tumors. *Pathol Annu* **15:**67, 1980

CHAPTER 149

HERITABLE DISORDERS OF CONNECTIVE TISSUE WITH SKIN CHANGES

Sheldon R. Pinnell and Victor A. McKusick

Heritable disorders of connective tissue are generalized defects involving primarily one element of connective tissue—collagen, elastin, or mucopolysaccharide—and are transmissible in a simple mendelian manner [1–3].

The Marfan syndrome

Summary description

Patients with the Marfan syndrome may have major abnormalities in three areas: the eye, especially dislocation of the lenses; the skeletal system, especially excessive length of extremities, loose-jointedness, kyphoscoliosis, and anterior chest deformity; and the cardiovascular system, especially aortic aneurysm (diffuse and/or dissecting) and mitral valve redundancy with regurgitation. The disorder is inherited as an autosomal dominant. Skin manifestations consist of striae distensae, a common finding, and elastosis perforans serpiginosa, a rare finding.

Clinical manifestations

Skeletal (Figs. 149-1 and 149-2). The skeletal features particularly impressed Marfan, who in 1896 described the syndrome which bears his name. Marfan's term for the disorder, *dolichostenomelia,* means "long narrow extremities." (Some [4] suggest that Marfan's patient, in fact, had congenital contractural arachnodactyly, a recently delineated entity, rather than the disorder we now call the Marfan syndrome.) The skeletal features were also the basis for Achard's designation, *arachnodactyly,* dating from 1902. Patients with the Marfan syndrome are excessively tall, or at least taller than unaffected relatives. The proportions are abnormal, with abnormally low ratio of upper segment to lower segment. The segments are measured below and above the top of the pubic symphysis. In practice, two measurements are made with the patient standing: height and lower segment (top of pubic symphysis to floor). In adult whites the mean ratio is about 0.92; in adult American blacks it is about 0.87. The excessive length of the extremities is primarily responsible for the abnormally low upper-segment-to-lower-segment ratio (US/LS) in the Marfan syndrome. Shortening of the trunk by kyphoscoliosis exaggerates the low US/LS and makes its interpretation difficult. Indeed, kyphoscoliosis of any cause usually results in an abnormally low US/LS. In the presence of more than minimal kyphoscoliosis, the US/LS should not be used in support of the diagnosis of the Marfan syndrome. The arm

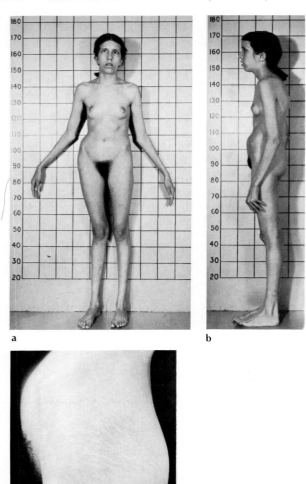

a   b

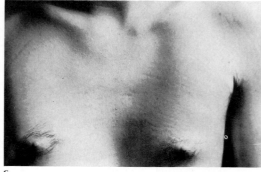

c

Fig. 149-1   The Marfan syndrome. (a and b) Frontal and lateral views of 15-year-old girl with the Marfan syndrome. Note tall stature, arachnodactyly, kyphoscoliosis, round shoulders, and strabismus. **(c)** Striae distensae over hips in same patient.

span of patients with the Marfan syndrome is often greater than the height. The metacarpal index based on the ratio of length to width of metacarpals is said to be useful, but requires a radiograph of the hands.

The ribs seem to undergo the same excessive longitudinal growth as do the bones of the extremities. Depression of the sternum (pectus excavatum) or projection (pectus carinatum) or an asymmetrical deformity of the anterior chest results.

Loose-jointedness is often striking in patients with the Marfan syndrome. Flat-footedness, hyperextensibility at the knees (genu recurvatum) and elbows, and dislocation of joints including congenital dislocation of the hip of the newborn are manifestations of the loose-jointedness. Because of both the loose-jointedness and the long extremities, the patient is often able to touch his umbilicus with the right hand passed around the back and approaching the umbilicus from the left. A relatively narrow palm of the

hand with long thumb and loose-jointedness is the basis for the Steinberg sign: the thumb opposed across the palm extends well beyond the ulnar margin of the hand.

Ocular. Most patients with the Marfan syndrome have myopia. It appears that the eyeball is abnormally long, as are the extremities. Probably about 70 percent of Marfan's syndrome patients have ectopia lentis. (Williams of Cincinnati described ectopia lentis in sibs with typical features of the Marfan syndrome in 1876, 20 years before Marfan's report.) Sometimes detection of mild abnormality requires full dilation of the pupils and slit-lamp examination for redundancy of the suspensory ligament of the lens. Most often the lens is displaced upward. With overt dislocation, the margin of the lens may be evident in the lower part of the pupil. An occasional tip-off to the presence of lens subluxation is iridodonesis, billowing of the iris curtain,

Fig. 149-2   The Marfan syndrome. (a and b) Frontal and lateral views of 20-year-old boy with the Marfan syndrome. Note tall stature, depressed sternum, scoliosis, and arachnodactyly. The father and a younger brother were also affected. This patient falls among the approximately 30 percent who do not have ectopia lentis. His brother, however, did have ectopia lentis. **(c)** Striae distensae over pectoral and deltoid areas.

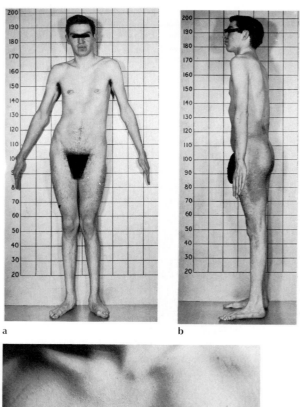

a   b

c

with quick motion of the eyeball due to lack of its usual support. Dislocation of the lens into the anterior chamber or trapping of the lens in the pupil sometimes occurs, and acute glaucoma can be a complication. Detachment of the retina is also an ocular complication of the Marfan syndrome. This is probably more than merely the detachment to which the long eyeball of myopia is subject.

Cardiovascular. The most frequent serious cardiovascular feature of the Marfan syndrome is a weakness of the aortic media which leads to diffuse aneurysm or dissecting aneurysm or a combination of the two. Aneurysm may develop in the first year or two of life or not until the fifth or sixth decade. Indeed, some patients live a respectable life span without developing aortic complications. The ascending aorta bears the main brunt even though the genetically determined defect is clearly generalized. The ascending aorta is subject to greater stress of a particular type, namely expansible pulsation, than any other part of the arterial tree; in combination with the genetic defect, the stress can lead sooner or later to structural fatigue in the aorta. Although the ascending aorta shows the main change, abdominal aneurysm without notable thoracic involvement has occurred in a few patients.

The first part of the aorta to undergo progressive dilation in the Marfan syndrome is usually that portion in the region of the sinuses of Valsalva. Since this is well within the radiographic silhouette of the heart, the patient may have outspoken aortic regurgitation without evident dilatation of the aorta. Echocardiography is a sensitive noninvasive diagnostic procedure for aortic root involvement and for estimating progression.

The mitral valve may be redundant, resulting in regurgitation. With mild abnormality, a murmur limited to late systole is produced, and cineangiographic studies show correlation with retrolapse of the posterior, or mural, leaflet of the mitral valve, producing regurgitation in the latter part of systole. With more advanced involvement of the mitral valve, the murmur is pansystolic and the regurgitation is of major functional significance.

Other features. The palate usually has a high arch and the anterior teeth may be crowded. Hernia is frequent in the Marfan syndrome. Pulmonary manifestations include cystic changes, emphysema, and "spontaneous" pneumothorax. Musculature is often underdeveloped and hypotonic.

Skin changes. These are not a conspicuous feature of the Marfan syndrome. Two types of changes have been observed. Most patients show striae distensae, particularly in the pectoral and deltoid areas and over the thighs. Although the authors have not seen this feature, elastosis perforans serpiginosa has been described in patients who appear to have the Marfan syndrome [5].

The basic defect

The precise nature of the gene-determined derangement in the Marfan syndrome is not known. A structural abnormality in the α_2 chain of type I collagen has been reported in a sporadic case of the Marfan syndrome [6]. Diminished type I collagen synthesis has been reported in tissue culture

of aortic media and adventitia in another sporadic case [7]. Diminished elastin content and desmosine cross-linking have been described in aortas from other patients with the Marfan syndrome [8,9]. These changes may reflect abnormal fibrillogenesis and do not necessarily reflect a primary elastin mutation.

Genetics

The Marfan syndrome is inherited as an autosomal dominant. About 15 percent of cases of the Marfan syndrome are sporadic, i.e., have normal parents and other ancestors, and arise apparently by a new mutation in the sperm or ovum. Once originated, the condition can be transmitted in an autosomal dominant pedigree pattern. In a number of dominantly inherited conditions, including this one, "paternal age effect" is demonstrated. The average age of fathers of sporadic cases of the Marfan syndrome is several years greater than that of all fathers. (Maternal age effect in several chromosomal aberrations, notably mongolism, is well known; paternal age effect in point mutations is less familiar.)

Considerable case-to-case variability in the severity of the Marfan syndrome is observed. Even sibs may vary in severity of affection, and some components of the syndrome, e.g., the ocular, may be missing in one sib, present in another. The variability is undoubtedly due both to exogenous (environmental or nongenetic) factors and to differences in the rest of the genotype of the individual and the genetic milieu in which the mutant gene operates. The "normal" allele with which the mutant allele is paired can be of diverse types; these are called isoalleles. This source of variability may account in part for the fact that dominant conditions are usually more variable than recessive ones. In addition, many modifier genes may be present at other loci. Observations of the Marfan syndrome in monozygotic twins who show closely similar type and degree of affection demonstrate the role of genetic modifiers. Variability in the Marfan syndrome is reminiscent of observations on single-gene syndromes in mice by Dunn and others: depending on the genetic background on which the particular mutant gene is placed, some features of the syndrome may disappear or be strikingly modified in severity.

Homocystinuria

Summary description

Homocystinuria is an inborn error in the metabolism of methionine. Activity of the enzyme cystathionine synthase is deficient. Clinical features include ectopia lentis, dolichostenomelia, and chest and spinal deformity as in the Marfan syndrome. Generalized osteoporosis, arterial and venous thrombosis, and mental retardation are features of homocystinuria not found in the Marfan syndrome. Homocystinuria is an autosomal recessive condition. The cutaneous manifestations include malar flush, wide-pored skin of the face, and cutis reticulata.

Clinical manifestations

Ocular. Most patients with homocystinuria have ectopia lentis by age 10. The dislocation of the lens is progressive

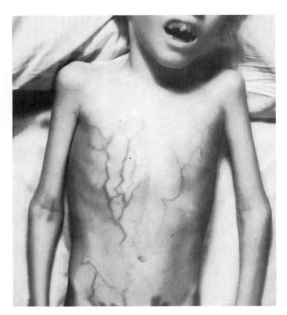

Fig. 149-3   Homocystinuric child, aged 7½ years. Collateral venous channels have developed secondary to thrombosis of the inferior vena cava.

so that the eyes may be found to be normal in the early years of life. It appears that the displacement of the lens is most often downward rather than upward as in the Marfan syndrome. Myopia is present in these patients also. Staphyloma, rupture of the sclera, has been observed.

Skeletal. Dolichostenomelia may be as striking as in the Marfan syndrome. Loose-jointedness, however, is usually inconspicuous; indeed, the joints sometimes show reduced mobility. The hand may, for example, have a "tight feel." Generalized osteoporosis is present in most cases. The vertebrae are often of "codfish" type from a hollowing out of the vertebral bodies by pressure of the expansile intervertebral disk. Fractures are frequent in homocystinuria.

Vascular. Although the aorta and heart (except for the coronary arteries) are not significantly affected in homocystinuria, serious, often fatal arterial and venous thromboses represent major problems (Fig. 149-3). Acute coronary occlusion, renal artery stenosis or occlusion with hypertension, bilateral thrombosis of the internal carotid arteries, and occlusion of arteries of the extremities have all been observed and may occur even in the first decade of life. Phlebothrombosis with pulmonary embolism, thrombosis of the inferior vena cava or of the portal vein, and intracranial venous and arterial thromboses have been described. The arterial thrombosis can sometimes be shown to have occurred episodically; a completely occluded vessel may show a process of several vintages.

Other features. Mental retardation of some degree occurs in a majority of patients. However, some patients escape this feature. Even among homocystinuric sibs, one may be retarded and another of normal intelligence.

Skin. Malar flush is common in homocystinuric patients but is usually, it seems, not as striking in the United States

as it is in Britain where homocystinuria was first described. Possibly the lack of central heating and the cool, damp climate of Britain bring out this feature. The authors observed a very strikingly red face in a 46-year-old man with homocystinuria who, because of his employment as a farmer in the northern part of the United States, was much exposed to the elements. With exertion in hot weather the face of homocystinuric children may become unusually flushed, and a violaceous flush may appear when the child is recumbent.

The skin of the face is usually wide-pored in teen-aged and older patients. The skin of the extremities and, to some extent, of the trunk is reticulated.

The basic defect

Because of deficiency in the activity of cystathionine synthase, the normal condensation of homocysteine and serine to form cystathionine is defective. As a result, homocysteine is converted to homocystine which appears in the urine, or is converted back to methionine which is also present in increased amount in the urine as well as in the serum. As a result of the block in the pathway from methionine to cystine, cystine is an essential amino acid in these patients.

Current thinking about the pathogenesis of the connective tissue manifestations, such as ectopia lentis and osteoporosis, centers around the effects of sulfhydryl-containing compounds on collagen. Harris and Sjoerdsma [10] demonstrated a decrease of cross-linking of collagen in skin from two patients with homocystinuria. Specifically, they found an excess of alpha, or monomer, collagen relative to the amount of beta, or dimer, collagen. In two other patients this abnormality was not found. Homocysteine bears a structural resemblance to penicillamine which has been found to affect cross-linking in collagen. A number of sulfhydryl-containing compounds accumulate proximal to the block in homocystinuria. Another manner in which abnormality may be produced in inborn errors of metabolism is relative deficiency of some substance distal to the block. Because cystathionine synthase and cystathionine are present in normal brain and absent in the brain of homocystinuric patients, and because they are found mainly in higher animals, the possibility has been entertained that they normally pertain to intellect and that a deficiency leads to mental retardation. (Intracranial thrombosis undoubtedly contributes to mental retardation.) Whether a deficiency of cystine contributes to the connective tissue defect is unclear. Collagen has little or no sulfur-containing amino acid although procollagen does contain cysteine. The basis for the thromboses is also not established.

Genetics

Like all other Garrodian inborn errors of metabolism, homocystinuria is inherited as an autosomal recessive. This conclusion is supported by segregation analysis, by the increased frequency of consanguinity of parental pairs, and by the finding in liver biopsy specimens from both parents of affected persons of a level of activity of cystathionine synthase which is intermediate between the normal and the very low level of the affected person. Males and females are affected equally often and the clinical manifestations are, on the average, equally severe in both sexes. Affected parent and child have not been observed, and although many of the affected persons have had children, the offspring have not been affected. Loading tests with methionine or homocystine fail to give results which identify the heterozygote with certainty.

Homocystinuria may have a frequency of about 1 in 20,000 births. Survival of homocystinuric patients as a group is reduced. Of 68 cases in a series, 15 have died at ages varying from 18 months to 28 years, all of thrombotic complications. Several of the 68 patients are now in their fifties. Many different ethnic extractions are represented in the series.

Heterogeneity in the category of homocystinuria has been found. One form tends to be clinically milder with, for example, normal intelligence, responds to administration of vitamin B_6 (pyridoxine) in doses of about 100 mg per day with clearing of homocystine from the urine and probably avoidance of thrombotic episodes and of lens dislocation (if such has not already occurred), and shows low but measurable residual activity of cystathionine synthase which increases after B_6 administration. In contrast, other cases are B_6 nonresponsive and show no measurable cystathionine synthase activity. Restriction of methionine in the diet is the mainstay of therapy for this form.

Homocystinuria, in a literal sense, occurs with certain rare genetic defects of folate and vitamin B_{12} metabolism. In these conditions, the conversion of homocysteine back to methionine is defective.

Osteogenesis imperfecta

Summary description

Although the presently preferred designation for this condition refers only to the skeletal feature of the disorder, abnormalities are often present in the eye (blue sclerae) and ear (deafness), as well as the joints (which are hyperextensible) and the skin (which tends to be thin and form unusually wide scars). Sillence [11] has divided this heterogeneous disorder into four clinical groups (Table 149-1). Marked clinical and biochemical variability occurs within each subtype. The condition may be inherited as an autosomal dominant or autosomal recessive. Sporadic mutations appear to be common.

Clinical manifestations

Skeletal. "Brittle bones" is a familiar and dramatic feature of osteogenesis imperfecta (OI). Sometimes fractures occur in utero and the antenatal diagnosis is possible by x-ray of the unborn child. In such cases the extremities are likely to be short and bent at birth. Other patients escape fractures although they have blue sclerae and deafness and may suffer rupture of the Achilles or patellar tendon. Brittle bones result from a defect in the collagenous matrix of bone. The skeletal aspect of OI is, therefore, a hereditary form of osteoporosis. "Codfish vertebrae" (hollowing out of vertebral bodies by pressure from expansile intervertebral disk) or flat vertebrae are observed in some patients, particularly older patients in whom senile or postmenopausal changes exaggerate the change, or in young patients who are immobilized after fractures or osteotomies. Usually the frequency of fractures decreases at puberty. Because of failure of union of fractures, pseudoarthroses, e.g., of humerus or femur, occur in some. Loose-jointedness is sometimes striking in OI patients. Dislocation of joints can be a problem. Teeth may be opalescent (dentinogenesis imperfecta).

Eyes. Blue sclerae represent a valuable clue to the diagnosis. However, the ocular features are not of great functional importance and, as discussed below, are absent in some forms of OI.

Ears. Deafness develops in many of the patients by the second decade of life. Audiologically the deafness is usually indistinguishable from that of otosclerosis, although some patients have an element of cochlear, or nerve, deafness.

The skin. Patients with OI may have thin, rather translucent skin. It may resemble the atrophic skin of the aged. A study of surgical incisions in these patients shows healing of skin wounds to result in wider scars than usual. Macular atrophy of the skin was described by Blegvad and

Table 149-1   Osteogenesis imperfecta

Type*	Inheritance	Major clinical features	Biochemical defect
I (blue scleral dominant) (16620)	Autosomal dominant	Mild bony fragility Blue sclerae and deafness Dentinogenesis imperfecta present in some families	Diminished type I collagen synthesis with an altered pro α_1(I) gene
II (perinatal lethal) (25940) (16621)	Autosomal recessive	Intrauterine or early infant death Marked tissue fragility Broad, crumpled thighs Beaded ribs	Diminished type I collagen synthesis Defective pro α_1 (I) gene
III (Progressive deforming) (25942)	Autosomal recessive	Moderate bony fragility Marked postnatal growth retardation Marked kyphoscoliosis Normal sclerae and hearing	Delayed secretion of type I collagen with altered mannosylation
IV (white scleral dominant) (16622)	Autosomal dominant	Kyphoscoliosis Postnatal growth retardation Light blue to normal sclerae, normal hearing Dentinogenesis imperfecta present in some families	Defective pro α_2(I) gene

* Numbers in parentheses refer to entry in McKusick's *Mendelian Inheritance in Man*, 6th ed. Baltimore, Johns Hopkins University Press, 1983.

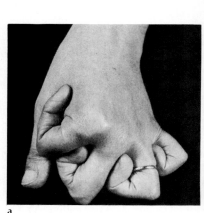
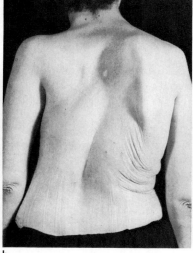
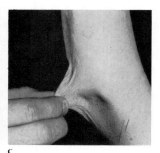

a   b   c

Fig. 149-4 The Ehlers-Danlos syndrome in a 37-year-old woman. (a) Loose-jointedness is demonstrated. (b) Note the severe scoliosis as well as the loose, puckered skin over the elbows. (c) Loose skin is demonstrated over the elbow. The patient is blind from retinal detachment as is also a brother with the Ehlers-Danlos syndrome.

Haxthausen [12]. Elastosis perforans serpiginosa has been described in OI.

Unusual bruisability occurs in some OI patients. This is probably due to a defect in the connective tissue in the walls of small blood vessels or in the supporting connective tissues. No consistent defect of the coagulation mechanism has been demonstrated.

The basic defect

Abnormalities in structure and synthesis of type I collagen have been demonstrated in OI. Collagen fiber bundles in skin and bone are diminished in size and decreased in number. Since type I collagen is the predominant collagen in these tissues, alteration in its synthesis might be expected to interfere with function. In type I OI, diminished type I collagen synthesis associated with one-half normal production of $\alpha_1(I)$ has been reported [13]. This may result from a deletion of one of the two pro $\alpha_1(I)$ alleles. Type I collagen production is also diminished in type II OI [3]. In one apparent new mutation, an internal deletion in the pro $\alpha_1(I)$ collagen gene has been reported [14]. A patient with type III OI has been described with excess mannosylation in the C-terminal propeptide of type I collagen [15]. Type IV OI has been described lacking $\alpha_2(I)$ collagen chain synthesis [16]. Another patient has been found with an apparent deletion in the $\alpha_2(I)$ chain [17].

Genetics

Inheritance may be autosomal dominant or autosomal recessive (see Table 149-1). Sporadic mutations undoubtedly occur in all types.

The Ehlers-Danlos syndromes

Summary description

The Ehlers-Danlos syndromes are a group of conditions sharing phenotypic features including hyperextensible skin and joints, poor wound healing, easy bruisability, and occasional fragility of large blood vessels and viscera [1–13]. At least 11 varieties of Ehlers-Danlos syndrome have been recognized on the basis of clinical and biochemical criteria. The syndrome may be inherited as an autosomal dominant, autosomal recessive, or X-linked recessive.

Clinical manifestations (Fig. 149-4).

Skin. The skin in the Ehlers-Danlos syndrome is thin, soft, velvety, and hyperextensible (Fig. 149-5). After stretching, the skin recoils promptly to its normal position (Fig. 149-4c); in later life this feature may lessen so that in some areas, such as the elbows, the skin may hang like dewlaps. In contrast to the rest of the body, skin over the palms and soles may be loose and redundant.

The skin may be excessively fragile and may split when subjected to minor, blunt trauma. Repairing such skin may be difficult since sutures often tear through the thin dermis; taping may result in the most satisfactory repair. Wound healing is delayed and scar tissue is thin "cigarette paper scar" and poorly retractile "fishmouth scar." Atrophic pigmented pretibial plaques in type VIII Ehlers-Danlos syndrome may resemble necrobiosis lipoidica diabeticorum [18]. So-called molluscoid pseudotumors occur over the elbows and knees (Fig. 149-6); these appear to represent herniations of fat through the dermis with subsequent encapsulation and calcification. Pea-sized calcified spherules occur subcutaneously over the extremities. Radiologically, the spherules are ovoid with a densely radiopaque shell surrounding diffuse calcification.

Easy bruisability is common, and this feature seems to be related to fragile blood vessels and the poor quality of the surrounding connective tissue. Clotting parameters are ordinarily normal. Acrocyanosis is a feature in some patients and varicosities may be prominent. Umbilical, hiatal, and inguinal hernias are common.

Skeletal. Hyperextensibility of joints is a cardinal feature of the Ehlers-Danlos syndrome. Joint dislocations are com-

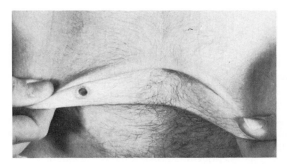

Fig. 149-5   Abnormally stretchable skin in the Ehlers-Danlos syndrome.

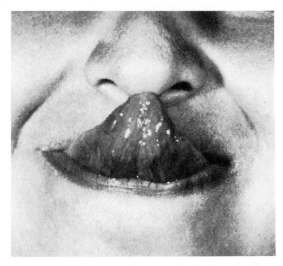

Fig. 149-7   The Ehlers-Danlos syndrome. Approximately 50 percent of patients can exhibit this ability compared to 10 percent of normals.

mon, and newborns often have dislocated hips. Osteoarthritis may develop after many years as a result of excessive mobility of large joints. Kyphoscoliosis is occasionally severe (Fig. 149-4b).

Internal manifestations. Rupture of a large artery and gastrointestinal perforation are the two most serious complications of the Ehlers-Danlos syndrome, often leading to death. Angiography is especially risky. Mitral valve prolapse is common. Surgery should be undertaken with caution since the tissues have been likened to wet blotting paper. Dehiscence of surgical wounds is common.

Other features. Premature birth with premature rupture of the fetal membranes occurs commonly. Since the fetal

Fig. 149-6   Atrophic scarring and a pseudotumor in the Ehlers-Danlos syndrome.

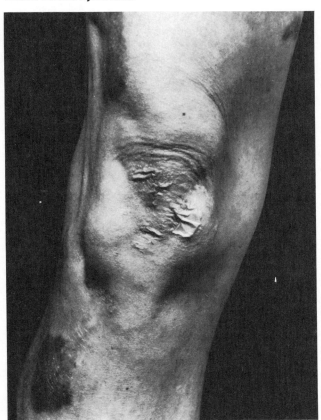

membranes are derived predominantly from the fetus, they share the same connective tissue fragility as the rest of the body. Pregnancy is undertaken with some risk in the Ehlers-Danlos syndrome; perineal lacerations and large hematomas are common, uterine rupture may occur, and forceps delivery is especially dangerous. Common ophthalmologic features include microcornea, blue sclera, and detachment of the retina. Severe, generalized periodontitis is a prominent feature distinguishing type VIII Ehlers-Danlos syndrome [14]. Some patients with the Ehlers-Danlos syndrome are able to touch the tip of their nose with the tongue (Gorlin's sign) (Fig. 149-7).

Basic defect

Abnormalities in collagen biosynthesis have been described in four of the eleven types of the Ehlers-Danlos syndrome [3]. Diminished levels of type III collagen have been demonstrated in tissues from patients with the ecchymotic form of the Ehlers-Danlos syndrome (type IV) [19]. Their skin fibroblasts produce diminished type III procollagen when compared to controls. One form of the disorder appears to be associated with a secretion defect for type III procollagen [20,21]. In hydroxylysine deficiency (type VI), hydroxylysine levels in collagen-containing tissues are diminished [22]. This disorder results from a deficiency of lysyl hydroxylase [23]. In type VII Ehlers-Danlos syndrome, procollagen conversion to collagen is abnormal. The incompletely cleaved procollagen is unable to participate in normal fibrillogenesis and collagen cross-linking. In most cases, the disorder results from a deficiency in procollagen aminoprotease [24]. One form appears to involve a structural mutation of the procollagen aminoprotease site of the α_2 chain of type I procollagen [25]. In type IX Ehlers-Danlos syndrome, an abnormality in copper metabolism results in deficient lysyl oxidase activity [26, 27]. This copper-dependent enzyme is necessary for collagen cross-linking. Lysyl oxidase deficiency has also been described in some patients with type V Ehlers-Danlos syndrome [28] but is normal in others [29]. In type X Ehlers-Danlos syndrome, abnormal platelet aggregation appears to be associated with a fibronectin abnormality [30].

Genetics

The Ehlers-Danlos syndrome, in its several forms, can be inherited as an autosomal dominant, autosomal recessive, or X-linked recessive (see Table 149-2). Accurate diagnosis depends on careful consideration of clinical, genetic, and biochemical features.

Pseudoxanthoma elasticum

Summary description

As in osteogenesis imperfecta, the preferred designation for this syndrome refers to only one aspect, the cutaneous one. Changes in the skin of the neck, axillary folds, and other areas usually develop in the second decade or later and are progressive. Other cardinal features are ocular (angioid streaks and retinal hemorrhages) and vascular (gastrointestinal hemorrhage and ischemic cardiac and peripheral arterial disease). Pseudoxanthoma elasticum (PXE) occurs in both autosomal recessive and autosomal dominant forms. The earliest detectable histologic lesion is accretion of elastic fibers with calcium. Later, fragmentation of elastic fibers in the skin and blood vessels and cracking of Bruch's membrane in the eye occur, producing the characteristic clinical features (Fig. 149-8).

Clinical manifestations

The skin. About the neck, in the axillary folds, around the umbilicus, in the inguinal area, in the antecubital fossae, and even on the penis and facial folds, the skin becomes loose and thickened in a pebbled or peau d'orange manner (Fig. 149-9). The infiltrative yellowish lesions in the antecubital fossae may alert the internist to the correct diagnosis when the blood pressure is taken. The pebbly lesions are yellowish, resembling xanthoma, leading to the name pseudoxanthoma. Although loose skin of the neck may be evident in most by the second decade of life, a few patients with angioid streaks and vascular lesions of PXE show, even in their forties and fifties, minimal skin lesions demonstrated chiefly by histologic study. The characteristic histologic change consists of fragmentation of elastic fibers which are calcified in the deeper layers of the dermis. Foreign-body giant cells are sometimes found in these areas, as well as a collagenous reaction. Sometimes calcification can be demonstrated in the skin lesions by radiography.

Another type of skin lesion found in some patients is perforating elastoma. The lesions may have a serpiginous distribution with points of perforation where material can be expressed (Fig. 149-10). Mucosal lesions, clinically and histologically similar to the skin lesions, are demonstrable by appropriate endoscopic methods on the inner aspect of the lower lip and in the rectum and vagina, as well as in the stomach and bladder. The labial lesion consists of a yellow patch with extensive vascularity. In mild form it may be distinguished with difficulty from Fordyce's condition (ectopic sebaceous glands), although the latter condition is usually more striking on the buccal mucosa than on the labial mucosa.

The eye. The ocular hallmark of PXE is the finding of angioid streaks. These streaks, wider than blood vessels, extend across the fundus in a distribution more or less radial from the optic disk. They are usually gray in color (Fig. A4-10). Crazing of an unusually brittle Bruch's membrane is responsible for angioid streaks which occur along lines of force in the eyes created by the pull of the muscles. Retinal hemorrhage is an acute complication which sometimes can be related to trauma to the eye. Scarring with or without preceding hemorrhage also endangers vision.

Vascular system. Gastrointestinal hemorrhage is the complication which most often brings the PXE patient to the attention of the internist. Lesions such as peptic ulcer or hiatal hernia are sometimes found and are aggravated by the presence of the vascular disease of PXE, but gastrointestinal bleeding often occurs in their absence. Recurrent hemorrhages may have their onset in the first decade of life. Bleeding from the urinary tract also has been observed. Submucosal vessels show changes, primarily in elastic fibers, comparable to those in the skin.

Hypertension results from involvement of the renal arteries. Hypertensive PXE patients of teen age have been reported.

Absent or reduced pulses in the extremities and arterial calcification, demonstrable radiographically, are found in a majority of PXE patients by age 30. Ischemic manifestations are uncommon, however. In the arms, neither the radial nor the ulnar pulse may be palpable, or they may be replaced by a pulsation anomalously situated in the middle of the wrist on its volar aspect; yet such patients usually have no signs or symptoms of deficient vascular supply to the hand. Arteriographic studies in such cases may show complete occlusion of the radial and ulnar arteries with the interosseous arteries unaffected; indeed, they may be dilated, giving at the wrist large terminal collaterals to the occluded radial and ulnar arteries and thereby providing adequate filling of the arteries in the hand. Biopsied arteries of the arm, shown arteriographically to have been occluded, exhibit fragmentation of the elastica of the media with surrounding reaction which has swollen the media and occluded the lumen of the artery. The medial lesion seems to be comparable to the pebbly lesion of the skin.

At autopsy the endocardium, especially that of the left atrium, and the pericardium have shown gross and histologic changes like those of the skin, but these are probably of no functional significance. Medial changes in the coronary arteries in PXE are probably the basis of, or at least a prominent contributing factor in, coronary occlusion in patients with PXE.

The basic defect

Skin biopsy reveals fragmentation and clumping of elastic fibers in the mid and lower dermis with calcification of the amorphous elastin core. The precise biochemical defect in PXE remains unknown. Ultrastructural studies have revealed abnormalities of both elastic tissue and collagen

Table 149-2   Ehlers-Danlos syndrome

Type*	Inheritance	Major clinical features	Biochemical defect
I (gravis) (13000)	Autosomal dominant	Prematurity associated with premature rupture of fetal membranes, marked skin fragility and poor wound healing Marked joint and skin hyperextensibility Easy bruisability	Unknown
II (mitis) (13001)	Autosomal dominant	Mild manifestations Joint hypermobility limited to digits	Unknown
III (benign hypermobile) (13002)	Autosomal dominant	Marked large joint hypermobility Mild skin features	Unknown
IV (ecchymotic) (22535)	Autosomal dominant	Marked bruisability, thin fragile skin, arterial rupture, intestinal perforation	Diminished type III collagen synthesis
	Autosomal recessive	Similar to IV autosomal dominant Marked bruisability, thin skin	Diminished type III collagen synthesis
	Unknown		Intracellular accumulation of collagen (? type III)
V (X-linked) (30520)	X-linked recessive	Short stature, hernias, mitral and tricuspid valve prolapse, moderate joint hypermobility	Lysyl oxidase deficiency
	X-linked recessive	Extensible skin, mild to moderate joint hypermobility	Unknown
VI (hydroxylysine deficient) (22540)	Autosomal recessive	Marked joint hypermobility, kyphoscoliosis, ocular fragility, hyperextensible and moderately fragile skin	Lysyl hydroxylase
VII (arthrochalasis multiplex congenita) (22541)	Autosomal recessive	Marked joint hypermobility, hip dislocation, short stature, moderate skin hyperextensibility	Procollagen amino-protease deficiency
	New dominant mutation	Marked joint hypermobility, hip dislocation	Probable structural mutation of pro α_2 (I)
VIII (periodontitis) (30415)	Autosomal dominant	Severe generalized periodontitis Marked skin fragility especially over shins	Unknown
IX (X-linked cutis laxa) (30415)	X-linked recessive	Hyperextensible skin, bony occipital horns, hernias	Abnormal copper metabolism Lysyl oxidase deficiency
X (fibronectin deficient) (22531)	Autosomal recessive	Easy bruisability, hyperextensible skin and joints	Abnormal fibronectin
XI (familial joint laxity) (14790)	Autosomal dominant	Marked joint laxity and dislocation Normal skin	Unknown

* Numbers in parentheses refer to entry in McKusick's *Mendelian Inheritance in Man*, 6th ed. Baltimore, Johns Hopkins University Press, 1983.

fibers [31]. In addition, the ground substance appears to be increased [32].

Genetics

Although previously considered exclusively an autosomal recessive trait, PXE is now known, particularly from the work of Pope [33–35], to exist in at least one dominant and one recessive form. Pope's type I dominant form is characterized by classic peau d'orange skin changes, by severe vascular complications such as angina, claudication, and hypertension, and by severe choroiditis. His type II dominant form, which he suggests is about 4 times more frequent than type I, is characterized by macular (or focal) changes in the skin, which is excessively stretchable, and by myopia, high arched palate, blue sclerae, and loose-jointedness in a significant number of cases [33]. Whereas Pope's recessive type I is the classic disorder, his type II is very rare, being present in only 3 of 121 probands in his extensive study in the United Kingdom. It is characterized by generalized skin changes with no blood vessel or ocular manifestations.

Other considerations

Cutaneous manifestations like PXE together with angioid streaks have been described with familial hyperphosphatemia [36]. Angioid streaks are rather frequently associated

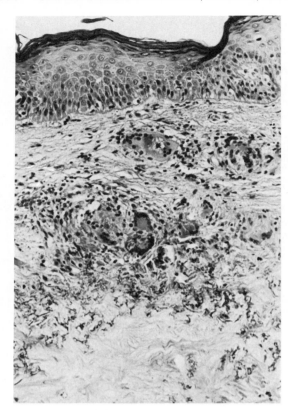

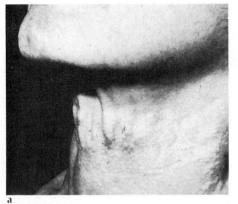

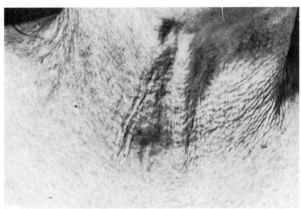

Fig. 149-8 Pseudoxanthoma elasticum. The pathology affects the connective tissue of most of the reticular dermis. Even in routine hematoxylin and eosin preparation one may see the tightly, but irregularly coiled, basophilic elastic fibers. The collagen associated with the fibrils is also abnormal; the broad collagen bundles so characteristic of the reticular dermis are replaced by irregular and rather confluent collagen fibrils. ×160. (Micrograph by Wallace H. Clark, Jr., M.D.)

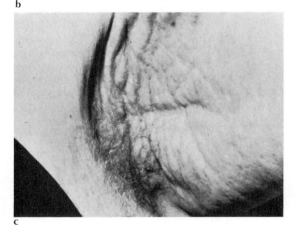

Fig. 149-9 Pseudoxanthoma elasticum. (a) Papules on the neck. There is a distinct yellowish hue. Loose, thickened skin with a pebbled appearance on the neck (b), and the axillae (c).

with Paget's disease of bone, and several have reported PXE changes of the skin, angioid streaks of the retina, and Paget's disease of bone in combination. The angioid streaks of Paget's disease are thought to reflect crazing of Bruch's membrane which has become brittle because of calcium deposition. (Iron deposit in Bruch's membrane may be responsible for the angioid streaks of sickle-cell anemia.) Possibly the PXE-like changes of Paget's disease are the result of damage to elastic fibers from metatopic calcification.

The appearance of the skin changes of actinic elastosis is somewhat similar to that of PXE but the distribution is quite different. The hands, almost never involved in PXE, are affected in actinic elastosis, whereas unexposed areas such as the axillae and groin are spared. The histologic appearance in actinic elastosis is different, being characterized by diffuse involvement in the superficial parts of the dermis, less intense basophilia of the connective tissue fibers than in PXE, and usually no fragmentation and granulization of the connective tissue fibers.

Elastosis perforans serpiginosa (also known as keratosis follicularis serpiginosa, and perforating elastoma) occurs as an asymptomatic cluster of keratotic papules often arranged, as the name implies, in an annular, serpiginous, or arciform pattern. Lesions appear during the first two dec-

ades of life. The lesions characteristically occur on the hairless regions of the nuchal area or less commonly on the cheeks and extremities (see Fig. 151-1). The conical or flattopped papules, which are 2 to 3 mm in diameter, contain a central keratotic plug and are light brown in color. Smith et al [37], in a review of this curious disorder, found an association of the skin changes with a heritable connective tissue disorder in 15 of 40 reported cases: osteogenesis imperfecta, the Ehlers-Danlos syndrome, the Marfan syndrome, pseudoxanthoma elasticum, Down's syndrome, and the Rothmund-Thomson syndrome. This

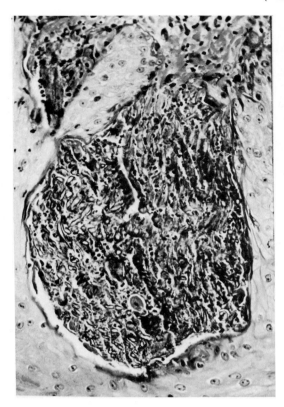

Fig. 149-10   Elastosis perforans serpiginosa. The clawlike epidermal—mesenchymal interaction shows a periphery of epidermal cells and a central area of fat bacillary-like orcein-ophilic fibers associated with inflammatory cell debris. × 256. (Micrograph by Wallace H. Clark, Jr., M.D.)

association was confirmed by Korting [38]. Histologic features are shown in Figs. 149-10 and 151-3.

Cutis laxa (dermatochalasia, generalized elastolysis)

Summary description

Cutis laxa is a rare group of disorders in which the skin hangs loosely in folds, resulting in a prematurely aged appearance. The disorder may be inherited (autosomal dominant, autosomal recessive, or X-linked recessive) or acquired.

Clinical manifestations

Skin. In cutis laxa the skin gives the appearance of being too large for the rest of the body. It tends to sag under the influence of gravity in areas where the skin is normally loose, e.g., around the face and eyes (Fig. 149-11). Sagging jowls may result in a "bloodhound" look. The skin may be excessively wrinkled and appear prematurely aged. At birth, the skin may be noticeably soft, loose, and hyper-extensible; in contrast to the Ehlers-Danlos syndrome, it returns slowly to its normal position after being stretched. Skin fragility, easy bruisability, joint hypermobility, and poor wound healing are not usually associated with cutis laxa. Cosmetic surgery can ordinarily be undertaken without complication.

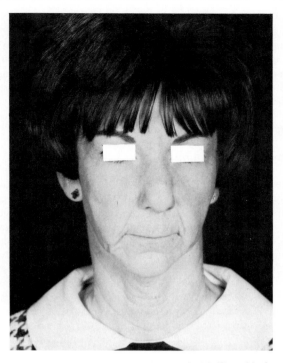

Fig. 149-11   Cutis laxa in a 15-year-old girl. The skin hangs in loose folds, giving the appearance of premature aging. (Courtesy of Dr. Peter Beighton, Johns Hopkins University School of Medicine.)

Other features. Beighton [39] pointed out characteristic facial features including a hooked nose, inverted nostrils, and a long upper lip. The cry of an affected infant may be hoarse, and a low-pitched voice is often associated with redundancy of the vocal cords. Hernias (inguinal, umbilical, and obturator) as well as diverticula of the gastrointestinal and genitourinary tracts are common. Angiographic studies in cutis laxa have revealed tortuous blood vessels with a particular corkscrew appearance [40]. Aortic dilatation and peripheral pulmonary artery stenosis have been described. The most severe manifestation of cutis laxa is progressive emphysema which may lead to early death from cor pulmonale. One form of cutis laxa is associated with growth retardation and congenital hip dislocation [41].

The basic defect

Elastic fibers are fragmented and diminished in number in cutis laxa skin [42,43]. In addition, collagen fiber morphology may be defective [44]. An X-linked form of cutis laxa associated with diminished lysyl oxidase activity and abnormal copper metabolism has been reclassified as type IX Ehlers-Danlos syndrome [26,27].

Genetics

Autosomal dominant, autosomal recessive, and X-linked recessive forms of cutis laxa are recognized. The dominant form of cutis laxa is basically a cosmetic problem and the prognosis is good. One autosomal recessive form of cutis laxa is associated with severe cardiorespiratory complications [42]. Another is characterized by growth retardation and ligamentous laxity [41]. X-linked cutis laxa (type IX Ehlers-Danlos syndrome) is characterized by mild joint laxity, bladder diverticula, hernias, and cranial occipital exostoses or horns [27]. Acquired forms of cutis laxa have been reported, often following an ill-defined febrile illness [45,46]. A rare autosomal recessive form of pseudoxanthoma elasticum may also resemble cutis laxa [34].

The genetic mucopolysaccharidoses

Summary description

The mucopolysaccharide storage diseases [47] or mucopolysaccharidoses, are clinically progressive, hereditary disorders characterized by the accumulation of mucopolysaccharides (glycosaminoglycans) in various tissues. Each of those outlined in Table 149-2 is caused by deficiency of a specific lysosomal enzyme normally involved in the degradation of one or more species of mucopolysaccharide. Ten enzymatically distinct types of mucopolysaccharidosis have been identified and most appear to have allelic variants. In most of these conditions the skin is diffusely thickened and hirsute. Pebbly lesions overlie the inferior end of the scapulae in the Hunter's syndrome (MPS II).

Pathophysiology

Lysosomes are the disposal and reclamation systems of the cell. The mucopolysaccharidoses (and some other conditions discussed in this book such as Fabry's disease) fulfill the criteria for lysosomal storage disease as defined by Hers [48].

1. As seen by electron microscopy, the cellular inclusions are bound by single membranes and stain positively for acid phosphatase.
2. The disorders are progressive.
3. Multiple organs are affected, e.g., liver, cornea.
4. The stored material is heterogeneous, e.g., both dermatan sulfate and heparan sulfate in MPS I and II.

The mucopolysaccharides consist of a protein core to which is attached multiple side chains made up of alternating uronic acid and hexosamine residues, some of which are sulfated. The side chains are digested by enzymes which work sequentially like a zipper. Thus even though different enzymes are deficient in the Hurler (MPS I) and Hunter (MPS II) syndromes, the same two mucopolysaccharides appear in excess in the urine because each of the two enzymes is involved at the distinct and different point in the degradation of these mucopolysaccharides.

With radioactive sulfate, Neufeld and her colleagues (for summary see [47]), in classic experiments with patients with one or another form of mucopolysaccharidosis, found that the radioactivity is retained for an abnormally long period. Furthermore, they could show that cocultivation of fibroblasts from different mucopolysaccharidoses led to mutual cross-correction of the defect in handling of ^{35}S. There were two surprises: (1) the Hurler and Scheie syndromes, previously considered separate entities called MPS I and V, respectively, were found not to cross-correct, indicating that they have the same defect; (2) phenotypically indistinguishable cases of the Sanfilippo syndrome (MPS III) were found to be of two (now four) different

types, on the basis of mutual cross-correction or lack thereof.

Eight separate classes of mucopolysaccharidoses are now identified through demonstration of deficiency of specific lysosomal enzymes. As shown in Table 149–3, these are MPS I, II, III A, III B, III C, IV, VI, and VII. For example, α-L-iduronidase is the enzyme deficiency in the MPS I group of conditions and includes the Hurler and Scheie syndromes which are thought to be allelic, i.e., due to homozygosity for different mutant genes at the same locus, like SS and CC diseases among the hemoglobinopathies. Several of these, in addition to MPS I, have seemingly allelic, severe and mild forms. In the case of the MPS I class, genetic compounds are suspected, i.e., patients who have a Hurler gene on one chromosome and a Scheie gene on the other; cases of an intermediate and to some extent unique phenotype that may represent the genetic compound at the α-L-iduronidase locus have been identified.

Clinical manifestations (Fig. 149-12)

These are given in Table 149-3 for each of the mucopolysaccharidoses. Clinical manifestations relate to the eye, heart, brain, bony skeleton, skin, and other systems.

Eye. Corneal clouding occurs in all except MPS II and III. It is a minor finding in MPS IV and can be severe in the others. A pigmentary retinal degeneration develops in the Scheie (MPS I S) and Hunter (MPS II) syndromes, and glaucoma is a complication particularly of MPS I S. Chronic papilledema is a feature of the Hunter syndrome (MPS II).

Heart. A pseudoatherosclerosis develops from intimal deposition of mucopolysaccharides, and coronary insufficiency (angina pectoris) may occur in children with the Hurler syndrome (MPS I H). The major cardiac problems, other than for cor pulmonale, are valvular and occur in most of the mucopolysaccharidoses. Aortic valve disease is a feature, for example, of the Scheie syndrome (MPS I S), and patients with the mild variety of MPS VI have required valve replacement. Patients with MPS IV have had aortic regurgitation.

Brain. Progressive deterioration of intellect is a cardinal feature in the Hurler (MPS I H) and Sanfilippo syndromes. In the Scheie (MPS I S) and the Maroteaux-Lamy syndromes (MPS VI) intellect is normal or near normal. In the mild form of the Hunter syndrome (MPS II) intellectual capacity is normal in some areas such as arithmetic function, but abnormal in other areas such as verbal performance; in the severe form of MPS II intellectual function is progressively and severely reduced.

Hydrocephalus, perhaps from "gumming up" of the meninges, is frequent in the MPS I and severe MPS II. Arachnoid cysts erode in the area of the sella turcica. In the case of the Hurler-Scheie compound, erosion into the nasal cavity with chronic spinal fluid rhinorrhea has been noted.

Skeleton. The changes in the bony skeleton are generically referred to as dysostosis multiplex. Running through most

Table 149-3   The genetic mucopolysaccharidoses

Number*	Eponym	Clinical	Genetics	Urinary MPS	Enzyme deficient
MPS I H (25280)	Hurler	Clouding of cornea, grave manifestations, death usually before age 10	Homozygous for MPS I H gene	Dermatan sulfate, heparan sulfate	α-L-Iduronidase
MPS I S	Scheie	Stiff joints, cloudy cornea, aortic valve disease, normal intelligence and (?) life span	Homozygous for MPS I S gene	Dermatan sulfate, heparan sulfate	α-L-Iduronidase
MPS I H/S	Hurler-Scheie	Intermediate phenotype	Genetic compound of MPS I H and MPS I S genes	Dermatan sulfate, heparan sulfate	α-L-Iduronidase
MPS II-XR, severe (30990)	Hunter, severe	No corneal clouding, milder course than in MPS I H, death before 15 years	Hemizygous for X-linked gene	Dermatan sulfate, heparan sulfate	Iduronate sulfatase
MPS II-XR, mild	Hunter, mild	Survival to 30s to 60s, fair intelligence	Hemizygous for X-linked allele	Dermatan sulfate, heparan sulfate	Iduronate sulfatase
?MPS II-AR (25285)	?Autosomal Hunter	Same as mild or severe MPS II-XR	Homozygous for autosomal gene	Dermatan sulfate, heparan sulfate	Iduronate sulfatase
MPS III A (25290)	Sanfilippo A	Indistinguishable phenotype: mild somatic, severe central nervous system effects	Homozygous for Sanfilippo A gene	Heparan sulfate	Heparan N-sulfatase
MPS III B (25292)	Sanfilippo B		Homozygous for Sanfilippo B gene	Heparan sulfate	N-Acetyl-α-D-glucosaminidase
MPS III C (25293)	Sanfilippo C		Homozygous for Sanfilippo C gene	Heparan sulfate	α-Glucosaminidase
MPS III D (23294)	Sanfilippo D		Homozygous for Sanfilippo D gene	Heparan sulfate	N-acetyl-α-D-glucosamide-6-sulfatase
MPS IV A (25300)	Morquio A	Severe, distinctive bone changes, cloudy cornea, aortic regurgitation	Homozygous for Morquio A genes	Keratan sulfate	Galactosamine-6-sulfate sulfatase
MPS IV B (25301)	Morquio B	Mild bone changes, cloudy cornea, hypoplastic odontoid	Homozygous for Morquio B gene	Keratan sulfate	β-Galactosidase
MPS VI, severe (25320)	Maroteaux-Lamy, classic severe	Severe osseous and corneal change; valvular heart disease, striking WBC inclusions; normal intellect; survival to 20s	Homozygous for Maroteaux–Lamy (ML) gene	Dermatan sulfate	Arylsulfatase B (N-acetylgalactosamine-4-sulfatase)
MPS VI, Intermediate	Maroteaux–Lamy, intermediate	Moderately severe changes	Homozygous for allele at ML locus or genetic compound	Dermatan sulfate	Arylsulfatase B (N-acetylgalactosamine-4-sulfatase)
MPS VI, mild	Maroteaux–Lamy, mild	Mild osseous and corneal change, normal intellect; aortic stenosis	Homozygous for allele at ML locus	Dermatan sulfate	Arylsulfatase B (N-acetylgalactosamine-4-sulfatase)
MPS VII (25322)	Sly	Hepatosplenomegaly dysostosis multiplex, mental retardation variable; WBC inclusions	Homozygous for mutant gene at β-glucuronidase locus	Dermatan sulfate, heparan sulfate	β-Glucuronidase

* Numbers in parentheses refer to entry in McKusick's *Mendelian Inheritance in Man*, 6th ed. Baltimore, Johns Hopkins Univ Press, 1983.

of the mucopolysaccharidoses are qualitatively similar features of skeletal x-rays with unique features superimposed in some of the individual conditions (e.g., the Morquio syndrome, MPS IV).

Skin. The only truly distinctive skin change of the MPSs is the ''pebbling'' (Fig. 149-13) over the inferior angle of the scapulas in MPS II (the Hunter syndrome). In addition, a generalized thickening of the skin is found in most of the conditions, although perhaps not in MPS IV (see below). Generalized hirsutism is also a striking feature of most, perhaps all, of the MPSs. Meyer et al [49] showed that rabbits injected with mucopolysaccharides grew hair in shaved areas more rapidly than did untreated rabbits.

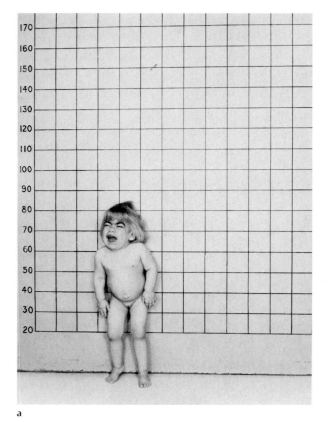

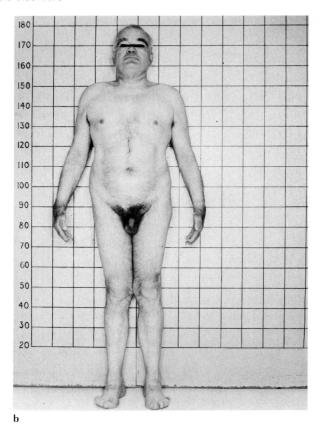

a

b

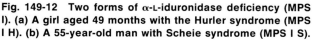

Fig. 149-12   Two forms of α-L-iduronidase deficiency (MPS I). (a) A girl aged 49 months with the Hurler syndrome (MPS I H). (b) A 55-year-old man with Scheie syndrome (MPS I S).

The skin in MPS IV may be rather loose—over the hand, for example. It is noteworthy that epithelium shows the abnormality in keratan sulfate metabolism more strikingly than do cultured skin fibroblasts.

Genetics

All the mucopolysaccharidoses are recessive and all except MPS II are autosomal recessive. The Hunter syndrome is classically X-linked recessive, but a less frequent autosomal recessive form may exist. The phenomenon has been observed of multiple allelic forms of individual mucopolysaccharidoses with different phenotypes (the Hurler-Scheie phenomenon) and that of the same phenotype resulting from different enzyme deficiencies (the Sanfilippo syndrome) as well as the phenomenon of genetic compounds when a patient inherited two different mutant alleles.

Pachydermoperiostosis

Synonyms

Idiopathic clubbing and periostosis, idiopathic hypertrophic osteoarthropathy, the Touraine-Solente-Golé syndrome, acropachyderma with pachyperiostitis, chronic hypertrophy of skin and long bones, osteodermatopathia hypertrophicans.

Summary description

The principal features are: clubbing of the digits; periosteal new bone formation, especially at the distal ends of the long bones; coarsening of the facial features with thickening, furrowing, and oiliness of the skin of the face and forehead; cutis verticis gyrata; and hyperhidrosis of the hands and feet. Onset occurs in the teens. Although inherited as an autosomal dominant, sex influence is demonstrated by more marked affection of males.

Clinical manifestations

Skin. The skin exhibits marked sebaceous hyperplasia with wide-open sebaceous pores filled with plugs of sebum. Ptosis, caused by hypertrophy of the eyelids, may be so severe as to obstruct vision. The skin over the hands and feet is often thickened as well. Skin biopsies show widening of the stratum corneum, marked hyperplasia of sebaceous glands, and perivascular round-cell infiltration.

Massive thickening of the scalp and forehead results in transverse folds and a picture designated cutis verticis gyrata. Hyperhidrosis of the hands and feet may be the main or only complaint.

Skeleton. The ends of the fingers and toes are bulbous and often grotesque. The clubbing is produced mainly by soft tissue hyperplasia that stops abruptly at the distal inter-

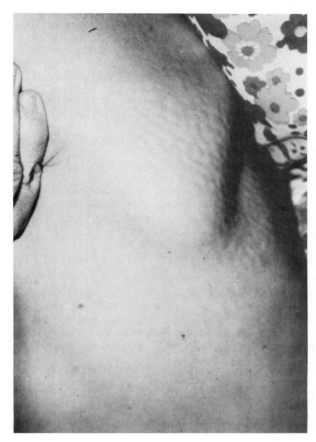

Fig. 149-13 "Pebbly" lesions on the back in a patient with the Hunter syndrome (MPS II).

phalangeal joint. The terminal phalanges often show no radiologic change, but may exhibit burs or atrophy.

The long bones, especially in the vicinity of the ankle and wrist, are increased in diameter by periosteal proliferation, which is bilaterally symmetrical. Enlargement of the distal extremities results from the changes in the bones as well as the overlying soft tissues and skin.

Radiologic examination shows irregular subperiosteal ossification over the long bones, primarily at the distal ends, more pronounced at the insertion of tendons and ligaments. The transverse diameter of the metacarpals, metatarsals, and proximal two phalanges may be increased by periosteal new bone. The clavicles, patellae, and pubis may be affected; the carpal and tarsal bones, sella turcica, and articular surface are spared.

The patient may complain of nonspecific neuromuscular or arthritic symptoms. Changes begin around puberty and slowly progress for about 10 years, being static thereafter.

The basic defect

The primary gene-determined defect is unknown. Simple clubbing has been shown to be accompanied by increased blood flow to the digits [50]. However, in patients with pachydermoperiostosis, Rimoin [51] found changes he interpreted as indicating reduced blood flow in the extremities: in arteriograms, signs of sluggish flow with vascular stasis and tortuosity and segmental narrowing of arteries,

reduced flow by plethysmography, and high arteriovenous oxygen differences. It is possible, of course, that these represent late stages in the process which was earlier hyperemic in nature.

Some of the manifestations of pachydermoperiostosis suggest hyperactivity of the autonomic nervous system; and observations in pulmonary osteoarthropathy, which resembles pachydermoperiostosis, suggest an important role of reflex neurogenic factors in pathogenesis.

Genetics

A majority of reported cases have been in males. For example, the first reported patients were the Hagner brothers, described by Friedreich in 1868 [52] and subsequently studied by Erb, Virchow, and Arnold. (These cases were thought to be examples of acromegaly. Early nosologic confusion is further indicated by the fact that, of the nine cases on which Marie based his original description of pulmonary hypertrophic osteoarthropathy, five, including the only patient he personally examined, were cases of pachydermoperiostosis.) Carefully studied families (e.g., [51]) have shown radiologic evidence of involvement of females who otherwise appeared to represent "skipped generations." Male-to-male transmission has been observed.

Other considerations

Simple clubbing has been described as an autosomal dominant trait in many families. It is likely that hereditary clubbing is, in most instances, an entity separate from pachydermoperiostosis.

Cutis verticis gyrata also occurs as an entity separate from pachydermoperiostosis. Its association with mental retardation seems to represent a distinct syndrome of probable genetic causation, possibly an autosomal recessive [53]. In five males in three sibships of two generations, Åkesson [54] observed the combination of cutis verticis gyrata, thyroid aplasia, and mental retardation. Only the proband was examined in full. Åkesson suggested X-linked inheritance but, as he indicated, this cannot be considered proved.

In a black family of Louisiana, Rosenthal and Kloepfer [55] described what may represent a "new" syndrome, consisting of acromegaloid changes, cutis verticis gyrata, and corneal leukoma. Thirteen persons in three generations were affected.

References

1. McKusick VA: *Heritable Disorders of Connective Tissue,* 4th ed. St. Louis, CV Mosby, 1972, p 292
2. Pinnell SR, Murad S: Disorders of collagen, in *The Metabolic Basis of Inherited Disease,* 5th ed, edited by JB Stanbury et al. New York, McGraw-Hill, 1982, p 1425
3. Hollister DW et al: Genetic disorders of collagen metabolism. *Adv Hum Genet* **12**:1, 1982
4. Haber J: Miescher's elastoma (elastoma intrapapillare perforans verruciforme). *Br J Dermatol* **71**:85, 1959
5. Harris ED Jr, Sjoerdsma A: Effect of penicillamine on human collagen and its possible application to treatment of scleroderma. *Lancet* **2**:996, 1966

6. Byers PH et al: Marfan syndrome: abnormal α_2 chain in type I collagen. *Proc Natl Acad Sci USA* **78**:7745, 1981

7. Halbritter R et al: Case report and study of collagen metabolism in Marfan's syndrome. *Klin Wochenschr* **59**:83, 1981

8. Halme T et al: Desmosines in aneurysms of the ascending aorta (annulo-aortic ectasia). *Biochim Biophys Acta* **717**:105, 1982

9. Abraham PA et al: Marfan syndrome: demonstration of abnormal elastin in aorta. *J Clin Invest* **70**:1245, 1982

10. Harris ED Jr, Sjoerdsma A: Effect of penicillamine on human collagen and its possible application to treatment of scleroderma. *Lancet* **2**:996, 1966

11. Sillence D: Osteogenesis imperfecta: an expanding panorama of variants. *Clin Orthop* **159**:11, 1981

12. Blegvad O, Haxthausen H: Blue sclerotics and brittle bones, with macular atrophy of skin and zonular cataract. *Br Med J* **2**:1071, 1921

13. Barsh GS et al: Type I osteogenesis imperfecta: a nonfunctional allele for pro α_1(I) chains of type I procollagen. *Proc Natl Acad Sci USA* **79**:3838, 1982

14. Chu M-L et al: Internal deletion in a collagen gene in a perinatal lethal form of osteogenesis imperfecta. *Nature* **304**:78, 1983

15. Peltonen L et al: A defect in the structure of type I procollagen in a patient who had osteogenesis imperfecta: excess mannose in the COOH-terminal propeptide. *Proc Natl Acad Sci USA* **77**:6179, 1980

16. Nicholls AC et al: Biochemical heterogeneity of osteogenesis imperfecta: new variant. *Lancet* **1**:1193, 1979

17. Byers PH et al: Abnormal α_2-chain in type I collagen from a patient with a form of osteogenesis imperfecta. *J Clin Invest* **71**:689, 1983

18. Nelson DL, King RA: Ehlers-Danlos syndrome type VIII. *J Am Acad Dermatol* **5**:297, 1981

19. Pope FM et al: Patients with Ehlers-Danlos syndrome type IV lack type III collagen. *Proc Natl Acad Sci USA* **72**:1314, 1975

20. Byers PH et al: Altered secretion of type III procollagen in a form of type IV Ehlers-Danlos syndrome. *Lab Invest* **44**:336, 1981

21. Holbrook KA, Byers PH: Ultrastructural characteristics of the skin in a form of the Ehlers-Danlos syndrome type IV. Storage in the rough endoplasmic reticulum. *Lab Invest* **44**:342, 1981

22. Pinnell SR et al: A heritable disorder of connective tissue: hydroxylysine deficient collagen disease. *N Engl J Med* **286**:1013, 1972

23. Krane SM et al: Lysyl-protocollagen hydroxylase deficiency in fibroblasts from siblings with hydroxylysine-deficient collagen. *Proc Natl Acad Sci USA* **69**:2899, 1972

24. Lichtenstein JR et al: Defect in conversion of procollagen to collagen in a form of the Ehlers-Danlos syndrome. *Science* **182**:298, 1973

25. Steinmann B et al: Evidence for a structural mutation of procollagen type I in a patient with the Ehlers-Danlos syndrome type VII. *J Biol Chem* **255**:8887, 1980

26. Byers PH et al: X-linked cutis laxa. Defective cross-link formation in collagen due to decreased lysyl oxidase activity. *N Engl J Med* **303**:61, 1980

27. Kaitila II et al: A skeletal and connective tissue disorder associated with lysyl oxidase deficiency and abnormal copper metabolism, in *Skeletal Dysplasias*, edited by CJ Papadatos, CS Bartsocas. New York, Alan R Liss, 1982, p 307

28. Di Ferrante N et al: Lysyl oxidase deficiency in Ehlers-Danlos syndrome type V. *Connect Tissue Res* **33**:49, 1975

29. Siegel RC et al: Cross-linking of collagen in the X-linked Ehlers-Danlos type V. *Biochem Biophys Res Commun* **88**:281, 1979

30. Arneson MA et al: A new form of Ehlers-Danlos syndrome. *JAMA* **244**:144, 1980

31. Danielsen L: Morphologic changes in pseudoxanthoma elasticum and senile skin. *Int J Dermatol* **21**:449, 1982

32. Pasquali-Ronchetti I et al: Pseudoxanthoma elasticum: biochemical and ultrastructural studies. *Dermatologica* **163**:307, 1981

33. Pope FM: Autosomal dominant pseudoxanthoma elasticum. *J Med Genet* **11**:152, 1974

34. Pope FM: Two types of autosomal recessive pseudoxanthoma elasticum. *Arch Dermatol* **110**:209, 1974

35. Pope FM: Historical evidence for the genetic heterogeneity of pseudoxanthoma elasticum. *Br J Dermatol* **92**:493, 1975

36. McPhaul JJ Jr, Engel FL: Heterotopic calcification, hyperphosphatemia and angioid streaks of retina. *Am J Med* **31**:488, 1961

37. Smith EW et al: Reactive perforating elastosis: features of certain genetic disorders. *Bull Johns Hopkins Hosp* **111**:235, 1962

38. Korting GW: Elastosis perforans serpiginosa as an ectodermal symptom in cutis laxa. *Arch Klin Exp Dermatol* **224**:437, 1966

39. Beighton P: The dominant and recessive forms of cutis laxa. *J Med Genet* **9**:216, 1972

40. Meine F et al: Radiographic findings in congenital cutis laxa. *Radiology* **113**:687, 1974

41. Sakati NO et al: Syndrome of cutis laxa, ligamentous laxity, and delayed development. *Pediatrics* **72**:850, 1983

42. Goltz RW et al: Cutis laxa: a manifestation of generalized elastosis. *Arch Dermatol* **92**:373, 1965

43. Hashimoto K, Kanzaki T: Cutis laxa: ultrastructural and biochemical studies. *Arch Dermatol* **111**:861, 1975

44. Marchase P et al: A familial cutis laxa syndrome with ultrastructural abnormalities of collagen and elastin. *J Invest Dermatol* **75**:399, 1980

45. Reed WB et al: Acquired cutis laxa. Primary generalized elastolysis. *Arch Dermatol* **103**:661, 1971

46. Verhagen AR, Woerdeman MJ: Post-inflammatory elastolysis and cutis laxa. *Br J Dermatol* **92**:183, 1975

47. McKusick VA et al: The mucopolysaccharide storage diseases, in *The Metabolic Basis of Inherited Disease*, 4th ed, edited by JB Stanbury et al. New York, McGraw-Hill, 1978, p 1282

48. Hers H: Inborn lysosomal disease. *Gastroenterology* **48**:625, 1965

49. Meyer K et al: Effect of acid mucopolysaccharides on hair growth in rabbit. *Proc Soc Exp Biol Med* **108**:59, 1961

50. Mendlowitz M: Cardiovascular shunts. *Am J Med* **22**:1, 1957

51. Rimoin DL: Pachydermoperiostosis (idiopathic clubbing and periostosis): genetic and physiologic considerations. *N Engl J Med* **272**:923, 1965

52. Friedreich N: Hyperostose des gesammten Skelettes. *Virchows Arch [Pathol Anat]* **43**:83, 1868

53. Åkesson HO: Cutis verticis gyrata and mental deficiency in Sweden. I. Epidemiologic and clinical aspects. *Acta Med Scand* **175**:115, 1964

54. Åkesson HO: Cutis verticis gyrata, thyroaplasia and mental deficiency. *Acta Genet Med Gemellol (Roma)* **14**:200, 1965

55. Rosenthal JW, Kloepfer HW: Acromegaloid, cutis verticis gyrata, corneal leukomia syndrome: new medical entity. *Arch Ophthalmol* **68**:722, 1962

CHAPTER 150

HERITABLE DISEASES WITH INCREASED SENSITIVITY TO CELLULAR INJURY

Kenneth H. Kraemer

A group of heritable diseases with differing clinical features share the common characteristics of in vitro or in vivo cellular hypersensitivity to damage by several physical or chemical agents [1–17]. Diseases with autosomal recessive, X-linked, and autosomal dominant inheritance fall into this group [18–20]. Clinical abnormalities in these disorders involve cutaneous, ocular, nervous, immune, hemopoietic, skeletal, or gastrointestinal systems. Some are associated with increased incidence of neoplasia. Several have a primary feature of progressive degeneration of previously normal bodily function [21]. This cellular hypersensitivity is often of diagnostic utility. Further, it may suggest pathogenic mechanisms and measures for therapeutic or prophylactic intervention. Very little is presently known of the molecular basis of the cellular hypersensitivity in most of these disorders. In this chapter the clinical features and cellular abnormalities found in each disorder will be described. The diseases listed in Table 150-1 will be discussed in terms of the systems affected, the cellular hypersensitivity, and the relevance of the cellular abnormality to the clinical symptoms. The major tests used to assess cellular hypersensitivity and to measure DNA repair are outlined in Chap. 13.

Xeroderma pigmentosum

Definition

Xeroderma pigmentosum (XP) serves as the prototype heritable disease with cellular hypersensitivity [1–11]. Xeroderma pigmentosum is an autosomal recessive disease with sun sensitivity, photophobia, early onset of freckling, and subsequent neoplastic changes on sun-exposed surfaces. There is cellular hypersensitivity to ultraviolet (UV) radiation and certain chemicals in association with abnormal DNA repair. Some of the patients have progressive neurologic degeneration.

Frequency

Xeroderma pigmentosum has been estimated to occur with a frequency of 1:250,000 in the United States and to be more common in Japan [1]. Patients have been reported worldwide in all races. Consanguinity is common.

Clinical features

Approximately half of the XP patients have a history of acute sunburn reaction on minimal UV radiation exposure.

Continued sun exposure causes the patient's skin to become dry and parchment-like and hence the name *xeroderma* ("dry skin") (Fig. 150-1a). Numerous, freckle-like, hyperpigmented macules appear, usually before two years of age (Fig. 150-1b). These are strikingly limited to sun-exposed areas. Signs and symptoms of the process begin by 1 year in 50 percent of patients and by 15 years in 95 percent. Premalignant actinic keratoses also develop at an early age (Fig. 150-1b) and patients have a greater than 1000-fold increased risk of basal cell or squamous cell cancer of the skin and eyes. The median age of onset of skin cancer reported in XP patients was 8 years in comparison to 60 years in the general population. The appearance of sun-exposed skin in children with XP is similar to that occurring in farmers and sailors after many years of extreme sun exposure. Multiple primary melanomas may occur. More rarely, primary neoplasms of the oral cavity (especially the tip of the tongue) and the brain and leukemia have been reported.

Ocular abnormalities are almost as common as the cutaneous abnormalities and are an important feature of XP [2,2a]. Photophobia is usually present and is associated with prominent conjunctival injection. Continued UV exposure of the eye may result in severe keratitis (Fig. 150-1c) and vascularization. The lids develop increased pigmentation and loss of lashes. Atrophy of the skin of the lids results in ectropion, entropion, or, in severe cases, complete loss of the lids. Benign conjunctival inflammatory masses or papillomas of the lids may be present. Epitheliomas, squamous cell carcinomas, and melanomas of UV-exposed portions of the eye are common.

Progressive neurologic degeneration has been reported in approximately 40 percent of the patients [2,2a]. Onset of neurologic abnormalities may be early in infancy or, in some patients, delayed until the second decade. The neurologic abnormalities may be mild (e.g., isolated hyporeflexia) or severe, with progressive mental retardation (Fig. 150-1d), sensorineural deafness, spasticity, or seizures. The most severe form, known as the DeSanctis-Cacchione syndrome, involves the cutaneous and ocular manifestations of classic XP plus additional neurologic and somatic abnormalities including microcephaly, progressive mental deterioration, low intelligence, hyporeflexia or areflexia, choreoathetosis, ataxia, spasticity, Achilles tendon shortening with eventual quadraparesis, markedly retarded growth, and immature sexual development. The complete DeSanctis-Cacchione syndrome has been recognized in very few patients; however, many XP patients have one or more of its neurologic features. The predominant neu-

Table 150-1 Heritable diseases with cellular hypersensitivity

Disease	Clinical abnormalities					Cellular abnormalities	
	Cutaneous	Ocular	Nervous	Hematopoietic	Neoplasia	Type	Mechanism
Autosomal recessive							
Xeroderma pigmentosum	Sun sensitivity, atrophy, freckling	Photophobia, UV conjunctivitis, UV keratitis	Deafness, progressive mental deterioration	Normal	BCC, SCC, melanoma	UV-induced: cell killing, mutagenesis, chromosome breakage, SCE	Abnormal DNA repair
Ataxia-telangiectasia	Telangiectasia, x-ray sensitivity	Conjunctival telangiectasia Oculomotor dyspraxia	Progressive ataxia	Humoral and cellular immune defects	Lymphoreticular, GI	Spontaneous chromosome breakage; x-ray-induced: cell killing, chromosome breakage	Abnormal DNA repair (?)
Fanconi's anemia	Hyperpigmentation	Normal	Normal	Anemia	Leukemia, liver	Spontaneous chromosome breakage; mitomycin C-induced: cell killing, chromosome breakage	Abnormal DNA cross-link repair
Cockayne's syndrome	Sun sensitivity, hyperpigmentation	Retinal pigmentation	Progressive mental deterioration	Normal	None	UV-induced: cell killing, SCE	?
Bloom's syndrome	Telangiectasia, sun sensitivity	Normal	Normal	Defective immunity	Leukemia, GI	Spontaneous chromosome breakage, SCE	?
Chédiak-Higashi syndrome	Pigment dilution, gray hair	Hypopigmented irises	Normal	Defective immunity	?	UV-induced: cell killing	?
X-linked							
Dyskeratosis congenita	Poikiloderma, nail dystrophy	Stenosis of lacrimal duct	Normal	Anemia	GI	Psoralen-induced: SCE	?
Autosomal dominant							
Familial dysplastic nevus syndrome	Dysplastic nevi	Normal	Normal	Normal	Cutaneous melanoma	UV-induced: cell killing, mutagenesis (some patients)	?
Gardner's syndrome	Cysts, desmoids	Normal	Normal	Normal	Colon polyps and carcinoma	X-ray induced: cell killing (some patients)	?
Basal cell nevus syndrome	Palmar pits, x-ray sensitivity	Cataract, coloboma	Mental retardation (some patients)	Normal	BCC, medulloblastoma, ovarian tumors	Spontaneous chromosome abnormalities (some patients)	?
Familial retinoblastoma	Normal	Retinoblastoma	Normal	Normal	Retinoblastoma Osteosarcoma	Chromosome deletion; x-ray-induced: cell killing	?
Tuberous sclerosis	White spots, shagreen patch, angiofibromas	Normal	Seizures	Normal	?	X-ray induced: cell killing	?
Huntington's disease	Normal	Normal	Adult-onset mental deterioration	Normal	None	X-ray induced: cell killing	?

Fig. 150-1 Xeroderma pigmentosum. (a) Pigmentary and atrophic changes in the skin of a 16-year-old patient. (b) Cheek of a 14-year-old patient with pigmentary abnormalities, actinic keratoses, and basal cell carcinoma. (c) Corneal clouding, prominent conjunctival blood vasculature, and loss of lashes. (d) A 26-year-old patient with deafness and mental retardation.

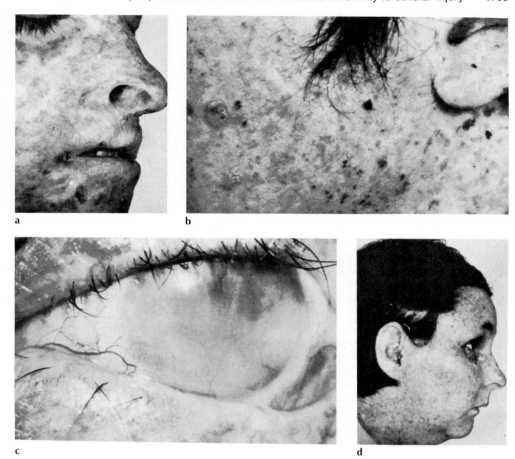

a   b

c   d

ropathologic abnormality found at autopsy in patients with neurologic symptoms is loss (or absence) of neurons, particularly in the cerebrum and cerebellum.

Laboratory abnormalities

There have been no consistent clinical laboratory abnormalities in patients with XP. Tests of cellular hypersensitivity, however, have shown uniformly abnormal results.

Cultured cells from XP patients generally grow normally when not exposed to damaging agents. The population growth rate is reduced to a greater extent than normal, however, following exposure to UV radiation (see Fig. 13-1) and cellular recovery is delayed. This delay in growth is paralleled by a similar delay in recovery of the rate of DNA synthesis following UV radiation exposure [2].

Single-cell survival, as measured by colony-forming ability following UV irradiation, is also reduced in XP cells [1,2,2a,21–23] (see Fig. 13-2). A range of post-UV colony-forming abilities has been found with fibroblasts from patients, some having extremely low post-UV colony-forming ability and others having nearly normal survival.

Xeroderma pigmentosum fibroblasts are deficient in their ability to repair some UV-damaged viruses to a functionally active state [1,2,2a,24]. This assay, known as host cell reactivation, has detected an abnormality in every form of XP tested. Adenovirus 2 host cell reactivation is the most sensitive test for the XP genetic defect.

Ultraviolet-irradiated XP fibroblasts produce more mutations per survivor than normal fibroblasts [2,2a]. This has been observed at several sites of mutation, including hypoxanthine-guanine phosphoribose transferase (HGPRT) and diphtheria toxin resistance. If prevented from dividing for an interval after irradiation, normal cells apparently repair the damage induced, with resultant increased survival and fewer mutants per survivor. This phenomenon has been called *potentially lethal damage recovery* and is analogous to "liquid holding recovery" in bacteria. XP fibroblasts exhibit diminished or absent potentially lethal damage recovery after UV irradiation, thereby indicating a defect in cellular recovery mechanisms.

Xeroderma pigmentosum cells generally are found to have a normal karyotype without excessive chromosome breakage or increased sister chromatid exchanges (SCEs). Following exposure to UV radiation, however, an abnormally large increase in chromosome breakage and in SCEs has been observed [1,2,2a,8,25]. The extent of this induced abnormality varies in different patients.

A number of DNA damaging agents other than UV radiation have been found to yield hypersensitive responses with XP cells (Table 150-2) [2,2a]. These hypersensitivities have been measured by studies of cell survival, host cell reactivation, mutagenesis, and chromosome integrity. These agents include drugs (psoralens, chlorpromazine), cancer chemotherapeutic agents [platinum, 1,3-*bis*-2,3-chloroethyl-1-nitrosourea (BCNU)], and chemical carcin-

Table 150-2 Xeroderma pigmentosum: DNA damaging agents inducing cellular hypersensitivity

Drugs
  Psoralens plus long-wavelength UV radiation (PUVA)
  Chlorpromazine
  Nitrofurantoin
  Mitomycin C
  Anthramycin
  Platinum
  Bis(chloroethyl)nitrosourea (BCNU)
Carcinogens
  Aflatoxin
  Benzo[a]pyrene derivatives
  Nitroquinoline oxide derivatives (4NQO)
  Acetoaminofluorene derivatives (AAF)
  Phenanthrene derivatives

ogens (benzo[a]pyrene derivatives). Presumably these agents induce DNA damage whose repair involves portions of the DNA repair pathways that are defective in XP.

The hypersensitivity of cultured XP cells to UV radiation damage was reported by Cleaver, in 1968 [26], to be the result of defective DNA repair. He found defective UV-induced repair replication, indicating a defect in the nucleotide excision repair system. In 1970, Epstein et al [27] demonstrated that the DNA repair defect was present in vivo as well as by measurements of unscheduled DNA synthesis in the skin of patients. The fact that the XP cells have a normal response to treatment with x-rays was interpreted as indicating that the UV DNA excision repair defect was at the level of endonuclease function. The other tests of nucleotide excision repair discussed in Chap. 13 have shown abnormalities with most XP cells and support the notion of the presence of defective UV endonuclease activity. However, up to 1985 no one has successfully isolated a UV endonuclease that is defective in XP. There is evidence that repair in XP may involve defects in accessibility of the damaged DNA within its chromatin covering [2].

In 1972, investigators in The Netherlands, by using cell fusion techniques (see Fig. 13-9), demonstrated genetic heterogeneity among the XP DNA repair defects [28]. They fused cultured fibroblasts from two different patients and then measured UV-induced unscheduled DNA synthesis. The unfused cells had the typical low level of UV-induced unscheduled DNA synthesis seen in most XP fibroblasts (see Fig. 13-8). Fusion of cells from certain pairs of patients

resulted in the presence of fused cells with nearly normal levels of unscheduled DNA synthesis (see Fig. 13-10). In these heterokaryons each cell provides components that the other was lacking, resulting in enhanced DNA repair. These "complementing cells" thus have different DNA repair defects. Fibroblasts from patients with the same DNA repair defect do not correct each other when fused and are said to be in the same complementation group. In 1975, Kraemer et al [29] reported that the first five complementation groups discovered had characteristic residual rates of UV-induced unscheduled DNA synthesis. They were thus named A through E, in order of increasing DNA repair activity. Groups F and G were discovered more recently [2,2a]. Their rates of unscheduled DNA synthesis overlap with groups C and A, respectively. Thus, assignment of cells to complementation groups must be based on fusion studies, not on the rate of DNA repair. Up to 1985, nine such complementation groups have been identified [2,2a,29a] (Table 150-3).

In 1971, Burk et al [30] reported a patient with clinically severe XP who had normal unscheduled DNA synthesis in his fibroblasts, lymphocytes, and even his tumor cells [1,2]. This patient subsequently was termed a xeroderma pigmentosum *variant* (Table 150-3). Studies of cellular hypersensitivity revealed a slightly increased sensitivity to UV-induced inhibition of cell growth and colony-forming ability, to adenovirus host-cell reactivation, and to UV-induced mutations in vitro [2,24]. DNA repair studies revealed the presence of a defect in a second DNA repair system [2,8], that of postreplication repair. Cells from this patient had a delayed rate of increase of the molecular weight of newly replicating DNA following UV irradiation. Further, these cells were especially sensitive to inhibition of this process by caffeine.

More recent studies have reported defective excision repair, due to altered AP endonuclease activity, and diminished photoreactivation repair in a few XP cell strains [2]. These observations have not been confirmed by other laboratories. Synthesis of poly(ADP-ribose), a possible intracellular regulator, is much less stimulated by UV radiation treatment in XP cells than in normal cells [31]. The significance of this finding is unclear at present.

Treatment

Management of patients with XP is based on early diagnosis, lifelong protection from UV radiation exposure, and

Table 150-3 Xeroderma pigmentosum: characteristics of DNA repair complementation groups

Complementation group	Skin cancer	Neurologic abnormalities	UDS, % of normal	Number of patients
A	+	+ and −	0.3–1.3	55
B	+	+	3–7	1
C	+	−	10–25	51
D	+	+	25–50	28
E	+	−	10–20	2
F	−	−	10–20	3
G	−	+	<5	2
H	+	+	30	1
I	+	+	15	2
Variant	+	−	100	45

early detection and treatment of neoplasms. Diagnosis rests on clinical features and is confirmed by laboratory tests of cellular hypersensitivity. Prenatal diagnosis has been reported by measuring UV-induced unscheduled DNA synthesis in cultured amniotic fluid cells [32].

Patients should be educated to protect all body surfaces from UV radiation by wearing protective clothing, glasses, and hair styles. They should adopt a life style to minimize UV exposure and use sunscreens with the highest sun protective factor (SPF) ratings daily. Patients should be examined frequently by a family member who has been instructed in recognition of cutaneous neoplasms. A set of color photographs of the entire skin surface with close-ups of lesions (including a ruler) is often extremely useful to both the patient and the physician in detecting new lesions. Patients should be examined by a physician, usually at intervals of three months. Premalignant lesions such as actinic keratoses may be treated by freezing with liquid nitrogen or with topical 5-fluorouracil. Larger areas have been treated with therapeutic dermatome shaving or dermabrasion to remove the more damaged superficial epidermal layers and permit repopulation by relatively UV-shielded cells from the follicles and glands.

Cutaneous neoplasms are treated in the same manner as in patients who do not have XP. XP patients are not abnormally sensitive to x-rays. Oral retinoids have been reported as being effective in preventing new neoplasms in a few patients [33].

The eyes should be protected by wearing UV-absorbing glasses with side shields. Methylcellulose eye drops or soft contact lenses have been used to keep the cornea moist and to protect against mechanical trauma in patients with deformed eyelids. Corneal transplantation has restored vision in patients with severe keratitis with corneal opacity. Neoplasms of the lids, conjunctiva, and cornea are usually treated surgically.

Clinical–laboratory correlations

Patients with XP are hypersensitive to UV radiation and so are their cultured cells. Cutaneous and ocular abnormalities are strikingly limited to UV-exposed areas and usually spare such UV-shielded locations as the axillae, buttocks, and retina.

At least ten different molecular defects are associated with the clinical abnormalities recognized as XP, as indicated by the existence of nine complementation groups and the variant form (Table 150-3) [2,2a,29a]. Complementation group A contains patients with the most severe neurologic and somatic abnormalities (the DeSanctis-Cacchione syndrome) as well as patients with minimal or no neurologic abnormalities. This form is seen in the United States, Europe, and the Middle East. It is the most common form of XP in Japan [2].

Complementation group B at present is composed of a unique patient who had the cutaneous abnormalities characteristic of XP (including neoplasms) in conjunction with neurologic and ocular abnormalities typical of Cockayne's syndrome. Her DNA repair defects were different from those of all the other patients tested to date [1,2,29].

Patients in complementation group C, with rare exceptions, have XP with skin and ocular involvement without neurologic abnormalities. This is the most common group

in the United States, Europe, and Egypt, and it has been found in one patient from Japan [1,2].

Patients in complementation group D may have a late onset of neurologic abnormalities in their second decade of life [1,2,21,23].

Complementation group E to date has been found in only one kindred in Europe. These two cousins had relatively mild cutaneous abnormalities without neurologic involvement. Their cultured cells had the unusual property of increasing their regional DNA repair rate with increasing UV exposure. Thus, at low doses the unscheduled DNA synthesis was very low while at high doses it was nearly normal [2].

Complementation group F patients have been found only in Japan. These three patients were free of neurologic abnormalities and had not had skin cancer [2].

Two patients in complementation group G have been identified in Europe. Both had neurologic abnormalities without skin cancer. Fibroblasts from one of the patients were found to be hypersensitive to killing by x-ray as well as to UV radiation [2].

Xeroderma pigmentosum variant cells have normal DNA nucleotide excision repair and thus do not fall into any of the complementation groups of cells with defective DNA excision repair. There is, however, defective postreplication repair. XP variants have been identified in the United States, Europe, and Japan. None of the variants so far identified has neurologic abnormalities. The cutaneous and ocular abnormalities have been severe in some patients and mild in others. A family with four affected individuals was described in Germany; they had had extensive sun exposure and late onset of cutaneous cancers. These individuals had originally been thought to represent a separate disorder (pigmented xerodermoid) [34]. Recent cellular studies showed the findings typical of XP variants.

The cutaneous and ocular changes in XP patients are consistent with the notion that repeated insults by environmental agents, particularly UV radiation, produce continual DNA damage. Because of defective DNA repair, this damage results in cell death, diminished cell growth, or somatic cell mutations. Through mechanisms that are not understood, these cellular alterations lead to atrophy, hyper- and hypopigmentation, and telangiectasia, as well as benign and malignant neoplasms. Thus XP provides strong support for the somatic mutation theory of carcinogenesis. Further, rigorous protection from UV radiation from early infancy in a few patients has been shown to prevent most of the serious cutaneous and ocular abnormalities.

Since cells from XP patients are also hypersensitive to environmental mutagens (such as benzo[a]pyrene found in cigarette smoke) (Table 150-2), the question arises as to whether they have an increased susceptibility to developing internal neoplasms which may be carcinogen-induced.

Review of the world literature has revealed a substantial number of cases of oral cavity neoplasm, particularly squamous cell carcinoma of the tip of the tongue [2,2a], including squamous cell carcinoma of the gum and the hard palate. Leukemia, and brain (sarcoma and medulloblastoma), lung, uterine, breast, and testicular tumors have been reported in XP patients. Overall, these reports suggest an approximate 10- to 20-fold increase in internal neoplasms in XP.

The neurologic abnormalities in XP demonstrate the clinical features of progressive degeneration [1,2,2a,21]. Severely affected patients lose their ability to walk and talk. Histologically, the picture is of loss (or absence) of neurons without evidence of vascular abnormality, deposition of abnormal material, or inflammatory reaction. It has been hypothesized, in analogy to the cutaneous degenerative changes, that the neurologic degeneration is a manifestation of unrepaired DNA damage. Since mature neurons do not divide, unrepaired DNA damage would lead to cell death without replacement by other neurons. This process would lead to progressive loss of neurologic function. The specific cause of such damage, whether by exogenous or endogenous agents, and the explanation of why some neurons are more severely affected than others is not known. The defects in XP patients with associated neurologic disease have been shown to correlate with the UV sensitivity of their skin fibroblasts [2,21,23]. Post-UV colony-forming ability is diminished to the greatest extent in fibroblasts from patients with XP who have severe neurologic abnormalities and to a much lesser extent in XP patients without neurologic abnormalities, both within and among complementation groups. Thus, this is evidence that patients having XP with neurologic abnormalities have a different defect in other tissues than patients without neurologic abnormalities.

Xeroderma pigmentosum heterozygotes (parents and some other relatives) are carriers of the gene for XP but are clinically normal. There is some epidemiologic evidence to indicate that these people have an increased risk of developing skin cancer [35]. Most tests of cell function or DNA repair yield normal responses with cells from XP heterozygotes. Unfortunately, up to 1985, no simple laboratory test has been developed that can reliably detect XP heterozygotes. Until such a test is available, these epidemiologic data may not be justifiably applied to individual persons at risk of being heterozygotes.

Ataxia-telangiectasia

Definition

Ataxia-telangiectasia (AT) is an autosomal recessive disease with progressive cerebellar ataxia, ocular and cutaneous telangiectasia, immune deficiency, and a high frequency of neoplasia [9,36–38]. There is clinical and laboratory evidence of x-ray hypersensitivity [3–17,39].

Frequency

Ataxia-telangiectasia is among the most common of the diseases described in this chapter. The frequency is approximately 1 patient (homozygote) per 40,000 births [36,40]. From this figure, one can estimate that the frequency of heterozygotes (carriers) would be on the order of 1 percent of the general population [40].

Clinical features

The onset of AT is usually in early childhood. Affected children develop progressive cerebellar ataxia resulting in loss of ability to coordinate movements. They have difficulty walking or using the upper extremities. Abnormal eye movements, called *oculomotor dyspraxia*, often develop. Intelligence is usually not affected. Deep tendon reflexes may be diminished or absent.

Frequent bacterial pulmonary or sinus infections may develop as a manifestation of immune deficiency. There is impairment of both humoral and delayed hypersensitivity. The thymus is rudimentary.

Cutaneous and ocular abnormalities usually occur after the onset of neurologic abnormalities. Telangiectasia of the bulbar conjunction may become prominent at 3 to 6 years of age, assisting in the differentiation of AT from other forms of ataxia. Telangiectasia may be prominent on the pinnae, malar area, eyelids, neck, dorsa of the hands, and antecubital and popliteal fossae. The telangiectasia is not limited to sun-exposed sites. Vitiligo, café au lait spots, and other macular hyperpigmentation may be present. Acanthosis nigricans has been noted in AT patients with occult and diagnosed neoplasms [9].

Insulin-resistant diabetes mellitus has been observed. Some of these patients have been found to have abnormal insulin receptors.

Approximately 10 percent of the patients develop neoplasms [9]. Eighty percent of the neoplasms develop before age 15. Lymphoproliferative disorders predominate, primarily lymphomas or lymphoblastic (not myeloid) leukemia. In a recent report from the Immunodeficiency Cancer Registry concerning 108 AT patients with neoplasia, 48 had non-Hodgkin's lymphoma, 26 had leukemia, 12 had Hodgkin's disease, and 22 had carcinomas (involving stomach, brain, skin, ovary, liver, larynx, parotid gland, and breast) [41]. Several AT patients have developed severe reactions to standard doses of radiotherapy for neoplasms. These reactions have included radionecrosis of the oropharynx and central nervous system deterioration leading to death. Thus, AT patients have clinical hypersensitivity to ionizing radiation.

Epidemiologic studies of family members suggest that heterozygotes (parents and other carriers of the AT genetic defect) who are clinically normal may have an increased risk of dying from neoplasms before age 45 [40]. The data suggest an increase in cancers of the ovary, stomach, and biliary tract. Since AT heterozygotes may comprise 1 percent of the general population, they may comprise more than 5 percent of all persons dying from these cancers before age 45. Confirmation of this potentially very important observation awaits development of a reliable test for detection of AT heterozygotes.

Laboratory abnormalities

Clinical laboratory abnormalities primarily relate to humoral or cellular immune dysfunction. There is often decreased or absent IgA (resulting from diminished IgA synthesis), decreased IgE, and decreased or absent IgG_2. An IgM macroglobin may be present. Other abnormalities include impaired delayed skin test reactivity, reduced ability to reject allogeneic skin grafts, reduced ability to be sensitized with dinitrochlorobenzene, reduced lymphocyte count, and poor lymphocyte mitogenic response to phytohemagglutinin, in vitro. There is also reduced helper T-cell function. Virtually 100 percent of the AT patients have elevated α-fetoprotein, a finding that may sometimes be very useful in differential diagnosis [38].

Neurologic testing commonly shows reduced nerve conduction velocity and a neuropathic electromyogram. These findings point toward a primary neurologic degeneration [9].

Karyotypic analysis of peripheral blood leukocytes frequently shows a high frequency of "spontaneous" breaks, gaps, and translocations [9,42,43]. A common abnormality in AT is a deletion or translocation involving a portion of chromosome 14. Several patients have been reported to have chromosomally distinct clones of abnormal circulating lymphocytes. In some patients those abnormal cells have been documented to increase in frequency and, in a few patients, to progress to leukemia. Increased spontaneous chromosome breakage has also been found in cultured skin fibroblasts, but, interestingly, not in lymphoblastoid cell lines.

Baseline SCE frequency is normal (see Fig. 13-5). X-ray treatment of cultured AT cells results in an abnormally large increase in chromosome breakage. However, there is a very small increase in SCEs following x-ray treatment in normal and AT lymphocytes.

The observation of clinical x-ray hypersensitivity prompted the laboratory study of survival of AT cells following x-irradiation. Cultured skin fibroblasts and lymphoblastoid cell lines (see Fig. 13-1b) were found to be hypersensitive to killing by x-ray. Hypersensitivity to killing was found also to treatments with the chemotherapeutic agent, bleomycin, or with the carcinogen, methylnitronitrosoguanidine (MNNG). These findings suggest that AT cells may be an x-ray analogue of XP [9]. There is one important difference, however: AT cells were found not to be hypermutable following x-ray.

The mechanism of the AT hypersensitivity to x-rays and to certain chemicals is only partially understood. As measured by loss of endonuclease-sensitive sites, repair replication, and BND (benzylated naphthylated DEAE) cellulose chromatography, some AT cells have been shown to have defective DNA repair following x-ray or MNNG. Other AT cell strains, equally as sensitive to killing by x-ray or MNNG, have no detectable DNA repair defects. Extracts of AT cells have diminished ability to repair x-ray-damaged DNA to an extent that the DNA may function as a template for bacterial DNA polymerase in vitro.

A number of other abnormalities have recently been reported in AT cells. Several laboratories independently discovered an apparent anomaly in that AT cells fail to slow their rate of DNA synthesis following treatment with x-rays despite increased sensitivity to killing x-rays. Normal cells do slow down DNA synthesis after x-ray injury. Probably this slowdown gives normal cells time to repair their damaged DNA before the next round of replication. The AT cells would thus be more likely to suffer injury by x-rays when DNA synthesis continues at a rapid rate. This abnormal control of DNA synthesis may be mediated by a defective poly(ADP-ribose) control mechanism [44]. The relationship of these DNA synthesis abnormalities to the DNA repair pathways is not clear at present.

Cell fusion studies of x-ray-treated AT cells, measuring repair replication or x-ray-induced inhibition of DNA synthesis, have indicated the existence of several complementation groups [5,12,38]. Other workers reported the presence of a "clastogenic factor" in serum and in medium from growing AT cells [45]. This factor induces chromosome breaks in normal lymphocytes. This test has been used for prenatal diagnsois of AT [46].

Clinical–laboratory correlations

Ataxia-telangiectasia, like XP, has clinical features of progressive degeneration, particularly in the central nervous system [9]. Histopathologically, there is loss (or absence) of neurons without deposition or inflammation. In AT, the major abnormalities are found in the cerebellum, particularly the loss of Purkinje cells. In contrast to XP, there is relative sparing of the cerebrum. Consequently, in AT, cerebellar symptoms (ataxia, incoordination) predominate, while XP patients with neurologic abnormalities may have early deterioration of intellectual functions and develop incoordination rather late. In both AT and XP, progressive loss of neurons may be the consequence of unrepaired DNA damage in cells that cannot be replaced by cell division [21]. The cause of the damage, whether from exogenous or endogenous factors, and the reason for the anatomic location of the affected cells is not known.

The clinical hypersensitivity to cancer-therapeutic doses of radiation is clearly correlated with the x-ray hypersensitivity of cultured cells. However, the role of x-radiation in the development of neoplasms is not as straightforward. One patient developed a carcinoma of the scalp 10 years after superficial radiation for tinea capitis [9]. However, the patient had a chronic radiodermatitis during the interval, which, in itself, might have induced the neoplasm. In contrast to XP where cultured cells are hypermutable to UV radiation, cultured AT cells have normal to low rates of x-ray-induced mutagenesis.

The lymphoreticular neoplasms (reticulum cell sarcoma, lymphoma, Hodgkin's disease) occurring in patients with AT are unusual in their early age of onset (before 15 years in comparison of the median age of 55 to 59 years in the U.S. white population) and greatly increased occurrence (6 percent of patients vs. 13 per million annual incidence in the U.S. white population) [9,41]. The 2 percent prevalence of leukemia is also much greater than the 42 per million incidence in the U.S. white population. Particularly notable is the complete absence of acute or chronic myeloid leukemia. This distribution of types of neoplasms is different from that of children without AT, where leukemia and central nervous system neoplasms are more common than lymphoma. The distribution of types of neoplasms seen in AT patients is not that expected from radiation exposure. Neoplasms most commonly observed in populations receiving high doses of radiation are leukemia (myelogenous and lymphoid) and thyroid, breast, lung, bone, and gastrointestinal carcinomas without an increase in lymphoreticular neoplasms. The predominance of lymphoreticular neoplasms in AT is similar to its predominance in other immunodeficiency diseases. Thus the immunodeficiency in AT may be a more significant factor contributing to the high frequency of neoplasms than is the cellular hypersensitivity to ionizing radiation.

The relationship of the cellular hypersensitivity to the immune defects is at present speculative. Immune deficiency is often present in early childhood. There is no evidence of progression of immunologic defects as with the neurologic abnormalities. Rather than being the result of repeated postnatal insults (as may be the case for neurologic degeneration), both the immune deficiency and the cellular hypersensitivity may be the result of separate (or linked) developmental defects.

Fanconi's anemia

Definition

Fanconi's anemia is an autosomal recessive disorder with anemia, developmental defects, and a high incidence of neoplasia. Approximately 300 patients have been reported in the literature [3–8,47–56].

Clinical features

Hemopoietic manifestations usually have their onset before the age of 10 years. These consist of a hypocellular bone marrow with progressive decrease in the number of circulating platelets, granulocytes, and erythrocytes.

Sixty-six percent of 129 patients with Fanconi's anemia had skeletal malformations [52]. These included aplasia or hypoplasia of the thumb, metacarpals, or radius; less frequently, hip dislocation or scoliosis was reported. Sixty percent of the patients had short stature; most had low birth weight. Malformations of other organ systems were also observed. Twenty-eight percent of the patients had renal deformities, including renal aplasia and horseshoe kidney. Twenty-one percent had ocular abnormalities, including strabismus and microphthalmia; 20 percent of the patients had hypogonadism. Central nervous system abnormalities (hyperreflexia and mild mental retardation) were observed in less than 20 percent of the patients. Deafness due to deformities of the ear anatomy was present in less than 10 percent of the patients. Heart defects (patent ductus arteriosis, aortic stenosis, auricular septal defect) were observed in eight patients.

Cutaneous abnormalities were present in almost 80 percent of the patients. Hyperpigmentation was present from birth or early childhood. The hyperpigmentation was diffuse and accentuated over the neck, joints, and trunk. Café au lait macules and achromic lesions were present. Following repeated blood transfusions, hyperpigmentation due to iron overloading may be present.

Patients with Fanconi's anemia have a high incidence of neoplasia, particularly nonlymphatic leukemia [49]. In recent years hepatomas have been noted with increasing frequency. There is some suspicion that these hepatomas may be a late effect of the anabolic steroids used to treat the anemia.

The course is often progressively downhill with death from infection, hemorrhage, or neoplasia.

Laboratory abnormalities

Clinical laboratory abnormalities reflect the bone marrow failure. There is a hypocellular marrow with thrombocytopenia, leukopenia, and anemia.

Fanconi's anemia is associated with a high frequency of spontaneous chromosomal abnormalities [49,55–57]. These include gaps, breaks, and translocations. With Fanconi's anemia cells the chromosomal abnormalities are increased to a greater extent than with normal cells following treat-

ment with diepoxybutane, mitomycin C, psoralen plus UVA, or isonicotinic acid hydrazide (INH) [51,55–58].

The baseline frequency of SCEs is normal. Following treatment with mitomycin C, the increase in SCEs in Fanconi's anemia lymphocytes was less than that induced in normal lymphocytes [59] but was greater than normal in fibroblasts [60].

Colony-forming ability of cultured fibroblasts and lymphoblasts is hypersensitive to inhibition by treatment with agents that form cross-links in DNA [4–8,47,48]. These include mitomycin C, busulfan, nitrogen mustard, and psoralen plus UVA. Colony-forming ability has a normal response to killing by UV radiation. Some Fanconi's anemia fibroblast strains are slightly hypersensitive to killing by x-radiation, while others have a normal response [13].

The mechanism of the cellular hypersensitivity to DNA cross-linking agents is thought to involve defective DNA repair [47]. A detailed understanding of this defect has not yet been attained. Some Fanconi's anemia fibroblasts have been reported to have defective removal of an x-ray-induced thymidine analogue, thymine glycol (see Table 13-3).

Cells from heterozygous carriers of Fanconi's anemia have a chromosomal response to damage with diepoxybutane [55] or with nitrogen mustard [56] intermediate between the homozygotes and normals.

Clinical–laboratory correlations

Fanconi's anemia is a progressive, degenerative disease with major involvement of the hematologic system. There is a high frequency of spontaneous chromosomal breakage in association with a high rate of neoplasia, particularly nonlymphatic leukemia. Immunodeficiency is not prominent. Cells are hypersensitive to killing and to induction of chromosome aberrations by DNA cross-linking agents. At present, incorporating these diverse observations into a unitary theory involves considerable speculation. The progressive nature of the disease is similar to XP and AT and suggests the presence of accumulated cellular damage. ''Spontaneous'' chromosomal breakage may be a manifestation of this damage. The neoplasia may be related to the chromosomal breakage. However, when considering two diseases with spontaneous chromosome breakage (Fanconi's anemia and AT), lymphoid leukemia is absent in Fanconi's anemia and predominant in AT. Nonlymphoid leukemia predominates in Fanconi's anemia and is absent in AT. Thus, other modifying factors, perhaps the immune defects in AT, may be at work. The postulated damage may be caused by agents similar to the DNA cross-linking agents to which the Fanconi's anemia cells are hypersensitive. It should be noted that almost 40 percent of a recent series of neoplasms in Fanconi's anemia were hepatomas [49]. These had not been observed prior to 1959, when effective treatment of the anemia with exogenous androgens was introduced. It is possible that the prolonged life has permitted expression of latent hepatomas or that the therapy has induced hepatic neoplasia.

Clinical symptoms in Fanconi's anemia have been observed to vary from mild to severe and to be similar in multiple affected children within a family. Similarly, cells from different patients have shown different degrees of sensitivity to x-radiation damage and repair. This suggests that genetic heterogeneity may exist within Fanconi's anemia.

The chromosomal aberrations induced by diepoxybutane have been used successfully as a test for prenatal diagnosis of Fanconi's anemia [57]. Many more chromosome aberrations are induced by diepoxybutane in cultured amniotic fluid cells from Fanconi's anemia than from normal fetuses.

Cockayne's syndrome

Definition

Cockayne's syndrome is an autosomal recessive, degenerative disease with cutaneous, ocular, neurologic, and somatic abnormalities [3–8,61,62]. Fewer than 50 patients have been described in the literature.

Clinical features

In 1936, Cockayne described a syndrome characterized by cachectic dwarfism, deafness, and pigmentary retinal degeneration with a characteristic "salt and pepper" appearance of the retina. The skin had photosensitivity and diffuse hyperpigmentation without the excessive pigmentary abnormalities seen in XP. There was marked loss of subcutaneous fat resulting in a "wizened" appearance with typical "bird-headed" facies. Additional ocular findings included cataracts and optic atrophy.

Neurologic abnormalities, in addition to deafness, include peripheral neuropathy, normal pressure hydrocephalus, and microcephaly. Birth weight and early development are usually normal. The disease onset is most often in the second year of life, with slowly progressive neurologic degeneration. Intellectual deterioration may be nonuniform with some functions preserved better than others.

X-ray examination may show a thickened skull. Bone age is usually normal. Height and weight are usually well below the third percentile for the age.

Cockayne's syndrome is not associated with an increased incidence of neoplasia.

Laboratory abnormalities

Clinical laboratory testing often shows sensorineural deafness, neuropathic electromyogram, and slow motor nerve conduction velocity [61]. The electroencephalogram may be abnormal. Computerized tomography may be diagnostically useful in the detection of normal pressure hydrocephalus [61].

As with XP, cultured cells (fibroblasts or lymphocytes) from Cockayne's syndrome patients are hypersensitive to UV-induced inhibition of growth and colony-forming ability [3–8,63,64]. They are also hypersensitive to killing by the carcinogen 4-nitroquinoline oxide (4NQO).

Host cell reactivation of UV-damaged adenovirus is reduced, although generally to a lesser extent than in XP [24]. Studies of induced mutations in Cockayne's syndrome cells have not been published.

Chromosome karyotype and SCE frequency is generally normal in untreated cells. Ultraviolet treatment of Cockayne's syndrome cells results in a greater than normal increase in SCEs [23,65].

These cellular abnormalities are similar to those of XP. However, the Cockayne's syndrome cells do not have the same DNA repair defects as in XP. There is, however, a prolonged decrease in the rate of DNA and RNA synthesis following UV radiation. These tests have been used to detect three complementation groups in Cockayne's syndrome [66,67]. Despite investigation in a number of laboratories, no mechanism has been found for the cellular abnormalities in Cockayne's syndrome.

Clinical–laboratory correlations

Cockayne's syndrome, like XP and AT, is a disease of progressive neurologic degeneration. Pathologically there is loss (or absence) of neurons without inflammatory reaction or deposition of material. This is consistent with the theory that the neurons are damaged repeatedly but do not recover fully and die [1,21]. Since mature neurons cannot divide, the dead neurons are not replaced, resulting in progressive loss of neurologic functioning. As in XP and AT, the cause of this damage and the reason for the precise anatomic location of the damage is not known.

Despite similar UV radiation hypersensitivity to cell killing in Cockayne's syndrome as in XP, patients with Cockayne's syndrome do not have an increased frequency of cutaneous (or internal) neoplasia. The only Cockayne's syndrome patient in the literature with multiple skin cancers also had XP [1,61]. This unusual patient also had a unique DNA repair defect and is the only patient in complementation group B (Table 150-3) [29]. Thus, cellular hypersensitivity, in the absence of a documented DNA repair defect, does not necessarily result in increased neoplasia.

Bloom's syndrome

Definition

Bloom's syndrome is an autosomal recessive disease characterized by sun sensitivity, facial telangiectasia, short stature, and a high frequency of neoplasia [3–8,49,68–70]. The Bloom's Syndrome Registry has documented 103 cases worldwide. Bloom's syndrome is most frequent among Ashkenazi Jews where the carrier rate has been estimated as 1:120 [71].

Clinical features

Facial erythema and telangiectasia superficially resembling lupus erythematosus often is present within the first few weeks after birth in the malar area, on the nose, and around the ears [69,70]. Sun exposure accentuates these abnormalities and may induce bullae with bleeding and crusting of the lips and eyelids. The telangiectatic lesions often involve the ears and dorsa of the hands but characteristically spare the trunk, buttocks, and lower extremities. The intensity of the facial lesions may vary from minimal telangiectasia around the lips to severe erythema of the malar area, cheeks, and nose (Fig. 150-2). Café au lait spots are common, at times accompanied by adjacent depigmented areas.

Affected children are generally born at full term but are of low birth weight, averaging approximately 2000 g. Patients are well-proportioned but small. Adult height is usually under 150 cm. Patients have a long, narrow head, with a characteristic facies consisting of a narrow prominent nose, relatively hypoplastic malar areas, and a receding chin. Major skeletal abnormalities are unusual. Neurologic abnormalities are uncommon and intelligence is generally normal.

Bloom's syndrome patients are predisposed to multiple severe infections of the respiratory or gastrointestinal tract. There is a tendency for the frequency of infections to decrease with advancing age. There is immune dysfunction [72].

Sexual development generally appears to be normal but male infertility due to defective sperm is the rule [73]. Approximately 20 percent of Bloom's syndrome patients have developed neoplasms—half occurred before the age of 20 years [49,71]. Bloom's syndrome patients have been estimated to have a 150- to 300-fold increased frequency of development of lymphatic and nonlymphatic leukemia, lymphosarcoma, lymphoma, and carcinomas of the oral cavity and digestive system.

Laboratory abnormalities

Laboratory studies of immunity have shown diminished immunoglobulin levels, reduced cellular proliferative response to mitogens, and decreased proliferation in the mixed leukocyte reaction [72].

Studies of gonadal function in males revealed azoospermia with a high follicle-stimulating hormone (FSH) response to luteinizing hormone-releasing hormone (LHRH) [73]. The studies indicated primary hypogonadism mainly affecting the tubular element of the testis. There was relative sparing of the androgen-secreting Leydig cells, resulting in normal puberty.

Cytogenetic abnormalities are found in cultured cells from virtually all patients with Bloom's syndrome [3–8,42,49,69,74,75]; these include a high frequency of chromosomal breakage and rearrangements, including isochromatid gaps and breaks, transverse breakage at centromeres, dicentric chromosomes, and acentric fragments. The most characteristic of these aberrations, the quadriradial configuration, was found in 0.5 to 14.0 percent of all dividing PHA-stimulated lymphocytes from Bloom's syndrome patients (see Fig. 13-4) [68]. Quadriradials are believed to be the result of a rearrangement before the onset of mitosis, resulting from the exchange of chromatid segments of two homologous chromosomes. The quadriradial is almost never found in cells from normal individuals. There is also a markedly elevated rate of spontaneous SCEs in Bloom's syndrome cells (see Fig. 13-6). Increased SCEs and the presence of quadriradials are considered essential for the diagnosis of Bloom's syndrome.

The carcinogen, ethylmethane sulfonate, induces a greater increase in SCEs in Bloom's syndrome lymphocytes than in lymphocytes from normals [69]. Bloom's syndrome cells show a normal increase in chromosome aberrations when treated with x-rays in the G_1 phase of the cell cycle but show a greater than normal increase when irradiated in G_2.

Fusion (see Fig. 13-9) of Bloom's syndrome fibroblasts with rodent cells, or with normal human fibroblasts, results in a normal rate of SCEs in the fused cells [74]. This result

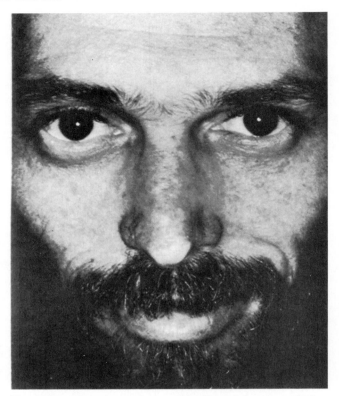

Fig. 150-2 Bloom's syndrome. Prominent telangiectasia in malar distribution.

implies that the defect in Bloom's syndrome cells is the consequence of the loss of a normal function rather than the acquisition of a new abnormal function.

Some Bloom's syndrome fibroblasts have been reported to be hypersensitive to killing by UV radiation. Other Bloom's syndrome strains have a normal response to UV radiation. Cells from three Japanese Bloom's syndrome patients were hypersensitive to killing by mitomycin C. Bloom's syndrome fibroblasts were reported to have an eight- to tenfold increase in the spontaneous mutation rate [76].

The molecular basis for these abnormalities remains elusive. No consistent DNA repair abnormalities have been documented. The rate of DNA chain elongation was found to be significantly slower than with normal fibroblasts [75]. Other studies found a markedly increased rate of interchange of DNA between newly synthesized and older DNA strands, consistent with the observed increase in SCEs.

Clinical–laboratory correlations

The clinical diagnosis of Bloom's syndrome is confirmed by the findings of increased SCEs and increased chromosome breakage, including the presence of quadriradials.

The high frequency of neoplasia in Bloom's syndrome may be related to the chromosome breakage or the immune deficiency (or both), as in AT. The observation of increased spontaneous mutation rate in cultured cells suggests that somatic mutations may play a role in the neoplasia. Homologous chromosome exchange (as in quadriradials) may be a mechanism whereby heterozygous (recessive) traits become homozygous within somatic cells and thereby result in mutation or neoplasia.

Variable UV radiation hypersensitivity among cell lines suggests the possibility of different defects in different patients with Bloom's syndrome.

Dyskeratosis congenita

Definition

Dyskeratosis congenita, the Zinsser-Engman-Cole syndrome, is an X-linked multisystem disease with cutaneous, mucosal, ocular, gastrointestinal, and hematologic abnormalities and an increased incidence of cancer. Approximately 70 cases are recorded in the literature, including some female patients [3–8,77–79].

Clinical features

The most common features are hyperpigmentation, dystrophic nails, and leukoplakia [77]. During the first decade of life patients develop reticulated poikiloderma of sun-exposed areas, with hyperpigmentation and occasionally bullae. Nail dystrophy is present in virtually all patients, beginning at approximately age 2 to 5 years. The nails initially split easily and then develop longitudinal ridging with irregular free edges. Eventually the nails become smaller, resulting in rudiments remaining. The fingernails are usually involved before the toenails. Other skin abnormalities include atrophic, wrinkled skin over the dorsa of hands and feet and hyperhydrosis and hyperkeratosis of the palms and soles with disappearance of dermal ridges (absence of fingerprints).

Leukoplakia may be present in any mucosal site [77]. The oral mucosa is the most frequent, but leukoplakia has also been found in the urethra, glans penis, vagina, and rectum. Mucosal surfaces such as the esophagus, urethra, and lacrimal duct may become constricted and stenotic, resulting in dysphagia, dysuria, and epiphora. Multiple dental caries and early loss of teeth are common. Approximately half of the patients have had subnormal intelligence. Patients may have multiple infections.

There is an increased incidence of neoplasia, particularly squamous cell carcinoma of the mouth, rectum, cervix, vagina, esophagus, and skin. In fact, patients with dyskeratosis congenita have been estimated to have a 100- to 700-fold increased frequency of digestive system, buccal cavity, and pharyngeal neoplasms [80]. Several patients have had multiple primary neoplasms. Most neoplasms occurred in the third or fourth decade. None of the patients had leukemia. Half of the patients developed anemia secondary to bone marrow failure in the second or third decade. Leukopenia and thrombocytopenia may also be present, resulting in a hematologic picture similar to Fanconi's anemia.

Laboratory abnormalities

Immune function was studied in only a small number of patients. Defects in immunoglobulin levels and in cell-mediated immunity were found in some patients [81].

Chromosomes are usually normal in untreated cells. There is a report of one patient with elevated spontaneous SCEs [79]. Treatment of peripheral blood leukocytes from two patients with psoralens plus UV radiation in vitro induced abnormally large increases in SCEs [78]. Survival studies showed increased cell killing after treatment with mitomycin C [82].

Clinical–laboratory correlations

Dyskeratosis congenita, like Fanconi's anemia, is associated with anemia and increased incidence of neoplasia. However, patients with dyskeratosis congenita do not have the developmental malformations or spontaneous chromosomal breakage seen in Fanconi's anemia. In both disorders, however, there is a suggestion of an abnormal chromosomal response to the DNA cross-linking induced by psoralens. In dyskeratosis congenita, abnormally large increases in numbers of SCEs were incuded in lymphocytes [78], while in Fanconi's anemia there was an abnormally small increase.

Like those with AT, patients with dyskeratosis congenita have an increased incidence of neoplasia and immune deficiency. However, the types of neoplasia most commonly seen in AT, lymphoma and leukemia, have not been reported in dyskeratosis congenita. The mechanism and the extent of cellular abnormalities in dyskeratosis congenita are presently not understood.

Dysplastic nevus syndrome

Definition

The familial dysplastic nevus syndrome is an autosomal dominant form of hereditary cutaneous melanoma [83–87a]. Affected individuals have distinctive pigmented nevi which in these families are markers of an increased risk for melanoma [88,89]. Individual dysplastic nevi occasionally progress to melanoma. This disorder has also been called the B-K mole syndrome [86], familial atypical multiple mole-melanoma (FAMMM) syndrome [90], large atypical mole syndrome, and expanded and activated melanocyte syndrome [91].

Incidence, genetics, and epidemiology

Ten percent of all melanoma patients have hereditary melanoma [83]. The familial form of the dysplastic nevus syndrome is the major form of hereditary cutaneous melanoma presently characterized. It is defined as a kindred in which at least two blood relatives have cutaneous melanoma and one or more dysplastic nevi. The frequency of the familial dysplastic nevus syndrome is not known, however nearly 150 families have been identified by the National Cancer Institute. Based on estimates from the Institute, there probably are more than 30,000 people with this syndrome in the United States [92].

Formal genetic analysis of 14 kindreds with the familial dysplastic nevus syndrome has demonstrated autosomal dominant inheritance of the cutaneous melanoma trait with reduced penetrance [87]. (The dysplastic nevus trait was more frequent than would be predicted by autosomal dominant inheritance, probably because of a high frequency of sporadic dysplastic nevi in the general population.) These features of reduced penetrance and sporadic phenocopies confound the determination as to whether an individual with dysplastic nevi and melanoma has the familial dysplastic nevus syndrome. Evaluation of the extended family (grandparents, uncles, aunts, and cousins) as well as parents and siblings may be necessary to classify an individual accurately.

Clinical features

In affected family members, dysplastic nevi are first observed in late childhood and continue to appear throughout adulthood [87a–89,93]. Some individuals experience bursts of activity of nevi at puberty and in pregnancy.

Dysplastic nevi are best recognized clinically by their characteristic color and morphology (Fig. 150-3 and Table 150-4). They have variegated coloration ranging from shades of dark brown to tan and pink distributed irregularly throughout the lesion. Areas of depigmentation may be present. The border is irregular, often angulated with portions fading into the surrounding skin. Dysplastic nevi are predominantly macular but may have central elevations. Skin surface markings are present and may show some disruption. There may be a fine scale. Dysplastic nevi frequently are 5 to 10 mm in diameter or larger, however, small dysplastic nevi have been documented. The number of dysplastic nevi also can be variable, with some individuals having only a few lesions and others more than 100. More than two-thirds of dysplastic nevi are found on the trunk with the back being the single site of the greatest number. However, dysplastic nevi have been observed on the entire skin surface including sun-shielded locations such as the scalp, buttocks, pubic area, and female breast.

Melanomas in individuals with the familial dysplastic nevus syndrome usually occur from progression of preexisting dysplastic nevi but may also occur de novo on apparently normal skin [85,89]. Clinically, early melanomas appear as black areas in dysplastic nevi. Patients may complain of itching of their nevi and this may be accompanied by increased redness of nevi. Melanomas in patients with the familial dysplastic nevus syndrome have the same clinical features as do patients with sporadic melanoma. These include increase in size, change in color (new black or red areas), altered shape, increased scaling or oozing of surface, and almost total disruption of skin markings.

More than 80 percent of the melanomas found in patients with familial dysplastic nevus syndrome were of the superficial spreading type [83,89]. Nodular, lentigo maligna, and acral lentiginous melanomas also were present. The trunk predominated in location of melanoma followed by arms and head/neck. Melanomas have been found in the scalp [93]. The median age at diagnosis of melanoma in familial dysplastic nevus syndrome was about 35 years [89]. This is considerably younger than the median age of 51 years in the general population. Multiple primary melanomas were present in nearly half of the familial dysplastic nevus syndrome patients with melanoma. Most of the melanomas were thin (less than 0.76 mm in depth). Melanoma deaths were due to metastatic spread in patients with thick melanomas of the trunk. In general, prognostic criteria for cure of melanomas in these patients appear to be related to the depth of invasion as with sporadic melanomas.

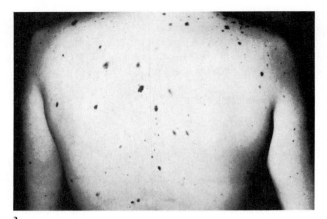

a

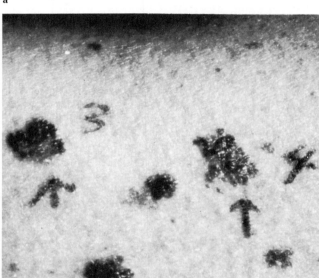

b

Fig. 150-3 Familial dysplastic nevus syndrome (B-K mole syndrome). (a) Back of a 27-year-old woman who had four primary cutaneous melanomas. Her back shows multiple dysplastic nevi. (b) Close-up photograph of right posterior shoulder of patient in (a) showing multiple dysplastic nevi. The dysplastic nevi have irregular borders, multiple colors (brown, tan, pink), and variable morphology from lesion to lesion. Inclusion of a ruler in photographs of dysplastic nevi aids in determination of size for follow-up examinations. (Photographs courtesy of Wallace H. Clark, Jr., M.D.)

Laboratory features

Histologic confirmation of dysplastic nevi is based on finding nuclear atypia (dysplasia) of melanocytes as evidenced by pleomorphism, hyperchromatism, and irregularities of nuclear membranes, in association with a dermal lymphocytic host response and lamellar fibroplasia [85]. Dysplastic melanocytes are usually located at the dermal-epidermal junction above a dermal lymphocytic infiltrate. Frequently associated melanocytic abnormalities include: lentiginous (basal, discontinuous) or ellipsoid, irregular, nested hyperplasia; epithelioid (cuboidal) epidermal melanocytic cells singly or grouped; small dermal melanocytic cells with impairment of maturation and pigment synthesis; and

Table 150-4   Familial dysplastic nevus syndrome: clinical features

Color
  Variegated tan, brown, and pink
  Often areas of depigmentation
  Focal black areas suggest malignant melanoma
  Lesion-to-lesion variability
Shape
  Irregular outline, frequently angulated
  Predominantly macular
  Border may fade into surrounding skin
  May have central papule
Size
  Frequently 5 to 10 mm or larger
Number
  Variable, few to more than 100
Distribution
  Predominantly back and trunk
  May occur on scalp, breast, buttock
Age of appearance
  Onset late childhood or adolescence
  New nevi may appear through adulthood (beyond age 35 years)
Family history
  Cutaneous melanoma and dysplastic nevi in at least 2 blood relatives
  Dysplastic nevi may have similar appearance in multiple family members
  Melanoma occurs virtually only in family members with dysplastic nevi

prominent junctional component. The dermal reaction may include neovascularization and numerous pigment-laden melanophages. Careful measurement of histologic sections of pigmented lesions has shown an increased frequency of melanocytes (dopa-reactive perikaryons) in dysplastic nevi and in superficial spreading melanomas in comparison to acquired nevi or solar lentigines. The diameter of basal unit melanocytes in dysplastic nevi was larger than melanocytes in acquired nevi but smaller than melanocytes in superficial spreading melanoma [94].

Limited studies of cultured dermal fibroblasts or E-B virus-transformed lymphoblastoid cell lines from patients with familial melanoma or familial dysplastic nevus syndrome have reported hypersensitivity to UV-induced cell killing and hypermutability induced by UV radiation [95,96]. No DNA repair abnormalities were detected; however, one group reported delayed recovery of DNA synthesis following UV radiation [95].

Treatment

Treatment is based on attempts to prevent melanoma occurrence combined with early detection and treatment of melanomas. The entire skin surface is examined for presence of nevi. Examination of the scalp may be facilitated by use of a hair dryer, at a cool setting, to blow hair away. Baseline color photographs (with a ruler next to the nevi) (Fig. 150-3b) greatly facilitate early detection of changes. Patients are instructed to monitor their nevi regularly and to be examined by a physician at least every six months. For initial diagnosis, a minimum of two clinically dysplastic nevi are excised for histologic verification. At any visit, lesions exhibiting signs of progression toward melanoma

(increased size, altered outline, new red or black areas, increased scaling or oozing of surface, redness or swelling of surrounding skin, new sensations in nevi such as itching, tenderness, pain) should be removed. Blood relatives should be examined for presence of dysplastic nevi or melanoma to confirm the diagnosis of familial dysplastic nevus syndrome.

Ultraviolet radiation is thought to play a role in melanoma development. Consequently, patients are encouraged to minimize exposure to UV radiation by using effective sunscreens, wearing hats and other protective clothing, and limiting sun exposure. Patients should also be particularly watchful of alterations in nevi at times of changes in hormone balance (puberty, pregnancy, or while using oral contraceptives or other hormones) since these have been associated with changes in nevi.

Clinical–laboratory correlations

The dysplastic nevus is believed to represent a formal precursor lesion to cutaneous melanoma [84,85,87a]. Dysplastic nevi have clinical features intermediate between common acquired nevi and malignant melanomas. Histologically the melanocyte frequency and size in dysplastic nevi are also intermediate between acquired nevocellular nevi and superficial spreading melanoma [94]. In prospective studies of families with the dysplastic nevus syndrome, new melanomas developed only in individuals with dysplastic nevi. In a few cases, individual dysplastic nevi have been photographically documented in progress to melanoma [88].

Epidemiologic studies indicate a several-hundred-fold increased risk of development of melanoma in individuals with the familial form of the dysplastic nevus syndrome [89]. Studies in progress suggest close to 100 percent lifetime risk of development of melanoma in those dysplastic nevus syndrome family members with dysplastic nevi. Family members without dysplastic nevi may have nearly normal risk of melanoma [89].

Linkage studies of 401 individuals in 14 kindreds with familial dysplastic nevus syndrome demonstrated autosomal dominant inheritance and suggest that the defective gene may be located on the short arm of chromosome 1 near the Rh locus [87].

Finding abnormalities in cultured fibroblasts or lymphoblasts from patients with familial dysplastic nevus syndrome suggests that they have a systemic defect not localized to the pigment cells. The types of abnormalities found (hypersensitivity to killing and hypermutability following UV radiation exposure) are similar to those seen in XP, although the small number of observations reported to date makes this conclusion tentative. There are clinical similarities between familial dysplastic nevus syndrome and XP: both have markedly increased risk of cutaneous melanoma in association with increased numbers of pigmented lesions. These clinical and laboratory similarities, if borne out, suggest that laboratory tests may be developed for early detection of the familial dysplastic nevus syndrome.

Pigmented lesions that are clinically and histologically indistinguishable from dysplastic nevi have been identified in at least 33 percent of people with cutaneous melanoma (most of whom had no family history of melanoma [85,97])

DYSPLASTIC NEVUS SYNDROME TYPE	DESCRIPTION	MELANOMA IN KINDRED?	DYSPLASTIC NEVI IN TWO OR MORE BLOOD RELATIVES?	MELANOMA RISK	NUMBER OF PEOPLE AFFECTED
A	Sporadic Dysplastic Nevi	−	−	LOW	MANY
B	Familial Dysplastic Nevi	−	+		
C	Sporadic Dysplastic Nevi with Melanoma	+	−		
D-1	Familial Dysplastic Nevi with Melanoma	+	+		
D-2		+ +*	+	HIGH	FEW

*AT LEAST TWO BLOOD RELATIVES WITH CUTANEOUS MELANOMA

Fig. 150-4 Classification of kindreds with the dysplastic nevus syndrome.

and in 2 to 5 percent of the adult population [92]. It is unlikely that these millions of individuals with dysplastic nevi all have the same melanoma risk. The assessment of the melanoma risk of an individual with dysplastic nevi appears to depend on his family history as well as his personal history. A classification of four types of kindreds with dysplastic nevi has been proposed based on putative increasing melanoma risk categories [92] (Fig. 150-4). Dysplastic nevus syndrome type A (sporadic dysplastic nevi) is a kindred with one person with dysplastic nevi without melanoma. Dysplastic nevus syndrome type B (familial dysplastic nevi) is a kindred with more than one blood relative with dysplastic nevi without melanoma. Dysplastic nevus syndrome type C (sporadic dysplastic nevi with melanoma) is a kindred with only one individual who has both dysplastic nevi and cutaneous melanoma and no other blood relatives with dysplastic nevi or melanoma. Dysplastic nevus syndrome type D (familial dysplastic nevi with melanoma) is a kindred with at least two blood relatives having dysplastic nevi and one (type D-1) or two or more (type D-2) blood relatives with melanoma. Dysplastic nevus syndrome type D-2 is the form described in this section; it is the group with the highest melanoma risk but is the smallest numerically. The melanoma risk of people with the other types of dysplastic nevus syndrome is not known at present but is under active investigation.

Gardner's syndrome

Defintion

Gardner's syndrome is an autosomal dominant form of familial adenomatous polyposis of the colon associated with multiple osteomas and soft tissue tumors. Patients have a high frequency of colonic carcinoma. Gardner's syndrome has been estimated to occur with a frequency of 1 in 14,000 persons [98].

Clinical features

The cutaneous and osseous abnormalities usually precede recognition of colonic polyps in patients with Gardner's syndrome. Cutaneous lesions consist of cystic lesions (sebaceous or epidermal inclusion cysts) which may occur all over the body surface but have a predilection for the scalp and face. They often occur with increasing frequency in children and stabilize later in life. Subcutaneous fibromas may be present.

Desmoid tumors may occur, particularly in surgical scars along the abdominal wall. They are believed to arise from the connective tissue of muscle. The desmoid tumors may be locally invasive, destroying muscle or occasionally forming massive "mesenteric fibromatosis." Histologically they may be mistaken for low-grade fibrosarcomas.

Bony abnormalities are found in at least half of the patients, mostly involving membranous bones of the calvaria and face [98]. They may be true osteomas or irregular cortical thickenings. They include odontomas, rudimentary or supernumerary teeth, osteodontomas, dentigerous cysts, and unerupted teeth. Dentures at an early age are common. Scoliosis is frequent.

The intestinal polyposis occurs mainly in the colon but may occasionally be present in the duodenum and elsewhere in the gastrointestinal tract. The adenomatous polyps are identical to those in familial multiple polyposis without extraintestinal involvement. At least half of the patients have polyps by the end of the third decade of life. There is a very high frequency of malignant degeneration of the polyps. In a recent series of patients with familial polyposis and colon cancer, approximately 60 percent had developed colon cancer by age 40 years [98]. This is at least 30 years earlier in life than the age of a comparable proportion of the colon cancer patients in the U.S. population. Other tumors reported in patients with Gardner's syndrome include adrenal carcinoma, thyroid carcinoma, ovarian tumors, melanoma, carcinoid tumors, and leiomyomas of the gastrointestinal tract and retroperitoneum.

Laboratory abnormalities

Abnormalities in routine laboratory tests relate to the bony alterations detected on x-ray examination and the polyps of the colon. There may be anemia associated with bleeding from the gastrointestinal tract.

Analysis of chromosomes from cultured fibroblasts from patients in two families with Gardner's syndrome showed an increased percentage of cells with a tetraploid number of chromosomes (11 to 35 percent in patients vs. 0 to 4 percent in normal controls) [99]. Other studies of growth of cultured Gardner's syndrome fibroblasts showed a lack of contact inhibition and a decreased serum requirement for growth [100]. The cells had a greatly increased susceptibility to transformation by the Kirsten murine sarcoma virus.

Studies of cell survival showed an increased sensitivity to inhibition of colony-forming ability by x-radiation, UV radiation, and mitomycin C in fibroblast cultures from an affected father and daughter [101]. The mechanism of this sensitivity was not determined.

Clinical–laboratory correlations

Patients with Gardner's syndrome have progressive degenerative changes in the colon and to a lesser extent in skin and bones. Exuberant muscle connective tissue fibroblast proliferation following surgery leads to desmoid formation. Skin fibroblasts grow very well in culture, often growing in criss-crossed layers, a property rarely seen with normal fibroblasts. They are readily transformed by murine sarcoma virus. Chromosomal tetraploidy is present. These cellular abnormalities may reflect the abnormal cell growth in vivo. The hypersensitivity to radiation, and, indeed, most of the other cellular abnormalities, have been described in very few affected individuals. A more complete explanation will require further studies.

Basal cell nevus syndrome

Definition

Basal cell nevus syndrome is a progressive degenerative multisystem disorder characterized by early onset of mandibular cysts and basal cell carcinomas. Inheritance is autosomal dominant with variable penetrance. There may be a high spontaneous mutation rate. The frequency of the basal cell nevus syndrome is not known but the disease is not rare [102,103].

Clinical features

The early features of the basal cell nevus syndrome usually do not involve the skin (Table 150-5). Patients may be born with congenital blindness (due to coloboma, cataracts, or glaucoma) or hydrocephalus. Multiple cysts of the mandible or maxilla with keratinized lining (keratocysts) may occur early in the disease. Patients have a characteristic facies with broad nasal root, frontal bossing, well-developed supraorbital ridges, hypertelorism, and mild mandibular prognathism. There may be lateral displacement of the inner canthi (dystopia canthorum).

The most common cutaneous abnormality is the presence of multiple basal cell carcinomas. These may occur early in life in sites shielded from sunlight as well as in sites exposed to sunlight. Patients may have a few to dozens or hundreds of basal cell carcinomas. The term *nevus* in basal cell nevus syndrome is an old medical term referring to any circumscribed lesion believed to arise under genetic influence. It referred to vascular or nonvascular growths and not just nevus cell nevi, or "moles," as in the terminology of today. The *nevi* in the basal cell nevus syndrome are true basal cell carcinomas.

Approximately 50 percent of the patients have minute pits (epidermal defects in keratin production) of the palms

Table 150-5 Basal cell nevus syndrome: clinical features

Cutaneous abnormalities:
  Multiple basal cell carcinomas
  Pits in palms and soles
  Benign lesions: milia, cysts, lipomas, fibromas
Characteristic facies:
  Broad nasal root
  Frontal bossing
  Hypertelorism
Osseous abnormalities:
  Oral: jaw cysts, defective dentition, ameloblastoma
  Ribs: bifid, splayed, pectus excavatum
  Brachymetacarpalism
Ocular abnormalities:
  Hypertelorism
  Dystopia canthorum
  Strabismus
  Congenital blindness: cataracts, coloboma, glaucoma
Neurologic abnormalities:
  Mental retardation
  Calcification of the dura
  Congenital hydrocephalus
  Medulloblastoma
Endocrine abnormalities:
  Male hypogonadism: absent or undescended testes
  Female: ovarian fibromas

and soles. There may be few to hundreds of these pits. They are more numerous on the lateral surfaces of the palms, soles, and fingers. Other cutaneous lesions include milia, multiple cysts, lipomas, and fibromas or desmoids.

The keratocysts of the jaws are lined with squamous epithelium. They have extensive keratinization and walls of connective tissue. They may range from a few millimeters to several centimeters in diameter. Recurrences after surgery are common. Teeth may be carious, misshapen, or in abnormal locations. Ameloblastomas, an oral analogue of the basal cell carcinoma, may occur.

Brachymetacarpalism (Albright's sign) consists of a short fourth metacarpal [104]. It is easily seen by examining the knuckles on the dorsum of a clenched fist and verified by hand x-ray (Fig. 150-5a). In addition to the basal cell nevus syndrome, Albright's sign is seen in pseudohypoparathyroidism, Turner's syndrome, and pseudopseudohypoparathyroidism. Rib or vertebral abnormalities are common. Lamellar calcification of the falx is often a valuable diagnostic sign (Fig. 150-5b).

Mental retardation is present in a minority of the patients. The electroencephalogram may show nonspecific abnormalities. Congenital abnormalities include agenesis of the corpus callosum and congenital hydrocephalus.

Other abnormalities in some patients include male hypogonadism with absent or undescended testes, infantile external genitalia, female pubic hair pattern, and scanty facial hair. Ovarian fibromas and pelvic calcification may be present. Lymphatic mesenteric cysts may necessitate laparotomy [102].

Patients with the basal cell nevus syndrome are subject to internal neoplasms as well as to cutaneous basal cell carcinomas. These include ameloblastomas of the oral cavity, fibrosarcoma of the jaw, ovarian fibromas, teratomas, or cystadenomas. Medulloblastoma of the brain has been present in several patients. Treatment of the medulloblas-

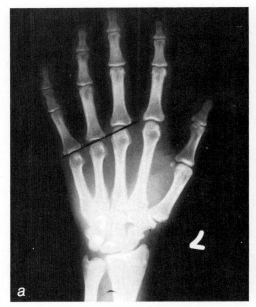 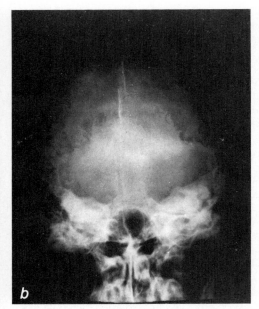

Fig. 150-5   Basal cell nevus syndrome. (a) Short fourth meta-carpal (Albright's sign). A line drawn through the distal ends of the fifth and fourth metacarpals intersects the third meta-carpal proximal to its end. (b) Lamellar calcification of the falx.

toma with standard dosage of radiotherapy has resulted in a remarkable phenomenon: Numerous basal cell carcinomas appeared in the skin within 4 years; these were strikingly limited to the portions of skin that were exposed in the radiotherapy field [105].

Laboratory abnormalities

Most standard clinical laboratory tests are normal in patients with basal cell nevus syndrome. Chromosome abnormalities have been found in a small number of patients [106]. Two patients in one family had an unusual group F chromosome (a "marker chromosome") with an unusually long pair of secondary constrictions in one pair of arms. Other cells from these patients showed deletions of portions of these chromosomes. In another study, two basal cell nevus syndrome patients had increased rates of chromosome breakage and rearrangement in cultured fibroblasts. Studies of induced breakage or of SCEs have not been published.

The clinical observation of the induction of numerous basal cell carcinomas in skin in the path of radiotherapy for treatment of central nervous system neoplasms prompted the study of x-ray sensitivity of cultured cells from patients with basal cell nevus syndrome. Studies of dermal fibroblasts have shown normal survival response following x-ray [4].

Clinical–laboratory correlations

Patients with basal cell nevus syndrome have features of progressive degeneration with occurrence of multiple jaw cysts and basal cell carcinomas. A few patients have chromosomal abnormalities, but this has not been studied systematically in a large series of patients.

There is striking clinical x-ray induction of basal cell carcinomas. However, a corresponding cellular radiohy-persensitivity has not been demonstrated. Perhaps the defect is limited to the epidermal basal cells and not found in the dermal fibroblasts that are usually cultured.

Retinoblastoma

Definition

Retinoblastoma is a childhood tumor of the retina. It occurs with a frequency of approximately 1 per 20,000 live births in a hereditary and a nonhereditary form [7,107–110].

Clinical features

Retinoblastoma is diagnosed most frequently in children between 2 and 6 years of age. Approximately 10 percent of patients are diagnosed at birth. About 60 percent of the cases are nonhereditary. Forty percent are hereditary, inherited in an autosomal dominant manner from an affected survivor or a nonaffected latent gene carrier, or due to a new germinal mutation in a healthy patient. Retinoblastoma is equally frequent in the left and right eyes and is bilateral in about 25 percent of cases. Rarely the pineal gland is also involved (so-called trilateral retinoblastoma). Overall, about 94 percent of all retinoblastoma cases, both hereditary and nonhereditary, are sporadic. All cases with bilateral retinoblastoma are hereditary and about 10 to 15 percent of the unilateral cases are sporadic, but due to a new germinal mutation. Approximately 25 percent of infants with $13q^-$ chromosome deletion syndrome have retinoblastoma [107].

The most frequent presenting symptom is the amaurotic "cat's eye" (Fig. 150-6) [107]. This results from a growing retinal tumor filling the vitreous humor and producing a white pupillary reflex (leukocoria) in the normally black pupillary opening. Another sign is turning the face toward

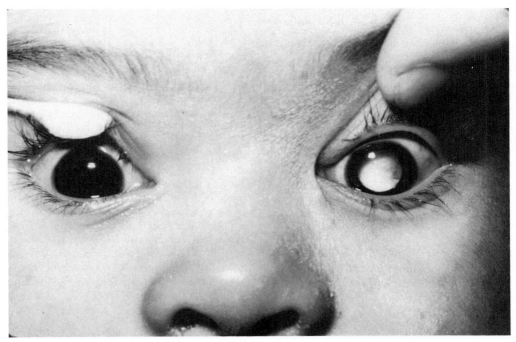

Fig. 150-6   Retinoblastoma. Amaurotic "cat's eye" in a child with retinoblastoma of the left eye. (Photograph courtesy of Jerry S. Shields.)

the side of the diseased eye when reading or looking at something in detail. This sign may be misinterpreted as a "tic" or torticollis. It results from use of the normal eye to compensate for deficient vision in the affected eye. Retinoblastoma may be associated with heterochromia of the iris, with the affected eye having the darker iris. Early lesions may present as decreased vision or strabismus.

The clinical diagnosis is made by fundoscopic examination. Early tumors may appear as one or more white, elevated retinal masses with indistinct borders. Tumor progression may involve the vitreous or the choroid, producing retinal detachment and a white pupillary reflex. Continued tumor growth may result in secondary glaucoma, photophobia, or hemorrhage.

Diagnosis of localized retinoblastoma may be suggested by fluorescein angiography. Masses may be localized by ultrasonography. Intraocular calcifications in children are highly suggestive of retinoblastoma.

The tumor most often metastasizes to subcutaneous tissue of the head and preauricular lymph nodes. Distant metastases may occur. The most common cause of death is brain metastasis.

Treatment consists mainly of surgical enucleation of the affected eye and/or local x-radiation. The five-year cure rate in the United States is above 80 percent, one of the highest for any childhood neoplasm [107].

Survivors of retinoblastoma have an increased risk of developing a second neoplasm, particularly osteosarcomas [111,112]. Osteosarcomas have occurred in sites not treated with radiation as well as in sites in the field of radiation therapy. Other second neoplasms have included rhabdomyosarcoma, leukemia, thyroid adenocarcinoma, and melanoma. In the hereditary form of retinoblastoma the risk of developing nonradiogenic osteosarcoma was increased 230-fold in carriers of the retinoblastoma gene (whether clinically affected or not) [112].

Laboratory abnormalities

Chromosome studies of cultured cells from some patients with retinoblastoma have shown a specific defect: deletion of the q14 band on the long arm of chromosome 13. A few patients with congenital abnormalities, including retinal lesions but without retinoblastoma, were found to have deletions in chromosome 13 not including the q14 region. Thus this region is suspected of containing genetic material responsible for prevention of development of retinoblastoma. Retinoblastoma tumors were found to have altered DNA sequences resulting in homozygosity of a mutant allele on chromosome 13 [112a].

Cultured fibroblasts from patients with retinoblastoma and deletion of a portion of chromosome 13 were found to be hypersensitive to inhibition of colony forming by x-radiation [16,17]. Fibroblasts from patients with hereditary retinoblastoma without chromosome deletion were mildly hypersensitive to x-ray-induced killing. Fibroblasts from patients with sporadic retinoblastoma had normal x-ray survival. Studies of x-ray-induced chromosome abnormalities or mutagenesis have not been published. The basis for the x-ray hypersensitivity in cultured cells from patients with hereditary retinoblastoma has been postulated to involve abnormal DNA repair. However, no DNA repair defect has yet been reported in these cells.

Clinical-laboratory correlations

The hereditary forms of retinoblastoma are unusually susceptible to development of multiple primary tumors in one retina, to bilateral retinoblastomas, and to other primary neoplasms at distant sites. These occur in sites receiving radiation as well as in nonradiated sites. Cells from patients with hereditary retinoblastoma are hypersensitive to killing by x-radiation. These observations have been cited as supporting a "two hit" model of carcinogenesis, as proposed by Knudson et al [113]. According to this theory, cancer is the result of two distinct mutations, each occurring with a frequency of about 1 in 1 million. Both mutations would thus occur by chance with a frequency of 1 in 10^{12}, an exceedingly rare event. Patients with hereditary retinoblastoma are assumed to have inherited the first mutation. This mutation is thus present in all their cells. The cells thus need only be subjected to a single mutation to develop cancer. Patients with hereditary retinoblastoma do develop retinoblastoma at a younger age than do patients with the spontaneous form. The x-ray hypersensitivity of all their cells may further predispose to the development of the second mutation in ocular and other tissues.

Other disorders

Investigations of a number of other disorders have led to publications describing cellular hypersensitivity (Table 150-1). Generally, each paper described abnormalities in a small number of affected individuals.

Fibroblasts from two tuberous sclerosis patients (of three tested) showed increased sensitivity to inhibition of colony-forming ability by hypoxic gamma radiation [12].

Lymphoblastoid cell lines from four patients with Huntington's disease were abnormally sensitive to x-ray inhibition of cell growth [114].

Lymphoblastoid cell lines from two patients with Chédiak-Higashi syndrome [115,116] were abnormally sensitive to growth inhibition by UV radiation and by treatment with the carcinogen 4-nitroquinoline oxide [117]. No defect in DNA repair was detected to explain this hypersensitivity.

Fibroblasts from a patient with juvenile dermatomyositis who developed a basal cell carcinoma of the eyelid at age 16 were found to be hypersensitive to x-ray and to 313-nm UV radiation [118]. No DNA repair defect was found.

Conclusion

Increased sensitivity to some physical and chemical agents has been recognized in a small number of heritable diseases in recent years (Table 150-1). Clinical hypersensitivity to sunlight or to radiotherapy has been shown to be manifested by a corresponding cellular hypersensitivity in XP, Cockayne's syndrome, and AT. In XP and in some patients with AT the cellular hypersensitivity has been shown to be related to defective DNA repair.

Spontaneous chromosomal breakage is a feature of AT, Bloom's syndrome, and Fanconi's anemia. As with most of these disorders, the molecular mechanisms involved in the chromosomal abnormalities are just beginning to be understood.

Recognition of the hypersensitivity of these disorders has significance for diagnosis of several of them. Diagnosis of Bloom's syndrome, Fanconi's anemia, and XP may be facilitated by examining chromosomal abnormalities or DNA repair. Prenatal diagnosis has been accomplished in

XP, Fanconi's anemia, and AT on the basis of cellular hypersensitivity to UV radiation [32], to diepoxybutane [57], and to induction of chromosome breaks [46], respectively.

Although these heritable diseases are rare, carriers of the affected genes can be calculated to comprise several percent of the general population. These individuals are usually free of clinical symptoms. However, epidemiologic studies have suggested that they may have an increased risk of neoplasia. In particular, heterozygous carriers of AT may have a fivefold increased risk of dying from ovarian, stomach, or biliary tract cancer before age 45 [40]. Since they may comprise 1 percent of the general population, they may thus represent 5 percent of the persons dying from these cancers before age 45 years. There is a similar suggestion that persons heterozygous for XP have an increased risk of developing skin cancer [35]. Asymptomatic carriers of the retinoblastoma genetic defect have a 200-fold increased risk of developing osteosarcoma [112]. Many of these individuals may be at an increased risk from exposure to environmental agents. There are thus implications for cancer control, preventive medicine, and occupational medicine. At present, however, there is no laboratory test that can reliably detect the asymptomatic carriers of most of these disorders.

There is a tantalizing link between these cellular abnormalities and certain common clinical features such as neoplasia, neurologic degeneration, and immune deficiency. Progressive cutaneous, neoplastic, or neurologic degeneration (as in XP, AT, Cockayne's syndrome, dyskeratosis congenita, basal cell nevus syndrome, retinoblastoma, Gardner's syndrome, or Huntington's disease) may be the result of impaired survival of cells subjected to damage by exogenous or endogenous physical or chemical agents. Immune deficiency is seen in AT, Bloom's syndrome, Chédiak-Higashi syndrome, and dyskeratosis congenita. The immune deficiency may be related to in utero damage, to defective DNA processing at a crucial stage of embryonic development, or to other, not presently identified, defects. A better understanding of the relationship between these clinical abnormalities and the cellular defects in these patients will undoubtedly provide insights to disease in normal individuals.

Appendix

In order to gather quantitative information on clinical abnormalities in several of these rare disorders and to provide insights into etiology, five registries have been established:

1. Patients with xeroderma pigmentosum should be reported to:

    Xeroderma Pigmentosum Registry
    c/o Department of Pathology
    Medical Science Building, Room C520
    CMDNJ—New Jersey Medical School
    100 Bergen Street
    Newark, NJ 07103
2. Patients with Bloom's syndrome should be reported to:

    Bloom's Syndrome Registry
    c/o Laboratory of Human Genetics
    The New York Blood Center
    310 East 67th Street
    New York, NY 10021

3. Patients wtih immunodeficiency (e.g., ataxia-telangiectasia) and cancer should be reported to:
   Immunodeficiency—Cancer Registry
   Box 609 Mayo
   University of Minnesota
   Minneapolis, MN 55455
4. Patients with Fanconi's anemia should be reported to:
   Fanconi Anemia International Registry
   c/o Dr. Arleen Auerbach
   Laboratory for Investigative Dermatology
   The Rockefeller University
   1230 York Avenue
   New York, NY 10021
5. Patients with Gardner's syndrome should be reported to:
   Familial Polyposis and Gardner's Syndrome Registry
   c/o Dr. Martin Lipkin
   Memorial Hospital for Cancer Research
   1275 York Avenue
   New York, NY 10021

References

*1. Robbins JH et al: Xeroderma pigmentosum: an inherited disease with sun sensitivity, multiple cutaneous neoplasms, and abnormal DNA repair. *Ann Intern Med* **80:**221, 1974
*2. Kraemer KH: Xeroderma pigmentosum, in *Clinical Dermatology,* vol 4, edited by DJ Demis et al. Hagerstown, Harper & Row, 1980, p 1
2a. Kraemer KH, Slor H: Xeroderma pigmentosum. *Clinics Dermatol* **2:**33, 1985
*3. Setlow RB: Repair deficient human disorders and cancer. *Nature* **271:**713, 1978
*4. Arlett CF, Lehmann AR: Human disorders showing increased sensitivity to the induction of genetic damage. *Annu Rev Genet* **12:**95, 1978
*5. Paterson MC: Environmental carcinogenesis and imperfect repair of damaged DNA in *Homo sapiens:* causal relation revealed by rare hereditary disorders, in *Carcinogens: Identification and Mechanisms of Action,* edited by AC Griffin, CR Shaw. New York, Raven Press, 1979, p 251
*6. Friedberg EC et al: Human diseases associated with defective DNA repair. *Adv Radiat Biol* **8:**85, 1979
*7. Gianelli F: DNA repair in human diseases. *Clin Exp Dermatol* **5:**119, 1980
*8. Lehmann AR, Karran P: DNA repair. *Int Rev Cytol* **72:**101, 1981
*9. Kraemer KH: Progressive degenerative diseases associated with defective DNA repair: xeroderma pigmentosum and ataxia telangiectasia, in *DNA Repair Processes,* edited by WW Nichols, DG Murphy. Miami, Symposium Specialists, 1977, p 37
*10. Cleaver JE: Xeroderma pigmentosum, in *The Metabolic Basis of Inherited Disease,* 5th ed, edited by JB Stanbury et al. New York, McGraw-Hill, 1983, p 1227
*11. Robbins JH et al: Hypersensitivity to DNA-damaging agents in abiotrophies: a new explanation for degeneration of nervous, photoreceptor, and muscle in Alzheimer, Parkinson, and Huntington diseases, retinitis pigmentosa and Duchenne muscular dystrophy, in *Muscular Basis of Aging,* Basic Life Science Series, edited by AD Woodhead et al. New York, Plenum Press, in press
*12. Paterson MC et al: Gamma ray hypersensitivity and faulty DNA repair in cultured cells from humans exhibiting familial cancer proneness, in *Radiation Research,* edited by S Okada et al. Tokyo, Toppan, 1979, p 484

13. Arlett CF, Harcourt SA: Survey of radiosensitivity in a variety of human cell strains. *Cancer Res* **40:**926, 1980
14. Smith PJ, Paterson MC: Abnormal responses to mid-ultraviolet light of cultured fibroblasts from patients with disorders featuring sunlight sensitivity. *Cancer Res* **41:**511, 1981
*15. Paterson MC, Smith PJ: Ataxia telangiectasia: an inherited human disorder involving hypersensitivity to ionizing radiation and related DNA-damaging chemicals. *Annu Rev Genet* **13:**291, 1979
16. Weichselbaum RR, Little JB: Familial retinoblastoma and ataxia telangiectasia: human models for the study of DNA damage and repair. *Cancer* **45:**775, 1980
17. Weichselbaum RR et al: X-ray sensitivity of fifty-three human diploid fibroblast cell strains from patients with characterized genetic disorders. *Cancer Res* **40:**920, 1980
*18. Mulvihill JJ: Genetic repertory of human neoplasia, in *Genetics of Human Cancer,* edited by JJ Mulvihill et al. New York, Raven Press, 1977, p 137
*19. Reed WB: Congenital and genetic skin disorders with tumor formation. *Australas J Dermatol* **16:**95, 1975
*20. Lynch HT, Frichot BC: Skin, hereditary and cancer. *Semin Oncol* **5:**67, 1978
*21. Robbins JH: Significance of repair of human DNA: evidence from studies of xeroderma pigmentosum. *J Natl Cancer Inst* **61:**645, 1978
22. Kraemer KH et al: Colony-forming ability of ultraviolet-irradiated xeroderma pigmentosum fibroblasts from different DNA repair complementation groups. *Biochim Biophys Acta* **442:**147, 1976
23. Robbins JH, Moshell AN: DNA repair processes protect human beings from premature solar skin damage: evidence from studies of xeroderma pigmentosum. *J Invest Dermatol* **73:**102, 1979
*24. Day RS: Human adenoviruses as DNA repair probes, in *DNA Repair Processes,* edited by WW Nichols, DG Murphy. Miami, Symposium Specialists, 1977, p 119
25. Chang WS et al: Ultraviolet light-induced sister chromatid exchanges in xeroderma pigmentosum and in Cockayne's syndrome lymphocyte cell lines. *Cancer Res* **38:**1601, 1978
26. Cleaver JE: Defective repair replication of DNA in xeroderma pigmentosum. *Nature* **218:**652, 1968
27. Epstein JH et al: Defect in DNA synthesis in skin of patients with xeroderma pigmentosum demonstrated in vivo. *Science* **168:**1477, 1970
28. De Weerd-Kastelein EA et al: Genetic heterogeneity of xeroderma pigmentosum demonstrated by somatic cell hybridization. *Nature* **238:**80, 1972
29. Kraemer KH et al: Genetic heterogeneity in xeroderma pigmentosum: complementation groups and their relationship to DNA repair rates. *Proc Natl Acad Sci USA* **72:**59, 1975
29a. Fisher E et al: A ninth complementation group in xeroderma pigmentosum, XPI, *Mutat Res* **145:**217, 1985
30. Burk PG et al: Ultraviolet stimulated thymidine incorporation in xeroderma pigmentosum lymphocytes. *J Lab Clin Med* **77:**759, 1971
31. Berger NA et al: Defective poly(adenosine diphosphoribose) synthesis in xeroderma pigmentosum. *Biochemistry* **19:**289, 1980
32. Ramsay CA et al: Prenatal diagnosis of xeroderma pigmentosum: report of the first successful case. *Lancet* **2:**1109, 1974
33. Braun-Falco O et al: Tumorprophylaxe bei Xeroderma pigmentosum mit aromatischem Retinoid (RO-109359). *Hautarzt* **33:**445, 1982
34. Hofmann H et al: Pigmented xerodermoid: first report of a family. *Bull Cancer (Paris)* **63:**347, 1978
35. Swift M, Chase C: Cancer in families with xeroderma pigmentosum. *J Natl Cancer Inst* **62:**1415, 1979

*36. Sedgwick RP, Boder E: Ataxia telangiectasia, in *Handbook of Clinical Neurology*, vol 14, edited by PJ Vinken, GW Bruyn. Amsterdam, North-Holland, 1972, p 267

*37. McFarlin DE et al: Ataxia telangiectasia. *Medicine (Baltimore)* **51**:281, 1972

*38. Waldman TA et al: Ataxia-telangiectasia: a multisystem hereditary disease with immunodeficiency, impaired organ maturation, x-ray hypersensitivity, and a high incidence of neoplasia. *Ann Intern Med* **99**:367. 1983

39. Henderson EE, Ribecky R: DNA repair in lymphoblastoid cell lines established from human genetic disorders. *Chem Biol Interact* **33**:63, 1980

40. Swift M et al: Malignant neoplasms in the families of patients with ataxia telangiectasia. *Cancer Res* **36**:209, 1976

*41. Spector BD et al: Epidemiology of cancer in ataxia-telangiectasia, in *Ataxia-Telangiectasia—A Cellular and Molecular Link Between Cancer Neuropathy and Immune Deficiency*, edited by BA Bridges, DG Harnden. New York, John Wiley & Sons, 1982, p 103

*42. Harnden DG, Taylor AMR: Chromosomes and neoplasia. *Ann Hum Genet* **9**:1, 1979

*43. Taylor AMR: Cytogenetics of ataxia-telangiectasia, in *Ataxia-Telangiectasia—A Cellular and Molecular Link Between Cancer, Neuropathy, and Immune Deficiency*, edited by BA Bridges, DG Harnden, New York, John Wiley & Sons, 1982, p 53

44. Edwards MJ, Taylor AMR: Unusual levels of (ADP-ribose)$_n$ and DNA synthesis in ataxia telangiectasia cells following gamma-ray irradiation. *Nature* **287**:745, 1980

45. Shaham M et al: A diffusable clastogenic factor in ataxia telangiectasia. *Cytogenet Cell Genet* **27**:155, 1980

46. Shaham M et al: Prenatal diagnosis of ataxia telangiectasia. *J Pediatr* **100**:134, 1982

47. Fujiwara Y et al: Cross-link repair in human cells and its possible defect in Fanconi's anemia cells. *J Mol Biol* **113**:635, 1977

48. Ishida R, Buchwald M: Susceptibility of Fanconi's anemia lymphoblasts to DNA cross-linking and alkylating agents. *Cancer Res* **42**:4000, 1982

*49. German J (ed): *Chromosome Mutation and Neoplasia*. New York, Alan R Liss, 1983

*50. Nilsson LR: Chronic pancytopenia with multiple congenital abnormalities (Fanconi's anemia). *Acta Paediatr Scand* **49**:518, 1960

51. Sasaki M, Tonomura A: A high susceptibility of Fanconi's anemia to chromosome breakage by DNA cross-linking agents. *Cancer Res* **33**:1829, 1973

*52. Gmyrek D, Syllm-Rapoport I: Fanconi's anemia: analysis of 129 described cases. *Z Kinderheilkd* **91**:294, 1964

*53. Schroeder TM et al: Formal genetics of Fanconi's anemia. *Hum Genet* **32**:257, 1976

54. Gozdasoglu S et al: Fanconi's aplastic anemia: analysis of 18 cases. *Acta Haematol (Basel)* **64**:131, 1980

*55. Auerbach AD, Wolman SR: Carcinogen-induced chromosome breakage in chromosome instability syndromes. *Cancer Genet Cytogenet* **1**:21, 1979

56. Berger R et al: Sister chromatid exchanges induced by nitrogen mustard in Fanconi's anemia: application to the detection of heterozygotes and interpretation of the results. *Cancer Genet Cytogenet* **2**:259, 1980

57. Auerbach AD et al: Pre- and postnatal diagnosis and carrier detection of Fanconi anemia by cytogenetic method. *Pediatrics* **67**:128, 1981

58. Schroeder TM, Stahl-Mauge C: Mutagenic effects of isonicotinic acid hydrazide in Fanconi's anemia. *Hum Genet* **52**:309, 1979

59. Latt SA et al: Induction by alkylating agents of sister chromatid exchanges and chromatid breaks in Fanconi's anemia. *Proc Natl Acad Sci USA* **72**:4066, 1975

60. Kano Y, Fujiwara Y: Roles of DNA interstrand crosslinking and its repair in the induction of sister-chromatid exchange and a higher induction in Fanconi's anemia cells. *Mutat Res* **81**:365, 1981

61. Brumback RA et al: Normal pressure hydrocephalus: recognition and relationship to neurological abnormalities in Cockayne's syndrome. *Arch Neurol* **35**:337, 1978

62. Riggs W, Seibert J: Cockayne's syndrome: roentgen findings. *Am J Roentgenol* **116**:623, 1972

63. Wade MH, Chu EHY: Effects of DNA damaging agents of cultured fibroblasts derived from patients with Cockayne's syndrome. *Mutat Res* **59**:49, 1979

64. Andrews AD et al: Cockayne's syndrome fibroblasts have increased sensitivity to ultraviolet light but normal rates of unscheduled DNA synthesis. *J Invest Dermatol* **70**:237, 1978

65. Marshall RR et al: Increased sensitivity of cell strains from Cockayne's syndrome to sister chromatid exchange induction and cell killing by UV light. *Mutat Res* **69**:107, 1980

66. Tanaka K et al: Genetic complementation groups in Cockayne syndrome. *Somatic Cell Genet* **7**:445, 1981

67. Lehmann A: Three complementation groups in Cockayne syndrome. *Mutat Res* **106**:347, 1982

68. German J, Schonberg S: Bloom's syndrome. IX. Review of cytological and biochemical aspects, in *Genetic and Environmental Factors in Experimental and Human Cancer*, edited by HV Gelboin et al. Tokyo, Japan Scientific Societies Press, 1980, p 175

*69. German J: Bloom's syndrome. II. The prototype of human genetic disorders predisposing to chromosome instability and cancer, in *Chromosomes and Cancer*, edited by J German. New York, John Wiley & Sons, 1974, p 601

70. Bloom D: Congenital telangiectatic erythema resembling lupus erythematosus in dwarfs. *Am J Dis Child* **88**:754, 1954

71. German J et al: Bloom's syndrome. VII. Progress report for 1978. *Clin Genet* **15**:361, 1979

72. Weemaes CMR et al: Immune responses in four patients with Bloom syndrome. *Clin Immunol Immunopathol* **12**:12, 1979

73. Kauli R et al: Gonadal function in Bloom's syndrome. *Clin Endocrinol* **6**:285, 1977

74. Alhadeff B et al: High rate of sister chromatid exchanges of Bloom's syndrome is corrected in rodent human somatic cell hybrids. *Cytogenet Cell Genet* **27**:8, 1980

75. Hand R, German J: Bloom's syndrome: DNA replication in cultured fibroblasts and lymphocytes. *Hum Genet* **38**:297, 1977

76. Gupta RS, Goldstein S: Diphtheria toxin resistance in human fibroblast cell strains from normal and cancer-prone individuals. *Mutat Res* **73**:331, 1980

77. Sirnavin C, Trowbridge AA: Dyskeratosis congenita: clinical features and genetic aspects. Report of a family and review of the literature. *J Med Genet* **12**:339, 1975

78. Carter DM et al: Psoralen-DNA cross-linking photoadducts in dyskeratosis congenita: delay in excision and promotion of sister chromatid exchange. *J Invest Dermatol* **73**:97, 1979

79. Burgdorf W et al: Sister chromatid exchange in dyskeratosis congenita. *J Med Genet* **14**:256, 1977

80. Feinberg AP, Coffey DS: Organ site specificity for cancer in chromosomal instability disorders. *Cancer Res* **42**:3252, 1982

81. Fudenberg HH et al: Active and suppressor T cells: diminution in a patient with dyskeratosis congenita and in first-degree relatives. *Gerontology* **25**:231, 1979

82. Nagasawa H, Little JB: Suppression of cytotoxic effect of mitomycin-C by superoxide dismutase in Fanconi's anemia and dyskeratosis congenita fibroblasts. *Carcinogenesis* **4**:795, 1983

83. Greene MH, Fraumeni JF: The hereditary variant of malig-

nant melanoma, in *Human Malignant Melanoma,* edited by WH Chark Jr et al. New York, Grune & Stratton, 1979, p 139

84. Elder DE et al: Acquired melanocytic nevi and melanoma: the dysplastic nevus syndrome, in *Pathology of Malignant Melanoma,* edited by AB Ackerman. New York, Masson, 1981, p 185

85. Elder DE et al: The dysplastic nevus syndrome: our definition. *Am J Dermatopathol* **4:**455, 1982

86. Clark WH Jr et al: Origin of familial malignant melanomas from heritable melanocytic lesions: the B-K mole syndrome. *Arch Dermatol* **114:**732, 1978

87. Greene MH et al: Familial cutaneous malignant melanoma—an autosomal dominant trait possibly linked to the Rh locus. *Proc Natl Acad Sci USA* **80:**6071, 1983

87a. Kraemer KH, Greene MH: Dysplastic nevus syndrome familial and sporadic precursors of cutaneous melanoma. *Dermatologic Clinics* **3:**225, 1985

88. Greene MH et al: Clinical recognition of acquired precursors of cutaneous melanoma: the familial dysplastic nevus syndrome. *N Engl J Med* **312:**91, 1985

89. Greene MH et al: The prospective diagnosis of malignant melanoma in a population at high risk: hereditary melanoma and the dysplastic nevus syndrome. *Ann Intern Med,* in press

90. Lynch HT et al: Tumour spectrum in the FAMMM syndrome. *Br J Cancer* **44:**553, 1981

91. MacKie R: Multiple melanoma and atypical melanocytic naevi—evidence of an activated and expanded melanocytic system. *Br J Dermatol* **107:**621, 1982

92. Kraemer KH et al: Dysplastic naevi and cutaneous melanoma risk. *Lancet* **2:**1076, 1983

93. Tucker MA et al: Dysplastic nevi on the scalp of prepubertal children from melanoma-prone families. *J Pediatr* **103:**65, 1983

94. Rhodes AR et al: Increased intraepidermal melanocyte frequency and size in dysplastic melanocytic nevi and cutaneous melanoma. A comparative quantitative study of dysplastic melanocytic nevi, superficial spreading melanoma, nevocellular nevi, and solar lentigines. *J Invest Dermatol* **80:**452, 1983

95. Ramsey RG et al: Familial melanoma associated with dominant ultraviolet radiation sensitivity. *Cancer Res* **42:**2909, 1982

96. Smith PJ et al: Abnormal sensitivity to UV-radiation in cultured skin fibroblasts from patients with hereditary cutaneous malignant melanoma and dysplastic nevus syndrome. *Int J Cancer* **30:**39, 1982

97. Elder DE et al: Dysplastic nevus syndrome: a phenotypic association of sporadic cutaneous melanoma. *Cancer* **46:**1787, 1980

*98. Lipkin M et al: Memorial Hospital registry of population groups at high risk for cancer of the large intestine: age of onset of neoplasms. *Prev Med* **9:**335, 1980

99. Danes BS: The Gardner syndrome: increased tetraploidy in cultured skin fibroblast. *J Med Genet* **13:**52, 1976

100. Kopelovich L: Hereditary adenomatosis of the colon and rectum: relevance to cancer promotion and cancer control in humans. *Cancer Genet Cytogenet* **5:**333, 1982

101. Little JB et al: Abnormal sensitivity of diploid skin fibroblasts from a family with Gardner's syndrome to the lethal effects of x-irradiation, ultraviolet light, and mitomycin C. *Mutat Res* **70:**241, 1980

*102. Berlin NI et al: Basal cell nevus syndrome. *Ann Intern Med* **64:**403, 1966

*103. Dunnick NR et al: Nevoid basal cell carcinoma syndrome: radiographic manifestations including cystlike lesions of the phalanges. *Radiology* **127:**331, 1978

104. Slater S: An evaluation of the metacarpal sign (short fourth metacarpal). *Pediatrics* **46:**468, 1970

105. Strong LC: Theories of pathogenesis: mutation and cancer, in *Genetics of Cancer,* edited by JJ Mulvihill et al. New York, Raven Press, 1977, p 401

106. Happle R, Hoehn H: Cytogenetic studies on cultured fibroblast-like cells derived from basal cell carcinoma tissue. *Clin Genet* **4:**17, 1973

*107. Shields JA, Augsburger JJ: Current approaches to the diagnosis and management of retinoblastoma. *Surv Ophthalmol* **25:**347, 1981

*108. Francois J: Costenbader Memorial Lecture: Genesis and genetics of retinoblastoma. *Adv Ophthalmol* **39:**181, 1979

109. Gaitan-Yanguas M: Retinoblastoma: analysis of 235 cases. *Int J Radiat Oncol Biol Phys* **4:**359, 1978

*110. Vogel F: Genetics of retinoblastoma. *Hum Genet* **52:**1, 1979

*111. Meadows AT et al: Patterns of second malignant neoplasms in children. *Cancer* **40:**1903, 1977

112. Matsunaga E: Hereditary retinoblastoma: host resistance and second primary tumors. *JNCI* **65:**47, 1980

112a. Cavenee WK et al: Expression of recessive alleles by chromosomal mechanisms in retinoblastoma. *Nature* **305:**779, 1983

113. Knudson AG et al: Mutation and childhood cancer: a probabilistic model for the incidence of retinoblastoma. *Proc Natl Acad Sci USA* **72:**5116, 1975

114. Moshell AN et al: Radiosensitivity in Huntington's disease: implications for pathogenesis and presymptomatic diagnosis. *Lancet* **1:**9, 1980

*115. Blume RS, Wolff SM: The Chédiak-Higashi syndrome: studies in four patients and a review of the literature. *Medicine (Baltimore)* **51:**247, 1972

*116. Wolff SM et al: The Chédiak-Higashi syndrome: studies of host defenses. *Ann Intern Med* **76:**293, 1972

117. Tanaka H, Orii T: High sensitivity but normal DNA-repair activity after UV irradiation in Epstein-Barr virus-transformed lymphoblastoid cell lines from Chédiak-Higashi syndrome. *Mutat Res* **72:**143, 1980

118. Smith PJ et al: In vitro radiosensitivity in a patient with dermatomyositis and cancer. *Lancet* **1:**216, 1981

* Indicates general references.

CHAPTER 151

ELASTOSIS PERFORANS SERPIGINOSA AND REACTIVE PERFORATING COLLAGENOSIS

Elisabeth C. Wolff-Schreiner

Elastosis perforans serpiginosa

Definition and synonyms

Elastosis perforans serpiginosa (EPS) is a rare, probably genetically determined, disorder of the skin characterized by the extrusion of dermal elastic tissue through the epidermis. Synonyms: keratosis follicularis serpiginosa, elastoma intrapapillare perforans verruciforme.

Historical aspects

Originally described as "porokeratosis" by Jones and Smith [1], EPS was recognized as an entity by Lutz [2] and Miescher [3]. More than 100 cases were reviewed in 1968 [4] and many more have been reported since. An association with genetically determined disorders of the connective tissue and mongolism was recognized more than 20 years ago [5–8] and more recently, EPS has been linked to long-term penicillamine treatment of Wilson's disease [9–14].

Etiology and pathogenesis

It has been proposed that in EPS altered elastic fibers of the upper dermis act as foreign material and are eliminated transepidermally [4]. The basic change is assumed to occur in the connective tissue; it is postulated that a decrease in the amount of mature cross-linked elastin and an increase in tropoelastin may be the primary pathogenic events [9].

It appears that three forms of EPS exist. (1) EPS occurs without underlying systemic disease. (2) EPS is associated with genetically determined disorders of the connective tissue in 26 [4] to 40 [8] percent of the reported cases. These disorders include Ehlers-Danlos syndrome, osteogenesis imperfecta, pseudoxanthoma elasticum, cutis laxa, Rothmund-Thomson syndrome, Marfan's syndrome, acrogeria [4–7,15–17], and mongolism [4–7]. In one study EPS was found in one percent of the patients with Down's syndrome in an institution for the mentally retarded [18]. Familial occurrence has been reported [19]. (3) Increasing numbers of patients are being reported who have developed EPS after prolonged treatment with penicillamine for Wilson's disease [9–14] and cystinuria [20,21]. On the other hand, EPS has not been described in untreated Wilson's disease and it is noteworthy that although penicillamine has been used in the treatment of a wide variety of other disorders, EPS has not been seen in these conditions. This, however, is related to the duration of treatment and the

total dose of penicillamine employed. Patients with Wilson's disease and EPS usually have received 1.5 to 2.0 g of penicillamine daily for 6 years or more.

Penicillamine chelates copper leading to copper depletion and it is known that copper deficiency produces vascular disease and changes in the elastic tissue in swine [22,23]. On the other hand, in Menkes' disease which is characterized by copper deficiency [24] and in which changes seen in the elastic tissue of vessels [25] closely resemble those in experimentally copper-deficient animals [26], EPS has so far not been observed. It has therefore been suggested that in penicillamine-treated Wilson's disease EPS may be due to deficiency of another trace metal which is removed by penicillamine [11]. Penicillamine has profound effects on fibroblasts, elastic and collagen fibers, the ground substance, and lymphocytes [27].

As far as collagen is concerned, current opinion holds that the penicillamine effect is due to an interference with the maturation of collagen, inhibiting the formation of insoluble collagen fibers from soluble collagen precursors [28,29]. This inhibition results in a net decrease of mature collagen and involves reversible interactions of aldehydes present in tropocollagen to form a thiazolidine complex [28]. It has been suggested that in low doses penicillamine blocks polyfunctional intramolecular cross-links of lysine [30]. The fact that penicillamine does not affect mature, insoluble collagen [31] may explain why it takes years for penicillamine-induced lesions to develop [27]. How this relates to the changes observed in the elastic tissue in penicillamine-induced EPS is not known, but it is noteworthy that the microscopic and ultrastructural appearance of the elastic tissue in the idiopathic form of EPS and that associated with connective tissue disorders differ from that in penicillamine-induced EPS [9,11,13].

Lesions clinically indistinguishable from EPS have also been observed in rare cases of morphea [32] and systemic sclerosis [33,34] not treated with penicillamine.

Clinical manifestations

The disorder starts most commonly during the second decade of life. Males are more frequently affected than females [4]. Lesions consist of small, skin-colored, slightly erythematous, keratotic papules arranged in serpiginous lines (Fig. 151-1) and circles or segments of circles (Fig. 151-2), but clustering of individual papules without particular configuration also occurs. Lesions enlarge by peripheral development of new papules and involute in the center which eventually becomes atrophic and slightly hypopigmented.

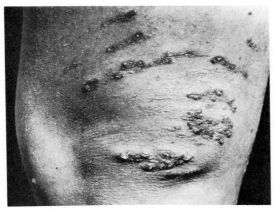

Fig. 151-1   Elastosis perforans serpiginosa on the knee.

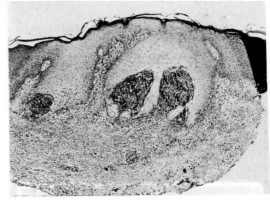

Fig. 151-3   Elastosis perforans serpiginosa. A clawlike epidermal downgrowth partially surrounds a mixture of mesenchymal debris. This distinctive histologic picture is per se not diagnostic of elastosis perforans serpiginosa, for it is a manifestation of an epidermal-mesenchymal reaction seen in a variety of similar disorders and termed transepidermal elimination. When associated with a great excess of elastic tissue, it is diagnostic of elastosis perforans serpiginosa. (Micrograph by Wallace H. Clark, Jr., M.D.)

Sites of predilection are the nape or the sides of the neck and the upper extremities; less frequently lesions also occur on the face, the lower extremities, and the trunk. In a high percentage of cases, the lesions are distributed symmetrically [35]. Although in most cases lesions tend to be localized to one particular area, widespread dissemination has been described both for the idiopathic form [36] and in patients with pseudoxanthoma elasticum and Down's syndrome [4,18].

The clinical course is unpredictable. Usually the lesions spread slowly by peripheral enlargement and central healing and persist over a number of years. Eventually, spon-

Fig. 151-2   Elastosis perforans serpiginosa in the antecubital fold of a patient on long-term penicillamine treatment for Wilson's disease. (Courtesy of Drs. G. Niebauer and W. Gebhart.)

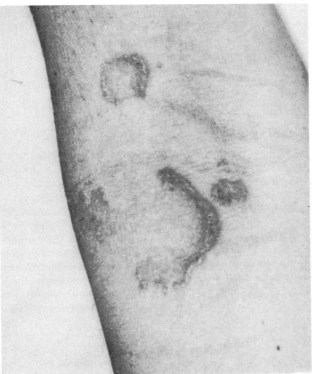

taneous involution occurs, resulting in atrophic, linear or retiform scars and slight hyperpigmentation.

Histopathology

The individual papules of EPS show a central plug of deeply basophilic material, which fills a straight or winding canal perforating the entire thickness of the acanthotic epidermis (Fig. 151-3). At the dermal end of the canal, the epidermis appears irregular and hyperplastic, often surrounding the basophilic debris in a clawlike fashion (Fig. 151-4); in the papillary dermis, more of the basophilic material is surrounded by an inflammatory infiltrate and foreign-body granulomas (Fig. 151-4). The basophilic plug consists of degenerated inflammatory cells, epidermal cells, and contains some coarse, brightly eosinophilic fibers; on the surface it is topped by parakeratotic horny material. With elastic tissue stains, the amount of elastic tissue in the dermis appears increased, individual fibers appearing coarser than in normal skin. The widened dermal papillae contain massive amounts of homogenous elastic material, and a stream of connective tissue with many elastic fibers and inflammatory cells appears to enter the canal, forming the plug [4] (Fig. 151-4). In healing lesions, the granulomatous tissue is replaced by fibrous tissue which leads to superficial scarring.

The microscopic appearance of the elastic fibers in idiopathic EPS and EPS associated with connective tissue disorders differs from that encountered in EPS due to penicillamine treatment. In the former, elastic fibers have been described as clumped, curly, granular, fragmented [7], and more refractile and broader than normal elastic fibers [15]. In penicillamine-induced EPS the elastic fibers have serrated, sawtooth-like contours [11,13] (Fig. 151-5) and, at the ultrastructural level, exhibit a concentric stratification into a core and cortical zones [11,13] with abundant, irregularly shaped, matrix material ("lumpy-bumpy" fibers

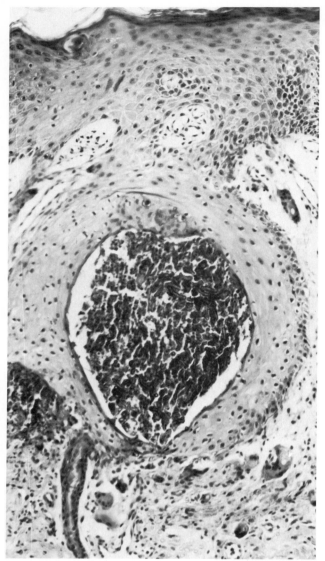

Fig. 151-4 **Elastosis perforans serpiginosa in penicillamine-treated Wilson's disease. Cellular and fibrous debris containing large amounts of elastic fibers are found at the lower end of the transepidermal perforation channel. Note granulomatous reaction in the dermis. *(From Bardach et al [13], with permission.)***

[13]). Similar changes of elastic tissue were observed in penicillamine-induced pulmonary lesions [13].

Differential diagnosis

Clinically, granuloma annulare, porokeratosis Mibelli, annular sarcoidosis, lupus vulgaris, and tinea have to be considered. The presence of a hyperkeratotic plug, the absence of the characteristic longitudinal furrow of porokeratosis Mibelli, predilection of certain regions of the body, the symmetry of lesions, and the age of the patient, as well as an associated disorder of the connective tissue, help to establish the proper clinical diagnosis. Histologically, reactive perforating collagenosis and Kyrle's disease have to be considered in the differential diagnosis.

Treatment

Various therapeutic measures have proved unsatisfactory. Cryotherapy or cellophane tape stripping can be beneficial [4,37]. Corticosteroids applied locally or intralesionally have been unsatisfactory, whereas electrodesiccation can result in keloid formation and should be avoided [4].

Reactive perforating collagenosis

Definition

First described by Mehregan in 1967 [38], reactive perforating collagenosis (RPC) is a peculiar pattern of cutaneous reactivity to superficial trauma characterized by the extrusion of degenerated connective tissue through the epidermis. Together with elastosis perforans serpiginosa it is grouped among the disorders characterized by the phenomenon of transepidermal elimination [39].

Etiology and pathogenesis

This rare disorder appears to have a genetic background as most observations have been made in siblings [39–42]. Two studies describe RPC occurring in two generations [41,42]. Eruptions usually start during childhood. Following superficial trauma, the connective tissue of dermal papillae becomes necrobiotic and is subsequently eliminated through the disrupted epidermis. Lesions can be produced experimentally in susceptible individuals by superficial abrasion or scratching but not by incisional wounds [41–43].

Recently, skin lesions indistinguishable from RPC both clinically and histologically have been described in six patients with severe diabetes, retinopathy, and peripheral vascular diseases, five of whom also had major renal failure [44]. Onset of disease was in adult life in these patients and it is not clear at present whether this condition is true RPC or a RPC-like reaction pattern related to diabetic nephropathy and the associated pruritus. The term *perforating disease of diabetes and renal failure* has been suggested for this group of patients [45] (see also Chaps. 51, 169, and 173).

Clinical manifestations

RPC preferentially affects children and persists into adult life. Predilection sites are the extremities, particularly the fingers, dorsal aspects of hands and forearms, but lesions may also occur on the face, trunk, and buttocks. They develop in response to superficial trauma and consist of pinhead-sized keratotic-appearing papules which are either discrete or arranged in a linear fashion that suggests a Koebner phenomenon. Within a few weeks the papules increase slowly in size to reach 5 to 10 mm in diameter and in the fully developed state they show a central umbilication containing a tightly adherent, leathery plug. Within another 2 to 4 weeks the lesions regress slowly and eventually transform into hypopigmented macules [38].

Histopathology

In early lesions, basophilic staining of the connective tissue in a dilated dermal papilla is associated with thinning of

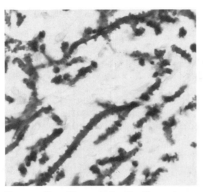

Fig. 151-5   Serrated outline of elastic fibers in pencillamine-associated elastosis perforans serpiginosa. *(From Bardach et al [13], with permission.)*

the overlying epidermis; in later stages, basophilic debris containing inflammatory cells and still-recognizable basophilic collagen bundles seem to be extruded through focal disruptions of the epidermis. In other lesions, the epidermis overlying the affected papilla forms a cup-shaped depression which contains masses of parakeratotic material, degenerated connective tissue, collagen bundles, and degenerated inflammatory cells [38]. In resolving lesions, the epidermis slowly regenerates at the base of the central plug which disappears as epidermal regeneration is complete.

Differential diagnosis

Prurigo, perforating granuloma annulare, Kyrle's disease, and elastosis perforans serpiginosa have to be taken into consideration. In the latter, the perforating, brightly eosinophilic elastic fibers can be recognized in hematoxylin and eosin-stained sections.

RPC also has to be differentiated from perforating folliculitis. This common eruption waxes and wanes, it affects all ages, and the lesions are erythematous follicular papules with a central keratotic plug containing a curled-up hair [46]. Histologically there is a dilated hair follicle filled with a parakeratotic keratin plug and eosinophilic debris which perforates into the dermis within its infundibular portion.

Treatment

The course is self-limited; therapeutic attempts to control existing and to prevent new lesions have been unsuccessful.

References

1. Jones PE, Smith DC: Porokeratosis. Review and report of cases. *Arch Dermatol Syphilol* **56:**425, 1947
2. Lutz W: Keratosis follicularis serpiginosa. *Dermatologica* **106:**318, 1953
3. Miescher G: Elastoma intrapapillare perforans verruciforme. *Dermatologica* **110:**254, 1955
4. Mehregan A: Elastosis perforans serpiginosa. A review of the literature and report of 11 cases. *Arch Dermatol* **97:**381, 1968
5. Woerdeman JJ, Scott FP: Keratosis follicularis serpiginosa (Lutz). *Dermatologica* **118:**18, 1959
6. Haber H: Miescher's elastoma (elastoma intrapapillare perforans verruciforme). *Br J Dermatol* **71:**85, 1959
7. Whyte HJ, Winkelmann RK: Elastosis perforans (perforating elastosis). The association of congenital anomalies, salient facts in the histology, studies of enzyme digestion and a report of necropsy in a case. *J Invest Dermatol* **35:**113, 1960
8. Smith EW et al: Reactive perforating elastosis: feature of certain genetic disorders. *Bull Johns Hopkins Hosp* **111:**235, 1962
9. Pass F et al: Elastosis perforans serpiginosa during penicillamine therapy for Wilson's disease. *Arch Dermatol* **108:**713, 1973
10. Guilaine J et al: Elastome perforant verruciforme chez un malade traité par pénicillamine pour maladie de Wilson. *Bull Soc Fr Dermatol Syphiligr* **79:**450, 1972
11. Kirsch N, Hukill PB: Elastosis perforans serpiginosa induced by penicillamine. *Arch Dermatol* **113:**630, 1977
12. Sfar Z et al: Deux cas d'elastomes verruciformes après l'adminstration prolongée de D-penicillamine. *Ann Dermatol Venereol* **109:**813, 1982
13. Bardach H et al: "Lumpy-bumpy" elastic fibres in the skin and lungs of a patient with a penicillamine-induced elastosis perforans serpiginosa. *J Cutan Pathol* **6:**243, 1979
14. Rosenblum GA: Liquid nitrogen cryotherapy in a case of elastosis perforans serpiginosa. *J Am Acad Dermatol* **8:**718, 1983
15. Hitch JM, Lund HZ: Elastosis perforans serpiginosa. *Arch Dermatol* **79:**407, 1959
16. Reed WB, Pidgeon JW: Elastosis perforans serpiginosa with osteogenesis imperfecta. *Arch Dermatol* **89:**342, 1964
17. Carey TD: Elastosis perforans serpiginosa. *Arch Dermatol* **113:**1444, 1977
18. Rasmussen JE: Disseminated elastosis perforans serpiginosa in four mongoloids. *Br J Dermatol* **86:**9, 1972
19. Woerdemann ML et al: Elastosis perforans serpiginosa: report of a family with a chromosomal investigation. *Arch Dermatol* **92:**559, 1965
20. Abel M: Elastosis perforans serpiginosa associated with penicillamine. *Arch Dermatol* **113:**1303, 1977
21. Hashimoto K et al: Ultrastructure of penicillamine-induced skin lesions. *J Am Acad Dermatol* **4:**300, 1981
22. Shields GS: Studies of copper metabolism: cardiovascular lesions in copper deficient swine. *Am J Pathol* **41:**603, 1962
23. Miller EJ et al: The biosynthesis of elastin crosslinks: the effect of copper deficiencies and a lathryogen. *J Biol Chem* **240:**3623, 1965
24. Matsuda I et al: Determination of apoceruloplasmin by radioimmunoassay in nutritional copper deficiency, Menkes' kinky hair syndrome, Wilson's disease, and umbilical cord blood. *Pediatr Res* **8:**821, 1974
25. Danks DM et al: Menkes' kinky hair syndrome: an inherited defect in copper absorption with widespread effects. *Pediatrics* **50:**188, 1972
26. Waisman J, Carnes WH: Cardiovascular studies on copper-deficient swine: the fine structure of the defective elastic membranes. *Am J Pathol* **51:**117, 1967
27. Levy RS et al: Penicillamine: review and cutaneous manifestations. *J Am Acad Dermatol* **8:**548, 1983
28. Nimni ME: Mechanism of inhibition of collagen cross-linking by penicillamine. *Proc R Soc Med* **70 (suppl):**65, 1977
29. Nimni ME: Collagen defect induced by penicillamine. *Fed Proc* **25:**715, 1966
30. Siegel RC: Collagen cross-linking: effect of D-penicillamine on cross-linking in vitro. *J Biol Chem* **252:**254, 1977
31. Herbert CM et al: Biosynthesis and maturation of skin collagen in scleroderma and effect of D-penicillamine. *Lancet* **1:**187, 1974
32. Barr RJ et al: Elastosis perforans serpiginosa associated with morphea. *J Am Acad Dermatol* **3:**19, 1980
33. Pai SH, Zak SH: Concurrence of pseudoxanthoma elasticum,

elastosis perforans serpiginosa and systemic sclerosis. *Dermatologica* **140**:54, 1970

34. May N, Lester RS: Elastosis perforans serpiginosa associated with systemic sclerosis. *J Am Acad Dermatol* **6**:945, 1982
35. Macaulay WL: Symmetry in elastosis perforans serpiginosa: its significance. *Arch Dermatol* **88**:215, 1963
36. Pedro SD, Garcia RL: Disseminate elastosis perforans serpiginosa. *Arch Dermatol* **109**:84, 1974
37. Rosenblum GA: Liquid nitrogen cryotherapy in a case of elastosis perforans serpiginosa. *J Am Acad Dermatol* **8**:718, 1983
38. Mehregan AH et al: Reactive perforating collagenosis. *Arch Dermatol* **96**:277, 1967
39. Mehregan AH: Perforating dermatosis—a clinicopathological review. *Int J Dermatol* **16**:19, 1977

40. Weiner AL: Reactive perforating collagenosis. *Arch Dermatol* **102**:540, 1970
41. Nair BKH et al: Reactive perforating collagenosis. *Br J Dermatol* **91**:399, 1974
42. Kanan MW: Familial reactive perforating collagenosis and intolerance to cold. *Br J Dermatol* **91**:399, 1974
43. Bovenmyer DA: Reactive perforating collagenosis. Experimental production of the lesions. *Arch Dermatol* **102**:313, 1970
44. Poliak SC et al: Reactive perforating collagenosis associated with diabetes mellitus. *N Engl J Med* **306**:81, 1982
45. Huntley AC: The cutaneous manifestations of diabetes mellitus. *Am J Acad Dermatol* **7**:427, 1982
46. Mehregan AH, Coskey RJ: Perforating folliculitis. *Arch Dermatol* **97**:394, 1968

SECTION 25

Cutaneous manifestations of diseases in other organ systems

CHAPTER 152

LUPUS ERYTHEMATOSUS

Richard D. Sontheimer, Naomi Rothfield, and James N. Gilliam*

Lupus erythematosus (LE) is a chronic, inflammatory disease of unknown etiology. It has been suggested that LE is an autoimmune disease since autoantibody production is a common finding in the systemic form of this disorder. Lupus erythematosus is an extremely heterogeneous disease that includes a broad spectrum of clinical forms in which cutaneous disease may occur with or without systemic involvement. For this reason it has been difficult to develop a unifying concept of LE and this has led to the practice of identifying subsets of LE patients that share similar clinical and/or laboratory abnormalities. Patients

within these LE subsets tend to follow a similar clinical course, often making it possible to anticipate which patients are at risk for more or less aggressive forms of the disease. This has obvious benefits from the standpoint of appropriate patient management since it is essential to tailor the treatment to the needs of the individual patient.

Lupus erythematosus is perhaps one of the best examples of a systemic disease in which a careful assessment of the cutaneous lesions can yield valuable diagnostic and prognostic information. Skin involvement is a major feature of LE, occurring in 70 to 85 percent of patients with this disease [1,2]. It has also been established that skin disease ranks second only to joint symptoms as the most

---

* Deceased June 6, 1984.

common initial manifestation of systemic LE. In the past, patients with LE have been classified clinically as having either systemic LE (i.e., a multisystem disease) or discoid LE (i.e., disease limited to the skin). This classification has always produced some degree of confusion since the term "discoid LE" has also been used to describe a particular clinical type of LE-specific skin lesion that can occur as an isolated manifestation of LE or as part of the multisystem disease process. Although cutaneous LE is the most common and easily recognized form of isolated disease, LE can occasionally be confined to any organ for prolonged periods. Thus, epilepsy, arthritis, glomerulonephritis, anemia, or thrombocytopenia may be the sole manifestation of LE for long periods before the disease can be diagnosed. The cutaneous lesions of LE have well-defined clinical and histologic features that are pathognomonic of LE whether confined to the skin or present as part of the more generalized systemic disease. Thus, the term "cutaneous LE" rather than "discoid LE" should be used in a generic sense to indicate skin disease caused by LE whether confined to the skin or present as a manifestation of systemic LE. A careful analysis and proper classification of the cutaneous findings in patients with LE can provide important insight into the general nature of this disease process.

Historical background

Lupus erythematosus was first recognized as a skin disease and for many years the systemic form of this disorder was unknown. In 1851, Cazenave introduced the name *lupus erythematosus* to distinguish patients with a nontuberculous form of lupus from those with lupus vulgaris. Thus, the name lupus (meaning to have the appearance of something that has been gnawed at by wolves) took its origin from the eroded quality of the destructive skin lesions sometimes seen in this disorder. Kaposi in 1872 is regarded as being the first to have recognized the systemic component of LE. Thereafter it became clear that the generalized systemic disorder did not spread from the skin as was believed earlier. It was also recognized that the skin disease seemed to bear little relation to the severity or extent of the systemic disease process. Indeed, it is now clear that the severity of the systemic disease is often inversely related to the chronicity and destructiveness of the condition in the skin. This relationship between chronic discoid and systemic LE has been the subject of numerous controversies and will be discussed in more detail later in this chapter.

Classification of LE-related skin disease

The cutaneous manifestations of LE can be classified as LE-specific (diagnostic) or LE-nonspecific (nondiagnostic). Routine histopathologic examination of biopsies from LE-specific skin lesions will give diagnostic information in most cases. This is not possible when biopsies of LE-nonspecific skin lesions are examined microscopically. Thus, LE-specific skin lesions are considered to be a manifestation of the lupus process in the skin and will be referred to as cutaneous LE. Cutaneous LE can be classified into three types based strictly upon the clinical appearance without consideration of extracutaneous or laboratory features of the disease. The three forms of cutaneous LE are: (1) chronic cutaneous LE which includes discoid LE; (2) subacute cutaneous LE; and (3) acute cutaneous LE. Subtypes of these major categories are listed in Table 152-1.

LE-specific skin disease

Chronic cutaneous LE (discoid LE)

The most common form of chronic cutaneous LE is discoid lupus erythematosus (DLE). DLE is a chronic, persistent disease which is usually confined to the skin. The skin lesions are characterized by scaling, erythematous papules and plaques with prominent follicular hyperkeratosis. Active lesions are erythematous with hyperpigmentation at the margin. Lesions gradually expand and eventually heal with central scarring and depigmentation. The lesions are most commonly located on the face, scalp, and ears. These chronic lesions persist for months to years. A number of clinical variants of the disease are recognized and will be described below.

Although the lesions are generally located above the neck (localized DLE), a number of patients have more extensive disease. When cutaneous involvement occurs both above and below the neck the term *generalized discoid LE* is used. Localized DLE is not usually associated with systemic disease, and patients presenting with this form of cutaneous LE are at little risk for developing systemic LE [3]. There is some evidence to suggest that patients with generalized DLE are more likely to develop overt systemic involvement.

The term *disseminated discoid LE* has also been used to describe patients with widespread chronic scarring cutaneous LE. This term should be avoided since it has also been used in the past to describe nonscarring forms of cutaneous LE (e.g., subacute cutaneous LE) and to indicate systemic disease (e.g., SLE).

Clinical features. The skin lesions of DLE are discrete, erythematous papules and plaques with a well-formed adherent scale which extends into dilated patulous follicles (Fig. 152-1). The most common site of involvement is the face, followed by scalp and external ear. DLE lesions can

Table 152-1 Clinical forms of LE-specific (histopathologically diagnostic) skin lesions

Chronic cutaneous LE:
  Localized discoid LE
  Generalized discoid LE (lesions above and below the neck)
  Hypertrophic discoid LE
  Lupus panniculitis (lupus profundus)
Subacute cutaneous LE (SCLE):
  Papulosquamous (psoriasiform) SCLE
  Annular-polycyclic (occasionally vesicular) SCLE
Acute cutaneous LE:
  Facial (malar) erythema
  Widespread macular or papular erythema of face, scalp, neck, upper chest, shoulders, extensor arms, and dorsa of hands
  Bullous, erythema multiforme-like, or toxic epidermal necrolysis-like lesions

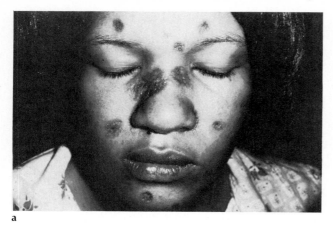

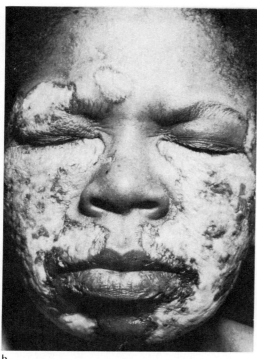

Fig. 152-1 (a) Early discoid lupus erythematosus. Lesions are discrete, hyperpigmented, and contain areas of focal atrophy. (With permission from W. B. Saunders Company Ltd.) (b) Late discoid lupus erythematosus. Lesions have become confluent, developed central depigmentation, and produced extensive, destructive atrophic scarring.

occur at any site; however, isolated discoid lesions below the neck without head or neck involvement are distinctly uncommon (less than 4 percent).

Mucous membrane lesions occur in approximately 15 percent with the buccal mucosa and gingivae being the most common sites. Conjunctival involvement can also occur. A silvery white appearance of the vermilion border of the lips is highly characteristic of LE. Thus, the lips and mouth of patients must be carefully examined for evidence of silvery-white scaling and ulceration. Squamous cell carcinoma can develop in long-standing mucosal DLE lesions.

The skin lesions begin as flat or slightly elevated, well-defined, violaceous papules with a rough, scaly surface.

Follicular involvement is a prominent early feature with scales accumulating in dilated follicles from which the hair is lost. When the scale is removed, examination of its undersurface will reveal the characteristic "carpet tack" appearance that is produced by the retained follicular keratin spikes. Hyperpigmentation is often seen in the initial phases; however, eventual loss of pigment occurs in the older scarred areas in the central zone of the lesions. Irreversible alopecia occurs due to follicular destruction (Fig. 152-2). The clinical diagnosis of DLE can be easily confirmed by routine light microscopic examination of a skin biopsy.

Clinical course. Most patients (90 to 95 percent) with chronic scarring DLE have a disease that remains confined to the skin. A careful history and physical examination coupled with routine laboratory testing will usually identify patients with significant extracutaneous disease. A history of excessive fatigue, recurrent low-grade fever, joint pain, diffused nonscarring alopecia, photosensitivity, pleurisy, or Raynaud's phenomenon should arouse suspicion regarding the possibility of systemic disease. The presence of diffuse alopecia, generalized lymphadenopathy, vasculitic skin lesions, unexplained anemia, leukopenia, a positive antinuclear antibody test at a significant titer, and immune deposits at the dermal-epidermal junction of clinically normal skin should also suggest the possibility of extracutaneous involvement.

The progression of patients who present with isolated DLE skin lesions to SLE is distinctly uncommon. However, approximately 15 percent of SLE patients have discoid skin lesions at the onset of their systemic disease and as many as 25 percent may develop typical chronic discoid skin lesions at some time during the course of their illness [2]. SLE patients with discoid skin lesions generally have a more benign form of systemic LE. Life-threatening complications such as diffuse proliferative glomerulonephritis are uncommon in these patients and survival is increased when compared to SLE patients without DLE lesions [4,5]. Thus, SLE patients with DLE skin lesions have been considered by some to form a distinct SLE subset [4]. This subset of SLE patients appears to have a higher incidence of Raynaud's phenomenon and vasculitis. Anti-DNA antibodies are uncommon in such patients; however, antibodies to ribonuclear protein (RNP) are relatively com-

Fig. 152-2 Chronic discoid lupus erythematosus of the scalp. Irreversible alopecia.

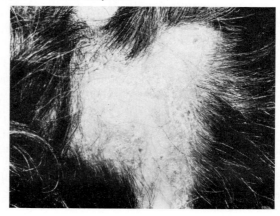

mon. Therefore, patients with clear-cut SLE who also have chronic cutaneous LE seem to have a better prognosis than SLE patients without such lesions [2].

The most important fact to keep in mind about the course and prognosis of patients who present with chronic cutaneous LE as their only symptom is that the great majority have a condition that remains confined to the skin and life-threatening complications from systemic involvement rarely occur. However, a small fraction of patients with SLE do have chronic cutaneous LE for periods up to 35 years before multisystem disease appears [6].

It is unfortunate that patients with chronic cutaneous LE are sometimes frightened when their physicians diagnose "lupus erythematosus" and fail to explain that they have a relatively self-limited disease which will probably not threaten their health. These patients should receive a thorough history and physical examination followed by laboratory studies which should include a complete blood count, an erythrocyte sedimentation rate, and an antinuclear antibody test. If no abnormalities are found the patients should be reassured and followed at appropriate intervals to care for their skin disease.

Histopathology. The interface between the epidermis and dermis (basement membrane zone) is the principal pathologic target in cutaneous LE. Morphologic changes noted by light, fluorescence, and electron microscopy suggest that the basal or germinal cell of the epidermis is a principal site of injury in cutaneous LE whether acute, subacute, or chronic in nature. In chronic cutaneous LE there is prominent hyperkeratosis and well-developed follicular plugging. The most characteristic changes, however, are seen along the basal layer of the epidermal and follicular epithelium (Fig. 152-3). There is loss of the normal organization and orientation of basal cells, edema with vacuole formation between and sometimes within basal cells, focal necrosis of basal cells, and interruption of pigment transfer leading to the accumulation of melanin in dermal macrophages. The focal hydropic degeneration of the basal layer,

which is also referred to as liquefaction degeneration, is the most diagnostic change of cutaneous LE. Lichen planus may show similar basal layer changes; however, clinical features usually allow one to distinguish lichen planus from DLE.

A dense mononuclear cell infiltrate composed predominantly of T lymphocytes is present around hair follicles, blood vessels, and scattered in the upper dermis. In chronic cutaneous LE this lymphocytic infiltrate is also present deep in the dermis and occasionally in the subcutaneous tissue. A few plasma cells are also present but polymorphonuclear leukocytes and other acute inflammatory cells are absent. The dermal changes in DLE are less specific and a similar patchy lymphocytic dermal infiltrate may be seen in lymphocytoma cutis, plaque type polymorphous light eruption, lymphocytic infiltration of the skin of Jessner, and lymphocytic lymphoma. In the absence of hydropic degeneration of the basal layer, the histologic changes in these conditions may be difficult to distinguish from DLE. However, in DLE the infiltrate usually impinges on the pilosebaceous structures, sometimes producing hydropic changes in the basal layer of the hair follicles.

Immunopathology. Direct immunofluorescence staining of biopsies taken from DLE skin lesions demonstrates a thick band of immunoglobulin along the dermal-epidermal junction in over 75 percent of cases (Fig. 152-4). Ultrastructural localization of these immune deposits using the immunoperoxidase technique confirms that most of them are on the upper dermal collagen fibers and along the lamina densa of the basement membrane zone (Fig. 152-5). The presence of immune deposits in the interface region between the epidermis and dermis has been taken as evidence that the injury at this site is mediated by antibody or antigen–antibody complexes and that this is the primary event in the production of LE skin disease. Several lines of investigation have cast doubt on this concept. It is now well known that subepidermal immunoglobulin deposits are

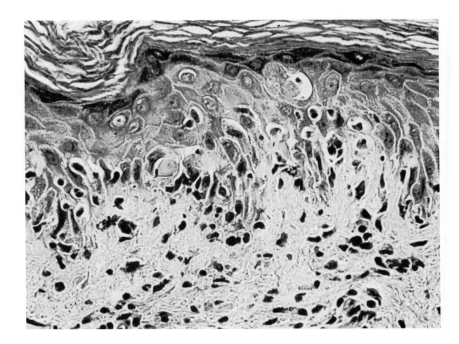

Fig. 152-3 Lupus erythematosus-specific skin disease. The characteristic changes occur at the dermal-epidermal junction. Cells of the epidermal basal layer lose their normal polarity and undergo vacuolar (liquefactive) degeneration. A lymphohistiocytic cellular infiltrate is present in the lower epidermis, at the dermal-epidermal junction, and in a perivascular distribution in the upper dermis. Melanin-containing macrophages are present in the upper dermis.

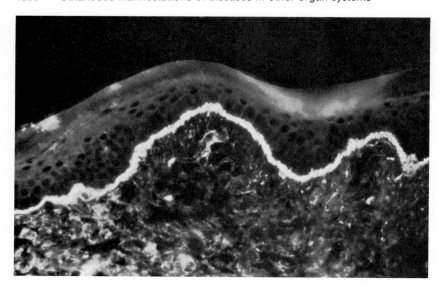

Fig. 152-4 Biopsy of flexor forearm nonlesional skin from a patient with systemic lupus erythematosus that has been reacted with a fluorescein isothiocyanate-conjugated goat antibody to human IgG. There is a granular deposition of IgG along the dermal-epidermal junction. IgA and IgM were also present. Cutaneous lupus erythematosus lesions frequently have a similar pattern of immunoglobulin deposition at the dermal-epidermal junction.

present in clinically normal skin of patients with SLE and that such deposits are not related to the presence or development of LE skin lesions [7]. In addition, the appearance of subepidermal immunoglobulin follows the inflammatory response in experimentally induced LE skin lesions by several weeks [8]. Finally, the histology of LE skin lesions is more consistent with cell-mediated immune injury similar to that seen in graft-versus-host skin disease [9,10].

Laboratory findings. A search for abnormal laboratory values in patients with chronic DLE is generally unrewarding [11–13]. A low-titer positive antinuclear antibody test may be seen in as many as 30 percent of these patients; however, less than 5 percent will have a positive antinuclear antibody test at a significant titer. A small percentage will show biologic false-positive tests for syphilis, positive rheumatoid factor test, slight depressions in serum complement levels, modest elevations in gamma globulin, and modest leukopenia. Therefore, unexplained anemia, significant leukopenia (particularly lymphopenia of less than 1000 cells per cubic millimeter), a persistently positive antinuclear antibody test at high titers, moderate to marked hypergammaglobulinemia and immune deposits along the dermal-epidermal junction of clinically normal skin (i.e., a positive Lupus Band Test) should lead one to suspect extracutaneous disease. A careful history and physical examination will usually identify patients with significant systemic involvement.

Diagnosis and differential diagnosis. The clinical features of chronic DLE are generally quite distinctive and do not present great difficulty in diagnosis. Occasionally DLE lesions may be confused with other diseases and require histopathologic and immunopathologic examination in order to rule out or to confirm the diagnosis. As mentioned earlier the histologic picture is usually diagnostic. The following diseases may occasionally be confused with DLE.

CHRONIC POLYMORPHOUS LIGHT ERUPTION. Plaque type polymorphous light eruption may closely resemble early lesions of DLE. These lesions occur on the face or other light-exposed areas of the body in the late spring or early summer months following exposure to the sun. The ab-

sence of hyperkeratosis, follicular plugging, and lack of dyschromia help in distinguishing these lesions from cutaneous LE. In addition, the lesions in chronic polymorphous light eruption do not produce atrophy and scarring.

LYMPHOCYTIC INFILTRATION OF THE SKIN (JESSNER-KANOF). These lesions primarily affect the face although occasionally they appear on other parts of the body. As with chronic polymorphous light eruptions, lymphocytic infiltration of the skin may be confused clinically with the early stages of chronic DLE. The lesions are erythematous, discoid in shape, and slightly elevated. They begin as small reddish papules and expand peripherally, occasionally with central clearing. There is no follicular hyperkeratosis and the lesions regress without scarring.

TINEA FACIA. Superficial fungal infections involving the face can occasionally simulate DLE. An elevated active erythematous margin with central clearing can cause some confusion. The absence of telangiectasia, central atrophy, follicular dilatation and plugging, and no alteration in skin pigmentation often make it possible to rule out the possibility of DLE.

LICHEN PLANUS. When the lesions of lichen planus involve the mucous membranes, lips, and hands, they may lack the characteristic shape and color of the lesions seen elsewhere. Lesions of the palms or dorsal surface of the hands may be difficult to diagnose unless they are accompanied by more typical lesions on the flexor surfaces of the wrist. Since the histopathologic feature of hydropic degeneration is also seen in biopsies from the lesions of lichen planus, it may be difficult to separate lupus from lichen planus histologically. In such cases the correct diagnosis usually depends upon identifying the more typical lesions of lichen planus at other sites.

SARCOIDOSIS. Cutaneous sarcoidosis can produce elevated erythematous lesions with advancing margins on the face, ears, scalp, arms, and upper trunk in a distribution similar to that seen in DLE. Histopathologic examination will promptly establish the correct diagnosis.

BASAL CELL EPITHELIOMA. A superficial or sclerosing basal cell epithelioma may simulate an isolated lesion of DLE. There is an advancing raised margin with telangiectasia and central atrophy similar to that seen in DLE. Follicular dilatation with plugging and the characteristic

Fig. 152-5 Cutaneous discoid lupus erythematosus lesional skin: electron microscopic immunoperoxidase method. Immunoglobulins are present on the basal lamina (asterisks) and in the subjacent dermis, where they form occasional aggregates (Ig). In some areas they extend to the very surface of the basal cell (arrows). HD = one of the half desmosomes which are coated by the deposits; BC = basal cell. ×104,000. *(From Wolff-Schreiner EC, Wolff K: Arch Dermatol Res 246:193, 1973.)*

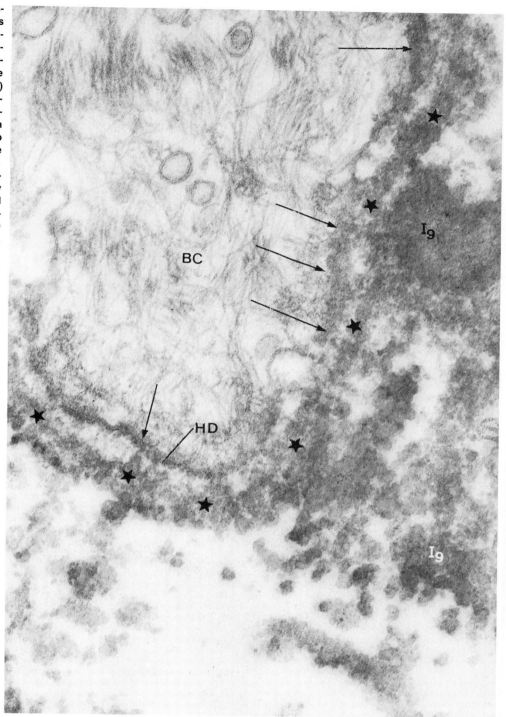

pigmentary changes of DLE are not present. A biopsy will be diagnostic.

FOCAL SCARRING ALOPECIA. Diseases that cause focal scarring alopecia may closely resemble old inactive lesions of DLE. Lichen planus, localized scleroderma, sarcoidosis, and trauma can cause such changes.

Other forms of chronic cutaneous LE. LUPUS PANNICULITIS (LUPUS PROFUNDUS). Kaposi originally described subcutaneous nodules in a patient with lupus erythematosus in 1883. Irgang introduced the term *lupus erythematosus pro-*

fundus in the English literature in 1940 [14]. This unusual variant of chronic cutaneous LE is characterized by the appearance of persistent, firm, well-defined nodules on the face, scalp, breast, upper portion of the arms, thighs, and buttocks. Grossly visible epidermal changes are not always present. Typical lesions of DLE may be present overlying these nodules, and ulcerations may occur. The inflammatory reaction in lupus panniculitis or profundus is in the deeper portion of the dermis and subcutaneous area. The histology is that of a trabecular and lobular lymphocytic panniculitis, and direct immunofluorescence staining of

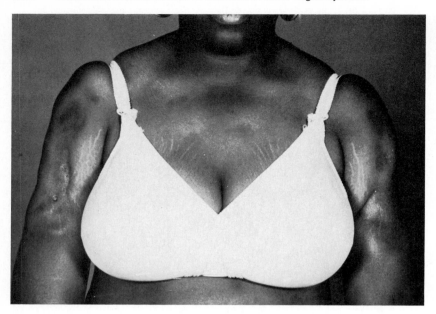

Fig. 152-6 Lupus panniculitis (profundus). Note the areas of dishlike atrophy over the shoulders and extensor arms.

biopsies from these lesions will show staining in the blood vessel walls in the lower dermis and subcutaneous fat. The overlying skin is attached to the firm subcutaneous nodular

Fig. 152-7 Facial lipoatrophy resulting from chronic activity of lupus panniculitis (profundus). Note discoid lupus erythematosus lesion on anterior scalp.

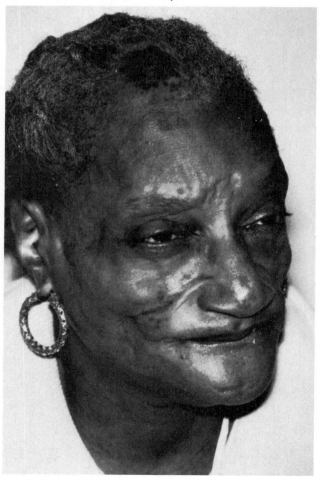

lesion and in time the surface is drawn inward to produce deep depressions (Fig. 152-6). Approximately 70 percent of the patients with this type of chronic cutaneous LE also have typical DLE lesions and 50 percent have mild systemic involvement. The lesions may ulcerate, particularly if traumatized or biopsied. Thus, one must be aware of this outcome when the lesions are subjected to any traumatic procedure. Lupus profundus lesions may involve the breast and mimic cancer. The lesions can be linear and at times difficult to differentiate from linear scleroderma. Lupus profundus may also be mistaken for morphea or morphea profundus. Extensive involvement of the face can result in an appearance resembling acquired lipoatrophy (Fig. 152-7).

HYPERTROPHIC DISCOID LE. Hypertrophic DLE is another unusual variant of chronic cutaneous LE. Uitto and coworkers [15] in 1978 emphasized that the verrucous hyperkeratotic character of these lesions could be mistaken for keratoacanthoma or hypertrophic lichen planus (Fig. 152-8). These lesions can usually be recognized by the presence of more typical DLE lesions elsewhere. Patients with hypertrophic DLE lesions may have, in addition, cutaneous lesions that have both clinical and histologic features suggestive of lichen planus. Patients with overlapping clinical and histologic features of LE and lichen planus have been well described by Romero and associates [16].

Treatment. LOCAL THERAPY. Since DLE often produces permanent scarring, these lesions are disfiguring and should be treated aggressively during the active inflammatory stage. Ointments containing potent fluorinated corticosteroids such as fluocinonide or betamethasone are helpful in many patients with DLE. These preparations should be used with caution on the face and intertriginous areas since they have the capacity in themselves to produce cutaneous erythema, telangiectasia, and atrophy. Occlusive treatments with corticosteroid-impregnated tape can also be useful.

The lesions of hypertrophic DLE are best treated with intralesional corticosteroid. Triamcinolone acetonide suspensions diluted to 2.5 mg per mL with either 1% Xylo-

Fig 152-8 Hypertrophic discoid lupus erythematosus lesions on the extensor forearm.

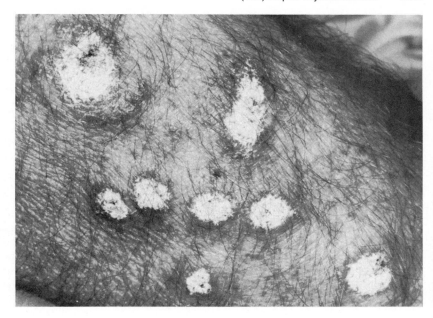

caine or normal saline can be used in the treatment of lesions on the face. For lesions elsewhere the initial strength should be 5.0 mg per mL. Since intralesional corticosteroids can in themselves produce cutaneous and subcutaneous atrophy, higher concentrations must be used with extreme caution. Intralesional therapy of LE panniculitis should be avoided since such therapy can result in breakdown of the lesions with ulcer formation.

SYSTEMIC THERAPY. If local measures are ineffective in controlling the lesions of DLE the most effective systemic medication is an aminoquinoline antimalarial agent. These agents are particularly useful in patients with widespread DLE and lupus profundus. Chloroquine phosphate (250 mg daily) or hydroxychloroquine sulfate (200 mg daily) are the antimalarial agents most commonly used. Hydroxychloroquine sulfate (Plaquenil) is preferred because it appears to produce less ocular toxicity. The usual approach is to give an initial loading dose of 2 tablets (400 mg) daily over a period of 3 to 4 weeks, followed by 1 tablet (200 mg) daily. The most serious side effect is retinal damage; however, this complication is unusual if the dose is kept to 1 tablet per day. A careful ophthalmologic examination should be performed prior to treatment and at 3- to 4-month intervals while taking these drugs. Other side effects include nausea, dizziness, headache, lichenoid drug eruptions, pigmentation of the palate, nails, and skin of the lower legs, bleaching of the hair of the scalp and mustache, neuropathy and neuromuscular atrophy.

Patients who fail to respond to either hydroxychloroquine or chloroquine may have a beneficial response with the addition of quinacrine. Quinacrine does not produce retinal toxicity; however, it can produce punctate corneal opacities as can hydroxychloroquine or chloroquine. These opacities represent accumulations of the drug in the cornea and are completely reversible with discontinuation of treatment. They are not usually associated with significant visual disturbance. Quinacrine may produce significant hemolysis in patients with glucose 6-phosphate dehydrogenase deficiency. In general, quinacrine is associated with a higher incidence of side effects such as headache, gastrointestinal intolerance, pruritus, lichenoid drug eruptions, and mucosal or cutaneous pigmentary disturbances than is either hydroxychloroquine or chloroquine. Quinacrine also commonly produces a yellowish discoloration of the entire skin and in fair-skinned individuals this may prove to be objectionable. This yellow discoloration is also completely reversible upon discontinuation of the drug. Children appear to be more susceptible to the serious toxic side effects of antimalarial agents and some authorities would consider young age a contraindication to the use of these drugs.

OTHER SYSTEMIC MEDICATIONS. Systemic corticosteroids are not indicated for patients with uncomplicated DLE. Some otherwise refractory patients will respond to aminodiphenylsulfone (Dapsone). A daily dose of 100 mg by mouth should be tried initially. The dose can be increased in a stepwise fashion to 300 mg per day if necessary. Other agents that have been reported to be beneficial in refractory cases include thalidomide and clofazimine, both of which are currently unavailable in the United States.

Subacute cutaneous LE

Subacute cutaneous lupus erythematosus (SCLE) is a widespread, nonscarring photosensitive form of histologically specific cutaneous LE [17]. This form of cutaneous LE can be distinguished from the generalized form of scarring DLE on clinical grounds alone. Patients with SCLE frequently have mild systemic illness marked by musculoskeletal complaints and characteristic serologic abnormalities. Approximately half of these patients can be classified as SLE by American Rheumatism Association preliminary criteria; however, serious central nervous system disease, progressive renal disease, or severe systemic vasculitis is uncommon.

The term *subacute cutaneous LE* was chosen to provide an acceptable name for this clinically distinct type of cutaneous LE that has been given many different names in the past (e.g., subacute LE, superficial disseminated LE, subacute disseminated LE, psoriasiform LE, autoimmune annular erythema, annular vesicular LE, disseminated

Table 152-2 Comparison of disease manifestations in patients with subacute cutaneous lupus erythematosus (SCLE) and a form of chronic cutaneous LE (DLE)

	SCLE	DLE
Clinical features:		
Thick, adherent scale	No	Yes
Delicate, easily detachable scale	Yes	No
Follicular changes	No	Yes
Atrophic scarring	No	Yes
Telangiectasia	Yes	Yes
Dyschromia	Yes	Yes
ARA* criteria for systemic LE ≥4	50%	10%
Histopathology:		
Liquefactive degeneration of epidermal basal cell layer	Yes	Yes
Basement membrane thickening	No	Yes
Periappendageal infiltrates	No	Yes
Deep dermal and subcutaneous infiltrates	No	Yes
Immunopathology:		
Dermal-epidermal junction immunoglobulin and complement		
Lesional	60%	90%
Nonlesional	25%	0%
Serology:		
ANA on a human substrate	75%	5%
Anti-SS-A/Ro antibodies	60%	3%
Antilymphocyte antibodies	30%	0%
Circulating immune complexes	60%	5%
Immunogenetics:		
HLA-B8	63%	34%
HLA-DR3	77%	

* American Rheumatism Association.

DLE, subacute DLE, and maculopapular photosensitive LE). As might be expected with any division of a disease continuum such as LE, overlapping features can be expected to occur. Thus, patients having both SCLE and DLE skin lesions have been seen. However, in most patients with cutaneous LE one type of skin involvement predominates so that patients have either DLE or SCLE as a manifestation of the lupus process in their skin. Since these cutaneous manifestations of LE are associated with

different clinical, serologic, histopathologic, and immunogenetic features (Table 152-2), it is justified to adhere to a strict and uniform classification that emphasizes the differences in these cutaneous expressions of LE.

Clinical features. Subacute cutaneous lupus erythematosus is a disease that usually affects young and middle-age white women. SCLE is uncommon in blacks or Hispanics of either sex. The exact incidence of this form of cutaneous involvement in patients with LE is unknown but it has been estimated to be 10 to 15 percent of the LE population.

Subacute cutaneous LE lesions assume a characteristic distribution affecting the shoulders, extensor surfaces of the arms, dorsal surface of the hands, upper back, and V area of the upper anterior chest. The face and scalp are much less commonly involved and the disease rarely occurs below the waist. There is striking sparing of the medial portion of the forearms and arms, axillary vault, and lateral aspect of the trunk. This distribution suggests a photoinduced or photoexacerbated process; however, the relative absence of facial involvement suggests that UV radiation is not an essential factor in the induction of SCLE lesions.

The early lesion is a slightly scaly erythematous papule. The lesions tend to enlarge and merge to form rather confluent areas of involvement. Some patients develop papulosquamous lesions that assume a psoriasiform appearance (Fig. 152-9), whereas in others annular lesions develop (Fig. 152-10). With merging of the papulosquamous lesions, a reticulate or retiform configuration results. Merging of the annular lesions leads to the formation of large polycyclic lesions. Occasionally annular SCLE lesions can present a target or irislike appearance (Fig. 152-11). Vesiculobullous changes are sometimes present at the active margin of annular lesions. Histologically the vesicular change is due to epidermal separation resulting from severe basal layer injury. The central zones of annular lesions often have a grayish hypopigmentation; however, atrophic scarring does not develop. Telangiectasia is a constant feature of both the early and later stages of the lesion. SCLE lesions have a delicate surface scale in contrast to the thicker and more adherent scale that is seen in the lesions of DLE. The characteristic dilatation and plugging

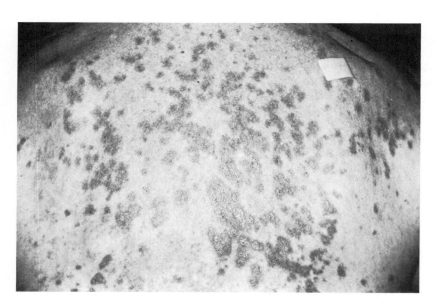

Fig. 152-9 Subacute cutaneous lupus erythematosus. Papulosquamous lesions on the upper back. (With permission from W. B. Saunders Company Ltd.)

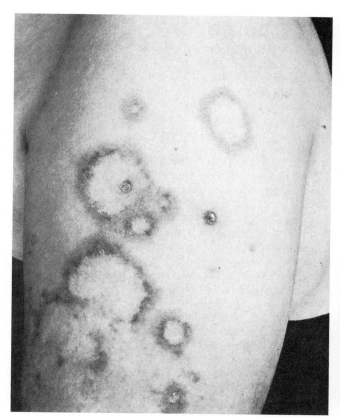

Fig. 152-10 Subacute cutaneous lupus erythematosus. Annular lesions on the shoulder and extensor arm. *(With permission from Little, Brown and Co.)*

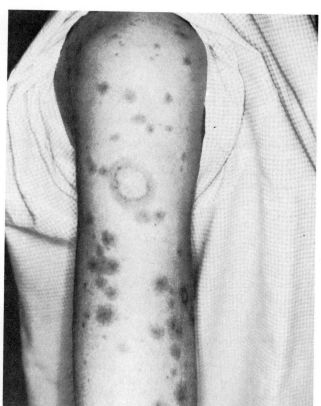

Fig. 152-11 Subacute cutaneous lupus erythematosus. The early lesions in this patient have an erythema multiforme-like appearance; however, the older lesions have become annular.

of follicles seen in DLE is not a feature of SCLE. As in other forms of cutaneous LE, pruritus is not a prominent feature.

Thus, SCLE and DLE share similar clinical features but there are definite differences. SCLE is nonscarring, has less prominent scaling and follicular plugging, is somewhat less persistent, and is more widespread in distribution than DLE. Individual SCLE lesions are less discrete and have a tendency to coalesce, forming large confluent areas of involvement. The pigmentary changes in SCLE may be prominent and depigmentation may remain for many months after the acute inflammatory changes have resolved. Unlike DLE this pigmentary change is not associated with dermal atrophy and is eventually reversible in many patients. Over half the patients with SCLE have diffuse, nonscarring alopecia which is not seen in uncomplicated DLE. In addition, photosensitivity is much more common in SCLE. LE lesions of the hard palate are present in 40 percent with SCLE and this is especially common in those with overt systemic manifestations. Livedo reticularis and periungual telangiectatic changes are seen in 20 percent of patients with SCLE; such changes are rarely found in DLE patients. Twenty percent of the SCLE patients also have typical localized scarring DLE lesions. These DLE lesions are usually located on the scalp and they often appear before the onset of SCLE by many years. Almost all patients with SCLE have mild systemic complaints, and approximately one-half have four or more ARA criteria for classification as SLE. In contrast, DLE

patients rarely have symptoms or findings of SLE. The most common extracutaneous manifestations in SCLE are joint pain, unexplained fever, and malaise. Severe central nervous system and renal disease are uncommon. These differences emphasize the importance of establishing a separate diagnostic category for SCLE.

Clinical course. Since SCLE has been recognized as a distinct clinical entity for only a relatively short period of time, the natural history of this disorder is not fully understood. Based on our current understanding it would seem that patients with SCLE and systemic involvement in general do relatively well when compared with SLE patients who do not have lesions of SCLE. As a group, SCLE patients do have more extensive disease than patients presenting with the chronic forms of cutaneous LE such as localized or generalized DLE. Thus, SCLE serves as a clinical marker for a subset of LE patients whose overall disease is different from the patients with chronic cutaneous LE. For the most part the systemic involvement that occurs in patients with SCLE tends to be relatively mild and for most SCLE patients the greatest problem is their skin disease rather than systemic symptoms. However, because a small percentage of these patients have developed significant clinical complications, each patient with SCLE must be followed carefully.

In most cases all of the cutaneous features of SCLE are completely reversible as the inflammatory process subsides. However, a small percentage of patients will develop seemingly permanent vitiligo-like depigmentation at previous sites of SCLE involvement. Ultraviolet radiation exposure aggravates the skin disease of most SCLE patients. However, some patients will experience flares of cutaneous activity as often during the winter as during the sunnier parts of the year. Some patients deny any relationship between sun exposure and worsening of their skin disease.

Histopathology. The histologic abnormalities in biopsies of SCLE lesions are characteristic of LE and thus similar to the changes described for DLE. However, there are several differences between the changes seen in SCLE and DLE. Follicular plugging, hyperkeratosis, and the density and depth of the cellular infiltrate are considerably less prominent in SCLE. The mononuclear cell infiltrate is usually restricted to the perivascular and periappendageal regions of the upper one-third of the dermis. The diagnostic changes along the basal layer of the epidermis are similar to those seen in all forms of LE-specific skin disease. Indeed, the hydropic degeneration in SCLE is often quite prominent, at times leading to epidermal separation.

Immunopathology. In contrast to the frequent finding of immunoglobulin deposits along the dermal-epidermal junction in DLE, 40 to 50 percent of SCLE lesions do not have immune deposits in this region on direct immunofluorescence examination. Thus, the absence of this finding cannot be used to exclude the diagnosis of SCLE. When present, these deposits occur in a granular bandlike array as in DLE lesions. Approximately one-fourth of patients with SCLE will have immune deposits at the dermal-epidermal junction of clinically normal skin. Patients with uncomplicated DLE rarely if ever have immune deposits in their clinically normal skin.

Laboratory findings. Antinuclear antibodies can be demonstrated by indirect immunofluorescence testing of serum in a majority of patients with SCLE (70 to 80 percent) if a sensitive antinuclear antibody substrate of human origin, such as KB or Hep-2 tumor cells, is used. The pattern of nuclear fluorescence is usually homogeneous or particulate. Antibodies to double-stranded DNA are relatively uncommon in these patients (15 to 25 percent) and when anti-DNA antibodies are detected they are usually present in low concentrations. Antibodies to the Ro/SSA antigen are common (greater than 60 percent), and abnormal levels of circulating immune complexes are present in approximately the same number [18]. Antibodies to the extractable nuclear antigens RNP and Sm have been rarely detected.

HLA typing of patients selected strictly on the basis of having SCLE has yielded a striking association with HLA-B8 and -DR3. HLA-DR3-positive individuals have a relative risk of 10.8 for developing SCLE of either the papulosquamous or annular type and a relative risk of 67.1 for the development of the annular variety of SCLE.

Diagnosis and differential diagnosis. In most cases, SCLE of either the annular or papulosquamous variety can be readily recognized by the characteristic morphology of the primary lesions in the typical widespread symmetrical distribution as described. The clinical impression can be readily confirmed by examination of biopsies by routine light microscopy. Since a significant number of these lesions will not show immune deposits at the dermal-epidermal junction, direct immunofluorescence staining of skin biopsies is not helpful.

The differential diagnosis of the papulosquamous form of SCLE would most often include psoriasis or dermatomyositis. Psoriasis can be readily distinguished by examining the histopathologic changes on a skin biopsy. Scalp and facial involvement, periorbital erythema and swelling, severe pruritus, and lesions on elbows, knees, and knuckles would suggest dermatomyositis. The annular form of SCLE can occasionally be confused with erythema annulare centrifugum or erythema multiforme. A skin biopsy would be helpful in making this distinction.

A number of patients with hereditary deficiencies of complement components associated with "DLE" have been described but the appearance of the cutaneous lesions in many of these publications suggests that these patients have SCLE [19]. The skin manifestations are often the presenting complaint in these patients. Additional features include early age at onset, marked photosensitivity, low titers of antinuclear antibodies, absence of anti-DNA antibodies, absence of immune deposits at the dermal-epidermal junction of normal and lesional skin, and a low frequency of severe lupus nephritis. There is some evidence to suggest that these patients also have a high frequency of anti-Ro/SSA antibodies [20]. Patients with this combination of features apparently represent a small portion of all patients with SCLE since we have not identified a homozygous complement deficiency state in any of over 60 SCLE patients. However, this possibility should be kept in mind when evaluating patients with SCLE.

Treatment. Since local treatment is usually unsuccessful in patients with SCLE, most patients will require some form of systemic therapy. The aminoquinoline antimalarials are the preferred drugs for inducing and maintaining remissions in patients with SCLE. After a pretreatment ophthalmologic examination, hydroxychloroquine sulfate, 400 mg per day, can be started. After 3 to 4 weeks the dose should be decreased to 200 mg per day. Four to six weeks are usually required before the full effects of antimalarials are seen. If necessary, quinacrine hydrochloride, 100 mg per day, can be added to this regimen. As mentioned earlier, such patients must be warned that a reversible yellow discoloration of the skin is likely to develop as a result of the quinacrine therapy. If the condition fails to respond to this regimen, benefit may be gained in some patients by substituting chloroquine for the hydroxychloroquine. Although more effective, chloroquine probably represents a greater risk for retinal toxicity than does hydroxychloroquine.

Low to moderate daily doses of oral corticosteroids such as prednisone, 20 to 30 mg per day, can be utilized in those patients by substituting chloroquine for the hydroxychloralone. Once remission has been achieved the drugs should be discontinued so that patients are not maintained on these agents for prolonged periods of time. Dapsone is occasionally useful in SCLE patients who fail to respond to the above-mentioned measures. In addition, there have been reports that thalidomide is effective in this form of cutaneous LE as in DLE.

Since photosensitivity is a common feature in SCLE,

patients should be encouraged to take a commonsense approach to avoid unnecessary sun exposure. In addition, effective sunscreen preparations should be applied regularly.

Acute cutaneous LE

Acute cutaneous LE appears almost exclusively in patients with active SLE. Thus, the signs and symptoms of active SLE usually overshadow this often subtle and transient form of cutaneous involvement.

Acute cutaneous LE has been recognized for many years by the characteristic facial butterfly erythema that is occasionally accompanied by edema and fine scale. The malar areas are usually most prominently involved, with the nasolabial folds being relatively spared. Some patients have a more diffuse erythema involving the face, upper chest, upper back, and extensor extremities. The lesions are abrupt in onset, last for hours to days, and frequently coincide with exacerbations of the systemic disease process. Patients with heavily pigmented skin can develop rather marked postinflammatory hyperpigmentation. Occasionally the facial involvement is extensive and includes the periorbital areas, simulating dermatomyositis.

Histopathology and immunopathology. The histologic findings in biopsies from lesions of acute cutaneous LE are often quite subtle. A careful examination may reveal a number of the basal layer changes described above as characteristic of LE. The dermal changes include a sparse cellular infiltrate and upper dermal edema. The histopathologic changes more closely resemble those of SCLE than DLE. Fibrinoid deposits in the connective tissue of the upper dermis are frequently present. Such fibrinoid deposits may also occasionally be seen in the walls of dermal capillaries. The fibrinoid deposits on the collagen and vascular walls sometimes give the upper dermis an homogenized appearance. Occasionally there is marked liquefaction degeneration of the basal layer and edema in the upper dermis which leads to vesiculobullous changes. Epidermal necrosis may occur in the most severe forms of acute cutaneous LE producing a toxic epidermal necrolysis-like histopathology. Examination of fresh biopsy specimens by direct immunofluorescence frequently demonstrates a granular band of immune deposits at the dermal-epidermal junction.

Laboratory findings. Patients with acute cutaneous LE often have positive antinuclear and anti-DNA antibody tests, low complement levels, anemia, leukopenia, hypergammaglobulinemia, proteinuria, hematuria, pyuria, and cylinduria.

Diagnosis and differential diagnosis. The diagnosis of acute cutaneous LE is usually not a problem since these patients frequently have clinical and serologic evidence of active SLE. The facial involvement may occasionally be difficult to distinguish from the skin lesions seen in patients with dermatomyositis. In such patients the most helpful clues come from the distribution of the skin lesions over the hands since the lesions of LE generally spare the skin over joints and the skin lesions of dermatomyositis tend to localize over joints. If vesicular changes develop, the diagnosis of pemphigus erythematosus or contact dermatitis may be entertained. The histopathology and immunopathology can be helpful in this situation. Facial erythema with slight scaling may suggest a diagnosis of seborrheic dermatitis; however, the distribution of the lesions of acute cutaneous LE is different from that of seborrheic dermatitis. Rosacea may occasionally simulate acute cutaneous LE. The persistence of this facial eruption and the presence of pustules should make it possible to arrive at the correct diagnosis. Facial involvement by cellulitis or Sweet's syndrome can occasionally cause confusion. The presence of polymorphonuclear leukocytes in large numbers in the biopsy specimens from these conditions largely excludes the diagnosis of cutaneous LE.

Treatment. Since patients with acute cutaneous LE have a very evanescent eruption that almost always occurs in the presence of active SLE, the treatment of the systemic disease will also alleviate the skin involvement. Therapeutic decisions in such patients are based on the type of systemic involvement. High doses of prednisone (greater than 50 mg per day) have been advocated for active lupus nephritis as well as for patients with active cerebritis. Patients who fail to respond are often given a second cytotoxic or immunosuppressive agent. This treatment must be carefully tailored to fit the needs of an individual patient and requires careful supervision by a physician with experience in managing complicated patients with multisystem diseases. SLE patients with less aggressive and non-life threatening forms of the disease are usually treated with low-dose glucocorticoid therapy, antimalarials, or nonsteroid inflammatory agents. The nonsteroid anti-inflammatory agents have been of particular value for the management of fever, pleurisy, and pericarditis. Arthritis, arthralgia, and myalgia may respond to salicylates administered every 4 to 6 h to maintain anti-inflammatory blood levels (14 to 25 mg/dL). Hepatotoxicity from salicylates may occur with increased frequency in patients with SLE. There is no evidence that the nonsteroidal anti-inflammatory agents or salicylates provide any benefits for the acute cutaneous LE lesions. Prednisone appears to shorten the course of the inflammatory process in the skin.

In summary, patients with acute cutaneous LE generally have active SLE and require systemic corticosteroid therapy. The dose and duration of treatment will be dictated by the nature of the systemic disease. Patients with severe and life-threatening complications require larger doses of corticosteroids and some patients must be given cytotoxic drugs for their steroid-sparing effect or to gain control of the disease. The therapeutic goal is to balance control of life-threatening SLE with life-threatening drug toxicities.

LE-nonspecific skin disease

Although not diagnostic or histologically specific, the identification of the nonspecific but disease-related skin lesions is important since their presence implies systemic disease and they are often useful indicators of systemic disease activity. One or more of these lesions are present at some point in the course of disease in 40 to 60 percent of patients with SLE. The different categories of LE-nonspecific skin lesions are shown in Table 152-3.

Table 152-3 The nonspecific but disease-related skin lesions in LE

Vascular lesions:
   Dermal vasculitis
   Thrombophlebitis
   Raynaud's phenomenon
   Livedo reticularis
   Chronic ulcers
   Rheumatoid nodules
   Peripheral gangrene
   "Degos-like" dermal infarcts or atrophie blanche lesions
   Urticaria
Alopecia:
   Frontal ("lupus hair")
   Diffuse (nonscarring)
Pigmentary abnormalities
Sclerodactyly
Calcinosis cutis
Bullous lesions

Vascular lesions

A variety of vascular lesions are seen that can be classified into one of the following categories: (1) dermal vasculitis, (2) thrombophlebitis, (3) Raynaud's phenomenon, (4) livedo reticularis, (5) chronic ulcers, (6) rheumatoid nodules, (7) peripheral gangrene, and (8) "Degos-like" dermal infarcts or atrophie blanche-like lesions.

Vasculitis involving the dermal arterioles and postcapillary venules produces papular, erythematous, and purpuric lesions which may become necrotic. Small-vessel vasculitis may produce dermal infarcts along the lateral nail fold or scattered purpuric papular lesions about the ankles, elbows, or hands. Tender papular lesions on the extensor forearms just distal to the elbows are common in SLE patients with small-vessel vasculitis. Ischemic infarcts are also relatively common, which may be explained by the tendency for arterioles to be involved. The most prominent pathologic changes are fibrinoid deposits and thrombosis in small dermal blood vessels, which may be accompanied by surprisingly little cellular infiltration.

Vasculitic lesions involving both small dermal vessels and larger subcutaneous vessels often coexist so that the same patient has a combination of papular purpuric lesions (small-vessel disease) coupled with peripheral gangrene, painful subcutaneous nodules, chronic and recurrent ulcers, and livedo reticularis (large-vessel disease). The presence of these cutaneous and subcutaneous vasculitic lesions should suggest the possibility of a more widespread visceral vasculitis. Cutaneous vasculitic lesions have been shown to correlate with the presence of central nervous system disease and thrombocytopenia [21].

Alarcon-Segovia and Osmundson [22] have emphasized that recurrent superficial and deep thrombophlebitis may be an early sign of SLE. This complication may be a prominent feature in some SLE patients who have false-positive serologic tests for syphilis and circulating anticoagulants [23]. Since these patients are at risk for recurrent thromboembolic episodes, it is important to recognize these associated features.

Raynaud's phenomenon occurs in approximately 30 percent of patients with SLE. It is often seen in patients who have other scleroderma-like features or features of the mixed connective tissue disease syndrome described by Sharp and associates [24]. Dimant and coworkers [25] have suggested that Raynaud's phenomenon is a good prognostic sign in SLE.

Urticarial eruptions in patients with active SLE should suggest the possibility of underlying necrotizing leukocytoclastic vasculitis. Indeed, when biopsies from such lesions are examined, histologic evidence of vasculitis is commonly found [26]. Erythema multiforme has been occasionally described in active LE; however, some of the early reports of LE patients with erythema multiforme were probably patients with either subacute or acute cutaneous LE.

Rheumatoid nodules occur in approximately 5 percent of SLE patients. These lesions may be clinically and histologically identical to the rheumatoid nodules in patients with rheumatoid arthritis; however, they are often more superficially located and may contain hematoxylin bodies. A deforming nonerosive arthritis may be seen in SLE patients with these lesions. SLE patients with this deforming nonerosive type of joint disease (Jaccoud's syndrome) also have a higher frequency of endocardial lesions which can produce clinically significant mitral stenosis in some patients [27].

Alopecia

Hair loss (alopecia) is one of the most common and nonspecific cutaneous signs of SLE. Alopecia can be classified as either scarring or nonscarring, depending upon whether the follicular structures are permanently destroyed by the disease process. Scarring alopecia is caused by the chronic forms of cutaneous LE. Diffuse nonscarring alopecia occurs during the acute toxic exacerbations of systemic disease. Frontal alopecia with increased hair fragility producing short broken-off hairs has been referred to as "lupus hair." The diffuse forms of alopecia are generally transient; however, occasionally patients will have diffuse nonscarring alopecia which is more persistent. This is especially common in those patients who have clinical and serologic features of the syndrome designated mixed connective tissue disease by Sharp et al [24].

Bullous lesions

Bullous lesions of several types occur in patients with LE. Subepidermal blisters may develop in the subacute and acute cutaneous LE lesions due to marked liquefactive degeneration at the basal layer. Case reports of the coexistence of SLE and bullous pemphigoid, dermatitis herpetiformis, acquired epidermolysis bullosa, and porphyria cutanea tarda have been published. SLE patients with a pemphigoid-like disorder who have immune deposits on and below the basal lamina have also recently been reported [28]. Other patients with SLE and bullous lesions have been described with skin biopsies showing neutrophilic papillary microabscesses resembling dermatitis herpetiformis but with immunofluorescence findings more consistent with the diagnosis of LE [29]. Barvie, Lazarus, and Barland described an SLE patient with a subepidermal blistering process and circulating antibodies that reacted with an epidermal basement membrane zone (BMZ) antigen which appeared to be distinct from the bullous pemphigoid antigen [30]. We have recently studied the serum and skin from a similar patient and found that the anti-BMZ antibody localizes to the lamina densa region of the BMZ. Thus, there appears to be a variety of bullous lesions that occur in patients with SLE. Some of them are LE-specific, others are not.

Miscellaneous nonspecific lesions

Diffuse cutaneous hyperpigmentation is occasionally seen in SLE but is more often present in patients with scleroderma or in those with a scleroderma-like disorder. The mechanisms for this diffuse hypermelanosis are unknown. Calcinosis cutis has been occasionally reported in patients with LE. This complication is much more common in patients with scleroderma or dermatomyositis, especially the childhood type. Subcutaneous calcification is also a common feature of lupus panniculitis.

Extracutaneous manifestations of lupus erythematosus

General manifestations

Fever, fatigue, weight loss, and generalized malaise are very common manifestations of SLE. At the time of diagnosis 68 percent of our patients had loss of weight, 83 percent had fever, and moderate to severe fatigue was present in 76 percent [31]. Fever may be low-grade or spiking. It is important to remember that fever may represent the presence of infection in a patient with SLE and that infection should therefore always be ruled out even in a recently diagnosed untreated SLE patient.

Joint manifestations

Joint involvement is the most common manifestation of SLE, occurring in 95 percent of patients. Arthritis with pain on motion, tenderness, or effusion is present in about 80 percent and arthralgia is present in an additional 51 percent of patients. The joints most commonly involved are the proximal interphalangeal, knee, wrist, and metacarpophalangeal joints. The joint involvement is usually strikingly symmetrical. Morning stiffness was present in 50 percent of our patients. Deforming arthritis does occur in SLE patients who may have typical swan neck deformities and ulnar deviation of the fingers [32]. These abnormalities, present in about 15 percent of patients with long-standing disease, are very similar to the abnormalities of rheumatoid arthritis. However, in SLE patients x-rays reveal no abnormalities whereas in rheumatoid arthritis these deformities are always associated with x-rays that reveal loss of cartilage and bony erosions. Such erosive disease is extremely rare in SLE. Rheumatoid nodules are also rarely found in SLE patients. Synovial fluid is usually clear with good viscosity and a low white blood cell count with a predominance of mononuclear cells. This type of fluid is unlike the cloudy, poorly viscous fluid with a high white blood count of polymorphonuclear leukocytes seen in rheumatoid arthritis effusions. Tendonitis is occasionally present and tendon rupture occasionally occurs. Aseptic necrosis of the femoral head, knee, or wrist may occur late in the disease in a corticosteroid-treated patient and should be distinguished from the joint pains due to the disease by the demonstration of aseptic necrosis by bone scan or x-ray.

Myalgia and myositis

At the time of diagnosis, myalgia was present in one-third of our patients. Pain and tenderness of muscles was much less common and muscle weakness was rare [33]. In SLE patients treated with corticosteroids for more than a few months in moderate to high doses (40 to 60 mg per day), weakness of the proximal muscles may occur due to the therapy. Chloroquine myopathy has also been described [34]. In rare instances, myasthenia gravis has been associated with SLE.

Renal disease

Clinically evident kidney involvement occurs in approximately 55 to 60 percent of SLE patients [2]. The overall prognosis depends on the type and severity of the renal lesions. Patients with mesangial hypercellularity usually have only mild proteinuria and have an excellent outcome as long as their systemic disease does not become active. Patients with diffuse proliferative nephritis usually have significant proteinuria, hematuria, and may have red cell casts [35]. Renal insufficiency may be present at the time that SLE is diagnosed. This type of renal disease is present in only about 20 percent of patients and may be associated with the nephrotic syndrome. At the present time, these patients have a good five-year survival without dialysis which is probably due to the more aggressive treatment used and to the use of serologic tests such as complement levels and antibodies to native DNA in monitoring the disease activity. Mild focal lupus nephritis is the most common form of renal disease and has an excellent prognosis [36]. These patients usually have mild to moderate proteinuria and may have hematuria as well, but are rarely nephrotic and do not have renal insufficiency. Serologic abnormalities such as anti-DNA antibodies and low serum complement levels may be present. The least common form of lupus nephritis is membranous nephritis, which is characterized by significant proteinuria, nephrotic syndrome, and, in some patients, hematuria. Although antibodies to DNA and low serum complement levels are less common in these patients, these serologic abnormalities may be noted. In all patients with lupus nephritis, hypertension is considered a poor prognostic sign and should be treated aggressively [37]. Elevations of serum creatinine, if mild, may return to normal.

Cardiopulmonary manifestations

The most common symptom is pleuritic chest pain, which is present in about 40 percent of patients. Pleural effusions are found somewhat less often. Pleural effusions are usually exudates, and in contrast to those found in patients with rheumatoid arthritis, do not have low glucose levels. Pulmonary infiltrates due to lupus pneumonitis occur in only about 10 percent of patients and the major manifestation is dyspnea. Rarely pulmonary hemorrhage may occur. It is very important to rule out infectious causes for any pulmonary infiltrate in a patient with SLE and such patients should be aggressively studied and treated for infectious pneumonitis until this is done.

The most common cardiac manifestation is pericarditis which occurs in about 25 percent of patients. Tachycardia, an enlarging heart, congestive heart failure, arrhythmias, and conduction defects are noted in an occasional patient. Coronary arteritis may lead to myocardial infarction in an occasional patient. More frequently coronary artery disease is noted late in the course of the disease in patients treated with corticosteroids and is due to atherosclerosis of coronary arteries. Chronic disease of the valves due to the pathologic abnormalities of Libman Sacks endocarditis in patients who have been successfully treated has been described. Aortic valvular insufficiency with perforations of the valves and mitral regurgitation rarely occurs. It is important to remember that subacute and acute bacterial endocarditis may be superimposed on a valve damaged by Libman Sacks endocarditis.

Nervous system manifestations

Peripheral neuropathy occurs in about 14 percent of patients and usually produces a mixed sensory-motor disturbance similar to mononeuritis multiplex. Guillain-Barré syndrome occasionally may be seen. Cranial nerve involvement is seen less commonly than peripheral neuropathy and optic neuritis may also be noted. Transverse myelitis occurs in less than 4 percent of patients.

Movement disorders such as chorea or choreoathetosis are rarely observed but may be the first manifestation of disease.

Seizures are noted in about 15 percent of patients and are usually grand mal seizures and present early in the disease. Other types of seizure disorders including Jacksonian seizures, psychomotor epilepsy, petit mal, and temporal lobe epilepsy are rare.

Organic brain syndromes are characterized by impairment of orientation, perception, memory, and intellectual function [21]. This type of psychosis is found early in the course of the disease and is very rare later in the course if the patient remains in remission after the initial treatment. The five-year survival was not influenced by the presence of organic brain syndrome at the time of diagnosis in our series of patients studied in New York at the Bellevue Hospital [38].

Severe headaches may occur in SLE patients and may be associated with organic brain syndrome or seizures. In addition, these headaches, which are usually clinically indistinguishable from classical migraine headaches, may be noted in patients with brain infarcts demonstrated by computerized axial tomography (CT scan). Arteritis of the cerebral arteries has been found in a small number of patients with severe headaches or evidence of cerebral vascular accidents who have been studied by arteriography.

Cerebrospinal fluid abnormalities were noted in 32 percent of the neuropsychiatric episodes in 37 patients reported by Feinglass et al [21]. Protein elevations occurred in one-half of the fluids and increased numbers of white blood cells were also noted in some of these fluids. The electroencephalogram is usually abnormal in patients with organic brain syndrome or seizure disorders but also may be abnormal in patients without central nervous system manifestations. Brain scans have been reported to be abnormal in patients with central nervous system disease and to eventually return to normal after treatment. These findings have not been noted in other series. CT scan is of more value in the work-up of a patient with central nervous system manifestations. Although cerebral atrophy is frequently reported, this finding may be nonspecific and should not be interpreted as evidence of central nervous system disease due to SLE.

Psychological abnormalities are very common in SLE patients, especially in recently diagnosed individuals. Disfigurement due to the disease (skin lesions, alopecia) and due to the corticosteroid therapy leads to significant reactive depression in many patients. In addition, most patients have significant anxiety about their prognosis and difficulty in understanding why their treatment causes so many problems. Unless the physician provides adequate psychological support and uses allied health professionals such as nurses or support groups, patients may be confused and noncompliant. It is very valuable to have the patients understand why treatment is necessary and why repeated visits and laboratory tests are needed. Patients who are depressed and/or anxious should be encouraged to verbalize and to seek additional help from a psychologist or psychiatrist, if necessary. The psychological abnormalities must be distinguished from organic brain syndrome and, of course, should not be considered as manifestations of the disease requiring increases in corticosteroid therapy.

Gastrointestinal manifestations

Gastrointestinal manifestations such as nausea, vomiting, or anorexia are present in about 20 percent of patients at the time of diagnosis or during periods of disease activity. Abdominal pain is uncommon, occurring in only 10 percent, but is a very important symptom. Crampy abdominal pain associated with localizing signs and rebound tenderness should be viewed as a surgical emergency. Perforation of the large or small bowel or infarction without perforation may occur as a manifestation of SLE and is due to mesenteric arteritis [39]. Such patients have other evidence of disease activity and should have the earliest surgical intervention possible since only those who have received surgery early have survived. Other abdominal pain may be due to non-SLE causes such as rupture of an ovarian cyst, tubal-ovarian abscess, or appendicitis. Early diagnosis and surgical intervention are crucial in these patients.

Ascites is rarely present in SLE patients. Dysphagia may be present and usually is associated with Raynaud's phenomenon. Pancreatitis occurs occasionally in patients with active systemic disease and is considered to be a manifestation of the disease. Hepatomegaly is noted in about 30 percent of patients and liver enzyme abnormalities may also be noted. Biopsy-proved chronic active hepatitis may be associated with active SLE. Splenomegaly is present in 20 percent of patients and is usually not associated with hemolytic anemia. Splenic atrophy has recently been described [40].

Lymphadenopathy

Enlarged lymph nodes are present in about one-half of patients during disease activity. These nodes may be moderately enlarged in children and may be associated with hepatosplenomegaly, suggesting a diagnosis of lymphoma.

Ocular manifestations

Conjunctivitis and episcleritis occur in about 15 percent of patients and are usually associated with extensive cutaneous lesions. Occlusion of the central retinal artery has been reported as well as blindness from retinal arteritis [41]. Cytoid bodies are present in about 8 percent of patients. These are hard white lesions adjacent to retinal vessels which appear during disease activity and are due to retinal artery vasculitis. Keratoconjunctivitis sicca may occur in SLE patients.

Parotid gland manifestations

Acute enlargement of one or both parotid glands occurs occasionally in SLE patients. The swelling may be painful and usually returns to normal as the systemic disease is controlled.

Menstrual abnormalities and pregnancy

Some patients report that they have an increase in SLE symptoms such as joint pain or rashes immediately prior to their menstrual periods. Cessation of menses usually occurs around the time of diagnosis and returns about six months later as the disease is controlled and corticosteroid dose lowered. Pregnancy is associated with a flare of the disease if the disease is active at the time of conception. Thus, pregnancy should be avoided for the first few years of disease or until the patient is well controlled on low corticosteroid doses. Postpartum flare of the disease can be controlled by increasing corticosteroid doses during labor.

Hematologic abnormalities

One or more hematologic abnormalities are present in nearly all SLE patients who have clinical evidence of active disease [42]. Most common is a mild to moderate normocytic normochromic anemia. Anemia with hematocrit values of less than 30 percent occurs in one-half of patients and hemolytic anemia with reticulocytosis occurs in only 10 percent of patients. Leukopenia with white blood cell counts of less than 4000 per cubic millimeter was present in only 17 percent of our 365 patients [38]. In most patients with active disease an absolute lymphopenia is noted.

Mild thrombocytopenia is present in one-third of SLE patients but significant thrombocytopenia (less than 100,000 platelets per cubic millimeter) occurs less frequently.

The lupus anticoagulant can be identified by the presence of a slight prolongation of the thomboplastin time and a more marked prolongation of the partial thromboplastin time. This prolongation of the partial thromboplastin time cannot be corrected by the addition of equal volumes of normal plasma to the patient's plasma at varying dilutions. The lupus anticoagulant does not appear to be associated with bleeding since renal biopsies and other procedures can be performed on patients without difficulty. Recent

evidence has suggested that there may be a relationship between the presence of the lupus anticoagulant and thrombosis. The lupus anticoagulant usually disappears with corticosteroid therapy. The lupus anticoagulant is frequently noted in patients with a false-positive test for syphilis.

Laboratory findings in systemic lupus erythematosus

Plasma protein abnormalities are extremely common in patients with SLE. Acute phase reactants are elevated during active phases of the disease, as reflected by an increased erythrocyte sedimentation rate. The serum globulin is also increased and serum protein electrophoretic analysis will demonstrate a polyclonal hypergammaglobulinemia. Serum complement levels are generally decreased in active SLE, especially in those patients with active nephritis. The first complement component to fall is generally C4, followed by C3, Clq, and the total hemolytic complement activity (CH_{50}). The C4 level usually remains depressed longest, although exceptions are observed [43]. Low complement levels are generally thought to result from complement consumption with fixation by antigen-antibody complexes. However, there is also some evidence that the major determinant of a low C3 level in some patients with SLE is decreased synthesis of this complement component [44]. In addition, an illness that resembles SLE has been described in a number of patients with congenital complement component deficiencies. The best method for detecting a complement component deficiency is the functional assay for total hemolytic complement (CH_{50}).

A broad spectrum of autoantibodies may be found in patients with SLE. For diagnostic purposes, antinuclear antibodies (ANA) are the most sensitive laboratory test for SLE. Patients with clinical characteristics of SLE and persistently negative antinuclear antibodies are rare and usually have other autoantibodies such as anti-single-stranded (ss) DNA, LE cells, or anticytoplasmic (Ro/La) antibodies. Antinuclear antibodies are usually detected by the fluorescent antinuclear antibody (FANA) test. For the demonstration of more specific antibodies to well-defined nuclear antigens, radioimmunoassays, immunodiffusion, or hemagglutination techniques are used. Considerable interest has developed in recent times in detecting specific nuclear antigen-antibody systems which seem to be related to rather well-defined clinical subsets (Table 152-4). Antibodies to native or double-stranded DNA seem to be closely linked to the development of significant lupus nephritis. High titers of antibodies to double-stranded DNA are essentially restricted to SLE. However, they are not always present, being detectable in only 65 to 70 percent of patients. Antibodies to single-stranded DNA also occur in SLE but are not specific. Antibodies to RNP are found in patients with lupus who have overlapping features of myositis and scleroderma. Antibodies to an acidic nuclear protein (Sm) have been identified almost exclusively in patients with SLE. Antibodies to the Ro/SSA antigen are particularly common in patients with SCLE.

Five nuclear staining patterns (peripheral, homogeneous, particulate, speckled, and nucleolar) are demonstrable by fluorescent antibody techniques (Table 152-5). Sera

Table 152-4   Immunospecificities of antinuclear antibodies

Antibody specificity	Disease subset
Double-stranded deoxyribonucleic acid (DNA)	Active SLE with nephritis
Single-stranded (denatured) DNA (purine and pyrimidine determinants)	Nonspecific, found in a variety of rheumatic and nonrheumatic diseases
Deoxyribonucleoprotein (DNP) Antigenic determinant consists of a complex of DNA and histones	LE-cell antibody, present primarily in idiopathic SLE and in drug-induced LE
Histones	Drug-induced LE
Nonhistone acidic nuclear protein antigens:	
Sm antigen	Diagnostic of SLE
Nuclear ribonucleoprotein (RNP)	High titers diagnostic of mixed connective tissue disease, low titers occur in other rheumatic diseases
SS-A (Ro), SS-B (La) and Ha antigens	High prevalence in Sjögren's syndrome sicca complex; common in SCLE, neonatal LE, and C2 deficiency with LE
Nucleolar antigens: Nucleolar 4S-6S RNA	Present in patients with Raynaud's phenomenon, majority have scleroderma-like features

from SLE patients generally show two or more of these patterns. The homogeneous pattern is characterized by diffuse nuclear staining which is produced by an antibody to a DNA-histone complex. The particulate patterns are produced by antibodies to saline-extractable nuclear antigens (ENA) which include RNP and the Sm antigen. The speckled (true fine-speckled) pattern is produced by antibodies to the centromeric region of the chromosomes. These antibodies are highly specific for the CREST syndrome and are rarely seen in patients with LE. The nucleolar pattern is characterized by fluorescence of each nucleolus, and this antibody is usually present in patients with Raynaud's phenomenon and other scleroderma-like features. The peripheral (membranous or shaggy) pattern results from the staining of the periphery of the nucleus. This pattern indicates the presence of antibodies to native DNA. Peripheral and homogeneous patterns are the most common patterns seen in active SLE.

Examination of the normal-appearing skin by direct immunofluorescence can also be useful in the diagnosis of patients with SLE. The presence of subepidermal immunoglobulin deposits in uninvolved skin of patients with cutaneous LE is evidence for systemic disease. Epidermal nuclear staining suggests the presence of antibodies to nuclear RNP and is usually seen in patients with overlap-

ping features of scleroderma, LE, and dermatomyositis. Vascular staining by immunofluorescence in biopsies from normal skin is commonly associated with cutaneous vasculitis or central nervous system disease. The presence of IgM alone at the dermal-epidermal junction of normal skin suggests benign, nonagressive disease, in contrast to more severe disease in patients with IgG, plus IgM, and/or IgA. Subepidermal immunoglobulin is found frequently in skin biopsies taken from the extensor aspect of the arm or exposed areas of skin in patients with SLE, and is of diagnostic, but not prognostic, significance. Subepidermal immunoglobulin deposits are usually present in SLE skin lesions. However, since subepidermal deposits may also be present in other inflammatory skin diseases, this finding is not as useful in a diagnostic sense, as the presence of deposits in otherwise normal nonexposed skin.

The clinical utility of the newer laboratory tests in patients with SLE is variable. Tests that measure antibodies to double-stranded DNA are clearly useful for both diagnosis and patient management. Their presence in high concentrations suggests active disease and an increased risk for nephritis. Antibodies to the Sm antigen are also useful in the diagnosis of LE because of their specificity for this disease. Antibodies to histones appear in procainamide-induced lupus, and antibodies to neuronal tissue may be

Table 152-5   Clinical significance of fluorescent antinuclear antibody (FANA) patterns

Pattern	Previous nomenclature	Associated disease
Particulate	Speckled, thready, fibrillar, reticular	Mixed connective tissue disease (MCTD), SLE, scleroderma, undifferentiated connective tissue disease, malignancy
Homogeneous	Diffuse, solid	Connective tissue disease; when present in high titer suspect SLE
Peripheral	Shaggy, rim, membranous	Active SLE (highly specific); common in SLE with nephritis
Speckled	True speckled "pepper dots"	Scleroderma/CREST, Raynaud's phenomenon (anticentromere antibody)
Nucleolar	Large discrete speckles	Scleroderma, Raynaud's phenomenon; uncommon in SLE, rare in MCTD

associated with the presence of CNS involvement. Antibodies of other specificities appear to have little practical value in the diagnoses or management of patients with LE.

Clinical course and prognosis of systemic lupus erythematosus

Systemic lupus erythematosus is a generalized, idiopathic, autoimmune disease which is relatively uncommon. Its natural course may be fulminant, leading to death within a few weeks, mild, or slowly progressive with exacerbations and remissions. Twenty-five years ago only half of SLE patients survived for four years after diagnosis. Today, 80 to 90 percent of patients survive for 10 to 15 years after diagnosis. Several factors account for this remarkable increase in survival. Greater medical awareness of LE has led to earlier diagnosis and more effective treatment of the disease. Mild cases of SLE are being detected earlier and corticosteroids are being used more appropriately, leading to less toxicity. Advances in our understanding of the proper medical management of infections and other complications such as hypertension have also contributed to this overall improved survival.

Renal failure remains the leading cause of death, while deaths from neurologic disease have become less common. Other causes of SLE-related deaths have emerged. These include death from massive pulmonary hemorrhage, colonic perforation due to vasculitis, mesenteric artery disease, coronary artery disease, and bizarre infections resulting from chemotherapeutic interventions.

The clinical spectrum of SLE varies widely. Many patients have a mild, recurring disease which is annoying, but not aggressive or life-threatening. Occasionally, patients present with severe central nervous system, cardiopulmonary, or renal disease which is rapidly fatal. Fortunately, most SLE patients have a disease that is intermediate in severity, with exacerbations and remissions occurring over a period of many years. Appropriate management requires adequate suppression of the disease during the active phases, with reduction or discontinuation of treatment during the periods of remission.

References

1. Dubois EL, Tuffanelli DE: Clinical manifestations of systemic lupus erythematosus. *JAMA* **190**:104, 1964
2. Estes D, Christian CL: The natural history of systemic lupus erythematosus studied by prospective analysis. *Medicine (Baltimore)* **50**:85, 1971
3. Millard LG, Rowell NR: Abnormal laboratory test results and their relationship to prognosis in discoid lupus erythematosus. A long-term follow-up study of 92 patients. *Arch Dermatol* **115**:1055, 1979
4. Prystowsky SD, Gilliam JN: Discoid lupus erythematosus as part of a larger disease spectrum. Correlation of clinical features with laboratory findings in lupus erythematosus. *Arch Dermatol* **111**:1448, 1975
5. Fries JF: The clinical aspects of systemic lupus erythematosus. *Med Clin North Am* **61**:229, 1977
6. Shearn MA, Pirofsky B: Disseminated lupus erythematosus. Analysis of 34 cases. *Arch Intern Med* **90**:790, 1952
7. Gilliam JN et al: Immunoglobulin in clinical uninvolved skin in systemic lupus erythematosus. Association with renal disease. *J Clin Invest* **53**:1434, 1975
8. Cripps DJ, Rankin J: Action spectra of lupus erythematosus and experimental immunofluorescence. *Arch Dermatol* **107**:563, 1973
9. Gilliam JN: Immunopathology and pathogenesis of cutaneous lupus erythematosus, in *Immunodermatology*, edited by B Safai, RA Good. New York, Plenum, 1981
10. Stastny P et al: Homologous disease in the adult rat, a model for autoimmune disease. *J Exp Med* **118**:635, 1963
11. Rothfield NF et al: Chronic discoid lupus erythematosus: a study of 65 patients and 65 controls. *N Engl J Med* **269**:1155, 1963
12. Prystowsky SD et al: Chronic cutaneous lupus erythematosus (DLE): a clinical and laboratory investigation of 80 patients. *Medicine (Baltimore)* **55**:1983, 1976
13. Schrager MA, Rothfield NF: Pathways of complement activation in chronic discoid lupus: serologic and immunofluorescence studies. *Arthritis Rheum* **20**:637, 1977
14. Irgang S: Lupus erythematosus profundus; report of example with clinical resemblance to Darier-Roussy sarcoid. *Arch Dermatol* **42**:97, 1940
15. Uitto J et al: Verrucous lesions in patients with discoid lupus erythematosus. Clinical, histological and immunofluorescence studies. *Br J Dermatol* **98**:507, 1978
16. Romero RW et al: Unusual variant of lupus erythematosus on lichen planus. Clinical, histopathologic and immunofluorescent studies. *Arch Dermatol* **113**:741, 1977
17. Sontheimer RD et al: Subacute cutaneous lupus erythematosus. A cutaneous marker for a distinct lupus erythematosus subset. *Arch Dermatol* **115**:1409, 1979
18. Sontheimer RD et al: Serologic and HLA associations of subacute cutaneous lupus erythematosus. *Ann Intern Med* **97**:664, 1982
19. Agnello V: Complement deficiency states. *Medicine (Baltimore)* **57**:1, 1978
20. Vandersteen PR et al: C_2 deficient systemic lupus erythematosus. *Arch Dermatol* **118**:584, 1982
21. Feinglass EJ et al: Neuropsychiatric manifestations of systemic lupus erythematosus: diagnosis, clinical spectrum, and relationship to other features of the disease. *Medicine (Baltimore)* **55**:323, 1976
22. Alarcon-Segovia D, Osmundson PJ: Peripheral vascular syndromes associated with systemic lupus erythematosus. *Ann Intern Med* **62**:907, 1965
23. Peck B et al: Thrombophlebitis in systemic lupus erythematosus. *JAMA* **240**:1728, 1978
24. Sharp GC et al: Association of autoantibodies to different nuclear antigens with clinical patterns of rheumatic disease and responsiveness to therapy. *J Clin Invest* **50**:350, 1971
25. Dimant J et al: The clinical significance of Raynaud's phenomenon in systemic lupus erythematosus. *Arthritis Rheum* **22**:815, 1979
26. O'Laughlin S et al: Chronic urticaria-like lesions in systemic lupus erythematosus. *Arch Dermatol* **114**:879, 1978
27. Bywaters EGL: Jaccoud's syndrome. A sequel to the joint involvement of systemic lupus erythematosus. *Clin Rheum Dis* **1**:125, 1975
28. Olansky AJ et al: Bullous systemic lupus erythematosus. *J Am Acad Dermatol* **7**:511, 1982
29. Hall RP et al: Bullous eruption of lupus erythematosus. *Ann Intern Med* **97**:165, 1982
30. Barvie A et al: Basement membrane antibody with skin bullae. *NY State J Med* **76**:2127, 1976
31. Rothfield HF: Clinical features of systemic lupus erythematosus, in *Textbook of Rheumatology*, vol 2, edited by WN Kelley et al. Philadelphia, WB Saunders, 1981, p 1106
32. Labowitz R, Schumacher HR: Articular manifestations of systemic lupus erythematosus. *Ann Intern Med* **74**:911, 1971
33. Tsokos GC et al: Muscle involvement in SLE. *JAMA* **246**:766, 1981
34. Itobashi HH, Kokman E: Chloroquine neuromyopathy. A reversible granulovacuolar myopathy. *Arch Pathol* **93**:209, 1972

35. Baldwin DS et al: The clinical course of the proliferative and membranous forms of lupus nephritis. *Ann Intern Med* **73**:929, 1970

36. Morel-Maroger L et al: The course of lupus nephritis: contribution of serial renal biopsies. *Adv Nephrol* **6**:79, 1976

37. Decker JL et al: Systemic lupus erythematosus: evolving concepts. *Ann Intern Med* **91**:587, 1979

38. Urman JD, Rothfield NF: Corticosteroid treatment in systemic lupus erythematosus: survival studies. *JAMA* **238**:2272, 1977

39. Zizic TM et al: Colonic perforation in systemic lupus erythematosus. *Medicine (Baltimore)* **54**:411, 1975

40. Dillon AM et al: Splenic atrophy in SLE. *Ann Intern Med* **96**:40, 1982

41. Copetto J, Lessell S: Retinopathy in SLE. *Arch Ophthalmol* **95**:794, 1977

42. Budman DR, Steinberg AD: Hematologic aspects of SLE. Current concepts. *Ann Intern Med* **86**:220, 1977

43. Schur PH, Austen KF: Complement in human disease. *Annu Rev Med* **19**:1, 1968

44. Sliwinski AJ, Zvaifler NJ: Decreased synthesis of the third component of complement (C3) in hypocomplementemic SLE. *Clin Exp Immunol* **11**:21, 1972

CHAPTER 153

DERMATOMYOSITIS

John A. Mills

Dermatomyositis is one of the major systemic inflammatory diseases of connective tissue. The principal pathology is an acute and chronic inflammation of striated muscle accompanied by segmental necrosis of myofibers. This process causes progressive muscle weakness that affects proximal more than distal muscles. A characteristic dermatitis occurs in about a half of the cases. When the dermatitis is not present the disease is referred to as polymyositis. The clinical and pathologic characteristics of the myositis appear to be the same in both instances, although some authorities disagree [1].

Myositis may be a prominent feature of other connective tissue diseases, especially lupus erythematosus and the closely related mixed connective tissue disease [2,3]. In some cases the cutaneous lesions are also very similar to those of dermatomyositis. Myositis can also occur in patients who have sclerodermatous skin changes, a condition that has been called sclerodermatomyositis [4]. Patients who have prominent myositis but also features of other connective tissue disease such as Sjögren's syndrome, mixed connective tissue disease, or even rheumatoid arthritis are usually classified separately [5]. They tend to have a more variable course than patients with simple polymyositis or dermatomyositis and to have the serum autoantibodies that occur in the other connective tissue diseases [6]. This chapter will not consider such syndromes in detail. Occasional cases with overlapping features defy precise categorization.

Historical aspects

Although the first detailed description of dermatomyositis was by Wagner in 1863, only sporadic reports appeared for almost the next century. In 1940 O'Leary and Waisman analyzed 40 cases from the Mayo Clinic [7] and in 1957 and 1958 clinical studies of two other patient groups appeared [8,9]. Systemic studies of the disease by Carl Pearson's group were published over the next decade and culminated in the analysis of 153 cases in 1977 [5].

Etiology and pathogenesis

Myositis occurs in a number of infectious diseases, particularly those of viral origin [10,11]. Attempts to identify an infectious etiologic agent in the muscle of patients with dermatomyositis or polymyositis have been unsuccessful. A myositis clinically similar to that of polymyositis may be seen in infections with *Toxoplasma gondii*. However, despite serologic evidence of recent infection with *Toxoplasma* in 5 to 10 percent of cases of polymyositis, the frequency of microscopic identification of the organism or its recovery in culture of muscle suggests that few cases are caused by *Toxoplasma* [12].

Autoimmunity to an antigen in muscle may be involved in the pathogenesis of dermatomyositis. Kakulas et al first reported that lymphocytes obtained from the blood of patients with the disease, but not from patients with other diseases, could damage human fetal myocytes maintained in tissue culture [13]. Dawkins and Mastaglia subsequently demonstrated a similar cytotoxicity using chick embryo myocytes as the target tissue [14]. However, not all investigators have been able to support these observations [15,16].

Immunization of young animals of several species with heterologous muscle combined in Freund's adjuvant can induce an acute myositis that can be transferred to another animal of the same species by peripheral blood lymphocytes [17]. The lymphocytes that infiltrate muscle in polymyositis are predominantly of the cytotoxic/suppressor subset [18]. Investigation of a case of polymyositis that seemed to be related to the taking of cimetidine showed that the drug could stimulate cytotoxic T cells [19].

These observations are evidence for the participation of a cell-mediated immune response in the pathogenesis of polymyositis. Cutaneous delayed-hypersensitivity responses to tumor extracts have been demonstrated in several patients whose myositis was associated with the presence of a tumor [17].

There is some indication that humoral factors may be

involved as well. Immune complexes have been demonstrated both in the affected muscle and in the serum of patients with active disease [20]. A number of different methods have been used to detect the immune complexes and have been variably successful in different laboratories. The therapeutic effectiveness of plasmapheresis [21] points to the importance of some circulating factor in the pathogenesis of polymyositis.

Arterial pathology is a prominent finding in some cases of juvenile dermatomyositis, and vascular damage may play a pathogenic role. Perifascicular fibers are usually the most severely affected, a pattern that may indicate an ischemic component [1].

Several connective tissue diseases including dermatomyositis occur in patients with congenital deficiencies of the second component of serum complement [22]. It has been speculated that such a deficiency might be genetically linked to other disorders of immune regulation or could be responsible for an abnormal response to a foreign antigen.

In spite of these observations, it must be concluded that knowledge of the etiology and pathogenesis of dermatomyositis and polymyositis is still largely conjectural.

Clinical manifestations

Progressive muscle weakness affecting the proximal or limb girdle muscles is the most important clinical manifestation and the first sign of the disease in nearly all patients with polymyositis. It is also the major feature in the majority of cases of dermatomyositis. The rest of the latter group present with the dermatitis and later develop muscle weakness [23]. In rare cases the myositis never occurs.

Typically, patients with limb girdle weakness first complain of difficulty climbing stairs, rising from low chairs, or raising their arms overhead to wash or brush their hair. Turning in bed becomes difficult. Although mild muscle tenderness may be present, only 20 percent of patients complain of muscle pain. Myalgia is more common in patients with the overlap syndromes or other diseases [24]. Rarely patients present with symptoms of distal weakness such as reduced grip strength or a flat-footed gait and are misdiagnosed as having motor neuron disease or muscular dystrophy [9].

Involvement of the facial or bulbar musculature occurs in about 5 percent of patients with dermatomyositis or polymyositis. They tend to be the more severe cases or those who have an associated tumor or myasthenia [25]. Dysphagia caused by weakness of the oropharyngeal muscles must be distinguished from that caused by smooth muscle dysfunction in the lower esophagus. The latter is more characteristic of scleroderma or overlap syndromes.

On examination the muscles may feel flabby and are tender in some patients. Muscle size is preserved out of proportion to the weakness, a feature which helps to distinguish polymyositis from the various limb girdle dystrophies wherein the opposite pertains. Patients whose weakness seems not inconsistent with other manifestations of a chronic illness usually turn out to have some other disease.

Tendon reflexes are preserved until late in the disease and muscle fasciculation is rarely seen. When signs of muscle denervation occur in patients with other features of dermatomyositis, a tumor-associated syndrome is almost certain. In some patients with polymyositis there is a myasthenic component to the weakness and a reduction in the number of acetylcholine receptors at motor end plates has been found [26].

Cutaneous manifestations

In cases of dermatomyositis the dermatitis may be the most striking feature of the disease or so minor as to be easily overlooked. In about a third of cases, the cutaneous manifestations occur first and weakness may not be appreciated until weeks or months later [25]. One of the more common and characteristic dermatologic features is a purplish-red periorbital discoloration most prominent on the upper lids, often described as a heliotrope erythema (see Fig. A2-5). In association with muscle weakness it is almost diagnostic and may be the only evidence of the dermal component (Fig. 153-1).

The usual dermatitis consists of an erythematous, scaly, macular and papular rash that involves the forehead, malar area, neck, and extensor surfaces of the extremities [6]. It is often localized to the knuckles, elbows, and knees giving a pathognomonic appearance called Gottron's sign [27] (Fig. 153-2). These cutaneous lesions may evolve into poikiloderma, plaquelike areas of atrophy, vitiligo, or hyperpigmentation. Erythema and infarction of dilated capillaries at the nail margins is a common finding but may be seen also in systemic lupus erythematosus and scleroderma [28]. The skin manifestations occasionally resemble lichen planus, erythema multiforme, pityriasis, or psoriasis [29]. The dermatitis, as in lupus erythematosus, may be activated by sunlight exposure. Mucous membrane involvement rarely occurs except in the overlap syndromes [5].

Other manifestations

Pathology in other organ systems occurs predominantly in patients with overlap syndromes. These manifestations in-

Fig. 153-1 Periorbital heliotrope erythema in a patient with tumor-associated dermatomyositis.

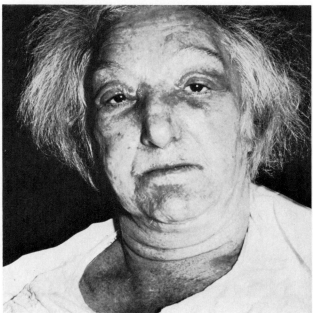

clude arthritis, esophageal and intestinal motility disorders, polyserositis, and Sjögren's syndrome [5,25]. A mild transient nonerosive polyarthritis may develop early in the course of either polymyositis or dermatomyositis [30]. Cardiac and pulmonary complications do occur in classical polymyositis or dermatomyositis. The incidence, which varies from 10 to 40 percent, depends on the sensitivity of the method used for their detection. The lower limit approximates their importance clinically. Cardiac manifestations reflect myocarditis and occur more often in cases of polymyositis than of dermatomyositis [31]. Arrhythmias including atrial and ventricular irritability and atrioventric-

ular block are among the more common findings but are rarely life threatening [32]. However, diffuse myocarditis ranks high among the causes of death from the disease. A rare form of myositis associated with a thymoma and often with myasthenia has a much higher incidence of myocarditis. Multinucleate giant cells are a distinctive histologic finding in the muscle of such cases [33].

Tests of pulmonary function may be abnormal in almost a third of patients and radiologic evidence of interstitial fibrosis occurs in 15 percent. Clinically important pulmonary fibrosis with hypoxia has been reported infrequently [34].

Juvenile dermatomyositis

Both polymyositis and dermatomyositis occur in children and have been reported in infants [35,36]. In children the disease has a number of special features, the most important of which is an arteritis [37]. This can be seen in muscle but is of more importance clinically in the gastrointestinal tract and peripheral nerve. Polyarthritis and dysphagia are more common in the juvenile form of the disease than in adults; and two features, glomerulonephritis and retinopathy, although present in less than 5 percent of cases, are unique to the childhood form [38].

Calcification in subcutaneous and fascial planes is a distressing late complication that occurs in about two-thirds of cases of juvenile dermatomyositis or polymyositis [39] (Fig. 153-3). It may progress even after the myositis remits and eventually become totally incapacitating. There is no effective therapy for this complication, which is referred to as *calcinosis universalis*.

Laboratory findings

Laboratory tests reveal only a few abnormalities but they are of great diagnostic help. In the more acute forms of the disease, a moderate leukocytosis is common. Anemia

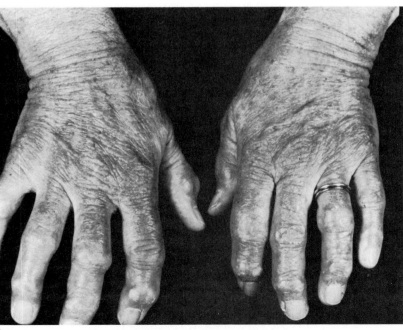

a

b

Fig. 153-2 (a) Papular erythema over knuckles (Gottron's sign). Note erythema on "V area" of neck and eyelids. (b) Diffuse telangiectatic erythema over the dorsa of the hands.

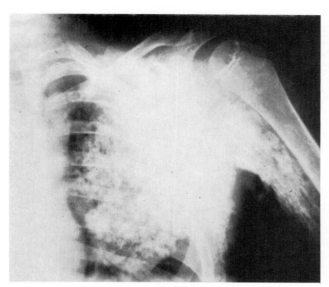

Fig. 153-3   Calcinosis universalis in pectoral muscles. A 6-year-old patient with dermatomyositis.

is absent or develops slowly in the course of chronic cases. More often than not, the sedimentation rate is normal.

The urinalysis during exacerbations frequently reveals a trace of protein. The passage of dark urine should alert one to the presence of myoglobinuria and possible renal tubular obstruction by myoglobin casts. Myoglobinuria is a complication of very acute myositis which is usually not seen in polymyositis or dermatomyositis. Most such cases are self limited and often follow virus infections or severe muscular exertion in individuals with metabolic myopathies [40].

Apart from muscle biopsy, the most useful laboratory studies are the serum levels of enzymes released from muscle by the disease process [41]. Of those commonly measured, the serum creatine phosphokinase is probably the most sensitive. Aldolase, glutamic oxalacetic transaminase, and lactic dehydrogenase are also often elevated during the active phase of the myositis, but there may be considerable discrepancy among the relative levels of these enzymes in individual cases. Red cells contain both aldolase and lactic dehydrogenase, so minor degrees of in vitro hemolysis of blood samples may falsely elevate serum levels. Creatine phosphokinase (CPK) is more specific for muscle disease. Isoenzyme analysis shows that most of the CPK is of the MM type. However, when levels are high, a significant amount of MB may be present. The levels of one or more of these enzymes will closely reflect the activity of the myopathy in most cases and variations in their levels usually precede changes in muscle strength by several weeks. They are a useful guide to therapy. Bed rest will substantially reduce the serum enzyme levels. They may also fall out of proportion to the return in muscle strength when steroid therapy is started but a return to normal levels indicates control of the myositis. Late in the disease, if severe muscle atrophy has occurred, enzyme levels may also return toward normal.

The excretion of creatine in the urine is increased during active disease. In adults, the normal 24-h creatine excretion is not more than 100 mg or about 12 percent of the urine creatinine excretion. Values in excess of 200 mg per 24 h are helpful diagnostically. As the disease becomes inactive, the creatine excretion falls. Substantial creatinuria in the absence of raised enzyme levels in a patient on corticosteroids suggests steroid myopathy. Children and pregnant women normally have higher and more variable creatine excretions and the test may be difficult to interpret in those instances.

Electromyography is useful to confirm the presence of a myopathy and to help exclude neuromyopathy [42,43]. The abnormalities found include unusual irritability on insertion of the electrodes and sometimes spontaneous fibrillation at rest. The latter finding, originally thought to be a specific mark of denervation, is now known to be present occasionally in dermatomyositis. Other characteristic features are the presence of pseudomyotonic discharges and positive sharp waves. These are of uncertain pathogenesis. A sustained interference pattern is obtained during voluntary activity but the potentials are of short duration and generally of low amplitude with an increased number of polyphasic potentials. The electromyogram may be normal in 20 to 30 percent of cases of dermatomyositis. Evidence of denervation such as fibrillation potentials and a grossly incomplete interference pattern with giant action potentials is usually not seen in uncomplicated cases. When such features are present, the coexistence of a tumor should be suspected.

Muscle biopsy remains the most definitive diagnostic test. However, a single biopsy taken at random may reveal normal muscle in one-fourth of cases eventually proven to be dermatomyositis [44]. The biopsy should always be obtained from a muscle of the shoulder or pelvic girdle and preferably one that is weak or tender. The muscles most commonly biopsied are the deltoid, supraspinatus, gluteus, or quadriceps. Electrode insertion sites should be avoided. Within the next few years needle biopsy may replace the classical surgical technique [45].

At biopsy, usually no gross abnormality is seen. The characteristic microscopic feature is a segmental necrosis within muscle fibers with loss of the cross-striations and a waxy or coagulative type of eosinophilic staining [1]. Both type I and type II fibers are affected. There may be considerable variation in fiber size, some being swollen above the normal diameter and others reduced to collapsed sarcolemmal membranes. Sarcolemmal nuclei appear to be increased in number due either to loss of myoplasm or to proliferation in areas of muscle regeneration which in themselves are very characteristic. Regenerating fibers show central migration and hypertrophy of the sarcolemmal nuclei and a distinctly basophilic myoplasm in routine histologic stains (Fig. 153-4).

Inflammatory cells may vary considerably in composition and intensity. The histiocyte or macrophage tends to predominate early in the process and there may be phagocytosis of degenerating muscle fibers. A variable infiltrate of lymphocytes and plasma cells is found in the interstitium, especially around venules. In some biopsies inflammation may be absent, others show many inflammatory cells with little myofiber necrosis. Additional biopsies may be helpful if the morphology is not diagnostic.

An important feature of biopsies in childhood dermatomyositis is the presence of vascular lesions [38]. These are found in small arterioles which show intimal hypertrophy and the deposition of fibrin and platelet material in the

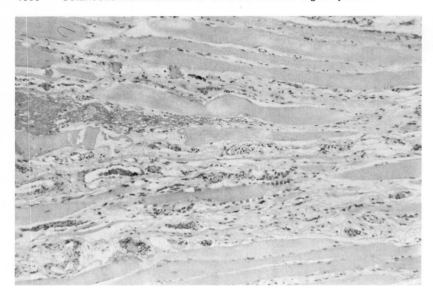

Fig. 153-4 Muscle biopsy showing segmental necrosis. Mild interstitial round cell infiltration and focal early muscle regeneration.

lumen that may lead to its occlusion. Whether the basic pathogenesis of the juvenile disease differs from the usual adult type of dermatomyositis is not clear [1].

The pathology in the skin is usually of a nonspecific character [46]. The epidermis may show mild acanthosis or atrophy with vacuolar degeneration of the basal cells. Capillary dilatation is prominent in the dermis and the vessels are often surrounded by a cuff of mononuclear inflammatory cells. Edema and the presence of mucous material and occasionally fibrin in the superficial dermis are characteristic features. Inflammatory cells are usually sparse.

The autoantibodies that characterize other connective tissue diseases are not found in polymyositis or dermatomyositis except in cases with overlapping features. A distinct antibody to a protein component of cell nuclei, PM1, has been identified in some patients with polymyositis. It seems to be present in only a minority [47].

Investigation of muscle disease by means of nuclear magnetic resonance may prove to be diagnostically valuable but is still in the experimental stage [48].

Diagnosis and differential diagnosis

The diagnosis of polymyositis for a patient with proximal muscle weakness requires that at least two of the three major laboratory criteria be met. Those are elevated serum "muscle enzyme" levels, characteristic electromyographic changes, or diagnostic muscle biopsy. Demonstration of muscle weakness on physical examination is helpful but muscle testing is not truly objective on the part of either patient or examiner and can be misleading. Furthermore, a person who was previously very strong can lose considerable strength before it is detectable.

When the typical skin rash is present in a patient who has proximal muscle weakness, the diagnosis of dermatomyositis is almost certain. As noted, less characteristic rashes resembling those of lupus erythematosus, scleroderma, or psoriasis may occur in patients with overlap syndromes. Whether these syndromes should be considered to be polymyositis with manifestations of another connective tissue disease or another connective tissue disease with prominent myositis is moot.

The serologic reactions that characterize other connective tissue diseases are not positive in more than 3 to 5 percent of patients with polymyositis or dermatomyositis. They are useful in patients with atypical presentations to help further define overlap syndromes. Muscle weakness is not present at the onset in about 20 percent of cases of dermatomyositis and occasional patients never develop myositis. The diagnosis then depends on the clinical and pathologic features of the rash itself [49].

A patient whose electromyogram shows evidence of denervation as well as myopathic features should be thoroughly investigated for the presence of a tumor. This applies also to any males when disease begins after age 50. In that group the incidence of an accompanying tumor approaches 40 percent [25].

Polymyositis must be distinguished from myositis of other causes including specific infectious agents, granulomatous diseases, and toxins. Inclusion body myositis is clinically similar to polymyositis. It can be distinguished only by muscle biopsy which reveals viruslike inclusions in muscle fiber nuclei when the tissue is examined by electron microscopy [50]. Extensive muscle involvement occurs occasionally in sarcoidosis and may be accompanied by a rash similar to that of dermatomyositis [51]. As noted previously, toxoplasmosis can also produce a syndrome that closely resembles dermatomyositis [52] as can trichinosis, although in the latter, myalgia is usually present out of proportion to weakness.

Diffuse or sometimes proximal muscle weakness can be caused by a number of drugs, among them penicillamine, chloroquine, clofibrate, and alcohol [53–55]. Severe phosphate depletion in patients with chronic alcoholism, some vascular bone tumors, malnutrition, or hemodialysis can also result in proximal muscle weakness [56]. Thyrotoxic myopathy should be ruled out by appropriate thyroid function tests.

The muscular dystrophies and a growing number of metabolic myopathies must be considered. The last group nearly always causes episodic weakness during or immediately after exertion whereas weakness in patients with myositis is constant. Motor neuron disease, spinal muscle atrophy and other generalized, predominantly motor neuropathies also enter the differential diagnosis [57].

Prominent oculobulbar involvement, particularly early in the course of the disease, usually points to a primary neurologic disorder—multiple sclerosis, motor neuron disease, or myasthenia. Muscle fasciculation, hyperactive reflexes, and muscle atrophy out of proportion to the weakness also indicate motor neuron disease. About a third of such patients may have moderately elevated muscle enzymes.

The serum muscle enzyme levels suggest myositis when they are greatly elevated (5 to 10 times the normal range) but are otherwise not helpful in differential diagnosis. In muscular dystrophies, levels may also overlap the broad range seen in the various myositis syndromes. Muscle biopsy helps to distinguish between inflammatory and noninflammatory disorders, provides additional evidence for the presence of a neuromyopathy when differential staining of fiber types is employed, and defines by electron microscopy, rare muscle disorders characterized by morphologic abnormalities [58]. Histochemical and classical biochemical analyses of biopsies may be necessary to diagnose certain metabolic myopathies of muscle metabolism that cause weakness related to exertion [59].

Polymyalgia rheumatica is a disease of elderly persons characterized by pain and stiffness of limb girdle muscles. Weakness is not present but the myalgia often makes testing difficult. Clinical and pathologic evidence of myositis is absent and there is no skin disease. The major laboratory features are a very high sedimentation rate and a dramatic response to small doses of corticosteroid, neither of which occurs in polymyositis.

Treatment

Active polymyositis or dermatomyositis should be treated with adrenocorticosteroid [5,60]. Prednisone is the drug of choice. The initial dose should be at the level of 0.5 to 1.0 mg/kg body weight per day. It can nearly always be given effectively in single daily dose. The dose should be increased to 1.5 mg/kg for at least 2 weeks if the lower dose proves ineffective. As soon as the muscle enzyme levels approach normal, tapering of the steroid dose should be started. Decrements of 15 percent of the existing dose can be made at weekly intervals. Bed rest and the initiation of steroid therapy may acutely lower muscle enzyme levels by up to 50 percent.

Improvement of muscle strength lags 2 to 4 weeks behind that of the muscle enzymes. Since corticosteroid-induced muscle weakness may begin to obscure progress after 4 to 6 weeks, in tapering the dose of corticosteroids one should not wait for a major improvement of muscle strength as long as the serum levels of muscle enzymes are normal or nearly so. Fluorinated corticosteroids, which may be particularly prone to cause myopathy, are best avoided. In some patients, despite a satisfactory return of strength, CPK and aldolase levels remain in the range of twice normal unless unacceptably high doses of prednisone are continued. It may be preferable in this situation to pursue lower-dose therapy if muscle strength is improving.

A satisfactory response to steroid therapy can be expected in about two-thirds of cases [25,60]. Patients with polymyositis or dermatomyositis respond equally well but the response rate is considerably less in patients whose disease is associated with a tumor.

If corticosteroid therapy proves effective, alternate-day therapy can be attempted once the daily dose has been reduced to the range of 30 mg of prednisone. The author prefers to wean the patients to an alternate-day dose. Another practice is to change abruptly to an alternate-day dose approximately twice the daily dose and continue tapering after a short period for stabilization. Unfortunately, less than half of those whose disease responds to daily steroid can be controlled on alternate-day therapy [60].

The benefit of physical rest is often overlooked and is extremely important during the active phase of disease. As noted, serum enzyme levels fall substantially with bed rest alone and control of the disease may be gained with much lower doses of steroid than would be possible otherwise. Physical therapy, except for gentle range of motion exercises done once daily to prevent contractures, is best not started until some control of the inflammatory process is obtained. Thereafter, light resistance exercise is given in bed and graded resistance added when enzyme levels have become normal or nearly so.

If enzyme levels are not controlled or strength improved after 4 to 6 weeks on prednisone doses in the range of 1.5 mg/kg per day, other therapy should be instituted. At the present time three options are available: cytotoxic drugs, plasmapheresis, or low-dose total-body radiation. The last of these is still highly experimental [61]. Methotrexate has been the most successfully used cytotoxic drug [62,63]. Hepatotoxicity may be reduced by giving it parenterally in a dose of 0.5 to 1.0 mg/kg body weight once a week. A clinical response may require 5 to 10 weeks of treatment. Intervals between doses are increased as the disease allows once muscle enzymes are normal. Of the other cytotoxic drugs, cyclophosphamide has been used successfully [60]. However, clinical studies in which azathioprine and corticosteroid therapy was compared to corticosteroid therapy alone failed to show any superiority for that combination [64].

Plasmapheresis has been used effectively in juvenile dermatomyositis and in some adult cases of both polymyositis and dermatomyositis. In one series, 32 of 35 cases improved after having received between 4 and 33 plasmapheresis treatments [21]; however all patients were simultaneously treated with corticosteroid and a cytotoxic agent. The component that is responsible for disease activity and that is removed by plasmapheresis has not been identified. Improvement is often not apparent until 2 to 3 weeks after plasmapheresis is started. It is general practice to continue corticosteroid therapy and often cytotoxic drugs during plasmapheresis.

Course and prognosis

The course of individual cases of polymyositis or dermatomyositis is unpredictable. About two-thirds of cases respond initially to corticosteroid and at least one-half have a favorable long-term result on either low doses of corticosteroid or none [5,25,60]. Fewer patients with tumor-associated myositis respond and the death rate is high, although usually from the tumor rather than the myositis itself.

In one large series of patients followed for a mean of 5 years the death rate in cases not associated with a tumor was approximately 20 percent for both polymyositis and dermatomyositis. Children fared somewhat better than adults [60]. When patients with tumors are excluded there is no difference in the prognosis of polymyositis and dermatomyositis. In general, patients with overlap syndromes have milder but often very chronic myositis.

Patients with weakness of bulbar musculature have a substantially worse prognosis, in part because they more often have an associated malignancy. These patients in particular, but also others with severe myopathy, may develop weakness of the muscles of respiration. This can happen insidiously and be manifest only by anxiety, hypertension, or simply unexplained acidosis. If there is any reason to suspect involvement of thoracic or diaphragmatic muscle, ventilation and arterial blood gases must be monitored. Nasogastric tube feeding is far preferable to intravenous nutrition if dysphagia is present. However since the weakness is of the pharyngeal muscles, a tracheostomy may be necessary also.

The dermal component of dermatomyositis may improve with systemic steroid therapy or remain more or less active despite improvement of the myositis. Topical corticosteroid is helpful but carries the risk of worsening the poikilodermatous changes that often follow the active dermatitis. It should be used sparingly. Sunlight exposure must be avoided.

There is no effective treatment for the distressing complication of calcinosis universalis that affects about 40 percent of children to some degree. Reports of a beneficial effect of chelation therapy with EDTA or the administration of diphosphonate have not been substantiated [65].

All patients over age 50 who develop dermatomyositis should be investigated for an associated malignancy. There is no specific tumor type, the common tumors being those most commonly associated with a myopathy [66,67]. Successful removal or treatment of a malignant tumor is often followed by improvement of the myositis. Adult celiac disease complicates a small number of cases of polymyositis [68].

References

1. Carpenter S, Karpati G: The major inflammatory myopathies of unknown cause. *Pathol Annu* 16:205, 1981
2. Isenberg DA, Snaith M: Muscle disease in systemic lupus erythematosus. *J Rheumatol* 8:917, 1981
3. Oxhandler R et al: Pathology of skeletal muscle in mixed connective tissue disease. *Arthritis Rheum* 20:985, 1977
4. Clements PJ et al: Muscle disease in progressive systemic sclerosis: diagnostic and therapeutic considerations. *Arthritis Rheum* 21:62, 1978
5. Bohan A et al: A computer assisted analysis of 153 patients with polymyositis and dermatomyositis. *Medicine (Baltimore)* 56:255, 1977
6. Ringel SP et al: Sjögren's syndrome and polymyositis or dermatomyositis. *Arch Neurol* 39:157, 1982
7. O'Leary PA, Waisman M: Dermatomyositis, a study of 40 cases. *Arch Dermatol Syphilol* 41:1001, 1940
8. Everett MA, Curtis AC: Dermatomyositis. *Arch Intern Med* 100:70, 1957
9. Walton JN, Adams RD: *Polymyositis.* Edinburgh, E & S Livingston, 1958
10. Swartz MN: Myositis, in *Principles and Practice of Infectious Diseases,* edited by GL Mandel et al. New York, John Wiley & Sons, 1979, p 818
11. Ruff RL, Secrist D: Viral studies in acute benign childhood myositis. *Arch Neurol* 39:261, 1982
12. Phillips PE et al: Increased *Toxoplasma* antibodies in ideopathic inflammatory muscle disease. *Arthritis Rheum* 22:209, 1979
13. Kakulas B et al: In vitro destruction of human fetal muscle cultures by peripheral blood lymphocytes from patients with polymyositis and lupus erythematosus. *Proc Aust Assoc Neurol* 8:85, 1971
14. Dawkins RL, Mastaglia FL: Cell mediated cytotoxicity to muscle in polymyositis. Effect of immunosuppression. *N Engl J Med* 288:434, 1973
15. Haas D: Absence of cell mediated cytotoxicity to muscle cultures in polymyositis. *J Rheumatol* 7:671, 1980
16. Iannaccone ST et al: Cell mediated cytotoxicity and childhood dermatomyositis. *Arch Neurol* 39:400, 1982
17. Smith PD et al: Current progress in the study of allergic polymyositis in guinea pig and man, in *Clinical Neuroimmunology,* edited by FC Rose. Oxford, Blackwell Scientific, 1979, p 146
18. Rowe DJ et al: Characterization of polymyositis infiltrates using monoclonal antibodies to human leukocyte antigens. *Clin Exp Immunol* 45:290, 1981
19. Watson AJS et al: Immunologic studies in cimetidine-induced nephropathy and polymyositis. *N Engl J Med* 308:142, 1983
20. Behan WMH et al: Detection of immune complexes in polymyositis. *Acta Neurol Scand* 65:320, 1982
21. Dau PC: Plasmapheresis in ideopathic inflammatory myopathy. Experience with 35 patients. *Arch Neurol* 38:544, 1981
22. Leddy J et al: Hereditary complement (C2) deficiency with dermatomyositis. *Am J Med* 58:83, 1975
23. Krain LS: Dermatomyositis in six patients without initial muscle involvement. *Arch Dermatol* 111:241, 1975
24. Morgan-Hughes J: Painful disorders of muscle. *Br J Hosp Med* 22:360, 1979
25. DeVere R, Bradley WG: Polymyositis: its presentation, morbidity and mortality. *Brain* 98:637, 1975
26. Pestronk A, Drachman DB: Reduction of acetylcholine receptors in polymyositis. *Neurology (NY)* 32:A120, 1982
27. Gottron H: Haut veranderungen bei Dermatomyositis, in *VIII Congres International de Dermatologie,* 1930, edited by S Lomholt. Copenhagen, Engelsen and Schroder, 1931, p 826
28. Spencer-Green G et al: Nailfold capillary abnormalities and clinical outcome in childhood dermatomyositis. *Arthritis Rheum* 25:954, 1982
29. Braverman IM: *Skin Signs of Systemic Diseases,* 2d ed. Philadelphia, WB Saunders, 1981, p 302
30. Schumacher HR et al: Articular manifestations of polymyositis and dermatomyositis. *Am J Med* 67:287, 1979
31. Haupt HM, Hutchins GM: The heart and cardiac conduction system in polymyositis-dermatomyositis. A clinicopathologic study of 16 autopsied patients. *Am J Cardiol* 50:998, 1982
32. Kehoe RF et al: Cardiac conduction defects in polymyositis. *Ann Intern Med* 94:41, 1981
33. Conley CL, Eggelston JC: Thymoma with myositis and myocarditis. *Johns Hopkins Med J* 140:69, 1977
34. Songcharoen S et al: Interstitial lung disease in polymyositis and dermatomyositis. *J Rheumatol* 7:353, 1980
35. Pachman LM, Cooke N: Juvenile dermatomyositis. A clinical and immunologic study. *J Pediatr* 96:226, 1980
36. Thompson C: Infantile myositis. *Dev Med Child Neurol* 24:30, 1982
37. Banker BO, Victor M: Dermatomyositis systemic angiopathy of childhood. *Medicine (Baltimore)* 45:261, 1966
38. Crowe WE et al: Clinical and pathogenetic implications of histopathology in childhood polydermatomyositis. *Arthritis Rheum* 25:126, 1982
39. Sewell RL et al: Calcinosis in juvenile dermatomyositis. *Skeletal Radiol* 3:137, 1978
40. Rowland LP, Penn AS: Myoglobinuria. *Med Clin North Am* 56:1233, 1972
41. Munsat TL et al: Serum enzyme alterations in muscular disorders. *JAMA* 226:1536, 1973

42. Warmolts JR: Electrodiagnosis in neuromuscular disorders. *Ann Intern Med* **95**:599, 1981

43. Sandstedt ER, Henriksson KG: Quantitative electromyography in polymyositis and dermatomyositis. *Acta Neurol Scand* **65**:110, 1982

44. Barwick DD, Walton J: Polymyositis. *Am J Med* **35**:646, 1963

45. Edwards R et al: Needle biopsy of skeletal muscle in the diagnosis of myopathy and the clinical study of muscle function and repair. *N Engl J Med* **302**:261, 1980

46. Janis JF, Winklemann RK: Histopathology of the skin in dermatomyositis. *Arch Dermatol* **97**:640, 1968

47. Wolfe JF et al: Antinuclear antibody with distinct specificity for polymyositis. *J Clin Invest* **59**:176, 1977

48. Edwards RHT et al: Clinical use of nuclear magnetic resonance in the investigation of myopathy. *Lancet* **2**:725, 1981

49. Keil H: The manifestations in the skin and mucous membranes in dermatomyositis with special reference to the differential diagnosis from systemic lupus erythematosus. *Ann Intern Med* **16**:828, 1942

50. Chad D et al: Inclusion body myositis associated with Sjögren's syndrome. *Arch Neurol* **39**:186, 1982

51. Itoh J et al: The rash of dermatomyositis in sarcoid myopathy. *Neurology (NY)* **30**:118, 1980

52. Topi GC et al: Dermatomyositis-like syndrome due to *Toxoplasma. Br J Dermatol* **101**:589, 1979

53. Lane RJM, Mastaglia FL: Drug-induced myopathies in man. *Lancet* **2**:562, 1978

54. Doyle DR et al: Fatal polymyositis in D-penicillamine treated rheumatoid arthritis. *Ann Intern Med* **98**:327, 1983

55. Martin FC et al: Alcoholic muscle disease. *Br Med Bull* **38**:53, 1982

56. Knochel JP: The pathophysiology and clinical characteristics of severe hypophosphatemia. *Arch Intern Med* **137**:203, 1977

57. Harrington TM et al: Elevation of creatine kinase in amyotrophic lateral sclerosis. *Arthritis Rheum* **26**:201, 1983

58. DiGirolami U, Smith TW: Muscle pathology—a teaching monograph. *Am J Pathol* **107**:231, 1982

59. Kar N, Pearson CM: Muscle adenylate deaminase deficiency. Report of six new cases. *Arch Neurol* **38**:279, 1981

60. Henriksson KG, Sandstedt P: Polymyositis—treatment and prognosis. A study of 107 patients. *Acta Neurol Scand* **65**:280, 1982

61. Engel WK et al: Polymyositis: remarkable response to total body irradiation. *Neurology (NY)* **32**:A120, 1982

62. Metzger AL et al: Polymyositis and dermatomyositis: combined methotrexate and corticosteroid therapy. *Ann Intern Med* **81**:182, 1974

63. Niakan E et al: Immunosuppressive agents in corticosteroid refractory childhood dermatomyositis. *Neurology (NY)* **30**:286, 1980

64. Bunch TW et al: Azathioprine with prednisone for polymyositis. *Ann Intern Med* **92**:365, 1980

65. Metzger AL et al: Failure of disodium etidronate in calcinosis due to dermatomyositis and scleroderma. *N Engl J Med* **291**:1294, 1974

66. Barnes B: Dermatomyositis and malignancy. *Ann Intern Med* **84**:68, 1976

67. Callen JP: The value of malignancy evaluation in patients with dermatomyositis. *J Am Acad Dermatol* **6**:253, 1982

68. Henriksson KG et al: Polymyositis and adult celiac disease. *Acta Neurol Scand* **65**:301, 1982

CHAPTER 154

SCLERODERMA

Arthur Z. Eisen, Jouni J. Uitto, and Eugene A. Bauer

Definition

Scleroderma is a chronic disease of unknown cause which may occur as a localized form, *morphea,* or as a systemic disease, *systemic sclerosis* (systemic scleroderma). Systemic sclerosis is a progressive and often fatal disorder characterized by diffuse involvement of the connective tissue of the dermis leading to induration and thickening of the skin and fibrous deposition in certain internal organs. Several clinical forms of localized scleroderma are recognized. The most common type is morphea, in which the lesions are usually single or few in number. A generalized form of morphea, frequently having symmetric and bilateral lesions, also occurs. The absence of Raynaud's phenomenon, acrosclerosis, and organ involvement differentiates it from systemic scleroderma. A guttate variant of morphea has been described, but its status is tenuous since it may be a variety of lichen sclerosus et atrophicus. A linear form of localized scleroderma also occurs in which the lesions are arranged in a bandlike linear distribution and may involve the deeper layers of the skin and underlying structures. Hemiatrophy and other deformities may be associated with linear scleroderma.

Epidemiology

Localized scleroderma is a relatively uncommon disorder. Women are affected approximately three times as often as men. From the reported cases, the disease appears to be much more common in whites than in blacks. In a large series [1], 75 percent of the cases of morphea had their onset between the second and fifth decades. In linear scleroderma, the age of onset is younger, a majority occurring before the age of 40 and a significant number in the first two decades of life.

Systemic scleroderma is also four times more common in women than in men, with the sex difference most evident during the child-bearing years. Although once thought to be more common in whites, it has now been shown that there are no significant racial differences in incidence. The disease does increase in frequency with age among white females, but the occurrence of the disease is relatively stable among black females throughout adulthood. Although the precise incidence of systemic sclerosis is unknown, it has been estimated that the average annual incidence of systemic scleroderma is 2.7 new patients per million population [2]. Although the disease may occur at almost any time in life, it is relatively uncommon in childhood. In a majority of patients, the onset is between 30 and 50 years of age.

In a large combined study of 309 patients from two different geographic areas of the country, the 7-year survival after entry into the study was 35 percent [3]. A significantly decreased survival rate was found in older patients of both groups after allowance was made for the natural increase in mortality with age. Females had a significantly better survival rate than males and the mortality from scleroderma for black females was significantly greater than for white females, a finding which differs from earlier observations [4]. In the large combined study [3] the survival for blacks was significantly worse than for whites during the first year of follow-up but not in subsequent years. It is not surprising that involvement of kidney, heart, and lung (in that order) significantly decreased the survival rate. Although the disease has been reported to be more common in underground coal and gold miners [5], it is not felt that silica exposure itself is a principal factor in the cause of the disease. An unusual syndrome characterized by Raynaud's phenomenon, morphea-like skin changes, capillary abnormalities of the nail fold (similar to those seen in systemic sclerosis), osteolysis of the distal phalanges, and hepatic and pulmonary fibrosis, has been reported in workers exposed to polyvinyl chloride [6,7]. The relationship of this disorder to systemic sclerosis remains unclear. The antitumor agent bleomycin has also been reported to produce cutaneous changes indistinguishable from systemic sclerosis [8] as well as pulmonary fibrosis and Raynaud's phenomenon [9]. The development of these changes appears to be dose-dependent and is reversible following discontinuation of the drug. Familial cases of systemic scleroderma have been reported but a clear-cut genetic predisposition for the disease has not been established [9,10].

Clinical manifestations

Localized morphea is characterized by circumscribed, sclerotic plaques with an ivory-colored center and a surrounding violaceous halo. The presence of the violaceous border signifies that the disease is in an active state. The lesion often begins as an erythematous area which may show some nonpitting edema. The center gradually becomes white or yellowish in color. Frequently, there is an absence of hair and a diminished sweat response within the lesion. The plaques, which may be either slightly elevated or depressed, are firm and indurated or hard but not bound to the deeper structures. Most commonly the lesions are single or few in number but in some cases they are multiple. Their size varies from 1 to 30 cm [7].

Generalized morphea, a severe form of the local disease, is characterized by widespread skin involvement with multiple indurated plaques, hyperpigmentation and, frequently, muscle atrophy. The lesions involve the upper trunk, abdomen, buttocks, and legs and, in the early stages, the plaques are often indistinguishable from localized morphea although they may be larger. Generalized morphea is not associated with systemic disease. Antinuclear antibodies, elevated immunoglobulins, and the presence of rheumatoid factor have been reported in all forms of localized scleroderma [11,12] but the overall incidence

has not been adequately determined. The prognosis is good, with the disease frequently becoming inactive in 3 to 5 years [1]. As with localized morphea, slight atrophy, often with hyperpigmentation, may be the only persisting evidence of previous skin involvement. In severe cases, disability may result from the muscle atrophy.

Guttate morphea is an uncommon variant of localized morphea. Considerable confusion still exists between this entity and lichen sclerosus et atrophicus. However, it should be emphasized that morphea and lichen sclerosus et atrophicus can occur simultaneously in the same patient. The authors have reported [13] the coexistence of these two disorders in 10 patients, with the same lesion frequently showing histologic evidence of both diseases. This suggests that these lesions may reflect similar etiologic events or closely related pathologic processes in the two diseases. Guttate morphea is characterized by multiple, small, chalk-white lesions primarily involving the anterior chest, neck, shoulders, and occasionally other areas of the body. The lesions do not have the firm sclerotic character of morphea.

Linear scleroderma is a form of the localized disease which appears in a linear bandlike distribution. The lesions are usually single and unilateral. The lower extremities are most frequently involved, followed by the upper extremities, frontal regions of the head, and anterior thorax [1]. Both the upper and lower extremities may be simultaneously involved, with the lesions being primarily homolateral in such cases. Calcinosis within a linear lesion may rarely occur. Frontal or frontal parietal linear scleroderma, *coup de sabre,* is characterized by atrophy and a furrow, or depression, that extends below the level of the surrounding skin. In severe cases the atrophic furrow may extend, producing facial hemiatrophy on the corresponding side. Atrophy of the tongue on the same side as the lesion may be present. Active plaques of morphea may occur on the homolateral side of the face in association with linear frontal lesions.

An important distinction between linear scleroderma and morphea is that linear scleroderma tends to involve not only the superficial but also the deeper layers of the skin, with fixation to underlying structures. Since the onset of linear scleroderma occurs most frequently during the first two decades of life, severe deformities, such as hemiatrophy of an extremity or a side of the face as well as contractures, may result [14]. Linear scleroderma may also be associated with anomalies of the vertebral column, the most common being spina bifida occulta [1,15]. *Melorheostosis,* an unusual linear, dense, cortical hyperostosis often affecting an involved limb, but occasionally widespread, may also rarely occur [16].

The *Parry-Romberg syndrome* (facial hemiatrophy) may well be a form of linear scleroderma but this has not been established (see Chap. 172). The facial hemiatrophy syndrome is characterized initially by hyperpigmentation followed by atrophy of the dermis, subcutaneous fat, muscle, and occasionally the underlying bone. The degree of atrophy is usually deeper than that associated with coup de sabre. Although the skin may be atrophic, it is less often bound down, but still it may not be possible to make a distinction between the two disorders. Whether scleroderma-like hemiatrophy involving the face, which may spread to involve the homolateral and occasionally the contralateral side of the body, represents a variation of the Parry-Romberg syndrome has not been established. It is of interest to note that one case of progressive facial hemiatrophy has been reported [17] with a positive ANA, rheumatoid factor, and elevated gamma globulins, findings which may also be associated with linear scleroderma.

In *systemic scleroderma* the clinical manifestations depend on the site of predominant involvement. The initial complaints usually are related either to Raynaud's phenomenon or to chronic, usually nonpitting, edema of the hands and fingers. As many as one-third of the patients may have initial pain and stiffness of the fingers and knee joints. A true polyarthritis, frequently migratory, may also occur and in some cases may represent the first manifestation of the disease. Severe erosive digital osteoarthritis (particularly in females with the CREST syndrome) may also occur [9]. Radiographically a high frequency of flexion contractures, digital tuft resorption, sclerodactyly, and subcutaneous calcification is seen. Additionally, joint space narrowing and focal erosions to the dorsal aspects of metacarpophalangeal or proximal heads, may also be present. Most commonly, skin changes precede visceral involvement by several years, but occasionally this is reversed [9].

The skin of the fingers and hands usually is involved first. Gradually, extension occurs to involve the upper extremities (Fig. 154-1), trunk, face (Fig. 154-2), and finally the lower extremities, which in some cases are spared. In the early stages there may be a peculiar, painless, slightly pitting type of edema frequently lasting several months before tightening of the skin occurs. Often the skin feels indurated and stiff, and as the disease progresses to the atrophic state, it becomes tense, smooth, hardened, and eventually firmly bound to the underlying structures (see Fig. A2-6b). The skin of the face becomes masklike and

Fig. 154-1 Scleroderma. The fingers and hands, which are usually involved first, develop a stiffness and the skin becomes firmly bound to the underlying structures so that it becomes impossible to completely flex the hand.

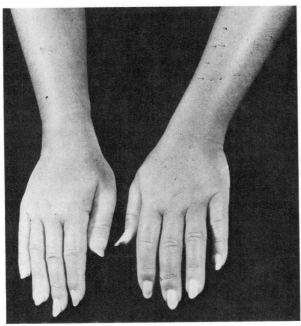

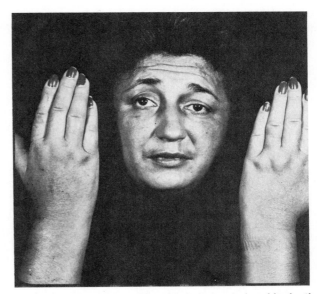

Fig. 154-2 Scleroderma. The skin is indurated and inelastic with a loss of normal facial lines.

expressionless with a loss of the normal facial lines and the skin of the forehead appearing smooth. However, isolated periorbital edema [18] may occur in the early edematous phase in patients with few other manifestations of systemic scleroderma. As the disease progresses, there is thinning of the lips, the opening of the mouth is constricted (microstomia) (see Fig. A2-6a), and radial furrowing around the mouth is not infrequent (Fig. 154-3). Uncommonly, the mucous membranes may be involved, with painful induration of the gums and tongue. Tightening of the skin over the nasal cartilage, giving the nose a small, sharp appearance, is a prominent feature (see Fig. A2-6a). Matlike telangiectases, particularly about the face and the upper trunk, may also develop. Occasionally there is a thinning or complete loss of hair and anhidrosis in the affected areas. Generalized hyperpigmentation, resembling Addison's disease but without biochemical evidence of adrenal insufficiency, can occur. The addisonian pigmentation may at times antedate the sclerotic changes and is not associated with elevated levels of plasma beta-MSH [19]. Focal hy-

Fig. 154-3 Radial furrowing around the mouth in a patient with systemic scleroderma.

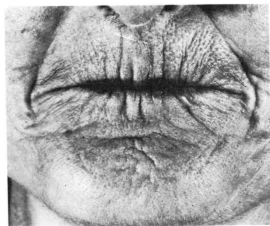

perpigmentation or hypopigmentation, perhaps representing a postinflammatory response, may be seen in areas of sclerosis.

Sclerodactyly may occur as the fingers become tapered with marked atrophy of the overlying skin (see Fig. A2-6b). Periungual telangiectasia, as in systemic lupus erythematosus (SLE) and dermatomyositis, can frequently be seen in cases of scleroderma. Capillary microscopy of the nail folds (which can be performed with an ophthalmoscope) may be useful in confirming the diagnosis of scleroderma [20]. Enlarged, dilated nail fold capillaries forming "giant" or sausage-shaped loops have been reported in as many as 75 percent of the cases of systemic sclerosis. The pattern seen in scleroderma cannot be distinguished from that seen in dermatomyositis but can clearly be distinguished from the capillary changes in SLE. Similar nail fold capillary changes have been reported in patients with Raynaud's disease in which a significant number have subsequently developed systemic sclerosis [21]. Thus, capillary microscopy may be of prognostic value in Raynaud's disease. Recurrent painful ulcerations of the fingertips, which frequently become secondarily infected, are a common problem (Fig. 154-4). Slow-healing ulcers over the knuckles may also be present. The ulcers can become chronic but often heal with stellate scarring. Gangrene, although rare, may develop. The fingers become stiff, and flexion contractures trouble many patients. Resorption of bone may result in complete dissolution of one or more terminal phalanges. Cutaneous calcification develops in some cases and is often particularly evident about the fingertips and bony prominences. It can occur in any area involved in the sclerodermatous process. The large calcified deposits may ulcerate, extrude calcified material, and reepithelialize very slowly.

Radiologic examination of the teeth of patients with systemic scleroderma often shows widening of the periodontal membrane and loss of the lamina dura. Bone reabsorption at the angle of the mandible, perhaps secondary to tightness of the facial skin and atrophy of the underlying muscles, can also occur.

Systemic involvement may manifest itself in a variety of ways. Esophageal dysfunction represents the most common internal manifestation (over 90 percent) found in patients with systemic scleroderma. Dysphagia due to diminished or absent peristalsis, particularly in the distal two-thirds of the esophagus, may readily be revealed by radiologic or manometric examination. Heartburn from reflux esophagitis, resulting from a loss of tone of the gastro-

esophageal sphincter, is another common manifestation, but esophageal hemorrhage is rare. Patients with dysphagia, often occurring long before the development of any skin involvement, have been described [22], giving rise to the concept of scleroderma sine scleroderma. Abnormal esophageal motility in patients with Raynaud's phenomenon in the absence of concomitant evidence of connective tissue disease, as well as in those with scleroderma, dermatomyositis, and in a few with lupus erythematosus has been reported [23]. The small intestine also may be involved and produce symptoms of constipation, diarrhea, abdominal bloating, and, in some, the malabsorption syndrome. Delayed transit, prolonged retention of barium, and distention of the small intestine, all secondary to atonia of the bowel, are frequent radiologic findings.

Pulmonary involvement is an extremely important feature of systemic scleroderma, resulting in pulmonary fibrosis in many patients. Exertional dyspnea is a frequent complaint, and small airway disease is often an early and sensitive indicator of pulmonary involvement, often preceding measurable impairment of gas diffusion [24]. Cardiac involvement, leading to conduction defects and heart failure, may also occur in systemic scleroderma. Pericarditis, often associated with pericardial effusion, occasionally leading to cardiac tamponade, is a common form of heart disease in scleroderma.

Renal involvement is a frequent occurrence and although some patients develop slowly progressive uremia, in the majority, renal failure is abrupt and often associated with a highly malignant form of arterial hypertension. Although there has been some suggestion that the development of acute renal failure and hypertension may be induced by the administration of corticosteroids, it should be made clear that these findings have occurred in patients who have never received steroid therapy [9].

CREST syndrome

A clinically recognized variant of scleroderma is the CREST syndrome, which refers to the presence of calcinosis cutis, Raynaud's phenomenon, esophageal dysfunction, sclerodactyly, and telangiectasia. Although the vascular lesions are most evident on the cutaneous surface, particularly the face, upper trunk, and hands, they also occur on the lips, oral mucous membranes, and throughout the entire gastrointestinal tract. Gastrointestinal bleeding is uncommon, but it does occur in the CREST syndrome. Generally the CREST syndrome is a more slowly progressive form of the disease, with the development of clinical features later in life than in systemic sclerosis, and thus, has a more favorable prognosis. It should not be regarded as a separate entity and is not an entirely benign syndrome as evidenced by the development of esophageal dysfunction, identical to that seen in systemic sclerosis, and occasionally the presence of pulmonary hypertension and biliary cirrhosis. In addition, these patients may show signs of Sjögren's syndrome. Antibodies to centromeric chromatin, anticentromere antibodies, have been reported to characterize the CREST syndrome [25]. These antibodies have been found in 50 to 96 percent of patients with CREST and in only 7 to 12 percent of individuals with systemic sclerosis [26]. It has been suggested that these autoantibodies may be of prognostic value since they may

Fig. 154-4   Ulceration of the fingertips in a patient with Raynaud's phenomenon and scleroderma.

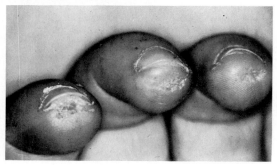

appear prior to the development of the full clinical picture of the CREST syndrome and are associated with longer duration of disease and less systemic involvement.

Patients with combined features of scleroderma, lupus erythematosus, and myositis have been grouped under the term *mixed connective tissue disease*. These patients have high titers of antibody to ribonucleoprotein, the so-called extractable nuclear antigen [27,28]. Patients with systemic scleroderma alone have not been found to have antibodies to this antigen [27].

Eosinophilic fasciitis

A scleroderma-like syndrome described by Shulman [29], in which the prognosis is clearly better than for systemic scleroderma, has now been named eosinophilic fasciitis (for review see [30]). Considerable question still exists as to whether eosinophilic fasciitis is a distinct entity or a variant of scleroderma. This syndrome may have its beginning after undue physical exertion, and often tends to have a seasonal onset with many cases beginning in the autumn. It is characterized by firm, often puckered skin that is tightly bound to underlying structures, considerable pain and swelling of the extremities but with sparing of the hands and feet, arthralgias, eosinophilia, hypergammaglobulinemia, fasciitis, and occasionally myositis. Trunk and facial involvement is uncommon. In addition, only 12 to 15 percent of patients have antinuclear or anti-DNA antibodies. The inflammatory infiltrate in the fascia and muscle is predominantly round cell in nature, consisting of plasma cells, lymphocytes, and occasional eosinophils, with the development of lymphoid follicles. The patients do not have Raynaud's phenomenon or evidence of visceral scleroderma. Although the natural history is unknown, the response to corticosteroids is often dramatic. In one case, cimetidine has been reported [31] to produce marked improvement in this syndrome. Whether this will prove to be an effective form of therapy, and the mechanisms whereby it produces this effect, must await further studies.

Cutaneous histopathology

The cutaneous pathologic features of morphea and systemic scleroderma, as seen in any single histopathologic preparation, depend upon the stage of the disease as well as the site from which the biopsy is obtained (Figs. 154-5 to 154-8). In morphea, specimens obtained from the peripheral violaceous border show a striking accumulation of inflammatory cells among collagen bundles of the lower two-thirds of the reticular dermis and among collagen bundles of the fibrous trabeculae of the subcutaneous tissue. In addition, inflammatory cells frequently are seen among the fat cells of the subcutaneous tissue. Usually lymphocytes and histiocytes are predominant, but in many instances large numbers of plasma cells may be seen and occasionally there is an increase in mast cells. The formation of typical lymphoid follicles with germinal centers has also been observed [32]. Mononuclear cell infiltrates are frequently less common in systemic sclerosis than in localized scleroderma (49 vs. 84 percent) and often less severe [33].

Associated with the inflammatory infiltrate are collagen changes which first occur in the lower third of the dermis

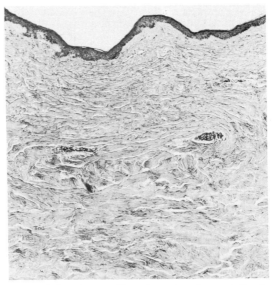

Fig. 154-5 Scleroderma. The changes of generalized scleroderma and localized scleroderma (morphea) overlap; the former, however, is dominated by dense, acellular sclerosis, and the latter shows varying degrees of inflammation with some extension into the subcutis. Figs. 154-5 and 154-6 show the pathologic changes of scleroderma and Figs. 154-7 and 154-8 the pathologic changes of morphea. In the above photomicrograph one sees broad collagen bundles which tend to parallel each other, diminished interbundle spaces, and few cells of any kind. × 40. (Micrograph by Wallace H. Clark, Jr., M.D.)

Fig. 154-6 Scleroderma. The collagen bundle pattern of the reticular dermis is virtually obliterated, and one cannot distinguish between papillary and reticular dermis. × 160. (Micrograph by Wallace H. Clark, Jr., M.D.)

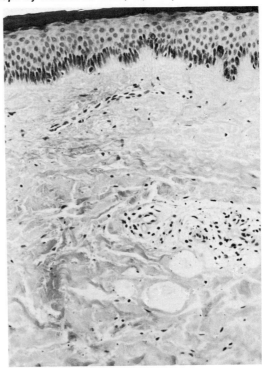

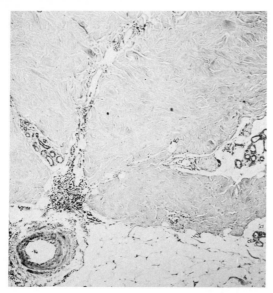

Fig. 154-7   Morphea. The connective tissue changes in morphea seem to extend from the lower reticular dermis outward and are usually indistinguishable from the changes of generalized scleroderma. Biopsies taken from the margins of morphea lesions, however, frequently show extensive inflammation; such inflammation may be patchy, as one sees here, or it may involve the reticular dermis rather diffusely, presenting some difficulty in histologic diagnosis. × 40. (Micrograph by Wallace H. Clark, Jr., M.D.)

and in the fibrous trabeculae of the subcutaneous tissues. In the later stages of the disease the changes extend to the upper portion of the dermis. These changes consist of a striking increase in collagen eosinophilia, broadening of the collagen bundles, and a decreased interbundle space, so that the normal shrinkage of collagen bundles characterized by formalin-fixed, paraffin-embedded material is obscured. Biopsies taken from the central region of well-developed lesions of morphea may show only the collagen

Fig. 154-8   Morphea. A higher magnification of an area of Fig. 154-7. × 160. (Micrograph by Wallace H. Clark, Jr., M.D.)

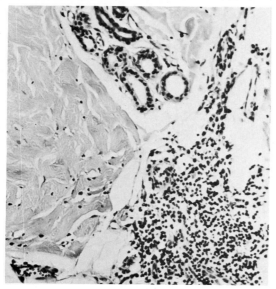

changes with little evidence of inflammation. In the late stages of morphea the pathologic process is similar to that of systemic scleroderma. The collagen bundle pattern tends to be altered so that most bundles appear to parallel the dermal-epidermal interface. The inflammatory stage is followed by the replacement of the subcutaneous tissue by hyalinized connective tissue [32]. Electron microscopic observations [34] indicate that the fibrous trabeculae of the subcutaneous tissue are increased in thickness due to the deposition of immature collagen fibrils with a much smaller diameter than normal, suggesting increased collagen synthesis in the subcutaneous tissue.

In systemic scleroderma, there is sclerosis of the lower two-thirds of the dermis as well as in the subcutaneous fibrous trabeculae. Indeed, the subcutaneous fat is virtually replaced by hyalinized connective tissue [35]. The replacement of fatty tissue by connective tissue is particularly evident around the eccrine sweat glands. These findings may be associated with a panniculitis that may be a prominent feature during the early stages of the disease. The collagen is pale and homogeneous in appearance and there is some swelling of collagen bundles. The collagen bundle swelling, enhanced eosinophilia, and inflammatory component are not as prominent as in morphea. A marked increase in ground substance, glycosaminoglycans, as demonstrated by special stains, has been reported [35]. In the late stages of systemic scleroderma, secondary changes such as absence of pilosebaceous units, eccrine ducts and glands, and effacement of the rete ridges of the epidermis may be evident. These abnormalities, which may at times be quite striking, are of little diagnostic significance except to indicate that the process is at a relatively advanced stage. Electron microscopic observations [35] have revealed the presence of randomly arranged "immature" collagen fibrils, ranging in diameter from 100 to 400 Å in contrast to the mature collagen fibers with a diameter of approximately 700 to 800 Å. Whether the "immature" collagen fibrils represent newly synthesized collagen remains speculative at this time.

Vascular involvement has been described as an important, although not necessarily consistent, feature of systemic scleroderma, and vessels of all sizes may be involved. In the early edematous stages, there may be only dilatations of capillaries and lymphatics. As the disease progresses, intimal proliferation and complete occlusion of the vessels may occur. Such changes may also be evident in muscle capillaries. Occlusive changes are not found in morphea, and although it is of interest to speculate that this may be related in some way to the spontaneous involution of the disease, the precise nature of this finding is not clear. In addition, the structure of skeletal muscle fibers underlying areas of affected skin in morphea may also show evidence of damage in the absence of changes in muscle capillaries [36].

Pathogenesis

The cause of scleroderma is unknown. However, it has been suggested [9] that immunologic abnormalities play a role and that they are the common denominator relating scleroderma to the rheumatic diseases (i.e., rheumatoid arthritis, SLE, and dermatomyositis). For example, scleroderma has been found in association with Hashimoto's thyroiditis and Sjögren's syndrome. In addition, hyperglobulinemia, usually moderate, with a diffuse nonspecific increase in gamma G globulin is present in about one-half the cases. Rheumatoid factor and antinuclear antibodies, frequently showing a speckled, or nucleolar, pattern have been demonstrated in as many as 95 percent of patients [37]. However, positive LE cell preparations are found in only about 5 percent. Antinucleolar antibodies [38] as well as antibodies to single-stranded RNA, which are specific for the uracil bases of RNA, have been found in sera of scleroderma patients [39]. Precipitating antibodies to a soluble 70,000 molecular weight nuclear protein called Scl 70 [40] have been found in approximately 20 percent of patients. These antibodies are immunochemically distinct from those found in SLE and may correspond to the antinucleolar antibodies [37]. Antibodies to DNA and antinuclear antibodies have been reported [41] in children and adults with both generalized and localized scleroderma (morphea).

It is of interest that antibodies to collagen types I and IV have been demonstrated in the sera of patients with systemic sclerosis who had diffuse interstitial lung disease [42]. The presence of these antibodies to types I and IV collagen correlated closely with the presence of abnormal, pulmonary diffusing capacity. The relationship of these findings to the fibrotic process and the vascular lesions in lung and other tissues remains to be determined. As already indicated, an extensive and intense inflammatory infiltrate composed of lymphocytes, histiocytes, and plasma cells is almost always present in the active areas from lesions of morphea and in systemic scleroderma. No correlation has been shown between the immunologic abnormalities and the presence or severity of the cellular infiltrates or with the duration of disease [43]. However, it has been demonstrated [44] that lymphokines from phytohemagglutinin-stimulated normal human peripheral blood mononuclear cells can cause increased collagen synthesis by human embryonic lung fibroblasts. In addition, phytohemagglutinin-stimulated normal human lymphocytes have been reported to increase collagen production in cultures of human skin fibroblasts [45]. Extracts of sclerodermatous skin can cause the release of macrophage-migration inhibition factor by lymphocytes from patients with scleroderma but not from normal subjects [46]. Thus lymphokines of patients with scleroderma have been shown to attract fibroblasts and to stimulate collagen production by these cells. Certain mitogens, such as platelet-derived growth factor, fibroblast growth factor, and nerve growth factor, do not have a selective effect on collagen synthesis in scleroderma fibroblasts [47]. However, scleroderma fibroblasts in culture are insensitive to the mitogenic effect of platelet-derived growth factor which does stimulate control skin fibroblasts [47], suggesting that perhaps in vivo exposure of scleroderma fibroblasts to platelet-derived growth factor has altered their ability to respond. It is also of interest that although normal human serum contains a factor(s) which markedly increases the production of type I and III procollagens by skin fibroblasts, the authors have found no evidence of a factor from the serum of patients with either systemic sclerosis or localized scleroderma which causes a further stimulation of procollagen synthesis [48].

Whether collagen serves as an autoantigen in the pathogenesis of scleroderma remains to be determined. However, it has been shown that peripheral blood leukocytes from patients with scleroderma, when cultured in the presence of type I collagen from normal human skin or with isolated alpha chains from chick skin collagen, elaborate a factor chemotactic for human monocytes and fibroblasts. In addition, 3 of 12 patients exhibited lymphocyte transformation in response to these antigens [49]. Thus far, however, it has not been possible to implicate immunologic changes directly in the pathogenesis of the disease, and it is important to point out that scleroderma not infrequently occurs in the absence of a demonstrable immunologic abnormality.

Although the lesions of morphea and systemic scleroderma have certain features in common, there are differences, as emphasized by the results of reciprocal skin transplantation experiments. Normal skin grafted into a lesion of morphea will become morphea-like over a period of 6 to 9 months [50]. Skin from a morphea lesion when grafted into an uninvolved region will transform to normal. In systemic scleroderma [51], when clinically normal skin was placed in a sclerodermatous bed it became involved with scleroderma. Scleroderma skin placed in a normal bed, however, remained sclerodermatous.

The initial concept that the connective tissue content in the skin and other tissues was increased in scleroderma was based largely on histologic observations in which the homogenization of collagen was equated with an increase in the total collagen content. Although electron microscopic studies have failed to demonstrate any consistent abnormality in the collagen fibers or the ground substance [52], they did suggest that there is an increased collagen biosynthesis in scleroderma skin [53]. Early studies showed that when the collagen content of skin punch biopsies from plaques of morphea was determined under a fixed area of skin, in results expressed as milligrams of collagen per square millimeter of skin [54], a significant increase in the collagen content was found, compared to control values. When expressed in terms of dry weight, the values for morphea were normal, emphasizing that relative expressions (i.e, milligrams of hydroxyproline or collagen per dry weight) do not represent an accurate reflection of the changes in total amounts of collagen in a given piece of skin. It has now also been clearly shown that in the skin of patients with systemic sclerosis there is marked increase in both skin thickness and dermal collagen content which is most striking in the indurative phase of the disease [55].

The evidence now indicates that the rate of collagen synthesis is increased in the skin of patients with active systemic sclerosis. This is based on the observation that the activity of prolyl hydroxylase, the enzyme that catalyzes the hydroxylation of proline in nascent peptide chains destined to be collagen, is increased in the skin of patients with active scleroderma [56–58]. In addition, the incorporation of radioactive proline and the synthesis of radioactive hydroxyproline in skin collagen is increased in skin biopsies obtained from patients during the active stage of scleroderma, when compared to normal controls [59,60]. In the rapidly progressive stages of scleroderma, skin collagen contains newly formed, labile cross-links, an observation consistent with excessive synthesis of new collagen [61].

Tissue culture studies employing fibroblasts from patients with scleroderma have also been used to assess collagen synthesis, but the results have been variable. LeRoy [62,63] first demonstrated that the synthesis of collagen by cultured fibroblasts from patients with scleroderma was increased on a per cell basis, as determined by measurements of total hydroxyproline synthesized by the fibroblasts. Although this finding was confirmed [64], others have indicated [65] that the synthesis of collagen by fibroblasts from scleroderma patients may be the same as that of normal control cells. Our studies [66], however, have also confirmed and extended those of LeRoy [62,63]. The results obtained indicate that the rate of procollagen synthesis by scleroderma skin fibroblasts in culture is indeed increased but that the ratios of type I/III procollagens in scleroderma cell lines do not differ from controls. Thus, the increased biosynthesis of procollagen by scleroderma fibroblasts is directed toward the synthesis of both type I and type III procollagens in the same relative ratio. These procollagens are also similar to the corresponding molecules synthesized by control fibroblasts. The demonstration of increased procollagen mRNA activity in scleroderma fibroblasts [67] adds further support to the concept that the accumulation of collagen in tissues in scleroderma is directly related to an increased rate of collagen biosynthesis. In addition to the increased accumulation of collagen in scleroderma, immunofluorescence studies have demonstrated a marked increase in fibronectin in the reticular dermis [68] which appears to parallel the distribution of collagen accumulation in the involved reticular dermis. It has also been shown that, in cultures, scleroderma skin fibroblasts derived from the lower portions of the dermis synthesize markedly increased levels of glycosaminoglycans [69]. Cells from the lower levels of the dermis were used because several studies have indicated that fibroblast cultures from this area synthesize increased amounts of collagen when compared to other levels of the skin [64,70,71]. Interestingly, the increased synthesis of glycosaminoglycans persists in culture for at least 10 generations; thus, this difference between normal and scleroderma cells can be propagated. These observations may account for the increased quantities of glycosaminoglycans that have been shown to be present in the skin of patients with systemic sclerosis [72].

The capacity of scleroderma cells as well as skin in organ culture to synthesize collagenase has also been examined [66]. No abnormalities in the synthesis of this enzyme were detected, thus the possibility that the increase in collagen in scleroderma is in part due to the absence of collagenase resulting in a decreased rate of collagen degradation [73] is not supported by these studies. It is not known, however, whether increased fibronectin, which can bind to the collagenase cleavage site in mammalian collagen [68], renders the substrate less susceptible to cleavage by collagenase.

Cultured human skin fibroblasts appear to be a heterogeneous population of cells, in that cells from the papillary dermis grow faster and longer than cells from the reticular dermis [74,75]. This suggests that selective factors may affect the final population of cells in a given area of skin in vivo. As a result of these and other studies [76] it has been postulated that the increased level of collagen production by cultured scleroderma fibroblasts represents in vivo selection of clones (from a heterogeneous fibroblast population) that have an increased capability to synthesize

collagen. Such a selection process would ultimately lead to an increased accumulation of connective tissue. There is, however, an intriguing alternative, namely that exposure of fibroblasts to mononuclear cell mediators in vivo may lead to a metabolic abnormality, such as increased collagen synthesis, that persists in vitro after multiple cell generations. That such effects can indeed occur has been shown by Korn [77] in studies of fibroblast prostaglandin E_2 synthesis. Exposing fibroblasts to mononuclear cell products in vitro resulted in a population of cells that produced abnormally high levels of prostaglandin E_2. This enhanced prostaglandin E_2 synthesis persisted in culture for as long as 20 weeks and 19 cell generations after the original exposure to mononuclear cell products.

Whether there is a specific abnormality in tryptophan metabolism in scleroderma remains unclear [78,79]. Serotonin in experimental animals causes localized fibrosis following repeated subcutaneous injections [80] but has not been identified as a significant factor in the pathogenesis of scleroderma. It has also been proposed [81] that there is impaired transformation of serotonin into 5-hydroxyindole acetic acid in subjects with scleroderma after tryptophan loading. It was suggested that the metabolism of biogenic amines derived from tryptophan in scleroderma is abnormal, perhaps as a result of impaired monoamine oxidase activity.

Vascular abnormalities have been implicated in the pathogenesis of scleroderma based on the frequent occurrence of Raynaud's phenomenon, which usually precedes skin changes, or the presence of periungual telangiectases, and on the histologic and ultrastructural capillary abnormalities in skin, muscle [82], and other viscera [83]. Patients with Raynaud's phenomenon also demonstrate a significantly decreased blood flow in their fingertips in both warm and cool environments unlike normal subjects who with body cooling show no change in capillary blood flow [84]. In addition, scleroderma patients, during a period of controlled cooling, were found to have a significantly reduced skin blood flow. Skin temperature during reflex warming was also subnormal in scleroderma despite a normal cutaneous blood flow [85]. Thus there is quantitative evidence of a disturbance of capillary function. Microscopically, the most prominent changes occur in small arteries or arterioles and consist of thickening of the walls as a result of intimal proliferation with luminal narrowing associated with hyaline or fibrinoid degeneration. Duplication of the basement membrane, which may be a feature of other collagen vascular diseases, is also frequently seen in scleroderma. In addition, autoradiographic studies [86] indicate an increase in [³H]thymidine labeling of endothelial cells of skin capillaries in systemic scleroderma, perhaps as an attempt to replace damaged cells. It is of interest that sera from some patients with scleroderma, but also patients with other connective tissue diseases, contain cytotoxic activity specific for endothelial cells [87,88]. This endothelial cell cytotoxic activity is abolished by serine protease inhibitors, suggesting that the cytotoxic activity is protease mediated [89]. In addition, these investigators also observed a functional deficiency of protease inhibitors in these scleroderma sera. Although vessel damage may be involved in the pathogenesis of scleroderma, the manner in which the vascular changes are related to the disturbance in the connective tissue remains to be defined.

It is evident that the lack of a natural animal model for

scleroderma (as would be true for many other diseases as well) has deterred progress in understanding the pathogenesis of the disorder. The tight-skin mouse, an autosomal dominant mutant [90], has been investigated as a potential animal model for scleroderma [91]. Both disorders share certain features in common such as hypertrophy of the dermis, particularly the hypodermis associated with an abundance of fibroblasts, firm anchoring of hypodermal connective tissue to deeper tissues, localized areas of homogenization or hyalinization of dermal connective tissue, and lastly, induration of the skin. However, there are also significant differences which include the presence of hyalinization in the more superficial dermis, the absence of vascular changes, normal-appearing skin appendages, and the fact that the tight-skin mutation is a heritable disorder while systemic sclerosis is usually acquired. Another genetically determined disorder occurring in chickens also has certain features similar to scleroderma [92]. These animals develop dermal and esophageal fibrosis, comb involution, antinuclear antibodies, and rheumatoid factor. The fibrosis differs in having its onset in the neonatal period and in the presence of an intense inflammatory process, frequently producing a severe perivasculitis. Lastly scleroderma-like skin changes also develop in homologous disease of rats, which are perhaps analogous to those seen in patients with graft-versus-host disease (for review see [93]). It is hoped that these animal diseases will provide new insights into the pathogenesis of systemic sclerosis.

Course

In patients with morphea or linear scleroderma, the disease may last from a few months to many years. In approximately one-half the cases, the lesions may disappear or soften, leaving areas of either hyperpigmentation or depigmentation. In some, the disease may involute completely. In the coup de sabre type of scleroderma, the lesions will remain unchanged or become more extensive [14]. The question of whether localized scleroderma ever progresses into systemic scleroderma remains unanswered although Curtis and Jansen [14] reported such a progression in 6 of 106 cases (5.7 percent) in their series. Tuffanelli et al [94] have reported three cases in which localized scleroderma with hemiatrophy was associated with SLE, systemic scleroderma, or a rheumatoid arthritis-like picture.

In systemic scleroderma, although the course may be extremely variable, evidence of visceral involvement will develop in most of the patients if they are followed long enough. In some cases, the disease may progress rapidly, and the eventual outcome will be determined by the severity of involvement of vital organs. The prognosis is particularly poor in those with cardiopulmonary involvement, in patients who develop hypertension and renal insufficiency, and in individuals 45 years or older at the time the initial diagnosis is made. In most cases the disease may reach a plateau or show signs of regression and result in only a moderate degree of disability. In support of this, the 10-year survival rate of 727 cases of systemic scleroderma reported by Tuffanelli and Winkelmann [95] was 58 percent and in only six cases was complete remission noted. Somewhat poorer survival rates have been reported by Medsger, Masi, and Rodnan [3]. In these studies the survival rate 7 years after initial diagnosis was only 45 percent.

Management

The treatment of localized scleroderma remains unsatisfactory. The use of topical corticosteroids and the intralesional injection of steroids into plaques of morphea have been unrewarding, in the authors' experience. The use of antimalarials, bismuth, and systemic corticosteroids is not indicated. Physiotherapy or surgery to prevent contractures may be helpful in linear scleroderma.

The management of systemic scleroderma is, at best, a frustrating problem. The list of drugs used in the treatment of systemic scleroderma is impressive, but most agents have not proved to be effective when studies have been well controlled. Enthusiasm for relaxin, EDTA, aminocaproic acid, dimethyl sulfoxide (DMSO), p-aminobenzoate (Potaba), colchicine, and immunosuppressive drugs has not continued, since these agents appear to be of little therapeutic value. Systemic corticosteroids may be of some benefit in the early stages of the disease but have not been helpful in altering visceral manifestations.

It has been suggested that penicillamine, which is a lathyrogen in animals and can produce an increase in soluble collagen in sclerodermatous skin [96], may be effective in treating systemic sclerosis. The results of a retrospective analysis [97] of 73 patients with systemic scleroderma treated with high-dose penicillamine, 500 to 1500 mg (median 750 mg) daily for an average of 24 months, are encouraging. Significant improvement however, was not noted in the treated patients until 19 to 42 months after the initiation of therapy. An impressive reduction in skin thickness and in the rate of new visceral organ involvement, especially for the kidney, was found in the treated group. In addition, patients treated with penicillamine had a greater 5-year cumulative survival rate, 88 percent vs. 66 percent, than the comparison group. These changes were not found in patients treated with colchicine or immunosuppressive agents. Fibroblast cultures from forearm skin biopsies of three patients obtained before and after they had shown a marked decrease in skin thickness during one year or more of penicillamine therapy have been examined for glycosaminoglycan and collagen production [98]. Interestingly, no differences were observed in the synthesis of these connective tissue components. These findings indicate that, although penicillamine has a clinical effect on the connective tissue, the fibroblasts from the thinned skin retain their potential for increased collagen and glycosaminoglycan synthesis.

Malabsorption has been successfully treated in some patients by means of long-term, broad-spectrum antibiotics. The rationale for such treatment is based on the fact that bacterial overgrowth occurring in the atonic loops of the bowel plays a major factor in malabsorption [99,100].

Patients with Raynaud's phenomenon should be carefully instructed about protecting their hands from thermal, chemical, and mechanical trauma. Application of emollients to the hands may be helpful in preventing drying and fissuring of the skin. The use of reserpine or phenoxybenzamine (Dibenzyline) may be beneficial in ameliorating Raynaud's phenomenon in patients with fissures and ischemic ulcerations of their fingertips. Beneficial results from intraarterial reserpine have been reported in patients with Raynaud's phenomenon associated with scleroderma; however, the authors' experience has not been as gratifying. Recently the calcium-channel blockers nifedipine and verapamil [101] have been used to treat Raynaud's phenomenon. Although there is variability in the response to therapy, and indeed some patients fail to respond, at least with nifedipine, 66 percent of the cases treated showed subjective symptomatic improvement in double-blind controlled clinical trials [101]. Sympathectomy is ineffective in the management of Raynaud's phenomenon secondary to scleroderma and should not be recommended [102].

References

1. Christianson HB et al: Localized scleroderma: a clinical study of two hundred thirty-five cases. *Arch Dermatol* **74**:629, 1956
2. Medsger TA Jr, Masi AT: Epidemiology of systemic sclerosis (scleroderma). *Ann Intern Med* **74**:714, 1971
3. Medsger TA et al: Survival with systemic sclerosis (scleroderma). *Ann Intern Med* **75**:369, 1971
4. Masi AT, D'Angelo WA: Epidemiology of fatal systemic sclerosis (diffuse scleroderma). *Ann Intern Med* **66**:870, 1967
5. Rodnan GP et al: The association of progressive systemic sclerosis (scleroderma) with coal miners' pneumoconiosis and other forms of silicosis. *Ann Intern Med* **66**:323, 1967
6. Maricq HR et al: Capillary abnormalities in polyvinylchloride production workers. Examination by *in vivo* microscopy. *JAMA* **236**:1368, 1976
7. Veltman G et al: Clinical manifestations and course of vinylchloride disease. *Ann NY Acad Sci* **245**:6, 1975
8. Finch WR et al: Bleomycin-induced scleroderma. *J Rheumatol* **7**:651, 1980
9. Rodnan GP: Progressive systemic sclerosis (scleroderma), in *Arthritis and Allied Conditions*, edited by DJ McCarty. Philadelphia, Lea & Febiger, 1979, p 762
10. Greger RE: Familial progressive systemic scleroderma. *Arch Dermatol* **111**:81, 1975
11. Hanson V et al: Some immunologic considerations in focal scleroderma and progressive systemic sclerosis in children. *Pediatr Res* **8**:806, 1974
12. Hanson V et al: Rheumatoid factor in children with focal scleroderma. *Pediatrics* **53**:945, 1974
13. Uitto J et al: Morphea and lichen sclerosus et atrophicus. *J Am Acad Dermatol* **3**:271, 1980
14. Curtis AC, Jansen TG: The prognosis of localized scleroderma. *Arch Dermatol* **78**:749, 1958
15. Rubin L: Linear scleroderma: association with abnormalities of spine and nervous system. *Arch Dermatol Syphilol* **58**:1, 1948
16. Soffa DJ et al: Melorheostosis with linear sclerodermatous changes. *Diagn Radiol* **114**:577, 1975
17. Hickman JW, Shiels WS: Progressive facial hemiatrophy. *Arch Intern Med* **113**:716, 1964
18. Dorwart BB: Periorbital edema in progressive systemic scleroderma. *Ann Intern Med* **80**:273, 1974
19. Smith AG et al: Immunoreactive beta-melanocyte stimulating hormone and melanin pigmentation in systemic sclerosis. *Br J Med* **3**:733, 1976
20. Minkin W, Rabhan NB: Office nail fold capillary microscopy using ophthalmoscope. *J Am Acad Dermatol* **7**:190, 1982
21. Maricq HR et al: Predictive value of capillary microscopy in patients with Raynaud's phenomenon. *Arthritis Rheum* **23**:716, 1980
22. Rodnan GP, Fennel RH Jr: Progressive systemic sclerosis sine scleroderma. *JAMA* **180**:665, 1962
23. Stevens MB et al: Aperistalsis of esophagus in patients with connective tissue disorders and Raynaud's phenomenon. *N Engl J Med* **270**:1218, 1964
24. Guttadauria M et al: Pulmonary function in scleroderma. *Arthritis Rheum* **20**:1071, 1977
25. Moroi Y et al: Antibody to centromere (kinetocore) in scleroderma sera. *Proc Natl Acad Sci USA* **77**:1627, 1980
26. Fritzler MJ et al: The CREST syndrome: a distinct serologic entity with anticentromere antibodies. *Am J Med* **69**:520, 1980
27. Sharp GC et al: Association of autoantibodies to different nuclear antigens with clinical patterns of rheumatic disease and responsiveness to therapy. *J Clin Invest* **50**:350, 1971
28. Sharp GC et al: Mixed connective tissue disease: an apparently distinct rheumatic disease syndrome associated with a specific antibody to an extractable nuclear antigen (ENA). *Am J Med* **52**:148, 1972
29. Shulman LE: Diffuse fasciitis with eosinophilia: a new syndrome? *Trans Assoc Am Physicians* **88**:70, 1975
30. Pincus SH, Wolff SM: Dermatologic diseases associated with eosinophilia, in *Update: Dermatology in General Medicine*, edited by TB Fitzpatrick et al. New York, McGraw-Hill, 1983, p 13
31. Solomon G et al: Eosinophilic fasciitis responsive to cimetidine. *Ann Intern Med* **97**:547, 1982
32. Fleischmajer R, Nedwich A: Generalized morphea. I. Histology of the dermis and subcutaneous tissue. *Arch Dermatol* **106**:509, 1972
33. Fleischmajer R et al: Cellular infiltrates in scleroderma skin. *Arthritis Rheum* **20**:975, 1977
34. Fleischmajer R, Prunieras M: Generalized morphea. II. Electron microscopy of collagen, cells, and the subcutaneous tissue. *Arch Dermatol* **106**:515, 1972
35. Fleischmajer R et al: Alteration of subcutaneous tissue in systemic scleroderma. *Arch Dermatol* **105**:59, 1972
36. Michalowski R: Ultrastructural study of skeletal muscle in morphea. *Br J Dermatol* **82**:137, 1970
37. Catoggio LJ et al: Serologic markers in progressive systemic sclerosis: clinical correlations. *Ann Rheum Dis* **42**:2327, 1983
38. Pinnas JL et al: Antinucleolar antibody in human sera. *J Immunol* **111**:996, 1973
39. Alarcon-Segovia D, Fishbein E: Immunochemical characterization of the anti-RNA antibodies found in scleroderma and systemic lupus erythematosus. I. Differences in reactivity with poly U and poly A-poly U. *J Immunol* **115**:28, 1975
40. Douvar AS: Identification of a nuclear protein (Scl-70) as a unique target of human antinuclear antibodies in scleroderma. *J Biol Chem* **254**:10514, 1979
41. Hanson V et al: DNA antibodies in childhood scleroderma. *Arthritis Rheum* **13**:798, 1970
42. Mackel AM et al: Antibodies to collagen in scleroderma. *Arthritis Rheum* **25**:522, 1982
43. Fleischmajer R et al: Cellular infiltrates in scleroderma skin. *Arthritis Rheum* **20**:975, 1977
44. Johnson RL, Ziff M: Lymphokine stimulation of collagen accumulation. *J Clin Invest* **58**:240, 1976
45. Spielvogel RL et al: Mononuclear cell stimulation of fibroblast collagen synthesis. *Clin Exp Dermatol* **3**:25, 1978
46. Kondo H et al: Cutaneous antigen-stimulating lymphokine production by lymphocytes of patients with progressive systemic sclerosis (scleroderma). *J Clin Invest* **58**:1388, 1976
47. LeRoy EC: Pathogenesis of scleroderma (systemic sclerosis). *J Invest Dermatol* **79** (**suppl**):87s, 1982
48. Tan EML et al: Human skin fibroblasts in culture: procollagen synthesis in the presence of sera from normal healthy subjects and from patients with dermal fibroses. *J Invest Dermatol* **76**:462, 1981
49. Stuart JM et al: Evidence for cell-mediated immunity to collagen in progressive systemic sclerosis. *J Lab Clin Med* **88**:601, 1976
50. Haxthausen H: Studies of the pathogenesis of morphea, vitiligo, and acrodermatitis atrophicans by means of transplantation experiments. *Acta Derm Venereol (Stockh)* **27**:352, 1946

51. Fries JF et al: Reciprocal skin grafts in systemic sclerosis (scleroderma). *Arthritis Rheum* **14**:571, 1971

52. Fisher ER, Rodnan GP: Pathologic observations concerning the cutaneous lesion of progressive systemic sclerosis: an electron microscopic, histochemical and immunohistochemical study. *Arthritis Rheum* **3**:536, 1960

53. Braun-Falco O, Rupec M: Collagen fibrils of scleroderma in ultra-thin skin sections. *Nature* **202**:708, 1964

54. Shuster S et al: Quantitative skin changes in skin collagen in morphea. *Br J Dermatol* **79**:456, 1967

55. Rodnan GP et al: Skin thickness and collagen content in progressive systemic sclerosis and localized scleroderma. *Arthritis Rheum* **22**:130, 1979

56. Uitto J et al: Protocollagen proline hydroxylase activity in scleroderma and other connective tissue disorders. *Ann Clin Res* **2**:235, 1970

57. Keiser HR et al: Increased protocollagen proline hydroxylase activity in sclerodermatous skin. *Arch Dermatol* **104**:57, 1971

58. Fleckman PH et al: A sensitive microassay for prolyl hydroxylase: activity in normal and psoriatic skin. *J Invest Dermatol* **60**:46, 1973

59. Keiser HR, Sjoerdsma A: Direct measurement of the rate of collagen synthesis in skin. *Clin Chim Acta* **23**:341, 1969

60. Uitto J et al: Skin collagen in patients with scleroderma: biosynthesis and maturation *in vitro*, and the effect of D-penicillamine. *Ann Clin Res* **2**:228, 1970

61. Herbert CM et al: Biosynthesis and maturation of skin collagen in scleroderma and effect of D-penicillamine. *Lancet* **1**:187, 1974

62. LeRoy EC: Connective tissue synthesis by scleroderma skin fibroblasts in cell culture. *J Exp Med* **135**:1351, 1972

63. LeRoy EC: Increased collagen synthesis of scleroderma skin fibroblasts *in vitro*. *J Clin Invest* **54**:880, 1974

64. Buckingham R et al: Increased collagen accumulation in dermal fibroblast culture from patients with progressive systemic sclerosis (scleroderma). *J Lab Clin Med* **92**:5, 1978

65. Perlish JS et al: Connective tissue synthesis by cultured scleroderma fibroblasts. I. *In vitro* collagen synthesis by normal and scleroderma dermal fibroblasts. *Arthritis Rheum* **19**:891, 1976

66. Uitto J et al: Scleroderma: increased biosynthesis of triple-helical type I and type III procollagens associated with unaltered expression of collagenase by skin fibroblasts in culture. *J Clin Invest* **64**:921, 1979

67. Graves PN et al: Increased procollagen mRNA levels in scleroderma skin fibroblasts. *J Invest Dermatol* **80**:130, 1983

68. Cooper SM et al: Increase in fibronectin in the deep dermis of involved skin in progressive systemic sclerosis. *Arthritis Rheum* **22**:983, 1979

69. Buckingham RB et al: Progressive systemic sclerosis dermal fibroblasts synthesize increased amounts of glycosaminoglycans. *J Lab Clin Med* **101**:659, 1983

70. Gay RE et al: Collagen types synthesized in dermal fibroblast cultures from patients with early progressive systemic sclerosis. *Arthritis Rheum* **23**:190, 1980

71. Fleischmajer R et al: Variability in collagen and fibronectin synthesis by scleroderma fibroblasts in primary culture. *J Invest Dermatol* **76**:400, 1981

72. Uitto J et al: Connective tissue in scleroderma. A biochemical study on the correlation of fractionated glycosaminoglycans and collagen in human skin. *Acta Derm Venereol (Stockh)* **51**:401, 1972

73. Brady AH: Collagenase in scleroderma. *J Clin Invest* **56**:1175, 1975

74. Harper RA, Grove G: Human skin fibroblasts derived from papillary and reticular dermis: differences in growth potential *in vitro*. *Science* **204**:526, 1979

75. Tajima S, Pinnell SR: Collagen synthesis by human skin fibroblasts in culture: studies of fibroblasts explanted from papillary and reticular dermis. *J Invest Dermatol* **77**:410, 1981

76. Botstein GR et al: Fibroblast selection in scleroderma. An alternative model of fibrosis. *Arthritis Rheum* **25**:189, 1982

77. Korn JH: Fibroblast prostaglandin E_2 synthesis. Persistence of an abnormal phenotype after short-term exposure to mononuclear cell products. *J Clin Invest* **71**:1240, 1983

78. Pinals RS: Tryptophan metabolism in rheumatic diseases. *Arthritis Rheum* **7**:662, 1964

79. Price JM et al: Scleroderma. II. Tryptophan metabolism before and during treatment of chelation (EDTA). *J Invest Dermatol* **29**:289, 1957

80. MacDonald RA et al: Dermal fibrosis following injections of serotonin creatinine sulphate. *Proc Soc Exp Biol Med* **97**:334, 1958

81. Stachow A et al: Five-hydroxytryptamine and tryptamine pathways in scleroderma. *Br J Dermatol* **97**:147, 1977

82. Norton WL et al: Evidence of microvascular injury in scleroderma and systemic lupus erythematosus: quantitative study of the microvascular bed. *J Lab Clin Med* **71**:919, 1968

83. D'Angelo WA et al: Pathologic observations in systemic sclerosis (scleroderma): a study of 58 autopsy cases and 58 matched controls. *Am J Med* **46**:428, 1969

84. Coffman JD, Cohen AS: Total and capillary fingertip blood flow in Raynaud's phenomenon. *N Engl J Med* **285**:259, 1971

85. LeRoy EC et al: Skin capillary blood flow in scleroderma. *J Clin Invest* **50**:930, 1971

86. Fleischmajer R, Perlish JS: ^{3}H-Thymidine labeling of dermal endothelial cells in scleroderma. *J Invest Dermatol* **69**:379, 1977

87. Kahaleh MB et al: Endothelial injury in scleroderma. *J Exp Med* **149**:1326, 1979

88. Shanahan WH Jr, Korn JH: Cytotoxic activity of sera from scleroderma and other connective tissue diseases. Lack of cellular and disease specificity. *Arthritis Rheum* **25**:1391, 1982

89. Kahaleh MB, LeRoy EC: Endothelial injury in scleroderma. A protease mechanism. *J Lab Clin Med* **101**:553, 1983

90. Green MC et al: Tight-skin, a new mutation of the mouse causing excessive growth of connective tissue and skeleton. *Am J Pathol* **82**:493, 1976

91. Menton DN et al: The structure and tensile properties of the skin of tight-skin (TSK) mutant mice. *J Invest Dermatol* **70**:4, 1978

92. Gershwin ME et al: Characterization of a spontaneous disease of white Leghorn chickens resembling progressive systemic sclerosis (scleroderma). *J Exp Med* **153**:1640, 1981

93. Farmer ER, Hood AF: Graft-versus-host disease, in *Update: Dermatology in General Medicine*, edited by TB Fitzpatrick et al. New York, McGraw-Hill, 1983, p 28

94. Tuffanelli DL et al: Linear scleroderma with hemiatrophy: report of three cases associated with collagen-vascular disease. *Dermatologica* **132**:51, 1966

95. Tuffanelli DL, Winkelmann RK: Systemic scleroderma. *Arch Dermatol* **84**:359, 1961

96. Harris ED, Sjoerdsma A: Effect of penicillamine on human collagen and its possible application to treatment of scleroderma. *Lancet* **2**:996, 1966

97. Steen VD et al: D-penicillamine therapy in progressive systemic sclerosis (scleroderma). A retrospective study. *Ann Intern Med* **97**:652, 1982

98. Shapiro LS et al: D-penicillamine treatment of progressive systemic sclerosis (scleroderma). A comparison of clinical and *in vitro* effects. *J Rheumatol* **10**:316, 1983

99. Kahn IJ et al: Malabsorption and intestinal scleroderma: correction by antibiotics. *N Engl J Med* **274**:1339, 1966

100. Cliff IS et al: Control of malabsorption in scleroderma. *J Invest Dermatol* **47**:475, 1966

101. Rodheffer RJ et al: Controlled double-blind trial of nifedipine in the treatment of Raynaud's phenomenon. *N Engl J Med* **308**:880, 1983

102. Gifford RW Jr et al: Sympathectomy for Raynaud's phenomenon: follow-up study of 70 women with Raynaud's phenomenon. *Circulation* **17**:5, 1958

CHAPTER 155

RELAPSING POLYCHONDRITIS

Stephen I. Katz

Definition

Relapsing polychondritis is a rare disease manifested by recurring episodes of inflammation in cartilaginous tissues throughout the body.

Historical aspects

The disease was first described by Jaksch-Wartenhorst in 1921 [1] and given the name polychondropathia in 1923 [2]. Pearson et al [3] suggested the name relapsing polychondritis in 1960 to emphasize its episodic nature leading to degeneration and replacement of cartilaginous structures by fibrous tissue. In 1976, McAdam et al reviewed 159 reported cases of relapsing polychondritis including 23 patients whom they had seen over the 15-year period 1960–1975 [4]. They also empirically defined diagnostic criteria, which included the most common clinical features.

Etiology and pathogenesis

Considerable evidence suggests that relapsing polychondritis is an autoimmune disease mediated by immunity to type II collagen. In humans, type II collagen is restricted to cartilage and constitutes over 50 percent of the proteins of cartilage.

The concurrence of relapsing polychondritis with various rheumatic and autoimmune diseases initially led to the suggestion that an immunologic dysfunction may play a role in the pathogenesis of relapsing polychondritis [4]. Indeed several investigators had reported abnormal cellular and humoral immunologic phenomena in relapsing polychondritis [5–10]. However, most of the reported findings lacked specificity for relapsing polychondritis, and the antigens used were not well characterized. More recently, Foidart et al detected antibodies to type II collagen in the sera of 6 of 23 patients with relapsing polychondritis [11]. All patients in whom antibodies were detected had active disease.

The demonstration of antibodies to type II collagen in sera of patients with relapsing polychondritis raises the question of whether these antibodies are functionally active in vivo or whether they simply represent an epiphenomenon secondary to injury to cartilage and consequent exposure to the relevant antigens. That the antibodies are directed mainly against native rather than denatured collagen would favor the former possibility [11]. Experimentally induced autoimmunity to type II collagen in rats [12,13] results in acute arthritis, suggesting that immune responses to type II collagen may play a role in inciting an inflammatory reaction in cartilage. Moreover, some rats sensitized with type II collagen also develop inflammatory ear lesions characterized by an intense, destructive chondritis which resembles relapsing polychondritis histologically [14]. The observation that relapsing polychondritis may be transferred from an afflicted mother to her newborn child and that the child may then recover completely from the disease [15] also suggests an important role for antibodies in the pathogenesis of relapsing polychondritis. Finally, the finding in vivo of deposits of immunoglobulin and complement in inflamed cartilage in two patients with relapsing polychondritis [16] supports the likelihood that immunity to type II collagen plays a role in the pathogenesis of relapsing polychondritis.

Clinical manifestations

The most frequent presenting symptom and sign is an auricular chondritis which is characterized by the sudden onset of redness, warmth, swelling, and tenderness limited to the cartilaginous portion of the external ears. Often only one ear is initially involved and the earlobe is typically uninvolved. The acute inflammation usually subsides spontaneously in one to two weeks. It is characterized by recurrences which appear after highly variable periods—from weeks to months. Eventually 90 percent of patients with relapsing polychondritis will develop auricular chondritis [4]. Nasal chondritis follows the same pattern as the auricular chondritis and eventually occurs in about 70 percent of patients. The recurrent episodes of chondritis usually result in the destruction of normal cartilaginous structures with fibrotic replacement. Clinically this results in floppy or cauliflower ears and nasal deformities (Figs. 155-1 and 155-2).

Arthritis, which may involve only one or many joints, either large or small, is the second most frequent presenting sign and is eventually manifest in approximately 80 percent of patients. At its onset, the arthritis is often migratory and is frequently associated with effusions, but it may be monoarticular and difficult to distinguish from gouty or infectious arthritis.

Other organ system involvement includes the eyes,

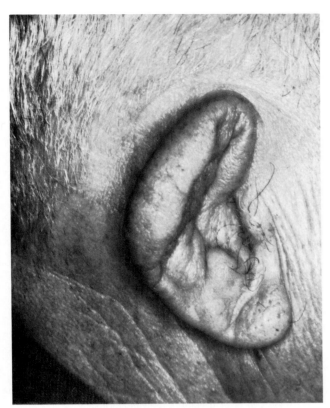

Fig. 155-1   Relapsing polychondritis. Cartilaginous portion of ear is deformed and fibrotic.

where the inflammation may affect almost every part of the eye and adnexal structures [4] manifesting as conjunctivitis, episcleritis, and keratitis (Fig.155-3); the respiratory tract, where symptoms may include hoarseness, aphonia, and dyspnea; the inner ear, where symptoms may include nausea, vomiting, tinnitus, and deafness as a result of

Fig. 155-2   Relapsing polychondritis. "Cauliflower" ear and nasal deformity.

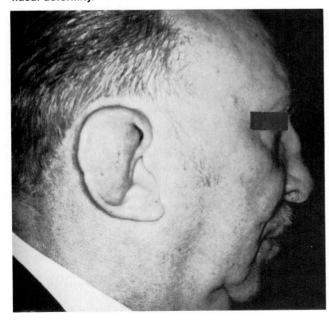

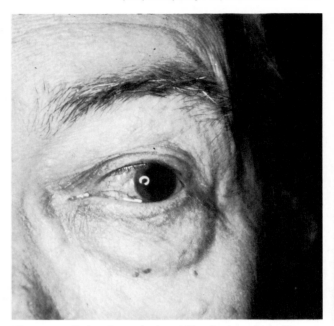

Fig. 155-3   Relapsing polychondritis. Acute episcleritis.

audiovestibular damage; and, less frequently, the cardiovascular system. Approximately 30 percent of patients have an associated rheumatic or autoimmune disease [4].

Laboratory findings

The only laboratory finding which is consistently abnormal is an elevated erythrocyte sedimentation rate. The white blood count is elevated and/or the hemoglobin or hematocrit is decreased in over half of patients [4]. Indirect immunofluorescence studies have detected circulating antibodies to collagen in about one-third of patients [11].

Pathology

Relapsing polychondritis is characterized by a loss of the normal basophilia of cartilage with a perichondral inflammatory infiltrate (Fig. 155-4). The earliest of the inflammatory cells are thought, by some, to be neutrophils and, by others, to be round cells. The end stage of the disease is characterized by the fibrocytic replacement of cartilage.

Diagnosis

McAdam et al suggested that the diagnosis of relapsing polychondritis can be made when three of the following criteria are present along with histologic confirmation of the chondritis [4].

1. Bilateral auricular chondritis
2. Noninvasive seronegative inflammatory polyarthritis
3. Nasal chondritis
4. Ocular inflammation
5. Respiratory chondritis
6. Audiovestibular damage

Ordinarily relapsing polychondritis presents little problem in diagnosis. However, there are patients who have only auricular and nasal chondritis and none of the other

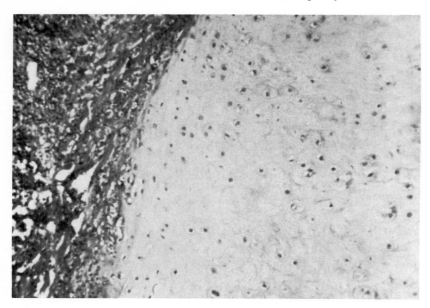

Fig. 155-4 Relapsing polychondritis. Histopathology showing loss of basophilic staining of cartilage and perichondral inflammatory infiltrate.

manifestations of relapsing polychondritis. If the histology shows perichondral inflammation and the loss of the normal cartilaginous basophilia and if other conditions are excluded, a diagnosis of relapsing polychondritis should be made.

Concurrent rheumatic diseases may, at times, obscure the diagnosis of relapsing polychondritis. Cellulitis of the ear or nose may rarely be confused with relapsing polychondritis; however, sparing of the earlobe favors the diagnosis of relapsing polychondritis.

Treatment

Because of the highly variable course of relapsing polychondritis, individualized therapy is the key to optimum management. Systemic corticosteroids are helpful in controlling the acute inflammation. Seventy-five percent of patients in McAdam's series required chronic corticosteroid therapy with an average dose of prednisone of 25 mg/day [4]. Immunosuppressive therapy may also be efficacious in severe progressive disease [4]. Dapsone has also been reported to be an effective treatment [17,18]; however, this author's experience with dapsone in relapsing polychondritis has been disappointing. The frequent spontaneous remissions that occur during the acute episodes have made evaluation of most treatments difficult. The more chronic manifestations of relapsing polychondritis can be managed with indomethacin in some patients.

Course and prognosis

The course of relapsing polychondritis is unpredictable. The acute chondritis in most patients lasts for 1 to 2 weeks; in a few cases it may be more prolonged. Some patients have a relatively mild course with few episodes of chondritis. Other patients may have multiple episodes of chondritis. The degree of tissue destruction and fibrosis is difficult to predict early in the course of the disease. About one-third of the patients die as a result of relapsing polychondritis, mainly of respiratory and cardiovascular complications. The most frequent cause of death is airway collapse or obstruction [4].

References

1. Jaksch-Wartenhorst R: Arztliche vortragsabende. *Prag Med Klin* **17**:342, 1921
2. Jaksch-Wartenhorst R: Polychondropathia. *Wein Arch Inn Med* **6**:93, 1923
3. Pearson CM et al: Relapsing polychondritis. *N Engl J Med* **263**:51, 1960
4. McAdam LP et al: Relapsing polychondritis. Prospective study of 23 patients and a review of the literature. *Medicine (Baltimore)* **55**:193, 1976
5. Herman JH, Dennis MV: Immunopathologic studies in relapsing polychondritis. *J Clin Invest* **52**:549, 1973
6. Rajapakse DA, Bywaters EGL: Cell-mediated immunity to cartilage proteoglycan in relapsing polychondritis. *Clin Exp Immunol* **16**:497, 1974
7. Dolan DL et al: Relapsing polychondritis. *Am J Med* **41**:285, 1966
8. Hundeiker M et al: Infiltrat und Knorpelzerstorung bei polychondritis (Histochemische und immunofluoreszenz-histologische Befunde). *Z Haut Geschlechtskr* **45**:437, 1970
9. Hughes RAC et al: Relapsing polychondritis. *Q J Med* **41**:363, 1972
10. Rogers PH et al: Relapsing polychondritis with insulin resistance and antibodies to cartilage. *Am J Med* **55**:243, 1973
11. Foidart JM et al: Antibodies to type II collagen in relapsing polychondritis. *N Engl J Med* **299**:1203, 1978
12. Trentham DE et al: Autoimmunity to type II collagen: an experimental model of arthritis. *J Exp Med* **146**:857, 1977
13. Trentham DE et al: Humoral and cellular sensitivity to collagen in type II collagen-induced arthritis in rats. *J Exp Med* **154**:535, 1981
14. Cremer MA et al: Auricular chondritis in rats: an experimental model of relapsing polychondritis induced with type II collagen. *J Exp Med* **154**:535, 1981
15. Arundell FW, Haserick JR: Familial chronic atrophic polychondritis. *Arch Dermatol* **82**:439, 1960
16. Valenzuela R et al: Relapsing polychondritis: value of immunomicroscopic examination of ear biopsy. *Hum Pathol* **11**:19, 1980
17. Barranco VP et al: Treatment of relapsing polychondritis with dapsone. *Arch Dermatol* **112**:1286, 1976
18. Martin J et al: Relapsing polychondritis treated with dapsone. *Arch Dermatol* **112**:1272, 1976

CHAPTER 156

SCLEREDEMA AND
PAPULAR MUCINOSIS

Raul Fleischmajer

Scleredema

Definition

Scleredema is a connective tissue disease which was recognized as a distinct entity by Buschke in 1902. The disease affects all races and appears to be more prevalent among females. In a review of 209 cases by Greenberg et al [1], 29 percent were children under 10 years, 22 percent were between 10 and 20 years old, and 49 percent were adults.

Pathogenesis

The cause of scleredema is unknown although the following hypotheses have been proposed: streptococcal hypersensitivity, injury of lymph channels, alterations of pituitary function, and peripheral nerve abnormalities, none of which has been substantiated. The dermis is markedly increased in thickness although it appears that this is due in part to the replacement of the subcutaneous tissue by connective tissue (Fig. 156-1). Chemical analysis of the dermis reveals an increase in hydroxyproline and hexosamines proportional to the increase in skin thickness. Fractionation of acid mucopolysaccharides shows a normal distribution of hyaluronic acid and dermatan sulfate. Water content of skin is normal [2]. Teller and Vester [3] noted, by electron microscopy, clumping of collagen fibrils, increase in ground substance, and collagen fibrils with re-

duced diameter. Urinary excretion of hydroxyproline and hydroxylysine appears normal [4]. More recently, a monoclonal gammopathy was noted in three cases of scleredema. In two cases, the immunoglobulins were of the IgG-kappa type while one patient had a paraproteinemia of the IgG-lambda type. Monoclonal immunoglobulins were not detected in the skin [5].

Clinical manifestations

Skin involvement may be preceded by a prodrome of low-grade fever, malaise, myalgia, and arthralgia. A few days to 6 weeks prior to the onset, 65 percent of patients develop an infection, usually of streptococcal origin [1]. The following have been observed: influenza, scarlet fever, measles, mumps, tonsillitis, pharyngitis, otitis, furuncles, erysipelas, and impetigo.

The onset is frequently sudden and consists of marked, nonpitting, symmetrical induration of the skin usually affecting the posterior and lateral aspects of the neck and then spreading to the face, shoulders, arms, and thorax (Fig. 156-2). The buttocks, legs, and abdomen are less frequently involved and hands and feet are affected in about 10 percent of the cases. The disease usually reaches maximal involvement in about 1 to 2 weeks although it may continue spreading for 2 to 3 additional months.

The induration is of wooden-like consistency, waxy white or shiny in appearance, and rather diffuse so that there is no sharp line of demarcation between involved and noninvolved areas as in localized scleroderma. Folding of the skin is almost impossible and the normal markings are lost. When the face is involved, there is lack of expression

Fig. 156-1 Scleredema skin from the back (top) and normal control. Note marked increase in thickness. (From Fleischmajer R et al [2].)

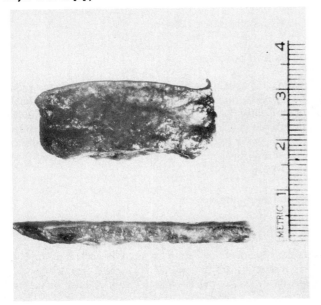

Fig. 156-2 Scleredema of 41-year duration affecting the neck and back.

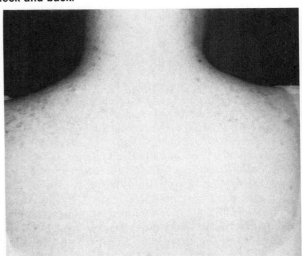

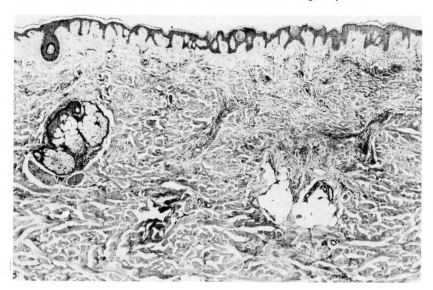

Fig. 156-3 Scleredema. Edematous papillary layer, mild perivascular cellular infiltrates and collagen bundles separated by large interfascicular spaces. H&E, ×18.

and often difficulties in opening the mouth. Curtis and Shulak [6] described a transient, erythematous, macular or papular eruption during the early stage of the disease. Pain is absent although paresthesias may occur. Heart abnormalities occur, and in children the most common are diastolic gallop without evidence of cardiac failure, a nonspecific S-T depression, and T-wave inversion, usually reverting to normal in 3 to 9 months. Carditis secondary to rheumatic fever has also been noted [4].

Recently, a new syndrome has been recognized consisting of scleredema of long duration, obesity, maturity onset, latent or overt diabetes, and a high incidence of cardiovascular disease [2,7]. Diabetic retinopathy is not uncommon [2,8]. Most patients are quite resistant to antidiabetic therapy, including insulin, chlorpropamide, and phenformin. Furthermore, antidiabetic therapy has no effect on the evolution of the scleredema.

Laboratory findings

Most laboratory tests are usually normal except for an increase in ASO titer in some patients [2]. A glucose tolerance test should be performed to rule out diabetes mellitus [2,7]. Hyperinsulinism may be present.

Pathology

The epidermis and its appendages are normal. The dermis reveals collagen bundles separated by large interfascicular spaces. The papillary layer is prominent and slightly edematous. In the upper dermis, there may be mild perivascular or scattered infiltrates consisting mostly of lymphocytes and histiocytic type cells (Fig. 156-3). An increase in mast cells also has been noted [6,9]. The secretory coils of the eccrine sweat glands are found in the upper third or mid dermis. The subcutaneous tissue is reduced, probably due to its replacement by connective tissue [2]. The ground substance reveals an increase in metachromatic material with toluidine blue [9] which also stains positive with alcian blue at pH 2.5. The alcian blue at pH 0.5, which stains

sulfated acid mucopolysaccharides, is negative [10]. Hyaluronidase digestion completely removes the alcian blue-positive material, suggesting an increase in hyaluronic acid. However, this increase is only temporary and not seen in all patients.

Differential diagnosis

Scleredema has to be differentiated from the early edematous stage of systemic scleroderma. However, in systemic scleroderma there is usually Raynaud's phenomenon, predilection for hands, abnormal pigmentation, telangiectasia, ischemia, and atrophic skin changes, not seen in scleredema. Scleredema should also be differentiated from trichinosis, dermatomyositis, scleromyxedema, myxedema, progeria, sclerema neonatorum, edema neonatorum, primary systemic amyloidosis, and edema from cardiac or renal origin.

Treatment

There is no effective treatment.

Course and prognosis

Prognosis is usually good and the disease undergoes spontaneous resolution in 6 months to 2 years. However, Curtis and Shulak [6] noted that 25 percent of the patients showed no tendency toward resolution. The disease persists indefinitely in those patients with associated diabetes mellitus. In the Fleischmajer et al (2) series, duration ranged from 2 to 41 years.

Papular mucinosis

Definition

Papular mucinosis or lichen myxedematosus is a rare disease characterized by a papular-lichenoid eruption, mucin deposition, and a paraproteinemia. A clinical variant of

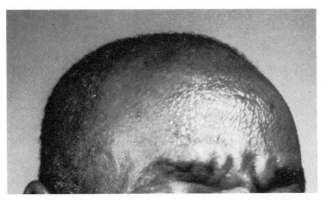

Fig. 156-4   Papular mucinosis. Note discrete papules on the forehead and longitudinal folding of the glabella. *(Courtesy of Dr. L. Shapiro.)*

papular mucinosis is scleromyxedema where the disease is more generalized and accompanied by erythema and sclerosis [11].

Pathogenesis

The pathogenesis of papular mucinosis remains unknown. This disease is frequently associated with a paraproteinemia which consists of a myeloma-like, homogeneous serum globulin of the IgG type, with predominantly lambda light chains, although kappa light chains have also been noted [12,13]. Less commonly, paraproteins of the IgM and IgA types have been identified. The paraprotein in papular mucinosis is a 7S, papain-sensitive globulin, which is strongly basic due to its high content in lysine [14]. It has a molecular weight of about 110,000 (normal IgG has a molecular weight of 160,000), thus suggesting that this IgG globulin is incomplete by missing a significant antigenic portion of the Fd fragment [15]. The initial suggestion that papular mucinosis represents a plasma cell dyscrasia has never been substantiated. Its association with multiple myeloma is rare, if it occurs at all. Furthermore, the paraprotein in multiple myeloma is usually a monoclonal IgG with kappa light chains. It has been shown that serum from papular mucinosis patients can "in vitro" stimulate DNA synthesis and proliferation of normal human fibroblasts [16]. However, removal of the paraprotein from culture media did not decrease fibroblast mitosis, thus suggesting that another serum factor may be responsible for this proliferative effect.

Clinical manifestations

The disease affects adults from 30 to 70 years of age, has no sex predilection, and usually runs a chronic course. The primary lesion is a dome-shaped papule, skin color or erythematous, 2 to 4 mm in diameter; the lesions may be densely grouped in a lichenoid fashion or may show a linear arrangement. The areas most frequently affected are the dorsa of the hands and fingers, axillary folds, and external surfaces of arms and legs. Coalescence of papules on the face, particularly in the glabella area, results in longitudinal folding, giving the appearance of leonine facies (Fig. 156-4). The lesions are usually asymptomatic, although mild pruritus may be present. In scleromyxedema, large parts of the body may be involved; the skin shows erythematous, scleroderma-like induration accompanied by reduced mobility of lips, arms, hands, and legs. Other skin lesions include urticaria, nodules, and cysts [17]. Although the disease primarily affects the skin, systemic manifestations have

Fig. 156-5   Scleromyxedema. Mucin and numerous plump fibroblasts in the upper dermis. Alcian blue, pH 2.5. *(Courtesy of Dr. L. Shapiro.)*

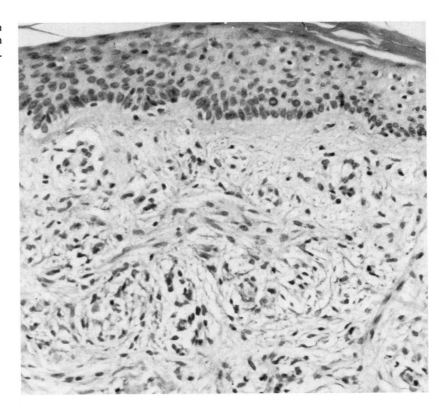

been described such as severe proximal myopathy, inflammatory polyarthritis [18,19], central nervous system symptoms resembling acute organic brain syndrome [20], esophageal aperistalsis, and hoarseness [21,22].

Laboratory findings

The paraproteinemia is present in most patients, particularly in those with the clinical form of scleromyxedema. Immunofluorescence microscopy of the skin lesions occasionally shows deposits of IgG with or without IgM in the papillary and upper reticular dermis [13,15]. However, others have failed to reproduce these findings [23]. Other inconsistent findings refer to elevated sedimentation rate, leukocytosis with eosinophilia, albuminuria, and plasma cell aggregates in the bone marrow.

Pathology

The most striking changes are in the upper dermis which shows a horizontal band of mucinous material between collagen bundles. This material is a glycosaminoglycan that stains with alcian blue at pH 2.5 and is susceptible to hyaluronidase digestion (Fig. 156-5). The epidermis may appear thinner due to pressure from the mucinous deposits. There is an increase in fibroblasts, which appear plump and stellate, and dermal fibrosis. Cellular infiltrates may be present around the small blood vessels and appendages and consist mostly of lymphocytes with some histiocytic types and polymorphonuclear cells [24]. An increase in plasma cells has also been noted [23]. Electron microscopy reveals fibroblasts with long cytoplasmic processes and dilated rough endoplasmic reticulum. In addition, there are numerous thin collagen fibrils, suggestive of young collagen [25]. Muscle biopsies reveal an atypical necrotizing myopathy with fiber necrosis, severe type II fiber atrophy, and vacuolization [19]. Mucin deposits have also been reported in the adventitia of blood vessels in kidney, heart, adrenal glands, pancreas, and kidney papillae. However, internal involvement in papular mucinosis still remains controversial [23]. Papular mucinosis has to be differentiated histologically from follicular mucinosis, amyloidosis, hyalinosis cutis et mucosae, scleredema, scleroderma, cutaneous focal mucinosis, pretibial myxedema, and colloid degeneration.

Diagnosis and differential diagnosis

Diagnosis is based on the presence of papular lesions, demonstration of mucin in the dermis, and the presence of paraproteinemia. Clinically, papular mucinosis should be differentiated from scleredema, scleroderma, amyloidosis, disseminated granuloma annulare, malignant lymphomas, and dermatomyositis. The more localized forms should be differentiated from colloid degeneration, lichen planus, morbus moniliformis, and epithelioma adenoides cysticum.

Treatment

The treatment of papular mucinosis remains unsatisfactory. Topical therapy is of no help. Complete clearance of lesions was reported with melphalan (1–10 mg per day) and cyclophosphamide (200 mg per day) alone or in combination with prednisone [26–29]. However, since side effects can be severe, these drugs should be restricted to patients with widespread disease.

Course and prognosis

The disease runs a chronic course and usually has no tendency toward spontaneous resolution. The prognosis for long-term survival is good, however. Reported causes of death appear to be unrelated to the disease and included tuberculosis, pneumonia, and vascular thrombosis.

References

1. Greenberg LM et al: Scleredema adultorum in children. *Pediatrics* **32**:1044, 1963
2. Fleischmajer R et al: Scleredema and diabetes mellitus. *Arch Dermatol* **101**:21, 1970
3. Teller H, Vester G: Elektronenmikroskopische Untersuchungsergebnisse an der Interzellularsubstanz des Coriums beim Skleroedema adultorum Buschke. *Z Haut Geschlechskr* **23**:142, 1957
4. Yogman M, Echeverria P: Scleredema and carditis: report of a case and review of the literature. *Pediatrics* **54**:108, 1974
5. Kovary PM et al: Monoclonal gammopathy in scleredema: observations of three cases. *Arch Dermatol* **117**:536, 1981
6. Curtis AC, Shulak BM: Scleredema adultorum. *Arch Dermatol* **92**:526, 1965
7. Cohn BA et al: Scleredema adultorum of Buschke and diabetes mellitus. *Arch Dermatol* **101**:27, 1970
8. Breinin GM: Scleredema adultorum: ocular manifestations. *Arch Ophthalmol* **50**:155, 1953
9. Braun-Falco O: Neueres zur Hispathalogie des Scleroedema adultorum (Buschke). *Dermatol Wochenschr* **125**:409, 1952
10. Fleischmajer R, Lara JV: Scleredema: a histochemical and biochemical study. *Arch Dermatol* **92**:643, 1965
11. Gottron HA: Skleromyxödem. (Eine eigenartige Erscheinungsform von Myxothesaurodermie). *Arch Dermatol Syphilol* **199**:71, 1954
12. Osserman EF, Takatsuki K: Role of an abnormal myeloma-type, serum gamma globulin in the pathogenesis of the skin lesions of papular mucinosis (lichen myxedematosus). *J Clin Invest* **42**:962, 1963
13. McCarthy JT et al: An abnormal serum globulin in lichen myxedematosus. *Arch Dermatol* **89**:446, 1964
14. Lawrence DA et al: Immunochemical analysis of the basic immunoglobulin in papular mucinosis. *Immunochemistry* **9**:41, 1972
15. Kitamura W et al: Immunochemical analysis of the monoclonal paraprotein in scleromyxedema. *J Invest Dermatol* **70**:305, 1978
16. Harper RA, Rispler J: Lichen myxedematosus serum stimulates human skin fibroblast proliferation. *Science* **188**:545, 1978
17. Wright RC et al: Scleromyxedema. *Arch Dermatol* **112**:63, 1976
18. McAdam LP et al: Papular mucinosis with myopathy, arthritis and eosinophilia: a histopathologic study. *Arthritis Rheum* **20**:989, 1977
19. Verity MA et al: Scleromyxedema myopathy: histochemical and electron microscopic observations. *Am J Clin Pathol* **69**:446, 1978
20. Ochitill HN, Amberson J: Acute cerebral symptomatology: a rare presentation of scleromyxedema. *J Clin Psychiatry* **39**:471, 1978
21. Braverman IM: *Skin Signs of Systemic Disease*. 2d ed. Philadelphia, WB Saunders, 1981, p 233

22. Alligood TR et al: Scleromyxedema associated with esophageal aperistalsis and dermal eosinophilia. *Cutis* **28**:60, 1981

23. Farmer ER et al: Papular mucinosis: a clinicopathologic study of four patients. *Arch Dermatol* **118**:9, 1982

24. Perry HO et al: Further observations on lichen myxedematosus. *Ann Intern Med* **53**:955, 1960

25. Lever WF, Schaumburg-Lever G: Lichen myxedematosus, in *Histopathology of the Skin,* 5th ed. Philadelphia, JB Lippincott, 1975, p 405

26. Feldman et al: Scleromyxedema: a dramatic response to melphalan. *Arch Dermatol* **99**:51, 1969

27. Harris RB et al: Treatment of scleromyxedema with melphalan. *Arch Dermatol* **115**:295, 1979

28. Jessen RT et al: Lichen myxedematosus: treatment with cyclophosphamide. *Int J Dermatol* **17**:833, 1978

29. Howsden SM et al: Lichen myxedematosus: a dermal infiltrative disorder responsive to cyclophosphamide therapy. *Arch Dermatol* **111**:1325, 1975

CHAPTER 157

SKIN MANIFESTATIONS OF RHEUMATIC DISEASE

Eric G. L. Bywaters

Rheumatic fever

The skin manifestations of rheumatic fever are of considerable diagnostic value, but little is known of their pathogenesis despite their ready accessibility for observation. They consist of subcutaneous nodules, erythema marginatum, and erythema papulatum; they appear in both children and adults.

Subcutaneous nodules

These are usually small, 2 to 5 mm in diameter, and multiple, occurring over bony prominences where there is friction between skin and bone, e.g., knuckles, olecranon processes, humoral epicondyles, and occiput; they are sometimes better seen than felt (Fig. 157-1). In a study by Bywaters and Thomas [1] they occurred in 34 percent of the total cases of rheumatic fever. Over the olecranon their appearance is preceded by a diffuse thickening in the neighborhood of the bursa. Nodules occur somewhat later in the course of the disease than do other acute manifestations and may both appear and persist after the erythrocyte sedimentation rate has returned to normal. Heart disease of considerable severity is often present [2]. Histologically, fibrinoid in latticelike formations separates groups of thick-walled vessels and a few lymphocytes; in a few cases an attempt at palisading by fibroblasts is seen,

but this is seldom as marked as in rheumatoid arthritis. In rheumatic fever the cells are always much plumper and there is much less fibrosis (Fig. 157-2). Cutaneous nodules like those of sarcoid or xanthomatosis have been described rarely (in two cases), but diagnosis of rheumatic fever was not fully established [3]. This author has seen none of this character in over 2000 cases of rheumatic fever.

Erythema marginatum (erythema annulare, erythema circinatum)

This is the specific rash of rheumatic fever and has been known for over 100 years [4]. Perry [5] and Keil [6] give good historical reviews. It is a rapidly spreading, ringed eruption, sometimes with raised margins (erythema marginatum) and sometimes flat (erythema annulare or circinatum). The eruption spreads rapidly (as traced in Fig. 157-3) before it dies out or is lost in a confluent and sometimes lightly pigmented area or becomes a tangle of apparently isolated active segments. The lesion may start as

Fig. 157-2 Histologic appearance of a nodule in a female aged 18 in her second attack of rheumatic fever. H&E, ×140.

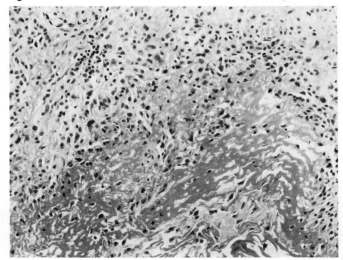

Fig. 157-1 Nodules in a girl aged 15 with rheumatic fever for 3 months, with erythema marginatum and severe carditis.

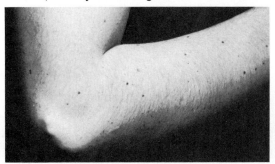

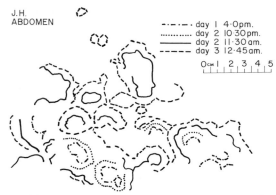

Fig. 157-3 Tracings of margins of erythema marginatum over a 3-day period, showing spread.

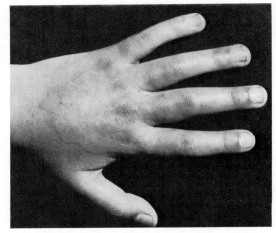

Fig. 157-5 Erythema marginatum on the hand in a girl aged 6 with rheumatic fever and mild carditis. The lesion was evanescent.

a small erythematous blotch or papule; as it spreads peripherally, it leaves a pale or sometimes pigmented and inactive center (Fig. 157-4). The essential feature is the rapid spread, which may be 2 to 10 mm in 12 h. These ringed eruptions occur usually on the trunk and on the limbs, and, contrary to what is often stated, they may invade the proximal areas of the hands (Fig. 157-5) or the face. The advancing periphery is usually circular initially but later may develop either smooth polycyclic or festooned outlines or a more irregular "geographical" outline (Figs. 157-6 and A3-11). Purpuric changes are very rare and may be associated with salicylate-induced vitamin K deficiency. In a few cases the whole central area is raised (urticarial) due to increased capillary exudation (Fig. 157-7), but itching is only rarely present. This rash should be sought in the axillary hollow; it is often to be found here alone and often also in only fragmentary form as a few isolated segments of the original circles (Fig. 157-8).

Often the least raised eruptions have the most pigmentation, perhaps because of less rapid pigment removal. Pigment is probably hematogenous due to gross capillary leakage. Polymorphs in various stages of necrosis may be seen (Fig. 157-9) in diffuse perivascular distribution similar in some ways to the appearances in Henoch-Schönlein purpura. However, the rash of allergic purpura [7] does

not spread and always has more extravasated erythrocytes (see Chap. 107).

These marginate rashes seldom last for more than several weeks. They seem unaffected by anti-inflammatory treatment (Fig. 157-10), although it is known that ACTH or steroid reduces the capillary permeability of inflammation.

The rash on occasion precedes joint involvement, and this author has seen some cases with carditis and rash but no joint symptoms. Usually the rash follows the onset of migratory arthritis by a few days and, in some instances, may appear on and off for prolonged periods (months or even a year). It is usually associated with carditis but may occasionally appear without it. Over a period of 10 years, 203 cases with erythema marginatum out of 1124 cases of rheumatic fever have been seen in the Rheumatism Research Unit, an incidence of 18 percent varying from 10 to 20 percent in any single year. (For other figurate erythemata, see Chap. 88.)

Erythema papulatum

This has become a rare but well-authenticated manifestation of rheumatic fever. Only three examples have been seen in over 2000 cases observed in the Rheumatism Research Unit. Papules—often indolent—appear on flexor

Fig. 157-4 Erythema marginatum in a boy aged 14 with mild carditis.

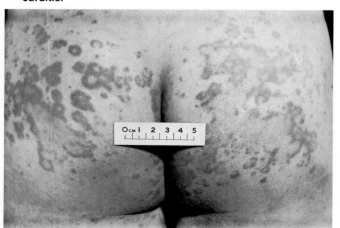

Fig. 157-6 Tracings of a rather irregular marginate rash of rheumatic fever over a 4-day period on the right arm.

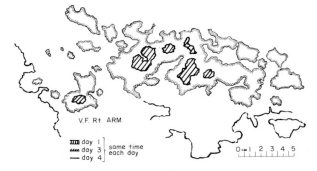

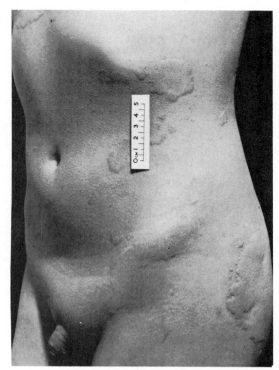

Fig. 157-7   Atypical erythema marginatum in a boy aged 12 with chorea and mild carditis for 3 months. More typical erythema marginatum occurred later.

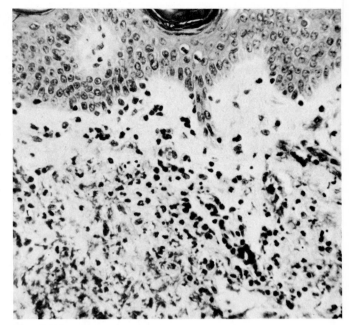

Fig. 157-9   Erythema marginatum biopsy in a girl aged 15 with rheumatic fever for 7 weeks and marginate rash for 6 weeks. H&E, × 275. Note the perivascular polymorph debris.

surfaces (usually the elbow or knee); these are marginal to a diffuse, perhaps frictional erythema (Fig. 157-11). The rash should be distinguished from that of granuloma annulare. It was described by Cockayne [8], later by Bass [9] with chorea, and Gadrat [10] (with biopsy findings). As Gadrat explains in a discussion of the same case [11], these are *not* subcutaneous nodules. They may reach 3 to 4 mm in diameter, may last 6 to 8 days, and are characterized by parakeratosis and edema of the basal layer.

Keil [6] reviews the older literature. Biopsies performed at the Rheumatism Research Unit (Fig. 157-12) showed well-defined focal perivascular collections of round cells

with some general diffuse cellular increases, quite distinct from the acute lesion of erythema marginatum.

Differential diagnosis

These rheumatic fever rashes need to be distinguished from other ringed eruptions. In a child with fever, joint pains, and carditis with a raised antistreptolysin titer, to cite only a few of the diagnostic criteria formulated by Jones [12], this is usually easy to do. If carditis is not present, differentiation from Still's disease may be difficult unless the rash persists long enough for spreading to be observed. In adults, other ringed eruptions may be seen. Syphilis and ringworm need scarcely be mentioned. Urticaria due to horse serum is seldom seen but has given rise to circinate

Fig. 157-8   Isolated segments of erythema marginatum in the same patient as in Fig. 157-4 at a later stage.

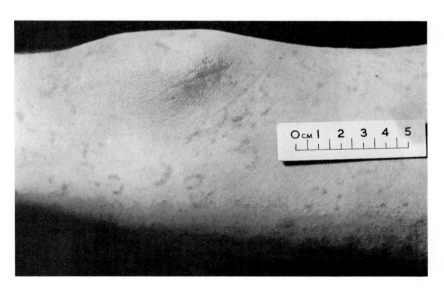

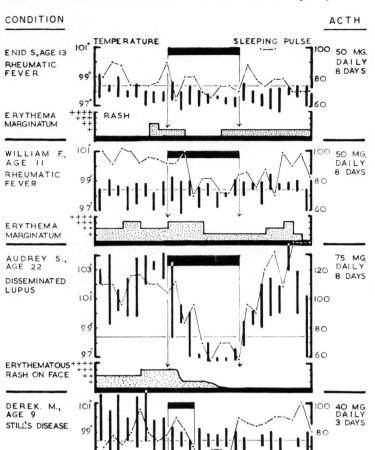

Fig. 157-10 Chart showing effect of ACTH in rashes of erythema marginatum, lupus erythematosus, and Still's disease.

rashes [13]. Urticaria is nowadays usually of food or drug origin and may also be accompanied by migratory joint involvement and fever but is only rarely marginate or circinate. Erythema multiforme, possibly of viral origin, sometimes of marginate configuration, may occasionally be accompanied also by joint symptoms and effusions; occasionally in mononucleosis with joint involvement, the skin rash (Fig. 157-13) may show central pallor and has on occasion been mistaken for rheumatic fever. In the tropics, circinate erythemas have been seen with trypanosomiasis [14], but no later descriptions have been found.

Erythema gyratum repens (possibly associated with carcinoma and disappearing with removal of the primary lesion) [15] and erythema gyratum perstans [16] are rare eruptions, as is erythema annulare centrifugum, which lasts for many months and is also sometimes associated with metastatic carcinoma [17] or with fungus ingestion [18] or fungal infection [19]. There is, in addition, a familial type of annular erythema [20] and a neonatal type [21]. In children with rheumatism, however, these dermatologic curiosities are seldom relevant, and the usual diagnostic difficulty is to distinguish from penicillin-induced or other urticaria or from a Still's disease rash (which may rarely show some central pallor). The essential difference from the latter is that the rheumatic fever rash spreads and the Still's disease rash does not. Occasionally, marginate rashes occur in childhood without other accompaniments of rheumatic fever [22].

Other rashes

Erythema nodosum is often regarded as "rheumatic." The author does not believe that this is so. Erythema nodosum,

Fig. 157-11 Erythema papulatum on the elbow in a boy aged 14 with severe carditis.

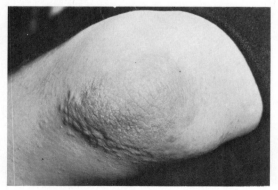

of which there are at least seven different known etiologic agents and probably a larger number of unknown etiologic agents (see Chap. 99), is often accompanied by arthralgia and occasionally by polyarthritis with effusion. The antistreptolysin titer may or may not be raised; usually it is not. It is wrong to label such cases as rheumatic fever. There is no cardiac involvement, and it is essentially a panniculitis. Erythema nodosum may coexist with rheumatic fever, but only rarely has this coincidence been seen.

The same argument applies to "rheumatic purpura"; joints are not infrequently involved; rarely, cardiac involvement may be seen [7], but this does not necessarily mean that the patient is suffering from rheumatic fever. In general, Henoch-Schönlein purpura, erythema nodosum, and rheumatic fever are three different nosologic entities in regard to age of onset, manifestations, and sequelae, although streptococcal infection may precede each of the former and invariably precedes rheumatic fever.

Pathogenesis

The marginate rash of rheumatic fever is nearly specific and must, like other manifestations of the disease, be related in some way to a group A beta streptococcal infection and the immunologic reaction thereto. Despite ready accessibility, its waywardness has dampened experiment; and despite an interest in this subject for over 20 years, the author has failed to gather any adequate data on the reasons for spread and the factors concerned in the genesis of the initial erythematous reaction. Kingston and Glynn [23] have shown a cross-reacting antibody between streptococcal antigen and stratum granulosum and fibroblasts of normal human skin, but no studies of antibodies or complement deposition in the rash of rheumatic fever have yet been traced.

Still's disease
(chronic juvenile polyarthritis with systemic onset)

One of the ironies of medical history is that George Frederic Still [24] did not mention the specific rash which characterizes Still's disease. As may be seen (Fig. 157-14), it occurs in 50 percent of cases with onset before the age of 2 and in nearly 33 percent of cases in subsequent years until puberty. Yet it was not until 1932 [25] and 1933 [26] that it was recognized. As may be seen from Fig. 157-15, the eruption usually consists of small erythematous macules, 3 mm or less in diameter, scattered over the limbs, the trunk, and the face, rarely becoming confluent in larger areas. At onset, some areas may be slightly raised. Central pallor may sometimes be seen in the larger macules, and some pallor due to deviation of blood flow is always seen surrounding the lesion. As noted in an earlier publication based on 46 children with rash and 7 adults with a similar disease [27], the rash does not spread (in contradistinction to the rash of rheumatic fever), is usually associated with fever, and is therefore most obvious toward afternoon or evening (Figs. 157-16 and A2-11), vanishing by morning. There is no sparing of previously involved areas. Mild trauma, as by a pajama cord, may tend to localize the eruption, and very rarely some of the rash is raised and itching (Fig. 157-17).

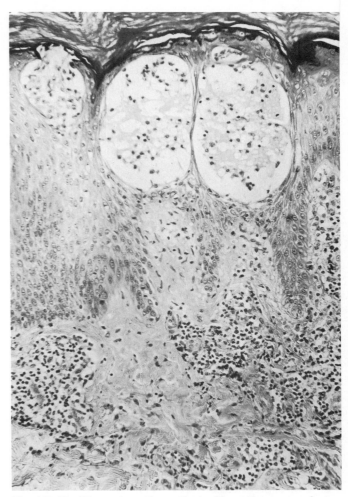

Fig. 157-12 Biopsy from the patient with erythema papulatum shown in Fig. 157-11. There is perivascular mononuclear cell infiltration and mononuclear cells in blister spaces. H&E, ×150.

Fig. 157-13 The rash of glandular fever in a girl aged 11.

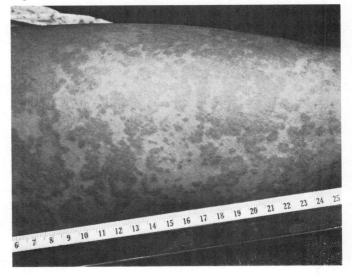

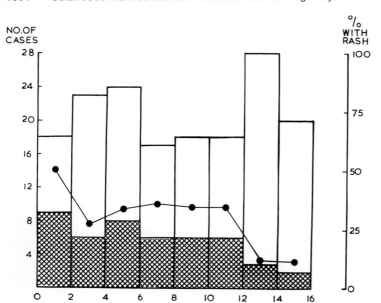

Fig. 157-14 Chart showing the incidence of rash in Still's disease.

The rash and fever may precede joint manifestations but usually accompany or follow them; the rash may last from a week to 11 years, often as long as the active stage of the disease. As may be seen from Table 157-1, it correlates with little except fever, though affected children also more commonly exhibit splenomegaly and lymphadenopathy. The Rose-Waaler test is positive in the same proportion of children with rash as of those without. Treatment with various drugs is without much effect.

Pathologically, biopsies show a sparse perivascular infiltration of polymorphs (Fig. 157-18), very different from the florid picture of erythema marginatum.

Adults aged 20 to 60 may occasionally be seen with a rash similar in appearance, behavior, and microscopic appearances, accompanied by a mild chronic polyarthritis. Seven such cases have been reported in detail [27], and others have been observed since; they are usually seronegative [28]. A follow-up study of 17 of these patients [29] for an average of 20 years has shown that the rash, fever, and arthritis may persist on and off in the majority. They will often show residual ankylosis in the carpus, tarsus [30], and neck (as in juvenile-onset cases), as well as distal interphalangeal involvement, and occasionally destructive lesions [31]. In the majority, the illness interferes only minimally with daily life activities.

Other macular rashes of childhood are associated with virus infection and seen sometimes in adults, but are usually fleeting and more diffusely distributed. Adenovirus and Coxsackie-associated arthritis of the juvenile type with rash, fever, splenomegaly, and recurrent arthritis lasting

between 8 months and 3 years have been described [32]. Eleven other such viral infections with rash, lymphadenopathy and arthritis are listed by Malawista and Steere [33] who have also, with others, described a new disease, mainly of children, with rash and arthritis—Lyme arthritis or erythema chronica migrans—caused by a deer tick-borne spirochete.

Perhaps the most important of these is rubella arthritis, either natural or postvaccinal, which may sometimes be mistaken for rheumatic fever or a Still's type juvenile arthritis, but is distinguished by the mononuclear character of the synovial exudate [34] as well as by other manifestations of the disease. In atypical cases, confusion may occur with drug reactions with rash and synovitis. Cases of Wissler's syndrome [35] and "subsepsis allergica" [36] are probably examples of Still's disease.

Familial diseases with rash and joint symptoms include: (1) familial cold "urticaria" first described by Kile and Rusk [37], with skin histologically resembling that of a rheumatic fever rash due to release of chymotrypsin enzyme [38]; (2) Muckle and Wells' syndrome [39], characterized by "aguey bouts" [40]; (3) hereditary inflammatory vasculitis with nodules [41]; (4) erythrokeratoderma with deafness [42]; (5) recurrent rash with episcleritis and rheumatism, described by Jones and Champion [43] in a mother and child and seen in a patient whom (with Professor Lachmann) we have investigated without success for complement deficiencies; and (6) other children with Still-like rashes and arthritis that we have seen, such as the familial arthropathy associated with rash, uveitis, mental retarda-

Table 157-1 Association of rash with other factors of Still's disease

	No.	Fever	Lymphad-enopathy	Spleno-megaly	Positive DAT*
Children with rash	46	85%*	67%*	50%†	26%
Children without rash	120	34%	35%	15%	28%

* Differential sheep cell agglutination titer for rheumatoid factor.
† Significant at $p < 0.001$.

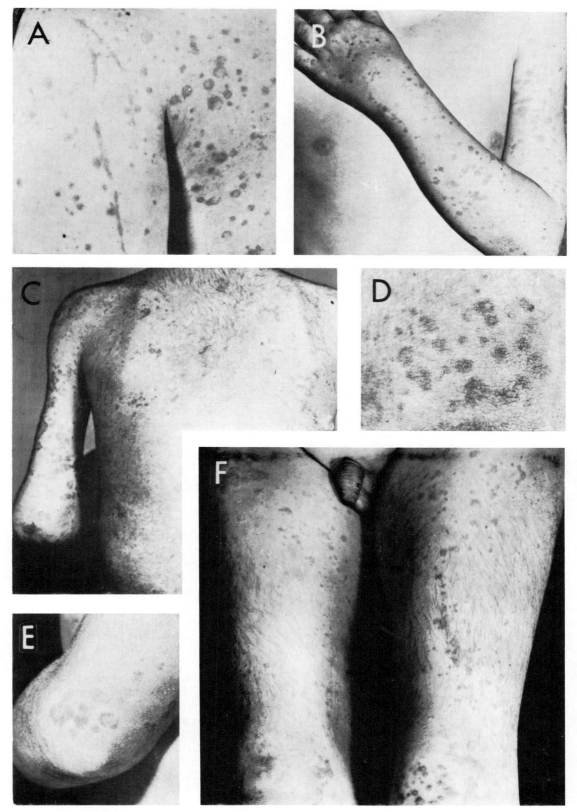

Fig. 157-15   Examples of rash in Still's disease. (From Isdale and Bywaters [27]. Reprinted by kind permission of the Clarendon Press, Oxford.)

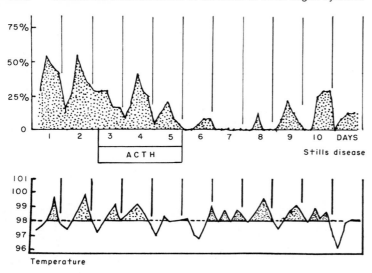

Fig. 157-16   Chart showing diurnal variation of Still's disease in relation to temperature and ACTH administration.

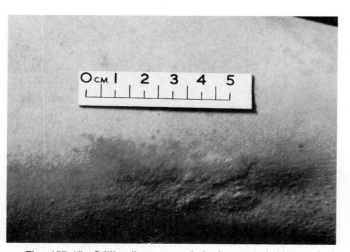

Fig. 157-17   Still's disease rash in boy aged 11, atypical because slightly raised in places.

Fig. 157-18   Biopsy of a rash in woman aged 23 with rheumatoid arthritis for 1 year and a rash typical of Still's disease. Rash lasted on and off over a period of 4 years, despite cortisone therapy. H&E, ×225.

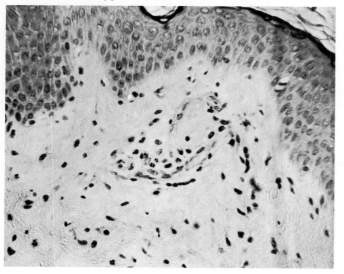

tion, and a most peculiar facies [44] to be differentiated from Lowe's syndrome [45]. Farber's storage disease must also be differentiated or, in adults, multicentric reticulo-histiocytosis, both with destructive arthropathy.

Other types of skin involvement occurring during the course of Still's disease are usually drug rashes or rashes due to intercurrent infection, e.g., pityriasis rosea. Only very rarely are vascular lesions seen in childhood rheumatoid arthritis, and these only in older seropositive (Rose-Waaler-positive) patients.

Psoriatic arthritis may occur during childhood, and, as in the adult, the synovitis may present years before the development of the skin lesion and sometimes even before the development of nail pitting.

In adults, Sweet's syndrome or acute febrile neutrophilic dermatosis needs to be differentiated [46].

Subcutaneous nodules are found predominantly in those cases of juvenile chronic polyarthritis with a positive Rose-Waaler test result and usually in teenagers. As has been shown in a review of 197 cases [47], these nodules, occurring in 9 percent, resembled more closely those of rheumatic fever than those of rheumatoid arthritis (Fig. 157-19) and lacked the highly organized division into necrotic center and peripheral cellular palisade. Thus, if a child is found to have subcutaneous nodules histologically resembling those of adult rheumatoid arthritis (e.g., [48]), the likelihood is that they are the nodules of granuloma annulare (Fig. 157-20), and, indeed, in some such cases the later development of the characteristic cutaneous lesion has been seen. Such subcutaneous nodules have been described as "benign rheumatoid nodules" [49] or as "pseudorheumatoid" (isolated) nodules with negative tests for antinuclear factor and rheumatoid factor [50]. However, more recently "hidden" rheumatoid factor has been found in the serum of such cases—19S IgM and complement-fixing [51].

Rheumatoid arthritis in the adult

Skin manifestations of adult rheumatoid arthritis are, with the exception of leg ulceration, usually confined to those patients with rheumatoid factor (Rose-Waaler) in the serum—a 19S macroglobulin with antibody-like action toward, and forming a complex with, altered 7S gamma globulin. It seems probable that the vasculitis is due to deposition of immune complex of a certain size in the vessel wall with complement activation: cryoprecipitate has been found associated with vasculitis [52]. Skin vessels in rheumatoid arthritis, even in normal areas, have been shown to contain IgM and C3 deposits [53]. The presence of IgM deposits and complement in the dermal-epidermal junction in 50 percent of rheumatoid cases (similar to those in SLE) [54] were not confirmed by DeBoer et al [55]. It seems to this author probable that the skin lesions in seropositive rheumatoid arthritis are due to vasculitis and that vasculitis itself is due to the presence of IgM and complement in the perivascular areas, the added insult of trauma increasing permeability and allowing complement to reach the area with subsequent activation and inflammation. Lesions in vessels shown by arteriography appear to be localized at the sites of mild trauma. Patients with cutaneous manifestations resulting from vasculitis usually have high titers of rheumatoid factor and show subcutaneous nodules on the elbows or elsewhere; lung lesions and episcleritis are common, and in some instances polyarteritis or arterial blockage in important visceral territories may develop (see [56]).

These vascular lesions first manifest themselves on the digits [57] (Fig. 157-21), usually as intracutaneous papules of the finger pulp, of the nail fold, or at the nail edges. They are sometimes painful, always at pressure sites, and progress from a pale to a red papule, then developing central staining and the formation of a brown scar with superficial flaking. These lesions can be initiated by trauma and occur only if the fingers are used. They disappear if the patient is brought into the indolent atmosphere of a hospital, although the underlying arterial obstructions may be seen also in the paralyzed limbs of hemiplegic rheu-

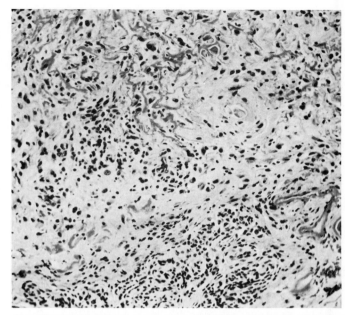

Fig. 157-19   Histologic appearance of Still's disease nodule in a girl aged 9. There is a resemblance to rheumatic fever, but the nuclei are not as plump. There is no palisading, despite the presence of a considerable amount of latticelike fibrinoid. H&E, ×120.

matoid patients [58]. In severe cases, pulp atrophy or even gangrene may ensue [59]; in milder cases, all that may be left is nail ridging resulting from vascular lesions of the nail fold. Arteriography will always show some digital arterial closures, and histologic examination shows a bland obliterative endarteritis [59].

Fig. 157-20   Granuloma annulare presenting as subcutaneous nodules (biopsy), with later appearance of cutaneous lesions in a boy aged 11.

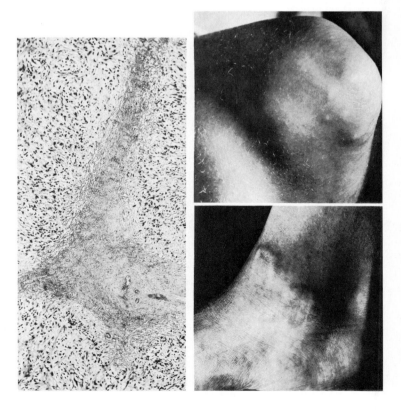

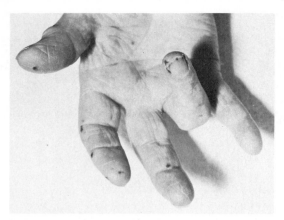

Fig. 157-21   Cutaneous vascular lesions in finger pulps and nail edges in a man aged 59 with seropositive rheumatoid arthritis for 11 years.

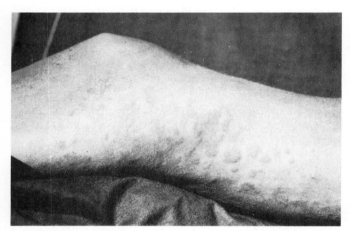

Fig. 157-22   Urticarial rash due to vasculitis in a woman aged 42 with seropositive rheumatoid arthritis for 14 years.

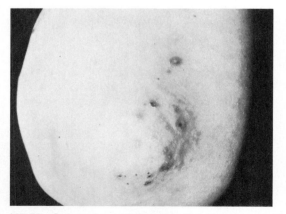

Fig. 157-23   Cutaneous nodules over the elbow in a woman aged 27 with seropositive rheumatoid arthritis since the age of 18, with episcleritis, lung nodules, and gangrene.

In other patients, wider ischemic changes are seen, with the formation of urticaria and erythematous areas or purpura. It is not uncommon to see in one patient over a period of time the whole gamut of changes, from nail fold,

nail edge, and pulp lesions, with later development of urticarial lesions in perhaps the forearm (Fig. 157-22), purpura on the legs (aided by gravity) with neuritis, and ulceration or gangrene of the extremities. In others, bullous lesions may appear, sometimes complicated by infection (''pyoderma gangrenosum''). Such a patient will often succumb finally to mesenteric thrombosis with infarction, and at autopsy obliterative arterial damage of a rheumatoid nature may be seen in many different organs. However, the prognosis is not wholly bad, and many patients with such changes have been followed over many years of remission and active useful life [60].

Other skin changes in rheumatoid arthritis which should be mentioned briefly include:

1. Skin atrophy. Most obvious in the elderly or in steroid-treated patients, it is present also in younger patients, not on steroid, with disuse due to pain.

2. ''Liver palms,'' or Dawson's palms. A bright red coloration of the contact surfaces of the palms and pulps, this is seen in rheumatoid arthritis, also in liver disease, and in a few normal individuals. Its significance is unknown.

3. A vivid yellow coloration of the skin [61]. This has sometimes been seen in severely crippled rheumatoid patients. This can be removed by vigorous washing and is due to inspissated sweat.

4. Cutaneous (dermal) nodules (Fig. 157-23). These may frequently be found, especially in those patients who have subcutaneous nodules (see below). Perhaps because of their superficial location, they are detected and biopsied earlier than the usual subcutaneous nodule and present a proliferating cellular lesion very different on first analysis from the indolent necrotic lesion of the subcutaneous nodule but are essentially the same [57].

5. The subcutaneous nodule of rheumatoid arthritis has been extensively reviewed by Collins [62], Keil [6], and Bennett et al [63]. These occur only in seropositive rheumatoid arthritis, and Sokoloff [64] believes they are due to the vascular changes seen in such patients. Rarely, nodules with this characteristic structure of central necrosis and peripheral palisade may be found in patients without clinical arthritis. In such instances, where the Rose-Waaler test is almost always negative, the lesions are usually those of the subcutaneous variant of granuloma annulare [57].

Other associations of joint and skin disease

Other diseases involving the skin are occasionally associated with arthritis, synovitis, or arthralgia, e.g., acne conglobata [65,66], scleroderma, both systemic (see Chap. 154) and localized [67], diffuse fasciitis [68], probably another variant, keratoderma blenorrhagica with Reiter's syndrome (see Chap. 159), the thickened skin and synovial effusions of hereditary osteoarthropathy or of acromegaly, dermatomyositis (see Chap. 153), and of course, systemic lupus erythematosus (see Chap. 152).

References

1. Bywaters EGL, Thomas GT: Bed rest, salicylates and steroid in rheumatic fever. *Br Med J* 1:1628, 1961
2. Bywaters EGL: Rheumatic fever and chorea, in *Textbook of the Rheumatic Diseases,* 3d ed, edited by WSC Copeman. Edinburgh, Livingstone, 1964, p 120

3. Burns RE et al: Cutaneous papules heralding rheumatic carditis (Rosenberg). *Arch Dermatol* **89**:334, 1964

4. Rayer P: *Theoretical and Practical Treatise on Diseases of the Skin,* 2d ed. London, Baillière, Tindall & Cox, 1835

5. Perry CB: Erythema marginatum (rheumaticum). *Arch Dis Child* **12**:233, 1937

6. Keil H: The rheumatic erythemas: a critical survey. *Ann Intern Med* **11**:2223, 1938

7. Bywaters EGL et al: Schönlein-Henoch purpura: evidence for a group A β-haemolytic streptococcal aetiology. *Q J Med* **26**:161, 1957

8. Cockayne EA: Rheumatic rashes and their significance. *Archives of Middlesex Hospital* **28(clin ser 11)**:28, 1912

9. Bass MH: The cutaneous manifestations of acute rheumatic fever in childhood. *Med Clin North Am* **2**:201, 1918

10. Gadrat J: Erythème papulaux rhumatismal: lésions dermiques du type Aschoff–Klinge. *Bull Soc Fr Dermatol Syphiligr* **44**:1782, 1937

11. Gadrat J: Sur les érythèmes rhumatismaux. *Ann Dermatol Syphiligr (Paris)* **9**:1045, 1938

12. Jones TD: The diagnosis of rheumatic fever. *JAMA* **126**:481, 1944

13. Goodall EW: Further observations on serum sickness, *Metropolitan Asylums Board (London) Annual Report 1924–1925,* p 160

14. Darré H: Les symptomes cutanés de la trypanosomiase humaine; étude clinique et anatomique des exanthèmes trypanosomiasiques. *Ann Dermatol Syphiligr (Paris)* **9**:673, 1908

15. Purdy MJ: Erythema gyratum repens: report of a case. *Arch Dermatol* **80**:590, 1959

16. Shammy HK: Bronchiolar carcinoma presenting as erythema gyratum perstans. *Proc R Soc Med* **56**:904, 1963

17. Summerly R: The figurate erythemas and neoplasia. *Br J Dermatol* **76**:370, 1964

18. Shelley WB: Erythema annulare centrifugum due to *Candida albicans. Br J Dermatol* **77**:383, 1965

19. Jillson OF: Allergic confirmation that some cases of erythema annulare centrifugum are dermatophytids. *Arch Dermatol* **70**:355, 1954

20. Beare JM et al: Familial annular erythema: an apparently new dominant mutation. *Br J Dermatol* **78**:59, 1966

21. Fried R et al: Erythema annulare centrifugum (Darier) in a newborn infant. *J Pediatr* **50**:66, 1957

22. Burke JB: Erythema marginatum. *Arch Dis Child* **30**:359, 1955

23. Kingston D, Glynn LE: A cross-reaction between *Str. pyogenes* and human fibroblasts, endothelial cells and astrocytes. *Immunology* **21**:1003, 1971

24. Still GF: On a form of chronic joint disease in children. *Med-Chir Tr (London)* **80**:47, 1897

25. Fahr T, Kleinschmidt H: Multiple chronische Gelenkerkrankung und rheumatische Infektion im Kindesalter. *Klin Wochenschr* **11**:708, 1932

26. Boldero HEA: Case of Still's disease. *Trans Med Soc Lond* **56**:55, 1933

27. Isdale IC, Bywaters EGL: The rash of rheumatoid arthritis and Still's disease. *Q J Med* **25**:377, 1956

28. Bywaters EGL: Still's disease in the adult. *Ann Rheum Dis* **30**:121, 1971

29. Elkon K et al: Adult-onset Still's disease: twenty year follow-up and further studies of patients with active disease. *Arthritis Rheum* **25**:647, 1982

30. Healey LA, Willkens RF: Tarsal arthritis with ankylosis in late-onset Still's disease. *Arthritis Rheum* **25**:1254, 1982

31. DeMulder PHM, Van der Putte LBA: Adult onset Still's disease: destructive distal interphalangeal arthritis associated with transient capsular calcification. *Ann Rheum Dis* **41**:544, 1982

32. Rahal JJ et al: Coxsackie virus and adenovirus infection: association with acute febrile and juvenile rheumatoid arthritis. *JAMA* **235**:2496, 1976

33. Malawista SE, Steere AC: Viral arthritis, in *Textbook of Rheumatology,* edited by WN Kelley et al. Philadelphia, WB Saunders, 1981, p 1586

34. Chambers RJ, Bywaters EGL: Rubella synovitis. *Ann Rheum Dis* **22**:263, 1963

35. Wissler H: Die chronische Polyarthritis des Kindes. *Rheumatismus* **24**:1, 1942

36. Böttiger LE, Landegren J: Wissler's syndrome. *Acta Med Scand* **174**:415, 1963

37. Kile RL, Rusk HA: Case of cold urticaria with an unusual family history. *JAMA* **114**:1067, 1940

38. Doeglas HMG, Bloemink E: Familial cold urticaria. *Arch Dermatol* **110**:382, 1974

39. Muckle TJ, Wells M: Urticaria, deafness, amyloidosis: a new heredo-familial syndrome. *Q J Med* **31**:235, 1962

40. Prost A et al: Rhumatisme intermittent revelateur d'un syndrome familial arthrite—éruption urticarienne—surdite: syndrome de Muckle et Wells sans amylose rénale. *Rev Rhum Mal Osteoartic* **43**:201, 1976

41. Reed WB et al: Hereditary inflammatory vasculitis with persistent nodules. *Br J Dermatol* **87**:299, 1972

42. Beare JM et al: Atypical erythrokeratoderma with deafness, physical retardation and peripheral neuropathy. *Br J Dermatol* **87**:309, 1972

43. Jones BR, Champion RH: Still's disease: rash in mother and daughter. *Br J Dermatol* **88**:202, 1973

44. Ansell BM et al: Familial arthropathy with rash, uveitis and mental retardation. *Proc R Soc Med* **68**:584, 1975

45. Athreya BH et al: Arthropathy of Lowe's (oculocerebrorenal) syndrome. *Arthritis Rheum* **26**:728, 1983

46. Krauser RE, Schumacher HR: The arthritis of Sweet's syndrome. *Arthritis Rheum* **18**:35, 1975

47. Bywaters EGL et al: Subcutaneous nodules of Still's disease. *Ann Rheum Dis* **17**:278, 1958

48. Taranta A: Occurrence of rheumatic-like subcutaneous nodules without evidence of joint or heart disease: report of a case. *N Engl J Med* **266**:13, 1962

49. Simons FER, Schaller JG: Benign rheumatoid nodules. *Pediatrics* **56**:29, 1975

50. Williams HJ et al: Isolated subcutaneous nodules (pseudorheumatoid). *J Bone Joint Surg [Am]* **59**:73, 1977

51. Moore TL et al: Complement-fixing hidden rheumatoid factor in children with benign rheumatoid nodules. *Arthritis Rheum* **21**:930, 1978

52. Weisman MH, Zwaifler NJ: Immunopathogenesis of the vasculitis of rheumatoid arthritis. *J Clin Invest* **52**:88a, 1973

53. Conn DL et al: Cutaneous vessel immune deposits in rheumatoid arthritis. *Arthritis Rheum* **19**:15, 1976

54. Donde R et al: Immune deposits in the dermo-epidermal junction in rheumatoid arthritis. *Scand J Rheumatol* **6**:57, 1977

55. DeBoer DC et al: Skin basement membrane immunofluorescence in rheumatoid arthritis. *Arthritis Rheum* **20**:653, 1977

56. Bywaters EGL, Scott JT: The natural history of vascular lesions in rheumatoid arthritis. *J Chronic Dis* **16**:905, 1963

57. Bywaters EGL: A variant of rheumatoid arthritis characterized by recurrent digital pad nodules and palmar fasciitis, closely resembling palindromic rheumatism. *Ann Rheum Dis* **8**:2, 1949

58. Thompson M, Bywaters EGL: Unilateral rheumatoid arthritis following hemiplegia. *Ann Rheum Dis* **21**:370, 1962

59. Bywaters EGL: Peripheral vascular obstruction in rheumatoid arthritis and its relationship to other vascular lesions. *Ann Rheum Dis* **16**:84, 1957

60. Bywaters EGL: Vasculitis and the rheumatoid nodule, in *Rheumatic Diseases,* edited by JJR Duthie, WRM Alexander. University of Edinburgh Pitzer Medical Monograph 3. Edinburgh, Edinburgh Univ Press, 1968

61. Spender JK: On some of the rarer complications of rheumatoid arthritis. *Br Med J* **1**:905, 1892

62. Collins DH: The subcutaneous nodule of rheumatoid arthritis. *J Pathol Bacteriol* **45**:97, 1937

63. Bennett GA et al: Subcutaneous nodules of rheumatoid arthritis and rheumatic fever: a pathologic study. *Arch Pathol* **30**:70, 1940

64. Sokoloff L: The pathophysiology of peripheral blood vessels in collagen diseases, in *The Peripheral Blood Vessels,* edited by JL Orbison, DE Smith. International Academy of Pathology Monographs in Pathology, Baltimore, Williams & Wilkins, 1963, p 297

65. Windom R et al: Acne conglobata and arthritis. *Arthritis Rheum* **4**:632, 1961

66. Bastin R et al: Manifestations rhumatismales de l'acne conglobata. *Nouv Presse Med* **7**:831, 1978

67. Ansell BM et al: Scleroderma in childhood. *Ann Rheum Dis* **35**:189, 1976

68. Shulman LE: Diffuse fasciitis with eosinophilia: a new syndrome. *Trans Assoc Am Physicians* **88**:70, 1975

CHAPTER 158

MULTICENTRIC RETICULOHISTIOCYTOSIS

Karl Holubar

Definition

Multicentric reticulohistiocytosis (MR) is a systemic granulomatous disease of unknown cause. The disease is rare and is characterized by a distinct histology.

Skin, mucosa, synovia, bone, and internal organs may be involved. Cutaneous nodules and destructive arthritis are the clinically most prominent features. A possible paraneoplastic character of MR is in consideration.

Historical aspects

Caro and Senear in 1952 [1] first studied sections of a patient with multiple cutaneous nodules for which they coined the term *reticulohistiocytic granuloma.* Ackerman in his textbook has recently reintroduced this designation [2]. The majority of authors [3–6], however, stick to the use of *multicentric reticulohistiocytosis*—originally employed by Goltz and Laymon in 1954—as the proper designation because it emphasizes the multifocal origin of the process and alludes to its systemic nature. There are at least a dozen synonyms in use in the literature [3–6], which include lipoid dermatoarthritis, giant cell histiocytosis, giant cell reticulohistiocytosis, giant cell reticulohistiocytoma, reticulohistiocytosis [3], nondiabetic cutaneous xanthomatosis, and others. These various terms reflect the insecurity as to the nature of this disease. In 1937, Weber and Freudenthal published a comprehensive study on one of their patients and during the ensuing years several more reports surfaced; by the early 1950s a new entity had emerged (for references see [4]). However, it took several more years until the systemic nature of the disease, its various clinical manifestations, and the occurrence of a destructive form of arthritis were accepted as constituting different aspects of the same disease process.

Epidemiology

Drawing from the two comprehensive reviews available to date [4,5] hardly more than about 80 cases have been reported, but it is probable that many cases have gone undiagnosed. There appears to be no geographic area of prevalence. Caucasians prevail but this may merely reflect the higher number of reports from North America and Europe; patients of African, Japanese, and American-Indian ancestry have also been reported [4,5]. According to Barrow and Holubar [4] women are more often affected than men, the ratio being about 3:1. Another review [5] reports on an equal distribution between the sexes; a third [7] again finds a greater number of women affected. Barrow and Holubar [4] calculated 43 years as the mean age of onset. After an average of about eight years, the disease burns out and becomes inactive.

Etiology and pathogenesis

Virtually nothing is known about the etiology of MR and only speculations can be made regarding its pathogenesis [4,5]. The hallmark of the disease is a granulomatous, proliferative process of histiocytes, some of which are multinucleated and laden with lipids. The stimulus is not known and no specific metabolic defect has been found; there is also no evidence of an infective agent and no data are available as to a possible compromise of the host's immune status. Anatomic proximity of lipid-laden histiocytes to blood vessels has repeatedly been observed and emphasized, but there is no evidence to permit inclusion of MR into one of the lipid storage diseases.

Clinical manifestations

Skin and joint symptoms dominate the clinical picture. Almost two-thirds of patients first note arthritis; about one-fifth note skin nodules first, and in one-fifth skin and joint changes appear simultaneously. About half of the cases eventually develop mucous membrane manifestations [4].

Skin changes

The face, particularly the nose and paranasal areas, hands (particularly the nail folds, Fig. 158-1), ears, forearms, scalp (particularly behind the ears), neck, and trunk are

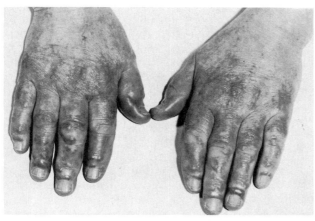

Fig. 158-1 Hands of a patient with active skin lesions of multicentric reticulohistiocytosis. Note the periungual array of some of the nodules. (From Barrow and Holubar [4], with permission of Hautarzt.)

involved in decreasing order of frequency. The hemispherical, nontender nodular lesions have a reddish brown hue; they vary in size from a few millimeters to conglomerate nodules measuring several centimeters. Ulceration normally does not occur. Pruritus may be a prominent symptom. Erythema may precede the formation of nodules.

Articular changes

There is symmetrical involvement of the interphalangeal joints, knees, shoulders, wrists, hips, ankles, feet, elbows, and vertebral joints, in decreasing order of frequency. The arthritic process is destructive (arthritis mutilans); bone and cartilage are destroyed and severe deformation of the joints ensues. The process progresses rapidly in the beginning, to taper off gradually and finally to "burn out." There is a marked discrepancy between the severity of the radiographic findings and the underlying bone destruction, and the relatively mild clinical symptomatology. In far-advanced cases the fingers are considerably shortened but can be pulled out to their full length. This has led to designations like "la main en lorgnette," opera-glass hand, telescope fingers, or concertina-hand. There is no periosteal reaction or osteoporosis.

Mucosal changes

Roughly half the patients have mucosal lesions [4]; the lips, buccal mucosa, tongue, gingiva, and nasal septum are most frequently involved. Physically, the nodules mimic those in the skin (Fig. 158-2).

Other clinical manifestations

Reports on other lesions include xanthelasmata, infiltrates along tendon sheaths, lesions in the myocardium and in the lungs [8], adenopathy, and pathologic fractures; hypertension and hyperextensible joints have also been noted. Flam et al [6] also observed a carpal tunnel syndrome, Dupuytren's contracture, and pleural effusion, but the histopathology of their case was atypical so that it must be left open as to whether their patient had MR or not. This

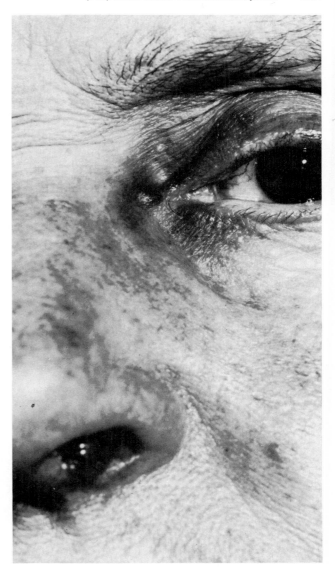

Fig. 158-2 Multicentric reticulohistiocytosis. Mucocutaneous nodular infiltrate on nasal mucosa and adjoining skin. (From Barrow and Holubar [4], with permission of Hautarzt.)

may also be the case in Fast's patient [8] presenting with cardiopulmonary complications, and another report on mixed aortic and mitral valvular disease where the authors [9] raise the question as to whether these changes may not have been of rheumatic origin. Piette et al [10] observed splenomegaly and pancytopenia in a patient with MR who did not have facial lesions; they suspected a possible relationship to a hematologic disorder, but could not solve the question because the patient was lost to follow-up. Randall et al [11] in their report on two cases of atypical MR, found an association with a gamma heavy-chain type of paraprotein. Neither case presented with any articular involvement. Again, it is questionable whether these two patients had MR or not. The same holds for the case of Furey et al [12], who exhibited salivary gland involvement and pericardial effusion. Gold et al [13] alluded to a possible causal relationship between MR and tuberculosis, and Chevrant-Breton [5] in her extensive review cites various authors who reported on ocular changes, neurologic and

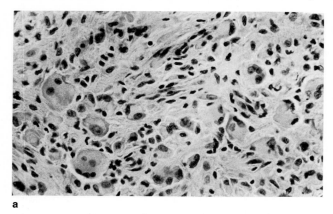

a

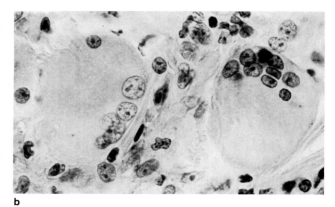

b

Fig. 158-3   Microphotograph of a lesion of the patient shown in Fig. 158-1. Note histiocytic infiltrate (a) and multinucleated giant cells with aggregated nuclei and "ground-glass" cy- toplasm (b). × 100 (a), × 250 (b). *(From Holubar and Mach [3], with permission of Hautarzt.)*

(terminal) hematologic manifestations. All these findings, however, are not substantiated by the presence of the specific histopathologic infiltrates and the question of a fortuitous association cannot be answered.

Laboratory findings

Only nonspecific findings have been reported: anemia, elevated sedimentation rate, leukocytosis and eosinophilia, hyper- and hypocholesterolemia, hypergammaglobulinemia. Cold agglutinins and cryoglobulins have been found in a few cases. Positive skin tests to tuberculin and negative serology have been seen with rheumatoid arthritis.

Pathology

Skin and mucous membrane lesions

The histopathology of skin lesions is fairly uniform [4,5,14–18]. The nodules are nonencapsulated, moderately well circumscribed, and occupy the entire dermis or parts of it. Frequently there is a narrow zone of noninfiltrated connective tissue between the infiltrates and the slightly atrophic epidermis. Lesions consist of histiocytic cells, irregular in size and shape (Fig. 158-3a). Many have transformed into multinucleated giant cells, generally up to about 250 μm in diameter, occasionally also larger (Fig. 158-3b). They contain up to 20 or more aggregated nuclei with a distinct nuclear membrane and prominent nucleoli. The cytoplasm is slightly eosinophilic, has a granular appearance ("ground-glass cytoplasm"), and occasionally may be foamy or show tiny vacuoles. There are no Tuton type giant cells [2,19] (Fig. 158-3a and b). MR nodules contain lymphocytes which are more numerous in early lesions, and plasma cells, eosinophils, mast cells, and occasionally, extravasated erythrocytes. With increasing age of the lesions, lymphocytes and giant cells decrease in number, fibroblasts appear, and there is fibrosis. Lesions are usually well vascularized and the capillaries show endothelial hypertrophy. At places, histiocytes and giant cells show a perivascular arrangement. Elastic fibers are fragmented, clumped, and thickened, particularly in the early lesions.

Histochemical investigations

The cytoplasm of histiocytes and giant cells is PAS-positive, hyaluronidase- and diastase-resistant, suggesting the presence of glycoproteins [4]; it contains phospholipids, neutral fats, and iron [4]. Biochemical studies by Barrow et al (for references see [4]) have failed to reveal an isolated enzyme defect responsible for the lipid accumulation in these cells.

Electron microscopy

There are no Birbeck granules (Langerhans cell granules) in the histiocytic cells. Both histiocytes and giant cells show lobulated nuclei with indented contours and margination of nuclear chromatin, an enlarged Golgi apparatus, and hyperplastic endoplasmic reticulum with dilated cysternae. Lipid-laden vacuoles are present and numerous small, electron-dense, ovoid or rod-shaped cytoplasmic granules, up to 250 nm in size have been described. Autophagic vacuoles are present and acid phosphatase activity has been detected in the rod-shaped granules and in the autophagic vacuoles [14,16]. Complex interdigitation of membranes of adjacent histiocytic cells has been described as a constant and characteristic feature. In addition, Caputo et al [20] have observed collagen phagocytosis.

The histiocytes which make up the infiltrate in MR have been characterized by their iron uptake, positivity for acid phosphatase and unspecific esterase, and for lysozyme [4,5,14,16,20,21].

Synovial lesions

The histopathology of the lesions is identical to that of skin. However, the number of giant cells and histochemical reactions has been reported to be variable [5].

Lesions in other tissues

The histopathology of lesions in other organs, e.g., the endocardium, myocardium, pleura, in the eyes, etc., are not typical for MR and it is not clear whether they signify involvement with MR or are due to other, concomitant disease factors.

Diagnosis and differential diagnosis

Typical cases should hardly be missed by anyone who is familiar with the syndrome. Morphology and localization of cutaneous nodules, the typical articular symptoms, and radiographic findings (symmetrical involvement, particularly of the distal interphalangeal joints) are highly suggestive. The histopathology of a mucocutaneous nodule will provide the diagnosis. A variety of disorders has to be differentiated from MR [4,5]: rheumatoid arthritis, the various types of xanthomas, Farber's disease (disseminated lipogranulomatosis), lepromatous leprosy, lipoid proteinosis, sarcoidosis, histiocytosis X, juvenile and adult xanthogranuloma, solitary reticulohistiocytoma, generalized eruptive histiocytoma, the congenital reticulohistiocytoma of Hashimoto and Pritzker [22], and Zayid's familial histiocytic dermatoarthritis [23]. MR is not familial or congenital. The absence of one of the typical features of MR such as acral or facial nodules, mutilating arthritis, characteristic histopathology, and history of the patient will rule out many of the above. Rheumatoid arthritis differs from MR with regard to the history of the patient, the rheumatoid serology, histopathology of the paraarticular nodules, and the absence of rapidly mutilating arthritis.

In generalized eruptive histiocytoma [24–26] lesions are confined to the skin, the distribution is symmetrical, typically confined to the trunk and upper extremities, and without concomitant articular lesions. The histopathology and ultrastructure are unlike MR and are diagnostic [25]. Differentiation from juvenile and adult xanthogranuloma [2,19] again rests on history, clinical presentation, absence of joint involvement, and histopathologic details. Xanthogranulomas abound in Tuton type giant cells but lack the MR type giant cell; the infiltrate is more "mixed" with lymphocytes, neutrophils, eosinophils, and fibroblasts. The cytoplasm of histiocytes in xanthogranuloma is foamy and has no "ground-glass" appearance as in MR. Histiocytosis X is easily separated from MR clinically, histopathologically, and by electron microscopy, because the MR histiocytes are not of the Langerhans cell type and lack Birbeck granules. Finally, differential diagnosis should consider diffuse cutaneous reticulohistiocytosis [27]; there was no arthritis in this single case of Goette et al and the skin eruption consisted of psoriatic lesions and asymptomatic, nonscaling papules which spread over the body and then partially involuted spontaneously. This patient developed leukemia.

Associated conditions

Various concomitant diseases have been mentioned [4]: thyroid disorders, tuberculosis, diabetes, hemoblastoses, and cancer. Patients with cancers of the colon, breast, bronchus, cervix, ovary, and stomach have been reported [4,17]. Incidence rates vary between 15 percent [4] and 27 and 24 percent [7,17]. An association with sarcoma and lymphoma has also been observed and prompted Caterall and White [17] to compare MR with dermatomyositis. However, the relationship between MR and an accompanying tumor is complex; the tumor may progress and MR may remit; on the other hand, MR may progress despite removal of the tumor. Many authors therefore remain skeptical with regard to the alleged paraneoplastic character of MR [5]. Whatever the relationship may be, a careful search in MR patients for occult neoplasms is warranted.

Treatment

Corticosteroids, ACTH, antimalarials, salicylates, indomethacine, pyrazolone, clofibrate, and various antimitotic compounds have been tried but controlled studies have not been performed. Recently, topical therapy with nitrogen mustard has also been advocated [28]. The administration of antimitotic agents such as nitrogen mustard, chlorambucil, vinca alkaloids, and cyclophosphamide, appears to be a rational approach but the possibility that MR may be a paraneoplastic condition must be taken into account. The employment of antimetabolites and cytostatics may have an inducer-enhancer effect on occult tumor growth and constitutes a potential additional risk for the patient.

Course and prognosis

Skin nodules and arthritis do not necessarily run parallel. Articular changes may wax and wane and finally evolve into mutilating arthritis, while skin nodules may not appear at all or erupt in successive crops with new infiltrates being superimposed on older, regressing ones. The course of MR is capricious; about half of the patients will eventually suffer from destructive arthritis as a prominent feature. Prediction as to the individual course is difficult.

As a rule, the disease burns out after five to eight years [4,5], the patient being left with severe articular deformations and related disfigurement of the hands, face, and scalp. Systemic involvement of other organs is even more difficult to assess and the course cannot be prognosticated. Biopsies of internal organs are not always available and where they are the histopathology may not allow an unequivocal correlation with the mucocutaneous lesions of MR.

Thanks are due to the Herman D. Oritsky Dermatology Research Fund, Jerusalem, and to Schering Berlin.

References

1. Caro MR, Senear FE: Reticulohistiocytoma of the skin. *Arch Dermatol* **65:**701, 1952
2. Ackerman AB: *Histologic Diagnosis of Inflammatory Skin Diseases.* Philadelphia, Lea & Febiger, 1978, p 472
3. Holubar K, Mach K: Histiocytosis giganto-cellularis. *Hautarzt* **17:**440, 1966
4. Barrow MV, Holubar K: Multicentric reticulohistiocytosis. *Medicine (Baltimore)* **48:**287, 1969
5. Chevrant-Breton J: La réticulo-histiocytose multicentrique. Revue de la littérature récente (depuis 1969). *Ann Dermatol Venereol* **104:**745, 1977
6. Flam M et al: Multicentric reticulohistiocytosis. *Medicine (Baltimore)* **52:**841, 1972
7. Catterall MD: Multicentric reticulohistiocytosis. A review of eight cases. *Clin Exp Dermatol* **5:**267, 1980
8. Fast A: Cardiopulmonary complications in multicentric reticulohistiocytosis. *Arch Dermatol* **112:**1139, 1976
9. Jessop S, Gordon W: Multicentric reticulohistiocytosis. *S Afr Med J* **49:**2191, 1975
10. Piette J-C et al: Réticulohistiocytome multicentrique avec

splénomégalie et pancytopénie. *Ann Dermatol Venereol* **109:**801, 1982

11. Randall JRS et al: Atypical multicentric reticulohistiocytosis with paraproteinemia. *Arch Dermatol* **113:**1576, 1977
12. Furey N et al: Multicentric reticulohistiocytosis with salivary gland involvement and pericardial effusion. *J Am Acad Dermatol* **8:**679, 1983
13. Gold KD et al: Relationship between multicentric reticulohistiocytosis and tuberculosis. *JAMA* **237:**2213, 1977
14. Coode PE et al: Multicentric reticulohistiocytosis: report of two cases with ultrastructure, tissue culture and immunology studies. *Clin Exp Dermatol* **5:**281, 1980
15. Burgdorf WHC et al: Immunohistochemical identification of lysozyme in cutaneous lesions of alleged histiocytic nature. *Am J Clin Pathol* **75:**162, 1981
16. Tani M et al: Multicentric reticulohistiocytosis. *Arch Dermatol* **117:**495, 1981
17. Catterall MD, White JE: Multicentric reticulohistiocytosis and malignant disease. *Br J Dermatol* **98:**221, 1978
18. Krmpotić L et al: Multizentrische Retikulohistiozytose. *Hautarzt* **31:**384, 1980
19. Ackerman AB et al: *Differential Diagnosis in Dermatopathology.* Philadelphia, Lea & Febiger, 1982, p 166
20. Caputo R et al: Collagen phagocytosis in multicentric reticulohistiocytosis. *J Invest Dermatol* **76:**342, 1981
21. Brégeon C et al: Réticulohistiocytose multicentrique. *Rev Rhum Mal Osteoartic* **49:**59, 1982
22. Hashimoto K, Pritzker MS: Electron microscopic study of reticulohistiocytoma. *Arch Dermatol* **107:**263, 1973
23. Zayid I, Farraj S: Familial histiocytic dermatoarthritis. A new syndrome. *Am J Med* **54:**793, 1973
24. Winkelmann RK, Muller SA: Generalized eruptive histiocytoma. *Arch Dermatol* **88:**586, 1963
25. Cramer H-J: Multiple Reticulohistiocytome der Haut ohne nachweisbare Zweiterkrankung. *Hautarzt* **14:**297, 1963
26. Muller SA et al: Generalized eruptive histiocytoma. Enzyme histochemistry and electron microscopy. *Arch Dermatol* **96:**11, 1967
27. Goette DK et al: Diffuse cutaneous reticulohistiocytosis. *Arch Dermatol* **118:**173, 1982
28. Brandt F et al: Topical nitrogen mustard therapy in multicentric reticulohistiocytosis. *J Am Acad Dermatol* **6:**260, 1982

CHAPTER 159

REITER'S SYNDROME

Frank C. Arnett, Jr.

Definition

Reiter's syndrome (disease) is classically defined as the triad of nongonococcal urethritis, conjunctivitis, and arthritis [1,2]. Its prominent mucocutaneous lesions constitute the rationale for considering it a clinical tetrad. More recent findings, however, have made broader definitions necessary. Many patients will not clinically express all features, including urethritis and/or conjunctivitis (incomplete Reiter's syndrome) [3]. The American Rheumatism Association recently has adopted the following definition: "an episode of peripheral arthritis of more than one month's duration occurring in association with urethritis and/or cervicitis"[4]. A more mechanistic concept is that of a *reactive arthritis* following enteric and possibly sexually transmitted infections in the genetically predisposed host.

Historical aspects

An association between urethritis (blennorrhagica) and arthritis was first reported in 1784 by Swediaur, but differentiation of Reiter's syndrome from gonococcal arthritis in early descriptions is impossible [5]; Brodie's may have been the first (1818) since conjunctivitis was a notable feature [5]. Keratodermia blennorrhagica was introduced as a term in 1896 and was long considered a lesion related to gonococcal infections [6]. In 1916 Fiessinger and Leroy observed a *conjunctivo-urethro-synovial* syndrome in four French soldiers following dysentery [6]. One week later Hans Reiter described the same syndrome along with dermatitis in a young German officer [1]. Bauer and Engleman

recorded the first American cases during World War II [2]. The link to *Shigella flexneri* was firmly established by Paronen's report of 344 cases of Reiter's syndrome evolving 1 to 4 weeks after an outbreak of bacillary dysentery among 150,000 Finnish soldiers in 1944 [7]. A smaller epidemic of 9 cases in 1962 was recorded by Noer [8] following shigellosis in 602 crew members of the American naval vessel, "Little Rock." A genetic predisposition was established in 1973 with the demonstration of a striking association between Reiter's syndrome and the histocompatibility antigen, HLA-B27 [9]. Infectious-genetic interplay in pathogenesis was further solidified by finding HLA-B27 in 78 percent of 50 survivors of the Finnish epidemic [10] and in 4 of 5 sailors from the shipboard outbreak [11].

Epidemiology

Reiter's syndrome occurs in two environmental settings [12]. The epidemic or postdysenteric form has been reported most frequently from continental Europe and North Africa. Endemic disease, often attributed to venereal exposure, constitutes the majority of cases described in the United States and the United Kingdom.

The disease affects predominantly males between the ages of 15 and 35 years. In fact, studies in military populations suggest that Reiter's syndrome may be the most common cause of peripheral inflammatory arthritis in young men [3,13]. Affected women account for only 5 to 10 percent in most series and they usually have the postdysenteric form. Caucasians, usually of northern European descent, are most commonly affected. The disease is rare in Orientals and African blacks but is encountered occa-

Table 159-1   Relationships with HLA antigens

	HLA-B27 positive*	Other HLA associations	References
Reiter's syndrome	63–75%	B7-Creg†	[9, 20–23]
With sacroiliitis	90%	—	
With uveitis	90%	—	
With aortitis	100%	—	
Ankylosing spondylitis	90%	Bw16 (Bw38, Bw39) B7-Creg†	[24–26]
Pustular psoriasis	56%	—	[27]
Psoriasis vulgaris	Not increased	B13, B17, B37, Cw6, ?DR7	[28]
Psoriatic arthritis Peripheral	Not increased	B16 (Bw38, Bw39), ?DR4	[28,29]
Spondylitis	50%	Bw16 (Bw38, Bw39)	[28,29]

* Normal Caucasian frequency 8 percent.
† Includes B7, Bw22, B40, and Bw42 (in addition to B27).

sionally in American blacks. A true prevalence is difficult to estimate given the sporadic occurrence of the disease, its often brief self-limited course, and underdiagnosis, especially of incompletely expressed cases [12].

Etiology and pathogenesis

Although genetic risk factors and infectious triggering agents have been identified, the mechanisms underlying the inflammatory processes seen in various tissues are unknown. Synovial fluid and cutaneous lesions are typically sterile, although earlier reports suggested recovery of *Chlamydia (Bedsonia)* and *Mycoplasma* organisms [14,15]. Furthermore, cause and effect has not been shown for these same organisms commonly cultured from the urethra. Therefore, immunologically mediated tissue injury is currently presumed.

Genetic predisposition

Reiter's syndrome, ankylosing spondylitis, psoriasis, and psoriatic arthritis demonstrate intimate clinical and genetic interrelationships [16]. Sacroiliitis, the hallmark of ankylosing spondylitis, occurs in approximately 20 percent of patients with Reiter's syndrome and 20 percent with psoriatic arthritis [16,17]. The concurrence of psoriasis and Reiter's syndrome has often been described [18]. In a family survey of 110 relatives of 35 probands with Reiter's syndrome Lawrence [19] found a significantly increased prevalence of ankylosing spondylitis (4 percent), bilateral sacroiliitis (12 percent), and psoriasis (13 percent) in male members. HLA antigen associations may explain several of these relationships [20–29] (Table 159-1).

HLA-B27 occurs in 63 to 75 percent of Caucasians with Reiter's syndrome and in 8 percent of normal whites [9,20]. A weaker correlation exists in blacks (14 to 37 percent) who also have a lower normal prevalence of the antigen (2 to 3 percent) [30]. B27-negative patients have significantly less sacroiliitis, uveitis, and carditis, and generally the disease pursues a milder course [9,20]. A 20 percent risk for Reiter's disease has been calculated for B27-positive individuals exposed to the causative enteric pathogens [11]. A similar frequency of ankylosing spondylitis exists among B27 positives [31].

Family studies indicate a 10 percent prevalence of Rei-

ter's disease among relatives of probands affected with the same disorder, similar to the 14 percent demonstrated in spondylitis families [32–34]. Disease almost invariably segregates with B27 in such families, although with incomplete penetrance. Reiter's syndrome and ankylosing spondylitis also tend to each "breed true" within families [32–34].

It is not known whether HLA-B27 itself is the primary gene or only a marker for another closely linked locus on chromosome 6 [35]. The former theory seems more likely since immunologically cross-reactive HLA-B locus antigens (B7-Creg) occur in the majority of B27-negative patients [21,22]. Molecular differences in B27 molecules, recently defined, may explain clinical and familial differences

Table 159-2   Demographic and clinical features*

Age at onset	
Range (years)	16–59
Mean (years)	25
Median (years)	22
Sex (% males)	88
Race (% white)	76
Antecedent diarrhea	7%
Genitourinary	93%
Ocular	61%
Uveitis	20%
Mucocutaneous lesions	56%
Keratodermia	24%
Circinate balanitis (males)	41%
Oral ulcers	22%
Nail changes	10%
Affected joints	100%
Upper limb only	0%
Lower limb only	41%
Upper/lower limbs	59%
Knees	66%
Ankles	49%
Feet	63%
Low back pain	61%
Sausage digits	54%
Heel pain	54%
Fever (≥39°C)	39%
Cardiac lesions	5%
Amyloidosis	2%

* Author's series of 41 patients with either urethritis or conjunctivitis; incomplete cases lacking both features were excluded [47].

between Reiter's syndrome and ankylosing spondylitis [36,37].

Infectious agents

Enteric pathogens that trigger a reactive arthritis include *Shigella flexneri* (but not *S. sonnei*); *Salmonella enteritidis, typhimurium,* and *heidelberg; Yersinia enterocolitica* and *pseudo-tuberculosis;* and *Campylobacter fetus* [7,8,38–40]. Urethritis and/or conjunctivitis usually trail the enterocolitis by 1 to 4 weeks and herald the arthritis by several days, at which time stool cultures are almost always negative. Although only certain species and serotypes have been implicated, an antigenic factor or effect common to each has not been identified. Preliminary in vitro data have shown that T lymphocytes from American patients can be selectively stimulated by a formalin-killed European strain of *Yersinia* which also adheres to the lymphocyte at the HLA antigen site [41].

Venereal transmission is a popular supposition but has never been proved. This hypothesis pivots on the presence of urethritis and the assumption that it is sexually acquired [42,43]. Urethral inflammation, however, is an inherent mucocutaneous manifestation of Reiter's disease occurring in postdysenteric cases including children with no evident sexual exposure. Although *Chlamydia trachomatis* can be cultured from urethral secretions in 37 percent of cases, it is also found in 35 percent of patients with nongonococcal urethritis alone [44] and in 5 to 17 percent of asymptomatic males [45].

Clinical features

The patient usually is a young white male presenting with an acute arthritis and often fever [46] (Table 159-2). Urethritis and/or conjunctivitis in most cases have preceded arthritis over the preceding several days or weeks. Only one-third of patients will have the complete triad, and 40 percent will have arthritis as the only feature of the triad (incomplete Reiter's syndrome) [47].

Genitourinary

Mild to moderate dysuria with a transient mucopurulent urethral discharge is usual. Prostatitis is often concurrent, while cystitis or seminal vesiculitis is rare. Prostatic massage is not recommended since articular flares may be induced. Instead, examination of a morning urine for sterile pyuria may yield the only evidence of genital tract inflammation. Diagnosis is more difficult in women and depends on sterile pyuria and/or cervicitis.

Ocular

The nonbacterial conjunctivitis is usually bilateral, mild, and evanescent. Acute anterior uveitis (iritis), identical to that occurring in ankylosing spondylitis, occurs in 20 percent of cases.

Mucotaneous lesions

Keratodermia blennorrhagica most often begins as erythematous, pinpoint, vesicular or macular lesions on the soles and palms. Enlargement and papule formation is ac-

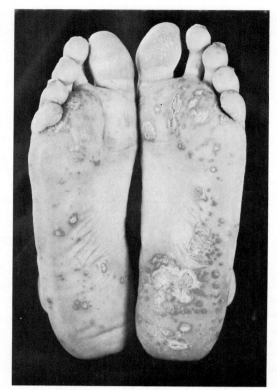

Fig. 159-1 Keratodermia blennorrhagica involving feet. *(From Renlund et al [46], by permission of The Johns Hopkins Medical Journal and University Press.)*

companied by a pustular center, thickening, hyperkeratosis, and crusting (Fig. 159-1). Heaped-up lesions may resemble mollusk shells (Fig. 159-2). Scaling plaques may develop on the scalp and over elbows, knees, buttocks, and any other area (Fig. 159-3). Erosive, exudative patches

Table 159-3 Laboratory and radiographic manifestations

	Frequency
Hematologic:	
Anemia (mild; normocytic, normochronic)	39%
Leukocytosis (10,000–20,000/mm³)	34%
Thrombocytosis (400,000–600,000/mm³)	31%
Elevated erythrocyte sedimentation rate	72%
Serologic:	
Rheumatoid factor, ANA	0%
Tissue typing:	
HLA-B27	73%
B7-Creg (B7, Bw22, B40, Bw42) in B27-negatives	70%
Synovial fluid:	
Leukocytosis (5,000–50,000/mm³)	Usual
Protein—elevated	Usual
Glucose—normal	Usual
Complement—elevated	Usual
"Reiter's cells"—macrophage containing ingested polymorphs	Rare
Bacterial cultures—negative	Usual
Radiographic:	
Periostitis	Frequent
Calcaneus ("lover's heel")	Frequent
Bony fusion across joints, especially feet	Frequent
Sacroiliitis, especially unilateral	Frequent
Syndesmophytes, especially asymmetrical	Frequent

Source: Author's series [47].

Fig. 159-2 Mollusk-like lesions of keratodermia.

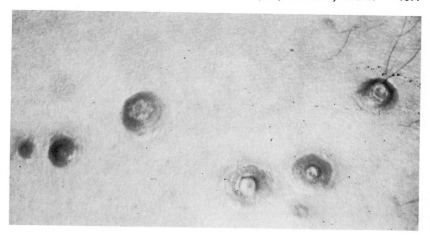

often are found on the penile shaft, especially at the scrotal junction. Involvement may be widespread and differentiation from pustular psoriasis impossible.

The clinical characteristics of *circinate balanitis* are variable. Crusting, desiccated plaques, similar to keratoderma, occur on the glans penis in the circumcised male (Fig. 159-4), while shallow, moist, serpiginous, painless ulcers with slightly raised borders, similar to oral lesions, are found in uncircumcised men (Fig. 159-5). Balanitis occurs independently of urethritis.

Oral mucous membrane ulcers of variable size, and typically painless, may be found on the tongue or hard palate (Fig. 159-6).

Nail changes include the development of small yellow pustules below the nail which enlarge, desiccate, and discolor (brownish). Thickening and opacification ensue with onycholysis and hyperkeratosis (Fig. 159-7), often with surrounding erythema and scaling of the skin (pseudoparonychia). Pitting is absent.

Musculoskeletal features

The arthritis is typically oligoarticular, involving one to six joints, and is asymmetrical (Table 159-2). Lower extremities are most often affected, usually the knees, ankles, and small articulations in the feet. Low back pain is common. Diffuse swelling (sausaging or dactylitis) characterizes toe and finger involvement (Fig. 159-8).

Fig. 159-3 Scaling plaques of keratodermia over the ankle resembling pustular psoriasis.

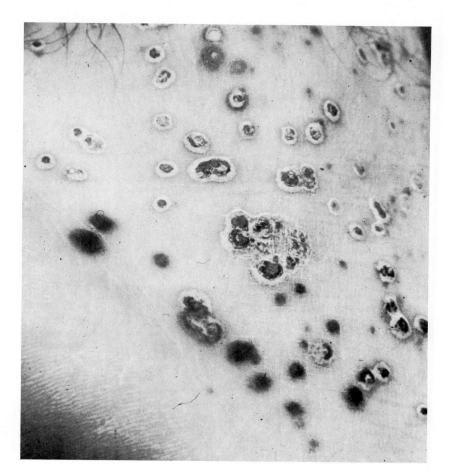

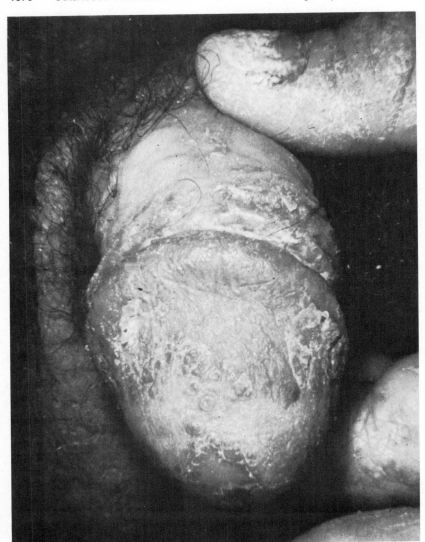

Fig. 159-4 Circinate balanitis in a circumcised male demonstrating dry keratodermia-like lesions.

Prominent inflammation at bony sites of tendon and fascial attachment (enthesopathy) gives rise to complaints in nonarticular areas such as ischial tuberosities, iliac crests, and over long bones and ribs. Heel pain reflecting involvement at plantar aponeurosis and/or Achilles tendon insertions is a common and disabling feature (Fig. 159-9).

Other features

Inflammatory involvement of aortic root, valve, and adjacent conducting system leads to significant aortic regurgitation and/or heart block in 5 percent of patients. Amyloidosis occurs rarely, either during acute fulminating illness or after a protracted course [48].

Laboratory features

There is no specific laboratory test for Reiter's syndrome. Potentially useful laboratory and radiographic findings are listed in Table 159-3. Specifically, typing for HLA-B27 is usually not necessary but may prove helpful in incomplete or atypical cases.

Pathology

Keratodermia is characterized by neutrophilic dermal and epidermal infiltration, elongation and hypertrophy of rete ridges, degeneration of epidermal cells whose remaining membranes and nuclei form microabscesses or spongiform pustules, and intense hyperkeratosis and parakeratosis leading to horny excrescences in the outer layers (Fig. 159-10). Dry penile lesions are histologically identical to lesions on the skin, and moist penile and oral ulcers show similar changes except for the absence of keratosis [49,50]. Histologic differentiation between keratodermia and pustular psoriasis is impossible. The synovium shows an intense nonspecific inflammatory reaction indistinguishable from many other arthritides [49,50].

Diagnosis and differential diagnosis

Diagnosis depends on the typical pattern of arthritis plus one or more other discriminating features, especially urethritis, conjunctivitis, a mucocutaneous manifestation, or heel pain. Gonococcal infection must be excluded by ap-

Fig. 159-5 Circinate balanitis in an uncircumcised male demonstrating moist shallow ulcers with raised borders.

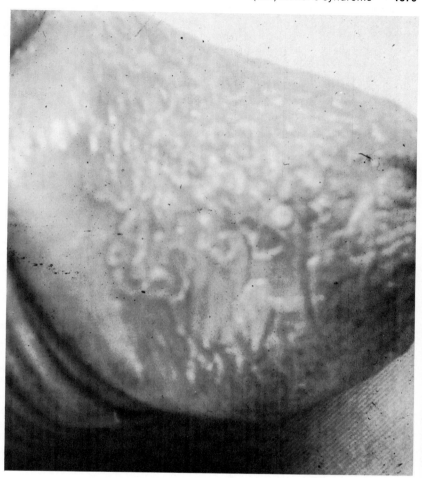

Fig. 159-6 Shallow painless ulcerations on tongue.

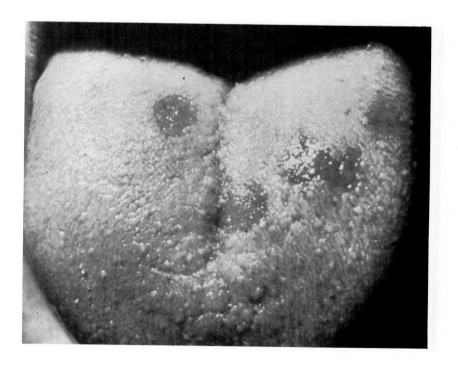

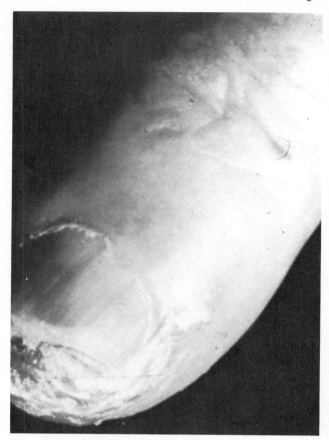

Fig. 159-7 Onychodystrophy of nail with opacification and hyperkeratosis.

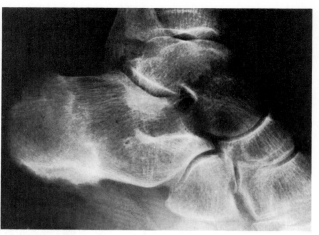

Fig. 159-9 Roentgenograph of os calcis showing periostitis typical of enthesopathy. (From Renlund et al [46], by permission of The Johns Hopkins Medical Journal and University Press.)

propriate urethral and synovial cultures since the two disorders may coexist. Gonococcal arthritis is more common in women and has different skin lesions. Psoriatic arthritis may be impossible to distinguish early; however, nail pit-

ting, distal interphalangeal finger involvement, and lack of fever may be useful differentiating features. Gout is unusual in the young age range typical of Reiter's syndrome; nonetheless, monosodium urate crystals should be sought in synovial fluid. Behçet's disease characteristically has deeper and more painful oral-genital ulcers, an erythema nodosum-like vasculitic rash, and "pathergic" pustulonecrotic skin lesions at venipuncture sites. Rheumatoid arthritis can be differentiated by its propensity to affect older people, a dominant upper extremity symmetrical polyarthritis, subcutaneous nodules, and seropositivity for rheumatoid factor.

Course

Arthritis is the most serious and disabling feature. The majority of patients (over 50 percent) experience a self-

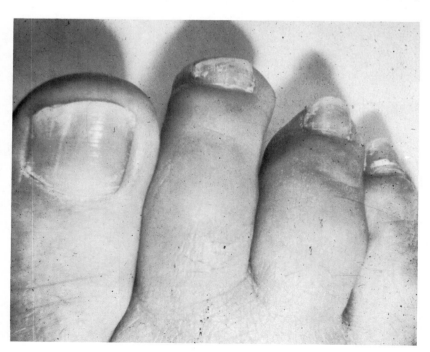

Fig. 159-8 Diffuse swelling (sausaging) of toes.

limited illness lasting 3 months to 1 year [47,51]. Another third have a relapsing course, often with many years separating the attacks. A chronic deforming arthritis, with or without accompanying dermatitis, occurs in 10 to 20 percent. Significant disability ensues in 10 to 15 percent, usually as a consequence of foot deformities, visual loss, or cardiac disease [52]. Death is rare but may result from heart involvement or amyloidosis.

Treatment

Therapy should be aimed at suppressing articular inflammation and preventing deformities. During the acute phase, bed rest and joint splinting may be necessary. Salicylates usually are not effective but may be worth trying. Nonsteroidal anti-inflammatory agents such as indomethacin, tolmetin, naproxen, and sulindac generally are more useful. Response to phenylbutazone 200 to 400 mg per day is often dramatic; however, potential hematologic toxicity should limit its use. Methotrexate in doses of 7.5 to 15 mg per week may be necessary to control severe skin and/or joint disease. As articular inflammation is suppressed and/or improves, physical therapy is desirable to maintain function and prevent deformity.

It is unclear whether antibiotics alter the course of urethritis or prevent any ensuing articular flares. Thus, a trial of tetracycline or erythromycin may be warranted.

References

1. Reiter H: Ueber eine bisher unerkannte Spirochäeteninfektion (Spirochaetosis arthritica). *Deutsch Med Wochenschr* **42**:1535, 1916
2. Bauer W, Engleman EP: A syndrome of unknown etiology characterized by urethritis, conjunctivitis and arthritis (so-called Reiter's disease). *Trans Assoc Am Physicians* **57**:307, 1942
3. Arnett FC et al: Incomplete Reiter's syndrome: discriminating features and HLA-W27 in diagnosis. *Ann Intern Med* **84**:8, 1976
4. Willkens RF et al: Reiter's syndrome: evaluation of preliminary criteria for definite disease. *Arthritis Rheum* **24**:844, 1981
5. Brodie BC: *Pathological and Surgical Observations on Diseases of the Joints.* London, Longman, Hurst, Rees, Orme and Brown, 1818, p 54
6. Benedek TG, Rodman GP: A brief history of the rheumatic diseases. *Bull Rheum Dis* **32**:59, 1982
7. Paronen I: Reiter's disease. Study of 344 cases observed in Finland. *Acta Med Scand [Suppl]* **212**:1, 1948

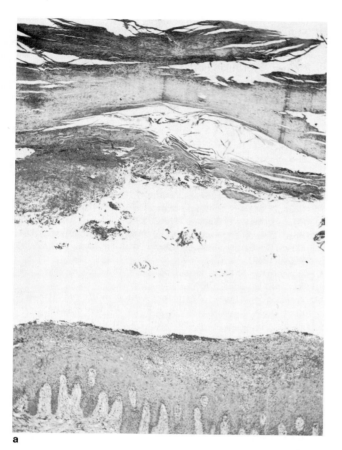

a

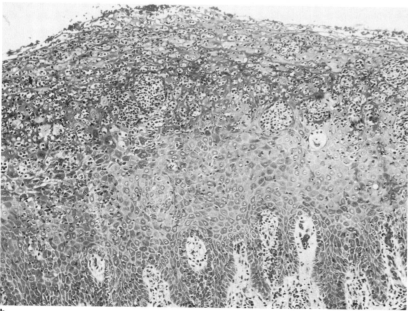

b

Fig. 159-10 (a) Histopathology from keratodermia involving sole, showing massive hyperkeratosis and psoriasiform epidermal hyperplasia with marked exocytosis of neutrophils. H&E, ×35. (Courtesy of Dr. Evan R. Farmer.) (b) Higher-power view of epidermis, demonstrating massive influx of neutrophils and formation of spongiform pustules. H&E, ×40. (Courtesy of Dr. Evan R. Farmer.)

8. Noer HR: An "experimental" epidemic of Reiter's syndrome. *JAMA* **198**:693, 1966

9. Brewerton DA et al: Reiter's disease and HL-A 27. *Lancet* **2**:996, 1973

10. Sairanen E, Tiilikainen A: HL-A 27 in Reiter's disease following shigellosis. *Scand J Rheumatol* **4(suppl 8)**: abstr 30-11, 1975

11. Calin A, Fries JF: An "experimental" epidemic of Reiter's syndrome revisited. Follow-up evidence on genetic and environmental factors. *Ann Intern Med* **84**:564, 1976

12. Masi AT, Medsger TA Jr: A new look at the epidemiology of ankylosing spondylitis and related syndromes. *Clin Orthop* **143**:15, 1979

13. West SG, Lawless OJ: The chronic disability of Reiter's syndrome in the US Army. *Arthritis Rheum* **24(suppl)**:S78, 1981

14. Schacter J et al: Isolation of bedsoniae from the joints of patients with Reiter's syndrome. *Proc Soc Exp Biol Med* **122**:283, 1966

15. Bartholomew LE: Isolation and characterization of mycoplasmas (PPLO) from patients with rheumatoid arthritis, systemic lupus erythematosus and Reiter's syndrome. *Arthritis Rheum* **8**:376, 1965

16. Moll JMH et al: Associations between ankylosing spondylitis, psoriatic arthritis, Reiter's disease, the intestinal arthropathies and Behçet's syndrome. *Medicine (Baltimore)* **53**:343, 1974

17. Good AR: Involvement of the back in Reiter's syndrome: follow-up of thirty-four cases. *Ann Intern Med* **57**:44, 1962

18. Wright V, Reed WB: The link between Reiter's syndrome and psoriatic arthritis. *Ann Rheum Dis* **23**:12, 1964

19. Lawrence JS: Family survey of Reiter's disease. *Br J Vener Dis* **50**:140, 1974

20. McClusky OE et al: HL-A27 in Reiter's syndrome and psoriatic arthritis. A genetic factor in disease susceptibility and expression. *J Rheumatol* **1**:263, 1974

21. Arnett FC et al: Cross-reactive HLA antigens in B27-negative Reiter's syndrome and sacroiliitis. *Johns Hopkins Med J* **141**:193, 1977

22. Schwartz BD et al: Public antigenic determinant on a family of HLA-B molecules. Basis for cross-reactivity and a possible link with disease predisposition. *J Clin Invest* **64**:938, 1979

23. Ruppert GB et al: Cardiac conduction defects in Reiter's syndrome. *Am J Med* **73**:335, 1982

24. Brewerton DA et al: Ankylosing spondylitis and HL-A27. *Lancet* **1**:904, 1973

25. Khan MA et al: A subgroup of ankylosing spondylitis associated with HLA-B7 in American blacks. *Arthritis Rheum* **21**:528, 1978

26. Khan MA et al: Genetic heterogeneity in primary ankylosing spondylitis. *J Rheumatol* **7**:383, 1980

27. Karvonen J: HLA antigens in psoriasis with special relevance to the clinical type, age of onset, exacerbations after respiratory infections and occurrence of arthritis. *Ann Clin Res* **7**:301, 1975

28. Murry C et al: Histocompatibility alloantigens in psoriasis and psoriatic arthritis. *J Clin Invest* **66**:670, 1980

29. Arnett FC, Bias WB: HLA-Bw38 and Bw39 in psoriatic arthritis: relationships and implications for peripheral and axial involvement. *Arthritis Rheum* **23**:649, 1980

30. Khan MA et al: Low association of HLA-B27 with Reiter's syndrome in blacks. *Ann Intern Med* **90**:202, 1979

31. Calin A, Fries JF: The striking prevalence of ankylosing spondylitis in "healthy" W27 positive males and females: a controlled study. *N Engl J Med* **293**:835, 1975

32. Hochberg MC et al: Family studies in HLA-B27 associated arthritis. *Medicine (Baltimore)* **57**:463, 1978

33. Yunus M et al: Family studies with HLA typing in Reiter's syndrome. *Am J Med* **70**:1210, 1981

34. Calin A et al: Familial aggregation of Reiter's syndrome and ankylosing spondylitis: a comparative study. *J Rheumatol* **11**:672, 1984

35. Woodrow JC: Histocompatibility antigens and rheumatic diseases. *Semin Arthritis Rheum* **6**:257, 1977

36. Grumet FC et al: Monoclonal antibody subdividing HLA-B27. *Hum Immunol* **5**:61, 1982

37. Breuning MH et al: Subtypes of HLA-B27 detected by cytotoxic T lymphocytes and their role in self-recognition. *Hum Immunol* **5**:259, 1982

38. Aho K et al: HL-A27 in reactive arthritis. A study of *Yersinia* arthritis and Reiter's disease. *Arthritis Rheum* **17**:521, 1974

39. Hakansson U et al: HL-A27 and reactive arthritis in an outbreak of salmonellosis. *Tissue Antigens* **6**:366, 1975

40. Kaslow RA et al: Search for Reiter's syndrome after an outbreak of *Shigella sonnei* dysentery. *J Rheumatol* **6**:562, 1979

41. Brenner MB et al: A new experimental approach to Reiter's disease. *Arthritis Rheum* **25**:S63, 1982

42. Ford DK, Rasmussen G: Relationships between genito-urinary infection and complicating arthritis. *Arthritis Rheum* **7**:220, 1964

43. Wright V: Arthritis associated with venereal disease. *Ann Rheum Dis* **22**:77, 1983

44. Keat AC et al: Role of *Chlamydia trachomatis* and HLA-B27 in sexually acquired reactive arthritis. *Br Med J* **1**:605, 1978

45. Jacobs NF et al: Nongonococcal urethritis: the role of *Chlamydia trachomatis*. *Ann Intern Med* **86**:313, 1977

46. Renlund DG et al: Reiter's syndrome. *Johns Hopkins Med J* **150**:39, 1982

47. Arnett FC: Incomplete Reiter's syndrome: clinical comparisons with classical triad. *Ann Rheum Dis* **38(suppl 1)**:73, 1979

48. Miller LD et al: Amyloidosis in Reiter's syndrome. *J Rheumatol* **6**:225, 1979

49. Kulka JP: The lesions of Reiter's syndrome. *Arthritis Rheum* **5**:195, 1962

50. Weinberger HW et al: Reiter's syndrome, clinical and pathologic observations: a long term study of 16 cases. *Medicine (Baltimore)* **41**:35, 1962

51. Csonka GW: The course of Reiter's syndrome. *Br Med J* **1**:1088, 1958

52. Fox R et al: The chronicity of symptoms and disability in Reiter's syndrome. An analysis of 131 consecutive cases. *Ann Intern Med* **91**:190, 1979

Bibliography

Bitter T (ed): Symposium on Reiter's Syndrome. *Ann Rheum Dis* **38(suppl 1)**:1, 1979

CHAPTER 160

SKIN MANIFESTATIONS OF SJÖGREN'S SYNDROME

Kenneth H. Fye and Norman Talal

In the waning decades of the nineteenth century and the first 30 years of the twentieth century, a number of observers noted the association of xerophthalmia and xerostomia, often in the presence of arthritis [1–5]. In 1933, Henrik Sjögren [6] published a monograph on his experience with 19 patients who had keratoconjunctivitis sicca and xerostomia (the sicca complex), 13 of whom also had arthritis. He felt that these patients represented a distinct clinical entity, and since then the triad of keratoconjunctivitis sicca, xerostomia, and rheumatoid arthritis has come to be known as Sjögren's syndrome. The sicca complex can be seen in association with a number of autoimmune disorders [7,8], including systemic lupus erythematosus [9], scleroderma [10], polymyositis [11], periarteritis nodosa [12], primary biliary cirrhosis [13], and chronic active hepatitis [14].

Although Sjögren's syndrome may be seen at any age in either sex, in general it affects middle-aged women [8,11, 12,15]. The clinical manifestations of Sjögren's syndrome are the result of decreased exocrine gland function throughout the body. Although ocular and oral mucosal glands are most commonly affected, nasal, pharyngeal, laryngeal, tracheobronchial, vulval, cervical, gastric, and probably intestinal mucosal glands are also involved [15]. Pancreatic exocrine gland function is decreased in some patients [15]. Keratoconjunctivitis sicca and xerostomia are the most common clinical findings in Sjögren's syndrome [11,12,16]. Symptoms associated with keratoconjunctivitis sicca include photophobia, burning and itching of the eyes, a "gritty" sensation in the eyes, and the inability to cry. Typical physical findings include an abnormal Schirmer's test, a shortened tear breakup time, the presence of debris over the surface of the eyes, and abnormal fluorescein and rose bengal staining demonstrating punctate erosions of the cornea and conjunctiva. Symptoms associated with xerostomia include oral dryness, polydipsia, dysphagia (particularly with dry foods), dysphonia, oral burning sensations, and complaints of a sore throat. Due to the polydipsia, many patients complain of polyuria and nocturia. On physical examination one usually sees erythema and dryness of the oral mucosa. The tongue is red and depapillated. Most patients report increased dental caries. Angular cheilosis, often associated with oral candidiasis, is common.

In some patients, lymphocytic infiltration into extraglandular tissues, such as lymph nodes, lungs, kidneys, or liver, may be seen [17]. Pulmonary lymphocytic infiltration may lead to interstitial fibrosis and eventual respiratory failure [18]. Renal involvement has been associated with renal tubular acidosis [19–21], nephrogenic diabetes insipidus [22,23], and the Fanconi syndrome [22]. In a few patients

with Sjögren's syndrome the lymphocyte aggressive process undergoes malignant degeneration, leading to either non-Hodgkin's lymphoma [24,25], or Waldenström's macroglobulinemia [17,24].

Although Sjögren's syndrome was classically defined by the presence of sicca symptoms, the advent of labial salivary gland biopsies has allowed us to define the syndrome histologically. The pathologic lesion is a lymphocyte and plasma cell infiltrate into exocrine gland tissues [26,27] (Fig. 160-1) with destruction and atrophy of normal structures. Talal et al [28] used anti-T-cell antibodies with indirect immunofluorescence and fluorescein-labeled anti-immunoglobulin to demonstrate the presence of both T and B cells in the pathologic lymphocytic infiltrate.

Sjögren's syndrome is considered to be an autoimmune disease. The autoimmune nature of the disorder is suggested by the prominence of lymphoid cells in the pathologic infiltrate. A wide variety of autoantibodies is found in patients with Sjögren's syndrome, including rheumatoid factor, antinuclear antibodies, anti-salivary duct antibodies, antithyroglobulin, and low-titer anti-double-strand DNA antibodies [29,30]. In addition, Alspaugh and Tan [31] found that patients with Sjögren's syndrome had precipitins directed against extracts of lymphocyte nuclei.

The antinuclear antibodies seen in Sjögren's syndrome are generally directed against one or more of a variety of acid-extractable nuclear antigens. Antibodies directed against the nuclear antigens SS-A and SS-B are characteristic of primary Sjögren's syndrome or Sjögren's syndrome associated with systemic lupus erythematosus [32–35]. Patients with Sjögren's syndrome and rheumatoid arthritis produce an antibody (rheumatoid arthritis precipitin, or RAP) directed against an antigen thought to be an Epstein-Barr virus-related antigen (rheumatoid arthritis nuclear antigen, or RANA) [36].

There is a definite genetic component in the etiology of Sjögren's syndrome. Fifty percent of patients have HLA-B8 and over 70 percent have HLA-DW3 [37–38]. Some investigators have suggested that patients with primary Sjögren's syndrome and Sjögren's syndrome associated with systemic lupus erythematosus tend to have HLA-B8, HLA-DW3, and HLA-DRW3, while patients with Sjögren's syndrome and rheumatoid arthritis have an increased incidence of HLA-DW4 and HLA-DRW4 [39].

Dermatologic manifestations (Table 160-1)

Dry skin and decreased sweating, often associated with pruritus, are common complaints among patients with Sjögren's syndrome [11,12,16,40–43]. Of 62 patients reported by Bloch et al [11], 67 percent complained of dryness of

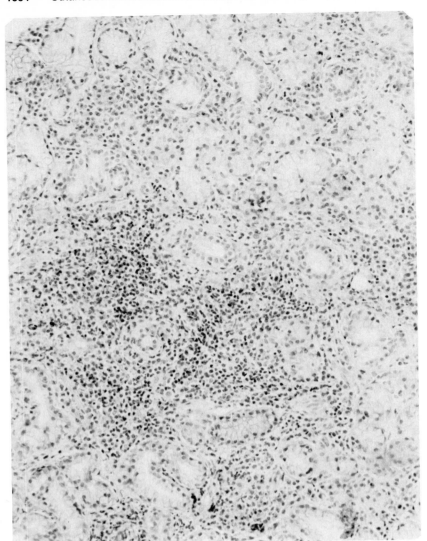

Fig. 160-1 Minor salivary gland biopsy from a patient with Sjögren's syndrome, demonstrating the characteristic lymphoid and plasma cell infiltrate. H&E, ×190.

the skin, and 27 percent had noticeably decreased sweating. Stolze et al [12], in a review of 248 patients with keratoconjunctivitis sicca, 139 of whom had clinical Sjögren's syndrome (not proved by biopsy), found that only 15 of 139 patients complained of dryness of the skin. Whaley et al [16] reported that 23 percent of their 171 Sjögren's patients complained of dryness of the skin. Among our own patients specifically queried about skin problems, 65 percent noted dryness of the skin with decreased sweating. A decreased sweating response to the administration of pilocarpine has been described in patients with Sjögren's syndrome [40].

One of the earliest pathologic descriptions of histologic changes in the skin seen in Sjögren's syndrome was published by Ellman et al [44]. They described a lymphocytic infiltration into sweat glands of a patient who died of Sjögren's syndrome with pulmonary involvement and superimposed bronchial pneumonia. In 1973, Whaley et al [16] biopsied 7 of their 40 patients who complained of dry skin. A nonspecific perivascular lymphocytic infiltration was seen in six. A mononuclear cell infiltrate of the sweat glands similar to that described by Ellman et al [44] was seen in one biopsy. The patient with the mononuclear cell

infiltrate in the sweat glands had a markedly decreased sweating response to both pilocarpine administration and thermal stimulation.

Feuerman [45] described the complete absence of sebaceous glands in a patient with severe skin dryness and atrophy of the sweat glands. That finding, however, has not been observed in skin biopsies done in a search for sweat gland abnormalities [11,16,39,44,46]. Apocrine gland dysfunction of the external auditory meatus was noted by Henkin et al [47]. Half of their patients had decreased cerumen, along with pruritus, scaling, and crusting of the external ear canal.

Dryness and crusting of the nasal passages are also common among patients with Sjögren's syndrome. Thirty-seven of the 62 patients studied by Bloch et al [11] had nasal dryness. One had nasopharyngeal crusting that was severe enough to block the eustachian tubes, leading to bilateral otitis media. Fifty-three of the 171 patients reported by Whaley et al [16] had comprehensive otorhino-laryngologic examinations. Forty-seven percent had dryness, 57 percent had crusting, 6 percent had mucosal atrophy, and 2 percent had nasopharyngeal crusting so severe that the eustachian tubes were blocked and hearing

Table 160-1 Dermatologic manifestations of Sjögren's syndrome

Keratoconjunctivitis sicca
Xerostomia
Nasal dryness and crusting
Vaginal dryness with dyspareunia
Dry skin
Hyper- and hypopigmentation
Patchy alopecia
Raynaud's phenomenon
Vasculitis:
  Hypergammaglobulinemic purpura
  Cryoglobulinemia
Thrombotic thrombocytopenic purpura

was impaired. Henkin et al [47] studied taste and smell in 29 patients with Sjögren's syndrome. Ninety-two percent had nasal dryness, 52 percent with crusting. Those patients with the most severe symptoms also had atrophy of the nasal mucosa with recurrent epistaxis. Forty-five percent of their patients complained of hyposmia and hypogeusia. Nasopharyngeal biopsy in patients with Sjögren's syndrome shows atrophy, mild fibrosis, and chronic inflammation of submucosal glands.

The prevalence of vaginal dryness in Sjögren's syndrome is a matter of some controversy. Whaley et al [16] reported that only 5 of 171 patients (3 percent) complained of vaginal dryness. In their review of 139 patients, Stoltze et al [12] found that 8 percent complained of vaginal dryness. Thirty-two percent of 62 patients with Sjögren's syndrome reported by Bloch et al [11] had vaginal dryness associated with dyspareunia and vaginal burning and pruritus. Eleven of those 20 patients were premenopausal. A postmenopausal biopsy and four postmortem examinations revealed histologic changes compatible with nonspecific vaginitis. The authors reported no vaginal biopsies of premenopausal patients. In our own experience, 33 percent of female patients specifically checked for vaginal problems had vaginal dryness, usually associated with dyspareunia.

Pigmentary changes consisting of localized areas of hypopigmentation or hyperpigmentation have been repeatedly noted in patients with Sjögren's syndrome [12,15,42]. Many patients develop hyperpigmented, frecklelike lesions over exposed areas.

Although most commonly associated with systemic lupus erythematosus, mixed connective tissue disease, and scleroderma, patchy alopecia can also be a manifestation of primary Sjögren's syndrome [7,12,48–50]. Decreases in head, body, and pubic hair have been noted [51].

Raynaud's phenomenon is seen in a number of rheumatic disorders, particularly scleroderma, mixed connective tissue disease, systemic lupus erythematosus, and cryoglobulinemia. Raynaud's phenomenon has also been described in approximately 20 percent of patients with Sjögren's syndrome [11,12,15].

The most dramatic cutaneous manifestations of Sjögren's syndrome are due to vasculitis. Histologically, the vasculitic lesion consists of a mononuclear cell perivascular infiltrate involving small vessels. Clinical lesions range from petechiae to palpable purpura to widespread ecchymoses. Thirty-three of the 62 patients reported by Bloch et al [11] had skin and muscle biopsies. Eight pa-

tients had histologic vasculitis not associated with purpura. In one, the vascular lesions were indistinguishable from those seen in periarteritis nodosa. Vascular lesions were noted in both muscles and nerves, as well as the skin. Mason et al [15] found that cutaneous vasculitic manifestations were commonly associated with vasculitis of the peripheral nerves and muscles. The overall prevalence of cutaneous vasculitis in patients with Sjögren's syndrome is estimated to be 20 to 30 percent [11,15,25].

Although vasculitis can be seen in Sjögren's syndrome in the absence of immunoglobulin abnormalities, vasculitic manifestations were generally associated with hypergammaglobulinemic purpura [11,15,19,23–25]. Cutaneous lesions of hypergammaglobulinemic purpura appear over dependent parts of the body and range from petechiae to palpable purpura. The hypergammaglobulinemia usually consists of diffuse elevations of immunoglobulins of all three major serum classes: IgA, IgM, and IgG. Hypergammaglobulinemia is seen in up to 80 percent of patients with Sjögren's syndrome [7,11,15,19,23–25,52–54] and is usually associated with significant systemic manifestations.

In addition to palpable purpura, hypergammaglobulinemia in Sjögren's syndrome has been associated with a number of renal disorders, including renal tubular acidosis, diabetes insipidus, and Fanconi's syndrome [19–23,52–54]. Five of the six patients with Sjögren's syndrome and renal disease studied by Talal et al [19] had purpuric lesions and hypergammaglobulinemia. However, there is some controversy as to the relationship between hypergammaglobulinemia per se and renal tubular acidosis. Shioji et al [21] found that 3 of 4 patients with Sjögren's syndrome and renal tubular acidosis had hypergammaglobulinemia. However, 7 of 10 patients with Sjögren's syndrome without renal tubular acidosis also had hypergammaglobulinemia. They found that the presence of renal tubular acidosis was always associated with renal interstitial lymphocytic infiltration, while patients without renal tubular acidosis had no renal infiltrative lesions. Extraglandular lymphocytic infiltration in Sjögren's syndrome, so-called pseudolymphoma, is also usually associated with hypergammaglobulinemic purpura [17,19,24,25]. In 8 patients with pseudolymphoma reported by Talal et al [24], 62 percent had purpura and 54 percent had vasculitis. Among their patients with Sjögren's syndrome who did not have pseudolymphoma, only 4 percent had purpura and 22 percent had cutaneous vasculitis.

Cryoglobulinemia is common in patients with Sjögren's syndrome [19,24,55]. In approximately 25 percent of cases with cryoglobulinemia, the cryoglobulins consist only of monoclonal immunoglobulins (type I cryoglobulinemia) [55]. IgM monoclonal cryoglobulins are the most common, but IgG and IgA monoclonal cryoglobulins have also been observed. Most cryoglobulins are mixed cryoproteins made up of immune complexes, usually IgM–IgG complexes [56–59]. The IgM component may be either monoclonal (type II cryoglobulinemia) or polyclonal (type III cryoglobulinemia), while the IgG component is always polyclonal [59,60]. Of 86 patients with cryoglobulinemia studied by Brouet et al [55], 8 had Sjögren's syndrome, 4 of whom had type II cryoglobulinemia while 4 had type III cryoglobulinemia. These patients had dependent vascular purpura, Raynaud's phenomenon, polyneuropathy, and necrotizing angiitis. Three had glomerulonephritis, an unusual complication in Sjögren's syndrome in the absence of cryoglobulinemia. Among the 8 patients with proved Sjögren's syndrome and pseudolymphoma reported by Talal et al [24], 4 had cryoglobulinemia, 3 had dependent purpura, and 2 had cutaneous vasculitis.

Although the association of Sjögren's syndrome with hypergammaglobulinemic purpura was known and reviewed in the late 1950s [61], the development of Waldenström's macroglobulinemia in patients with Sjögren's syndrome was not definitely demonstrated until the 1960s [24,25]. Two of the eight patients with pseudolymphoma reported by Talal et al [24] had primary macroglobulinemia; neither patient had purpura or documented vasculitis at the time the macroglobulinemia was discovered. Another patient in their series later developed Waldenström's macroglobulinemia and was reported in a subsequent publication [19]. Whitehouse et al [62] described a patient with a monoclonal IgM macroglobulinemia of Waldenström whose skin manifestations included livedo annularis, intermittent diffuse mottling, purpura, and biopsy-proved vasculitis. Hyperviscosity syndrome and constitutional manifestations, however, are more common than skin changes in patients with Sjögren's syndrome and Waldenström's macroglobulinemia. Amyloidosis involving the skin is a complication of longstanding Waldenström's macroglobulinemia, with or without Sjögren's syndrome [63].

Thrombotic thrombocytopenia purpura is a clinical triad consisting of thrombocytopenic purpura, hemolytic anemia, and neurologic manifestations [64]. Although it usually presents as a primary disorder, it has been described in rheumatoid arthritis [65,66], polyarteritis nodosa [67], and both discoid [68] and systemic [68,69] lupus erythematosus. Steinberg et al [70] described three patients with Sjögren's syndrome and thrombotic thrombocytopenic purpura. The authors hypothesized that an underlying vasculitis led to platelet consumption and thrombosis in involved vessels. Presumably, only patients with Sjögren's syndrome and widespread vasculitis would develop the full syndrome of thrombotic thrombocytopenic purpura.

Since both Sjögren's syndrome and dermatitis herpetiformis are associated with HLA-B8 and HLA-DW3, it is not surprising that the two disorders have occasionally been observed in the same patient [71]. Sjögren's syndrome has also been described in association with Sweet's syndrome, a dermatologic disorder characterized by the presence of dull-red macules over the trunk and limbs and defined histologically by perivascular polymorphonuclear infiltration and leukocytoclasis in the papillary and upper reticular dermis [72]. The final disease association that should be mentioned is that between Sjögren's syndrome and chronic graft-versus-host disease [73]. Lawley et al reported one such patient who developed both scleroderma-like cutaneous sclerosis and Sjögren's syndrome after undergoing bone marrow transplantation as part of the treatment for acute myelogenous leukemia [73].

Treatment

At present there is no cure for Sjögren's syndrome. The treatment modalities presently available are aimed at symptomatic relief of the manifestations of the disease. Good oral hygiene and intermittent fluoride treatments help to prevent the rampant dental caries commonly seen in these patients. Sugarless gum or candy to stimulate salivary flow and frequent sips of water help alleviate the symptoms of dry mouth. The frequent oral candidal infections can be treated with nystatin mouthwashes or tablets. Artificial tears are the mainstay of the treatment of the ocular manifestations of Sjögren's syndrome. The most successful artificial tear preparations include long-chain polysaccharides, such as hydroxyethylcellulose or methylcellulose, to more closely simulate natural tear composition. Water-miscible lubricants are helpful in treating vaginal and nasal dryness and crusting. Many patients find that lanolin-based skin creams help alleviate dryness and pruritus of the skin.

Steroids, cytotoxic agents, and radiation have been used in patients with severe, life-threatening disease. High doses of daily steroids (60 mg prednisone per day or its equivalent) are used only in pseudolymphoma or severe systemic vasculitis. Cytotoxic agents, such as cyclophosphamide, chlorambucil, or azathioprine, have been used in patients with pseudolymphoma who have not responded adequately to steroid therapy, or in patients who have gone on to develop diffuse histiocytic lymphoma or Waldenström's macroglobulinemia.

References

1. Hadden WB: On "dry mouth" or suppression of the salivary and buccal secretions. *Trans Clin Soc London* **21**:176, 1888
2. Houwer AWM: Keratitis filamentosa and chronic arthritis. *Trans Ophthalmol Soc UK* **47**:88, 1927
3. Albrich K: Die Keratitis filiformis und die Sekretion der Tranenduse. *Arch Ophthalmol* **121**:402, 1928
4. Chamberlin WB: Xerostomia. *JAMA* **45**:470, 1930
5. Critchley M, Meadows SP: Xerostomia and xerophthalmia. *Proc R Soc Med* **26**:306, 1933
6. Sjögren H: Zur Kenntnis der Keratoconjunctivitis sicca (Keratitis filiformis bei Hypofunktion der Trandendrusen). *Acta Ophthalmol (Kbh)* **11 (suppl 2):1,** 1933
7. Ehrich GE: Oculocutaneous manifestations of rheumatic diseases: introduction: of syndromes and interfaces. *Rheumatology* **4**:1, 1973
8. Shearn MA: Sjögren's syndrome, in *Major Problems in Internal Medicine,* vol II, edited by LH Smith Jr. Philadelphia, WB Saunders, 1971
9. Alarcon-Segovia D et al: Sjögren's syndrome in systemic lupus erythematosus. *Ann Intern Med* **81**:577, 1974
10. Shearn MA: Sjögren's syndrome in association with scleroderma. *Ann Intern Med* **52**:1352, 1960
11. Bloch KJ et al: Sjögren's syndrome. A clinical, pathological and serological study of sixty-two cases. *Medicine (Baltimore)* **44**:187, 1965
12. Stoltze CA et al: Keratoconjunctivitis sicca and Sjögren's syndrome. Systemic manifestations and hematologic and protein abnormalities. *Arch Intern Med* **106**:513, 1960
13. Alarcon-Segovia D: Features of Sjögren's syndrome in primary biliary cirrhosis. *Ann Intern Med* **79**:31, 1973
14. Golding PL et al: Multisystem involvement in chronic liver disease. *Am J Med* **55**:772, 1973
15. Mason AMS et al: Sjögren's syndrome—a clinical review. *Semin Arthritis Rheum* **2**:301, 1973
16. Whaley K et al: Sjögren's syndrome. I. Sicca components. *Q J Med* **166**:279, 1973
17. Anderson LG, Talal NP: The spectrum of benign to malignant lymphoproliferation in Sjögren's syndrome. *Clin Exp Immunol* **10**:199, 1972
18. Tomasi TB et al: Possible relationship of rheumatoid factors and pulmonary disease. *Am J Med* **33**:243, 1962

19. Talal N et al: Renal tubular acidosis, glomerulonephritis and immunologic factors in Sjögren's syndrome. *Arthritis Rheum* **6**:774, 1968

20. Kaltreider BH, Talal N: Impaired renal acidification in Sjögren's syndrome and related disorders. *Arthritis Rheum* **12**:538, 1969

21. Shioji R et al: Sjögren's syndrome and renal tubular acidosis. *Am J Med* **48**:456, 1970

22. Shearn MA, Tu WH: Nephrogenic diabetes insipidus and other defects of renal tubular function in Sjögren's syndrome. *Am J Med* **39**:312, 1965

23. Kahn M et al: Renal concentrating defect in Sjögren's syndrome. *Ann Intern Med* **36**:883, 1962

24. Talal N et al: Extrasalivary lymphoid abnormalities in Sjögren's syndrome (reticulum cell sarcoma, "pseudolymphoma," macroglobulinemia). *Am J Med* **43**:50, 1967

25. Bunim JJ, Talal N: The association of malignant lymphoma with Sjögren's syndrome. *Trans Assoc Am Physicians* **26**:45, 1963

26. Greenspan JS et al: The histopathology of Sjögren's syndrome in labial salivary gland biopsies. *Oral Surg* **37**:217, 1974

27. Daniels TE et al: The oral component of Sjögren's syndrome. *Oral Surg* **39**:875, 1975

28. Talal N et al: T and B lymphocytes in peripheral blood and tissue lesions in Sjögren's syndrome. *J Clin Invest* **53**:180, 1974

29. Fischer CJ et al: Sjögren's syndrome. Electrophoretic and immunological observations on serum and salivary proteins of man. *Arch Oral Biol* **13**:257, 1968

30. Notman DD et al: Profiles of antinuclear antibodies in systemic rheumatic diseases. *Ann Intern Med* **83**:464, 1975

31. Alspaugh MA, Tan EM: Antibodies to cellular antigens in Sjögren's syndrome. *J Clin Invest* **55**:1067, 1975

32. Alspaugh M, Maddison P: Resolution of the identity of certain antigen-antibody systems in systemic lupus erythematosus and Sjögren's syndrome: an interlaboratory collaboration. *Arthritis Rheum* **22**:796, 1979

33. Martinez-Lavin M et al: Autoantibodies and the spectrum of Sjögren's syndrome. *Ann Intern Med* **91**:185, 1979

34. Scopelitis E et al: Anti-SS-A antibody and other antinuclear antibodies in systemic lupus erythematosus. *Arthritis Rheum* **23**:287, 1980

35. Manthrope R et al: Antibodies to SS-B in chronic inflammatory connective tissue diseases. *Arthritis Rheum* **25**:662, 1982

36. Alspaugh MA et al: Precipitating antibodies to cellular antigens in Sjögren's syndrome, rheumatoid arthritis and other organ and non-organ specific autoimmune diseases. *Ann Rheum Dis* **37**:244, 1978

37. Fye KH et al: Association of Sjögren's syndrome with HLA-B8. *Arthritis Rheum* **19**:883, 1976

38. Fye KH et al: Relationship of HLA-DW3 and HLA-B8 to Sjögren's syndrome. *Arthritis Rheum* **21**:337, 1978

39. Moutsopoulos HM et al: Genetic difference between primary and secondary sicca syndrome. *N Engl J Med* **301**:761, 1979

40. Behrman HT, Lee KK: Sjögren's syndrome. *Arch Dermatol Syphilol* **61**:63, 1950

41. Raffle RB: Sjögren's disease associated with a nutritional deficiency syndrome. *Br Med J* **1**:1470, 1950

42. Rothman S et al: Sjögren's syndrome associated with lymphoblastoma and hypersplenism. *Arch Dermatol Syphilol* **63**:642, 1951

43. Allington HV: Dryness of the mouth. *Arch Dermatol Syphilol* **62**:829, 1950

44. Ellman P et al: A contribution to the pathology of Sjögren's disease. *Q J Med* **20**:33, 1951

45. Feuerman EJ: Sjögren's syndrome presenting as recalcitrant generalized pruritus. Some remarks about its relation to collagen diseases and the connection of rheumatoid arthritis with the sicca syndrome. *Dermatologia* **137**:74, 1968

46. Szanto L et al: On Sjögren's disease. *Rheumatism* **13**:60, 1957

47. Henkin RI et al: Abnormalities of taste and smell in Sjögren's syndrome. *Ann Intern Med* **76**:375, 1972

48. Reader SR et al: Sjögren's disease and rheumatoid arthritis. *Ann Rheum Dis* **10**:288, 1951

49. Georgiades G: Gougerot-Houwer-Sjögren's syndrome: 2 cases. *Ann Rheum Dis* **12**:62, 1953

50. Thompson M, Eadie S: Keratoconjunctivitis sicca and rheumatoid arthritis. *Ann Rheum Dis* **15**:21, 1956

51. Cadman EFB, Robertson AJ: The treatment of Sjögren's syndrome with A.C.T.H. *Br Med J* **1**:68, 1952

52. Mason AM, Golding PL: Hyperglobulinaemic renal tubular acidosis: a report of nine cases. *Br Med J* **1**:143, 1970

53. McCurdy DK et al: Hyperglobulinemic renal tubular acidosis. *Ann Intern Med* **67**:110, 1967

54. Pasternack A, Linder E: Renal tubular acidosis: an immunopathological study on four patients. *Clin Exp Immunol* **7**:115, 1970

55. Brouet JC et al: Biologic and clinical significance of cryoglobulins. *Am J Med* **57**:775, 1974

56. LoSpalluto J et al: Cryoglobulinemia based on interaction between a gamma macroglobulin and 7S gamma globulin. *Am J Med* **32**:142, 1962

57. Metzger N: Characterization of a human macroglobulin. V. A Waldenström macroglobulin with antibody activity. *Proc Natl Acad Sci USA* **57**:1490, 1967

58. Stone MJ, Metzger H: Binding properties of a Waldenström macroglobulin antibody. *J Biol Chem* **243**:5977, 1968

59. Meltzer M, Franklin EC: Cryoglobulinemia. A study of twenty-nine patients: IgG and IgM cryoglobulins and factors affecting cryoprecipitability. *Am J Med* **40**:828, 1966

60. Meltzer M et al: Cryoglobulinemia. A clinical and laboratory study. II. Cryoglobulins with rheumatoid factor activity. *Am J Med* **40**:837, 1966

61. Strauss WG: Purpura hyperglobulinemia of Waldenström. *N Engl J Med* **260**:857, 1959

62. Whitehouse AC et al: Macroglobulinemia and vasculitis in Sjögren's syndrome. Experimental observations relating to pathogenesis. *Am J Med* **43**:609, 1967

63. Husby G et al: Amyloid fibril protein subunit, "protein AS": distribution in tissue and serum in different clinical types of amyloidosis including that associated with myelomatosis and Waldenström's macroglobulinemia. *Scand J Immunol* **2**:395, 1973

64. Amorosi EL, Ultmann JE: Thrombotic thrombocytopenic purpura: report of 16 cases and review of the literature. *Medicine (Baltimore)* **45**:139, 1966

65. Beigelman PM: Variants of the platelet thrombosis syndrome and their relationship to disseminated lupus. *Arch Pathol* **51**:213, 1951

66. Blackman NS et al: Thrombotic thrombocytopenic purpura: report of a case. *JAMA* **143**:546, 1952

67. Benitez I et al: Platelet thrombosis with polyarteritis nodosa. *Arch Pathol* **77**:116, 1964

68. Meacham GC et al: Thrombotic thrombocytopenic purpura: a disseminated disease of arterioles. *Blood* **6**:706, 1951

69. Levine S, Shearn MA: Thrombotic thrombocytopenic purpura and systemic lupus erythematosus. *Arch Intern Med* **113**:826, 1964

70. Steinberg AD et al: Thrombotic thrombocytopenic purpura complicating Sjögren's syndrome. *JAMA* **215**:757, 1971

71. Fraser NG et al: Dermatitis herpetiformis and Sjögren's syndrome. *Br J Dermatol* **100**:213, 1979

72. Prystowski SD et al: Acute febrile neutrophilic dermatosis associated with Sjögren's syndrome. *Arch Dermatol* **114**:1234, 1978

73. Lawley TJ et al: Scleroderma, Sjögren-like syndrome, and chronic graft-versus-host disease. *Ann Intern Med* **87**:707, 1977

CHAPTER 161

SARCOIDOSIS OF THE SKIN

D. Geraint James

Definition

Sarcoidosis is one member of a large family of granulomatous disorders in which the common denominator is the histology of epithelioid cell granulomas (Table 161-1). Like many other members of this loose-knit family, its etiology is unknown.

Sarcoidosis is a multisystem disorder that most commonly affects young adults, presenting with intrathoracic, skin, and eye lesions. The diagnosis is most secure when clinicoradiographic findings are supported by histologic evidence of widespread noncaseating epithelioid cell granulomas in more than one system or by a positive Kveim-Siltzbach skin test. There is immunologic evidence of depression of delayed-type hypersensitivity with impairment of thymus-mediated suppressor T cells in the peripheral blood but with evidence of an increased number and activity of T helper cells in lung and bronchoalveolar fluid. There is simultaneous evidence of lymphoproliferation with overactivity of B cells and in particular of the lambda and kappa light chains. Other common features are circulating immune complexes and also hypercalciuria with or without hypercalcemia.

The course and prognosis correlate with the mode of onset: an acute onset with erythema nodosum heralds a self-limiting course and spontaneous resolution, while an insidious onset may be followed by relentless progressive fibrosis (Table 161-2). Corticosteroids relieve symptoms and suppress inflammation and granuloma formation.

Pathology and pathogenesis

The central histologic feature is that of noncaseating epithelioid cell granulomas in all tissues. In recent years, emphasis has shifted away from the static morphology of the sarcoid granuloma to its more vital metabolic activity. Instead of counting the inclusion bodies we are endeavoring to quantitate its secretory products. The enzymes secreted by the granuloma include angiotensin-converting enzyme, lysozyme, glucuronidase, collagenase, and elastase. The serum angiotensin-converting enzyme activity has been harnessed for clinical use and it has proved helpful in monitoring the activity of sarcoidosis. The sarcoid granuloma consists of focal, tightly packed, interdigitating collections of modified macrophages, epithelioid cells (which often fuse to form multinucleate Langhans' type giant cells), and closely admixed lymphocytes. Central necrosis is usually absent or present in minimal amounts. As the lesions age, the granuloma is infiltrated by fibroblasts with deposition of reticulin and hyalinized collagen. Cellular inclusions, chiefly Schaumann and asteroid bodies, are frequent and increase in number with aging. Schaumann bodies are composed of concentric, laminated, aggregated spherules, conchoidal bodies, made up of cal-

cium/iron-impregnated lipomucoglycoproteins with central birefringent, possibly calcite crystals. They are densely basophilic and when fully formed look like a mulberry or raspberry. They form within epithelioid and giant cells and later become extracellular and invoke a foreign-body giant cell reaction. They are probably the end result of autophagocytic activity, are a kind of "residual" body, and are not considered to contain any causative agent.

An antigenic insult, whether by an infective agent or chemical or even vegetable matter, or by an immune complex, is met by a reticuloendothelial response in which thymus-derived (T) cells, plasma (B) cells, and macrophages participate [1]. Committed T cells produce lymphokines, B cells produce immunoglobulins, and activated macrophages secrete prostaglandins and a variety of T-cell activators, which aggregate into highly active epithelioid cells. Macrophage migration is inhibited by lymphokines thereby contributing to the dense packing of epithelioid cell granulomas. If the antigenic insult is airborne, this cellular interaction commences as an intense inflammatory alveolar alveolitis which metamorphoses into sarcoid granulomas and eventually to pulmonary fibrosis. Bronchoalveolar lavage provides an increased yield of macrophages with prominent pseudopodia and vesiculation in pulmonary sarcoidosis but, unfortunately, does not yield the epithelioid cells seen in tissue specimens. Alveolar macrophages have increased angiotensin-convertase activity and this is probably related to prostaglandin synthesis. It is likely that the beneficial effects of both corticosteroids and prostaglandin inhibitors are directed at this early stage of inflammation. B-cell humoral overactivity is particularly evident in certain ethnic groups due to loss of B-cell immunoregulation caused by a significant decrease in the number of suppressor T cells. This decrease may be due to an absolute reduction or a result of blocking of surface receptors by immune complexes with consequent interference of recognition. Trypsin releases the binding of immune complexes to suppressor T cells with a consequent increase in their number.

Etiology

The cause of sarcoidosis is unknown, so theories abound. Granuloma formation is the final common pathway of several different and unrelated disorders. It is not known whether sarcoidosis is one disease resulting from one cause or whether it is a multicausal syndrome. Claims that it is an infection are long-standing; the most popular infective agents that have been implicated are mycobacteria, fungi, and viruses. Even human foreskin fibroblast has been used for tissue culture of sarcoid lymph nodes, but no viral cytopathic effect was observed.

The occasional occurrence of familial sarcoidosis suggests possible genetic influences. We have observed 16

Table 161-1   A classification of granulomatous disorders

Infections	Neoplasia	Leukocyte oxidase defect
Fungi:	Carcinoma	Chronic granulomatous
Histoplasma	Reticulosis	disease of childhood
Coccidioides	Pinealoma	**Extrinsic allergic alveolitis**
Blastomyces	Dysgerminoma	Farmers' lung
Sporothrix	Seminoma	Bird fanciers'
Aspergillus	Reticulum cell sarcoma	Mushroom workers'
Cryptococcus	Malignant nasal granuloma	Suberosis (cork dust)
Protozoa:	**Chemicals**	Bagassosis
Toxoplasma	Beryllium	Maple bark strippers'
Leishmania	Zirconium	Paprika splitters'
Metazoa	Silica	Coffee bean
Toxocara	Starch	**Other**
Schistosoma	**Immunologic aberration**	Whipple's disease
Spirochetes:	Sarcoidosis	Pyrexia of
Treponema pallidum	Crohn's disease	unknown origin
Treponema pertenue	Primary biliary cirrhosis	Radiotherapy
Treponema carateum	Wegener's granulomatosis	Cancer chemotherapy
Mycobacteria:	Giant cell arteritis	Panniculitis
M. tuberculosis	Peyronie's disease	Chalazion
M. leprae	Hypogammaglobulinemia	Sebaceous cyst
M. kansasii	Systemic lupus erythematosus	Dermoid
M. marinum	Lymphomatoid granulomatosis	Sea urchin spine injury
M. avian	Histiocytosis X	
BCG vaccine	Hepatic granulomatous disease	
Bacteria:	Immune complex disease	
Brucella	Rosenthal-Melkersson syndrome	
Other infections:	Churg-Strauss allergic	
Cat scratch	granulomatosis	
Lymphogranuloma		

families, in whom 33 persons had sarcoidosis. The group comprised eleven brother–sister, four mother–offspring, and one uncle–niece relationships, and it was also once noted in a husband and wife. The clinical, radiographic, and other features of the disorder are similar in familial and sporadic sarcoidosis, but the course of one sister was considerably worse than that of her brother, suggesting adverse hormonal factors. Four of these families were from the West Indies, suggesting a racial predisposition to familial sarcoidosis. Prof. Jude Turiaf (personal communication) has also noted a greater incidence in French West Indians from Martinique; he finds familial sarcoidosis in 1 percent of white Europeans, but in 8 percent of Martiniques, living in Paris. The evidence suggests a recessive mode of inheritance for sarcoidosis susceptibility. It is likely that there are many contributory factors (Fig. 161-1).

Immunology

Sarcoidosis is characterized and perpetuated by helper T cells at sites of activity and by overactive B cells [2]. Activated macrophages and T helper cells are conjointly responsible for activation of B lymphocytes and immunoglobulin synthesis at sites of activity, such as the lungs in sarcoidosis (or the synovium in rheumatoid arthritis or the skin in mycosis fungoides). Associated features are the presence of circulating immune complexes, various changes in serum complement levels, enhanced K and NK cell activity, and certain HLA correlations. There is increased recognition of cell types in blood and bronchoalveolar fluid, and also the enzymes and proteins associated with these cell types; some are proving to be helpful markers of activity (Table 161-3).

Cellular immunity

Monoclonal antibody techniques have enabled the proportion of helper (Tm) to suppressor (Tg) cells to be assessed at sites of disease activity. The T helper:suppressor ratio is 10.5:1 in bronchoalveolar fluid of active pulmonary sarcoidosis compared with 1.4:1 in inactive disease. The Italian school [3] is extending these observations to the redistribution of T cells throughout the body, in keeping with the multisystem nature of the disease. The excess helper T cells also seem to be present in skin, lymph nodes, conjunctival follicles, aqueous humor, and liver.

Beta$_2$-microglobulin is a low-molecular-weight (11,800) protein that constitutes part of the HLA antigens on cell membranes. Activated T cells release it so that a significant elevation is noted in 40 percent of patients with active sarcoidosis.

Ia antigens, usually present on lymphoid cells of non-T origin, are also expressed in a small proportion of circulating T cells. They may be identified by indirect immunofluorescence using a monoclonal antibody; they are significantly increased in active sarcoidosis.

Activated macrophages and epithelioid cells

Following an antigenic stimulus, monocytes become activated macrophages, which play an important role in T-lymphocyte differentiation and B-lymphocyte stimulation.

Table 161-2   Features differentiating acute from chronic sarcoidosis

	Acute (transient)	Chronic (persistent)
Age (years)	< 30	> 40
Onset	Abrupt	Insidious
Chest x-ray	Bilateral hilar lymphadenopathy	Pulmonary infiltration/ fibrosis
Eyes	Acute iritis, conjunctivitis, conjunctival nodules	Keratoconjunctivitis, chronic uveitis, glaucoma, cataract
Skin	Erythema nodosum, vesicles, macular and papular rash	Lupus pernio, plaques, scars, keloids
Parotitis Lymphadenopathy Splenomegaly Bell's palsy	Usually transient	Rarely permanent
Bone cysts	No	Yes
Histology	Epithelioid and giant cells	Hyaline fibrosis, interstitial pneumonitis
Acid phosphatase Leucine aminopeptidase	Increased	Normal
Calcium metabolism	Hypercalcemia, hypercalciuria	Nephrocalcinosis
Urinary hydroxyproline	Increased	Normal
Kveim-Siltzbach test	Positive	May be negative
Tuberculin test	Negative	+
K and NK cells	High	Unchanged
Gallium-67 uptake	High	Low
Macrophages in alveoli	High	Low
Angiotensin-converting enzyme	High	May be raised
Serum lysozyme	Increased	May be increased
Crystal's alveolitis	High intensity	Low intensity
Protein L1	Increased	Normal
Beta$_2$-microglobulin	High	May be raised
Circulating immune process	+ +	±
T helper:suppressor ratio in:		
Lungs	10.5:1	1.4:1
Blood	0.8:1	1:1
Radioactive imipramine or propranolol reveal lung cell mass	Increased	Normal
Free light chains of immunoglobulins	Normal	Elevated
Lactoferrin	Increased	Normal
Serum collagenase	Elevated	Normal
Spontaneous remission	Frequent	Rare
Steroid therapy	Abortive effect	Symptomatic relief
Alternative drugs	Oxyphenbutazone	Chloroquine: POTABA methotrexate
Recurrence after steroid therapy	Rare	Frequent
Prognosis	Good	Poor

They present antigens to lymphocytes with the production of important soluble products. The macrophage secretes prostaglandins which activate T suppressor cells to release peptides which, in turn, suppress T- and B-cell mitogen responses.

Activated macrophages clump together into giant and epithelioid cells which are indistinguishable in sarcoidosis, Kveim granulomas, beryllium disease, and extrinsic allergic alveolitis. Depending upon the activating stimulus and the defense mechanisms in the host, these epithelioid cells may be phagocytic or secretory. They secrete angiotensin-converting enzyme, muramidase, lysozyme, collagenase, and several other important enzymes necessary for the success of an inflammatory reaction.

The experimental epithelioid cell granuloma is profoundly affected by cyclosporin A, a fungal metabolite with interesting immunosuppressant properties. It acts selectively on immunocompetent T lymphocytes at an early

Fig. 161-1   Background factors contributing to sarcoidosis.

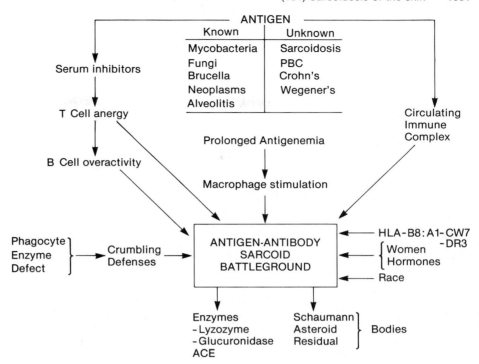

stage of the stimulation, interfering with leukotriene production and preventing organ transplantation. Cyclosporin A prevents the formation of epithelioid cell granulomas or the development of caseous necrosis. Macrophages accumulate at the local site and in the regional lymph node without generalized dissemination of the antigenic stimulus. This experimental observation may have profound therapeutic implications not only in sarcoidosis but in many mycobacterial disorders [4].

Humoral immunity

Whereas there may be both impairment and enhancement of cellular immunity, there is always enhanced humoral immunity with raised immunoglobulin levels and nonspecific increased circulating antibody titers. The immunoglobulin levels can be measured by radioimmunoassay of kappa and lambda free light chains. They provide a marker of chronic persistent, rather than acute, sarcoidosis.

Table 161-3   Markers of activity of sarcoidosis

Clinical	Biochemical	Immunologic
Erythema nodosum	Hypercalcemia	β_2-microglobulins
Uveitis	Hypercalciuria	Tm helper cells in BAL
Macular and papular rash	SACE	Increased CKT4:CKT8 ratio (in
Dactylitis	LACE	BAL)
Polyarthralgia	Serum lysozyme	Decreased OKT4:OKT8 ratio (in
Myopathy	Serum collagenase	blood)
Neuropathy	Urinary hydroxyproline	Kappa and lambda light chains
Granulomatous scars	Glucuronidase	(by radioimmunoassay)
Splenomegaly		
Lymphadenopathy		
Salivary and lacrimal gland enlargement		
Cardiac arrhythmia		
Changing chest x-ray		
Transfer factor		
Exercise KCO		
Fluorescein angiography		
Tuberculin skin test		
Kveim-Siltzbach skin test		
Biopsies		
Radioactive gallium scan		
Thallium-201 myocardial scan		
24-Hour ECG tape		
Bronchoalveolar lavage		

Circulating immune complexes

Various techniques have been employed to detect circulating immune complexes. They are most evident at the stage of erythema nodosum, iritis, polyarthralgia, and bilateral hilar lymphadenopathy in which C3 activation products have been found within the first six weeks [5]. During this early stage of acute sarcoidosis there is activation of the complement system due to circulating immune complexes. These tests for circulating complexes subside as the acute skin lesions disappear. At the present time, all tests for circulating complexes are crude, and it is necessary to use a battery of different techniques. Whenever they are detectable, the sedimentation rate is very high so this remains the least expensive bedside indicator of these complexes.

HLA antigens. In our series, British patients have a significantly increased frequency of HLA-B8, -CW7, and -DR3. The B8/CW7/DR3 haplotype is significantly associated with erythema nodosum, polyarthralgia, short duration of the disease, and a good prognosis. This finding does not hold for West Indians attending the same clinic (Table 161-4).

Kveim-Siltzbach skin test. Williams and Nickerson [6] pioneered the test but an important additional observation was provided by Kveim [7]: by means of intracutaneous inoculations of a heat-killed suspension of a sarcoid lymph node he obtained, in 1 to 4 weeks, lesions histologically consistent with sarcoidosis in 12 of 13 patients with sarcoidosis. Simultaneous control injections of Frei antigen and tuberculin did not produce this response. Since this reaction did not occur in normal subjects, nor in patients with lupus vulgaris, he concluded that the papules were specific lesions due to an unknown agent and that the test served to differentiate sarcoidosis from tuberculosis. Siltzbach and Ehrlich [8] described it as a simple, safe, and specific outpatient technique for providing histologic proof of sarcoidosis and an index of activity and progress of the disease.

Since those early days there has been a generation of experience with the course and prognosis of sarcoidosis around the world. A world survey indicates that the Kveim test remains reliable and helpful in three continents [9]. It was positive in 1714 of 2189 (78 percent) patients, with insignificant false reactions.

Epidemiology

Sarcoidosis has a worldwide distribution but it is more frequently seen in sophisticated communities. Whenever tuberculosis or leprosy is rampant, sarcoidosis is in eclipse, but as they are brought under control, so will sarcoidosis become more evident. It is 10 times more frequent in the black than in the white population in the United States, and there is a similar preponderance in the black population in South Africa. Nonetheless it is commonly seen in the fair-haired Scandinavian and the red-headed Irish. In a world survey of sarcoidosis in 11 cities there is a variable incidence of skin involvement, but overall there is an extraordinary parallelism when it is realized that the 3676 patients in this series are of differing ethnic groups and

Table 161-4   HLA types and their significance in sarcoidosis

HLA type	Significance in sarcoidosis
B8/A1	Sarcoid arthritis, erythema nodosum
B13	Chronicity
CW7	Sarcoidosis in English
B8/CW7/ DR3	Good prognosis in sarcoidosis in English
DR3	Short duration of disease
B7	Symptomatic tuberculin-negative in Swedish
BW15	Black Americans

from different climates and environments (Table 161-5). To this worldwide series may now be added a strikingly similar comparison of sarcoidosis in Eastern Europe (Table 161-6).

Clinical features

In a special Sarcoidosis Clinic we have kept a series of 818 patients with histologically confirmed multisystem sarcoidosis under close supervision. This series includes 251 patients presenting with erythema nodosum and 147 with other skin lesions which includes 35 patients with lupus pernio [5,10] (Table 161-6). It is seen that sarcoidosis overall is slightly more frequent in women and usually presents in patients 20 to 40 years of age.

Lupus pernio

Lupus pernio, or purple lupus, was first described by Ernest Besnier in 1889 as a chronic, persistent, violaceous skin lesion with a predilection for the nose, cheeks, and ears. Manifestations range from a few small buttonlike lesions or nodules under the tip of the nose to exuberant plaques covering the nose and spreading across both cheeks. There may be similar nodules on the eyelids and ears and associated plaques on the arms, buttocks, and thighs.

We have compared the features of lupus pernio with sarcoidosis overall (Table 161-7). Whereas sarcoidosis overall usually presents in three-quarters of those under 40 years old, lupus pernio usually does so in those over 40. Lupus pernio is twice as common in females as in males and it predominates in those from the West Indies. It is associated with chronic fibrotic sarcoidosis in many other systems. Compared with sarcoidosis overall, lupus pernio has a closer affinity with sarcoidosis of the upper respiratory tract (SURT), bone cysts, lacrimal gland involvement, and renal sarcoidosis. It is less often associated with erythema nodosum than in the overall series. The serum angiotensin-converting enzyme (SACE) was elevated in 19 (55 percent) patients.

Lupus pernio is an indicator of chronic fibrotic sarcoidosis. It develops insidiously and progresses indolently over the years. It is complicated by nasal ulceration and septal perforation, which may be aggravated disastrously by the well-meaning intervention of nasal and plastic surgeons. Intrathoracic pulmonary infiltration progresses to fibrosis with little tendency to resolution. It is best kept under control by repeated courses of prednisolone and weekly methotrexate.

Table 161-5 Incidence of involvement of sarcoidosis of the skin in a series of 3676 patients in 11 cities

City	Investigator	No. of patients	Female, %	Age at presentation, % under 40	Erythema nodosum		Other skin lesions	
					No.	%	No.	%
London	D. G. James E. Neville	537	56	67	167	31	135	25
New York	L. E. Siltzbach	311	68	71	33	11	59	19
Paris	J. Turiaf J. P. Battesti	350	45	72	22	7	39	12
Los Angeles	O. P. Sharma	150	67	69	14	9	31	27
Tokyo	Y. Hosoda R. Mikami M. Odaka	282	47	74	10	4	33	12
Reading	A. Karlish	425	62	64	134	32	55	13
Lisbon	T. G. Villar	89	44	72	11	12	16	18
Edinburgh	A. C. Douglas W. Middleton	502	64	72	167	33	34	7
Novi Sad	B. Djuric	285	60	37	31	11	12	4
Naples	A. Blasi D. Oliveiri	624	53	77	38	6	3	0.4
Geneva	D. Press	121	47	79	13	11	7	6
Total		3676	57	68	640	17	324	9

Source: James et al [9].

Experimental model

Lupus pernio is a good experimental therapeutic model because in a single patient there are three features that may be observed and the response to treatment noted serially:

1. The very obvious clinical skin lesions. Serial photography records the response to treatment. Effective therapy is followed by improvement in a matter of 8 to 12 weeks.

2. Serial histology of nasal mucosa which always reveals sarcoid tissue. Effective treatment will convert sarcoid granulomas into a nonspecific inflammatory reaction in the course of 6 months.

3. Nasal bone erosion is slow to develop and slow to heal, but this may be expected in the course of years.

Corticosteroid therapy and methotrexate are effective treatments of lupus pernio, but, unfortunately, relapses follow withdrawal of treatment. Long-term administration of chloroquine is followed by a moderate response in the course of 9 to 12 months. Antituberculous drugs and levamisole fail to influence lupus pernio.

Before embarking on a large-scale, long-term, double-blind clinical trial of any new drug for the treatment of sarcoidosis, consider lupus pernio as a therapeutic screen. It will provide helpful data on the clinical response within a few weeks and on the histologic response within a few months. To these measures may be added serial measurement of SACE. If there is no clinical or histologic response and SACE does not fall as a response to treatment, then it can be assumed that the drug is of little value in overcoming sarcoidosis. It will certainly provide guidance for any prospective and expensive long-term trials.

Erythema nodosum

We have observed erythema nodosum due to sarcoidosis in 251 patients. It may be present in any season but is predominant in the spring. The characteristic red, hot, tender, shining and symmetrical lesions on the shins are also frequently seen on the calves, knees, buttocks, and sometimes on the arms. Some constitutional disturbance is usual at the onset, with swinging fever accompanied by

troublesome polyarthralgia. The development of the skin lesions, from the onset through the play of colors to the end of bruising, takes 3 weeks but ranges from 1 to 20 weeks.

Recurrences are seen in 10 percent of patients usually

Table 161-6 Comparisons of sarcoidosis around the world (percentages given for ease of comparison)

Features	Western worldwide*	Eastern Europe†
Total number	3676 (100%)	2066 (100%)
Women	57	57
Black	10	0.3
Age at presentation under 40 years	68	70
Onset		
Routine chest x-ray	40	64
Chest x-ray 0	8	4
I	51 (65)‡	58 (65)
II	29 (49)	30.5 (31)
III	12 (20)	7.5 (3)
Total % resolution	(54)	(55)
Intrathoracic	87	96
Lymph nodes	22	8
Erythema nodosum	17	11
Eyes	15	4
Other skin lesions	9	5
Spleen	6	1
Parotid	4	1.5
Nervous system	4	1
Bone cysts	3	3.5
Positive Kveim-Siltzbach test	78	73
Negative tuberculin	64	58
Hyperglobulinemia	44	44
Hypercalcemia	11	12
Treated with steroids	47	59.5
Mortality due to:		
Sarcoidosis	2.2	1
Other causes	1.4	1

* From James et al [9].
† From Djuric et al [11].
‡ Percentage resolution of chest x-ray changes at each stage in parentheses.

Table 161-7   Features of 818 patients with histologically confirmed sarcoidosis compared with 35 patients with lupus pernio attending the Royal Northern Hospital, London

Features	Sarcoidosis overall		Lupus pernio	
	No. of patients	%	No. of patients	%
Total	818	100	35	100
Women	500	61	24	69
Presentation under 40 years	604	74	13	40
Intrathoracic	700	86	29	83
Peripheral lymphadenopathy	225	27	2	6
Splenomegaly	101	12	3	9
Erythema nodosum	251	31	3	9
Other skin lesions	147	21	9	26
Ocular lesions	224	27	8	23
Nervous system	77	9	2	6
SURT	53	6	20	57
Parotid	52	6	4	11
Lacrimal	22	3	3	9
Bone	31	3	6	17
Heart	27	3	0	—
Kidney	10	1	2	6
Positive Kveim-Siltzbach skin test	430/658	65	16/35	46
Negative tuberculin skin test	488/702	70	32/35	91
Hyperglobulinemia	161/526	31	1	3
Hypercalcemia	99/547	18	1	3
Corticosteroid therapy	344	42	29	80
Mortality due to:				
Sarcoidosis	25	3	0	
Other causes	23	3	0	

within 3 months but rarely up to 12 months later. Polyarthralgia, usually of the ankles and knees, but sometimes generalized, is experienced by over one-half of patients; it most commonly occurs during the 2 weeks preceding or following the onset of erythema nodosum, but it may appear up to 6 weeks before the eruption. Polyarthralgia preceding erythema nodosum may be indistinguishable from acute rheumatism since the distribution of flitting pains, fever, sweating, and a grossly elevated sedimentation rate are common to both. The absence of a cardiac murmur and normal electrocardiographic findings are helpful differential points; the subsequent appearance of erythema nodosum, bilateral hilar lymphadenopathy, and a positive Kveim-Siltzbach test are decisive. Accompanying bilateral hilar lymphadenopathy subsides in most patients within a year or so. There are numerous causes of erythema nodosum [11] (Table 161-8).

Irrespective of the precipitating cause, the ultimate development of polyarthralgia and erythema nodosum depends upon racial or constitutional predisposition, hormonal and even geographical factors. It is common in women of childbearing years and in association with pregnancy and lactation. It is particularly evident among Irish women in London, Puerto Rican migrants to New York, and Martinique women in Paris. It presents as histoplasmosis in Ohio, coccidioidomycosis in California, leprosy in Africa, and tuberculosis in India. In Europe polyarthralgia and erythema nodosum are common presentations of sarcoidosis. The oral contraceptive may precipitate its development. In his pioneer studies, Lofgren [12] emphasized this interplay of factors, particularly with pelvic inflammation, pregnancy and lactation, gallbladder disease, and streptococcal infection.

Erythema nodosum pinpointed the onset of sarcoidosis in 600 of 3676 (10 percent) patients in a worldwide sarcoidosis survey. The distribution was interestingly uneven, for it occurred in one-third of each of the three British series (London, Edinburgh, and Reading) and was less evident elsewhere. It was never a presenting feature of sarcoidosis in Tokyo. This may be due to differing HLA antigen frequencies in various ethnic groups. In British sarcoidosis patients (as distinct from West Indian patients), erythema nodosum is most likely to occur in those who are HLA-B8, -A1, -CW7, or -DR3.

Macular and papular eruptions

Transient macular and papular or vesicular eruptions may herald the onset of the disease, coinciding with acute (rather than chronic) uveitis or parotid gland enlargement. These features are sufficiently alarming and sudden in onset for patients to seek early medical advice and investigation. Intrathoracic involvement likewise appears at an earlier stage than in patients with lupus pernio or persistent plaques. The eruption occurs at various sites including the trunk, face, arms, thighs, calves, ears, or fingers. It usually resolves within a month but it may recur with exacerbations of iridocyclitis. It is possible that these transient recurrent multisystem features reflect a circulating immune complex.

Table 161-8 Conditions associated with erythema nodosum

Associated disease	Age, yr	Clinical features	X-ray	Skin test	Laboratory confirmation
Sarcoidosis	20–40 Rare below 20	Female preponderance Lymphadenopathy Uveitis or conjunctivitis	Bilateral hilar adenopathy +/− pulmonary infiltration	Kveim–Siltzbach test: positive Tuberculin test: negative	Histology of inflamed scar tissue
Streptococcal infection	Any	Preceding upper respiratory tract infection	——	——	Beta-hemolytic streptococcus in throat Raised antistreptolysin titer
Tuberculosis	Under 20	Close contact with tuberculosis Primary complex	Unilateral hilar adenopathy Ghon focus	Tuberculin conversion to high degree of positivity	Isolation of *Mycobacterium tuberculosis*
Drugs	Any	Transfer factor Sulfonamides Oral contraceptives Sulfones Penicillin	——	——	Recurs when rechallenged with drug
Histoplasmosis	Any	From Ohio Respiratory symptoms Lymphadenopathy	Miliary mottling	Histoplasmin	Complement-fixation test Fungal hyphae in sputum or lung biopsy
Coccidioidomycosis	Any	From California Respiratory symptoms Flu-like illness	Miliary mottling Hilar glands or cavitation	Coccidioidin	Complement-fixation test Fungus in sputum or lung biopsy
Leprosy (lepromatous)	Any	From "Tropics" Symmetrical nodular rash Iridocyclitis Patchy sensory loss	Normal	——	Isolate *M. leprae*: skin or nerve biopsy
Ulcerative colitis	15–40	Diarrhea	Barium enema	——	Rectal biopsy
Crohn's disease	15–40	Abdominal pain, fever Fistulas	Barium follow-through	Depression of delayed-type hypersensitivity	Intestinal biopsy
Yersinia infection	Any	Particularly from France and Scandinavia Abdominal pain Diarrhea	Barium enema Normal chest radiograph and barium studies	——	Stool culture: *Y. enterocolitica* Raised agglutinin titers
Pregnancy	15–40	First trimester	——	——	Recurs with next pregnancy
Behçet's disease	20–40	Orogenital ulceration Thrombophlebitis Arthritis	——	——	Think of it if erythema nodosum occurs in men

Scars

Scars may draw attention to or provide histologic evidence of the disease. They include scars on the abdomen or neck, or on cutaneous venesection and tuberculin skin test sites. In all instances these previously atrophic scars suddenly become purple and livid, proclaiming some inflammatory change, and biopsy reveals active sarcoid tissue. There is no explanation for this phenomenon, first noted by Lofgren [12], in which the sarcoid process seems to creep into and light up these scars, but it suggests a hypersensitivity reaction of skin to erythema nodosum and may indicate a circulating immune complex. Inoculation sites such as Mantoux test sites may also contain sarcoid tissue, so they should be scrutinized in the same way as Kveim sites, after a month, for evidence of palpable nodules. Intrathoracic involvement seems to be long-standing, suggesting that the reaction in the scars is not an initial manifestation of the disease but rather an exacerbation late in its course. Some scars become livid and inflamed. The scar phenomenon is also observed at the onset of erythema nodosum, but it is then a transient and early feature rather than longstanding and recurrent.

Persistent plaques

Hutchinson [13] first recognized and described elevated purple patches (Figs. 161-2 and A2-14), often bilateral and

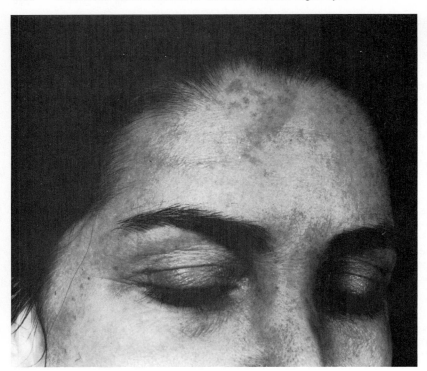

Fig. 161-2 Annular, reddish purple plaque on the forehead in sarcoidosis.

nearly symmetric, commonly situated on the limbs (Fig. 161-3) and buttocks. Whereas lupus pernio is associated with upper respiratory tract mucosal lesions, chronic uveitis, and bone cysts, persistent plaques are more prone to be associated with lymphadenopathy and splenomegaly. They share a similar chronic fibrotic intrathoracic sarcoidosis.

Biochemistry

Acute exudative disease is characterized by hydroxyprolinuria, increased serum angiotensin-converting enzyme, hypercalcemia, hypercalciuria, and raised immunoglobulins IgG, IgA, and IgM. These biochemical abnormalities tend to revert to normal when activity subsides or when

Table 161-9 Skin tests in which a sarcoid granuloma develops 1 month after inoculation

Useful skin tests	Antigen	How done	Read at	Positive result	Negative result	Interpretation of results and remarks
Kveim–Siltzbach	Human sarcoid tissue from spleen or lymph node	Intradermal	1 month	Palpable nodule biopsy reveals sarcoid tissue	Suggests either sarcoidosis not present or it is inactive	Positive test in 80 percent of patients with sarcoidosis. It also indicates activity
Zirconium	1:10,000 solution zirconium chloride or nitrate	Intradermal	1 month	Palpable nodule biopsy reveals sarcoid tissue	Rules out zirconium hypersensitivity	Specific for zirconium hypersensitivity
Beryllium	1% beryllium sulfate or nitrate	Patch	2 days and 1 month	Palpable nodule biopsy reveals sarcoid tissue	Rules out beryllium hypersensitivity	Specific for beryllium hypersensitivity. At 2 days eczematous rash present at patch test site
Lepromin: Fernandez	Skin bacilli	Intradermal	2 days	Tuberculin-like	Negative in lepromatous leprosy	Aid to classification and prognosis rather than diagnosis of leprosy
Mitsuda	Extract of nodules of lepromatous leprosy	Intradermal	1 month	Biopsy of palpable nodule reveals sarcoid tissue		

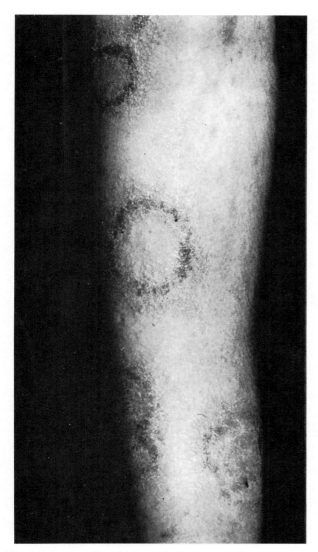

Fig. 161-3 Annular, dusky red plaques on the arm in sarcoidosis.

the disease assumes a chronic fibrotic course, although hypercalciuria and hyperglobulinemia may persist. Hyperuricemia reflects renal failure rather than bone and joint involvement [14].

Markers of activity

During the last hundred years there were very few markers of activity or criteria of cure. Now in the last 10 years, we have been inundated with new markers of activity—so many that it is difficult to choose the most helpful. They may be grouped as bedside and clinical, biochemical, and immunologic techniques.

Bedside and clinical techniques

Fluorescein angiography provides a fresh dimension of leakage of dye indicating active retinal vasculitis associated with posterior uveitis. Other clinical features of activity are dactylitis, polyarthralgia, myopathy, neuropathy, scars, splenomegaly, lymphadenopathy, and enlargement of salivary and lacrimal glands.

Biochemical techniques

Hydroxyprolinuria, hypercalcemia, hypercalciuria, and raised serum angiotensin-converting enzyme (SACE) levels all denote active disease. SACE is raised in 60 percent of patients with sarcoidosis and in 10 percent with other diseases. It is not a particularly good diagnostic test but it is most beneficial as a monitor of progress. It remains high when sarcoidosis is active, but it falls to normal with steroid therapy; rising levels herald a relapse of sarcoidosis [14].

Immunologic techniques

These include the presence of circulating immune complexes, a high sedimentation rate, raised $beta_2$-microglobulins, radioimmunoassay of kappa and lambda chains, and increased T helper:suppressor ratio at the sites of disease activity.

Diagnosis

The clinical diagnosis should be confirmed by histologic proof of the presence of sarcoid tissue by organ biopsy or by the Kveim-Siltzbach skin test. The earlier that histologic confirmation is sought, the more likely will a positive biopsy be obtained. At the late stage of hyaline fibrosis, it may be difficult to find the characteristic epithelioid granulomas which characterize the earlier stages of sarcoidosis.

The Kveim-Siltzbach skin test is a reliable, safe, specific, and simple outpatient technique for delineating multisystem sarcoidosis from the numerous other causes of nonspecific sarcoid tissue reactions. It is positive in about 80 percent of patients around the world whereas the tuberculin skin test is negative in about 66 percent of patients [9]. There are other specific skin tests which distinguish zirconium and beryllium hypersensitivity (Table 161-9). These zirconium and beryllium skin tests are negative in sarcoidosis, just as the Kveim-Siltzbach test is negative in beryllium and zirconium hypersensitivity.

Other useful diagnostic tests indicating acute sarcoidosis are hydroxyprolinuria and serum angiotensin-converting enzyme.

Treatment

Corticosteroids are the sheet anchor of treatment, particularly indicated for uveitis, worsening chest roentgenogram, breathlessness, persistent hypercalciuria, disfiguring skin lesions, myocardial and neurologic involvement, and for involvement of salivary and lacrimal glands and hypersplenism.

There are alternative treatments when steroids are contraindicated or have proved ineffective, but the choice depends on whether it is acute or chronic sarcoidosis. Oxyphenbutazone controls acute exudative sarcoidosis, whereas chloroquine and potassium para-aminobenzoate are indicated for chronic fibrotic sarcoidosis. Azathioprine may be considered for its temporary steroid-sparing effect

Table 161-10   Response of lupus pernio to various drugs

Treatment	Dose	Months	Results
Prednisolone	Smallest possible	Shortest possible	Good
Chloroquine	250 mg alternate days	9	Moderate
Methotrexate	5 mg weekly	3	Very effective
Potassium para-aminobenzoate	12 g daily	12	Slight
Levamisole	150 mg daily	1	Unchanged
Antituberculous	Full	6	Unchanged

when otherwise massive doses of steroids would be necessary.

Persistent hypercalciuria may require a low calcium diet and drugs that chelate with calcium in the intestine—sodium phytate and inorganic phosphate.

Methotrexate in an adult dose of 5 mg once weekly for 3 months is effective in the treatment of lupus pernio and other skin lesions (Table 161-10). This small weekly dose is sufficient and prevents the development of hepatic fibrosis. Cyclosporin A may become a treatment of the future.

Certain treatments which used to be popular but are now contraindicated include radiotherapy, calciferol, and antituberculous drugs.

References

1. James DG, Jones WW: Immunology of sarcoidosis. *Am J Med* **72**:5, 1982
2. Crystal RG et al: Pulmonary sarcoidosis: a disease characterised and perpetuated by activated lung T-lymphocytes. *Ann Intern Med* **94**:73, 1981
3. Semanzato G, Pezzutto A: Insights into the immunopathogenesis of sarcoidosis. *Immunol Clin Sper* **1**:35, 1982
4. Muller-Hermelink HK et al: Modulation of epithelioid cell granuloma formation to apathogenic mycobacteria by cyclosporin A. *Pathol Res Pract* **175**:80, 1982
5. James DG, Jones WW: *Sarcoidosis and Other Granulomatous Disorders*. Philadelphia, WB Saunders, 1985
6. Williams RH, Nickerson DA: Skin reactions in sarcoid. *Proc Soc Exp Biol Med* **33**:403, 1935
7. Kveim A: En ny og spesifikk kirtan reaksjon ved Boeck's sarcoid. *Nord Med* **9**:169, 1941
8. Siltzbach LE, Ehrlich JC: The Nickerson-Kveim reaction in sarcoidosis. *Am J Med* **16**:790, 1954
9. James DG et al: A worldwide review of sarcoidosis. *Ann NY Acad Sci* **278**:321, 1976
10. James DG, Studdy PR: *Colour Atlas of Respiratory Disorders*. London, Wolfe Medical Publications, 1982
11. Djuric B et al: Sarcoidosis in six European cities, in *Sarcoidosis and Other Granulomatous Diseases*. Cardiff, Alpha Omega Publishing Ltd, 1980, p 527
12. Lofgren S: Erythema nodosum. Studies on etiology and pathogenesis in 185 adult cases. *Acta Med Scand* **[Suppl 174] 124**:1, 1946
13. Hutchinson J: Case of papillary psoriasis, in *Illustrations of Clinical Surgery*. London, Churchill, 1877, p 42
14. Studdy PR et al: Biochemical findings in sarcoidosis. *J Clin Pathol* **33**:528, 1980

CHAPTER 162

THE MASTOCYTOSIS SYNDROME

Robert A. Lewis and K. Frank Austen

The similarity in normal pulmonary mast cells and cutaneous mastocytosis cells of histamine and heparin content and capacity to generate prostaglandin D_2 (PGD_2) suggests that much of the recent information concerning human pulmonary mast cells may be relevant to understanding the full complex of symptoms and signs in mastocytosis. In addition, it is possible to offer a rationale for and clinical experience with new therapeutic interventions in mastocytosis, namely cromolyn, cimetidine, and nonsteroidal anti-inflammatory drugs.

Definition

Mastocytosis is an uncommon disease of mast cell proliferation, which occurs in both cutaneous and systemic forms. Since the mast cell is a connective tissue cell, the systemic disease has been reported to involve directly virtually all organs except the central nervous system. The most common locations for excess mast cells are skin, bone, gastrointestinal tract, liver, spleen, and lymph nodes. Mast cells in lesional sites are generally identifiable by their

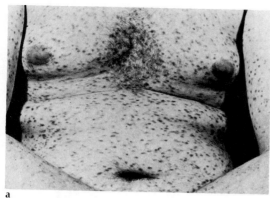

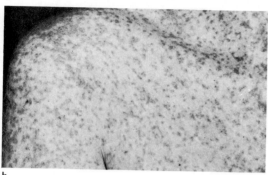

Fig. 162-1   Pigmented macular and papular lesions of generalized urticaria pigmentosa in an adult.

metachromatic granules when histologic sections are stained with basic thionine dyes.

Incidence and prevalence

Fewer than 1000 cases of mastocytosis have been reported in the literature. As the hallmark of this disease is based on cutaneous manifestations, over 95 percent of mastocytosis patients are said to have skin lesions [1]. However, the actual percentage of patients with visceral mastocytosis and lacking the dermatologic stigmata may be underestimated, based upon the recent description of patients with cardiovascular manifestations and no fixed cutaneous lesions [2,3]. The first occurrence of cutaneous lesions is more prevalent in early childhood than after maturity and is not sex-linked for any age of onset [4]. Visceral disease is not commonly associated with skin lesions arising in infancy or early childhood. However, approximately one-quarter of individuals with adult-onset cutaneous lesions have visceral involvement [1].

Cutaneous manifestations

Mastocytosis lesions of the skin are designated urticaria pigmentosa. The lesions may be isolated mastocytomas or generalized and multiple (Fig. 162-1), and they are generally reddish brown and plaquelike or nodular. Much less common are the telangiectatic and the doughy-feeling erythrodermic forms. When a cutaneous lesion is stroked firmly, it often becomes pruritic and raised with surrounding erythema (Darier's sign). Stroked cutaneous lesions of very young children with the disease may vesiculate. In up to 50 percent of patients, stroking of macroscopically uninvolved skin produces a wheal of dermographia due to microscopic dermal mastocytosis. However, generalized pruritus and flushing may occur with or without cutaneous lesions.

Systemic symptoms of an acute nature (Table 162-1) reflect a sudden and greatly elevated level of released mast cell mediators. An acute symptomatic systemic episode may focus on the vasculature and present with headache, flushing, dizziness, tachycardia, hypotension, syncope and even frank shock, rarely irreversible and fatal, and/or on the gastrointestinal tract, causing anorexia, nausea, vomiting, and diarrhea. Occasionally rhinorrhea and, rarely, audible wheezing occur, reminiscent of the signs of rhinitis and asthma, respectively.

More chronic problems include ill-defined neuropsychiatric symptoms, ranging from malaise to decreased attention span and irritability, and such gastrointestinal manifestations as malabsorption [5] or even a possible predilection for peptic ulceration [1]. Malabsorption with or without steatorrhea may be due to the chronic release of mediators from mast cells infiltrating small bowel mucosa and lamina propria. Hepatomegaly or hepatosplenomegaly occurs in about 5 to 10 percent of patients and is directly related to infiltrative disease of those organs [6]. Biopsy specimens in patients with hepatomegaly may reveal periportal proliferation of mast cells, eosinophil infiltration, and fibrosis [7], and these findings may account for the rare manifestations of portal hypertension and gastroesophageal varices. More than 10 percent of all mastocytosis patients, and a greater proportion of those with systemic disease, are estimated to have osseous lesions [8], most commonly in the pelvis, ribs, vertebrae, skull, and proximal long bones. Bone pain may occur with or without pathologic fractures. Anemia, leukopenia, thrombocytopenia, and even mast cell leukemia have been rarely reported in association with severe bone marrow infiltration by mast cells.

Pathobiology

When human mast cells degranulate in response to a physiologic, IgE-dependent stimulus, they both release their preformed granule-associated mediators [9] and generate PGD_2 as well as sulfidopeptide leukotrienes (LTs) [10–12]. Mast cells are abnormal in number in mastocytosis (Fig. 162-2), but not in the types or concentrations of preformed mediators contained per mast cell [13]. The apparent ease with which the cells degranulate in response to physical stimuli, such as gentle stroking (Darier's sign) and moderate heat or cold, and to chemical stimuli known to be histamine releasers, such as codeine and radiopaque dyes, is most likely due to the quantities of products released by the increased mast cell numbers rather than some unusual fragility or responsiveness. Once a skin lesion urticates, it requires up to 3 days to regenerate adequate granule histamine to form a second wheal at that site.

The heparin released from concentrations of mastocytoma cells has been implicated in the prolonged local bleed-

Table 162-1   Clinical manifestations of mastocytosis

Cutaneous	Reddish-brown papules
	Flush
Cardiovascular	Tachycardia, hypotension, and syncope (rarely fatal)
Gastrointestinal	Nausea, vomiting, diarrhea (exacerbated by alcohol)
	Malabsorption (rare)
	Portal hypertension (rare)
Bone	Pain
Neurologic	Neuropsychiatric symptoms (malaise, irritability)
Respiratory	Rhinorrhea, wheezing (rare)
Hematologic	Anemia, leukopenia, thrombocytopenia (rare)
	Eosinophilia
	Coagulopathies
	Leukemia (rare)

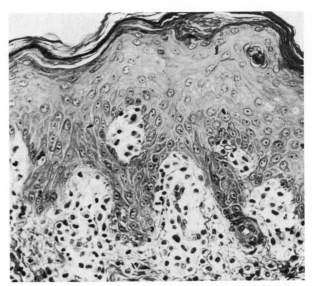

Fig. 162-2   Mast cells in papillary dermis, urticaria pigmentosa. In hematoxylin and eosin preparations mast cells present oval, uniformly staining, dark blue nuclei without recognizable nucleoli or clumping of chromatin. Such nuclei are surrounded by an abundance of dark pink cytoplasm, which may show faint granulation. With care one may usually recognize mast cells in routine preparations, but errors are made and metachromatic stains should always be used when a specific diagnosis is dependent upon the recognition of mast cells. H&E, ×256. (Photomicrograph by Wallace H. Clark, Jr., M.D.)

ing time at the sites of excised lesions, the occasional purpura underlying cutaneous mastocytomas, and the rare incidence of significant gastrointestinal bleeds related to local mast cell infiltration. The moderate eosinophilia noted in 10 to 20 percent of mastocytosis patients does not have a mechanistic explanation at present, while the prominent association of tissue eosinophilia with mastocytosis lesions in bone and in periportal spaces most likely reflects the action of eosinophilotactic granule peptides [14,15] and the generation from arachidonate of monohydroxyeicosatetraenoic acids (HETEs) [16,17] and leukotriene B₄ [18–20]. The development of osseous lesions which are porotic and sclerotic [21] may relate to the action of mast cell tryptase [22,23] and acid hydrolases [23,24] on extracellular proteoglycans. Hepatic periportal fibrosis may also be a result of the action of these enzymes.

Prior to the recognition of the lipid mediators, the majority of the manifestations of mastocytosis were ascribed to effects of released histamine. The primacy of histamine in causing local cutaneous whealing and pruritus as well as rhinitis, when it occurs, remains likely. However, the causative mediators of vasodilatation and of the spectrum of gastrointestinal symptoms in this disease are likely multiple. Because the combined use of antihistamines of both the classical H_1 antagonist group, such as chlorpheniramine maleate, and the more recently described H_2 antagonists, exemplified by cimetidine, has failed to control either the gastrointestinal symptoms or the hypotension in some mastocytosis patients, the identification of a vasodilating prostaglandin (PGD_2) may be relevant to both pathophysiology and therapy (Table 162-2).

Arachidonic acid, a 20-carbon fatty acid with four olefinic bonds, is released from perturbated mast cell plasma membrane phospholipid stores by the actions of one or more acyl hydrolases, as exemplified by phospholipase A_2 [25]. The free fatty acid is then metabolized via the cyclooxygenase pathway in rat peritoneal mast cells to PGD_2 and prostacyclin (PGI_2) (Fig. 162-3), with the former being the predominant product by almost an order of magnitude [10,11]. In human mast cells dispersed from lung parenchyma, only PGD_2 is generated via the cyclooxygenase pathway after immunologic activation with anti-IgE antibody [11]. Further, elevated levels of PGD_2 metabolites have been detected in urines obtained from mastocytosis patients with flushing, hypotension, and even shock in the

absence of cutaneous lesions [2,3]. An initial report described measurement by gas chromatography-mass spectrometry (GC-MS) of one urinary metabolite, 9α-hydroxy-11,15-dioxo-2,3,4,5-tetranorprostane-1,20-dioic acid (PGD-M_1) (Fig. 162-3) from two such patients, as contrasted to the undetectable levels of this metabolite in urines of over 200 normal individuals [26]. Elevated urinary excretion of a second metabolite, 9α-hydroxy-11,15-dioxo-2,3,18,19-tetranorprost-5-ene-1,20-dioic acid (PGD-M_2) (Fig. 162-3), also described in the first two patients, was quantitated from an additional 18 mastocytosis patients with attacks of flushing and dizziness and was elevated in 13, to as much as 150-fold above normal [3]. Since PGD_2 has been shown to be potent as both a vasodilator and bronchoconstrictor in the dog [27], the release of the compound from lesional mast cells may be causatively related to the flushing and hypotension and the less common wheezing described in patients with this disease. Since these same

Table 162-2   Pathobiologic factors in mastocytosis

Histamine	Urticaria
	Gastrointestinal symptoms
PGD_2	Flush
	Cardiovascular symptoms
	Gastrointestinal symptoms
Heparin	Bleeding at biopsy site
	Purpura and hemorrhage (rare)
Neutral protease and acid hydrolases	Patchy hepatic fibrosis
	Bone lesions

Fig. 162-3 Mast cell pathways of oxidative metabolism of arachidonic acid. Products identified from rodent mast cells (†), human mast cells (*), and mastocytosis patient urines (**).

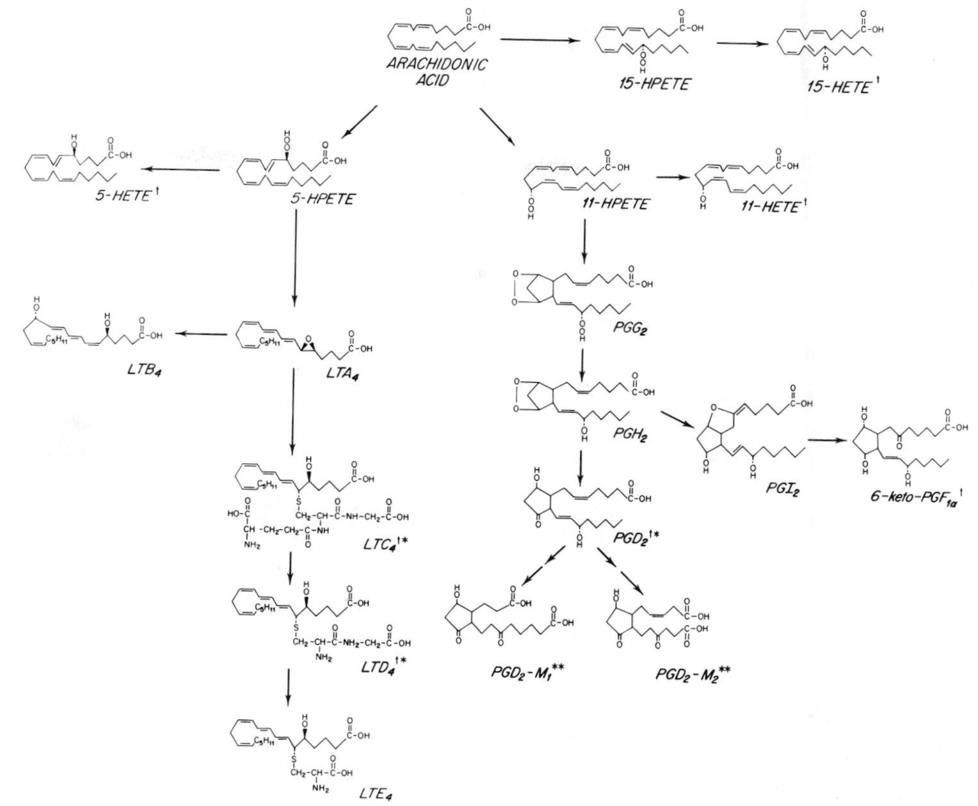

patients also excreted amounts of histamine, the relative clinical effects of histamine and PGD_2 can only be surmised from data on therapeutic intervention noted below. Further, the importance of quantities of histamine and PGD_2 released in the tissue locations of mastocytosis is not known, and they do not necessarily correlate with those levels of each compound measured in the urine.

In addition to PGD_2, a number of other biologically active oxidative metabolites of arachidonic acid have been appreciated in extracts and release supernatants of rat serosal mast cells incubated with the calcium ionophore A23187 and of mouse bone marrow-derived mast cells either activated with A23187 or sensitized with antigen-specific monoclonal IgE and activated by specific antigen. Among these compounds are included several products of the 5-lipoxygenase pathway: the granulocyte-chemotactic lipids 5(S)-hydroxy-6,8,11,14-eicosatetraenoic acid (5-HETE) and 5(S),12(R)-dihydroxy-6,14-cis-8,10-trans-eicosatetraenoic acid (LTB4) as well as the slow-reacting substance LTs 5(S)-hydroxy-6(R)-S-glutathionyl-7,9-trans-11, 14-cis-eicosatetraenoic acid (LTC4) and 5(S)-hydroxy-6(R)-S-cysteinylglycyl-7,9-trans-11,14-cis-eicosatetraenoic acid (LTD4) [20,28–31] (Fig. 162-3). LTC4 and LTD4 have been generated from both mast cell-containing human lung fragments and purified human lung mast cells by IgE-dependent activation for histamine release [12,32]. Both LTC4 and LTD4 evoke peripheral airway bronchospasm in guinea pigs and humans [33–35] and also increase vasopermeability in both species [33,36]. The 15-lipoxygenase product 15-HETE and 11-HETE, which is a cyclooxygenase metabolite and possibly a product of a specific lipoxygenase, are both modest granulocyte chemotactic factors and are produced by ionophore-stimulated rat mast cells

[37]. None of these compounds or their known metabolites has been measured in biologic fluids from patients with mastocytosis. It is nonetheless possible that administration of nonsteroidal anti-inflammatory drugs to these patients may not only decrease PGD_2 generation by inhibiting the cyclooxygenase, but also increase the biosynthesis of lipoxygenase products by redirecting available arachidonic acid as substrate for the latter pathways.

Diagnosis

While the cutaneous lesions in conjunction with Darier's sign are pathognomonic, especially with biopsy confirmation of mastocytosis (Fig. 162-4), additional criteria are helpful in establishing the diagnosis, especially in the absence of skin lesions (Table 162-3). Osseous infiltration by mast cells may be suspected from radiologic lesions with adjacent areas of osteoporosis and mottled osteosclerosis and proved by bone marrow biopsy, demonstrating areas of abnormally high mast cell numbers, along with rarefaction of the spongiosa or, alternatively, myelofibrosis and sclerosis. In the absence of radiologic abnormalities, ^{99}Tc bone scans may define areas of increased radionuclide uptake [38]. Bone marrow aspiration or biopsy may be positive for increased numbers of mast cells even without localizing laboratory findings. Histaminuria of 2 to 3 times normal 24-h levels (36 ± 15 μg) [39] is common among patients with extensive cutaneous involvement with or without acute symptoms of visceral disease, although both episodic normal values and striking elevations of over 1000 μg per 24 h occur. Further, due to interference with radioenzymatic quantitation of histamine in urine specimens,

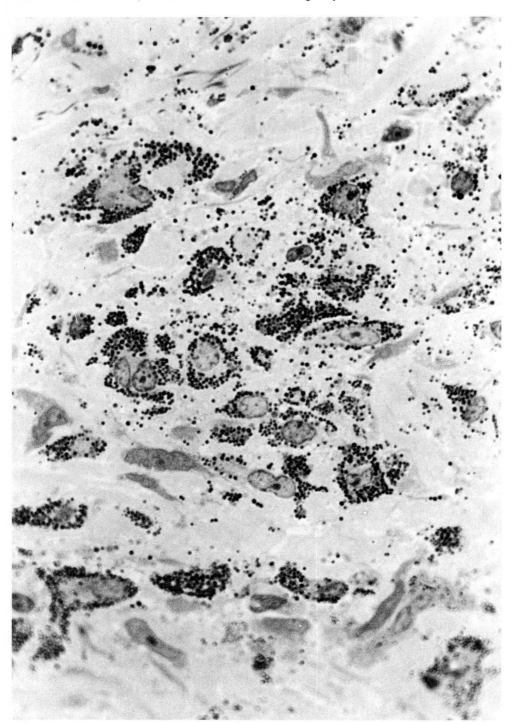

Fig. 162-4 A 1-μm Epon-embedded, Giemsa-stained lesional skin biopsy specimen, showing mast cell proliferation in the dermis. ×520. *(Photomicrograph by John P. Caulfield, M.D.)*

some apparently normal levels of histamine may actually be elevated; these levels may be correctly measured by a more precise mass-spectrometric method (L. J. Roberts II, personal communication). Twenty-four-hour urinary excretions of 9α-hydroxy-11,15-dioxo-2,3,18,19-tetranor-prost-5-ene-1,20-dioic acid, even during asymptomatic periods, may range from 1.5- to 150-fold above normal levels of 286 ± 75 ng [2,3].

For the patient with flushing, intermittent hypotension, diarrhea, tachycardia, and possibly hepatomegaly and peptic ulceration, the main differential diagnosis is with the carcinoid syndrome. The most direct criterion is a biopsy demonstrating mast cell proliferation, as opposed to argentaffin cell infiltration in an involved organ. Failing this, the measurement of grossly elevated levels of histamine and its metabolites in the urine favors mastocytosis, while elevated urinary levels of 5-hydroxyindoleacetic acid (5-HIAA) are noted in carcinoid syndrome. However, it should be recalled that gastric carcinoids lead to increased urinary excretion of both histamine and 5-HIAA [40] and that elevated urinary levels of 5-HIAA have been reported in mastocytosis, although rarely [41].

Table 162-3 Diagnosis of mastocytosis

Darier's sign
Tissue biopsy enriched for mast cells
  Skin
  Bone marrow
24-H urine collection
  Histamine
    Increased to > 50 μg/24 h
  9α-Hydroxy-11,15-dioxo-2-3,18,19-tetranorprost-5-ene-
    1,20-dioic acid
    Increased to > 350 ng/24 h
  5-Hydroxyindoleacetic acid
    Generally normal

Treatment

Treatment of patients with asymptomatic cutaneous lesions may be unnecessary or limited to H_1 antihistamines if pruritus and whealing are bothersome and can be controlled by such an agent. The addition of an H_2 blocker, cimetidine, has been reported to be helpful [42], but the efficacy of a combination of H_1 and H_2 blockers has not been established by any controlled studies or objective measurements.

Drugs known to cause mast cell degranulation, such as alcohol, morphine, and codeine, are to be prohibited. The former is well described to exacerbate diarrhea, occasionally to the extent of a malabsorption syndrome, in patients with intestinal mastocytosis. It is particularly for the gastrointestinal symptoms that oral therapy with disodium cromoglycate (cromolyn), given at 100 mg 4 times daily, has been effective in a double-blind controlled trial [39]. While the mode of cromolyn action is incompletely defined, it is thought to prevent mast cell degranulation by interfering with cellular calcium flux [43]. As less than 2 percent of the drug is known to be absorbed, a local action on the gastrointestinal mast cell proliferative infiltrate seems likely. It is less convenient to explain the therapeutic effects of this agent in decreasing cutaneous symptoms of pruritus, whealing, and flushing, as well as normalization of some of the neuropsychiatric complaints [39]. Cromolyn may prove useful in combination with antihistamines and aspirin, but this is unproved and the introduction of a nonsteroidal agent requires the precautions noted below.

Since aspirin and other nonsteroidal anti-inflammatory drugs (NSAIDs) inhibit prostaglandin synthesis, it is reasonable to relax judiciously the previous prohibition of aspirin use in these patients, with careful monitoring and pretreatment with H_1 and H_2 blockers. The occasional reports of hypotensive episodes induced by administration of aspirin and other NSAIDs seem valid on the basis of a repetitive episode with a second administration [44,45]. Thus, because of the theoretical possibilities of effecting increases in both lipoxygenase product synthesis by diversion of arachidonate and mast cell histamine release by augmentation of secretion with NSAIDs, it is advisable to administer therapeutic doses of both H_1 and H_2 antihistamines prior to the use of aspirin and then to employ very small initial doses of the latter agent. In a recently employed protocol for use in adult mastocytosis patients, therapy was initiated with 8 mg chlorpheniramine maleate and 300 mg cimetidine 4 times daily. After 2 days, aspirin therapy was added at initial doses of 16 mg (0.25 gr) 4

times daily, and the dose doubled on each subsequent day until either symptomatic relief was achieved or the side effect of tinnitus required maintenance at that dose [2,3,26]. In these patients, the minimum therapeutic aspirin dose, in combination with the antihistamines, is then maintained chronically. Of eight patients treated on this protocol for 1 to 15 months, none has reported severe flushing or hypotensive episodes while on therapy [2]. If severe hypotension occurs, either spontaneously or in response to aspirin, pressor therapy with intravenous epinephrine, 4 to 15 μg/min, may successfully reverse the episode, whereas dopamine, up to 20 μg/kg/min, fails to do so [46].

Isolated cutaneous mastocytomas of infancy commonly involute spontaneously; when this does not occur, the single lesions may be excised surgically. None of the recently recognized medical therapies [26,39] effects involution of either cutaneous or visceral lesions. In a preliminary report, the use of oral 8-methoxypsoralen and long-wave ultraviolet irradiation (PUVA) has been purported to effect a partial involution of cutaneous lesions [47].

Malignant mastocytosis is a very rare disorder with high mortality within 2 years of diagnosis. It may occur either as a cutaneous or a systemic disease and reportedly may appear by malignant transformation of a benign neoplasm, especially of the systemic variety. Histopathologic analysis utilizing special staining procedures, such as the naphthol-AS-chloracetate esterase technique, may be necessary to detect the immature granules of malignant cells [48,49]. No particular cytotoxic drug protocol has been established or recommended. Leukemias associated with mastocytosis may be monocytic, mastocytic, or myeloid, in approximately equal frequencies, of which the sum appears in few of all mastocytosis patients. The relationship of mastocytosis to such leukemias has been unclear but possibly may relate to the recent evidence that mast cells, at least in some portion, are derived from bone marrow stem cells [50–53].

References

1. Sagher F, Even-Paz Z: *Mastocytosis and the Mast Cell.* Chicago, Year Book Medical Publishers, 1967
2. Roberts LJ II et al: Shock syndrome associated with mastocytosis: pharmacologic reversal of the acute episode and therapeutic prevention of recurrent attacks. *Adv Shock Res* 8:145, 1982
3. Roberts LJ II et al: Mastocytosis without urticaria pigmentosa. A frequently unrecognized cause of recurrent syncope. *Trans Assoc Am Physicians* 95:36, 1982
4. Shaw JM: Genetic aspects of urticaria pigmentosa. *Arch Dermatol* 97:137, 1968
5. Scott BB et al: Involvement of the small intestine in systemic mast cell disease. *Gut* 16:918, 1975
6. Cryer PE, Kissane JM: Clinicopathologic conference: systemic mastocytosis. *Am J Med* 61:671, 1976
7. Capron JP et al: Portal hypertension in systemic mastocytosis. *Gastroenterology* 74:595, 1978
8. Lucaya J et al: Mastocytosis with skeletal and gastrointestinal involvement in infancy. *Pediatr Radiol* 131:363, 1979
9. Austen KF: Biologic implications of the structural and functional characteristics of the chemical mediators of immediate hypersensitivity. *Harvey Lect* 73:93, 1979
10. Roberts LJ II et al: Prostaglandin, thromboxane and 12-hydroxy-5,8,10,14-eicosatetraenoic acid production by iono-

phore-stimulated rat serosal mast cells. *Biochim Biophys Acta* **575**:185, 1979

11. Lewis RA et al: Preferential generation of prostaglandin D₂ by rat and human mast cells, in *Biochemistry of the Acute Allergic Reactions, 4th International Symposium,* edited by EL Becker et al. New York, Alan R Liss, 1981, p 239

12. MacGlashan DW Jr et al: Generation of leukotrienes by purified human lung mast cells. *J Clin Invest* **70**:747, 1982

13. Metcalfe DD et al: Identification of sulfated mucopolysaccharides, including heparin, in the lesional skin of a patient with mastocytosis. *J Invest Dermatol* **74**:210, 1980

14. Goetzl EJ, Austen KF: Purification and synthesis of eosinophilotactic tetrapeptides of human lung tissue: identification as eosinophil chemotactic factor of anaphylaxis. *Proc Natl Acad Sci USA* **72**:4123, 1975

15. Boswell RN et al: Intermediate molecular weight eosinophil chemotactic factors in rat peritoneal mast cells: immunologic release, granule association, and demonstration of structural heterogeneity. *J Immunol* **120**:15, 1978

16. Goetzl EJ et al: The regulation of human eosinophil function by endogenous monohydroxyeicosatetraenoic acids (HETEs). *J Immunol* **124**:926, 1980

17. Goetzl EJ et al: Modulation of human neutrophil function by monohydroxyeicosatetraenoic acids. *Immunology* **39**:491, 1980

18. Borgeat P, Samuelsson B: Metabolism of arachidonic acid in polymorphonuclear leukocytes. Structural analysis of novel hydroxylated compounds. *J Biol Chem* **254**:7865, 1979

19. Goetzl EJ, Pickett WC: The human PMN leukocyte chemotactic activity of complex hydroxyeicosatetraenoic acids (HETEs). *J Immunol* **125**:1789, 1980

20. Mencia-Huerta J-M et al: Immunological and ionophore-induced generation of leukotriene B₄ from mouse bone marrow-derived mast cells. *J Immunol* **30**:1885, 1983

21. Gagnon JH et al: Mastocytosis: unusual manifestations: clinical and radiologic changes. *Can Med Assoc J* **112**:1329, 1975

22. Montagna W: Histology and cytochemistry of human skin. XI. The distribution of β-glucuronidase. *J Biophys Biochem Cytol* **3**:343, 1957

23. Schwartz LB et al: Acid hydrolases and tryptase from secretory granules of dispersed human lung mast cells. *J Immunol* **126**:1290, 1981

24. Glenner GG, Cohen LA: Histochemical demonstration of a species-specific trypsin-like enzyme in mast cells. *Nature* **185**:846, 1960

25. Hirata F et al: Concanavalin A stimulates phospholipid methylation and phosphatidyl serine decarboxylation in rat mast cells. *Proc Natl Acad Sci USA* **76**:4813, 1979

26. Roberts LJ II et al: Increased production of prostaglandin D₂ in patients with systemic mastocytosis. *N Engl J Med* **303**:1400, 1980

27. Wasserman MA et al: Bronchopulmonary and cardiovascular effects of prostaglandin D₂ in the dog. *Prostaglandins* **13**:255, 1977

28. Yecies LD et al: Slow reacting substance (SRS) from ionophore A23187-stimulated peritoneal mast cells of the normal rat. *J Immunol* **122**:2083, 1979

29. Falkenhein SF et al: Effect of the 5-hydroperoxide of eicosatetraenoic acid and inhibitors of the lipoxygenase pathway on the formation of slow reacting substance by rat basophilic leukemia cells: direct evidence that slow reacting substance is a product of the lipoxygenase pathway. *J Immunol* **125**:163, 1980

30. Razin ER et al: Generation of leukotriene C₄ from a subclass

of mast cells differentiated *in vitro* from mouse bone marrow. *Proc Natl Acad Sci USA* **79**:4665, 1982

31. Razin ER et al: IgE-mediated release of leukotriene C₄ chondroitin sulfate E proteoglycan, β-hexosaminidase, and histamine from cultured bone marrow-derived mast cells. *J Exp Med* **157**:189, 1983

32. Lewis RA et al: Slow reacting substances of anaphylaxis: identification of leukotrienes C-1 and D from human and rat sources. *Proc Natl Acad Sci USA* **77**:3710, 1980

33. Drazen JM et al: Comparative airway and vascular activities of leukotrienes C-1 and D *in vivo* and *in vitro*. *Proc Natl Acad Sci USA* **77**:4354, 1980

34. Weiss JW et al: Bronchoconstrictor effects of leukotriene C in human subjects. *Science* **216**:196, 1982

35. Weiss JW et al: Airway constriction in normal humans produced by inhalation of leukotriene D. Potency, time course, and effect of aspirin therapy. *JAMA* **249**:2814, 1983

36. Soter NA et al: Local effects of synthetic leukotrienes (LTC₄, LTD₄, LTE₄, and LTB₄) in human skin. *J Invest Dermatol* **80**:115, 1983

37. Lewis RA et al: Generation of oxidative metabolites of arachidonic acid from rat serosal mast cells (abstr). *J Allergy Clin Immunol* **63**:220, 1979

38. Sostre S, Handler HL: Bony lesions in systemic mastocytosis: scintigraphic evaluation. *Arch Dermatol* **113**:1245, 1977

39. Soter NA et al: Oral disodium cromoglycate in the treatment of systemic mastocytosis. *N Engl J Med* **301**:465, 1979

40. Oates JA, Sjoerdsma A: The unique syndrome associated with secretion of 5-hydroxytryptophan by metastatic gastric carcinoids. *Am J Med* **32**:333, 1962

41. Demis DJ: The mastocytosis syndrome: clinical and biological studies. *Ann Intern Med* **59**:194, 1963

42. Gerrard DM, Ko C: Urticaria pigmentosa: treatment with cimetidine and chlorpheniramine. *J Pediatr* **94**:843, 1979

43. Foreman JC, Garland LG: Cromoglycate and other antiallergic drugs: a possible mechanism of action. *Br Med J* **1**:820, 1976

44. Brogren H et al: Urticaria pigmentosa (mastocytosis). *Acta Med Scand* **163**:223, 1959

45. Hamrin B: Release of histamine in urticaria pigmentosa. *Lancet* **1**:867, 1957

46. Turk J et al: Intervention with epinephrine in hypotension associated with mastocytosis. *J Allergy Clin Immunol* **71**:189, 1983

47. Christopher E et al: PUVA-treatment of urticaria pigmentosa. *Br J Dermatol* **98**:701, 1978

48. Leder LD: Subtle clues to diagnosis by histochemistry in mast cell disease. *Am J Dermatopathol* **1**:261, 1979

49. Lennert K, Parwaresch MR: Mast cell neoplasia: a review. *Histopathology* **3**:349, 1979

50. Razin E et al: Growth of a pure population of mouse mast cells *in vitro* with conditioned medium derived from concanavalin A-stimulated splenocytes. *Proc Natl Acad Sci USA* **78**:2559, 1981

51. Schrader JW et al: The persisting (P) cell: histamine content, regulation by a T cell-derived factor, origin from a bone marrow precursor, and relationship to mast cells. *Proc Natl Acad Sci USA* **78**:323, 1981

52. Tertian G et al: Long term *in vitro* culture of murine mast cells. 1. Description of a growth factor-dependent culture technique. *J Immunol* **127**:788, 1981

53. Nabel G et al: Another inducer T cell function: synthesis of a factor that stimulates proliferation of cloned mast cells. *Nature* **291**:332, 1981

CHAPTER 163

SKIN CHANGES IN THE CARCINOID SYNDROME

Seymour J. Gray

The carcinoid syndrome is a constellation of clinical signs and symptoms in which the cutaneous manifestations are often dominant. The syndrome includes episodic flushing of the skin, patchy cyanosis, telangiectasia, pellagra-like skin lesions, diarrhea, asthma, and valvular heart disease occurring in patients with carcinoid tumors [1]. Recognition of the syndrome began in 1953 with Lembeck's discovery that carcinoid tumors of the intestine (argentaffinomas) contained considerable quantities of serotonin (5-hydroxytryptamine), a powerful smooth-muscle stimulant formed predominantly within the argentaffin cells of the gastrointestinal tract. One year later, Thorson, Biörck, Björkman, and Waldenström described the clinical picture of the "carcinoid syndrome" in patients suffering from malignant carcinoid tumors of the ileum with massive liver metastases, and implicated an overproduction of serotonin in the pathogenesis of the syndrome. More recently, variant syndromes have been described in which the primary carcinoid tumors arise outside the small intestine.

Although an excess of serotonin remains as the chemical hallmark of the carcinoid syndrome, other unrelated pharmacologically active agents are elaborated by the carcinoid tumors which may contribute to the production of the cutaneous flushes. These include (1) a powerful vasodilator peptide, bradykinin, (2) histamine, and (3) adrenocorticotropic hormone (ACTH) which are produced, stored, and released in varying amounts.

Pathology

Oberndorfer in 1907 first proposed the term *carcinoid* to emphasize the malignant appearance but slow growth of the tumor. Carcinoid tumors of the intestine arise from the argentaffin cells of the intestinal mucosa (Kulchitsky cells) near the bases of the crypts of Lieberkühn. These cells contain cytoplasmic granules with an affinity for silver compounds, yield a positive argentaffin reaction (hence "argentaffinoma"), and secrete serotonin. Carcinoid tumors are yellow, firm on section, and consist of clumps of epithelial cells in a fibrous stroma.

The typical functioning malignant carcinoid develops from a primary lesion in the region of the ileocecal valve, principally in the appendix and terminal ileum where 80 to 95 percent are found, although they may be located anywhere from the stomach to the rectum. Carcinoids may be found in the small intestine, colon, gallbladder, bile ducts, pancreatic ducts, ampulla of Vater, stomach, bronchus, or in a Meckel's diverticulum; they are multiple in 15 to 25 percent of cases. Occasionally a carcinoid may arise from an ovarian or testicular teratoma. Appendiceal carcinoids metastasize rarely, if at all. Carcinoid tumors involving the ileum, cecum, colon, or stomach metastasize more frequently, usually to the liver and regional lymph nodes and occasionally to the ovaries, lungs, and bones. Bronchial carcinoids are usually benign but metastasize occasionally. Carcinoids of the bronchus, stomach, and pancreas tend to metastasize to liver, bone, and skin. Metastatic lesions may appear late, grow slowly, and assume massive proportions.

Associated abnormalities are found primarily in the skin and heart. Widely dilated capillaries and small veins are observed in the skin, representing telangiectasia during life. Pigmentation of the skin is caused by an increase in melanin pigment in the basal layer and by a broad layer of iron-containing granules in the subpapillary connective tissue. Pigmented patches covering a network of wide and tortuous veins also have been reported.

Characteristically, the involvement of the heart is primarily, but not exclusively right sided, with the pulmonic and tricuspid valves presenting a pearly gray fibrosis with sclerosis, thickening, and retraction of the chordae tendinae, resulting in stenosis and regurgitation. Plaquelike deposits on the endocardial surface of the heart produce the valvular deformities. In some instances the mural endocardium becomes markedly thickened. With bronchial carcinoids, the valvular lesions may involve only the mitral and aortic valves. When cardiac involvement appears in association with carcinoid tumors of the ileum, hepatic metastases are invariably present.

Serotonin metabolism

An excess secretion of serotonin by the carcinoid tumors and a disturbance in tryptophan metabolism characterize the carcinoid syndrome although other physiologically active substances also are involved in its pathogenesis [2].

Serotonin is derived from the essential amino acid, tryptophan, by hydroxylation to 5-hydroxytryptophan (5-HTP) and decarboxylation to 5-hydroxytryptamine (5-HTA) or serotonin, which in turn is metabolized to 5-hydroxyindoleacetic acid (5-HIAA) by monoamine oxidase and excreted in the urine (Fig. 163-1). Increased production of serotonin from tryptophan in the tumor and its subsequent degradation to 5-HIAA result in an increased excretion of 5-HIAA in the urine [2,3].

Approximately 1 percent of dietary tryptophan is normally metabolized by this 5-hydroxyindole pathway, whereas in the carcinoid syndrome 60 percent of the dietary tryptophan may be diverted into the serotonin pathway by the carcinoid tumor. This excessive shunting of tryptophan away from the kynurenine-niacin pathway leaves less available for the formation of niacin and protein which, along with the diarrhea and decreased food intake, may result in the development of a pellagra-like picture and protein deficiency.

Approximately 90 percent of the total body serotonin is

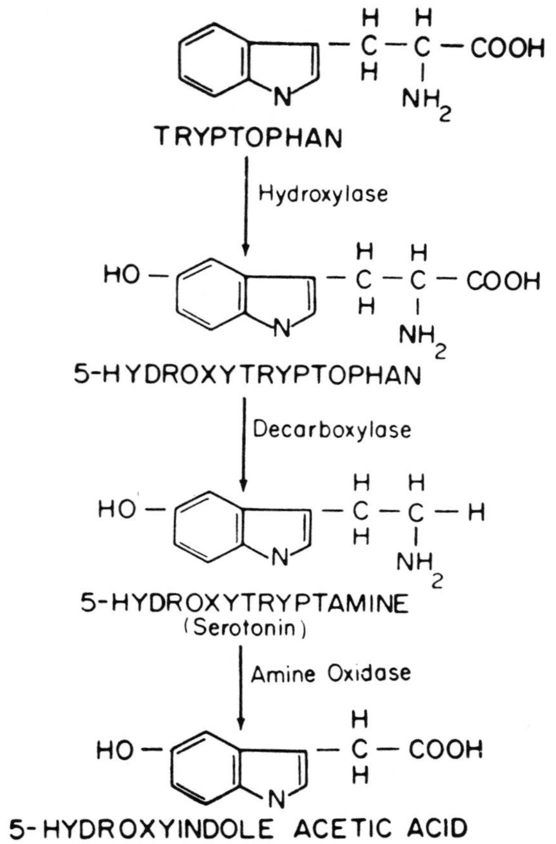

Fig. 163-1 Metabolic pathway of serotonin. (*Principles of Internal Medicine*, 5th ed, edited by TR Harrison et al. New York, McGraw-Hill, 1966, p 546.)

stored within the argentaffin cells of the gastrointestinal tract. Smaller amounts are present in the brain and blood platelets, as well as in the spleen, lungs, and other tissues.

Clinical manifestations

The spectrum of symptoms which makes up the carcinoid syndrome often extends over a period of years and may be evanescent in onset in view of the slow growth of the carcinoid tumors [2,3]. Carcinoids occur at any age from childhood to extreme old age although the carcinoid syndrome is most commonly seen in the older age groups, equally among the sexes. The clinical features of the carcinoid syndrome become evident only after hepatic metastases have occurred or when the primary tumor is a bronchial carcinoid or a carcinoid arising in an ovarian teratoma where the venous drainage bypasses the hepatic circulation [1,5].

Vasomotor—the cutaneous flush

Episodic flushing of the face and the neck is the most distinctive and often the earliest symptom of the carcinoid syndrome. Facial flushing may be the only presenting symptom. The appearance of the frequent, brief, acute episodes of cutaneous flushing warrants a thorough search for a carcinoid tumor. The flush exhibits a panorama of colors ranging from pinkish orange to bright red to violaceous to blue to blanching white. It may be red to begin

with, changing quickly to pink or salmon-red, leaving blue lakes interspersed with white normal skin. At first only the face is involved, then the flush may spread to the neck and later to the shoulders, chest, and arms (Fig. A2-17). The back and abdomen are rarely affected. The ordinary flush is of brief duration, starting abruptly without premonitory signs and lasting for only a few minutes. The flushing episodes generally begin insidiously, are faint and infrequent at first, but later increase in frequency, intensity, and duration as the disease progresses. Some patients with a long history of flushing experience a succession of flushes, each of which may persist for 10 min or longer, fading first from the face and then from the trunk. Attacks may occur daily, recur 10 to 20 times or more during the day, or appear at variable unpredictable intervals. Emotional disturbances, physical exertion, defecation, colonic enemas, manual manipulation or compression of the tumor, and food or alcohol intake may precipitate a flushing episode. Periorbital edema, tachycardia, abdominal pain, diarrhea, or wheezing often accompany the more severe episodes.

With progression of the disease, permanent hyperemia of the face and neck may ensue. Cutaneous capillaries and venules become chronically dilated producing patchy cyanosis of the face, although the arterial oxygen saturation remains normal. Widened tortuous veins on the nose and cheeks may appear and become permanent. After several years, localized miliary and gross telangiectasia may develop on the cheeks, nose, or forehead, and more rarely on the upper trunk. In some instances the telangiectases disappear after complete removal of the tumor.

The cutaneous flush is the manifestation of a generalized hemodynamic alteration in the vasomotor system as a whole, as demonstrated by ballistocardiograms taken during the flushing episode. The peritoneum observed during abdominal laparotomy reveals flushing as well. Increased pressure in the pulmonary vessels, a well-documented serotonin effect, has been demonstrated during flushing by cardiac catheterization.

Cutaneous hyperpigmentation has been observed in a limited number of patients with the carcinoid syndrome. Pellagra-like lesions, characterized by hyperkeratosis with dry scaling and grayish-black pigmentation on the legs, forearms, or trunk, have been described in a few patients, one of whom presented with a fiery red glossitis. These lesions may improve or disappear after niacin therapy. A second type of pigmentation, consisting of cutaneous patches of a yellow-brown or brown-gray color without hyperkeratosis (Fig. 163-2), has been observed on the forehead, back, wrists, and thighs. The pigmented areas vary in size up to that of the palm of a hand, are not raised above the surface, and occasionally appear atrophic. They are observed later than the flush, and disappear or regress after removal of the tumor. The chemical nature of the pigment is unknown.

Gastrointestinal

Abdominal discomfort and chronic, recurrent diarrhea are among the most frequent manifestations of the syndrome, and may be the presenting complaints. Nausea, vomiting, and diarrhea often accompany the flushing. Borborygmi, colicky abdominal pain, and other signs of hyperperistalsis are common. An enlarged liver usually signifies metastases, although metastatic involvement may be present in the absence of hepatomegaly. An increased incidence of peptic ulcer and intestinal malabsorption with steatorrhea have been reported.

Carcinoids of the appendix may obstruct the lumen and produce the clinical picture of appendicitis, or in the small bowel may cause symptoms of intestinal obstruction. In rare instances tumors obstructing the biliary system produce jaundice.

Cardiovascular

Right-sided cardiac involvement appears late in the disease when metastasis to the liver has already occurred; it is seen in about half of the advanced cases. The tricuspid and pulmonic valves are most commonly involved. Valvular damage generally produces incompetency or stenosis, alone or in combination. Cardiac murmurs depend upon the location and extent of valvular involvement. Right-sided heart failure may supervene. Brawny edema of the lower extremities is common in the early phase of the carcinoid syndrome. Hypotension may be associated with episodes of flushing or diarrhea, and syncope may occur.

Respiratory

Attacks of dyspnea and asthmatic wheezing occur in some patients, particularly during flushing episodes, presumably related to the bronchiolar constriction. Recurrent paroxysms of coughing also may be noted.

Other symptoms

Other symptoms include arthritis with swelling and stiffness of the joints, sudden localized edema of the hands or face, dependent edema, and weight loss. Rarely a malabsorption syndrome or scleroderma may accompany the carcinoid syndrome.

Variant syndromes

Carcinoids arising from the bronchus may be accompanied by unusually severe and prolonged flushing episodes, facial and periorbital edema, excessive lacrimation, salivation, tachycardia, and hypotension. There may be protracted nausea, vomiting, explosive diarrhea, and bronchial constriction associated with severe anxiety and disorientation. Widespread bone and skin metastases occur.

Metastatic gastric carcinoids produce vivid, bright-red erythematous patches with sharp serpentine borders. As the blush heightens, the patches may coalesce. Skin flushes are more likely to occur after meals. Gastric carcinoids may secrete large amounts of histamine and 5-HTP. The incidence of peptic ulceration is increased.

Pathologic physiology and pharmacology

The major depot of serotonin is the carcinoid tumor which generally contains 1.0 to 3.0 mg 5-HTA per gram of tumor. The serotonin pool in the body of a patient with malignant carcinoidosis approximates 2800 mg. Elevated levels of 5-HIAA in the urine (50 to 1000 mg per day) are characteristic of the carcinoid syndrome in the presence of hepatic metastases or with bronchial or ovarian carcinoids. The

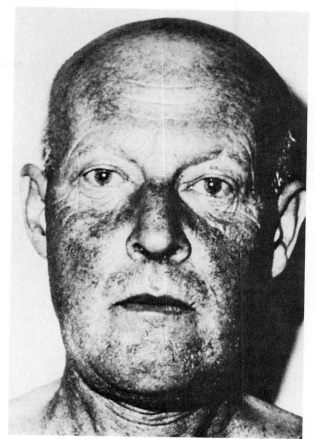

Fig. 163-2   A 62-year-old male with brownish-gray pigmentation of the face in carcinoid syndrome with metastases.

blood and urinary levels of serotonin are also increased to 0.5 to 3.0 μg/mL and 0.5 to 12 mg daily, respectively [2].

Carcinoid tumors arising in the bronchus, stomach, or pancreas tend to secrete more 5-HTP and less serotonin than carcinoids elsewhere. Multiple endocrine adenomas and hyperadrenocorticism may be found more frequently. Metastases to bone and skin are more common in this group.

Serotonin causes venoconstriction and arteriolar dilatation. Infusion of the amine decreases blood flow, increases vascular volume, and produces flushing and cyanosis of the skin. It also induces intense spasm of the infused vein. Serotonin has been reported to increase cardiac output and may elevate pulmonary artery pressure. Its effect on systemic blood pressure is variable although there is usually a fall in blood pressure during spontaneous or induced flushes. The bronchoconstriction, intestinal hyperperistalsis, and diarrhea have been attributed to the pharmacologic action of serotonin in inducing smooth-muscle spasm. The cardiac lesions as well have been considered serotonin induced.

Mechanism of the carcinoid flush

No single cause for the carcinoid flush has been established. Although an overproduction of serotonin characteristically attends the syndrome, the flushing reaction cannot be attributed solely to serotonin [4]. It has not been possible to demonstrate a consistent increase in blood

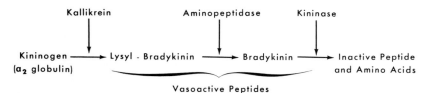

Fig. 163-3   The kallikrein-kinin system. (From Mason and Melmon [6].)

serotonin or in urinary 5-HIAA during spontaneous or induced flushing. While intravenous injections of epinephrine produce flushing attacks in malignant carcinoidosis identical to those occurring spontaneously, the levels of serotonin in the hepatic vein blood during the flush are usually unaltered. Moreover, while the infusion of serotonin into the brachial artery produces a deep flush in the injected area, the characteristic facial flush is not induced consistently in normal subjects or in patients with malignant carcinoid. Finally, decarboxylase inhibitors capable of reducing serotonin synthesis, and serotonin antagonists do not control the flushing.

Bradykinin has been implicated in the production of the carcinoid flush and other manifestations of the syndrome [5,6]. Bradykinin is a powerful dilator of both arterioles and veins, and may also produce diarrhea and wheezing by its stimulating action on smooth muscle of the bronchi and intestines. This kinin-peptide is capable of altering endothelial permeability and initiating inflammatory reactions which could play a role in the production of lesions in the endocardium.

Epinephrine, norepinephrine, and a variety of sympathomimetic amines when administered intravenously provoke the typical flush in patients with malignant carcinoid by triggering the release of proteolytic enzymes, kallikreins, from the carcinoid tumors into the peripheral circulation. These enzymes in turn act upon a specific substrate formed in the liver and found abundantly in the plasma (kininogen—an alpha$_2$ globulin), thereby liberating bradykinin and other vasoactive kinin peptides which then produce vasodilatation and the typical cutaneous flush (Fig. 163-3). Infusion of bradykinin in normal subjects and in patients with carcinoid disease produces the typical facial flushes and hypotension, accompanied by dilatation of arterioles and veins. Moreover, large amounts of kallikrein capable of catalyzing the production of bradykinin have been demonstrated in hepatic metastases of carcinoid tumors and in the hepatic vein blood of carcinoid patients during catecholamine-induced flushes. An increase in bradykinin has also been demonstrated in the blood of these patients during spontaneous or epinephrine-induced flushing, clearly implicating the kinin-generating system in the production of the carcinoid flush.

Bradykinin release, however, cannot be demonstrated in all patients during flushing. It has been postulated that bradykinin, serotonin, or histamine may contribute to the production of the varied types of flushes seen in the carcinoid syndrome. The presence of still another flush substance, not yet identified, cannot be excluded.

Diagnosis

The diagnosis may be evident from the clinical symptoms when the syndrome is fully manifest, but is more difficult in the early stages when the symptoms are evanescent or limited. A single sign such as cutaneous flushing or diarrhea may be the only evidence of a malignant carcinoid. Induction of the flush by intravenous epinephrine (1 to 10 μg) is a useful test. The diagnosis can be established by demonstrating an increased urinary excretion of 5-HIAA (above 25 mg per day) by quantitative assay. A simple screening test for 5-HIAA, consisting of a purple color when a nitrosonaphthol solution is added to urine, becomes positive when the daily excretion of 5-HIAA exceeds 40 mg. Marked increases of 5-HIAA do not occur except in carcinoidosis, although a slight elevation may be observed in some patients with nontropical sprue and, transiently, after the administration of reserpine. The ingestion of bananas, which contain significant amounts of serotonin (4 mg per banana), or pineapples can also increase the urinary excretion of 5-HIAA. Decreased excretion has been noted in renal insufficiency and in some instances of phenylketonuria. Medications containing mephenesin carbamate and phenothiazines interfere with the determination. Guaiacolate in cough syrups may cause falsely high values.

The level of 5-HIAA in the urine is a measure of the extent of the functioning tumor mass and may be helpful in following the clinical course of the patient after surgery or other therapy. It returns to normal when the carcinoid is completely removed if no metastases are present. Other diagnostic aids include the demonstration of elevated levels of serotonin in the blood or urine.

Prognosis

In view of the slow growth of the carcinoid tumor, patients may live as long as 10 to 20 years after the symptoms appear. The immediate prognosis is variable but is not necessarily poor in spite of metastases. Death results from heart failure, metastatic liver disease, malnutrition, or intercurrent infection.

Management

Surgical resection of the primary carcinoid tumor and palliative removal of liver metastases should be attempted, whenever feasible, since it may relieve the symptoms of the carcinoid syndrome, reduce serotonin production and 5-HIAA excretion, and prolong life for many years. Local complications such as intestinal obstruction can be prevented, and removal of a solitary bronchial or ovarian carcinoid may prove curative.

Regional arterial perfusion of the tumors with 5-fluorouracil is under investigation. Irradiation is generally ineffective.

There is no specific treatment for the symptoms of the syndrome. Certain drugs tend to relieve flushing while others are more effective in controlling diarrhea or bronchoconstriction. Individualization of dose schedules is essential although relief of symptoms is quite variable. A bland diet with vitamin supplements including niacin is recommended. Corticosteroids have proved to be unusually effective in controlling the flushes in some patients with bronchial carcinoids, and may combat anorexia in others. Phenothiazines decrease the severity of the flush in some instances by acting as an antagonist to the vascular effects of bradykinin. Propranolol, a beta-receptor blocking agent, has been noted to diminish the frequency and severity of the flushing reaction [6].

Methysergide (Sansert), a serotonin antagonist, is useful in controlling severe diarrhea in some instances. The tryptophan hydroxylase inhibitor, *p*-chlorophenylalanine, which blocks serotonin synthesis, may also improve the diarrhea.

References

1. Thorson AH: Studies on carcinoid disease. *Acta Med Scand* **161 (suppl 344)**:1, 1958
2. Sjoerdsma A et al: A clinical, physiologic and biochemical study of patients with malignant carcinoid (argentaffinoma). *Am J Med* 21:520, 1956
3. Resnick RH, Gray SJ: Serotonin metabolism and the carcinoid syndrome: a review. *Med Clin North Am* 44:1323, 1960
4. Robertson JIS et al: The mechanism of facial flushes in the carcinoid syndrome. *Q J Med* 31:103, 1962
5. Oates JA, Butler TC: Pharmacologic and endocrine aspects of carcinoid syndrome. *Adv Pharmacol* 5:109, 1967
6. Mason DT, Melmon KL: New understanding of the mechanism of the carcinoid flush. *Ann Intern Med* 65:1334, 1966

CHAPTER 164

THE SKIN AND THE HEMATOPOIETIC SYSTEM

Michael B. Brodin and Dorothea Zucker-Franklin

Purpura

Purpura (from Latin and Greek roots signifying purple) occurs when blood extravasates into the skin. A classification of purpura is given in Table 164-1. It should be remembered that purpura is often a sign of abnormal bleeding produced by an underlying disease and that the underlying disease may cause far more serious bleeding in sites other than the skin, such as the optic fundi, gastrointestinal tract, joints, and central nervous system.

The appearance of purpura varies greatly. Small red macules (petechiae) may range in size from a pinpoint to a pinhead, whereas ecchymoses, the common black-and-blue spots, are larger and of variable shape and color. Vibices (singular, vibex) are linear hemorrhages often due to trauma. If bleeding is sufficiently severe it can result in a blood-filled blister. The color of purpura depends upon its severity, location, and duration; the hue, chroma, and intensity will change as pigments are broken down in the skin. One may see shades of red, orange, brown, violet, purple, and green.

Purpura must be distinguished from erythema and telangiectasia. One way to do this is by diascopy, but this method is not foolproof because vessels cannot always be emptied. It is also important to decide whether purpura is palpable, for palpability almost always signifies vasculitis. On occasion, however, the lesions of vasculitis are not grossly palpable, and one must search diligently with delicate touch or careful side lighting in order to detect subtle elevations.

In general one should rely upon laboratory investigations to reveal the etiology in an individual case of purpura, but there are exceptions in which clinical appearance is important:

1. *Bateman's (actinic or senile) purpura* is found on sun-damaged skin in the elderly. Lesions are usually on the backs of the hands and forearms. The skin is thin and finely wrinkled, looking flimsy. Large erosions due to shearing are sometimes seen because the skin is so fragile. These purpuric lesions are due to diminished strength of blood vessel walls and form with mild trauma. The macules may be small or very large and are usually irregularly shaped.

2. The purpura of *scurvy* is usually petechial, perifollicular, but may be ecchymotic, and is found on the lower legs.

3. *Progressive pigmentary purpuras* collectively show grouped petechiae on the lower extremities and occasionally elsewhere that are asymptomatic or cause mild itching. New lesions unpredictably appear in weeks to years. The most striking clinical feature may be brown pigmentation due to the presence of heme pigments, although erythema and eczematous changes may be seen. The pathologic basis is a capillaritis. The clinical and eponymic designations that are used for these disorders are probably unsound and should be abandoned. They usually refer to one of the variable morphologic features. Various terms with their eponyms are given here for reference purposes: (a) peculiar progressive pigmentary disease, or progressive pigmentary dermatosis (Schamberg); (b) pigmented purpuric lichenoid dermatitis (Gougerot and Blum); (c) purpura annularis telangiectodes (Majocchi). The typical location of the lesions

Table 164-1 Classification of purpura

Hematologic (Platelet defects)
  Quantitative (thrombocytopenia)
    Increased platelet destruction
      Immunologic
        Autoimmune thrombocytopenic purpura (ITP)
        Drug hypersensitivity
        Posttransfusion
      Nonimmunologic
        Infection
        Prosthetic heart valves
        Disseminated intravascular coagulation
          Generalized stimulus
          Localized stimulus (Kasabach-Merritt syndrome)
        Thrombotic thrombocytopenic purpura
    Decreased platelet formation
      Direct injury to bone marrow
      Replacement of bone marrow
      Aplastic anemia
      Vitamin deficiencies
      Wiskott-Aldrich syndrome
    Platelet sequestration
      Splenomegaly
      Hypothermia
  Functional platelet disorders
    von Willebrand's disease
    Storage pool disease
    Bernard-Soulier syndrome
    Glanzmann's thrombasthenia
Vascular-extravascular
  Vasculitis
  Capillary fragility
  Actinic damage (Bateman's purpura)
  Steroid purpura
  Ehlers-Danlos syndrome
  Gardner-Diamond syndrome
  Factitial trauma
  Scurvy
  Amyloid
  Increased intravascular pressure
  Progressive pigmentary purpura

in areas of increased hydrostatic pressure suggests that an extravascular tissue deficit or abnormality could play a role.

4. *Acute purpura* due to sudden raising of intravascular pressure presents a striking clinical picture. The patient usually states that he was startled to awake with a shower of red marks on his neck and face. Examination reveals that the marks are petechiae, and upon further questioning the patient admits to a night of heavy drinking and severe retching. The lesions form during the Valsalva maneuver.

5. Many pruritic skin lesions and eruptions can become purpuric from scratching or rubbing. This is particularly true of insect bites, especially flea assaults on the lower legs, which can become so traumatized that they mimic allergic vasculitis.

6. *Factitial or iatrogenic purpura* is often distinctive, bearing evidence of the device responsible and the method of its deployment. One type seen in Asians is due to "cupping," in which a device producing negative pressure is applied to the skin, leaving numerous purplish red circles over the trunk.

7. *Gardner-Diamond syndrome* (painful bruising syndrome, autoerythrocyte sensitization syndrome) is a rare disorder of uncertain etiology. Many cases cannot be dis-

cerned from factitial purpura, particularly since marked psychological disturbance is a prominent feature of both syndromes. Ninety-five percent of patients are adult females, but the syndrome has been reported in males and children [1]. Clinical lesions often appear after trauma, venipuncture, surgery, or emotional upset. They begin as nodules which first become red and then ecchymotic (Fig. 164-1). Symptoms begin with tingling or itching which then progresses to pain and tenderness. The extremities are most commonly involved. Histology shows vasculitis, dermal edema, a lymphocytic and monocytic perivascular infiltrate, and extravasation of red blood cells [2]. Initially it was thought that extravasated blood stimulated the formation of a skin-sensitizing antibody [3], but immunofluorescence is negative. Skin tests with autologous blood cells have been reported to reproduce the clinical lesions, but positive results are inconsistent, and in certain cases may have even been the result of factitial intervention by the patient. Prognosis is highly variable, some patients clearing spontaneously in a few months while symptoms in others continue for many years [4]. Treatment is usually unsuccessful, but in certain cases psychotherapy seems to be of value [1].

If the foregoing disorders have been eliminated, the investigating physician should undertake a laboratory study to discover the cause of purpura. Although theoretically any disorder of hemostasis may produce bleeding anywhere in the body, the following rule of thumb should be noted: coagulation defects (for example, hemophilia) produce problems with large-vessel hemostasis, whereas platelet defects produce problems with small-vessel hemostasis. This is because platelet plugs by themselves effectively stop bleeding from capillaries and small blood vessels but are incapable of stopping hemorrhage from larger vessels. Thus, since purpura is produced by leakage from small cutaneous vessels, it is almost always due to some platelet disorder, *when it is due to a hematologic disease.* As has been stated, purpura is not always hematologic in origin.

Platelet defects may be divided into two groups, quantitative and qualitative. More common by far is the former, thrombocytopenia, which is defined as a platelet count of less than 100,000. But even at this level there continues to be virtually normal hemostasis. When the platelet count falls below 40,000, bleeding occurs with minor trauma. At a count of 10,000 to 20,000 there may be spontaneous bleeding without trauma. The three major causes of thrombocytopenia are: (1) decreased or faulty production, (2) increased destruction, and (3) sequestration.

Decreased or faulty production of platelets may be caused by direct injury to the bone marrow by cytotoxic drugs, chemicals, radiation, or infection. Similar results occur if the marrow is replaced by neoplasms or fibrosis. There may also be faulty platelet production in aplastic anemia due to acquired or congenital marrow failure, vitamin B_{12} and folic acid deficiencies, and in the Wiskott-Aldrich syndrome.

The Wiskott-Aldrich syndrome [5,6] consists of thrombocytopenic purpura, recurrent infections, and skin lesions. Infections are due to defective processing of microbial polysaccharide antigens. Skin lesions are identical to those of atopic dermatitis but in addition are often purpuric and infected. Since the disease is X-linked only boys are affected. Patients also usually have a Coombs'-positive

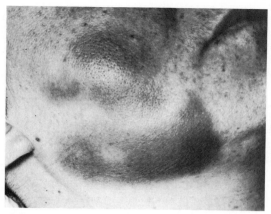

Fig. 164-1 Purpuric lesions in a woman with autoerythrocyte sensitization.

hemolytic anemia, a leukocyte chemotactic defect, and immunoglobulin deficiencies. They commonly die in childhood from bleeding, infection, or a lymphoreticular malignancy.

Thrombocytopenia due to *increased destruction of platelets* may come about immunologically or nonimmunologically.

In autoimmune thrombocytopenic purpura, antibodies to platelets can be demonstrated. The condition is frequently associated with connective tissue diseases such as systemic lupus erythematosus, or with chronic lymphatic leukemia, but most often the disorder is idiopathic (ITP). ITP can be acute or chronic. In both instances the main clinical sign is purpura of the skin and mucous membranes.

Acute ITP occurs mainly in children between the ages of two and six, but is occasionally seen in adults. Purpura develops quickly and is most severe at the onset of the disease. At this time there may be bleeding into the central nervous system and fatal cerebral hemorrhage may ensue. Acute ITP usually lasts a few days but sometimes persists. If thrombocytopenia lasts longer than six months the disease is considered chronic. Chronic ITP is seen most often in women between the ages of 20 and 40. It is believed to be an autoimmune disease. The plasma of most patients will cause thrombocytopenia when transfused into healthy recipients. Platelet transfusions are to no avail since the transfused platelets, like the patient's own platelets, will be sensitized by the circulating antibody. Autoimmune thrombocytopenia is usually accompanied by subclinical hemolysis [7]. When ITP is associated with frank hemolytic anemia it is referred to as Evan's syndrome [8].

Thrombocytopenia may also result from drug hypersensitivity, especially to sulfonamides, quinine, and quinidine. In this case, the mechanism of action is thought to be due to the formation of an antigen–antibody complex with an affinity for platelets, the platelets being injured as innocent bystanders [9].

Thrombocytopenic purpura due to drug hypersensitivity may occur shortly after a drug is started or may occur in patients who have taken the same drug with impunity for long periods of time. In either case, it resolves quickly after drug administration has been discontinued [10]. Immunologic purpura may also be the consequence of sensitization to alloantigens acquired transplacentally or during blood transfusion.

Nonimmunologic causes of increased platelet destruction include those seen in infection (secondary to the direct action of the organism or toxin) and in malfunctioning prosthetic heart valves (due to increased turbulence and mechanical injury to platelets). Nonimmunologic thrombocytopenic purpura is also seen in cases of increased platelet consumption, as in disseminated intravascular coagulation (DIC).

DIC has diverse etiologies, the precise natures of which are often elusive. The stimulus to widespread intravascular coagulation may be generalized or localized. When DIC complicates hypovolemic or cardiogenic shock, gram-negative sepsis or other infections, the clinical presentation is usually fulminant. There is extensive bleeding from multiple sites in addition to purpura of the skin. Purpura fulminans is a variant of DIC seen mostly in children and occurring after a latent period following a bacterial or viral infection. Treatment is difficult and must be directed toward the underlying disease in addition to the coagulation abnormality. Replacement of coagulation factors is futile since they too will be consumed. In a few instances heparinization prior to replacement therapy has proved helpful [11,12]. Optimal replacement therapy is achieved by administration of platelet concentrates, fresh frozen plasma, and cryoprecipitate in order to reconstitute platelets, coagulation factors, and fibrinogen, respectively.

In contrast to the above, the stimulus for disseminated coagulation is localized in the Kasabach-Merritt syndrome. In this disorder a congenital hemangioma triggers generalized intravascular coagulation. The syndrome consists of thrombocytopenia, hypofibrinogenemia, and elevated levels of fibrinopeptide A, a fibrinogen degradation product. Peak incidence is in early infancy. The hemangioma is very large at the outset or else small and rapidly growing; it usually involves a limb but may be truncal or even visceral [13]. Older patients may experience sudden episodes of thrombocytopenic purpura, and there are reports of the syndrome being precipitated by surgery, angiography, and parturition. Unlike generalized forms of DIC, those due to the Kasabach-Merritt syndrome may be mild and chronic. Treatment always depends upon the clinical picture, since moderate thrombocytopenia may be tolerated quite well over long periods. The well-known tendency for most congenital hemangiomas to resolve suggests that the majority of cases are self-limited. If DIC is fulminant, however, the administration of systemic steroids appears to be beneficial.

Thrombotic thrombocytopenic purpura (TTP, Moschcowitz syndrome) [14–16] is a syndrome manifesting, in addition to purpura, a Coombs'-negative hemolytic anemia, fever, renal failure, and protean neurologic symptoms. It is usually fulminant, and often fatal. Inhibitors of platelet function and large doses of prednisone are used for treatment. In recent years, plasma exchange transfusions have achieved remissions in a substantial number of patients. Heparin is reserved for patients whose condition is complicated by DIC.

Sequestration of platelets leads to a relative rather than to an absolute thrombocytopenia. Patients with splenomegaly sometimes have low platelet counts owing to this mechanism. In health, approximately 30 percent of available platelets are stored in the spleen, but splenic enlargement may increase this number to more than 80 percent, thus producing a relative decrease of platelets in the peripheral blood. This form of thrombocytopenia, however, is almost never severe enough to produce purpura. A similar form of thrombocytopenia may be produced by hypothermia during anesthesia.

Defects in platelet function

The most important function of platelets is their ability to form plugs in injured vessels. The plugs form in a series of steps. First, platelets adhere to injured endothelium. This is followed by aggregation, a process which is accompanied by degranulation and the release of numerous substances with diverse physiologic effects. In the final stage platelets mediate clot contraction. A malfunction at any of these stages will produce a defect in hemostasis. The underlying diseases are suspected when there is a normal platelet count in conjunction with a prolonged bleeding time or positive tourniquet test. Von Willebrand's disease is by far the most common condition associated with impaired hemostasis. It is inherited as an incompletely dominant autosomal trait, and its expression is extremely variable. Actually, von Willebrand's disease may be due to a qualitative or quantitative abnormality of factor VIII which is required for normal platelet adhesion. Clinical manifestations are usually limited to epistaxis, easy bruisability, and somewhat prolonged bleeding with minor injuries. The laboratory diagnosis is usually made by finding that the patient's platelets do not aggregate when exposed to the antibiotic ristocetin.

In storage pool disease [17] platelets also adhere poorly. In most instances, the problem is attributable to a reduced level of adenosine diphosphate (ADP) stored in platelet granules, but in some cases the release mechanism is also defective. A reduction in the number of dense bodies, believed to store serotonin, and abnormalities in platelet lipids have also been described [18]. When storage pool disease is associated with albinism it is called the Hermansky-Pudlak syndrome [19,20].

Other rare diseases due to platelet dysfunction are the Bernard-Soulier syndrome [21] and Glanzmann's thrombasthenia [22]. Both disorders are due, in part, to deletions of membrane glycoproteins which are critical to normal platelet function.

The Bernard-Sovlier syndrome is extremely rare. Thrombocytopenia is mild, but purpura may be severe. A routine blood smear reveals the characteristic giant platelets. The platelets are defective in binding coagulation factors, but they do aggregate with ADP.

Glanzmann's thrombasthenia is more common. In this syndrome, platelets fail to adhere or aggregate. They do not react with fibrinogen and appear to have low intrinsic levels of this protein. The membrane abnormalities have been well defined [23]. Since most of the qualitative platelet defects are inherited, a thorough history may be helpful. A prolonged bleeding time or positive tourniquet test in the face of a normal platelet count warrants a workup by an expert.

Disorders associated with white blood cells

Leukocytes include granulocytes (neutrophils, eosinophils, and basophils), mononuclear phagocytes (monocytes and macrophages), and lymphocytes. Leukocytes become in-

volved in all cutaneous and systemic infections; each type of cell may provide a specialized function which depends upon the type of infection and its duration.

Neutrophilia

An increase in the circulating level of neutrophils is commonly seen in acute infections, particularly in generalized bacterial infections due to cocci. Localized bacterial infections such as furuncles, carbuncles, and cellulitis may also elicit this response, as do infections with certain fungi, spirochetes, and parasites. The effect of viruses is variable, but most viruses do not cause neutrophilia. Herpes zoster and varicella may produce either leukopenia or leukocytosis. On occasion the presence of neutrophilia in a viral infection signifies a superimposed bacterial infection.

Skin diseases that often show a prominent leukocytosis are Sweet's syndrome and von Zumbusch pustular psoriasis. Neutrophilia is also caused by systemic steroids, so that it may be difficult to assess leukocytosis in a dermatologic patient who has been receiving corticosteroids chronically.

Neutropenia

Numerous infectious agents and chemicals may cause a decrease in the level of circulating white cells. Infections of dermatologic interest associated with leukopenia are: measles, chickenpox, rubella, rickettsialpox, Rocky Mountain spotted fever, and leishmaniasis. Some drugs, especially antimetabolites, consistently cause leukopenia and granulocytopenia. In general this effect is dose related, although idiosyncratic reactions occur. Some diseases are associated with neutropenia for unknown reasons. These include lupus erythematosus, anaphylactic shock, and cyclic neutropenia. Splenomegaly for any reason may be associated with neutropenia either because neutrophils are sequestered in the organ, or because the spleen exerts a suppressive effect on the bone marrow. Splenectomy may be beneficial.

There are certain rare diseases characterized by neutropenia that frequently exhibit skin manifestations, especially skin infections. These include familial benign chronic neutropenia, the lazy leukocyte syndrome, isoimmune neonatal neutropenia, autoimmune neutropenia, and chronic granulocytopenia of childhood.

Leukocyte dysfunction

Diseases caused by abnormal function of phagocytes are of relatively recent discovery. Theoretically, there are four possible types of defects [24]:

1. Intrinsic defects in the leukocyte causing it to fail to migrate from blood to exudate
2. Normal killing of organisms with defective chemotactic factors
3. Defective killing of organisms due to lysosomal enzyme deficiencies
4. Defective killing of organisms due to other metabolic leukocyte defects

Leukocyte dysfunction causes difficulty in handling infections, and patients with these diseases exhibit skin infections.

Chronic granulomatous disease of childhood (CGD)

Leukocytes of patients with CGD ingest bacteria normally but fail to kill them. The defect in bactericidal function is due to the inability of the cells to generate hydrogen peroxide and free oxygen radicals [25,26]. This implies that some bacteria, for example streptococci, whose killing does not seem to be dependent on this pathway are combated normally. Because the usual mode of inheritance is X-linked, males are most often affected, but females with similar clinical features have been recognized [27]. This subject is well reviewed by Tauber et al [28].

Patients develop infections at multiple sites, including lymph nodes, liver, lung, and bone. Skin lesions initially are purulent and eczematous but gradually become granulomatous as infections smolder. Diagnosis is most readily accomplished by means of the nitrobluetetrazolium (NBT) dye test, in which diseased leukocytes are unable to reduce the colorless NBT dye to blue-black. Treatment should be directed toward combating infections with antibiotics and surgery. Granulocyte transfusions and bone marrow transplantation have been used successfully. Without treatment most patients die in early childhood after a protracted downhill course.

Chédiak-Higashi anomaly

This is an autosomal recessive disorder which is associated with abnormal granulation of neutrophils as well as other granulated cells throughout the body [29]. The granules are many times their normal size and fail to fuse with phagocytic vacuoles, or do so poorly. Clinical manifestations correlate with the type of cell involved. Thus, uneven distribution and function of melanosomes within melanocytes result in light-colored hair and photophobia, whereas the analogous abnormality in leukocytes predisposes patients to multiple infections. Since the granules of platelets are also affected, and since release of platelet granules is necessary for normal function, these patients also suffer bleeding abnormalities. Prognosis is poor. Many affected individuals die in childhood and even those who survive ultimately succumb after a rapid downhill course. There are reports of successful treatment with cyclic GMP, cholinergic agonists [30], and ascorbate [31], but the results have not been long-lived.

Job's syndrome

Job's syndrome was named for its seeming resemblance to the biblical Job, who is thought to have suffered from furunculosis [32].

The first report described two unrelated girls who had recurrent infections, eczematous skin lesions, and fair skin with red hair. The precise nature of the defect is not known, but defective chemotaxis and increased levels of IgE have been demonstrated in several laboratories [33]. Leukocyte function is otherwise normal [34].

Disorders associated with red blood cells

Anemia

Pallor, which is generally thought to be the classic cutaneous sign of anemia, is actually not reliable. It may be masked by a ruddy complexion, dermatitis, or telangiectasia from solar damage. Better indicators are the mucous membranes (especially conjunctivae), nail beds, and palmar creases. The pallor of anemia results both from reduction in the mass of hemoglobin and shunting of blood from superficial vessels to the vital organs.

Chronic anemia also disturbs epithelial structures: there is loss of the normal skin elasticity and tone, sparseness and thinning of the hair, fragility and ridging of the nails, and hyperpigmentation. The skin may become dry and wrinkled. In pernicious anemia and iron-deficiency anemia in particular there may be mucosal changes.

Anemia may be associated with several dermatologic diseases, although mostly it is an incidental finding. Anemia, as a consequence of cutaneous disease, may be observed in psoriasis, because of chronic skin loss of iron and folate, and in dermatitis herpetiformis. In scleroderma there is a 25 percent incidence of anemia attributable to chronic inflammatory disease, bleeding mucosal telangiectases, intestinal malabsorption, and microangiopathic hemolysis [35].

Iron-deficiency anemia

This is by far the most common cause of anemia. In adults it is almost always due to chronic blood loss, rarely to malnutrition. It is important to note that a state of iron deficiency may exist without obvious anemia, that is, in the presence of a normal hematocrit. Suspected cases of iron deficiency may require not only blood counts, but also bone marrow aspiration, serum ferritin, serum iron, and total iron binding capacity determinations to assess iron storage. In cases of doubt a Prussian blue stain of the bone marrow will be diagnostic. Mucosal changes in iron-deficient states are common—sore tongue, absence of filiform papillae, and lesser degrees of papillary atrophy occur in 39 percent of cases [36]. The nail content of iron has been shown to correlate well with total iron stores [37]. Flattening or spooning of the nails is seen in 28 percent of cases. Nail changes such as fragility and ridging may be present but are nonspecific since they also result from trauma or advancing age. In infancy spooning of nails correlates very well with iron-deficiency anemia [38] but is less reliable in adults, since it may be the result of chronic exposure to caustics.

Fanconi's anemia

Fanconi's anemia, also known as congenital pancytopenia, is a recessively inherited condition whose salient features are pancytopenia, skeletal abnormalities, chromosomal instability, and increased risk of malignancy. Numerous associated congenital defects have been reported, and the clinical course is highly variable.

The most frequent skin manifestation is a disturbance in pigmentation. The overall impression is one of mottling, with hypopigmented macules interspersed within hyperpigmented patches [39]. There are two patterns, the first of which has a predilection for sun-exposed areas. Histologically, it is characterized by atypical keratinocytes. The other type is more diffuse and is accentuated in the body folds, especially the perineum [40].

Fanconi's anemia may be confused with dyskeratosis congenita, which also has a variable clinical picture, pigmentary changes, pancytopenia, and an increased risk of malignancy. Dyskeratosis congenita is also usually X-linked, although it has been described in one family as autosomal dominant [41]. In contradistinction to Fanconi's anemia, however, patients with dyskeratosis congenita have poikiloderma, hair and nail abnormalities (hypotrichosis and nail hypoplasia), and mucosal changes (leukoplakia, erosions, and atrophic papillae) [38]. Nonetheless there are certain transitional cases which seem to defy accurate classification, probably because of genetic heterogeneity.

Polycythemia

Polycythemia rubra vera is a neoplastic myeloproliferative disease which involves erythrocytes, leukocytes, and platelets. Facial plethora is common and other cutaneous findings include ecchymoses and pruritus in 15 percent of patients [42]. Pruritus is seen particularly after a bath or shower, is often sudden in onset and may be of limited duration, suggesting that it is due to the activation or release of a humoral factor triggered by a decrease in body temperature [43]. Since the disease is almost always associated with peripheral basophilia and increased mast cells in the marrow, pruritus has been attributed to the release of histamine by these cells. Urticaria [44] may also be present, and may be due to the same pathologic mechanism. Purpura is sometimes seen [45] along with easy bruisability and is due either to the distended vasculature or to intrinsic platelet dysfunction. Cholestyramine [46] and aspirin [43] have been used to relieve pruritus.

An *absolute* increase in the mass of red blood corpuscles in the presence of normal oxygen saturation is virtually diagnostic. Individuals who live at high altitudes or patients with cardiac or pulmonary disease may have an expanded red cell mass in the face of hypoxemia.

Hemolytic anemias

In hemolytic anemia the lifespan of the red blood cell is shortened; defects may be genetic or acquired, intrinsic or extrinsic to the erythrocyte. Jaundice is frequent. The most common congenital hemolytic anemia and the one with the highest incidence of associated skin abnormalities is sickle cell anemia. The sickling tendency is due to HbS, an inherited molecular variant of hemoglobin, which, when deoxygenated, forms tactoids which distort the red cell into a rigid crescent. Normal blood flow depends upon the red cell's pliable biconcave disc shape which is capable of negotiating small vessels. Sickled red cells occlude vessels and cause local hypoxia. The process of sickling is usually reversible, but if prolonged it can become permanent.

Leg ulcers are extremely common in sickle cell disease, occurring in up to 75 percent of patients who live in tropical areas [47]. They are often bilateral and may be multiple, healing slowly and often recurring. Bed rest, avoidance of trauma, attention to infection, and gentle debridement with hydrogen peroxide are useful in treatment. Transfusions will hasten healing, and there are reports of oral zinc being of help [48]. Skin grafts have been used in refractory cases.

The hand-foot syndrome is a form of sickle cell crisis which occurs in children. Attacks lasting one to two weeks consist of exquisitely painful, swollen distal extremities,

sometimes associated with fever and leukocytosis. Bone necrosis can result [49]. Other cutaneous signs of sickle cell anemia include pruritus [50], alopecia, and tattoos [51]. The tattoos or keloidal scarifications are seen in Africa, being designed specifically by medicine men for sufferers of sickle cell disease. Many otherwise primitive tribes have made accurate observations on sickle cell disease for centuries.

Leg ulcers are seen also in other hemolytic anemias, such as thalassemia [52,53] and congenital spherocytosis [54].

The hemolytic anemia caused by deficiency of glucose 6-phosphate-dehydrogenase (G6PD) is of particular importance to dermatologists because of the frequent use of dapsone in treating diseases of the skin. Dapsone is one of a number of drugs that interfere with the ability of red blood cells to regenerate reduced glutathione, a process mediated by G6PD. G6PD is an enzyme with more than 100 genetic variants, not all of which are functional. Normally, patients with low levels of functional G6PD do not exhibit hemolysis except when their red cells are stressed with oxidizing agents, such as dapsone. Among drugs that have been implicated in precipitating hemolysis are sulfonamides, sulfones, nitrofurans, antipyretics, and analgesics. The list is too long for enumeration here. There are conflicting reports regarding the ability of various sulfonamide drugs to produce this phenomenon [55–57].

Oxidizing drugs such as dapsone may also produce a complication known as methemoglobinemia. Methemoglobin is a form of hemoglobin in which ferrous ions have been oxidized to the ferrous state; it is nonfunctional, being unable to carry either oxygen or carbon dioxide. Cyanosis results when the level of methemoglobin reaches 1.5 g/dL but is reversible upon administration of suitable reducing agents such as methylene blue or ascorbic acid. Some patients are extremely sensitive to the development of methemoglobin, which may be due to defects in the level of NADH-methemoglobin reductase. Other drugs and chemicals are also liable to cause methemoglobinemia, such as aniline dyes, aniline derivatives (such as acetanilid and phenacetin), sulfonamides, nitrates, and nitrites (such as amyl nitrite and nitroglycerin).

Sulfhemoglobin is another nonfunctional type of hemoglobin that may be formed by any of these drugs. This condition is similar to methemoglobinemia except that sulfhemoglobin is an *irreversible* derivative and the threshold for cyanosis is less (0.5 g/dL). Spectroscopic analyses can distinguish among these hemoglobin derivatives. HbM can also be identified on electrophoresis under appropriate conditions.

Pernicious anemia

Classically, pernicious anemia is marked by weakness, sore tongue, and numbness and tingling of the extremities. In addition to glossitis there may be generalized stomatitis and atrophy of the filiform papillae. The skin may be dry and inelastic or velvety and smooth; it often has a lemon-yellow tint. Diffuse or blotchy hyperpigmentation may be seen in both whites [58] and blacks [59]. Patients tend to have fair skin and light-colored hair because pernicious anemia is found with greater frequency in persons of northern European extraction; southern Europeans, blacks, and

Orientals are affected less often. There is a high incidence of prematurely gray hair and light blue or gray eyes [60]. Pernicious anemia is associated with a very high incidence of autoantibodies directed against parietal cells, thyroid cells, and intrinsic factor. It is of interest that pernicious anemia is often associated with other autoimmune diseases, such as autoimmune thyroiditis, hypoparathyroidism, and Addison's disease [61]. A greater than chance association with vitiligo has also been found, with incidences as high as 10.6 percent [62].

Patients with pernicious anemia have a megaloblastosis which shares features with folic acid deficiency. Folic acid deficiency may show widespread mucosal changes similar to those of pernicious anemia. Neurologic manifestations, however, are absent, and patients are apt to appear wasted; in contradistinction, those with pernicious anemia usually appear flabby. Folic acid deficiency may be due to gastrectomy, intestinal malabsorption, intestinal parasites, malnutrition, cirrhosis, alcoholism, or pregnancy.

Acquired hemolytic anemias

Most acquired hemolytic anemias are immunologic, the antibodies being directed either against an intrinsic red cell antigen or one that is attached to its surface [63]. Antibodies may be formed as a result of sensitization with isoantigens, as is the case in transfusion reactions and pregnancy, or may be induced by foreign agents such as drugs (penicillin, alpha methyl dopa) and microorganisms. In most cases, however, these anemias are idiopathic, and more is known about the mechanisms of red cell destruction than about the origin of the antigenic stimulus.

Antibodies are frequently divided into "warm" and "cold" types. Warm antibodies are those reactive at normal body temperature and are usually of the IgG (sometimes IgA) class. Connective tissue diseases and lymphoproliferative states are often associated with idiopathic autoimmune hemolytic anemias of this type. Cold antibodies react only at low temperatures (below 32°C), are usually of the IgM class, and react with the I antigen of red cells.

The cold agglutinin syndrome is of this type. It is mostly a disease of the elderly and often accompanies occult malignancies. Clinically, there is acrocyanosis with painful, suffused swellings of the nose, ears, and distal extremities because of the cooler temperatures at these sites. If the condition is chronic, trophic changes of the extremities and even gangrene may develop. Such severe alterations, however, are more likely to occur in the presence of cryoglobulins. Acrocyanosis is due both to agglutination and to hemolysis. In younger individuals hemolytic anemia caused by cold agglutinins is seen in *Mycoplasma* pneumonia, infectious mononucleosis, and lymphomas.

Mycoplasma pneumoniae pneumonia is by far the most common cause of cold agglutinin disease. A few patients with infectious mononucleosis have also been described. The antibodies, which are usually of the IgM class, have specificity for the I-i antigens of red cells. They fix complement and can be shown to lyse red cells in vitro. The syndrome is usually self-limited and subsides within a few weeks. The idiopathic form of cold agglutinin disease is chronic. It occurs mostly in the elderly and is associated with malignancies. In this case the antibodies are usually monoclonal.

Paroxysmal cold hemoglobinuria is caused by the Donath-Landsteiner antibody, a 7S IgG which binds to the red cell in the cold, fixes complement, and acts as a powerful hemolysin subsequent to warming. Although this antibody is found primarily in association with syphilis, it is also seen in viral infections such as measles and mumps. Skin manifestations of this disease are absent; the symptoms include hemoglobinemia, hemoglobinuria, fever, chills, malaise, and muscle pains.

Cold agglutinin disease must be distinguished from cryoglobulinemia; both disorders may have the same skin manifestations upon exposure to low temperatures. Signs of cryoglobulinemia include Raynaud's phenomenon, acrocyanosis, malleolar leg ulcers (which occur in about 30 percent of cases), livedo reticularis, cold urticaria, and purpura. These are due to the intravascular precipitation of cryoglobulins. Although this syndrome is most commonly related to the M-component in patients with multiple myeloma, the so-called mixed cryoglobulinemias are seen in immune complex disease of disparate etiologies, such as rheumatoid arthritis and viral hepatitis.

References

1. Campbell AN et al: Autoerythrocyte sensitization. *J Pediatr* **103**:157, 1983
2. Nelson CT: Autoerythrocyte sensitization. *Arch Dermatol* **103**:549, 1971
3. Gardner FH, Diamond LK: Auto-erythrocyte sensitization: a form of purpura producing painful bruising following autosensitization to red blood cells in certain women. *Blood* **10**:675, 1955
4. Ratnoff OD: The psychogenic purpuras: a review of auto-erythrocyte sensitization, autosensitization to DNA, hysterical and factitial bleeding and religious stigmata. *Semin Hematol* **17**:192, 1980
5. Baldini MG: Platelet defect in Wiskott-Aldrich syndrome. *N Engl J Med* **281**:107, 1969
6. Blaese RM et al: Immunodeficiency in the Wiskott-Aldrich syndrome. *Birth Defects* **11**:250, 1975
7. Zucker-Franklin D, Karpatkin S: Red cell and platelet fragmentation in idiopathic autoimmune thrombocytopenic purpura. *N Engl J Med* **297**:517, 1977
8. Evans RS et al: Primary thrombocytopenic purpura and acquired hemolytic anemia. *Arch Intern Med* **87**:48, 1951
9. Shulman NR: Immunoreaction involving platelets. IV. Studies on the pathogenesis of thrombocytopenia in drug purpura using test doses of quinidine in sensitized individuals; their implication in idiopathic thrombocytopenic purpura. *J Exp Med* **107**:711, 1958
10. Miescher PA: Drug induced thrombocytopenic purpura. *Semin Hematol* **10**:311, 1973
11. Corrigan JJ Jr: Disseminated intravascular coagulopathy. *Pediatrics* **64**:37, 1979
12. Bell WR: Disseminated intravascular coagulation. *Johns Hopkins Med J* **146**:289, 1980
13. Esterly NB: Kasabach-Merritt syndrome in infants. *J Am Acad Dermatol* **8**:504, 1983
14. Moschowitz E: An acute febrile pleiochromic anemia with hyaline thrombosis of terminal arterioles and capillaries—an undescribed disease. *Arch Intern Med* **36**:89, 1925
15. Casala LA: Thrombotic thrombocytopenic purpura. Report of a case and review of 157 cases. *Hawaii Med J* **25**:93, 1965
16. Amorosi EL, Ultman JE: Thrombotic thrombocytopenic purpura. *Medicine (Baltimore)* **45**:139, 1966
17. Holmsen H, Weiss HJ: Hereditary defect in the platelet re-

lease reaction caused by a deficiency in the storage pool of platelet adenine nucleotides. *Br J Haematol* **19:**643, 1970

18. Weiss HJ et al: Heterogeneity in storage pool deficiency. Studies on granule-bound substances in 18 patients including variants deficient in α-granule, platelet factor 4, β-thromboglobulin, and platelet-derived growth factor. *Blood* **54:**1296, 1979

19. Hermansky F, Pudlak P: Albinism associated with hemorrhagic diathesis and unusual pigmented reticular cells in the bone marrow. *Blood* **14:**162, 1959

20. Logan LJ et al: Albinism and abnormal platelet function. *N Engl J Med* **284:**1340, 1971

21. Jamieson GA et al: Platelet membrane glycoproteins in thrombasthenia, Bernard-Soulier syndrome and storage pool disease. *J Lab Clin Med* **93:**652, 1979

22. Hardisty RM et al: Thrombasthenia. *Br J Haematol* **10:**371, 1964

23. Phillips DR, Agin PP: Platelet membrane defects in Glanzmann's thrombasthenia. *J Clin Invest* **60:**535, 1977

24. Douglas SW, Adamson JW: The anemia of chronic disorders: studies of marrow regulation and iron metabolism. *Blood* **45:**55, 1975

25. Bridges RA et al: A fatal granulomatous disease of childhood: the clinical, pathological and laboratory features of a new syndrome. *Am J Dis Child* **97:**387, 1957

26. Douglas SD et al: Granulocytopathies: pleomorphism of neutrophil dysfunction. *Am J Med* **46:**901, 1969

27. Holmes B et al: Chronic granulomatous disease in females. *N Engl J Med* **283:**217, 1970

28. Tauber AI et al: Chronic granulomatous disease: a syndrome of phagocyte oxidase deficiencies. *Medicine (Baltimore)* **62:**286, 1983

29. Blume RS, Wolff SM: The Chédiak-Higashi syndrome: studies in four patients and a review of the literature. *Medicine (Baltimore)* **51:**247, 1972

30. Oliver JM: Impaired microtubule correctable by cyclic GMP and cholinergic agonists in the Chédiak-Higashi syndrome. *Am J Pathol* **85:**395, 1976

31. Boxer LA: Correction of leukocyte function in Chédiak-Higashi syndrome by ascorbate. *N Engl J Med* **295:**1041, 1976

32. Donabedian H, Gallin JI: The hyperimmunoglobin E recurrent infection (Job's) syndrome. *Medicine (Baltimore)* **62:**195, 1983

33. Hill HR et al: Defect in neutrophil granulocyte chemotaxis in Job's syndrome of recurrent "cold" staphylococcal abscesses. *Lancet* **2:**617, 1974

34. Schopfer K et al: Staphylococcal IgE antibodies, hyperimmunoglobulinemia E and *Staphylococcus aureus* infections. *N Engl J Med* **300:**835, 1979

35. Frayha RA et al: Hematological abnormalities in scleroderma. A study of 180 cases. *Acta Haematol* **64:**25, 1980

36. Beveridge BR: Hypochromic anemia. *Q J Med* **34:**145, 1965

37. Sobolewski S et al: Human nails and body iron. *J Clin Pathol* **31:**1068, 1978

38. Hogan GW, Jones B: The relationship of koilonychia and iron deficiency in infants. *J Pediatr* **77:**1054, 1970

39. Steier W et al: Dyskeratosis congenita: relationship to Fanconi's anemia. *Blood* **39:**510, 1972

40. Johansson E et al: Fanconi's anemia. Tumor-like warts, hyperpigmentation associated with deranged keratinocytes, and depressed cell-mediated immunity. *Arch Dermatol* **118:**249, 1982

41. Tchou PK, Kohn T: Dyskeratosis congenita: an autosomal dominant disorder. *J Am Acad Dermatol* **6:**1034, 1982

42. Winklemann RK, Muller SA: Pruritus. *Annu Rev Med* **15:**53, 1964

43. Fjellner B, Hagermark O: Pruritus in polycythemia vera: treatment with aspirin and possibility of platelet involvement. *Acta Derm Venereol (Stockh)* **59:**505, 1979

44. Small P, Lerman S: Hyperthyroidism and polycythemia vera with chronic urticaria and angioedema. *Ann Allergy* **46:**256, 1981

45. Redding KG: Thrombocythemia as a cause of erytermalgia. *Arch Dermatol* **113:**468, 1977

46. Chanarin I, Szur L: Relief of intractable pruritus in polycythemia rubra vera with cholestyramine. *Br J Haematol* **29:**669, 1975

47. Serjeant GR: Leg ulceration in sickle cell anemia. *Arch Intern Med* **133:**690, 1974

48. Serjeant GR et al: Oral zinc sulfate in sickle cell ulcers. *Lancet* **2:**891, 1970

49. Karayalcin G: Sickle cell anemia—clinical manifestations in 100 patients and review of the literature. *Am J Med Sci* **269:**51, 1975

50. Wilkin JK: Pruritus in sickle cell disease: response to cholestyramine. *J Natl Med Assoc* **69:**325, 1977

51. Konotey-Ahulu FID: The sickle cell diseases. Clinical manifestations of sickle cell diseases including "the sickle cell crisis." *Arch Intern Med* **133:**611, 1974

52. Samitz MH et al: Leg ulcers in Mediterranean anaemia. *Arch Dermatol* **90:**567, 1964

53. Kinatender J: Leg ulcers in beta-thalassemia (Ulcus cruris bei Beta-Thalassamie). *Hautarzt* **31:**273, 1980

54. Beinhauer LG, Gruhn JG: Dermatologic aspects of congenital spherocytic anemia. *Arch Dermatol* **75:**642, 1957

55. Allen SD, Wilkerson JL: The importance of glucose-6-phosphate dehydrogenase screening in a urologic practice. *J Urol* **107:**304, 1972

56. Seeler RA et al: Adriamycin and trimethoprim-sulfamethoxazole in G6PD deficiency: absence of hemolysis in two cases. *Am J Pediatr Hematol Oncol* **2:**187, 1980

57. Beutler E: *Hemolytic Anemia in Disorders of Red Cell Metabolism.* New York, Plenum Press, 1978

58. Baker SJ et al: Hyperpigmentation of the skin. A sign of vitamin B12 deficiency. *Br Med J* **1:**1713, 1963

59. Ogbuawa O et al: Hyperpigmentation of pernicious anemia in blacks. *Arch Intern Med* **138:**388, 1978

60. Callender ST et al: Blood groups and other inherited characters in pernicious anemia. *Br J Haematol* **3:**107, 1957

61. Chanarin I: *The Megaloblastic Anemias.* Philadelphia, FA Davis, 1969

62. Howitz J, Schwartz M: Vitiligo, achlorhydria and pernicious anemia. *Lancet* **1:**1331, 1971

63. Garratty G, Petz T: *Acquired Immune Hemolytic Anemias.* New York, Churchill Livingston, 1980

CHAPTER 165

CUTANEOUS ASPECTS OF INTERNAL MALIGNANT DISEASE

David I. McLean and Harley A. Haynes

An internal malignant neoplasm may have external manifestations in the skin. Recognition of these cutaneous signs may lead to the diagnosis of a previously unknown malignancy. Often these manifestations are rather nonspecific, and many can be quite subtle. Hypertrichosis lanuginosa acquisita can be a marker for many different malignant neoplasms. Some are quite specific, such as necrolytic migratory erythema for a glucagon-producing tumor of the pancreas. The most specific cutaneous signs, of course, are metastatic deposits from the internal malignancy.

An attempt has been made to classify these manifestations (Table 165-1). Unfortunately our lack of knowledge does not allow us to classify these alterations by a pathophysiologic approach in all cases. Indeed, there is a very large group where the biochemical or immunologic relationship to the neoplasia is not yet understood. Groupings of these signs have been made according to the major clinical manifestations, for example, bullous disorders.

A second problem relates to proving an association of a cutaneous eruption with a tumor. This is not difficult where the supposed manifestation is very rare and the tumor is also very uncommon. It becomes a major problem where the manifestation is very common, such as seborrheic keratoses in the sign of Leser-Trelat, and the presumed association is with a wide spectrum of commonly occurring neoplasms. In this situation the literature becomes replete with anecdotal reports, which may or may not be a true indication of an association with the malignant neoplasm.

Color changes secondary to the deposition of substances in the skin

Icterus (see also Chap. 167)

Icterus as a manifestation of internal malignancy is generally a late sign. It is usually secondary to obstruction of the bile duct or gross intrahepatic obstruction. Extrahepatic obstruction can be secondary to malignant disease of the gallbladder, pancreas, bile duct, or adjacent bowel.

Icterus must be distinguished from other causes of yellow skin such as carotenemia and lycopenemia. Carotenemia, which can produce a carotenoderma, differs from icterus in that it is often uneven in its coloration. It is usually darkest in areas of hyperkeratotic skin such as the palms and soles. Deposition is also quite prominent on the face. The sclerae are not stained by carotene. Lycopenemia also produces a yellow color. This yellow color is also produced by carotenoids, but these are generally derived from tomatoes and tomato juice.

Melanosis (see also Chap. 79)

Melanosis is a condition caused by the abnormal deposition of melanin pigments in tissue. It is manifested clinically by a gray-brown pigmentation of the skin, but the pigment can be deposited in most of the organs of the body. Darkening of the skin due to hormonal stimulation of melanocytes may be seen with adrenal insufficiency, either primary or secondary to infiltration of the glands by a malignancy, or be seen with tumors that are themselves ACTH-producing [1,2]. Adrenal insufficiency is associated with an elevation in α-MSH and ACTH, which has a terminal amino acid sequence similar to α-MSH.

Diffuse melanosis can also be secondary to pigment deposition by malignant melanoma. The pigment of the skin has been attributed to free melanin [3] and to the presence of single-cell metastases from the primary melanoma [4–6]. Diffuse micrometastases can also appear in the nail matrix, leading to pigment streaks in the nail plate [7]. Patients with melanosis may also have increased melanogenesis, possibly secondary to circulating tyrosinase [5,8]. Circulating tumor cells have been found in patients with melanosis [9]. Melanuria is frequently associated with melanosis of the skin. Urine from patients who have melanuria is usually not black when voided, but gradually darkens to a deep brown and later a black color when exposed to the air for several hours [4]. The intermediary metabolites of tyrosine are oxidized spontaneously to melanin.

Andreev and Petkov have noted a melasma-like hyperpigmentation on the face in five patients with "brain tumors" [10]. In three patients the hyperpigmentation resolved after the surgical removal of the tumor.

A diffuse gray-brown pigmentation of the skin can also be produced by hemochromatosis.

Hemochromatosis

Hemochromatosis is an iron-storage disorder resulting predominantly from increased iron absorption from the gut. There is deposition of iron in the form of hemosiderin in many tissues. A third of untreated patients will develop hepatocellular carcinoma [11]. The pigment seen in hemochromatosis does not appear to be the increased tissue iron, but rather the increased melanin produced in these patients. Vitiligo in a patient with hemochromatosis causes

Table 165-1 Classification of cutaneous signs of internal malignancy

I. Lesions secondary to the deposition of substances in the skin
   A. Icterus
   B. Melanosis
   C. Hemochromatosis
   D. Xanthomas
   E. Systemic amyloidosis
II. Vascular and blood abnormalities
   A. Flushing
   B. Palmar erythema
   C. Telangiectasia
   D. Purpura
   E. Vasculitis
   F. Cutaneous ischemia
   G. Thrombophlebitis
III. Bullous disorders
   A. Bullous pemphigoid
   B. Pemphigus vulgaris
   C. Dermatitis herpetiformis
   D. Herpes gestationis
   E. Erythema multiforme
   F. Epidermolysis bullosa acquisita
IV. Infections and infestations
   A. Herpes zoster
   B. Herpes simplex
   C. Bacterial infections
   D. Fungi and yeast infections
   E. Scabies
V. Disorders of keratinization
   A. Acanthosis nigricans
   B. Acquired ichthyosis
   C. Palmar hyperkeratosis
   D. Erythroderma
   E. Paraneoplastic acrokeratosis of Bazex
VI. Collagen-vascular disease
   A. Dermatomyositis
   B. Lupus erythematosus
   C. Progressive systemic sclerosis
VII. Skin tumors and internal malignant disease
   A. Muir-Torre syndrome
   B. Gardner's syndrome
   C. Cowden's disease
   D. Mucosal neuroma syndrome
   E. Neurofibromatosis
VIII. Hormone-related conditions
IX. Disorders associated with primary skin cancer
   A. Nevoid basal cell carcinoma syndrome
   B. Arsenical manifestations
X. Various disorders associated with internal malignant disease
   A. Pruritus
   B. Erythema gyratum repens
   C. Subcutaneous fat necrosis
   D. Sweet's syndrome
   E. Hypertrichosis lanuginosa acquisita
   F. Necrolytic migratory erythema
   G. Clubbing
   H. Leukoderma
   I. Peutz-Jeghers syndrome
   J. Tuberous sclerosis
   K. Wiskott-Aldrich syndrome
   L. Multiple eruptive seborrheic keratoses
   M. Porphyria cutanea tarda
XI. Direct tumor involvement in the skin

a complete loss of pigment, indicating that the iron per se is a negligible contributory factor in the skin color [12].

Xanthomas (see also Chap. 145)

The predominant type of xanthoma associated with internal malignant disease is the plane xanthoma. The most common association of diffuse plane xanthoma is with multiple myeloma. Patients have been described with xanthomas and multiple myelomas of many types, including IgG L Type [13,14], IgG K Type [15], and IgA Type multiple myeloma [16]. Xanthomas, as well as atypical eruptive histiocytosis with lipid deposition, have also been associated with myelocytic leukemia, myelomonocytic leukemia, leukemic lymphocytic reticuloendotheliosis, and diffuse histiocytic lymphoma [17–21]. Juvenile xanthogranuloma can be associated with juvenile chronic myeloid leukemia [22] but such an association must be very rare.

Patients with xanthomas may be normolipemic, or they may have a hyperlipoproteinemia. Type 2A hyperlipoproteinemia has been described in association with IgG Type L myeloma [13], as have Type 4 and Type 5 hyperlipoproteinemia [14]. Type 3 (broad beta) and pre-beta hyperlipoproteinemia have been described in association with IgA myeloma [16].

Purpura may be a feature of diffuse plane xanthomas associated with malignant disease. Pinch purpura has been noted within xanthomatous plaques in a normolipemic patient with myeloma [23].

Hemorrhagic bullae have been associated with xanthoma disseminatum and IgG K Type multiple myeloma [24]; this patient was normolipemic. Xanthoma disseminatum should be carefully distinguished from diffuse plane xanthomas.

Systemic amyloidosis (see also Chap. 142)

Systemic amyloidosis of both the primary type and that associated with multiple myeloma commonly have skin lesions. It is important to differentiate skin lesions of systemic amyloidosis from the far more commonly seen purely cutaneous variants of amyloidosis. The typical lesions of systemic amyloidosis consist of raised waxy papules and plaques commonly involving eyelids, eyebrows, and paranasal skin, as well as lesions which can be diffusely present over the body surface. Purpura is generally seen mixed with these waxy papules. The purpura can be within the papules, or large ecchymotic patches can be seen on clinically normal-appearing skin. The purpura in these patients is presumably secondary to amyloid deposition in the walls of dermal blood vessels, leading to increased fragility. The purpura occurs secondary to very minor trauma of these vessels. Other changes include alopecia, macroglossia, and pallor [25]. All patients with skin lesions of systemic amyloidosis should be thoroughly investigated for multiple myeloma.

Intradermal bullae have been associated with myeloma-related amyloidosis [26]. These bullae were probably the result of extensive dermal infiltration with amyloid, resulting in cleavage of the uppermost dermis from the lower dermis.

Although macular amyloidosis, a form of amyloidosis

most commonly seen limited to the skin of the upper trunk and characterized by pruritic macular pigmented patches, generally has no association with internal malignant disease, it has been reported in a patient with myelofibrosis and myeloid metaplasia [27].

Vascular and blood abnormalities

Flushing (see also Chap. 163)

Acquired pronounced flushing, usually of the central face and upper trunk, may be a manifestation of carcinoid syndrome, caused by carcinoid tumors [28]. These tumors may arise from bronchus, stomach, pancreas, and thyroid, and less often from teratomas. Metastatic tumors from the small bowel are most likely to produce flushing. Flushing, often immediately after food intake, can be produced by a carcinoid tumor of the stomach. Bronchial carcinoid can produce a particularly prolonged flushing and can be associated with periorbital edema.

When fading, the flushing of carcinoid syndrome can become gyrate. After many episodes, telangiectasia and chronic diffuse erythema can develop. Uncommonly, skin sclerosis can occur. A pellagra-like dermatosis, secondary to tryptophan diversion from niacin to serotonin production, can also occur.

The flushing of carcinoid syndrome is secondary to the release of vasoactive substances from the tumor.

Palmar erythema (see also Chap. 167)

Palmar erythema can be associated with advanced liver failure. Such liver failure may be secondary to either primary or metastatic tumor in the liver. The palmar erythema in these patients can possibly be secondary to decreased estrogen metabolism or to a high-output cardiac state [29].

Telangiectasia

Localized, grouped telangiectatic vessels on the anterior chest wall may be a marker for breast cancer [30]. There is often a clinically palpable, indurated, warm, subcutaneous plaque immediately beneath the telangiectatic area. Telangiectatic vessels may also be the first evidence of distant subcutaneous metastases of breast cancer, as well as other malignant tumors.

Generalized telangiectasia can be a presenting factor of malignant angioendotheliomatosis. Biopsy of the telangiectatic vessels will show malignant endothelial cells to be present within them, in contrast to normal cells seen in the telangiectatic vessels associated with breast cancer, and other non-blood-vessel tumors [31].

Progressive telangiectases have been associated with carcinoid tumors (see above), and with adenocarcinoma of the hepatic bile duct [32].

Telangiectasia may also be a manifestation of a genodermatosis, which in turn can be associated with systemic malignant disease such as lymphoma. These genodermatoses include ataxia-telangiectasia, Bloom's syndrome, and xeroderma pigmentosum and its variant, the De Sanctis-Cacchione syndrome. Ultraviolet radiation sensitivity

would appear to be the cause of the telangiectasia in all but the ataxia-telangiectasia.

Purpura (see also Chap. 164)

Lymphoma is the most common cause of idiopathic thrombocytopenic purpura (ITP) associated with malignant disease. Hodgkin's disease is the most common associated lymphoma, and the diagnosis of ITP may precede other evidence of lymphoma.

Disseminated intravascular coagulation (DIC) as a cause of purpura in malignant disease is most commonly associated with acute lymphocytic or myelomonocytic leukemia, in particular T-cell acute lymphocytic leukemia [33]. Many patients may not have full-blown DIC, but only biochemical or mild clinical manifestations of the process.

Purpura can also be associated with the hyperglobulinemia seen in multiple myeloma or lymphoma. In purpura secondary to cryoglobulins, lesions are often found in acral areas, and may be associated with Raynaud's phenomenon. Benign hyperglobulinemic purpura can be associated with Sjögren's syndrome, which in turn can be associated with malignant disease [34].

Purpura is also seen secondary to thrombocytopenia due to bone marrow infiltration by leukemia or carcinoma.

Vasculitis (see also Chap. 107)

Leukocytoclastic vasculitis, such as can be seen in Henoch-Schönlein purpura, can be associated with malignant neoplasms. The vasculitis seen in patients with malignant neoplasms does not differ clinically from that which occurs much more commonly secondary to non-neoplastic causes. It can be a presenting sign in squamous cell carcinoma, particularly of the bronchus [35–37]. Leukocytoclastic vasculitis can also be associated with malignant lymphoma [38,39].

A periarteritis nodosum-like syndrome has been reported in association with hairy cell leukemia, acute lymphocytic leukemia, and multiple myeloma [40–43].

Cutaneous ischemia (see also Chap. 171)

Evidence of compromised peripheral circulation can be a marker for many malignant neoplasms. It is frequently manifested by evidence of digital ischemia either as Raynaud's phenomenon or frank gangrene. Peripheral ischemia has been associated with many malignant neoplasms including carcinoma of the pancreas, stomach, small bowel, ovary, and kidney, as well as lymphoma and leukemia [44–46]. There may be associated splinter hemorrhages of the nail bed, suggestive of an underlying vasculitic process. The etiology, however, is rarely apparent. The peripheral cutaneous ischemia of polycythemia rubra vera appears to be secondary to the increased viscosity of the peripheral circulation associated with this disease [47,48]. The increased viscosity may lead to frank venous thrombosis.

Similarly, the ischemia seen in cryoglobulinemia appears to be secondary to increased blood viscosity. Cryoglobulinemia may be associated with multiple myeloma, or with lymphoma [49].

Thrombophlebitis (see also Chap. 171)

Isolated vein thrombophlebitis is not commonly associated with internal malignant disease. Multiple-lesion "migratory" superficial thrombophlebitis is much more often seen in association with cancer, and when this syndrome is present, the patient should be examined carefully for occult malignant disease. The association of peripheral thrombophlebitis (phlebothrombosis) with gastric carcinoma was noted by Trousseau in the nineteenth century. Migratory superficial thrombophlebitis as a marker for cancer has been confirmed, and the association has been extended to include tumors of the pancreas, prostate, lung, liver, bowel, gallbladder, and ovary, as well as lymphoma and leukemia. The migratory nature of the thrombophlebitis probably relates to a generalized hypercoagulable state.

Mondor's disease is thrombophlebitis of the anterior chest wall presenting as a tender or nontender cord. Usually benign, it may be associated with breast cancer [50].

Bullous disorders

Bullous pemphigoid

There is probably no significantly increased risk of malignant tumor in patients with bullous pemphigoid [51]. However. isolated patient reports have shown that some patients with bullous pemphigoid clear when a concomitant tumor is treated, indicating a possible causal relationship in the rare patient [52,53]. In a patient with bullous pemphigoid and chronic lymphocytic leukemia, studies have failed to show the production of specific antibody by the neoplastic lymphocytes [54].

It has not yet been shown that the immunosuppressive treatment of bullous pemphigoid has led to any increased risk of neoplasia.

Pemphigus vulgaris

Pemphigus vulgaris can be associated with Hodgkin's disease [55], in which case the two diseases can run a parallel course [56]. A patient with lymphoma and pemphigus vulgaris had a high titer of pemphigus antibody in a tumor homogenate [57]. Pemphigus vulgaris has also been associated with Kaposi's sarcoma [58,59].

The relationship of solid tumors to pemphigus vulgaris is less well defined. Pemphigus vulgaris has been reported in association with many solid tumors, but these have been small series or isolated case reports. It has not been possible from these studies to decide whether there is a greater than expected incidence of pemphigus in these patients.

There is a well-defined association of pemphigus vulgaris with thymoma, with or without clinical myasthenia gravis [60–63]. Pemphigus foliaceus has also been reported in association with thymoma and myasthenia gravis [64].

Pemphigus erythematosus may be associated with bronchial carcinoma [65].

Dermatitis herpetiformis (see also Chap. 60)

Dermatitis herpetiformis is associated with intestinal lymphoma [66–71]. It is associated with gluten sensitivity, and the presumed etiology of the lymphoma is the resulting chronic antigenic stimulation. The lymphoma, when it occurs, is usually a diffuse histiocytic lymphoma [67,72].

Many solid tumors have also been described in association with dermatitis herpetiformis, but the reports have been isolated cases or small series. There is no indication that there is a greater than expected number of patients with dermatitis herpetiformis developing tumors other than intestinal lymphoma.

Herpes gestationis (see also Chap. 58)

Herpes gestationis has been described in association with hydatidiform mole [73,74]. Hydatidiform mole can evolve into choriocarcinoma.

Erythema multiforme

Erythema multiforme is not a specific marker for any internal neoplasm. It has been reported in association with many tumors, but few studies have shown an incidence of erythema multiforme to be higher than expected. Erythema multiforme appears to occur more frequently in patients with acute leukemia, but whether this relates to the leukemia or to its treatment has not been well defined. Occurrence with monocytic and lymphocytic leukemia is more common than with granulocytic leukemia [75]. Although erythema multiforme may be an early marker of a malignant disease such as acute leukemia, it usually appears late in the course of the malignant disease.

Erythema multiforme can also occur in cancer patients secondary to drug or radiation therapy [76].

Epidermolysis bullosa acquisita

Epidermolysis bullosa acquisita is a very rare disorder that has been associated with carcinoma of the bronchus [77] and with amyloidosis and multiple myeloma [78].

Infections and infestations

Herpes zoster (see also Chap. 191)

Only a small percentage of patients with localized herpes zoster have a concurrent malignant disease and investigation for malignant disease in otherwise healthy patients is not indicated [79]. Patients with leukemia or lymphoma do have an increased risk of herpes zoster, but the herpes zoster usually occurs late in the course of their disease. The incidence of herpes zoster in patients with lymphoma is approximately 10 percent, possibly even higher in patients with Hodgkin's disease [80]. There may be an increased risk of herpes zoster in splenectomized lymphoma patients [81]. Localized herpes zoster can also occur in association with solid tumors such as breast cancer; in this instance, the dermatomal distribution of the herpes zoster may indicate involvement of the nerve root area with metastatic tumor. Segmental herpes zoster can also occur post irradiation therapy, presumably secondary to nerve damage, with subsequent viral activation.

Disseminated herpes zoster is commonly associated with underlying malignant disease. Any patient with disseminated herpes zoster otherwise unexplained should be carefully examined for evidence of cancer. The most commonly associated malignant diseases are lymphoma and leukemia. Chemotherapy of cancer also has increased the risk of disseminated herpes zoster appearing in a cancer patient, presumably through suppression of the patient's immune response to the virus.

The development of herpes zoster can be evidence of a lymphoma recurring. Other evidence of the recurrence of Hodgkin's disease after remission has been preceded by herpes zoster. This sign is of particular value in patients who develop the herpes zoster more than six months after clinical remission [80]. The dermatome of the herpes zoster has also been found to be associated with Hodgkin's disease recurrence in that or an adjacent dermatome [80,82].

Herpes simplex (see also Chap. 190)

While typical localized herpes simplex is rarely a marker for cancer, extensive, often chronic, local herpes simplex, generalized cutaneous herpes simplex, or disseminated systemic herpes simplex is indeed associated with malignant disease, which is often far advanced. Lymphoma and leukemia are most often the associated cancers, but any advanced malignant tumor can produce the compromised host immune response associated with these conditions [83].

Generalized cutaneous herpes simplex can also be associated with extensive skin involvement by the tumor, even in the presence of a reasonably intact immune system. Such generalization, called Kaposi's varicelliform eruption and most commonly seen in patients with eczema, has been reported in association with mycosis fungoides [84].

Bacterial infections

Bacterial infection of the skin as a marker for the diagnosis of internal malignancy is very uncommon, and when it is associated with malignancy it is usually associated with very advanced disease. Skin lesions of a septicemia, often gram-negative, occur in cancer patients, but again generally late in the disease as a manifestation of reduced host immunity. These skin lesions are nonspecific for the malignant disease, and include pustules, nodules, vasculitic lesions, and, in *Pseudomonas* septicemia, ecthyma gangrenosum.

Fungi and yeast

Dermatophyte infections of the skin are not associated with internal malignant disease. Deep fungal infections, with their associated skin lesions, can be associated with malignant disease. Similarly, mucosal candidiasis usually indicates a severely compromised host immune response, which can be secondary to advanced malignant disease, or to chemotherapy.

Scabies

Norwegian scabies, a severe generalized form of scabies, is associated with the leukemia-lymphoma group of neoplasms, but it can be seen in any severely immune-compromised host. The scabies is frequently manifested by a minimal inflammatory response, and should always be considered in patients who have advanced malignant disease associated with pruritus.

Disorders of keratinization

Acanthosis nigricans

Acanthosis nigricans can be classified into two major groups: benign and malignant. The benign group embraces idiopathic (including obesity-associated acanthosis nigricans), endocrine (including insulin-resistant diabetes, Stein-Leventhal syndrome, Addison's disease, pituitary tumors, and pinealoma), and drug-related (including nicotinic acid, glucocorticoids, and diethylstilbestrol) disease. The acanthosis nigricans malignant group includes those cases associated with a malignant tumor [85].

Acanthosis nigricans, as the name implies, is a gray-brown thickening of the skin. It is manifested as symmetrical, velvety, papulomatous plaques, with increased skin fold markings. The most common sites of involvement are the axilla, base of the neck, groin, and antecubital fossa, but the dorsum of the hand, elbow, periumbilical skin, and the mucous membranes can also be involved. There may be an associated pruritus, particularly with malignant acanthosis nigricans. Malignant acanthosis nigricans usually is of sudden onset and is rapidly progressive, but it is otherwise indistinguishable from benign acanthosis nigricans.

Malignant acanthosis nigricans is usually secondary to an adenocarcinoma (Figs. 165-1, 165-2, and A2-16). The adenocarcinoma is usually intraabdominal (70 to 90 percent) and it is usually gastric (55 to 61 percent) [86,87]. Nonadenocarcinoma tumors such as squamous cell carcinoma and lymphoma have been reported to be associated with malignant acanthosis nigricans, but this is uncommon [85,87–89]. The appearance of the acanthosis nigricans may precede other evidence of the internal malignant disease.

Most patients with malignant acanthosis nigricans have tumors in the APUDoma group [90]. Malignant acanthosis nigricans may be secondary to peptide production by the tumor [87].

Malignant acanthosis nigricans will frequently remit following extirpation of the tumor.

Acquired ichthyosis

The sudden onset of ichthyosis in an adult may indicate an occult malignant tumor, most often lymphoma (Fig. 165-3). The ichthyosis is a true hyperkeratosis, and can be differentiated clinically and histologically from simple dry skin (xerosis). While the ichthyosis usually occurs as a late manifestation of a lymphoma, it may precede the diagnosis by several years [91]. In addition to Hodgkin's disease, ichthyosis has been reported in association with mycosis fungoides, other lymphomas, and multiple myeloma. Other

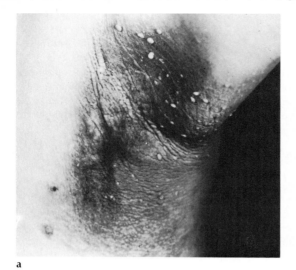

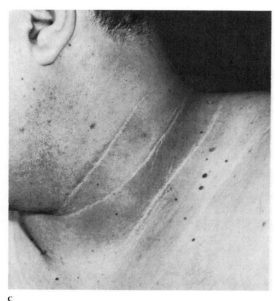

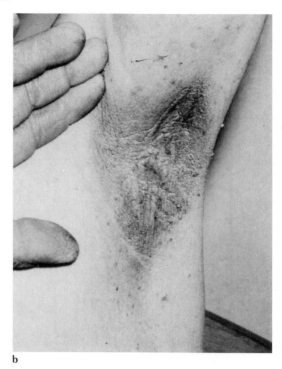

Fig. 165-1 (a and b) Malignant acanthosis nigricans. (c) Pseudo acanthosis nigricans.

tumors reported in association with acquired ichthyosis have included cancer of the breast, cervix, and lung as well as Kaposi's sarcoma and leiomyosarcoma [92–94].

Follicular hyperkeratosis has been reported in association with multiple myeloma [95,96]. Horny follicular spicules stud the forehead, cheeks, nose, and chin, and can extend to invade the upper back and arms. Microscopically one sees a hyperkeratotic mass in the follicle mouth. Amyloid deposition is not seen histologically in these myeloma patients.

Palmar hyperkeratosis

There are two groups of patients with palmar hyperkeratosis and associated malignant tumors: those with diffuse palmar hyperkeratosis and those with punctate palmar hyperkeratosis.

Diffuse hyperkeratosis, or tylosis, was reported by Howel-Evans in 1958 to be associated in two families with an almost certain development of esophageal carcinoma by age 65 [97]. The tylosis in these patients can be separated clinically from the benign form in that that found in the latter occurs at an earlier age (early childhood), has sharply delimited edges, and is of uniform thickness. In addition to the Howel-Evans families, there would appear to be a greater than expected incidence of esophageal carcinoma in other families with a pedigree of tylosis [98].

The second type of palmar hyperkeratosis that may be associated with neoplasia consists of discrete hyperkeratotic papules on the palms. These patients have been reported to have a greater than expected risk of cancer of the breast, uterus, lung, bladder, and colon, among other tumors [99–102]. Arsenic, known to be associated with punctate palmar hyperkeratosis and an increased risk of cancer, may be responsible for this apparently increased risk of malignant disease [103]; although studies have failed to show increased arsenic exposure on history [101]. Some authors question the existence of the relationship of punctate palmar hyperkeratosis and internal cancer [104–107]. It appears that the association, if present, is not very strong.

Erythroderma (see also Chap. 44)

Erythroderma, a diffuse erythema of the skin surface, usually associated with induration and scaling of the skin, is most commonly associated with the hematologic malignancies, in particular leukemia and lymphoma. These lymphomas are most frequently of the T-cell type and include the Sézary syndrome and mycosis fungoides [108,109].

Among solid tumors, erythroderma has been associated

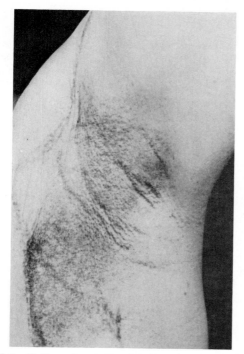

Fig. 165-2   Malignant acanthosis nigricans in a female patient with metastatic cancer of the breast. The presentation is unusual in that there is very little hyperplasia but marked pigmentation.

with carcinoma of the lung, liver, prostate, thyroid, colon, pancreas, and stomach [108]. The erythroderma occurring from solid tumors usually occurs at a relatively late stage of the disease. The eruption may resolve after resection of the tumor [110].

The erythroderma seen in the T-cell lymphomas and leukemias is associated with an infiltrate of the neoplastic T cells in the affected skin. The etiology of the erythroderma associated with solid tumors is not known.

Fig. 165-3   Acquired ichthyosis.

Paraneoplastic acrokeratosis of Bazex

Paraneoplastic acrokeratosis of Bazex is a symmetrical dermatosis that most commonly affects the hands, feet, ears, and nose with an erythematous psoriasiform eruption. The eruption is of a bluer hue than in psoriasis [111]. Later changes involve the cheeks, elbows, and knees, with still later changes often involving the central trunk where bullae may be seen. Acanthosis nigricans can also be associated. The nails are involved early, and severely. There is subungual hyperkeratosis, as well as a flaky white surface to the nail. The nails may be shed. The distal digits show an erythematous scaling eruption, often fissured, and often with suppuration [112–114]. Biopsy of the skin lesions of one patient showed diffuse deposition of IgA, IgM, and IgG along the basement membrane [115].

Bazex syndrome is associated with neoplasia of the upper respiratory system, lungs, tongue, and esophagus. Patients with this syndrome have a virtual certainty of a tumor being present. Frequently the eruption predates other evidence of the cancer [111].

This syndrome should not be confused with another Bazex syndrome which is completely unrelated to internal neoplasia and which consists of follicular atrophoderma associated with basal cell carcinoma, hypotrichosis, and localized or generalized hypohidrosis [116].

Collagen-vascular diseases

Dermatomyositis (see also Chap. 153)

Dermatomyositis can be a marker for internal neoplasia, and the development of the dermatomyositis can predate the diagnosis of the cancer. In reviewing the world literature, Andreev reported that bronchogenic carcinoma is the most common tumor seen in association with dermatomyositis, with breast, ovary, cervix, and gastrointestinal tract tumors also reported in a large percentage of patients [117]. In addition to these neoplasms, almost all other

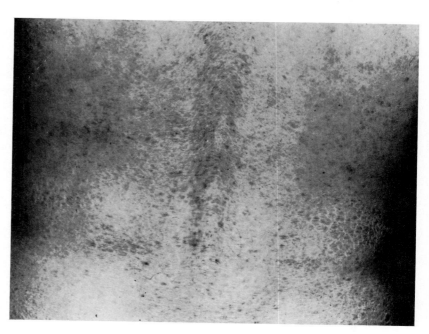

malignant tumors have been reported at least once in association with dermatomyositis. The true incidence of malignant tumors in association with dermatomyositis is quite difficult to define. Bohan et al assessed 153 patients with polymyositis-dermatomyositis and found an associated malignant tumor in 8.5 percent of the total, and in 19.2 percent of men over the age of 50 years [118]. Approximately 37 percent of the 650 patients with dermatomyositis reported in the literature have had an underlying malignancy [117]. Callen et al noted a 26 percent incidence of malignancy in their patients with dermatomyositis; they found that while there appeared to be a significantly increased risk of cancer in older patients with dermatomyositis, there did not seem to be a significant relationship of polymyositis to cancer [119]. The cancers are usually identifiable by history and physical examination [120]. It would appear that adults with dermatomyositis, but not polymyositis, should be examined thoroughly for evidence of an associated malignant tumor.

The clinical manifestations of dermatomyositis are the same with and without a malignant tumor. There is a suggestion that there is a male preponderance of patients with dermatomyositis with malignant tumors, but this has not been verified. Previous reports that biopsied muscle from patients with malignancy associated with dermatomyositis lacks an inflammatory infiltrate have recently been called into question [118].

A patient with dermatomyositis and metastatic melanoma cleared with extirpation of a known tumor, but dermatomyositis recurred simultaneously with evidence of further metastases [121].

Dermatomyositis has been reported in association with Eaton-Lambert syndrome in a patient with breast cancer [122].

Lupus erythematosus (see also Chap. 152)

Systemic lupus erythematosus (SLE) is only rarely associated with malignant neoplasia. In the majority of reported cases such an association was probably fortuitous. In one series, only 4 percent of SLE patients had neoplasia vs. 26 percent of patients from the same institution with dermatomyositis [119]. In a single case report, SLE associated with ovarian dysgerminoma cleared after extirpation of the tumor [123]. In another two patients, SLE developed during the course of melanoma [124]. Despite reports such as these it would appear that, with the exception of thymoma and lymphoma, SLE is not commonly associated with internal neoplasia.

There is a clearly recognized association between SLE and thymoma [125,126]. A feature of many cases is erythroid aplasia [127,128]. Pemphigus erythematosus has been noted in association with malignant thymoma and myasthenia gravis [129], as has a pemphigus vulgaris-like eruption and positive LE cell test [127].

There is an association of SLE and lymphoma [130–132]. The exact incidence and types of lymphoma associated with SLE have not been defined, but the association is probably real. In these lymphoma patients, the SLE may precede, coincide with, or follow first evidence of the lymphoma [132].

Progressive systemic sclerosis (see also Chap. 154)

Progressive systemic sclerosis is not commonly associated with internal malignancy. In 727 cases of systemic scleroderma only 2.6 percent had an internal malignant lesion [133]. The only tumor that has been found to be consistently associated with progressive systemic sclerosis is carcinoma of the lung [134–139]. Almost all patients with associated lung tumors have very advanced progressive systemic sclerosis. The association is most likely one of a lung tumor developing secondary to the chronic pulmonary fibrosis.

Sclerodermatous skin changes have been reported in association with the carcinoid syndrome. Presumably the sclerotic changes are secondary to the effect of an increased level of serotonin-like substances. These skin changes can be indistinguishable from the skin changes associated with progressive systemic sclerosis. Similar scleroderma-like changes have also been reported in a patient with myeloma [140].

Werner's syndrome of accelerated aging with sclerodermatous skin changes is associated with a broad range of malignant neoplasms [141].

Skin tumors and internal disease

Muir-Torre syndrome

First described by Muir et al in 1967 and by Torre in 1968, the essential features of the Muir-Torre syndrome are sebaceous tumors of the skin, with or without keratoacanthomas, in association with visceral neoplasms which are often multiple [142,143]. The sebaceous tumors are usually on the face or trunk, are usually multiple, and, while most are sebaceous adenomas, can include sebaceous hyperplasia, sebaceous epithelioma, and sebaceous carcinoma. Often the same patient will have the complete histologic spectrum of sebaceous tumors. The keratoacanthomas can be very large [144].

The visceral neoplasms are often multiple. They include tumors of a wide variety of tissues. Colon cancers are particularly common, and they may be associated with colonic polyposis [143,145–147]. Other neoplasms include other tumors of the gastrointestinal tract as well as tumors of the larynx and endometrium [145]. There has been one report of an associated lymphoma [148]. Patients with the Muir-Torre syndrome appear to have a reasonably good survival rate, despite the profusion of neoplasms [149–151].

Inheritance patterns have not been well defined, but the Muir-Torre syndrome appears to be autosomal dominant [152]. There is an association of the Muir-Torre syndrome with cancer family syndrome [153,154].

Gardner's syndrome (see also Chap. 150)

The essential features of Gardner's syndrome are intestinal polyposis (usually colonic), with a high rate of malignant transformation; epidermoid cysts, particularly of the face, scalp, and trunk; osteomatosis of the maxilla, mandible, and cranial bones; and fibromas, desmoids, and other fibrous tumors of the skin and subcutaneous tissue [155–157]. The epidermoid cysts may show areas of pilomatrix-

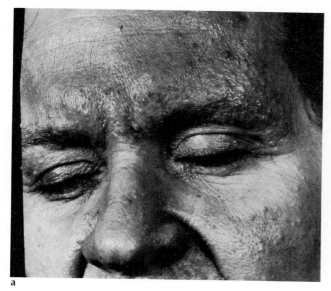
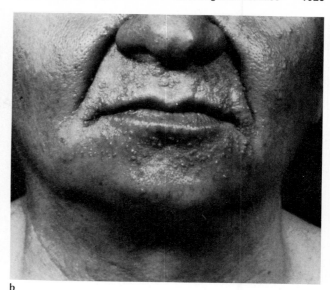

a
b

Fig. 165-4 Cowden's disease in a patient with associated adenocarcinoma of the breast. Note the multiple tricholemmomas around the eyes (a) and the mouth (b).

oma histologically [158]. The desmoids often occur in the wounds and can be deeply invasive. At times erroneously called sebaceous cysts, the epithelioid cysts of Gardner's syndrome often precede the development of bowel cancer. There is a virtual certainty of malignant transformation of the gastrointestinal tract polyps. Some of the polyps are almost always visible by proctoscopic examination, but they can be found up to the stomach [159]. There may be some overlap of the features of Gardner's syndrome and nevoid basal call carcinoma syndrome [160]. Gardner's syndrome is inherited as an autosomal dominant condition.

Cowden's disease

Cowden's disease, or multiple hamartoma syndrome, was first described in 1963 by Lloyd and Dennis, and was named after the propositus [161]. Inherited as an autosomal dominant trait, the distinctive cutaneous lesions are multiple tricholemmomas [157]. These lesions are grouped around the mouth, nose, and ears, and resemble warts clinically (Fig. 165-4). Some patients also show closely set papules with a cobblestone pattern that have a fibromatous histology [162]. Small keratotic lesions resembling plane warts occur on the acral skin. Patients may have an adenoid facies and high arched palate [163]. Other cutaneous lesions can include lipomas, hemangiomas, neuromas, vitiligo, café au lait lesions, and acromelanosis [164–167]. Angioid streaks may be present in the retina [167].

Patients with Cowden's disease have a greatly increased risk of breast and thyroid carcinoma. The breast changes seen in women with this syndrome range from fibrocystic disease to adenocarcinoma, and can occur at a young age. Prophylactic mastectomy may be indicated [168]. Thyroid adenoma is the most common thyroid tumor in this group, but thyroid carcinoma can develop [166]. There may be an increased risk of gastrointestinal malignancy. One patient has been reported with a T-lymphocyte defect, and even-

tually developed acute myelogenous leukemia [169]. Female reproductive tract hamartomas and benign tumors are common. Squamous carcinoma of the tongue and basal cell carcinoma of the perianal skin have been reported [170].

Mucosal neuroma syndrome

Mucosal neuroma syndrome is probably a variant of multiple endocrine neoplasia, Type II (MEN II or IIA, Sipple's syndrome). Also designated multiple endocrine neoplasia, Type III (MEN III or IIB), the typical features include oral, nasal, upper gastrointestinal tract, and conjunctival neuromas, associated with medullary thyroid carcinoma (MTC) and pheochromocytoma. The appearance of the neuromas usually precedes the development of cancer, but the MTC can appear in early childhood. The major cause of death in patients with MEN III is the MTC, as metastases are common. The pheochromocytomas are often bilateral. Unlike MEN II, parathyroid hyperplasia is rare [171].

In addition to the mucosal neuromas, other abnormalities can include "blubbery" lips, a marfanoid habitus, lax joints, kyphoscoliosis, lentigines, café au lait lesions, medullated corneal nerve fibers, diverticulosis, and megacolon [172,173].

Neurofibromatosis (see also Chap. 172)

Von Recklinghausen's neurofibromatosis has many associated malignant tumors. Malignant schwannoma is the most common, perhaps occurring in 29 percent of patients [174,175]. These patients are usually over the age of 30. Other tumors include fibrosarcoma [176], rhabdomyosarcoma [177], nephroblastoma (Wilms' tumor) [178], and acute and chronic myelogenous leukemia [179,180]. There is an increased incidence of ocular melanoma [181], although probably not an increased incidence of cutaneous melanoma [182]. Benign neural tumors, peripheral and intracranial, are common.

Hormone-related conditions

Malignant tumors may release hormones into the circulation, and such hormones can produce skin manifestations. The manifestation of such hormone excess is not specific to the tumor, and can occur secondarily from an excess of that hormone from any cause.

Hirsutism may be a manifestation of an increase in circulating androgen. Such androgen excess is most typically seen with testicular or ovarian tumors. Non-androgen-related hair increase, hypertrichosis, can result from porphyria cutanea tarda associated with internal malignancy, or can appear as hypertrichosis lanuginosa acquisita also secondary to internal malignant disease.

Gynecomastia in the male can be produced by an excess of estrogens. Such estrogens may be produced by a tumor of the testis. Lung tumors can also produce gynecomastia [183].

Cushing's syndrome is generally secondary to excessive ACTH production. Tumors from widely diverse sites can produce excessive ACTH. Many of these are derived from APUD tissue. The most common tumor site is the lung, with the pancreas the next most common site [184].

Acne can be caused by the same tumors that produce hirsutism. Acne may also be a marker for internal malignancy in another way. Female patients with severe acne show an apparent increase in the incidence of breast cancer [185]. Patients with breast cancer have increased sebum production [186,187]. It may well be that the stimulus for breast cancer and for increased sebum production is similar.

Disorders associated with primary skin cancers

Nevoid basal cell carcinoma syndrome (see also Chap. 76)

Nevoid basal cell carcinoma syndrome consists of multiple nevoid basal carcinomas, jaw cysts, skeletal abnormalities, and a tendency to malignant disease. Both benign and malignant tumors have been described in association with nevoid basal cell carcinoma syndrome. Benign tumors have included leiomyomas [188] and fibromas of the ovary [189,190]. The most common malignant tumor is medulloblastoma [191,192]. These tumors can occur in patients without any cutaneous basal cell carcinomas but with a family history of nevoid basal cell carcinoma syndrome [189]. Other tumors of the CNS include astrocytomas, meningiomas, and craniopharyngiomas [193]. The CNS tumors can occur at a very early age, sometimes in the first year of life [194]. Fibrosarcoma has also been reported in association with nevoid basal cell carcinoma syndrome [189,193], as has carcinoma of the maxillary antrum.

Arsenical intoxication (see also Chap. 75)

Chronic arsenic toxicity can be manifested by arsenical melanosis, plantar and palmar keratoses, and Bowen's disease. There would also appear to be an increased risk of internal neoplasia. The risk of internal neoplasia is probably increased if the Bowen's disease is on non-sun-exposed skin [195], possibly secondary to previous arsenic intake. The increased cancer risk may be up to nine times the expected incidence [196]. It has been estimated that approximately one-third of patients with Bowen's disease develop an internal malignancy six to ten years after the initial diagnosis of the Bowen's disease [195,197]. Malignancies have included tumors of the urogenital region, mouth, esophagus, and lung [198]. Airborne arsenic pollutants may account for an increased lung cancer rate in an industrial setting [199]. Against the many small series that have been reported showing an increased rate of internal malignancy, there is evidence that not all patients with Bowen's disease, including both sun-exposed and unexposed sites, have an increased risk of internal malignancy. When a large series of general Bowen's disease was compared to controls, no significant difference in systemic malignancy was found [200]. Arsenical keratoses on the palms and soles, a more specific finding, did correlate with an apparent increase in internal malignancy [201].

Various disorders associated with internal malignant disease

Pruritus (see also Chap. 8)

Pruritus, often accompanied by excoriations, is a nonspecific marker of internal malignant disease. Although often associated with xerosis, the pruritus of malignant disease can occur in apparently normal skin. It can be continuous or paroxysmal. It is usually generalized.

When occurring with malignant disease, pruritus is most commonly associated with leukemia and lymphoma. The pruritus of Hodgkin's disease often starts on the legs, is usually continuous, and may be associated with a burning sensation [202]. Pruritus is one of the most common cutaneous manifestations of leukemia, probably exceeded only by purpura. The pruritus of leukemia is usually less severe than that associated with lymphoma, and is more often generalized [203,204]. While the pruritus of both leukemia and lymphoma can precede the diagnosis of the malignancy, usually it is a sign of late disease. The severity of the pruritus tends to parallel the course of the disease, with severe pruritus heralding a poor prognosis [205].

Pruritus associated with bathing is a marker for polycythemia rubra vera (PRV), and is present in half of patients [206]. This itch can be severe and paroxysmal. Patients with PRV can also have chronic continuous pruritus unrelated to bathing. Severe pruritus can be a feature of Fanconi's anemia [207] and myeloma [208].

Pruritus associated with visceral neoplasia is most commonly associated with pancreatic and stomach tumors [204], but it can also be associated with most other solid tumors. The appearance of pruritus after treatment of the primary tumor may herald a tumor recurrence [209]. Renal and liver involvement with primary or metastatic cancer can also produce pruritus secondary to the accumulation in the skin of pruritogenic metabolites. Severe pruritus of the nostrils is evidence for a CNS tumor [210].

Itch can also be a feature of specific tumor infiltrates in the skin. In this instance, the skin does not usually appear normal [211].

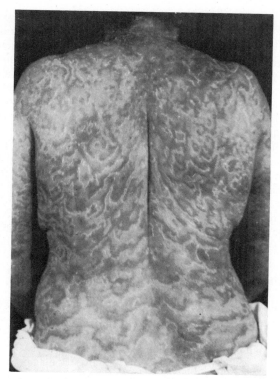

Fig. 165-5 Erythema gyratum repens in a woman with adenocarcinoma of the breast with metastases. (From Curth HO: Arch Dermatol 71:95, 1955, with permission.)

Erythema gyratum repens

Erythema gyratum repens is a cutaneous eruption consisting of concentric raised erythematous bands moving in waves over the body surface in a "wood-grain" pattern [212] (Fig. 165-5). Almost all patients with this eruption have an internal malignant neoplasm. The erythematous bands in erythema gyratum repens may be flat or raised; they are frequently surmounted by a fine marginal desquamation. The erythematous bands may move at a speed of approximately one centimeter per day [212]. Removal of the malignant tumor usually results in complete resolution of erythema gyratum repens within six weeks.

Almost all cases of erythema gyratum repens are associated with internal malignancy. Although first described with carcinoma of the breast [212–214], it has also been found in association with tumors of the lung [215–217], bladder [218], prostate [218], cervix [219,220], stomach, esophagus [221], and multiple myeloma [222]. All cases of erythema gyratum repens should be thoroughly investigated for an internal malignant disease.

Subcutaneous fat necrosis

Subcutaneous fat necrosis is a cutaneous marker for acinar cell carcinoma of the pancreas. Identical lesions can also occur with pancreatitis [223]. Subcutaneous fat necrosis associated with pancreatic disease frequently is associated with polyarthralgia, which can affect most of the joints of the body. Ankle involvement is common [223]. The polyarthralgia is presumably the result of fat necrosis of the periarticular tissue. There is frequently a concomitant associated fever and eosinophilia [224–226].

The lesions of subcutaneous fat necrosis can be painful or painless subcutaneous nodules which can occur anywhere on the body, but which are most common on the legs, buttocks, and trunk. The nodules may be fluctuant, and skin-colored to violaceous. Clinically they resemble the lesions of panniculitis or erythema nodosum. The skin lesions are presumably secondary to the effects of increased serum levels of lipase, amylase, or trypsin on the subcutaneous fat.

Sweet's syndrome (see also Chap. 111)

In 1964 Sweet described the syndrome which he termed *acute febrile neutrophilic dermatosis* [227]. This syndrome consists of painful, red, raised plaques and nodules that can appear anywhere on the skin surface but occur most commonly on the face and extremities. They are often asymmetric. Vesicles or pustules may cover the surface of the plaques. The plaques often expand peripherally with central clearing. Uncommonly, lesions may resemble lesions of pyoderma gangrenosum [228–230]. There is frequently an associated arthritis, conjunctivitis, and episcleritis [231]. There is often a history of preceding respiratory tract infection [232].

Sweet's syndrome is commonly associated with leukemia. It is most often seen with acute myelocytic leukemia [233,234], but may also be seen in acute myelomonocytic leukemia [235]. Much less commonly Sweet's syndrome is seen with solid tumors which include adenocarcinoma [236] and embryonal carcinoma of the testis [237].

Hypertrichosis lanuginosa acquisita

Hypertrichosis lanuginosa acquisita (HLA) is an acquired excessive growth of lanugo (vellus) hairs (Fig. 165-6). Soft downy hairs initially cover the face and ears, but eventually all hair-bearing skin may be involved. Associated abnormalities include a glossitis, which is often painful. The tongue is studded with red papules [238]. Fully expressed HLA usually occurs secondary to a malignant tumor, but excessive lanugo hair growth also can be caused by drugs such as exogenous steroids, phenytoin, diazoxide, streptomycin, penicillamine, and minoxidil [239] or by conditions such as anorexia nervosa.

HLA secondary to malignancy is usually abrupt in its onset and is rapidly progressive. Tumors reported in association with HLA include tumors of the colon [238,240] including carcinoid tumors [241], tumors of the rectum [240,242,243], bladder [244], lung [239,245,246], pancreas [247], gallbladder [248], uterus [249], and breast [250], and lymphoma [249]. The excessive lanugo hair growth is presumably secondary to a circulating factor produced by the tumor. Most of the tumors capable of producing HLA would appear to be of the APUD group.

Necrolytic migratory erythema (see also Chap. 168)

Necrolytic migratory erythema is a marker for an alpha-2-glucagon-producing islet cell tumor of the pancreas [251–254]. It is manifested by erythema, vesicles, pustules, bullae, and erosions which typically involve the face and

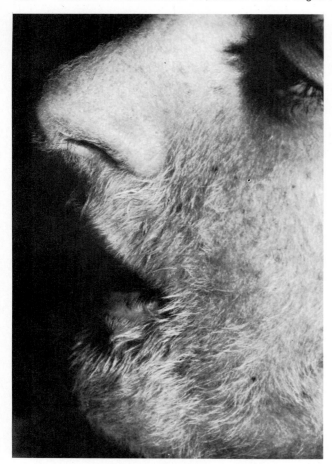

Fig. 165-6   Hypertrichosis lanuginosa acquisita in a 19-year-old woman with pancreatic carcinoma.

intertriginous areas such as the groin. The eruption can also involve the shins, ankles, and feet, as well as the fingertips. The vesicles are often very superficial and tend to become confluent. Differential diagnosis includes atypical psoriasis and mucocutaneous candidiasis. There can be brownish-red papules scattered over much of the skin surface [255,256]. Associated abnormalities include a glossitis, stomatitis, dystrophic nails, alopecia, weight loss, anemia, and diabetes [257].

Most patients with necrolytic migratory erythema have a pancreatic tumor of the glucagon-producing type, and resection of the tumor clears the eruption, sometimes within 48 h [253,256,258]. These patients have high blood glucagon levels. It would appear, though, that the dermatitis is secondary to low serum amino acid levels, rather than the elevated glucagon levels, as infusion of amino acids clears the dermatitis [259]. The dermatitis has also occurred in patients without cancer but with hepatic cirrhosis and hyperglucagonemia [260], with pancreatitis [261] or with celiac sprue [262].

Clubbing (see also Chap. 170)

Clubbing is a soft tissue enlargement of the tips of the fingers and toes which can be associated with neoplasms of the lung. It can also occur secondary to chronic lung lesions such as bronchiectasis and lung abscesses. Club-

bing is manifested by an enlargement of the distal digits. Clubbing accompanied by subperiosteal new bone formation is called *hypertrophic osteoarthropathy*. A more florid expression of this, accompanied by acromegalic features, is called *pachydermoperiostosis*. Patients with the latter two conditions can have diffusely painful bones. Pachydermoperiostosis is usually idiopathic, but can be secondary to lung cancer [263]. The clubbing and associated bone changes can be either insidious or abrupt.

The most common tumor associated with clubbing is bronchogenic carcinoma. Five to ten percent of patients with bronchogenic carcinoma develop clubbing [264]. Mesothelioma can also produce similar changes. Clubbing can also be produced by other solid tumors metastatic to the thorax. It has also been reported in Hodgkin's disease of the lung [265]. Clubbing can also be seen with diffuse intestinal lymphoma [263].

Leukoderma (see also Chap. 79)

Leukoderma is the acquired complete loss of normal skin pigment. The most common cause of leukoderma is vitiligo. Vitiligo is usually unassociated with malignant disease, but has been reported uncommonly in association with thyroid carcinoma [266]. Far more significant is the association of leukoderma and malignant melanoma (Fig. 165-7). Depigmentation of the skin has long been known to be associated with melanocytic tumors, both benign and malignant. The halo nevus and halo melanoma are typical examples of this. Ectopic depigmentation can also occur with malignant melanoma. The appearance of leukoderma in patients post resection of their primary tumor may herald occult metastatic disease. Despite this, there is growing evidence that melanoma patients with metastatic disease and leukoderma may have a relatively prolonged survival [267,268]. Uveitis may be an associated abnormality in patients with leukoderma and melanoma [269]. Leukoderma may also be associated with ocular melanoma [270].

Peutz-Jeghers syndrome (see also Chaps. 79 and 168)

First described by Hutchinson in 1900 [271], the association of cutaneous and muscosal hyperpigmentation with gastrointestinal tract polyposis is now well known [272]. These GI tract polyps can be associated with the development of malignant tumors. The pigmentary changes involve both the skin and mucous membrane. The skin hyperpigmented macules usually are present at birth or early infancy, and frequently fade at puberty. They can be typically grouped around the mouth, eyes, and nostrils, with pigmented macules also being found on the fingers, palms, toes, periumbilical skin, or diffusely over the skin surface [273]. Mucosal pigmented lesions are similar to the skin lesions, but persist for life. Buccal mucosal pigmented papillomas have also been described [274].

The most common malignancy associated with Peutz-Jeghers syndrome is duodenal carcinoma. These malignant tumors are frequently associated with hamartomatous polyps [275]. The lifetime risk of a patient with Peutz-Jeghers syndrome developing an upper GI tract malignancy is 2 to 3 percent [276]. Granulosa cell tumors may be present in as many as 20 percent of females with the Peutz-Jeghers

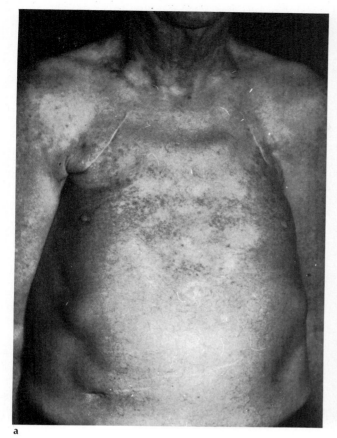

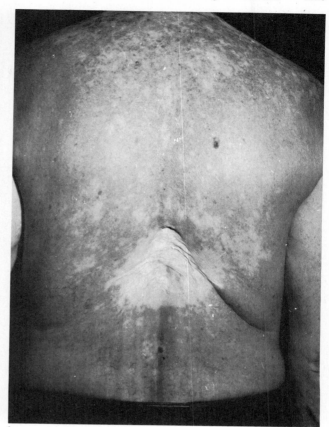

a

b

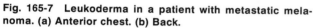

Fig. 165-7   Leukoderma in a patient with metastatic melanoma. (a) Anterior chest. (b) Back.

syndrome [277]. Granulosa-theca cell tumors of the ovary may be associated with precocious puberty [278]. The Peutz-Jeghers syndrome is inherited as an autosomal dominant condition.

Tuberous sclerosis (see also Chap. 172)

Tuberous sclerosis can be associated with tumors of many organ systems. Most of these tumors are hamartomatous, and some of these can become malignant. The malignant change occurring within hamartomas is usually sarcomatous. Metastatic lesions are uncommon [277]. Malignant transformation in tuberous sclerosis occurs in probably no more than 5 percent of patients [278]. Tumors of the kidney are frequently embryonal. Neural tumors are many and include glioblastoma multiforme, and ependyomas [279,280]. Death can result from the growth of histologically benign lesions within the CNS.

Wiskott-Aldrich syndrome

Wiskott-Aldrich syndrome is associated with the development of malignant neoplasms. The vast preponderance of these are of the lymphoreticular system [281,282]. Tumors have included reticulum cell sarcoma, other lymphosarcomas, as well as leukemia, leiomyosarcoma, and astrocytoma [281].

Multiple eruptive seborrheic keratoses

Multiple eruptive seborrheic keratoses, also known as the sign of Leser-Trelat, have been mentioned in association with multiple internal malignancies. These malignant tumors have included tumors of the stomach [283], breast [284], prostate [285], lung [286], colon [287,288], as well as many references to its occurrence in lymphoma [289–292]. It has also been mentioned in association with hyperkeratosis of the palms and soles associated with malignant disease [283] and with acanthosis nigricans [293]. The presumed relationship of seborrheic keratoses to malignant disease is in doubt. Seborrheic keratoses are very common. A hallmark of many patients with so-called eruptive seborrheic keratoses is a cutaneous eruption which is also inflammatory [294–296]. It may well be that the inflammatory dermatosis is centering around skin papillomas and seborrheic keratoses making them suddenly "appear." Indeed it is common clinical experience to see an increase in the prominence of seborrheic keratoses in patients with generalized dermatitis from any cause.

Porphyria cutanea tarda (see also Chap. 143)

Porphyria cutanea tarda, clinically manifested by hypertrichosis, increased skin fragility, and bulla formation, particularly in sun-exposed skin, has been associated with the

Table 165-2 Heritable diseases with skin manifestations and propensity to develop internal malignancy

Disorder	Skin signs	Alterations of other systems	Predominant malignancy
Dominant inheritance:			
Multiple hamartoma syndrome (Cowden's disease)	Acral verrucous papules, trichilemmomas of face, fibromas of oral mucosa	Multiple hamartomas, lipomas, hemangiomas, fibrocystic disease of breast, thyroid adenomas, neuromas	Thyroid carcinoma, breast carcinoma
Gardner's syndrome	Epidermal cysts, sebaceous cysts, dermoid tumors, lipomas, fibromas	Polyposis of colon, osteomas	Colonic adenocarcinomas (very high incidence, unless colectomy done)
Multiple mucosal neuromas	Neuromas on eyelids, lips, tongue, nasal or laryngeal mucosae	Parathyroid adenomas, hypertension	Pheochromocytoma, medullary carcinoma of thyroid (high incidence)
Neurofibromatosis (von Recklinghausen's)	Neurofibromas, café au lait spots, axillary "freckles," giant nevi	Acoustic and spinal neuromas, meningiomas, osseous fibrous dysplasia	Malignant neurilemmoma (5% incidence), pheochromocytoma (uncommon), astrocytoma, glioma (uncommon)
Nevoid basal cell carcinoma syndrome	Multiple basal cell carcinomas, epidermoid cysts, "pits" on palms and soles	Jaw cysts, rib and vertebral abnormalities, short metacarpals, ovarian fibromas, hypertelorism	Medulloblastoma, fibrosarcoma of jaw (low incidence)
Palmar-plantar hyperkeratosis (tylosis)	Hyperkeratosis of palms and soles (onset usually after age 10)	None	Esophageal carcinoma (95% incidence)
Peutz-Jeghers syndrome	Pigmented macules on lips, oral mucosa, digits	Intestinal polyposis (predominantly small intestine)	Gastric, duodenal, and colonic adenocarcinomas (low incidence, 2–3%)
Tuberous sclerosis	Hypopigmented macules, shagreen patches, adenoma sebaceum, subungual fibromas	Epilepsy, mental retardation, hamartomas in brain, kidneys, heart	Astrocytomas, glioblastomas (low incidence)
Autosomal recessive:			
Ataxia-telangiectasia	Telangiectasia (neck, malar, antecubital fossae, popliteal fossae, ears)	Cerebellar ataxia, sinopulmonary infections, IgA deficiency, ± IgE deficiency	Lymphoma, leukemia (10% incidence)
Bloom's syndrome	Telangiectasia of sun-exposed skin, photosensitivity	Short stature, fine features, dolichocephaly	Leukemia (high incidence)
Chédiak-Higashi syndrome	Dilution of skin and hair color, recurrent pyoderma, giant melanosomes	Recurrent infections, azurophilic leukocytic inclusions, nystagmus, iris translucence, photophobia, pancytopenia	Lymphoma (high incidence)
Fanconi's anemia	Patchy hyperpigmentation	Bone anomalies, chromosomal aberrations	Leukemia (high incidence)
Werner's syndrome (adult progeria)	Premature aging, scleroderma-like changes, graying hair and baldness, leg ulcers	Arteriosclerosis, cataracts	Sarcoma, meningiomas
Sex-linked recessive:			
Bruton's sex-linked agammaglobulinemia	Recurrent infections	Recurrent infections, agammaglobulinemia	Leukemia, lymphoma (5% incidence)
Dyskeratosis congenita	Reticulate hyperpigmentation, leukoplakia of mucosae, loss of nails, hyperkeratosis of palms and soles, atrophy of skin of extensor surfaces	Pancytopenia	Carcinomas (high incidence), leukemia (occasional)
Wiskott-Aldrich syndrome	Eczematous dermatitis, petechial purpura, recurrent pyoderma	Decreased IgM, thrombocytopenia	Leukemia, lymphoma (10% incidence)

development of malignant tumors, predominantly of the liver. Porphyria cutanea tarda can predate or antedate the apparent development of the primary liver tumor [297–301]. One patient coincidentally also had evidence of multiple ''eruptive'' seborrheic keratoses associated with bullae on the skin [301]. Porphyria has also been reported in a patient with lymphoma and an apparently normal liver [302].

Other syndromes with skin manifestations and a cancer association (Table 165-2)

Direct tumor involvement in the skin

Solid tumors

Direct involvement of the skin by metastatic spread from a distant primary tumor is unquestionably a marker for internal malignancy. Generally such a metastatic lesion is obvious, being an erythematous cutaneous, or subcutaneous mass; and is frequently rapidly growing. At times, though, it can be difficult to diagnose metastatic lesions. This is especially true with metastases from breast cancer.

Most commonly breast cancer lesions metastasize to the anterior chest wall. They can typically show up as small nodules ranging from 1- to 2-mm lesions to large masses of tumor. The tiny nodules can be erythematous or can be frankly hemorrhagic. The hemorrhage can be present within the nodules, or in the field surrounding the nodules. Metastatic breast cancer can also present as erysipelas-like eruption. A diffuse, warm, indurated plaque appears on the skin surface. Frequently it is asymptomatic, but can be painful. Even more uncommon is the leather-like skin change of sclerosing metastatic breast cancer known as carcinoma en cuirasse. Carcinoma en cuirasse can be progressive for many years, even decades, in the absence of any apparent systemic involvement.

Metastases from malignant melanoma are usually pigmented. Often there is a bluish tint to the lesion. Although the primary tumor may be pigmented, the metastases can be amelanotic. The reverse is also true.

Other tumors that commonly metastasize to skin include lung, stomach, kidney, and ovary. The scalp is quite commonly involved by metastases from lung, kidney, and breast. Alopecia may result. The face and neck may be involved by metastases from oropharyngeal carcinomas.

Metastases to the skin can appear many years after extirpation of the primary tumor. Progression, as in the case of carcinoma en cuirasse, can be very slow, and may indeed not appreciably shorten life expectancy. Generally, though, cutaneous metastases herald a poor prognosis, as evidence of systemic spread to other sites is usually quickly apparent.

Metastases from renal and thyroid carcinomas may be pulsatile and may have a bruit.

Lymphoma–leukemia

Involvement of the skin with lymphoma cells is quite common, particularly in the case of a T-cell lymphoma. Indeed mycosis fungoides and Sézary syndrome are usually heralded by a cutaneous eruption. Like T-cell lymphomas, T-cell leukemias frequently have skin involvement. This in-

volvement may manifest itself as a diffuse erythroderma as is seen in Sézary syndrome. Alopecia can also be caused by lymphoma. Alopecia mucinosa is involvement of hair follicles by lymphoma with associated mucin deposition.

B-cell lymphomas can also involve the skin, with Hodgkin's disease being the most common. B-cell lymphoma involvement of the skin is usually manifested by the development of one or more papules or nodules. The nodules may be ulcerated, or may, as they clear in the center and spread peripherally, form arcuate lesions.

Aside from the erythroderma seen in T-cell leukemia, other lymphocytic and myeloid leukemias can have cutaneous manifestations. The most common of these are the infiltrations of the skin produced by monocytic or myelomonocytic leukemia, which can produce a leonine facies, in addition to other infiltrative plaques. The infiltrated skin frequently has a plum-colored hue. Involvement of the skin can be a presenting feature in myelomonocytic leukemia, although it generally occurs late in the course of the disease.

Multiple myeloma can appear as small red nodules on the skin surface with a diagnostic myeloma histology.

It is important when assessing a solitary nodule which is histologically lymphoma, in the absence of any definable systemic disease, to consider the benign cutaneous lymphoid infiltrates in the differential diagnosis.

Paget's disease (see also Chap. 103)

Paget's disease of the nipple is an erythematous scaling eruption which indicates ductal carcinoma of the underlying breast. Extramammary Paget's disease, which can occur in the anogenital skin, similarly is associated with an underlying adenocarcinoma. The underlying carcinoma may be of apocrine or eccrine sweat gland origin, or can be from the rectum or urethra. Paget's disease, both mammary and extramammary, closely resembles eczema. It is important to consider Paget's disease in a differential diagnosis of any eczema involving the breast or perineum that is not clearing well with appropriate eczema therapy.

Histiocytosis X (see also Chap. 166)

The classical skin lesions of Letterer-Siwe disease are fine erythematous papules surmounted by a scale. These small papules are frequently on the scalp, but can be generalized. On cursory examination the diagnosis of seborrheic dermatitis is suggested, but unlike seborrheic dermatitis the eruption of histiocytosis X is papular and can be hemorrhagic. The red-brown papules can tend to become confluent, forming a greasy scale. Frequently there are erosions, particularly in the flexures. Frank ulcers may occur behind the ears, and in the groin. While virtually all patients with Letterer-Siwe disease have these papular skin lesions, only 30 to 50 percent of those with Hand-Schüller-Christian disease have skin lesions.

Skin lesions of eosinophilic granuloma are uncommon, but when they occur they are usually identical to those seen in Letterer-Siwe disease. Larger papules and nodules may also occur.

Xanthomas of the skin can also be a manifestation of histiocytosis X.

References

Color changes secondary to the deposition of substances in the skin

1. Nelson DH et al: ACTH-producing pituitary tumors following adrenalectomy for Cushing's syndrome. *Ann Intern Med* **52**:560, 1960
2. Haugen HN, Köken AC: Carcinoma of the hypophysis associated with Cushing's syndrome and addisonian pigmentation. *J Clin Endocrinol Metab* **20**:173, 1960
3. Adrian RM et al: Diffuse melanosis secondary to metastatic malignant melanoma. *J Am Acad Dermatol* **5**:308, 1981
4. Fitzpatrick TB et al: Pathogenesis of generalized dermal pigmentation secondary to malignant melanoma and melanuria. *J Invest Dermatol* **22**:163, 1954
5. Silberberg I et al: Diffuse melanosis in malignant melanoma. *Arch Dermatol* **97**:671, 1968
6. Konrad K, Wolff K: Pathogenesis of diffuse melanosis secondary to malignant melanoma. *Br J Dermatol* **91**:635, 1974
7. Retsas S, Samman PD: Pigment streaks in the nail plate due to secondary malignant melanoma. *Br J Dermatol* **108**:367, 1983
8. Sohn N et al: Generalized melanosis secondary to malignant melanoma. *Cancer* **24**:897, 1969
9. Goodall P et al: Malignant melanoma with melanosis and melanuria, and with pigmented monocytes and tumour cells in the blood. *Br J Surg* **48**:549, 1961
10. Andreev VC, Petkov I: Skin manifestations associated with tumours of the brain. *Br J Dermatol* **92**:675, 1975
11. Powell LW, Isselbacher KJ: Hemochromatosis, in *Harrison's Principles of Internal Medicine*, 10th ed, edited by RG Petersdorf et al. New York, McGraw-Hill, 1983, p 530
12. Perdrup A, Poulsen H: Hemochromatosis and vitiligo. *Arch Dermatol* **90**:34, 1964
13. Marien KJC, Smeenk G: Plane xanthomata associated with multiple myeloma and hyperlipoproteinaemia. *Br J Dermatol* **93**:407, 1975
14. Moschella SL: Plane xanthomatosis associated with myelomatosis. *Arch Dermatol* **101**:683, 1970
15. Wilson DE et al: Multiple myeloma, cryoglobulinemia and xanthomatosis. *Am J Med* **59**:721, 1975
16. Roberts-Thomson PJ et al: Polymeric IgA myeloma, hyperlipidaemia and xanthomatosis: a further case and review. *Postgrad Med J* **51**:44, 1975
17. Lynch PJ, Winkelmann RK: Generalized plane xanthoma and systemic disease. *Arch Dermatol* **93**:639, 1966
18. Haqqani MT, Hunter RD: Normolipemic plane xanthoma and histiocytic lymphoma. *Arch Dermatol* **112**:1470, 1976
19. Mays JA et al: Juvenile chronic granulocytic leukemia. *Am J Dis Child* **134**:654, 1980
20. O'Donnell J et al: Acute myelomonocytic leukaemia presenting as a xanthomatous skin eruption. *J Clin Pathol* **35**:1200, 1982
21. Statham B et al: Atypical eruptive histiocytosis—a marker of underlying malignancy? *Br J Dermatol* **110**:103, 1982
22. Cooper PH et al: Association of juvenile xanthogranuloma with juvenile myeloid leukemia. *Arch Dermatol* **120**:371, 1984
23. Weber G, Pilgrim M: Contribution to the knowledge of normolipaemic plane xanthomatosis. *Br J Dermatol* **90**:465, 1974
24. Maize JC et al: Xanthoma disseminatum and multiple myeloma. *Arch Dermatol* **110**:758, 1974
25. Brownstein MH, Helwig EB: The cutaneous amyloidoses. *Arch Dermatol* **102**:20, 1970
26. Westermark P et al: Bullous amyloidosis. *Arch Dermatol* **117**:782, 1981
27. Coskey RJ: Macular amyloidosis. *Arch Dermatol* **111**:929, 1975

Vascular and blood abnormalities

28. Thorn GW et al (eds): *Harrison's Principles of Internal Medicine*, 8th ed. New York, McGraw-Hill, 1977
29. Jeffries GH: Diseases of the hepatic system, in *Cecil-Loeb Textbook of Medicine*, 13th ed. Philadelphia, WB Saunders, 1971, p 1377
30. Weber FP: Bilateral thoracic zosteroid spreading marginate telangiectasia—probably a variant of "carcinoma erysipelatodes" (C. Rasch)—associated with unilateral mammary carcinoma, and better termed "carcinoma telangiectaticum." *Br J Dermatol* **45**:418, 1933
31. Kauh YC et al: Malignant proliferating angioendotheliomatosis. *Arch Dermatol* **116**:803, 1980
32. Rosenbaum FF et al: Essential telangiectasia, pulmonic and tricuspid stenosis, and neoplastic liver disease: a possible new clinical syndrome. *J Lab Clin Med* **42**:941, 1953
33. French AJ, Lilleyman JS: Bleeding tendency of T-cell lymphoblastic leukemia. *Lancet* **2**:469, 1979
34. Goltz RW, Good RA: Benign hyperglobulinemic purpura. *Arch Dermatol* **83**:26, 1961
35. Cairns SA et al: Squamous cell carcinoma of bronchus presenting with Henoch-Schönlein purpura. *Br Med J* **2**:474, 1978
36. Maurice TR: Carcinoma of bronchus presenting with Henoch-Schönlein purpura. *Br Med J* **2**:831, 1978
37. Mitchell DM, Hoffbrand BI: Relapse of Henoch-Schönlein disease associated with lung carcinoma. *J R Soc Med* **72**:614, 1979
38. Sams WM et al: Necrotising vasculitis associated with lethal reticuloendothelial diseases. *Br J Dermatol* **80**:555, 1968
39. Jellinger K et al: Primary malignant lymphoma of the CNS and polyneuropathy in a patient with necrotizing vasculitis treated with immunosuppression. *J Neurol* **220**:259, 1979
40. Best WR, Fine G: Periarteritis nodosa and multiple myeloma: report of simultaneous occurrence in a patient receiving stilbamide. *Ann Intern Med* **34**:1472, 1951
41. Elkon KB et al: Hairy-cell leukaemia with polyarteritis nodosa. *Lancet* **2**:280, 1979
42. Hughes GRV et al: Polyarteritis nodosa and hairy-cell leukaemia. *Lancet* **1**:678, 1979
43. Gerber MA et al: Periarteritis nodosa, Australia antigen and lymphatic leukemia. *N Engl J Med* **286**:14, 1972
44. Hawley PR et al: Association between digital ischaemia and malignant disease. *Br Med J* **3**:208, 1967
45. Palmer HM: Digital vascular disease and malignant disease. *Br J Dermatol* **91**:476, 1974
46. Palmer HM, Vedi KK: Digital ischaemia and malignant disease. *Practitioner* **213**:819, 1974
47. Brown GE, Giffin HZ: Peripheral arterial disease in polycythemia vera. *Arch Intern Med* **46**:705, 1930
48. Fagrell B, Mellstedt H: Polycythemia vera as a cause of ischemic digital necrosis. *Acta Chir Scand* **144**:129, 1978
49. Narita H et al: A case of cryoglobulinemic gangrene in myeloma with fatal outcome despite successful skin grafting. *Dermatologica* **160**:125, 1980
50. Vieta JO, Heymann AD: Mondor's disease. *NY State J Med* **77**:120, 1977

Bullous disorders

51. Stone SP, Schroeder AL: Bullous pemphigoid and associated malignant neoplasms. *Arch Dermatol* **111**:991, 1975
52. Rook AJ: A pemphigoid eruption associated with carcinoma of the bronchus. *Trans St Johns Hosp Dermatol Soc* **54**:152, 1968
53. Goodnough LT, Muir A: Bullous pemphigoid as a manifestation of chronic lymphocytic leukemia. *Arch Intern Med* **140**:1526, 1980
54. Cuni L: Bullous pemphigoid in chronic lymphocytic leukemia with the demonstration of antibasement membrane antibodies. *Am J Med* **57**:987, 1974

55. Naysmith A, Hancock BW: Hodgkin's disease and pemphigus. *Br J Dermatol* **94**:695, 1976
56. Sood VD, Pasricha JS: Pemphigus and Hodgkin's disease. *Br J Dermatol* **90**:575, 1974
57. Saikia NK: Extraction of pemphigus antibodies from a lymphoid neoplasm and its possible relationship to pemphigus vulgaris. *Br J Dermatol* **86**:411, 1972
58. Pisanty S, Garfunkel A: Kaposi's sarcoma. *J Oral Med* **25**:89, 1970
59. Rosenmann E: Kaposi's disease in a patient with pemphigus vulgaris. *Isr J Med Sci* **2**:269, 1966
60. Peck SM et al: Studies in bullous disease. *N Engl J Med* **279**:951, 1968
61. Stillman MA, Baer RL: Pemphigus and thymoma. *Acta Derm Venereol (Stockh)* **52**:393, 1972
62. Vetters JM et al: Pemphigus vulgaris and myasthenia gravis. *Br J Dermatol* **88**:437, 1973
63. Safai B et al: Pemphigus vulgaris associated with a syndrome of immunodeficiency and thymoma: a case report. *Clin Exp Dermatol* **3**:129, 1978
64. Imamura S et al: Pemphigus foliaceus, myasthenia gravis, thymoma and red cell aplasia. *Clin Exp Dermatol* **3:285, 1978**
65. Saikia NK, MacConnell LES: Senear-Usher syndrome and internal malignancy. *Br J Dermatol* **87**:1, 1972
66. Andersson H et al: Malignant mesenteric lymphoma in a patient with dermatitis herpetiformis, hypochlorhydria and small bowel abnormalities. *Scand J Gastroenterol* **6**:397, 1971
67. Fowler JM, Thomas DJO: Lymphoma in dermatitis herpetiformis. *Br Med J* **2**:757, 1976
68. Gould DJ, Howell R: Dermatitis herpetiformis and reticulum cell sarcoma, a rare complication. *Br J Dermatol* **96**:561, 1977
69. Freeman HJ et al: Primary abdominal lymphoma. *Am J Med* **63**:585, 1977
70. Brandt L et al: Lymphoma of the small intestine in adult coeliac disease. *Acta Med Scand* **204**:467, 1978
71. Jenkins D et al: Histiocytic lymphoma occurring in a patient with dermatitis herpetiformis. *J Am Acad Dermatol* **9**:252, 1983
72. Reunala T et al: Lymphoma in dermatitis herpetiformis: report on four cases. *Acta Derm Venereol (Stockh)* **62**:343, 1982
73. Dupont C: Herpes gestationis with hydatidiform mole. *Trans St Johns Hosp Dermatol Soc* **60**:103, 1974
74. Tillman WG: Herpes gestationis with hydatidiform mole and chorion epithelioma. *Br Med J* **1**:1471, 1950
75. Cormia FE, Domonkos AN: Cutaneous reactions to internal malignancy. *Med Clin North Am* **49 (suppl 3)**:655, 1965
76. David J, Pack GT: Erythema multiforme following deep x-ray therapy. *Arch Dermatol* **66**:41, 1952
77. Reed WB et al: Epidermal neoplasms with epidermolysis bullosa dystrophica with the first report of carcinoma of the acquired type. *Arch Dermatol Res* **253**:1, 1975
78. Trump DL et al: Epidermolysis bullosa acquisita. *JAMA* **243**:1461, 1980

Infections and infestations

79. Ragozzino MW et al: Risk of cancer after herpes zoster. *N Engl J Med* **307**:393, 1982
80. Wilson JF et al: Herpes zoster in Hodgkin's disease. *Cancer* **29**:461, 1972
81. Monfardini S et al: Herpes zoster-varicella infection in malignant lymphoma. Influence of splenectomy and intensive treatment. *Eur J Cancer* **11**:51, 1975
82. Mill WB, Frisse ME: Herpes zoster in Hodgkin's disease. *Mo Med* **75**:515, 1978
83. Shneidman DW et al: Chronic cutaneous herpes simplex. *JAMA* **241**:592, 1979
84. Segal RJ, Watson W: Kaposi's varicelliform eruption in mycosis fungoides. *Arch Dermatol* **114**:1967, 1978

Disorders of keratinization

85. Brown J, Winkelmann RK: Acanthosis nigricans: a study of 90 cases. *Medicine (Baltimore)* **47**:33, 1968
86. Curth HO: Significance of acanthosis nigricans. *Arch Dermatol* **66**:80, 1952
87. Rigel DS, Jacobs MI: Malignant acanthosis nigricans: a review. *J Dermatol Surg Oncol* **6**:923, 1980
88. Schwartz RA: Acanthosis nigricans, florid cutaneous papillomatosis and the sign of Leser-Trelat. *Cutis* **28**:319, 1981
89. Azizi E et al: Generalized malignant acanthosis nigricans and primary fibrinolysis. *Arch Dermatol* **118**:955, 1982
90. Hage E, Hage J: Malignant acanthosis nigricans—a paraendocrine syndrome? *Acta Derm Venereol (Stockh)* **57**:169, 1977
91. Stevanovic DV: Hodgkin's disease of the skin. *Arch Dermatol* **82**:96, 1960
92. Krakowski A et al: Acquired ichthyosis in Kaposi's sarcoma. *Dermatologica* **147**:348, 1973
93. Majekodunmi AE, Femi-Pearse D: Ichthyosis: early manifestation of intestinal leiomyosarcoma. *Br Med J* **3**:724, 1974
94. Flint GL et al: Acquired ichthyosis. *Arch Dermatol* **111**:1446, 1975
95. Braverman IM: *Skin Signs of Systemic Disease,* 2d ed. Philadelphia, WB Saunders, 1981
96. Kovary PM, Macher E: Hautkrankheiten und monoklonale Gammopathien. *Z Hautkr* **54**:1002, 1979
97. Howel-Evans W et al: Carcinoma of the oesophagus with keratosis palmaris et plantaris (tylosis). *Q J Med* **27**:413, 1958
98. Harper PS et al: Carcinoma of the oesophagus with tylosis. *Q J Med* **39**:317, 1970
99. Dobson RL et al: Palmar keratoses and cancer. *Arch Dermatol* **92**:553, 1965
100. Millard L, Gould D: Hyperkeratosis of the palms and soles associated with internal malignancy and elevated levels of immunoreactive human growth hormone. *Clin Exp Dermatol* **1**:363, 1976
101. Mortimer P et al: Palmar keratoses and internal malignancy. *Br J Dermatol* **109**:21, 1983
102. Bennion S, Patterson J: Keratosis punctata palmaris et plantaris and adenocarcinoma of the colon. *J Am Acad Dermatol* **10**:587, 1984
103. Andreev VC: Skin manifestations in visceral cancer, in *Current Problems in Dermatology.* Series editor, H Mali. Basel, S Karger, 1978
104. Bean SF et al: Palmar keratoses and internal malignancy. *Arch Dermatol* **97**:528, 1968
105. Stolman LP et al: Are palmar keratoses a sign of internal malignancy? *Arch Dermatol* **101**:52, 1970
106. Rhodes EL: Palmar and plantar seed keratoses and internal malignancy. *Br J Dermatol* **82**:361, 1970
107. Gilbertsen VA et al: Palmar keratoses and visceral cancer. *Arch Dermatol* **105**:222, 1972
108. Nicolis GD, Helwig EB: Exfoliative dermatitis. *Arch Dermatol* **108**:788, 1973
109. Abrahams I et al: 101 cases of exfoliative dermatitis. *Arch Dermatol* **87**:96, 1963
110. McGaw B, McGovern VJ: Exfoliative dermatitis associated with carcinoma of the lung. *Australas J Dermatol* **3**:115, 1956
111. Jacobsen F et al: Acrokeratosis paraneoplastica (Bazex syndrome). *Arch Dermatol* **120**:502, 1984
112. Bazex A, Griffiths A: Acrokeratosis paraneoplastica—a new cutaneous marker of malignancy. *Br J Dermatol* **102**:301, 1980
113. Baran R: Paraneoplastic acrokeratosis of Bazex. *Arch Dermatol* **113**:1613, 1977
114. Bazex A et al: Paraneoplastic acrokeratosis. *Excerpta Med* **248**:53, 1972

115. Pecora A et al: Acrokeratosis paraneoplastica (Bazex syndrome). *Arch Dermatol* **119**:820, 1983
116. Bazex A et al: Génodermatose complexe de type indéterminé associant une hypotrichose, un état atrophodermique généralisé et des dégénérescences cutanées multiples (épithéliomas basocellulaires). *Bull Soc Fr Dermatol Syphiligr* **71**:206, 1964

Collagen-vascular disease

117. Andreev VC: Skin manifestations in visceral cancer, in *Current Problems in Dermatology*. Series editor, H Mali. Basel, S Karger, 1978
118. Bohan A et al: A computer-assisted analysis of 153 patients with polymyositis and dermatomyositis. *Medicine (Baltimore)* **56**:255, 1977
119. Callen JP et al: The relationship of dermatomyositis and polymyositis to internal malignancy. *Arch Dermatol* **116**:295, 1980
120. Callen JP: The value of malignancy evaluation in patients with dermatomyositis. *J Am Acad Dermatol* **6**:253, 1982
121. Sunnenberg TD, Kitchens CS: Dermatomyositis associated with malignant melanoma. *Cancer* **51**:2157, 1983
122. Artigou C et al: Dermatomyosite et syndrome de Lambert-Eaton. *Ann Dermatol Venereol* **109**:737, 1982
123. Kahn MF et al: Systemic lupus erythematosus and ovarian dysgerminoma: remission of the systemic lupus erythematosus after extirpation of the tumour. *Clin Exp Immunol* **1**:355, 1966
124. Herstoff JK, Bogaars HA: Cutaneous lupus erythematosus associated with melanoma and BCG vaccine therapy. *Arch Dermatol* **115**:856, 1979
125. Singh BN: Thymoma presenting with polyserositis and the lupus erythematosus syndrome. *Aust Ann Med* **18**:55, 1969
126. Larsson O: Thymoma and systemic lupus erythematosus in the same patient. *Lancet* **2**:665, 1963
127. Kough RH, Barnes WT: Thymoma associated with erythroid aplasia, bullous skin eruption, and the lupus erythematosus cell phenomenon. *Ann Intern Med* **61**:308, 1964
128. Takigawa M, Hayakawa M: Thymoma with systemic lupus erythematosus, red blood cell aplasia, and herpes virus infection. *Arch Dermatol* **110**:99, 1974
129. Beutner EH et al: Autoimmunity in concurrent myasthenia gravis and pemphigus erythematosus. *JAMA* **203**:845, 1968
130. Green JA et al: Systemic lupus erythematosus and lymphoma. *Lancet* **2**:753, 1978
131. Fournie GJ et al: Systemic lupus erythematosus and malignant histiocytosis. *Lancet* **2**:1305, 1978
132. Wyburn-Mason R: SLE and lymphoma (letter). *Lancet* **1**:156, 1979
133. Tuffanelli DL, Winkelmann RK: Systemic scleroderma. *Arch Dermatol* **84**:359, 1961
134. Montgomery RD et al: Bronchiolar carcinoma in progressive systemic sclerosis. *Lancet* **1**:586, 1964
135. Richards RL, Milne JA: Cancer of the lung in progressive systemic sclerosis. *Thorax* **13**:238, 1958
136. Tomkin GH: Systemic sclerosis associated with carcinoma of the lung. *Br J Dermatol* **81**:213, 1969
137. Collins DH et al: Scleroderma with honeycomb lungs and bronchiolar carcinoma. *J Pathol Bacteriol* **76**:531, 1958
138. Caplan H: Honeycomb lung and malignant pulmonary adenomatosis in scleroderma. *Thorax* **14**:89, 1959
139. Haqqani MT, Holti G: Systemic sclerosis with pulmonary fibrosis and oat cell carcinoma. *Acta Derm Venereol (Stockh)* **53**:369, 1973
140. Huriez CL et al: Une génodysplasie non encore individualisée: la génodermatose scléro-atrophiante et kératodermique des extremités fréquemment dégénérative. *Sem Hop Paris* **44**:481, 1968
141. Hrabko RP et al: Werner's syndrome with associated malignant neoplasms. *Arch Dermatol* **118**:106, 1982

Skin tumors and internal disease

142. Muir EG et al: Multiple primary carcinomata of the colon, duodenum and larynx associated with kerato-acanthomata of the face. *Br J Surg* **54**:191, 1967
143. Torre D: Multiple sebaceous tumors. *Arch Dermatol* **98**:549, 1968
144. Bakker PM et al: Multiple sebaceous gland tumours with multiple tumours of internal organs. *Dermatologica* **142**:50, 1971
145. Housholder MS, Zeligman I: Sebaceous neoplasms associated with visceral carcinomas. *Arch Dermatol* **116**:61, 1980
146. Schwartz RA et al: The Torre syndrome with gastrointestinal polyposis. *Arch Dermatol* **116**:312, 1980
147. Fahmy A et al: Muir-Torre syndrome: report of a case and re-evaluation of the dermatologic features. *Cancer* **49**:1898, 1982
148. Descalzi ME, Rosenthal S: Sebaceous adenomas and keratoacanthomas in a patient with malignant lymphoma. *Cutis* **28**:169, 1981
149. Bitran J, Pellettiere EV: Multiple sebaceous gland tumors and internal carcinoma: Torre's syndrome. *Cancer* **33**:835, 1974
150. Rulon DB, Helwig EB: Multiple sebaceous neoplasms of the skin. *Am J Clin Pathol* **60**:745, 1973
151. Leonard DD, Deaton WR: Multiple sebaceous gland tumors and visceral carcinomas. *Arch Dermatol* **110**:917, 1974
152. Reiffers J et al: Hyperplasies sebacées, kérato-acanthomes, épithéliomas du visage et cancer du colon. *Dermatologica* **153**:23, 1976
153. Fusaro RM et al: Torre's syndrome as phenotypic expression of cancer family syndrome. *Arch Dermatol* **116**:986, 1980
154. Banse-Kupin L et al: Torre's syndrome: report of two cases and review of the literature. *J Am Acad Dermatol* **10**:803, 1984
155. Fitzgerald GM: Multiple composite odontomes coincidental with other tumorous conditions: report of a case. *J Am Dent Assoc* **30**:1408, 1943
156. Gardner EJ: A genetic and clinical study of intestinal polyposis, a predisposing factor for carcinoma of the colon and rectum. *Am J Hum Genet* **3**:167, 1951
157. Lever WF, Schaumburg-Lever G: *Histopathology of the Skin*, 6th ed. Philadelphia, JB Lippincott, 1983
158. Cooper PH, Fechner RE: Pilomatricoma-like changes in the epidermal cysts of Gardner's syndrome. *J Am Acad Dermatol* **8**:639, 1983
159. Golitz LE: Heritable cutaneous disorders which affect the gastrointestinal tract. *Med Clin North Am* **64**:829, 1980
160. Lynch PJ: Nevoid basal cell carcinoma syndrome with features of Gardner's syndrome. *Cutis* **16**:905, 1975
161. Lloyd KM II, Dennis M: Cowden's disease. *Ann Intern Med* **58**:136, 1963
162. Weary PE et al: Multiple hamartoma syndrome (Cowden's disease). *Arch Dermatol* **106**:682, 1972
163. Salem OS, Steck WD: Cowden's disease (multiple hamartoma and neoplasia syndrome). *J Am Acad Dermatol* **8**:686, 1983
164. Gentry WC et al: Multiple hamartoma syndrome (Cowden's disease). *Arch Dermatol* **109**:521, 1974
165. Nuss DD et al: Multiple hamartoma syndrome. *Arch Dermatol* **114**:743, 1978
166. Thyresson HN, Doyle JA: Cowden's disease (multiple hamartoma syndrome). *Mayo Clin Proc* **56**:179, 1981
167. Aram H, Zidenbaum M: Multiple hamartoma syndrome (Cowden's disease). *J Am Acad Dermatol* **9**:774, 1983
168. Brownstein MH et al: Cowden's disease. *Cancer* **41**:2393, 1978
169. Ruschak P et al: Cowden's disease associated with immunodeficiency. *Arch Dermatol* **117**:573, 1981

170. Camisa C et al: Cowden's disease. *Arch Dermatol* **120**:677, 1984

171. Petersdorf RG et al (eds): *Harrison's Principles of Internal Medicine,* 10th ed. New York, McGraw-Hill, 1983

172. Gorlin RJ et al: Multiple mucosal neuromas, pheochromocytoma and medullary carcinoma of the thyroid—a syndrome. *Cancer* **22**:293, 1968

173. Khairi MRA et al: Mucosal neuroma, pheochromocytoma and medullary thyroid carcinoma: multiple endocrine neoplasia type 3. *Medicine (Baltimore)* **54**:89, 1975

174. Das Gupta TK, Brasfield RD: von Recklinghausen's disease. *Cancer* **21**:174, 1971

175. Lee CW et al: Malignant degeneration of thoracic neurofibromata. *NY State J Med* **75**:347, 1975

176. Crowe FW et al: *A Clinical, Pathological and Genetic Study of Multiple Neurofibromatosis.* Springfield, IL, Charles C Thomas, 1956

177. McKeen EA et al: Rhabdomyosarcoma complicating multiple neurofibromatosis. *J Pediatr* **93**:992, 1978

178. Stay EJ, Vawter G: The relationship between nephroblastoma and neurofibromatosis (von Recklinghausen's disease). *Cancer* **39**:2550, 1977

179. Bader JL, Miller RW: Neurofibromatosis and childhood leukemia. *J Pediatr* **92**:925, 1978

180. Bestak M et al: Juvenile chronic myelogenous leukemia and dermal histiocytosis. *Am J Dis Child* **133**:831, 1979

181. Wiznia RA et al: Malignant melanoma of the choroid in neurofibromatosis. *Am J Ophthalmol* **86**:684, 1978

182. Mastrangelo MJ et al: Cutaneous melanoma in a patient with neurofibromatosis. *Arch Dermatol* **115**:864, 1979

Hormone-related conditions

183. Omenn GS: Ectopic polypeptide hormone production by tumours. *Ann Intern Med* **72**:136, 1970

184. Liddle GW et al: The ectopic ACTH syndrome. *Cancer Res* **25**:1057, 1965

185. Lerner MR, Lerner AB: Relationship between carcinoma of the breast and acne. *Cancer* **6**:870, 1953

186. Krant MJ et al: Sebaceous gland activity in breast cancer. *Nature* **217**:463, 1968

187. Burton JL et al: Increased sebum excretion in patients with breast cancer. *Br Med J* **1**:665, 1970

Disorders associated with primary skin cancer

188. Kahn LB, Gordon W: The basal cell naevus syndrome—report of a case. *S Afr Med J* **41**:832, 1967

189. Jackson R, Gardere S: Nevoid basal cell carcinoma syndrome. *Can Med Assoc J* **105**:850, 1971

190. Clendenning WE et al: Basal cell nevus syndrome. *Arch Dermatol* **90**:38, 1964

191. Gorlin RJ et al: The multiple basal cell nevi syndrome. *Cancer* **18**:89, 1965

192. Graham JK et al: Nevoid basal cell carcinoma syndrome. *Arch Otolaryngol* **87**:90, 1968

193. Tamoney HJ: Basal cell nevoid syndrome. *Am Surg* **35**:279, 1969

194. Moynahan EJ: Basal cell naevus syndrome. *Trans St Johns Hosp Dermatol Soc* **50**:187, 1964

195. Peterka ES et al: An association between Bowen's disease and internal cancer. *Arch Dermatol* **84**:623, 1961

196. Hugo NE, Conway H: Bowen's disease: its malignant potential and relationship to systemic cancer. *Plast Reconstr Surg* **39**:190, 1967

197. Graham JH, Helwig EB: Bowen's disease and its relationship to systemic cancer. *Arch Dermatol* **80**:133, 1959

198. Sommers SC, McManus RG: Multiple arsenical cancers of skin and internal organs. *Cancer* **6**:347, 1953

199. Blot WJ, Fraumeni JF: Arsenical air pollution and lung cancer. *Lancet* **2**:142, 1975

200. Andersen SLC et al: Relation between Bowen's disease and internal malignant tumors. *Arch Dermatol* **108**:367, 1973

201. Reymann F et al: Relationship between arsenic intake and internal malignant neoplasms. *Arch Dermatol* **114**:378, 1978

Various disorders associated with internal malignant disease

202. Cormia FE, Domonkos AN: Cutaneous reactions to internal malignancy. *Med Clin North Am* **49** (**suppl 3**):655, 1965

203. Wiener K: *Skin Manifestations of Internal Disorders.* London, H Kimpton, 1947

204. Newbold PCH: Skin markers of malignancy. *Arch Dermatol* **102**:680, 1970

205. Feiner AS et al: Prognostic importance of pruritus in Hodgkin's disease. *JAMA* **240**:2738, 1978

206. Wasserman LR: The treatment of polycythemia vera. *Semin Hematol* **13**:57, 1976

207. Swift MR, Hirshhorn K: Fanconi's anemia. *Ann Intern Med* **65**:496, 1966

208. Erskine JG et al: Pruritus as a presentation of myelomatosis. *Br Med J* **1**:687, 1977

209. Shoenfeld Y et al: Generalized pruritus in metastatic adenocarcinoma of the stomach. *Dermatologica* **155**:122, 1977

210. Andreev VC, Petkov I: Skin manifestations associated with tumors of the brain. *Br J Dermatol* **92**:675, 1975

211. Czarnecki DB et al: Pruritic specific cutaneous infiltrates in leukemia and lymphoma. *Arch Dermatol* **118**:119, 1982

212. Gammel JA: Erythema gyratum repens. *Arch Dermatol Syphilol* **66**:494, 1952

213. Purdy MJ: Erythema gyratum repens. *Arch Dermatol* **80**:590, 1959

214. Jacobs R et al: Carcinoma of the breast, pemphigus vulgaris and gyrate erythema. *Int J Dermatol* **17**:221, 1978

215. Schneeweiss J: Erythema gyratum repens. *Proc R Soc Med* **52**:367, 1959

216. Gold SC: Erythema gyratum repens. *Proc R Soc Med* **52**:367, 1959

217. Solomon H: Erythema gyratum repens. *Arch Dermatol* **100**:639, 1969

218. Thomson J, Stankler L: Erythema gyratum repens. *Br J Dermatol* **82**:406, 1970

219. Duperrat B et al: Erythema gyratum en rapport avec un carcinome cervical métastatique. *Bull Soc Fr Dermatol Syphiligr* **68**:20, 1961

220. Van Dijk E: Erythema gyratum repens. *Dermatologica* **123**:301, 1961

221. Barrière H et al: Erythema gyratum repens et ichtyose acquise associée avec un carcinoma oesophagien. *Ann Dermatol Venereol* **105**:319, 1978

222. Thivolet J et al: Une dermatose paranéoplastique méconnue: l'erythema gyratum repens. *Rev Lyonn Med* **19**:789, 1970

223. Hughes PSH et al: Subcutaneous fat necrosis associated with pancreatic disease. *Arch Dermatol* **111**:506, 1975

224. Belsky H, Cornell NW: Disseminated focal fat necrosis following radical pancreatico-duodenectomy for acinous carcinoma of head of pancreas. *Ann Surg* **141**:556, 1966

225. MacMahon HE et al: Acinar cell carcinoma of the pancreas with subcutaneous fat necrosis. *Gastroenterology* **49**:555, 1965

226. Mullin GT et al: Arthritis and skin lesions resembling erythema nodosum in pancreatic disease. *Ann Intern Med* **68**:75, 1968

227. Sweet RD: An acute febrile neutrophilic dermatosis. *Br J Dermatol* **76**:349, 1964

228. Goldin D, Wilkinson DS: Pyoderma gangrenosum with chronic myeloid leukaemia. *Proc R Soc Med* **67**:1239, 1974

229. Sheps M et al: Bullous pyoderma gangrenosum and acute leukemia. *Arch Dermatol* **114**:1842, 1978

230. Burton JL: Sweet's syndrome, pyodermal gangrenosum and acute leukemia. *Br J Dermatol* **102**:239, 1980

231. Krauser RE, Schumacher HR: The arthritis of Sweet's syndrome. *Arthritis Rheum* **18**:35, 1975

232. Gunawardena DA et al: The clinical spectrum of Sweet's

syndrome (acute febrile neutrophilic dermatosis) a report of eighteen cases. *Br J Dermatol* **92**:363, 1975

233. Klock JC, Oken RL: Febrile neutrophilic dermatosis in acute myelogenous leukemia. *Cancer* **37**:922, 1976

234. Goodfellow A, Calvert H: Sweet's syndrome and acute myeloid leukaemia. *Lancet* **2**:478, 1979

235. Spector JI et al: Sweet's syndrome. *JAMA* **244**:1131, 1980

236. Greer KE et al: Acute febrile neutrophilic dermatosis (Sweet's syndrome). *Arch Dermatol* **111**:1461, 1975

237. Shapiro L et al: Sweet's syndrome (acute febrile neutrophilic dermatosis). *Arch Dermatol* **103**:81, 1971

238. Hegedus SI, Schorr WF: Acquired hypertrichosis lanuginosa and malignancy. *Arch Dermatol* **106**:84, 1972

239. Knowling MA et al: Hypertrichosis lanuginosa acquisita associated with adenocarcinoma of the lung. *Can Med Assoc J* **126**:1308, 1982

240. Van der Lugt L, Dudok de Wit C: Hypertrichosis lanuginosa acquisita. *Dermatologica* **146**:46, 1973

241. Davies RA et al: Acquired hypertrichosis lanuginosa as a sign of internal malignant disease. *Can Med Assoc J* **118**:1090, 1978

242. Fretzin DF: Malignant down. *Arch Dermatol* **95**:294, 1967

243. Hensley GT, Glynn KP: Hypertrichosis lanuginosa as a sign of internal malignancy. *Cancer* **24**:1051, 1969

244. Lyell A, Whittle CH: Hypertrichosis lanuginosa, acquired type. *Proc R Soc Med* **44**:576, 1951

245. Potter B, Fretzin DF: Hypertrichosis lanuginosa and anaplastic carcinoma. *Arch Dermatol* **94**:801, 1966

246. Ikeya T et al: Acquired hypertrichosis lanuginosa. *Dermatologica* **156**:274, 1978

247. McLean DI, Macaulay JC: Hypertrichosis lanuginosa acquisita associated with pancreatic carcinoma. *Br J Dermatol* **96**:313, 1977

248. Herzberg JJ et al: Hypertrichose lanugineuse acquise. *Ann Dermatol Syphiligr (Paris)* **96**:129, 1969

249. Samson MK et al: Acquired hypertrichosis lanuginosa. *Cancer* **36**:1519, 1975

250. Wadskow S et al: Acquired hypertrichosis lanuginosa. *Arch Dermatol* **112**:1442, 1976

251. McGavran MH et al: A glucagon-secreting alpha-cell carcinoma of the pancreas. *N Engl J Med* **274**:1408, 1966

252. Wilkinson DS: Necrolytic migratory erythema with carcinoma of the pancreas. *Trans St Johns Hosp Dermatol Soc* **59**:244, 1973

253. Mallinson CN et al: A glucagonoma syndrome. *Lancet* **2**:1, 1974

254. Montenegro-Rodas F, Samaan NA: Glucagonoma tumors and syndrome. *Curr Probl Cancer* **6**:3, 1981

255. Church RE, Crane WAJ: A cutaneous syndrome associated with islet-cell carcinoma of the pancreas. *Br J Dermatol* **79**:284, 1967

256. Sweet RD: A dermatosis specifically associated with a tumour of pancreatic alpha cells. *Br J Dermatol* **90**:301, 1974

257. Shupack JL et al: The glucagonoma syndrome. *Dermatol Surg Oncol* **4**:242, 1978

258. Kahan RS et al: Necrolytic migratory erythema. *Arch Dermatol* **113**:792, 1977

259. Norton J et al: Amino acid deficiency and the skin rash associated with glucagonoma. *Ann Intern Med* **91**:213, 1979

260. Doyle J et al: Hyperglucagonaemia and necrolytic migratory erythema in cirrhosis—possible pseudoglucagonoma syndrome. *Br J Dermatol* **100**:581, 1979

261. Thivolet J: Necrolytic migratory erythema without glucagonoma. *Arch Dermatol* **117**:4, 1981

262. Goodenberger D et al: Necrolytic migratory erythema without glucagonoma: report of two cases. *Arch Dermatol* **115**:1429, 1979

263. Braverman IM: *Skin Signs of Systemic Disease,* 2d ed. Philadelphia, WB Saunders, 1981

264. Petersdorf RG et al (eds): *Harrison's Principles of Internal Medicine,* 10th ed. New York, McGraw-Hill, 1983

265. Kuritzky P et al: Cavitary pulmonary Hodgkin's disease. *JAMA* **234**:1166, 1975

266. Ortonne J-P et al: *Vitiligo and Other Hypomelanoses of Hair and Skin.* New York/London, Plenum Medical Book Co, 1983

267. Nordlund JJ et al: Vitiligo in patients with metastatic melanoma: a good prognostic sign. *J Am Acad Dermatol* **9**:689, 1983

268. Koh HK et al: Malignant melanoma and vitiligo-like leukoderma: an electron microscopic study. *J Am Acad Dermatol* **9**:696, 1983

269. Sober A, Haynes H: Uveitis, poliosis, hypomelanosis, and alopecia in a patient with malignant melanoma. *Arch Dermatol* **114**:439, 1978

270. Albert DM et al: Vitiligo or halo nevi occurring in two patients with choroidal melanoma. *Arch Dermatol* **118**:34, 1982

271. Jackson R: Hutchinson's archives of surgery revisited. *Arch Dermatol* **113**:961, 1977

272. Jeghers H et al: Generalized intestinal polyposis and melanin spots of the oral mucosa, lips and digits. *N Engl J Med* **241**:993, 1949

273. Dormandy TL: Gastrointestinal polyposis with mucocutaneous pigmentation (Peutz-Jeghers syndrome). *New Engl J Med* **256**:1093, 1141, 1186, 1957

274. Lowe NJ: Peutz-Jeghers syndrome with pigmented oral papillomas. *Arch Dermatol* **111**:503, 1975

275. Cochet B et al: Peutz-Jeghers syndrome associated with gastrointestinal carcinoma. *Gut* **20**:169, 1979

276. Reid JD: Intestinal carcinoma in the Peutz-Jeghers syndrome. *JAMA* **229**:833, 1974

277. Schimke RN: *Genetics and Cancer in Man.* London, Churchill Livingston, 1978

278. Christian CD et al: Peutz-Jeghers syndrome associated with functioning ovarian tumor. *JAMA* **190**:935, 1964

279. Marshall D et al: Tuberous sclerosis. *N Engl J Med* **261**:1102, 1959

280. Horton WA: Genetics of central nervous system tumors. *Birth Defects* **12**(1):91, 1976

281. Heidelberger KP, LeGolvan DP: Wiskott-Aldrich syndrome and cerebral neoplasia: report of a case with localized reticulum cell sarcoma. *Cancer* **33**:280, 1974

282. Model LM: Primary reticulum cell sarcoma of the brain in Wiskott-Aldrich syndrome. *Arch Neurol* **34**:633, 1977

283. Millard LG, Gould DJ: Hyperkeratosis of the palms and soles associated with internal malignancy and elevated levels of immunoreactive human growth hormone. *Clin Exp Dermatol* **1**:363, 1976

284. Lynch HT et al: Leser-Trelat sign in mother and daughter with breast cancer. *J Med Genet* **19**:218, 1982

285. Gitlin MC, Pirozzi DJ: The sign of Leser-Trelat. *Arch Dermatol* **111**:792, 1975

286. Doll CD et al: Sign of Leser-Trelat. *JAMA* **238**:236, 1977

287. Walter JA et al: Eruptive basal cell papillomata with carcinoma of caecum. *Proc R Soc Med* **65**:595, 1972

288. Kovary PM et al: Monoclonal gammopathy in scleredema. *Arch Dermatol* **117**:536, 1981

289. Safai B et al: Cutaneous manifestation of internal malignancies (11). The sign of Leser-Trelat. *Int Soc Trop Dermatol* **17**:494, 1978

290. Halevy S et al: The sign of Leser-Trelat in association with lymphocytic lymphoma. *Dermatologica* **161**:183, 1980

291. Wagner RF, Wagner KD: Malignant neoplasms and the Leser-Trelat sign. *Arch Dermatol* **117**:598, 1981

292. Dantzig PI: Sign of Leser-Trelat. *Arch Dermatol* **108**:700, 1973

293. Ballin DB: Acanthosis nigricans. *Arch Dermatol* **71**:746, 1955

294. Berman A, Winkelmann RK: Seborrheic keratoses. *Arch Dermatol* **118**:615, 1982
295. Brown F: Sign of Leser-Trelat. *Arch Dermatol* **110**:129, 1974
296. Bruckner N et al: Pemphigus foliaceus resembling eruptive seborrheic keratoses. *Arch Dermatol* **116**:815, 1980
297. Meynadier PRJ, Giulhou JJ: La porphyrie cutanée tardive. *Sem Hop Paris* **49**:719, 1973
298. Keczkes K, Barker DJ: Malignant hepatoma associated with acquired hepatic cutaneous porphyria. *Arch Dermatol* **112**:78, 1976
299. Thompson RPH et al: Cutaneous porphyria due to a malignant primary hepatoma. *Gastroenterology* **59**:779, 1970
300. Waddington RT: A case of primary liver tumour associated with porphyria. *Br J Surg* **59**:653, 1972
301. Harrington CI: Leser-Trelat sign with porphyria cutanea tarda and malignant hepatoma. *Arch Dermatol* **112**:730, 1976
302. Maughan WZ et al: Porphyria cutanea tarda associated with lymphoma. *Acta Derm Venereol (Stockh)* **59**:55, 1979

CHAPTER 166

THE HISTIOCYTOSIS SYNDROMES

Allen C. Crocker

The stimulation for proliferation and aggregation of histiocytes (also known as reticuloendothelial cells, fixed macrophages, etc.) in lesions appears to have many origins. These widely distributed and relatively undifferentiated cells are one of the major reactive elements in many types of tissue injury and infection, and hence the basic term *histiocytosis* really must be viewed as nonspecific. Most commonly, histiocytic infiltration is accompanied by simultaneous collection of other cells also involved in defense and reaction (polymorphonuclear leukocytes, lymphocytes, etc.). Giant cell formation and/or evolution into lipid-laden foam cells are often part of the phenomenon.

The word histiocytosis is usually employed, however, to identify a definite group of syndromes of rather predictable natural history, where idiopathic histiocytic granulomas are the principal lesions (localized and nodular or diffusely infiltrative). The justification for presenting juvenile xanthogranuloma, xanthoma disseminatum, and the Letterer-Siwe group under one generic heading is to acknowledge that they all share equally unknown initiating mechanisms, a comparable histiocytic proliferation in lesions, and potential spontaneous reversibility of lesion formation. Further, one is struck by finding occasional patients belonging to the above syndromes for whom classification is difficult because of the presence of manifestations which cross over the usual separate syndrome lines [1]. At the moment, it would appear that humility is appropriate regarding rigidity of nosology, and the categories listed here are designed for clinical utility.

Juvenile xanthogranuloma

Definition and historical aspects

Juvenile xanthogranuloma has become the accepted name for the common orange-colored nodular cutaneous granulomas seen in otherwise healthy infants. This term, proposed by Helwig and Hackney [2], has logically supplanted the earlier name of *nevoxanthoendothelioma*, since there is no evidence for relationship to nevi as such. Many other synonyms exist (juvenile xanthoma, possibly some instances recorded as histiocytoma, etc.), and the present author erroneously employed the term *xanthoma disseminatum* for these lesions (see preferred use for this nomenclature later in this contribution) in an early paper [3].

Incidence

In any large pediatric or well-baby service, lesions of this sort are seen regularly although infrequently. The children are well nourished and develop normally, with no special predisposing factors (except as noted below).

Clinical manifestations

Typically, these skin xanthomas are seen first in the newborn period or during the first 6 months of life, rapidly developing from small red papules into discrete 2- to 8-mm orange, golden, or brown nodules, without specific local symptoms (Fig. 166-1). There may be as few as one or two lesions, or as many as several hundred, with a characteristic axial distribution (scalp, face, trunk, and proximal portions of extremities) [4,5]. They are found also on mucous membranes or at mucocutaneous junctions (palate, vaginal orifice, perianal area). There is an increase in size and number until the patient is about 1 to 1½ years of age, and then begins an orderly involution (Fig. 166-1). In their declining phases, the lesions first lose mass, with wrinkling of the surface and a more brown color noted, and they then shrink until a flat, or even depressed, scar is formed (by the time the patient is 3 to 5 years old). Skin texture at these sites may remain abnormal for many years (for example, with protrusion if local edema or inflammation occurs from other causes). Without treatment the final cosmetic result is not objectionable.

The clinical story of these patients would really be quite unremarkable (as noted above) were it not for some recently appreciated relationships to more generalized dis-

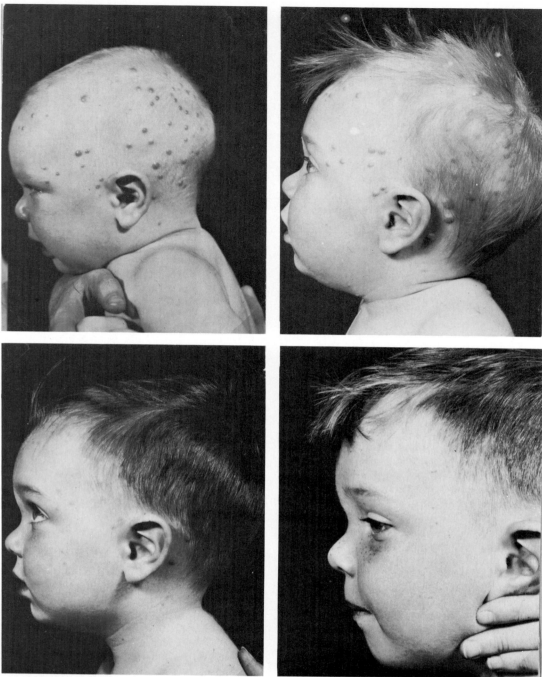

Fig. 166-1 Typical involvement of the scalp and face in juvenile xanthogranuloma. Prominent lesions are noted at 5 months of age (upper left) and 1 year (upper right), with gradual involution by 2 years of age (lower left) and 3 years (lower right).

ease. The vast majority (possibly 90 percent or more) of juvenile xanthogranuloma patients have self-limited cutaneous disease only. Retrospective survey of this patient group, however, has revealed that the majority have café au lait macules, or have relatives who do. With the common base of juvenile xanthogranuloma lesions, café au lait macules, and a family history of some type of neurofibromatosis involvement, one then sees the following kinds of additional difficulties:

1. Further complications of neurofibromatosis (subcutaneous masses, laryngeal tumors, etc.)
2. Minor signs of visceral involvement, probably of a histiocytic type (slight hepatomegaly, minimal pulmonary infiltration, anemia, leukocytosis)
3. More severe signs of myeloproliferative disease, with a peripheral blood picture of monomyeloid leukemia, major hepatosplenomegaly, pulmonary infiltration, etc., occasionally with fatal outcome of a leukemic type

4. Special complications from the xanthomatous lesions, including in the eye (uveal tract, cornea—see [1]), bone, or lung

It is thus evident that normocholesteremic skin xanthomas in infants and young children may have a sporadic origin, resembling that of benign cutaneous tumors, or may arise in a setting of peculiar constitutional disease (related in some fashion to neurofibromatosis). For almost all cases of the latter, the neurofibromatosis is of no clinical importance. For a few patients, however, the final picture may be of critical severity. From the prognostic point of view, one can state that the hematologic abnormalities (and, hence, the threat to survival) will be evident by 1 year of age if this is ever to be expressed. Although the involvement of other family members with features of neurofibromatosis is common, a familial expression of the xanthoma diathesis is extremely rare (less than 1 percent in the author's experience).

Serum lipid measurements in these patients have been uniformly normal, but one may find an increase in blood carotenoid level (perhaps enhancing the orange coloration of the xanthoma lesions) as is common in the infant age group [3,6].

Pathology

The cutaneous lesions show the usual configuration of xanthomas, with a nodular histiocytic proliferation, in a subepidermal location, usually with frank foam cell formation. Direct tissue lipid analysis has shown 1 to 2 percent of the wet weight as cholesterol, with unremarkable phospholipid and glycolipid content. When the fibromatous masses have been studied, their histology has been that of conventional neurofibromatosis.

Differential diagnosis

The appearance of the cutaneous lesions of juvenile xanthogranuloma is so characteristic that biopsy is seldom necessary for diagnosis. No other discrete orange nodular skin lesions occur in this age group. Homozygously abnormal patients with familial hypercholesterolemia may have skin xanthomas as early as 1 year of age, but the distribution of the lesions is quite different (heels, knees, buttocks), and the family history is obvious. Analogous lesions occur in some Letterer-Siwe syndrome patients (perhaps also in reticulohistiocytoma or lipoid dermatoarthritis), but other features of involvement serve to identify the primary problem.

Treatment

No treatment is indicated for the cutaneous xanthomas. Their natural involution produces a much more satisfactory final result than that obtained from any type of operative interference. Radiotherapy is not justified. For the child with very extensive lesions, considerable reassurance may be required. In the rare situation where hematologic abnormalities are present, the program is best directed along conventional lines for leukemia management, particularly involving the use of antitumor agents. This kind of care requires the guidance of specialists.

Xanthoma disseminatum

Definition and historical aspects

The name *xanthoma disseminatum* is properly reserved for a rare syndrome with disseminated nodular xanthomatous lesions of rather particular distribution. These lesions tend to be brown, occurring in clusters in flexor skin folds, as well as in special sites of notable symptomatic significance—the mucosa of the mouth and respiratory tract, the cornea and sclera, and the meninges. Reports of this syndrome also have appeared under the name of xanthoma multiplex. Turner [7] emphasized the severity of the mucosal lesions in a particularly well-illustrated report. The meningeal xanthomas, which often produce the manifestation of diabetes insipidus, have caused some patients of this sort to be reported under the name of Schüller-Christian disease, and a direct analogy is probably appropriate.

Incidence and course

Patients with the fully developed manifestations of this syndrome are infrequently encountered, the result to date totaling fewer than 30 cases. The usual onset of lesions is from early childhood to young adult life, the active course lasting no more than several years. No instances of familial involvement have been reported. The random nature of the syndrome's occurrence and its rarity have allowed no meaningful conjectures to be developed about etiology or conditioning circumstances. Association with neurofibromatosis has not been noted.

Clinical manifestations

The expression of this disease can be clearly divided into regions. The *cutaneous* lesions, usually hundreds in number, are moderately disfiguring or mechanically interfering but not otherwise the source of symptoms (Fig. 166-2) [5,8]. They are firm and of moderate mass (up to 7 to 8 mm in diameter) when freshly developed, later involuting to flattened or even excavated lesions or tablike scarred remnants. The *ocular* lesions are characteristically epibulbar, within the substance of the sclera and/or cornea, and present in these areas as fleshy orange growths (Fig. 166-3). They may extend into the region of central vision and can produce an obstructive blindness [1]. Lesions in the mucosa of the *mouth and upper respiratory tract* are found as pink or orange nodules, occasionally of sufficient number and size to cause hoarseness (larynx) or interference with the airway (trachea and bronchi). The *meningeal* lesions are notable for their strategic infiltration at the base of the skull, where they may produce clinical diabetes insipidus. Seizures, growth retardation, and increases in spinal fluid protein also have been found. Patients qualifying for this diagnosis have not been known to have significant internal visceral involvement.

Pathology

Biopsy studies show a histopathology again of the standard, rather nonspecific xanthoma type—histiocytic proliferation with variable degrees of foam cell formation, and histochemical evidence of moderate intracytoplasmic cho-

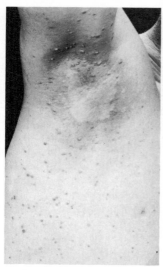
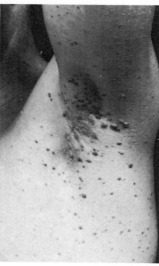

Fig. 166-2   Axillary lesions of xanthoma disseminatum in a 15-year-old male. The depigmented patch in the left axilla signifies a region of temporary suppression of lesions by superficial radiotherapy. This young man also had lesions in the groin, on the eyelids, and on the trunk.

lesterol accumulation. Direct chemical analysis of mature lesions has shown a cholesterol content of about 0.5 percent of the wet weight.

Differential diagnosis

The unique distribution pattern of these xanthomatous nodules (flexor skin creases, especially), plus the special involvement often seen in the eye, mouth, and upper respiratory tract, makes the diagnosis of xanthoma disseminatum obvious in the typical patient. In the early stages, however, one could confuse the skin lesions with verru-

Fig. 166-3   A more extensive distribution of xanthoma disseminatum lesions, with occurrence of xanthomatous nodules in skin creases around the chin, neck, and eyes, plus scleral and corneal involvement in the left eye (see [1]), at age 4 years.

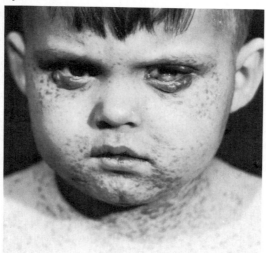

cous growths or molluscum contagiosum. In the adult patient, several other rare syndromes with nodular xanthoma-like lesions of uncertain nosology but with some clinical similarity to xanthoma disseminatum have been described. These include multiple "common histiocytomas," generalized eruptive histiocytoma [9], and disseminated xanthosiderohistiocytosis [10].

Treatment

Xanthoma disseminatum lesions have been difficult to control by antitumor chemotherapy, although theoretically they should be affected by drugs such as the alkylating agents (chlorambucil, etc.). Corticosteroids have not been useful. Superficial radiotherapy will reduce lesion size, but this is not practical for widely distributed involvement. Older lesions can be modified with dermabrasion techniques. The problems attendant upon the corneal involvement present a special challenge [1]. In most instances, the natural involution of lesions provides the most satisfactory result, although the threatening aspect of ocular or respiratory tract pathologic changes may justify a more aggressive approach.

The Letterer-Siwe/Schüller-Christian syndromes

Definition and historical aspects

The most provocative type of histiocytic proliferative disease occurs in those patients qualifying for the "idiopathic" classification of eosinophilic granuloma of bone, Schüller-Christian syndrome, or Letterer-Siwe syndrome. Here one sees a spectrum of increasing extension of histiocytosis, with the final clinical expression determined by largely unknown host factors.

The definition of these disease pictures involves the tabulation of some positive and a number of negative aspects. Basically, one is speaking of a disseminated granulomatous process, where the most significant cytologic participant is the histiocyte. Sharing in the tissue reaction are a number of other responsive cellular classes, including lymphocytes, polymorphonuclear leukocytes (often especially eosinophils), and fibroblasts. A familiar pattern of clinical presentation, seen repeatedly, offers support for this diagnosis, with lesions found especially in the medullary cavity of bone, in nodes, in the skin, and in liver, lung, spleen, and meninges. Inasmuch as the formation of a granuloma can often suggest possible slow osteomyelitis, septic adenopathy, chronic bacterial or fungal pulmonary disease, or secondary hepatic or splenic inflammation, it is mandatory that a consideration of, and search for, possible primary microorganisms be undertaken. The granulomatous disease, as presented here, has never been found to be familial—which suggests that contagion and definite hereditary factors are not pertinent and renders all the more puzzling the variations in patient response. The "idiopathic" aspects of the process are further emphasized by the considerable range in types of disease course and by the potential spontaneous reversibility of even rather severe types of lesion formation.

The original description of this disease process presented individual patients with, respectively, more chronic courses, especially with notable involvement in bone

(Schüller-Christian), or rapid, fatal pictures, with serious internal visceral disease and hematologic abnormalities (Letterer-Siwe). It remained for a series of careful analytic studies in the 1930s and 1940s [11–14] to demonstrate that the pathologic alterations were actually of one basic nature in the acute disease, the chronic, multiple-lesion patient, and even the child with solitary eosinophilic granuloma of bone. This unitary hypothesis has received general acceptance, and the histiocytosis, or reticuloendotheliosis, mantle now customarily covers all patients conforming to the basic pathologic or clinical picture [15]. As will be outlined below, the eponymic designations have limited utility and are based on clinical course only. Taken in the sum, patients of this type are uncommon, but by no means rare, in pediatric practice; adult incidence is infrequent. Males outnumber females by a ratio of about 2:1. There is a universal geographic occurrence of such patients, with no specific epidemiologic aspects.

Clinical manifestations and course

When all patients with so-called idiopathic histiocytic granulomatous disease of bone or viscera are reviewed, one finds a number of recurring clinical pictures, suggesting rather equilibrated expression at a series of levels. Although instances of progression from lesser to more extensive forms of disease are seen, it should be noted that most patients settle into their final level of involvement within the first months, and prognostication about eventual status is ordinarily possible at a relatively early stage [16]. In the absolute sense, there is a nearly continuous spectrum of intensity of disease expression when a large series of patients is surveyed, but some groupings are justified for classification purposes.

1. In about half of the total patient group, lesions develop in the medullary cavity of *bone only* (eosinophilic granulomas), either solitary or multiple. There is some parallel in the distribution of these bone lesions to that of the cutaneous involvement of juvenile xanthogranuloma—namely, that they are primarily axial in orientation (skull, spine, shoulder girdle, and pelvis), and they also occur in the more proximal portions of the extremity bones (femora and humeri).

2. Another group of patients shows comparable *lesions in bone, plus minor evidence of systemic participation* in the granulomatous process (anemia, lesions of skin or mucous membranes, and/or basal meningeal involvement leading to the development of diabetes insipidus). Such patients usually are identified as having Schüller-Christian syndrome.

3. A relatively frequent clinical picture is that of *bone lesions, plus moderate visceral involvement*. In this class, one often finds evidence of pulmonary infiltration (by x-ray), mild hepatomegaly, some adenopathy, destructive lesions around the orbit, middle ears, and base of the skull, limited cutaneous lesions, involvement of the mucous membranes of the mouth, and a seborrhea-like eruption on the scalp. Children with this picture would be labeled as having Schüller-Christian syndrome by some observers or a mild form of Letterer-Siwe syndrome by others.

4. In the most devastating form of clinical expression, signs of *serious visceral disease* develop rather rapidly, with major hepatomegaly or splenomegaly, generalized lymphadenopathy, pulmonary infiltration, fever, anemia, thrombocytopenia, often a leukocytosis (in the earlier phases), and troubling cutaneous eruptions (vesicular, papular, petechial, etc.). These children have a very poor prognosis, and commonly expire with a picture of bone marrow failure and secondary bacterial sepsis. The Letterer-Siwe syndrome terminology is regularly employed in the situation. Destructive lesions of bone may develop, but often the spreading granulomatous involvement of the medullary cavity is documented only by autopsy study.

5. A small group of patients show unusually *aggressive granulomatous disease in a special location,* with relatively mild generalized involvement. Particular problems are seen with localized lateral cervical adenopathy, debilitating reactions in the lungs (with cysts, pneumothorax, etc.), or special involvement of the hepatic parenchyma (with jaundice, pruritus, and hyperlipidemia). For patients of this sort, the Letterer-Siwe syndrome terminology is pertinent.

Within the pediatric age group, there is a tendency for the youngest individuals to show the poorest containment of the reactive pathology—the infant patients commonly showing generalized involvement, the toddlers a moderate type of process, and the older child a bone lesion picture only. Paradoxically, when the disease is expressed in the newborn period the outlook is often quite good. In adult life, the prognostic interpretation is much more difficult, and prolonged courses of indefinite outcome are not infrequent.

Cutaneous lesions

The variety of appearance of the cutaneous manifestations of the generalized histiocytosis syndromes is prodigious. Not infrequently the skin problems are the presenting manifestation, and they may be among the most troubling issues as the course proceeds, as well. The major types of cutaneous involvement are:

1. Small scaly papules, or vesicles, usually seen on the trunk or scalp. They may be of minor nature, easily overlooked, or of more serious degree (Fig. 166-4).
2. Intertriginous eruption, with coalescence, and loss of epidermis in the groin, axillae, behind the ears, etc. These lesions, usually moist and pruritic, are very troublesome, and do not respond to local measures of control (Fig. 166-5).
3. Petechiae, often at first as a light distribution on the trunk (representing multiple small perivascular infiltrations) and then later in a heavy fashion as a thrombocytopenic complication of the papular and vesicular eruption (Fig. 166-6).
4. Scaly and exudative eruption of the scalp, present in mild degree in many patients and severe in some (Fig. 166-7). This annoying and odoriferous involvement, with a moist, inflamed base, also does not respond well to local therapy.
5. Special difficulties in the ear canals, in the perianal area, and at the vaginal orifice, with wet, exudative, pruritic eruption, commonly with superimposed bacterial infection. Involvement of the gingivae also occurs, with inflammation, necrosis, retraction of soft tissues, and loosening of teeth, usually correlating with simultaneous disease of the mandible and maxilla.

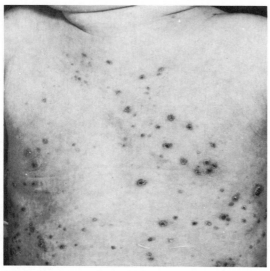

Fig. 166-4 Papular and vesicular lesions on the trunk of a typical Letterer-Siwe syndrome patient, at age 5 months. This is the same child discussed in [17].

6. Xanthomas are found on the skin of these patients, usually relatively late in the course (Fig. 166-5), and ordinarily as de novo nodular lesions [18]. Such xanthomas are clinically indistinguishable from juvenile xanthogranuloma lesions and represent an intriguing demonstration of the underlying correlates in the various histiocytosis syndromes.

Pathology

The cellular pathologic change appears fundamentally reactive rather than inflammatory or malignant. First on a more circumscribed basis and then in many patients in broader distribution, there is evidence of evocation of a histiocytic response. Localized granuloma formation can give way to a diffuse infiltrative proliferation, reminiscent on occasion of the compounding overresponse of an immunologically altered host. Again as mentioned, there is simultaneously a mobilization of eosinophils, other polymorphonuclear leukocytes, lymphocytes, and, to a lesser extent, plasma cells. Some "echelons" of bodily involvement are apparently present—participation of skin, medullary cavity, liver, and lung seem of milder implication, while the activation of significant histiocytosis in deep nodes, intestine, and spleen represents a major phenomenon of more serious importance.

Under favorable circumstances the process can abate, with a fibrotic repair and eventual total involution (as also seen after radiotherapy of a lesion). Microorganisms are found only when the clinical picture also suggests secondary infection. Extensive culturing of fresh lesions by all techniques has not yielded infectious agents. The cellular pathologic process of these idiopathic histiocytosis syndromes requires careful correlation with the clinical findings before a final diagnosis is reached, since no absolute, specific pathologic condition can be claimed. Lesions within the skin (and mucosal areas) show a relatively more diagnostic configuration, with the characteristic clustering

of histiocytes immediately beneath the epidermis. It is considered by most pathologists that the presence of Langerhans-like cells (with Birbeck granules) is a critical element in the diagnosis of idiopathic histiocytosis lesions, particularly in the skin.

There is a tendency in some locations toward the evolution of the histiocytes into lipid-laden foam cells. In both the acute and chronic forms of the syndromes, one can occasionally find extraordinary development of xanthomatous masses in bone, the dura, and thymus. Direct tissue analysis can yield results of up to 5 to 10 percent of the wet weight as cholesterol; triglycerides are also increased, but phospholipid and glycolipid levels are normal. The liver, spleen, lung, and lymph nodes do not share in the lipid modification of the lesions. At the moment, no special interpretations can be given to this remarkable xanthomatosis, and it must be listed merely as an intriguing curiosity, obviously secondary and not of critical diagnostic significance.

Differential diagnosis

The diagnosis of the patient with fully expressed Schüller-Christian or Letterer-Siwe syndrome presents no problem; more puzzling can be the classification of the child with isolated or atypical involvement (see group 5, under "Clinical Manifestations and Course"). In these instances careful attention is needed to rule out the possibility of unusual infection (fungal, atypical acid-fast bacilli, etc.). On occasion there may be temporary confusion with the lymphomas or metastatic solid tumors in children. There are also reticuloendotheliosis syndromes somewhat paralleling the picture of Letterer-Siwe disease, but of familial nature, with serious central nervous system aspects, rapidly fatal courses, and other special signs (see the review in [19]). Cutaneous involvement has not been of a true Letterer-Siwe type in these diseases.

Treatment

There is no specific treatment for the histiocytosis syndromes. For the patient with mild involvement, the course can be expected to be self-limited. Radiotherapy is reserved for the suppression of diabetes insipidus, and for the management of osseous lesions which are unusually large, painful, or in threatening weight-bearing locations. Control of skin lesions cannot be accomplished by local measures, although electron-beam therapy will produce temporary amelioration.

For the patient with disseminated disease, there is no agreement on the most useful treatment plan. Modern supportive therapy, with attention to control of infection and use of transfusion when needed, will assist and may be sufficient. Historically much effort has been given to the use of antitumor agents, and some clinical effects can be achieved in this fashion. Later review has raised doubts about the sustained value of these potentially dangerous medications [20]. If such trials are desired, vinblastine appears to be the most useful (used sparingly), with alkylating agents less so. Combinations of drugs are probably not justified. For the child with serious visceral lesions

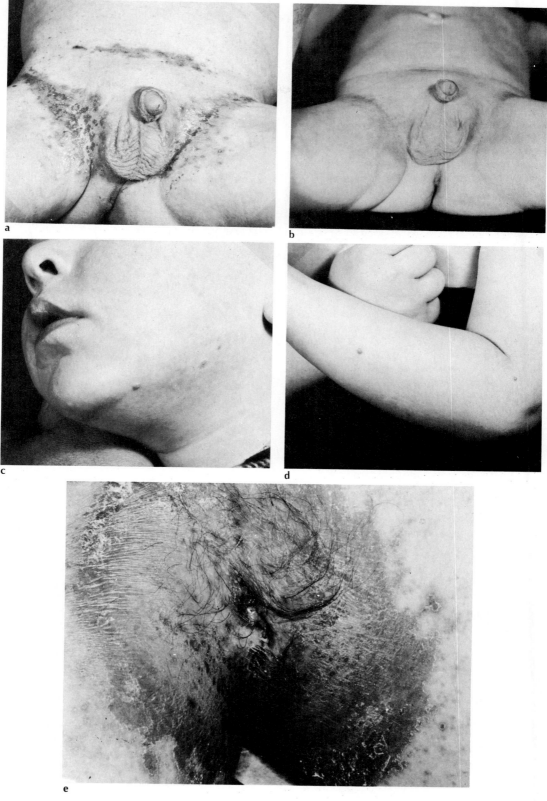

Fig. 166-5 The intertriginous eruption in the groin of a Letterer-Siwe patient at 14 months (a) with healing of these lesions after chlorambucil therapy at 19 months (b). This same boy later showed several isolated cutaneous xanthomas on the chin (c) and forearm (d) at 3 to 3½ years. He is now well, at 21 years of age, except for the persistent handicap of diabetes insipidus. (e) A 53-year-old male who presented with an intertriginous eruption of the axilla. Note the ulceration in the axillary vault. Biopsy of the ulcer revealed histiocytosis. The patient also had eosinophilic granuloma of the vertebra and diabetes insipidus. Treatment with cytotoxic agents arrested the vertebral process and therefore prevented collapse of the vertebra.

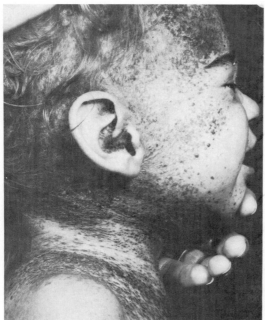
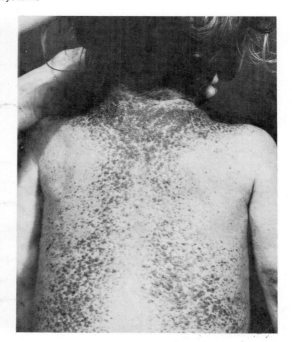

Fig. 166-6 Heavy cutaneous involvement (scaly papules, petechiae) in a 17-month-old child in the terminal phases of Letterer-Siwe syndrome.

(such as major splenomegaly), it is regrettably true that no currently known regime will alter the outcome.

Lipogranulomatosis (Farber's disease)

Definition, historical aspects, and incidence

Farber first reported in 1952 and later described in more detail [21] an unusual syndrome in which histiocytic gran-

Fig. 166-7 Severe exudative and crusting lesions of the scalp in a 5-year-old boy with a clinical diagnosis of Schüller-Christian syndrome. Extensive lesions of bone were also present.

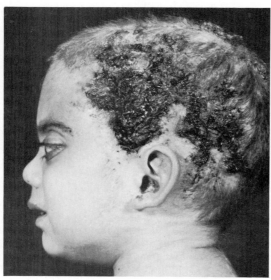

ulomas are found but in which there is an additional inborn error of metabolism. The earliest patients with so-called lipogranulomatosis died in infancy, but it is now known that longer survival is possible. Twenty-seven patients have been reported, two of whom are siblings [22], with a possible increased gene frequency in Azores Islands Portuguese (but not in Portugal). The syndrome has now been shown to have autosomal recessive inheritance.

Clinical manifestations and course

Irritability and hoarseness, plus other signs of arthralgia and arthropathy, usually begin in the early months of life, as does formation of peculiar subcutaneous masses over the wrists and ankles. For these infants growth was poor, gradual general deterioration of condition developed (Fig. 166-8), and death occurred by 4 years of age with inanition and infection. Additional children have shown slower courses, long survival, and more definite cutaneous lesions. One, the patient of Zetterström (Fig. 166-9), died at 16 years of age with serious joint deformities, persistence of his tracheostomy, borderline intelligence (IQ about 80), and the presence of unusual cutaneous nodules [23]. A boy reported in detail from the Children's Hospital in Boston [22] is now 24 years of age, with good growth and no evidence of nervous system involvement, but with masses over the wrists and ankles, some joint restriction, and a peculiar pebbly texture of his skin (Fig. 166-10).

Pathology

As is immediately obvious, there is an intriguing two-phase aspect to the pathology of lipogranulomatosis. On the one hand, there are the basically granulomatous lesions, pre-

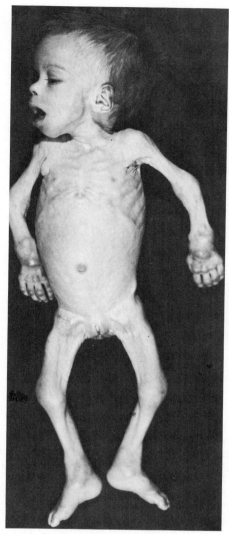

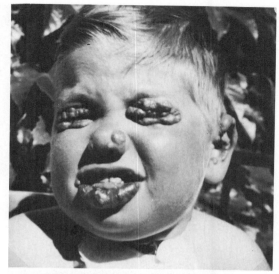

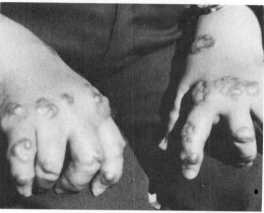

Fig. 166-8   The advanced clinical picture of the lipogranu-lomatosis syndrome, with debility, nutritional failure, and subcutaneous masses over the wrists and ankles, at 13 months of age (death occurred 1 month later). (Reproduced by courtesy of Pergamon Press, Oxford, from [22]).

Fig. 166-9   Appearance of an unusual patient with lipogran-ulomatosis, at 9 years of age, showing cutaneous nodules, joint deformities, and persistent tracheostomy. (Courtesy of Dr. Rolf Zetterström of Stockholm.)

dominantly histiocytic, seen in the skin, subcutaneous tis-sue, tendon sheaths, synovium, and, to some degree, in the viscera (lymph nodes, kidney, liver, and spleen). In these loci, one also finds some foam cell formation, with an accumulation of ceramide, and a specific deficiency of tissue acid ceramidase levels [24]. In addition, however, there is the central nervous system pathology of distended neurons in gray matter and retina, of the type characteristic of the inborn error metabolic syndromes [22].

It is now felt that the entire syndrome is best explained as an expression of acid ceramidase deficiency. This en-zymatic aberration has been found consistently in cultured skin fibroblasts and in white blood cells. Partial deficiency has been identified in obligate heterozygotes, and prenatal diagnosis has been possible by studies on fetal cells. The origin of the histiocytic granuloma formation (skin, tendon sheaths, etc.) is puzzling; one hypothesis considers these to be reactive to local ceramide accumulation.

Differential diagnosis

The presence of the characteristic subcutaneous masses over the wrists and ankles remains a unique diagnostic feature of this syndrome. A limited similarity can be seen in lipoid dermatoarthritis or reticulohistiocytoma, but no serious confusion would exist. The specific diagnosis is established by analysis for acid ceramidase in white blood cells or cultured skin fibroblasts.

Treatment

No rational approach to the therapy of lipogranulomatosis exists at this time. It is unlikely that the fundamental bio-chemical abnormality will be correctable by current meth-ods. The possibility exists that the integumental and syn-ovial histiocytic granulomas may be suppressed by antitumor chemotherapy (e.g., chlorambucil; see [22]); corticosteroid therapy and radiotherapy have not been use-ful.

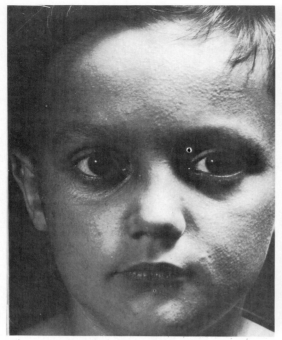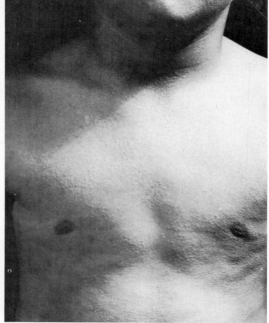

Fig. 166-10   Irregular texture of the skin in a 7-year-old boy with a relatively mild involvement in the lipogranulomatosis syndrome (see [22]).

References

1. Liebman SD et al: Corneal xanthomas in childhood. *Arch Ophthalmol* **76:**221, 1966
2. Helwig EB, Hackney VC: Juvenile xanthogranuloma (nevo-xantho-endothelioma). *Am J Pathol* **30:**625, 1954
3. Crocker AC: Skin xanthomas in childhood. *Pediatrics* **8:**573, 1951
4. Nomland R: Nevoxantho-endothelioma: benign xanthomatous disease of infants and children. *J Invest Dermatol* **22:**207, 1954
5. Thannhauser SJ: *Lipidoses: Diseases of the Intracellular Lipid Metabolism,* 3d ed. New York, Grune & Stratton, 1958
6. Crocker AC: Pigmentation in the lipidoses, in *Pigments in Pathology,* edited by M Wolman, New York, Academic Press, 1969, p 287
7. Turner AL: A case of xanthoma tuberosum with extensive distribution of the xanthomatous nodules on the mucous membrane of the respiratory tract. *J Laryngol Otol* **40:**249, 1925
8. Braun-Falco O, Braun-Falco F: Zum Syndrom "Diabetes insipidus und disseminierte Xanthome." *Z Laryngol Rhinol Otol* **36:**378, 1957
9. Winklemann RK, Muller SA: Generalized eruptive histiocytoma. *Arch Dermatol* **88:**586, 1963
10. Halprin KM, Lorincz AL: Disseminated xanthosiderohistiocytosis. *Arch Dermatol* **82:**63, 1960
11. Fraser J: Skeletal lipoid granulomatosis (Hand-Schüller-Christian's disease). *Br J Surg* **22:**800, 1935
12. Green WT, Farber S: "Eosinophilic or solitary granuloma" of bone. *J Bone Joint Surg* **24:**499, 1942
13. Farber S: The nature of "solitary or eosinophilic granuloma" of bone. *Am J Pathol* **17:**625, 1941
14. Wallgren A: Systemic reticuloendothelial granuloma: non-lipoid reticuloendotheliosis and Schüller-Christian disease. *Am J Dis Child* **60:**471, 1940
15. Crocker AC: The histiocytosis syndromes, in *Textbook of Pediatrics,* 11th ed, edited by VC Vaughan III et al. Philadelphia, WB Saunders, 1979, p 1983
16. Avery ME et al: The course and prognosis of reticuloendotheliosis (eosinophilic granuloma, Schüller-Christian disease, and Letterer-Siwe disease). *Am J Med* **22:**636, 1957
17. Griesemer R, Crocker AC: Letterer-Siwe disease. *Arch Dermatol* **92:**474, 1965
18. Altman J, Winkelmann RK: Xanthomatous cutaneous lesions of histiocytosis X. *Arch Dermatol* **87:**164, 1963
19. Miller DR: Familial reticuloendotheliosis: concurrence of disease in five siblings. *Pediatrics* **38:**986, 1966
20. Greenberger JS et al: Results of treatment of 127 patients with systemic histiocytosis. *Medicine (Baltimore)* **60:**311, 1981
21. Farber S et al: Lipogranulomatosis: a new lipo-glyco-protein storage disease. *J Mount Sinai Hosp NY* **24:**816, 1957
22. Crocker AC et al: The "lipogranulomatosis" syndrome, in *Inborn Disorders of Sphingolipid Metabolism,* edited by SM Aronson, BW Volk. Oxford, Pergamon Press, 1966, p 485
23. Zetterström R: Disseminated lipogranulomatosis (Farber's disease). *Acta Paediatr* **47:**501, 1958 (plus personal communication, 1966)
24. Moser HW, Chen WW: Ceramidase deficiency: Farber's lipogranulomatosis, in *The Metabolic Basis of Inherited Disease,* 5th ed, edited by JB Stanbury et al. New York, McGraw-Hill, 1983, p 820

CUTANEOUS MANIFESTATIONS OF HEPATOBILIARY DISEASE

Imrich Sarkany

An association has been well recognized for centuries between the skin and the liver (Fig. 167-1). It has been taken over by folklore, which in the Middle Ages labeled females with various vascular skin blemishes as witches, still accepts a "bottle-nose" as a sign of an alcoholic with liver trouble, and describes a variety of pigmented skin lesions as "liver spots." Even the term *spider* is said to have originated in the New York underworld where barmaids spotted "spiders" as evidence of advanced liver disease in their customers.

It must be stressed that the vascular, pigmentary, allergic, nail, and hair changes found in the skin of patients with hepatobiliary disease may also occur in its absence or in association with physiologic states. For example, spider nevi may be seen in normal children and in pregnancy. Conversely, there may be no visible skin changes in patients with severe or advanced liver disease and dramatic cutaneous manifestations may be seen with minimal hepatic dysfunction. Severe itching may antedate other features of biliary cirrhosis by months or years. In chronic alcoholics with little or no liver disease, hypogonadism may be responsible in male alcoholics for a number of abnormal sexual changes including reduced beard growth, loss of libido and potency, testicular atrophy, and reduced fertility. Similarly, hyperestrogenism in male alcoholics, even in the absence of cirrhosis, may manifest itself with gynecomastia, vascular spiders, and changes in body hair and fat distribution [1].

Several types of interaction between the skin and the liver are possible:

1. Liver disease may cause skin changes. Primary disorders of hepatic synthetic, excretory, conjugating, or regulatory functions may induce structural and functional changes in the skin and its appendages. Jaundice, itching, pigmentary abnormalities, and alterations in nails and hair fall into this category. These are the cutaneous changes best recognized by physicians as contributing to an early diagnosis of disease of the hepatobiliary tract.

2. Skin disease may cause liver abnormalities. Disturbances of metabolism as a consequence of skin disease are less well known but they have been documented. Abnormalities of serum proteins in erythroderma, gynecomastia, and hepatomegaly in exfoliative dermatitis are consequent upon severe skin involvement. These changes have been aptly called the metabolic cost of skin disease. Serum protein abnormalities commonly found in erythroderma from eczema or psoriasis have for long been thought to be associated with some concurrent systemic disorder, particularly hepatic dysfunction. On the other hand, hypoalbuminemia was considered to be the result of excessive protein loss due to scales shed in exfoliative disease [2,3]. The first convincing evidence that protein abnormalities were due to the skin disease was given by Bauer [4] when he showed that they could be reversed by treatment of the rash. However, Shuster and Wilkinson [5] suggested that the low serum albumin in these cases was due to dilution of the plasma volume consequent on the hemodynamic changes induced by skin disease, and only to a lesser extent due to protein loss through the skin and gut. They, therefore, claimed that significant albumin depletion did not occur in these patients and that the most important factor in the production of their hypoalbuminemia was dilution in the plasma and expansion of the extravascular albumin space. Decreased serum albumin and increased serum globulin concentrations were not considered to be the result of hepatic abnormality. Similarly, folic acid deficiency in patients with skin disease has recently been shown not to be due to hepatic dysfunction in which urinary FIGLU (formiminoglutamic acid) may also be increased. In patients with liver disease the abnormal FIGLU excretion cannot be corrected by folate administration, whereas in patients with skin disease, FIGLU excretion returns to normal after resaturation with folic acid [6,7], suggesting that the skin patients have a true folate deficiency.

3. The skin and liver are involved by the same pathologic process, as seen, for example, in xanthomatosis or histiocytosis.

4. Inherited factors can be responsible for involvement of the liver, skin adnexa, and other organs, as in argininosuccinic aciduria or some reported cases of xeroderma pigmentosum.

5. Skin, liver, and bone can be affected by exposure to chemicals, as seen in vinyl chloride disease, leading to scleroderma-like cutaneous changes, hepatitis, angiosarcoma of the liver, and acroosteolysis. When skin lesions occur in association with liver disease, they are generally not specific of any particular type of hepatic pathology, but the most florid cutaneous lesions are generally seen in patients with chronic active hepatitis and in alcoholics.

Jaundice

Jaundice, or icterus, is the generalized yellow or ocher coloration of skin, mucous membranes, and other body tissues imparted by the bile pigment bilirubin. Both jaundice and pigmentation are most prominent with obstruction and primary biliary cirrhosis. Clinically detectable jaundice is always indicative of disease and must, therefore, be distinguished by clinical examination and chemical methods from simple olive or sallow skin complexions, benign carotenemia, and the yellowish skin pigmentation pro-

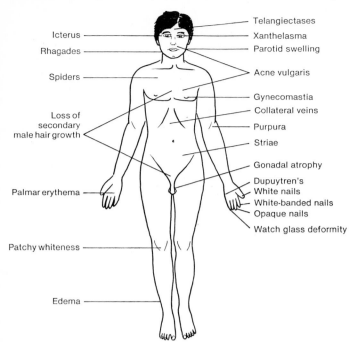

Icterus

Rhagades

Spiders

Loss of
secondary
male hair growth

Palmar erythema

Patchy whiteness

Edema

Telangiectases

Xanthelasma

Parotid swelling

Acne vulgaris

Gynecomastia

Collateral veins

Purpura

Striae

Gonadal atrophy

Dupuytren's

White nails

White-banded nails

Opaque nails

Watch glass deformity

Fig. 167-1   Main skin changes in liver disease.

duced by quinacrine and busulfan. Finally, prolonged ingestion of large volumes of tomato juice may produce lycopenemia, a benign orange staining of skin, palms, and soles due to deposition of lycopene, a carotene-like pigment. Overt jaundice may appear in the course of any disease that produces significant hyperbilirubinemia, as noted below, but most often accompanies disorders of the hepatobiliary system.

Pathogenesis

Jaundiced skin, varying in hue from faint golden to dark greenish yellow, results from increased local cellular or connective tissue binding of the tetrapyrrole bilirubin (or its metabolites). The tissue pigment, which has a special affinity for elastin, is derived from the perfusing blood and lymph, circulating almost exclusively as a tightly bound complex with serum albumin (2 moles of bilirubin per mole of protein). The elevated serum bilirubin level results, in turn, from a dynamic imbalance between overall pigment production and excretion, varying rapidly and widely as the balance changes in the course of disease or therapy.

The tissue–serum equilibration, or exchange, is slower, however, and the intensity of clinical icterus often fails to reflect accurately the concurrent serum bilirubin level. This simple fact explains the observations that hyperbilirubinemia may antedate the onset of detectable jaundice in acute hepatitis or biliary obstruction by one or more days and that, conversely, scleral and cutaneous icterus may persist despite falling or normal serum bilirubin levels. Local changes in vascular permeability may "sequester" bile pigment or impair its equilibration with the general circulation—hence, the occasional finding of jaundice of different intensity in areas of edema. The correlation between cutaneous staining and serum pigment levels is especially poor in newborn infants.

Finally, further discrepancy between tissue and serum pigment levels in infants may result from the administration of drugs such as sulfisoxazole and salicylates, compounds which apparently uncouple protein-bound bilirubin and favor its passage into body tissues [8]. Clinically detectable jaundice appears, therefore, when sufficient bilirubin has become tissue bound, generally implying in adults that total serum levels have exceeded 2.5 to 3.0 mg/dL (normally less than 1.5 mg/dL) over a period of days. Jaundice is often not obvious in newborn infants until serum levels reach 6.0 to 8.0 mg/dL (1 mg = 17 μmol/L).

Etiology

Significant elevations in serum bilirubin levels precede clinical jaundice and imply an imbalance between pigment production and excretion. Between 80 and 90 percent of bilirubin entering the circulation of normal adults is derived from red cell hemoglobin degradation within the reticuloendothelial system; the remainder arises from red cell precursors in the marrow and from nonhemoglobin heme compounds in the liver. This newly formed pigment is albumin-bound, unconjugated, and reacts only slightly (and "indirectly") with the standard diazo reagent. Within the normal adult liver, which has a metabolic reserve that permits disposal of fivefold increases in pigment production without the development of jaundice, unconjugated and albumin-free pigment is coupled by microsomal enzymes with glucuronic acid, transported to bile canaliculi, and excreted actively as the water-soluble diglucuronide that reacts "directly" with the diazo reagent [9].

No current etiologic classification of jaundice is complete or physiologically sound, but a functional approach based on the simple diazo measurement (Van den Bergh reaction) of conjugated and total serum bilirubin concentrations has some merit (Table 167-1). Thus, most types of clinical jaundice are caused either predominantly by overproduction or underconjugation of bilirubin (with less than 15 percent conjugated, or "direct-reacting," pigment in the serum) or predominantly by liver cell damage and impaired excretion (with greater than 15 percent conjugated pigment in the serum).

Clinical features

Jaundice is a cardinal sign of disease and always requires careful evaluation. Its onset, evolution, and implications depend on the underlying disease process. Hyperbilirubinemia and cutaneous icterus produce neither symptoms nor harmful effects in adults.

Slight jaundice is frequently unremarked by patients and family; poor lighting, dark skin coloration, and subtle progression often combine to delay the clinical diagnosis for days or weeks. Careful inspection of peripheral ocular sclerae in natural or bluish light is the best clinical method for detecting minimal jaundice, the high elastic tissue content of the sclerae apparently accounting for this preferential staining. Prolonged and deep jaundice may assume a greenish-tan quality, the result perhaps of melanosis and partial oxidation of bilirubin to biliverdin.

Finally, the intensity of jaundice and levels of serum bilirubin in patients with biliary atresia, acquired bile duct obstruction, or defective bilirubin conjugation tend to sta-

Table 167-1 Functional classification of jaundice

Unconjugated ("indirect") hyperbilirubinemia:
  Newborn and infant
    "Physiologic"—functional hepatic immaturity
    Hemolysis—Rh, ABO, sepsis, drug factors
    Prematurity
    Transient familial hyperbilirubinemia—maternal steroid
      inhibitors
    Crigler-Najjar—glucuronyl transferase deficiency
      (hereditary)
  Adult
    Excess bilirubin production
      Hemolysis
        Congenital
        Acquired
      Dyserythropoietic—"shunt" hyperbilirubinemia
    Deficient conjugation
      Familial
        Constitutional hepatic dysfunction (Gilbert's
          syndrome)
        Crigler-Najjar type II
      Acquired
        Posthepatic
        Associated disease—cardiac, enteric, metabolic
        Drug-induced
  Diagnostic features
    Serum-conjugated bilirubin less than 15 percent of total
    Absence of bilirubinuria
    Low to normal urine urobilinogen
    Absence of other liver function disturbances
    Normal morphologic features of liver
Conjugated ("direct-reacting") hyperbilirubinemia:
  Hepatic cell damage
    Acute—viral, toxic, anoxic, metabolic
    Chronic—cirrhosis, metabolic
  Impaired bile excretion
    Extrahepatic obstruction
    Intrahepatic cholestasis—atresias, viral, drugs,
      hormones, pregnancy, benign recurrent cholestasis
    Familial (defect confined to bilirubin excretion)
    Dubin-Johnson—excretory defect and cell pigment
    Rotor—excretory defect and no pigment
  Diagnostic features
    Serum-conjugated bilirubin more than 15% of total
    Bilirubinuria common
    Urine urobilinogen often elevated
    Other liver functions often abnormal in hepatic cell
      damage and impaired bile excretion
    Characteristic morphologic abnormalities of liver

bilize despite continued pigment production; the fate or disposition of the excess pigment is still uncertain. Some degradation of bilirubin has been shown to occur with exposure to ultraviolet radiation. This is the basis for phototherapy of babies to prevent kernicterus in severe neonatal jaundice. It is suggested that the colorless breakdown products are excreted in the urine. The urine becomes dark yellow and then tea colored as conjugated serum bilirubin exceeds an inconstant "threshold" value of 0.4 to 0.6 mg/dL and escapes into the urine. Bilirubinuria is not a feature of unconjugated hyperbilirubinemic states. Since most of the brown color of normal feces is produced by urobilins derived from degradation of bilirubin in the intestine, the jaundice of impaired pigment excretion or bile obstruction is associated typically with gray or tan "clay-colored" stools.

Diagnosis

The precise diagnosis of jaundice requires methodical consideration of all factors that may induce hyperbilirubinemia by overproduction, impaired transport and/or conjugation, faulty secretion, or blocked excretion of bilirubin (Table 167-1). Careful history and clinical examination should indicate the underlying disease in 60 to 70 percent of cases; cautious interpretation of a selected group of liver function tests should afford a diagnosis in another 10 to 15 percent; special procedures such as needle biopsy of the liver, radiographic studies of the biliary tree, measurement of red blood cell survival, ultrasound, CT scan and possibly laparoscopy may be required to establish a definitive diagnosis in the remainder.

Treatment and course

Jaundice relating to acute hepatitis will resolve spontaneously and no specific measures are needed. A small percentage of patients with acute hepatitis, predominantly those with hepatitis type A, may enter a cholestatic phase with jaundice and severe itching. These patients may be "whitewashed" by a short course of systemic steroids which does not in any way affect the healing of the liver lesion, but will make the patients feel considerably better. The jaundice of chronic liver disease may also improve when the underlying liver involvement improves. In the alcoholic, this is achieved by abstinence from alcohol, so that jaundice is only rarely seen in alcoholics with inactive cirrhosis. Equally, patients with chronic active hepatitis will lose their jaundice to a large extent following successful therapy with steroids. Patients with primary biliary cirrhosis may also show lessening of jaundice following treatment with penicillamine. The jaundice of biliary obstruction will resolve when the obstruction is relieved. In addition to phototherapy in babies, help may be offered to patients with Gilbert's and the Crigler-Najjar syndromes. In these, benign unconjugated hyperbilirubinemia is found in association with otherwise normal liver function. Treatment with microsomal enzyme inducers, such as phenobarbitone, will result in a lowering of the bilirubinemia and subsequent cosmetic benefit.

Melanosis

Apart from the yellow color of jaundice and the deep green of long-standing jaundice, there are other color changes of diagnostic value in chronic liver disease. These may be diffuse or circumscribed. A *diffuse* darkening of the skin giving rise to a muddy gray color in patients with long-standing cirrhosis is essentially due to melanin deposition in the epidermis, especially in the basal layer. This diffuse grayish pigmentation may assume a yellowish tinge in the presence of jaundice and the deposition in the skin of hemosiderin.

Melanin pigmentation of the skin in primary biliary cirrhosis initially involves exposed areas but gradually becomes generalized. It is a common feature in this disease, it may be an early presenting sign, and it can become clinically obtrusive [10]. This impressive pigmentation rarely occurs in other forms of chronic liver disease and is not a feature of secondary biliary cirrhosis. Blotchy circumscribed areas of dirty brown pigmentation in irregular distribution are also occasionally seen. Accentuation of normal freckling and of areolar pigmentation may appear. Localized linear pigmentation may be found in the creases of the fingers and of the palms. A special form of *circumscribed* pigmentation may occur in perioral and periorbital areas where darkening of the skin resembles chloasma of pregnancy and has been described by older clinicians as chloasma hepaticum and which the French call *masque biliaire* [11]. Facial chloasma in a man or a nonpregnant woman should alert the clinician to the possibility that it may be a manifestation of liver disease. Other etiologic factors must, of course, be borne in mind, which in women include pigmentation caused by the contraceptive pill and exogenously induced pigmentation from certain photosensitizing chemicals contained in facial creams and perfumes.

Patchy depigmentation [12] refers to white pea-sized flecks—guttate hypomelanosis on the skin of the buttocks, back, thighs, and forearms which is sometimes seen in cirrhosis and which may be associated with spiders. These paler patches may be uniformly depigmented or there may be a central spider. It has been suggested that these pale flecks are analogous to the white flecks seen in individuals with spiders, including pregnant women who may develop white patches in areas of vascular spiders due to vasoconstriction as a response to cold.

Hemochromatosis is an inherited condition in which excess iron is deposited in the liver, pancreas, heart, and joints. Skin pigmentation is striking in this condition to such an extent that its alternative name is bronze diabetes. The metallic gray or bronze-brown color of hemochromatosis is usually generalized [13] and buccal mucosal and conjunctival pigmentation may also be present in 20 percent of cases.

Etiology and pathogenesis

The etiology and pathogenesis of various forms of hyperpigmentation in chronic liver disease are obscure. The generalized brownish pigmentation, usually gradual in onset, slowly progressive, and related to advancing liver disease, suggests a humoral mechanism, perhaps comparable to that seen in spontaneous or experimental ACTH or MSH excess [14] although MSH levels are not raised in liver disease.

A different mechanism for pigmentation in biliary cirrhosis was postulated by Burton and Kirby [15]. They showed that bile salts caused itching when applied to blister bases in normal subjects and postulated that cytotoxic properties of bile salts caused the release of proteolytic enzymes which are known to be potent pruritogens. Proteolytic enzymes are also known to activate epidermal tyrosinases, possibly by splitting a small blocking peptide from the inactive precursor, prototyrosinase, and this may produce pigmentation. They suggested that the continued release of low concentrations of proteolytic enzymes in the skin due to nonspecific cytotoxic effects of bile salts could account for both the pigmentation and the pruritus of patients with chronic obstructive jaundice.

In a recent study of the relation of bile acids to pruritus, no correlation was found between serum or interstitial fluid total bile acid or individual bile acid concentrations and pruritus. A decrease in serum bile acid concentrations achieved by percutaneous transhepatic biliary drainage had little or no effect on pruritus and it was concluded that bile acids had no causative role in the pruritus of cholestatic liver disease [16].

A histologic and ultrastructural study of cutaneous pigmentation in primary biliary cirrhosis [17] has claimed that the pigmentation was due to excess melanin which is widely dispersed throughout the epidermis, often accumulating into giant compound melanosomes, and frequently spilling over into the dermis. No deposits of stainable iron were observed. Similar changes were seen in one patient with alcoholic cirrhosis and skin pigmentation. Compared with skin from matched sites from control patients with alcoholic cirrhosis and no pigmentation, the melanocyte:keratinocyte ratio was not significantly higher in primary biliary cirrhosis. However, in the latter, melanosomes persisted to unusually high levels in the epidermis and were packaged in larger membrane-bound clusters than in controls. It was not clear whether the excess melanin resulted from increased melanogenesis or defective melanin degradation. No hormonal (β-MSH and ACTH) or chemical (bile salt irritation) stimuli were shown to increase melanogenesis.

In hemochromatosis, faulty intestinal absorption of iron and a failure of the mucosal block results in increased absorption of iron and its deposition in the skin, liver, heart, pancreas, and endocrine organs. The darkening is generalized but is most marked over sun-exposed areas and in traumatized skin. The mucosal surfaces of the mouth and eyes are occasionally affected. The pigmentation is not caused by the presence of hemosiderin in the skin, but is produced by melanin. In the skin, iron, melanin, and lipofuscin are histochemically demonstrable. Hemosiderin granules are seen inconstantly in macrophages within the dermis and its appendages, perhaps contributing to the slate-gray quality of hemochromatotic skin [18]. Others [13] have stressed the high incidence of ichthyosis-like states and koilonychia, and the presence of siderosis in eccrine sweat glands has been claimed to be of diagnostic help. Postphlebotomy, histologic siderosis, and clinical skin pigmentation decreased, whereas melanosis remained histologically unchanged.

Hepatic iron stores and markers of iron overload in alcoholics and in patients with idiopathic hemochromatosis were investigated [19] and it was concluded that liver iron concentration remained the best way of assessing iron stores in these two groups of patients. It was shown that liver iron concentrations were elevated in approximately one-third of alcoholics, irrespective of liver damage, but there was no overlap with values found in patients with idiopathic hemochromatosis.

Perdrup and Poulsen [20] provided further evidence that increased pigmentation in hemochromatosis was caused by melanin and not iron. In a patient who had both vitiligo and hemochromatosis, they showed that while histochemically there was iron in the white area of vitiligo as well as in the remainder of the skin, the vitiliginous areas remained completely white due to the absence of melanin in them while the remainder of the skin showed hyperpigmentation as a result of excess melanin pigment.

Other cutaneous pigmentary changes associated with liver disease may be due to derangement of porphyrin or cholesterol metabolism. In porphyria cutanea tarda, the light-exposed parts of the body, particularly the face, neck, and dorsa of the hands, are subject to blister formation, bruising, and excoriations. The healed sites show residual pigmentation which is usually accompanied by various degrees of general melanin hyperpigmentation on the face and hands. Hypertrichosis in the periorbital and malar regions and ecchymoses on the forearms are often present. The yellow- and orange-colored lesions of xanthomatosis and xanthelasma are common in biliary cirrhosis, especially in the primary form. These changes are also frequently seen in the absence of liver disease. While pigmentation is usually seen late in the course of liver disease, this is not invariable. The main exceptions are primary biliary cirrhosis and hemochromatosis, which show pigmentation early. However, both have a relatively good prognosis.

Diagnosis and management of pigmentation

In the differential diagnosis of generalized pigmentation related to hepatobiliary disease, certain endocrinopathies and chronic debilitating diseases should be considered. Primary adrenal insufficiency (Addison's disease) and certain pituitary tumors may produce weakness, wasting, pigmentary changes of the skin and mucous membranes, hair loss, etc. Appropriate tests showing intact endocrine function and the presence of physical signs and liver-function abnormalities should confirm the association of the melanosis with cirrhosis. Similarly, debilitating diseases such as lymphoma, tuberculosis, and malabsorption syndromes may produce weakness, pigmentation, and hepatic dysfunction. Awareness of these associations and appropriate tests should help to ascertain whether the liver disease is the primary cause of the skin changes. Liver biopsy is essential in making the diagnosis, and in a number of conditions, as, for example, in iron-storage disease, liver biopsy specimens stained for hemosiderin are much more certain indicators of iron storage than are skin, marrow, or urinary sediment preparations. Chemical estimations of liver iron are the surest guide to diagnosis [19].

Once the liver is chronically damaged as in cirrhosis, it will never regain normal structure [21]. However, the liver cells retain such an enormous regenerative capacity that functional compensation may be attained. Bed rest in acute cases, control of alcoholism, improved nutrition, selective use of steroid hormones, and surgical correction of mechanical biliary obstruction may arrest or reverse the severity of the secondary cutaneous changes.

Vascular changes

The skin of patients with chronic liver disease often shows telangiectatic changes, mainly over the areas of the body exposed to light, i.e., the face, neck, forearms, and hands. They resemble the vascular changes not infrequently seen in, for example, sailors and farmers whose skin is damaged by the sun and wind. Numerous tiny telangiectases sometimes give the impression of a diffuse, almost exanthematic redness [12] and are known as "dollar paper markings," since they resemble the small threads in paper money held up against light. These fine telangiectatic changes fade on pressure with a glass slide and rarely pulsate. Minimal

dilatation of venules is the most likely cause of these diffuse vascular changes.

Spider nevus

The vascular spider, arterial spider, or spider angioma is the most representative and classical vascular lesion of chronic liver disease, although it may be seen also in alcoholics without liver involvement [1]. It derives its name from its resemblance to a spider because it consists of a central arteriole which is represented by a red point from which numerous small twisted vessels radiate outward. The arterial spider is bright red and ranges in size from a pinhead to 2 cm (Fig. 167-2). When sufficiently large it can be seen or felt to pulsate, especially when pressed with a glass slide. Pressure on the central arteriole with the head of a pin or a matchstick causes blanching of the whole lesion, including its branches, as would be expected from an arterial structure. Because the spider contains red arterial blood, it is not demonstrable by infrared photography [21]. Spider nevi are most commonly present on the face, the necklace area, forearms, hands, and the upper part of the chest, i.e., mainly over the region drained by the superior vena cava, and only rarely below a line joining the nipples. They are rarely found in mucous membranes of the nose, mouth, and pharynx. They fade after death [22,23]. Spider nevi may be seen in 10 percent of the

Fig. 167-2 Reconstruction of a spider nevus.

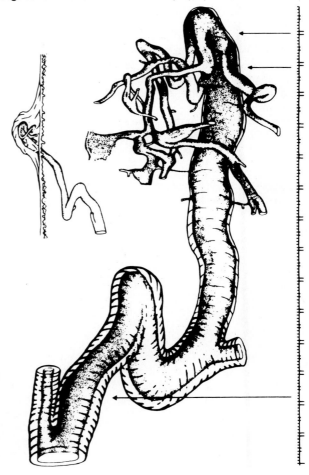

normal general population and not infrequently in children of all ages, but mostly just before puberty. In children, 1 to 3 lesions are common. The most usual site is on the nose or just below the eye. They may appear in large numbers in pregnancy and generally disappear rapidly after parturition, although some lesions may persist. With or without palmar erythema, they may also be seen in thyrotoxicosis, rheumatoid arthritis, with estrogen therapy, and after taking the contraceptive pill. A familial incidence of spider nevi without underlying disease has also been reported. Regression of spiders in liver disease is possible with improvement of the underlying condition. Persistence of the lesions is more likely. However, spiders are functionally reversible. It is not clear whether the central artery is obliterated when they disappear or whether it persists morphologically but simply fails to fill because the filling pressure in it is no longer sufficient. In some patients with hereditary hemorrhagic telangiectasia (Osler's disease), cirrhosis may also be present. A number of cases of unilateral nevoid telangiectasia associated with chronic liver disease are on record, although this vascular anomaly may also be of congenital origin or it may be related to pregnancy, hormonal changes, and estrogen therapy. It has also been suggested that unilateral nevoid telangiectasia and liver disease could be manifestations of a disease involving skin and liver vessels, as in hereditary hemorrhagic telangiectasia [24]. The selective distribution of vascular spiders is not understood. Traditionally, vascular spiders and palmar erythema [21] have been attributed to estrogen excess. They are also found in pregnancy when circulating estrogens are increased. Estrogens have an enlarging, dilating effect on the spiral arterioles of the endometrium and this mechanism may explain the closely similar cutaneous spiders in men [25], although this does not usually occur, when estrogen therapy is given for prostatic carcinoma. Although the liver inactivates estrogens, there are many difficulties in explaining the relationship of the vascular spiders in liver disease.

The blood pressure in these small arteries has been measured at 50 to 70 mm Hg; the temperature is 2 to 3°C higher than that of surrounding skin. Morphologic studies with the help of reconstruction methods [26] have demonstrated that spiders represent an arterial end organ in which five separate parts can be distinguished: (1) a cutaneous arterial net, (2) the central spider arteriole, (3) a subepidermal ampulla, (4) a star-shaped arrangement of efferent spider vessels, and (5) capillaries. Martini and Staubesand [27] have demonstrated that the central spider comes from the subcutis, winds up to the epidermis, and there branches out as an end artery. The efferent branches of the dilated arteriole show no evidence of a transition into veins. The spider is not to be considered, therefore, an arteriovenous anastomotic structure. The structure of the wall of the central artery is striking in that its media is considerably thicker on one side than on the opposite side. The muscular component of the vessel wall disappears as it approaches the surface; it gradually resembles a vein, and just below the epidermis it gives the impression of a dilated vascular bed whose wall is formed by a thin endothelial tube.

Palmar erythema

Palmar erythema or liver palm occurs in two clinical forms. In the first variety (Fig. 167-3), there is an exaggeration of normal mottling, the hands are warm and bright red in color especially in the palm, dorsa of the hands, fingers, and base of nails. The second type shows well-demarcated redness of the hypothenar eminence which gradually spreads to other parts of the hand [28]. The soles of the feet may show similar changes. The mottling blanches on pressure and, when a glass slide is pressed on the palm, it flushes synchronously with the pulse rate [21]. The patient may complain of throbbing or tingling palms. "Liver palms" occur not only in liver disease, but similar appearances are also seen in pregnancy and in a number of chronic diseases such as chronic polyarthritis, chronic lung disease, and subacute bacterial endocarditis, i.e., in diseases with a marked increase in globulins [12]. Palmar erythema has also been reported with chronic febrile diseases, chronic leukemia, and thyrotoxicosis. It has been suggested that palmar erythema in liver disease and pregnancy is due to hyperestrogenism. Liver palms are less

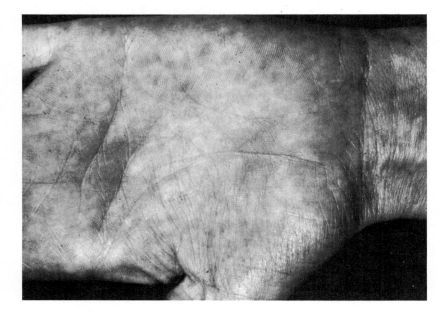

Fig. 167-3 Palmar erythema or "liver palms" showing the characteristic mottling and blotchy redness.

common in chronic liver disease than are spider nevi. Occasionally, palmar erythema has been ascribed to the ingestion of the higher-estrogen-content contraceptive pill. In a number of individuals, the characteristic mottling and blotchy redness are of no clinical significance and no abnormality can be demonstrated. Finally, palmar flushing may be familial and unassociated with liver disease.

Other vascular changes

Corkscrew scleral vessels, i.e., tortuous small arteries that traverse the margins of the ocular sclerae, have been described in many patients with chronic liver disease and have been thought to indicate increased local cutaneous arterial perfusion and vasodilatation [W. A. Tisdale and R. C. Williams, unpublished observations, 1960]. The pathogenesis of all the vascular changes in cirrhosis is not understood, but it has been claimed that cardiac output is frequently increased, total peripheral resistance may be decreased, and arteriovenous shunting may occur within the lungs, liver, and extremities [29]. The various vascular phenomena such as spiders, palmar erythema, etc., could be explained on the basis of actual structural arteriovenous shunts or as a result of functional alterations.

In portal hypertension, whether associated with cirrhosis or noncirrhotic liver disease or with portal vein block, portal systemic collateral vessels may develop and may be an important clue to the existence of portal hypertension. Often the umbilical vein will be dilated and visible in the epigastrium. This is seen more commonly than the often quoted *caput medusae*.

Purpuric lesions ranging from pinpoint manifestations to large ecchymoses are not uncommonly associated with acquired clotting defects of liver disease. They occur mainly on the lower limbs, may be transient and recurrent, and are sometimes accompanied by follicular hyperkeratosis. They are usually not associated with demonstrable vitamin C deficiency. Bruising, especially at the sites of venipuncture, may often be seen.

Hormone-induced changes of the skin

Hormonal disturbances have been claimed to be responsible for a variety of skin and hair changes in cirrhosis. There is occasionally a complaint of a decrease in the rate of growth of facial hair in men, but loss of forearm, axillary, and pubic hair may occur in both sexes. Pectoral alopecia and female pubic hair distribution may be seen in men. Loss of libido and potency, testicular atrophy, and oligospermia are generally accepted associations in men. Striae distensae occur in both sexes in association with chronic liver disease, not only on the abdomen but also on the thighs. They arise in the absence of ascites or systemic steroid therapy, but they may of course accompany either of these. They are usually found only in patients with chronic active hepatitis of the lupoid type. Dupuytren's contracture and swelling of the parotid gland, as well as gynecomastia, are more frequently seen in chronic cirrhosis. It has been generally assumed that gynecomastia and many other hormonally induced changes are due to hyperestrogenism as a result of inability of the liver to inactivate estrogens in chronic liver disease. Martini [12] has pointed out that many of these so-called hormonal changes, including gynecomastia, Dupuytren's contracture, and parotid swelling, occur more commonly in patients with cirrhosis in countries where alcohol consumption is high, and he wonders whether they could be the result of dietary deficiencies rather than due to measurable hormonal abnormalities. In chronic alcoholics, there are other definite effects on the endocrine system, even in the absence of liver disease [30]. These include facial mooning, truncal obesity, and proximal muscle wasting, i.e., features reminiscent of Cushing's syndrome. This alcohol-related "pseudo-Cushing's syndrome" reverts to normal when alcohol intake is discontinued.

The precise endocrine abnormality responsible for gynecomastia is unknown and a number of different hormonal disturbances have been invoked, including increased secretion of estrogen, increased conversion of androgen to estrogen, altered binding of androgen by globulins, decreased estrogen metabolism, increased production of growth hormone and other pituitary hormones, and altered local tissue response to a normal hormonal environment. Some of these concepts are more plausible than others. Thus, for example, the suggestion that gynecomastia may be due to an increased concentration of sex hormone binding globulin found in chronic liver disease is worthy of consideration. Since testosterone is more tightly bound to sex hormone binding globulin than estradiol, an increase in the concentration of sex hormone binding globulin causes a greater increase in the binding of testosterone than of estradiol and thus increases the ratio of free estradiol to free testosterone in the plasma. This may lead to the development of secondary female sexual characteristics. Shuster and Marks [31] have investigated estrogen metabolism in patients with erythroderma showing evidence of gynecomastia. They found hyperestrogenism and increased urinary estrogen excretion in a number of these cases. They postulated that even skin disease itself might lead to hyperestrogenism resulting occasionally in gynecomastia.

In view of the hormone-induced skin changes seen in pregnancy and their association with an increase in serum and urinary estrogens, a similar presumptive mechanism has been accepted in cirrhosis. An exuberant growth of condylomata acuminata of the vulva and vagina has been described in women with cirrhosis [32] and has been likened to the occasional appearance of large moist warts in pregnancy, presumably as a result of increased urinary estrogens.

Chemically induced changes of the skin

Porphyria cutanea tarda and erythropoietic protoporphyria are dealt with in detail in Chap. 143. Liver disease is invariably associated with the former and the liver is the source of fecal protoporphyria in the latter. In porphyria cutanea tarda, fragility of the skin and bulla formation in sun-exposed areas are often accompanied by purpuric and ecchymotic lesions, scarring, hyperpigmentation, and a sclerodermoid quality of the skin. Hypertrichosis, particularly over the malar and periorbital regions, may be present. In erythropoietic protoporphyria, the most striking skin changes are small atrophic scars on the nose, on the malar eminences, the pinnae, and occasionally on the dorsa of the fingers.

A wide range of xanthomatous lesions may be seen in biliary cirrhosis and other hyperlipemic states. These are described in detail in Chap. 145.

Immunologic manifestations of liver disease

Abnormalities of the immunologic mechanisms have been implicated in some forms of hepatitis and cirrhosis, especially chronic active hepatitis and biliary cirrhosis. While these liver diseases may show evidence of nonspecific cutaneous involvement characterized by vascular, pigmentary, nail, hair, and other manifestations encountered in other forms of hepatic dysfunction, they may, more interestingly, be accompanied by allergic skin changes which form part of a multisystem autoimmune disease.

In a study of the premonitory phase of hepatitis B in 100 patients over a period of 2 weeks before the onset of the disease, Veyre and Brette [33] found that 33 percent of the patients developed urticaria and, to a lesser extent, various erythemas and purpura. They considered that these cutaneous as well as premonitory joint changes were based on an immune mechanism and thus resembled serum sickness.

Exacerbation of chronic urticaria following ingestion of aspirin is well recognized [34,35]. This reaction is apparently unrelated to food or drug allergy. In a few patients aspirin reactivity in chronic urticaria is complicated by jaundice and the liver histology shows changes of atypical portal cirrhosis [36]. It is possible that this phenomenon is yet another allergic cutaneous manifestation of liver disease.

One patient with localized scleroderma and chronic active hepatitis and three patients with scleroderma in association with biliary cirrhosis have been seen by this author. Scleroderma and primary biliary cirrhosis were also noted by others [37–40], and Reynolds et al [41] found six cases of systemic sclerosis among 41 patients with primary biliary cirrhosis.

Chronic active hepatitis and the skin

In chronic active hepatitis, Read et al [42] found that in about one-quarter of their series of 81 patients there were, in addition to the usual cutaneous stigmata seen in liver disease, cutaneous striae even before steroid therapy and a number of skin eruptions, including acne, "erythematous" rashes, lupus erythematosus-type changes, localized scleroderma, purpura, and splinter hemorrhages under the nails and at the nail bases. An allergic capillaritis of the skin in juvenile cirrhosis (chronic active hepatitis) was described by Sarkany [43]. The skin changes are clinically recognizable. The chronic skin eruption is mainly on the trunk and less marked on the limbs (Fig. 167-4). It may persist for years but fluctuates with the severity of the disease and with response to therapy. There are active inflammatory papules with a central pustular element, later forming a crust and eventually leading to atrophy and formation of a characteristically depressed scar. Eventually, the pink color fades and a persistent, pale, depressed, circular or oval lesion remains which resembles a postvaccination scar. In fresh cases only the inflammatory papule with pus or a crust in the center may be present, while later all elements or the residual scars only may be seen. Systemic steroids have a suppressive effect and the skin

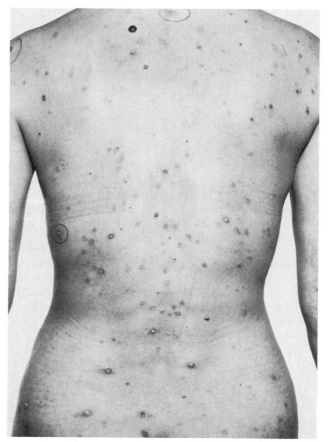

Fig. 167-4 Eruption of red papules with central crusts and depressed scars caused by allergic capillaritis of skin in chronic active hepatitis.

changes may not necessarily correspond to the severity of the liver disease.

Histologically, the epithelium contains a crater in which there is a parakeratotic plug. In the subbasal region there are patchy quantities of fibrin and there is a dermal infiltrate consisting of lymphocytes, histiocytes, and eosinophils. Many capillaries show edema and cuffing with fibrin-like material giving a positive stain with periodic acid-Schiff. There appears to be increased permeability of small vessels associated with endothelial swelling, permeation of plasma, fibrin formation, and resulting hyalinosis. The microscopic changes are characteristic of an allergic response. This eruption is due to an allergic capillaritis which corresponds to histopathologic changes affecting other parts of the body in chronic active hepatitis.

Chronic active hepatitis, when not associated with the hepatitis B virus, is also known as juvenile cirrhosis, lupoid hepatitis, and plasma cell hepatitis [44–46]. Although originally thought to occur in nonalcoholic young women, causing facial mooning, acne, abdominal striae, amenorrhea, and irregular nodular cirrhosis with plasma cell and lymphocyte infiltration, it is now known to affect all age groups (Fig. 167-5). Jaundice and fever may be accompanied by other diseases, due to a disturbance of immunologic mechanisms, in particular ulcerative colitis, rheumatoid arthritis, glomerulonephritis, or Hashimoto's disease. The number of diseases associated with active

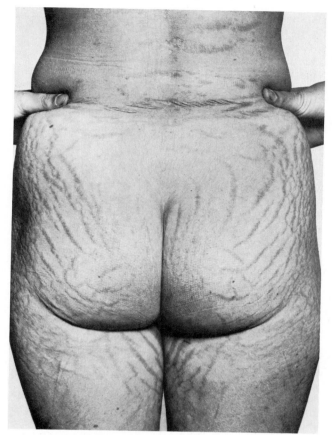

Fig. 167-5 Widespread stretch marks in a boy of 16 with chronic active hepatitis.

chronic hepatitis continues to increase. Now pyoderma gangrenosum has been added [47–49]. In view of the well-known occurrence of pyoderma gangrenosum in ulcerative colitis and in other diseases based on a disturbance of the immune system, the absence of the expected combination of pyoderma gangrenosum and active chronic hepatitis from previously reported series was surprising. Respiratory infections are also frequent complications of this form of cirrhosis. Raised serum transaminases, positive sero-flocculation and lupus erythematosus cells, and high levels of antinuclear factors and other autoantibodies are found [50]. The liver histology shows cell damage with rosette formation and hepatic fibrosis leading to postnecrotic cirrhosis with infiltration by lymphocytes and plasma cells. The allergic capillaritis of the skin fits into this overall picture of a liver disease associated with wide-ranging autoimmune phenomena. Exactly similar clinical and histologic findings have been reported from other centers [51]. Treatment with systemic steroids improved the liver disease and suppressed the skin changes. Reduction of the dose of cortisone led to relapse of the eruption. In a wider range of cases of acute and chronic hepatitis [52], less uniform clinical and histologic skin reaction patterns were found. These included urticarial, macular, and papular rashes as well as raised (palpable) purpuric lesions. Corresponding histologic features were various degrees of cutaneous vasculitis, some showing a primarily lymphocytic venulitis with focal necrosis, while the purpuric lesions noted in chronic hepatitis were represented by neutrophilic

necrotizing vasculitis involving small vessels. The finding of vascular deposits of immunoglobulins, complement, and fibrin in skin, as well as hypocomplementemia in these patients suggested that these cutaneous lesions associated with liver disease resulted from immune complex-mediated vascular injury.

Cutaneous manifestations and primary biliary cirrhosis

An association of primary biliary cirrhosis, cutaneous capillaritis, and IgM-associated membranous glomerulonephritis has been reported [53]. The finding of capillaritis associated with IgM and C3 in the skin lesions suggests that immunologic and possibly complement-mediated events have contributed to the itching of the papules and vesicles on the skin. It was further postulated that deposition of circulating immune complexes including IgG and IgM might account for both the renal glomerular lesion and the cutaneous capillaritis.

Lichen planus. The diagnosis of primary biliary cirrhosis is based on a typical clinical picture, liver function tests suggestive of cholestasis, antimitochondrial antibodies, and characteristic histology. Nonspecific skin changes usually associated with liver disease, cutaneous capillaritis, and occasionally scleroderma and systemic sclerosis have for long been accepted as cutaneous associations of this form of cirrhosis. Recently, lichen planus has been added to this list, and positive cutaneous immunofluorescence findings in primary biliary cirrhosis have strengthened the ties between this liver disease and the skin.

A group of five patients with lichen planus and primary biliary cirrhosis reported from a single center [54] suggested that this coexistence of the two diseases was more than coincidental and that it was most likely due to the fact that both conditions were based on alteration of immune mechanisms. Earlier reports [55] claimed an association between erosive lichen planus and cirrhosis, but there was no precise documentation of the cirrhotic disease. Lichen planus-like lesions with primary biliary cirrhosis have also been described and were claimed to be due to concurrent therapy with penicillamine [56], but this association was probably coincidental rather than causative.

Immunopathologic mechanisms play an important part in both lichen planus and primary biliary cirrhosis. The clinical and investigative evidence for this has been carefully reviewed [54]. It has also been claimed that primary biliary cirrhosis has features in common with chronic graft-versus-host disease [57] in which the grafted lymphoid cells mount, in the liver, an immune response against the recipient's tissue antigens primarily directed against the epithelium of the bile ducts. Similar damage to the lacrimal and salivary glands gives rise to the dry eyes and mouth of the sicca syndrome [57]. In these respects chronic graft-versus-host disease closely resembles primary biliary cirrhosis. Furthermore, lichen planus is the skin disease that most closely resembles the graft-versus-host reaction. Here too an alteration in epithelial antigenicity is responsible for the donor lymphoid cells mounting an immune reaction on the recipient's epidermal cells. There is thus an additional similarity between primary biliary cirrhosis and chronic graft-versus-host disease in that lichen planus may occur in association with both conditions and a clear pathogenetic link between lichen planus, primary biliary cirrhosis and chronic graft-versus-host disease is established.

Cutaneous immunofluorescence. Immune deposits have been found in skin of patients with primary biliary cirrhosis [58–60]. IgM was found at the basement membrane zone and around blood vessels; C3, fibrin, IgA, and IgG were seen less frequently. The pattern of immune deposition was similar or identical to that seen in lupus erythematosus. It is important because it represents an additional accessible immunologic marker and possible diagnostic aid in primary biliary cirrhosis. The positive immunofluorescence was not related to the presence of high serum IgM levels and it was therefore not just a washout effect [61]. Although it has been claimed that the immunofluorescence could be altered or abolished by penicillamine and that this offered a means of assessing the efficacy of this therapy [58], this has not been confirmed by others [60]. On the other hand, IgA deposits in skin in alcoholic liver disease, particularly in superficial dermal capillaries, were shown to correlate with characteristic deposition of IgA in the liver [62].

Nail changes in liver disease

Although a variety of nail changes has been described, it must be stressed that the nails of many patients with liver disease are normal and that nail abnormalities are a less constant physical sign than, for example, spiders or liver palms. However, in cirrhotic patients, clubbing, white nails, watch-glass deformity, flat nails, white bands, striations, and brittleness may be found.

While clubbing of the fingers is primarily a sign of lung and heart disease, it is also frequently associated with all forms of cirrhosis, especially primary biliary. The exact incidence of clubbing in lung and heart disease is not known, but figures as high as 80 percent and as low as 10 percent in pulmonary disease have been quoted. A 60 percent incidence has been claimed in subacute bacterial endocarditis, and no precise figures for extrapulmonary disease, especially cirrhosis and ulcerative colitis, are available based on large series [63]. However, in a series of 106 patients with biliary cirrhosis and chronic active hepatitis, clubbing was present in 18 cases (16 percent) (M. J. Whelton, personal communication) and in 35 cases of active chronic hepatitis, Cook [64] found 5 patients with clubbing and 2 with opaque white nails. Martini [65] noted an association between the incidence of clubbing and palmar erythema and pointed out that the latter was also common in pregnancy. Cirrhosis, pregnancy, and lung disease have in common an increased blood flow [66]. The exact pathogenesis of clubbing, spiders, and palmar erythema is not understood, but Bean [28] believes that they may all be the result of the same forces that operate in liver disease.

The essential anatomic basis of clubbing is an increased thickness of the nail bed caused by edema, cellular infiltration, and increased vascularity. While the change in the nail bed is largely responsible for the characteristic shape of the clubbed digit, other vascular and tissue changes may be contributory factors in determining the generalized expansion of the terminal phalanx that occurs in the advanced case [63].

The actual changes of clubbing are, therefore, the result of an increase in connective tissue between the nail and bone, and the increase in peripheral blood flow is not always equally marked and is probably an essential feature but not a primary cause of clubbing. It has been suggested that there is a type of clubbing principally associated with lung disease characterized mainly by an increase in amount of connective tissue and a second variety due mainly to increased blood flow in the distal portion of the finger. Mendlowitz [67–69] examined patients with clubbing who were suffering from chronic lung and gut diseases and found that the blood flow of the distal portion of the fingers in patients with clubbing was greater than in normal digits and that the gradient of pressure normally diminishing toward the periphery of the finger was lost. In all cases of clubbing there was a marked increase in blood pressure in the digital arteries as compared with controls. Increased digital blood flow may also occur without producing clubbing, as in pregnancy. On the other hand, however, it has been shown that the disappearance of clubbing was followed by a reduction in blood flow. It must be concluded, therefore, that the rise in peripheral blood flow is not the only prerequisite but one of a number of factors concerned in the formation of clubbing. The development of clubbing secondary to lung or heart disease has also been blamed on the action of reduced ferritin which was said to result from inadequate oxidation in the pulmonary capillaries. The reduced ferritin dilated the arteriovenous anastomoses in the finger tips by antagonizing the vasoconstrictor effect of circulating adrenaline. The demonstration of portopulmonary anastomoses bypassing the pulmonary capillary bed in postmortem studies of patients with cirrhosis has been taken as evidence of a right-to-left shunt in cases of clubbing secondary to cirrhosis [70], but there was no correlation between the incidence of clubbing and arterial desaturation, or the presence of portopulmonary anastomoses demonstrated in life in a group of patients with cirrhosis [71]. Reid [72] postulated, nevertheless, that cyanosis and finger clubbing in patients with hepatic cirrhosis were due to arteriovenous pleural shunts or pleural "spider nevi." The (convex) watch-glass deformity of the nail has been considered to be simply a milder form of clubbing and is occasionally combined with some of the other features of this condition. It may be seen in patients who also have palmar erythema.

White nails may be seen occasionally in normal people and in a variety of diseases, especially in patients with cryoglobulinemia, Raynaud's syndrome, and systemic scleroderma. However, intensely white nails are characteristic of cirrhosis. Terry [73] reported white nails in 82 of 100 patients with cirrhosis. The white color was not within the nail plate but was due to opacification of the nail bed since the whiteness did not move with nail growth nor did it alter when blood was forced into the subungual tissue by compression of digital vessels. In severe cases all fingernails may be affected and show a ground-glass opacity of almost the entire nail bed. There may be a zone of normal pink at the distal edge of the nail. The white nail is probably due to overgrowth of connective tissue between the nail and the bone and this reduces the amount of blood in the subcapillary plexus. Watch-glass deformity

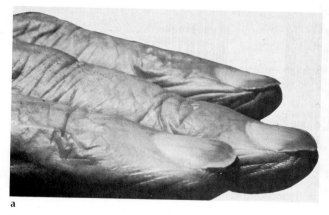

a

Fig. 167-6 (a) Flat white nails with slight convex watch-glass deformity showing a distal pink band in a patient with liver disease. (b) Terry's white nails in cirrhosis.

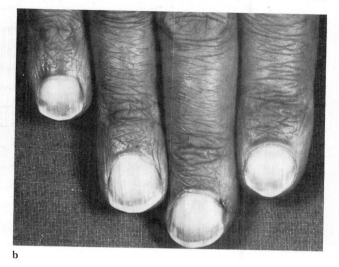

b

may accompany white nails (Fig. 167-6a and b). In a patient with alcoholic liver disease, all the fingernails showed multiple transverse white bands which later disappeared and turned into typical white nails [74]. The changes were located in the nail bed and were thought to be due to vascular effects. Opaque nails [75] and thinned nail folds with a wide cuticle [76] have also been reported in chronic liver disease due to alcohol.

Flat or spoon nails [77] are less common in liver disease. They are the opposite of the convex watch-glass deformity, are either flat or concave, pale in color, and frequently show longitudinal ridging. In idiopathic hemochromatosis, koilonychia [13] was said to be the most common of the nail abnormalities but was not related to anemia, either before or induced by treatment, even though koilonychia is classically described in hypochromic anemia. A deficit of sulfhydrated amino acids metabolized by the liver has been suggested and vitamin C deficiency has been postulated to be involved in the mechanism of development of the nail change. Faulty iron metabolism has been incriminated in the development of koilonychia in other forms of liver disease. Brittle nails have also been blamed on liver disease, often without adequate documentation.

Azure lunules, a bluish color of the lunular portion of nails, occur in hepatolenticular degeneration or Wilson's disease [78]. The Kayser-Fleischer ring, a thin greenish-gold opalescent band situated along the limbus of the cornea, often most marked in its superior and inferior aspects, is pathognomonic of Wilson's disease. It should be carefully looked for, especially in children and young adults with unexplained cirrhosis, by direct inspection and by slit-lamp examination. This author has also seen azure lunules and corneal changes resembling Kayser-Fleischer rings in a patient with argyria [79] described subsequently by Whelton and Pope [80].

Itching

Pruritus is one of the most common and distressing symptoms associated with diseases of the hepatobiliary tract. It may be mild and transient or so severe and prolonged that it dominates the clinical picture of the disease. The exact incidence of pruritus in liver disease is not known, but

Wüst [81] found evidence of intensive pruritus as judged by the presence of excoriations or sleep disturbance in 40 percent of a series of 1000 patients with liver disease. Now more sophisticated methods of measurement of itch with sensitive limb movement meters exist [82].

Itching may precede the visible onset of jaundice in primary biliary cirrhosis. In hepatitis, it may affect selectively the lower limbs and is frequently missed as an early sign of the disease, but occasionally pruritus occurs in the later icteric phase of the illness. It may be transient or last 4 to 6 weeks. In viral hepatitis itching was found in 40 percent of adults but in only 3 percent of children [81]. Most marked on the extremities, it may affect severely the trunk, rarely the neck and face, and hardly ever the genitalia. It may be troublesome and even debilitating in primary biliary cirrhosis, and in mechanical biliary obstruction. Pruritus is the presenting symptom in over 50 percent of cases of biliary cirrhosis and it may precede jaundice by months or even a year or two. As parenchymal destruction of cirrhosis increases and hepatocellular failure supervenes, itching may subside spontaneously.

Pathogenesis of pruritus

The physiologic basis of pruritus is not completely known. While there are no specific receptors for itch, there is a rich cutaneous nerve network in the superficial papillary dermis which subserves this sensation. The itch stimulus is carried by slow-conducting C fibers to the spinal cord and from there in the anterolateral spinothalamic tracts to the thalamus and the posterior central gyrus of the cortex. Mechanical, electrical, and thermal stimuli can cause itching by their effects on the skin; irritant and allergic processes in the skin may cause histamine release which may cause itching, but, in addition to histamine, proteolytic enzymes and prostaglandins have been shown to be involved in the chemical mediation of pruritus.

The mechanism of itching in jaundice is still not known, although it has been suggested that it is due to bile salt retention causing irritation of cutaneous sensory nerves. Bile acids have been identified in the skin of patients with pruritus, but no association has been found with the concentration of any particular conjugated or free bile acid and the presence or absence of itching. The correlation between bile acid levels in cholestasis and the presence of pruritus has been studied. A great overlap of values of bile acid levels has been shown in patients with cholestasis with and without pruritus. There is strong evidence against the hypothesis of a direct causative role for retained bile acids in pruritus associated with cholestasis [83]. Moreover, in terminal liver failure when pruritus is lost, serum bile acids may still be increased [21]. The association of itching with the absence of bile from the feces, whether as a result of cholestasis or hepatitis, suggests that pruritus is due to some substance normally excreted in the bile. Intrahepatic cholestasis may itself be made worse by methyl testosterone, previously used in the management of pruritus. Other drugs that may induce cholestasis are erythromycin, oral contraceptives, phenothiazines, chlorpropamide, para-aminosalicylic acid, and nitrofurantoin. Relief of itching by the bile-salt chelating resin cholestyramine also suggests that bile salts are implicated. The disappearance of itching when liver cells fail indicates that whatever is responsible is manufactured by the liver.

It has also been suggested that the poor correlation between serum bile salt concentration and pruritus may be due to variation in bile salt composition. The pruritic effect of purified bile salts has been tested by applying them to blister bases [84]. All the salts tested were pruritogens, but the dihydroxy salts (especially unconjugated chenodeoxycholate) were more effective than the trihydroxy salts. Chemical mediators of itching may act by directly depolarizing cutaneous nerves or by releasing endogenous pruritogens such as histamine or proteolytic enzymes. Although bile salts liberate small amounts of histamine on perfusion of animal skin [85] and blood histamine levels increase in experimental obstructive jaundice [86], the poor correlation between pruritus and plasma histamine in liver disease [87] and the poor therapeutic response to antihistamines suggest that histamine is not the major mediator of pruritus [84].

Clinical features

In liver disease, itching implies cholestasis or unrelieved mechanical biliary obstruction. Pruritus is significant in primary biliary cirrhosis, cholestatic hepatitis, benign recurrent cholestasis, cholestasis of pregnancy or induced by the birth control pill, and sclerosing cholangitis. Itching in hepatobiliary disease may be transient or continuous and may or may not be accompanied by jaundice. It is usually generalized. It occurs in hepatitis, obstructive and cholestatic jaundice, and all forms of cirrhosis. There may be no visible skin change, but more often there are scratch marks and excoriations, sometimes complicated by crusting and secondary infection. Macular, papular, or urticarial lesions may be present, and in long-standing cases lichenified plaques or the nodules of prurigo are found on the trunk, the extensor surfaces of the limbs, and the buttocks. Histologically, these changes are nonspecific. In the differential diagnosis, the whole range of systemic diseases and skin conditions in which pruritus may be a predominant symptom must be considered. Itching of pregnancy has been found to be associated with cholestasis with or without jaundice and has tended to recur in subsequent pregnancies in half the cases. An increased incidence of cholelithiasis was discovered in these [88]. Apart from reticuloses such as Hodgkin's disease, pruritus in thyrotoxicosis may cause difficulties in diagnosis, especially because the latter's cutaneous manifestations of hyperpigmentation, onycholysis, and palmar erythema may have some resemblance to those seen in liver disease [89].

Management

The itching of acute viral hepatitis and mild drug-induced cholestasis requires only sympathetic understanding and reassurance, mild sedation, and local applications such as calamine lotion with 1% phenol or 0.25% menthol or both for their soothing effect. Persistent and troublesome itching of primary biliary cirrhosis may require more effective topical antipruritics such as Eurax cream or lotion (crotamiton 10%), topical steriods, or phenothiazines. Systemic androgens have been tried but they are not used now because they tend to produce deepening jaundice. More effective in the treatment of pruritus is the basic anion-exchange resin cholestyramine, which sequesters bile acids within the intestine and lowers serum (and tissue) levels. It is given in 5- to 10-g doses per day. It is best to give cholestyramine approximately one-half hour before breakfast. In many patients up to 6 sachets per day are used, starting one-half hour before and giving more one-half hour after the meal, when serum bile acids are at their lowest and the largest amount of bile acids reaches the intestine. Serum bile acids reach their peak after the evening meal and it has been suggested that the high levels of bile acids in the serum after dinner are responsible for the itching of jaundice being worst at night. Patients taking cholestyramine to control their itching have been found to have low vitamin C concentrations. Although this may be a causal relationship, patients with cirrhosis are, in any case, well known to have deficiencies of many water- and fat-soluble vitamins [90]. Cholestyramine is known to bind to vitamin C and precipitate it out of the diet [91]. For this reason, any other medication that has to be administered concurrently should be given between and away from cholestyramine because this preparation binds to many other drugs too. An ideal alternative to cholestyramine is Colestipol. Itching due to mechanical obstruction of bile requires corrective surgical treatment or establishment of a functioning biliary-enteric fistula to relieve the effects of obstruction. More recently, plasmapheresis has been tried in the treatment of cholestatic pruritus with variable results. Patients with uncontrollable pruritus secondary to cholestatic liver disease were subjected to plasma perfusion in an attempt to remove "toxins" considered to be responsible for this symptom. The improvement in a high proportion of patients was said to be dramatic and surprisingly long-lasting. Serum bile acid levels fell in the patients in whom the pruritus improved, but not in a patient who responded less favorably [92,93].

Indirectly associated liver and skin changes

Many systemic diseases may involve both the skin and liver, but the association is not a regularly occurring one and the two organs, though involved by the same pathology, may suffer damage which is separated by an interval of months or years. For example, a cutaneous chancre may antedate hepatitis by months and hepatic gummata by years. However, true syphilitic hepatitis in secondary syphilis has been well documented [94], the disease presenting itself with pruritus and cholestatic jaundice. Liver biopsy showed centrilobular cholestasis with liver cell swelling and pleomorphism. Rapid disappearance of jaundice, itching, and all other symptoms and signs followed treatment with penicillin. Several other case reports of the association of secondary lues with liver disease have been published.

Drug-induced hepatic lesions may be characterized by cholestasis and the associated skin component by erythema. Cholestatic jaundice possibly associated with a generalized hypersensitivity reaction has resulted from erythromycin estolate. However, erythromycin laurolate is not associated with hepatitis. Intrahepatic cholestasis and cutaneous bullae associated with glibenclamide therapy [95] and a bullous eruption with chronic active hepatitis and glomerulonephritis [96] have suggested possible associations of bullous skin changes in liver disease. Drugs frequently used in the management of liver disease may also produce cutaneous side effects. Vitamin K_1 (phytomenadione) is used widely as an antidote to anticoagulants and in hypoprothrombinemic states. Erythematous, tender, indurated plaques at the site of intramuscular injections of vitamin K_1 administered to patients with liver disease have been described [97]. Liver involvement may also be encountered in patients with severe systemic lupus erythematosus. This association is more common than previously recognized. In a retrospective study of 238 patients with systemic lupus erythematosus, 43 patients were found to have liver disease [98]. In most patients, a specific viral or drug etiology could not be implicated and the changes included cirrhosis, chronic active hepatitis, and steatosis. In one patient, granulomatous hepatitis appeared and subsided simultaneously with an exacerbation of the systemic lupus erythematosus [99]. At autopsy, multiple nodular hyperplasia of the noncirrhotic liver was found in some patients with systemic lupus erythematosus and these changes were taken to be a regenerative-hyperplastic process [100].

Cutaneous granulomata have been seen rarely in patients with primary biliary cirrhosis. In one case, granulomata in the lungs were also found; in another, cholestyramine cleared up the skin lesions. On the other hand, granulomata in the liver have been diagnosed in tuberculosis, sarcoidosis, glandular fever, syphilis, and as a result of administration of phenylbutazone, sulfonamides, and allopurinol, and also in association with lichen amyloidosis.

Hepatitis and the skin—special risks and associations

Virus-induced hepatitis is divided into three main forms: A, B, and non-A, non-B. The hepatitis A virus (HAV) is the cause of infectious hepatitis, is classed with the enteroviruses, and is transmitted mainly by the fecal–oral route. The only form of prophylaxis so far available against it is passive immunization with standard immune serum globulin.

The most common form of posttransfusion hepatitis is due to an agent or agents which have not been properly characterized and which are called non-A, non-B. At present, there are no serologic tests or details of its viral structure and immune response, but it is known that acute non-A, non-B or subclinical non-A, non-B hepatitis can result in chronic liver disease [21].

The virus of hepatitis B (HBV) is the cause of serum hepatitis and is of particular medical and public health interest, for, in contrast to hepatitis A, it can give rise to a carrier state and to chronic liver disease. Moreover, it is probable that chronic HBV infection is a cofactor in the genesis of primary liver carcinoma [101]. Important progress has been made in the prevention of hepatitis B by means of active and passive immunization. The hepatitis B virus is transmitted by whole blood and its products. The virion or Dane particle is composed of double-stranded DNA, the core antigen (HBcAg), DNA polymerase, the "e" antigen, and the surface antigen (HBsAg). HBsAg has been detected in various body fluids, including semen, saliva, tears, urine, and impetiginized skin lesions [102]. It has been calculated that there are more than 200 million chronic carriers of the hepatitis B surface antigen worldwide [101]. The morbidity, mortality, and economic burden of acute hepatitis B and its chronic sequelae are enormous [103].

Dermatologic risks of hepatitis B and their prevention

Although hepatitis B virus is usually transmitted parenterally, infection may also occur in the absence of overt parenteral exposure and in these cases penetration of virus into the body has been postulated through cutaneous or mucosal microlesions. In an attempt to assess the role of skin lesions due to diseases such as psoriasis and eczema as possible routes of entry for hepatitis B virus, a group from Italy [104] tested patients and controls for HBsAg, anti-HBs, and anti-(HBc) by radioimmunoassay. They showed that in patients with chronic skin disease, there was a higher risk of infection with hepatitis B virus. They concluded that skin lesions facilitated penetration of the virus, especially in regions where there was a prevalence of HBsAg in the general population.

The medical profession, laboratory workers, dialysis and oncology personnel, dentists, physicians, and surgeons are at increased risk of acquiring hepatitis B [103], and dermatologists have been warned of the risks of hepatitis B virus infection as a result of carrying out various minor surgical procedures without gloves [105]. Special care should be taken by all who take blood or carry out any investigative or surgical procedures on patients who have hepatitis B. It should not be forgotten that many patients may be unsuspected carriers of the hepatitis B virus and "routine" bloodletting can never be considered to be entirely without risk of hepatitis B infection. Details of safe methods for venipuncture [106] and other codes of practice for prevention of infection have been described [107].

A proportion of patients with hepatitis B fail to clear the virus and become chronic carriers. The carriage rate is high among the indigenous population in parts of the world such as Asia, Africa, and South America. Additionally, a high carriage rate is found in individuals who are immunocompromised, have chronic disease, or who are drug addicts or homosexuals.

A vaccine for medical, nursing, and laboratory staff who work among populations with high HBsAg carriage rates has recently become commercially available (Thomas Morson Pharmaceuticals) and no doubt others will be produced. The recommended procedure is 3 doses, the boosters being given 1 month and 6 months after the initial dose. Immunity is predicted to last about 5 years. This may also be used together with hyperimmune globulin to protect individuals exposed to potential infection, e.g., spouses of patients with acute type B hepatitis, homosexuals, and neonates born to a HBsAg-positive mother. Hyperimmune globulin is also available for use in patients who are going into areas where there is a high incidence. It can be used to confer passive immunization in a person who either has been in contact with someone suffering from acute type B hepatitis or has been inoculated with HBsAg-positive blood.

Skin manifestations of hepatitis B

Circulating immune complexes contribute to the pathogenesis of extrahepatic manifestations of type B viral hepatitis. The best-documented cutaneous associations of hepatitis B are:

1. Urticaria
2. Essential mixed cryoglobulinemia
3. Polyarteritis nodosa
4. Gianotti-Crosti syndrome (papular acrodermatitis of childhood)

Urticaria may be the predominant or sole feature of the transient prodromal serum-sickness-type syndrome which occurs in about 20 to 30 percent of patients with acute hepatitis B virus infection. Usually there are skin changes, polyarthralgia, and arthritis in this phase, but the urticaria may occur in anicteric hepatitis or in the preicteric stages days or weeks before jaundice and may last several days [52,108]. Deposition of immune complexes containing HBsAg in involved cutaneous vessels, C3, and IgM have been found [108–110], and therefore many of the extrahepatic manifestations of viral hepatitis B have been attributed to its association with antigen-antibody-complement complexes.

Essential mixed cryoglobulinemia is yet another immune-complex-mediated illness related to hepatitis B, which is characterized by purpura, arthralgia, and weakness, often accompanied by renal involvement [111,112].

Polyarteritis nodosa and hepatitis B virus association has been documented [113,114] by finding circulating immune complexes composed of HBsAg and immunoglobulin as well as electron microscopically by finding particles thought to represent the virion of hepatitis B virus. It has also been suggested [103,115] that leukocytoclastic vasculitis which involves smaller vessels may be associated with the presence of the type B virus antigen.

Gianotti-Crosti syndrome, or papular acrodermatitis of childhood, is characterized by an erythematous papular rash on the limbs and face of children. It is said to be slightly infectious, nonrelapsing, and lasts some 3 weeks. It may be associated with a reactive reticulohistiocytic lymphadenitis and acute hepatitis, usually anicteric, which commonly lasts about 2 months [116]. Hepatitis B surface antigen has been claimed to be invariably present in the blood of patients with the exanthem and hepatitis [117]. In Italy, this disease was found to be HBV subtype ayw,

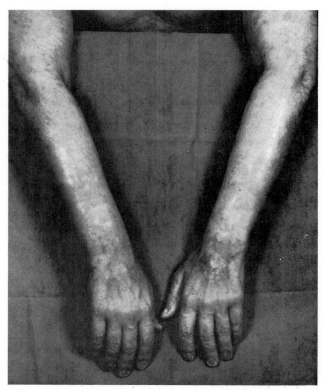

Fig. 167-7 Sclerodermatous changes affecting upper limbs of a patient in the late chronic phase of graft-versus-host disease.

whereas the small number of cases of papular acrodermatitis with hepatitis in North America with HBs antigenemia were of a different subtype and were related to HBV and Epstein-Barr virus infections [118]. HBs antigenemia persists for months or years in more than one-third of patients and is accompanied by persistently elevated liver enzymes.

Skin manifestations of graft-versus-host disease
(see also Chap. 114)

Bone marrow transplantation is used increasingly in the treatment of serious hematologic disorders, especially leukemia and aplastic anemia. The main complications of bone marrow transplantation are graft-versus-host disease (GVHD), infection, and pneumonitis. The skin, the gastrointestinal tract, and the hepatobiliary system are the main targets of a graft-versus-host reaction (GVHR) in which immune-competent cells of the graft mount an immunologic attack on tissue of an immunosuppressed, histoincompatible recipient. In acute GVHD, the liver changes are those of hepatitis, whereas in chronic GVHD the picture is strikingly similar to the pathologic manifestations of the liver in primary biliary cirrhosis. The skin is thus a primary target organ for GVHD and early recognition of the cutaneous changes is important [119]. The skin changes are often the first and predominant finding or they may be associated with the clinical features of a GVHR. Recognition of the cutaneous picture and histologic confirmation of the diagnosis enables the responsible clinician to institute rapid treatment aimed at suppressing the unwanted side effects of bone marrow transplantation.

Clinical features

The severity of GVHD is variable, and chronologically three separate stages are recognized. The *acute phase* starts soon after the transplant, usually between 7 and 30 days, but it may occur both earlier and later. An *early chronic phase* generally starts after the hundredth posttransplant day and a *late chronic phase* may occur months later [119,120].

The acute stage is characterized by fever, hepatic involvement with elevated enzymes and jaundice, diarrhea of different degrees of severity, and a rash.

An erythematous macular and papular or scarlatiniform eruption, with or without a purpuric element, may start within a few days of the transplant. It starts on the sides or the back of the neck and the cheeks and spreads to the palms, soles, and other parts of the body. The rash may be mild and fluctuant, but skin involvement may be severe and generalized in the form of a toxic erythema or epidermal necrolysis which may result in the patient's death [121,122]. If the patient survives and the acute phase of GVHD settles, desquamation occurs, followed by residual pigmentation. Later, a new and different cutaneous eruption may develop which is called chronic GVHD [120] and this too may be associated with damage to or involvement of other organ systems in addition to the skin.

The early chronic phase of GVHD generally appears

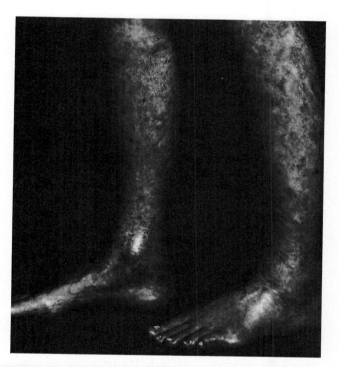

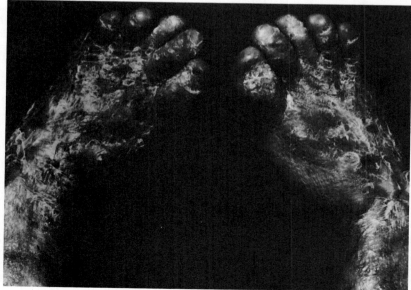

Fig. 167-8 Lower limbs with morpheic changes in late graft-versus-host disease.

after the hundredth posttransplant day and may or may not have been preceded by the acute stage. The eruption is lichenoid or completely resembles lichen planus, including the characteristic oral mucous membrane changes. The chronologic separation of the acute and chronic phases is stressed by some authors [120], but others [117,123] have suggested a less rigid separation and time sequence between the acute and early chronic stages, allowing for an earlier transition of the early into the chronic stage, the absence of a disease-free interval, and the absence of an acute phase.

Finally, the late chronic phase sets in, represented by pigmented, reticulate, and atrophic changes of the skin [119]. Violaceous plaques may occur on this poikilodermatous background. This may continue for months but eventually sclerodermatous changes may develop leading to extensive morphea with or without skin ulceration, with limitation of joint mobility, the sicca syndrome, and eye symptoms. However, sclerosis and Raynaud's syndrome are absent and the picture is not that of systemic sclerosis (Figs. 167-7 and 167-8) [120,124–126].

The clinical states of human GVHD may thus be viewed as a progressive immune attack resulting from the donor lymphocytes mounting an attack upon recipient cells and producing at first a macular and papular rash, later lichen planus-like changes, poikiloderma, and eventually sclerosis. It has been suggested [120] that while it seems convenient to consider GVHD as occurring in acute, early, and late chronic stages, there are many patients whose clinical course is not punctuated by separate phases, and that it is more realistic to view GVHD as a continuum, starting in the skin with relatively nonspecific skin changes which progress through the typical lichenoid picture and may end in a late sclerodermatous pattern.

Histology

The early changes of acute GVHD affect the basal cell and malpighian layers. Loss of polarity, focal hyperkeratosis, the presence of a few vacuoles, and lymphocytes at the dermal-epidermal junction are signs of satellite cell dyskeratosis or necrolysis [119,127]. The early chronic phase histology is that of lichen planus, but the density of the dermal lymphocytic infiltrate is less intense than that of the idiopathic lichen planus variety. The late chronic phase resembles scleroderma histologically, but the sclerosis of GVHD begins in the upper dermis [119,120].

Ultrastructurally [128], the early oral and cutaneous lichenoid phase shows damage to the basement membrane and keratinocytes of the basal layer and low spinous layers. The presence of epidermal regenerative cells is a feature common to the lichenoid phase of chronic GVHD and idiopathic lichen planus. The late sclerotic phase of GVHD, with persistence of basal cell injury, normal periodicity and structure of collagen fibers and active fibroblasts in the upper third of the dermis, distinguishes GVHD from scleroderma. The localization in the papillary dermis of both lymphocytes and active fibroblasts favors the "descending process" theory of dermal sclerosis in GVHD.

The presence of cutaneous immunoglobulin and complement was investigated in a group of patients with and without GVHD after transplantation of bone marrow from HLA-identical siblings for the treatment of acute leukemia or aplastic anemia [129]. Dermal-epidermal IgM deposits and complement were found in acute and chronic cutaneous GVHD. Humoral immunity was held to be responsible for the development of GVHD.

References

1. Morgan MY: Sex and alcohol. *Br Med Bull* **38**:43, 1982
2. Pegum JS: Exfoliative dermatitis associated with liver changes and hypoproteinaemia. *Guy's Hospital Reports* **100**:304, 1951
3. Tickner A, Basit A: Serum proteins and liver function in exfoliative dermatitis. *Br J Dermatol* **72**:138, 1960
4. Bauer F: Generalized exfoliative dermatitis and liver function. *Aust J Dermatol* **2**:69, 1953
5. Shuster S, Wilkinson P: Protein metabolism in exfoliative dermatitis and erythroderma. *Br J Dermatol* **75**:344, 1963
6. Knowles JP et al: Folic-acid deficiency in patients with skin disease. *Lancet* **1**:1138, 1963
7. Knowles JP et al: Folic-acid metabolism in liver disease. *Clin Sci* **24**:39, 1963
8. Diamond I, Schmid R: Experimental bilirubin encephalopathy: the mode of entry of bilirubin-^{14}C into the central nervous system. *J Clin Invest* **45**:678, 1966
9. Arias IM: Hepatic aspects of bilirubin metabolism. *Annu Rev Med* **17**:257, 1966
10. Schaffner F: Primary biliary cirrhosis, in *Cirrhosis*, edited by H Popper. *Clin Gastroenterol* **4**:351, 1975
11. Bohnstedt RM: Haut und Leber, in *Leber, Haut und Skelett*, edited by L Wannagat. Stuttgart, George Thieme, 1964
12. Martini GA: Leber und Haut, in *Leber, Haut und Skelett*, edited by L Wannagat. Stuttgart, George Thieme, 1964
13. Chevrant-Breton J et al: Cutaneous manifestations of idiopathic hemochromatosis. *Arch Dermatol* **113**:161, 1977
14. Lerner AB, McGuire JS: Melanocyte-stimulating hormone and adrenocorticotrophic hormone. *N Engl J Med* **270**:539, 1964
15. Burton JL, Kirby J: Pigmentation and biliary cirrhosis. *Lancet* **1**:458, 1975
16. Bartholomew TC et al: Bile acid profiles of human serum and skin interstitial fluid and their relationship to pruritus studied by gas chromatography–mass spectrometry. *Clin Sci* **63**:65, 1982
17. Mills PR: Melanin pigmentation of the skin in primary biliary cirrhosis. *J Cutan Pathol* **8**:404, 1981
18. Finch SC, Finch CA: Idiopathic hemochromatosis, an iron storage disease. A. Iron metabolism in hemochromatosis. *Medicine (Baltimore)* **34**:381, 1955
19. Chapman RW et al: Hepatic iron stores and markers of iron overload in alcoholics and patients with idiopathic hemochromatosis. *Dig Dis Sci* **27**:909, 1982
20. Perdrup A, Poulsen H: Hemochromatosis and vitiligo. *Arch Dermatol* **90**:34, 1964
21. Sherlock S: *Diseases of the Liver and Biliary System,* 6th ed. Oxford, Blackwell, 1981
22. Bean WB: The cutaneous arterial spider: a survey. *Medicine (Baltimore)* **24**:243, 1945
23. Bean WB: The arterial spider and similar lesions of the skin and mucous membrane. *Circulation* **8**:117, 1953
24. Capron JP et al: Unilateral nevoid telangiectasia and chronic liver disease. *Am J Gastroenterol* **76**:47, 1981
25. Bean WB: *Vascular Spiders and Related Lesions of the Skin.* Oxford, Blackwell, 1959
26. Schirren C: Hautveränderungen bei inneren Erkrankungen, in *Handbuch der Haut- und Geschlechtskrankheiten,* edited by HA Gottron. Berlin, Springer-Verlag, 1967, p 569
27. Martini GA, Staubesand J: Zur Morphologie der Gefässpinnen ("vascular spiders") in der Haut Leberkranker. *Virchows Arch [Pathol Anat]* **324**:147, 1953

28. Bean WB: *Vascular Spiders*. Oxford, Blackwell, 1958
29. Kontos HA et al: General and regional circulatory alterations in cirrhosis of the liver. *Am J Med* 37:526, 1964
30. Morgan MY: Alcohol and the endocrine system. *Br Med Bull* **38**:35, 1982
31. Shuster S, Marks J: *Systemic Effects of Skin Disease*. London, Heinemann, 1970
32. Blank H: Common viral diseases of the skin. *Med Clin North Am* 43:1401, 1959
33. Veyre B, Brette R: L'hépatite B à la phase prémonitoire. *Nouv Presse Med* 4:1349, 1975
34. Calnan CD: Release of histamine in urticaria pigmentosa. *Lancet* 1:996, 1957
35. Warin RP: The effect of aspirin in chronic urticaria. *Br J Dermatol* 72:350, 1960
36. Moore-Robinson M, Warin RP: Effect of salicylates in urticaria. *Br Med J* 4:262, 1967
37. Murray-Lyon IM et al: Scleroderma and primary biliary cirrhosis. *Br Med J* 3:258, 1970
38. Rau R et al: Liver involvement in scleroderma. *Schweiz Med Wochenschr* **104**:1877, 1974
39. McCoy DG: Spontaneous rupture of the liver in a case of scleroderma. *J Irish Med Assoc* **60**:474, 1967
40. De Graaf P et al: Primaire biliaire cirrose med sclerodermie en hypothyreidie. *Tijdschr Gastroenterol* 18:151, 1975
41. Reynolds TB et al: Primary biliary cirrhosis with scleroderma, Raynaud's phenomenon and telangiectasis. New syndrome. *Am J Med* 50:302, 1971
42. Read AE et al: Active "juvenile" cirrhosis considered as part of a systemic disease and the effect of corticosteroid therapy. *Gut* 4:378, 1963
43. Sarkany I: Juvenile cirrhosis and allergic capillaritis of the skin. A hepato-cutaneous syndrome. *Lancet* 2:666, 1966
44. Mackay IR et al: Lupoid hepatitis and the hepatic lesions of systemic lupus erythematosus. *Lancet* 1:65, 1959
45. Good RA: Plasma-cell hepatitis, and extreme hypergammaglobulinaemia in adolescent females. *Am J Dis Child* **92**:508, 1956
46. Page AR, Good RA: Plasma-cell hepatitis, with special attention to steroid therapy. *Am J Dis Child* **99**:288, 1960
47. Byrne JPH et al: Pyoderma gangrenosum associated with active chronic hepatitis. *Arch Dermatol* 112:1297, 1976
48. Norris DA et al: Pyoderma gangrenosum. Abnormal monocyte function corrected in vitro with hydrocortisone. *Arch Dermatol* 114:906, 1978
49. Burns DA, Sarkany I: Active chronic hepatitis and pyoderma gangrenosum: report of a case. *Clin Exp Dermatol* 4:465, 1979
50. Bouchier IAD et al: Serological abnormalities in patients with liver disease. *Br Med J* 1:592, 1964
51. Kurwa A (for Waddington E): Hepato-cutaneous syndrome (juvenile cirrhosis, allergic capillaritis of the skin, proctocolitis and arthritis). *Br J Dermatol* 80:839, 1968
52. Popp JW et al: Cutaneous vasculitis associated with acute and chronic hepatitis. *Arch Intern Med* 141:623, 1981
53. Rai GS et al: Primary biliary cirrhosis, cutaneous capillaritis, and IgM-associated membranous glomerulonephritis. *Br Med J* 1:817, 1977
54. Graham-Brown RAC et al: Lichen planus and primary biliary cirrhosis. *Br J Dermatol* 106:699, 1982
55. Rebora A et al: Erosive lichen planus and cirrhotic hepatitis. *Ital Gen Rev Dermatol* 15:123, 1978
56. Seehafer JR et al: Lichen planus-like lesions caused by penicillamine in primary biliary cirrhosis. *Arch Dermatol* 117:140, 1981
57. Epstein O et al: Primary biliary cirrhosis is a dry gland syndrome with features of chronic graft-versus-host disease. *Lancet* 1:1166, 1980
58. Randle HW et al: Cutaneous immunofluorescence in primary biliary cirrhosis. *JAMA* 246:1679, 1981
59. Hendricks AA et al: Cutaneous immunoglobulin deposition in primary biliary cirrhosis. *Arch Dermatol* 118:634, 1982
60. Graham-Brown RAC, Sarkany I: Positive cutaneous immunofluorescence in primary biliary cirrhosis. Personal observations, 1983
61. Lindgren S et al: IgM deposition in skin biopsies from patients with primary biliary cirrhosis. *Acta Med Scand* **210**:317, 1981
62. Swerdlow MA et al: IgA deposits in skin in alcoholic liver disease. *Arch Dermatol* **118**:950, 1982
63. Ginsburg J: Clubbing of the fingers. *Circulation* 3:2377, 1965
64. Cook GC: Active chronic hepatitis and its response to corticosteroid therapy. MD thesis. University of London, 1965
65. Martini GA: Über Gefässveränderungen der Haut bei Leberkranken. *Z Klin Med* 153:470, 1955
66. Martini GA, Hagemann JE: Über Fingernagelveränderungen bei Lebercirrhose als Folge veränderter peripherer Durchblutung. *Klin Wochenschr* 34:25, 1956
67. Mendlowitz M: Some observations on clubbed fingers. *Clin Sci* 3:387, 1938
68. Mendlowitz M: Measurements of blood flow and blood pressure in clubbed fingers. *J Clin Invest* 20:113, 1941
69. Mendlowitz M: *Digital Circulation*. New York, Grune & Stratton, 1954
70. Calabresi P, Abelmann WH: Porto-caval and porto-pulmonary anastomoses in Laennec's cirrhosis and in heart failure. *J Clin Invest* 36:1257, 1957
71. Shaldon S et al: The demonstration of porto-pulmonary anastomoses in portal cirrhosis with the use of radioactive krypton (Kr^{85}). *N Engl J Med* 265:410, 1961
72. Reid L: Cyanosis and finger clubbing in liver disease explained? *Med Trib Int Ed (Gr Brit)* 2(2):25, 1967
73. Terry RB: White nails in hepatic cirrhosis. *Lancet* 1:757, 1954
74. Jenssen O: White fingernails preceded by multiple transverse white bands. *Acta Derm Venereol (Stockh)* 61:261, 1981
75. Lewin K: The finger nail in general disease. A macroscopic and microscopic study of 87 consecutive autopsies. *Br J Dermatol* 77:431, 1965
76. Young AW: Cutaneous stigmata of alcoholism. *Alcohol Health Res World*, p 24, Summer 1974
77. Kleeberg J: Flat finger-nails in cirrhosis of the liver. *Lancet* 2:248, 1951
78. Bearn AG, McKusick VA: Azure lunulae: an unusual change in the fingernails in two patients with hepatolenticular degeneration (Wilson's disease). *JAMA* 166:904, 1958
79. Sarkany I: The skin lesions associated with liver disease. *Prog Dermatol* 4:1, 1969
80. Whelton MJ, Pope FM: Azure lunules in argyria. *Arch Intern Med* 121:267, 1968
81. Wüst H: Zur Klinik und Therapie des Pruritus bei Lebererkrankungen, in *Leber, Haut und Skelett*, edited by L Wannagat. Stuttgart, George Thieme, 1964
82. Summerfield JA, Welch ME: The measurement of itch with sensitive limb movement meters. *Br J Dermatol* 102:275, 1981
83. Freedman MR et al: Pruritus in cholestasis: no direct causative role for bile acid retention. *Am J Med* 70:1011, 1981
84. Kirby J et al: Pruritic effect of bile salts. *Br Med J* 4:693, 1974
85. Schachter M: The release of histamine by pethidine, atropine, quinine and other drugs. *Br J Pharmacol* 7:646, 1952
86. Anrep GV, Barsoum GS: Blood histamine in experimental obstruction of the common bile duct. *J Physiol (Lond)* 120:427, 1953
87. Mitchell RG et al: Histamine metabolism in diseases of the liver. *J Clin Invest* 33:1199, 1954
88. Furhoff A-K: Itching in pregnancy: a 15-year follow-up study. *Acta Med Scand* 196:403, 1974

89. Barnes HM et al: Pruritus and thyrotoxicosis. *Trans St Johns Hosp Dermatol Soc* **60**:59, 1974

90. Leading article: Liver disease and vitamin C. *Br Med J* **1**:735, 1977

91. Beattie AD, Sherlock S: Ascorbic acid deficiency in liver disease. *Gut* **17**:571, 1976

92. Carey WD et al: Pruritus of cholestasis treated with plasma perfusion. *Gastroenterology* **76**:330, 1981

93. Lauterburg BH et al: Treatment of pruritus of cholestasis by plasma perfusion through USP-charcoal-coated glass beads. *Lancet* **2**:53, 1980

94. Sarkany I: Pruritus and cholestatic jaundice due to secondary syphilis. *Proc R Soc Med* **66**:237, 1973

95. Wongpaitoon V et al: Intrahepatic cholestasis and cutaneous bullae associated with glibenclamide therapy. *Postgrad Med J* **57**:244, 1981

96. Breathnach SM et al: A severe bullous eruption occurring in a patient with chronic active hepatitis and glomerulonephritis. *Arch Dermatol* **116**:1061, 1980

97. Barnes HM, Sarkany I: Adverse skin reaction from vitamin K₁. *Br J Dermatol* **95**:653, 1976

98. Runyon BA et al: The spectrum of liver disease in systemic lupus erythematosus. *Am J Med* **69**:187, 1980

99. Feurle GE et al: Granulomatous hepatitis in systemic lupus erythematosus. Report of a case. *Endoscopy* **14**:153, 1982

100. Kuramochi S et al: Systemic lupus erythematosus associated with multiple nodular hyperplasia of the liver. *Acta Pathol Jpn* **32**:547, 1982

101. Roggendorf M, Deinhardt F: Recent results on the pathogenesis of hepatitis B and characterization of the agent. *Triangle* **21**:123, 1982

102. Gerity RJ: Hepatitis B transmission between dental or medical workers and patients. *Ann Intern Med* **95**:229, 1981

103. Rogers RB et al: Hepatitis and the skin. *J Am Acad Dermatol* **7**:552, 1982

104. Guadagnino V et al: Risk of hepatitis B virus infection in patients with eczema or psoriasis of the hand. *Br Med J* **284**:84, 1982

105. Graham Smith J Jr: A glove upon that hand. *Br J Dermatol* **107**:12, 1982

106. Welsby PD: How to take blood from patients who have hepatitis B. *Br Med J* **282**:1052, 1981

107. *Code of Practice for the Prevention of Infection in Clinical Laboratories and Post-mortem Rooms* (Howie Report). London, HMSO, 1978

108. Dienstag JL et al: Urticaria associated with acute viral hepatitis type B. Studies of pathogenesis. *Ann Intern Med* **89**:34, 1978

109. Marwick C: The epic of hepatitis B. *Med World News*, p 50, Oct 26, 1981

110. Neumann HAM et al: Hepatitis B surface antigen deposition in the blood vessel walls of urticarial lesions in acute hepatitis B. *Br J Dermatol* **104**:383, 1981

111. Dienstag JL et al: Hepatitis B and essential mixed cryoglobulinemia. *N Engl J Med* **297**:946, 1977

112. Levo Y et al: Association between hepatitis B virus and essential mixed cryoglobulinemia. *N Engl J Med* **296**:1501, 1977

113. Goche DJ et al: Association between polyarteritis and Australia antigen. *Lancet* **2**:1149, 1970

114. Trepo CH, Thivolet J: Antigène Australien, hépatite A virus et périartérite noueuse. *Presse Med* **78**:1575, 1970

115. Gower RG et al: Small vessel vasculitis caused by hepatitis B virus immune complexes. *J Allergy Clin Immunol* **62**:222, 1978

116. Gianotti F: Papular acrodermatitis of childhood. An Australia antigen disease. *Arch Dis Child* **48**:794, 1973

117. Colombo M et al: Immune response to hepatitis B virus in children with papular acro-dermatitis. *Gastroenterology* **73**:1103, 1977

118. San Joaquin VH, Marks MI: Gianotti disease or Gianotti-Crosti syndrome? *J Paediatr* **101**:216, 1982

119. Saurat JH: Cutaneous manifestations of graft-versus-host disease. *Int J Dermatol* **20**:249, 1981

120. Shulman HM et al: Chronic cutaneous graft-versus-host disease in man. *Am J Pathol* **91**:545, 1978

121. Peck GL et al: Toxic epidermal necrolysis in a patient with graft-vs-host reaction. *Arch Dermatol* **105**:561, 1972

122. Betzold J, Hong R: Fatal graft versus host disease after small leucocyte transfusion in a patient with lymphoma and varicella. *Pediatrics* **62**:63, 1978

123. Roujeau JC et al: Graft versus host reactions, in *Recent Advances in Dermatology*, no 5, edited by A Rook, J Savin. Edinburgh, Churchill Livingstone, 1980, p 131

124. Van Vloten WA et al: Localised scleroderma-like lesions after bone marrow transplantation in man. *Br J Dermatol* **96**:337, 1977

125. Gratwohl AA et al: Sjögren-type syndrome after allogeneic bone-marrow transplantation. *Ann Intern Med* **87**:703, 1977

126. Graham-Brown RAC, Sarkany I: Scleroderma-like changes due to chronic graft-versus-host disease. *Clin Exp Dermatol*, in press

127. Rappeport J et al: Acute graft-versus-host disease in recipients of bone marrow transplants from identical twin donors. *Lancet* **2**:717, 1979

128. Janin-Mercier A et al: The lichen planus-like and sclerotic phases of the graft-versus-host disease in man: ultrastructural study of six cases. *Acta Derm Venereol (Stockh)* **61**:187, 1981

129. Mang-So T et al: Deposition of IgM and complement at the dermoepidermal junction in acute and chronic cutaneous graft-vs-host disease in man. *J Immunol* **120**:1485, 1978

CHAPTER 168

THE SKIN AND DISORDERS OF THE ALIMENTARY TRACT

Janet Marks and Sam Shuster

Diseases of the skin and alimentary tract coexist more often than would be expected by chance. It is often assumed that when both systems are involved the alimentary disease is the primary one, but this is not necessarily so and the following possibilities exist [1]:

1. The alimentary disease is the cause of the skin disease
2. The skin disease is the cause of the alimentary disease
3. The skin and alimentary diseases have a common cause or common pathology
4. There is an indirect relationship between the two as in the genetic cutaneoalimentary syndromes

Some alimentary–cutaneous relationships cannot at present be defined in terms of these groups because knowledge is insufficient, but most can, and identification of the relationship is important both for understanding and for clinical management.

Because of the skin's unique position abnormal physical signs are easily detected there, and just as examination of the whole patient should be part of a dermatologic assessment, it is important to examine the skin when a patient presents with a gastrointestinal problem. This is particularly so in gastrointestinal emergencies such as bleeding or severe abdominal pain where skin signs may give clues relevant to whether or not surgical intervention is necessary. In less urgent situations skin signs may be present before there is any other indication of illness and this can be important in malignant gastrointestinal disease, though often spread of malignancy has occurred by then.

In this section we shall deal with changes in the skin which are associated with disease in the pharynx, esophagus, stomach, intestine, and pancreas, and their presenting signs and symptoms will be listed.

Dysphagia and the skin

Immunologic and hyperkeratotic disorders
  Bullous dermatoses
  Lichen planus
  Acanthosis nigricans
  Darier's disease
Oro-oculo-genito-cutaneous syndromes
  Stevens-Johnson syndrome
  Behçet's disease
Carcinoma of the esophagus
  Plummer-Vinson syndrome
  Tylosis
  Celiac disease and dermatitis herpetiformis
Collagen vascular diseases
  Systemic sclerosis
  Dermatomyositis

Immunologic and hyperkeratotic disorders

Skin diseases such as pemphigus, pemphigoid, dermatitis herpetiformis, lichen planus, acanthosis nigricans, and Darier's disease can also involve mucous membranes including the pharynx and esophagus. Of the skin infections that extend to the esophagus, candidiasis is the most common, especially in immunosuppressed individuals. Probably the most serious esophageal involvement of all occurs in the recessive, dystrophic form of epidermolysis bullosa: in small babies blistering can be severe enough to interfere with feeding, and scarring later leads to stricture formation. Very large doses of corticosteroid followed by reconstructive surgery enable some badly affected children to survive [2]. Phenytoin has been used for its anti-collagenase action and is reported to improve some of the skin lesions but its effect on the esophagus is not known. Now that the condition can be diagnosed in utero by fetoscopy and biopsy [3] it may be more appropriate to consider abortion in severely involved cases.

Oro-oculo-genito-cutaneous syndromes

In Stevens-Johnson syndrome and Behçet's disease dysphagia may result from ulceration of buccal and pharyngeal mucosae. In the former there is usually also crusting and ulceration of the lips. In the latter the ulcers probably represent one extreme end of the spectrum of aphthous ulceration; intestinal involvement, probably of an arteritic nature, sometimes coexists in Behçet's disease.

Carcinoma of the esophagus

In the Plummer-Vinson (Patterson-Kelly) syndrome a postcricoid web is associated with koilonychia, angular stomatitis, and a sore tongue: the common cause is iron deficiency with or without anemia. About 5 to 10 percent of patients with a postcricoid web develop carcinoma at the site. Tylosis is another marker of esophageal cancer. It is a not uncommon disease of palms and soles. Its association with carcinoma of the esophagus, though much talked of, is excessively rare, but the skin lesions are a reliable indicator, the cancer occurring only in those who have them. Two families have been described where the tylosis and cancer were inherited as autosomal dominant traits; the cancer, which appeared from 30 years upward and after the tylosis, occurred eventually in 95 percent of those with the skin condition [4]. Patients with celiac disease have been shown to have an increased risk of developing gastrointestinal malignancies including carcinoma of the esophagus [5]. It might be expected, therefore, that dermatitis herpetiformis with its strong association with celiac disease would carry a similar risk. Finally, treatments used for dermatologic conditions can increase the risk of malignancy, and this was particularly so in the case of medicinal arsenic [6].

Collagen vascular diseases

Vasculitic ulcers in the mouth and pharynx occur infrequently in systemic lupus erythematosus and probably in other diseases of this group as well. Dysphagia also occurs, particularly in systemic sclerosis and dermatomyositis, and is caused by changes in the esophageal and pharyngeal wall.

Systemic sclerosis. The esophagus is probably the internal organ most commonly involved in systemic sclerosis. Symptoms, especially dysphagia and heartburn, occur frequently, and radiologic or manometric abnormalities can be detected in up to 70 percent of cases [7]. The basis of the esophageal abnormalities which result in decreased peristalsis, dilatation, and stricture formation is thought to be fibrosis similar to that in the skin, though muscle and nerve may be affected as well. Abnormalities at the gastroesophageal junction lead to acid regurgitation and peptic ulceration and are another cause of dysphagia.

Dermatomyositis. In this collagen vascular disease, and occasionally in others, the muscles of swallowing can be affected in a similar fashion to the proximal skeletal muscles. Regardless of whether or not there is an underlying neoplasm, a myopathy, especially when it involves muscles of swallowing, is an indication for urgent treatment with adequate doses of systemic corticosteroids and possibly azathioprine as well.

Gastrointestinal bleeding and dermatologic disease

Vascular abnormalities
    Hereditary hemorrhagic telangiectasia
    Blue rubber bleb nevus syndrome
    Kaposi's sarcoma
Inherited defects of connective tissue
    Ehlers-Danlos syndrome
    Pseudoxanthoma elasticum
Gastrointestinal tract cancer
Polyposis
Vasculitis
Ulcerative colitis and Crohn's disease

The main groups of diseases in which skin signs are present and may help to elucidate the cause of bleeding are the vascular malformations and the inherited diseases of connective tissue; conditions like polyposis, vasculitis, inflammatory bowel disease, and malignant disease that also cause bleeding will be dealt with separately.

Vascular abnormalities

Hereditary hemorrhagic telangiectasia. The vascular dilatations that characterize the condition occur particularly on skin and on oral, nasal, and gastrointestinal mucosa, and may bleed at any of these sites. They are similar to the mat telangiectases of systemic sclerosis although these do not bleed. Although the condition is inherited as an autosomal dominant trait, lesions may not be apparent until young adult life. Treatment with estrogens reduces bleeding at some sites [8] perhaps by increasing keratinization of the mucosa, but this is unlikely to be relevant to the majority of gastrointestinal bleeds. When bleeding is severe, inhibition of fibrinolysis, e.g., by epsilon aminocaproic acid, is a suggested method of treatment but as with estrogens there are no controlled trials to support its usefulness in this condition.

Blue rubber bleb nevus syndrome. This is another condition associated with gastrointestinal bleeding and also inherited as an autosomal dominant trait. The lesions are cavernous hemangiomata which in the skin look and feel as their name suggests, and in the bowel project as submucous tumors into the lumen particularly of the small intestine.

Kaposi's sarcoma. This tumor of vascular endothelium and pericapillary cells presents clinically with vascular papules and nodules. It runs a fairly benign course in the elderly men it most commonly affects, but in younger African blacks it has long been known to be aggressive and to spread from the skin of the extremities it most commonly affects to other organs, including the gastrointestinal tract, where it causes bleeding. More recently this more aggressive spread has been seen in homosexual men as part of AIDS (see Chap. 209) and patients having immunosuppressive therapy [9,10]. Genetic, infective, and immune factors have been implicated in the pathogenesis.

Inherited defects of connective tissue

These involve both collagen and elastic fibers and the mode of inheritance varies. Careful examination of the skin for signs of these defects again may help to elicit the cause of a gastrointestinal bleed.

Ehlers-Danlos syndrome. There are now known to be at least eight types of this disease and they probably represent defects in the different enzymes concerned with collagen formation and degradation, though the precise abnormality has not been defined in all cases. Rupture of vessels in the gastrointestinal tract and elsewhere occurs mainly in type IV where the variety of collagen (type III) found in skin, gastrointestinal tract, and blood vessels is defective [11]. Diverticula and hiatus and inguinal hernias occur in addition to bleeding and perforation in the gastrointestinal tract.

Pseudoxanthoma elasticum. Here the defect is in elastic fibers and the disease will probably turn out to be a series of enzyme defects as with the Ehlers-Danlos syndrome: as yet four types have been described [12]. Gastrointestinal bleeds and signs from blockage of major arteries are clinical features.

Abdominal pain and the skin

Herpes zoster
Porphyrias
Fabry's disease
Urticaria and angioedema
Vasculitis

Rare instances where skin signs help in diagnosis include herpes zoster, porphyria, and Fabry's disease. Urticaria and angioedema, including the familial hereditary form, can produce a variable amount of abdominal pain from intestinal edema. Abdominal pain is also a feature of vasculitis and this will be discussed elsewhere.

Herpes zoster

This may produce pain before the blisters which, when they do appear, are usually of dermatomal distribution (T_7-L_1). Postherpetic neuralgia can result in prolonged pain. Motor complications are unusual at these levels but involvement of the sacral roots can produce, as well as perineal pain, difficulty with defecation [13].

Porphyrias

It is in the rarer variegate porphyria and hereditary coproporphyria that gut and skin changes occur together. The skin changes resemble those of porphyria cutanea tarda, although in this condition abdominal crises do not occur. Diagnosis entails measurement of urinary, fecal, or erythrocyte porphyrins. The abdominal signs are of pain, vomiting, and constipation. A number of drugs including estrogen and barbiturates precipitate attacks and must therefore be avoided [14], and in some forms impaired liver function, especially if it is caused by alcohol, makes the skin lesions worse. Rarely hepatic tumors produce porphyrins and present with clinical porphyria [15].

Fabry's disease

In this rare lysosomal storage disease which is inherited as a sex-linked recessive trait, unexplained pains are frequently the presenting feature: usually these are in the limbs, but they may be in the abdomen, and a diagnosis of a neurosis is easily made if other signs are not elicited. The skin lesions do not appear until adolescence and even then can be very unimpressive. The signs and symptoms are due to deposits of a lipid which result from the deficiency of the enzyme α-galactosidase A; vomiting and diarrhea are explained on the basis of involvement of the myenteric plexus. Exceptionally, renal and bone marrow transplants have been used in treatment.

Skin signs of vasculitis of intestinal vessels

Anaphylactoid purpura—leukocytoclastic vasculitis
Collagen vascular diseases
   Acute
   Chronic
Malignant atrophic papulosis

There are many cases of acute vasculitis and mesenteric vessel obstruction where similar disease affects the skin. Skin signs are also associated with chronic mesenteric vessel obstruction.

Anaphylactoid purpura

This leukocytoclastic vasculitis, manifest by "palpable purpura," especially on the legs and buttocks, is accompanied by joint swellings, hematuria, and abdominal colic.

In children the illness often follows an infection with *Streptococcus pyogenes* but other infections and drugs can also be responsible. Bleeding from the gut, abdominal pain, and, in children, intussusception occur.

Collagen vascular diseases

Acute involvement of different-sized vessels in small and large intestine occurs in this group of diseases and occasionally such an episode is the cause of death. The skin signs of small-vessel disease are likely to be present as well. Chronic obliteration of small intestinal vessels in these diseases can result in malabsorption [16].

Malignant atrophic papulosis [17]

It is difficult to know whether this subacute vasculitis of skin, brain, and gut vessels is a separate disease entity or whether it is a variety of one of the more common collagen vascular diseases, but the histologic finding of an endarteritis with thrombosis is said to be diagnostic. The scars in the skin take on a porcelain-like appearance and the patient usually dies from vascular disease or perforation of the bowel. Although a bad prognosis is the rule, skin lesions can present for years with apparent fitness in other respects [18].

Polyposis and dermatologic disease

Gardner's syndrome—adenomas
Peutz-Jeghers syndrome—hamartomas
Canada-Cronkhite syndrome—inflammatory
Neurofibromatosis
Ulcerative colitis—inflammatory

True polyps are adenomatous tumors with malignant propensity: they are rare except in the colon and rectum. Polypoid lesions, which are hamartomatous or inflammatory, occur in all parts of the gut [19]. All may have dermatologic associations.

Gardner's syndrome [20]

Here adenomatous polyps with a high risk of malignancy occur in association with multiple epidermoid cysts, fibromas, and lipomas, as well as osteomas of the facial bones. The syndrome is inherited as an autosomal dominant trait; epidermoid cysts and polyposis coli also occur separately in families and the relationship of these cases to Gardner's syndrome is uncertain.

Peutz-Jeghers syndrome [21]

In this syndrome the polyps are hamartomatous and occur mainly in the small intestine. As with other hamartomas, the histologic appearance may suggest malignancy but the risk of malignant behavior with metastases is probably not increased. The skin changes comprise small dark freckles around the mouth, on the lips, and on the distal parts of the fingers and toes; patchy pigmentation occurs inside the mouth. With increasing age the characteristic freckles tend to disappear, leaving a mouth pigmentation which may be indistinguishable from that due to racial factors or to Addison's disease. The syndrome is inherited as an autosomal dominant trait but some members of the families seem to have the skin or intestinal changes alone.

Canada-Cronkhite syndrome

In this rare acquired disease with alopecia and abnormal nails, inflammatory polyps are present in the stomach as well as the bowel; a protein-losing enteropathy is part of the syndrome but the hair and nail changes precede the bowel trouble and so do not seem to be the result of protein lack. The alopecia is patchy and the nail changes are characteristic but not diagnostic [22]. The inverted triangle of normal nail with surrounding dystrophy is possibly due to the growth of what embryologically is the ventral nail.

Neurofibromatosis

This fairly common dominantly inherited skin disease is occasionally associated with polypoid bowel tumors.

The skin in ulcerative colitis and Crohn's disease

Pyoderma gangrenosum
Granulomas
Erythema nodosum
Aphthous ulcers
Malnutrition
Rashes at ileostomy and colostomy sites
Annular erythema, erythema multiforme, lichen planus, vascular thromboses

Skin complications are similar in the two conditions but the relative frequencies with which they occur are different. In particular, pyoderma gangrenosum (PG) is much more common in ulcerative colitis (UC) while granulomata are more common in Crohn's disease.

Pyoderma gangrenosum (Figs. 168-1 and 168-2)

This, like most of the other skin signs of UC, is usually related to the activity of the bowel disease and regresses when the bowel improves. Half the patients with PG have UC but less than 10 percent of patients with UC have PG and very few of those with Crohn's disease have PG [23]. It has been suggested that the underlying mechanism is a Schwartzmann reaction, and other conditions in which PG occurs are rheumatoid disease and myeloma. In the absence of an obvious cause, the bowel should always be investigated, for in some cases of PG UC is asymptomatic. Topical corticosteroids, if necessary under occlusion, can be a very effective form of treatment, but occasionally systemic corticosteroids, salazopyrine, or dapsone are required for the skin.

Granulomas

Granulomas occur in the mouth in Crohn's disease where they may coalesce to give a cobblestone appearance or may cause diffuse thickening of the lips. Granulomas also occur around the anus, at colostomy and ileostomy sites, and in association with scars, sinuses, and fistulae. So-called metastatic granulomas occur at sites remote from the bowel [24].

Erythema nodosum

UC and Crohn's disease are relatively uncommon causes of this rash.

Aphthous ulcers

Aphthous ulcers are reported to occur in 8 percent of patients with UC [25] and 6 percent of patients with Crohn's disease [26]. They may be the presenting feature of either of these conditions or of celiac disease; therefore, in intractable mouth ulcers, investigation of the bowel should be considered. It is sometimes difficult to differentiate Crohn's disease with mouth ulcers from Behçet's disease with bowel involvement.

Malnutrition

Various skin signs of specific and nonspecific deficiencies can arise from inflammatory bowel disease or its treatment with elemental diets and these will be described elsewhere.

Rashes at colostomy and ileostomy sites

These can occur, especially in poorly fashioned ileostomies, from digestion of the skin by gut enzymes. Irritant and allergic contact dermatitis, and, in the genetically susceptible, psoriasis also occur.

Other skin abnormalities

Annular erythemas, vascular thromboses, erythema multiforme, and lichen planus have also been described. It is not always clear that they are caused by the bowel condition, especially in cases where drugs are being given.

Atopy and the gut

The role of ingested allergens in atopic eczema is a controversial one and outside the scope of this chapter. Gross edema and hypoalbuminemia from protein-losing enterop-

Fig. 168-1 Pyoderma gangrenosum of the arm.

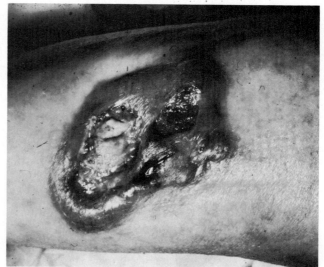

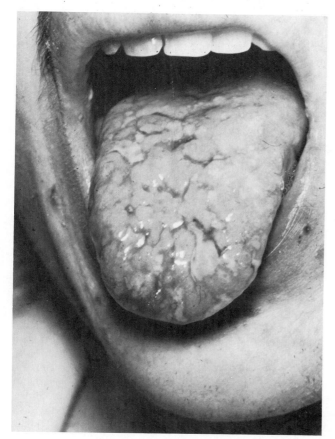

Fig. 168-2 Ulceration of the tongue in a patient with ulcerative colitis.

athy occur occasionally in atopic subjects. Protein is lost into the gut as a result of an immediate hypersensitivity reaction in the gut wall. Treatment is by elimination of the offending food; it has also been suggested that disodium cromoglycate given by the oral route may be effective.

Skin signs of pancreatic disease

Fibrocystic disease and sweat sodium
Acute pancreatitis and extravasation of blood
Fat necrosis
Superficial thrombophlebitis
Glucagonoma
Hemochromatosis
Diabetes mellitus

Fibrocystic disease

Although the main clinical signs are alimentary and pulmonary, circulatory collapse from hyponatremia can occur during excessive sweating as these patients are unable to conserve sodium in sweat. The mechanism is thought to be a sweat duct defect in absorption, and the measurement of sodium in sweat is useful in diagnosis.

Pancreatitis

Acute pancreatitis leads to extravasation of blood into the skin of the flanks, the abdominal wall, and around the umbilicus. Chronic pancreatitis, presumably by liberating lipolytic enzymes into the circulation, results in fat necrosis with painful subcutaneous nodules.

Carcinoma of pancreas

Migratory superficial thrombophlebitis occurs in neoplasia, particularly carcinoma of the pancreas. The rash of glucagonoma will be described later.

Hemochromatosis

Two of the organs in which iron is deposited are the pancreas, leading to diabetes, and the skin, leading to hyperpigmentation.

The skin and peritoneal disease

Serosal surfaces, including the peritoneum, can be involved in collagen vascular diseases, especially systemic lupus erythematosus. The most severe peritoneal involvement of dermatologic interest, however, occurred in patients given the cardioselective β-blocker practolol in the 1970s [27] and some of these patients had antinuclear factor in the serum as well as a rash with some features of lupus erythematosus. The sclerosing peritonitis presented with recurrent intestinal obstruction, and pericarditis, pleurisy, and Sjögren's syndrome with corneal scarring also occurred with serious consequences. Although the drug is no longer available the syndrome is described because of the need to be alert to complications of newer β-blocking drugs: although the majority of patients involved had taken practolol itself, a few cases of a similar cutaneous syndrome were seen with oxyprenolol.

Skin disease and malabsorption

Skin changes due to malabsorption
  Nonspecific
    Acquired ichthyosis
    Hair and nail abnormalities
    Hyperpigmentation
    Skin texture and elasticity
    Eczematous and psoriasiform rashes
    Intestinal bypass syndrome
  Lack of specific nutrients
    Zinc—acrodermatitis enteropathica
    Essential fatty acids
    Vitamins A, B, C, and K
    Folic acid and iron
    Protein
Malabsorption due to skin disease
  Dermatogenic enteropathy
Collagen vascular diseases
Dermatitis herpetiformis and celiac disease

Many skin changes occur in association with malabsorption, some as a result of it, some due to a disease process that affects the bowel as well as the skin, and some because of a genetic susceptibility to two different diseases; in addition, skin disease can actually cause malabsorption [1].

Skin changes due to malabsorption

Some of these are quite specific, e.g., the rash of zinc deficiency, while others are nonspecific, e.g., those that occur as a result of wasting or of illness in general.

Nonspecific cutaneous effects. These do not depend upon the nature of the underlying disease and, although they are most common in patients who have lost weight, for example from malabsorption or malignant disease, they are not necessarily confined to this group. Usually by the time the skin is involved it is apparent that the patient is systemically ill, but this is not invariable; for instance, patients with malignant lymphoma may have pruritus long before they have clinical evidence of underlying disease.

ACQUIRED ICHTHYOSIS. The skin of sick people often feels dry; this is one of the main causes of the itch about which they may complain. The skin resembles that seen in dominantly inherited ichthyosis of mild degree. It is not known whether a genetic predisposition is necessary for the development of the acquired form, but the frequency with which it occurs makes this doubtful. The cracks in the skin often become eczematized and the resulting clinical picture, on the shins particularly, is described as crazy-paving eczema. The presence of this, not only in malabsorption, but in cancer, chronic renal disease, and chronic hepatic disease as well, led the authors to postulate that malabsorption was the common factor and that this in turn was due to flattening of the intestinal mucosa such as has been described in malignant disease. The possibility has not been investigated systematically, but we did find villous atrophy with acquired ichthyosis due to lymphoma [28]. More likely is the possibility of essential fatty acid (EFA) deficiency or a comparable defect due either to malabsorption or to abnormal metabolism within the skin. Although preliminary studies show a decrease in plasma linoleic acid in wasting disease, they do not show an increase in plasma 5,8,11-eicosatrienoic acid which is thought to be the metabolic marker of severe EFA deficiency (see below).

HAIR AND NAILS. Hair and nails are frequently abnormal in poorly nourished people. Deficiencies of specific nutrients such as protein, iron, zinc, and folic acid may be found, but in the majority of cases the mechanism is not known and is likely to be multifactorial. Changes in hair and nails in malnourished patients whose main dietary deficiency is protein have been studied in kwashiorkor [29], and include reduction in both linear growth and diameter of the shaft with liability of the hair to break; there is also an increase in the percentage of hairs in telogen at any one time. Thus the clinical picture is that of chronic telogen effluvium.

Nails are generally poor and brittle in these patients and there may be episodic slowing of growth resulting in horizontal ridges (Beau's lines). When koilonychia occurs in malnutrition, it usually indicates iron deficiency with or without anemia. The transverse white bands that appear in the nails in hypoalbuminemia remain unexplained.

SKIN COLOR. One of the most interesting skin changes in malabsorption as well as in malignant disease is hyperpigmentation due to melanin. This may be gross and indistinguishable from that of Addison's disease with hyperpigmentation in the palmar creases and buccal mucosa. It is not due to an increase in circulating MSH peptide.

SKIN TEXTURE AND ELASTICITY. In the course of wasting diseases the skin becomes thinner from loss of collagen. This occurs in anorexia nervosa and after experimental dietary deprivation in the rat. The effect may be exaggerated clinically by the loss of subcutaneous fat. The skin is also less elastic and does not spring back normally after stretching.

ECZEMATOUS AND PSORIASIFORM RASHES DUE TO MALABSORPTION. These occur in malabsorption regardless of its cause, although most observations have been done in patients with celiac disease and tropical sprue [30–32]. A number of specific deficiencies, including EFA deficiency, have been postulated as causes, but these have not been substantiated in the group as a whole. Treatment of the malabsorption is always effective in curing the rash. Although atypicality of the eczematous and psoriasiform rashes has been stressed in the past, there do not seem to be any special diagnostic features in the rashes that these authors have seen from malabsorption. Associated acquired ichthyosis and hyperpigmentation were other points stressed, but neither is confined to patients wasting from malabsorption. Furthermore, hyperpigmentation is common in extensive rashes and in these patients it is not related to the presence or absence of malabsorption. In the absence of clear indications, investigation of the bowel in such cases is not necessary: no cases of celiac disease were found by small-intestinal mucosal biopsy of 100 unselected consecutive patients with eczema and psoriasis (personal observation). This is of course in direct contrast to dermatitis herpetiformis, where biopsy leads to the discovery of many previously unsuspected cases of celiac disease.

JEJUNOILEAL AND JEJUNOCOLIC ANASTOMOSES. The increase in the number of patients with obesity treated by these by-pass operations has led to the recognition of certain metabolic consequences, most of which are of unknown etiology. Apart from dryness of the skin and hair loss, which are presumably due to malabsorption, inflammatory and vasculitic skin lesions occur together with fever, leukocytosis, and arthralgia [33].

Cutaneous effects of malabsorption of specific nutrients. ZINC DEFICIENCY AND ACRODERMATITIS ENTEROPATHICA. Zinc deficiency can occur from malabsorption in celiac disease and inflammatory bowel disease; it was relatively common when elemental feeds were deficient in zinc. A congenital abnormality of zinc absorption occurs in acrodermatitis enteropathica. Although there are reasons for believing deranged zinc metabolism, due to malabsorption or not, might have adverse effects on the skin, it has been difficult to prove that common skin conditions are associated with zinc deficiency. Low plasma zinc concentrations have been found in psoriasis and leg ulcers as well as in many other unrelated diseases [34]. This does not mean that there is a deficiency in the body as a whole or that zinc is helpful in therapy. More dynamic studies of zinc metabolism using Zn-65 have been few and show there is a wide variation of absorption and reexcretion into the bowel and no evidence of overall zinc deficiency in patients with stasis leg ulcers [35].

Acrodermatitis enteropathica presents, usually at the time of weaning, with a blistering rash on the hands, feet, and around the mouth and anus; alopecia and "failure to thrive" are other features. All are reversed by treatment with zinc though this has to be continued indefinitely. Absorption of zinc is impaired [36] although the mechanism is not understood. Moynahan [37] suggests that dietary zinc is chelated in the bowel by an abnormal small-molecular-weight substance. Large doses of oral zinc result in sufficient absorption to overcome the defect although it is not known how.

ESSENTIAL FATTY ACID DEFICIENCY. The appearance of a scaly rash in experimental animals with EFA deficiency is well known, and a dry skin with cracking of the horny layer has been reported in children fed on diets low in linoleic acid. Most is known about the patients who have a scaly skin as the result of malabsorption from small-gut resection [38]. They have a low linoleic acid, and an abnormal metabolite 5,8,11-eicosatrienoic acid in the plasma. Clinically their skin is improved by topical linoleic acid such as is found in sunflower-seed oil. In other wasting conditions, including celiac disease, plasma linoleic acid is again low but the abnormal metabolite is not found: it is not certain how specific this is to EFA deficiency but it seems reasonable to treat patients with a scaly skin which may be due to this with sunflower-seed oil.

How the scaliness of EFA deficiency is brought about is not clear. Barrier function is impaired and there is an increase in transepidermal water loss; it is difficult to explain why the horny layer cracks as if it were poorly hydrated, yet percutaneous water movement is increased. As in other scaly dermatoses, there is an increase in total lipid synthesis in the skin with as yet incompletely defined qualitative changes in the different lipid classes. EFA deficiency impairs prostaglandin synthesis and topical prostaglandin (PGE_2) will improve the skin changes in animals.

MALABSORPTION OF VITAMINS AND OTHER NUTRIENTS. The rashes due to deficiency of vitamins A, B, C, and K, usually in combination, occur in severe small-bowel abnormalities. In addition, malabsorption of vitamin K occurs in obstructive jaundice. Deficiency of vitamin A, whether due to malabsorption or not, is no longer thought to be a causal factor in pityriasis rubra pilaris and other scaly dermatoses as was once thought. The mechanism of action of the vitamin A-related aromatic retinoids in some of these conditions is not understood but it is thought not to involve the bowel. Folate, iron, and zinc deficiency may contribute to the poor hair growth of malnutrition. Malabsorption of protein, or protein-losing enteropathy, leads to edema of the skin, which is common in kwashiorkor. In this condition, however, there are many deficiencies in addition to that of protein and it is difficult to attribute the physical signs to a specific one. There is a recent suggestion that an alfatoxin from fungi growing on cereals in humid climates may be as important as malnutrition.

Malabsorption due to skin disease

Dermatogenic enteropathy [39]. A large proportion of patients with extensive skin disease exhibits mild secondary malabsorption as a result; in one study we found steatorrhea in 22 of 30 patients with erythroderma. Malabsorption of fat has been most studied in eczema and psoriasis, where it has been shown that the steatorrhea is proportional to the extent of the skin disease, and responds rapidly to topical treatment of the rash. It is not related to gluten sensitivity or celiac disease, and structural changes, if they occur at all, are minimal [40]. The mechanism of its production is unknown, but it is one of the systemic effects of skin disease [1]; similar malabsorption appears to occur in other chronic diseases. Symptoms of dermatogenic enteropathy are rare, and the importance lies in the confusion that can occur if it is not recognized for what it is in a patient with a rash and malabsorption. If in doubt, a small-intestinal biopsy can be done, and a flat biopsy will exclude it and point to celiac disease; treatment of dermatogenic enteropathy, other than by clearing the rash, is not necessary, and, in particular, a gluten-free diet should not be given.

Malabsorption in collagen vascular diseases

This can occur as a result of poor peristalsis from changes in the small-intestinal wall in systemic sclerosis, or by chronic obliteration of mesenteric vessels in polyarteritis and other forms of vasculitis [16]. The small-intestinal changes in systemic sclerosis are stucturally similar to those that occur in the esophagus and the large bowel; in the latter case they are accompanied by saccules or wide-mouthed diverticula found on barium enema examination in a large proportion of patients [41]. The structural changes in the small bowel which result in malabsorption seem to do so by allowing bacterial colonization higher up the bowel than is usual and producing, in effect, a blind loop syndrome. Clinical symptoms and signs of diarrhea and steatorrhea are severe in some cases but can be improved at least for a time by broad-spectrum antibiotics such as lincomycin.

Dermatitis herpetiformis

Dermatitis herpetiformis (DH) is perhaps the most important and interesting skin disease associated with malabsorption. When malabsorption occurs it is due to celiac disease (CD). Diagnosis of DH thus has gastrointestinal implications, and it is important that such a diagnosis should not be made without its specific features. An itchy rash predominantly affecting extensor surfaces with grouped papules and small tense blisters is characteristic, but atypical forms occur, including large blister forms. The exacerbation of the rash by iodides, its response to treatment with sulfones and sulfonamides and the histologic finding of papillary-tip microabcesses in recent (nonblistered) lesions all help in diagnosis but are not totally specific. The finding of IgA deposits in clinically uninvolved skin is likewise not completely specific [42]; it is nevertheless the most valuable single criterion in reliable hands. When facilities are not available, or their quality is in doubt, the authors have shown that a combination of clinical and histologic features and response to treatment is sufficient. In particular it is inadvisable for nondermatologists to label a rash DH from the immunofluorescence findings alone [43]. It is most usual for the IgA deposits to be granular and fibrillary and localized to the papillary dermis. A linear pattern is also found and it is still uncertain in this small subgroup whether the clinical features including the prevalence of enteropathy are the same [44].

Celiac disease in dermatitis herpetiformis. Although there was initially some difficulty in accepting the possibility that the enteropathy of DH was CD [45], this is no longer the case. Doubt arose mainly because of the mildness of the enteropathy in DH compared with that of CD as it usually

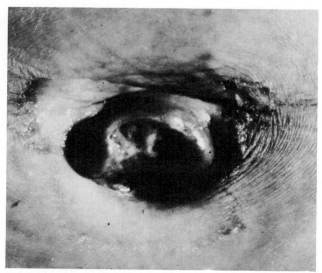

Fig. 168-3 Secondary deposit in umbilical skin from adenocarcinoma of the colon.

presents to the gastroenterologist. Cases of severe CD do occur in DH but are rare, most cases being mild, subclinical, or latent. CD can usefully be considered as the proverbial iceberg with a submerged zone of subclinical disease of unknown, but probably considerable, dimension; thus it is to be expected that, by selecting cases for small-intestinal mucosal biopsy which present to the dermatologist with what we now know is a marker of CD, much of the CD discovered will indeed be subclinical. The structural abnormalities are, as in CD, worse in the proximal small bowel and responsive to gluten withdrawal.

Diagnosis and incidence of celiac disease in dermatitis herpetiformis. Although the exact incidence of DH in CD is not known it is unlikely to be high, for 10 to 20 percent of patients have rashes and only a proportion of these are DH. By contrast, the proportion of patients with DH who have CD is high. The precise number depends on the criteria used for diagnosing CD. Only 33 percent of the authors' series [42] have clinical or biochemical evidence of CD, but 58 percent have structural abnormalities on stereomicroscopic or histologic examination. Attempts have been made to extend the diagnostic criteria of CD, and, if we take a raised interepithelial lymphocyte count in the small bowel even in the absence of other abnormalities as indicating CD, as others have done [46], the incidence in our patients with DH becomes 81 percent. Whatever criteria are used for diagnosis, the percentage of patients with DH who have CD always falls short of 100 percent.

Relationship of dermatitis herpetiformis and celiac disease. The nature of this relationship remains unknown. In particular, the the presence of CD is obviously not necessary for the development of DH; despite many statements to the contrary [47], malabsorption cannot be the cause of the rash. Likewise, the role of gluten, which is generally thought to be important in the production of the rash, is not known. Although the gut almost always responds to gluten withdrawal, the response of the skin is less clear

and its time course is remarkably prolonged. Moreover, the response of skin and gut can occur independently of one another [48]. Patients with DH and CD have a significant increase in the incidence of HLA B8 and related antigens. This occurs even in the patients with DH who do not have CD, and suggests a genetic association. Although the consensus is that the rash as well as the bowel defect is caused by gluten sensitivity, we believe that the evidence is still not entirely convincing.

Treatment of DH with a gluten-free diet. There are several reasons why one may want to treat DH with a gluten-free diet. Obviously patients with clinical and biochemical evidence of CD should be treated this way. It is more difficult to advise people with DH who have only structural changes in the small-bowel mucosa. Where malignant disease, especially lymphoma of the gastrointestinal tract, occurs in DH it is usually in conjunction with CD, and, even in CD, it is not certain that a gluten-free diet protects against malignancy. Consequently it is difficult to insist on the diet in patients with subclinical CD.

Quite apart from prescribing a gluten-free diet for the bowel in DH, there is the question of prescribing it for the skin. A number of patients develop DH when they are on a gluten-free diet for CD and when their enteropathy is, as a result, well controlled. Nevertheless, the general view is that a strict gluten-free diet enables the rash to be controlled without dapsone, or with a much reduced dose of dapsone, in a significant proportion of patients with DH, although this may take months or years.

Skin disease and malignancy

Signs of wasting
Signs of malignant disease
   Secondary deposits
   Dermatomyositis
   Acanthosis nigricans
   Hypertrichosis lanuginosa
   Nonspecific rashes
Signs of specific gastrointestinal tumors
   Carcinoma of esophagus
   Carcinoma of stomach
   Small bowel tumors
      Carcinoid
      Mastocytosis
      Lymphoma
   Carcinoma of large bowel
   Carcinoma of pancreas—glucagonoma

In malignancy, as in malabsorption, some of the skin manifestations are very specific to a particular tumor, e.g., the rash of a glucagonoma, while others can occur in different malignancies, and still others are common to all wasting diseases. As with malabsorption, too, there are three possible causal relationships between skin changes and systemic diseases.

Signs of wasting

Most of the points have already been discussed in connection with malabsorption.

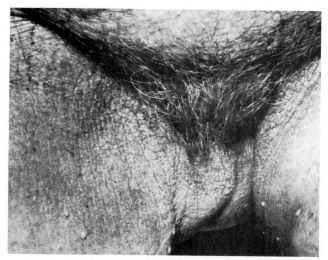

Fig. 168-4   Acanthosis nigricans in a patient with jejunal carcinoma.

Hyperpigmentation. Though common to both wasting and malignancy, this has been studied more in malignant disease. Ectopic production of hormones which contain the melanocyte-stimulating heptopeptide sequence is a rare cause of hyperpigmentation in malignant disease. In other situations concentrations of melanocyte-stimulating peptides (immunoreactive α- and β-MSH and β-LPH) are not increased in the circulation.

Dryness and itch. The dryness that has been described in malabsorption is a major factor in the production of itch in lymphoma and other malignant disease, although some of these patients itch without any visible abnormality of their skin. The mechanism is not understood. It is not known, for instance, whether unconjugated bile salts like chenodeoxycholate, which are important in the itch of bilary obstruction, are important here also. The investigation for malignant disease of a patient who is apparently well and yet suffers from pruritus is an exercise of few returns. Most people itch because of a common skin disease, and others because their skin is dry for nonmalignant reasons. Hypoferremia is a rare cause of itch. This is related to the decreased iron concentration itself rather than to any accompanying anemia, for it disappears within hours of intravenous administration of iron. A group of male patients with itch and hypoferremia who subsequently developed lymphoma has been described [49], and so a patient with unexplained itch in these circumstances may be worth further investigation.

Signs of malignancy

Secondary deposits in skin. These occur in the skin from tumors in all internal organs including the gastrointestinal tract, and the scalp skin is a common site. Sister Joseph's nodule is the name given to metastatic carcinoma at the umbilicus from intraabdominal adenocarcinoma, usually of the stomach or large bowel (Fig. 168-3).

Secondary deposits in internal organs. A number of skin tumors metastasize to the gut. Malignant melanoma does

so relatively commonly and can produce bleeding as a result. Kaposi's sarcoma has already been mentioned in connection with alimentary bleeding.

Dermatomyositis. This collagen vascular disease, when it occurs in adults, may be due to underlying malignant disease and 7 to 52 percent of cases are said to show such an association [50]. The associated tumors are the ones most prevalent in a particular population: gastric and colonic cancers feature less often than bronchogenic ones in Europe and North America and in the Chinese, in whom nasopharyngeal carcinoma is a common tumor; this is also one most often associated with dermatomyositis. There is no doubt that the rash and myopathy can regress after removal of the tumor and, as dermatomyositis may be a relatively early sign of internal malignancy, its recognition is potentially lifesaving. Overall, however, investigation of patients with dermatomyositis for malignancy gives a poor return of diagnosis of treatable disease. This should temper the vigor of investigation in the individual case, e.g., the question of speculative laparotomy. The degree of investigation to which patients have in the past been subjected, as well as the acceptance of different criteria for diagnosis, is partly responsible for the great variation in incidence of malignant disease quoted in the different series.

Acanthosis nigricans (Fig. 168-4). This is a generic term for three separate disorders: (1) genetodevelopmental or nevoid, (2) due to friction and maceration as in obesity, (3) epidermotrophic, e.g., in acromegaly. Here we are con-

Fig. 168-5   Ear of a patient with hypertrichosis lanuginosa.

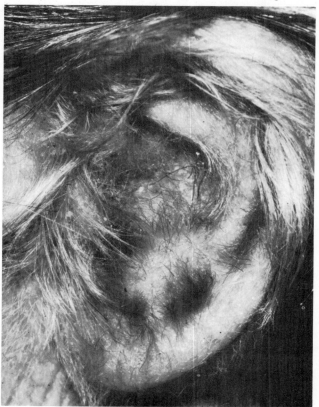

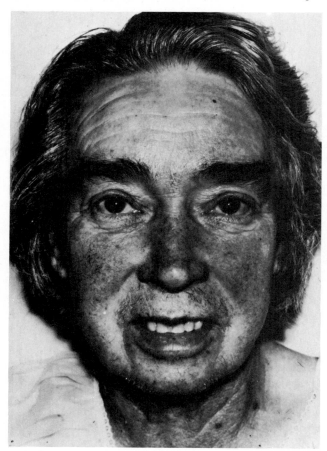

Fig. 168-6 Face of a patient with carcinoid tumor with liver metastases.

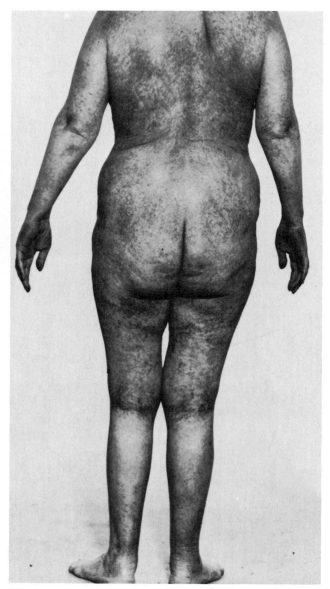

Fig. 168-7 Rash of urticaria pigmentosa. The patient also had malabsorption and celiac disease.

cerned only with the form seen in malignancy, and it seems likely that eventually a circulating epidermotrophic factor will be found. In this context it is interesting that in two-thirds of the patients with acanthosis nigricans and cancer the tumor is gastric, and that urogastrone, which is a potent physiologic inhibitor of gastric secretion, is similar in structure to human epidermal growth factor. It is rare for a tumor not to be found in this type of acanthosis nigricans and the rash may regress if the tumor, usually an adenocarcinoma, is removed. However, recognition of the disorder is more important diagnostically than therapeutically, since the tumor is already well established in 80 to 90 percent of patients at the time of diagnosis of the rash.

Hypertrichosis lanuginosa (Fig. 168-5). This excessive growth of lanugo hair, which may cover the whole body, is a rare complication of malignant disease, including gastrointestinal cancer. The mechanism of its production is not understood but it is suggested that inappropriate cortisol production is to blame.

Nonspecific rashes. Urticarias, erythemas, and vasculitis are among the nonspecific rashes that occur occasionally, apparently as a result of malignant disease, although much more often the same diseases have a less sinister cause. A special relationship of pemphigoid to neoplasia remains unproved.

Signs of special gastrointestinal tumors

Carcinoma of the esophagus. These signs have already been discussed under "Dysphagia and the Skin."

Carcinoma of the stomach. Vitiligo is a rare presenting sign of carcinoma of the stomach. The association is through atrophic gastritis and pernicious anemia which themselves have an association with vitiligo. A similar, comparatively increased chance of developing carcinoma of the stomach might be expected in patients with dermatitis herpetiformis and lichen sclerosus who also have an increased incidence of parietal cell antibodies.

Small-bowel tumors. CARCINOID (Fig. 168-6). The characteristic carcinoid flush is not as a rule seen in carcinoid tumors confined to the gastrointestinal tract, e.g., those of the appendix, for the vasoactive substances do not reach

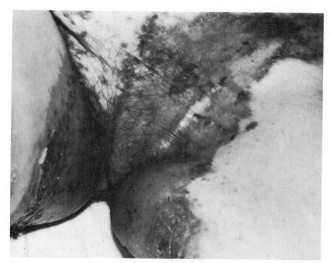

Fig. 168-8 Migratory epidermal necrolysis in a patient with glucagonoma of the stomach.

the systemic circulation; the cutaneous effects can occur in tumors of other tissues, e.g., the ovary and lung, and when liver metastases are present and are due to the serotonin, histamine, prostaglandins, and kinins they produce [51]. A pellagra-like rash occurring on light-exposed areas has been attributed to tryptophan deficiency associated with the increased serotonin production. The flush has a cyanotic tinge and can be intermittent initially, but later it becomes permanent and associated with telangiectasia, hyperpigmentation, and scarring. Diagnosis is confirmed by finding 5-hydroxyindoleacetic acid in the urine, though occasionally this is episodic as well.

MASTOCYTOSIS (Fig. 168-7). Most mast cell infiltrates are benign. The major effects of benign and malignant tumors are due to the histamine they produce. Urticaria pigmentosa may involve organs other than the skin: the rarer diffuse mast cell infiltration of the skin is usually accompanied by widespread infiltration of internal tissues. Small bowel and pancreas are among the organs affected and malabsorption can result. Celiac disease has been described in patients with mastocytosis [52] and is another cause of malabsorption in these patients. Osteomalacia can occur in consequence and it may be difficult to differentiate this from the osteoporosis which sometimes results from the liberation of heparin-like substances from the mast cells. Not all the gastrointestinal effects of mastocytosis are due to infiltration by mast cells, for the liberation of large amounts of pharmacologically active substances from the skin lesions, e.g., during bathing, can lead to diarrhea and abdominal pain.

LYMPHOMA. The occurrence of lymphoma with dermatitis herpetiformis has already been mentioned. When a lymphoma occurs in a patient with celiac disease, with or without dermatitis herpetiformis, it can be difficult to diagnose early on, since the clinical signs are often vague and nonspecific. "Ulcers, nodules and skin rashes" have been described as arising at the onset of the lymphoma in one series of cases [53].

Patients with lymphomas, including those of the bowel, are prone to skin complications of immunosuppression, whether this is due to the disease or its treatment. There is increased susceptibility to infection with viruses, bacteria, fungi, and protozoa, including those that are not normally pathogenic. Herpes simplex and herpes zoster may occur, and tend to be widely disseminated, and *Candida albicans* infection may be systematized or accompanied by granuloma formation.

Carcinoma of the large bowel. The skin signs that occur in conjunction with the potentially malignant forms of polyposis, and those that occur in ulcerative colitis which is to be regarded as a premalignant condition have been described. Paget's disease in the perianal skin is, like mammary Paget's disease, associated with an underlying carcinoma. This tumor is not always in adjacent tissue, but most commonly does arise in rectal mucosa, apocrine glands, or cloacal remnants. A rare presentation in the last case is as a chronic anal fistula.

Carcinoma of the pancreas (glucagonoma). Apart from the rather nonspecific skin signs of carcinoma of the exocrine cells already mentioned, the rash of particular interest is the migratory necrolysis of glucagonoma. This rare but distinctive rash occurs in flexures (Figs. 168-8 and A2-15) and around orifices, with blistering, hyperpigmentation, gyrate configuration, and necrolysis. Although a specific association with glucagon-producing tumors is described [54], it seems likely that similar rashes occur rarely with other gastrointestinal peptides. Glucagon and related peptides, such as vasoactive intestinal peptide and gastric inhibitory peptide, are produced in excess by tumors of the pancreas and other parts of the gastrointestinal tract, and occasionally by tumors elsewhere. The cause of the skin lesions is not known, but therapeutic administration of glucagon to patients with pancreatitis has been reported to have produced a similar rash in one patient. Moreover, the rash of one of our patients with a glucagonoma showed some improvement when she was treated with the α-cell inhibitor streptozotocin. In addition to their high circulating levels of glucagon, these patients have many other metabolic abnormalities including severe malabsorption, gross hypoaminoacidemia, and a low serum zinc concentration. The resemblance of the rash to acrodermatitis enteropathica and the apparent response of one patient to treatment with zinc (personal observation) raises the question of whether zinc deficiency is important in the production of the rash.

References

1. Shuster S, Marks J: *Systemic Effects of Skin Disease.* London, Heinemann, 1970
2. Moynahan E: The treatment and management of epidermolysis bullosa. *Clin Exp Dermatol* **7**:665, 1982
3. Eady R et al: Prenatal diagnostic studies in epidermolysis bullosa: observations in five cases. *Br J Dermatol* **107(suppl 22)**:9, 1982
4. Howel-Evans W et al: Carcinoma of the oesophagus with keratosis palmaris et plantaris (tylosis). *Q J Med* **27**:413, 1958
5. Harris O et al: Malignancy in adult coeliac disease and ideopathic steatorrhoea. *Am J Med* **42**:899, 1967
6. Robson AO, Jelliffe AM: Medicinal arsenic poisoning and lung cancer. *Br Med J* **2**:207, 1963
7. Weihrauch TR, Korling GW: Manometric assessment of

oesophageal involvement in progressive systemic sclerosis, morphoea and Raynaud's disease. *Br J Dermatol* **107**:325, 1982

8. Harrison DF: Familial haemorrhagic telangiectasia: 20 cases treated with systemic oestrogen. *Q J Med* **33**:25, 1964

9. Brennan RD, Durack DT: Gay compromise syndrome. *Lancet* **2**:1338, 1981

10. Gange W, Jones EW: Kaposi's sarcoma and immunosuppressive therapy: an appraisal. *Clin Exp Dermatol* **3**:135, 1978

11. Pope FM et al: Patients with Ehlers-Danlos syndrome type IV lack type III collagen. *Proc Natl Acad Sci USA* **72**:1314, 1975

12. Pope FM: Autosomal dominant pseudoxanthoma elasticum. *J Med Genet* **11**:152, 1974

13. Jellinek EH, Tulloch WS: Herpes zoster with dysfunction of bladder and anus. *Lancet* **2**:1219, 1976

14. Moore MR et al: Drugs and the acute porphyrias. *Trends Pharmacol Sci* **2**:330, 1981

15. Thompson RPG et al: Cutaneous porphyria due to a malignant primary hepatoma. *Gastroenterology* **59**:779, 1970

16. Carron DB, Douglas AP: Steatorrhoea in vascular insufficiency of the small intestine. *Q J Med* **34**:331, 1963

17. Degos R et al: Dermatite papulosquameuse atrophiante. *Bull Soc Fr Dermatol Syphiligr* **52**:60, 1942

18. Hall-Smith P: Malignant atrophic papulosis (Degos' disease). *Br J Dermatol* **81**:817, 1969

19. Bussey H, Morson B: Familial polyposis coli, in *Gastrointestinal Tract Cancer,* edited by M Lipkin, R Good. New York, Plenum Press, 1978, p 275

20. Gardner EJ: A genetic and clinical study of intestinal polyposis, a predisposing factor for carcinoma of the colon and rectum. *Am J Hum Genet* **3**:167, 1951

21. Jeghers H et al: Generalised intestinal polyposis and melanin spots of the oral mucosa, lips and digits. *N Engl J Med* **241**:993, 1961

22. Cunliffe W, Anderson J: Case of Cronkhite-Canada syndrome with associated jejunal diverticulosis. *Br Med J* **4**:601, 1967

23. Stathers GM et al: Pyoderma gangrenosum in association with regional enteritis. *Arch Dermatol* **95**:375, 1967

24. McCallum DI, Kinmont PDL: Dermatological manifestations of Crohn's disease. *Br J Dermatol* **80**:1, 1968

25. Edwards FC, Truelove SC: The course and prognosis of ulcerative colitis. *Gut* **5**:1, 1964

26. Croft CB, Wilkinson AR: Ulceration of the mouth, pharynx and larynx in Crohn's disease of the intestine. *Br J Surg* **59**:249, 1972

27. Brown P et al: Sclerosing peritonitis, an unusual reaction to a β-adrenergic blocking drug (practolol). *Lancet* **2**:1477, 1974

28. Shuster S: The gut and the skin, in *Third Symposium on Advanced Medicine. Proceedings of a Conference Held at Royal College of Physicians, London,* edited by AM Dawson. London, Pitman, 1967, p 349

29. Sims RT: Hair as an indicator of incipient and developed malnutrition and response to therapy—principles and practice, in *An Introduction to the Biology of the Skin,* edited by RH Champion et al, Oxford/Edinburgh, Blackwell, 1970, p 387

30. Cooke WT et al: Symptoms, signs and diagnostic features of idiopathic steatorrhoea. *Q J Med* **22**:59, 1953

31. Badenoch J: Steatorrhoea in the adult. *Br Med J* **2**:879, 1960

32. Wells GC: Skin disorders and malabsorption. *Br Med J* **2**:937, 1962

33. Kennedy C: The spectrum of inflammatory skin disease following jejuno-ileal bypass for morbid obesity. *Br J Dermatol* **105**:425, 1981

34. Greaves MW, Boyd TRC: Plasma-zinc concentrations in patients with psoriasis, other dermatoses and venous leg ulceration. *Lancet* **2**:1019, 1967

35. Hawkins T et al: Whole body monitoring and other studies of zinc 65 metabolism in patients with dermatological disease. *Clin Exp Dermatol* **1**:243, 1976

36. Lombeck et al: Akrodermatitis enteropathica eine Zinkstoffwechselstorung mit Zinkmalabsorption. *Z Kinderheilkd* **120**:181, 1975

37. Moynahan EJ: Acrodermatitis enteropathica; a lethal inherited human zinc-deficiency. *Lancet* **2**:399, 1974

38. Prottey C et al: Correction of the cutaneous manifestations of essential fatty acid deficiency in man by application of sunflower seed oil to the skin. *J Invest Dermatol* **64**:228, 1975

39. Shuster S, Marks J: Dermatogenic enteropathy—a new cause for steatorrhoea. *Lancet* **1**:1367, 1965

40. Marks J, Shuster S: Small-intestinal mucosal abnormalities in various skin diseases—fact or fancy. *Gut* **11**:281, 1970

41. Harper R, Jackson DC: Progressive systemic sclerosis. *Br J Radiol* **38**:825, 1965

42. Marks J: Dogma and dermatitis herpetiformis. *J Clin Exp Dermatol* **2**:189, 1977

43. Karlsson I et al: Absence of cutaneous IgA in coeliac disease without dermatitis herpetiformis. *Br J Dermatol* **99**:621, 1978

44. Leonard J et al: Linear IgA disease in adults. *Br J Dermatol* **107**:301, 1982

45. Weinstein WM et al: What is coeliac sprue? in *Coeliac Disease. Proceedings of an Internal Conference Held at the Royal Postgraduate Medical School, London, 1969,* edited by CC Booth, RH Dowling. Edinburgh, Churchill Livingstone, 1970, p 232

46. Fry L et al: Lymphocytic infiltration of epithelium in diagnosis of gluten-sensitive enteropathy. *Br Med J* **3**:371, 1972

47. Katz SI et al: Dermatitis herpetiformis: the skin and gut. *Ann Intern Med* **93**:857, 1980

48. Fry L et al: Long-term follow up of dermatitis herpetiformis with and without gluten withdrawal. *Br J Dermatol* **107**:631, 1982

49. Vickers CFH: Nutrition and the skin, in *Tenth Symposium on Advanced Medicine,* edited by JGG Ledingham. London, Pitman, 1974

50. Rowell NR: Lupus erythematosus, scleroderma and dermatomyositis, in *Textbook of Dermatology,* 3d ed, edited by A Rook et al. Oxford, Blackwell, 1979, p 1238

51. Graham-Smith DD: The carcinoid syndrome. *Gut* **11**:189, 1970

52. Scott BB et al: Involvement of the small intestine in systemic mast cell disease. *Gut* **16**:918, 1975

53. Austad WI et al: Steatorrhea and malignant lymphoma. *Am J Dig Dis* **12**:475, 1967

54. Mallinson CN et al: A glucagonoma syndrome. *Lancet* **2**:1, 1974

CHAPTER 169

CUTANEOUS ASPECTS OF RENAL DISEASE

Barbara A. Gilchrest and John W. Rowe

Dermatologic concomitants of renal disease fall into two general categories: (1) a variety of inherited and acquired disorders with specific or characteristic renal and cutaneous manifestations, and (2) the nonspecific pathologic and clinical changes that accompany renal insufficiency regardless of its etiology. The first category includes diseases in which the same basic process leads to clinical manifestations in both skin and kidney, such as deposition of abnormal globulins in dysproteinemia, or immunoglobulins in systemic lupus erythematosus, abnormal lipids in Fabry's disease, and amyloid in amyloidosis, as well as disorders in which the cutaneous and renal involvements appear histologically unrelated, such as developmental disorders (tuberous sclerosis, nail patella syndrome) and a larger group of diseases of unknown etiology (scleroderma, familial Mediterranean fever). Examples from this category are listed in Table 169-1, and a more detailed discussion of the dermatologic findings in each disease can be found elsewhere in this text.

The remainder of this chapter concerns the second category, cutaneous manifestations of uremia.

Historical aspects

In the last century, pathognomonic skin changes of uremia were widely accepted. Uremic frost, although first described in patients dying of cholera [1], was recognized by Hirschsprung in 1865 as an agonal finding in uremia [2]. Erythema papulatum uremicum, an eruption believed to occur only in uremia, was reported in up to 15 percent of patients in some series and frequently presaged death. The characteristic erythematous nodules on palms, soles, forearms, and occasionally face coalesced, became hemorrhagic, and sometimes ulcerated over a period of several weeks. The condition was considered rare by the twentieth century [1] and is no longer recognized. Several other dermatologic conditions such as uremic erysipeloid and uremic roseola have also disappeared, undoubtedly through reassignment to more specific pathophysiologic categories.

Clinical features

Diffuse hyperpigmentation, accentuated in sun-exposed areas, is characteristic of uremic patients. Melanogenesis is increased in the epidermis as a result of increased tissue levels of β-MSH, which is poorly dialyzable and not excreted normally in uremia [3,4]. The sallow, yellow cast commonly seen in uremia is attributed to retained carotene, urochromes, and other yellow pigments, as well as to a relative lack of red tones in this severely anemic population. Linear hyperpigmentation commonly results from scratching. Scattered ecchymoses and petechiae reflect the increased vascular fragility and the platelet dysfunction associated with uremia. Xerosis is common and often associated with perifollicular hyperkeratosis [5]. Body hair is sparse [2].

Uremic frost remains a distinctive terminal finding among patients in severe renal failure. The numerous white to tan granules are most prominent on the nose, beard area, and neck, and represent crystallization of urea from sweat [2].

A self-limited bullous dermatosis has been reported in patients undergoing chronic dialysis and appears to affect up to 16 percent of the dialysis population [6–9]. The bullae strongly resemble those of porphyria cutanea tarda (PCT), but porphyrin concentrations are normal in the plasma, stool, urine, and erythrocytes. Clinically, the bullae and cutaneous fragility are identical to those seen in PCT, but milia formation, facial hirsutism, periorbital suffusion, and other stigmata of PCT occur rarely if at all. One-micron-thick histologic sections reveal noninflammatory subepidermal bullae with thickened venular walls in the papillary dermis and prominent hypogranulation of mast cells, indistinguishable from PCT. Focal immunoglobulin deposition may be present perivascularly or along the floor of the blister cavity [6]. In some patients the eruption can be attributed to furosemide or nalidixic acid [7–13], but persistent bullae have been well documented in the absence of all recognized exogenous photosensitizers [6]. Photosensitization due to retention of an endogenous nonporphyrin compound is likely, but has not been documented.

True PCT also occurs in patients undergoing chronic hemodialysis [14–16] and is probably more common than in the general population. Because urinary output is often insignificant, correct diagnosis relies on plasma and fecal porphyrin determinations. PCT in dialysis patients is characterized by extremely high plasma levels of uroporphyrin [17–19] which appears not to cross the dialysis membrane, and even asymptomatic nonporphyric dialysis patients may have mildly elevated levels [17,18]. Suppression of uroporphyrin decarboxylase activity as well as reduced porphyrin excretion may contribute to this increase [18]. Therapeutic phlebotomy is contraindicated by the usually severe anemia in this patient population, and even low-dose chloroquine treatment is complicated by poor, uncertain excretion of this drug. Use of a large-pore dialysis membrane [16] or actual plasma exchange [20] may be justified, but for most patients sun avoidance alone appears most prudent. Customary nonopaque sunscreens are ineffective since they do not block the porphyrin-activating wavelengths in the visible portion of the solar spectrum.

Kyrle's disease, hyperkeratosis follicularis et parafollicularis in cutem penetrans, is characterized clinically by hyperpigmented, often pruritic, papules and nodules with

Table 169-1   Multisystem diseases with major renal and cutaneous findings

Disease	Renal manifestations	
	Histologic	**Clinical and laboratory**
Amyloidosis	Glomerular deposition of amyloid	Proteinuria, nephrotic syndrome, chronic renal failure
Angiokeratoma corporis diffusum universale (Fabry's disease)	Glomerular deposition of glycosphingolipid	Proteinuria, hematuria, chronic renal failure in males
Diabetes mellitus	Glomerulosclerosis, papillary necrosis	Proteinuria, nephrotic syndrome, chronic renal failure, renal infection
Dysproteinemias	Glomerulonephritis	Proteinuria, hematuria, acute and chronic renal failure
Familial Mediterranean fever	Glomerular deposition of amyloid	Proteinuria, nephrotic syndrome
Gout	Interstitial nephritis	Nephrolithiasis, mild proteinuria, hematuria, slowly progressive chronic renal failure
Henoch-Schönlein purpura	Glomerulonephritis (focal and diffuse)	Hematuria, proteinuria, occasional acute renal failure
Nail-patella syndrome	Glomerulonephritis	Proteinuria, hematuria, generally benign course
Scleroderma	Renal vascular abnormalities, some glomerular changes	Proteinuria, accelerated hypertension, renal failure
Sickle cell anemia	Interstitial nephritis, papillary necrosis, glomerulonephritis (uncommon)	Hematuria, urine concentrating defect, nephrotic syndrome (uncommon)
Syphilis (secondary)	Glomerulonephritis	Nephrotic syndrome
Systemic lupus erythematosus	Glomerulonephritis (variable in severity and histologic type)	Hematuria, proteinuria, chronic renal failure
Tuberous sclerosis	Renal hamartoma (angiomyolipoma)	Renal masses, hematuria, hemorrhage

a central keratin plug. Although once considered rare, the condition is now diagnosed not infrequently at large hemodialysis units and was present in 9 of 200 patients examined at one center [21]. A vast majority of reported patients have had both diabetes mellitus and end-stage renal disease, but Kyrle's disease may occur in association with either condition alone [21–29]. Blacks may be affected disproportionately [21,29]. Treatment with topical retinoic acid reduces pruritus and flattens lesions [19,29], but is too irritating for some patients. Etiology is unknown.

Cutaneous calcification is relatively uncommon in uremia and virtually restricted to patients with overt hyperparathyroidism. It may present as a diffuse flesh-colored to erythematous, sometimes tender, papular eruption; as nodules at sites of injection or other traumas; as subcutaneous, often periarticular, plaques, with or without local tenderness; or as soft cystic masses [30]. Any of these lesions may ulcerate and discharge a chalky material.

The half-and-half nail, which has been emphasized as a marker for uremia, consists of a proximal white band and a distal red-brown band, occupying 20 to 60 percent of the nail plate [31]. In Lindsay's series, 25 of 1500 hospitalized medical patients had this finding and 21 of these 25 were azotemic. In later studies, half-and-half nails were noted in 12 of 34 (35 percent) and 5 of 25 (20 percent) patients with varying degrees of renal failure [5,32], and in fewer than 2 percent of nonuremic patients [32]. The pathophysiology is unknown.

Oral manifestations of uremia include xerostomia, gingival friability, and ulcerative stomatitis [33]. Xerostomia is most common and probably secondary to mouth breathing or dehydration in most patients. Stomatitis rarely appears before the blood urea level reaches 300 mg/dL, responds promptly to dialysis, and is probably an ammoniacal burn due to bacterial decomposition of salivary urea. Alkaline solutions such as Scholl's solution administered by mouth to treat uremic acidosis may also cause oral chemical burns [34].

Treatment of pruritus associated with renal insufficiency

Generalized pruritus is the most important dermatologic symptom of renal insufficiency. It affects up to 86 percent of uremic patients and is sometimes disabling [35]. Of 237 patients undergoing maintenance dialysis, 37 percent reported "prolonged bothersome itchiness" at the time surveyed, and an additional 41 percent had previously been affected [36]. Discomfort occurred only during or soon after dialysis in 25 percent of pruritic patients and was most severe at those times in an additional 42 percent. Overall, pruritus was rated as mild, moderate, and severe by approximately equal numbers of patients. Usually no cause but uremia itself can be implicated, although other etiologies deserve consideration. Uremic patients are frequently on numerous medications, and drug reactions including generalized pruritus are not uncommon. Xerosis often contributes to the pruritus and this component may be relieved by topical emollients.

Relief from itching after partial parathyroidectomy in uremic patients with secondary hyperparathyroidism has been reported [37], although remissions are inconstant and often short-lived. The response of uremic pruritus to hemodialysis is unpredictable. In some cases, pruritus is relieved as the general condition of the patient improves. In other cases, however, pruritus begins only after dialysis is instituted, with an average delay of nearly 1.5 years in one series of 38 patients [38]. Pruritus may worsen while patients are on chronic hemodialysis, whether or not there is evidence of secondary hyperparathyroidism, and in the absence of other known causes of pruritus. At present, the most widely employed therapeutic agents for uremic pruritus are oral antihistamines, which are generally ineffective except for their sedative effects. Intravenous administration of lidocaine during dialysis is effective in relieving uremic pruritus for up to 24 h in some patients [39]. It is particularly helpful for patients with pruritus limited to the period of dialysis, but entails the potential side effect of hypotension and cardiac arrhythmias. Maintenance hemodialysis patients with persistent pruritus have benefited from phototherapy with sunburn-spectrum artificial ultraviolet radiation. Eight treatments over a 1-month period caused remissions lasting weeks to months in 9 of 10 patients in one controlled trial [40]. In two later studies, 32 of 38 [38] and 8 of 10 [41] patients improved after similar courses of phototherapy and approximately half experienced prolonged remissions. Oral cholestyramine resin [42] and oral charcoal [43] have also been reported to decrease the severity of uremic pruritus. The pathogenesis is unknown, but present data suggest the gradual accumulation of a circulating toxin which can be chelated in the gut or deactivated by ultraviolet irradiation.

Pathology

Histopathologic changes in the skin vary with the duration and severity of renal failure [5,44]. Major epidermal findings include a marked thickening of the stratum corneum, flattening of the dermal-epidermal junction, a reduction in the number of prickle cell layers, and cytologic changes including pyknotic nuclei and vacuolated cytoplasm. Dermal findings generally parallel epidermal ones in severity. Dilation of capillaries and lymphatics with endothelial swelling, seen in mild azotemia, progresses in advanced renal failure to dermal atrophy with loss of blood vessels, hair follicles, and sebaceous and sweat glands. Remaining sweat glands are shrunken, but there is no consistent relationship between size and degree or cause of uremia [45]. Histologic examination of normal-appearing skin of 27 patients with varying degrees of renal failure revealed endothelial cell activation and/or necrosis, basement membrane zone thickening, and reduplication of the basal lamina involving both venules and arterioles in all specimens. The microangiopathy was severe in 18 of 24 (75 percent) of the uremic specimens, but severity correlated poorly with serum creatinine levels, hemodialysis status, and known duration of renal failure, except that it was less severe in the first 2 years. In contrast, the microangiopathy was very much less severe in transplant recipients than in patients on hemodialysis and, in one patient studied both before and after transplantation, changes regressed from severe to moderate within 2 months. Mast cell alterations, modest perivenular lymphocytic infiltrates, elastic fiber fragmentation, and intravascular erythrocyte compaction and rouleaux formation were present in many specimens, but did not correlate with vessel changes [5]. The increase in dermal elastin described in uremic skin appears to be related to chronic acidosis rather than to uremia per se [2].

Calcium content in biopsies of normal-appearing skin is slightly elevated in those uremic patients without clinical and laboratory evidence of secondary hyperparathyroidism and markedly elevated in those patients with documented hyperparathyroidism [46]. Frank calcification, associated clinically with papules or nodules, may occur between dermal collagen fibers or within epidermal appendages. Electron microscopy may be necessary to visualize the calcium crystals [30]. Subclinical calcification of the skin appears to be rare in dialysis patients, even those with documented metastatic calcification in other body sites and/or an elevated calcium-phosphate solubility product [47].

References

1. Chargin L, Keil H: Skin disease in nonsurgical renal disease. *Arch Dermatol Syphilol* **26**:314, 1932
2. Scoggins RB, Harlan WR Jr: Cutaneous manifestations of hyperlipidemia and uraemia. *Postgrad Med* **41**:537, 1967
3. Gilkes JJH et al: Plasma immunoreactive melanotrophic hormones in patients on maintenance hemodialysis. *Br Med J* **1**:656, 1975
4. Smith AG et al: Role of the kidney in regulating plasma immunoreactive beta-melanocyte-stimulating hormone. *Br Med J* **1**:874, 1976
5. Gilchrest BA et al: Clinical and histological skin changes in chronic renal failure: evidence for a dialysis-resistant, transplant-responsive microangiopathy. *Lancet* **2**:1271, 1980
6. Gilchrest BA et al: Bullous dermatosis of hemodialysis. *Ann Intern Med* **83**:480, 1975
7. Thivolet J et al: La pseudoporphyrie cutanée tardive de hémodialysis. *Ann Dermatol Venereol* **104**:12, 1977
8. Griffon-Euvrard S et al: Recherche de la pseudo-porphyrie cutanée tardive chez 100 hémodialyses. *Dermatologica* **155**:193, 1977
9. Brivet F et al: Porphyria cutanea tarda-like syndrome in hemodialyzed patients. *Nephron* **20**:258, 1978
10. Kennedy AC, Lyell A: Acquired epidermolysis due to a high-dose furosemide. *Br Med J* **1**:1509, 1976
11. Burry JN, Lawrence JR: Phototoxic blisters from high furosemide dosage. *Br J Dermatol* **94**:495, 1976
12. Keczkes K, Farr MJ: Cutaneous bullae and furosemide in chronic renal failure (letter). *Br Med J* **2**:236, 1976
13. Heydenreich G et al: Bullous dermatosis among patients with chronic renal failure of high dose furosemide. *Acta Med Scand* **202**:61, 1977
14. Poh-Fitzpatrick MB et al: Porphyria cutanea tarda in two patients treated with hemodialysis for chronic renal failure. *N Engl J Med* **299**:292, 1978
15. Poh-Fitzpatrick MB et al: Porphyria cutanea tarda associated with chronic renal disease and hemodialysis. *Arch Dermatol* **116**:191, 1980
16. Garcia Parilla J et al: Porphyria cutanea tarda during maintenance haemodialysis. *Br Med J* **280**:1358, 1980
17. Poh-Fitzpatrick MB et al: Porphyrin levels in plasma and erythrocytes of chronic hemodialysis patients. *J Am Acad Dermatol* **7**:100, 1982
18. Day RS, Eales L: Porphyrins in chronic renal failure. *Nephron* **26**:90, 1980
19. Topi GC et al: Porphyria and pseudo-porphyria in hemodialyzed patients. *J Biochem* **12**:963, 1980
20. Drisler P et al: Treatment of hemodialysis-related porphyria cutanea tarda with plasma exchange. *Am J Med* **72**:989, 1982
21. Hood AF et al: Kyrle's disease in patients with chronic renal failure. *Arch Dermatol* **118**:85, 1982
22. Abele DC, Dobson RL: Hyperkeratosis penetrans (Kyrle's disease). *Arch Dermatol* **83**:277, 1961
23. Aram H et al: Kyrle's disease. *Arch Dermatol* **100**:453, 1969
24. Ephraim AJ, Barbanti BJ: Kyrle's disease. *Arch Dermatol* **101**:704, 1970

25. Pajarre R, Alavaikko M: Kyrle's disease. *Acta Derm Venereol (Stockh)* **54**:505, 1973

26. Petrozzi JW, Warthan TL: Kyrle's disease: treatment with topical tretinoin. *Arch Dermatol* **110**:762, 1974

27. Stone RA: Kyrle-like lesions in two patients with renal failure undergoing dialysis. *J Am Acad Dermatol* **5**:707, 1981

28. Brand A, Brody N: Keratotic papules in chronic renal disease. *Cutis* **28**:637, 1981

29. Hurwitz RW et al: Perforating folliculitis in association with hemodialysis. *Am J Dermatopathol* **4**:101, 1982

30. Parfitt PM: Soft-tissue calcification in uremia. *Arch Intern Med* **124**:544, 1969

31. Lindsay PG: The half and half nail. *Arch Intern Med* **119**:583, 1967

32. Stewart WK, Raffle EJ: Brown nail-bed arcs and chronic renal disease. *Br Med J* **1**:784, 1972

33. Grunskin SE et al: Oral manifestations of uremia. *Minn Med* **53**:495, 1970

34. Newell GB, Stone PJ: Irritant contact stomatitis in chronic renal failure. *Arch Dermatol* **109**:53, 1974

35. Young AW et al: Dermatologic evaluation of pruritus in patients on hemodialysis. *NY State J Med* **73**:2670, 1973

36. Gilchrest BA et al: Clinical features of pruritus among patients undergoing maintenance hemodialysis. *Arch Dermatol* **118**:154, 1982

37. Hampers CL et al: Disappearance of "uremic" itching after subtotal parathyroidectomy. *N Engl J Med* **279**:695, 1968

38. Gilchrest BA et al: Ultraviolet phototherapy of uremic pruritus. *Ann Intern Med* **91**:17, 1979

39. Tapia L et al: Pruritus in dialysis patients treated with parenteral lidocaine. *N Engl J Med* **296**:261, 1977

40. Gilchrest BA et al: Relief of uremic pruritus with ultraviolet phototherapy. *N Engl J Med* **297**:136, 1977

41. Shultz BC, Roenigk HH Jr: Uremic pruritus treated with ultraviolet light. *JAMA* **243**:1836, 1980

42. Silverberg DS et al: Cholestyramine in uremic pruritus. *Br J Med* **1**:752, 1971

43. Pederson JA et al: Relief of idiopathic generalized pruritus in dialysis patients treated with activated oral charcoal. *Ann Intern Med* **93**:446, 1980

44. Rosenthal SP: Uremic dermatitis. *Arch Dermatol Syphilol* **23**:934, 1931

45. Cawley EP et al: The eccrine sweat glands of patients in uremia. *Arch Dermatol* **84**:51, 1961

46. Massry SG et al: The effect of calcemic disorders and uremia on the mineral content of skin. *Isr J Med Sci* **7**:514, 1971

47. De Graaf P et al: Metastatic skin calcification: a rare phenomenon in dialysis patients. *Dermatologica* **161**:28, 1980

CHAPTER 170

CUTANEOUS ASPECTS OF CARDIOPULMONARY DISEASE

Andrew G. Franks, Jr.

Descriptions of abnormalities of the skin in association with diseases of the heart and lungs are among those first recorded in medical antiquity. While many are familiar and easily recognizable by the physician, others are unique and may remain a diagnostic challenge. The purpose of this chapter is to present the cutaneous manifestations of selected cardiopulmonary diseases in which the skin contributes to the clinical picture.

There are a number of situations in which the skin and the cardiopulmonary system are involved that have been described elsewhere in this volume. These include pruritus associated with cardiac failure or pulmonary insufficiency (see Chap. 8), pigmentary changes associated with hemochromatosis or endocrine abnormalities (see Chap. 79), the hyperlipidemias (see Chap. 145), the mucocutaneous lymph node syndrome (see Chap. 199), lipoid proteinosis (see Chap. 147), and amyloid (see Chap. 142).

Alterations in skin quality

The skin may be warm in high-output states such as erythroderma or exfoliative dermatitis with or without high-output congestive failure. Hyperthyroidism with increased cardiac output and vasodilation may lead to increased skin temperature. Conversely, the temperature may be reduced in hypothyroidism and low-output congestive failure secondary to atherosclerotic disease or myocardial infarction.

The texture of the skin may be coarse and dry in myxedema, coarse in acromegaly, and smooth, satiny, and moist in hyperthyroidism. The texture of the skin may be waxy in amyloidosis and when stroked may become hemorrhagic. Amyloidosis may be associated with conduction disturbances, myocardial disease, and orthostatic hypotension.

Hyperelastic velvety skin that rebounds to the original position after being stretched, "cigarette-paper" scars, and hyperextensible joints are characteristic of the Ehlers-Danlos syndrome (Fig. 170-1). Mitral and tricuspid prolapse, dilatation of the aorta and pulmonary artery, arterial rupture, a variety of congenital heart diseases, and panacinar emphysema may accompany this syndrome [1].

A progressive looseness of skin with pendulous folds and droopy eyelids can be a clue to cutis laxa (Fig. 170-2). This may be associated with generalized hyperelastosis that may cause aortic dilatation and rupture, congestive heart failure, cor pulmonale with pulmonary artery stenosis, and progressive emphysema [2].

The skin in pseudoxanthoma elasticum is thick, lax, and

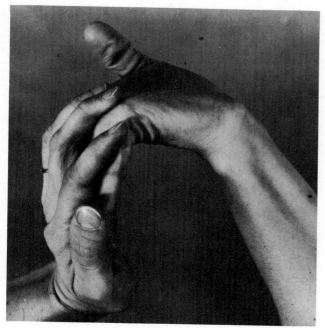

Fig. 170-1 Hyperextensive joint in Ehlers-Danlos syndrome. *(Courtesy of New York University, Department of Dermatology.)*

yellowish, especially over the axillae, antecubital area, and the neck (Fig. 170-3). The skin around the mouth may sag. Yellow patches may occur on mucous membranes, especially the labia. The arteries may be calcified, and the aortic and mitral valves thickened. Angina pectoris and claudication are frequent symptoms [3].

In Werner's syndrome the skin appears atrophic and tight; there is marked loss of subcutis, with ulcerations of the legs and severe coronary atherosclerosis with frequent death by myocardial infarction at an early age [4].

Changes in skin color

Changes in skin color are due to a number of variables including: hemoglobin, melanin, carotene, vasoactivity (reflectance), metals, and miscellaneous other phenomena.

Fig. 170-2 Marked looseness of the skin in cutis laxa. *(Courtesy of New York University, Department of Dermatology.)*

Cyanosis

An increase in the absolute amount of unoxygenated (reduced) hemoglobin results in a purplish or bluish discoloration of the skin. By definition, cyanosis is divided into "central" and "peripheral" types, the latter being the more common. For practical purposes, the terms refer to the level of arterial oxygen saturation present, and not to the anatomic source of the cyanosis. Thus, central cyanosis occurs in states which produce low arterial oxygen saturation, such as congenital heart or pulmonary disease with intracardiac or intrapulmonary right-to-left shunting, as well as pneumonia and chronic pulmonary disease. Peripheral cyanosis occurs in states that have normal arterial oxygen saturation but have reduced blood flow, such as low-output cardiac failure, valvular heart disease, and local vasospastic phenomena. Pulmonary infarction may result in a combination of central cyanosis due to intrapulmonary shunting, as well as peripheral cyanosis due to low cardiac output.

Central cyanosis is usually present on the warm areas of the skin such as the tongue, oral mucosae, and conjunctivae. Peripheral cyanosis is usually seen on the cool areas such as the nose, lips, earlobes, and fingertips. However, this distinction is not absolute since both central and peripheral cyanosis may affect any of the aforementioned areas of the body. Detection of cyanosis may be difficult, even to the experienced observer. Although the tongue is probably the area where it is most easily detected, a number of false-positive evaluations may occur. Therefore, examination of the fingertips and conjunctivae, while less sensitive, may reflect the underlying condition more clearly. In the anemic patient, detection of cyanosis may be impossible since the absolute amount of reduced hemoglobin is not increased. In order to avoid confusion with staining of the skin, either topically or from systemic increases of heavy metals or other chemicals, it is important to note that cyanosis will fade on pressure since the color is within the blood vessels [5].

Cyanosis of the fingers of more intensity than of the toes suggests complete transposition of the great vessels, with either a preductal coarctation or complete interruption of the aortic arch, pulmonary hypertension, and a reversed shunt through a patent ductus arteriosus. If the cyanosis

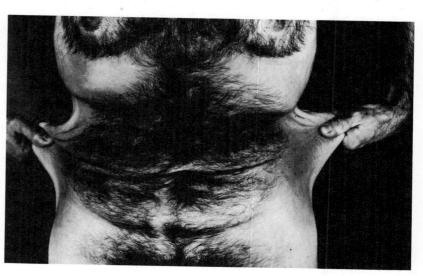

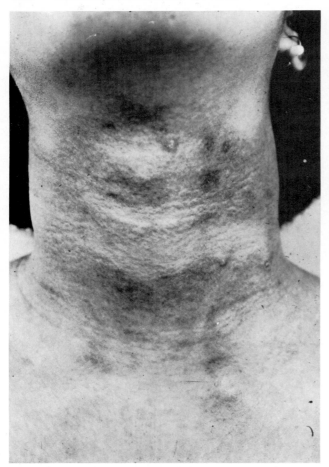

Fig. 170-3 Thickened, yellow patches in pseudoxanthoma elasticum. *(Courtesy of New York University, Department of Dermatology.)*

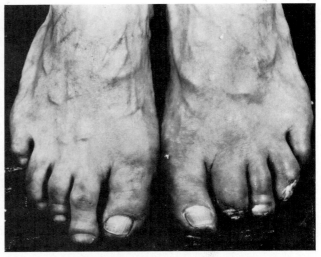

Fig. 170-4 Erythremia of the toes in polycythemia vera. *(Courtesy of New York University, Department of Dermatology.)*

is slightly more on the right hand, coarctation of the aorta is more likely. Equal cyanosis of both hands suggests complete aortic interruption [6].

Cyanosis and clubbing of the toes associated with cyanosis in the left hand and a normal right hand suggests pulmonary hypertension with a reversed shunt through a patent ductus arteriosus bringing unsaturated blood to the left arm and both legs [7].

Redness/flushing

Redness of the skin may be due to an increase in the amount of oxygenated hemoglobin, an increase in the diameter or actual number of skin capillaries, or a combination of these.

Erythroderma or exfoliative dermatitis with intense redness may be associated with capillary dilatation of such proportion that high-output cardiac failure occurs, especially in compromised patients [8].

Polycythemia may produce the characteristic "ruddy" complexion, but may also cause a peculiar coloration termed *erythremia*, which is a combination of redness and cyanosis. The tongue, lips, nose, earlobes, conjunctivae, and fingertips especially demonstrate this latter feature (Fig. 170-4). Erythremia is the result of the increased amounts of oxygenated hemoglobin producing the redness, as well as the increased amounts of unoxygenated hemoglobin producing cyanosis due to the inability of the body to fully oxygenate the increased absolute amounts of hemoglobin. Of note, the absence of nail clubbing may help to differentiate patients with polycythemia vera from those patients with cardiopulmonary disease who develop secondary polycythemia. In addition, the hypervolemic state of polycythemia vera is associated with an increased stroke volume and may lead to high-output cardiac failure, while pulmonary infarction may result from venous thrombosis and embolization secondary to hyperviscosity [9].

Paroxysmal intense flushing of the face, neck, chest, and abdomen, often with telangiectases of the face and neck, may occur with carcinoid tumors that have metastasized to the liver, thereby producing increased amounts of serotonin. Serotonin and histamine are responsible for the bronchospasm seen in this syndrome. Fibrosis of the right side of the heart may lead to a combination of stenosis and regurgitation at the tricuspid valve and pulmonary stenosis. If cyanosis occurs, the combination of flushing and cyanosis may produce the reddish, cyanotic erythremia seen in some patients with polycythemia. Occasionally, patients who develop this syndrome have a patent ductus arteriosus or foramen ovale, and metastases occur in the lung. In this setting, left-sided cardiac lesions may also occur [10].

Systemic mastocytosis may produce flushing as a result of vasodilatation, and may be associated with telangiectasia (Fig. 170-5). Histamine release from degranulated mast cells is the pathogenetic mechanism. Cardiopulmonary alterations include hypotension and bronchospasm [11].

Pheochromocytoma may cause flushing of the face and forehead as well as redness and cyanosis of the hands. Generalized, extreme flushing, mimicking carcinoid, may occur in Sipple's syndrome, in which prostaglandin and serotonin are increased in addition to catecholamines [12].

Edema of the face, arms, and hands associated with redness and/or cyanosis may indicate the presence of ob-

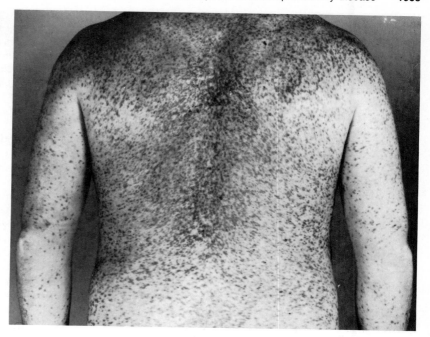

Fig. 170-5 Flushing and telangiectasia in systemic mastocytosis. (Courtesy of New York University, Department of Dermatology.)

struction of the superior vena cava due to mediastinal disease.

Erythromelalgia (labile hyperthermia). Besides the idiopathic variety, atherosclerosis, hypertension, and polycythemia may produce this peculiar pattern of erythema on the hands and feet. During the episodes, the patient will complain, especially when exposed to heat, of pain, warmth, and swelling of the areas, which sometimes extend to the elbows and knees. The pulses are either normal or slightly increased in intensity [13].

Palmar erythema. Palmar erythema may occur in many healthy women, but when of recent onset or increased intensity, the possibility of liver involvement should be considered. This may be associated with high-output cardiac failure. The erythema primarily involves the hypothenar eminence, but may also affect the thenar eminence and the fingertips. Other factors, including pregnancy and hyperthyroidism, may cause this condition [5].

Jaundice

Hyperbilirubinemia and jaundice may occur in heart failure as a result of raised intrahepatic pressure due to passive congestion. Hemorrhagic pulmonary infarction with destruction of red cells and hemoglobin may also produce jaundice, especially when passive congestion of the liver is present. Constrictive pericarditis and tricuspid valvular disease may produce jaundice secondary to cardiac cirrhosis. Under fluorescent light, jaundice may be difficult to assess [4].

Alterations in sweat

Sweating may be prominent in a number of cardiopulmonary states such as acute myocardial infarction, cardio-

genic shock, left ventricular failure, massive pulmonary emboli, and pulmonary edema. Pallor and clamminess or coldness of the extremities and exposed surfaces are also often found. Excessive sweating when associated with hypertension may suggest pheochromocytoma. There may also be additional features such as flushing, most prominent in those patients with Sipple's syndrome where prostaglandin and serotonin production by the tumor may simulate carcinoid. Myocardial infarction may occur, or cardiac failure may develop due to a metabolic cardiomyopathy. Neurofibromatosis and café au lait macules have been found in up to 10 percent of patients, especially those with bilateral pheochromocytoma [12].

An increase in the sodium and chloride content of sweat is present in cystic fibrosis and may lead to an increase in skin wrinkling after immersion, as when bathing [14].

Alterations of nails, hands, and arms

Nail clubbing

Nail clubbing and osteoarthropathy are distinct entities which may be associated with significant cardiopulmonary abnormalities (Fig. 170-6).

Clinically, nail clubbing has various manifestations. Beaking or distal curvature of the nail may occur. There may be loss of the normal 15° angle between the nail and cuticle (unguophalangeal angle). Sponginess or "floating" of the nail when pressure is applied is also characteristic. Finally, an increase in the size of the terminal tuft may occur. The latter may be quantified by measuring the depth of the finger at the base of the nail and dividing by the depth of the finger at the distal interphalangeal (DIP) joints. The ratio should normally be less than 1.0.

Clubbing most commonly occurs in bronchogenic carcinoma, suppurative lung disease, endocarditis, and congenital heart disease, but it may be idiopathic [4].

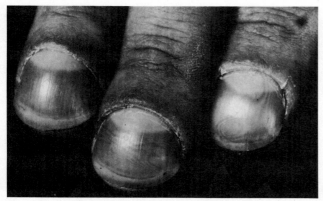

Fig. 170-6   Clubbing of the fingernails. *(Courtesy of New York University, Department of Dermatology.)*

Quincke pulse

Flushing of the nail beds synchronous with the heartbeat is one sign of aortic regurgitation called Quincke pulsations [7].

In addition, the fingernail beds may be used to evaluate the microcirculation. Capillary "fill" is estimated by pressing down on the nail bed until blanching occurs. Following release, there should be immediate filling and a pink appearance. However, perfusion of the skin may not reflect perfusion of internal organs.

Hypertrophic osteoarthropathy

Hypertrophic osteoarthropathy often has clubbing as a feature, but in addition there is an associated arthralgia and/or arthritis of the fingers, wrists, knees, and ankles, as well as painful periostitis revealed as subperiosteal new bone formation on x-ray. Suffusion of the digits may be prominent, with pitting edema. Shiny skin with increased sweating and paronychial thickening are sometimes noted.

Although it is most often associated with malignant tumors of the chest, there are numerous other disorders that may produce this syndrome. In addition, some cases are primary or idiopathic. Pachydermoperiostosis, a primary form, is frequently familial, with onset around puberty, and with a number of cutaneous manifestations. Distinctive thickening and furrowing of the skin of the scalp, forehead, and cheeks may present as leonine facies. Other features include excessive sweating, especially of the hands and feet, a severe seborrhea of the scalp and face, and a dermatitis of the hands and feet [15]. Familial clubbing alone may also be found and may represent a partial expression of this syndrome. Thyroid acropachy may mimic osteoarthropathy but is most often painless.

Shoulder-hand syndrome

The shoulder-hand syndrome is a painful periarthritis or adhesive capsulitis of the shoulder ("frozen shoulder"), usually on the left, associated with erythema, sweating, shiny induration, edema, tenderness, pain, and immobility of the ipsilateral hand. Neurotrophic ulcerations of the fingers and thickening of the palmar aponeurosis with nod-

ules and/or Dupuytren's contracture may be late sequelae. This syndrome was observed in up to 15 percent of patients with myocardial infarction in the past when bed rest was prolonged, but it is now uncommon. Other predisposing conditions include arterial embolization, cerebrovascular accidents, and protective disuse of the arms for any reason [16].

The heart and the skin

Coronary heart disease

Familial hyperlipidemia. The risk of coronary artery disease (CAD) may increase with elevation of plasma cholesterol and triglyceride concentrations [17,18]. Familial hyperlipidemias comprise a group of metabolic disorders with elevated plasma cholesterol and/or triglyceride, and some may be associated with a high incidence of CAD. Xanthomatosis may be present in these disorders, and they have been associated for many years with a high incidence of CAD [19]. As noted previously, the lipidoses are discussed in Chap. 145.

Earlobe crease. A number of reports relate coronary artery disease to the presence of a diagonally positioned skin crease along the earlobe [20–23]. These may be unilateral or bilateral. It is not known whether such creases are congenital or acquired, nor is the mechanism of their formation known (Fig. 170-7).

Their association with other risk factors including hyperlipidemia has not been evaluated. However, their presence suggests an increased risk for CAD based upon clinical [24], angiographic [25], and postmortem [26] studies.

Cholesterol emboli. In patients with advanced atherosclerosis of the abdominal aorta, cholesterol crystals may microembolize to the lower extremities. The pulses may remain normal [27,28]. In addition to the systemic complaints of pain in the legs, buttocks, and low back, myalgia, restless legs, or abdominal symptoms, various skin lesions develop [29]. Livedo reticularis affecting the lower abdomen and back, buttocks, legs, and feet may occur [30].

Ulcerations on the legs and feet, described as surrounded by an erythematous or violaceous halo and a small scab, are present [31]. Cyanosis and digital gangrene may simulate necrotizing vasculitis [32,33].

Indurated plaques and nodules have been noted as well [34], and their association with livedo reticularis and ulceration may mimic polyarteritis nodosa [35]. These plaques and nodules are firm, violaceous, painful, and necrotic in the center. They are most prominent on the thighs and calves. Superficial skin biopsy is often nondiagnostic while a deep skin and muscle biopsy revealing the intraarteriolar site of pathology is more useful [36,37]. The characteristic findings are arterioles occluded by multinucleated foreign-body giant cells and fibrosis surrounding biconvex, needle-shaped forms, leaving clefts corresponding to the cholesterol crystal microemboli [38].

Post-bypass surgery skin changes. Coronary artery bypass surgery is commonly performed using the superficial veins of the legs as donor-graft sites. A dermatitis has been

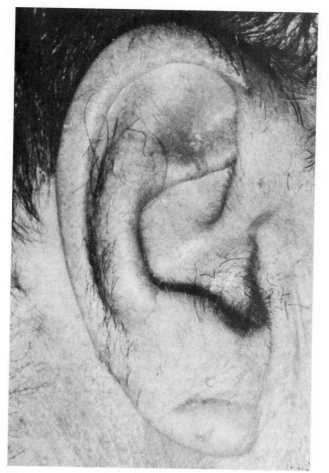

Fig. 170-7 Earlobe crease and ear-canal hair. *(From Wagner RF Jr et al: N Engl J Med 311:1317, 1984.)*

reported to occur along the saphenous vein graft scar on the medial aspect of the legs [39,40]. Patients with this problem have no prior history of venous stasis, thrombophlebitis, ankle edema, or skin disease. Examination generally reveals a reddish-brown, slightly scaling, and fissured dermatitis along the distal part of a well-healed saphenous vein graft scar. Each case has developed two to six months after surgery as the patients returned to full activity. Although the cause is unclear, possibly relating to the high incidence of postoperative thrombophlebitis [41] and resultant stasis dermatitis, it responds to topical steroids. Recurrence is usual and most patients have required continued treatment. Interestingly, one patient [39] had two episodes of secondary infection with coagulase-positive *Staphylococcus aureus* at the vein graft site which cleared with antibiotics. In one large series of over 2000 patients undergoing coronary revascularization with the saphenous vein, 1 percent developed leg wound complications at the vein graft site within the immediate postoperative period. The majority developed either *S. aureus* or mixed gram-negative infections, primarily in the thigh area [42].

Another group of patients developed recurrent cellulitis in the healed vein graft site many months after surgery. These patients present with fever and chills; erythema may extend along the entire vein graft site, with pain and ten-

derness. Swelling may be significant, and often the patients are initially considered to have thrombophlebitis. Although cultures are not always positive, beta-hemolytic streptococcus was isolated in a number of cases. Treatment with intravenous antibiotics followed by oral antibiotics caused resolution, but recurrence was not unusual [43].

The presence of an associated tinea pedis in patients with this complication was reported [44] as well. These authors recommend that all patients considered for vein graft surgery be examined carefully for evidence of tinea infections of the feet, which, if found, should be treated vigorously with antifungal medication prior to surgery. Vein graft dermatitis with the subsequent secondary infection may also play a role in the development of cellulitis.

Cardiomyopathy

Cutaneous abnormalities may aid in the diagnosis and subsequent treatment of some types of cardiomyopathy. These disorders of the myocardium affect ventricular function and may produce cardiac failure. A useful classification divides cardiomyopathies into dilated, nondilated, and hypertrophic types. It has recently been stressed that each type of cardiomyopathy has a distinct differential diagnosis and that little etiologic overlap occurs [45].

Thus, a specific cutaneous finding in conjunction with the appropriate studies to determine the type of cardiomyopathy may be very important for the correct diagnosis. Either radionuclide ventriculography or two-dimensional echocardiography estimates ventricular volume and left ventricular ejection fraction. These measurements are utilized to distinguish among the three types of cardiomyopathy. Tables 170-1 and 170-2 list the causes of cardiomyopathy according to type.

Myxoma

Atrial myxomas, the most common primary tumors of the heart, are benign hamartomatous intracardial tumors, which may produce a wide variety of clinical symptoms and signs, and may simulate a number of disease states.

The cardiopulmonary findings reviewed in one series of 24 cases [46] included, in order of frequency: congestive heart failure (54 percent), mitral murmur (38 percent), chest pain (29 percent), pulmonary edema (25 percent), and embolic phenomena (21 percent).

Additionally, valvular insufficiency, constrictive pericarditis, conduction blocks, arrhythmias, and intracardiac shunts may occur. Variable murmurs may be an important clue.

Pulmonary emboli and pulmonary hypertension may also occur, in addition to other systemic findings including: fever, cachexia and malaise, arthralgia, arthritis, clubbing, hypergammaglobulinemia, anemia or polycythemia, thrombocytosis or thrombocytopenia, and leukocytosis [46].

The cutaneous manifestations of atrial myxomas may be quite dramatic. In addition to biphasic digital color changes on cold exposure [47], various cutaneous lesions have been described which simulate collagen vascular disease or vasculitis: tender, violaceous, nonblanching, annular and serpiginous lesions of digital pads, as well as splinter hemorrhages presenting as a systemic vasculitis [48] or

Table 170-1   Causes of cardiomyopathy by type

Dilated:
    *Coronary artery disease with multiple infarcts
    *Alcoholic
     Peripartum
    *Valvular
    *Infectious acute inflammatory myocarditis
    *Chagas' disease
    *Sarcoid
     Doxorubicin toxicity
    *Uremia
    *Hemochromatosis
    *Pheochromocytoma
     Hypocalcemia
    *Diabetes mellitus
     Nutritional (? selenium)
     Idiopathic
Nondilated:
    *Amyloid heart disease
     Endomyocardial diseases:
       *Loeffler's disease
       *Pseudoxanthoma elasticum
       Endomyocardial fibrosis (Davies' disease)
    *Neoplastic:
       *Melanoma
     Ventricular thrombosis:
       *Polycythemia vera
       Mitral valve prosthesis
     Idiopathic
Hypertrophic:
     Genetic form (? autosomal dominant)
     Acquired or secondary forms:
       *Neurofibromatosis
       *Lentiginosis
       *Hyperthyroidism
       *Hypothyroidism
       *Noonan's syndrome
       Hypertension
       Valvular or subvalvular obstruction of left ventricular
         outlet tract
       Pompe's disease
       Friedreich's ataxia
       In infants of diabetic mothers

* May have significant cutaneous features
Modified from Johnson and Palacios [45].

infective endocarditis. Others have reported characteristic pruritic, erythematous papules as well as cyanosis and ecchymosis of the extremities [49]. A reddish-violet malar flush along with macular erythema and cyanosis of digits simulated acute rheumatic fever in one patient [50].

Another patient with arthritis and nonblanching erythema was thought to have rheumatoid arthritis [51]. The diagnosis may be made by biopsy of the skin and subcutaneous tissue in an area of embolic infarct. Myxomatous emboli with large pale-staining cytoplasms and stellate nuclei may be found along occluded blood vessels [46].

Prior to 1960, over 80 percent of patients were undiagnosed at postmortem since echocardiography was unavailable. However, the diagnosis may now be made earlier and more frequently, allowing successful surgical intervention.

Recently, the association of atrial myxoma with mucocutaneous pigmented lesions, including lentigines, nevomelanocytic nevi, and blue nevi, as well as dermal myxo-matous nodules, has been described and termed either the NAME [52] or LAMB [53] syndrome depending on the acronym chosen.

Leopard syndrome

Multiple lentigines syndrome, an autosomal dominant disorder, has been associated with numerous abnormalities of variable clinical expression including disturbances of the heart [54,55]. Each letter of the mnemonic "leopard" represents a feature of the syndrome: L, lentigines, multiple; E, electrocardiogram conduction defects; O, ocular telorism; P, pulmonary stenosis; A, abnormalities of genitalia; R, retardation of growth; D, deafness, sensorineural [55] (Fig. 170-8).

Other malformations and related disorders have also been reported [56]. Multiple lentigines, which are usually present at birth, are the most characteristic feature of the syndrome. They vary in size, shape, and shades of brown to black. While the entire body, including the palms and soles may be covered, the oral mucosa and lips are spared [55,56].

The abnormal pigmentation may also be found in the iris [57] and retina [58]. There is a tendency for the lentigines to increase with age, especially around puberty, but they are not affected by sun exposure, appearing in areas normally not exposed to sunlight [55–57].

Giant melanosomes were found in dermal melanophages, melanocytes, and keratinocytes in all epidermal layers in a patient with the multiple lentigines syndrome [59].

The disorder may arise in the neuroectoderm [57]. Involvement of the neural crest in the development of the inner ear and the sympathetic nervous system may explain some features of the syndrome [56].

The types of cardiac involvement include electrocardiographic conduction disturbances and anatomic malformation. Axis deviation [56], prolonged P-R intervals [60], left anterior hemiblock [56], bundle branch block [61], and complete heart block [58] have been reported.

Hypertrophic cardiomyopathy appears to be the most common anatomic abnormality [57,62]. Subaortic stenosis is the most common valvular lesion [57]. Although earlier reports suggested that pulmonary stenosis was frequent [55], some of the clinical and physiologic features of hypertrophic cardiomyopathy mimic pulmonary stenosis and were clarified only after catheterization [62] or echocardiograms [63].

The clinical expression of the conduction disturbances and the anatomic malformation vary in onset and severity, suggesting that frequent cardiac evaluation be performed [64–66].

Subacute bacterial endocarditis

The cutaneous manifestations of bacterial endocarditis are important clues to the diagnosis. They include Osler's nodes, Janeway lesions, subungual splinter hemorrhages, purpura, and petechiae. These findings are less common than in the preantibiotic era.

Clinical differences noted between Osler's nodes and Janeway lesions included the fact that the former were exquisitely painful and tender and present on the digital tufts, whereas Janeway lesions were nontender and located

Table 170-2   Infectious causes of acute dilated cardiomyopathy*

Coxsackie virus B	Cytomegalovirus
Coxsackie virus A	Mumps
Echo virus	Psittacosis
Poliovirus	*Cryptococcus neoformans*
Arbovirus (dengue, chikungunya fever)	*Candida albicans*
Toxoplasma gondii	*Trichinella spiralis*
Trypanosoma cruzi	*Schistosoma mansoni*
Mycoplasma pneumoniae	*Corynebacterium diphtheriae*
Varicella	*Neisseria meningitidis*
Variola	Leptospira
Influenza	Polymicrobial bacterial
Rabies	myocarditis

* Most have cutaneous features
Modified from Johnson and Palacios [45].

on the palmar and plantar surfaces [67,68]. While suppuration occurs primarily with Osler's nodes, other differences are more variable. Osler's original description in 1885 did not specify the tenderness of these lesions [69], but a later report [70] did emphasize the qualities with which we are familiar today.

Histologically, Osler's nodes are a perivasculitis or necrotizing vasculitis without microabscess formation or other evidence for infection or emboli [71–74]. However, Osler

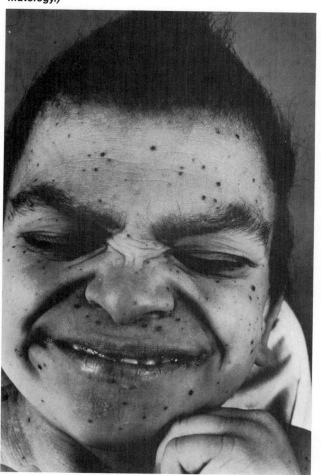

Fig. 170-8   Ocular telorism and lentigines in the leopard syndrome. (Courtesy of New York University, Department of Dermatology.)

himself considered them septic emboli [69]. Cultures have generally been negative, although more recent reports have reemphasized the possibility of septic microemboli with microabscess formation [75]. Janeway lesions have also been described histologically as vasculitis with microabscess formation [76].

Other criteria such as color, nodularity, size, location, and duration are variable [77]. As noted, both Osler's nodes and Janeway lesions are vasculitic [78]. In addition, the petechiae and Roth spots in the eye may be of similar pathogenesis [79]. The reason for the differences in appearance and tenderness is unknown, although this may be related to the location since Osler's are mostly on digital tufts and Janeway lesions are most often on palms and soles where the density of tissue and nerves is less.

The popular theory with regard to the pathogenesis of both Osler's nodes and Janeway lesions is immunologic or allergic due to immune complex deposition [80,81], but some reports dispute this concept, suggesting that the initial event is a septic microembolus, which subsequently causes the endothelial swelling and perivasculitis seen in older lesions [75]. Thus, organisms may be occasionally cultured initially, but later the lesions become sterile.

Splinter hemorrhages (Fig. 170-9) have been associated with endocarditis as well [82,83]. Infected arterial catheters have been reported to precipitate clinical lesions comparable to Osler's nodes, Janeway lesions, and splinter hemorrhages, supporting the concept that these are infectious in etiology [84–86]. Osler's nodes and Janeway lesions have been found to occur in other conditions, particularly systemic lupus erythematosus, gonococcemia, hemolytic anemia, and typhoid fever [87–89]. Splinter hemorrhages are also considered to be nonspecific in up to 20 percent of patients, being induced by trauma, *Trichinella*, and other disorders [90].

Petechiae are the most common mucocutaneous manifestation of bacterial endocarditis, the incidence varying from 20 to 40 percent of patients with both acute and subacute bacterial endocarditis [91,92]. Small, red or violaceous macules that do not blanch subsequently become brownish and fade. Purpuric lesions, both flat and elevated, have also been associated with subacute endocarditis without evidence of platelet dysfunction, and may represent a leukocytoclastic vasculitis [93,94]. The petechiae may be observed on the skin, especially on the heels, shoulders, and legs, but the conjunctiva and oral mucosa must also be evaluated [95].

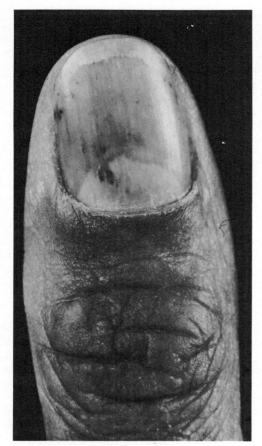

Fig. 170-9 Splinter subungual hemorrhages in subacute bacterial endocarditis. *(Courtesy of New York University, Department of Dermatology.)*

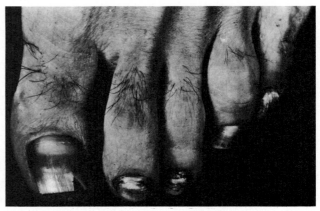

Fig. 170-10 Nail changes in the yellow nail syndrome. *(Courtesy of New York University, Department of Dermatology.)*

An unusual presentation of endocarditis caused by *Erysipelothrix*, with bullae of the hand initially mimicking herpes zoster, has been noted [96]. This organism, while rare, is sometimes seen in butchers and fish handlers and is responsible for erysipeloid. In contrast to the "cutaneous only" form, the systemic infection may lead to endocarditis. Early diagnosis of the offending organism may be made by the exposure history to meats and fish and the bullous eruption on the violaceous base. Of importance, the bullae that are subepidermal are usually sterile. Diagnosis can be made by culturing the tissue [97]. Erysipeloid is caused by *E. rhusiopathiae,* which is a slender, curved, nonmotile, non-spore-forming, gram-positive bacillus. It is a facultative anaerobe that produces alpha hemolysis on sheep blood agar.

The lungs and the skin

Yellow nail syndrome

Yellow nails with primary lymphedema were described in 1964 [98]. Separately, primary lymphedema and pleural effusion were reported [99]. The triad of yellow nails, primary lymphedema, and pleural effusion was then recognized [100], followed by a number of reports with partial or complete features [101].

The characteristics of the nails include thickening, trans-verse ridging, diminished growth, increased curvature with a "hump," and onycholysis. The lunulae and cuticles may be absent. The color may vary from a pale yellow to green [102,103] (Fig. 170-10). The nail changes are secondary to congenitally hypoplastic lymphatics [104].

The lymphedema in this disorder is also due to congenitally hypoplastic lymphatics [98]. It is characteristically slowly progressive and somewhat asymmetric, with induration and hyperkeratosis extending to the thighs. Periodic lymphangitis is frequent and may contribute to the swelling [100].

Respiratory findings include sinusitis, bronchiectasis, and pleural effusions, unilateral or bilateral. Symptoms vary from mild to severe, with some patients requiring repeated thoracentesis, treatment for pneumonia secondary to bronchiectasis, and drainage of the sinusitis. Patients may have a cough, both productive and nonproductive, dyspnea, frequent upper respiratory infections, and pneumonia. Chest x-rays may be normal but generally reveal evidence of fibrosis and/or effusion at the bases [104].

Pulmonary features and lymphedema may not occur until late in the course; therefore, follow-up of patients who present with this type of nail dystrophy is recommended [104]. Finally, a number of patients have developed lymphomas or sarcomas with metastases [104].

Pulmonary arteriovenous fistulas

Pulmonary arteriovenous fistulas are congenital abnormalities of capillary development that may not become clinically apparent until late adolescence [105]. Osler-Weber-Rendu syndrome (hereditary hemorrhagic telangiectasia), an autosomal dominant trait, may be present in one-third to one-half of such patients [106]. It is characterized clinically by punctate, linear, or spiderlike telangiectasia of the skin, especially the upper body, oral and nasal mucous membranes, and nail beds. The radiating arms about an elevated punctum are the most characteristic feature, especially on the lips and tongue. They are distinguished from true spider telangiectasia since they do not pulsate [107]. Recurrent epistaxis is the most frequent presenting symptom and may begin in early childhood or adolescence. Other organ systems besides the lung may be involved, including the liver, gastrointestinal and genitourinary tracts, and central nervous system, and recurrent hemorrhage may result. Bleeding may be enhanced by an associated von Willebrand's disease [108].

The pulmonary findings present in those patients with an arteriovenous fistula of the lungs include dyspnea, hemoptysis, cyanosis, clubbing, polycythemia, and pulmonary bruits accentuated by inspiration. Chest x-rays reveal nodular ''coinlike'' lesions, sometimes initially considered to be metastatic disease.

Asthma-eczema complex (atopy)

The association of atopic (infantile) eczema, asthma, and hay fever is well known. While infants with eczema are at increased risk to develop asthma and hay fever, there appears to be a difference in prevalence of each component. Different hereditary patterns probably exist, with some patients developing only one or two components of the atopic diathesis.

The early onset of eczema, its severity, and its duration past the age of two years all appear to favor the later development of asthma and/or hay fever.

Mediators of the atopic inflammatory response may be released by sensitized IGE-mast cell complexes present along the tracheobronchial tree. Dust, pollen, and dander may initiate this response.

Although asthma may be divided into the extrinsic and intrinsic types, most patients have overlapping clinical features. The extrinsic group has known external allergies (dust, pollen, dander), a higher incidence of associated eczema and hay fever and a higher incidence of positive atopic family history [109].

Cutaneous findings in chronic pulmonary diseases

Chronic obstructive pulmonary disease (COPD) is actually a group of disorders resulting from chronic bronchitis, pulmonary emphysema, or asthma. The incidence and mortality of COPD have increased recently and approach that of heart disease in the United States. Smoking habits as well as increased longevity of the population may be responsible, in part, for this increase. Genetic, infectious, occupational, and environmental factors also contribute.

Two basic types of COPD have been described: Type A or emphysematous and Type B or bronchial. Clinically both may present with dyspnea, cough, wheezing, and recurrent respiratory infections. Type A patients have been termed ''pink puffers'' since they usually hyperventilate and maintain arterial oxygen tension. Type B patients have been termed ''blue bloaters'' since they frequently are hypoxic with cyanosis and associated congestive heart failure. These patients, especially if young, should be evaluated for the possibility of cystic fibrosis.

Cigarette stains on the fingertips may be helpful in determining etiologic factors when the patient's history is unclear [110].

Cystic fibrosis

Cystic fibrosis is an autosomal recessive disorder of the exocrine glands which subsequently involves the tracheobronchial tree, pancreas, and gastrointestinal tract. The basic alteration of mucus is unknown, with viscid mucous

plugs causing fecal impaction, intussusception, and rectal prolapse in infancy. Pancreatic insufficiency may subsequently predominate but it is the pulmonary disease that is the most significant feature. Progressive lung disease with chronic bronchitis, emphysema, and cor pulmonale from cystic fibrosis is the leading cause of death among all genetic disorders in the United States. As patients live longer with appropriate antibiotic care and tracheobronchial toilet, other features such as cirrhosis, hemoptysis, and pneumothorax have been noted [111].

The cutaneous features of this disorder result from increased amounts of electrolyte in the sweat, which leads to excessive skin wrinkling when the palms and soles are immersed in water. Although this feature is not always present, it may be a valuable clue to the disease. Parents are often aware of, but not disturbed by, the wrinkling [112].

Larva migrans and pulmonary involvement

Cutaneous larva migrans or creeping eruption may occasionally cause minimal respiratory symptoms and be associated with transient pulmonary infiltrates and a peripheral eosinophilia (Loeffler's syndrome). The skin lesions are initially nonspecific and highly pruritic, and subsequently progress to erythematous, serpiginous, tunnellike tracks. Older lesions are frequently excoriated and crusted (Fig. 170-11).

Visceral larva migrans or toxocariasis may lead to granulomatous involvement of the liver, lungs, heart, muscle, brain, and eyes. Marked eosinophilia, hyperglobulinemia, pneumonitis with wheezing, recurrent bronchitis, fever and tender hepatomegaly frequently occur. Skin lesions may present as patchy urticaria or erythematous papular eruptions [113].

Fig. 170-11 Serpiginous tracks in larva migrans. (Courtesy of New York University, Department of Dermatology.)

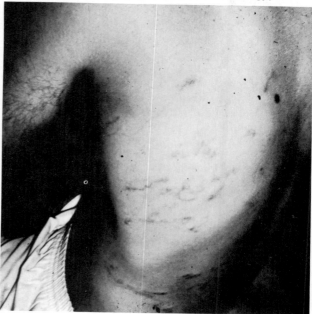

Fat embolism syndrome

Petechiae, respiratory insufficiency, and cerebral dysfunction after long bone fracture are termed the fat embolism syndrome. Petechiae alone after fractures should suggest this syndrome. Histologically, the presence of fat globules within the dermal and pulmonary vessels is reported. Additional factors such as hyperglycemia, diabetes, or elevated beta-lipoproteins may play a contributing role.

The petechiae are most commonly on the neck, axillae, shoulder, chest, and conjunctivae, and often appear prior to other manifestations. They begin about the second or third day after injury, appear in crops, and are almost never found on the face or posterior aspects of the body. When widespread, they tend to herald more significant cerebral and pulmonary dysfunction. Cyanosis may be prominent [114].

The respiratory involvement may begin with dyspnea, tachypnea, or hemoptysis. Tachycardia and fever may be found. Pulmonary edema may occur. X-rays may show patchy densities or linear streaks [115].

Cerebral dysfunction includes restlessness, irritability, delirium, and coma. Additional features include jaundice, renal involvement, anemia, thrombocytopenia, and elevated sedimentation rate.

Selected diseases affecting the cardiopulmonary system

Lipoid proteinosis

Affected individuals are homozygous for a mutant recessive autosomal gene [116], with normal chromosome findings [117]. The disease is worldwide in distribution. Deposition of the amorphous "hyalin," while primarily affecting the mucous membranes and skin, has also been found in other organ systems including the respiratory tract and heart [118].

Oropharyngeal and laryngeal mucous membranes are usually affected early in the course of the disease, being present in infancy and childhood. Hoarseness due to laryngeal infiltration is often the initial finding and may be present at birth [119]. Laryngeal and tracheal infiltration may progress and cause respiratory insufficiency requiring tracheostomy [120]. The trachea and main-stem bronchus may be thickened and studded with wartlike hyaline projections [119]. An increased risk of aspiration pneumonia has been reported [121], as well as repeated upper respiratory infections [122]. Cardiovascular involvement is rare, but conduction defects and arrhythmias have been reported [119].

The skin abnormalities usually appear in childhood shortly after the onset of mucous membrane changes. These consist of waxy, translucent induration, followed by papules, nodules and plaques, characteristically on the face, which are easily traumatized [123]. A beadlike pattern on the palpebral margins and angles of the mouth is common [124] (Fig. 170-12).

Additional cutaneous manifestations include pitted acnelike scarring, alopecia, hyperkeratosis, and onychodystrophy [119].

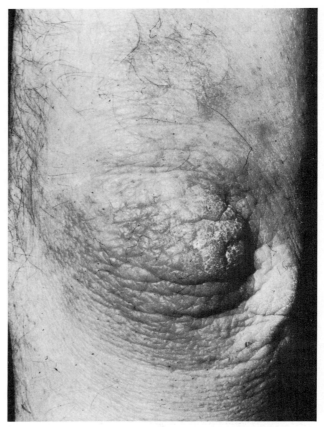

Fig. 170-12   Waxy papules on the arm in lipoid proteinosis. (Courtesy of New York University, Department of Dermatology.)

Multicentric reticulohistiocytosis

Multicentric reticulohistiocytosis (MRH) is an uncommon disorder presenting with characteristic mucocutaneous lesions and a deforming arthritis [125,126] in association with systemic symptoms such as fever, malaise, weight loss, and myopathy [127–129]. The cardiopulmonary complications include pulmonary infiltrates [130], pleural effusions [128,131], pericarditis [125], cardiomegaly [125], congestive heart failure [125], angina pectoris [125], myocardial infarction [132], and pulmonary infarction [132].

The eruption is composed of yellow to brown, firm papules and nodules especially localized about the hands and face. The dorsum of the hand is more common than the palm, and the paronychial zone and lateral aspects of the digits with accentuation about the finger joints are most often affected [127] (Fig. 170-13). Involvement of the scalp, ears, and nose may coalesce, resulting in a leonine appearance [133]. The mucous membranes are also involved and infiltration of the lips, gingiva, tongue, and pharynx are reported [127]. Histologically, these lesions are composed of histiocytic, multinucleated giant cells which are PAS-positive and sudanophilic [130]. The PAS-positive material is thought to represent a mucoprotein or glycoprotein and the sudanophilic material may represent a combination of triglycerides, cholesterol, neutral fat, phospholipids, and glycolipids [134].

Fig. 170-13 Papules on the hand in multicentric reticulohistiocytosis. *(Courtesy of New York University, Department of Dermatology.)*

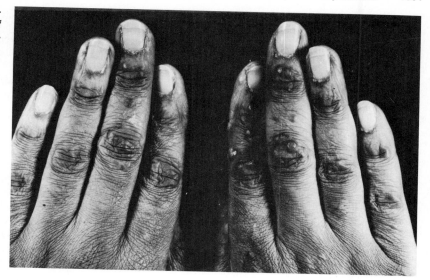

The arthritis is frequently inflammatory in type [126] and, when associated with the nail dystrophy which occurs in the disease [135], it may mimic psoriatic arthritis. There is early involvement of the DIP joints. Rheumatoid arthritis may be considered, but MRH patients are seronegative [135].

An association of MRH with malignancy has been recorded in a few reports [127,130,136], suggesting the need for complete evaluation of these patients [136].

Sarcoidosis

Sarcoidosis is a multisystem granulomatous disease of unknown cause with widespread manifestations [137]. Cardiac involvement may be occult, but it is clinically evident in about 20 percent of patients [138]. Ventricular arrhythmias and conduction disturbances are responsible for the palpitations, presyncope, and syncope reported [139]. Congestive heart failure and chest pain occur less frequently and may be due to cor pulmonale [140]. Additionally, prolapsed mitral valves, papillary muscle dysfunction, and aneurysm formation may be found rarely [141]. The prognosis for patients with cardiac involvement is unfavorable [139].

Sarcoidosis affects the pulmonary system most commonly [142]. Intrathoracic sarcoid affects both the lymph nodes and lung parenchyma in about 90 percent of patients [142]. Respiratory failure is often the most difficult clinical problem, characterized by shortness of breath, dyspnea, and hypoxemia [143].

The cutaneous features of sarcoidosis may not be clinically apparent at the time of cardiac involvement but occur in about 30 percent of patients [137]. Lesions are found especially about the eyes, nose, nasolabial folds, and mouth.

The quality of clinical lesions varies considerably, but such features as a distinctive red color, translucency, and central atrophy with ringed borders should suggest the diagnosis. Flattopped papules with or without scale are also common [137]. These lesions, when biopsied, reveal a granulomatous pattern with noncaseating epithelial tu-

bercles and giant cells. Additionally, erythema nodosum and erythema multiforme may occur as nonspecific reactive phenomena [143]. Although sarcoid lesions generally are not pruritic and do not ulcerate, exceptions have been documented [144,145].

While there are at least two forms of sarcoidosis, acute (transient) and chronic (persistent), no definite correlation between skin and internal involvement has been made. However, those patients who present abruptly with hilar adenopathy and nonspecific skin involvement, such as erythema nodosum (Lofgren's syndrome), appear to respond to steroid therapy, have less frequent recurrence, and a more favorable prognosis [143].

Amyloidosis (see Chap. 142)

Involvement of the heart may occur in all three systemic forms of amyloidosis, but appears clinically predominant in the primary and myeloma-associated types [146]. Senile amyloidosis may also affect the heart but is often asymptomatic [147]. Clinical findings include dizziness, palpitations, syncope, orthostatic hypotension, and congestive heart failure. Chest x-ray may reveal cardiomegaly. EKGs may show low-voltage, abnormal Q waves, conduction defects, and arrhythmias [148]. Echocardiography may reveal a restrictive cardiomyopathy with enlargement of the left ventricular wall and obstruction of the outflow tract. Pathologically, infiltration of the endocardium, myocardium, pericardium, valves, and coronary vessels may occur [148].

Upper and lower respiratory tract involvement also occurs in all systemic forms of amyloidosis, but is clinically predominant in primary and myeloma-associated types. Macroglossia may impede respiration, especially when complicated by bleeding. The larynx and trachea may become infiltrated, causing hoarseness, cough, and respiratory stridor. Bronchial and lung parenchymal involvement may cause asthmalike symptoms, hemoptysis, and severe restrictive pulmonary disease [149]. Chest x-rays may reveal interstitial type involvement and occasionally amyloid nodules may mimic a malignant tumor [150]. Pulmonary function studies may reveal a deficit in diffusing capacity as well as various types of tubular disease [149].

Cutaneous involvement occurs most often in the primary and myeloma-associated types and, therefore, serves as a marker for cardiopulmonary involvement [151]. Translucent papules and plaques on the eyelids, nasolabial folds, mouth, neck, and upper trunk may be found. A sclerodermoid appearance may occur with extensive involvement, especially with the myeloma-associated type [151].

Areas of petechiae, purpura, and hemorrhage (pinch purpura) occur readily due to early involvement of dermal blood vessels. This may occur in areas of previously involved skin or in areas that are clinically normal in appearance, suggesting the high incidence of dermal blood vessel involvement. Therefore, a skin biopsy of clinically normal skin in a patient suspected of having amyloidosis may demonstrate deposition within the vessels in as many as 50 percent of patients [151,152].

Lymphomatoid granulomatosis

This infiltrative systemic disease affects the skin, lungs, central nervous system, kidneys, and other organs in a characteristic histologic pattern [153]. Pulmonary involvement may begin with transient alveolar or interstitial infiltrates and effusions on chest x-ray, which subsequently may progress to nodular, masslike densities. These lesions may cavitate and be responsible for profuse hemoptysis [154]. Although many patients remain asymptomatic, cough, dyspnea, and chest pain may be found [153]. Cardiac involvement is uncommon and when present may involve the coronary vessels with subsequent myocardial ischemia [155].

Skin lesions are found in up to half of all patients and are varied in appearance, often not suggestive of vasculitis. Erythematous papules, nodules, and plaques are found which sometime ulcerate (Fig. 170-14). These lesions usually reveal the characteristic histologic pattern of lymphoreticular cells surrounding and infiltrating blood vessels [156].

Collagen vascular diseases

The cardiopulmonary complications of the various collagen vascular diseases may sometimes be associated with a specific cutaneous sign or constellation of features.

Rheumatoid arthritis

Extraarticular manifestations of rheumatoid arthritis, especially in the pulmonary system, appear to correlate with subcutaneous nodules and vasculitic skin lesions. The nodules may become necrobiotic and ulcerate, causing pain, secondary infection, and poor healing. The vasculitic lesions include palpable purpura, splinter hemorrhages, digital pitting, ulceration or gangrene, sometimes in association with Raynaud's phenomenon, and pyoderma gangrenosum [157–159].

In addition, laboratory evidence of high-titer rheumatoid factor, hypocomplementemia, cryoimmunoglobulinemia, and hypereosinophilia may be associated with the extraarticular manifestations including cardiopulmonary disease [154,160–162]. These manifestations occur more commonly in men with long-standing disease, but they may not necessarily correlate with arthritis activity at the time [163]. The pulmonary disease may be asymptomatic. Complaints include dyspnea, cough, pleuritic chest pain, and hemoptysis. Cardiac involvement may not be clinically apparent, although autopsy studies have revealed a high incidence of cardiac lesions related to granuloma or vasculitis [164].

Systemic lupus erythematosus

Cutaneous manifestations of systemic lupus erythematosus (SLE) appear in over 75 percent of patients during the course of their disease. While the extent of cutaneous features in SLE may not correlate with the severity of visceral disease, the trend toward serologic and clinical subsets has suggested certain associations.

Photosensitive dermatitis, discoid type lesions, Raynaud's phenomenon, and polyarthritis are associated with an increased incidence of serositis, including pleurisy, pericarditis, and noninfectious peritonitis [165]. The incidence of significant serositis may be higher in drug-induced SLE syndromes, particularly with procainamide [166].

Pleuropulmonary disease in SLE. Pleuritis may be present during the course of disease in about half of SLE patients. Chest pain may become subacute or chronic secondary to adhesions and may be confused with costochondritis. Pleural effusions with or without a friction rub may also occur [165]. Parenchymal lung involvement in SLE is usually due to secondary factors such as infections or pulmonary emboli [167]. Primary lung involvement in SLE may be classified as follows: (a) diffuse interstitial pneumonitis, (b) acute pneumonitis, (c) intrapulmonary hemorrhage, (d) diaphragm dysfunction with decreased lung volume (shrinking lung syndrome), (e) pulmonary hypertension with cor pulmonale, and (f) fibrosing alveolitis [168–173].

Respiratory difficulty may also be due to acute epiglottitis, necrotic and ulcerative laryngitis, and tracheobronchitis [174].

Cardiac involvement in SLE is frequently subclinical [165]. Pericarditis may be more common in those patients with drug-induced syndromes or those in whom photosensitive discoid lesions are found [165]. Chest pain may be present, especially when associated with effusion. A friction rub may be heard. The EKG changes primarily are T-wave abnormalities [175].

Myocarditis is often undiagnosed and may be associated with prolonged P-R intervals, heart block, and arrhythmias [176]. Since the introduction of steroid therapy an increased incidence of atherosclerotic-related myocardial infarction has been reported [176].

Valvular heart disease in SLE is most often of the Libman-Sacks type and is manifested by systolic murmurs which may occur in almost one-half of all patients. These are rarely clinically significant [176]. Although diastolic murmurs may occur due to noninfectious mitral stenosis or aortic insufficiency, the onset of a new diastolic murmur should provoke a search for subacute bacterial indocarditis (SBE) [177]. The cutaneous clues of SBE, such as splinter hemorrhages, Osler's nodes, Janeway lesions, and Roth spots, should be searched for, although these may occur

Fig. 170-14 Erythematous papules and ulcer in lymphomatoid granulomatosis. *(Courtesy of New York University, Department of Dermatology.)*

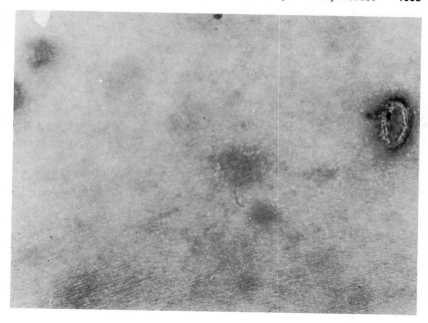

in SLE without infection. It appears that SLE, as well as other cutaneous vascular diseases, may be associated with complete heart block in newborn infants. In SLE, this may be due to placental transfer of maternal antibodies, especially anti-Ro antibody [178]. The newborn infants of SLE patients may also have distinctive evanescent cutaneous eruptions including prominent telangiectasia and periorbital erythema [179].

Progressive systemic sclerosis

Microvascular abnormalities are among the earliest pathologic changes seen in progressive systemic sclerosis patients, supporting the concept of a primary vascular defect in the disease [180]. Characteristically the vascular lesions reveal intimal proliferation with loose connective tissue at the internal elastic membrane, medial thinning, and adventitial fibrosis [181].

Many of the cutaneous features of this disorder are directly attributable to vascular abnormalities. Vasospastic episodes (Raynaud's) are often the first cutaneous findings. Telangiectases, also found early in the disease, are typically polygonal and sharply defined, commonly appearing as "mats" about the malar area of the face and upper trunk. Nail fold capillary change also occurs early in the disease as dilated and distorted capillary loops alternating with avascular areas on wide-field capillary microscopy [182]. Skin involvement generally follows three stages: edematous, fibrotic, and atrophic.

Pulmonary abnormalities. Dyspnea on exertion is usually the most common symptom occurring in about half the patients. Chronic, nonproductive cough and pleuritic chest pain may also occur. Examination may reveal dry rales, especially at the bases, as well as diminished breath sounds and pleural rubs. Chest x-ray may show a diffuse reticulonodular interstitial pattern and cystic changes, as well as calcification. Pulmonary function tests reveal diminished diffusing capacity, decreased volume, and decreased compliance [183].

Abnormalities of the respiratory system may not be due only to parenchymal lung disease. Thus, pulmonary hypertension with cor pulmonale and congestive heart failure may develop independently of parenchymal disease. Biopsies of the lung show the typical changes described earlier about the small pulmonary arteries and arterioles [184]. Esophageal dysmotility may cause aspiration pneumonia and acute respiratory insufficiency [154]. Finally, the finding of fairly abrupt changes in respiratory function suggests the possibility of a bronchiolar carcinoma in association with long-standing pulmonary fibrosis [183].

Cardiovascular disease in progressive systemic sclerosis. Acute and chronic pericarditis is an important feature of the disease, and, when associated with congestive heart failure, may be a marker for incipient renal failure. Pericardial effusions may be occult, and constrictive pericarditis and tamponade may occur [185].

Transient vasospasm may involve the coronary vessels and cause myocardial ischemia with angina. Additionally, small-vessel involvement of the myocardium may lead to fibrosis (scleroderma heart) [186].

Fibrosis of the conduction system may cause arrhythmias and sudden death. Right ventricular hypertrophy due to cor pulmonale with congestive failure and pulmonary hypertension is observed [187]. The presence of the CREST variant may be associated with biliary cirrhosis and may not imply diminished cardiopulmonary or renal involvement in all cases as originally described.

Recently an attempt to correlate nail fold capillary abnormalities with visceral manifestation has been reported. The presence of increased tortuosity of capillaries and areas of avascularity suggests an increased probability of cardiopulmonary and renal disease [182].

Relapsing polychondritis

Relapsing polychondritis is characterized by inflammation and destruction of cartilage and connective tissues including those of the cardiopulmonary system. The pathogenesis is unknown, although it appears to be an autoimmune process frequently associated with other immunologic disorders such as systemic lupus erythematosus and rheumatoid arthritis [188].

Clinically, auricular chondritis with pain, swelling, and redness of the pinna but complete sparing of the lobes is characteristic. Nasal chondritis may be associated with rhinorrhea and epistaxis and progress to "saddle-nose" deformity. Ocular involvement includes episcleritis and iritis. Various skeletal complaints including arthralgias, polyarthritis, costochondritis, and manubriosternal arthritis may be found [189]. Vasculitis involving multiple-size vessels may occur and simulate giant cell arteritis or polyarteritis nodosa. Cutaneous involvement includes dermal vasculitis sometimes associated with panniculitis. Additional cutaneous manifestations include postinflammatory hyperpigmentation, alopecia, nail dystrophy, and subcutaneous fat necrosis [190].

Respiratory tract involvement may begin with hoarseness or tenderness of the anterior trachea. Degeneration of the laryngeal, tracheal, and/or bronchial rings may lead to progressive insufficiency or sudden collapse requiring emergency tracheostomy. Adequate ventilatory support may not be possible if advanced scarring and deformity are present [189].

Cardiac involvement includes degeneration of the aortic ring with valvular insufficiency and aneurysmal dilatation. "Floppy" mitral valve syndrome also occurs. Pericardial and myocardial abnormalities have been reported [191].

References

1. Cupo LN et al: Ehlers-Danlos syndrome with abnormal collagen fibrils, sinus of valsalva aneurysms, myocardial infarction, panacinar emphysema and cerebral heterotopias. *Am J Med* **71:**1051, 1981

2. Merten DF, Rooney R: Progressive pulmonary emphysema associated with congenital generalized elastosis (cutis laxa). *Pediatr Radiol* **113:**691, 1974

3. Lebowohl MG et al: Pseudoxanthoma elasticum mitral-valve prolapse. *N Engl J Med* **307:**228, 1982

4. Silverman ME, Hurst JW: Inspection of the patient, in *The Heart, Arteries and Veins,* 5th ed. New York, McGraw-Hill, 1982, p 165

5. DeGowin EL, DeGowin RL: *Bedside Diagnostic Examination,* 4th ed. New York, Macmillan, 1981

6. Chesler E et al: Anatomic basis for delivery of right ventricular blood into localized segments of the systemic arterial system. *Am J Cardiol* **21:**72, 1968

7. Silverman ME, Hurst JW: The hand and the heart. *Am J Cardiol* **22:**718, 1968

8. Hecht HH: On cardiocutaneous syndromes. *Trans Assoc Am Physicians* **80:**91, 1967

9. Cobb LA et al: Circulatory effects of chronic hypervolemia in polycythemia vera, *J Clin Invest* **39:**1722, 1960

10. Engelman K: The carcinoid syndrome, in *Textbook of Medicine,* 16th ed, edited by JB Wyngaarden, LH Smith Jr. Philadelphia, WB Saunders, 1982, p 1312

11. Schosser RH et al: Mastocytosis, in *Cutaneous Aspects of Internal Disease,* edited by JP Callen. Chicago, Year Book Medical Publishers, 1981, p 539

12. Gifford FW et al: Clinical features, diagnosis and treatment of pheochromocytoma. *Mayo Clin Proc* **39:**281, 1964

13. Babb RR et al: Erythermalgia: review of 51 cases. *Circulation* **29:**136, 1964

14. Johns MK: Skin wrinkling in cystic fibrosis. *Med Biol Illus* **25:**205, 1975

15. Altman RD, Tenenbaum J: Hypertrophic osteoarthropathy in *Textbook of Rheumatology,* edited by WN Kelley et al. Philadelphia, WB Saunders, 1981, p 1647

16. Steinbrocker O: The shoulder-hand syndrome: present perspective. *Arch Phys Med Rehabil* **49:**388, 1968

17. Kannel WB et al: Serum cholesterol, lipoprotein, and the risk of coronary heart disease. The Framingham study. *Ann Intern Med* **74:**1, 1971

18. Carlson LA, Bottiger LE: Ischaemic heart disease in relation to fasting values of plasma triglycerides and cholesterol. Stockholm prospective study. *Lancet* **1:**865, 1972

19. Muller C: Angina pectoris in hereditary xanthomatosis. *Arch Intern Med* **64:**674, 1939

20. Frank ST: Aural sign of coronary artery disease (letter). *N Engl J Med* **289:**327, 1973

21. Lichstein E et al: Diagonal ear lobe crease: incidence and significance as a coronary risk factor (abstr). *Clin Res* **21:**949, 1973

22. Lichstein E et al: Diagonal ear-lobe crease: prevalence and implications as a coronary risk factor. *N Engl J Med* **290:**615, 1974

23. Christiansen J et al: Diagonal ear-lobe crease in coronary heart disease (letter). *N Engl J Med* **293:**308, 1975

24. Wyre H: The diagonal ear-lobe crease: a cutaneous manifestation of coronary artery disease. *Cutis* **23:**328, 1979

25. Sternlieb JJ et al: The ear crease sign in coronary artery disease (abstr). *Circulation* **50:**152, 1974

26. Lichstein E et al: Diagonal ear-lobe crease and coronary artery sclerosis. *Ann Intern Med* **85:**337, 1976

27. Fisher ER et al: Disseminated atheromatous emboli. *Am J Med* **29:**176, 1960

28. Carvajal JA et al: Atheroembolism: an etiologic factor in renal insufficiency, gastrointestinal and peripheral vascular diseases. *Arch Intern Med* **119:**593, 1967

29. Leroy D: Les manifestations cutanées des embolies de cristaux de cholestérol. A propos d'une observation simulant une péri-artérite-noueuse. Thèse médécine, Rouen, 1975, p 56

30. Moldveen-Geronimus M, Merriam JC: Cholesterol embolization. From pathological curiosity to clinical entity. *Circulation* **35:**946, 1967

31. Stewart WM et al: Les manifestations cutanées des embolies de cristaux de cholestérol. *Ann Dermatol Venereol (Paris)* **104:**5, 1977

32. Crane C: Atherothrombotic embolism to lower extremities in arteriosclerosis. *Arch Surg* **94:**96, 1967

33. Calhoun P: Cholesterol emboli causing gangrene of the extremities. *Arch Dermatol* **111:**1373, 1975

34. Fischer DA, Kistner RL: Athero-thrombotic emboli in the lower extremities. *Arch Dermatol* **104:**533, 1971

35. Deschamps P et al: Livedo reticularis and nodules due to cholesterol embolism in the lower extremities. *Br J Dermatol* **97:**93, 1977

36. Maurizi CP et al: Atheromatous emboli. A postmortem study with special references to the lower extremities. *Arch Pathol* **86:**528, 1968

37. Anderson WR, Richard AM: Evaluation of lower extremity muscle biopsies in the diagnosis of atheroembolism. *Arch Pathol* **86:**535, 1968

38. Anderson WR: Necrotizing angiitis associated with embolization of cholesterol. *Am J Clin Pathol* **43:**65, 1965

39. Carr RD, Rau RC: Dermatitis at vein graft site in coronary artery bypass patients. *Arch Dermatol* **117:**814, 1981

40. Bart RS: Dermatitis at vein graft site (letter). *Arch Dermatol* **119:**97, 1983

41. Timmis GC: *Cardiovascular Review: 1980.* Baltimore, Williams & Wilkins, 1980, pp 220, 251

42. Giacomo A et al: Leg wound complications associated with coronary revascularization. *J Thorac Cardiovasc Surg* **81**:403, 1981

43. Baddour LM, Bisno AL: Recurrent cellulitis after saphenous venectomy for coronary bypass surgery. *Ann Intern Med* **97**:493, 1982

44. Greenberg J et al: Vein-donor cellulitis after coronary artery bypass surgery. *Ann Intern Med* **97**:565, 1982

45. Johnson RA, Palacios I: Dilated cardiomyopathies of the adult. *N Engl J Med* **307**:1051,1119, 1982

46. Bullkley BH, Hutchins GM: Atrial myxomas: a fifty year review. *Am Heart J* **97**:639, 1979

47. Kounis NG: Left atrial myxoma presenting with intermittent claudication and Raynaud's phenomenon: echocardiographic patterns of tumor size. *Br J Med* **56**:356, 1977

48. Byrd WE et al: Left atrial myxomas presenting as a systemic vasculitis. *Arthritis Rheum* **23**:240, 1980

49. Huston KA et al: Left atrial myxoma simulating peripheral vasculitis. *Mayo Clin Proc* **53**:752, 1978

50. McWhirter WR, Tetteh-Lartey EV: A case of atrial myxoma. *Br Heart J* **36**:839, 1974

51. Currey HLF et al: Right atrial myxoma mimicking a rheumatic disorder. *Br Med J* **1**:547, 1967

52. Atherton DJ et al: A syndrome of various pigmented lesions, myxoid neurofibromata and atrial myxoma: the NAME syndrome. *Br J Dermatol* **103**:421, 1980

53. Rhodes AR et al: Mucocutaneous lentigines, cardiomucocutaneous myxomas, and multiple blue nevi: the "LAMB" syndrome. *J Am Acad Dermatol* **10**:72, 1984

54. Moynahan EJ: Multiple symmetrical moles with psychic and somatic infantilism and genital hypoplasia. *Proc R Soc Med* **55**:959, 1962

55. Gorlin RJ et al: Multiple lentigines syndrome. *Am J Dis Child* **117**:652, 1969

56. Norlund JJ et al: The multiple lentigines syndrome. *Arch Dermatol* **107**:259, 1973

57. Polani PE, Moynahan EJ: Progressive cardiomyopathic lentiginosis. *Q J Med* **41**:205, 1972

58. Smith RF et al: Generalized lentigo: electrocardiographic abnormalities, conduction disorders and arrhythmia in three cases. *Am J Cardiol* **25**:501, 1970

59. Weiss LW, Zelickson AS: Giant melanosomes in multiple lentigines syndrome. *Arch Dermatol* **113**:491, 1977

60. Matthews NL: Lentigo and electrocardiographic changes. *N Engl J Med* **278**:780, 1968

61. Walther RJ et al: Electrocardiographic abnormalities in a family with generalized lentigo. *N Engl J Med* **275**:1220, 1966

62. Somerville J, Bonham-Carter RE: The heart in lentiginosis. *Br Heart J* **34**:58, 1972

63. Hopkins BC et al: Familial hypertrophic cardiomyopathy and lentiginosis. *Aust NZ J Med* **5**:359, 1975

64. Voron DA et al: Multiple lentigines syndrome. *Am J Med* **60**:447, 1976

65. Selmanowitz VJ et al: Lentiginosis profusa syndrome (multiple lentigines syndrome). *Arch Dermatol* **104**:393, 1971

66. Seuanez H et al: Cardiocutaneous syndrome (the "leopard" syndrome). *Clin Genet* **9**:266, 1976

67. Libman E: The clinical features of subacute streptococcal (and influenzal) endocarditis in the bacterial stage. *Med Clin North Am* **2**:117, 1918

68. Janeway E: Certain clinical observations upon heart disease. *Med News* **75**:257, 1899

69. Osler W: Gulstonian lectures on malignant endocarditis. *Lancet* **1**:415, 459, 505, 1885

70. Osler W: Chronic infectious endocarditis. *Q J Med* **2**:219, 1909

71. Merklen P, Wolf M: Participation des endotheliiites arteriocapillaries au syndrome de l'endocardite maligne lente. *Presse Med* **36**:97, 1928

72. Lian C et al: Histopathologie de nodule d'Osler, étude sur l'endothéliite de l'endocardite maligne à évolution lente. *Presse Med* **37**:497, 1929

73. Von Gemmengen GR, Winkelmann RK: Osler's nodes of subacute bacterial endocarditis. *Arch Dermatol* **95**:91, 1967

74. Cornil L et al: Contribution a l'étude histologique du nodule d'Osler. *Ann Anat Pathol* **13**:675, 1936

75. Alpert JS et al: Pathogenesis of Osler's nodes. *Ann Intern Med* **85**:471, 1976

76. Kerr A: *Subacute Bacterial Endocarditis*. Springfield, IL, Charles C Thomas, 1956, p 101

77. Farrior JB, Silverman ME: A consideration of the differences between a Janeway's lesion and an Osler's node in infectious endocarditis. *Chest* **70**:239, 1976

78. Ruiter M, Mandema E: New cutaneous syndrome in subacute bacterial endocarditis. *Arch Intern Med* **113**:283, 1964

79. Kennedy JE, Wise GN: Clinicopathologic correlation of retinal lesions, subacute bacterial endocarditis. *Arch Ophthalmol* **74**:658, 1965

80. Weinstein L: "Modern" infective endocarditis. *JAMA* **223**:260, 1975

81. Weinstein L, Schlesinger JJ: Pathoanatomic, pathophysiologic and clinical correlation in endocarditis. *N Engl J Med* **291**:832, 1122, 1974

82. Horder T: Clinical significance and course of subacute bacterial endocarditis. *Br Med J* **2**:301, 1920

83. Blumer G: The digital manifestations of subacute bacterial endocarditis. *Am Heart J* **1**:257, 1926

84. Michaelson ED, Walsh RE: Osler's node—a complication of prolonged arterial cannulation. *N Engl J Med* **283**:472, 1970

85. Matthews J, Gibbons RB: Embolization complicating radial artery puncture. *Ann Intern Med* **75**:87, 1971

86. Fanning L, Aronson M: Osler node, Janeway lesions and splinter hemorrhages: occurrence with an infected arterial catheter. *Arch Dermatol* **113**:648, 1977

87. Rudusky BM: Recurrent Osler's nodes in systemic lupus erythematosus. *Angiology* **20**:33, 1969

88. Keil H: The rheumatic subcutaneous nodules and simulating lesions. *Medicine (Baltimore)* **17**:261, 1938

89. Howard EJ: Osler's nodes. *Am Heart J* **59**:633, 1960

90. Gross N: Clinical significance of splinter hemorrhages. *Br Med J* **2**:1496, 1963

91. Pankey GA: Subacute bacterial endocarditis at the University of Minnesota Hospital, 1939 through 1959. *Ann Intern Med* **55**:550, 1961

92. Pankey GA: Acute bacterial endocarditis at the University of Minnesota Hospital, 1939 through 1959. *Am Heart J* **64**:583, 1962

93. Horwitz LD, Silber R: Subacute bacterial endocarditis presenting as purpura. *Arch Intern Med* **120**:483, 1967

94. Rubenfeld S, Kyung-What M: Leukocytoclastic angiitis in subacute bacterial endocarditis. *Arch Dermatol* **113**:1073, 1977

95. Myall RW et al: Mucosal and dermal lesions seen in bacterial endocarditis. *J Am Dent Assoc* **78**:120, 1969

96. Park CH et al: Erysipelothrix endocarditis with cutaneous lesion. *South Med J* **69**:1101, 1976

97. Grieco MH, Sheldon C: *Erysipelothrix rhusiopathiae*. *Ann NY Acad Sci* **174**:523, 1970

98. Samman PD, White WF: The "yellow nail" syndrome. *Br J Dermatol* **76**:153, 1964

99. Hurwitz PA, Pinals DJ: Pleural effusion in chronic hereditary lymphedema (Nonne, Milroy, Meige's disease): report of two cases. *Radiology* **82**:246, 1964

100. Emerson PA: Yellow nails, lymphoedema, and pleural effusions. *Thorax* **21**:247, 1966

101. Marks R, Ellis JP: Yellow nails: a report of six cases. *Arch Dermatol* **102**:619, 1970

102. Runyon BA: Pleural-fluid kinetics in a patient with primary

lymphedema, pleural effusions and yellow nails. *Am Rev Respir Dis* **119:**821, 1979

103. Awerbuch MS: The yellow nail syndrome, bronchiectasis and Raynaud's disease—a relationship. *Med J Aust* **2:**829, 1976

104. Hiller E et al: Pulmonary manifestations of the yellow nail syndrome. *Chest* **61:**452, 1972

105. Shumacker HB Jr, Waldhausen JA: Pulmonary arteriovenous fistulas in children. *Ann Surg* **158:**713, 1963

106. Dines DE et al: Pulmonary arteriovenous fistulas. *Mayo Clin Proc* **58:**176, 1983

107. Harrison DF: Familial haemorrhagic telangiectasia. *Q J Med* **33:**25, 1964

108. Conlon CL et al: Telangiectasia and von Willebrand's disease in two families. *Ann Intern Med* **89:**921, 1978

109. Meijer A: Asthma predictors in infantile atopic dermatitis. *J Asthma Res* **12:**181, 1975

110. Burrows B: Chronic airways diseases, in *Textbook of Medicine,* 16th ed, edited by JB Wyngaarden, LH Smith Jr. Philadelphia, WB Saunders, 1982, p 363

111. Di Sant'Agnese PA, Davis PB: Cystic fibrosis in adults. *Am J Med* **66:**121, 1979

112. Johns MK: Skin wrinkling in cystic fibrosis. *Med Biol Illus* 25:205, 1975

113. Katz R et al: The natural course of creeping eruption and treatment with thiabendazole. *Arch Dermatol* **91:**420, 1965

114. Tachakra SS: Distribution of skin petechiae in fat embolism rash. *Lancet* **1(7954):**284, 1976

115. Cole WG, Oakes BW: Skin petechiae and fat embolism. *Aust NZ J Surg* **42:**401, 1973

116. Gordon H et al: Lipoid proteinosis in an inbred Namaqualand community. *Lancet* **1:**1032, 1969

117. Burnett JW, Marcy SM: Lipoid proteinosis. *Am J Dis Child* **105:**81, 1963

118. Caplan RM: Visceral involvement in lipoid proteinosis. *Arch Dermatol* **95:**149, 1967

119. Hofer PA: Urbach-Wiethe disease: a review. *Acta Derm Venereol (Stockh)* **53(suppl 71):**1, 1973

120. Caplan RM: Lipoid proteinosis: a review including some new observations. *Univ Mich Med Bull* **28:**365, 1962

121. Weidner WA et al: Roentgenographic findings in lipoid proteinosis: a case report. *Am J Roentgenol* **110:**457, 1970

122. Sanderson KV: Lipoid proteinosis. *Proc R Soc Med* **63:**888, 1970

123. Heyl, T: Lipoid proteinosis. I: The clinical picture. *Br J Dermatol* **75:**465, 1963

124. Jensen AD et al: Lipoid proteinosis. *Arch Ophthalmol* **88:**273, 1972

125. Warin RP et al: Reticulohistiocytosis (lipoid dermato-arthritis). *Br Med J* **1:**1387, 1957

126. Bortz AI, Vincent M: Lipoid dermato-arthritis and arthritis mutilans. *Am J Med* **30:**951, 1961

127. Barrow MV, Holubar K: Multicentric reticulohistiocytosis: a review of thirty-three patients. *Medicine (Baltimore)* **48:**287, 1969

128. Ehrlich GE et al: Multicentric reticulohistiocytosis (lipoid dermato-arthritis): a multisystem disorder. *Am J Med* **52:**830, 1972

129. Anderson TE et al: Myositis and myotonia in a case of multicentric reticulohistiocytosis. *Br J Dermatol* **80:**39, 1968

130. Orkin M et al: A study of multicentric reticulohistiocytosis. *Arch Dermatol* **89:**640, 1964

131. Flam M et al: Multicentric reticulohistiocytosis: report of a case with atypical features and electron microscopic study of skin lesions. *Am J Med* **52:**841, 1972

132. Fast A: Cardiopulmonary complications in multicentric reticulohistiocytosis. *Arch Dermatol* **112:**1139, 1976

133. Braverman IM: In *Skin Signs of Systemic Disease,* 2d ed. Philadelphia, WB Saunders, 1981, p 208

134. Barrow MV et al: Identification of tissue lipids in lipoid dermatoarthritis (multicentric reticulohistiocytosis). *Am J Clin Pathol* **47:**312, 1967

135. Barrow MV: The nails in multicentric reticulohistiocytosis. *Arch Dermatol* **95:**200, 1967

136. Catterall MD, White JE: Multicentric reticulohistiocytosis and malignant disease. *Br J Dermatol* **98:**221, 1978

137. James DG et al: A worldwide review of sarcoidosis. *Ann NY Acad Sci* **278:**321, 1976

138. Matsui Y et al: Clinicopathological study on fatal myocardial sarcoidosis. *Ann NY Acad Sci* **278:**455, 1976

139. Stein E et al: Clinical course of cardiac sarcoidosis. *Ann NY Acad Sci* **278:**470, 1976

140. Lorell B et al: Cardiac sarcoidosis. *Am J Cardiol* **42:**143, 1978

141. Roberts WC et al: Sarcoidosis of the heart. *Am J Med* **63:**86, 1977

142. Mitchell DN et al: Sarcoidosis: state of the art. *Am Rev Resp Dis* **110:**774, 1974

143. Jones Williams W. Davies BH: *Eighth International Conference on Sarcoidosis and Other Granulomatous Disease.* Cardiff, Wales, Alpha Omega Publishing Ltd, 1980

144. Fong YW, Sharma OP: Pruritic maculopapular skin lesions in sarcoidosis. *Arch Dermatol* **111:**362, 1975

145. Schiffner V, Sharma OP: Ulcerative sarcoidosis. *Arch Dermatol* **113:**676, 1977

146. Meaney E et al: Cardiac amyloidosis, constrictive pericarditis and restrictive cardiomyopathy. *Am J Cardiol* **38:**347, 1976

147. Westermark P et al: Senile cardiac amyloidosis: evidence of two different amyloid substances in the aging heart. *Scand J Immunol* **10:**303, 1979

148. Kyle RA, Bayrd ED: Amyloidosis: review of 236 cases. *Medicine (Baltimore)* **54:**271, 1975

149. Celli BR et al: Patterns of pulmonary involvement in systemic amyloidosis. *Chest* **74:**543, 1978

150. Brauner GJ et al: Acquired bullous disease of the skin and solitary amyloidoma of the lung. *Am J Med* **57:**978, 1974

151. Rubinow A, Cohen AS: Skin involvement in generalized amyloidosis. *Ann Intern Med* **88:**781, 1978

152. Brownstein MH, Helwig EB: The cutaneous amyloidoses: II. Systemic forms. *Arch Dermatol* **102:**20, 1970

153. Liebow AA et al: Lymphomatoid granulomatosis. *Hum Pathol* **3:**457, 1972

154. Hunninghake GW, Fauci AS: Pulmonary involvement in the collagen vascular diseases. *Am Rev Respir Dis* **119:**471, 1979

155. Israel HL et al: Wegener's granulomatosis, lymphomatoid granulomatosis and benign lymphocytic angiitis and granulomatosis of the lung: recognition and treatment. *Ann Intern Med* **87:**691, 1977

156. Minars N et al: Lymphomatoid granulomatosis of the skin. *Arch Dermatol* **111:**493, 1975

157. Gordon DA et al: The extra-articular features of rheumatoid arthritis: a systemic analysis of 127 cases. *Am J Med* **54:**445, 1973

158. Gardner DL et al: Pulmonary hypertension in rheumatoid arthritis: report of a case with intimal sclerosis of the pulmonary and digital arteries. *Scott Med J* **2:**183, 1957

159. Stolman LP et al: Pyoderma gangrenosum and rheumatoid arthritis. *Arch Dermatol* **111:**1020, 1975

160. Mongan ES et al: A study of the relation of seronegative and seropositive rheumatoid arthritis to each other and to necrotizing vasculitis. *Am J Med* **47:**23, 1969

161. Winchester RJ et al: Observations on the eosinophilia of certain patients with rheumatoid arthritis. *Arthritis Rheum* **14:**650, 1971

162. Weisman M, Zvaifler N: Cryoimmunoglobulinemia in rheumatoid arthritis. *J Clin Invest* **56:**725, 1975

163. Hurd ER: Extraarticular manifestations of rheumatoid arthritis. *Semin Rheum Dis* **8:**151, 1979

164. Bonfiglio T, Atwater E: Heart disease in patients with sero-

positive rheumatoid arthritis; a controlled autopsy study and review. *Arch Intern Med* **127**:714, 1969

165. Fries JF, Holman HR: *Systemic Lupus Erythematosus: A Clinical Analysis.* Philadelphia, WB Saunders, 1975, p 64

166. Byrd RB, Schanger B: Pulmonary sequelae in procaine amide induced lupus-like syndrome. *Dis Chest* **55**:170, 1969

167. Dubois EL, Tuffanelli DL: Clinical manifestations of systemic lupus erythematosus. *JAMA* **190**:104, 1964

168. Eisenberg H et al: Diffuse interstitial lung disease in systemic lupus erythematosus. *Ann Intern Med* **79**:37, 1973

169. Matthay RA et al: Acute lupus pneumonitis: response to azathioprine therapy. *Chest* **63**:117, 1973

170. Eagen JW et al: Pulmonary hemorrhage in systematic lupus erythematosus. *Medicine (Baltimore)* **57**:545, 1978

171. Gibson GJ et al: Diaphragm function and lung involvement in systemic lupus erythematosus. *Am J Med* **63**:926, 1977

172. Perez HD, Kramer N: Pulmonary hypertension in systemic lupus erythematosus: report of four cases and review of the literature. *Sem Arthritis Rheum* **11**:177, 1981

173. Sperryn PN: Systemic lupus erythematosus with fibrosing alveolitis. *Proc R Soc Med* **64**:58, 1971

174. Toomey JM et al: Acute epiglottitis due to systemic lupus erythematosus: *Laryngoscope* **84**:522, 1974

175. Ropes MW: *Systemic Lupus Erythematosus.* Cambridge, MA, Harvard Univ Press, 1976

176. Bulkley BH, Roberts WC: The heart in systemic lupus erythematosus and the changes induced in it by corticosteroid therapy. A study of 36 necropsy patients. *Am J Med* **58**:243, 1975

177. Dubois EL: *Lupus Erythematosus: A Review of the Current Studies of Discoid and Systemic Lupus Erythematosus,* 2d ed. Los Angeles, Univ of Southern California Press, 1976

178. McCue CM et al: Congenital heart blocks in newborns of mothers with connective tissue disease. *Circulation* **56**:82, 1977

179. Vonderheid EC et al: Neonatal lupus erythematosus. Report of four cases with review of the literature. *Arch Dermatol* **112**:698, 1976

180. Campbell PM, LeRoy ED: Pathogenesis of systemic sclerosis: a vascular hypothesis. *Semin Arthritis Rheum* **4**:351, 1975

181. D'Angelo WA et al: Pathologic observations in systemic sclerosis (scleroderma): a study of 58 autopsy cases and 58 matched controls. *Am J Med* **46**:428, 1969

182. Maricq HR et al: Skin capillary abnormalities as indicators of organ involvement in scleroderma (systemic sclerosis), Raynaud's syndrome and dermatomyositis. *Am J Med* **61**:862, 1976

183. Young RH, Mark GJ: Pulmonary vascular changes in scleroderma. *Am J Med* **64**:998, 1978

184. Hurwitz AL et al: Esophageal dysfunction and Raynaud's phenomenon in patients with scleroderma. *Am J Dig Dis* **21**:601, 1976

185. McWhorter JE, LeRoy EC: Pericardial disease in scleroderma (systemic sclerosis). *Am J Med* **57**:566, 1974

186. Gupta MF et al: Scleroderma heart disease with skin flow velocity in coronary arteries. *Chest* **67**:116, 1975

187. Bulkely BH et al: Myocardial lesions of progressive systemic sclerosis: a cause of cardiac dysfunction. *Circulation* **53**:483, 1976

188. Arkin CR, Masi AT: Relapsing polychondritis: review of current status and case report. *Semin Arthritis Rheum* **5**:41, 1975

189. Herman VH: Polychondritis, in *Textbook of Rheumatology,* edited by WN Kelley et al. Philadelphia, WB Saunders, 1981, p 1500

190. Bergfeld WF: Relapsing polychondritis with positive direct immunofluorescence. *Arch Dermatol* **114**:127, 1978

191. Cipriano PR et al: Multiple aortic aneurysms in relapsing polychondritis. *Am J Cardiol* **37**:1097, 1976

CHAPTER 171

CUTANEOUS CHANGES IN PERIPHERAL VASCULAR DISEASE

Edward A. Edwards and Jay D. Coffman

Organic arterial disease

The most common peripheral arterial problem confronting a vascular specialist is undoubtedly arteriosclerosis of the major arteries of the lower extremeties. By contrast, the dermatologist more frequently sees the effects of obstruction of the smaller inflow vessels of the upper extremities with symptoms which are often episodic, whether or not organic disease is present. Nevertheless this discussion will gain clarity if we first consider organic major artery disease.

Etiology and pathogenesis

Table 171-1 gives a comprehensive list of pathologic entities causing major artery obstruction. Arteriosclerosis is

by far the most common. Chronic obstruction is produced by the progressive growth of the atheromas, with sudden worsening by thrombosis of the involved segment. The thrombus causing peripheral embolism usually originates in the heart. Atrial fibrillation is a contributing factor, especially in rheumatic valvular disease. Fibrillation is of less importance when embolism complicates myocardial infarction [1]. In the latter instance it may originate in a ventricular aneurysm. In some cases the thrombus may originate on a proximal arteriosclerotic plaque or within an aneurysm. This latter episode is particularly prone to occur with popliteal aneurysms. Small bits of atheroma may also produce "atheromatous emboli" (Fig. 171-1).

Contrary to its manifestations in the nondiabetic, in patients with diabetes arteriosclerosis develops at an early age, not sparing young women, and with an intensity de-

Table 171-1   Causes of organic major peripheral artery obstruction

Arteriosclerosis and diabetic variations
Buerger's disease (thromboangiitis obliterans)
Miscellaneous lesions:
   Arterial cannulation, external trauma, infection
   Systemic lupus erythematosus and other "collagen diseases"
   Takayasu's arteritis (aortic arch syndrome)
   Giant cell arteritis (temporal or cranial arteritis)
   Fibromuscular dysplasia
Peripheral arterial embolism

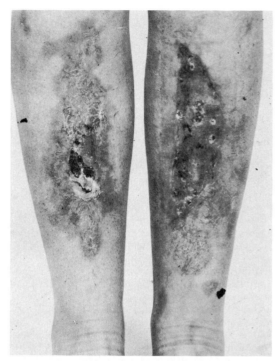

Fig. 171-2   Necrobiosis lipoidica diabeticorum in a young diabetic woman.

pending not on the severity of the diabetes but rather on its duration; it has a greater tendency to include the small arteries in its development; it tends to be more rapidly progressive. Arteriosclerosis is but one of four conditions in the diabetic patient that can produce ulceration alone or in combination. The other three are infection, neuropathy with trauma to an insensitive foot, and necrobiosis lipoidica diabeticorum (Fig. 171-2; see also Figs. 173-9 and A2-3).

Buerger's disease is an inflammatory disorder of arteries and veins of uncommon incidence. It affects predominantly young men, often in their twenties, rarely beginning after 40 years of age; it is exceedingly rare in women. The radial or ulnar arteries are often attacked along with the arteries of the lower limbs. A migrating superficial thrombophlebitis is frequent. Inflammation and fibrosis spread beyond the vessels to adjacent nerves. Tobacco sensitivity is generally accepted as the cause. A recent study [2] suggests that a sensitivity to collagen exists in the disease.

There is ample evidence that systemic lupus erythematosus (SLE) can produce focal lesions in major arteries, including the aorta, and in veins, in addition to its involvement of small distal vessels. Scleroderma attacks not only the digital arteries but also the arterial arches of the hand; rarely the ulnar or radial pulses are lost.

Injury by arterial cannulation as for cardiac catheterization has superseded embolism as the most common cause of major artery obstruction in the upper limb. The other

miscellaneous conditions listed in Table 171-1 are rarely encountered in the extremities.

The effects of organic arterial disease depend on the lowering of the pressure and flow of blood as presented to the capillaries of the part. When the small distal vessels are diffusely involved or when acral arteries, such as the digitals, are occluded, little blood will reach the capillaries, and the part dies. Gangrene of all the toes may thus be produced in the presence of excellent pedal pulses, as in patients with panarteritis nodosa. Contrariwise, if truly localized major artery obstruction is present and good collaterals are available (as often happens in brachial artery embolism), the pressure and flow in the major artery may be reduced, but there will be no further hindrance to the blood in its passage to the capillaries.

Most organic disorders present a combination of proximal and distal occlusion. Even in arteriosclerosis, the obstruction in the major arteries is accompanied by a variable degree of diffuse distal small artery involvement [3]. Blood flow, already lowered by the stenosis, thus meets a second resistance in the distal vessels. When that distal resistance is great, it may be more significant than the major artery stenosis in limiting blood flow.

The various tissues of the limb react to the ischemia in a fashion dictated partly by the steadiness of their needs for blood. With the arteries moderately obstructed, but with the limb at rest, all the tissues may be adequately supplied with blood. With activity, it is the muscles, which in exercise require about 20 times more blood than at rest, that may be the first to signal a low blood flow through the symptom of cramp or fatigue.

Anatomically, the various tissues of the limb possess a relatively circumscribed arterial inflow; that is, their arteries make few collateral connections with those of neigh-

Fig. 171-1   Atheromatous embolism. Resolution of small infarcts of the heel.

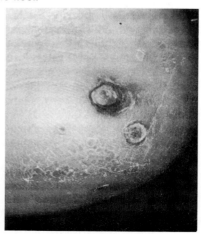

boring structures. This is true of the individual muscles and, as regards functional needs, of the nerve trunks as well. While the arteries to the skin do show numerous collateral connections, one or more arteries to a particular region may be dominant, and occlusion of such a vessel may give rise to localized ischemia and infarction. This is particularly true of a digit, but examples can be shown of such localized problems in the leg as well [4].

Clinical manifestations

The major symptoms are those of ischemia. As implied above, moderate chronic ischemia may produce only symptoms of intermittent claudication, that is, a limitation of walking due to pain or excessive fatigue in the muscles of the limb. This may be localized to the foot in tibial artery disease but proceeds as high as the thigh or buttock in aortoiliac stenosis. Characteristically the discomfort is present only on walking and is relieved in minutes on resting. This may be accompanied by muscle atrophy of the foot, calf, or thigh.

The patient may complain of coldness and hypesthesia of the foot. With high-grade obstruction, constant pain may be felt in the feet, especially at night, with relief sought by hanging the feet over the edge of the bed, walking about, or sleeping in a chair. This so-called rest pain occurs during elevation, because the patient loses the assistance which hydrostatic pressure on standing adds to the pressure presented to the capillaries. It is thought that this heightened pressure on standing is not offset by hydrostatic influence in the veins; first, because the resultant stretching of arterioles, capillaries, and venules lowers the peripheral resistance, and, secondly, because muscular motion against the valved veins tends to empty them, leaving a net increase of the artery-to-vein pressure head.

The foot is usually cold. Its color depends on position, as discussed below under "Special Findings on Examination." The skin is apt to be atrophic, dry, and shiny. Hair usually present on the feet or toes of males may be missing, and nail growth is impeded [5] (Fig. 171-3). Atrophy of the fat pads of the heel and toes may be noted.

Severe ischemia of the skin results in ulceration. This most often starts at the tips of the fingers or toes. It is characteristically extremely painful—except when a neuropathy coexists, as in diabetes. The ulcers are shallow,

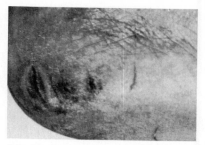

Fig. 171-4   Arteriosclerosis. Necrotic "cracks" of the heel.

with a sloughing gray or black base. The heel may show a characteristic "crack" which surmounts a small round zone of cyanosis that may slowly ulcerate (Fig. 171-4). Acral ulceration can, of course, extend onto the foot, but ulceration occasionally starts on the leg itself [6]. Spontaneous ulceration of this sort occurs most often in the diabetic. It starts as a dark pustule which slowly ulcerates to the characteristic "cutaneous infarct." The ulcer usually shows an eschar sitting loosely on necrotic tissue undergoing purulent softening. It is surrounded by a zone of cyanosis where microscopic examination discloses an advancing small vessel thrombosis. The ulceration progresses through the cyanosis, which itself advances. At the same time the ulceration deepens, and, when the deep fascia is entered, infection reaches the depth of the limb, which is then doomed.

"Cutaneous infarction" may occur in an arteriosclerotic limb which is generally only moderately ischemic. In a variant called "hypertensive ischemic ulceration" described by Hines and Farber [7], arteriolitis is demonstrated or presumed. These ulcers are unusually painful, again with black areas of necrosis. They tend to be multiple. They are usually seen at the ankle (Fig. 171-5) but may be present anywhere on the body.

An uncommon form of ulceration is due to atheromatous emboli. These tend to be small and multiple, and often come in recurrent bouts of painful blue toes, petechiae, or livedo reticularis. Pulses are often present (Fig. 171-1).

Ulceration in an ischemic limb may be precipitated by the patient or the physician in a variety of ways (Figs. 171-6 and 171-7). Ulceration in a diabetic patient deserves special consideration. As noted, infection is more prominent. Small chronic ulcerations may overlie sinuses leading to septic joints. Interdigital infections are apt to be associated with infection of flexor tendon sheaths and fascial spaces. Acute spreading cellulitis with septicemia is then a constant threat. The increased frequency of cutaneous infarction has been noted. Some neuropathy is probably always present in the diabetic, and it is not unusual to find the foot insensitive to the presence of an ulceration. An uncommon form, mal perforant, or neuropathic foot, is characterized by ulceration on the ball of the foot in the center of a heavy button of callus. The x-ray shows dissolution of one or more bones and joints (Charcot's joints), while there may be little or no ischemia. Necrobiosis lipoidica diabeticorum is a disease which occurs on the feet or legs of diabetic, prediabetic, or normal persons and may lead to ulceration spontaneously or after trauma (Fig. 171-2). It is not related to ischemia.

Acute arterial obstruction by embolism or thrombosis

Fig. 171-3   Buerger's disease. New nail growth during improvement of ischemia. (From Edwards [5], with permission.)

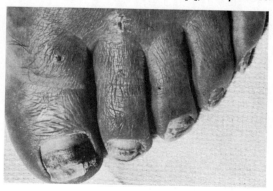

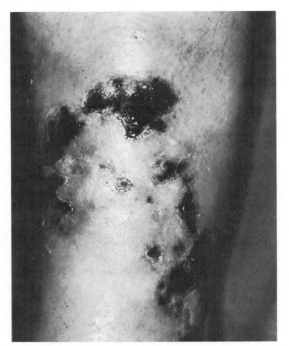

Fig. 171-5   Hypertensive ischemic ulceration at the ankle.

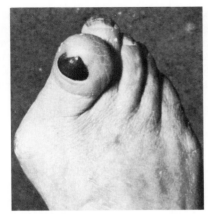

Fig. 171-7   Arteriosclerosis. Necrosis of the nail bed produced by removal of the nail for ischemic pain.

produces sudden limb pain (often described as a sustained muscle cramp), coldness, numbness, and tingling of the hand or foot. In extreme instances the patient cannot move the fingers or toes or even more proximal parts. Demarcated coldness and pallor often reach several inches below the highest level of obstruction.

Special findings on examination

One must first establish that there is major artery obstruction. Palpation of the peripheral pulses should include those of the hand and foot as well as the proximal arteries. When the ulnar pulse cannot be palpated, the radial compression test of E. V. Allen may demonstrate its patency: the patient clenches his fists and the examiner compresses the radial arteries. On unclenching the fists, redness returns to the palm if the ulnar artery is open, but remains blanched if it is not (Fig. 171-8). If bilateral blanching is obtained, the arteries may simply lack an anatomic communication.

In the foot, one must palpate for the posterior tibial pulse as well as the dorsalis pedis pulse. In some, the anterior tibial artery ends above the ankle and the perforating branch of the peroneal (located somewhat more laterally) continues onto the dorsum of the foot. One of these pulses may be lacking normally; if so, the pattern tends to be bilaterally symmetric.

Instrumental confirmation of the status of the pulses is usually done by examination with a Doppler instrument. One of us (EAE) prefers oscillometric measurement at two levels (as calf and ankle), noting maximal amplitude and pressure. An aneroid manometer can substitute. Finally, auscultation of the major arteries often reveals a systolic murmur at places of partial stenosis [8,9].

A significant drop in arterial pressure beyond stenosis is also shown by blanching on elevation and a cyanotic redness on dependency. The timing of delay in appearance of this redness and of filling of the veins on return to the horizontal quantifies the severity of ischemia. Sometimes the redness is paradoxically vivid. It is accompanied by coldness of the part; therefore, it does not signify hyperemia. In such cases one of us (EAE) has demonstrated through spectrophotometry that the cutaneous hemoglobin

Fig. 171-8   Radial artery compression in a patient with Buerger's disease, demonstrating occlusion of his right ulnar artery.

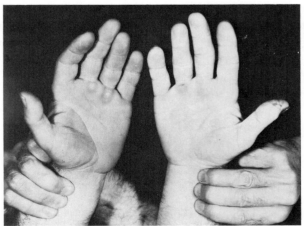

Fig. 171-6   Buerger's disease. Necrosis produced by salicylic acid corn cure. (From Edwards EA: N Engl J Med 221:251, 1939)

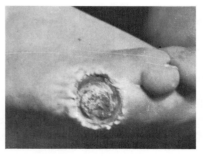

Table 171-2 Probable frequency of causes of arterial obstruction in the upper extremity

1. Operative trauma (cardiac catheterization, arteriography)
2. Embolism
3. Scleroderma, systemic lupus erythematosus
4. Arteriosclerosis
5. Buerger's disease
6. Neurovascular compression of upper limb (shoulder-girdle syndrome)

is inappropriately rather highly oxygenated. An abnormality of transfer of oxygen to the tissue is suggested.

The severity of the ischemia in acute arterial obstruction may be gauged by the presence and degree of anesthesia and of fine-muscle movement. In the severest cases the muscle may be in rigor, relaxing with improvement or going on to autolysis with flail passive motion if ischemia persists for a day or two.

There are few laboratory findings of significance except for arteriography, which actually delineates the arterial disease. Since arteriography carries some risk of morbidity, it is not ordinarily carried out unless needed for the planning of surgical procedures. It is sometimes helpful in making the diagnosis, especially to differentiate between embolism and thrombosis. The demonstration of arterial calcification on the plain film is significant only in establishing the presence of an aneurysm, since calcification bears little relation to the presence or degree of arterial obstruction. Special procedures to differentiate the various causes of obstruction will be noted below.

Diagnosis and differential diagnosis

The diagnosis of arterial obstruction will have been suggested by a history of intermittent claudication with or without symptoms of tissue ischemia (pain, coldness, ulceration) usually located in the hand or foot. It will be confirmed by the demonstration of stenosis through the pulse palpation, auscultation, Doppler or oscillometric examination, and distal signs of blanching on elevation, with redness on dependency and retarded venous filling after elevation.

"Rest pain" is significant as a sign of severe ischemia, but it is identified only if it is alleviated by dependency and accompanied then by a severe degree of redness, often with a cyanotic tint.

The most common nonarterial cause of limb pain, paresthesias, or night cramps is lumbosacral nerve plexus irritation due to arthritis of the spine, poor posture, herniated disk, or fatigue [10]. Pain in a diabetic patient is often caused by neuritis alone. Characteristically, it bears no relation to activity, and examination discloses some abnormality in sensation or reflexes. Neuropathic ulceration is accompanied by a diminished sensation of pain and the absence of tendon reflexes, especially the ankle jerks.

Once ischemia is diagnosed, the identity of the causative process can be sought. Diabetes is diagnosed by the usual laboratory tests. The most frequent causes of ischemia in the upper limb are noted in Table 171-2. Ischemias of a transient or recurrent nature are discussed under "Vasospastic Diseases," below. Buerger's disease need not be considered unless a patient is a young male smoker; it is

exceedingly rare in women. Thrombophlebitis may be present simultaneously, and a biopsy of a superficial vein may disclose the characteristic intraluminal granuloma. Buerger's disease, because of the involvement of the nerves in inflammation and scarring, is apt to be a particularly painful malady. The young person with chronic major arterial disease who is a nonsmoker, especially a woman, most likely suffers from systemic lupus erythematosus (see Chap. 152). Trauma, when causative, is usually identified.

Peripheral arterial embolism should be suspected in all instances of acute obstruction, since the ischemia is usually reversible through embolectomy. Study in one clinic [1] indicates that auricular fibrillation is present in three-fourths of rheumatic cases but only one-fourth of the patients in whom arteriosclerotic heart disease is responsible, and that there is a substantial incidence of emboli of unusual source, mainly from unrecognized mural thrombi in proximal large arteries [1]. An embolus has a predilection for lodgment at an arterial bifurcation, which is somewhat at variance with thrombosis. The pulse just above it may be exaggerated, as in instances of femoral artery embolism. Arteriography should be resorted to readily if there is any confusion as between embolism and thrombosis.

The varied causes of ischemic ulceration and the special forms found in diabetes are described above. It may be useful to note here conditions to be considered when ulceration or necrosis of toes or fingers is noted in the presence of palpable pulses (Table 171-3). Further considerations in this category are discussed under "Vasospastic Diseases," below.

Vasospastic diseases

Raynaud's phenomenon

Raynaud's phenomenon is characterized by episodic attacks of digital ischemia on exposure to cold and, sometimes, emotional stress. When no underlying cause can be found, it is termed *Raynaud's disease*, There are many secondary causes of Raynaud's phenomenon (Table 171-4); often these patients also have persistent vasospasm in addition to the episodic attacks. Attacks are characterized by well-demarcated blanching or cyanosis of the fingers or toes, extending from the tip to varying levels of the digit. The finger distal to the line of ischemia is white or blue and cold, while the proximal skin is pink and warmer. The fingers are usually numb during this phase of decreased to absent blood flow. On rewarming, the blanched digits may become cyanotic due to the slow blood flow. At the end

Table 171-3 Differential diagnosis of digital necrosis with palpable pulses

Embolism from:
  Heart
  Proximal aneurysm
  Proximal atheroma
Cutaneous infarction
Digital vasculitis
Intravascular agglutination from:
  Polycythemia vera
  Frostbite

Table 171-4   Causes of Raynaud's phenomenon

Collagen-vascular disease:	Drugs:
Scleroderma	Tobacco
Systemic lupus	Beta-adrenergic blockers
erythematosus	Ergot
Dermatomyositis	Methysergide
Rheumatoid arthritis	Bleomycin
Polyarteritis and vasculitis	Clonidine
Sjögren's syndrome	Trauma:
Obstructive arterial disease:	Vibratory tools
Arteriosclerosis obliterans	Pianists, typists
Thromboangiitis obliterans	Meat cutters
Arterial embolism	Hematologic causes:
Neurologic disorders:	Cryoproteins
Thoracic outlet syndrome	Cold agglutinins
Carpal tunnel syndrome	Macroglobulins
Hemiplegia	Polycythemia
Poliomyelitis	Hormonal:
Multiple sclerosis	Hypothyroidism
Syringomyelia	

of the attack the digits return to normal color or display a bright red, reactive hyperemic phase. Throbbing pain and some swelling may occur at this time. Attacks may last minutes to hours. When pain is a prominent symptom, especially of the ischemic phase, a secondary cause should be suspected.

Hyperhidrosis, the presence of excessive sweating of hands, feet, or axillae, may or may not accompany vasospasm. It is discussed separately in Chap. 69.

Raynaud's disease (primary or idiopathic Raynaud's phenomenon)

Raynaud's disease is usually seen in young people and is overwhelmingly the most common cause of episodic digital vasospasm [11]. It occurs about five times more frequently in women than men. One study has reported an incidence of 22 percent among young women [12]. Symptoms may first claim the patient's attention at the time of menopause. The episodic attacks occur more often in the upper extremities; the feet are involved in approximately 40 percent of patients. Rarely the tip of the nose, earlobes, or the tongue may be involved. Blanching or cyanosis may occur in only one or two digits at the onset of the disease but later the attacks involve all of the digits. The thumbs are often spared.

Fig. 171-9   Raynaud's disease. Pterygium of the nails.

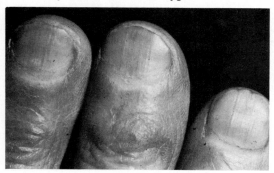

Some patients require an intense body and extremity cold exposure to induce attacks while others experience attacks with only slight provocation such as holding a cold glass. Patients may experience one or two attacks per cold season or multiple attacks per day. The digits appear normal between attacks but may be cool and moist with excess perspiration. Patients may show the nail change known as pterygium, which refers to a cuticle widened to several millimeters with the proximal skin fold thin and merging with the cuticle (Fig. 171-9) [5]. The incidence of trophic changes with tense and atrophic skin, clubbing and deformity of nails, scarring and shortening of the terminal phalanges (sclerodactyly) in Raynaud's disease is about 10 percent [13]. Sclerodactyly is not always a permanent disability but may improve in some patients. Less than 1 percent of patients develop gangrene of the tips of the fingers or lose part of a digit. Raynaud's disease may spontaneously improve or fail to recur in about 16 percent of patients, while the disease progresses in about one-third of patients.

Secondary Raynaud's phenomenon

The collagen vascular diseases are the most common cause of secondary Raynaud's phenomenon. Eighty to ninety percent of patients with scleroderma manifest Raynaud's phenomenon and/or persistent vasospasm. It is the presenting symptom in about one-third of patients and may be the only manifestation of the disease for years. Sclerodactyly with painful ulcerations and fissures of the skin of the fingers may become incapacitating. Sequestration of the terminal phalanges or the development of gangrene may lead to autoamputation of fingertips. Sometimes the skin ulcerations are due to subcutaneous calcifications instead of vasospasm; radiographs will disclose the subcutaneous calcium deposits. Multiple telangiectases of the skin and mucous membranes are common in patients with sclerodactyly as well as finger ulcerations, calcinosis, esophageal involvement, and Raynaud's phenomenon (the CREST syndrome). Raynaud's phenomenon occurs in 10 to 35 percent of patients with systemic lupus erythematosus and about 30 percent of those with dermatomyositis. It is also sometimes present in rheumatoid arthritis and the vasculitides. In rheumatoid arthritis, cold hands with mottled red and white areas are more common. Arteriograms in patients with collagen vascular diseases usually show digital and sometimes ulnar or radial artery obstructions (Fig. 171-10).

Raynaud's phenomenon may be of occupational origin and is especially common in people who use vibratory tools to cut stones or wood. Approximately 30 percent of chainsaw users in forestry develop the phenomenon, and it is clearly related to the duration of the exposure [14]. Traumatic vasospastic disease also occurs in a variety of other workers such as pianists, typists, riveters, and butchers. Arteriograms have shown digital, radial, ulnar, or palmar arch thromboses.

Any neurologic condition that produces permanent disuse of a limb can produce a sympathetic nervous system disturbance to that limb. This is usually manifested by persistent vasospasm with coldness, paleness, or cyanosis and even ulcerations, but Raynaud's phenomenon may occur. Nerve root pressure or nerve entrapment may pro-

Fig. 171-10 Raynaud's disease. Digital artery obstructions. *(From Edwards [3], with permission.)*

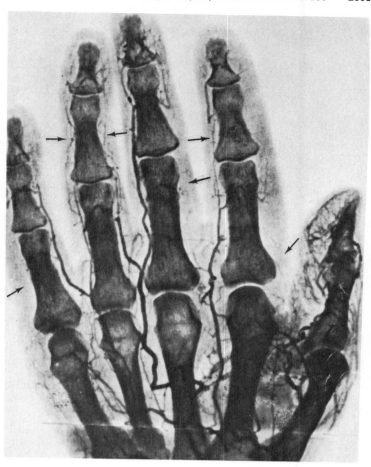

duce Raynaud's phenomenon. It is often present in the carpal tunnel syndrome and then may involve only the index and middle fingers; atrophy of the thenar muscles may be present. Tapping of the median nerve at the wrist may produce shooting pain in the distribution of the median nerve (Tinel's sign). Demonstration of a prolonged conduction time in the median nerve is the definitive test. Raynaud's phenomenon may be secondary to the neurovascular compression at the thoracic outlet (Figs 171-11 to 171-13). The latter may be due to cervical ribs, abnormalities of the scalenus anticus muscle, bony abnormalities of the cervical vertebrae, clavicle, or first rib, or the shoulder compression syndromes (the costoclavicular or hyperabduction syndrome). Assumption of postures to exaggerate the abnormality must reproduce the symptoms or produce a pale hand with disappearance of the radial pulse for diagnosis. Results of this test and those of nerve conduction should not be considered as absolutely diagnostic.

Several drugs have been implicated as causing Raynaud's phenomenon. Propranolol, one of the most widely used beta-receptor blockers in cardiovascular diseases and migraine headaches, is probably the most frequent offender [15]. Ergot preparations and methysergide used in the treatment of migraine headaches may also cause the phenomenon. Ergotamine is a powerful alpha-receptor vasoconstrictor agent and may produce gangrene of the fingers [16]. Methysergide, a serotonin antagonist, produces peripheral vascular symptoms or signs in about 7 percent of

patients [17]. It potentiates the effect of catecholamines on blood vessels but vasospasm may occur as a result of sensitivity reaction after small doses of this drug. Industrial exposure to vinyl chloride polymerization processes may produce acrosteolysis of the distal phalanges of the fingers in a small percentage of workers and Raynaud's phenomenon may also occur. Arteriograms in these patients show digital artery obstruction [18]. Bleomycin, a chemotherapeutic agent, also may cause the phenomenon [19]. The abuse of methylamphetamine has been followed by vasospasm. Intraarterial use of many medications may lead to vasospasm and gangrene of the fingers.

Patients with cold-precipitable plasma proteins, macroglobulins, and polycythemia can exhibit Raynaud's phenomenon probably secondary to rheologic disturbances or actual occlusion of small vessels (Fig. 171-14). Cold agglutinins may occasionally cause the syndrome due to blockage of the vessels by agglutinated erythrocytes; an associated vasospastic condition has not been found [20]. Similarly, cryoglobulins can induce ischemic episodes in digits. These are usually associated with monoclonal, particularly macroglobulinemia, or polyclonal gammopathies (e.g., rheumatoid arthritis). Cryoglobulins are most commonly seen in multiple myeloma but they also occur in leukemia, lymphoblastoma, or, rarely, as an idiopathic condition.

The most common hormonal disease causing Raynaud's phenomenon is hypothyroidism and the condition usually

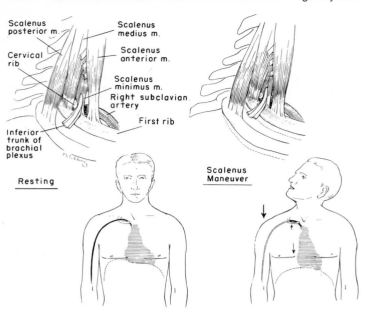

Fig. 171-11 Scalenus maneuver to demonstrate subclavian artery obstruction by a cervical rib or a scalenus muscle. The subject tilts the head backward and toward the opposite shoulder, rotating the chin toward the affected side. He takes a deep breath while the examiner pushes down the shoulder. In a positive result the radial pulse disappears, or if the subclavian is partly constricted, a systolic murmur is heard over the subclavian. *(From Edwards and Levine [9], with permission.)*

remits with thyroid replacement. Manifestations of peripheral vasospasm may also be seen in pheochromocytoma and carcinoid tumors.

Pathophysiology

The normal physiologic control of the digital circulation is different from other cutaneous areas of the body. An important factor in its distinction is the presence of a large number of arteriovenous anastomoses (AV shunts) besides a capillary circulation. Otherwise, the regulation of the digital blood flow depends on the sympathetic nervous system, vascular tone, humoral substances, and hemorheologic factors. Vasomotor tone increases progressively from the trunk to the digits; the hands, and particularly the feet, are colder than the trunk. Individuals vary in degree of tone, and women tend to have colder hands and feet than do men. There are several levels of control of vascular

tone in the brain besides the spinal cord and periphery (Fig. 171-15) [21].

Local digital cooling produces vasoconstriction as in other skin areas. However, unlike most other cutaneous vasculature, digital vessels are innervated only by sympathetic adrenergic vasoconstrictor fibers; a neurogenic vasodilator mechanism has never been demonstrated. Therefore, sympathetic nervous vasodilatation occurs only by the withdrawal of sympathetic activity. Body cooling or cold applied to most areas of the body induces reflex vasoconstriction in the digits via the sympathetic nervous system. This vasoconstriction involves mainly the AV shunts in normal subjects and is evidently a mechanism to retain body heat [22]. The shunts, but not the capillaries, have also been shown to possess beta receptors that are apparently excited only by circulating catecholamines and not by sympathetic nerves [23].

The pathogenesis of Raynaud's phenomenon or episodic vasospastic attacks is unknown but the above normal circulatory controlled mechanisms have been studied in pa-

Fig. 171-12   The hyperabduction syndrome. A Statue of Liberty position of the arm presses the axillary artery against the pectoralis minor and coracoid process. A murmur may be heard here. *(From Eaton LM: Surg Clin North Am 26:810, 1946, with permission.)*

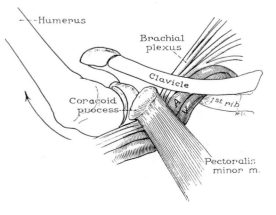

Fig. 171-13   The costoclavicular syndrome. Squaring of the shoulders squeezes the artery between the clavicle and first rib. *(From Eaton LM: Surg Clin North Am 26:810, 1946, with permission.)*

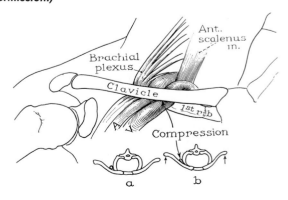

Fig. 171-14 Secondary effects of organic arterial disease on acral flow. *(From Edwards [21], with permission.)*

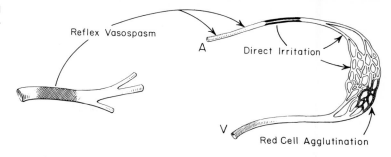

tients to determine whether abnormalities exist. The following are some of the most important findings reported since 1929:

1. Ischemic attacks can be produced in single fingers by local cooling and in sympathetically denervated or blocked fingers [24].

2. Local cooling of the hand augments the reflex sympathetic vasoconstriction induced by cooling of the nape of the neck in patients with Raynaud's disease but not in normal subjects [25]. Sensitization of alpha receptors by cold exposure was hypothesized.

3. Plasma levels of catecholamines are probably not increased in the venous drainage of the hands of patients with Raynaud's disease [26].

4. Systolic pressures at the brachial, proximal digit, and distal fingertip in a cool environment are significantly lower in patients with Raynaud's disease than in normal subjects [27].

5. Krahenbuhl et al [28] recorded the distal systolic pressure in single fingers as a measurement of hyperemia caused by prior arterial occlusion. Exposure to cold vi-

Fig. 171-15 Levels of control of vascular tone. *(From Edwards [21], with permission.)*

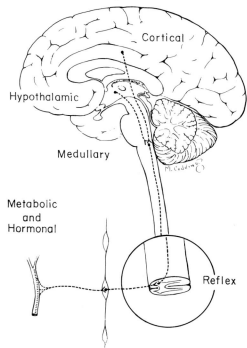

tiated this reaction in subjects with Raynaud's disease but not in warm-handed persons.

6. During body cooling to induce reflex digital vasoconstriction, capillary blood flow significantly decreased in patients with Raynaud's disease and phenomenon compared to normal subjects [29]. The reduced capillary blood flow is reversed by body warming.

The first three findings support the theory that there may be a local fault in which the blood vessels are abnormally sensitive to cold rather than the alternative theory of an overactivity of the sympathetic nervous system leading to an increased vasoconstrictor response to normal stimuli in Raynaud's disease. The second point indicated it may be at the receptor level. Other studies have failed to demonstrate an increased reflex sympathetic vasoconstriction to a cold stimulus or an abnormal thermoregulatory response in patients with Raynaud's phenomenon [30]. Although a heightened digital vasomotor tone perhaps due to increased sympathetic neural discharge exists in some patients, there is not an increased sensitivity to intravenous norepinephrine [31].

Concerning the fourth point, the intravascular pressure not only provides the potential energy for blood to flow but it also maintains blood vessel patency. In many of the secondary causes of Raynaud's phenomenon, there are vascular obstructions that would produce a low distal blood pressure. Under these circumstances, a normal vasoconstrictor sympathetic stimulus could lead to vessel closure and an ischemic attack. In Raynaud's disease, digital arteries are often normal by arteriogram; however, if the digital systolic pressures are lower than normal, the same sequence of events could occur. This would explain the finding described in point 5.

The decreased capillary flow in a cool environment (point 6), often to extremely low levels, helps explain the pathogenesis of ischemic attacks, for this is the nutritional blood flow. The sympathetic nervous system can be implicated since the decreased capillary flow during body cooling is partially reversible with body warming. However, if the vessel walls were hypertrophied, a normal degree of sympathetic stimulation would lead to a smaller vessel lumen than in a vessel with a normal wall thickness.

A study of the pathology of the radial, ulnar, and digital arteries in patients with Raynaud's syndrome was published by Lewis [32] in 1938 and remains unique to this day. He scrutinized the vascular state of patients suffering from "incurable diseases," both warm-handed and those exhibiting the Raynaud's phenomenon. He then examined the radial, ulnar, and digital arteries of those who came to autopsy. Intimal thickenings, increasing with age, were found equally in both groups. Thrombosis of digital arteries was associated with fingertip necrosis in patients he labeled as those with Raynaud's disease or those with scleroderma.

Serotonin has been incriminated as important in the induction of ischemic attacks in Raynaud's disease, for a serotonin inhibitor reduced the intensity and duration of the response of patients to immersion of their hands in cold water [33]. However, these studies have not been confirmed, and antiserotonin agents have not proved of value in treatment. The development of specific serotonin blocking agents may clarify this picture.

Measurements of blood viscosity by several investigators have yielded inconsistent results [34–36]. It may be raised in patients with systemic sclerosis and Raynaud's phenomenon. Consistent abnormalities in plasma fibrinogen, cold agglutinins, or cryoglobulins have not been demonstrated in Raynaud's disease but are important in certain secondary causes. Thus, aberrations in hemorheology in the idiopathic disease have not been documented. Platelets may be involved in the pathogenesis of the phenomenon; plasma β-thromboglobulin has been reported to be increased in patients [37]. Serial plasmapheresis has been reported as a useful treatment in severe Raynaud's disease, leaving the hemorheology theory open for further investigation.

Diagnosis

The diagnosis is usually made from the history of typical episodic attacks of demarcated vasospasm of the digits on cold exposure. Attacks are very difficult to induce in patients with idiopathic disease despite immersion of the hands in ice water during total-body cooling. Patients with sufficient symptoms to seek a physician's advice should have a complete workup to exclude secondary causes. The history will elicit symptoms of collagen vascular disease (arthralgias, arthritis, dysphagia, heartburn, facial rash from the sun, persistent tans), a drug etiology, symptoms of obstructive arterial disease (intermittent claudication, migratory thrombophlebitis), and exposure to vibratory tools or continuous finger trauma. Physical examination should carefully note all pulses, blood pressure in both arms, telangiectases, subcutaneous nodules, swollen or deformed joints, skin texture, discoloration of the eyelids, bruits in the neck, thyroid size, relaxation time of reflexes, neurologic deficits, and organomegaly. The thoracic outlet maneuvers should be performed (Figs. 171-11 to 171-13) and Tinel's sign sought. Blood analyses for anemia, polycythemia, leukopenia, sedimentation rate, serum protein electrophoresis, antinuclear antibodies, rheumatoid factor, cryoglobulins, and cold agglutinins are necessary. A urinalysis should be done, especially looking for proteinuria and red blood cell casts. A chest film will rule out the presence of cervical ribs. The history, examination, and tests should all be normal before a patient is reassured that the benign, idiopathic disease is probably the diagnosis.

Treatment

Most patients with Raynaud's disease respond to reassurance that they have a benign disease, to instructions to wear loose-fitting warm clothes covering as much of the body as possible to prevent reflex sympathetic vasoconstriction, and to avoid cold, especially with pressure on the digits. Tobacco smoking should be discouraged for nicotine induces cutaneous vasoconstriction; smokers are more numerous among patients with Raynaud's disease [12] and with traumatic vasospastic disease [14]. The underlying cause must be treated in patients with secondary Raynaud's phenomenon. In obstructive arterial disease, the large-vessel involvement must be corrected. In traumatic vasospastic disease, avoidance of the instigating cause will ameliorate, but not always completely cure, the symptoms. Drug-induced ischemic attacks usually respond to withdrawal of the offending agent, but in acute episodes of severe vasoconstriction, intravenous or intraarterial nitropusside may be needed. Shoulder shrugging exercises are often successful in the thoracic outlet syndromes and should be tried for several months before surgery is considered. Vascular symptoms or nerve deficit caused by cervical rib constitute a strong indication for removal of that structure. Hematologic abnormalities often respond to treatment of the underlying disease. The collagen vascular diseases usually must be treated symptomatically.

Drug therapy can be used in the more severe cases of the disease or phenomenon but is successful only in about 50 percent of patients [38]. Drugs that interfere with the action of the sympathetic nerves have had the most success. Both reserpine and guanethidine have been shown to increase capillary blood flow during cold exposure in patients and have the advantage of once-a-day administration. Painful ulcerations or gangrene have been reported to respond to intraarterial reserpine but one controlled study found no benefit compared to saline injections [39]. Other sympatholytic drugs including prazosin, methyldopa, phenoxybenzamine, and tolazoline have also been recommended. The calcium channel blocking agent nifedipine induces improvement in some patients but must be taken three times daily [40]; diltiazem may help patients with traumatic vasospastic disease [41]. Nitrates or their ointments have their proponents but are usually used in combination with other agents. Parenteral prostaglandins have been reported of benefit but oral preparations are not available [42]. Oral forms of other direct-acting agents such as niacin and papaverine are not useful nor are the drugs that are principally muscle vasodilators, nylidrin and isoxsuprine [38].

The painful and often ulcerated digits of scleroderma are usually amenable to the application of the long self-heating insulated sleeve suggested by Claff and Crane [43]. If the oft-quoted statement were true that the digital vessels cannot dilate because of the sclerosis, such heating—even to the modest temperature of the blood—would be contraindicated (as it is in arteriosclerosis with ulceration). However, studies by Edwards et al [44] have shown that the digital pulses respond to vasodilating influences, including heat, in all but the most extreme cases of scleroderma. Applications of the sleeve for several hours also serve to diminish the trauma to ulcerated digits.

Stanozolol, a fibrinolytic agent, has been shown to increase hand blood flow in patients but evidently does not act by decreasing blood viscosity [36]. Serial plasmapheresis has been reported to ameliorate the disease in more severely afflicted patients; its mode of action is undetermined [37]. Either biofeedback [45] or Pavlovian conditioning [46] may provide some benefit to patients, but the magnitude of warming is no more than that provided by insulated gloves or gauntlets. Sympathectomy is rarely needed in primary Raynaud's disease and is of uncertain benefit in the secondary cases.

Acrocyanosis

Patients with acrocyanosis complain of a persistently blue or reddish discoloration of the digits of hands or feet, extending sometimes as far proximally as the wrists or ankles. The digits are cool and often sweat excessively. The color abnormality is intensified by cold or emotional upset. It is usually relieved by warming the affected parts. The nose, cheeks, chin, and pinna may rarely manifest the cyanosis. Puffiness and numbness of the digits may accompany the cyanosis but pain and trophic changes do not occur. It is more common in females and sometimes a family history can be elicited.

The etiology and pathogenic factors in acrocyanosis are unknown. It is postulated that vasospasm of the small cutaneous arteries and arterioles leads to a decreased blood flow while a secondary dilatation of the capillaries and subpapillary venous plexus enhances the cyanotic color [47]. Skin blood flow is markedly reduced and probably capillary pressure is low. However, since these changes are reversible, gross structural changes of the vasculature have not been considered to be present. A heightened arteriolar tone at average room temperature was found in one study [48]. During sleep, the cyanosis may disappear and local cooling fails to produce vasoconstriction [49]. Pathologic studies are rare; minimal hypertrophy of the medial coats of cutaneous arterioles has been described. Capillary dilatation and abnormalities have been reported by microscopy of the nail beds.

Clinically, acrocyanosis can be distinguished from Raynaud's phenomenon by the lack of episodic, well-demarcated color changes, and from generalized cyanosis by the discoloration being limited to the hands and feet and by a normal arterial blood oxygen. A state of persistent cyanosis, sometimes of one limb, may occur in scleroderma, obstructive arterial disease, and other secondary causes of Raynaud's phenomenon; these diseases must be ruled out as in the workup for Raynaud's phenomenon. In acrocyanosis, all pulses should be present, trophic changes should not be apparent on the digits, and there should be bilateral involvement.

A more severe form of this disease has been termed *remittent necrotizing acrocyanosis* and is of unknown cause [50]. It usually appears suddenly in late adult life without regard for season and lasts for weeks to months. It may occur as only a single attack in some patients or it may recur in a few years. The cyanosis of the fingers extends with a mottled pattern to the hands and feet, and ulcers and gangrene of the fingers often occur. It is distinguished from benign acrocyanosis only by the presence of pain. Biopsies have shown small-artery and arteriolar occlusion by cellular proliferation or hyaline thrombi. It is probably different from the symmetrical cyanosis and gangrene found in acute infections.

Treatment of acrocyanosis is usually unnecessary since it is mainly a cosmetic problem. It does respond to drugs that interfere with sympathetic nerve activity such as reserpine.

Livedo reticularis

Livedo reticularis is characterized by a reddish blue mottling of the skin in a "fish net," reticular pattern (Fig. 171-16). The skin within the webs of the net is normal or pale in color.

It is most commonly seen accompanying vasospastic conditions such as primary and secondary Raynaud's phenomenon, acrocyanosis, and vasculitis. It is often a manifestation of an underlying disease and may be a clue to its diagnosis. It has been reported in association with obstructive arterial diseases, collagen vascular diseases, endocrine disorders, neurogenic diseases, drug reactions, hyperviscosity states, and hypertension. It has been shown to be induced by amantadine, a drug used for Parkinson's disease and influenza. It is an important manifestation of the diagnostic picture in atheromatous microembolization, described above.

The idiopathic mild variety, also called *cutis marmorata*, is aggravated by cold exposure and attenuated by warming [51]. It occurs predominantly on the extremities and only rarely on the trunk. The condition is most common in women less than 40 years of age. A more severe form has a widespread body distribution. It is also more common in young women but may occur at any age and does not disappear on warming. Cutaneous ulcerations of the lower extremities may develop during the winter months or sometimes during the summer [52].

The skin appearance is believed to be due to vasospasm of the perpendicular arterioles that perforate the dermis from below. The bluish red periphery of each web of the net is caused by deoxygenated blood in the surrounding horizontally arranged venous plexuses. Elevation of the limb decreases the intensity of the color, probably by improved drainage of the venules. Excess activity of the sympathetic nervous system is probably not at fault, for the skin pattern has persisted following regional sympathectomy. The pathology of the skin in patients with ulcerations shows arteriolar intimal proliferation with dilated numerous capillaries and thickening of the walls of venules; lymphocytic perivascular infiltration may also be present.

Causalgia and reflex sympathetic dystrophy

Vasospasm is a feature of true causalgia, a complication of major nerve injury in which extreme acral hyperesthesia is prominent [53]. The mechanism is unknown. Similar features, including moderate edema, seen after a variety of traumatic events are generally known as sympathetic dystrophy, minor causalgia [54], or (after myocardial infarction) as shoulder-hand syndrome. A reflex constriction is postulated, but disuse and dependency of the limb are significant factors. Many of the posttraumatic patients are hysterical (Charcot's *oedème bleu*), and some are malingerers [55–57].

First attempts at treatment consist of active physical therapy. If sympathetic ganglion block gives temporary relief, the block should be repeated with active exercises strongly encouraged during the hours or days of amelioration of the pain. In some cases such a program will give a reasonable cure. Surgical sympathectomy appears curative after injury of the sciatic or median nerves. We have

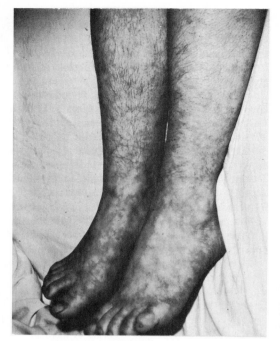
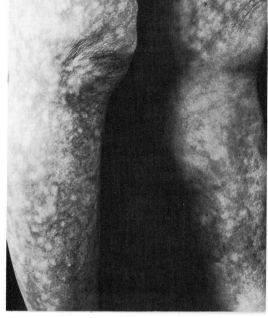

Fig. 171-16   The reticular pattern of livedo reticularis.

found the procedure disappointing in instances of so-called minor causalgia occurring after injury of other sorts. Sympathectomy has sometimes been helpful in these cases if each of a series of blocks has given good, although temporary, relief. The operation should be followed by strongly encouraged active exercises. Other helpful adjuncts to treatment are the settling of litigation surrounding the initiating trauma and the use of psychotherapy with or without mood-elevating drugs.

Frostbite

Frostbite gives rise to manifestations somewhat similar to those of burns and can therefore be categorized in first, second, and third degrees. Cold exposure short of freezing in trench or immersion foot gives rise to symptoms resembling first-degree frostbite, i.e., redness and pain. Changes are probably due to the anoxia secondary to the retardation of liberation of oxygen from cold oxyhemoglobin. When true frostbite sets in, the red color of cold exposure is succeeded by whiteness presumably due to an extreme vasospasm. Thawing is first characterized by hyperemia, which may persist with evidence of sympathetic paralysis (Fig. 171-17). This is also true in trench or immersion foot. In frostbite severe enough to give rise to tissue injury, the hyperemia is soon succeeded by obstruction to small-vessel flow caused by severe red cell agglutination [58]. At this time edema sets in, and, if the frostbite is of second degree, blistering is common. The blisters usually turn hemorrhagic. Hemorrhage also occurs beneath the nail plates. In some weeks, a dark eschar lifts off containing the old dried blisters and the affected nail plates, leaving live tissue behind if frostbite has been of second-degree, but including also actual necrotic tissue if some of the areas have been of third-degree severity.

In cases where major vascular disease such as arteriosclerosis was present prior to the frostbite, true fibrin thrombosis may occur in the larger arteries and veins and gangrene of a considerable extent may ensue.

The one significant advance in the treatment of frostbite in this century has been the use of rapid thawing of the part in warm air or water at a temperature no higher than blood heat. Thereafter the part is rested at usual room temperature. Mountain climbers have cautioned that the boots not be removed from frostbitten feet if the subject must walk out on his own; otherwise, the swelling after thawing will be too great for the boots to be put on again [59].

Rest, surgical cleanliness of the part, tetanus toxoid, and antibiotics will be needed. Vasodilator drugs or sympathetic nerve block have proved of no use. Heparin is of uncertain value unless thrombosis of the major vessel is probable. Dextran, given intravenously, has given ambiguous results in animals and has not had wide trial in humans [60,61].

Pernio or "chilblains" is a nodular and ulcerating form of vasculitis resulting from frequent exposures to cold (Fig. 171-18).

Erythermalgia (erythromelalgia)

Erythermalgia is a rare syndrome characterized by pain in the extremities associated with an increase in blood flow evidenced by large pulses and an increase in skin temperature. The present name for this malady, erythermalgia, indicating redness, heat, and pain, supercedes Mitchell's (1878) original term, erythromelalgia, which indicates only redness and pain in an extremity (*melos*, "limb"). Characteristic of this condition is an intolerance to heat, which indeed provokes the attack.

Fig. 171-17   Frostbite. Sweat pattern outlined by ferric chloride and tannic acid. (a) Five weeks after freezing. The left hand, more severely frozen, shows hyperemia (sympathetic paralysis); the right hand is moderately hyperhidrotic. (b) Fourteen weeks after freezing. The left fingers now show the tapering, shiny appearance of acrosclerosis and fail to share in the hyperhidrosis of the palm. (From [58], with permission.)

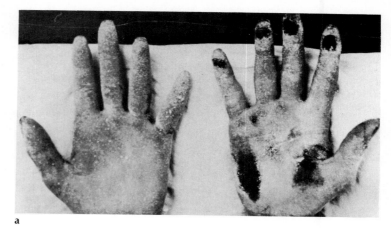

a

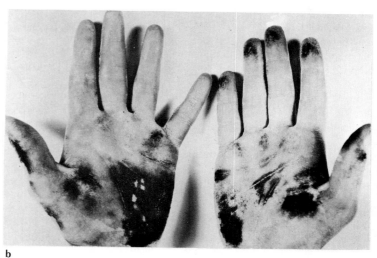

b

Etiology and pathogenesis

Idiopathic and secondary varieties are recognized. In a review of 51 cases seen at the Mayo Clinic, Babb et al [62] found 30 to be primary, or idiopathic. Twenty-one were considered secondary to other diseases, notably polycythemia vera and hypertension (Table 171-5). The erythermalgia preceded the diagnosis of myeloproliferative disease by as long as 12 years and preceded SLE, in one patient, by 5 months. The patients reported by Babb et al were mostly of middle age, the patients with secondary cases all 40 years or over, those with the primary variety ranging from the first to the eighth decades.

The early recovery phases of the moderately frostbitten hand or foot and of trench or immersion foot have not usually been characterized as exhibiting erythermalgia, but the syndrome then seen does satisfy the criteria for this condition. In these patients it is associated with damage to somatic and sympathetic nerve fibers [63], thought to be due in part to injury directly by the cold. Sympathetic paralysis can be demonstrated (Fig. 171-17).

Clinical manifestations

The condition attacks the fingers and toes; it may include the hands or feet; exceptionally it extends to the knees. It is usually bilateral in extent; occasionally it may be present in one or all four extremities.

The painful redness occurs in attacks brought on by warming of the extremities. These are therefore more frequent in warm weather. They last from minutes to hours, rarely for days. The pain is characterized as burning and

Fig. 171-18   Pernio. Ulcerating lesions in a young woman. (From Kinmonth [56], with permission.)

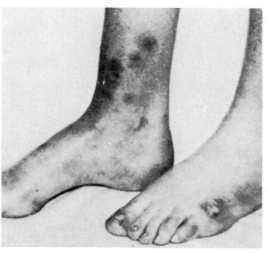

Table 171-5 Disorders associated with "secondary" erythermalgia*

Disorder	No. of cases
Myeloproliferative disease:	10
Polycythemia	9
Myeloid metaplasia	1
Hypertension	6
Postphlebitic varices	1
Diabetes mellitus	2
Systemic lupus erythematosus	1
Rheumatoid arthritis	1
Total	21

* From Babb et al [62].

throbbing. Examination shows bounding pulses, redness, and heat of the part. Vasoconstriction between attacks is unusual [64]. Relief is characteristically sought by exposing the part to cold, as by standing on a cold tile floor or dipping the hand in a basin of cold water. The pain of trench foot, as seen in World War II, was considerably relieved by rest, with the feet elevated and exposed to an electric fan. Smith and Allen noted that relief by small doses of acetylsalicylic acid was also characteristic.

Diagnosis and differential diagnosis

The diagnosis depends on pain in association with exposure to warmth and with examination disclosing a hot, red limb and bounding pulses. Relief should be given by elevation and cooling and perhaps by the use of acetylsalicylic acid.

A variety of conditions may present burning pain with increased temperature, but are not usually called erythermalgia. These include gout in its acute attack, as well as transient vasodilatation in the course of rheumatoid arthritis, or early posttraumatic dystrophy. Smith and Allen were led to search by biopsy for Kaposi's sarcoma in one of their cases. A warm, almost mottled hand may be seen in idiopathic palmar erythema, usually arising during pregnancy [65], as well as in portal cirrhosis or hyperthyroidism, but the hand is not painful in these conditions.

Frequently, patients with arteriosclerosis or other ischemic states will complain of burning pain and may obtain relief by cooling, but the presence of ischemia rules out erythermalgia.

A syndrome of "burning feet" has been observed in nutritional deficiency. Glusman [66], who saw the disease in American soldiers of World War II who were prisoners of the Japanese, named it nutritional melalgia. The feet were always tender, with paroxysms of pain precipitated by heat and relieved by cold; however, while the feet were often pink, they were not hot to touch, and proximal hyperesthesia was prominent, along with the distal hyperesthesia.

In true causalgia, after sciatic or median nerve injury, the patient characteristically keeps the part wrapped in a cold wet cloth, but hyperemia is not a feature, while signs of the nerve injury are apparent.

Infantile acrodynia (erythredema, pink disease) might be confusing from the evidence of extreme pain and the pink color of the extremities. In that condition, however, the parts are cool, and the prone photophobic and hypotonic posture of the child are said to be characteristic [67].

Thrombophlebitis

The dermatologist is more interested in the local effects of thrombophlebitis than in the complication of pulmonary embolism. Of special concern is the etiologic significance of thrombophlebitis when it occurs in unusual circumstances or locations.

Chronic postphlebitic effects will be discussed under "Varicose Veins and Chronic Venous Stasis" below.

Etiology and pathogenesis

Categories arranged by cause are shown in Table 171-6. All may be assumed to rest on one or more of the three basic factors in thrombus production enunciated by Welch: changes in the vessel wall, changes in the blood itself, and slowing of the bloodstream. The identification of these roles in each clinical situation is far from certain. Infection at the site of thrombophlebitis is not a factor except in frankly purulent processes such as septic endometritis or pylephlebitis or around indwelling catheters as for parenteral nutrition [68].

Thrombophlebitis of the deep veins of the calf in prolonged recumbency is the most common variety, and it is the most common cause of pulmonary embolism. Middle and old age predispose to the thrombosis and the embolism. Medical causes, such as heart failure, acute infections, or cerebrovascular accidents, are the most numerous. Long sitting constitutes recumbency adequate to produce thrombosis as in the "shelter leg" of the London bombings of World War II or the thrombosis produced by a long airplane trip. Common surgical causes are operations, childbirth, and trauma. Trauma may be minor as after a sprained ankle or, in the case of the upper limb, after arduous use of the part ("effort thrombosis" of the subclavian and axillary veins). Pulmonary embolism is extremely rare from an upper-limb process.

Malignancy predisposes to recumbency thrombophlebitis. In addition, malignant infiltration of the lymphatics or of the vein itself, as at the root of the upper or lower limb, can cause thrombophlebitis. Finally, visceral carcinoma is associated with a rare form of migrating thrombophlebitis (Fig. 171-19) which may be the first hint of the malignant disorder [69]. Andrasch et al [70] and Sack et al [71] report cases in which arterial emboli are produced in this setting.

Table 171-6 Etiologic categories of thrombophlebitis

Common or known causes	Apparently idiopathic entities
Recumbency	Overlooked varicosity
Varicosity	Oral contraceptive medication
Trauma	Buerger's disease
Malignant infiltration	Blood dyscrasia (polycythemia vera)
Infection (septic thrombophlebitis)	Vasculitis (SLE, rheumatoid arthritis, rheumatic fever)
	Carcinoma
	Marasmus
	"Idiopathic thrombophlebitis"

Clinical manifestations

Swelling of the limb, with warmth, pitting edema, and with full veins and cyanosis, are typical signs. Occasionally edema may be slight and detectable only by careful measurement of limb circumference. When the process is high, as at the iliac level, there will be prominence of the veins of the flank and hip. Subclavian vein thrombosis gives swelling of the upper limb with prominence of veins on the dorsum of the hand and over the pectoral and scapular regions. The local venous pressure is high. The superior vena cava syndrome includes great swelling of the upper limbs, head, and face, with proptosis. Impeded outflow of intracranial blood and cerebral spinal fluid may produce headache. The edema is greater if the process is secondary to malignant disease, present in about three-fourths of the cases [72], since then the lymphatics are usually infiltrated.

Unusually, petechiae are seen if the thrombosis is diffuse and the capillaries fragile.

Pain in deep thrombophlebitis is usually slight and may be absent. Tenderness with or without induration may be felt deep in the calf. Pain here on dorsiflexion of the foot indicates a deep process and in proper circumstances points to the diagnosis of thrombophlebitis. The thrombosed axillary vein may be palpated as a tender cord.

Venous gangrene is threatened if pain and cyanosis are unusually severe (phlegmasia cerulea dolens).

Thrombophlebitis of a superficial vein, varicosed or otherwise, is evidenced by painful induration of the vein with inflammation of the overlying skin. Edema may be marked over the vessel but is generally not present at the ankle unless that is the location of the varix or unless deep extension has occurred. Localized sweating is sometimes seen in the vicinity of a clump of thrombosed varices [68]. In one woman a growth of hair appeared over a thrombosis of varices of some weeks' duration [73].

Entities capable of producing a thrombophlebitis which at first glance may be apparently idiopathic are shown in Table 171-6. A truly idiopathic thrombophlebitis does exist. It attacks young adults as often as older patients. The deep or superficial veins of the upper or lower limbs or of the abdominal viscera may be involved. Attacks during the patient's lifetime may number from 1 to perhaps 30. Often multiple attacks occur over a period of some months, after which there may be freedom for some years. Pulmonary embolism occurs with fair frequency when the attacks are located in the deep veins of the lower limbs, and a goodly number of these patients go on to develop cor pulmonale.

Mondor's disease or thrombophlebitis of the breast is a rare disorder in which an inflamed subcutaneous cord appears on the breast (Fig. 171-21) sometimes extending to the abdomen or uncommonly to the arm. It does not appear to be a component of any generalized disease. It is most often seen in breast clinics where its presence has sug-

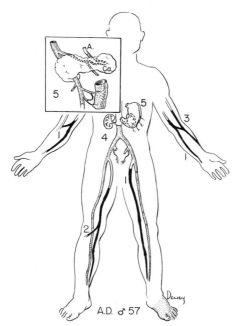

Fig. 171-19   Migrating thrombophlebitis of pancreatic carcinoma. Numbers indicate sequence of attacks of thrombophlebitis in the 3 months prior to death. There was venous gangrene of the left foot.

The occlusion of the vein by thrombus imposes a block to venous return, and the rise of venous pressure produces cyanosis and edema. Since the major lymphatics of the limbs are perivenous in location, they are apt to be compressed and thrombosed in the acute stages of the thrombophlebitis; this contributes to the edema. Some weeks are required for the interference to venous return to be alleviated by recanalization and collateral formation. Lymphangiography shows that the perivenous lymph trunks return to patency.

A deep thrombophlebitis may block the circulation sufficiently to cause gangrene, either when the process is unusually diffuse, as in the rare migrating thrombophlebitis of visceral carcinoma (Fig. 171-19), or when venous thrombosis supervenes in an arteriosclerotic limb, where the arteriole-to-venule pressure head is already lowered (Fig. 171-20).

Thrombophlebitis occurring in the varicosed saphenous vein or its tributaries is the second most common clinical form. It is capable of extending, especially if the patient is put to bed, into the deep veins of the calf or to the femoral vein and may thus give rise to embolism.

An apparently idiopathic thrombophlebitis is well known in young women. It is currently believed that this process may be caused by the oral administration of estrogenic contraceptive medication.

Fig. 171-20   Venous gangrene precipitated by venous thrombosis in an arteriosclerotic limb.

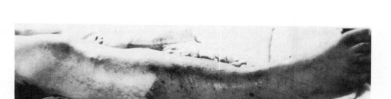

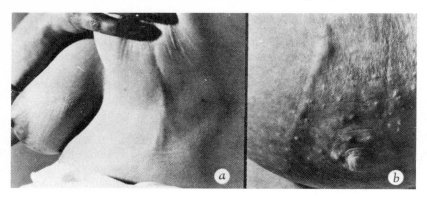

Fig. 171-21 Mondor's disease. (a) Bifurcating cords below left breast. (b) Cord on anterior part of another breast. (From Bircher et al [78], with permission.)

gested the possibility of malignancy. Farrow [74] reported 58 cases from such a clinic.

Mondor in 1939 [75] and Jönssen in 1955 [76] found inflammation along a vessel thought to be a lymph trunk. Certainly the most common pathology is that of a thrombophlebitis as seen in a biopsy reported by Mondor in 1944 [77] and abundantly by Bircher et al [78] and Johnson et al [79]. Duff [80] has reviewed the recent literature confirming this pathology.

Marked perivascular scarring is a peculiar sequel to the thrombophlebitis, which by shortening of the linear structure results in a depression and puckering of the skin (Fig. 171-21a). Abramson [81] suggests this can be relieved by subcutaneous cutting of the "string" and its disruption by forcible manipulation.

Diagnosis and differential diagnosis

The diagnosis of deep thrombophlebitis is almost certain when calf tenderness and swelling develop during some other illness. Three noninvasive tests are available to confirm the clinical diagnosis. These are: finding free flow in the major veins of the limb by Doppler examination, or by impedance plethysmography, or by the localization in the leg of intravenously administered [^{125}I]fibrinogen. X-ray venography has generally been considered a final and definitive test. However, commenting on a comparison of these tests, Hull et al [82] state: "Indeed, if, as our results suggest, the true risk of induced venous thrombosis after a negative venogram is as high as 4.1% then this may be greater than the risk of extension or of pulmonary embolism in patients with negative non-invasive test results." Rarely, a cellulitis or acute lymphangitis needs to be ruled out; occasionally secondary skin changes may obscure the underlying venous disease [83]. The development of painful induration of obvious varices allows an easy diagnosis of varicose thrombophlebitis.

If the usual background for deep thrombophlebitis is lacking, one must rule out a variety of pathologic states in tissues other than the veins. The confused picture of muscle conditions has included hematoma from injury, myositis, especially that of panarteritis nodosa and trichinosis, and sarcoma of the muscle. Various forms of panniculitis need to be considered. In middle-aged women the bolsters of fat on the medial side of the knee may periodically become inflamed, usually along with osteoarthritis of the knee joint. In young women one or more attacks of pain

and inflammation in the linear distribution near the saphenous vein may on biopsy prove to be inflamed fat. Occasionally there may be an epidemic of painful lumps of subcutaneous fat in young nurses, diagnosed as phlebitis by them or the medical staff. Weber-Christian-Schüller disease, erythema nodosum and induratum, nodular vasculitis, cold panniculitis, and localized myxedema have been referred for consultation as thrombophlebitis.

If one is satisfied that deep or superficial thrombophlebitis has occurred without the common precursors, one may be dealing with truly idiopathic thrombophlebitis. Some characteristics may still distinguish the process as being secondary to known entities. A tortuous saphenous vein, if not very wide, may yet be varicosed. Venous thrombosis secondary to polycythemia is most often a deep process. A spontaneous superficial thrombophlebitis of a nonvaricosed vein is most often due to vasculitis of Buerger's disease or other types. This is especially true for the dorsal venous arch of the foot. It may smolder here or in the saphenous vein for months or years [84].

The migrating thrombophlebitis of visceral carcinoma is painful, widely disseminated, and rapidly migrating. Carcinomas of the pancreas, lung, or stomach, with at least local metastases, are the most common precursors [69]. The diagnosis can probably be disregarded if the patient has survived a year from the onset of the phelebitis, unless the tumor has been removed by surgical treatment or radiation. There are patients in whom this type of thrombophlebitis has led to a search for a previously unrecognized visceral carcinoma with apparent cure after surgical treatment. In most patients, however, death occurs in a few months from extension of the tumor or from pulmonary embolism.

Varicose veins and chronic venous stasis

To speak of varicose veins, with or without the adjectives "primary," "congenital," or "idiopathic," is to refer to a disorder of the lower limbs in which the superficial veins are dilated and tortuous and in which the tissues of the limb show changes attributed to venous stasis. Abnormally large or tortuous veins found elsewhere are due to hemangioma, collateral formation, or stretching through local venous hypertension. Venous stasis of the leg is, however, not primarily related to the size of the veins, since in the postphlebitic limb (postphlebitic, or secondary, varices), where venous stasis is most severe, the superficial veins may be quite small and sclerotic. The one factor causing the venous stasis both in primary and in postphlebitic varices is the loss of competence of the local venous valves.

Etiology and pathogenesis

A hereditary influence in some patients with primary varicose veins is suggested by the presence of the disorder in many members of the same family, the appearance of the varices during adolescence, an unusual severity, and, in some, by the characteristics of hemangioma (see below). The frequency of unilateral enlargements speaks against any general predisposition. A favored theory is of venous widening from above downward through hydrostatic influence exerted in the great saphenous vein and based on the congenital absence of a valve in the femoral or external iliac veins above the saphenous termination. The absence of such a valve does not always correlate with the presence of varicose veins. Some have postulated that the saphenous vein destined to become varicosed is congenitally devoid of normal valves. Edwards and Edwards [85], however, have shown that the valves are present and that the first abnormality is a weakening at the commissures of the valves with dilatation leading to relative incompetence.

Some primary varices present signs suggesting that they are based on congenital hemangioma, even omitting cavernous hemangioma with gross arteriovenous shunts or extensive vascular nevi. In these apparently ordinary varices, subfascial dissection reveals deep angiomatous masses connecting with the varices, and angiography demonstrates small arteriovenous communications in their vicinity [86].

Pregnancy worsens primary varices through vein relaxation, expansion of the blood volume, and increase in venous pressure in the iliac and thus in the femoral and saphenous system. Burwell [87] showed that this venous-pressure increase is due mainly to the arteriovenous fistula-like nature of the placenta which allows a high-pressure flow into the uterine and iliac veins.

Venous stasis of the severest degree is found in the postphlebitic limb. Recanalization is the rule after venous thrombosis. This, plus the wealth of potential collaterals at the root of the limb, makes it unlikely that lack of deep channel often plays much of a part. Valve destruction occurs routinely, however, in the deep veins after phlebitis [88] and may extend to the many communicating and superficial veins. It is probably the major factor in local venous regurgitation and stasis. Primary varices which have undergone attacks of phlebitis or become recanalized after injection treatment take on the character of the postphlebitic state by reason of valve damage. Mention was made previously that an early obstruction may exist in the lymphatics lying on the major veins. Lymphangiography has failed to demonstrate lymphatic obstruction in the postphlebitic limb, except in the sense that the fine cutaneous lymphatics may be blocked in the immediate vicinity of an ulcer or scar.

The exact mechanism of spontaneous ulcer formation in varices is a matter of conjecture. A reasonable explanation would be that there is ischemia in the erect state by venous back pressure along the venules, thus preventing capillary flow. This is associated with the tendency toward edema formation with the high venular pressure. Very large ulcers may show considerable cellulitis as evidenced by improvement to pin the blame for varicose ulceration on fungal infection, but their consultant dermatologists have not been able to find fungi. Contrariwise, treatment directed to the basic cause of the ulceration by adequate surgical procedures has cured the ulcers without recourse to fungicidal treatment. It is reasonable to conclude that fungi play no role in the causation or continuance of most varicose ulcers.

In the ulcer bed, secondary changes of fibrosis and local reactive endarteritis or arteriosclerosis give rise to recalcitrance to healing or to recurrence. Either epidermoid or

Fig. 171-22   Varicose veins. Demonstration of venous reflux by the Trendelenburg test. (a) Elevation of the leg empties the varices. (b) While the patient is standing, varices remain empty until the tourniquet is removed, showing reflux from the saphenous vein. (c) Reflux takes place via communicating veins prior to removal of the tourniquet, with additional reflux from the saphenous vein when the tourniquet is removed.

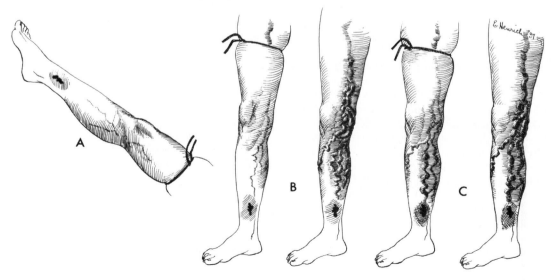

basal cell carcinoma can develop in a stasis ulcer of many years' duration. Tenopyr and Silverman [89] found an incidence of 4 such malignant tumors in 1000 varicose ulcers. This is probably a higher than usual figure [90,91].

Clinical manifestations

Symptoms of venous stasis include an aching discomfort in the limb or veins, some edema of the ankle in the course of the day, and frequent nocturnal muscle cramps.

The varices themselves, stemming from the enlarged great or small saphenous vein or both, are prominent in primary varicose disease. Examination by the Trendelenburg test demonstrates the valve incompetence (Fig. 171-22).

A hemangiomatous basis is suggested by a youthful onset, a strong family history, formation of many fine superficial cutaneous veins with a tendency to spontaneous rupture, and an unusual location of vein enlargement such as in the arch of the foot, the toes, or the posterior thigh.

Signs of venous stasis are not always present in primary varices. They include edema, enlargement of the cutaneous veins (especially at the ankle), pigmentation and scaling of the skin, or dermatitis and ulceration (see Fig. 171-23). Edema occurs each day below the knee. It pits readily on pressure and diminishes overnight. The skin changes are most marked on the ankle and are often limited to the medial side. They may encroach somewhat on the foot. The pigmentation is located in the dermis. It is derived from the breakdown of red cells which pass through the smaller vessels. The dermatitis is characterized by small erosions of the skin, often surmounted by abrasions from scratching. There is apt to be considerable crust formation whether or not ulceration is present. The dermatitis may be complicated by a sensitization to applied medication, and a dermatitis medicamentosa may be found widely distributed over the body.

The varicose ulcer is typically located at the medial side of the ankle (see Fig. A1-13), but one precipitated by trauma may be found higher on the leg though never above the knee. Ulceration may be multiple. Crusting is usually heavy. The ulcer is not generally deep or undermined. Its base is usually red. Even large ulcers may have epithelialized well from their edges and from more central parts.

Thrombophlebitis, a frequent complication of varices, exhibits a characteristic tender induration which in weeks or months may disappear, leaving hard areas where organization has occurred. Calcification may occur in a "pipestem" fashion in varices that have not thrombosed.

Hemorrhage is usually not strictly spontaneous. It is apt to follow a scratch or rough handling of a very superficial varix at the ankle. Varices most prone to recurrent bleeding are those of the angiomatous variety in which there is a tendency toward proliferation of small friable cutaneous veins, mostly at the ankle but sometimes as high as the knee.

The postphlebitic limb is characterized by larger ulcerations than are seen with idiopathic varices and especially by the development of a fibrosing panniculitis, felt as a firm subcutaneous induration at the medial side of the ankle, sometimes extending somewhat above the midleg. The induration often feels like an ovoid subcutaneous plaque, its long dimension in the long axis of the leg. The skin overlying it is usually heavily pigmented and always

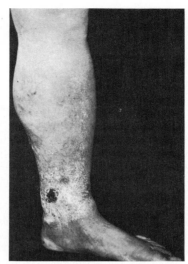

Fig. 171-23 Stasis dermatitis. An eczematous eruption occurring in individuals with chronic venous insufficiency; the lesions are most common over the region of the medial malleolus; exogenous factors, especially the injudicious use of irritating topically applied medicaments, undoubtedly are operative; generalized autoeczematization may occur.

bound down to the subcutaneous tissue. Postphlebitic ulceration is generally located over the plaque. The fibrosing process is usually wider than the plaque, so that the leg may show a firm retracted narrowing of its lower third, with pitting edema above it. Sometimes this engirdling gives rise to a lymphedema of the foot. On incising the panniculus, one can see a gradual reduction from above downward in the size of the subcutaneous fat lobules, with a corresponding increase in hard connective tissue, often with calcium deposit. In some cases droplets of milky lymph fluid ooze out from the involved fat.

Unusually the postphlebitic limb may present small, very painful superficial ulcerations scattered below the lateral or medial malleolus. The author has called this condition "ulcerating phlebitis" [73], since an active thrombophlebitis of small varices was found underlying the ulceration.

Diagnosis and differential diagnosis

The diagnosis of primary varicose disease rests primarily on seeing or palpating the varices and the enlargement of the great or small saphenous veins. It is important to determine whether these trunks are widened so as to plan proper surgical treatment, An occasional patient may show an isolated varix without this enlargement of the saphenous trunks.

The special features that indicate a hemangiomatous basis for primary varices have been described above. Such varices show a special tendency to recurrence. Hemangiomas in which large arteriovenous fistulae are present may be diagnosed through special signs such as the presence of venous pulsations, thrills, and the continuous murmur over the fistulae.

The special features of the postphlebitic limb may be present without a history of phlebitis; their presence nevertheless indicates that the limb has undergone valvular damage in the deep and communicating veins.

Many patients complain of the disfigurement of prominent, multiple, fine, cutaneous veins, especially on the thighs. These "angioids," or "spider bursts" are not part of ordinary varicose disease and often exist without any enlargement of the subcutaneous veins.

The differential diagnosis of thrombophlebitis of the varices has been discussed in the previous section. The differential diagnosis of edema is discussed earlier under "Thrombophlebitis" and below under "Lymphedema."

A diagnosis of stasis dermatitis or ulcer can hardly be considered unless the ankle shows the pigmentation and small-vein enlargement of venous stasis with or without the presence of primary varices or the special induration of the postphlebitic limb. The extension of stasis ulceration in arteriosclerosis was discussed earlier, under "Organic Arterial Disease." Malignant degeneration must be considered when stasis ulcer of long duration shows an exuberant growth of its base or an induration of its border.

Atrophie blanche, a disorder mainly of women, occurs on the ankles and legs. It begins as purpuric areas which undergo partial necrosis leading to white scars surrounded by telangiectases. In some patients this transpires in a setting of livedo reticularis—"livedoid vasculitis"—with summertime ulceration. Many [92–94] classify this as a clinical entity, microscopic examination showing a hyalinizing vasculitis with masses of hyaline material in the dermis, with or without ulceration and blanching. Others deny the specificity of this disease, noting that the same events occur in a setting of venous stasis [95–97] and that similar pathology may be found in any disorder that obstructs the cutaneous blood supply. Spontaneous healing of the ulceration is the rule. Heat and bed rest are advised. Steroid therapy is used by some but Winkelmann and Su [94] do not think it helpful.

Other conditions causing ulceration of dermatitis which may be confused with that of venous stasis are listed in Table 171-7 and illustrated in Figs. 171-24 and 171-25. Helpful discussions of ulceration due to other causes are given by Brunsting [98], Pascher and Keen [99], Chernoff et al [100], and Foley et al [101].

Treatment

The definitive treatment of varicose veins and their complications is surgical. The dermatologist may be called upon to treat acute hemorrhage from a varix. This is best done by an immediate sclerosing injection of the vein feeding the ulcer using 0.5 to 1 ml of sodium tetradecyl sulfate

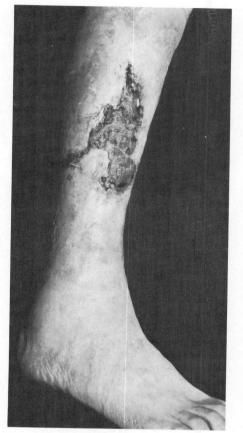

Fig. 171-24 Ulcerating gumma of the leg.

(Sotradecol). Stasis dermatitis usually yields to the application of corticosteroids in cream or ointment along with an elastic bandage. A stasis ulcer may be temporarily controlled by twice daily application of sterile gauze wet with tap water beneath a firm, wide elastic bandage from foot to knee. A bandage cast of the Unna type may be used. We find no value in home bed rest. Bed rest with repeated saline dressings may be used in the hospital, prior to operation on the veins or for excision and skin graft of the ulcer.

Fig. 171-25 Ulcers of the feet due to recurrent cellulitis.

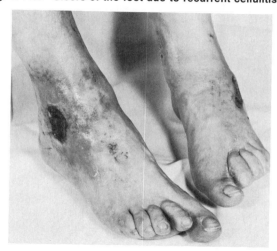

Table 171-7 Causes of ulceration of lower extremities other than venous stasis

Erythema induratum
Bacterial infection, trauma, hyperimmune states (pyoderma, pyoderma gangrenosum)
Syphilis
Mycotic infection (blastomycosis, leishmaniasis)
Malignancy (epidermoid, basal cell carcinoma, malignant melanoma)
Organic disease of large and small arteries
Vasospastic diseases (Cooley's and sickle-cell anemias, cryoglobulinemia, Sjögren's disease)
Metabolic disorders (necrobiosis lipoidica)
Pernio ("chilblains")
Atrophie blanche

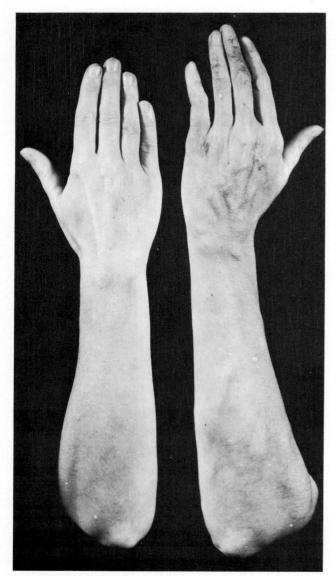

Fig. 171-26 Congenital AV fistulae in the right hand and wrist of a young woman. Note the increased length and prominent veins in the fingers, hand, and forearm.

Arteriovenous fistula

Arteriovenous fistula (AV fistula) is an abnormal communication between an artery and vein. The category does not include normal small arteriovenous shunts. AV fistulae may be acquired or congenital. The first is the result of trauma such as a knife or bullet wound. In the congenital form multiple fistulae exist almost invariably as features of hemangiomas. In these instances fistulae are not only located in the hemangiomas proper but may also occur as additional lesions elsewhere in the viscera [102].

Clinical features

A fistula is manifested by:

1. A thrill and murmur over the lesion. The murmur is often characterized as a "machinery hum" murmur since it is continuous across the pulse cycle with a systolic ac-

centuation. The murmur is loudest over the fistula but is well transmitted by way of adjacent bone. The patient may be aware of the thrill, and in case of an intracranial fistula may hear the murmur. The murmur is also transmitted along the vein, sometimes all the way to the heart [103]. Figs. 171-26 and 171-27 show such an instance. The application of digital or tourniquet occlusion of the limb at progressively more proximal places will indicate the part of the limb where the fistula is located and the murmur generated.

2. A dilatation of the artery leading to the fistula.

3. A palpable pulsation in the vein leading from the fistula.

4. An increased oxygen content in that vein when the fistula outflow constitutes a large proportion of the vein's content.

5. Evidence of direct arteriovenous flow by angiography.

6. There are certain general circulatory changes that result from the fistula. These consist of an increase in heart rate, cardiac output, and blood volume. These findings are in reaction to the loss of systemic pressure through the lowered resistance of the fistula. This can be demonstrated by a bradycardia in response to temporary occlusion of the feeding artery (Fig. 171-27). In time, cardiac hypertrophy and heart failure may result—the larger the fistula the surer and more rapid is this result. It appears that a fistula which can be seen only by angiography and is too small to give rise to an audible murmur is not capable of cardiac consequences.

7. There is relative ischemia of the part distal to the shunt. It is easier for arterial blood to enter the low venous resistance and flow back to the heart than to fight the resistance of the capillary bed distally.

8. External hemorrhage from an acquired AV fistula is uncommon, the high pressure of the arterial blood being relieved by easy admission to the vein. This is not invariable and the patient with such an injury should be operated on without too great a delay. However, if the condition has existed for some months or longer, operative treatment can be planned at leisure.

Hemangiomas give rise to some special manifestations (see Chap. 95). When external, the tumor is evident. It was noted earlier in this chapter that some varices represent minor hemangioma. If the fistulae are large, the part is hypertrophied and lengthened (Fig. 171-26). Episodes of thrombosis occur and give rise to painful indurations. The thromboses may be extensive and result in a hemorrhagic tendency secondary to platelet consumption [104,105]. Angiomas located in the viscera may bleed [102]. Anemia of unrecognized origin may result from such gastrointestinal bleeding.

Diagnosis

In acquired AV fistula there is usually a history of a wound, sometimes with considerable initial bleeding. Auscultation will reveal the characteristic "machinery hum" murmur, in contrast to a systolic murmur of arterial aneurysm or pseudaneurysm. If the fistula is large the abnormal pulsation of the affluent vein will be noted. The oxygen content of the vein will be increased and the carbon dioxide diminished, when compared with venous blood elsewhere. When the fistula is small, angiography will be required to

Fig. 171-27 Same patient as in Fig. 171-26. Proximal artery compression causes disappearance of the murmur and slowing of the heart rate, from the original rate of 72 to 63. The murmur over the effluent vein all but disappears on compression of the distal fistula. The small groups of persistent systolic vibrations are apparently caused by the entrance of blood from a few small fistulae of the forearm. *(From Edwards and Levine [103], with permission.)*

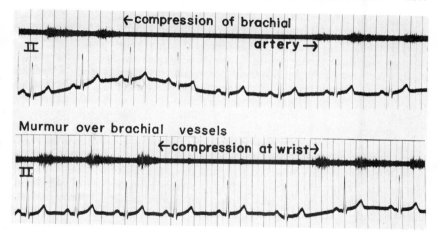

reveal it. This is usually the case in instances of visceral hemangiomas and fistulae.

Treatment

Surgical closure of the fistula is the treatment of choice. Ligation of the feeding artery only results in ischemia of the distant part, collateral blood flowing to the fistula and vein by preference over the capillary route. We have had no experience with other forms of treatment except for sclerosing injection of varices of the hemangiomatous type. In the case of congenital hemangioma, surgery should not be undertaken lightly. If the hemangioma is small, total excision can usually be done with little difficulty. It should be kept in mind that the AV fistulae of hemangioma are always multiple and any portions of the tumor left behind in bone, muscle, nerve, or skin are subject to later enlargement of the fistulae. We know of one instance of a hand and forearm hemangioma similar to that shown in Fig. 171-26 where an excellent surgeon found it impossible to close his surgical wound because of arterial bleeding from the skin and deep tissues, and terminated the procedure by amputating the limb.

Two principles of the pathology need to be kept in mind when planning surgery: (1) Planned excision must involve areas of major cutaneous involvement and some variety of skin graft needs to be planned. (2) The formation of the hemangioma is based on the persistence of the primitive vascular network. The AV fistulae represent portions where reduction to a capillary bed has not occurred. In addition, extensive hemangioma has a tendency to be formed along vessels of the embryo that normally regress. In the upper limb two such arteries are the median and the palmar part of the anterior interosseus. One of us (EAE) has successfully removed extensive hemangiomas with large fistulae from the hand and forearm of three patients. In each case a large median artery plexus existed displacing the fasciculi of the median nerve, and the anterior interosseus supplied a large plexus in the depth of the palm.

An important new development in the treatment of fistulae is their closure by introducing a small balloon or other foreign object via a transcutaneous arterial catheter. This is a rapidly developing field often subsumed under the term interventional radiology [106,107].

Platelet consumption coagulopathy is treated by anticoagulant therapy [104].

Lymphedema

The expression *lymphedema* connotes chronic or lasting swelling of a part due to obstruction of lymph outflow. The lower limbs, occasionally with the genitalia, are most frequently involved. The upper limbs are affected uncommonly except after radical mastectomy [108]; other parts such as the face become lymphedematous rarely. Kinmonth's book [109] constitutes the most comprehensive work available on the subject.

Etiology and pathogenesis

Women are more commonly affected than men. In roughly half of the cases the cause is unknown. Of these primary cases (Tables 171-8), the idiopathic nonfamilial type is overwhelmingly the most common. Kinmonth's lymphangiographic studies have led him to postulate a congenital aplasia or dysplasia of the lymphatic trunks in all the varieties of primary lymphedema. Varicosities and valve inadequacy were also demonstrable in some. He explains a late adult origin, in either the familial or nonfamilial type, by the inability of the inadequate system to remove the

Table 171-8   Varieties of lymphedema by cause

Primary:
  Congenital
  Familial (Milroy's disease)
  Idiopathic—nonfamilial
    Variant with yellow nails and pleural effusions*
Secondary:
  Infection
    Pyogenic
    Filarial
    Viral (cat-scratch fever)
  Ablation (radical lymph node excision or surgical scarring)
  Immune response (?)
  Malignant infiltration
  Fibrosis
    Overexposure to x-rays
    Stasis
    Localized myxedema
    Panniculitis
    Idiopathic retroperitoneal fibrosis
    Pharmacologic retroperitoneal fibrosis (methysergide)

* JJ Dilley et al, *JAMA 204*:122, 1968.

increased lymph that may be occasioned by such an incident as trauma. This trauma may be trivial, such as a sprained ankle. One of us (EAE) has seen both lymph node fibrosis and endolymphangitis in seemingly idiopathic disease, which brings up the possibility of an unrecognized initiating obstructive process in these patients. Forty-eight cases of Dilley's triad have been collected by Runyon et al [110].

Streptococcal or, less frequently, staphylococcal lymphangitis and adenitis are the most commonly known causes of the secondary variety; a viral infection (cat-scratch fever) has also produced lymphedema [111]. Usually a portal of entry is known, such as an abrasion or the erosion of athlete's foot. Some students of lymphedema believe that lymphedema will not develop in such obstructive diseases as filariasis [112] or after mastectomy [113] unless pyogenic infection supervenes. Other factors of importance in postmastectomy edema include the ablation of the lymphatics, surgical and postirradiation scarring, concomitant axillary vein obstruction (excision, scarring, or thrombosis), and local tumor recurrence [114].

Malignant infiltration at the root of a limb may or may not be associated with thrombosis of the adjacent major vein. Cancer of the lung, prostate, ovary, or uterus is a frequent example. Almost any type of panniculitis which is extensive may cause enough fibrotic reaction to produce some lymphedema. It is common distal to stasis panniculitis, and it has been seen when localized myxedema involves much of the ankle or foot (see Figs. 173-1 to 173-3). Retroperitoneal fibrosis of the truly idiopathic variety occasionally chokes off the lymphatics of the lower limb to give rise to lymphedema [115]. Methysergide therapy for migraine has occasioned an apparently identical process [17].

The obstruction to lymph flow produces a distal accumulation which not only distends all available lymphatics, mainly of the cutaneous and subcutaneous tissues, but enlarges the tissue spaces as well. Ultimately, fibroblastic growth is stimulated and adds a solid component to the swelling.

Recurrent bouts of inflammation and fever are frequent in lymphedematous patients. These attacks are commonly of frank erysipelas. The same organism, either a streptococcus or, less often, a staphylococcus, can be identified in all the attacks and may be the identical one which gave rise to an initiating lymphatic infection in the secondary variety. Each attack naturally produces more lymphatic destruction and more edema. Similar infection may supervene on the edema of idiopathic or of filarial origin.

In a second group, symptoms of recurrent infection occur, but bacteria cannot be isolated (pseudoerysipelas) [116]. In some of these patients there is no preexisting lymphedema, but each attack produces edema lasting 3 or 4 months. Dermatophytosis is almost invariably present. Two alternative mechanisms are postulated: the first, that streptococcal infection is responsible, in spite of the organisms not being found; the second, that attacks represent an immune response to the bacteria or the fungi of the usually present dermatophytosis. There are of course significant therapeutic connotations of each theory [116,117].

A malignant tumor, lymphangiosarcoma, may develop after many years of massive swelling [118]. It is exceedingly rare, arising in less than 1 percent of postmastectomy lymphedema, which is its most common setting.

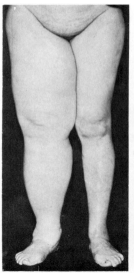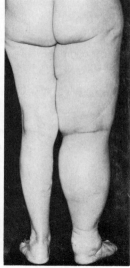

Fig. 171-28 Lymphedema initially idiopathic but augmented by several bouts of infection and later femoral vein ligation (scar) and lumbar sympathectomy. Note circumferential edema and absence of usual signs of venous stasis.

Clinical manifestations

Swelling of the limb may be limited to the most distal part. In early cases it may first involve a proximal area such as the thigh. This is especially true in malignant infiltration. Congenital lymphedemas may be associated with lymphangiomas. The edema in Milroy's disease may be present at birth; on the other hand, it may not be evident until late adult life (see Chap. 95). Idiopathic familial lymphedema arises most commonly in early adult life. It often first appears on the foot after a sprained ankle. The swelling may diminish in months or years, but new episodes of edema arise in the same or both limbs. The edema progressively increases in extent and severity until it may involve the entire extremity. A vague discomfort may be felt in the popliteal or femoral areas, but without distinct signs of adenitis. At first there may be some diminution in swelling overnight; later, when the condition is sufficiently massive to be termed elephantiasis, there is little change except after bed rest for several days.

Characteristically the limb shows a pale swelling circumferentially distributed, involving the toes and foot as well as the leg (Fig. 171-28). Pitting on pressure is present early but becomes minimal or absent late in the course. The skin is cool, and unless there have been episodes of infection, it is remarkably normal looking without induration or increased pigmentation. There may be a verrucous change, especially over the toes and particularly in response to infection [118]. Tiny vesicles of lymph may form here and there. An isolated fistula is sometimes seen. Rarely, this will leak a milky lymph (chylous reflux) through connections with retroperitoneal trunks.

Signs of infection are characteristically absent early in primary lymphedema. Episodes of secondary infection are ushered in by a chill, high fever, erysipelas, or cellulitis of the part, and tender lymph nodes. Epidermophytosis is evident in most of these patients. Recurrent infection may give rise to verrucous change. In extreme cases ulceration

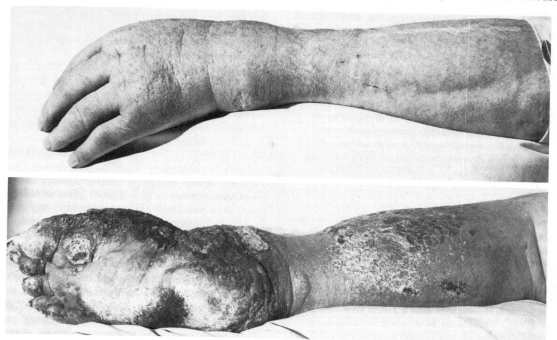

Fig. 171-29 Lymphedema secondary to staphylococcal infection via biopsy incision of the right calf. After 4 years of continued infection controlled only by antibiotics, the infected and useless elephantiasic right leg was amputated with no further infection; the edema of the left hand persisted. *(From Edwards [116], with permission.)*

with crusting and brown pigmentation occurs (Fig. 171-29). The development of lymphangiosarcoma is signaled by local swelling and tenderness and the presence of ecchymoses, bullae, or flat cyanotic nodules—the appearance being similar to that of Kaposi's sarcoma [119].

Lymphangitis and adenitis will be a prominent part of the history when pyogenic infection initiates the edema. The organisms are apt to reside as a resting infection in these cases, commonly giving rise to recurrent attacks as described above.

Malignant infiltration of the lymphatics of the lower limbs is often manifest years after the primary treatment of a pelvic malignant tumor. A gradual onset is unusual; a sudden onset or increase in swelling indicates concomitant venous thrombosis. In that case cyanosis and superficial vein enlargement will also be seen. Pain due to malignant involvement of the nerves is a prominent feature. When this process involves the root of the upper limb, Horner's syndrome may be added to the other features.

Constriction by fibrosis generally produces a mild lymphedema except for the postirradiation type seen in the upper limb after radical mastectomy, but, as noted earlier,

Table 171-9   Differential diagnosis of lymphedema

Idiopathic edema
Postphlebitic edema
Posttraumatic edema
Obesity and old age edema
Edema of constitutional disease
"Relative fat pattern" (fat legs)
Arthritis and synovitis of foot and ankle
Panniculitis
Localized myxedema

other mechanisms are additionally responsible in these limbs.

Diagnosis and differential diagnosis

The diagnosis rests mainly on the relative constancy of the edema. It differs from the postphlebitic variety by involving the toes and foot as well as the leg; by the lack of pigmentation, cyanosis, induration, and small-vein enlargement; by a usual lack of easy pitting on pressure; and, when present, by verrucous change, lymph blebs, or fistula. In special cases lymphangiography or phlebography may be necessary to define the diagnosis.

Filariasis is suggested by a prior residence in endemic zones, by involvement of the external genitalia along with the lower limbs, and by the history of a febrile illness at the beginning of the edema. It is difficult to establish this diagnosis with certainty except by biopsy, by the finding of the filaria in the blood at night during febrile episodes, or possibly by skin reactions to material prepared from known parasites [120].

Conditions other than lymphedema that should be kept in mind in making the diagnosis are given in Table 171-9. Idiopathic or periodic edema occurs almost exclusively in women. It commonly involves the ankles but may be part of a generalized water retention. Thorn [121] postulates that it begins in response to the cyclic hormonal changes of the female but may continue into the menopause as a conditioned response. Its fluctuation separates it from lymphedema. Similar inconstancy is characteristic of the edemas of constitutional disease or of obese older patients. In the latter, inactivity and dependence are probably responsible.

Persistent edema after trauma may be due to disuse and

dependency, but lymphedema and thrombophlebitis need to be excluded. Local thickenings can be due to hematoma or fat necrosis. Edema accompanied by vasospasm and acral hyperesthesia suggest reflex sympathetic dystrophy (see "Vasospastic Diseases" above).

The patient with normal but unusually fat legs or arms may complain of so-called swelling. The symmetry of the enlargement and the lack of other abnormal signs easily identifies this condition [122]. Careful examination will establish the periarticular swelling of arthritis or chronic synovitis (especially common at the ankles of middle-aged women) or of various forms of panniculitis or localized myxedema.

References

1. Edwards EA et al: Causes of peripheral embolism and their significance. *JAMA* **196**:133, 1966
2. Adar R et al: Cellular sensitivity to collagen in thromboangiitis obliterans. *N Engl J Med* **308**:1113, 1983
3. Edwards EA: Postamputation radiographic evidence for small artery obstruction in arteriosclerosis. *Ann Surg* **150**:177, 1959
4. Edwards EA: Localized ischemia in the lower extremities. *GP* **9**:40,1954
5. Edwards EA: Nail changes in functional and organic arterial disease. *N Engl J Med* **239**:362, 1948
6. Edwards EA: Necrotic lesions of the leg in arteriosclerosis. *N Engl J Med* **239**:571, 1948
7. Hines EA, Farber EM: Ulcer of the leg due to arteriosclerosis and ischemia occurring in the presence of hypertensive disease (hypertensive-ischemic ulcers): preliminary report. *Mayo Clin Proc* **21**:337, 1946
8. Edwards EA, Levine HD: Peripheral vascular murmurs. Mechanism of production and diagnostic significance. *Arch Intern Med* **90**:284, 1952
9. Edwards EA, Levine HD: Auscultation in the diagnosis of compression of the subclavian artery. *N Engl J Med* **247**:79, 1952
10. Edwards EA: Anatomic and clinical comments on shoulder girdle syndromes, in *Surgical Treatment of Peripheral Vascular Disease,* edited by WF Barker. New York, McGraw-Hill, 1962, chap 6
11. Coffman JD, Davies T: Vasospastic disorders: a review. *Prog Cardiovasc Dis* **18**:123, 1975
12. Olsen N, Nielsen SL: Prevalence of primary Raynaud phenomenon in young females. *Scand J Clin Lab Invest* **37**:761, 1978
13. Gifford RW, Hines EA: Raynaud's disease among women and girls. *Circulation* **16**:1012, 1957
14. Theriault G et al: Raynaud's phenomenon in forestry workers in Quebec. *Can Med Assoc J* **126**:1404, 1982
15. Marshall AJ et al: Raynaud's phenomenon as a side effect of beta-blockers in hypertension. *Br Med J* **1**:1498, 1976
16. Cranley JJ et al: Impending gangrene of four extremities secondary to ergotism. *N Engl J Med* **269**:727, 1963
17. Graham JR: Methysergide for prevention of headache. *N Engl J Med* **270**:67, 1964
18. Falappa P et al: Angiographic study of digital arteries in workers exposed to vinyl chloride. *Br J Ind Med* **39**:169, 1982
19. Teutsch C et al: Raynaud's phenomenon as a side effect of chemotherapy with vinblastine and bleomycin for testicular carcinoma. *Cancer Treat Rep* **61**:925, 1977
20. Marshall RJ et al: Vascular responses in patients with high serum titres of cold agglutinins. *Clin Sci* **12**:255, 1953
21. Edwards EA: Varieties of digital ischemia and their management. *N Engl J Med* **250**:709, 1954
22. Coffman JD: Total and nutritional blood flow in the finger. *Clin Sci* **42**:243, 1972
23. Cohen RA, Coffman JD: Beta-adrenergic vasodilator mechanism in the finger. *Circ Res* **49**:1196, 1981
24. Lewis T: Experiments relating to the peripheral mechanism involved in spasmodic arrest of the circulation in the fingers: a variety of Raynaud's disease. *Heart* **15**:7, 1929
25. Jamieson GG et al: Cold hypersensitivity in Raynaud's phenomenon. *Circulation* **44**:254, 1971
26. Kontos HA, Wasserman JA: Effect of reserpine in Raynaud's phenomenon, *Circulation* **39**:259, 1969
27. Cohen RA, Coffman JD: Reduced transmural systolic pressure promotes arterial closure in Raynaud's disease. *Clin Res* **30**:179A, 1982
28. Krahenbuhl B et al: Closure of digital arteries in high vascular tone states as demonstrated by measurement of systolic blood pressure in the fingers. *Scand J Clin Lab Invest* **37**:71, 1977
29. Coffman JD, Cohen AS: Total and capillary fingertip blood flow in Raynaud's phenomenon. *N Engl J Med* **285**:259, 1971
30. Downey JA et al: Thermoregulation and Raynaud's phenomenon. *Clin Sci* **40**:211, 1971
31. Mendlowitz M, Naftchi N: The digital circulation in Raynaud's disease. *Am J Cardiol* **4**:580, 1959
32. Lewis T: The pathological changes in the arteries supplying the fingers in warm-handed people and in cases of so-called Raynaud's disease. *Clin Sci* **3**:287, 1938
33. Halperin A et al: Raynaud's disease, Raynaud's phenomenon and serotonin. *Angiology* **11**:151, 1960
34. Pringle R et al: Blood viscosity in Raynaud's phenomenon. *Lancet* **1**:1086, 1965
35. Johnsen T et al: Blood viscosity and local response to cold in primary Raynaud's phenomenon. *Lancet* **2**:1001, 1977
36. Ayres ML et al: Blood viscosity, Raynaud's phenomenon and the effect of fibrinolytic enhancement. *Br J Surg* **68**:51, 1981
37. Zahavi J et al: Plasma exchange and platelet function in Raynaud's phenomenon. *Thromb Res* **19**:85, 1980
38. Coffman JD: Vasodilator drugs in peripheral vascular disease. *N Engl J Med* **300**:713, 1979
39. McFadyen IJ et al: Intra-arterial reserpine administration in Raynaud's syndrome. *Arch Intern Med* **132**:526, 1973
40. Smith CD, McKendry RJR: Controlled trial of nifedipine in the treatment of Raynaud's phenomenon. *Lancet* **2**:1299, 1982
41. Matoba T et al: Diltiazem and Raynaud's syndrome. *Ann Intern Med* **97**:455, 1982
42. Clifford PC et al: Treatment of vasospastic disease with prostaglandin E$_1$. *Br Med J* **281**:1031, 1980
43. Claff CL, Crane C: Self-heating insulated sleeve to replace the conventional hot pack poultice. *Am J Surg* **81**:695, 1951
44. Edwards EA et al: Pulse registration as a means of evaluating peripheral vascular patency and vasomotor activity. *Am J Cardiol* **4**:572, 1959
45. Sappington JT et al: Biofeedback as therapy in Raynaud's disease. *Biofeedback Self Regul* **4**:155, 1979
46. Jobe JB et al: Induced vasodilation as treatment for Raynaud's disease. *Ann Intern Med* **97**:706, 1982
47. Lewis T, Landis EM: Observations upon vascular mechanisms in acrocyanosis. *Heart* **15**:29, 1930
48. Larsson Y: The vasoconstrictor tone of the cutaneous arterioles in acroasphyxia, hypertension, and in the cold pressor test. *Acta Med Scand [Suppl]* **130**:146, 1948
49. Day R, Klingman W: Effect of sleep on skin temperature reactions in case of acrocyanosis. *J Clin Invest* **18**:271, 1939
50. Edwards EA: Remittent necrotizing acrocyanosis. *JAMA* **161**:1530, 1956
51. William CM, Goodman H: Livedo reticularis: a peripheral arteriolar disease. *JAMA* **85**:955, 1925

52. Feldaker M et al: Livedo reticularis with summer ulcerations. *Arch Dermatol* **72**:31, 1955

53. Mitchell SW et al: *Gunshot Wounds and Other Injuries of Nerves.* Philadelphia, JB Lippincott, 1864

54. Homans J: Minor causalgia: a hyperesthetic neurovascular syndrome. *N Engl J Med* **222**:870, 1940

55. Belenger M, Vander Elst E: L'œdème chronique du dos de la main. *Acta Chir Belg* **59**:203, 1960

56. Kinmonth JB et al: *Vascular Surgery.* Baltimore, Williams & Wilkins, 1963

57. Shaw RC: Pathologic malingering: the painful disabled extremity. *N Engl J Med* **271**:22, 1964

58. Edwards EA, Leeper RW: Frostbite: an analysis of 71 cases. *JAMA* **149**:1199, 1952

59. Houston CS: *Going High. The Story of Man and Altitude.* New York, American Alpine Club, 1980

60. Mundth ED et al: Treatment of experimental frostbite with low molecular weight dextran. *J Trauma* **4**:246, 1964

61. Penn I, Schwartz SI: Evaluation of low molecular weight dextran in the treatment of frostbite. *J Trauma* **4**:784, 1964

62. Babb RR et al: Erythermalgia: review of 51 cases. *Circulation* **29**:136, 1964

63. White JC: Vascular and neurologic lesions in survivors of shipwreck. I. Immersion-foot syndrome following exposure to cold. *N Engl J Med* **228**:211, 1943

64. Smith LA, Allen EA: Erythermalgia (erythromelalgia) of the extremities: a syndrome characterized by redness, heat, and pain. *Am Heart J* **16**:175, 1938

65. Bean WB: Vascular changes of the skin in pregnancy. *Surg Gynecol Obstet* **88**:739, 1949

66. Glusman M: The syndrome of "burning feet" (nutritional melalgia) as a manifestation of nutritional deficiency. *Am J Med* **3**:211, 1947

67. Bilderbeck JB: Infantile acrodynia, in *Brenneman's Practice of Pediatrics.* Hagerstown, MD, Prior, 1968, chap 17, part I, sec III

68. Edwards EA: Observations on phlebitis. *Am Heart J* **14**:428, 1937

69. Edwards EA: Migrating thrombophlebitis associated with carcinoma. *N Engl J Med* **240**:1031, 1949

70. Andrasch RH et al: Digital ischemia and gangrene preceding renal neoplasm. *Arch Intern Med* **136**:486, 1976

71. Sack GH et al: Trousseau's syndrome and other manifestations of chronic disseminated coagulopathy in patients with neoplasms. *Medicine (Baltimore)* **56**:1, 1977

72. Parish JM et al: Etiologic considerations in superior vena cava syndrome. *Proc Mayo Clin* **56**:407, 1981

73. Edwards EA: Thrombophlebitis of varicose veins. *Surg Gynecol Obstet* **66**:236, 1938

74. Farrow JH: Thrombophlebitis of superficial veins of the breast and anterior chest wall (Mondor's disease). *Surg Gynecol Obstet* **101**:63, 1955

75. Mondor H: Tronculite sous-cutanée subaiguë de la paroi thoracique antero-latèrale. *Mem Acad Chir* **65**:1271, 1939

76. Jönssen G et al: Subcutaneous cords on the trunk. *Acta Chir Scand* **108**:351, 1955

77. Mondor H: Phlebite en cordon de la paroi thoracique. *Mem Acad Chir* **70**:96, 1944

78. Bircher J et al: Mondor's disease: a vascular rarity. *Proc Staff Mayo Clin* **37**:651, 1962

79. Johnson WC et al: Superficial thrombophlebitis of the chest wall. *JAMA* **180**:103, 1962

80. Duff P: Mondor disease in pregnancy. *Obstet Gynecol* **58**:117, 1981

81. Abramson DJ: Mondor's disease and string phlebitis. *JAMA* **196**:135, 1966

82. Hull R et al: Replacement of venography in suspected venous thrombosis by impedance plethysmography and I_{125} fibrinogen leg scanning. *Ann Intern Med* **94**:12, 1981

83. Swanson P et al: Dermatologic aspect of superior vena cava syndrome. *Arch Dermatol* **98**:628, 1968

84. Edwards EA: Phlebitis and the diagnosis of thromboangiitis obliterans. *Ann Intern Med* **31**:1019, 1949

85. Edwards JE, Edwards EA: The saphenous valves in varicose veins. *Am Heart J* **19**:338, 1940

86. Edwards EA, O'Conner JF: Ordinary varicose veins as an expression of congenital hemangioma. *Surg Gynecol Obstet* **122**:1245, 1966

87. Burwell CS: The placenta as a modified arteriovenous fistula, considered in relation to the circulatory adjustments to pregnancy. *Am J Med Sci* **195**:1, 1938

88. Edwards EA, Edwards JE: The effect of thrombophlebitis on the venous valve. *Surg Gynecol Obstet* **65**:310, 1937

89. Tenopyr J, Silverman I: The relation of chronic varicose ulcer to epithelioma: based on records of over 1000 chronic leg ulcers. *Ann Surg* **95**:754, 1932

90. Rubenfield S: Epithelioma developing on varicose ulcer. *Am J Surg* **26**:372, 1934

91. Taylor GW et al: Epidermoid carcinoma of the extremities with reference to lymph node involvement. *Ann Surg* **113**:268, 1941

92. Gray HR et al: Atrophie blanche: periodic painful ulcers of lower extremities. *Arch Dermatol* **93**:187, 1966

93. Lever WF, Schaumburg-Lever G: *Histopathology of the Skin,* 5th ed. Philadelphia, JB Lippincott, 1975

94. Winkelmann RK, Su WPD: Vascular diseases of the skin, in *Peripheral Vascular Diseases,* 5th ed, edited by JL Jeurgens et al. Philadelphia, WB Saunders, 1980, p 655

95. Moschella SL et al: *Dermatology.* Philadelphia, WB Saunders, 1975

96. Braverman IM: *Skin Signs of Systemic Disease,* 2d ed. Philadelphia, WB Saunders, 1981

97. Pinkus H, Mehregan A: *A Guide to Dermatohistopathology,* 3d ed. New York, Appleton-Century-Croft, 1981

98. Brunsting HA: Pyoderma gangrenosum in association with chronic ulcerative colitis. *Ohio Med J* **50**:1150, 1954

99. Pascher F, Keen R: Ulcers of the leg in Cooley's anemia. *N Engl J Med* **256**:1220, 1957

100. Chernoff AL et al: Therapy of chronic ulceration of the legs associated with sickle cell anemia. *JAMA* **155**:1487, 1954

101. Foley JF et al: Anticoagulant therapy of cryoglobulinemic ulcers in a case of Sjögren's syndrome. *JAMA* **176**:149, 1961

102. Dines DD et al: Pulmonary arteriovenous fistulas. *Mayo Clin Proc* **58**:176, 1983

103. Edwards EA, Levine HD: The murmur of peripheral arteriovenous fistula. *N Engl J Med* **247**:502, 1952

104. Rodriguez-Erdmann F et al: Kasabach-Merritt syndrome: coaguloanalytical observations. *Am J Med Sci* **261**:9, 1971

105. Miale JB: *Laboratory Medicine Hematology,* 6th ed. St. Louis, CV Mosby, 1982

106. Keller FS et al: Percutaneous angiographic embolization: a procedure of increasing usefulness. Review of a decade of experience. *Am J Surg* **142**:5, 1981

107. Greenfield AJ: Transcatheter vessel occlusion: selection of methods and materials. *Cardiovasc Intervent Radiol* **3**:222, 1980

108. Britton RC, Nelson PA: Causes and treatment of postmastectomy lymphedema of the arm: report of 114 cases. *JAMA* **180**:95, 1962

109. Kinmonth JB: *The Lymphatics: Surgery, Lymphography and Diseases of the Chyle and Lymph Systems.* Baltimore, E Arnold, 1982

110. Runyon BA et al: Pleural-fluid kinetics in a patient with primary lymphedema, pleural effusions, and yellow nails. *Am Rev Respir Dis* **119**:821, 1979

111. Filler RM et al: Lymphedema after cat-scratch fever. *N Engl J Med* **270**:244, 1964

112. Matas R: Surgical treatment of elephantiasis and elephantoid

states dependent upon chronic obstruction of the lymphatic and venous channels. *Am J Trop Dis* **1**:60, 1913

113. Halsted WS: Swelling of arm after operations for cancer of breast: elephantiasis chirurgica—its cause and prevention. *Bull Johns Hopkins Hosp* **32**:309, 1921

114. Danese C, Howard JM: Post-mastectomy lymphedema. *Surg Gynecol Obstet* **120**:797, 1965

115. Mahoney EM, Edwards EA: Spontaneous regression of leg edema and hydronephrosis following idiopathic retroperitoneal fibrosis. *Am J Surg* **103**:514, 1962

116. Edwards EA: Recurrent febrile episodes and lymphedema. *JAMA* **184**:858, 1963

117. Babb RR et al: Prophylaxis of recurrent lymphangitis complicating lymphedema: preliminary observations. *Mayo Clin Proc* **37**:485, 1962

118. Reiss F: Lymphostatic verrucosa (letter to the editor). *JAMA* **156**:274, 1954

119. Eby CS et al: Lymphangiosarcoma: a lethal complication of chronic lymphedema. *Arch Surg* **94**:223, 1967

120. Temkin O: *A Report on the Medicinal Treatment of Filariasis bancrofti.* Washington, DC, US Government Printing Office, 1945

121. Thorn GW: Approach to the patient with "idiopathic edema" or "periodic swelling." *JAMA* **206**:333, 1968

122. Garn SM: Relative fat patterning: an individual characteristic. *Hum Biol* **27**:75, 1955

CHAPTER 172

NEUROCUTANEOUS DISEASES

Raymond D. Adams

General considerations

A search for a conceptual framework for the neurocutaneous diseases invites several logical possibilities, the most appealing of which is one based on histologic and pathogenic relationships. In pursuit of this idea, of first order of importance would be a grouping of diseases the common feature of which would be an underlying developmental fault, originating in the embryonic period and affecting cells of both skin and nervous system. The abnormalities in the two organ systems, once developed, would coexist and progress in parallel without having any direct interaction. Bourneville's tuberous sclerosis, von Recklinghausen's neurofibromatosis, and Sturge-Weber cranial hemangioma conform to this criterion.

A second category might include all the diseases in which some property common to the cells of skin and nervous system has rendered them simultaneously vulnerable to the same pathogenic agent. The latter might be a microbe (such as a virus, bacterium, or spirochete), a bacterial toxin, an exogenous poison, a deficiency state, or a metabolic (biochemical or endocrine) abnormality. Each of these agencies might be taken as a subdivision of this class of disease.

Next, one might consider as a separate group all the disorders of skin consequent on a real or hypothetical abnormality of the nervous system. Syringomyelia, congenital analgesia, polyneuropathy, and tabes dorsalis, to take the most familiar examples, by depriving the skin of sensory fibers which serve to protect it from injury, could result in inadvertent traumatism and chronic ulceration or unhygienic condition. And, once the skin is injured, a loss of the autonomic control of cutaneous vessels might interfere with natural healing processes, as happens in decubitus ulcerations secondary to diseases of the spinal cord.

Finally, there would be a logical position in such a clas-sificatory scheme for cutaneous diseases in which the primary abnormality resides in the skin, the nervous system being secondarily affected. Reference is made here to the cutaneous furuncle that gives rise to an epidural spinal abscess; a viral exanthema that induces a postinfectious encephalomyelitis; an infected wound through which is introduced a toxin that acts by disinhibiting the motor neurons in the spinal cord, giving rise to tetanus; a cutaneous melanoma that may seed neoplastic cells through the brain without itself appearing to be in an active phase of growth.

However one might conceive of them from a practical standpoint, the neurocutaneous diseases serve to emphasize the importance of expert examination of the skin in obtaining clues as to the origin of obscure neurologic diseases and of knowing something about the way the nervous system may affect the skin and give rise to cutaneous diseases. The neurologic cases secondary to a dermatologic abnormality have no special characteristics and, being known to every student of dermatology, will not be considered further in this chapter.

This, then, is the basis of the following classificatory scheme, which it is hoped will have the heuristic value of facilitating critical thinking and of putting into logical order the horde of maladies that implicate skin and nervous system either simultaneously or successively (Table 172-1).

Pathogenic mechanisms

A general consideration of the probable causes and mechanism of neurocutaneous diseases seems a useful theoretical introduction to our subject.

Dr. Wm. B. Reed (deceased) contributed to the original chapter in the first edition of this text. Requiescat in pace.

Pathologic derangements in the embryogenesis of the cellular elements of the neural crest

It has been shown that the symmetrically placed cells of the neural crest which, during embryonic life, lie dorsolateral to the neural tube are the common anlage of the dorsal or posterior root ganglion cells, sympathetic ganglion cells, Schwann cells, chromaffin cells, and melanocytes. Less certain is the neural crest origin of meningeal fibroblasts, endoneurial fibroblasts, and chrondrocytes. Most probably they arise from mesoderm. The neural crest is said also to be involved in the formation of dental enamel.

Theoretically, then, a developmental failure or retardation of the growth and differentiation of the neural crest could result in a corresponding deficiency in all the cellular elements derived from this structure. That such a state exists has been postulated by a number of writers [1] who cite cases in which an infant or child is observed to lack sensation over the entire body, to have blond or nonpigmented hair, blue-green irides, aplasia of dental enamel, and autonomic dysfunction (manifested by pupillary and eye abnormalities ranging from a partial to complete Horner's syndrome, neurogenic anhidrosis with normal sweat glands, vasomotor instability, and urinary excretion of abnormal quantities of homovanillic and vanillylmandelic acids.) This constellation of effects in the infant has been called "the syndrome of the neural crest."

Lesser degrees of impairment of these functions, affecting variably the somatic sensory as well as the autonomic systems, have also been observed. The congenital sensory (analgesic) neuropathy with selective absence of small dorsal root ganglion cells and myelinated fibers is one example and the Riley-Day disease, a type of partial congenital dysautonomia, is another. These partial syndromes might relate to some extent to the timing of the action of the pathogenic agency, since not all the derivatives of the neural crest form and migrate at the same time during embryonic life.

Disturbances of Schwann cell–endoneurial fibroblast relationships

The Schwann cell proves to be one of the most interesting of the neural crest derivatives. Its nucleus resembles that of the fibroblast but is shorter and more oval, and its cytoplasm encloses segments of the myelin of peripheral nerves, or enfolds groups of nonmyelinated axons (Remak fibers). Thus, an intimate relationship to the axon of nerve cells stands as one of its most distinctive characteristics. The laminated myelin sheath, formed by circular infoldings of the Schwann cell cytoplasmic membrane (the molecules of lipid and protein of which the myelin sheath is constructed lie in relation to this membrane), probably is necessary for the rapid transmission of nerve impulses. Destruction of the axon results in degeneration of the myelin segments and leads to a proliferation of Schwann cells; and destruction of Schwann cells leaving the axon intact results in demyelination and interferes with axonal transmission.

Schwann cells are important in another respect—that of influencing the orientation of endoneurial fibroblasts (sheath of Henle) that surround each medullated axon. Crude lesions which interrupt the tubes of Schwann cells (bands of Bungner) disturb the spatial orientation of endoneurial fibroblasts. Similarly, fibrosis and scarring block the regeneration of injured nerve by interfering with the linear growth of Schwann cells.

Thus, there is normally a fixed relationship between axons, Schwann cells, and fibroblasts, not only in number but in spatial arrangement. Together with the axons of nerves they form an efficient neural pathway from skin to central nervous system and back. They also provide a channel along which infective agents and toxins may pass. The quantitative aspects of Schwann cells are also interesting. Because of the repeated branching and rich plexuses of nerves in the skin, the latter harbors more Schwann cells and endoneurial fibroblasts than any other organ in the human body. Any fundamental disorder of these cells might be expected to reflect itself maximally in the nerves of the skin.

The dermatologist's interest in Schwann cells and endoneurial fibroblasts emanates from the large variety of dermal lesions to which these cells give rise in neurofibromatosis. In this disease, endoneurial fibroblasts and Schwann cells undergo a limited multifocal hyperplasia (most active around puberty) in cutaneous nerve twigs and form the large number and variety of tumors to be described later in this chapter. Pigmentary changes are also induced, causing either café au lait spots or freckle-like macules. The pathogenesis of these curious focal hyperplasias of fibroblasts, Schwann cells, and melanocytes in neurofibromatosis has never been elucidated. Of course, their genetic basis is known, but what is the mechanism? One might speculate that some locally acting biochemical agent, necessary for the inhibition of the natural processes of proliferation and migration of Schwann cells and fibroblasts, is lacking during a certain period in embryonic life. Embryologists only recently have become aware of the timed sequences of natural biochemical inhibitors of cell proliferation. Probably something has gone awry with this process. This pathogenic mechanism is not without implications in brain development as well, because there is a high incidence of cerebral dysgenesis and also of mental retardation in patients with neurofibromatosis. And in oncology it assumes importance because these benign overgrowths of tissue in nerves and brain, after years of quiescence, have a small but significant potential for malignant neoplastic transformation.

Disturbances of melanocytes

The precursor of this cell, the melanoblast, is believed to migrate from the neural crest to the skin, to the cerebrospinal meninges, to the choroid of the eye and the inner ear (see Chap. 21). Melanin formation occurs also in certain neurons of the brainstem (substantia nigra, locus ceruleus, and other nuclei) but these cells are of different embryonal origin, and the pigment also differs from that of epidermal melanocytes. Interestingly, the nerve cells retain their pigment in the human albino, whereas the melanosomes of melanocytes in the skin and hair are deficient in melanin.

Disorders of pigmentation are discussed fully in Chap. 79. Here only a few diseases in which pigmentary disturbances are associated with a neurologic disorder will be cited to exemplify these types of neurocutaneous diseases.

1. Simultaneous defect in melanocytes and developmental defect in the central nervous system. In Bourneville's

Table 172-1   Classification of neurocutaneous diseases

I. Congenital and developmental neurocutaneous diseases
  A. The congenital benign neoplasms and vascular formations
    *1. Tuberous sclerosis (Bourneville's disease)
    *2. Neurofibromatosis of von Recklinghausen
    *3. Cutaneous angiomatosis with abnormalities of the central nervous system
      *a. Craniofacial or trigeminocranial angiomatosis with cerebral calcification (Sturge-Weber-Dimitri disease)
      †b. Dermatomal hemangiomas with spinal vascular malformations (sometimes with limb hypertrophy as in Klippel-Trénauney-Weber syndrome)
    †4. Hemangioblastoma of cerebellum and retina (Lindau-von Hippel syndrome)
    †5. Familial telangiectasis (Osler-Rendu-Weber disease)
    †6. Ataxia-telangiectasia (Louis-Bar disease)
  B. Developmental neurocutaneous diseases (developmental anomalies of skin and nervous system)
    †1. Congenital skin defects with gross anomalies of the nervous system (spina bifida, cranium bifidum)
      a. Focal congenital skin defects and dermal hypoplasias
  C. Congenital somatic abnormalities, including those of the nervous system and skin
    ‡1. Somatic abnormalities with chromosomal changes (mongolism, or Down's syndrome; Patau's syndrome; Edward's syndrome; cri-du-chat syndrome; Turner's syndrome; Kleinfelter's syndrome)
    *2. Somatic abnormalities with normal chromosome pattern (Papillon-Psaume syndrome, Rubenstein-Taybi syndrome, Hallerman-Streiff syndrome, de Lange's Amsterdam dwarf syndrome, Russell-Silver dwarf state)
  D. Congenital eruptive diseases with nervous disorders
    *1. Incontinentia pigmenti (Bloch-Sulzberger syndrome)
    ‡2. Epidermolysis bullosa
    ‡3. Poikiloderma congenitale of Rothmund and Thomson
    ‡4. Anhidrotic ectodermal dysplasia
    ‡5. Hidrotic ectodermal dysplasia
    ‡6. Sebaceous and epithelial nevi
    ‡7. Basal cell nevus syndrome
  E. Congenital pigmentary disorders with anomalous development of the nervous system
    †1. Moynahan's syndrome
    †2. Giant pigmented nevus with concurrent involvement of meninges and malignant melanoma
    ‡3. Familial generalized melanoderma
    †4. Waardenburg-Klein and related syndromes of deafness
    †5. Chédiak-Higashi disease
  F. The congenital ichthyotic forms of nervous disease (congenital ichthyosis, xeroderma, hyperkeratosis)
    ‡1. Sex-linked ichthyosis (Rud's syndrome)
    ‡2. Xerodermic idiocy and ataxia (Laubenthal's syndrome)
    ‡3. Ichthyotic idiocy with retinitis and muscular atrophy (Stewart's syndrome)
    ‡4. Ichthyotic idiocy with spastic paraplegia (Sjögren-Larsson syndrome)

  G. Looseness, redundancy, and loss of elasticity of skin (dermatochalasis, generalized elastolysis)
    ‡1. Cutis laxa
    ‡2. Pterygium colli in Turner-Bonnevie-Ullrich syndrome
    ‡3. Leprechaunism
    ‡4. Cutis verticis gyrata
    ‡5. Melkersson-Rosenthal syndrome
II. Diseases which simultaneously affect the cells of skin and nervous system
  A. Metabolic abnormalities (including those of vitamin deficiency and endocrine diseases)
    †1. Cretinism
    †2. Pellagra
    †3. Phenylketonuria (PKU) (Følling's disease)
    ‡4. Homocystinuria
    ‡5. Argininosuccinic aminoaciduria
    †6. Hartnup disease
    ‡7. Hydroxykynureninuria
    ‡8. Monilethrix (trichorrhexis nodosa)
    ‡9. Kinky hair disease
    ‡10. Gargoylism (Hunter-Hurler syndrome) and other mucopolysaccharidoses
    ‡11. Xerodermic idiocy of de Sanctis and Cacchione
    ‡12. Myoclonic epilepsy of Unverricht and Lundborg
    ‡13. Albinism and the oculocerebral syndrome of Cross and McKusick
    ‡14. Congenital lipodystrophic diabetes (leprechaunism) and the Prader-Willi and Laurence-Moon-Biedl syndromes
    ‡15. Hypercholesterolemia with tendon xanthomatoses and neurologic abnormality (van Bogaert-Epstein-Scherer syndrome)
    ‡16. Refsum's syndrome, acanthocytosis, and Tangier disease
    ‡17. Lipoid proteinosis (Urbach-Wiethe disease)
    ‡18. Cryoglobulinemic polyneuropathy
    ‡19. Angiokeratoma corporis diffusum
    †20. Variegate porphyria
    †21. Familial hyperuricemia with self-destructive biting, mental retardation, cerebral palsy, and choreoathetosis (Lesch-Nyhan syndrome)
    †22. Hypoparathyroidism with superficial moniliasis, keratoconjunctivitis, and hypoadrenalism
    ‡23. Familial dysautonomia (Riley-Day syndrome)
    †24. Cockayne's syndrome
    25. Genetic myotonia syndromes
  B. Toxic disorders
    ‡1. Arsenic intoxication
    †2. Mercury acrodynia
    ‡3. Thallium poisoning
  C. Infective states, proved or suspected types
    †1. Meningococcemia, rickettsial infections, viral infections, and mycotic infections
    †2. Vogt-Koyanagi-Harada syndrome
    ‡3. Behçet's syndrome
III. Dermatologic disorders secondary to diseases of the nervous system
  †A. Trophic changes in skin due to sensory denervation
    1. Decubitus ulcerations, i.e., due to spinal cord trauma
    †2. Syringomyelia
    †3. Chronic sensory polyneuropathies
    †4. Congenital insensitivity to pain
  B. Factitious ulcers in hysteria and malingering
  C. Infections spreading from nervous system to skin
    †1. Herpes zoster

Table 172-1   Classification of neurocutaneous diseases (continued)

IV. Primary dermatologic diseases leading to abnormalities of nervous system	‡C. Diphtheritic wound infections
‡A. Tetanus	‡D. Tick and black widow spider bites
‡B. Rabies	†E. Herpes simplex
	‡F. Cutaneous melanomas

* Major.
† Mention, but not in detail.
‡ Optional, mention only.

tuberous sclerosis the earliest skin lesions are the ash leaf-shaped areas of hypopigmentation and the nervous system lesions: proliferations of abnormal astrocytes and nerve cells in the brain (tubers). In von Recklinghausen's neurofibromatosis, foci of hyperpigmentation (café au lait spots) due to enlarged melanosomes in cells of the malpighian layer are associated both with schwannomas of the peripheral nerves and gliotic foci in the brain.

2. Nevi of hyperpigmentation associated with melanomatosis of meninges, hydrocephalus, and a variety of anomalies of development of the brain and spinal cord.

3. Bloch-Sulzberger incontinentia pigmenti in which hyperpigmentation follows recurrent inflammation of skin and is associated with focal necroses of the brain.

4. Moynahan's syndrome in which multiple symmetrical lentigines are associated with mental retardation, dwarfism, genital hypoplasia, and mitral stenosis.

5. Waardenburg-Klein syndrome in which a white forelock is conjoined to anomalies of eyelids, eyebrows, root of nose, and deafness.

6. Chédiak-Higashi syndrome in which partial albinism, photophobia, and leukocytic inclusions are combined with a polyneuropathy.

7. Melanoma of skin with metastases to the brain and sometimes the meninges.

8. Various forms of albinism and mental deficiency.

9. Addison's adrenal insufficiency with leukodystrophy (adrenoleukodystrophy).

In several of these varieties of disease the melanoblasts are deficient, the melanocytes are reduced in number, melanosome formation is abnormal, or the transfer of melanosomes from melanocyte to malpighian cell (keratinocyte) is blocked. The number and variety of these disorders and their frequent conjunction with neurologic lesions strongly support the neurogenic derivation of melanocytes.

Developmental derangements of vascular structures in skin and nervous system

The development of blood vessels during embryonic life occurs in a series of steps, as outlined by Streeter in the *American Embryologist.* Beginning with a complex network (rete mirabile), arteries and veins emerge and form the familiar patterns in each organ. This involves a series of regressive steps and tends to follow a metameric pattern. It is not surprising, therefore, that abnormalities of blood vessels and vascular malformations (hemangiomas), which abound in the skin and brain, might coexist if certain of these embryonic regressions failed to occur in particular regions.

Probably the most dramatic form of neurocutaneous

hemangioma is exemplified by *Sturge-Weber-Dimitri disease,* a port-wine stain or nevus flammeus (feuermal, tache de feu) which occurs in association with cerebral meningeal hemangioma, cortical calcification, and glaucoma. Other examples are: the segmental *cutaneous hemangioma of the thorax* which may be combined with a *hemangioma of the spinal meninges* in corresponding segments (Cobb's syndrome), the brachial hemangioma and hypertrophy with a cervical spinal vascular malformation (Trénauney-Weber syndrome), and the cirsoid retinal aneurysm which is conjoined to vascular malformation of the brainstem (Bonnet-Dechaume syndrome).

Another pathogenic mechanism must account for the *familial telangiectasia of Osler-Rendu-Weber,* where minute capillary angiomas of skin and mucous membranes evolve and (rarely) implicate parts of the cerebrum and spinal cord. In *ataxia telangiectasia,* clusters of finely traced vessels in conjunctivae, skin of ears, and anterior thorax follow at some interval of time after degenerative changes in cerebellum and basal ganglia. The vessels appear to form as part of an inflammatory reaction or skin sensitivity. In Fabry's disease a defect in ceramide dihexosidase results in skin lesions and abnormalities in endothelial and perithelial cells of vessels in the peripheral nervous system. A fault in connective tissue in skin and blood vessels appears to underlie the diseases known as elastosis perforans serpiginosa and pseudoxanthoma elasticum.

The hereditary nature of several of these neurovascular disorders is revealed in the genealogies of large families. However, chromosomal studies have yielded little information. Local factors must account for interference with the natural vascular regression of the embryonal rete mirabile. The concurrence of lesions in the nervous system and corresponding skin segments indicates an involvement of the anlage of both tissues.

It should be emphasized that neurocutaneous vascular diseases need not be based on a developmental fault. The vessels of the two organ systems may be the seat of an inflammatory process (in viremia, bacteremia, or septicemia) or an allergic vasculitis. The latter group of diseases assumes different forms, depending in part on the size of vessels involved. Such diseases demonstrate both similarities and differences between the vasculature of the brain and spinal cord and of nerves and skin. For example, in disseminated lupus erythematosus small cerebral vessels are often affected in the more advanced stages of the disease while those of the spinal cord and nerves tend to be spared. However, there are many exceptions to this rule. In polyarteritis nodosa, which affects larger arteries, the vessels of the skin and cerebrospinal structures usually escape while the vessels of peripheral nerves are regularly damaged. In the disease known as granulomatous or giant-cell arteritis of the brain, cerebral vessels alone are usually involved. Of the several types of cutaneous angiitis, represented by erythema nodosum, the vessels of peripheral nerves, spinal cord, and brain are usually left untouched. In Degos' malignant necrotizing papulosis, skin lesions predominate, with frequent involvement of intestinal tract (see Chap. 168), but there may be lesions in the vessels of the spinal cord, brain, and peripheral nerves.

Disturbed lipocyte–nerve relationships

Nerve fibers exert trophic effects on fat cells—a fact long suspected from the remarkable segmental distribution of the lipodystrophic syndromes. Here all the fat cells may vanish from part of the body, for example one side of the face (Romberg's hemiatrophy), leaving the skin wrinkled and aged in appearance, or all the fat cells may disappear in a band which encircles the torso in a neurodermatomal distribution. That peripheral nerve does affect fat cells was established years ago by Sidman and Fawcett [2], who showed alteration in the appearance and chemical properties of the brown fat of animals following denervation. The relevance of these observations to humans has not been further clarified. Interruption of human nerves does not cause a loss of cutaneous fat, nor have nerve, root, or spinal lesions been demonstrated in human lipodystrophy. Yet, failure of grafts of fat tissue to survive in areas of lipoatrophy (in cases of segmental lipodystrophy) has led certain writers to postulate a defect in autonomic innervation, an idea that receives some support from the occasional finding of Horner's syndrome and blue or variegated iris coloration (attributed to a defect in autonomic innervation) in cases of Romberg's hemiatrophy of the face. Usually subdermal structures are not affected. The cases of Tedesco et al of atrophy of fat cells in the skin with scleroderma and localized myopathy are exceptions to this statement. Their cause is unknown. Similarly, the basis of excessive deposits of fat, so striking in some women, also remains obscure. This whole question of precisely what nerve contributes to the metabolism of fat cells awaits further study.

Universal derangements of biochemistry of cells, including those of skin and nervous system

Modern biochemical research has brought to light more than a hundred genetically determined metabolic diseases of the human nervous system. Some of these lead to progressive degeneration of particular systems of neurons. Interestingly, the enzymatic defects that account for the changes in neurons usually affect the cells of skin, blood, and other tissues, though not to a degree that alters their function. The changes in the latter structures, nevertheless, may be demonstrated by delicate biochemical tests and are visible under the electron microscope. Other diseases such as pellagra, Hartnup disease, and variegate porphyria express themselves by syndromes comprised of both cutaneous and neurologic abnormalities. Another example is phenylketonuria where a measurable increase in phenylalanine interferes in some unexplained way with the natural myelination of the brain in the first years of post-natal life, and, by competitively inhibiting tyrosinase, pre-

vents normal pigmentation of skin and hair. An example of a purely exogenous neurocutaneous toxin is organic arsenic; its ingestion leads to an exfoliative dermatitis that is accompanied by polyneuropathy and hemorrhagic encephalopathy. Here the neurocutaneous link is probably the affinity between As with sulfhydryl (S–H) radicals in skin, axons of nerves, and the capillary endothelium of the cerebral white matter. The involved structures are known to be unusually rich in mercaptans (S–H-containing proteins).

Further research will surely reveal other common chemical attributes of epithelial cells and neurons. And from such data it will be possible, ultimately, to construct a more complete conceptual framework for all neurocutaneous diseases. These few examples should suffice at present to persuade the student of dermatology of the promising rewards of research in this field.

Effects of denervating the skin

In the context of neurocutaneous diseases it is well to have clearly in mind the skin changes consequent on interruption of somatic motor, sensory, and autonomic nerves. Since the effects of autonomic or visceromotor and somatic sensory-motor nerves differ, they should be considered separately even though in many diseases of the peripheral nervous system both types of fibers are affected.

Somatic sensory-motor denervation

Most peripheral nerves are of mixed type, i.e., they contain both sensory and motor as well as postganglionic autonomic fibers (see Figs. 172-1 and 172-2). Interruption of only motor fibers may result from lesions that destroy anterior horn cells, anterior roots, and motor axons in nerves, and sensory denervation can be produced by the destruction of posterior roots, sensory ganglia, and sensory axons in nerves. Since the postganglionic sympathetic fibers arise from the sympathetic ganglia they too can be selectively paralyzed by diseases that strike the lateral horn cells of the spinal cord, the sympathetic ganglion cells, or rami communicantes. The pathogenic agents in certain of the peripheral nerve diseases tend more or less to selectively affect one or another of these systems of motor, sensory, or autonomic nerve cells or their axons.

In complete somatic motor denervation of a limb from loss of anterior horn cells (as in poliomyelitis) there results a flaccid paralysis of muscles which then proceed to undergo severe atrophy (75 to 80 percent of their normal bulk is lost in the first 3 months). The skin is usually cool, pale, and moist, indicating preserved autonomic activity. Dependency and poor venous return due to paralysis may lead to complaint of coldness and to edema of dermal structures; but the change is nonspecific, for hysterical paralysis has the same effect. There is no change in sudomotor, pilomotor, or sebaceous activity, and responses to skin stroking and histamine injection are normal.

With sensory denervation there is a disappearance within a few days of the free nerve endings in the skin and of the plexuses of cells around the hair shafts. However, the specialized endings such as Krause's end bulbs, Ruffinian plumes, and Meissner's and pacinian corpuscles remain in a recognizable form for a long time. Denervation

Fig. 172-1   Distribution of the sensory spinal roots on the surface of the body. (From Holmes G: Introduction to Clinical Neurology. Edinburgh, Livingstone, 1946.)

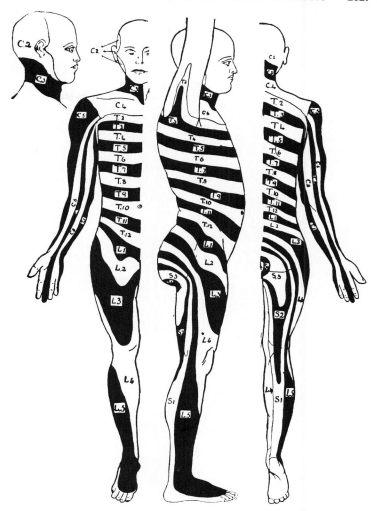

leads to no definite morphologic changes in sweat glands, hairs, blood vessels, or malpighian and other cutaneous cells.

Complete sensory denervation abolishes all forms of sensation (touch, pain, pressure, thermal, postural). Sensory stimuli fail also to evoke spinal segmental reflex effects. After Wallerian degeneration of the sensory nerves has occurred throughout their length, a vigorous stroke of the skin still elicits immediate pallor followed by a red line of dilated capillaries in the center of the pale band. But the two changes are not followed by spreading peripheral rubor, i.e., only part of the normal *triple response* occurs. This latter response depends on the integrity of vasodilator fibers in the sensory nerves and is said to persist as long as the peripheral sensory axons are intact, even though no afferent impulses reach the spinal cord. This is called the *axonal reflex.*

Partial sensory denervation leaves the skin paresthetic and sometimes painful. The equilibrium between patterns of sensory impulses as they act on the posterior horn cells of the spinal cord is disturbed. Impulses no longer arrive in proper temporal sequence to elicit natural common sensations. Slight forms of skin stimulation induce perverted sensory experiences. For example, activation of touch fibers leads to tingling, of pressure fibers to a sense of

tightness, of superficial pain and thermal fibers to prickling, smarting, or burning. In these, and more particularly in the *causalgic* syndrome of burning pain and tactile hyperpathia, the area supplied by the injured nerve may be cool and may sweat profusely or be dry, warm, and glossy, depending on whether structures under autonomic control are hyperactive or paralyzed. The sensitivity may be so severe that simple care of skin and nails is intolerable. Yellowish brown crusts then form in the territory of the nerve due to the accumulation of sebum, sweat, and dirt. The nails grow long and convex and show vertical ridging. Hair growth may increase (?effect of vasodilatation). Since the painful limb is held motionless for long periods of time, the bones lose calcium and become osteoporotic, and the muscles undergo disuse atrophy. This combination is sometimes called *Sudeck's atrophy.*

Ulceration of the denervated skin may occur as a consequence of repeated inadvertent injury, and once an ulcer is formed, the healing seems to be retarded. In the face, ulceration may extend deep into the cartilaginous structure of the nose, and infection of the cornea or entire eye may result from interruption of the first division of the trigeminal nerve. These trophic changes are initiated by trauma but may be self-induced when the patient abrades tissue because of itching and unpleasant paresthesias.

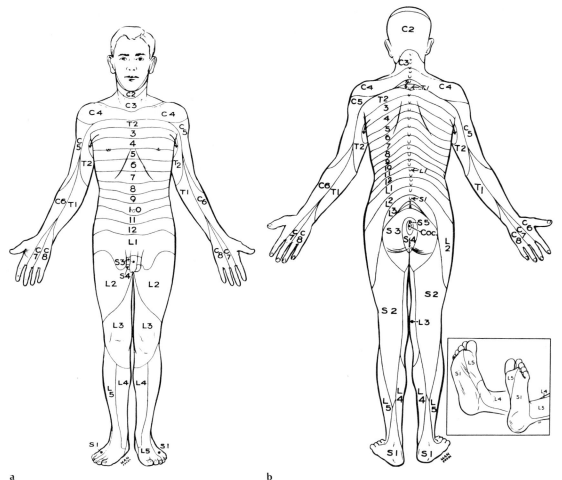

a   b

Fig. 172-2 The cutaneous fields of peripheral nerves. (a) The segmental innervation of the skin from the anterior aspect. The uppermost dermatome adjoins the cutaneous field of the mandibular division of the trigeminal nerve. The arrows indicate the lateral extensions of dermatome 13. (b) The dermatomes from the posterior view. Note the absence of cutaneous innervation by the first cervical segment. Arrows in the axillary regions indicate the lateral extent of dermatome T3; those in the region of the vertebral column point to the first thoracic, the first lumbar, and the first sacral spinous processes. *(From Haymaker W, Woodhall B: Peripheral Nerve Injuries. Philadelphia, WB Saunders, 1945.)*

Lesions of the autonomic nervous system interrupt the innervation of smooth muscles, sweat glands, and pilo-erector muscles. Diseases affecting preganglionic neurons may leave the postganglionic ones untouched and vice versa. Interruption of either the pre- or postganglionic neurons of the sympathetic system cause vasomotor paralysis (rubor and orthostatic hypotension) and anhidrosis (warm and dry skin), but after a time (weeks to months) the effector organs on which postganglionic neurons terminate become hypersensitive to circulating noradrenaline (Cannon-Rosenbleuth phenomenon). As a result, there occur Raynaud's phenomenon and excessive sweating. The tendency for this to happen is less with preganglionic lesions. Even after postganglionic fibers degenerate, the sweat glands and smooth muscles are relatively little changed, though the possibility of atrophy has not been well studied. Sebaceous glands are not influenced by autonomic innervation and any diseases involving them, e.g., seborrheic dermatitis and the greasy skin of Parkinson's disease, are only indirectly related to the nervous system. Probably the

neurologic abnormality interferes with proper skin hygiene. Diseases affecting the parasympathetic nervous system paralyze the pupil and accommodative mechanism of the eye, reduce tearing and salivation, paralyze the bladder and bowel, and cause impotence. Denervation hypersensitivity occurs here as well, at least in structures such as the pupil.

Descriptions of the neurocutaneous diseases

In order to facilitate exposition of the many maladies which possess in common the property of implicating the skin and the nervous system and to offer practical guidance in their recognition, the author has chosen, perhaps out of ignorance of underlying cause and pathogenesis, to present them as four major groups (Table 172-1), according to whether the lesions of skin and nervous system appear to be relatively independent of one another and related to some indefinable common property or whether the lesions of one organ (either skin or nervous system) are dependent upon diseases in the other. This obviously leaves the largest proportion of the diseases in the first category, and these have had to be subdivided further in accordance with current concepts of probable cause and pathogenesis. The author has yielded to tradition on another point as well—that of presenting neurofibromatosis, tuberous sclerosis, and craniocerebral hemangioma, the most familiar examples of neurocutaneous diseases, at the beginning of the chapter.

Diseases with independent, sometimes casually related, lesions in the skin and the nervous system

Congenital and developmental neurocutaneous diseases

Under this heading two major classes of disease have been placed: one in which a dermal abnormality of relatively stationary type is present at, or soon after, birth; the other in which it is inconspicuous at birth but continues to evolve as a series of quasi-neoplastic lesions during the early years of life. The latter, to which the term *phakomatoses* has been inappropriately applied (a term originally given the retinal lesions by van der Hoeve in 1920 [3]—from the Greek word *phakos,* meaning mother spot, mole, or freckle), includes tuberous sclerosis, neurofibromatosis, craniocerebral angiomatosis, and retinocerebellar hemangiomatosis. These diseases have been shown to possess many common features such as hereditary causation, tendency toward the formation of benign tumors or hamartomas, slow evolution of lesions in childhood and adolescence, and in some instances disposition to fatal malignant transformation. Since these are the most familiar of all the neurocutaneous diseases, discussions of them will be given more space than all the others.

The congenital benign neoplasms and vascular malformations. TUBEROUS SCLEROSIS (BOURNEVILLE'S DISEASE)

Definition [4]. Tuberous sclerosis is a congenital disease of manifestly hereditary type in which a variety of lesions arise in the skin, nervous system, heart, kidney, and other organs due to a limited hyperplasia of ectodermal and mesodermal cells. The most frequent clinical manifestations constitute a triad of adenoma sebaceum, epilepsy, and mental retardation.

History. It is stated that Virchow had recognized scleromas of the cerebrum in the 1860s and that von Recklinghausen had reported a similar case combined with multiple myomata of the heart in 1862, but Bourneville's articles, appearing between 1880 and 1900, presented the first systematic account of the disease and related the cerebral lesions to those of the skin of the face. These latter were first described in detail by Balzer and Menetrier in 1885, and by Pringle in 1890. Vogt, in 1908, fully appreciated the significance of the neurocutaneous relationship and formally delineated the classic triad of adenoma sebaceum, epilepsy, and mental retardation [5,6]. *Epiloia,* a term introduced by Sherlock in 1911, specifies the ensemble of convulsions, mental retardation, adenoma sebaceum, and tumors of the brain and other organs, but has never gained acceptance.

Epidemiology. The incidence of the disease is estimated to be approximately 5 to 7 per 100,000. Reports of cases have been forthcoming from all over the world, and there seems to be no difference in frequency among Caucasians, blacks, and Orientals, and the two sexes are affected alike. Hereditary is evident in approximately one-third of reported cases (a dominant autosomal gene of variable penetrance). The remaining cases are attributed to a gene mutation, the frequency of which is calculated at 1 in 20,000 to 1 in 50,000. The disease involves many organs aside from skin and brain and may assume a diversity of forms, the least severe of which, i.e., the forme fruste, is difficult to diagnose; hence, the true incidence cannot be fully ascertained from observations of the usual clinical syndrome. Among the feebleminded in institutions, the frequency ranges from 0.1 to 0.7 percent. Increasing numbers of patients whose mentality is preserved and who have never had convulsions are to be found in the recent medical literature. Probably incidence data drawn from surveys of mental hospital populations have tended to magnify the overall incidence of mental retardation in this disorder [5,7].

Etiology and pathogenesis. The cause of tuberous sclerosis is genetic; only its pathogenesis remains unknown. The chromosomes are morphologically unchanged. As was said earlier, the lesions involve cells derived from ectoderm as well as mesoderm. The cellular elements within the lesions are abnormal with respect to number and size. The tumor-like growths in different organs may include cells of more than one type, e.g., fibroblast and angioblast or glioblast and neuroblast, and their number is locally excessive. Something has gone awry with the proliferative process in embryologic development, yet it is usually kept under control, and only rarely does the growth undergo malignant transformation and metastasize. Highly specialized cells within the lesions may attain giant size; neurons 3 to 4 times normal size may be observed in the cerebral scleroses. These facts emphasize the blastomatous character of the process and suggest that some inhibitory growth factor must be lacking at crucial moments, in embryonic life and later, to account for both the hyperplasia and the hypertrophy of well-differentiated cells, Moolton [8] conceives of the abnormality as a disturbance, at an embryologic level, of cellular differentiation, dependent, so he believes, on the relationship between cell competence for specialization and the amount of an organizer substance which normally provides the inductive stimulus for differentiation. How the trait underlying this disease is genetically transmitted remains a mystery. The focal character of the pathologic process would argue against a systemic metabolic abnormality.

Clinical manifestations. The disease may be present at the time of birth (the diagnosis has been made pathologically in neonatal fatalities), but more often the infant is judged at first to be normal. Attention is initially drawn to the disease by the occurrence of disordered nervous function in the form of focal or generalized seizures or by retarded psychomotor development. As with any condition leading to mental retardation, the first suspicion is raised by evidence of delay in reaching the successive milestones of natural maturation, but whatever the initial symptom, within 2 to 3 years the convulsive disorder and mental retardation become more prominent and are combined. The facial cutaneous abnormality, the so-called adenoma sebaceum, appears later in childhood, usually between the fourth and tenth years, and thereafter progresses.

As the years pass, the seizures, which may at first have been focal, change pattern. In the first year to two they take the form of typical salaam spasms or flexion myoclonus with hypsarrhythmia (irregular dysrhythmic bursts of high-voltage spikes and slow waves in the EEG); later the seizures convert to more typical generalized motor, psychomotor, and at times brief attacks, occasionally petit mal. Mental function continues to deteriorate slowly. Seizures are always the most reliable index of the cerebral lesions, and focal neurologic abnormalities (paraplegia, quadriplegia, hemiplegia, extrapyramidal disorders, or visual field, sensory, and speech defects), such as might be expected from the number and size of the cerebral lesions, are distinctly uncommon. Exceptionally, a spastic weakness or mild choreoathetosis of the limbs becomes manifest, and in a few cases there is associated obstructive hydrocephalus. Caron [9] and van Bogaert et al [10] described cases with cerebellar incoordination, but they are rare in our experience. In Busch and Busch's [11] series of 12 cases, only one had a spastic hemiparesis. Donegani et al [12] comment on the rarity of cerebral diplegia and quadriplegia. Speech development is often delayed but not more so than with other forms of mental retardation.

As in any state of imbecility or idiocy, a variety of nonspecific motor peculiarities and behavioral deviations, such as crying, muttering, rocking and swaying movements and digital mannerisms, may be noted. Characterologic and affective derangements may be added to intellectual deficiency and result in a primary type of psychosis.

The lack of parallelism between the epilepsy, mental deficit, and dermal abnormality has been noted by all experienced clinicians who have access to neurologic patients in general hospitals. Not a few patients are subject to recurrent seizures while retaining relatively normal mental function; in other cases, only a few trivial skin lesions or a retinal phakoma may suggest the diagnosis. In these incomplete forms of disease, diagnosis may elude competent neurologists and dermatologists.

Limitations of space do not allow more than a mere catalog of other visceral abnormalities. Gray or yellow plaques (single or multiple) may be found in the retina, in or near the optic disk or at a distance from it in about 50 percent of cases. It is from this lesion, called *phakoma,* meaning mother spot, that van der Hoeve derived the term sometimes applied to all neurocutaneous diseases of this class. Benign rhabdomyomas of the heart have a linkage with tuberous sclerosis (50 percent of all recorded cases are associated with this disease), and other benign tumors have been found in the kidneys (hamartomas of mixed cell type), liver, thyroid, testes, and gastrointestinal tract. Cysts of pleura and lungs, bone cysts in digits, zones of marbling or densification in bones complete the picture.

In approximately 85 percent of the patients with tuberous sclerosis congenital white macules are present (Figs. A8-7 and A8-8). These lesions, called hypomelanotic macules (formerly partial albinism or vitiligo), appear before any of the other skin lesions and have unique clinical and histologic features [13]. They are located in the skin over the trunk or limbs and range in size from a few millimeters to several centimeters; their orientation is often linear, the configuration being oval with one end round and the other

pointed in the shape of an ash leaf. They vary in number from a few to 75 or more (Figs. 172-3 to 172-5).

A Wood's lamp which emits light waves of 360 nm facilitates the demonstration of these lesions; the visualization is improved because the melanin absorbs most of the light waves of this frequency, thereby exposing areas deficient in melanin. Close examination of the skin shows no alteration of skin markings; the vascular responses to stroking appear to be normal, and there is no change in sensation or sweating. Unlike vitiligo they are seldom completely devoid of pigment, and the presence of a vascular response to cold distinguishes them from nevus anemicus, the two lesions with which they may be confused. Poliosis of scalp hair and eyelashes may also be noted. Although recognized long ago, Gold and Freeman [14] and Fitzpatrick et al [13] have more recently emphasized their frequency and their value in the diagnosis of tuberous sclerosis during infancy before the other cutaneous lesions of this disease appear (see Chap. 79).

The well-developed facial lesions, pathognomonic of tuberous sclerosis, are present in 90 percent of patients over 4 years of age [5,6,15]. Although called *adenoma sebaceum,* these tumors are actually angiofibromas; the sebaceous glands are only passively involved. Typically they are red to pink nodules with a smooth, glistening surface, localized to the nasolabial folds, cheeks, chin, and sometimes the forehead and scalp (see Fig. 172-6a). The earliest manifestation of facial angiofibromatosis may be a mild erythema over cheeks and forehead, which is intensified by crying. The occurrence of large plaques of connective tissue on the forehead is usually expressive of an especially severe form of the disease (Fig. 172-6b).

A characteristic lesion that appears on the trunk is the shagreen patch (described first by Hallspean and Leredde in 1895) found most often in the lumbosacral region (Fig. A8-8C). It appears most often as a flat, slightly elevated area of skin with a "pigskin," "elephant hide," or "orange peel" appearance. Such areas, which are in reality plaques of subepidermal fibrosis, usually retain a flesh color; they vary from less than 1 cm in diameter to the size of the palm.

Another common site of fibromatous involvement is the nail bed. In some patients extensive subungual fibromas disrupt the entire nail bed. They usually appear at puberty and continue to develop with age. Gingival fibromas also occur.

Other skin changes seen not infrequently, but not in themselves diagnostic, include fibroepithelial tags (soft fibromas), café au lait spots, and port-wine hemangiomas.

Pathology. Grossly, the brain exhibits a number of anomalies of structure that are at once diagnostic. Broadening, unnatural whiteness, and firmness of parts of some of the cerebral convolutions are simulated by no other disease. These are the "tubers" after which the disease is named. They range from 5 mm up to 2 or 3 cm in surface diameter, and their cut surface reveals a lack of demarcation of gray cortex from white matter and the presence of white flecks of calcium salts, the latter often visible in x-rays of skull and called *brain stones.* The floors of the lateral ventricles may be encrusted with white or pinkish white masses resembling the gutterings of a candle. When calcified, they appear in radiographs as curvilinear opacities which follow the outline of the ventricle. Nodules of

Fig. 172-3 (a) Numerous "ash-leaf" spots in mother and son with tuberous sclerosis. Also notice the diffuse 1- to 2-mm hypomelanotic macules on the legs. These are highly characteristic of tuberous sclerosis. (b) Typical lance-ovate hypomelanotic macule. Note also the shagreen patch above and slightly to the right.

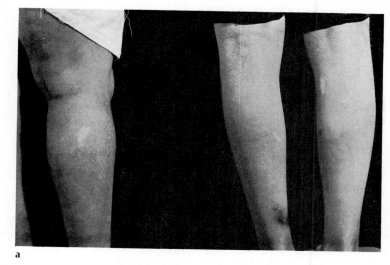

a

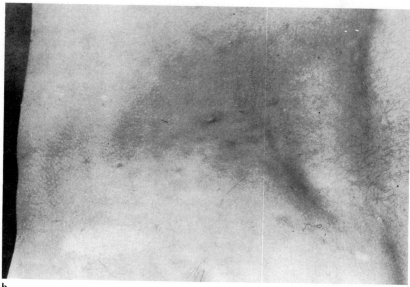

b

abnormal tissue are observed but rarely in the basal ganglia, thalamus, cerebellum, brain-stem, and spinal cord.

Under the microscope the whitish tubers are most often seen to be composed of interlacing rows of plump fibrous astrocytes (much like an astrocytoma). Derangements of cortical architecture result from abnormal-appearing glial cells. Monstrous neurons and glial cells, often difficult to distinguish, and displaced normal-sized neurons contribute to the chaotic histologic appearance of cerebral cortex and ganglionic structures. Gliomatous deposits may block the aqueduct or floor of the fourth ventricle causing the obstructive hydrocephalus. Neoplastic transformation of abnormal glial cells is a not infrequent occurrence and usually takes the form of a large-cell astrocytoma, but glioblastomas and even meningiomas may develop.

The phakomas of the retina are composed mainly of neuronal and glial components, but occasionally there is an admixture of fibrous tissue.

The microscopic changes of the various skin lesions are essentially of interlacing strands of fibroblasts and collagen

with numerous blood vessels, to which the name hamartoma has been given. A better name for the facial lesion would be angiofibroma. The ungual lesions present also the characteristics of an angiofibroma. The shagreen plaque is composed of a relatively avascular, dense, sclerotic mass of bundles of collagen fibers. In the white macules, there appears to be a reduction in the tyrosinase activity of the melanocytes compared to the normal pigmented skin surrounding the white macules (Fig. A8-11). Electron microscope studies have confirmed the findings of light microscopy, that melanocytes are present in the usual number but contain few melanosomes. This is in direct contrast to vitiligo, in which there is an absence of identifiable melanocytes. Thus it is not correct to speak of the white macules present in tuberous sclerosis as "vitiligo."

Diagnosis and differential diagnosis. When the full combination of mental, convulsive, and dermal abnormalities are conjoined, the diagnosis is self-evident. It is the early stages of the disease and the more common forme fruste

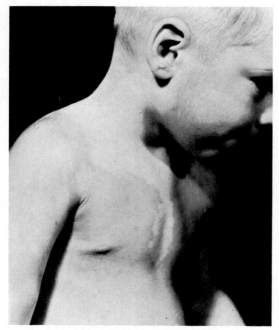

Fig. 172-4 **Dermatomal hypomelanosis in tuberous sclerosis.**

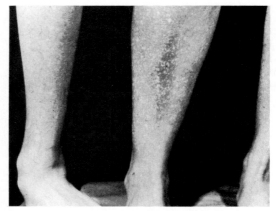

Fig. 172-5 **Confetti-like hypomelanosis in mother and son with tuberous sclerosis.**

that give trouble, and here the experienced dermatologist can be of the greatest help to the neurologist. Epilepsy, i.e., flexion spasms in infancy, and delay in psychomotor development are by no means diagnostic of tuberous sclerosis, since they occur in many diseases. It is in these cases and also in every sizable population of the epileptic or mentally retarded, especially when the family history is unrevealing, that a search for the dermal equivalents of the disease—hypomelanotic nevus, the adenoma sebaceum, the collagenous patch, the phakoma of retina, or subungual or gingival fibroma—is so rewarding. The finding of any one of these lesions provides confirmation of the partial and atypical case. Adenoma sebaceum is easily confused with acne vulgaris in the adolescent and may occasionally occur alone. The elicitation of a history of epilepsy and/or the demonstration of a dull mentality is helpful but not necessary for the diagnosis of tuberous sclerosis [7]. X-ray of the skull, a search for multiple calcific densities within the brain and localized patches of hyperosteosis on the inner surface of skull, CT scan to show ventricular deformity and tumor deposits along the striothalamic borders, and electroencephalography are useful laboratory measures for corroborating the neurologic features of the disease.

Treatment. Nothing can be offered in the way of prevention other than counsel against childbearing by affected individuals whose children may be more severely affected than they. The medical profession does not possess the means of halting the slow march of the disease once it has begun. Anticonvulsant therapy of the standard types (phenobarbital, Dilantin, etc.) suppresses the convulsive tendency more or less effectively in many patients and should be applied assiduously. ACTH is recommended for infantile spasms and hypsarrhythmia (mountainous slow waves in the EEG). It is rather pointless to attempt to excise tumors, especially in individuals who are severely affected. The main indications for neurosurgery are intra-

cranial hypertension and hydrocephalus. In a few instances excision of an epileptogenic focus has been beneficial. Radiotherapy is indicated for malignant neoplasms. However, there are many patients not mentally deficient who can be benefited by dermabrasion of their facial lesions, with the knowledge that they will slowly regrow.

Course and prognosis. In general, the disease progresses so slowly that years must elapse before one is sure of the advancing course. Of the severe cases, approximately 30 percent die before the fifth year and 50 to 75 percent before attaining adult age. Worsening is mainly in the mental sphere. Status epilepticus accounted for many deaths in the past, but improved anticonvulsant therapy has reduced this hazard. Neoplasias take their toll, and several such patients who died of malignant gliomas arising in striothalamic zones have been seen [7].

NEUROFIBROMATOSIS OF VON RECKLINGHAUSEN. *Definition.* Neurofibromatosis is a comparatively uncommon hereditary disease in which the skin, nervous system, bones, endocrine glands, and sometimes other organs are the sites of a variety of congenital abnormalities, tumors, and hamartomas. The typical clinical picture, usually identifiable at a glance, consists of multiple circumscript areas of increased skin pigmentation accompanied by dermal and neural tumors of various sizes and shapes.

History. The condition known as multiple idiopathic neuroma was the subject of a monograph by R. W. Smith in 1849, and even at that time he referred to examples of the same disease previously recorded by other writers. But it was von Recklinghausen who, in 1882, gave the definitive account of its clinical and pathologic features and who deserves the credit for its complete identification as a nosologic entity. The monograph of Alexis Thomsen, which appeared in 1900, contains useful statistical data on a large series of cases and a full bibliography. The report of Crowe et al [16] provides the most complete analysis of the genetic data. A more recent review of the subject has been written by Canale and Bebin [17].

Incidence and epidemiology. Neel and his associates in the Institute of Human Biology at the University of Michigan calculate the frequency of the disease to be 30 to 40 per 100,000 and expect one case of it in every 2500 to 3300 births. Approximately half of their cases have affected relatives, and in all instances the distribution of cases

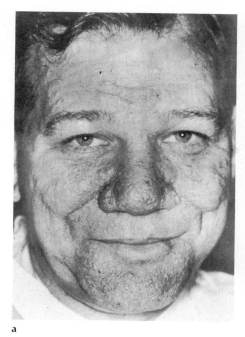 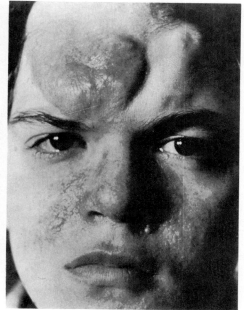

a   b

Fig. 172-6   Tuberous sclerosis with adenoma sebaceum.

within a family is consistent with autosomal dominant type of inheritance. They advance evidence of a mutation to the dominant gene in the remaining sporadic cases. The disease has been observed in all races in different parts of the world, and males appear to be affected somewhat more frequently than females.

Cause and pathogenesis. The cause has been established; it is the result of the action of an abnormal gene. Its location in the human karyotype of chromosomes remains unknown. Chromosome counts and morphology do not deviate from normal. The pathogenesis remains obscure. Cellular elements derived from neural crest, i.e., Schwann cells, melanocytes, and possibly endoneurial fibroblasts, the natural components of skin and nerves, multiply excessively in multiple foci, and the melanocytes function abnormally, but the time when this begins and the mechanism of it are as unclear as in tuberous sclerosis.

Clinical manifestations. In the majority of patients, spots of hyperpigmentation and cutaneous and subcutaneous tumors are the basis of clinical diagnosis. These appear in increasing numbers during late childhood and adolescence. Exceptionally, a neurofibroma of a spinal or cranial nerve root, disclosed during neurosurgical intervention, may be the initial manifestation of the disease. In the study of a large series of cases of neurofibromatosis, approximately one-third of the patients were discovered to have the cutaneous manifestations of the disease while being examined because of symptoms relating to some other disease; that is to say, the neurofibromatosis was asymptomatic and incidental. Of the remainder, many consulted a physician because of the cosmetic problem produced by the tumors or for the reason that some of the neurofibromas were producing symptoms. Seldom are the more peripheral tumors of nerve or skin painful or distressing.

Canale et al [18] noted that in the cases in which neurologic symptoms had led to hospital admission, numbering

one-third of their series of 92, the offending tumor in most instances was central. Typical syndromes were traced most often to unilateral or bilateral tumors of the eighth cranial nerve (nerve deafness, dizziness, headache, and staggering), trigeminal neuromas (facial pain and numbness), jugular foramen syndrome of IX, X, XI cranial nerves (vocal cord paralysis, dysphagia, paralysis of sternomastoid and trapezius muscles), hypoglossal nerve tumor (weakness and hemiatrophy of tongue), optic nerve gliomas (progressive monocular blindness and sometimes proptosis), other cranial nerve involvement, spinal root tumors with or without compression of the spinal cord, and multiple cranial or spinal meningiomas.

Mental deficiency, seizures, precocious puberty, and obscure pain were observed in a syndrome described by Yakovlev and Guthrie [19]. Mental retardation, ascribed to heterotopias of cerebral neurons [20], occurs in an estimated 7 to 8 percent of patients with neurofibromatosis but is usually not profound. Of mentally retarded epileptics in institutions, approximately 10 percent are said to have cutaneous manifestations of the disease. The mental retardation may become evident before the skin lesions.

Convulsions are far less frequent than in tuberous sclerosis and have been correlated by Yakovlev and Guthrie [19] and Canale et al [18] with heterotopias of glial and neural elements, hamartomas, and (rarely) glial tumors of the cerebrum. The seizures may be generalized or focal.

Precocious puberty in a child, like optic nerve astrocytoma, should always raise suspicion of neurofibromatosis. Both boys and girls have been seen with this condition, beginning at the age of 5 or 6 years. In several well-studied cases small hamartomas composed of abnormally situated neurons and glial cells have been found in the tuberal part of the hypothalamus. Urinary gonadotropin is elevated in some cases.

Concerning the dermatologic feature of the disease,

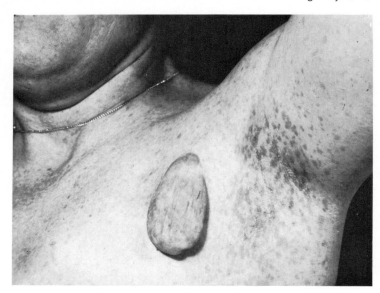

Fig. 172-7 Axillary freckle-like pigmentation in neurofibromatosis.

patches of cutaneous pigmentation, appearing shortly after birth and occurring any place on the body, constitute the most striking clinical expression (Fig. A8-20). They vary in size from a millimeter or two to many centimeters and in color from a light to dark brown (café au lait) and are rarely associated with any other pathologic state. In a survey of pigmented spots in the skin, Neel and his associates found that 10 percent of the normal population had one or more lesions of this type, but any patient with more than six spots exceeding 1.5 cm in diameter nearly always proved to have von Recklinghausen's disease. Of their 223 patients with neurofibromatosis, 95 percent had at least one spot, and no less than 78 percent had more than six large ones. Freckle-like or diffuse pigmentation of the axillae is characteristic and almost a pathognomonic feature of the syndrome (Fig. 172-7) [21].

Multiple cutaneous tumors stand as the other principal dermatologic manifestation of the disease. These appear in late childhood or early adolescence and may be divided into two groups, according to their location: (1) cutaneous, and (2) subcutaneous. The cutaneous tumor is situated in the dermis or next to it and forms a discrete, soft or firm papule (often called molluscum fibrosum because of its soft character—the Latin *molluscus* meaning soft). It varies in size from a few millimeters to a centimeter or more. In shape it may assume many forms—flattened, sessile, pedunculated, conical, lobulate, etc. It tends to be flesh-colored or violaceous and often has a comedo at its top. When pressed, the soft tumors tend to invaginate through a small opening in the skin, giving the feeling of a seedless raisin or a scrotum without a testicle. Crowe et al [16] speak of this phenomenon as "button-holing" and find it a most useful sign in distinguishing the lesions of this disease from other tumors, e.g., multiple lipomas. The number of dermal tumors in any given patient may range from a few to as many as 9000 (Fig.172-8). Probably every case of von Recklinghausen's disease has at least a few of them. The subcutaneous tumors, which are also multiple, take two forms: (1) firm, discrete nodules, often attached to a nerve, or (2) a great overgrowth of subcutaneous tissue sometimes reaching enormous size *(le tumeur royale)* (Fig. 172-9). The latter occur most often in the face, cranium,

neck, and chest and may cause hideous disfigurement. When palpated, these growths, which are called *plexiform neuromas,* also *pachydermatocele* or *elephantiasis neurofibromatosa,* feel like a bag of worms or strings. The underlying bone may enlarge. Nerve tumors (most frequent on ulnar and radial) may cause pain, muscle weakness, atrophy, and slight sensory loss. In the author's experience, they are less frequent than tumors of spinal and cranial nerve roots.

Other skin lesions such as multiple pigmented nevi and cutis laxa, similar to the skin in Ehlers-Danlos disease, have been reported, but it is doubtful whether they have any meaningful association with neurofibromatosis.

Bony skeletal abnormalities also occur with regularity and several of them have neurologic implications. In the Mayo Clinic series of Hunt and Pugh [22] a radiologic abnormality of bone was found in nearly 40 percent of their cases. Kyphoscoliosis is one of the most frequent, and the deformity may reach such a sharp angularity as to compromise the spinal cord. It is due not to the paralytic effects of spinal neurons but to dysgenesis of vertebral bodies. Intrathoracic meningocele is another associated abnormality; usually it is asymptomatic, but it must at times be distinguished from a symptomatic dumbbell tumor. The most diagnostically puzzling cranial abnormality is a defect in the posterior wall of the orbit, resulting in a pulsating exophthalmos. One may mistake this condition for an orbital tumor.

The other clinical features of neurofibromatosis are bone cysts, pathologic fractures, bone hypertrophy, pheochromocytoma, syringomyelia, nodules or abnormal glial cells in brain and spinal cord, ependymomas of spinal cord, obstructive hydrocephalus due to overgrowth of glial tissue, and malignant astrocytoma.

A separate but closely related syndrome in which multiple, large zones of macular pigmentation are combined with bone cysts and precocious puberty has been described by Albright (see Chap. 79).

Pathology. The cutaneous tumors which correspond clinically to the violaceous papule are characteristic. Beneath the rather thin epidermis whose basal layer may or may not be pigmented, the collagen and elastin of dermis

Fig. 172-8   Multiple cutaneous tumors in neurofibromatosis.

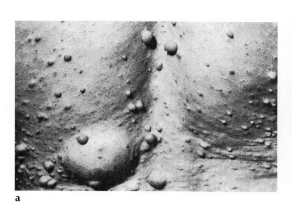

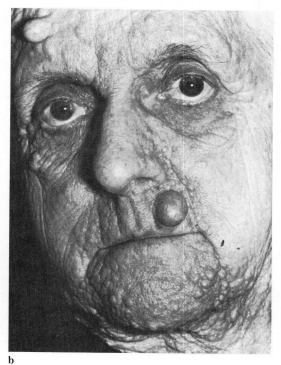

a

b

is replaced by a bluish gray gelatinous-appearing connective tissue. Under the microscope, that cutaneous tumor consists of a loose arrangement of elongated connective tissue cells. It lacks the support of the normal dermal collagen, which accounts for the palpable opening in the skin. The endoneurial fibroblasts are distinguished from the fibroblasts of a typical fibroblastoma only by their tendency to palisade and by the presence of axis cylinders among them. The accumulation of collagen within the tumor suggests that some of the cells are indeed fibroblasts. Mast cells are frequent.

The macular pigmented lesions contain only the normal numbers of melanocytes and the darkness of skin is due to an excess of melanosomes in the malpighian cells. Abnormally large melanosomes, measuring up to several microns in diameter, appear in some of the basal cells of the epidermis (Fig. A8-22) (see Chap. 79). Benedict et al [23], who first described these giant melanosomes, report that they do not occur in the closely related syndrome of Albright.

The nerve tumors are also composed of a mixture of fibroblasts and Schwann cells, except the optic nerve tumors, which contain a combination of astrocytes and fibroblasts. Occasionally one may find a tumor made up of partially or completely differentiated nerve cells (a typical ganglioneuroma). Special arrangements of cells (palisading of nuclei, tightly arranged whorls or Verocay bodies, and loose networks of vacuolated cells) differentiate the schwannoma from a fibroblastoma. Clusters of abnormal glial cells may be found in the brain and spinal cord and, according to Bielschowsky [24], form the link with tuberous sclerosis. Clinically, however, the two diseases seem to be relatively independent.

There has been an endless debate concerning the cellular origin of these nerve tumors, whether from Schwann cells, endoneurial or perineurial fibroblasts. All cell types are

found. Some pathologists insist that the main cell type is the precursor of the Schwann cell and that the fibroblast is only a reactive interstitial element. I agree with Rubinstein [25] that, in practice, the terms schwannoma, neu-

Fig. 172-9   Enormous plexiform neuromas.

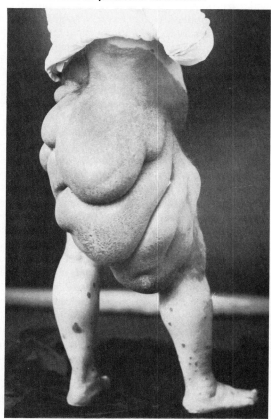

rofibroma, and neurilemmoma all refer to the same tumor and that there is no real difference among them.

Malignant degeneration of the tumors is found in 2 to 5 percent of cases; peripherally they become sarcomas and centrally, astrocytomas or glioblastomas. Meningiomas are also frequent.

Diagnosis and differential diagnosis. The cardinal features of the disease are the skin tumors and café au lait spots; if these are numerous, the identification of the disease occasions no difficulty. Positive family history in antecedent and collateral members makes recognition even more certain. Difficulty arises most often in cases of bilateral acoustic or other cranial or spinal neurofibromas (schwannomas) with only a few scattered skin lesions. This tendency for the central forms of neurofibromatosis to be accompanied by fewer skin lesions is well recognized. Plexiform neuromas with muscle weakness due to nerve involvement and abnormalities of underlying bone may be confused with other tumors, especially in children who, at a young age, tend always to have fewer café au lait spots and discrete cutaneous tumors. Enormous hypertrophy of a limb, which may occur, requires differentiation from other developmental anomalies.

Crowe and associates [16] believe that 80 percent of all patients with von Recklinghausen's neurofibromatosis can be diagnosed by the presence of more than six café au lait spots. Of the remaining 20 percent, those over 21 years of age will usually be found to have multiple cutaneous tumors and a few pigmented spots; those under 21, with no dermal tumors and but few café au lait spots, will be the most difficult. In these latter, a positive family history and x-ray demonstration of bone cysts will be helpful in some instances. Collateral evidence of feeblemindedness, precocious puberty, signs of involvement of cranial nerves (acoustic neuroma or optic glioma) and/or spinal nerves, centrally or peripherally, the latter with plexiform neuroma, aid the dermatologist in interpreting the skin lesions if they are otherwise unimpressive. The finding of a few café au lait spots and typical cutaneous tumors may help the neurologist diagnose a progressive spinal syndrome, a cerebellopontine angle syndrome, bilateral deafness, an optic nerve or chiasmal astrocytoma, precocious puberty, hydrocephalus, or mental retardation.

Treatment. The skin tumors should not be excised unless they are cosmetically objectionable or show suspicious increase in size suggesting malignant change. Response of the benign lesions to x-ray has been too feeble to justify the risk of heavy exposure. Plexiform neuromas about the face offer difficult problems. Here one must resort to plastic surgery, but the results are not always satisfactory, because the growths may involve cranial nerves superficially (with risk of greater paralysis after surgical excision) or alter the underlying bone, the latter being either eroded from pressure or hypertrophied from increased blood supply. Cranial and spinal neurofibromas are amenable to corrective surgical treatment, and the gliomas and meningiomas usually demand partial or complete extirpation once intracranial pressure is increased. The techniques of computerized axial tomography (CT scan), pneumoencephalography, arteriography, and radioactive isotope localization assist in localization.

Course and prognosis. The principal cutaneous lesions are rarely present at birth. Instead they appear with increasing prominence during childhood and adolescence. The mortality rate is higher than in nonaffected individuals, owing principally to malignant degeneration, usually during adult life, and to involvement of the central nervous system. Affected individuals should be advised not to have children, a precaution that is not always necessary, for their fertility seems to be reduced by the disease, especially that of the males.

CUTANEOUS ANGIOMATOSIS WITH ABNORMALITIES OF THE CENTRAL NERVOUS SYSTEM. There are six diseases in which a cutaneous vascular anomaly is associated with an abnormality of the nervous system: (1) craniofacial, or trigeminocranial, angiomatosis with cerebral calcification (Sturge-Weber-Dimitri syndrome); (2) dermatomal hemangiomas with spinal vascular malformations (sometimes with limb hypertrophy as in Klippel-Trénauney-Weber syndrome); (3) hemangioblastoma of cerebellum and retina (Lindau-von Hippel disease); (4) familial telangiectasia (Osler-Rendu-Weber disease; (5) ataxia-telangiectasia (Louis-Bar disease; (6) angiokeratosis corporis diffusum (Fabry's disease).

Craniofacial, or trigeminocranial, angiomatosis with cerebral calcification (Sturge-Weber-Dimitri disease). In this condition an extensive vascular nevus (port-wine stain, nevus flammeus) is observed at birth to cover a large part of the face and cranium on one side (in the territory of the ophthalmic division of the trigeminal nerve. The extent of it varies from a lesion involving only the upper eyelid to one covering the entire head and even other parts of the body (Fig. 172-10). The nevus is deep red, and its margins may be raised or flat; soft or firm papules, evidently composed of vessels, cause surface elevations and irregularities. The orbital tissue may be involved, (choroidal an-

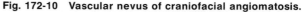

Fig. 172-10 Vascular nevus of craniofacial angiomatosis.

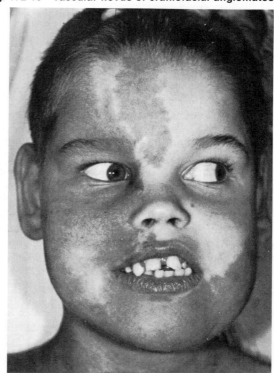

gioma) and congenital glaucoma (buphthalmos) may develop later in the eye on that side, accounting for blindness. The increased cutaneous vascularity may result in overgrowth of connective tissue and underlying bone, giving rise to a deformity similar to that of the Klippel-Trénauney-Weber syndrome. Indications of cerebral involvement appear later in childhood; the most frequent clinical manifestations are spastic hemiparesis with smallness of arm and leg, focal or unilateral seizures, hemisensory defects, and homonymous hemianopia, all on the side contralateral to the trigeminal nevus. X-rays of the skull, usually negative soon after birth, some years later reveal a characteristic "tram-line calcification" which outlines the convolutions of the parietooccipital cortex.

Parkes Weber was one of the first to show the association of cerebral lesion with the facial angioma, and Krabbe demonstrated that the calcification lay in the second and third layers of the cortex, which were gliotic, and not in the large numbers of surface veins and arteries in the meninges. The cortical lesion appears to be progressive and is thought to be caused by hypoxia and ischemia from the meningeal vascular malformation.

It must not be thought, however, that all cranial hemangiomas affect the cerebrum. Facial vascular nevi may occur without brain involvement, and, rarely, a cerebral meningeal angiomatosis of this type may be present without skin lesions. When the nevus lies entirely below the ophthalmic division, i.e., below the upper eyelid and nose, the cerebral lesions are usually absent, although in a few instances a hemangioma at the base of the skull and lower face has been associated with a vascular malformation of meninges overlying the brainstem and cerebellum. While of congenital origin, the cause and pathogenesis are unknown. Alexander and Norman [26] postulate a persistence of the primordial vascular plexus of the embryonal period of life. Familial coincidence has been observed but is exceptional. The chromosomes appear to be normal. The magnitude of the lesion usually contraindicates a neurosurgical approach even when the epilepsy is recalcitrant to anticonvulsant therapy. However, Alexander and Norman [26] report favorable results from surgical resection of the pathologic lobe of the brain early in the course of the disease. X-ray therapy of the facial nevus offers no hope of reducing the unsightly skin blemish, and sensitive patients usually try to hide it with cosmetics.

Dermatomal hemangiomas with spinal vascular malformations (sometimes with limb hypertrophy as in Klippel-Trénauney-Weber syndrome). Hemangiomas of the spinal cord may rarely be accompanied by vascular nevi in the corresponding dermatome of skin, as was pointed out by Cobb [27]. These lesions differ in no important way from the cranial hemangiomas and, like them, tend to conform to a dermatomal pattern. They are, as a rule, unilateral and are most frequent in the arm and trunk. When the cutaneous lesion involves an arm or leg, there may be enlargement of the entire limb or of fingers in combination with underdevelopment of certain parts (Klippel-Trénauney-Weber syndrome).

Among the dermatomal malformations should also be included that described by van Bogaert [28]. The clinical and pathologic features of this syndrome are angiomatosis of the skin in association with diffuse meningocortical angiomatosis. The neurologic expression is mental de-

fect, hemianopia, epilepsy, and both pyramidal and extrapyramidal disorders. The congenital poikiloderma of the skin is attributed to the cutaneous vascular abnormality. Also Brégeat [29] has described an oculoorbital angiomatosis with a thalamoencephalic involvement and a cutaneous angioma. It is manifested clinically by a nonpulsatile exophthalmos, photophobia, headaches, and mental retardation. Ulman's name is attached to a syndrome of cutaneous angiomatosis with similar lesions in the central nervous system and viscera [30].

Also a congenital angiomatous malformation, affecting the eye and upper brainstem (diencephalon), has been described by Bonnet et al [31]. The retinal lesion, a cirsoid aneurysm, is conjoined to an arteriovenous malformation of the thalamus. There may be a cutaneous facial telangiectasia, sometimes extending to the mucous membranes. Hemianopia, oculomotor palsy with contralateral pyramidal signs, and other cranial nerve palsies occur when the vascular malformation bleeds. The condition is thought to be related to the disease of Sturge-Weber and of von Hippel-Lindau (see below).

Hemangioblastoma of cerebellum and retina (Lindau-von Hippel syndrome). This condition, often affecting two or more successive generations of a family, consists of a benign cerebellar tumor composed of a mass of capillaries surrounded by a cyst. The vascular nodule and its cyst slowly increase in size during childhood and adolescence and produce a cerebellar syndrome with increased intracranial pressure. One or both retinas may be the site of a tangle of small vessels, visible some distance from the optic disk, as was first pointed out by von Hippel. These retinal angiomas may lead to blindness through retinal detachment or proliferation and hemorrhage; later they may calcify. Familial incidence has been recorded many times, the transmission being as an autosomal dominant trait. Lindau, who studied the pathology of all benign cerebellar cysts, noted the frequent association of the cerebellar tumor with cysts of pancreas, angiomas of liver, and hypernephromas of the kidney. The cerebellar tumor was later shown to sometimes elaborate an erythropoietic-like substance, which accounts for an accompanying polycythemia.

The majority of cases of Lindau's disease have no retinal lesions (retinal angiomas are found in only about 20 percent of cases) and are without cutaneous vascular nevi. The latter may be present, however, as was pointed out by Hall [32], and tend to be localized to the occipitocervical region. These cases appear to provide the link between this disease and the Sturge-Weber-Dimitri syndrome.

Familial telangiectasia (Osler-Rendu-Weber disease). This, a vascular anomaly transmitted as a simple dominant trait, affects the skin, the mucous membranes, the gastrointestinal and genitourinary tracts, and occasionally the nervous system (see Chap. 168). The basic lesion is probably a defect in the vessel walls, analogous in some respects to Fabry's angiokeratoma corporis diffusum, in which a hereditary defect in ceramide metabolism has been found. The lesions range from the size of a pinhead to 3 mm or more, are of bright red or violaceous color, and blanch under pressure. Some of them form small vascular papules 2 to 3 mm in diameter. Located sparsely in the skin of any part of the body, they first appear during childhood, enlarge during adolescence, and may assume spidery forms resembling, in late adult life, the cutaneous telan-

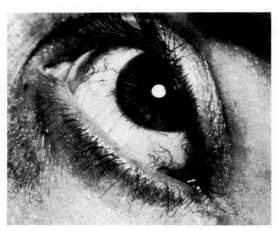

Fig. 172-11   Conjunctival telangiectases in ataxia-telangiectasia.

giectases of cirrhosis. The lesions cause trouble only because of their hemorrhagic tendency. During adult years they may give rise to severe and repeated epistaxis or gastric or intestinal or urinary tract hemorrhages. Chronic blood loss may result in an iron-deficiency anemia.

The angiomas of this disease form in either the spinal cord or brain and here can produce apoplectic syndromes; or an intermittently progressive cerebral syndrome may result from a succession of small hemorrhages. Diagnosis of an unexplained gastrointestinal, genitourinary, intracranial, or intraspinal hemorrhage warrants a search for these small cutaneous lesions, which are easily overlooked. Pulmonary fistulas constitute another important feature of the generalized vascular dysplasia. Such patients are peculiarly subject to brain abscesses. The treatment may require the application of oxidized cellulose (Oxycel or Gelfoam). While cautery eradicates a bleeding lesion, satellite ones tend to re-form. Prophylaxis has proved to be unsatisfactory.

Ataxia-telangiectasia (Louis-Bar disease). This hereditary disease, first described by Syllaba and Henner in 1926 [33], takes the form of oculocutaneous telangiectases com-

bined with cerebellar ataxia, choreoathetosis, and recurrent pulmonary infections with bronchiectasis. The recurrent respiratory infections are presumably related to an associated hypoglobulinemia (immune globulin A and possibly others) resulting from hypoplasia of the thymus. The pattern of inheritance is autosomal recessive. Ataxia of voluntary movements, often with choreathetosis, is the initial symptom, recognizable as a rule during early childhood long before the skin and conjunctival abnormalities become evident. Once fully developed, the syndrome includes slow, dysarthric speech, nystagmus, occasionally myoclonic jerks of the limbs, difficulty in maintaining ocular deviation from the central position, and poor voluntary control of eye movements (apraxia of gaze). Tendon reflexes are diminished or absent; intelligence may deteriorate as the disease advances; growth is retarded.

The telangiectases of conjunctivae consist of numerous tortuous vessels which issue from the canthal regions and fan out over the eyeball (Fig. 172-11); the lower tarsal conjunctiva is also involved. Similar traceries of fine vessels are observed inside the helix and over the backs of the ears, on the sides of the neck, and sometimes in a butterfly area over the face, in the cubital and popliteal fossae (Fig. 172-12), and dorsa of hands and feet. The pattern of telangiectasia appears in some patients to conform to the areas of greatest exposure to sunlight. In time the skin becomes tight and inelastic (patients are hidebound) like that of scleroderma. The hair and skin tend to be dry and coarse with gray hair appearing in some patients.

In a study of 22 patients, café au lait spots were also observed in four and areas of hypopigmentation in eight. Several examples of cutaneous malignancy developed after the age of 21. Also, resistance to skin and pulmonary infections (bacterial, viral, fungal) is reduced. Typical atopic dermatitis was noted in two patients and nummular eczema in another.

Autopsy findings indicate that more than half the patients die from pulmonary disease, while most of the remainder succumb to lymphoreticular malignant tumors. The thymus is absent or hypoplastic, and the spleen may be reduced

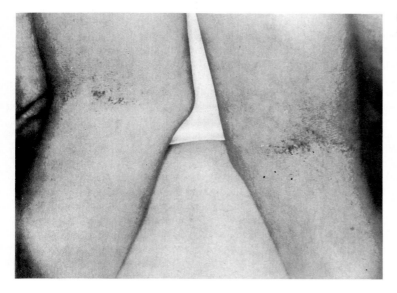

Fig. 172-12   Telangiectases in the cubital fossae in ataxia-telangiectasia.

in size. The significant pathologic abnormalities in the central nervous system are severe degeneration in the cerebellar cortex, loss of myelinated fibers in the posterior columns, and degenerative cell changes in the posterior root and sympathetic ganglia [34].

Neurocutaneous neurolipomatosis. As a general rule one or a few subcutaneous lipomas have no neurologic significance. However, lipomas of the brain do occasionally occur and there are instances in which they are conjoined to facial, axial, visceral, and skull lipomatosis, as described by Scherrer et al [35] and van Bogaert [36]. Also Krabbe and Bartels [37] have written a monograph on the subject of multiple cutaneous painless lipomas associated with pigmented skin nevi, cutaneous fibromas, mental retardation, neuropathy, and cerebellar atrophy. I have never observed such cases. Not to be confused with lipomas are the nodules of subcutaneous fat which may be extremely sensitive as in Dercum's so-called lipodystrophy.

PATHOGENESIS OF THE PHAKOMATOSES. Common to all the diseases described above is a genetic etiology. They appear to be caused by an abnormal gene with pleiotropic potentialities, i.e., capable of affecting the development of several tissues and organs simultaneously. The hereditary patterns are usually autosomal with regular or variable penetrance. The abnormal gene either acts directly on embryonic germinal layers or interferes with induction of the primary organization centers or multiple secondary ones. The variable manifestations of the phakomatoses appear to be determined by three factors: (1) specific affinity of the abnormal gene for a particular germinal layer and its derivatives; (2) the period of embryonic development when the gene intervenes; (3) the period of teratogenic sensitivity of multiple embryonic derivatives which are simultaneously damaged [30].

Developmental neurocutaneous diseases (developmental anomalies of skin and nervous system). Of the various so-called classic neurocutaneous diseases thus far discussed, only the Sturge-Weber-Dimitri craniofacial angioma and possibly the hypomelanotic nevus of tuberous sclerosis are present at birth or during the first days of infancy. In contrast, many of the other congenital neurocutaneous diseases in this group are apparent at, or soon after, birth and, like the neurologic disorders with which they are associated, tend to remain more or less stationary through life.

Since in this category of neurocutaneous diseases the dermal abnormality attracts notice at birth or soon thereafter, the dermatologist may be called to the nursery to assist in its interpretation long before the symptoms and signs of nervous disease become evident. Dermatologic diagnosis, if accurate, may serve, therefore, to warn the pediatrician and neurologist of impending neurologic abnormality and encourage a search for the earliest signs of cerebral disease. Of course, recognition of these early skin anomalies requires a familiarity with the skin of the newborn. A diffuse erythema lasting a few days (an almost universal finding in Caucasian infants) should not be confused with erythroedema. Extreme mottling of skin (livedo reticularis) must not be mistaken for scleredema or some other congenital lesion. Unnatural dryness, cracking, and flaking of skin, so typical of the postmature state (infants born beyond term) must not be misidentified as xerosis,

xeroderma, or ichthyosis. Indentations, hemorrhagic areas, linear erythema, or superficial erosions in the skin over the head due to pressure of a foot against the head in utero or to injury from the application of forceps must not be taken as signs of congenital anomalies of skin.

CONGENITAL SKIN DEFECTS WITH GROSS ANOMALIES OF THE NERVOUS SYSTEM (SPINA BIFIDA, CRANIUM BIFIDUM). Areas of the body may fail to be completely covered by skin, leaving underlying structures exposed. This dermal deficiency may be associated with other developmental defects or malformations involving bones, teeth, nails, and hair.

The most frequent examples are to be found in association with the various forms of rachischisis (spina bifida with meningocele or meningomyelocele or cranium bifidum with encephalocele). The skin may be missing or hypoplastic. Such lesions are usually midline and posterior or dorsal, and so obviously involve all tissues that they are not regarded as dermatologic problems. The least severe of them, associated with an occult defect of vertebra or cranial bone, may be revealed only by an abnormal tuft of hair or a dimple in the lumbosacral region, where there is also an absence of subcutaneous fat or dermal collagen.

Focal congenital skin defects and dermal hypoplasias. Campbell, in 1826, described focal skin defects of congenital origin in parent and child, and numerous confirmations of this finding are to be found in the medical literature since that time. The defect may involve epidermis alone or in combination with dermis, and it may extend into the subcutaneous tissue, even to underlying bone. The defect may be smooth, dry or moist, pale or red, or granular. Its borders are sharply circumscribed. The defect is gradually repaired from adjacent tissues and its appearance varies with age of lesion, viz., its stage of healing. Some are already cicatrized at birth. Most often they are located over the scalp, especially the occiput, but they may occur also over trunk and limbs. Theories as to origin are speculative. The notion of inflammation of amnion with the formation of adhesions between amnion and skin (Simonart's bands) is rejected by most pathologists in favor of an arrested development.

Closely related is *hypoplasia* of skin where the congenital anomaly is also circumscript and confined to dermis. The overlying skin is extremely thin and delicate. The subcutaneous fat may herniate out through the dermal defect because of the lack of connective tissue in the dermis. The mucous membranes show a similar tendency, with papilloma formation, and the teeth and fingernails are often defective. Telangiectases and linear streaks of pigmentation appear later in the thin epidermis.

These subcutaneous abnormalities are often associated with syndactyly, spina bifida, scoliosis, microcephaly, microphthalmia, strabismus, and colobomas of iris and choroid. Some of the affected children are later found to be mentally enfeebled. Familial coincidence due to a hereditary factor has been remarked in only a few instances.

Congenital somatic abnormalities, including those of the nervous system and skin. Unlike the first group of congenital diseases, in which defects of nervous system and skin present themselves at the moment of birth as obvious and arresting anomalies, in the following category of diseases it is a constellation of nonnervous somatic abnormalities

Table 172-2 Special developmental syndromes with somatic, neurologic, and cutaneous abnormalities

	Mongolism	13, 15 trisomy (Patau)	17, 18 trisomy	Turner's syndrome	Klinefelter's syndrome	Treacher-Collins syndrome
Intelligence	Reduced	Reduced	Reduced	Normal or reduced	Slightly reduced	Reduced
Eyes	Epicanthal fold Brushfield spots	Epicanthus variable	Epicanthus variable	Normal	Normal	Notched eyelids Antimongoloid slant
Nose	Broad low bridge	Defective		Normal	Normal	Normal
Ears	Deformed	Primitive		Normal	Normal	Grossly malformed Deaf
Lips and palate	Big tongue	Cleft		Normal	Normal	Normal
Jaws	Normal	Micrognathia	Maxilla small	Normal	Normal	Imperfectly developed
Cranium	Small brachycephalic	Small		Normal	Normal	Normal
Body growth	Stunted	Underdeveloped		Dwarfism	Tall	Normal
Psychomotor development	Delayed	Delayed		Average	Slow	Normal or delayed
Dermatoglyphics	Simian line Distal axial triradius Loop patterns	Abnormal	Abnormal	Normal	Normal	Normal
Other skin anomalies	Mongolian spots	Hemangiomas		Webbed neck	None	Congenital dermal sinuses
Heredity	21, 22 trisomy Normal	13, 15 trisomy	17, 18 trisomy	One X in karyotype Normal	Double XXY Normal	Autosomal dominant
Miscellaneous	Clumsy		Rocker-bottom feet	Only females	Only males	

that predominates. The skin, if altered at all, usually is not deranged in any characteristic fashion, except as part of a more general morphologic change of nose, eye, ear, lips, neck, and digits, and always the disorder is more than a purely dermal affection. The nervous system abnormality is even more elusive, being ordinarily not manifest until months or years after birth when the child fails to attain developmental milestones at the expected times. That the involvement of the nervous system should be one of the most consistent abnormalities in these many diverse syndromes, both in those conditions with as well as in those without demonstrable chromosomal aberrations, probably relates to the span of time required and the complexity of cerebral development which render it vulnerable at many different stages of maturation.

Occurring with monotonous frequency as common denominators in the dozen or more identifiable syndromes are microcephaly and deformities of cranium, eyes, ears, bridge of nose, jaws, lips, and digits of extremities. Certain of these regions of the body such as inner canthus of eyes, root of nose, and maxilla are known to be sites of intense embryologic organization, which probably explains their unusual susceptibility to genetic and teratogenous influences.

Interestingly, the skin, if it is to be affected in any particular way, nearly always exhibits eccentricities of ridges and other markings in the palms and soles of feet which are determined also by genetic factors. The recognition of this fact has led to the study of anomalies of fingernails and palmar and plantar lines and creases, the scientific

Table 172-2   Special developmental syndromes with somatic, neurologic, and cutaneous abnormalities (Continued)

Papillon-Psaume syndrome	Pierre Robin syndrome	Rubenstein-Taybi syndrome	Russell-Silver dwarf syndrome	de Lange's Amsterdam syndrome	Hallermann-Streiff (also François syndrome)	Fanconi's syndrome
Reduced	Normal or reduced	Reduced	Reduced	Reduced	Reduced	Reduced
Canthi malformed	Retinal separation, Congenital glaucoma	Antimongoloid slant	Normal	Optic atrophy and other ocular defects	Congenital cataracts, microphthalmia in some	Normal
Alar cartilage defective	Normal	Long and beaked	Normal	Upturned	Beaked	Normal
Normal	Deafness	Normal	Normal	Normal or malformed	Normal	Normal
Defects	Cleft palate	Normal	Inverted U-shaped mouth	Beaked upper lip, notched lower	Normal	Normal
Pseudo clefts	Receding chin	Normal	Normal	Small	Normal	Normal
Microcephaly	Normal or small	Microcephaly	Normal	Microcephaly	Microcephaly	Microcephaly
Normal or dwarfism	Normal or small	Dwarfed	Small	Dwarfed	Dwarfed	Dwarfed
Delayed	Normal or delayed	Delayed	Delayed	Delayed	Delayed	Delayed
Normal	Normal	Normal	Dwarfed	Normal	Normal	Normal
Granular skin, Frontal alopecia	Normal	Hirsutism, Hemangiomas	Café au lait spots	Bushy eyebrows to midline, Excess body hair, Marbled skin	Atrophy, Deficient hair	Brown reticulated pigmentation of skin
Autosomal dominant	?	Occasional chromosomal abnormalties	None, chromosomes normal	Autosomal recessive		Recessive (?)
Lethal in males—only females alive, Hypertrophied buccal frenula, Webbed fingers, Familial trembling	Anomalies of fingers and toes	Broad thumbs and toes	Precocious puberty, Small triangular face, Webbed toes, Clinodactyly, One leg hypertrophic	Hands and feet small and imperfect, Genitalia imperfect, Hypoplastic nipples, umbilicus		Abnormality of thumbs, Absence of radial bones, Renal malformation, Hypoplastic bone marrow

study of which is called *dermatoglyphics*. The student of dermatology who seeks a thorough grasp of developmental disorders of the skin must acquaint himself with the basic principles of this relatively new field. This group of diseases provides evidence, once again, of the manner in which the developmental plan of both the brain and the skin may relate to some more fundamental disturbances in embryogenesis.

The list of special syndromes in which there occurs a major abnormal deviation in somatic structure has become so lengthy that even pediatricians and pediatric neurologists concerned with developmental medicine have trouble keeping them in mind, and the number increases each year. In this discussion of them, instead of presenting a kind of catalog, the author has chosen to call attention to only a few of their main characteristics which are listed in Table 172-2.

Congenital eruptive diseases with nervous disorders. This motley group of disorders is characterized by a striking variety of skin lesions which declare their existence soon after birth or within the first weeks of life. Unlike the preceding category of diseases, where a congenital defect is all too obvious at birth, here the skin becomes, after an interval, the site of a disease process. It may mimic any one of a broad spectrum of eczematoid and vesicular eruptions and, through repeated exacerbations, combine in acute, subacute, and chronic forms which inevitably raise questions of infection, allergy, photosensitivity, etc. Scarring, hyperkeratosis, anhidrosis, pigmentation, inflammation, and ulceration are often present, and it is not always easy to decide whether they are primary or secondary. Only when the condition is viewed in longitudinal profile against a background of abnormalities of hair, teeth, eyes, ears, and other tissues does the pediatrician begin to think in terms of the syndromes outlined below. Familial incidence may shed light on the diagnostic puzzle, and as months and years pass, mental retardation and other disorders of nervous function provide additional clues. Early diagnosis is nonetheless advantageous, even though it does not lead to effective therapy, because the physician and parents are then alerted to the possibility of involvement of the nervous system and defects of certain senses.

Presented below are the main features of the best known of these congenital dermal eruptions. The list is not complete; rare ones are omitted and new ones will probably be discovered and eventually find their place in the group.

INCONTINENTIA PIGMENTI (BLOCH-SULZBERGER SYNDROME). The condition known as incontinentia pigmenti (see also Chap. 79) is rare. More than one case may occur in a family. Of the more than 200 cases on record, only a half dozen or so were in males. The first skin lesions are vesicular or bullous. The lesions tend to localize on the flexor surfaces of the extremities and the lateral aspects of the trunk; they are linearly arranged or grouped. The healing stage leaves the skin atropic and pigmented, with the resultant formation of curious whorls, streaks, and patches of geographic configuration. The streaks, which are of slate or brown color, resemble veins in marble. There is delayed dentition, and the teeth are conical. The nails are defective and hair scanty. Mental retardation, epilepsy, microcephaly or hydrocephalus, and spastic paralysis have later appeared in an undefined proportion of the patients with these skin lesions. Optic atrophy, squints, cataracts and corneal opacities, nystagmus, and blue sclerae are often added to the clinical picture.

EPIDERMOLYSIS BULLOSA. This stands as a closely related, dominantly or recessively inherited condition in which vesicles develop at sites of pressure on the wrists, elbows, feet, and knees soon after birth. Upon rupture they leave bleeding ulcers, which heal with the formation of thin scars. Oral bullae and hyperkeratotic plaques are common. Not infrequently the nails are malformed, the teeth absent or undeveloped, and the tongue adherent to the floor of the mouth. Physical and mental retardation occur in some cases (see Chap. 64).

POIKILODERMA CONGENITALE OF ROTHMUND AND THOMSON. This is a closely related syndrome consisting of atrophy of skin and telangiectasia, hypo- or hyperpigmentation, cataracts (developing during the juvenile period), skeletal abnormalities (dwarfism, frontal bossing, absence or rudimentary development of the bones of extremities), faulty dentition, and hypogonadism (Fig. 172-13). Alopecia and dystrophy of nails are present in some cases. Light sensitivity also may become evident at a later age, and there is a tendency toward cutaneous malignant tumors. In many of the cases, microcephaly and oligophrenia become manifest during childhood. The inheritance is autosomal recessive.

ANHIDROTIC ECTODERMAL DYSPLASIA. This disorder does not simulate congenital ichthyosis. The condition is a sex-linked recessive one occurring only in males. From birth the serious nature of it is suspected from the altered cranial physiognomy, with abnormalities about the eyes and, later, near absence of teeth in both dentitions. The skin is dry, thin, and shiny, with prominence of the subcutaneous vessels. There is absence of the eccrine sweat glands but not the apocrine sweat glands. Later, hair over the head may be scanty and, at puberty, axillary and genital hair does not appear. As to the neurologic aspect, a considerable proportion of the affected children have been able to attain upright stature and locomotion. The neuropathology has not been studied.

HIDROTIC ECTODERMAL DYSPLASIA. An autosomal dominant disorder, hidrotic ectodermal dysplasia is characterized by subtotal alopecia and dystropic nails. The sweat glands are normal. There may be hyperkeratosis of the palms and soles. Mental deficiency, epilepsy, and neural deafness have occurred in several of these patients.

SEBACEOUS AND EPITHELIAL NEVI. Brain involvement has been noted with linear sebaceous nevus and epithelial nevus. These patients may have multiple defects elsewhere in the body [38,39]. Of 23 patients with extensive epithelial nevi, 18 had skeletal abnormalities; 10, central nervous system abnormalities; and 9, both the skeletal and central nervous system abnormalities including arteriovenous malformations, mental retardation, epilepsy, and peripheral nerve disorders [40].

Another dozen or more patients have been described, all of whom have had a triad of linear midline sebaceous nevus, seizures, and mental retardation. A variety of other ectodermal and mesodermal abnormalities have also been reported. The nevus sebaceous lesion, known since the original description by Jadassohn in the last century, consists of "characteristic unctous yellow nodules with granular surfaces pitted with hypertrophic sebaceous glands" [39]. It is localized, often linear, and sometimes (rarely) generalized, usually on the face or scalp. The skin lesion may be present at birth or appears in early childhood. Unsightly and of cosmetic importance, the lesions are of concern to dermatologists because of their potential for malignant change. From birth to puberty they remain small and hairless only to become more verrucous, pitted, and unsightly during adolescence. Approximately 20 percent give rise to basal cell carcinomas in adult years. The mental retardation is of variable degree and has been absent in a few cases. The seizures usually begin in the first year of life and persist. The basis of the mental retardation and seizures has never been established. Rarely the CSF protein is increased; there are no intracranial calcifications.

BASAL CELL NEVUS SYNDROME. This syndrome comprises nevoid basal cell hyperplasia leading to carcinoma, palmar dyskeratoses, cysts of the jaw, lateral displacement of the inner canthi (hypertelorism), and other skeletal abnormalities (spina bifida, spade-shaped and bifid ribs). Concurrence of a variety of neurologic disorders (mental deficiency, medulloblastoma, and hydrocephalus) has been documented in several articles, and the disorders have been incorporated into a syndrome [41–43]. These writers refer to the familial basal cell nevus-medulloblastoma syndrome as the "fifth phakomatosis." However, the neurocutaneous relationships need further statistical validation, for their pathology does not yet provide an indubitable linkage (see Chap. 76). A closely related disorder is that described by Murphy and Tenser [44] in which nevoid basal cell carcinoma is associated with epilepsy.

Fig. 172-13 Poikiloderma congenitale of Rothmund and Thomson. *(Courtesy of José M. de Moragas, M.D., Barcelona.)*

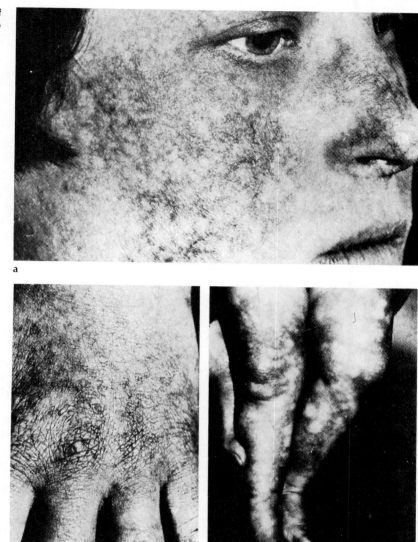

a

b

c

Congenital pigmentary disorders with anomalous development of the nervous system. GIANT PIGMENTED NEVUS WITH CONCURRENT INVOLVEMENT OF MENINGES AND MALIGNANT MELANOMA. This congenital disorder presents with one, a few, or many circumscribed, flat or raised, cutaneous pigmented nevi (color varies from light yellow to chocolate brown or black) (Fig. 172-14). The skin lesions tend to be oval or circular in contour, and sometimes their borders are irregular, bearing some resemblance to the outline of an animal; hence the popular belief that they are caused by a distressing maternal experience during pregnancy which has left its mark on the fetus. They may be present at birth, but some appear during the first year of life. The face, neck, trunk, thighs, buttocks, and external genitalia are common sites. The lesions may become less pigmented by the time of puberty, and age has another effect—to make them more elevated and corrugated or verrucous. Most of the lesions are covered with hair and a few contain cartilage. In one study of 55 patients, the dermatomal distribution of the lesions was noteworthy.

They tended to originate in the posterior part of the body, near the midline; the vortex of the nevus was near the center of the spine.

Some of the more extensive elevated pigmented nevi are associated with such an exuberant growth of tissue as to resemble the elephantiasic form of neurofibromatosis, and, like the lesions in this latter condition, the tissue of the nevus reacts positively to cholinesterase stains [45]. Likewise, anomalies of skeleton (spina bifida and clubfeet), atrophy or hypertrophy of the underlying musculature or bony structures, and a tendency toward malignant degeneration are common to both giant pigmented nevus and the elephantiasic form of neurofibromatosis. The giant nevus differs, however, in that it is not hereditary and benign tumors of the nerves are conspicuously absent.

Among the recorded examples of this disease it is to be remarked that in one series of 39 cases of pigmented nevi, 18 were in males and 29 in females. The tumors were present at birth in 8 and appeared between the ages of 1 and 5 years in 12, from 6 to 10 years in 4, from 11 to 20

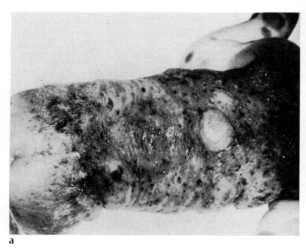
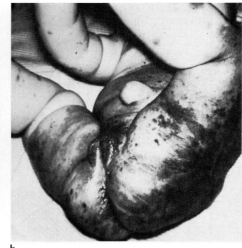

a   b

Fig. 172-14   Giant pigmented nevus with concurrent involvement of meninges and malignant melanoma.

years in 3, and over 20 years in 12. In the 13 autopsied cases (of the 23 that died) no less than 9 had metastatic melanotic carcinoma in the brain, and 2 had a diffuse melanocytosis of the leptomeninges. This last state is of particular interest insofar as many of the fully documented examples in the medical literature have been associated with extensive cutaneous nevi. The melanocytes are usually found to have proliferated abundantly. Death is usually due to communicating hydrocephalus (Fig. 172-15) which is caused by obliteration of the subarachnoid space, interfering with the circulation of cerebrospinal fluid from the posterior cranial fossa to its absorptive surface over the cerebral hemisperes [46–48]. Hypo- and hyperpigmentation of the skin have been observed in conjunction with familial spastic paraplegia.

FAMILIAL GENERALIZED MELANODERMA. This is another closely related condition which appears soon after birth. The skin, according to Berlin [49], who has described the condition in four siblings, is dry, thin, and mottled with brown or gray spots. Dwarfism and mental retardation are conjoined. Thin legs, flat nose, and defective dentition add to the grotesque appearance. In males, the penis and testicles are underdeveloped; in females, sexual development is normal. Retardation in mental development occurred in all cases.

WAARDENBURG-KLEIN AND RELATED SYNDROMES OF DEAFNESS (Fig. 172-16). Waardenburg [50] and Klein [51] have described a syndrome (Fig. 172-16), inherited in an autosomal dominant pattern, in which developmental anomalies of eyelids, eyebrows, and root of nose are associated with a neural type of deafness. The inner canthi of the eyes are displaced laterally, the eyebrows are excessively heavy, the irides are heterochromic or isochromic (pale blue). The iris may be hypoplastic, and the fundi are sometimes lacking in pigment. About half the patients have a white forelock, and a few have white areas elsewhere on the body [52]. The hair may turn gray prematurely. Piebaldness with deafness may be a closely related disorder; another is partial albinism and deafness (see Chap. 79).

CHÉDIAK-HIGASHI DISEASE (Fig. A8-13). This syndrome is a rare autosomal recessive disorder with the cardinal features of partial albinism, photophobia, repeated pyogenic infections, terminal hepatosplenomegaly, and leukocyte inclusions in the peripheral blood and bone marrow. Terminally, there may be associated cerebral lesions. Page et al [53] found cytoplasmic lipid inclusions in the histocytic infiltrations of the brain at autopsy. Stegmaier and Schneider [54] suggest that blood smears taken from albino infants should be examined for these peculiar granulations. Electron microscopic studies of the melanocytes have revealed giant melanosomes, a probable cause of the pigmentary changes seen in these patients (see Chap. 79).

MOYNAHAN'S SYNDROME. Moynahan reported a condition associated with multiple symmetric lentigines, genital hypoplasia, dwarfism, congenital mitral stenosis, psychic infantilism, and mental deficiency. Moynahan believes that this is a disorder of the development of the cellular derivatives of the neural crest [55–57] (see Chap. 79).

The congenital ichthyotic forms of nervous disease (congenital ichthyosis, xeroderma, hyperkeratosis). Ichthyosis of the common variety (ichthyosis vulgaris) does not usually appear until the second year of life, but there are a number of other states variously designated as congenital ichthyosis, xeroderma, ichthyosiform erythroderma, etc., which are apparent at birth or during the neonatal period. The time of onset of these conditions proves not to be well documented in the literature, and, indeed, some of the neurologic syndromes with which ichthyosis is associated have been observed only in the adult, the exact beginning of the skin lesion not being known (Table 172-3). The most completely described variety was presented in 1957 by Sjögren and Larsson [58] but prior to that time, Rud [59], de Sanctis and Cacchione [60], and others had called attention to clinical cases in which ichthyosis or xerosis had been variously combined with dwarfism, endocrine abnormalities, poor muscular development, convulsions, idiocy, psychosis, and retinal lesions. Xerodermic idiocy of de Sanctis and Cacchione, despite its name, is associated

Fig. 172-15 Giant pigmented ne-vus and hydrocephalus.

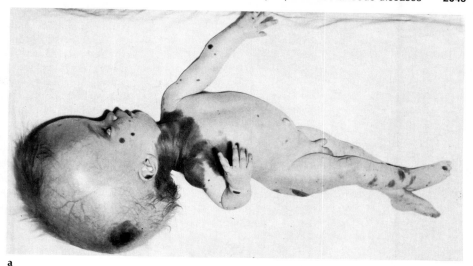

a

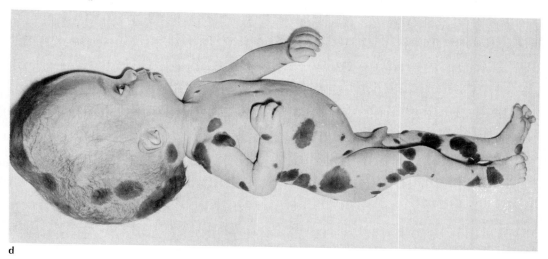

d

with xeroderma pigmentosum, a malignant cutaneous disorder (see Table 172-4).

SEX-LINKED ICHTHYOSIS (RUD'S SYNDROME). Congenital ichthyosis with infantilism, dwarfism, genital atrophy, diabetes mellitus, tetany, epilepsy, oligophrenia, polyneuropathy, and macrocytic anemia make up this syndrome. For a number of years little information was available as to the nature and time of onset of ichthyosis. In more recent writings ([61]; R. D. Wells, unpublished data), however, in which there is a tendency to call any neurocutaneous syndrome that combines ichthyosis, oligophrenia, epilepsy, dwarfism, and hypogonadism Rud's syndrome, the ichthyosis, inherited in a sex-lined pattern, had been present at birth.

XERODERMIC IDIOCY AND ATAXIA (LAUBENTHAL'S SYNDROME). This syndrome comprises ichthyosis, small stature, delayed dentition, mental retardation with tremor, cerebellar ataxia, and, in one instance, athetotic movements of the fingers. (The first cases were monozygotic twins.)

ICHTHYOTIC IDIOCY WITH RETINITIS AND MUSCULAR ATROPHY (STEWART'S SYNDROME). This is a syndrome the elements of which are congenital ichthyosis, idiocy, infantilism, epilepsy, arachnodactyly, muscular atrophy or hypoplasia, and atypical retinitis pigmentosa.

ICHTHYOTIC IDIOCY WITH SPASTIC PARAPLEGIA (SJÖGREN-LARSSON SYNDROME). In this disease, congenital ichthyosis indistinguishable from ichthyosiform erythroderma, there occur, after an interval of a year or more, manifest spastic weakness of legs, atypical retinitis pigmentosa, and in some instances epilepsy. Dentition may be abnormal—a true dysplasia of dental enamel. The disease is known to be inherited in an autosomal recessive pattern. Sjögren and Larsson [58] calculate that all the cases in their series from northern Sweden could be explained by the single mutation of a gene that occurred in a heterozygote about 600 years ago. The neuropathology has never been studied completely. In one case a developmental abnormality of the globus pallidus and frontal lobes was reported. Skin biopsies have revealed a picture consistent with congenital ichthyosiform erythroderma of the nonbullous type. A dermatologic study of 11 patients was made by Heijer and Reed [62]. These patients showed generalized ichthyosis but had normal scalp hair and nails. There was scaling, but no keratoderma of the palms and soles (Fig. 172-17). The severity of the skin involvement appears to be unrelated to the severity of the neurologic signs.

Looseness, redundancy, and loss of elasticity of skin (dermatochalasia, generalized elastolysis [see Chap. 149]). CUTIS LAXA. In this category of developmental abnormalities the

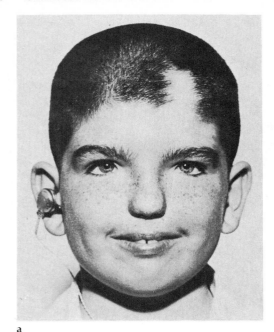

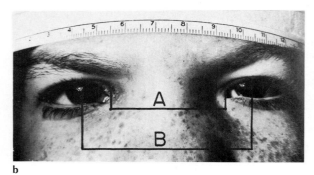

Fig. 172-16 Waardenburg-Klein syndrome. The interpupillary distance (B) is normal, but there is lateral displacement of the inner canthi (A).

natural turgor of the skin and its tight attachments to subcutaneous tissue are lacking. As a consequence, redundancy and laxity of dermis permit extreme wrinkling, and folds of it may be lifted from the underlying tissues. The skin is inelastic and when released does not at once return to its normal position. In some respects it resembles the skin of an aged person. The whole cutaneous surface may be involved, or only restricted regions such as neck (pterygium colli), scalp, or tongue. The condition has various clinical accompaniments such as pulmonary artery stenosis or ovarian agenesis. Hypothyroidism (cretinism) should be suspected when general laxity of skin is present in the first days of life, for it may be one of the few indications of this disease. Of course, it is important to recognize the latter condition, for a delay in treatment might result in irreparable impairment of the nervous system. The cause of cutis laxa is unknown in most instances; both familial (autosomal dominant) and nonfamilial examples have been recorded.

PTERYGIUM COLLI IN TURNER-BONNEVIE-ULLRICH SYNDROME. In the Turner-Bonnevie-Ullrich syndrome of ovarian dysgenesis in the female, redundancy of the skin of the sides of the neck (pterygium colli) is accompanied by short stature, infantile sexual development, and multiple congenital defects including coarctation of the aorta. The cells contain only 45 chromosomes, one of the X pair being absent. Although the majority of the patients have had no neurologic abnormalities, the author has observed an unusual incidence of low-normal mentality. Since this may not be evident during infancy and early childhood and the short stature may occur only after puberty, the webbing of the skin of the neck may provide the earliest clue to the syndrome and prompt the clinician to undertake confirmatory chromosomal studies.

LEPRECHAUNISM. A notable example of cutis laxa is observed in the syndrome known as *leprechaunism*. This is a term given a condition in which infants of low birth weight and deficient nutrition are observed to suffer an anomaly consisting of looseness of skin including cutis gyrata, muscular wasting, retarded bone age, broad nose, and facial hair. The hands and feet are too large for the body. Subcutaneous fat is deficient. Sexual organs are excessively large, and signs of precocious puberty may appear. There is a mild general aminoaciduria and a low serum alkaline phosphatase level, according to Patterson and Watkins [63]. The IQ is low. Some patients may have lipodystrophic diabetes.

CUTIS VERTICIS GYRATA. This disorder of the scalp is characterized by the presence of folds and furrows, giving a corrugated appearance to the skin. It looks as though the head were not large enough to fill out the scalp. No satisfactory pathologic studies of the dermal condition have been forthcoming. Approximately one-fourth of the patients later exhibit mental retardation and epilepsy. Deformities of cranium, eye defects, and acromegaly may coexist.

MELKERSSON-ROSENTHAL SYNDROME. This condition, inherited as an autosomal dominant, is featured by plication of the tongue (lingus plicata), paresis or paralysis of the muscles of facial expression on one side (like Bell's palsy), and a curious brawny edema of the lips or face on that side. The condition has usually been observed during adolescence or adult life, and its pathogenesis is unknown; therefore, unlike the other congenital and developmental neurocutaneous conditions discussed, it raises no problems during infancy.

Diseases that simultaneously affect the cells of skin and nervous system

Metabolic abnormalities (including those of vitamin deficiency and endocrine diseases)

No single unifying characteristic can be used to group the following diseases other than the fact that some metabolic, biochemical, or endocrine abnormality, in each instance, has affected both the skin and the nervous system. The reader's attention is drawn to the most important ones, but admittedly the list is not complete, and new diseases or syndromes are being reported every month or two. Doubtless some of the diseases already described under "Congenital and Developmental Neurocutaneous Diseases" will be brought into this group as new biochemical data are obtained. A recent reference on this subject is the monograph by Adams and Lyon [64]. The metabolic or endo-

Table 172-3   Classification of ichthyosiform dermatoses

Disorder	Presence at birth	Inheritance	Associated features of importance
Ichthyosis vulgaris	No	Autosomal dominant	Atopy sometimes
Sex-linked ichthyosis	Yes	Sex-linked	Corneal changes
Congenital ichthyosiform erythroderma—bulbous type ("epidermolytic hyperkeratosis")	Yes	Autosomal dominant	
Congenital ichthyosiform erythroderma—nonbullous type	Yes	Autosomal recessive	
Sjögren-Larsson syndrome	Yes	Autosomal recessive	Mental deficiency, tetraplegia, retinal degeneration
Conradi's syndrome (chondrodystrophia calcificans congenita)	Yes	Autosomal recessive	Stippled epiphyses, contractures, shortened proximal long bones, cataracts, etc.
Netherton's disease	Yes	? Autosomal recessive	Mental deficiency, bamboo hair deformity, atopic background
Erythrokeratoderma variabilis	Sometimes	Autosomal dominant	
Sex-linked ichthyosis with mental deficiency and hypogonadism	Yes	Sex-linked	Mental deficiency, hypogonadism
Lamellar ichthyosis	Yes	Autosomal recessive	
Porcupine man (Lambert family)	Yes	Autosomal dominant	
Unilateral congenital ichthyosiform erythroderma	Yes	Unknown ? teratogenic	Unilateral bony deformities
Ichthyosis with Down's syndrome	No	Chromosomal	Clinical signs of mongolism

crine abnormality in each instance has been present since birth or even before, but an interval of time usually elapses before the full clinical syndrome, especially that part relative to disorder of the nervous system, becomes manifest.

Cretinism. This was the first neurocutaneous metabolic disease to be identified. Two types of thyroid abnormality have been delineated, one an inherited defect in thyroid metabolism, the other an acquired iodine deficiency in individuals living in regions deficient in this element. The typical physical features of cretinism are not present at birth or in the first weeks of life, and the diagnosis may be delayed unless the condition is suspected because the mother is known to be hypothyroid or has had previous cretinoid children. Prolonged jaundice, an unusual degree of inactivity, and, as was mentioned above, dryness and laxity of skin and coarseness of hair are the earliest indications. Only as weeks and months pass do the thickness of lips, large tongue and open mouth, low-bridged nose, narrow brow, broad hands and stubby fingers, hoarse low-pitched cry, constipation, and delay in psychomotor development become manifest. Thus the dermatologist is in a particularly favorable position to assist the pediatrician in reaching an early diagnosis.

Pellagra (see Chap. 136). Formerly one of the most universal afflictions, this condition, now known to be due to a deficiency in nicotinic acid and other B vitamins (tryp-

Table 172-4   Ichthyotic disorders with neurologic disease

Sjögren-Larsson syndrome	Spastic paralysis
	Mental deficiency
	Epilepsy
	Retinitis pigmentosa-like changes
Conradi's syndrome	Mental deficiency
Rud's syndrome	Mental deficiency
	Epilepsy
Refsum's syndrome	Hypertrophic polyneuropathy
	Retinitis pigmentosa
	Neural deafness
	Cerebellar ataxia
Sex-linked ichthyosis	Mental deficiency
	Epilepsy

Fig. 172-17   Sjögren-Larsson syndrome.

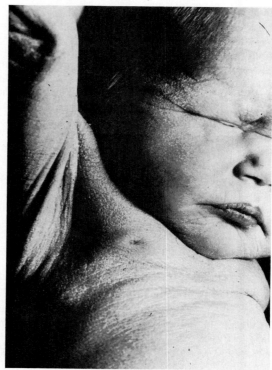

tophan deficiency may also be a factor), has been virtually eradicated in the Occidental world. This great advance in public health has been achieved by the fortification of the wheat flour in bread by nicotinic acid. It is still endemic in remote areas where green vegetables and red meat are unobtainable for parts of each year, and in chronic alcoholics and food faddists.

The skin lesions are evoked by exposure to sunlight, which leads to erythema, vesiculation, often with bullous formation, and then crusting and desquamation. The lesions appear mainly on the exposed parts of the body—backs of hands, forehead, cheeks, bridge of nose and shins. Sebaceous plugging of skin over nose, cheeks, and brow, and rhagades, or cracks, at the corners of the mouth are often found, but some research workers ascribe them to an associated riboflavin deficiency. The tongue and oral mucous membranes become red and smooth (lingual filiform papillae are effaced) and stomatitis (see Chap. 101) and vaginitis, with fusospirochetal infections, are frequent. Later the skin becomes lichenified and pigmented.

With the skin lesions there is often a moderately severe diarrhea. Macrocytic anemia and hypochlorhydria coexist. The earliest signs of involvement of the central nervous system are general weakness and fatigability (called neurasthenia), irritability, and suspiciousness, followed within days or weeks by a confusional psychosis (incorrectly termed *dementia,* to give an alliterative term to the symptom triad of dermatitis, diarrhea, and dementia). There may be an associated polyneuropathy. Babinski signs, sucking and grasping reflexes, and fluctuating rigidity of the limbs appear late, almost terminally. Nicotinic acid, given by injection or orally, will prevent and cure the disease. Since parts of the syndrome may be due to lack of other B vitamins (pyridoxine, riboflavin, thiamine, pantothenic acid, folic acid, and B_{12}), it is best to prescribe a balanced diet supplemented by the whole B complex. Pellagra should not be confused with Hartnup disease in which the skin lesions are identical.

Phenylketonuria (PKU) (Følling's disease). This, the most common of the metabolic disorders found among patients in mental institutions, is characterized by mental deficiency, epilepsy, and minor skin changes. The latter consist of decreased pigmentation of hair and skin, particularly noticeable among members of dark-skinned races, whose hair may then be brown instead of black (see Chap. 79), and a tendency in infants toward atopic dermatitis. Partington [65] noted that six of his patients developed a generalized eczema between the first and fourth month of life, and five others had dry skin and persistent nondescript rashes. Sensitivity to sunlight may prove a problem and lead to recognition of patients in a mental retardation hospital. It is said that Følling would find PKU patients by asking for all the patients who had an unusual degree of sensitivity to sunlight. Some patients also exhibit abnormal reactions to phenothiazine compounds.

The mental deficiency varies in degree; many children are profoundly retarded, eking out an existence in homes for the mentally enfeebled. They sit in idleness, manifesting digital mannerisms and rocking movements, making no effort to communicate by sign or word. Exceptionally, they exhibit flexion (salaam spasms) in infancy, and their limbs may be mildly spastic with increased tendon reflexes and

Babinski signs. The majority show no other major neurologic abnormalities. Considering the disease in toto, the skin alterations are of relatively little importance and are seldom of value in diagnosis with one exception—in the Asiatic races there is a dilution of hair color; the scalp hair is normally *black,* while in PKU the hair is dark brown and is easily recognized as abnormal (see Chap. 79) (Figs. A8-5 and A8-6). Patients have been reported with sclerodermoid changes in the skin associated with myositis. Lowering the phenylalanine level by diet in early life prevents mental retardation and leads to improvement in skin and behavior.

Homocystinuria. First recognized by Carson and her collaborators in 1965 [66], this syndrome has become widely recognized among pediatricians and neurologists. It is characterized by an excessive urinary excretion of homocystine, in association with fine sparse hair, malar flush, livedo reticularis, prominent joints, bilateral inguinal hernias, mental retardation convulsions, and, later, spastic weakness of the legs (see Chap. 139).

Argininosuccinic aminoaciduria. In this hereditary disease, in which mental dullness, epilepsy, and intermittent cerebellar ataxia are related to excesses of arginine and ammonia, the hair tends to be dry and brittle. When the hair is examined with a hand lens, nodose swellings and constrictions are seen along the shaft (trichorrhexis nodosa), an abnormality distinguishable from that in monilethrix (see Chap. 139).

Hartnup disease. This condition is named after the family in which four of eight children had a hereditary pellagralike skin rash aggravated by sunlight, a fluctuant cerebellar ataxia, and slight to moderate mental deficiency. These children were the result of a first-cousin marriage. One of the patients reported by the Halvorsens had premature graying of the hair [67]. The disease is extremely rare, having been identified only a few times in the United States (see Chap. 139).

Hydroxykynureninuria. This is a disease due presumably to a deficiency of kynureninase in which the nervous symptoms are much like those of Hartnup disease and congenital tryptophanuria. Sensitivity to sunlight and skin rash are associated with mental dullness and episodic ataxia.

Monilethrix (trichorrhexis nodosa). These patients are born without hair or lose it in early infancy. The remaining hair is dry, coarse, and fragile. Alopecia is usually not complete, whether in the scalp or elsewhere. Some patients exhibit defective dentition, cataracts, koilonychia, ichthyosis simplex, and mental deficiency. Monilethrix differs from pili torti, another inherited abnormality of the hair in which the shafts are flattened and twisted. (See Chap. 65 for a discussion of the metabolic disorder and its relation to argininosuccinic acid.)

Kinky hair disease. This disease was described in 1962 by Menkes et al [68] as a sex-linked hereditary disorder occurring only in females (probably lethal in males). Born normally from an unaffected mother after a normal gestation, the sparse kinky hair first attracts notice. Soon thereafter developmental delay of maturing nervous functions becomes apparent. The retardation and failure to thrive are of such severity that most of the patients have died in the first year of life but a few live on for a few years. Aguilar et al [69] in 1966 presented a more complete account of the disease, and details of the pathology have been amplified by Hirano et al [70] and others. (See Chap. 65.)

The abnormality of hair is not fully differentiated from monilethrix and pili torti (twisted hair), and from diseases such as were described by Robinson and Miller [71] in which kinky hair was associated with dysplasia of dental enamel, and by Bjornstad with nerve deafness (Bjornstad's syndrome). The underlying biochemical mechanism is a failure of absorption of copper (Cu) from the intestinal tract, due to a missing enzyme. Presumably lack of Cu in the neonatal and infantile tissues (probably interfering with the action of enzymes in which Cu is a trace element) is responsible for the severe nutritional and growth defect.

Neuronal loss and gliosis, myelin degeneration, deformities of Purkinje cells in the cerebellum with lack of development of proper somatic synapses underlie the neurologic abnormalities.

Tightly curled scalp hair is an early feature of congenital lipodystrophic diabetes.

The mucopolysaccharidoses: gargoylism (Hunter-Hurler) and other syndromes. The distinctive, grotesque appearance of patients with gargoylism reflects changes in nearly every part of the body due to the abnormal deposition of a mucopolysaccharide and a glycolipid. Recently, several new variants of the disease have been described. The typical patient shows dwarfism, skeletal abnormalities (beaked vertebrae), opacification of corneas, and mental retardation. There are two distinctive patterns of heredity: the form of the disease inherited as an autosomal recessive features clouding of the cornea and dwarfism; the sex-linked forms usually have no corneal opacities and less mental retardation and dwarfism. Most of these patients show generalized hirsutism over the body, papules, nodules, and a peculiar orange-peel appearance of the skin. A second type of skin involvement occurs in the hands, where the fingers may be semiflexed due to pseudocontracture. The skin over the hands may be thickened, lar-

daceous, and inelastic. Mucopolysaccharide deposition in the cytoplasm of the epidermal cells and in the fibrocytes of the dermis has been reported. Persistent tinea capitis infections, resistant to therapy, may occur, suggesting perhaps a reduced defense against infection. (See Chap. 149.)

Xerodermic idiocy of de Sanctis and Cacchione. Here xeroderma pigmentosum is combined with retarded skeletal development, mental retardation, dwarfism, and testicular hypoplasia (Fig. 172-18). Despite the name xeroderma, the skin changes result from the effect of solar ultraviolet irradiation leading to a thickened dry skin (see Chap. 150). This was first described in three brothers [60], and other similar families have been found since the original report. Elsässer et al [72] noted that 41 of the 286 patients with xeroderma pigmentosum reported in the literature have had evidence of mental and physical retardation; Larmande and Timsit [73], among their 20 patients, found two-thirds to have stunted growth, mental backwardness, and electroencephalographic abnormalities. The examination of the brain in one case revealed microencephaly with loss of neurons in the frontal and temporal lobes, but the details of the neuropathologic process await further case studies. There is a defective DNA repair after ultraviolet irradiation in cultured fibroblasts from the skin.

Albinism and the oculocerebral syndrome of Cross and McKusick. Universal albinism, another autosomal recessive disorder, classically shows absence or marked dilution of pigment in the skin, the hair, and the eye. Nystagmus is frequent. There is a tendency toward early cutaneous malignant tumors. These "moon children," as they have been called, may be found even among American Indians and the aborigines of western Australia. Albinism is the result of a genetically determined deficiency of tyrosinase in the melanocytes (see Chap. 79).

As a rule, human albinos exhibit no abnormalities of nervous function, though obviously their striking appearance sets them apart and taxes their powers of social adjustment. However, Cross et al [74] have described a family by the name of Mast, in which three living siblings are afflicted with mental retardation, spastic diplegia, cutaneous hypopigmentation, multiple ocular anomalies, microphthalmia, small opaque corneas, and coarse nystag-

Fig. 172-18 Xerodermic idiocy of de Sanctis and Cacchione.

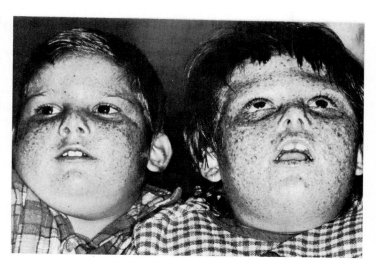

mus. The inheritance was autosomal recessive in this inbred Amish family. The author has also noted other patients with albinism with mental deficiency, epilepsy, and deafness, but without the anomalies of the eyes.

Congenital lipodystrophic diabetes (leprechaunism) and the Prader-Willi and Laurence-Moon-Biedl syndromes. Seip [75] described a congenital syndrome of lipodystrophy with rapid growth and advanced bone age, hepatomegaly, generalized muscular overdevelopment, hypertrichosis, and hyperpigmentation. All of his patients were young children at the time of the publication of his article. Insulin-resistant diabetes developed later. Hyperlipemia usually preceded the diabetes and resulted in eruptive xanthomas of the skin. Retarded psychomotor development was shown to be related to dilatation of the cerebral ventricles in five of his patients.

Reed et al studied three such patients, all mental defectives (one with epilepsy) [76]. In all these patients with definite neurologic deficits, the lipodystrophy had appeared early in life. Schwartz et al [77] first called attention to the presence of acanthosis nigricans in this condition and found two other examples in the medical literature.

Hypercholesterolemia with tendon xanthomatosis and neurologic abnormality (van Bogaert-Epstein-Scherer syndrome). Whereas familial hypercholesterolemia is seldom associated with nervous disorder, there has now been described a series of cases marked by prominent xanthelasma, tendon xanthomas and progressive spastic weakness, and cerebellar ataxia of the limbs. Intellectual deterioration may be added. First described in a monograph by van Bogaert et al [78], in recent years the discovery of other cases has established its existence as a clinicopathologic entity. Heavy deposit of crystalline cholesterol in the cerebellum, brainstem, and basal ganglia variably destroys parenchymal elements and excites an intense gliotic reaction. Familial coincidence attests to an inherited metabolic defect.

Refsum's syndrome, acanthocytosis, and Tangier disease. Heredopathic atactica polyneuritiformis (Refsum's syndrome) [79] is a hereditary disorder in which retinitis pigmentosa, deafness, and sensorimotor polyneuropathy are combined and may be accompanied occasionally by exceptional dryness and scaling of skin or frank ichthyosis. The skin disease, like that of the nervous system, is probably linked to the inability to degrade phytanic acid, an exogenous fatty acid which accumulates throughout the body [80]. For the dermatologist, the diagnosis is clarified by the discovery of sensorimotor paralysis and areflexia of the limbs in patients presenting with dry, scaling skin. For the neurologist, the skin changes in a patient with chronic progressive polyneuropathy should always suggest Refsum's syndrome.

An alpha-lipoproteinemia (Tangier disease) has been found among the inhabitants of Tangier Island in the Chesapeake Bay [81,82]. The characteristics are very large tonsils which are covered with orange-yellow deposits and enlarged liver, spleen, and lymph nodes. Patients with this disorder have the lowest amounts of plasma alpha-lipoproteins found in any disease (see Chap. 145).

Tangier disease resembles Refsum's disease in its clinical neurologic manifestations. Dermal deposition of cholesterol esters was found in cutaneous papules (xanthomas) or more diffusely in the skin in one case, but the skin has been clinically normal in four or five of the known living patients with Tangier disease.

Lipoid proteinosis (Urbach-Wiethe disease). Lipoid proteinosis is a rare autosomal recessive disease, typified by widespread papules, nodules, indurated plaques, and ulcerated lesions involving the skin and the mucous membranes. Hoarseness is a prominent symptom, due to involvement of vocal cords and the upper respiratory tract. Lipid, protein, and carbohydrate have been demonstrated in the extracellular deposits and walls of blood vessels; hence, the designation of the disease as a lipoglycoproteinosis. Epilepsy, mental impairment, and indifference to pain are the reported neurologic features of this metabolic defect (see Chap. 147).

Angiokeratoma corporis diffusum (Fabry's disease). This disease (see Chap. 146) was first described by Anderson and Fabry in 1898. It comprises a rash (small vascular lesions), inexplicable pains in the extremities (often lancinating and with paresthesias) indicative of a polyneuropathy, irregular fever, superficial corneal opacities, tortuosity of retinal vessels, a high incidence of cerebrovascular accidents at an early age, and cardiac and renal failure. The skin lesions may be present from childhood but usually appear later, evolving slowly but antedating the other symptoms. Typically the lesions are more or less symmetric, being marked most over bony prominences, particularly below the waist. They tend to cluster. In size they vary from a pinpoint to 3 to 4 mm; the smaller lesions are red, the larger black. Keratinized macules and papules also occur. The mucous membranes of the lips and the skin of the genitalia are involved in some cases. The vascular lesions consist of dilated vessels, but only the smaller ones blanch on pressure. Capillary dilatations cause a peculiar mottling of the palms. The general physique is, in some patients, poor, with slender limbs, stooped posture, and some degree of fixation of joints and even the spine. The muscles are thin and weak, possibly from atrophy of disuse occasioned by the limitation of movement and pain. The pattern of inheritance is usually that of a mendelian sex-linked trait [83].

Studies by Sweeley and Klionsky [84] suggest there may be a defect in glycolipid synthesis resulting in an accumulation of an unidentified substance, principally in the walls of blood vessels and glomeruli. The major part of the stored material is thought to be ceramide dihexoside and trihexoside. Exceptionally, small deposits of a storage material appear in the neurons of the brain, particularly in patients whose mental capacities have declined. In this respect, the disease falls into the class of lipidoses.

The pain, acroparesthesias, and burning (chiefly of the hands), the hypersensitivity to temperature, and the anhidrosis may be due to lipid infiltration of the vessels of the peripheral and autonomic nervous systems [85]. Dependent edema is part of the picture of cardiac decompensation. The vascular lesions in the brain, which may begin in adolescence or early adult life, are either embolic from

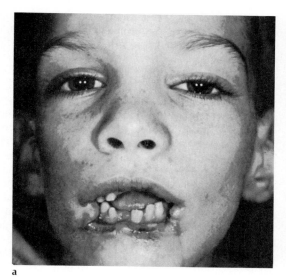

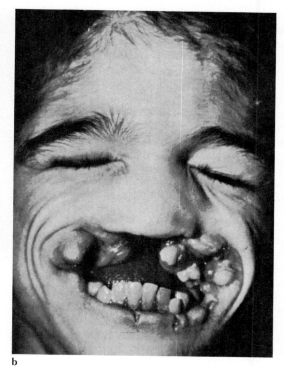

Fig. 172-19 Lesch-Nyhan syndrome showing severe self-mutilation.

heart or thrombotic. The female carrier may show only corneal opacities. Diagnosis is facilitated by the demonstration of the glycolipids (polaroscopy) in the urinary sediment. Most patients die of uremia or heart failure. The only known treatment is symptomatic. Neurologically, the disease is best listed with familial polyneuropathies, probably of vascular pathogenesis.

Variegate porphyria. In this autosomal dominant disorder, the cutaneous changes of porphyria cutanea tarda are combined with the severe neurologic crises of acute intermittent porphyria. This type of porphyria is very common among the Boers of South Africa [86]. These patients develop easy abrasion, bullae, hypertrichosis, scarring (scleroderma) and hyperpigmentation on the sun-exposed areas of the body. Intolerance to barbiturates and the sulfonamides has been demonstrated. Fecal and urinary coproporphyrin and porphobilinogen are increased. Goldberg [87] points out that the most striking clinical features are neurologic. (See Chap. 143.)

Familial hyperuricemia with self-destructive biting, mental retardation, cerebral palsy, and choreoarthetosis (Lesch-Nyhan syndrome). This sex-linked recessive syndrome occurs in young males who have a persistent hyperuricemia without other signs of clinical gout. The neurologic disorder takes the form of extensor spasms of the trunk, dysarthria, choreoathetosis, brisk tendon reflexes, and Babinski's signs. These have appeared during the first months of life. Mental deficiency and retarded growth have been noted in all reported cases. The blood uric acid ranges from 5 to 15 mg/dL due to a deficient activity of hypoxanthine-guanine phosphoribosyltransferase. Lowering uric acid by the use of allopurinol does not alter the course of the illness. Picking and rubbing of the skin results in mutilation of the face, particularly the lower lip, and of the hands unless the patient is restrained. Sometimes it is necessary to extract the teeth to prevent biting. Tophi and gouty arthritis occur later in some cases.

The severe self-mutilation which may result in a child literally devouring the whole lower lip has not been explained (Fig. 172-19). It is more pronounced and consistent than the self-injury of some low-grade mental defectives in whom biting of the back of the hand may be provoked during a moment of frustration or a temper tantrum. There seems to be no loss of sensation as in congenital familial sensory neuropathy with anhidrosis. At the time when the self-destructive behavior begins (usually about the age of 2 years), the uric acid content of the saliva is not greater than at other times.

Hypoparathyroidism with superficial moniliasis, keratoconjunctivitis, and hypoadrenalism. Most of the patients with this disorder follow a definite clinical sequence. The idiopathic hypoparathyroidism with tetany and calcification of the basal ganglia and, finally, adrenal and sometimes thyroid insufficiency, develops after an infantile moniliasis of buccal mucosa and nails which continues into adult life. Chronic keratoconjunctivitis, usually not monilial, is another important feature. At autopsy the parathyroid glands are usually absent, and the adrenal glands atrophied. The disorder appears to be familial.

Familial dysautonomia (Riley-Day syndrome). The essential features of familial autonomic dysautonomia are defective lacrimation leading to corneal ulceration, blotching of the skin, excessive sweating, and excessive drooling. Less constant findings are emotional instability, blood pressure lability, pain indifference, and faulty speech. This is an autosomal recessive disorder in which there is an enzyme defect in the metabolism and function of the catecholamines. Nearly all the patients have been of Jewish descent.

Cockayne's syndrome. Cockayne's syndrome has so far been described only in English patients. Macdonald et al [88] summarized the criteria for diagnosis as clinical onset in the second year of life after a normal infancy, microencephaly, dwarfism with kyphosis and ankylosis, disproportionately long extremities, long hands and feet, lipodystrophy of the face, mental deficiency, light sensitivity, retinitis pigmentosa, partial deafness, cerebellar ataxia, cyanotic extremities, and carious teeth. The neurologic disorder progresses relentlessly and terminates in blindness, deafness, and paralysis.

The most thorough neuropathologic study to date [89] has shown microgyria, cerebral atrophy (460 g compared with 1400 g in the normal brain) due to insufficiency of nerve cells in the cerebral cortex, as well as capillary encrustations of iron and calcium, and a patchy loss of myelin and axons in subcortical regions. Fewer lesions of the same type were observed in sections of lenticular nuclei and thalamus. Corticospinal and other descending tracts had degenerated. Also the inner granule cell layer of the cerebellum was depleted (cerebellopetal atrophy). The lesions were thought to be similar to those of one of the patchy, familial demyelinative diseases of the type described by Pelizaeus and Merzbacher. The author has observed similar lesions in one case of Seckel's bird-headed dwarfism with mental retardation.

A dermatitis affects the parts of the body exposed to the sun. The "butterfly area" of the face is the most severely involved, an appearance which suggests lupus erythematosus, congenital porphyria. Hartnup disease, and xerodermic idiocy.

Bloom [90] has described a disease that is so similar to Cockayne's syndrome that it probably cannot be distinguished from it. However, Bloom's patients were, for the most part, of Jewish extraction, and the nervous system was not involved.

Parry-Romberg hemiatrophy (Fig. 172-20) [91]

This condition falls in the category of partial progressive lipodystrophies (described in Chap. 100) of which Romberg's facial hemiatrophy is one of the most conspicuous syndromes. Usually all the lipocytes of one half of the face, or some other segment of the body, progressively disappear. The face is left shrivelled and wrinkled, like that of an aged person. There are usually no associated changes in the nervous system. Sensation is intact and muscles contract normally. Rarely, with the Romberg hemiatrophy, an abnormality of the autonomic innervation has been reported. The iris may be variegated blue-brown (from a congenital sympathetic defect), or the pupil may be dilated, or sweat and vasomotor reactions may be diminished.

Toxic disorders

Arsenic intoxication. Lead arsenate is the source of most of the trouble, being used in certain rural areas as an insecticide in sprays or as a powder for the extermination of boll weevils. Exposure leads to a syndrome which indicates involvement of many organs including skin (raindrop hyperpigmentation and keratosis), hair, nails, gastrointestinal tract (nausea and vomiting), bone marrow (anemia and leukopenia), liver (jaundice), and peripheral

and central nervous system (subacute sensorimotor polyneuropathy and convulsions and coma). Prevention of further ingestion and chelation with British antilewisite (BAL) have been the most effective treatment in the majority of patients.

Mercury and acrodynia. Mercury intoxication causes a variety of symptoms. In Minamata disease (resulting from ingestion of an organic methylated mercurial), cerebellar ataxia and sometimes blindness develop acutely. There is no skin lesion. In young children, a syndrome known as *acrodynia* (erythrodermic neuralgia, or pink disease) has been ascribed to poisoning by this element. Irritability, photophobia, confusion, and drowsiness, the initial symptoms, are followed by a fairly typical skin eruption in 2 to 4 weeks. The hands and feet become cold, cyanotic, erythematous, and swollen. The limbs are weak. The patient constantly rubs the hands and feet, and self-mutilation may occur, as in juvenile gout, perhaps from intense pain. Stomatitis has been observed, with loss of teeth. In most of the recently reported cases, mercury has been found in the urine. The source is said to be paint or exposure to the metallic form of the element.

Thallium poisoning. The use of thallium, formerly used as a depilatory, may result in a painful acute polyneuropathy, sometimes fatal. Loss of hair precedes or accompanies the peripheral nerve involvement.

Infective states, proved or suspected types

Meningococcemia and rickettsial, viral, and mycotic infections. In a variety of infections of the nervous system, the skin lesions may be among the earliest signs of a neurocutaneous syndrome. In meningococcemia, rickettsemia (Rocky Mountain spotted fever, or typhus), and some of the Coxsackie and echo viruses, the skin of the trunk and limbs may be flecked with petechiae or involved in a macular and papular rash, and only later will an infective meningitis develop. In such cases a systemic infection appears to underlie a generalized disease that may affect the skin

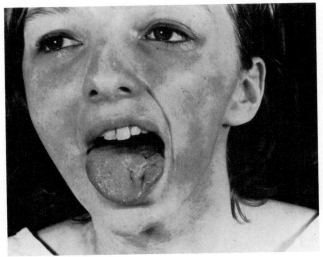

Fig. 172-20 Parry-Romberg hemiatrophy. Note shriveled tongue and obvious hemiatrophy of the left side of the face.

and other organs, including the cerebrospinal meninges. The skin disease seems not to be primary.

The postexanthematous encephalomyelitides (after rubeola, variola, vaccinia, etc.) are better regarded as systemic rather than primary dermatologic diseases. However, it seems probable that affection of cutaneous structures and skin lesions might be the conditioning stimulus to an autoallergic reaction in the central nervous system. Probably antirabies treatment provides the best example, for here cutaneous or subcutaneous inoculation seems to be the most effective means of sensitizing the organism to the essential antigen. Fungal infections which may attack the nervous system with regularity are rarely primary in the skin; the only examples the author has encountered are exceptional cases of torulosis (cryptococcosis), coccidioidomycosis, actinomycosis, moniliasis, and North American blastomycosis.

Vogt-Koyanagi-Harada syndrome. In this strange disease, presumably viral, the skin around the eyes, including the eyelashes (poliosis) and eyebrows, becomes depigmented (vitiligo). There may also be scattered depigmented macules on the trunk. The uveal tract is affected. Headache and mild stiffness of neck call attention to intracranial extension, and lumbar puncture reveals a pleocytosis (lymphocytic) and an elevated protein level in cerebrospinal fluid. There may be dysacousia or deafness. The course is subacute or chronic, and the process finally subsides. No treatment is known (see Chap. 79).

Behçet's syndrome. This is another presumed viral infection which affects mucous membranes (oral or genital), lungs, and cerebrum. The condition should be considered when ulcerations of mucous membranes are followed by systemic symptoms. Approximately one-quarter of the patients will have neurologic signs such as seizures, and a variety of other focal cerebral disturbances (mild hemiparesis, hemianesthesia, aphasia, ataxia, etc.). The neurologic signs are of a type which indicate involvement of the gray and white matter of the brain (i.e., tracts and nuclear structure), and the cerebrospinal fluid usually gives evidence of the inflammatory nature of the illness in that it contains lymphocytes and a protein exudate. The disease is rarely fatal, and no treatment is known to be effective. Corticosteroid therapy may be beneficial. (See Chap. 102.)

Dermatologic disorders secondary to diseases of the nervous system

Trophic changes in skin due to insensitivity

Decubitus ulcerations. Here the disease of the nervous system obviously dominates the clinical picture, and the skin lesion represents essentially a complication of it. It would be a mistake to assume the nervous system disorder is essential, for decubiti may develop in infirm, debilitated patients at any age. Usually some combination of immobility with prolonged pressure of skin against bony prominences must occur, but insensitivity to pain and hypotension are also important factors in the pathogenesis.

Syringomyelia. In this disease, in which cavitation of the cervical spinal cord forms during adult life, often in relation to congenital malformations of the cervical spine, skull, and cerebellum, two types of dermal abnormalities may be identified: (1) dysplasia of cutaneous and osseous structures of skull and neck; (2) trophic changes in skin and subcutaneous tissues of hands and arms. The former, present from early life long before the typical neurologic syndrome (segmental loss of pain and temperature sensation over shoulders and arms, amyotrophy with loss of reflexes) appears, may have evinced little interest or comment. The abnormalities take the form of low hairline of scalp, short neck, asymmetric or otherwise misshapen face, and kyphoscoliosis, and they indicate the existence of a congenital disturbance of cerebrocranial relationships. Less often, other structural abnormalities have been recorded, hypertrophy being the best known.

The patient may first become aware of the syringomyelic state when a burn or cut of the hand is sustained without causing pain. The odor of the burned flesh may attract attention before the patient notices that the object being grasped is scalding hot and has already seared or blistered the skin. Repeated injuries of this type may result in thickenings and callosities of skin, especially over the fingers and knuckles, and in painless sores (formerly called whitlows). The nails may become deformed. Repeated injuries may cause the terminal phalanges to be absorbed or drop off. More often, hands are merely edematous and swollen (*la main succulente,* of French writers) and the skin may be cold or warm, red or pale, and scaly. Many of these changes correspond to the syndrome of Morvan, in which an analgesic panaris with dermal changes of these types affects the upper extremities. The idea is now prevalent among neurologists that its basis is, in most instances, either syringomyelia or, more likely, a bibrachial sensory polyneuropathy. The resemblance to leprosy is so close that the latter must always be considered.

Tabes dorsalis (syphilitic radiculitis). This disease and also chronic polyneuropathies and congenital insensitivity to pain are other causes of painless ulcerations of skin.

Factitious ulcers in hysteria and malingering

Before concluding this section on dermatologic disorders secondary to nervous system diseases it is necessary to comment on the patient whose skin inexplicably breaks down repeatedly or persistently ulcerates in places where the circulation is ample. This may happen in the legs over the tibia in middle and late adult life consequent to stasis and a marginally reduced circulation, the latter being difficult to evaluate. But when it occurs over the volar surface of forearms or hands, especially in adolescent or adult women or after a compensable injury in either a man or a woman, it always should raise suspicion of self-inflicted injury. Usually a careful history will disclose other equally dubious past illnesses in a woman—the classic form of hysteria. To make the problem more difficult, a physician who has already examined cutaneous sensation in the involved part of the body may have induced an anesthesia by suggestion, even though sensory loss almost never is found in naïve hysterical individuals when first seen. Characteristically the patient states rather blandly that upon awakening she finds an area of redness and swelling of the skin and that an ulcer forms later. All signs of injection of a corrosive chemical or of picking at the skin with a sharp object may be obscured by the time of examination, and questions as to whether such an injury was accidentally or deliberately inflicted are denied vehemently.

The diagnosis can be difficult and depends upon the establishment of a hysterical pattern of behavior with multiple bizarre illnesses in the past and the finding of a lesion in an accessible part of the body that looks as though it had been produced by the fingernail or some sharp instrument. If the physician is uncertain as to the nature of the lesion, the application of a large cast, so that the patient cannot reach the area in question, may show that healing proceeds normally (see Chap. 3).

Infections spreading from nervous system to skin

Herpes zoster. This is the classic example of a viral infection arising in the nervous system and spreading to the skin along the branches of one or more peripheral nerves. The proof of this sequence of events is to be obtained from the clinical condition itself, where pain in one region of the body (always unilateral) almost always precedes by several days the appearance of groups of vesicles (with an erythematous base) in that region (see Chap. 191).

Primary dermatologic diseases leading to abnormalities of the nervous system

Infections and infestations

Tetanus. The wound that induces tetanus is nearly always located in the skin or subcutaneous tissues; only exceptionally has an operative site or an infection developing from the intestinal tract been the source. The inoculation of tetanus bacilli or their spores into abraded skin or beneath the skin by a puncture wound (rusty nail, infected hypodermic needle) seldom excites much inflammatory reaction. In fact, the skin lesion may appear so innocent as to be entirely forgotten by the patient, and even if remembered it may appear to be quite trivial by the time the first symptoms of the nervous disorder develop—usually 5 to 15 days later. In such circumstances only the trained eye of the dermatologist may succeed in finding the primary site of dermal invasion. To locate it, however, is not without importance, for its excision and the neutralization of the residual bacilli it harbors by local injection of antitoxin is necessary if the source of toxin is to be eradicated.

The nervous disease, which consists of involuntary spasms of striated muscle, is entirely the result of the toxin elaborated by the organism.

Rabies (see also Chap. 206). This disease is usually contracted from the bite of an infected carnivore (usually a dog), though scratches and abrasions and even the penetration of a mucous membrane by infected saliva from rabid animals may be the means of transmitting the viral infection. The disease is usually fatal. It can be prevented by human diploid vaccine.

Diphtheritic wound infections. Although diphtheritic infections seldom need to be considered in the Occidental world (since most children have been vaccinated against diphtheria), a chronic wound covered by a shaggy gray exudate should always be searched for Klebs-Loeffler (K-L) bacilli.

Contamination of the skin lesion by these organisms may cause the ulcer and its surrounding skin to become insensitive to touch and pinprick. The adjacent muscles may become palsied. The ulcer more often occurs on the pharyngeal wall rather than the skin, though in one case seen by the author it was on the buccal surface and was followed by numbness of the cheek, and palsy of facial and pharyngeal muscles (Bell's palsy and dysphagia). Only after several weeks have passed (4 to 8) does a symmetric, diffuse sensorimotor polyneuropathy develop. The protein level in the cerebrospinal fluid is elevated. Death is usually due to myocardiopathy. (see Chap. 178).

Tick and black widow spider bites (chronic atrophic acrodermatitis). The bite of a certain tick (*Dermacentor andersoni*), especially in the area of the head and neck, may be followed within a few hours by rapid pulse, hyperpnea, and later, flaccid paralysis of the legs, trunk, and arms. The paralysis is believed to be due to a toxin, for removal of the tick results in recovery within a few hours. However, the tick bite may be followed by an erythematous rash, erythema chronicum migrans, which lasts for months and spreads.

In Middle and Eastern Europe, Schaltenbrand [92] and others have observed a clinical entity which they call *acrodermatitis chronica atrophicans*. The usual sequence of events has been an insect bite on the trunk or limbs followed by local erythema, and then, after a few days to a few weeks, a sensory disturbance and weakness of muscles in the segments involved. The weakness may lead to muscle atrophy and reflex loss. Spread of the neurologic disorder to other parts of the body (a generalization of the radiculitis) may follow, and in a few cases signs of disease of pyramidal tracts have indicated involvement of the spinal cord. There has been a low-grade meningitis (lymphocytes in the cerebrospinal fluid with increased protein) in some cases. Recovery is the rule with variable residual signs. Pathologic verification has not been achieved. Postulation of a viral agent introduced by the arthropod similar to that of Czechoslovakian, or Russian, spring–summer encephalitis remains unproved.

In contrast, the bite of the black widow spider results in painful spasms of the muscles of the trunk and limbs. Again, a toxin appears to be responsible. Appearing within a few hours and frightening in their intensity, the spasms fortunately subside within a few days and leave no sequelae. Only symptomatic treatment is necessary.

Herpes simplex. Herpes simplex virus, the cause of ubiquitous low-grade, recurrent lesions in the oral and genital regions, may be induced to flare up upon exposure of lips to wind and sun, trauma, and fever (particularly that accompanying certain infections such as meningococcus meningitis). Occasionally the virus passes along nerve fibers (perhaps olfactory) to reach the central nervous system, where it induces an encephalitis. Viremia is another and more likely mode of spread, especially in infants where lesions in lungs, liver, and other viscera indicate hematogenous dissemination (see Chap. 190).

Primary neoplasms of the skin

Cutaneous melanomas. The patient with a metastatic melanoma may present himself or herself at a medical or neurologic service with symptoms and signs of increased intracranial pressure or a focal cerebral lesion. Melanoma becomes one of the most frequent metastatic lesions in the brain (following lung, breast, and gastrointestinal tract in frequency), and should always be suspected in an adult with a brain tumor. Often the patient will have forgotten about the cutaneous melanoma that was removed years before, and only by inquiring about each dermal scar may the cause be ascertained. Examination of the urine for melanin by-products may confirm the diagnosis, but only if metastatic lesions in the liver are numerous (see Chap. 81).

A clinical approach to the neurocutaneous disease

From this lengthy survey one cannot but be impressed with the number and variety of neurocutaneous diseases. Indeed, it would seem that the nervous system is more often implicated in dermatologic disease than any other organ in the human body. The reasons why this might be so were brought out in the discussion of pathogenic mechanisms.

It occurs to the author that if this large compilation of data is to be useful, it must be systematized. For the novice as well as the seasoned clinician, only some type of reordering of these facts could make them immediately applicable to the common problems likely to be encountered in the clinic. This the author has attempted to do in the following pages, considering in succession the clinical situations where a systematic knowledge of the dermatologic or neurologic aspects of these diseases might clarify the most frequently encountered medical problems.

An infant born with, or developing in the first weeks of life, a visible abnormality of skin

Here is a situation where accurate dermatologic diagnosis might serve in predicting whether the nervous system is, or will later prove to be, abnormal. One must keep in mind that clinical methods for assessing the immature nervous system at, or shortly after, birth are not wholly dependable. Since the human cerebrum is undeveloped and functioning imperfectly, the neurologic examination perforce must be limited to the testing of reflexes and the demonstration of certain segmental and postural automatisms, which serve only to establish the integrity of spinal cord and brainstem and peripheral sensorimotor structures. Warned through the dermatologic manifestations of an impending neurocutaneous disease, the clinician seeks the neurologic disorder more carefully.

Congenital defects of skin and other structures. Of course the gross defects of spine and/or cerebrum, such as meningomyeloceles, meningoencephaloceles, or anencephalic states, which are always associated with some abnormality of the skin and subcutaneous structures, pose no diagnostic problem. It is the minor blemishes, i.e., malformations of skin and hair or subcutaneous cystlike structures that give trouble. Many of these are of no significance and may disappear soon. Others, seemingly innocent, are of more dire significance. The observant mother who wants to know about every imperfection in her newborn infant may press for their removal. Excision without the guidance of x-ray has been a common mistake. If the defect is in the

midline posteriorly, one must always consider the possibility of a small meningocele with a fistulous connection between the subcutaneous cyst and meninges. An x-ray will show the opening in the skull through which it connects with interior structures or a defect in the pedicles and spine of vertebrae. Later such lesions may call attention to a cerebellar defect if occipital in location, or to a radicular or spinal cord abnormality of delayed onset if spinal in location. Since they may serve also as a pathway for the entrance of bacterial pathogens which give rise to brain abscess or recurrent meningitis, they should be sought in all children with intraspinal or intracranial suppuration.

Peculiarities of skin in conjunction with malformations of cranium, eyes, nose, lips, jaws, and ears. They may take many forms, which deserve study and differentiation. One group in which the eyes, nose, and lips fail to form is so striking that the configuration at once reveals the nature of the associated brain anomaly, i.e., cyclopia, or arrhinencephalis. The low, beetling brow, heavy eyebrows which fuse in midline, the upturned nose, and small head betray the cerebral abnormality of de Lange's dwarf state with almost certain development of mental retardation. One group of these disorders is associated with a demonstrable chromosomal abnormality: in mongolism, the epicanthic folds are observable at birth and, if combined with large tongue, open mouth, round head, transverse palmar creases, displaced triradii (dermatoglyphic abnormality), short curved fifth fingers, etc., should indicate an examination of the karyotype for presence of 21 trisomy, the 13,15 and 17,18 trisomies, 4,5 deletion syndrome, mosaicism of 18, and other abnormalities. In these and all the other craniofacial anomalies, cerebral development tends also to be curtailed, and mental retardation can be predicted. Caution is advised in the interpretation of single abnormalities, such as epicanthic folds, for they may occur in individuals who later turn out to have normal intelligence. Table 172-2 summarizes some of the principal syndromes.

Vascular malformations of skin. Cutaneous hemangiomas are to be numbered among the most frequent of all somatic abnormalities. Most of all the small midline hemangiomas bear no relation to abnormalities of the nervous system, nor does the spreading nevus flammeus, which develops a few days or weeks after birth. Many of them disappear after a few months or years. Only the large cranial hemangioma or the truncal-brachial or crural ones are of significance. Those of the ophthalmic–trigeminal area indicate the possibility of a concomitant meningeal angioma that will almost certainly become the basis of a neurologic syndrome consisting of convulsions, contralateral hemiplegia, etc., within a few years. A brachial–cervical hemangioma with hypertrophy of the arm (Klippel-Trénauney-Weber syndrome) should alert one to the later appearance of a spinal cord vascular malformation. As to the other neurologic disorders associated with vascular anomalies of skin such as familial telangiectasia, ataxia-telangiectasia, and Fabry's disease, the dermal vascular lesion, as a rule, appears much later in life (late childhood or adolescence) and, in the case of ataxia-telangiectasia, long after the development of neurologic symptoms.

Table 172-5   Differential diagnosis of pigmentary changes of skin with neurologic disorders

	Skin criteria	Neurologic disorders
Tuberous sclerosis	Hypomelanotic patches, adenoma sebaceum, subungual fibromas, shagreen patches	Epilepsy, mental retardation
Neurofibromatosis	Café au lait patches, cutaneous fibromas	Signs of cranial nerve root, spinal cord, or nerve involvement
Ataxia-telangiectasia	Telangiectasia of conjunctivae, ears, neck; white patches	Choreoathetosis, ataxia, mental retardation
Chédiak-Higashi disease	Albinism	Signs of cerebral disease
Waardenburg-Klein syndrome	White forelock (piebaldness), lateral displacement inner canthi, heterochromic irides	Deafness
Vogt-Koyanagi-Harada syndrome	Hypomelanotic macules, poliosis	Signs of lymphocytic meningitis
Sex-linked deafness of Ziprowski	Hyper- and hypomelanotic macules	Deafness
Total albinism and syndrome of Cross and McKusick	Cutaneous hypopigmentation, ocular abnormalities	Mental retardation, spastic diplegia epilepsy, deafness
Melanoderma	Generalized pigmentation	Mental deficiency
Giant pigmented nevi	Large pigmented nevi	Hydrocephalus
Phenylketonuria	Dilution of hair and iris pigmentation	Epilepsy and mental retardation
Adrenoleukodystrophy	Brownish pigmentation (diffuse)	Signs of leukodystrophy; male sex-linked disease

The ichthyoses and related disorders. The group of ichthyotic states must not be confused with the simple scaling of the skin (so often seen in the postmature infant), the desquamation which follows an intrauterine rash (as in syphilis), or the dermal abnormalities of cretinism. Some of the xerodermic and ichthyotic states do not appear until weeks or months after birth. Nevertheless, they usually are noted earlier than the common variety of a hereditary ichthyosis vulgaris (onset at 1 to 2 years of age). Unlike the latter they portend dwarfism, mental retardation, and a variety of generalized spastic, ataxic, and choreoathetotic states, listed under the eponyms of Rud's, Laubenthal's, Stewart's, and Sjögren-Larsson syndromes. Refsum's syndrome has also later developed in some patients with hereditary dryness of skin. The diseases listed in Table 172-4 should be considered in the differential diagnosis of ichthyotic idiocy.

Pigment disorders of skin. The giant pigmented nevi may present at this age as solitary congenital abnormalities, yet among such cases the incidence of mental retardation has been higher than in otherwise normal individuals. Moreover, there is risk in later childhood of melanoma or melanosis of the meninges, and of medulloblastoma. Scattered hyperpigmentation of the skin may result from chronic inflammatory states such as incontinentia pigmenti and occurs also in congenital melanoderma. Impairment of pigmentation may be observed in some patients with phenylketonuria. Hypomelanotic nevi may also appear in the first weeks of life and should warn the pediatrician of tuberous sclerosis, a diagnosis which may be confirmed early by the concatenation of other abnormalities (see Table 172-5).

Laxity of skin. This too may be detected early, though probably not in infancy. When observed, it raises suspicion of Turner-Bonnevie-Ullrich syndrome (confirmed by search for Barr bodies and deletion of an X chromosome) or the Ehlers-Danlos cutis elastica syndrome. If limited to the scalp, obvious delay in psychomotor development may be expected early in life. Some girls with Turner's syndrome will later be found to exhibit a mild degree of subnormal mental development without other neurologic abnormality.

Table 172-6   Hair changes with neurologic disorders

Argininosuccinic aciduria	Fragile hair, trichorrhexis nodosa
Homocystinuria	Fragile, lighter than normal siblings
Methioninuria or methionine absorption syndrome	White hair, fragile hair
Phenylketonuria	Blond hair, or usually lighter hair than in normal siblings
Bjornstad's syndrome of deafness	Pili torti
Kinky hair syndrome	Pili torti, easily broken hair
Ectodermal dysplasias: Anhidrotic Hidrotic	Sparsity and fragility of hair, lighter than in normal siblings
Lipodystrophic diabetes	Kinky hair, hirsutism
Dilantin ingestion	Hirsutism
Gargoylism (Hunter-Hurler syndrome)	Hirsutism Body hair, bushy eyebrows
Cornelia de Lange's syndrome	Hirsutism, bushy eyebrows
Thallium poisoning	Total loss of hair

Excessive hairiness of skin. Many congenital nevi are tufted with a growth of hair, and in lumbosacral dysraphism a tuft of hair may cover an underlying neural abnormality. Early hirsutism of face and trunk should suggest the Amsterdam dwarf syndrome of de Lange and also congenital lipodystrophic diabetes. Later in life hirsutism loses its significance, for chronic illness of any type during childhood may be attended by excessive growth of hair over the face and limbs. Hirsutism and gingival hyperplasia are

Table 172-7 Sensory syndromes with anhidrosis and often analgesia

	Congenital sensory neuropathy	Hereditary radicular neuropathy	Congenital indifference to pain	Syringomyelia, syringobulbia	Familial dysautonomia	Diabetic multiple neuropathy
Intelligence	Defective	Normal	Normal	Normal	Defective	Normal
Heredity	Recessive or dominant	Dominant	None	None	Recessive	None
Age of onset	Birth	Childhood	Birth	Adulthood	Birth	Late life
Distribution of sensory loss	Universal	Distal extremities, especially legs	Universal	Cervical segments	Universal	Asymmetrical legs
Pain and temperature perception	Absent	Absent	Absent	Absent	Reduced	Reduced
Touch	Present or diminished	Absent	Normal	Normal	Normal	Reduced
Axon reflex	None	None	None	Present	None	Reduced
Tendon reflexes	Hypoactive	Diminished or absent	Normal	Diminished or absent	Diminished	Absent
Motor function	Delayed	Weakness	Normal	Reduced or normal	Normal	Weakness or paralysis
Lesion	Nerve fibers reduced or absent	Loss of nerve fibers	Normal	Skin and nerve biopsy negative	Normal nerve endings	Loss of fibers in nerves and root

frequently observed in epileptic infants who have received Dilantin therapy. Dilantin itself will stimulate hair growth as well as hyperplasia of gums and breast tissue, but some of these changes are at times seen in children who have never received Dilantin (e.g., mannosidosis).

The most typical hair changes in neurologic disorders are listed in Table 172-6.

Abnormalities of sweating, lacrimation, salivation, etc. These are common to all the extensive hypoplastic or dysplastic congenital diseases of the skin. Anhidrotic ectodermal dysplasia, Fabry's disease, and incontinentia pigmenti are examples. If the skin is otherwise normal, the most likely possibility in the child is the Riley-Day dysautonomia syndrome or one of several familial or acquired polyneuropathies, including one type of congenital analgesia. The majority of the children will later be shown to have abnormalities of the peripheral nervous system, and not a few will prove to be mentally backward. In the adult, diseases of the peripheral nervous system (Shy-Drager syndrome), diabetic polyneuropathy, or one of the other familial polyneuropathies may produce a similar syndrome by affecting fibers of the autonomic nervous system.

Table 172-7 contains a listing of principal anhidrotic syndromes and their differential characteristics.

Light sensitivity with or without bullous formation. This phenomenon ordinarily does not become manifest until months have passed, since small babies are usually protected from sunlight. When present, it should always suggest one of the following diseases: Hartnup disease, hydroxykynurenuria, pellagra, Rothmund-Thomson syndrome, Cockayne's disease, phenylketonuria, xerodermic idiocy, variegate porphyria, phenothiazine reaction.

Thickening and colorless papules of skin. During infancy

and early childhood, cutaneous lesions of this type provide useful confirmation of Hunter-Hurler disease. Xanthomas may be the earliest sign of congenital lipodystrophic diabetes.

Miscellaneous disorders. The disorders listed earlier as focal dermal hypoplasia, incontinentia pigmenti, epidermolysis bullosa, congenital melanoderma, congenital poikiloderma, basal cell nevus syndrome, orofaciodigital syndrome, and anhidrotic ectodermal dysplasia become manifest early in life and must be distinguished one from another, for they each have slightly different neurologic implications. In focal dermal hypoplasia, anomalies of other organs and nervous system (syndactyly, spina bifida, microcephaly, coloboma, etc.) are frequently conjoined. However, the impairment of brain development may not declare itself until later, by lesions of the nervous system which are of the acquired type leading to microcephaly and mental retardation. In the closely related syndromes of incontinentia pigmenti, epidermolysis bullosa, and congenital poikiloderma, the microcephaly, mental retardation, epilepsy, and spastic paralysis of the legs may also be delayed in their appearance, but awareness of skin lesions will have alerted the pediatrician to these possibilities.

Some of the congenital neurocutaneous diseases result in a premature aging of the skin and tumor formation. These are listed in Table 172-8. In the author's experience the most difficult problem in the diagnosis of these diffuse skin lesions, some of which have vesicular, bullous, or erythematous features, has been to differentiate them from the skin lesions of congenital syphilis, rubella, cytomegalic inclusion disease, and herpes simplex. In the latter, the affection of the nervous system is almost always accompanied by signs of disease of the liver (hepatomegaly and jaundice) and other organs, and the cerebrospinal fluid

Table 172-8   Neurologic disorders resulting in premature aging of the skin and hair

Ataxia-telangiectasia
Xerodermic idiocy of de Sanctis and Cacchione
Myotonia congenita
Werner's syndrome
Rothmund-Thomson syndrome (poikiloderma congenitale)
Progeria
Mongolism (Down's syndrome)
Klinefelter's syndrome

contains cells, increased protein, and sometimes the infective agent. Later, during early infancy, these congenital skin lesions must be distinguished from eczematous dermatitis.

A child or adult with a disorder of the nervous system in which dermatologic study may clarify diagnosis

An infant or child, previously regarded as normal, in whom seizures have developed (massive flexion spasms in infancy, grand mal in childhood). As has been pointed out, during the first two years of life the onset of flexion, or salaam, spasms may be due to a variety of pathologic processes, some identifiable during life, others only at autopsy. In this respect this type of epilepsy differs in no important way from that which begins at a more advanced age; it merely signifies a cerebral pathologic condition without indicating the specific causative disease. Here, finding three or more white macules over trunk or limbs or focal hypomelanosis of eyelashes is highly suggestive of tuberous sclerosis, a diagnosis which, if once considered, may then be confirmed by x-rays of skull, CT scans, studies of heart, kidneys, etc., even at this early age. Here the Wood's lamp is indispensable. (Occasionally such a lesion may presage ataxia-telangiectasia. Vitiligo and nevus anemicus must be distinguished.)

Multiple café au lait spots will suggest neurofibromatosis. Here the point also to be noted is that pigmented patches in the skin may precede any recognizable neurologic disorder and should forewarn the dermatologist that an observed seizure or a slight backwardness may be the first and only neurologic expression of these diseases, easily missed if not sought.

Psychomotor retardation or seizures without other neurologic abnormality should suggest the possibility of an underlying phenylketonuria, histidinuria, or homocystinuria. Since all these diseases interfere to some degree with tyrosinase activity, any change in pigmentation of skin or hair must be accorded special notice. Also, the presence of a stubborn eczematous dermatitis is a notable accompaniment of some cases of phenylketonuria in infancy or childhood. Epilepsy with sensitivity to sunlight always raises the question of Hartnup disease.

Later in life, generalized seizures, especially when accompanied by retarded mental development, should prompt a careful search for the other skin manifestations of tuberous sclerosis as well as a variety of other metabolic derangements, such as argininosuccinic aminoaciduria, Hartnup disease, or phenylketonuria, any one of which may cause seizures.

A child brought to the clinic with retarded psychomotor development. This, one of the most frequent of all problems in the pediatric age group, has again multiple causation, the most common being developmental faults, obstetric accidents, and a wide variety of acquired infective, traumatic, and metabolic states. Once again the dermatologist must recall the dire portent of the group of idiopathic, vesicular, ulcerating, and fibrosing skin lesions arising in early life and leading to scaling, pigmentation, atrophy, and keratosis of the skin, and of the xerodermic, ichthyotic lesions and giant pigmented nevi. Mongolism and the other trisomic chromosomal abnormalities form another large group (some 10 percent of patients admitted to institutions for the feebleminded) where dermatologic clues have singular prominence. Epicanthic folds, abnormal palmar marking, and fingerprint patterns stand as the identifiable characteristics of mongolism. Other abnormalities of the cranium, nose, eyes, jaw, and palate indicate the possibility of one of the other chromosomal abnormalities or of cerebral developmental anomalies without chromosomal defect (arrhinencephalia, cyclops abnormality, etc.).

The metabolic disorders constitute another small but important group of diseases, several of which can be suspected by examination of skin and hair. In cretinism the skin is cool and dry, and the hair is sparse and coarse. An erythematous scaling rash on exposed surfaces should suggest ichthyosiform erythroedema in the neonate, and later, if persistent and recurrent, Hartnup disease, hydroxykynurenuria, Cockayne's disease, or pellagra. Sensitivity to sunlight is a prominent feature of these diseases, but this trait also occurs in some cases of phenylketonuria, lipid proteinosis, and variegate porphyria. Pale nodules or papules may provide the clue to tuberous sclerosis, gargoylism, or the lipid proteinosis of Urbach-Wiethe.

An aspect of dermatology, recently brought to medical attention, is the use of skin biopsy in the diagnosis of hereditary metabolic diseases of the nervous system. In an easily accessible specimen of skin, prepared for electron microscopic study, one may discover subcellular particles characteristic of a disease whose only or principal manifestations are neurologic. Martin et al [93] have reported their successes in the diagnosis of the following diseases: infantile and tardive forms of ceroid lipofuscinosis, mucopolysaccharidosis (Hurler, Sanfilippo A), mucolipidosis (I cell disease), acid maltase deficiency (Pompe's disease), and infantile metachromatic leukodystrophy.

The examination of hair, a relatively neglected part of dermatologic study, may give important leads, for a number of important metabolic neurocutaneous diseases express themselves through this appendage of skin. There may be abnormalities in growth of hair. Hirsutism is a feature of lipodystrophic diabetes and the de Lange dwarf syndrome; a beaked nose, antimongoloid slant of eyes, and small head open the possibility of the Rubenstein-Taybi syndrome. Sparse, coarse hair is found in hypothyroidism and in anhydrotic ectodermal dysplasia. Dilution of hair color favors the diagnosis of phenylketonuria, histidinuria, and homocystinuria; the virtual absence of pigmentation favors albinism.

A white forelock should alert the clinician to the possibility of Waardenburg-Klein syndrome (with associated deafness), but it is sometimes a solitary abnormality. Depigmentation around the eyes and tufts of hair raise the question of tuberous sclerosis or Chédiak-Higashi disease, and in later life it suggests Vogt-Koyanagi-Harada disease. In argininosuccinic aminoaciduria a vertical splitting occurs between nodosities of the hair shaft (trichorrhexis nodosa); in the kinky hair syndrome the shaft is also of uneven caliber and twisted; and in monilethrix it is flattened and twisted. A hand lens permits distinctions to be drawn among these three abnormalities of hair.

Dwarfism with mental retardation and other slowly evolving major neurologic abnormalities such as athetosis, dystonia, ataxia, and spastic diplegia. Here the neurologic disorder tends to dominate the clinical picture. The child is obviously stunted, and both his head circumference and body weight are down to the first percentile or below. Failure to attain the usual milestones of development in motor control, locomotion, speech, and perception can be noted even on cursory examination. Stiffness and hyperreflexia or, in the older child, tremor, ataxia, or rigidity and athetosis point to extensive involvement of motor cortices, basal ganglia, or cerebellum. Oddly enough, patients with such florid neurologic abnormalities seldom are found to have chromosomal abnormalities or biochemical disturbances. Developmental fault, a cerebral dysgenesis, or destruction of the cerebral hemispheres by hypoxia, kernicterus, or an antenatal or natal infection are the more frequent associated disease states and they seldom have dermatologic accompaniments. When there is a skin anomaly, it most often takes the form of ichthyosis or poikiloderma, which should not be difficult to recognize.

Dwarfism should raise suspicion of ataxia-telangiectasia, Cockayne's syndrome, xerodermic idiocy, generalized lentigines, and poikiloderma congenitale. Of these diseases, poikilodermatous changes in the skin (hyper- and hypopigmentation with atrophy and telangiectasia) are the most common.

Familial hyperuricemia, the syndrome of Cross et al [74] of mental deficiency, spasticity, athetosis and hypopigmentation of the skin, Hallervorden-Spatz progressive athetosis or dystonia, and Wilson's disease must also be included in the differential diagnosis. Self-mutilation suggests familial hyperuricemia, while hypermelanosis may indicate some of the other diseases.

A child or adult with cerebellar ataxia. Episodic ataxia, incoordination of limbs, and unsteadiness of gait, lasting usually for a few days after the occurrence of one or more convulsions, represents one of the more puzzling syndromes in pediatric neurology. Its differentiation taxes clinical acumen. In the very young child any convulsive illness which confines the patient to bed for days or weeks results in weakness and unsteadiness which may be difficult to distinguish from true cerebellar ataxia. Close inspection of the limbs will show none of the usual features of cerebellar ataxia, i.e., dysmetria, lack of synergism of component muscle groups involved in skilled acts, hypotonia, or intention tremor.

Sensory ataxia can be excluded by lack of sensory deficit (particularly vibratory and position senses) and retention of tendon reflexes which are nearly always abolished in diseases of the peripheral nervous system. Also finger

ataxia (pseudoathetosis of outstretched fingers with eyes closed) and positive Romberg's sign are present. Ataxia from an overdose of Dilantin or phenobarbital given for the control of the seizures, often accompanied by a pruritic macular and papular eruption, may also produce an episodic ataxia of cerebellar type. This diagnosis can be confirmed by measuring the blood levels of these drugs and observing the recession of the ataxia as the dose is reduced.

Recurrent episodic ataxia should always raise suspicion of Hartnup disease or hydroxykynurenuria and other of the hyperammonemias (e.g., argininosuccinic aminoaciduria and citrullinemia). Here the dematologic findings of skin erythema and blistering on exposure to sunlight and infrared rays are helpful to the neurologist, for they indicate Hartnup syndrome or hydroxykynurenuria. Blond coloration of hair, not concordant with race and parentage, and brittleness of hair point to argininosuccinic aminoaciduria. Urine analyses for these amino acids will confirm the clinical impression. A single attack of an acute cerebellar ataxia appearing in the wake of an infectious exanthematous disease such as chickenpox, vaccinia, or measles is most compatible with postinfectious encephalomyelitis.

The gradual development of a persistent ataxia of cerebellar type, appearing in the first few years of life, should alert the clinician to ataxia-telangiectasia. As mentioned previously, oculomotor apraxia and a movement disorder like choreoathetosis are other components of the syndrome. The characteristic tracery of small vessels over conjunctivae, ears, neck, etc., provides the obvious clue to diagnosis. This skin change may not appear for some years, but an expectant attitude facilitates its early recognition. Tremulous ataxia combined with xeroderma, small stature, and mental retardation, sometimes with athetotic movements of the fingers, comprise the Laubenthal syndrome of xerodermic idiocy. Cerebellar ataxia with tendon xanthomatoses occurs in the van Bogaert-Epstein-Scherer form of cholesterinosis. Cerebellar ataxia with dwarfism, mental deficiency, partial deafness, and retinitis pigmentosa comprise Cockayne's syndrome.

In Cockayne's syndrome (dwarfism with kyphosis and ankylosis, mental deficiency, deafness, and retinitis pigmentosa) a cerebellar ataxia may appear early in the illness. Suspicion should be raised by the finding of a dermatitis in the "butterfly area" of the face (suggestive of lupus erythematosus). Lipodystrophy of the face is another frequent finding. The onset is at about 2 years of age, and the disease is slowly progressive, ending in blindness, deafness, idiocy, and paralysis.

Cerebellar ataxia in combination with symptoms of intracranial tumor (headaches, papilledema, vomiting) developing in childhood may, rarely, be clarified by the finding of a basal cell nevus. Additional clues are provided by the presence of hypertelorism, other skeletal anomalies, and cysts of the jaw. The cerebellar tumor proves usually to be a medulloblastoma. Giant pigmented nevi may produce a similar syndrome by metastasis of melanotic melanoma to the cerebellum or by a basal meningeal melanomatosis with hydrocephalus and a cerebral type of ataxia. In the adolescent or young adult, a cerebellar tumor, especially if familial and with coincident polycythemia, should lead to a search for von Hippel's retinal angioma. Such findings corroborate the clinical impression of Lindau's cerebellar hemangioblastoma. Ataxia is also present in some cases of cretinism, manifested early in life by excessive livedo reticularis and later by dry, cool, lax, coarse skin and thick, sparse hair.

Progressive ataxia during childhood, adolescence, or adult life with areflexia of the limbs and other signs of peripheral nerve disease receives clarification by the finding of dryness and scaling of the skin, a combination typical of Refsum's heredopathia atactica polyneuritiformis. The presence of xanthomas of the skin suggests at once the diagnosis of congenital lipodystrophic diabetes, Tangier disease, and Urbach-Wiethe lipid proteinosis.

A child or adult with spastic paraparesis. Spastic weakness of the legs, out of proportion to affection of arms or cranial and trunk musculature, often presents as a relatively discrete syndrome. It may be combined with mental retardation. In its nonprogressive form the reader will recognize its identity with cerebral palsy or cerebral spastic diplegia. Not infrequently the condition becomes manifest toward the end of the first year of life, remaining thereafter rather stable. Presumably, development to the stage of standing and stepping have exposed a preexistent congenital defect.

The finding of congenital ichthyosis in conjunction with mental retardation and spastic paraparesis establishes, in most instances, the diagnosis of Sjögren-Larsson syndrome. In a case of the author's, however, autopsy disclosed a "globoid body" form of leukodystrophy (a hereditary disease of the cerebral white matter developing in the early years of life). Spastic weakness of the legs has been associated in some instances with homocystinuria.

Spastic paraparesis presenting in childhood or adolescence, if combined with cutaneous hypopigmentation (albinism) and multiple ocular anomalies, conforms to the Mast syndrome described by Cross et al [74].

Chronic pigmentation of the skin with adrenal insufficiency and spastic weakness as well as other signs of progressive leukodystrophy (dementia, blindness, etc.) in boys and male adults are indicative of adrenoleukodystrophy.

An infant, child, or adult with an acute illness consisting of disorder of cerebral function or meningeal irritation in association with a rash. This clinical problem, a frequent source of perplexity to the medical staff of every large hospital, requires consideration of a variety of disease states. For one thing, there are a number of idiosyncratic reactions to a drug such as Dilantin or phenobarbital, where a pruritic macular and papular eruption on the trunk and limbs may be combined with drowsiness, confusion, ataxia, or coma (the effects produced by the direct action of the drug on the nervous system).

The macular and papular rash with a lymphocytic ("aseptic") meningitis may provide the clue to one of the Coxsackie or echo viral infections and, in certain parts of the world, to a rickettsial disease.

A fading macular and papular or a vesicular eruption may be the residue of rubeola, rubella, or varicella infection which has been complicated by a postinfectious encephalomyelitis. Here history of exposure during an epidemic, details of the clinical state, and the lymphocytic pleocytosis of the cerebrospinal fluid are the main diag-nostic features. The hemorrhagic rash of meningococcemia aids in the recognition or anticipation of meningococcus meningitis, and the salmon-colored mottling of the limbs, of the Waterhouse-Friderichsen syndrome.

Specific sensory defects in which the diagnosis is aided by dermatologic study

Deafness. One of the first responsibilities of the pediatrician or pediatric neurologist in examining a child whose psychomotor development appears to be lagging is to make sure that the whole trouble is not a lack of hearing. It is obvious enough that the auditory and visual senses are the main avenues for receiving information about the world and also that early speech development is dependent upon hearing. Deaf children show disinterest in sounds and music, do not babble in an elaborate way or imitate their mothers, and do not acquire words. They may develop their own language (idioglossia), but usually grow up as deaf-mutes.

The dermatologist may be helpful in the diagnosis of such cases. Congenital deafness, which may be either of two types, conductive or neural, may be associated with a number of disorders of keratinization and pigmentation of skin and of craniofacial development. In the Waardenburg-Klein syndrome, attention will be called to the condition by the lateral displacement of the inner canthi, hypertrichosis of the eyebrows, heterochromia of irides, and white forelock. Also, the retinal pigment of the affected eye is decreased. Albinism and deafness constitute another syndrome, the inheritance tending to follow an autosomal recessive or sex-linked pattern. Some deaf children are piebald (autosomal dominant). In some patients with sensory nerve deafness there is pili torti, onychodystrophic nerve deafness, keratosis palmaris et plantaris, acanthosis nigricans, and ainhum. Pili torti, in which hair grows in a twisted configuration, and a cochlear type of deafness are part of Bjornstad's syndrome.

Neural deafness constitutes an element also in Refsum's syndrome, Fabry's disease, Cockayne's syndrome, xeroderma pigmentosum, Laurence-Moon-Biedl syndrome, Werner's syndrome, and Hunter-Hurler syndrome. Also, the conduction type of deafness appears conjoined with a number of craniofacial deformities such as the mandibulofacial dysostosis (Treacher Collins syndrome); maldevelopment of ears (only ear pits appearing); Hallerman-Streiff, Cornelia de Lange's, and Turner's syndromes; and E trisomy, Dysacousia and deafness of nerve type may also complicate the Vogt-Koyanagi-Harada syndrome and congenital syphilis.

Blindness. Obvious visual defects occasioned by microphthalmia, coloboma, retrolental fibrodysplasia, and chorioretinitis are usually unattended by dermatologic abnormality. Ophthalmic diagnosis in other very young patients proves most difficult. There may be uncertainty as to whether disinclination to follow moving objects, a failure to peer at the mother's face, or failure to recognize her represents an inadequacy of the peripheral visual mechanism or a cerebral disease (cortical blindness). As the months pass, however, repeated examinations usually leave little doubt as to the existence of visual impairment. In these cases a clue as to an oncoming gargoylism, the osseous features of which become evident in the second and third years, may be a mistiness or cloudiness of cornea or hirsutism and an orange-peel quality of the skin. Similarly Refsum's syndrome and the Laurence-Moon-Biedl syndrome may be suspected by the expert dermatologist before the retinal pigmentation is certain. Optic atrophy as a cause of blindness will at once be recognized as the Stewart syndrome if a congenital ichthyosis is noted. Blindness from glaucoma receives clarification when there is recognition of a craniofacial hemangioma—Sturge-Weber-Dimitri syndrome. Also, a certain number of cases of glioma of the optic nerve and chiasm will become obvious once the dermatologist confirms the presence of the skin lesions of neurofibromatosis.

References

1. Brown JW, Podosin R: A syndrome of the neural crest. *Arch Neurol* **15**:294, 1966
2. Sidman RS, Fawcett D: Effect of peripheral nerve section on brown fat. *Anat Rec* **118**:487, 1954
3. Van der Hoeve I: Eye symptoms of tuberous sclerosis of the brain. *Trans Ophthalmol Soc UK* **40**:329, 1920
4. Gomez MR: *Tuberous Sclerosis.* New York, Raven Press, 1979, p 246
5. Reed WB et al: Internal manifestations of tuberous sclerosis. *Arch Dermatol* **87**:715, 1963
6. Nickel WR, Reed WB: Tuberous sclerosis. *Arch Dermatol* **85**:209, 1962
7. Lagos JE, Gomez MR: Tuberous sclerosis: reappraisal of a clinical entity. *Mayo Clin Proc* **42**:26, 1967
8. Moolton SE: Hamartial nature of the tuberous sclerosis complex and its bearing on the tumor problem. *Arch Intern Med* **69**:589, 1942
9. Caron P: Contribution à l'étude clinique de la sclérose tubéreuse. Thesis, Paris, 1939
10. Van Bogeart L et al: Etude sur la sclérose tubéreuse de Bourneville à forme cérébelleuse. *Rev Neurol (Paris)* **98**:673, 1958
11. Busch KT, Busch G: Neuro-opthalmologische Befunde bei der tuberösen Sklerose. *Klin Monatsch Augenheilkd* **141**:388, 1962
12. Donegani G et al: Contribution à l'étude de la maladie de Bourneville. *Bull Int Serv Sante Arm* **1**:359, 1963
13. Fitzpatrick TB et al: White leaf-shaped macules, earliest visible sign of tuberous sclerosis. *Arch Dermatol* **98**:1, 1968
14. Gold AP, Freeman JM: Depigmented nevi, the earliest sign of tuberous sclerosis. *Pediatrics* **35**:1003, 1965
15. Butterworth T, Wilson M Jr: Dermatologic aspects of tuberous sclerosis. *Arch Dermatol Syphilol* **43**:1, 1941
16. Crowe FW et al: *A Clinical, Pathological and Genetic Study of Multiple Neurofibromatoses.* Springfield, IL, Charles C Thomas, 1956
17. Canale D, Bebin J: Von Recklinghausen's neurofibromatosis, in *Handbook of Clinical Neurology.* Amsterdam, North-Holland, 1972, p 132
18. Canale D et al: Neurologic manifestations of von Recklinghausen's disease of the nervous system. *Confin Neurol* **24**:359, 1964
19. Yakovlev PI, Guthrie RH: Congenital ectodermatoses (neurocutaneous syndromes) in epileptic patients. *Arch Neurol Psychiat* **26**:1145, 1931
20. Rosman NP, Pearce J; The brain in neurofibromatosis. *Brain* **90**:829, 1967
21. Crowe FW: Axillary freckling as a diagnostic aid in neurofibromatosis. *Ann Intern Med* **61**:1142, 1964
22. Hunt JC, Pugh DG: Skeletal lesions in neurofibromatosis. *Radiology* **76**:1, 1961
23. Benedict PH et al: Melanotic macules in Albright's syndrome and in neurofibromatosis. *JAMA* **205**:618, 1968
24. Bielschowsky M: Über tuberöse Sklerose und ihre Beziehungen zur Recklinghausenchen Krankheit. *Z Gesamte Neurol Psychiat* **26**:133, 1914
25. Rubinstein L: *Tumors of the Central Nervous System.* Washington, DC, Armed Forces Institute of Pathology, 1972
26. Alexander GL, Norman RM: *The Sturge-Weber Syndrome.* Bristol, John Wright & Son, 1960
27. Cobb S: Haemangioma of the spinal cord associated with skin naevi of the same metamere. *Ann Surg* **62**:641, 1915
28. Van Bogaert L: Pathologie des angiomatoses. *Acta Neurol Psych Belg* **50**:525, 1950
29. Brégeat P: Brégeat syndrome, in *Handbook of Clinical Neurology,* vol 14, *The Phakomatoses,* edited by PJ Vinken, GW Bruyn. Amsterdam, North-Holland, 1972, p 474
30. Haborland C: The phakomatoses, in *Handbook of Clinical Neurology,* vol 31, edited by PJ Vinken, GW Bruyn. Amsterdam, North-Holland, 1977, p 1
31. Bonnet B et al: L'anevrysme cirsoide de la rétine. *J Med Lyon* **18**:165, 1937
32. Hall GS: Blood vessel tumors of brain with particular reference to the Lindau syndrome. *J Neurol Psychopathol* **15**:305, 1935
33. Syllaba L, Henner K: Contribution à l'indépendance de l'athétose double idiopathique et congénital. *Rev Neurol (Paris)* **1**:541, 1926
34. Aguilar MJ et al: Pathological observations in ataxia-telangiectasia: report of 5 cases. *J Neuropathol Exp Neurol* **27**:659, 1968
35. Scherrer JR et al: Thrombocytopenie associée à un hemangioblastome cérébelleux. *Schweiz Med Wochenschr* **95**:1456, 1965
36. Van Bogaert L: Les dysplasies à tendance blastomaleuse, in *Traité de Médecine,* vol XVI. Paris, Masson, 1949
37. Krabbe H, Bartels ED: *La Lipomatose Circonscrite Multiple.* Copenhagen, Munksgaard, 1944
38. Marden PM, Venters HD Jr: A new neurocutaneous syndrome. *Am J Dis Child* **112**:79, 1966
39. Feuerstein RC, Mims LC: Linear nevus sebaceous with convulsions and mental retardation. *Am J Dis Child* **104**:675, 1962
40. Solomon LM et al: The epidermal nevus syndrome. *Arch Dermatol* **97**:273, 1968
41. Gorlin RJ et al: Multiple nevoid basal cell carcinoma, odontogenic keratocysts and skeletal anomalies. *Acta Derm Venereol (Stockh)* **43**:39, 1963
42. Herzberg JJ, Wiskemann A: Die fünfte Phakomatose: Baselzellnaevus mit familiärer Belastung und Medulloblastom. *Dermatologica* **126**:106, 1963
43. Hermans EH et al: Naevus epitheliomatoides multiplex een vijfde facomatose. *Ned Tijdschr Geneeskd* **103**:1795, 1959
44. Murphy N, Tenser L: Nevoid basal cell carcinoma syndrome and epilepsy. *Ann Neurol* **11**:372, 1982
45. Winkelmann RK, Johnson LA: Cholinesterases in neurofibromas. *Arch Dermatol* **85**:106, 1962
46. Reed WB et al: Giant pigmented nevi, melanoma and leptomeningeal melanocytosis: a clinical and histopathological study. *Arch Dermatol* **91**:100, 1965
47. Henschen F: Tumoren des Zentralnervensystems und seiner Hüllen, in *Handbuch der speziellen pathologischen Anatomie und Histologie: Ekrankungen des zentralen Nervensystems,* vol XIII, edited by O Lubarsch et al. Berlin, Springer-Verlag, 1955
48. Fanconi A: Neurocutane Melanoblastose mit Hydrocephalus communicans bei zwei Säuglingen. *Helv Paediatr Acta* **11**:376, 1956
49. Berlin C: Congenital generalized melanoleucoderma associ-

ated with hypodontia, hypotrichosis, stunted growth and mental retardation occurring in two brothers and two sisters. *Dermatologica* **123**:227, 1961

50. Waardenburg PJ: A new syndrome combining developmental anomalies of the eyelids, eyebrows and nose root with pigmentary defects of the iris and head hair and with congenital deafness. *Am J Hum Genet* **3**:195, 1951

51. Klein D: Albinisme partiel (leucisone) accompagné de surdité d'osteomyodysplasie de l'autres malformations congénitales. *Arch Klaus Stift Vererbrungsforsch* **22**:336, 1947

52. Reed WB et al: Pigmentary disorders in association with congenital deafness. *Arch Dermatol* **95**:176, 1967

53. Page AR et al: The Chédiak-Higashi syndrome. *Blood* **20**:330, 1962

54. Stegmaier OC, Schneider LA: Chédiak-Higashi syndrome. *Arch Dermatol* **91**:1, 1965

55. Moynahan E: Multiple symmetrical moles with psychic and somatic infantilism and genital hypoplasia: first male case of a new syndrome. *Proc R Soc Med* **55**:959, 1963

56. Walther RJ et al: Electrocardiographic abnormalities in a family with generalized lentigo. *N Engl J Med* **275**:1220, 1966

57. Mathews NL: Lentigo and electrocardiographic changes. *N Engl J Med* **278**:780, 1968

58. Sjögren T, Larsson T: Oligophrenia in combination with congenital ichthyosis and spastic disorders. *Acta Psychiatr Scand [Suppl]* **113**:9, 1957

59. Rud E: Et tilfaelde af infantilisme med tetani epilepsi, polyneuritis ichtyosis og anaemi af perniciøs type. *Hospitalstid* **70**:525, 1927

60. De Sanctis C, Cacchione A: L'idiozia xerodermica. *Riv Sper Freniatr* **56**:269, 1932

61. Lynch HT et al: Secondary male hypogonadism and congenital ichthyosis: association of two rare genetic diseases. *Am J Hum Genet* **12**:440, 1960

62. Heijer A, Reed WB: Sjögren-Larsson syndrome. *Arch Dermatol* **92**:545, 1965

63. Patterson JH, Watkins WL: Leprechaunism in a male infant. *J Pediatr* **60**:730, 1962

64. Adams RD, Lyon G: *Neurology of Hereditary Diseases of Children.* New York, McGraw-Hill, 1982

65. Partington MV: The early symptoms of phenylketonuria. *Pediatrics* **27**:465, 1961

66. Carson NAJ et al: Homocystinuria: clinical and pathological review of 10 cases. *J Pediatr* **66**:565, 1965

67. Halvorsen K, Halvorsen S: Hartnup disease. *Pediatrics* **31**:29, 1963

68. Menkes JH et al: A sex-linked recessive disorder with retardation of growth, peculiar hair and focal cerebral and cerebellar degeneration. *Pediatrics* **29**:764, 1962

69. Aguilar MJ et al: Kinky hair disease. *J Neuropathol Exp Neurol* **25**:507, 1966

70. Hirano A et al: Fine structure of the cerebellar cortex in Menkes kinky-hair disease. *Arch Neurol* **34**:52, 1977

71. Robinson GC, Miller JR: Hereditary enamel hypoplasia: its association with characteristic hair structure. *Pediatrics* **37**:498, 1966

72. Elsässer G et al: Das Xeroderma pigmentosum und die "xerodermische Idiotie." *Arch Dermatol Syphilol* **188**:651, 1955

73. Larmande A, Timsit EA: A propos de 20 cas de xéroderme pigmentosum. *Acta XVII Concil Ophtalmol (1954)* **3**:1643, 1955

74. Cross HE et al: A new oculocerebral syndrome with hypopigmentation. *J Pediatr* **70**:398, 1967

75. Seip M: Lipodystrophy and gigantism with associated endocrine manifestations: new diencephalic syndrome? *Acta Paediatr* **48**:556, 1959

76. Reed WB et al: Congenital lipodystrophic diabetes with acanthosis nigricans. *Arch Dermatol* **91**:326, 1965

77. Schwartz R et al: Generalized lipoatrophy, hepatic cirrhosis, disturbed carbohydrate metabolism and accelerated growth (lipoatrophic diabetes). Longitudinal studies and metabolic studies. *Am J Med* **28**:973, 1960

78. Van Bogaert L et al: *Une Forme Cérébrate de la Cholestérinose Généralisée.* Paris, Masson, 1937

79. Steinberg D et al: Refsum's disease: a recently characterized lipidosis involving the nervous system. *Ann Intern Med* **66**:365, 1967

80. Mize CE et al: Phytanic acid storage in Refsum's disease due to defective alpha-hydroxylation. *Clin Res* **16**:346, 1968

81. Waldorf DS et al: Cutaneous cholesterol ester deposition in Tangier disease. *Arch Dermatol* **95**:161, 1967

82. Fredrickson DS: The inheritance of high-density lipoprotein deficiency (Tangier disease). *J Clin Invest* **43**:228, 1964

83. Opitz J et al: The genetics of angiokeratoma corporis diffusum (Fabry's disease) and its linkage with the X$_g$ locus. *Am J Hum Genet* **17**:325, 1965

84. Sweeley CC, Klionsky B: Fabry's disease: classification as a sphingolipidosis and partial characterization of a novel glycolipid. *J Biol Chem* **238**:3148, 1963

85. Rahman AN et al: Angiokeratoma corporis diffusum universale. *Trans Assoc Am Physicians* **74**:366, 1961

86. Dean G: *The Porphyrias: A Story of Inheritance and Environment.* Philadelphia, JB Lippincott, 1963

87. Goldberg A: Acute intermittent porphyria: a study of 50 cases. *Q J Med* **28**:183, 1959

88. Macdonald WB et al: Cockayne's syndrome. *Pediatrics* **25**:997, 1960

89. Moossy J: The neuropathology of Cockayne's syndrome. *J Neuropathol Exp Neurol* **26**:654, 1967

90. Bloom D: Congenital telangiectatic erythema resembling lupus erythematosus in dwarfs. *Am J Dis Child* **88**:754, 1954

91. Tedesco AS et al: Myopathy associated with sclerodermal facial hemiatrophy. *Arch Neurol* **38**:592, 1981

92. Schaltenbrand G: Radikulomyelomeningitis nach Zeckenbiss. *Münch Med Wochenschr* **104**:829, 1962

93. Martin JJ et al: Contributions de la biopsie cutanée au diagnostique des encéphalopathies métaboliques. *Rev Neurol (Paris)* **132**:639, 1976

CUTANEOUS MANIFESTATIONS OF ENDOCRINE DISORDERS

Ruth K. Freinkel and Norbert Freinkel

General consideration of cutaneous expression of endocrine disorders

Hormones regulate physiologic processes by modifications of existing activities rather than by initiation of reactions de novo. Thus, in the skin as elsewhere, excesses or deficiencies of hormones generally result in quantitative rather than qualitative changes in cutaneous function and morphology. However, the expression of altered hormonal balance is determined to some extent by intrinsic properties of skin in various areas. The capacity of cutaneous structures to respond, local hemodynamics, and extrinsic factors such as light and trauma will influence the distribution as well as the quantity of hormonally induced changes in the skin.

The expression of endocrine disorders in the skin may reflect both alterations in total body economy and direct actions on cutaneous structures. For example, abnormalities in fluid and electrolyte balance resulting from endocrine imbalance may be evidenced in changes in skin turgor. As a major site for dissipation and preservation of heat, the skin may reflect derangements in thermogenesis in endocrine disease; skin temperature, vascular dilatation, and sweating may afford a visual index of such generalized derangements.

Intermediary metabolism is controlled by balanced actions of hormones. Control is exerted by direct effects on cells as well as by indirect effects via circulating fuels and other regulatory substances. Expression of hormonal effects at the cellular level is a function of circulating levels of the hormone and the ability of the tissue to respond. Excessive amounts of hormone accentuate activities of a cutaneous structure to the degree that it can respond. Deficiency of hormone may be expressed by diminished function in a responsive structure or by the unbalanced or excessive activity of other hormonal principles (e.g., ACTH excess in adrenal cortical deficiency).

For certain hormones the skin displays the responsiveness of a specific target tissue (e.g., sex hormones). For others it shares in overall effects in terms of those metabolic activities that affect its structure and function (e.g., thyroid hormone). For still other hormones the skin displays little if any direct response (e.g., adrenal mineralocorticoids). However, inasmuch as rapid cell turnover, synthesis of structural proteins such as keratin and collagen, lipids, and mucopolysaccharides, and a vast vasculature network are affected by hormonal action, the skin affords a sensitive barometer of endocrine disease. In subsequent sections the effects of various endocrinopathies on the skin will be considered in detail. In keeping with the concept that hormones regulate rather than initiate function, the discussion will be formulated in terms of too little or too much of a given hormone. This formulation is particularly appropriate in the face of increasing instances of iatrogenic endocrinopathy such as those induced by pharmacologic use of such hormones as corticosteroids and sex steroids. In these instances the cutaneous effects tend to mimic naturally occurring disease but may be exaggerated or qualitatively different because of the pharmacologic alterations in the natural hormone.

Finally, not all of the cutaneous manifestations of endocrine disorders can be directly attributed to hormonal effects. Thus, fungal infections in parathyroid deficiency and vitiligo in Graves' disease appear to reflect pathologic processes that initiate the endocrinopathy.

In the subsequent sections where information is sufficient, we will attempt to link cutaneous changes to actions of hormones as well as other pathophysiologic processes.

Thyroid hormone

Effects of thyroid hormone on the skin

"The most clearly definable function of thyroid hormone appears to be the establishment of a fundamental rate of energy turnover" [1]. This may be expressed in processes that culminate in growth and development as well as the maintenance of cellular activities at a physiologic level. The precise mechanism of action of thyroid hormone has not been elucidated. Triiodothyronine (T_3) appears to be the most active of the thyroid hormones and arises in part in the thyroid and in part from peripheral deiodination of thyroxine (T_4). T_3 is bound by specific nuclear receptors and stimulates synthesis of RNA; recent evidence indicates that there are T_3 receptors at other subcellular sites. Specific receptors have not as yet been demonstrated in skin but direct effects of T_3 in epidermal cells and fibroblasts have been demonstrated in vitro [2,3].

Available data suggest that thyroid hormone plays a pivotal role in embryonic development of mammalian skin as well as in the maintenance of normal cutaneous function in adult skin. Ablation of the thyroid gland of sheep in utero retards the formation of hair follicles and other adnexal structures as well as development of the dermis and epidermis [4]. Extrapolation from experiments in amphibian skin suggests that the effects of thyroid hormone on fetal development involve stimulation of mitotic activity and facilitation of differentiation. Studies of mammalian, including human, skin suggest a continuing role for thyroxine in the mature organism. Oxygen consumption [5], epidermal mitotic activity, and protein synthesis [6] are increased by thyroid hormone. Thyroid hormone appears to be necessary for both the initiation and maintenance of hair growth [7] and for normal secretion of sebum [8].

Thyroid hormones affect production of collagen and mucopolysaccharides by dermal fibroblasts. Acid-soluble collagen is increased and insoluble collagen decreased by thyroid hormones, while they apparently retard the accumulation of glycosaminoglycans.

Lack of thyroid hormone is expressed by changes in all of the above functions in the epidermis and dermis. However, excessive amounts of thyroxine do not correlate with abnormal acceleration.

Thyroid hormones also appear to have effects on pigmentation and both hyper- and hypopigmentation are seen in hyperthyroid states in humans. The precise nature of these effects is not clear and may be in part mediated through interactions of thyroid hormones with neurohumors.

Some of the actions of thyroid hormones on skin are indirectly mediated by generalized effects on heat production and altered cardiovascular dynamics. Excessive sweating and increased cutaneous blood flow result from excessive levels of thyroid hormone. To what extent these phenomena impinge on the local metabolic activity of the skin cannot be assessed.

Finally, it should be pointed out that not all of the cutaneous changes in thyroid disease can be directly attributed to the relative deficiencies or excesses of thyroid hormones. There is precedent for direct actions of pituitary tropic hormones on cutaneous structures (see below). Thus, excessive pituitary thyrotropin (TSH) may play a role in some of the changes noted with primary thyroid failure. Altered activity of neurohumors may be responsible for some of the actions that appear to result from excessive or deficient thyroid hormone. The more generalized disorders, including autoimmunity, underlying Graves' disease and Hashimoto's thyroiditis may be responsible for some of the more striking cutaneous changes that occur.

Cutaneous manifestations of too much thyroid hormone

Thyrotoxicosis is the syndrome that results from excessive amounts of thyroid hormone. It may be due to Graves' disease (see below), toxic nodular goiter, administration of excessive amounts of thyroid hormone, or as a transient phase in subacute thyroiditis.

The skin is above all warm, moist, soft, and smooth, resembling the texture of infant skin. The warmth, which is due to peripheral vasodilatation and increased blood flow, is often accompanied by a persistent flush of the face, redness of the elbows, and palmar erythema. There is excessive sweating generally, but this is particularly pronounced on the palms and soles where eccrine glands are under sympathetic control. Other evidence of vasomotor instability is seen in evanescent blushing over the head and neck.

The epidermis is thin but not atrophic; the stratum corneum appears well hydrated. Scalp hair tends to be fine and soft. Altered texture and diffuse alopecia are commonly observed by patients. Effects on sebaceous glands

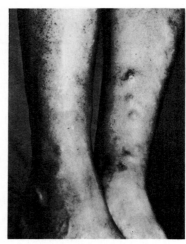

Fig. 173-1 Nodular pretibial myxedema.

are not readily apparent, but the skin seems less oily. Nails exhibit a characteristic onycholysis in which the free edge of the nail becomes undulated and curves upward (Plummer's nail). This finding, however, is not pathognomonic for thyrotoxicosis.

Other cutaneous manifestations may include generalized pruritus, chronic urticaria, and alopecia areata [9]. It is not clear whether these features are present only in patients with Graves' disease or may occur in other forms of thyrotoxicosis.

Hyperpigmentation of a diffuse or patchy type is not uncommon and generally occurs on the face. Vitiligo occurs in approximately 7 percent of patients with Graves' disease but is not abnormally more frequent in other forms of hyperthyroidism [10]. The depigmentation may antedate the endocrine disorder and is not improved by treatment of the thyrotoxicosis. A high percentage of such patients demonstrate autoantibodies to fractions of thyroid tissue.

Graves' disease. Graves' disease is a more generalized disorder in which autoimmune mechanisms seem to play a

Fig. 173-2 Extensive verrucous plaques of pretibial myxedema.

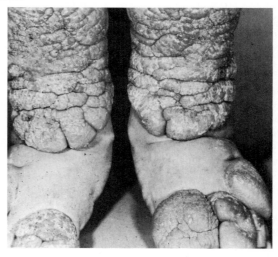

pathogenic role. The disorder may include thyrotoxicosis and goiter, ophthalmopathy, acropachy, and so-called pretibial myxedema. These various manifestations can occur independently of each other, and medical or surgical treatment to correct thyrotoxicosis has no effect on the progression of pretibial myxedema. The incidence of pretibial myxedema in Graves' disease is less than 5 percent. About 50 percent of cases develop during active thyrotoxicosis and the remainder occur after the patients have been rendered euthyroid. Pretibial myxedema is not pathognomonic for Graves' disease, having been reported as well in primary hypothyroidism and Hashimoto's thyroiditis [11].

The lesions occur most frequently on the anterior tibia and dorsa of the feet and are morphologically varied. They are usually bilateral but not symmetrical. Most commonly, lesions consist of pink, flesh-colored, or purplish nodules (Figs. 173-1 and A2-4). Diffuse, brawny, nonpitting edema may be present without nodules. Less common is an elephantiasis nostras variant where the extremity may become enlarged and covered with verrucous nodules (Figs. 173-2 and 173-3). Thickening of the skin of the extensor surface of the forearm has also been reported and dubbed preradial myxedema [12].

The changes in the dermis are identical to those in myxedema. Excessive amounts of hyaluronic acid and chondroitin sulfate are present in lesions and in clinically normal skin as well [13].

While the cause of these lesions is not known, factors in sera of affected patients have been shown to stimulate mucopolysaccharide synthesis by dermal fibroblasts [14].

Treatment of the disorder is not satisfactory. Neither systemic nor local corticosteroids afford relief. Plasmapheresis has been tried without clear-cut results, as have cytotoxic agents.

Cutaneous manifestations of too little thyroid hormone

Thyroid hormone deficiency may occur when (1) loss or atrophy of thyroid tissue results in decreased production of hormone despite maximal stimulation by thyrotropin (thyroprivic hypothyroidism); (2) there is inadequate stimulation of the gland due to pituitary or hypothalamic failure (trophoprivic hypothyroidism); (3) there is an absolute or relative impairment in biosynthesis of thyroid hormones

due to either intrinsic or extrinsic factors (goitrous hypothyroidism). The resultant endocrine disorder derives one of its names, myxedema, from its most prominent manifestations in the skin.

The skin in hypothyroidism is cold, dry (xerotic), and pale. The coldness is due to the reduced core temperature and cutaneous vasoconstriction. The xerosis is caused not only by absence of sweating but also by a change in skin texture. The epidermis is thin and hyperkeratotic, and there is follicular plugging. The changes are generalized and therefore may be differentiated from similar alterations in atopic individuals, seasonal changes, keratosis pilaris, etc., which are more prominent on the extremities. Fine wrinkling imparts a parchment-like quality, especially in hypothyroidism of pituitary origin.

Skin tends to be pale due in part to the increased content of water and mucopolysaccharides in the dermis which change the refraction of incident light. It may also have a yellowish hue which is accentuated on the palms, soles, and nasolabial folds. This is due to accumulation of carotene in the stratum corneum. Carotenemia in hypothyroidism has been ascribed to a defect in the hepatic conversion of β-carotene to vitamin A.

The hair is dry, coarse, and brittle. Hair growth is slow in the scalp, beard, and sexual areas. Patchy alopecia as well as diffuse thinning of scalp hair, loss of the outer third of the eyebrows, and diminished body hair are often seen. Massive effluvium may occur when there is abrupt onset of hypothroidism. Estimations of anagen/telogen ratios have shown that there is an increase in the percentage of hairs in telogen. The chronology of changes induced by administration of thyroxine to hypothyroid individuals suggests that hair loss is due to both the early arrest of anagen and failure of initiation of hair growth [15]. Hypothyroid patients, especially children, also frequently develop excessive growth of long lanugo-like hair on the upper back, shoulders, and extremities. The cause of this change is obscure.

Diminished sebum secretion contributes to the coarseness of the scalp hair, which loses the sheen and manageability imparted to it by scalp oil. Nails become brittle and grow slowly.

The most striking change in the skin is due to the dermal accumulation of mucopolysaccharides (myxedema). The entire skin is puffy with a boggy nonpitting edema that is more readily felt than seen. Unlike other forms of edema, the distribution is not affected appreciably by such factors as dependency. However, the accumulations are more striking in acral parts, where the lack of subcutaneous tissue tends to make dermal changes more prominent. Although myxedema is a diffuse phenomenon, multiple focal mucinous papules, responsive to L-thyroxine, have been reported in hypothyroidism.

The facial changes are especially characteristic (Fig. 173-4). The nose is broadened and lips are thickened. The tongue is large, smooth, red, and clumsy. There may be sticky secretions on the eyelids, which show a fine wrinkling and a flaccid, somewhat translucent puffiness. Drooping of the upper lids may occur even in the absence of edematous changes and has been ascribed to decreased sympathetic stimulation of the superior palpebral muscle. At rest, the face lacks expressiveness, and in full-blown myxedema, changing emotions are registered slowly be-

Fig. 173-3 Pretibial myxedema with hypertrophic changes, resembling elephantiasis nostras.

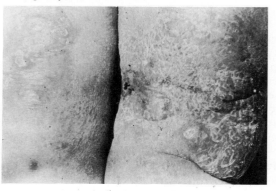

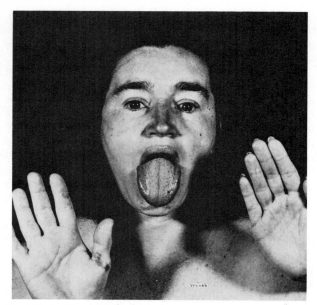

Fig. 173-4 Myxedema and macroglossia: characteristic facial changes.

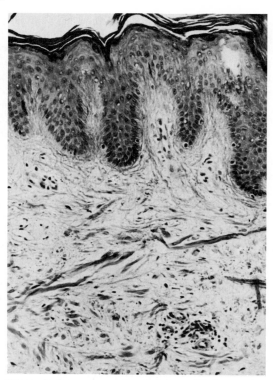

Fig. 173-5 Cutaneous mucinosis (of pretibial myxedema). A variety of processes may be associated with the accumulation of excess amounts of ground substance in the dermis. In H & E preparations the dermal mucin appears as delicate, basophilic fibrils between separated and narrow collagen bundles. The excess mucin is metachromatic, and when its presence is suspected, the tissue should always be stained with toluidine blue. x160. (Micrograph by Wallace H. Clark, Jr., M.D.)

cause of the concomitant lethargy; the facies is almost pathognomonic and may be simulated only in the nephrotic syndrome or untreated pernicious anemia.

The hypothyroid skin heals poorly, and this tendency is proportional to the degree of thyroid hormone deficiency.

The mucopolysaccharides that accumulate in the dermis are chondroitin sulfate and hyaluronic acid. The materials appear first in the papillary dermis and are most prominent around hair follicles and vessels. The mucopolysaccharides cause separation of collagen bundles, and some degeneration of collagen may occur secondarily (Fig. 173-5).

All the changes are reversible by judicious use of thyroid hormone. Mobilization of myxedematous deposits may be the earliest indication of thyroid hormone action and is characterized by a rise in the serum sodium level and a fall in the hematocrit [16]. Presumably, this is due to the conjoint release of water and electrolytes bound to the hydrophilic mucopolysaccharides.

The mechanism responsible for myxedema is not clear. There is evidence in animals and in tissue culture supporting action of thyroid hormone on both restraint of synthesis and increased catabolism of mucopolysaccharides. The putative role for IgG in pretibial myxedema and the fact that crude thyrotropin causes dermal accumulation of mucopolysaccharides [17] suggest pituitary peptides may play some role. However, while myxedema is less prominent in trophoprivic hypothyroidism, it need not be absent. It is thus likely that the lack of thyroid hormone is the primary factor in accumulation of dermal mucopolysaccharides but that interaction with pituitary and/or hypothalamic factors and other hormones plays a facilitating role.

Parathyroid hormone

Effects of parathyroid hormone on the skin

The hormone of the parathyroid gland regulates the flux of calcium and phosphate between extra- and intracellular

compartments in responsive tissues (i.e., renal tubules and bone) and the metabolism of vitamin D: a role for this hormone in the skin has not been identified. In fact, even though calcium deposition in the dermis is common in certain inflammatory conditions of the skin, hypercalcemia with or without hyperparathyroidism is not commonly associated with evident calcification in the skin. On the other hand, clinical experience [18] has suggested that abnormality of calcium and phosphate per se produces profound changes in the skin, attesting to the importance of circulating levels of these ions in normal skin physiology.

Cutaneous manifestations of excessive parathyroid hormone

Primary hyperparathyroidism is not associated with any cutaneous abnormalities except, rarely, pruritus which is apparently linked to microscopic deposits of calcium in the dermis [19]. Similarly, intractable pruritus in severe renal disease has been attributed to secondary hyperparathyroidism. An increased quantity of calcium has been reported in the skin of such patients and some have experienced relief of itching following parathyroidectomy [20]. However, it should be noted that such patients are usually being treated with chronic hemodialysis and that itching is frequently intensified during or immediately after treatments. This fact, plus failure of surgical ablation of parathyroid glands to relieve the pruritus in some patients, suggests that the mechanism for pruritus in chronic renal disease has not yet been entirely elucidated.

Cutaneous manifestations of too little parathyroid hormone

Hypoparathyroidism most commonly occurs due to ablation of the parathyroids as a complication of thyroidectomy. Primary failure of the parathyroids (i.e., idiopathic hypoparathyroidism) is a less common cause. It may occur as an isolated endocrinopathy or as part of the syndrome of multiple endocrine failure. In the latter disorder parathyroid failure may be associated with hypothyroidism (Hashimoto's thyroiditis), Addison's disease, ovarian failure, or pernicious anemia. Alopecia areata and vitiligo may occur. The least common cause of hypoparathyroidism is peripheral refractoriness to the action of parathyroid hormone (pseudohypoparathyroidism).

In all types of hypoparathyroidism the skin may be dry, scaly, hyperkeratotic, and puffy. Nails may become opaque and brittle and develop transverse ridges. Hair is coarse and sparse and there may be patchy alopecia. Eczematous dermatitis, exfoliative dermatitis, hyperkeratotic and macular and papular eruptions have been reported. These changes are all reversible when calcium values are normalized. They thus appear to relate to an abnormality of circulating calcium rather than to the level of parathyroid hormone.

Primary hypoparathyroidism, as opposed to other forms of the disease, is also frequently associated with chronic mucocutaneous *candidiasis,* as first reported by Sutphin et al [21]. The infection commonly involves the nails and oral mucosa, but vulvovaginitis and infection of intertriginous areas is frequently present. On other areas of skin, candidiasis often presents as an annular or arcuate scaling eruption which resembles dermatophytosis.

These infections are not altered by regulation of blood calcium and phosphorus levels and are attended by defects in cellular immunity. Moreover, they may antedate the onset of hypoparathyroidism by some years. The presence of autoantibodies to parathyroid tissue in 30 percent of cases as well as autoantibodies to melanocytes [22], various other endocrine tissues, and gastric parietal cells has suggested primary hypoparathyroidism results from a disturbed immune system [23].

Glucocorticoids

Effects of glucocorticoids on the skin

The effects of glucocorticoids on the skin are best appreciated by observation of the changes produced by excess hormone. Although endogenous hypercortisolism is uncommon, the iatrogenic disease has become all too familiar due to the common use of pharmacologic doses of synthetic corticosteroids in nonendocrine disorders.

The actions of corticosteroids on skin have been extensively studied both in vivo and in vitro using cell culture systems. Cortisol decreases the mass of dermal connective tissue due to direct effects on dermal fibroblasts. The hormone may decrease synthesis as well as accumulation of glycosaminoglycans and alter their relative composition [24,25]. The hormone increases collagen cross-linking, decreases activity of collagenase [26,27] but probably does not affect the relative proportions of types III and I collagen. It is not clear whether corticosteroids inhibit production of collagen [28] or whether the decrease in collagen content of the dermis reflects diminished numbers of active fibroblasts [29].

Corticosteroids appear to regulate diurnal variations in mitotic activity of the epidermis [30]. Mitotic peaks correlate inversely with serum cortisol levels [31] and these effects may be mediated via the adenylcyclase system. Differentiation of epidermal cells is accelerated by corticosteroids in vitro [32,33].

Hair growth is retarded in experimental animals, possibly due to effects on initiation of anagen [34] and mitotic activity. However, excessive glucocorticoids produce hypertrichosis, and loss of axillary hair in glucocorticoid deficient states suggests that corticosteroids play a physiologic role in maintaining hair growth, at least in some sites. There is little clear evidence to suggest that sebaceous glands are directly stimulated by glucocorticoids but follicular hyperkeratosis is frequently observed. It seems likely that the alteration of follicle walls plays the major role in the acne accompanying glucocorticoid excess rather than excessive sebum production.

The anti-inflammatory effects of corticosteroids in the skin are complex. Sensitization of the vascular walls to adrenergic agonists results in vasoconstriction and diminished permeability. Suppression of cells of the immune system may play a major role in anti-inflammatory effects. Stabilization of lysosomes by corticosteroids may also provide anti-inflammatory effects by inhibiting release of proteases and other mediators [35]. A more relevant action may be the reduction of cutaneous prostanoid synthesis from arachadonic acid due to inhibition of phospholipase A by corticosteroids [36].

That the skin is a major site for degradation and interconversions of glucocorticoids as well as other steroidal hormones has been established by numerous studies. In particular, the interconversion of cortisone and cortisol [37,38] is relevant to the effect of corticosteroid excess of both endogenous and exogenous origin. Cortisol has profound antiphlogistic effects, including those cited above on epidermal and dermal proliferation, while cortisone is relatively ineffective. Exquisite regulation of the rates of interconversion, which has been shown in such physiologic mechanisms as wound healing, may provide control of proliferative events [39].

Despite all of the above, it is not clear what role glucocorticoids play in the maintenance of normal structure and functions in the adult skin. In contrast to the effects of excess hormone, its lack seems to result in no clinically discernible changes in cutaneous integrity. However, the protean nature of the effects of glucocorticoids on skin suggests they play a regulatory role here as elsewhere. Indeed, high-affinity receptors for these hormones have been demonstrated in dermal fibroblasts and keratinocytes. It has also been shown that structural modifications in synthetic corticosteroids affect their binding affinity and that these changes appear to correlate with clinical efficacy [40]. Perhaps the absence of gross structural and functional changes in the face of too little glucocorticoid attests to the ability of the skin to function without fine tuning of such varied activities as mitotic division and collagen catabolism.

Effects of ACTH on the skin

Effects of glucocorticoids on skin cannot be discussed without mentioning the extraadrenal actions of pituitary corticotropin. Although corticosteroids do not directly affect pigmentation, corticotropin and its structurally related pituitary peptides α- and β-MSH/lipotropin stimulate melanogenesis. These hormones belong to two series of peptides that arise from a prohormone (pro-opimelanocortin) and which also include endorphin. In addition to stimulation of melanocytes, ACTH may also directly influence sebum production presumably via stimulation of lipogenesis [41].

Cutaneous manifestations of too much glucocorticoids (hypercortisolism)

Endogenous glucocorticoids. Endogenous hypercortisolism can arise from (a) functioning benign or malignant tumors of the adrenal cortex (Cushing's syndrome), (b) inappropriate secretion of ACTH by the pituitary (Cushing's disease), or (c) production of ACTH by nonpituitary neoplasia (ectopic ACTH syndrome). In all three types the effects of excess glucocorticoids may be mixed to varying degrees with those of excess mineralocorticoids and androgenic steroids.

The skin becomes generally atrophic. The epidermis is thin and shiny, and may have slight scaling. The dermis is also thin and loose, especially over the extremities where subcutaneous fat is diminished. The skin becomes friable and easily damaged. Wound healing is markedly impaired; even slight injuries may fail to heal and become ulcerated and infected secondarily. Patients are prone to develop dermatophytosis as well as tinea versicolor.

There is increased vascular fragility, and patients often display ecchymoses and petechiae from pressure or slight trauma, especially in dependent parts. Decreased vascular tone is evident in purplish mottling of the lower extremities (cutis marmorata).

Among the characteristic lesions of glucocorticoid excess are the broad, purple striae which usually appear in areas of stretch on the trunk but may be encountered elsewhere. They differ from the commonly found striae of adolescence, pregnancy, and obesity only with respect to their inordinate depth and breadth and intense color. The color fades when the disease is arrested, but the atrophy tends to remain. The lesion represents another index of the loss of integrity of the dermal connective tissue and the failure of normal regenerative powers.

Hyperpigmentation is unusual in Cushing's syndrome, but may occur in Cushing's disease where production of ACTH (and related peptides) is increased. Acanthosis nigricans occurs but is usually mild.

Plethora is common and is accompanied by appearance of telangiectasia on the face. Although this has been traditionally ascribed to associated polycythemia, the authors have seen numerous instances in which neither hemoconcentration nor increased red cell mass could be demonstrated.

Mild hirsutism and acne are common. The hypertrichosis is usually most marked on the face with development of coarse hair on the upper lip, chin, and lateral cheeks. Intense hirsutism involving body hair as well and accompanied by male-pattern alopecia is sufficiently unusual in bilateral adrenal hyperplasia to justify suspicion of an adrenal tumor.

One of the striking features of excess glucocorticoids is the change in appearance and body habitus. Excessive deposits of fat over the clavicles and back of the neck (buffalo hump) and abdomen may be accompanied by loss of subcutaneous fat over the extremities. In addition, there is deposition of fat in the cheeks, giving the face a rounded appearance (moon facies). The central obesity may be associated with muscle wasting. The factors which determine the deposition of this fat at pathognomonic sites are unknown. Reduced height and kyphosis as a result of osteoporosis and compression fractures of the vertebrae may add to the altered appearance.

Exogenous glucocorticoids. Because pharmacologic doses of synthetic glucocorticoids are frequently employed to treat cutaneous disorders, iatrogenic hypercortisolism is perhaps the most common endocrine disease encountered by the dermatologist.

The cutaneous manifestations of systemic administration of corticosteroids are quite similar to those of endogenous Cushing's syndrome. The major difference is the lack of those effects which may be ascribable to the elaboration of adrenal androgens. Although hypertrichosis is also seen in iatrogenic hypercorticism, it is usually confined to fine, long, lanugo-like hair, especially on the lateral cheeks. Acne is a common feature of iatrogenic Cushing's syndrome, especially in children and younger adults. The acne is dominated by closed comedones and uniformly small papulopustular lesions. It responds poorly to routine acne treatments, especially antibiotics, and therapy should be directed at the follicular hyperkeratosis (e.g., with topical retinoic acid).

The administration of ACTH produces fewer and less severe effects. However, acne is more common with ACTH therapy (possibly due to the stimulation of adrenal androgens), and hyperpigmentation is occasionally elicited [42]. The difference between the effects of ACTH and glucocorticoids may be more apparent than real. Even at seemingly equivalent doses, as judged by the 24-h excretion of urinary steroids, the oral administration of corticosteroids at fixed intervals results in oscillations between very high and low plasma levels, while more sustained and constant plasma concentrations of glucocorticoids are achieved by parenteral treatment with long-acting preparations of ACTH in gel.

The development of iatrogenic Cushing's syndrome and its severity depends upon the dose of drug, duration of therapy, and age of the patient. Adverse side effects are more frequent and more severe in older patients. At moderate to high doses for a protracted period some features of hypercortisolism are inevitable. With low doses administered clinically or high doses given for short periods, the appearance of signs and symptoms is highly variable. It is perhaps superfluous to point out that the enormous potential hazards and the unpredictability of the effects (even with low doses) must be carefully weighed against the potential benefits of steroid administration.

Administration of corticosteroids even in relatively low doses provides an additional hazard, i.e., suppression of the adrenal–pituitary axis. Although adrenal function returns rather promptly even after prolonged suppression, the ability of the pituitary to provide ACTH in response to acute demands may be persistently diminished [43]. Such diminished pituitary reserve constitutes a threat of adrenal insufficiency during stress such as infection, surgery, or other intercurrent disease. It is now well established that adverse effects of pituitary suppression and excessive glucocorticoids can be minimized by intermittent administration of corticosteroids. When it is clinically feasible and irrespective of the size of the dose, alternate-day therapy is preferable to daily administration during chronic use of corticosteroids.

Topical or intracutaneous administration of corticosteroids may produce a localized hypercortisolism characterized by atrophy, striae, epidermal thinning, and telangiectasia and a rosacea-like dermatitis. Such effects are rarely seen with hydrocortisone, but frequently follow prolonged use of fluorinated steroids. Differences in the relative rates of absorption probably account for the greater sensitivity of facial, axillary, and perineal skin to these adverse effects, especially in children [44].

In addition, administration of topical steroids may result in sufficient systemic absorption to cause adrenal suppression and systemic hypercortisolism. The amount of topically applied, biologically active steroid that becomes available systemically depends on a number of variables, e.g., concentration and potency of the corticosteroid, integrity of the stratum corneum, surface area exposed, use of occlusive plastic film. Thus it was shown that prolonged exposure of only 20 percent of normal skin to 0.1% triamcinolone under occlusion resulted in adrenal suppression [45]. Numerous subsequent reports confirm that adrenal suppression is not uncommon when potent topical corticosteroids are applied to relatively large areas of diseased skin even without occlusion. Such suppression is not permanent after treatment is stopped and lingering compromise of the pituitary–adrenal axis does not appear to occur except rarely [46]. Cushing's syndrome has been reported in a small number of cases, usually in treatment of extensive psoriasis with very potent topical steroids, and may eventuate without the use of occlusion [47]. Systemic hypercortisolism has also been reported in infants treated for extensive skin disease and in patients with severe impairment of liver function treated with topical corticosteroids [48,49]. More recently, attention has been drawn to the more common occurence of mild hypercortisolism (as evidenced by impaired carbohydrate tolerance and leukocytosis) in treatment of extensive psoriasis with potent topical steroids [50].

Cutaneous effects of too little glucocorticoid

Deficient formation of glucocorticoids (i.e., Addison's disease) can occur when adrenocortical parenchyma is (1) insufficient for normal hormonal biosynthesis (e.g., in primary adrenal failure due to idiopathic destructive atrophy, tuberculosis, etc.; status postadrenalectomy); (2) inadequately stimulated by ACTH (e.g., in secondary adrenal failure); or (3) thwarted via endogenous blockade of the biosynthetic sequence (e.g., in adrenogenital syndrome). Although the clinical manifestations of these disorders vary to some extent with the causative factors, glucocorticoid deficiency is common to all. Except in adrenogenital syn-

drome there is also lack of adrenal androgen. This produces clinical stigmata of androgen deficiency only when gonadal function is also diminished (e.g., in menopause).

While large amounts of glucocorticoids have a marked effect on the skin, their absence causes surprisingly little change. Unless the patient is markedly debilitated, the texture of the skin and its surface appear normal. Loss of body hair, however, is common; this may be diffuse but usually is most striking in the axilla. Since physiologic replacement doses of cortisone may restore axillary hair partly, some of the effect may be ascribable to the loss of glucocorticoids per se. Except for fibrosis and calcification of the pinna, mesenchymal changes are not apparent in the dermis.

The most striking cutaneous change of chronic adrenal insufficiency is hyperpigmentation, which occurs almost uniformly (Fig. A8-25). In 20 to 40 percent of cases it is the first sign of the disease [51]. The pigmentary change that results from excess ACTH (and of related peptides) is one of the chief differentiating features between adrenal insufficiency due to pituitary disease and that due to primary adrenal failure.

The hyperpigmentation is generalized and represents an accentuation of the normal distribution of melanin in the skin. Often it is first noted as the persistence of a tan acquired in the summer, and it is always darker in sun-exposed areas. Darkening occurs in areas of trauma, such as recent scars, and points of pressure and friction (elbows, knees, skin folds, and palmar creases). Skin in sexual areas (nipples, areola, axilla, perineum, and genitalia) takes on a darker color. In parous females the linea alba becomes darkened. Hair becomes darker, and longitudinal pigmented bands are observed on the nails. Pigmentation appears on mucosal surfaces, especially the buccal mucosa, gums, and tongue. Such pigmentation is normally present in non-Caucasians and will darken and become more extensive. From the above description it is obvious that the hyperpigmentation is relative and can be evaluated only in terms of the patient's previous skin color. Replacement therapy with corticosteroids produces a gradual diminution of the hyperpigmentation. In the treated addisonian patient, a waxing and waning in the intensity of pigmentary change may be one of the most sensitive indices of changing requirements in the maintenance dose of steroids and so may provide the patient with an objective criterion for increasing his medication during intercurrent infections, etc.

Other pigmentary changes are also observed. An early and sometimes prominent change is darkening of pigmented nevi and the appearance of intensely pigmented lentigo-like lesions. Vitiligo is associated with primary adrenal failure in as many as 15 percent of cases and may precede clinical manifestations of adrenal insufficiency. Recent studies suggest that vitiligo in Addison's disease is limited to those patients with multiglandular deficiencies [52]. Similarly, mucocutaneous candidiasis is associated with Addison's disease in patients with multiglandular insufficiency.

One of the more unusual variants of hyperpigmentation due to pituitary stimulation occurs after the performance of bilateral adrenalectomy for adrenal hyperplasia. This relatively uncommon syndrome [53] is characterized by marked hyperpigmentation, amenorrhea, and local pressure signs of an expanding pituitary lesion. Indeed, the color change may constitute the first indication that such a tumor is developing. The hyperpigmentation in this disorder exceeds that encountered in any other condition and is also associated with the highest blood levels of ACTH and MSH. Since the neoplasms are usually not observed prior to surgical intervention, present theories have ascribed their development to the loss of restraining feedback which follows loss of glucocorticoids after adrenalectomy.

Sex hormones

Effects of sex hormones on the skin

Androgenic hormones have trophic actions on the skin as a whole but certain parts of the skin such as sexual zones are particularly sensitive. Moreover, hair follicles and sebaceous glands appear to be particularly responsive. Under the influence of androgenic hormone mitotic activity, cell turnover time and thickness of epidermis are increased. Growth of sebaceous glands is enhanced; indeed, measurements of sebum production are sensitive indices of androgenicity [54]. Hair growth is markedly affected by androgens (see Chaps. 19 and 65). Pigmentation is increased by androgens not only in sexual skin but generally. This effect appears to be due, at least in part, to direct effects on the synthesis of melanin [55] and on packaging of melanosomes [56]. Androgens also cause thickening of the dermis with demonstrable increase in skin collagen content [57].

The nature of effects appears to be identical for all androgenic hormones irrespective of their source (adrenal or gonadal). Of circulating hormones, testosterone is the most potent. However, other androgens have trophic effects on cutaneous structures and may be quantitatively more important either because they are more abundant in the circulation (as may be be the case for adrenal androgens in females) or because of target tissue sensitivity.

A detailed review of the mechanism of action of androgens and other steroid hormones is beyond the scope of this chapter. According to the current theory, testosterone and other steroid hormones circulate in association with transport proteins and diffuse passively into cells in free form. Within cells, testosterone may be converted to dihydrotestosterone (DHT) by 5α-reductase. Conversions of other androgens by reductases, dehydrogenases, and isomerases produce intermediates which may be converted to DHT. For skin, it would appear that androgenic responsiveness depends more upon the availability of DHT rather than testosterone itself or other of its metabolites.

DHT and other active steroids are bound to specific high-affinity receptor proteins in the cytosol and translocated into the nucleus. Once the receptor–hormone complex is bound to nuclear proteins, synthesis of RNA is initiated and cell machinery for anabolic activity is set into motion. Although activity of the α-reductase for testosterone may correlate with certain aspects of androgen responsiveness, it appears clear that there are other events in this complex sequence that may determine both specificity of tissue response and potency of various androgenic hormones. These include the availability of cytoplasmic receptor protein as well as of nuclear protein binding sites. However,

conversion of adrenal or ovarian androgens, such as androstenedione and dehydroepiandrosterone to testosterone and DHT, may be a more important source of androgenic stimulation for the skin of the female than the limited amount of circulating testosterone [58]. Moreover, a considerable body of research suggests marked differences in the sensitivities of various portions of the skin to androgenic stimulation. These differences may reside in differences in the activity and distribution of androgen-metabolizing enzymes such as hydroxysteroid dehydrogenases and isomerases as well as 5α-reductases [59].

Extensive studies in animals have provided evidence that anterior pituitary hormones may facilitate the effects of testosterone. Although the mechanism remains controversial, animal studies have suggested that pituitary hormones facilitate the uptake and/or conversion of testosterone to DHT [41,60]. To what extent anterior pituitary or other central nervous system hormones interact with androgenic hormones on human skin is not clear.

Estrogens, likewise, have significant effects on skin, mainly in sexual zones. Animal studies have suggested that they accelerate the rate of maturation of epidermal cells [61] even as they induce cornification of human vaginal mucosa. It has been demonstrated that there are increases in mitotic division as well as thickness of epidermis in estrogen-treated women after castration [62] and alterations in collagen formation in the skin [63,64].

For the most part, however, the effect of estrogens on skin under physiologic conditions remains poorly defined. The suppression of sebaceous glands by pharmacologic amounts of estrogens is a well-known phenomenon which can be only partially explained by suppression of the pituitary–ovarian axis and reduced production of various androgens. Some direct effect on the target tissue must be invoked to explain the increased response of sebaceous glands to dosages of estrogen in excess of those required for suppression of ovarian function. Presence of high-affinity estrogen receptors in human skin suggests a role for direct effects of these hormones.

Cutaneous manifestations of diseases characterized by too much sex hormone

Too much androgen. The clinical manifestations of androgen excess are recognized as virilization when they occur in the adult female and as precocious puberty with virilization when present in preadolescent children. While the cutaneous changes are similar for various endocrine disorders in which virilization occurs, diagnostic differentiation can be made on the basis of additional features.

In virilizing syndromes, the skin becomes thickened and coarse. Pores on the face enlarge, and there is excessive oiliness. Typical acne vulgaris may develop. In children, the straight hairline is molded to conform to the adult configuration (calvities frontalis adolescentium); temporal recession and male-pattern alopecia may develop. Growth of body hair is accelerated. Coarse hair appears on the extremities, on the anterior chest, and in the beard area. Pubic and axillary hair develop in children. The genitalia show masculinization. Clitoral enlargement occurs in the female, and prepuberal males display hypertrophy of the penis and increased folding of scrotal skin. If virilization occurs during fetal life in females, pseudohermaphroditism may result. Hyperpigmentation of the perineum, external genitalia, axillae, and areolae and nipples is present.

In addition to the changes in the skin, effects on musculature and bone alter the body habitus.

In children, accelerated growth of long bones leads first to accelerated growth and ultimately, because of premature closure of the epiphyses, to a relatively short stature. The concurrence of somatic and skeletal maturation effects a masculine type of muscle development. In both children and adult females, the classic accumulation of subcutaneous fat around the girdle and shoulders disappears.

Specific virilizing disorders are:

1. Congenital adrenogenital syndrome. This disorder is a hereditary disease that may be evident at birth or become manifest later. The biochemical lesion is a defect in the synthesis of glucocorticoids and mineralocorticoids, most commonly due to defective hydroxylation of carbon-21 or -11 in the steroid nucleus. The relative absence of hydroxylated steroids precludes the normal homeostatic regulation of ACTH secretion by negative feedback. As a consequence, the pituitary secretion of ACTH is unrestrained, and an increased synthesis of adrenal androgens supervenes. The disorder is thus characterized by virilization, with varying degrees of insufficiency in the biosynthesis of glucocorticoids and mineralocorticoids. If the inborn defect in adrenal hydroxylations is pronounced, enough ACTH may be elaborated to effect a generalized increase in pigmentation of the addisonian type. Thus the pigmentary changes can parallel the severity of the salt-losing syndrome. Partial deficiencies in 11- or 21-hydrolysase activity may induce excessive androgenization of responsive cutaneous tissue and may thus induce hirsutism and recalcitrant acne in women [65].

2. Other virilizing syndromes. A number of syndromes have been described in which hirsutism and acne vulgaris occur and for which the pathogenesis is not clearly established. Elevations of circulating levels of free testosterone, dehydroepiandrosterone, and urinary ketosteroids have been variously reported in women with so-called idiopathic hirsutism, suggesting the presence of subtle endocrine abnormalities even in the absence of polycystic ovaries.

Too much estrogen. Excess estrogens may result from estrogen-producing tumors of the ovaries or testes or, rarely, from hypothalamic disorders. Endogenous increases in estrogens result in precocious puberty in the female with development of the genitalia, breasts, axillary and pubic hair, and early closure of the epiphyses. In males, gynecomastia, usually characterized by ductal proliferation, may be the only reflection of estrogen excess. However, in some instances, testicular atrophy may follow, and androgen-dependent functions may diminish as a consequence.

The widespread use of oral contraceptive agents containing various combinations of synthetic estrogens and progestins has introduced a spectrum of iatrogenic cutaneous manifestations due to excessive prolonged exposure to sex hormones [66]. Many of these manifestations are similar to the cutaneous disorders encountered in pregnancy. Thus vaginal candidiasis is frequent, hair loss may occur after withdrawal as well as concurrently with ad-

ministration of contraceptive agents, and about 5 percent of patients develop melasma. While some of the agents produce amelioration of acne, others cause worsening due to the type and quantity of the progestational component. Telangiectasia and spider angiomata may appear. Other cutaneous disorders are occasionally precipitated or exacerbated by oral contraceptive agents, e.g., erythema nodosum, porphyria cutanea tarda, herpes gestationis, or systemic lupus erythematosus.

Cutaneous manifestations of too little sex hormone

Absolute or relative lack of sex hormone may result from (1) congenital disorders in which the gonads fail to develop; (2) end organ unresponsiveness due to defects in metabolizing enzymes or hormone receptors in target tissues; (3) castration or suppression of gonadal function following administration of estrogens to the male; (4) diseases of the urogenital tract which destroy the gonads; or (5) disturbances in the hypothalamic–pituitary regulation of gonadotropin (panhypopituitarism or isolated trophic hormone defects).

The skin changes that result from lack of androgens depend, in large measure, upon the age at which the deficits occur and the sex of the patient. If males are deprived of testosterone before puberty, the fully developed picture of eunuchoidism or infantilism results: the skin remains thin and fine, and sebaceous glands, apocrine glands, and the follicles of sexual hair remain dormant. Facial pores are small; there is no oiliness, and acne vulgaris is absent. However, as time goes on, the skin around the eyes and lips develops the fine wrinkling characteristic of aging. The hairline remains straight over the forehead and low over the temples in male prepuberal castrates, and male-pattern baldness does not appear. Beard, axillary hair, and pubic hair are not present. Pallor of the skin is an outstanding feature. Not only is there lack of pigment in the skin of the sexual zones, but there is less pigment generally. Reduced cutaneous blood flow contributes to the pallor.

The penis remains small, and scrotal skin retains its relatively smooth contours. The body habitus is juvenile. Delayed somatic maturation is expressed in poor muscular development and excessive subcutaneous fat in the pectoral and girdle region. Delayed closure of epiphyses of long bones results in slow but prolonged growth, so that normal height may be achieved ultimately by virtue of the disproportionate length of the extremities.

The picture is modified if deprivation of androgen occurs after puberty. Although the initiation of terminal hair growth on the body and face requires testosterone, maintenance of such hair is much less dependent on androgens. Thus, in the male postpuberal castrate, hair in the axillae and perineum usually persists, although it becomes very sparse.

Coarse hair on the extremities, trunk, and beard area shows even less change. Although the necessity for regular shaving of the beard persists, the intervals become less frequent. Gross functional changes are most readily detected in sebaceous glands. By virtue of the requirement of the sebaceous glands for continuous androgenization, sebum secretion is markedly reduced so that the skin and hair are not oily. The texture of the skin is less coarse and shows facial wrinkling but does not revert to its prepuberal state.

All the above changes are reversible by replacement therapy with androgens.

Pituitary hormones

The adenohypophysis and neurohypophysis are the source of a number of hormones, some of which regulate endocrine structures such as adrenocorticotropin (ACTH), gonadotropins, and thyrotropin (TSH). They also include somatotropin (growth hormone, GH), prolactin, melanocyte-stimulating hormone (MSH), and lipotropin which do not appear to stimulate endocrine tissues directly. Peptides that are immunologically indistinguishable from their pituitary counterparts may be produced ectopically by certain solid tumors.

The implications of disordered adenohypophyseal function for the skin must be formulated in terms of direct actions mediated via target gland hormones whose elaboration is conditioned by the tropic stimulation from the pituitary. The latter introduces multiple potentialities, so that the alterations of the skin in pituitary disorders usually present a composite of endocrine effects. For example, too much hormone of one sort may be accompanied by too little of another variety (e.g., too much growth hormone with too little sex hormone).

Direct effects of pituitary hormones on the skin have not been convincingly demonstrated in humans with the exception of MSH and ACTH in relation to pigmentation. However, numerous studies in animals have suggested that somatotropin (GH), prolactin, TSH, ACTH, MSH, and lipotropins may facilitate responses of sebaceous glands to androgenic stimulation, suggesting that there may be subtle effects of pituitary peptides directly on the skin.

The subsequent section will deal with two disorders of pituitary functions which are well defined and which illustrate the complexity of composite endocrine effects on the skin: too much GH (acromegaly) and too little of all anterior pituitary hormones (panhypopituitarism).

Cutaneous manifestations of too much growth hormone (acromegaly)

Excessive growth hormone elaboration is commonly associated with eosinophilic adenomas of the pituitary. Although pituitary elaboration of other hormones, such as the gonadotropins, may be compromised, the preponderant changes in the skin and the rest of the body are those of excessive stimulation with growth hormone. In the skin, these changes are most pronounced in the connective tissue of the dermis. There is an increase in the content of glycosaminoglycans with proportional increases in chondroitin and dermatan sulfate [67]. The characteristic hyperplasia may be due not only to increased mucopolysaccharide but to the attendant retention of water by these hygroscopic substances. Whether or not collagen is increased or altered remains controversial. Most effects of growth hormone on skeletal tissues are mediated via stimulation of somatomedins; whether this is true of skin as well remains to be determined.

In acromegaly there is also hyperplasia of epidermis and dermal appendages. However, there is presently no evidence that this effect is on the epidermis per se, although that possibility cannot be excluded, it is equally conceivable that the alterations in the connective tissue of the dermal anlage indirectly stimulate growth of epidermal cells and appendages. For example, in certain nonendocrine conditions characterized by very similar mesenchymal hyperplasia, the changes in the epidermis and appendages are quite analogous, e.g., pachydermoperiostosis.

Growth hormone may also exert effects on pilosebaceous structures by potentiating the effectiveness of available androgen. However, while such actions have been demonstrated in animals, data in humans are not definitive. Thus, isolated deficiency of GH in sexual ateliotic dwarfs may not be associated with significant depression of sebaceous gland activity [54] and enhanced function of dermal appendages is usually sustained in acromegaly when hypogonadism develops.

Clinically, the effect on the integument can best be described as "too much skin." The entire skin is thickened and has a doughy feel; this is most marked over the face and on the extremities, where the skeletal changes are also most prominent (hence: acromegaly). Furrowing and accentuation of the folds contribute to the coarsening of the features (Fig. 173-6). Deepening of creases on the forehead and in the nasolabial area gives the patient a scowling, somber expression. In extreme cases, the overgrowth of the dermis results in a bizarre ridging of the skin of the scalp (cutis verticis gyrata). The eyelids are thick and edematous. The lower lip is enlarged and protruding, and there is macroglossia. The nose becomes elongated, and the exuberant hypertrophy of soft tissue usually exceeds the cartilaginous overgrowth. Increased soft tissue in the alae nasi gives the nose an unmistakable triangular configuration. Similar changes are easily recognized on the hands and feet as well as the abdominal skin. Over the bony prominences of the hands, the folds are accentuated. The pads of the digits become fleshy, and the fingers assume a blunted shape, and heel pads are thickened. The overgrowth of fibrous tissue leads to the production of small sessile or pedunculated fibromas which occur in 20 to 30 percent of cases [68].

There is thickening of the epidermis with accentuation of markings and enlarged pores. Nails become thickened and hard. Excessive eccrine and apocrine sweating occurs in the majority of patients and may be implicated in the heightened incidence of abscesses in the axillae and intergluteal cleft. Although breast tissue often becomes atrophic along with other stigmata of gonadal dysfunction, galactorrhea may occur.

Hypertrichosis is common, occurring in about half of patients. Excessive hair growth, however, differs from that associated with virilizing syndromes in that it is confined to the extremities, chest, sacral area, pubis, and axilla. The scalp and bearded area are not affected. The skin is said to be oily; acne, however, is not common.

Hyperpigmentation has been observed in about 40 percent of patients. The increase in color is usually not marked and occurs diffusely in the normal distribution of pigment (i.e., exposed parts, skin folds, sexual areas, and pressure points).

As activity of the disease diminishes, the skin changes become stationary. Occasionally, in the late stages of the disease, actual loss of body hair may occur, presumably

Fig. 173-6 Acromegalic changes.

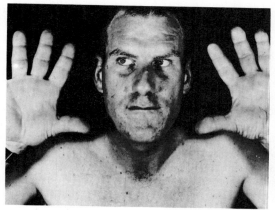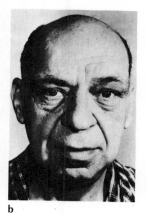

a   b

because hypogonadism predominates and androgens are insufficient. With effective tumor therapy and lowering of the excessive levels of GH, rapid regression of soft tissue changes has been observed.

The major cause of the grossly altered appearance in this disorder is change in bony and cartilaginous tissue. Since epiphyseal closure limits the longitudinal growth of long bones, the effects of too much growth hormone in adult life are primarily exerted on the skull, the hands and feet, and cartilage. The patient presents the characteristic features of such growth; accentuation of the frontal bosses and supraorbital ridges, enlargement of the lower jaw (prognathism) in which the teeth become more widely spaced, and enlarged ears. The rib cage may be deformed with resulting kyphosis. In extreme instances, grossly enlarged hands and feet are appended to arms and legs of normal girth, adding to the grotesque appearance. If the disease develops prior to closure of the epiphyses, the features of acromegaly are superimposed on gigantism.

Acanthosis nigricans is associated with acromegaly in a significant number of cases. Ten percent of a large series of patients with this peculiar epidermal hyperplasia had pituitary tumors with acromegaly [69].

Effects of too little of all pituitary hormones (panhypopituitarism)

A variety of conditions may compromise the anterior pituitary and, thereby, the elaboration of all pituitary hormones. Acute infarction may occur following postpartum hemorrhage (Sheehan's syndrome). Slower failure via destruction of the gland by chronic infection (e.g., syphilis, tuberculosis), granulomatous inflammation (sarcoid), neoplastic invasion (e.g., histiocytoses, metastatic malignancy), or by tumors arising within the pituitary (e.g., chromophobe adenoma) or in contiguous structures (craniopharyngiomas).

The alterations of the skin in panhypopituitarism depend upon the amount of pituitary tissue that has been destroyed and the integrated deprivation of those hormones which have been considered singly in earlier portions of the text. However, certain modifying factors warrant consideration. First, the individual hormonal deficits may not be as pronounced as in primary failure of the target glands, since some autonomous function of the target glands may persist

even in the absence of trophic stimulation. Second, the effects of the lack of one particular hormone may be modified by the lack of other hormones. For example, although the patient with panhypopituitarism may have marked hypothyroidism, the cutaneous myxedema is often mild. This may conceivably be due to the lack of other hormones which may stimulate mucopolysaccharide synthesis.

Cutaneous manifestations of too little pituitary hormone

Pallor of the skin is prominent. There is often a yellow tinge similar to that seen in hypothyroidism. The melanin content is apparently diminished. While this is most evident in the sexual areas, the phenomenon is generalized, and there is an increased sensitivity to sunlight and less pigmentation of traumatized or inflamed skin. Lack of a normal capillary flush of the face, earlobes, and palms contributes to the pallor, but mucous membranes retain their normal hue unless there is concomitant anemia. The texture of the skin is dry but smoother and softer than in primary hypothyroidism. There is, however, frequently some puffiness of the face, characteristic of myxedema. The facies tend to be expressionless because of a diminution of normal facial folds. The thinness of the skin and subcutaneous tissues results in fine wrinkling around the eyes and mouth, giving the appearance of advanced age.

Loss of body hair occurs in all patients and is found early. The axillae are affected first, and a reduced need for axillary shaving in the female may constitute the initial expression. Pubic hair loss takes longer to develop and is less consistent. Beard growth diminishes but is not lost altogether in adult males. Scalp hair tends to be fine and dry, and there may be generalized thinning. Sebaceous secretions also diminish, and sweating is decreased.

Diabetes mellitus

Diabetes mellitus is a metabolic disorder characterized by disturbances in the traffic of fuels. These arise via several pathogenic mechanisms which have been classified into two major groups: insulin-dependent diabetes, IDDM (type I) and non-insulin-dependent diabetes, NIDDM (type II) [70]. In IDDM, which begins in childhood most frequently, there is an absolute lack of pancreatic and circulating insulin. Autoimmune phenomena, circulating islet cell antibodies, antecedent viral infections, and distinctive patterns of histocompatibility antigens are present. NIDDM occurs in older populations and has a stronger familial frequency; pancreatic and circulating insulin are not lacking but the availability of insulin is inappropriate to peripheral needs (relative insulin insufficiency). Peripheral resistence to insulin action may be enhanced in the 60 to 70 percent of all NIDDM who are obese.

In all types of diabetes, disposition of ingested nutrients is faulty and there is poorly restrained recall of endogenous fuel stores. As a result, catabolism is inappropriate in the fasted state and anabolism is improperly synchronized in the fed state. While the common denominator is usually an absolute or relative lack of circulating insulin, the disturbances are in some instances due to peripheral factors that inhibit hormone action at the tissue level [71]. Rare syndromes have been described in which insulin action is blocked either by autoantibodies against insulin receptors or by defects in the receptors themselves [72]. Certain instances of NIDDM due to mutant insulins have also been described recently [73].

Acute, gross metabolic disturbance resulting in high blood sugar, hypertriglyceridemia, ketoacidosis, and classic symptomatology is usually correctable by appropriate therapy. However, all forms of diabetes are also associated in the longer term with multisystem degenerative disorders involving the cardiovascular and nervous systems, eyes, kidneys, and skin. These delayed changes have now been attributed to effects of chronic metabolic derangements which, until recently, were not rectified by available therapeutic strategies. Whether strict regulation of glycemia (so-called tight control) will entirely prevent these degenerative complications cannot yet be assessed. However, recent reports have described regressions of capillary basement membrane thickening in IDDM [74] and NIDDM [75] following prolonged rectification of hyperglycemia.

The skin shares in both the effects of acute gross metabolic derangements and chronic degenerative changes of diabetes. This is not surprising since the skin is an actively metabolizing tissue dependent on circulating fuels for biosynthetic activity.

Insulin affects the utilization of glucose by whole skin [76] even though it is not required to facilitate the entry of glucose into epidermal cells [77]. The amount of glucose in whole skin is greater than can be attributed to distribution in extracellular fluid. The ratio of glucose/g skin to glucose/ml blood is increased in diabetic skin, suggesting that insulin regulates intracellular disposition of glucose in the skin [78].

Insulin profoundly affects various components of the skin. It is required for growth and differentiation of keratinocytes in culture systems. Experimental wound healing, which involves both epidermal and dermal elements, is delayed in diabetic animals until they are treated with insulin. However, the most pronounced effects may be those on dermal fibroblasts. In experimental diabetes there is less acid-soluble dermal collagen and it is more cross-linked [79]. These changes parallel the findings in dermal collagen of human diabetics which show a decrease in acid-soluble collagen and more glycosylation than in age-matched controls [80].

Consideration of the cutaneous manifestations of diabetes may be divided into (a) those that accompany acute, gross metabolic disturbances and (b) those that correlate with the presence of chronic degenerative complications. In addition, there are a number of dermatologic disorders (c) that occur more frequently in diabetics but that do not correlate with either gross metabolic derangements or degenerative changes.

Cutaneous manifestations correlated with gross derangements of intermediary metabolism

Certain cutaneous disorders occur in diabetic patients specifically in relation to hyperglycemia and hyperlipidemia and are reversible when these abnormalities are corrected.

Infections. Poorly controlled or undiagnosed diabetes may be associated with bacterial and fungal infections of the skin. The infections most frequently encountered are staphylococcal pyodermas, candidiasis, erythrasma, and epidermophytosis. While the prevalence of the latter two appears to be definitely increased in diabetics, such a correlation has not been well established for staphylococcal and candidal infections. Moreover, it is not clear whether the diabetic host is more susceptible to infections or less able to deal with an infection once it is established.

Abnormalities in leukocyte function including diminished chemotaxis, phagocytosis, and killing of organisms have been demonstrated in diabetics and appear to relate to the degree of hyperglycemia [81]. This effect may be due in part to the hyperosmolality of the hyperglycemic serum [82]. Diminished leukocyte response may also be due to the inability of leukocytes to migrate through thickened capillary walls as well as diminished diffusion of insulin and nutrient substrates to sustain extravascular leukocytes. Furthermore, repair of minor trauma may be affected both by delayed wound healing and by compromised dermal vasculature, thereby providing access for pathogenic organisms. On the other hand, evidence for altered immune responses in diabetics has not been confirmed.

Vulvovaginitis due to *Candida albicans* is a common complication of diabetes. Involvement of other intertriginous skin (Fig. A1-19) and nails (Fig. A1-18) is frequently seen together with the genital infection.

The candidiasis responds readily to control of the hyperglycemia and does not occur more frequently in aglycosuric diabetics than the normal population. While generalized pruritus is not a feature of diabetes, vulvar itching with candidiasis should alert the clinician to the possible presence of diabetes unless other obvious precipitating causes such as pregnancy, oral contraceptives, or broad-spectrum antibiotics can be invoked.

Pyodermas, especially furunculosis, were formerly a serious complication of diabetes. The advent of antibiotics and tighter control of diabetes has lessened both the incidence and morbidity of such infections. Population surveys have shown no increased incidence of septic skin infections in the diabetic population. Nonetheless, pyogenic infections do occur more frequently in poorly controlled diabetics and control of well-regulated diabetes can be interrupted by intercurrent cutaneous infection. Sommerville and Lancaster-Smith [83] have shown that this cannot be attributed to a higher incidence of nasal carriers of *Staphylococcus* in controlled diabetes, as was earlier reported.

However, the carrier rate in uncontrolled disease has not been critically examined.

Infections of the lower extremities constitute a particular hazard for the diabetic patient. The presence of atherosclerosis and peripheral neuropathy leads to ulceration and gangrene as well as poor wound healing. The damaged and devitalized skin provides a fertile breeding ground for secondary infections. Moreover, the increased incidence of epidermophytosis of the feet provides portals of entry for pathogenic organisms.

Prevention of such infections requires meticulous care of the feet, which should be incorporated into every diabetic regimen. This includes the regular services of a podiatrist, well-fitting shoes to prevent pressure points, twice daily foot washing with tepid water followed by thorough drying and use of emollients. Prompt attention to foot wounds, blisters, minor infections, and epidermophytosis is indicated.

Xanthomatosis. Although plasma free-fatty acids and ketones may vary on a moment-to-moment basis with alterations in the utilization of glucose, a more sustained hyperlipidemia involving triglycerides and cholesterol more than phospholipids is common in diabetics even with rather mild elevations of blood glucose.

Xanthomas, secondary to chylomicronemia are characteristically multiple and tend to occur rapidly in crops. Small reddish-yellow nodules up to 0.5 cm in diameter present in clusters, primarily on extensor surfaces and buttocks (Fig. A2-1a). They may be pruritic initially and are much smaller and more inflammatory than the tendon and tuberous xanthomas associated with hypercholesterolemia. These eruptive xanthomas are clinically indistinguishable from those secondary to other states associated with chylomicronemia. Histologically, the lesions are laden with neutral lipid-rich histiocytes. Ultrastructural and chemical studies have demonstrated that the chylomicrons migrate through dermal capillary walls and are phagocytosed by tissue macrophages and perithelial cells. In freshly erupted xanthomas the lipid composition of the lesion reflects that of plasma chylomicrons, containing about 45 percent triglycerides. Resolving or evolving lesions gradually lose triglyceride and become relatively richer in cholesterol [84]. Rapid regression occurs when the hyperlipidemia is brought under control.

Xanthelasma occurs in most hyperlipidemic states including diabetes but may occur without any demonstrable abnormality of plasma lipids. Xanthelasma, however, does not usually regress when therapy for diabetes is instituted. Hyperlipidemia, even in the absence of xanthomatosis is sometimes accompanied by yellowish discoloration of the palms, soles, and nasolabial folds due to the deposition of carotene.

Cutaneous manifestations of diabetes correlated with chronic degenerative complications

It is now generally accepted that microangiopathy characteristic of diabetes occurs in the dermal vasculature as well and may result in decreased cutaneous blood flow [85]. In addition to changes in blood vessels, there are changes in dermal connective tissue and probably in cutaneous innervation. Thus, certain of the cutaneous manifestations which appear to correlate with multisystem degenerative complications may be attributable to the presence of biochemical and anatomic disturbances within the skin. Moreover, they appear to occur in both IDDM and NIDDM.

Diabetic dermopathy. This group of lesions was first described [86] as atrophic, circumscribed, brownish lesions of the lower extremities. The presence of small-vessel changes led to the term "diabetic dermopathy" [87] although the pathogenic significance of vascular changes in relation to the lesions remains to be established. The lesions are asymptomatic, irregularly shaped patches occurring primarily over the anterior lower legs; their surfaces are depressed and they have a light brown color. Lesions appear in crops and gradually resolve over $1\frac{1}{2}$ to 2 years; however, the constant appearance of new lesions gives the impression of a stationary course. Although Melin failed to observe antecedent cutaneous changes, other authors [87–89], have noted the presence of red patches, sometimes with scaling and erosion, prior to the development of the pigmented atrophic patches. Despite their resemblance to scars, recall of antecedent trauma is seldom elicited.

Histologically, dermal arterioles and capillaries display intimal thickening and deposition of PAS-positive fibrillar material in vessel walls. Capillaries show basement membrane thickening with focal deposition of PAS-positive material. Hemosiderin and extravasated red cells are often present and accumulation of leukocytes around vessel walls has been described (Figs. 173-7 and 173-8).

While these lesions are not clinically distinguishable from posttraumatic scarring on the legs of older patients with compromised circulation, they appear more frequently and in greater number in diabetics. They are more common in men than women (2:1) and are often accompanied by evidence of significant microangiopathy elsewhere, i.e., retinal microaneurysms, nephropathy, and neuropathy (50 percent or more of patients).

Erythema and necrosis. Reddening of the face (rubeosis facei) and of the extremities has been described in long-standing diabetes. More recently, attention has been called to erysipelas-like areas in the lower legs and feet which may or may not eventuate in frank necrosis and destructive lesions of underlying bone [90]. These painless areas are often edematous and do not differ clinically from the erythema that accompanies gangrene of the toes and feet due to arterial insufficiency in diabetes. Cardiac decompensation, unilateral edema from venous occlusion, and arterial insufficiency have been cited as precipitating factors. It is likely that these findings are manifestations of severe atherosclerosis.

Bullous lesions. Although appearance of bullae in diabetics was noted earlier, the first carefully studied series of 15 patients was presented in 1963 [91]. In this and subsequently reported series of patients the bullae appeared spontaneously, usually on the extremities, especially the feet. Generally the bullae heal in several weeks without significant scarring, although they may occasionally recur. The localization of the lesions has been disputed. Early reports suggested the bullae were intraepidermal without acantholysis. More recently, careful studies demonstrate

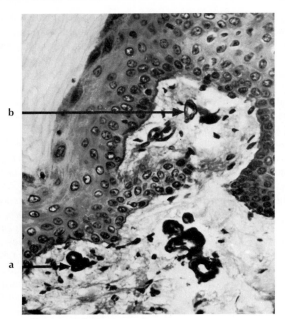

Fig. 173-7 "Thickened" (a), and "normal" (b) capillaries in the skin of the toe of a diabetic patient (PAS stain).

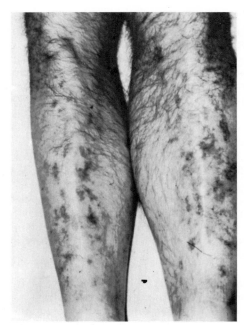

Fig. 173-8 Diabetic dermopathy.

that they are subepidermal with early reepithelialization spuriously giving an intraepidermal location. Ultrastructural studies in one case demonstrated the plane of separation in the basement membrane zone above the basal lamina [92]. Although in some cases distribution of the lesions in light-exposed areas suggests a resemblance to porphyria cutanea tarda, abnormalities or porphyrin metabolism have not been demonstrated. Moreover, neither trauma nor immunologic mechanisms have been implicated.

The cause of this rare manifestation of diabetes is unknown. Seventy-five percent or more of affected patients have significant diabetic retinopathy and in a reported series of three patients dermopathy and cutaneous microangiopathy were present [88]. The localization of the plane of separation suggests that weakness or injury in the basement zone is the underlying lesion. That this may indeed be the case is suggested by reports of a reduced threshold to formation of suction blisters on the forearms of insulin-dependent diabetics [93] and of reduplication and the thickening of the basement membrane zone [94].

Scleredema adultorum. This well-defined entity has been recognized as a cutaneous manifestation of diabetes only in the last two decades. It consists of cutaneous induration beginning on the posterior and lateral neck. The painless swelling gradually spreads to the face, shoulders, anterior neck, and upper torso; and may eventually involve the abdomen, arms, and hands. The affected skin is hard and does not pit on pressure. Demarcation from normal skin may be sharp or poorly defined.

The histologic findings consist of thickened collagen bundles and deposition of glycosaminoglycans, chiefly hyaluronic acid, in the dermis.

A more familiar form of this disorder has long been recognized as occurring subsequent to infections, usually

streptococcal. This syndrome resolves spontaneously in a period of months. In contrast, scleredema associated with diabetes may not remit for years. The scleredema, which may have systemic involvement, appears to occur primarily in obese patients with long-standing diabetes and evidence of vascular complications [95,96]. It is possible that these massive changes in dermal connective tissue represent the extreme example of a more common phenomenon. Rosenbloom et al [97] have reported the presence of limited motility of large and small joints together with waxy (indurated) skin of the extremities in 30 percent of a large series of insulin-dependent diabetics. The findings correlated positively with duration of the diabetes and appeared to be predictive of microvascular disease. While the underlying mechanism of these connective tissue abnormalities remains to be elucidated, it seems reasonable to postulate that they represent the clinical manifestations of altered metabolism of collagen and glycosaminoglycans due to insulin deprivation.

Peripheral neuropathy. Autonomic disturbances may accompany the sensory neuropathy, a common degenerative complication. An uncommon manifestation of autonomic neuropathy in diabetes is anhidrosis, which may be localized, as in the legs, or more generalized [98]. Involved areas of the skin show abnormalities in autonomic fibers adjacent to eccrine sweat glands [99].

Cutaneous disorders that are more common in diabetes without regard to metabolic derangement or degenerative changes

Although the literature abounds with reports of well-defined cutaneous disorders in more frequent association with diabetes, only a few of these have withstood careful examination.

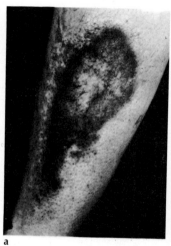

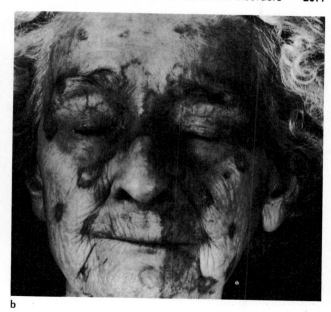

Fig. 173-9 Necrobiosis lipoidica diabeticorum. (a) Typical site on the shin. (b) Unusual location on the face with marked disfigurement.

Necrobiosis lipoidica diabeticorum. This very distinctive skin disease is perhaps the best example of such an association. These relatively asymptomatic lesions, which occur three times more often in women, are characteristically found on the anterior and lateral surfaces of the lower legs. They may occur, however, on the arms and trunk. There may be one or several lesions either unilaterally or bilaterally. The lesion begins as a small, dusky-red, elevated nodule with a sharply circumscribed border (Fig. A2-3). It slowly enlarges, becoming irregular in outline, flattened, and eventually depressed as the dermis becomes atrophic.

The color becomes brownish yellow except for the border, which may remain reddened. Coalescing or enlarging individual lesions may in time encompass the entire anterior tibial areas. The epidermis is smooth or slightly scaly and atrophic. Delicate vessels can be seen through the surface. The lesions of necrobiosis lipoidica diabeticorum (NLD) are chronic and indolent; shallow, often painful ulcerations frequently appear in long-standing lesions (see Fig. 171-2). In the early stages the lesion may resemble granuloma annulare or sarcoid, but the well-developed lesion is characteristic and easily recognized (Fig. 173-9). It dif-

Fig. 173-10 Necrobiosis lipoidica diabeticorum. The disorder results in pathologic changes in most of the dermis, from basement membrane to subcutis. In this photomicrograph, presumably from an active or early lesion, there are acellular, intensely eosinophilic areas of necrosis bordered by inflammation. x40. (Micrograph by Wallace H. Clark, Jr., M.D.)

Fig. 173-11 Necrobiosis lipoidica diabeticorum. Most of the reticular dermis is sclerotic; the usual collagen bundle pattern is obliterated. An ill-defined area of inflammation usually borders the sclerotic zone, outwardly toward the epidermis and inwardly toward the subcutis. x40. (Micrograph by Wallace H. Clark, Jr., M.D.)

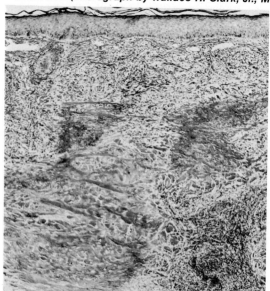

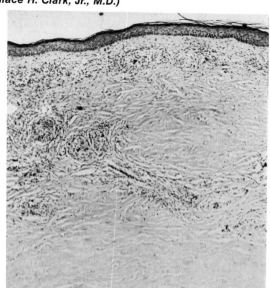

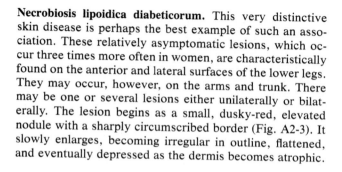

fers from the previously described atrophic patches in the striking degree of atrophy of the dermis and epidermis, in its sharply circumscribed border and greater size, and in its characteristic yellow-brown color.

The primary pathologic changes are in the lower dermis, where collagen is markedly altered, with focal areas of loss of normal structure, swelling, basophilia, and distortion of the bundles (necrobiosis) (Figs. 173-10 to 173-12). There is also loss and fragmentation of elastic fibers. In these areas there are aggregations of inflammatory cells including epithelioid cells, histiocytes, and multinucleated giant cells, sometimes containing asteroid bodies. The late appearance of foam cells accounts for the designation lipoidica. The vasculature is always involved. There is endothelial proliferation and sometimes occlusion of the lumina of arterioles and arteries. Capillary walls are thickened with focal deposits of PAS-positive material, which may be found in the lumina as well.

The relationship of these lesions to diabetes has not been clarified fully. NLD was first described in patients with well-established diabetes but subsequently was seen in patients without evident diabetes. The picture has been confused further by the description of a similar lesion (granulomatosis disciformis chronica progressiva) apparently unrelated to diabetes. Most investigators, however, now agree that NLD may present with varying clinical appearance depending on the degree of granulomatous response.

The precise correlation between NLD and diabetes remains controversial. In a study of 171 patients, the majority had diabetes when NLD developed; in most of the others, diabetes developed later, or there were other stigmata such as a close relative with diabetes or an abnormal cortisone-glucose tolerance test. Only about 10 percent of patients with NLD do not fall into any of these categories [100]. The induction of abnormal carbohydrate tolerance with glucocorticoids has been demonstrated in the majority of patients with NLD and without evident diabetes [101].

Thus, despite the lack of full concordance, NLD seems to be a valid marker for diabetes. However, the nature of the association remains as unclear as does the pathogenesis of these characteristic lesions. Since it occurs in both IDDM and NIDDM its pathogenesis cannot be related to genetic factors, underlying autoimmune disorders, or other causes of diabetes. It can be reasonably assumed that the granulomatous response is secondary to an alteration in dermal collagen. The controversy concerns the degenerative change in collagen. It is not clear whether this is secondary to an underlying vascular disease or whether it develops independently. The latter would ascribe the changes in dermal collagen and vasculature to some primary disorder of connective tissue, as yet unknown. However, the invariable presence of arteriolar changes deep to and within the areas of collagen degeneration suggests some interrelation between the two components of NLD. It has been hypothesized that increased platelet aggregation may be the triggering factor in the vascular changes. The demonstration of immune globulins, complement (C3), and fibrinogen in blood vessel walls further confuses the picture and raises the possibility of an immunologic process as a pathogenic component [102].

Treatment of NLD is not very satisfactory. Progression of the lesions does not correlate with normalization of the hyperglycemia by insulin or oral hypoglycemic agents. Local therapy with application of steroid creams under oc-

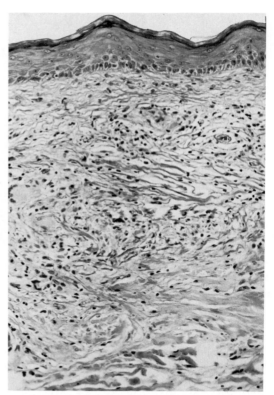

Fig. 173-12   Necrobiosis lipoidica diabeticorum. The outer inflammatory zone bordering the sclerotic collagen is shown; there are lymphocytes, histiocytes, and ill-formed giant cells. x160. (Micrograph by Wallace H. Clark Jr., M.D.)

clusive dressings or intralesional injections of steroids may afford some improvement. There have also been several enthusiastic reports on the use of aspirin and dipyridamole. While these have not been confirmed in a more rigorous double-blind trial [103], it has also been pointed out that the dose of aspirin may be a critical factor in achieving the optimal effect on platelet aggregation [104]. These authors have found favorable effects with very small doses of aspirin (3.5 mg/kg every 48 to 72 h).

Granuloma annulare. The similarity between pathologic features of NLD and granuloma annulare has led to an intensive search for the presence of abnormal carbohydrate metabolism in the latter disease. There is little evidence to support the association of overt diabetes with granuloma annulare but several authors have reported abnormal carbohydrate tolerance after cortisone administration in patients with granuloma annulare. This has been disputed by Williamson and Dykes [105] who failed to confirm abnormal oral glucose tolerance or insulin secretion with or without cortisone stress in patients with typical disease. A reported association of carbohydrate intolerance with atypical or generalized granuloma annulare also has not yet been convincingly confirmed [106]. On the basis of present evidence it appears unlikely that this benign and self-limited disorder represents a true manifestation of latent diabetes.

Vitiligo. Vitiligo occurs with a greater incidence than expected (4.8 percent) in patients with maturity-onset diabetes [107]. Vitiligo may precede the onset of clinically evident diabetes and also occurs more frequently in families of diabetics. Vitiligo has also been reported in association with IDDM; in one study, autoantibodies to adrenal, thyroid, or gastric parietal cells were also present in 4 out of 5 children with vitiligo diabetes [108]. Such autoantibodies have not been demonstrated in patients with NIDDM and vitiligo in the absence of other endocrine deficiency states. The association of the pigmentary disorder and diabetes thus requires further clarification.

Acanthosis nigricans. This disorder is characterized by velvety papillomatous hyperplasia of the epidermis with intense hyperpigmentation most prominently displayed in axillary, inguinal, inframammary, and neck creases. In its most developed form, it may be accompanied by verrucous patches on knuckles and other extensor surfaces, hyperkeratoses of the palms and soles, and other benign hyperplasias of the skin. Acanthosis nigricans is associated with three types of disorders. The most fully developed form is frequently found in patients with advanced malignant tumors, usually adenocarcinomas. Acanthosis nigricans is also seen in association with a variety of endocrine disorders [69] including acromegaly, Cushing's syndrome (especially when induced by exogenous glucocorticoids), and patients with diabetes and insulin resistance. In the latter circumstances acanthosis nigricans is part of the syndrome irrespective of the nature of the insulin receptor defect. In addition, acanthosis nigricans occurs in obese individuals who may have Stein-Leventhal syndrome, NIDDM, or no evident endocrine disorder. In this latter group, the skin changes tend to be limited to axillary and neck folds.

Kyrle's disease/reactive perforating collagenosis. This is an uncommon skin disease characterized by hyperkeratotic follicular and parafollicular papules. The pathologic process involves transepidermal elimination of material from the dermis that may have represented altered collagen. An inflammatory reaction is generally present. The perforating disorder occurs in diabetics with renal failure but also in renal failure without diabetes [109,110].

The condition is often pruritic, adding to the more generalized pruritus present in patients with chronic renal failure on dialysis. Treatment with topical retinoids or with ultraviolet radiation may be beneficial.

Glucagonoma syndrome. An unusual and striking cutaneous syndrome has recently been described in patients with glucagon-secreting tumors of the pancreatic islets. Although hyperglycemia as a consequence of excessive glucagon levels is usually present, the syndrome cannot be accurately classified as a manifestation of diabetes.

The glucagonoma syndrome was first recognized as such by Mallinson et al [111]; however, an undiagnosed dermatitis was present in the first confirmed case of glucagonoma in 1966 [112]. Typical features have been characterized in several series [113]. Although the eruption may begin as a recalcitrant, nonspecific, dry eczema with a faint papular component, the more characteristic pattern consists of migrating marginated areas of erythema with central blisters which crust and heal with hyperpigmentation. The eruption waxes and wanes and is more pronounced in the lower abdomen, buttocks, perineum, and legs. A beefy-red tongue, angular cheilitis, and nail dystrophy may be present. The somewhat diverse clinical features may also suggest Hailey-Hailey disease, pemphigus foliaceous, subcorneal pustulosis, pustular psoriasis, or acrodermatitis enteropathica. The most prominent feature of the histologic picture consists of spongiosis, necrosis, and cleft formation without acantholysis in the upper epidermis.

This clinical-histologic picture, now known as necrolytic migratory erythema, is considered to be characteristic for presence of an underlying glucagonoma. However, the relation of the cutaneous lesions to the neoplasm is still obscure. About 75 percent of the associated tumors are malignant and most patients have had widespread metastases when diagnosed. Removal of the tumor usually results in regression of the cutaneous signs, and somatostatin, which depresses elevated glucagon levels, may also suppress the skin lesions [114]. Nonetheless, it is not likely that glucagon per se causes the skin lesions since they are lacking in many glucagonomas with very elevated circulatory levels of hormone. Moreover there have been reports that administration of diiodoquin as well as zinc may improve skin lesions.

It appears likely that some other factor(s) secreted by or associated with these tumors is responsible. It could be another peptide since there are often different cell types present. In this regard, a report of necrolytic migratory erythema in two patients with normal glucagon levels, without pancreatic tumor and with small-bowel disease, is of interest [115].

References

1. Barker SB: In *The Thyroid Gland*, vol 1, edited by R Pitt-Rivers, WR Trotter. London, Butterworth, 1964, p 226
2. Holt PJ: In vitro responses of epidermis to tri-iodothyronine. *J Invest Dermatol* **71**:202, 1978
3. Smith TJ et al: The effect of thyroid hormone in glycosaminoglycans accumulation in human skin fibroblasts. *Endocrinology* **108**:2397, 1981
4. Chapman RE et al: The effects of fetal thyroidectomy and thyroxin: a demonstration on the development of skin and wool follicles of sheep fetuses. *J Anat* **117**:419, 1974
5. Freinkel RK: Effect of thyroxine administration on the metabolism of guinea pig skin. *J Invest Dermatol* **38**:31, 1962
6. Holt PJA, Marks R: The epidermal response to change in thyroid states. *J Invest Dermatol* **68**:299, 1977
7. Ebling FJ: Hormonal control and methods of measuring sebaceous secretions. *J Invest Dermatol* **62**:161, 1974
8. Goolmali SK et al: Thyroid disease and sebaceous gland function. *Br Med J* **1**:432, 1976
9. Barrow MV, Bird ED: Pruritus in hyperthyroidism. *Arch Dermatol* **93**:237, 1966
10. Ochi Y, deGroot LJ: Vitiligo in Graves' disease. *Ann Intern Med* **71**:935, 1969
11. Lynch PJ et al: Pretibial myxedema and nonthyrotoxic thyroid disease. *Arch Dermatol* **107**:107, 1973
12. Wortsman J et al: Preradial myxedema in thyroid states. *Arch Dermatol* **117**:635, 1981
13. Biererwaltes WH, Bollet AJ: Mucopolysaccharide content of skin in patients with pretibial myxedema. *J Clin Invest* **38**:945, 1959
14. Cheung HS et al: Stimulation of fibroblast biosynthetic activity by serum of patients with pretibial myxedema. *J Invest Dermatol* **71**:12, 1978
15. Freinkel RK, Freinkel N: Hair growth and alopecia in hypothyroidism. *Arch Dermatol* **106**:349, 1972
16. Ingbar SH, Freinkel N: Hypothyroidism. *DM*, September 1958

17. Dyrbe MO et al: Effect of thyroxine, thyrotrophic and somatotrophic hormones on skin of dwarf mice. *Proc Soc Exp Biol Med* **102**:417, 1959

18. Hirano K et al: Cutaneous manifestations in idiopathic hypoparathyroidism. *Arch Dermatol* **109**:242, 1975

19. Aurbach GD et al: Parathyroid hormone, calcitonin, and the calciferols, in *Textbook of Endocrinology,* 6th ed, edited by RH Williams. Philadelphia, WB Saunders, 1981, p 965

20. Kleeman CR et al: The disappearance of intractable pruritus after parathyroidectomy in uremic patients with secondary hyperparathyroidism. *Trans Assoc Am Physicians* **81**:203, 1968

21. Sutphin A et al: Five cases (three in siblings) of idiopathic hypoparathyroidism associated with moniliasis. *J Clin Endocrinol* **3**:625, 1943

22. Hertz KC et al: Autoimmune vitiligo: detection of antibodies to melanin producing cells. *N Engl J Med* **297**:634, 1977

23. Blizzard RM, Gibbs JH: Candidiasis: studies pertaining to its association with endocrinopathies and pernicious anemia. *Pediatrics* **42**:231, 1968

24. Dorfman A, Schiller S: Effects of hormones on the metabolism of acid mucopolysaccharide of connective tissue. *Recent Prog Horm Res* **14**:427, 1958

25. Sarnstrand B et al: Effect of glucocorticoids on glycosaminoglycans metabolism in cultured skin fibroblasts. *J Invest Dermatol* **79**:412, 1982

26. Oxlund H et al: Changes in the mechanical properties, thermal stability, reducible cross-links and glycosyl-lysines in rat skin induced by corticosteroid treatment. *Acta Endocrinol (Copenh)* **101**:312, 1982

27. Koob TJ et al: Hormonal interactions in mammalian collagenase regulation. Comparative studies in human skin and rat uterus. *Biochim Biophys Acta* **629**:13, 1980

28. Asboe-Hansen G, Blumenkrantz N: Cortisol effects on collagen biosynthesis in embryonic explants and in vitro hydroxylation of procollagen. *Acta Endocrinol (Copenh)* **83**:665, 1976

29. Booth BA et al: Steroid induced dermal atrophy: effects of glucocorticosteroids on collagen metabolism in human skin fibroblast cultures. *Int J Dermatol* **21**:333, 1982

30. Fisher LB, Maibach HI: Effect of corticosteroids on human epidermal mitotic activity. *Arch Dermatol* **103**:39, 1971

31. Schell H et al: Evidence of diurnal variation of human epidermal cell proliferation. *Arch Dermatol Res* **271**:41, 1981

32. Sugimoto M, Endo H: Effect of hydrocortisone on keratinization of chick embryonic skin cultured in chemically defined medium. *Nature* **222**:1270, 1969

33. Laurence EB, Christophers E: Selective action of hydrocortisone on postmitotic epidermal cells in vivo. *J Invest Dermatol* **66**:222, 1976

34. Morrill SD, Herrmann F: Influence of systemically administered cortisone on hair growth in mice. *J Invest Dermatol* **37**:243, 1961

35. Weissmann G, Thomas L: The effects of corticosteroids upon connective tissue and lysosomes. *Recent Prog Horm Res* **20**:215, 1964

36. Galey CI et al: Activation of phospholipase A$_2$ and C in murine keratinocytes by phorbol ester 12-0-tetradecanoyl-phorhol-13-acetate. *Clin Res* **31**:567A, 1983

37. Hsia SL, Hao YL: Transformation of cortisone to cortisol in human skin. *Steroids* **10**:489, 1967

38. Malkinson FD et al: In vitro studies of adrenal steroid metabolism in the skin. *J Invest Dermatol* **32**:101, 1959

39. Nabors CJ, Berliner DL: Corticosteroid metabolism during wound healing. *J Invest Dermatol* **52**:465, 1969

40. Ponec M: Glucocorticoids and cultured human skin cells: specific intracellular binding and structure relationships. *Br J Dermatol* **107 (suppl 23)**:24, 1982

41. Shuster S, Thody AJ: The control and measurement of sebum secretion. *J Invest Dermatol* **62**:172, 1974

42. Treadwell BLJ et al: Side-effects of long-term treatment with corticosteroids and corticotrophin. *Lancet* **1**:1121, 1964

43. Graber AL et al: Natural history of pituitary-adrenal recovery following long-term suppression with corticosteroids. *J Clin Endocrinol* **25**:11, 1965

44. Greaves MS: The in vivo catabolism of cortisol by human skin. *J Invest Dermatol* **57**:100, 1971

45. Scoggins RB, Kliman B: Relative potency of percutaneously absorbed corticosteroids in the suppression of pituitary-adrenal function. *J Invest Dermatol* **45**:347, 1965

46. James VHT et al: Pituitary-adrenal function after occlusive topical therapy with betamethasone valerate. *Lancet* **2**:1059, 1967

47. Himathongkam T et al: Florid Cushing's syndrome and hirsutism induced by desoximethasone. *JAMA* **239**:430, 1978

48. Keipert J, Kelly R: Temporary Cushing's syndrome from percutaneous absorption of betamethasone 17-valerate. *Med J Aust* **1**:542, 1971

49. Burton TT et al: Complications of topical corticosteroid therapy in patients with liver disease. *Br J Dermatol* **91 (suppl 10)**:22, 1974

50. Garden JM, Freinkel RK: Prospective evaluation of hypercorticism during treatment of psoriasis with topical steroids. *Clin Res* **32**:584A, 1984

51. Soffer LJ et al: *The Human Adrenal Gland.* Philadelphia, Lea & Febiger, 1961

52. McGregor BC et al: Vitiligo and multiglandular insufficiencies. *JAMA* **219**:724, 1972

53. Nelson DH et al: ACTH-producing pituitary tumors following adrenalectomy for Cushing's syndrome. *Ann Intern Med* **52**:561, 1960

54. Pochi PE, Strauss JS: Endocrinological control of the development and activity of the human sebaceous gland. *J Invest Dermatol* **62**:191, 1974

55. Wilson MJ, Spaziane E: The melanogenic response to testosterone in scrotal epidermis: effects on tyrosinase activity and protein synthesis. *Acta Endocrinol (Copenh)* **81**:435, 1970

56. Glimcher ME et al: Ultrastructure of normals and castrates and the effects of testosterone and ultra violet (UVLB) irradiation on scrotal skin of rates. *J Exp Zool* **207**:249, 1979

57. Black MM et al: Osteoporosis, skin collagen and androgens. *Br Med J* **4**:773, 1970

58. Hodgins MB, Hay JB: Steroid metabolism in human skin: its relation to sebaceous gland growth and acne vulgaris. *Biochem Soc Trans* **4**:605, 1976

59. Hay JB, Hodgins MB: Distribution of androgen metabolizing enzymes in isolated tissues of human forehead and axillary skin. *J Endocrinol* **79**:29, 1978

60. Ebling FJ: Hormonal control and methods of measuring sebaceous secretions. *J Invest Dermatol* **62**:161, 1974

61. Ebling FJ: Endocrine factors affecting cell replacement and cell loss in the epidermis and sebaceous glands of the female albino rat. *J Endocrinol* **12**:38, 1955

62. Punnonen R: Effect of castration and peroral estrogen treatment on the skin. *Acta Obstet Gynecol Scand [Suppl]* **21**:3, 1972

63. Smith QT, Allison DJ: Changes of collagen content in skin, femur, and uterus of 17β estradiol benzoate treated rats. *Endocrinology* **79**:486, 1966

64. Yang SL et al: The effect of estrogens on collagen synthesis at the site of a skin graft. *Am J Obstet Gynecol* **116**:694, 1973

65. Rose LI et al: Adrenocortical hydroxylase deficiencies in acne vulgaris. *J Invest Dermatol* **66**:324, 1976

66. Jelineck JE: Cutaneous side effects of oral contraceptives. *Arch Dermatol* **101**:181, 1970

67. Matsuoka LY et al: Histochemical characterization of the cutaneous involvement of acromegaly. *Arch Intern Med* **142**:1820, 1982

68. Davidoff LM: Studies in acromegaly. III. The anamnesis and

symptomatology in one hundred cases. *Endocrinology* **10**:461, 1926

69. Brown J, Winklemann RK: Acanthosis nigricans: a study of 90 cases. *Medicine (Baltimore)* **47**:33, 1968

70. National Diabetes Data Group: Classification and diagnosis of diabetes mellitus and other categories of glucose intolerance. *Diabetes* **28**:1039, 1979

71. Reaven GM: Insulin resistance in noninsulin dependent diabetes mellitus. Does it exist and can it be measured? *Am J Med* **74 [suppl 1A]**:3, 1983

72. Flier JS et al: Antibodies that impair insulin receptor binding in an unusual diabetic syndrome with severe insulin resistance. *Science* **190**:63, 1975

73. Shoelson S et al: Three mutant insulins in man. *Nature* **302**:1, 1983

74. Raskin PR et al: The effect of diabetic control on the width of skeletal muscle capillary basement membrane in patients with type I diabetes mellitus. *N Engl J Med* **309**:1546, 1983

75. Camerini-Davlos RA et al: Drug induced reversal of early diabetic microangiopathy. *N Engl J Med* **309**:1551, 1983

76. Hsia SL: *Essays in Biochemistry, vol 7, Potentials in Exploring the Biochemistry of Human Skin*. New York, Academic Press, 1971, p 1

77. Halperin KM, Ohkawara A: Glucose entry into human epidermis. *J Invest Dermatol* **49**:561, 1967

78. Peterka ES, Fusaro RM: Cutaneous carbohydrate studies. IV. The skin glucose content of fasting diabetics with and without infection. *J Invest Dermatol* **46**:459, 1966

79. Chang KJ et al: Increased cross linkages in experimental diabetes. *Diabetes* **29**:778, 1980

80. Schnider SL, Kohn RR: Effects of age and diabetes mellitus on the solubility and nonenzymatic glucosylation of human skin collagen. *J Clin Invest* **67**:1630, 1981

81. Sabin JA: Bacterial infections in diabetes mellitus. *Br J Dermatol* **91**:481, 1974

82. Drachman RH et al: Studies on the effect of experimental nonketotic diabetes mellitus on antibacterial defense. *J Exp Med* **124**:227, 1966

83. Sommerville DA, Lancaster-Smith M: The aerobic cutaneous microflora of diabetic subjects. *Br J Dermatol* **89**:395, 1973

84. Parker F, Short JM: Xanthomatosis associated with hyperlipoproteinemia. *J Invest Dermatol* **55**:71, 1970

85. Faris IB, Lassen NA: Increased vascular resistance in vasodilated skin an indicator of diabetic microangiopathy? *Cardiovasc Res* **16**:607, 1982

86. Melin H: An atropic circumscribed skin lesion in the lower extremities of diabetics. *Acta Med Scand [Suppl]* **423**:1, 1964

87. Binkley GW: Dermopathy in the diabetic syndrome. *Arch Dermatol* **92**:625, 1965

88. Kurwa A et al: Concurrence of bullous atrophic skin lesions in diabetes mellitus. *Arch Dermatol* **103**:670, 1971

89. Bauer M, Levan NE: Diabetic dermangiopathy. *Br J Dermatol* **83**:528, 1970

90. Lithner F: Lesions of the legs in diabetics. *Arch Med Scand [Suppl]* **589**:1, 1976

91. Rocca FF: Pereyra E: Phlyctenar lesions in the feet of diabetic patients. *Diabetes* **12**:220, 1963

92. Bernstein JE et al: Bullous eruptions of diabetes mellitus. *Arch Dermatol* **115**:324, 1979

93. Bernstein JE et al: Reduced threshold to suction-induced blister formation in insulin dependent diabetics. *J Am Acad Dermatol* **8**:790, 1983

94. Braverman IM: Ultrastructural features of aging in the skin of normal adults and juvenile diabetics. *Clin Res* **28**:247A, 1980

95. Fleischmajor R, Lara JV: Scleredema adultorum: a histochemical and biochemical study. *Arch Dermatol* **92**:643, 1965

96. Cohen BA et al: Scleredema adultorum of Buschke and diabetes mellitus. *Arch Dermatol* **101**:27, 1970

97. Rosenblum AL et al: Limited joint mobility in childhood diabetes indicates increased risk for microvascular disease. *N Engl J Med* **23**:191, 1981

98. Goodman JI: Diabetic anhydrosis. *Am J Med* **41**:831, 1966

99. Faerman I et al: Autonomic neuropathy in the skin: a histological study of the sympathetic nerve fibers in diabetic anhydrosis. *Diabetologica* **22**:96, 1982

100. Mueller SA, Winklemann RK: Necrobiosis lipoidica diabeticorum, a clinical and pathological investigation of 171 cases. *Arch Dermatol* **93**:272, 1966

101. Narva WM et al: Necrobiosis lipoidica diabeticorum: with apparently normal diabetic tolerance. *Arch Intern Med* **115**:718, 1965

102. Ullman S, Dahl MV: Necrobiosis lipoidica, an immunofluorescence study. *Arch Dermatol* **113**:1671, 1977

103. Statham B et al: A randomized double blind comparison of an aspirin-dipyridamole combination versus a placebo in the treatment of necrobiosis lipoidica. *Acta Derm Venereol (Stockh)* **61**:270, 1981

104. Karkavitsas K et al: Aspirin in the management of necrobiosis lipoidica. *Acta Derm Venereol (Stockh)* **62**:183, 1982

105. Williamson DM, Dykes RW: Carbohydrate metabolism in granuloma annulare. *J Invest Dermatol* **58**:400, 1972

106. Hiam S et al: Generalized granuloma annulare: relationship to diabetes mellitus as revealed in 8 cases. *Br J Dermatol* **83**:302, 1970

107. Dawber RPR: Vitiligo in mature-onset diabetes. *Br J Dermatol* **80**:275, 1968

108. Macaron C et al: Vitiligo and juvenile diabetes mellitus. *Arch Dermatol* **113**:1515, 1977

109. Poliak SC et al: Reactive perforating collagenosis associated with diabetes mellitus. *N Engl J Med* **306**:81, 1982

110. Zarate AR et al: Hyperkeratosis penetrans (HKP) a rare dermatological disease with high incidence in patients on hemodialysis. *Proceedings of the Dialysis Transplant Forum*, 1978, p 99

111. Mallinson CN et al: A glucagonoma syndrome. *Lancet* **2**:1, 1974

112. McGavran MH et al: A glucagon secreting α cell carcinoma of the pancreas. *N Engl J Med* **274**:1408, 1966

113. Binnick GN et al: The glucagoma syndrome. *Arch Dermatol* **113**:749, 1977

114. Sohier J et al: Rapid improvement of skin lesions in glucagonomas with intravenous somatostatin infusions. *Lancet* **1**:40, 1980

115. Goodenberger DM et al: Necrolytic migratory erythema without glucagonoma. *Arch Dermatol* **115**:1429, 1979

CHAPTER 174

SKIN CHANGES AND DISEASES IN PREGNANCY

Thomas J. Lawley

Cutaneous changes and eruptions during pregnancy are exceedingly common and in some cases a cause for substantial anxiety on the part of the prospective mother. These alterations may range from normal cutaneous changes which occur in almost all pregnancies, to common skin diseases that are not associated with pregnancy, to eruptions that appear to be specifically associated with pregnancy. Likewise the concerns of the patient may range from cosmetic appearance, to the chance of recurrence of the particular problem in a subsequent pregnancy, to its potential effects on the fetus in terms of morbidity and mortality. In this chapter the cutaneous changes that are specifically associated with pregnancy will be discussed.

Hormonal changes

Pregnancy is a time of great and complex changes in the physiology of a woman. Some of these changes are due to the de novo production of a variety of protein and steroid hormones by the fetoplacental unit as well as by the increased activity of the maternal pituitary, thyroid, and adrenal glands. The currently recognized hormones produced by the placenta include the protein hormones human chorionic gonadotropin (HCG), human placental lactogen (HPL) or human somatomammotropin, human chorionic thyrotropin, and human chorionic corticotropin, as well as the steroid hormones progesterone and estrogen [1,2]. A description of the chemistry, function, and metabolism of these hormones is beyond the scope of this chapter, but it should be kept in mind that the production and the serum levels of these hormones are dynamic. For instance HCG levels peak between the 10th and 12th weeks of gestation although they remain elevated throughout pregnancy. The levels of progesterone and estrogen rise throughout the first and second trimesters of pregnancy and plateau during the third trimester. The levels of these hormones are of diagnostic significance in certain obstetrical conditions and complications but their exact impact on cutaneous physiology as well as their influence on the immunology of the skin and the inflammatory response are essentially unknown.

Cutaneous changes commonly associated with pregnancy

While the influences that the individual hormones have on the skin are incompletely understood, it is thought that they are responsible, either primarily or secondarily, for many of the cutaneous changes that are normally seen during pregnancy.

Pigmentation. The nipples, areolae, and external genitalia become hyperpigmented during pregnancy. The linea alba becomes the pigmented linea nigra. Occasionally hyperpigmentation is noted in the axillae and the proximal medial portions of the thighs. The most noticeable pigmentary change during pregnancy is the development of a masklike hyperpigmentation of the face known as chloasma or melasma in over 50 percent of women [3]. This tendency is exacerbated by sun exposure in susceptible individuals and may also be exacerbated by birth control pills in nonpregnant women. Additionally, preexisting nevi or ephilids frequently darken during pregnancy. The degree of hyperpigmentation tends to be related to the skin type of the individual, with lightly complected individuals developing less intense pigmentation. In all of these instances there is usually partial, and at times complete, regression of the hyperpigmentation which occurs gradually following termination of pregnancy. The physiology of the hyperpigmentation appears to be related to the increased production of estrogens and perhaps to increased levels of progesterone or melanocyte-stimulating hormone.

Hair. Mild to moderate hirsutism is frequently seen during pregnancy. This is due to an increased number of hairs in the anagen phase. The hirsutism tends to resolve shortly after delivery or in some instances in the third trimester. Usually the hirsutism gradually and imperceptibly disappears but in a few instances the resulting telogen effluvium may be severe, resulting in significant hair loss from one to five months postpartum. In these instances regrowth, usually within one year, is the rule.

Connective tissue. The most common change is the development of striae distensae over the abdomen, hips, buttocks, and sometimes the breasts. Striae distensae occur in up to 90 percent of pregnant women [4]. The exact cause of striae is unknown although a combination of increased adrenal cortical activity associated with increased lateral stress on the connective tissue due to increased size of the various portions of the body are thought to be important. Striae distensae initially appear as pink to purple atrophic bands sometimes associated with mild pruritus. Following delivery they become pale and less apparent. There is no known effective treatment that will resolve striae distensae. Skin tags, sometimes known as molluscum fibrosum gravidarum, often appear on the lateral portions of the neck and axillae during pregnancy and may persist following delivery.

Vascular. Hyperemia is physiologic during pregnancy. This combined with a tendency toward vascular proliferation results in a number of common cutaneous changes during pregnancy. Up to two-thirds of women will develop palmar erythema and/or spider angiomas during pregnancy [5]. Vascular distention resulting in part from increased intraabdominal pressure is thought to be responsible for the edema and venous varicosities that commonly occur on the legs and feet. Hemorrhoids also occur for the same reasons. Vascular tumors such as glomus tumors or hemangiomas may appear or enlarge during pregnancy. The pregnancy tumor of the gingiva is a pyogenic granuloma that may appear in the second or third trimester and resolves shortly after delivery.

Well-defined dermatoses associated with pregnancy

A variety of cutaneous diseases have been reported to be associated with pregnancy (Table 174-1). Most of these "diseases" are poorly characterized both clinically and pathophysiologically. In a number of instances their very existence as disease entities is in doubt. Even with diseases that are reasonably well-defined clinically, there is dispute with regard to nomenclature. The section that follows is an attempt to describe the best known and most common of these diseases.

Herpes gestationis (see also Chap. 58)

Definition. Herpes gestationis is an extremely pruritic, recurrent, bullous dermatosis of pregnancy and the immediate postpartum period. Its name is a total misnomer since it is not known to be related to any viral infectious agent. Herpes gestationis is currently thought to be immunologically mediated.

History. Milton first used the term *herpes gestationis* in 1872 [6]. In 1973 Provost and Tomasi demonstrated that herpes gestationis is a distinct, immunologically mediated disease [7].

Clinical manifestations. Herpes gestationis is an extremely pruritic eruption that may occur at any time during pregnancy or immediately postpartum. The primary lesions of herpes gestationis are small papulovesicular lesions which are often grouped and frequently occur on a background of erythema and/or urticaria (Fig. 174-1). These lesions often develop into frank vesicles and in some instances into bullae (Fig. 174-1). As these lesions are extremely itchy, it is also common to see numerous crusts and excoriations. The eruption may be widespread but the most frequent areas of initial involvement are the abdomen, particularly the periumbilical area, and the extremities. The eruption frequently spreads to involve palms, soles, chest, and back. Mucous membrane lesions are rare.

The eruption may begin at any time during pregnancy.

Table 174-1 Dermatoses of pregnancy

Well-defined eruptions:
  Herpes gestationis
  Pruritic urticarial papules and plaques of pregnancy (PUPPP)
  Recurrent cholestasis of pregnancy
  Impetigo herpetiformis
Poorly defined eruptions:
  Prurigo gestationis (Besnier)
  Papular dermatitis of pregnancy (Spangler)
  Follicular eruption of pregnancy
  Autoimmune progesterone dermatitis

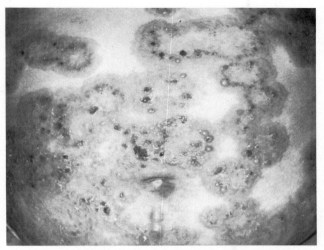

Fig. 174-1 Abdomen of a patient with herpes gestationis showing erythematous plaques with serpiginous borders. Numerous vesicles and crusts are visible in the plaques.

In a survey of 41 immunologically proven cases of herpes gestationis, 8 cases began in the first trimester, 15 cases in the second trimester, 12 in the third trimester, and 6 cases began immediately postpartum [8]. Flares of controlled disease are also especially prone to occur at or near the time of delivery. In this survey, 46 percent of patients had an exacerbation of disease shortly after delivery. Therefore 61 percent of patients in this study flared or developed herpes gestationis in the postpartum period.

Histopathology. An early lesion of herpes gestationis is characterized by edema of the dermal papillae with an infiltrate of eosinophils, lymphocytes, and a few neutrophils (Fig. 174-2). The epidermis may show spongiosis and focal necrosis of basal cells over the tips of the dermal papillae. There is also a superficial and middermal perivascular infiltrate of eosinophils, lymphocytes, and histiocytes. The accumulation of edema may result in the formation of teardrop-shaped dermal papillae. In older lesions frank vesicular or bullous changes may be present.

Immunology. DIRECT IMMUNOFLUORESCENCE. Direct immunofluorescence of perilesional or normal skin of herpes gestationis patients reveals the presence of the third component of complement (C3) deposited along the basement membrane zone in a linear band (Fig. 174-3). The diagnosis of herpes gestationis should not be made without this finding. Deposits of IgG are found in the same area in 40 to 50 percent of patients [8]. Other immunoreactants occasionally found at the basement membrane zone in herpes gestationis are IgM, IgA, Clq, C4, C5, and factor B. C3 deposits have persisted for more than one year after the cutaneous lesions have resolved. C3 deposits have also been found in the skin of infants of affected mothers.

INDIRECT IMMUNOFLUORESCENCE. Circulating IgG antibasement membrane zone antibodies are demonstrable in only about 25 percent of herpes gestationis patients, using conventional techniques. The use of a complement-binding technique will demonstrate the presence of "HG factor" in about 75 percent of patients. It has been clearly shown that the HG factor is simply an IgG anti-basement mem-

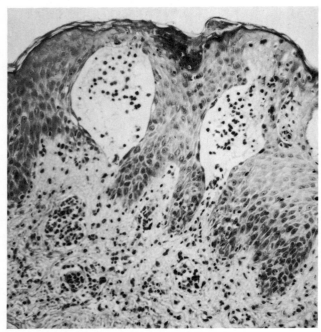

Fig. 174-2   Biopsy of an early lesion of herpes gestationis showing microvesicle formation. The inflammatory infiltrate consists of lymphocytes and eosinophils with an admixture of polymorphonuclear neutrophils.

brane zone antibody that is present in low titer [9,10]. C3 deposits are more readily detected than the IgG deposits because two IgG molecules activating complement will result in the deposition of 500 to 1000 C3 molecules at the site of activation, in this case the basement membrane zone. HG factor has also been detected in the cord blood of some infants born to affected mothers.

IMMUNOELECTRON MICROSCOPY. The deposits of C3 at the basement membrane zone have been shown to be located in the lamina lucida [11,12]. Immunoreactants may also be deposited along the dermal side of the basal cell plasma membrane [11].

Although the etiology of herpes gestationis is unknown and the exact pathophysiology is unclear, one plausible hypothesis is that circulating anti-basement membrane zone antibodies formed against some antigen present in pregnancy are bound in the skin, either primarily or through cross reaction, and activate complement, resulting in the influx of inflammatory cells.

Course. As mentioned above, herpes gestationis may begin any time during pregnancy but tends to remit spontaneously within a few weeks of delivery. There is a tendency for it to recur in subsequent pregnancies and it usually begins earlier in the subsequent pregnancy than it did in the first. Exacerbation of the disease may be induced by birth control pills.

One study has indicated an increased incidence of fetal morbidity and mortality in herpes gestationis [8], but another large study did not confirm this [13]. Rarely, infants may be born with cutaneous lesions of herpes gestationis which resolve over several weeks.

Treatment. The treatment of patients with herpes gestationis is aimed at relief of symptoms and amelioration of maternal cutaneous disease. Systemic corticosteroids are the most frequently used treatment and are usually quite effective in doses of 20 to 40 mg per day of prednisone in relieving pruritus and suppressing new lesion formation. The corticosteroid should be tapered as tolerated by the patient. In some instances it can be stopped even before delivery. In view of the frequency of postpartum disease exacerbations, the physician must be prepared to quickly reinstitute or increase therapy at the time of delivery. In very mild cases of herpes gestationis, vigorous use of topical corticosteroids will sometimes suffice. Infants born of mothers treated with prolonged courses of high-dose systemic corticosteroids should be monitored for adrenal insufficiency. It is not known whether maternal therapy decreases the risk of fetal morbidity or mortality.

Pruritic urticarial papules and plaques of pregnancy

Definition. Pruritic urticarial papules and plaques of pregnancy (PUPPP) is a common, intensely pruritic dermatosis which usually occurs late in the third trimester of pregnancy.

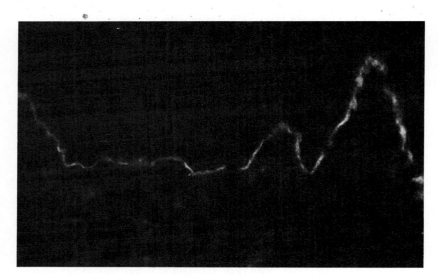

Fig. 174-3   Direct immunofluorescence of a biopsy of perilesional skin in a patient with herpes gestationis. C3 deposits are present at the basement membrane zone.

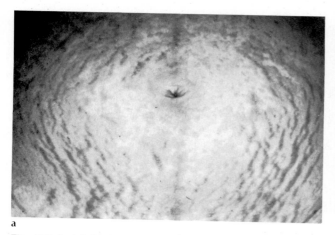

a

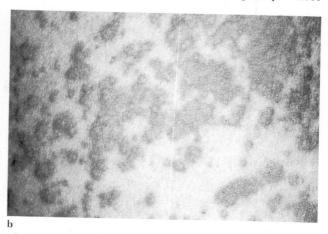

b

Fig. 174-4 **(a) Abdomen of a patient with PUPPP showing marked erythema and urticarial papules and plaques occurring within and outside of striae distensae. (b) Close-up view** of urticarial papules, both singly dispersed and confluent, in a patient with PUPPP.

History. The eruption was first described in detail and named by Lawley et al in 1979 [14]. Previously Nurse [15] and Bourne [16] reported similar eruptions that probably represented PUPPP. Nurse termed these eruptions *prurigo of pregnancy—late type* while Bourne used the term *toxemic rash of pregnancy.* Subsequently Holmes et al have used the name *polymorphous eruption of pregnancy* to describe this group of patients [13].

Clinical features. PUPPP is characterized by the onset of tiny (1- to 2-mm) erythematous papules on the abdomen, most often in the latter part of the third trimester of pregnancy [14,17–19]. The papules frequently begin in the striae distensae but soon coalesce to form large erythematous plaques centered around the umbilicus (Fig. 174-4). The lesions are extraordinarily itchy and patients frequently are unable to sleep at night. Curiously, despite the intense pruritus, excoriations are extremely unusual. The urticarial papules and plaques spread over the course of a few days to involve the buttocks and thighs. The morphology of the lesions as well as their anatomic progression is in general rather uniform from patient to patient. In some instances lesions will also occur on the arms, forearms, and legs. Lesions on or above the breasts are rare and lack of involvement of the face is a consistent feature. Close observation of the primary erythematous papules often reveals a surrounding narrow pale halo. Occasionally some papules are so edematous as to appear as papulovesicles.

Almost all reported cases have begun in the third trimester and most after the 35th week. The onset of PUPPP in the immediate postpartum period is rare. Although this eruption can occur in any pregnancy, it is most frequently seen in primigravidas. In our experience at NIH with 25 patients, 19 (76 percent) were primigravidas [17]. All of these patients had their onset of disease in the third trimester except one, who developed lesions in the immediate postpartum period. The average time of onset was the 36th week of gestation while the most frequent week of onset was the 39th. In all 25 patients the lesions began on the abdomen, and nearly one-half specifically indicated onset in their abdominal striae distensae.

Histopathology and immunofluorescence. The histopathologic findings in PUPPP are not specific. Biopsy of skin reveals a superficial and often middermal perivascular lymphohistiocytic infiltrate associated in some cases with a variable number of eosinophils and edema of the papillary dermis. Epidermal changes may include mild focal spongiosis and parakeratosis.

Direct immunofluorescence of lesional or perilesional skin is routinely negative.

Course. The natural history of PUPPP appears to be spontaneous resolution of most cases within a few days of delivery. Unlike herpes gestationis, postpartum onset or excaberation of PUPPP is exceptional. There does not appear to be a tendency for it to recur in subsequent pregnancies, nor does there appear to be an increased fetal morbidity or mortality associated with it [17,17a]. There is only one report of an infant being born with lesions. In our series of PUPPP patients, follow-up revealed that eight patients had subsequent pregnancies and none was complicated by PUPPP [17].

Differential diagnosis. In most instances the diagnosis of PUPPP is not difficult. The classic presentation is a primigravida late in the third trimester with an extraordinarily pruritic eruption of papules and plaques that began in the striae distensae on the abdomen and spread to involve the buttocks and thighs, sparing the upper chest and face. Herpes gestationis must be considered as a diagnostic possibility in some instances, although usually prominent vesicular and/or bullous lesions are found in these patients. Direct immunofluorescence of perilesional skin should be performed if herpes gestationis is considered.

It must also be kept in mind that all of the eruptions that occur in nonpregnant individuals may also occur in pregnancy and should not be confused with those dermatoses that are apparently pregnancy-specific. Thus erythema multiforme, drug eruptions, contact dermatitis, and insect bites can at times be confused with pregnancy-related dermatoses.

Treatment. Intense (5 to 6 times per day) therapy with potent topical corticosteroids seems to provide symptomatic relief in almost all cases. New lesions will usually stop appearing within 2 to 3 days and most patients can then begin to taper the frequency of applications. In many instances patients will be able to stop all therapy prior to delivery. Brief tapering courses of systemic corticosteroids will also provide relief. H_1 antihistamines do not appear to be effective.

Recurrent cholestasis of pregnancy (prurigo gravidarum)

Definition. Recurrent cholestasis of pregnancy, also known as prurigo gravidarum or benign recurrent intrahepatic cholestasis, is a hepatic condition usually occurring late in pregnancy and first manifested by severe generalized pruritus followed by the appearance of clinical jaundice. It is thought to be hormonally induced in susceptible individuals. Its incidence has been estimated at 0.02 to 2.4 percent of pregnancies [20].

History. Recurrent cholestasis of pregnancy was first separated from other causes of jaundice in pregnancy by Svanborg and Ohlsson [21].

Clinical features. Recurrent cholestasis of pregnancy has no primary cutaneous lesions although secondary excoriations may occur. The first symptom of recurrent cholestasis of pregnancy is pruritus. The severity may vary from moderate to severe and in the early stages may manifest itself only at night. Although often localized at first, the pruritus tends to become generalized [22]. The pruritus may precede the onset of clinical jaundice by up to four weeks although, rarely, it can be much longer. The patient also may complain of fatigue and anorexia. In some instances the patient may develop nausea and vomiting. Most cases occur during the third trimester although the onset has been reported as early as the first trimester. In fully developed cases numerous excoriations may be seen in conjunction with icterus. The patient may complain of right quadrant fullness or tenderness as well as dark urine and light-colored stools.

Course. The pruritus associated with recurrent cholestasis of pregnancy usually remits within a few days after delivery. There is a tendency for recurrent cholestasis of pregnancy to recur in subsequent pregnancies, and there have been reports of several members of families being affected, suggesting a genetic predisposition in some instances [23]. There have also been documented instances where patients who had developed recurrent cholestasis of pregnancy also developed cholestatic jaundice while taking synthetic estrogens and progestational agents for contraception [23]. It is not entirely clear whether estrogen or progesterone is the primary inciting agent and it may be that they work synergistically. Also the precise pathophysiology of the cholestasis is unknown. Finally, there have been patients who have been diagnosed as having recurrent cholestasis of pregnancy who did not develop clinical jaundice.

There appears to be an increased incidence of prematurity and low birth weights in the offspring of patients with recurrent cholestasis of pregnancy. In addition, post-partum hemorrhage is also more likely in these women. The incidence of untoward events seems to be highest in patients with both jaundice and pruritus [24].

Treatment. Attempts should be made to control pruritus with bland emollients and topical antipruritic regimens. In many instances these will provide adequate relief to the patient. The addition of antihistamines is at times of some benefit. Therapy with cholestyramine may occasionally be effective [25].

Impetigo herpetiformis

Definition. Impetigo herpetiformis is a form of pustular psoriasis which occurs during pregnancy and may be life threatening. It is exceedingly rare and only approximately 100 cases have been reported. This disease is not restricted to pregnancy and has been reported to occur in nonpregnant females as well as in males [26].

History. This disorder was first reported in 1872 by Hebra in five pregnant women, four of whom died [27].

Clinical manifestations. Impetigo herpetiformis tends to occur in the third trimester of pregnancy, although cases have been reported as early as the first trimester. Many of the affected women have had no personal or family history of psoriasis. Cases recurring in subsequent pregnancies have been reported.

The earliest lesions are erythematous patches occuring in the groin, axillae, and anterior and posterior neck [28]. At their margins these erythematous patches are studded with tiny superficial pustules. The lesions expand by peripheral extension, with new pustules occurring at the leading edges, while the old pustules at the interior of the expanding lesions break down, resulting in crusting or in some cases impetiginization. Pruritus is unusual in impetigo herpetiformis. Large areas of the body may be affected eventually and in flexural areas the lesions may become vegetative. In some cases mucous membranes may be affected and subungual pustules can cause onycholysis.

Most patients also have constitutional signs and symptoms, the most common being fever and chills accompanied at times by nausea, vomiting, and diarrhea. In the past, delirium, convulsions, and tetany secondary to hypocalcemia were often reported, but these complications as well as bacterial sepsis are infrequently seen in the modern era.

Histology. The histopathology of impetigo herpetiformis is the same as that of pustular psoriasis. The characteristic finding in an early lesion is the presence of collections of polymorphonuclear neutrophils in spongiotic foci in the epidermis, known as spongiform pustules of Kogoj. In mature lesions, the spongiform pustules become quite large and may assume a subcorneal location. Parakeratosis and elongation of rete ridges are also often found.

Laboratory results. Elevated white blood cell counts and sedimentation rates are quite common in impetigo herpetiformis. When these occur in the presence of fever, infection must be ruled out. The unopened pustules are sterile, but the skin may become secondarily infected. Decreased serum calcium and decreased serum albumin are sometimes found.

Course. The disease tends to remit promptly after delivery but may recur in subsequent pregnancies [29]. There may be an increased risk of fetal morbidity and mortality associated with placental insufficiency.

Treatment. Systemic corticosteroids are the treatment of choice in impetigo herpetiformis, with prednisone in doses of up to 60 mg per day being necessary at times to control the eruption [29–32]. Once under control, the prednisone can be tapered judiciously but there is a risk of sudden exacerbation of disease if tapered too rapidly.

Patients should be monitored for systemic and cutaneous infections and treated with appropriate antibiotics when indicated. Serum calcium and albumin levels should also be followed and replacement therapy undertaken if levels become too low.

Poorly defined eruptions associated with pregnancy

Prurigo gestationis (Besnier)

Prurigo gestationis is a pruritic dermatosis which may occur any time in the fourth to ninth month of gestation, but has peak incidence between the 20th and 34th weeks of pregnancy. It is characterized by the occurrence of small papules, most of which are excoriated, on the proximal limbs and upper trunk. In some instances the limb lesions tend to be distributed on extensor surfaces. Although Costello estimated a 2 percent incidence of prurigo gestationis in otherwise normal pregnancies, this is clearly a large overestimation [33]. Nurse [15] has suggested an incidence of 0.5 percent, but this too is probably much too high since 25 percent of Nurse's series of patients probably had PUPPP.

The eruption tends to resolve quickly after delivery although postinflammatory hyperpigmentation may persist for some time. Therapy with topical corticosteroids is apparently helpful. It is uncommon for prurigo gestationis to recur in subsequent pregnancies and there is no known increased incidence of fetal morbidity and mortality associated with this disease.

Papular dermatitis of pregnancy

Papular dermatitis of pregnancy is a rare, controversial eruption described by Spangler et al in 1962 [34]. The very existence of this disease is in doubt owing to the paucity of subsequent reports of well-described cases. Spangler estimated the incidence to be 1 case in 2400 pregnancies, but this is surely a vast overestimation.

Clinical manifestations. As described by Spangler, papular dermatitis of pregnancy is a pruritic eruption that may begin at any time during pregnancy. It is characterized by the appearance of small erythematous papules usually 3 to 5 mm in diameter which are often surmounted by a 1- to 2-mm central papule or central crust. Spangler indicated that the lesions were excoriated so rapidly that it was extremely rare to find an intact papule. The distribution of the lesions was generalized with no predilection for any area.

Histology. Spangler did not report biopsies of any of his cases. A biopsy of an unexcoriated papule in a case reported by Michaud et al showed hyperkeratosis, spongiosis, exocytosis, elongation of the rete ridges, and a perivascular infiltrate of lymphocytes in the papillary dermis [35]. Direct immunofluorescence for deposits of IgG, IgA, IgM, and C3 was negative.

Laboratory results. Patients with papular dermatitis of pregnancy have markedly elevated levels of urinary chorionic gonadotropin. Some patients also have low levels of urinary estriol [36] and plasma hydrocortisone. The half-life of plasma hydrocortisone is also decreased for the group as a whole.

Treatment. Therapy with systemic corticosteroids is reported to be effective in controlling the eruption [4,20]. At times doses of up to 100 mg of prednisone per day are necessary. Diethylstilbestrol, once recommended by Spangler and Emerson [36], should not be used due to the increased risk of vaginal carcinoma of offspring born to mothers treated with this agent. Spangler himself later [37] withdrew this therapeutic recommendation.

Course. The disease has been reported to recur in subsequent pregnancies. Spangler reported a 27 percent incidence of fetal death in untreated cases, while there was no fetal loss in treated cases. A recent careful reevaluation of these data has demonstrated a 12 percent incidence of fetal loss in patients with papular dermatitis of pregnancy [3]. The previously reported higher incidence was caused by the inclusion of fetal wastage in pregnancies in which there was no cutaneous eruption. Several of these mothers would almost surely be classified as habitual aborters today.

Miscellaneous disorders

Six patients with an eruption termed *pruritic folliculitis of pregnancy* were recently described by Zoberman and Farmer [38]. The onset of their eruption ranged from the fourth to the ninth month of gestation and their lesions consisted of 3- to 5-mm excoriated, erythematous papules. The lesions were generalized in five patients and confined to the extremities and abdomen in one. The striking feature of the histopathology of five of these cases was the presence of folliculitis with the hair follicles showing intraluminal pustule formation. The skin biopsy of one patient did not reveal folliculitis but only a mild perivascular infiltrate in the upper dermis and parakerotosis at the edges of the acrotrichium. Direct immunofluorescence was negative in all four patients tested. Two patients reported similar eruptions in previous pregnancies. All of the offspring born of these pregnancies were healthy. Of the five patients available for follow-up, two had the eruption resolve at delivery, two had it resolve one month after delivery, and in one patient it resolved spontaneously within a week of onset.

An eruption termed *autoimmune progesterone dermatitis of pregnancy* has been reported in one patient [39]. The eruption was characterized by the appearance of papules and pustules on the extensor surfaces of the thighs, arms, forearms, hands, and buttocks. The eruption began early in pregnancy and the patient experienced a spontaneous abortion in the third month. The patient reported a similar eruption associated with a previous pregnancy that also terminated in a spontaneous abortion in the second month. The eruption was exacerbated by an oral contraceptive. Intradermal skin tests with aqueous progesterone produced delayed-hypersensitivity reactions whose histology was similar to that found in naturally occurring lesions. However, the patient did not develop any exacerbation of her skin lesions premenstrually, a time during which progesterone levels are elevated. The exact relation of progesterone to this eruption as well as the existence of autosensitivity to progesterone is unclear.

References

1. Jaffe RB: Endocrine physiology of normal pregnancy, in *Obstetrics and Gynecology,* edited by DN Danforth. Philadelphia, Harper & Row, 1982, p 342

2. Osathanondh R, Tulchinsky D: Placental polypeptide hormones, in *Maternal-Fetal Endocrinology,* edited by D Tulchinsky, KJ Ryan, Philadelphia, WB Saunders, 1980, p 17

3. Winton GB, Lewis CW: Dermatoses of pregnancy. *J Am Acad Dermatol* 6:977, 1982

4. Scoggins RB: Skin changes and diseases in pregnancy, in *Dermatology in General Medicine,* 2d ed, edited by TB Fitzpatrick et al. New York, McGraw-Hill, 1979, p 1363

5. Demis DJ: Skin conditions during pregnancy, in *Clinical Dermatology,* edited by DJ Demis et al. Hagerstown, MD, Harper & Row, 1980, 12:25, p 1

6. Milton JL: *The Pathology and Treatment of Diseases of the Skin.* London, Robert Hardwicke, 1872, p 205

7. Provost TT, Tomasi TB Jr: Evidence for complement activation via the alternate pathway in skin diseases: herpes gestationis, systemic lupus erythematosus and bullous pemphigoid. *J Clin Invest* 53:1779, 1973

8. Lawley TJ et al: Fetal and maternal risk factors in herpes gestationis. *Arch Dermatol* 114:552, 1978

9. Jordon RE et al: The immunopathology of herpes gestationis: immunofluorescent studies and characterization of "HG factor." *J Clin Invest* 57:1426, 1976

10. Katz SI et al: Herpes gestationis: immunopathology and characterization of the HG factor. *J Clin Invest* 57:1434, 1976

11. Yaoita H et al: Herpes gestationis: ultrastructure and ultrastructural localization of in vivo-bound complement: modified tissue preparation and processing for horseradish peroxidase staining of skin. *J Invest Dermatol* 66:383, 1976

12. Hönigsmann H et al: Herpes gestationis: fine structural pattern of immunoglobulin deposits in the skin in vivo. *J Invest Dermatol* 66:389, 1976

13. Holmes RC et al: A comparative study of toxic erythema of pregnancy and herpes gestationis. *Br J Dermatol* 106:499, 1982

14. Lawley TJ et al: Pruritic urticarial papules and plaques of pregnancy. *JAMA* 241:1696, 1979

15. Nurse DS: Prurigo of pregnancy. *Australas J Dermatol* 9:258, 1968

16. Bourne G: Toxemic rash of pregnancy. *Proc R Soc Med* 55:462, 1962

17. Yancey KB et al: Pruritic urticarial papules and plaques of pregnancy (PUPPP): clinical experience in 25 patients. *J Am Acad Dermatol,* 10:473, 1984

17a. Ulhin SR: Pruritic urticarial papules and plaques of pregnancy. *Arch Dermatol* 117:238, 1981

18. Ahmed AR, Kaplan R: Pruritic urticarial papules and plaques of pregnancy. *J Am Acad Dermatol* 4:679, 1981

19. Callen JP, Hanno R: Pruritic urticarial papules and plaques of pregnancy (PUPPP). A clinicopathologic study. *J Am Acad Dermatol* 5:401, 1981

20. Sasseville D et al: Dermatoses of pregnancy. *Int J Dermatol* 20:223, 1981

21. Svanborg A, Ohlsson S: Recurrent jaundice of pregnancy. *Am J Med* 27:40, 1959

22. Holzbach RT: Jaundice in pregnancy. *Am J Med* 61:367, 1976

23. DePagter AGF et al: Familial benign recurrent intrahepatic cholestasis. *Gastroenterology* 71:202, 1976

24. Johnston WG, Baskett TF: Obstetric cholestasis: a 14-year review. *Am J Obstet Gynecol* 133:299, 1979

25. Laatikainen T: Effect of cholestyramine and phenobarbital on pruritus and serum bile levels in cholestasis pf pregnancy. *Am J Obstet Gynecol* 132:501, 1978

26. Braverman IM: Pregnancy and the menstrual cycle, in *Skin Signs of Systemic Disease.* Philadelphia, WB Saunders, 1981, p 761

27. Hebra F von: On some affections of the skin occurring in pregnant and puerperal women. *Wien Med Wochenschr* 48:1197, 1872. Abstracted in *Lancet* 1:399, 1872

28. Baker H, Ryan TJ: Generalized pustular psoriasis: a clinical and epidemiological study of 104 cases. *Br J Dermatol* 80:771, 1968

29. Beveridge GW et al: Impetigo herpetiformis in two successive pregnancies. *Br J Dermatol* 78:106, 1966

30. Sauer G: Impetigo herpetiformis. *Arch Dermatol* 83:119, 1961

31. Oosterling RJ et al: Impetigo herpetiformis or generalized pustular psoriasis. *Arch Dermatol* 114:1527, 1978

32. Oumeish OY et al: Some aspects of impetigo herpetiformis. *Arch Dermatol* 118:103, 1982

33. Costello MJ: Eruptions of pregnancy. *NY State Med J* 41:849, 1941

34. Spangler AS et al: Papular dermatitis of pregnancy. *JAMA* 181:577, 1962

35. Michaud RM et al: Papular dermatitis of pregnancy. *Arch Dermatol* 118:1003, 1982

36. Spangler AS, Emerson K: Estrogen levels and estrogen therapy in papular dermatitis of pregnancy. *Am J Obstet Gynecol* 110:534, 1971

37. Spangler AS: Letter to the editor. *Am J Obstet Gynecol* 113:570, 1972

38. Zoberman E, Farmer E: Pruritic folliculitis of pregnancy. *Arch Dermatol* 112:1534, 1976

39. Bierman SM: Autoimmune progesterone dermatitis. *Arch Dermatol* 107:896, 1973

PART FIVE

DISORDERS DUE TO MICROBIAL AGENTS

Section 26

Bacterial Diseases with Cutaneous Involvement

CHAPTER 175

GENERAL CONSIDERATIONS OF BACTERIAL DISEASES

Arnold N. Weinberg and Morton N. Swartz

The patient with a fever and cutaneous lesions presents one of the most challenging and frequently rewarding problems in medicine (see Atlas 3). The question of a treatable etiology (bacterial, fungal, herpes virus) should always be raised initially. The physician must actively and thoughtfully consider these possibilities and seek confirmation by appropriate studies to insure early optimal antimicrobial therapy.

Bacterial infection involving the skin may manifest itself in either of two major forms: (1) as a primarily cutaneous process, or (2) as a secondary manifestation in some other organ. The cutaneous changes associated with infection are not always suppurative, but may present as a vasculitis or a hypersensitivity response (e.g., lesions in subacute bacterial endocarditis or erythema nodosum).

The importance of the skin as a mirror of systemic infection cannot be overemphasized, especially when classical clinical findings are distorted as in immunocompromised patients. The timely recognition of the cutaneous clues of bacteremia may provide the early warning to consider life-threatening infections due to organisms such as *Pseudomonas aeruginosa*, *Salmonella typhi*, *Staphylococcus aureus*, and *Neisseria meningitidis*.

Natural resistance of the skin

The normal skin of healthy individuals is highly resistant to invasion by the wide variety of bacteria to which it is constantly exposed. It is difficult to produce localized infections such as impetigo, furunculosis, or cellulitis in laboratory animals [1] or human volunteers [2] if the integument is intact. Pathogenic organisms such as *Streptococcus pyogenes* (group A streptococcus) and *S. aureus* produce characteristic lesions of cellulitis and furunculosis in the absence of any obvious impairment of host defenses via disruption of the intact integument, i.e., by alcohol sponging, insect bites, an abrasion, or the introduction of a foreign body. For example, Elek [3] demonstrated that the presence of a silk suture reduces by a factor of 10,000, in the case of *S. aureus,* the number of organisms needed to produce an abscess in the human skin. Treatment with immunosuppressive agents can predispose patients to infections by the same organisms or by others of much lower intrinsic pathogenicity. The basis for this enhanced susceptibility of the compromised host is not understood, but undoubtedly involves specific and non-specific factors such as immunocompetence, nutritional state, and integrity of the cutaneous barrier [4].

Bacteria are unable to penetrate the keratinized layers of normal skin and, when applied to the surface, rapidly decrease in number [2]. The nature and the relative importance of the factors thought to be involved in this local resistance to bacterial multiplication and to infection are not clear [5]. *The low pH* (approximately 5.5) *of the skin environment* has been suggested as one of these properties, but it does not appear to have an important role. Many virulent bacteria are capable of growing at pHs below that of normal skin. The presence of *natural antibacterial substances* in the sebaceous secretions may be a factor in bacterial elimination from the skin. Streptococci appear to be particularly sensitive, in vitro, to the unsaturated long-chain fatty acids of the skin lipids, but in controlled studies in humans *Strep. pyogenes* (gpA) grows equally well in high- or low-lipid-containing regions [2]. Areas such as the palms and soles, lacking in sebaceous glands, remain relatively free of streptococci as well. The role of *circulating immunoglobulins, cellular immunity,* and *delayed hypersensitivity* in the defense of the skin against certain organisms is under intense investigation, especially the relationship of the thymus to Langerhans and epidermal cells and their contribution to stimulation and function of T lymphocytes [6]. IgM has not been found in normal sweat and IgA, IgG, and IgD have been found only in minute amounts (0.01 percent of the level in serum). However, the greater frequency with which a specific cutaneous and mucous membrane mycotic infection, moniliasis, occurs in patients with severe combined immunodeficiency (e.g., Swiss type of congenital lymphopenic agammaglobulinemia) suggests a relationship. Experimental and clinical observations, summarized by Kligman et al [5], consistently support the importance of moisture content and the indigenous cutaneous microflora in limiting colonization of the skin by potential pathogens. The *relative dryness* of normal skin contributes to the marked limitation of growth of bacteria, especially gram-negative bacilli with their higher moisture requirements (*Escherichia coli, Pseudomonas, Proteus*). *Bacterial interference* (the suppressive effect of one bacterial strain or species on colonization by another) exerts a major influence on the overall complexion of the skin flora. Although this effect is somewhat difficult to define, its relevance, at least in the case of colonization of the nose and skin by *S. aureus,* appears clear [7]. Profound changes in these bacterial interactions may be effected by the use of antibiotics.

The summation of these factors allows certain bacterial species to successfully colonize the skin surface while others are rapidly excluded. The organisms that characteristically survive and multiply in various ecologic niches of the skin constitute the "normal cutaneous flora." An appreciation of the composition of this flora and the attributes of its major elements is important in understanding and treating many bacterial infections of the skin.

Normal cutaneous flora

The skin is sterile at birth and for only a very short period thereafter. For example, *S. aureus* colonization of the umbilicus occurs in about 25 percent of infants during the first day of life, and this figure steadily increases from day to day over the first week. Paradoxically, this colonization occurs as the pH of skin falls from 7.0 to 5.5.

As a common convention, members of the normal skin flora have been divided into two principal categories: "transient" and "resident." Organisms capable of multiplication, as well as survival, are classed as resident flora, and are predictably found as the dominant constituents in almost all skin areas. The transient flora has been considered as simply deposited on the skin from mucous membrane "fallout" or from the environment. This sharp distinction, although possibly reasonable, is limited by a paucity of available quantitative ecologic data, which are difficult to obtain due to sampling problems. Variations in numbers of organisms from site to site, or from time to time, on the skin surface may blur this distinction between transient and resident flora [8]. Certainly many organisms isolated from the skin cannot be assigned unequivocally to one or another class. In recent years the changing complexion of the nature of infecting agents in hospitalized patients has focused attention on so-called opportunistic pathogens. Some of these bacteria and fungi (e.g., *S. epidermidis* and *Rhizopus* spp.) are nonpathogenic members of the resident or transient skin flora and produce infections in debilitated or otherwise compromised hosts [4].

Variations with anatomic areas

As summarized by Marples [9] and Noble et al [10], the available evidence suggests considerable anatomic variation in the composition of the flora. For convenience, these areas may be divided into three locations: (1) the exposed regions such as the face, neck, and hands; (2) moister areas of the body, such as the axillae, perineum, and toe webs; and (3) the remainder, consisting of the upper arms, trunk, and legs. The exposed areas have a higher bacterial density, and *S. aureus* is found more frequently there than on the skin of the trunk and legs. Gram-negative bacilli more often colonize the moist axillary and groin niches than drier regions of the skin.

Components of the resident flora

Propionibacterium acnes. This is the prototype anaerobic diphtheroid, uniformly found in large numbers associated with the sebaceous follicles of the skin in moist areas. Its presence in particularly high numbers in the lesions of acne probably does not indicate a causative role but merely a consequence of physiologic and anatomic changes of the underlying disease. These organisms have considerable lipolytic activity, and the resulting release of free fatty acids in and about sebaceous glands may contribute to the inflammatory component in acne. On rare occasions *P. acnes* has been an "opportunistic" pathogen (e.g., prosthetic valve endocarditis). (See also Chap. 67.)

Aerobic diphtheroids. Several species of aerobic diphtheroids are part of the normal flora. They are regularly found in the axilla and the interdigital skin of the foot; their numbers reach maximum levels where the skin has a high moisture content. Two gross categories have been described: lipophilic (those whose growth is enhanced by the oleic acids in the sebum) and nonlipophilic diphtheroids. *Corynebacterium tenuis* causes the condition trichomycosis axillaris, characterized by yellow or orange nodules on axillary or pubic hair. Another diphtheroid, *Corynebacterium minutissimum*, is responsible for a superficial infection, erythrasma, occurring in the groin or axilla.

Staphylococcus epidermis. This organism is uniformly present on the normal skin, in contrast to *S. aureus*, which is found on the exposed skin of only 20 percent of individuals. The extensive occurrence of *S. epidermidis* in large numbers undoubtedly exerts a suppressive effect on colonization of the skin by other organisms. *S. epidermidis* is an important pathogen in prosthetic valve endocarditis and in infections about indwelling venous catheters, central nervous system shunts, and other "foreign bodies."

Micrococci and peptococci (anaerobic staphylococci). These cocci are constantly present, usually only in small numbers and unlike other staphylococci do not increase in numbers in dermatologic diseases.

Gram-negative bacilli. Gram-negative organisms are uncommon on normal human skin except about the moist intertriginous areas of the groins, axillae, and toe webs. The effect of moisture on the nature of the skin flora can be illustrated in the case of the bacterial composition of the forearm surface. Normally, this area is too dry to support the growth of gram-negative bacilli. However, when an area is occluded with a plastic wrap, the gram-negative flora increases and may account for approximately 10 percent of the total bacterial population. These bacteria include *E. coli*, *Proteus*, *Enterobacter*, *Alcaligenes*, and *Pseudomonas*. *Acinetobacter calcoaceticus* var. *anitratum* (*Herellea*) and var. *lwoffi* (*Mima*), organisms, which in recent years have been increasingly implicated in nosocomial infections (e.g., bacteremias secondary to infected indwelling venous catheters), are normally carried in the axillae and toe webs of 10 to 25 percent of individuals. None of the aforementioned gram-negative organisms is a predominant component of the skin flora, and their density is well below that of the aerobic gram-positive species.

Transient flora

Aerobic spore-forming organisms (*Bacillus* spp., etc.), streptococci of various groups, and *Neisseria* may be visitors for short periods of time on the skin surface. The gram-negative bacilli of the intertriginous areas can be found transiently in other areas.

Although coagulase-negative staphylococci (*S. epidermidis*) are found in large numbers (10^2 to 10^6 organisms per square centimeter of skin surface) in essentially 100 percent of the population, coagulase-positive staphylococci (*S. aureus*) are found on the normal skin of only a small percentage (20 percent) of individuals who do not work in hospitals. Their presence is associated with nasal or perineal carriage of the same phage type in the majority of these instances. The concept that the maintenance of the skin carrier state of *S. aureus* depends on continued seeding from these areas is supported by studies which have shown a considerable reduction in the numbers of *S. aureus* on the skin when antibiotics have been applied locally to the noses of staphylococcal carriers [11]. A number of orally administered antibiotics, including rifampin, have been shown to effectively eradicate *S. aureus* from chronic nasal carriers [12]. Among hemodialysis patients the colonization of skin overlying the vascular access site by *S. aureus* is closely related to nasal carriage of organisms of the same phage type [13]. In addition to its role as a superficial transient, *S. aureus* may also colonize deeper skin areas and become, for a period at least, part of the resident flora. The skin of the perineum may be such an area. Dermatitic skin is especially susceptible to colonization and secondary infection by *S. aureus*, and even healthy skin may be inhabited profusely in individuals with conditions like eczema [8]. A number of studies in recent years have documented a similar ecology for *Strep. pyogenes* (gpA). Higher rates of nasal and anal ring carriage have been associated with increasing numbers of isolates, as transients or pathogens, on the skin of the upper and lower extremities, respectively. However, the colonization of skin may occur primarily, followed by spread, via hands, to the anterior nasal vestibule [14,15].

Pathogenesis of bacterial infection of the skin

The host–bacteria relationship in infections of the skin, as in infectious disease in general, involves three major elements: (1) the pathogenic properties of the organism, (2) the portal of entry, and (3) the host defense and inflammatory response to microbial invasion of the anatomic region.

Pathogenicity of the microorganism

The disease-producing capacity of bacteria is determined to a large measure by (1) the invasive potential (often based on antiphagocytic surface components), and (2) the toxigenic properties of the organism. A few species of bacteria (e.g., pneumococcus) appear to owe their pathogenicity solely to their ability to multiply extensively and invade tissues while resisting phagocytosis. No definable extracellular products or toxins that might contribute to their invasiveness have been discovered. Conversely, a few species have toxigenic properties that account for the local lesion (*Corynebacterium diphtheriae*, *Bacillus anthracis*) or systemic manifestations (*Clostridium tetani*) of a local infection. In the case of *Clostridium perfringens*, elaboration of a variety of extracellular toxins and enzymes (alpha toxin or lecithinase, proteases, collagenases) appears to play an important role in the rapidly spreading histotoxic lesions and systemic manifestations of clostridial myonecrosis. Though it is useful to distinguish between these two major pathogenic mechanisms whenever possible, most bacterial infections result from invasive and toxigenic properties of the organism. Local invasiveness (dependent to a considerable extent on the antiphagocytic M protein of the bacterial cell envelope) is an important element in streptococcal pharyngitis, but the clinical features of scarlet fever result from the elaboration of the erythrogenic toxin. For most disease-producing bacteria, including *S.*

aureus suppurative lesions, understanding of the basis for pathogenicity is lacking. The increasing prevalence of serious infections in compromised hosts, due to "traditionally" nonpathogenic bacteria that include the resident skin flora, supports the concept that pathogenicity is the resultant of microorganism and host interactions.

Gram-negative bacteria (*E. coli, S. typhi, N. meningitidis, N. gonorrhoeae, Brucella melitensis,* and others) contain complex phospholipid-polysaccharide macromolecules (endotoxins) as an integral part of the bacterial cell envelope. Endotoxins, unlike exotoxins, are released only upon breakdown of the bacterial cell. Their toxicity appears to be linked principally to the lipid fraction, while their antigenic determinants reside with the polysaccharide component [16]. Although the biologic effects of endotoxin in experimental animals are numerous (shock, fever, gastrointestinal hemorrhages, leukopenia, abortion) and well studied, their role in the pathogenesis of bacterial diseases remains ill defined [17]. The ability of endotoxin to induce leukocyte-fibrin deposition in the Shwartzman phenomenon has been suggested as the mechanism for the development of the hemorrhagic necrotic skin lesions (without bacterial invasion) sometimes seen in the course of certain gram-negative bacteremias (see below).

Changing patterns of bacterial infections of the skin. In addition to the usual pathogens, a variety of "nonpathogenic" members of the cutaneous, intestinal, or respiratory tract flora are capable of producing acute disease in debilitated patients and in individuals with altered humoral or cellular defenses and with a variety of skin defects. A patient receiving immunosuppressive therapy, for example, may have an atypical streptococcal or staphylococcal lesion due to impairment of the normal inflammatory response, or an unusual organism may be causal. Pain can be the most prominent feature, and etiologic considerations should include, in addition to streptococci and staphylococci, members of the Enterobacteriaceae (*E. coli, Klebsiella-Enterobacter-Serratia, Proteus* spp.); a variety of nonfermentative gram-negative bacilli (*Pseudomonas, Aeromonas, Acinetobacter* spp., etc.); and the indigenous anaerobic flora (peptostreptococci, *Bacteroides* spp., *C. perfringens,* etc.) [4,18,19].

Portal of entry

In laboratory animal models the pathogenic potential of many microorganisms depends, to a considerable extent, on the route of administration. Similarly, the character of the cutaneous inflammatory response to certain bacteria will be influenced by how the organisms reached the involved area. Thus, the vascular wall is often the primary site of skin involvement during bacteremic infection; hemorrhage or thrombosis with infarction is the initial manifestation. This is followed somewhat later by the cellular reaction expected from direct inoculation of the bacteria into the skin. Local inflammation and suppuration commonly accompany direct bacterial invasion of the skin, and these may, in turn, give rise to systemic spread via the rich cutaneous vascular network. Certain bacteria can produce bacteremia or distant lesions without evoking an obvious inflammatory response at the portal of entry [e.g., *Yersinia pestis, Streptobacillus moniliformis* (rat-bite fever)] even in a nonimmunosuppressed host. Occasionally a devastat-

ing *Strep. pyogenes* septicemia has followed closely upon an innocuous pinprick or abrasion that has not induced a significant local lesion. Table 175-1 lists those bacterial species most frequently involved in pyogenic infections of the skin.

Specific features of host inflammatory response to cutaneous infection

Morphologic aspects. In view of the relatively few cell types present in the skin, it is surprising that such a variety of rather distinctive clinical responses to various bacterial infections has been catalogued. In most instances it is the anatomic site of the infection and the attendant inflammatory response pattern, rather than the specific pathogen, that provides the characteristic clinical picture. The following brief examples are expanded upon in Chap. 176.

IMPETIGO. The very superficial location of the infection, with vesicopustule formation just beneath the stratum corneum, is the specific clinical feature.

FOLLICULITIS. This represents a circumscribed infectious process which originates in the hair follicle and is defined by its anatomic features. It may be located superficially in the follicle or may extend more deeply to produce perifollicular inflammation.

FURUNCLE (BOIL). This infection either complicates an antecedent folliculitis or develops as a deep-seated nodule about a hair follicle. The distinctive pathologic change results from its relation to the hair follicle; thus it does not occur in glabrous areas such as the palms. The deep location and its containment by the relatively thick dermis prevent spontaneous early drainage to the surface, and contribute to the hard, nodular, painful character of the lesion.

CARBUNCLE. This is a larger, more deep-seated extension of a furuncle with infection spreading under and between fibrous tissue septums, forming a whole series of interconnected abscesses. Drainage occurs through a number of projecting necrotic points in the skin.

CELLULITIS. This is an acute, inflammatory process in the skin, particularly in the deeper subcutaneous tissues. Because of the subcutaneous location, the borders of the lesion are usually indistinct, in contrast to the sharply defined margin of erysipelas (see below).

Interplay of morphology and specific bacterial properties

Erysipelas. This is a superficial inflammatory process of the skin and subjacent lymphatics, characterized by marked edema of the dermis and extensive invasion of connective tissue usually, but not exclusively, caused by *Strep. pyogenes* (gpA). The rapid progression of the process and the prominence of edema of the affected skin relate to the involvement of superficial lymphatics and the biologic properties of the microorganisms.

Influence of hypersensitivity to bacterial antigens on inflammatory reaction in skin

Although the introduction of certain bacteria in large numbers into the skin will elicit a local inflammatory reaction, the character and extent of this response may be modified by various host factors (e.g., leukopenia). In the case of

Table 175-1 Bacteria involved in cutaneous infection*

I. Primary cutaneous inflammation
- A. Gram-positive bacteria
  1. *Staphylococcus aureus*
  2. Streptococci
     - a. Group A
     - b. Other than group A (groups B, C, D, G, particularly)
     - c. Anaerobic streptococci (peptostreptococci) alone or mixed infection
  3. *Bacillus anthracis*
  4. *Corynebacterium diphtheriae*
  5. Anaerobic diphtheroids *(Propionibacterium acnes)*
  6. Aerobic diphtheroids *(Corynebacterium minutissimum)*
  7. *Clostridium perfringens*
  8. *Erysipelothrix insidiosa* (erysipeloid)
  9. *Borrelia burgdorferi* (Lyme disease)
- B. Gram-negative bacteria
  1. *Francisella tularensis* (tularemia)
  2. *Pasteurella multocida* (infected animal bites)
  3. Enterobacteriaceae *(Escherichia coli, Klebsiella-Enterobacter)*
  4. Nonfermentative gram-negative bacilli *(Pseudomonas, Acinetobacter, Aeromonas)*
  5. *Malleomyces mallei* (glanders)
  6. *Bacteroides* spp.
  7. *Hemophilus influenzae*
  8. Halophyllic vibrios *(Vibrio parahemolyticus, V. vulnificus,* etc.)

II. Bacteremic spread to skin
- A. Gram-positive bacteria
  1. *Staphylococcus aureus*
  2. Group A streptococci
  3. In bacterial endocarditis (acute)
     - a. *Staphylococcus aureus*
     - b. Streptococci (group A, group D especially)
  4. *Listeria monocytogenes*
  5. Histotoxic clostridia
- B. Gram-negative bacteria
  1. *Neisseria meningitidis*
  2. *Neisseria gonorrhoeae*
  3. *Pseudomonas aeruginosa*
  4. *Salmonella typhi*
  5. *Brucella* spp.
  6. *Hemophilus influenzae*
  7. *Streptobacillus moniliformis*
  8. *Pseudomonas pseudomallei* (melioidosis)

III. Bacteremia or systemic manifestation from innocuous skin portal
- A. Gram-positive bacteria
  1. Group A streptococci
  2. *Staphylococcus aureus*
  3. *Bacillus anthracis* (rarely)
  4. *Clostridium tetani*
  5. *Leptospiriae interrogans* serotypes
- B. Gram-negative bacteria
  1. *Yersinia pestis* (plague)
  2. *Francisella tularensis*
  3. *Streptobacillus moniliformis* (rat-bite fever)
  4. *Brucella* spp.

* Exclusive of mycobacterial and treponemal infections.

skin infection due to *S. aureus*, the tendency to recur is often quite striking. Initial lesions are usually suppurative and localized, whereas subsequent infections, when due to the same antigenic strain, may have more prominent sur- rounding cellulitis. The immunologic response to *S. aureus* has been suggested as a factor in this altered inflammatory response [20].

Vasculitis as a cutaneous response to systemic infection

Inflammatory changes in and about small blood vessels in the skin may occur in a variety of bacteremic infections in the absence of obvious localization of bacteria at these sites. The macular, papular, nodular, and petechial lesions of chronic meningococcemia show such histologic changes. The lesions of erythema nodosum have a prominent element of vasculitis even though the initiating infection (e.g., streptococcal pharyngitis) is distant and has a suppurative character. The Osler nodes and petechiae of subacute bacterial endocarditis (SBE), due to viridans streptococci, probably provide the best examples of this association of small-vessel vasculitis with bacteremia. Histologically, these lesions are more suggestive of vasculitis than of emboli. The occasional development of such lesions in profusion, localized to the lower extremities, supports the concept of cutaneous vascular inflammation rather than embolization.

Shwartzman phenomenon in gram-negative bacteremia

The experimental production of a characteristic hemorrhagic necrotic reaction in the skin and in certain other organs (e.g., kidney) of the rabbit has been a subject of considerable interest for many years [21–23]. This interest has been heightened because of the gross similarity of these lesions to those that occur during the course of meningococcemia. The Shwartzman reaction is divided into two types: local and generalized. In the former, an initial cutaneous injection of endotoxin (or endotoxin-containing bacteria), followed in some hours by an intravenous injection, produces gross hemorrhage and necrosis at the original skin site. The initial (''preparatory'') skin injection and the second (''eliciting'' or ''provocative'') intravenous injection may consist of endotoxin from different bacterial sources. It has even been possible to elicit the reaction when the second injection has consisted of certain nonbacterial materials such as washed antigen-antibody precipitates. Following the preparatory injection, there is polymorphonuclear leukocyte ''cuffing'' about the small veins locally. The intravenous eliciting reaction produces peripheral vasoconstriction, particularly in the veins at the prepared skin site. Leukocyte-rich thrombi form, with ensuing occlusion of capillaries and small veins, producing necrosis of vessel walls and resulting hemorrhage. This form of response may represent a type of hypersensitivity to endotoxin which can be neutralized by homologous antiserum [24]. Results of treatment of gram-negative bacteremia with human antiserum to endotoxin (lipopolysaccharide core) have been encouraging in a limited clinical study [25].

The generalized Shwartzman reaction occurs in rabbits when both the preparatory and the eliciting injections have been given intravenously, approximately 24 h apart. The typical histologic lesion consists of fibrin deposition within capillaries. This is particularly striking in the kidney, where

Table 175-2 Bacterial infections involving the skin*

I. Primary pyodermas
   A. Impetigo—group A streptococci and *Staphylococcus aureus* (see Chap. 176)
      1. Impetigo contagiosa—primarily due to Group A streptococci
      2. Impetigo bullosa—primarily due to *S. aureus* of phage group II
   B. Folliculitis (see Chap. 65)
      1. Superficial
         a. Follicular impetigo (Bockhart's impetigo)—usually due to *S. aureus* but in conditions of lowered host resistance (corticosteroid and antibiotic therapy, etc.) may be due to a variety of opportunistic organisms (gram-negative coliform bacilli, particularly). The lesions consist of small globular pustules, each located about a hair.
         b. *Pseudomas aeruginosa*—associated with water exposure (see Chap. 177)
      2. Deep
         a. Sycosis barbae (usually *S. aureus*)
         b. Pyoderma faciale (usually *S. aureus*)
         c. Folliculitis decalvans—rare condition, producing a scarring type of alopecia, attributed to chronic infection with *S. aureus,* but this etiologic role is not clearly established
   C. Furuncles and carbuncles *(S. aureus)* (see Chap. 176)
   D. Paronychia—usually of bacterial origin due to *S. aureus* or group A streptococci; rarely, a chronic form of the disease is due to *Pseudomonas aeruginosa*
   E. Ecthyma—group A streptococci initially (see Chap. 176); may also be due to *Pseudomonas* (see Chap. 177)
   F. Erysipelas—group A streptococci (see Chap. 176)
   G. Cellulitis—group A streptococci, *S. aureus,* and, less commonly, a variety of other organisms, especially in compromised hosts (see Chap. 176)
   H. Lymphangitis—usually group A streptococci, but occasionally *S. aureus* and other organisms (see Chap. 176)
   I. Erythrasma—*Corynebacterium minutissimum* (see Chap. 176)
II. Secondary bacterial infections
   A. Complicating preexisting skin lesions, such as:
      1. Burns (see information in Chap. 122)
      2. Eczematous dermatitis, including exfoliative erythrodermas—*S. aureus* or group A streptococci (see Chap. 116)
      3. Chronic ulcers (varicose, traumatic—these are particularly liable to invasion by gram-negative organisms *[Escherichia coli, Proteus, Pseudomonas]* as well as by anaerobic streptococci, *Bacteroides* or *Clostridium perfringens* [either alone or as a "synergistic" infection])
      4. Dermatophytoses—usually a *S. aureus* or group A streptococcal infection
      5. Traumatic lesions (abrasions, infestations, insect bites, etc.)—*Pasteurella multocida, Corynebacterium diphtheriae, S. aureus,* gpA streptococcus
      6. Vesicular or bullous eruptions (varicella, pemphigus, etc.)—*S. aureus,* gpA streptococcus
   B. Distinctive dermatologic clinical entities
      1. Secondary folliculitis
         a. Acne conglobata—*Propionibacterium acnes, S. aureus, Proteus,* and other coliforms (particularly after antibiotic therapy)
         b. Hidradenitis suppurativa—*S. aureus, Proteus* and other coliforms, peptostreptococci, *Bacteroides*
      2. Infectious eczematous dermatitis (usually *S. aureus;* occasionally group A streptococci)
      3. Intertrigo (*S. aureus;* occasionally group A streptococci)
      4. Pilonidal and sebaceous cysts—in addition to coliform organisms, particularly in infected pilonidal cysts, there is a high incidence of anaerobic streptococci and *Bacteroides* spp.
      5. Infectious gangrene
         a. Clostridial gas gangrene (see Chap. 176)
         b. Streptococcal gangrene (see Chap. 176)
         c. Fusospirochetal gangrene—a synergistic necrotizing infection due to anaerobic organisms such as *Fusobacteria, Bacteroides, Peptostreptococcus,* and usually associated with malnutrition, agranulocytosis, and other debilitating diseases or local injury
         d. Gangrenous balanitis and perineal phlegmon—an acute cellulitis with gangrene located in the area of the genitalia, usually due to group A streptococci, enteric bacteria *(E. coli, Klebsiella, Proteus)* or anaerobes, and most commonly seen in diabetic patients

characteristic bilateral renal cortical necrosis occurs. Alterations in levels of fibrinogen and other clotting factors have been found, and it appears that intravascular coagulation is the initiating event in this generalized phenomenon. Polymorphonuclear leukocytes appear to have a central role in the pathogenesis of this process, since prior induction of leukopenia with nitrogen mustard will prevent both the local and generalized reaction. Circulating fibrin monomers and inhibition of fibrinolysis appear to be essential since their absence will obviate the reaction [22]. It is possible to substitute cortisone for the preparatory injection of endotoxin in the production of the generalized Shwartzman reaction. This role of corticosteroids in the experimental Shwartzman reaction has raised questions regarding the use of these agents as adjuncts in the treatment of shock in acute meningococcemia and other gram-negative bacteremias.

It is tempting to attribute the hemorrhagic necrotic lesions that occur in meningococcemia (and other gram-negative bacteremias) to this phenomenon. However, as yet, clear proof of the occurrence of a true Shwartzman reaction in the course of disease in humans is lacking.

Table 175-2   Bacterial infections involving the skin (Continued)

6. Necrotizing ulcers
   a. Pyoderma gangrenosum (see Chap. 168)—many organisms (*S. aureus,* microaerophilic streptococci, *Proteus, E. coli,* and *Pseudomonas*) may be found secondarily in such lesions, which complicate ulcerative colitis. Proof of a primary bacterial cause of the lesions of pyoderma gangrenosa is lacking. In fact, cultures of early lesions are usually sterile.
      (1) Pyoderma vegetans—a variant of pyoderma gangrenosa with hypertrophic lesions
   b. Progressive bacterial synergistic gangrene (Meleney) (see Chap. 176)—peptostreptococci or microaerophilic streptococci plus a second organism *(S. aureus, Proteus)*
   c. Synergistic necrotizing cellulitis—mixed anaerobic and facultative infection often involving skin and muscle in addition to fascia, seen in diabetic and debilitated elderly patients
   d. Decubitus ulcer (*S. aureus,* coliforms, *Pseudomonas, Bacteroides, Clostridium perfringens*) (see Chap. 172)
   e. Tropical ulcer
   f. Phagedenic ulcers—small, circumscribed ulcers with black necrotic centers and erythematous areolas complicating preexisting lesions (e.g., varicella); lesions look like end stage of ecthyma; usually *S. aureus* or *Pseudomonas* cultured from lesions
7. Necrotizing fasciitis due to gpA streptococci or to mixed anaerobic and facultative bacteria (*Bacteroides,* peptostreptococci, coliforms, etc. (see Chap. 176)

III. Cutaneous involvement in systemic bacterial infections (exclusive of venereal diseases and mycobacterial infections)
   A. Bacteremia (see II in Table 175-1)
   B. Cutaneous lesions without direct microbial involvement of the skin
      1. Bacterial endocarditis (see Chap. 176)
         a. Subacute (usually viridans streptococci or other non-group A streptococci): petechiae, Osler's nodes, Janeway lesions
         b. Acute (most commonly *S. aureus*)
      2. Streptococcosis (group A)
         a. Scarlet fever (see Chap. 176)
         b. Purpura fulminans (see Chap. 176)
      3. Chronic meningococcemia—a variety of sterile macular, papular, nodular, and hemorrhagic lesions occurring intermittently (see Chap. 177)
      4. *S. aureus* including toxin-mediated syndromes—"scalded-skin" (see Chap. 176) and "toxic shock" (see Chap. 176)
      5. Erythema nodosum (see Chap. 99) associated with a variety of drugs and infections; among the latter are those due to group A streptococci, *Mycobacterium tuberculosis, M. leprae, Yersinia enterocolitica, Legionella pneumophila*
      6. Bacterids
      7. Purpura

IV. Infections due to unusual organisms (see Chap. 178)
   A. Cutaneous diphtheria
   B. Listeriosis *(Listeria monocytogenes)*
   C. Bartonellosis (Carrion's disease)—due to *Bartonella bacilliformis*
   D. Animal-borne or associated diseases
      1. *Bacillus anthracis*—cutaneous anthrax (malignant pustule)
      2. Pasteurelloses and related organisms
         a. *Francisella tularensis* (tularemia)
         b. *Pasteurella multocida*—produces infection at site of animal (usually cat) bite
         c. *Yersinia pestis* (plague)
      3. *Brucella (abortus, suis,* or *melitensis*)—skin lesions are rare in this systemic disease
      4. Rat-bite fever
         a. *Streptobacillus moniliformis* (Haverhill fever)
         b. *Spirillum minus* (sodoku)—exanthem with primarily erythematous macules, some papules, and nodules
      5. Erysipeloid *(Erysipelothrix insidiosa)*
      6. Leptospirosis, including Weil's disease—*Leptospira interrogans* serotypes
      7. Glanders *(Pseudomonas mallei)*
      8. Meliodosis *(Pseudomonas pseudomallei)*

* The localization and morphologic changes seen often constitute the initial clue in arriving at a specific etiologic cause of the skin lesion(s).

Classification of bacterial infections of the skin

The introduction, over the past three decades, of a variety of specific antibiotic and chemotherapeutic agents has effected rather striking changes in the management of bacterial infections. Indeed, with the availability of these drugs, the focus of attention has been on the determination of the specific bacterial cause so that the proper choice of antibacterial agent can be made. This has rendered unnecessary, and even obsolete, descriptions of some of the dermatologic entities whose status depended on imprecise morphologic criteria rather than on etiologic considerations. Consequently, from the pragmatic (therapeutic) viewpoint the approach has been to consider and classify these infections by bacterial causation, e.g., infections due to gram-positive organisms and infections due to gram-negative organisms. Although the foregoing classification is helpful from the therapeutic point of view, there is still need for a system of categorizing bacterial infections of the skin so that the dermatologic picture will provide the basis for consideration of the most likely bacterial etiologies. To this end, the classification of skin infections as (1)

Table 175-3   Selection of antibiotics

Infecting agent	Drug of choice[a,b] First	Alternatives
Gram-positive cocci:		
Staphylococcus aureus or *epidermidis*		
Non-penicillinase-producing	Penicillin G or V[c]	Cephalosporin,[d] erythromycin,[e] vancomycin,[f] clindamycin[g]
Penicillinase-producing	Penicillinase-resistant penicillin[h]	Same as above for non-penicillinase-producing strains
Methicillin-resistant[i]	Vancomycin (± rifampin or gentamicin)[j]	Trimethoprim-sulfamethoxazole[k]
Streptococci		
Groupable (e.g., group A)	Penicillin G or V	Erythromycin, clindamycin, cephalosporin
Group D (enterococcus)[l] (systemic infection)	Penicillin G (or ampicillin) + gentamicin	Vancomycin + gentamicin
Nongroupable (viridans streptococci, etc.)	Penicillin G	Cephalosporin, erythromycin, vancomycin
Anaerobic	Penicillin G	Clindamycin, erythromycin, chloramphenicol,[m] cephalosporin
Gram-positive bacilli:		
Bacillus anthracis (anthrax)	Penicillin G	A tetracycline,[n] erythromycin
Borrelia burgdorferi (Lyme disease spirochete)	Tetracycline	Penicillin G
Clostridium perfringens (gas gangrene)	Penicillin G	Chloramphenicol, metronidazole,[o] clindamycin
Corynebacterium, including *C. diphtheriae*	Erythromycin	Pencillin G
Erysipelothrix insidiosa	Penicillin G	Erythromcyin
Leptospira spp.	A tetracycline	Pencillin G
Listeria monocytogenes	Ampicillin ± penicillin G or gentamicin	Chloramphenicol, tetracycline, erythromycin
Gram-negative cocci:		
Neisseria gonorrhoeae (gonococcus)	Penicillin G followed by tetracycline	Ampicillin, spectinomycin, cefoxitin,[p] or cefotaxime
Neisseria meningitidis (meningococcus)	Penicillin G	Chloramphenicol, a sulfonamide (only if sulfonamide susceptibility of organism is proved by appropriate quantitative methods), cefuroxime, cefotaxime
Gram-negative bacilli:		
Aeromonas hydrophilia	Gentamicin	Chloramphenicol
Escherichia coli (systemic infection)	Aminoglycoside[q]	Ampicillin, cephalosporin, broad-spectrum penicillin;[r] trimethoprim-sulfamethoxazole, chloramphenicol
Francisella tularensis (tularemia)	Streptomycin[s]	Chloramphenicol, a tetracycline
Hemophilus influenzae (systemic infection)	Chloramphenicol ± ampicillin initially	Cefuroxime, cefotaxime, trimethoprim-sulfamethoxazole
Klebsiella pneumoniae	Aminoglycoside	Cephalosporin, chloramphenicol, trimethoprim-sulfamethoxazole
Klebsiella rhinoscleromatis	Tetracycline followed by trimethoprim-sulfamethoxazole	Streptomycin
Legionella pneumophila	Erythromycin	Add rifampin

primary infections (pyodermas), (2) secondary infections, and (3) cutaneous manifestations of systemic bacterial disease seems warranted. Primary bacterial infections are produced by the invasion of ostensibly normal skin by a *single* species of pathogenic bacteria. In such infections there is usually no doubt as to the primary etiologic role of the specific agent in the pathogenesis of the lesion.

Treatment aimed at the bacterial pathogen almost universally results in cure of the lesion. Impetigo, erysipelas, and furunculosis are familiar examples of primary cutaneous infections. Contrastingly, secondary infections develop in areas of already damaged skin. Although the bacteria present did not produce the underlying skin disorder, their proliferation and subsequent invasion of surrounding areas

Table 175-3   Selection of antibiotics (Continued)

Infecting agent	Drug of choice[a,b]	
	First	**Alternatives**
Pasteurella multocida	Penicillin G	A tetracycline, cephalosporin
Proteus mirabilis	Ampicillin	Cephalosporin, gentamicin, trimethoprim-sulfamethoxazole
Proteus—other species	Gentamicin	Cefotaxime, broad-spectrum penicillin, chloramphenicol, trimethoprim-sulfamethoxazole
Pseudomonas aeruginosa (systemic infection)	Tobramycin ± broad-spectrum penicillin[f]	Ceftazidime; amikacin
Pseudomonas mallei (glanders)	Sulfadiazine	Chloramphenicol + streptomycin
Pseudomonas pseudomallei (melioidosis)	Trimethoprim-sulfamethoxazole + cephalosporin	Chloramphenicol, a tetracycline
Salmonella typhi	Chloramphenicol	Ampicillin, trimethoprim-sulfamethoxazole
Salmonella spp.	Ampicillin (amoxicillin)	Chloramphenicol, trimethoprim-sulfamethoxazole
Streptobacillus moniliformis (rat-bite fever)	Penicillin G ± streptomycin	Cephalosporin, a tetracycline
Yersinia pestis	Streptomycin	Chloramphenicol, a tetracycline

[a] Drug sensitivity testing of bacterial isolates should be performed coincident with the initial choice of an antibacterial agent. Dosages of drugs of choice are given in Chaps. 176 to 178.

[b] Not all drugs listed are approved by the Food and Drug Administration for treatment of that infection.

[c] When used in low doses, hypersensitivity reactions (5 to 8 percent) are the major problem. Massive therapy (10 to 50 million units daily) for life-threatening gram-positive coccal infections or sepsis due to certain gram-negative bacilli may produce toxicity from hyperkalemia, central nervous system irritation (seizures), and Coombs-positive hemolytic anemia.

[d] A first-generation cephalosporin is preferred. Gram-negative organisms resistant to first-generation cephalosporins *may* be sensitive to second- or third-generation agents. Hypersensitivity reactions, reversible neutropenia, and, very rarely, nephrotoxicity at high doses are chief toxic problems.

[e] Side effects are uncommon except for gastrointestinal disturbances. Rarely, hypersensitivity reactions (fever or rash) and hepatotoxicity occur (with the oral erythromycin estolate preparation). Administered orally or intravenously.

[f] Causes phlebitis and fever, hypersensitivity reactions; and in the presence of renal failure or excessive dosage, ototoxicity. Should be given slowly (~1 h) i.v. to avoid histamine-like systemic effects.

[g] Gastrointestinal irritation (diarrhea) is common; rare pseudomembranous colitis and granulocytopenia.

[h] The semisynthetic penicillins (oxacillin, nafcillin, cloxacillin, dicloxacillin) cross-react with penicillin G in evoking hypersensitivity reactions.

[i] Methicillin-resistant strains are *always* cephalosporin-resistant too.

[j] Nephrotoxic and ototoxic, especially in the aged and in the presence of preexisting renal disease. Administered under the closest medical supervision with monitoring of renal (blood levels), auditory, and vestibular function.

[k] Trimethoprim-sulfamethoxazole may cause bone marrow toxicity due to either, or to combined drug effects. Hypersensitivity reactions, gastrointestinal upset, hepatitis, and anemias (megaloblastic and hemolytic) are occasionally encountered.

[l] For endocarditis or other serious infection.

[m] Chloramphenicol may depress bone marrow function, one or all elements being affected. This drug should be given only under close medical surveillance; check differential smear and white blood count look for a rise in serum iron levels as an indication of toxicity. Associated with the "gray syndrome" when administered without appropriate reduction in dosage to premature infants or neonates.

[n] All the tetracyclines are potent antianabolic drugs, gastrointestinal irritants; potentially hepatotoxic when doses exceed 2.0 g daily parenterally; discolor and alter organogenesis of primary and secondary teeth; photosensitizing. Outdated preparations may be nephrotoxic. All tetracyclines stimulate changes in the indigenous microflora favoring emergence of infections due to yeast and resistant staphylococci and gram-negative bacilli.

[o] Bactericidal for *Bacteroides* and *Clostridia* but variably effective in anaerobic and microaerophilic streptococcal infections.

[p] Second- (cefoxitin, cefamandol) and third- (cefotaxime, ceftazidime, moxalactam, cefaperazone) generation cephalosporins are occasionally drugs of choice, guided by sensitivity testing, for selected infections. In addition to cross-hypersensitivity with first-generation agents, they may cause superinfections due to their broad-spectrum activity and some may cause bleeding complications.

[q] Gentamicin has been used as a prototype aminoglycoside. In many situations tobramycin (or amikacin) may be selected, depending on the in vitro susceptibility of the organism involved or on known nosocomial patterns of aminoglycoside resistance.

[r] Includes carbenicillin, ticarcillin, piperacillin, azlocillin, mezlocillin, which have similar toxic and hypersensitivity effects to penicillin. In addition they may cause bleeding, due to platelet dysfunction, as well as add a significant sodium load.

[s] Vestibular toxicity, especially in the aged and those with renal failure, as well as hypersensitivity reactions.

[t] Tobramycin (or gentamicin) and broad-spectrum penicillins should not be mixed in the same intravenous infusion. Tobramycin has toxicity identical to gentamicin.

may aggravate and prolong the disease. Such secondary infection may occur when the skin has been broken or bruised, primarily involved with mycotic or viral infections, or altered by sensitivity reactions or medications. In contrast to the primary infections, the secondary infections often show a *mixture* of organisms on culture, and not infrequently it is impossible to determine which plays the major role. Pathogenic organisms such as *S. aureus* and *Strep. pyogenes* (gpA), generally considered transients on the skin, can colonize such lesions and sometimes produce active secondary infection. The appearance of these lesions is not characteristic, in comparison to the primary pyodermas, but is largely dependent on the nature of the underlying skin condition. The result of antibacterial treatment is much less clear-cut, since it has no effect on the underlying process.

Table 175-2 presents an outline of infections involving the skin in a classification based upon the appearance of the lesions. In this outline, specific entities that will be discussed elsewhere in detail are described only by the appropriate chapter reference, and the more common bacterial etiologic agents are noted. This table refers exclusively to bacterial infections.

Diagnostic strategies

Direct examination of aspirates and biopsies

Identification of bacteria from skin lesions may provide important information as to the cause of cutaneous infections, whether primary or secondary to systemic processes. The presence of "normal skin flora" can confuse interpretation of these cultures. All too often, the finding of a potential pathogen such as *S. aureus* or *Ps. aeruginosa* is equated with the presence of disease. It is important to recall that damaged skin (operative incisions, exudative dermatoses, etc.) provides a medium for proliferation of certain bacteria. Only by correlating the clinical appearance of the lesion (local suppuration, cellulitis, etc.) with the bacteriologic data can one reach the proper decision concerning the presence of a bacterial disease. Examination of a Gram-stained smear of material from a suspected skin infection can guide decisions on early antibiotic therapy before a cultural diagnosis is made. For these reasons, bacteriologic investigation is an important part of the initial evaluation of patients with skin lesions, and includes: (1) appropriate sampling, (2) interpretation of Gram-stained smears, and (3) use of selective growth media for culturing.

Gram's stain provides a very rapid method for examining a sample for number and type of bacteria, as well as for the character of the inflammatory exudate. Skin contaminants are usually recognized by being present in low concentration, often clumped in characteristic microcolonies (growth in skin crypts) and usually not associated with polymorphonuclear leukocytes. Obtaining an appropriate specimen for microscopic study and culture requires care to avoid contamination. Results of needle aspiration of superficial erysipelas lesions has been generally unrewarding. Our personal experience is in accord with published results for sampling *deeper* cellulitic lesions and bullae associated with acute infections [26]. Findings on needle aspiration are often positive, and an immediate useful guide to therapy. If sterile saline is injected into a lesion that initially yields no aspirate, bacteriostatic agent-free solutions should be employed. In circumstances where no data are available from needle aspiration, a surgical biopsy may yield information that is life-saving. Local lesions of the skin and subcutaneous tissues in immunocompromised patients should always be biopsied if aspiration fails to define a pathogen [4]. Encouraging results have been reported in a series of patients with suspected necrotizing fasciitis who had biopsies done to confirm the diagnosis early in the course of this devastating infection [27].

Methods of culture of skin material

All samples for culture should be planted routinely on blood agar and inoculated into a tube of thioglycollate (anaerobic) broth. Additional media should be used as indicated by clinical findings and evaluation of the Gram-stained smear and frozen sections if a biopsy is done. If cutaneous diphtheria is a consideration, Loeffler or tellurite agar should be inoculated. When gram-negative rod infection is suspected, an EMB or MacConkey plate is used; a chocolate agar or Thayer-Martin plate incubated in a CO_2 atmosphere is indicated for suspected meningococcal or gonococcal lesions; a blood agar plate incubated in an oxygen-free atmosphere should be used if anaerobic streptococci, clostridia, or *Bacteroides* is suspected. When the skin lesions are thought to be part of a generalized infection, blood cultures should also be obtained prior to institution of antibiotic therapy.

Other diagnostic procedures

Fluorescent antibody. The practical use of this procedure in bacterial diseases of the skin is of limited availability at this time. Spirochetes can be demonstrated (by the direct or indirect techniques) in chancres. *N. gonorrhoeae*, *Actinomyces israelii*, *Legionella* spp., and mycobacterial isolates have been identified by this rapid method. At the present time these techniques are still in the stage of experimental development for identifying the etiologic agent in most infections of the skin.

Other immunologic methods. A variety of serologic tests may be helpful in the diagnosis of bacterial infections of the skin, particularly in those where the cutaneous manifestations are secondary to systemic disease (e.g., "rose spots" of typhoid fever). In general, these tests have proved of value in confirming a diagnosis that has already been made by direct bacteriologic identification of the offending organism (e.g., *Salmonella* agglutination, *Brucella* agglutination, agglutination reaction for tularemia, leptospirosis complement fixation or agglutination tests). As in any serologic test, a fourfold or greater rise in titer during the course of the illness is considered significant.

Antibiotic therapy

The selection of the appropriate antibiotic should be made initially on the basis of the appearance of the skin lesion, the characteristics of any systemic illness, and a Gram-stained smear of material from a lesion if available to sample. Culture results and sensitivity testing of the isolated pathogen(s) are usually available within 48 h (Table 175-3).

Dosage: methods of administration; excretion

Primary cutaneous infections of mild to moderate severity can be treated with local measures, topical drugs, oral antibiotics, or by a combination of these methods. Extensive infections of the skin, with or without systemic manifestations, should be vigorously treated with parenteral antibiotics in adequate dosage.

A number of factors must be considered in administering antibiotics: oral treatment may be limited by absorption and gastrointestinal disturbances; hypotension, severe thrombopenia, and extensive skin disease can prohibit the intramuscular route; the proper drug selected may be suitable for administration only by a specific route. Caution must be exercised in administering intramuscular medications to avoid sterile or infected abscesses. When the intravenous route is used, a needle or "heparin-lock" is preferred. Percutaneous catheters should be changed frequently (every 2 to 3 days) and all line-skin sites kept clean with a topical antibiotic ointment and sterile dressing that is changed daily.

The excretory pattern of a given antibiotic should always be considered in order to avoid toxic accumulation in the face of specific organ malfunction (e.g., use of aminoglycosides or vancomycin in the presence of renal impairment).

Toxicity

The toxicity of antibiotics should be considered on an individual basis, but some problems are applicable to all antibiotics. Hypersensitivity reactions are relatively common and may include skin rashes, fever, or more severe manifestations such as acute anaphylaxis or exfoliative erythrodermas. The penicillins and sulfonamides are particularly likely to produce these problems. Questions regarding previous drug allergy should be asked whenever any antibiotic is to be administered. All antibiotics alter the relative kinds and absolute numbers of the indigenous flora, and superinfection may result from their use, especially with broad-spectrum agents like the cephalosporins. Gastrointestinal disturbances and oral mucous membrane lesions are the major nonspecific types of problems encountered with alteration of the flora, although changes also occur on burn surfaces and other lesions. There are numerous other untoward reactions (renal, hematologic, hepatic, nervous system) to antibiotics which may represent acceptable risks if the reasons for use of these drugs are compelling (see footnotes, Table 175-3). The responsibility is the physician's, however, to be aware of the usual and unusual manifestations of toxicity of any of the antibiotics used, and to be alert to possible novel effects in individual patients.

Antibiotic resistance due to "R" factors

Transferable resistance to multiple antibiotics has emerged as a widespread problem. Extrachromosomal genetic elements (R plasmids) in bacteria are the basis for such resistance [28]. Prolonged antibiotic therapy, especially in a closed environment like a hospital, may select R-factor-carrying members of the indigenous flora (e.g., in the gastrointestinal tract), which may subsequently transfer this property to a recently acquired organism. In this way, antibiotic resistance to chloramphenicol, tetracycline, and kanamycin conferred by a plasmid in *E. coli* can be transferred during mating to a *Klebsiella* or *Salmonella* strain. As a consequence, organisms with greater intrinsic pathogenicity can become antibiotic-resistant as well. This phenomenon and its practical consequences have been verified in a number of studies [29].

R plasmids (R factors) have been found in most pathogenic gram-negative bacteria, including *E. coli, Klebsiella, Proteus, Pseudomonas, Salmonella,* and *Shigella.* They are responsible also for high-level resistance to the penicillins (penicillinase plasmids) and cephalosporins.

In recent years R-factor-associated antibiotic resistance has been identified in group A and group D streptococci

as well as *Hemophilus influenzae* and *N. gonorrhoeae,* all important pathogens in skin as well as systemic infection.

Topical antibacterial agents

Topical antibacterial agents frequently have been used to prevent, as well as to suppress, bacterial growth in burns and other open lesions. Their greatest usefulness has been when employed along with strict aseptic techniques in preventing percutaneous line sepsis. These agents are capable of inhibiting the local flora, but, as is true of all antibiotics, they have a relatively limited spectrum of activity, which favors the emergence of bacterial resistance during treatment. In addition, topical drugs may precipitate contact dermatitis and can be absorbed to toxic levels. Furthermore, there has been very little evidence that they add a great deal therapeutically [30]. An exception to this is the result, in burn patients, of the use of sulfamylon acetate or 0.5% silver nitrate solutions. However, even with these broad-spectrum agents, resistant species, such as *Clostridium perfringens, Klebsiella,* and *Enterobacter,* may emerge as the dominant potential pathogen of the local flora.

Among the most useful topical antibacterial agents are acetic acid (1 to 5%) for *Pseudomonas* nail and toe web infections, and bacitracin (500 units per milliliter or gram) for selected superficial *S. aureus* and streptococcal lesions. Neomycin (0.5% ointment) and gentamicin (0.17% cream) may be useful in selected patients when mixed gram-negative bacteria require local suppression. A number of broad-spectrum antiseptics are also available for topical use, combining antibacterial with nonirritating properties. Povidone-iodine (Betadine) is effective against most gram-positive and gram-negative bacteria, but does not persist in the skin to provide a residual action. Chlorhexidine gluconate (4% solution) is an antiseptic which combines broad antibacterial properties with prolonged action due to local accumulation. An alcoholic preparation is especially effective, is not appreciably absorbed into the blood, and generally is not irritating to the skin [31,32]. These broad-spectrum antiseptics can be used prophylactically or to treat local wounds and superficially infected dermatoses.

The topical therapy of burns is discussed in Chap. 122.

References

1. Johnson JE II et al: Studies on the pathogenesis of staphylococcal infection. I. The effect of repeated skin infection. *J Exp Med* **113**:235, 1961
2. Leyden JJ et al: Experimental infections with group A streptococci in humans. *J Invest Dermatol* **75**:196, 1980
3. Elek SD: Experimental staphylococcal infections in the skin of man. *Ann NY Acad Sci* **65**:85, 1956
4. Wolfson JS et al: Dermatologic manifestations of infection in the compromised host. *Annu Rev Med* **34**:205, 1983
5. Kligman AM et al: Bacteriology. *J Invest Dermatol* **67**:160, 1976
6. Sauder DN: Immunology of the epidermis: changing perspectives (editorial). *J Invest Dermatol* **81**:185, 1983
7. Shinefield HR et al: Bacterial interference, in *Skin Bacteria and Their Role in Infection,* edited by HI Maibach, G Hildick-Smith. New York, McGraw-Hill, 1965, chap 17
8. Bibel DJ et al: Skin flora maps: a tool in the study of cutaneous ecology. *J Invest Dermatol* **67**:265, 1976
9. Marples MJ: *The Ecology of the Human Skin.* Springfield, IL, Charles C Thomas, 1965

10. Noble WC et al: *Microbiology of Human Skin*. London, WB Saunders, 1974
11. Varga DT, White A: Suppression of nasal, skin, and aerial staphylococci by nasal application of methicillin. *J Clin Invest* **40**:2209, 1961
12. McAnally TP et al: Effect of rifampin and bacitracin on nasal carriers of *Staphylococcus aureus*. *Antimicrob Agents Chemother* **25**:422, 1984
13. Goldblum SE et al: Nasal and cutaneous flora among hemodialysis patients and personnel: quantitative and qualitative characterization and patterns of staphylococcal carriage, *Am J Kidney Dis* **2**:281, 1982
14. Taplin D et al: Prevalence of streptococcal pyoderma in relation to climate and hygiene. *Lancet* **1**:501, 1973
15. Richman DD et al: Scarlet fever and group A streptococcal surgical wound infection traced to an anal carrier. *J Pediatr* **90**:387, 1977
16. Elin RJ et al: Biology of endotoxin. *Annu Rev Med* **27**:127, 1976
17. Wolff SM: Biological effects of bacterial endotoxins in man. *J Infect Dis* **128**:S259, 1973
18. Bornstein DL et al: Anaerobic infections—review of current experience. *Medicine (Baltimore)* **43**:207, 1964
19. Fields BN et al: The so-called "paracolon" bacteria: a bacteriologic and clinical reappraisal. *Am J Med* **42**:89, 1967
20. Cluff LE: The inflammatory response of skin to bacterial invasion, in *Skin Bacteria and Their Role in Infection*, edited by HI Maibach, G Hildick-Smith. New York, McGraw-Hill, 1965, p 95
21. Thomas L: The effects of cortisone on bacterial infection and intoxication, in *Effects of ACTH and Cortisone upon Infection and Resistance*, edited by G Shwartzman. New York, Columbia Univ Press, 1953, Chap 12
22. Lipinski B et al: The organ distribution of ^{125}I-fibrin in the generalized Shwartzman reaction and its relation to leucocytes. *Br J Haematol* **28**:221, 1974
23. Horn RG: Evidence for participation of granulocytes in the pathogenesis of the generalized Shwartzman reaction: a review. *J Infect Dis* **128**:S134, 1973
24. Braude AI et al: Treatment and prevention of intravascular coagulation with antiserum to endotoxin. *J Infect Dis* **128**:S157, 1973
25. Ziegler EJ et al: Treatment of gram-negative bacteremia and shock with human antiserum to a mutant *Escherichia coli*. *N Engl J Med* **307**:1225, 1982
26. Uman SJ et al: Needle aspiration in the diagnosis of soft tissue infections. *Arch Intern Med* **135**:959, 1975
27. Stamenkovic I et al: Early recognition of potentially fatal necrotizing fasciitis. The use of frozen-section biopsy. *N Engl J Med* **310**:1689, 1984
28. Elwell LP et al: Plasmid-mediated factors associated with virulence of bacteria to animals. *Annu Rev Microbiol* **34**:465, 1980
29. Falkow S: *Infectious Multiple Drug Resistance*. London, Pion, 1975
30. Editorial: Topical antibiotics. *Br Med J* **1**:1494, 1977
31. Editorial: Chlorhexidine and other antiseptics. *Med Lett Drug Ther* **18**:85, 1976
32. Lilly HA et al: Detergents compared with each other and with antiseptics as skin "degerming" agents. *J Hyg (Lond)* **82**:89, 1979

Bibliography

Abramowicz M (ed): The choice of antimicrobial drugs. *The Medical Letter*. New York, 1984

Davis BD et al (eds): *Microbiology*, 3d ed. New York, Harper & Row, Hoebner Medical Division, 1980

Goodman LS, Gilman A: *The Pharmacologic Basis of Therapeutics*, 6th ed. New York, Macmillan, 1980

Mandell GL et al (eds): *Principles and Practice of Infectious Diseases*, 2nd ed. New York, John Wiley & Sons, 1985

Rosebury T: *Microorganisms Indigenous to Man*. New York, McGraw-Hill, 1962

CHAPTER 176

INFECTIONS DUE TO GRAM-POSITIVE BACTERIA

Morton N. Swartz and Arnold N. Weinberg

The majority of the primary pyodermas are due to infection with either group A streptococci or *Staphylococcus aureus*. A variety of clinical pictures may be presented by infections due to these organisms, depending on local anatomic considerations and on host factors.

Streptococcal skin infections

General features

Bacteriology and pathogenic aspects. In view of the association of specific groups of streptococci with certain types of infections and postinfectious sequelae [1], an understanding of the various categories of streptococci has practical value. The presence of many varieties of streptococci as commensals on mucous membranes, in the intestinal tract, and occasionally on the skin makes difficult the assessment of the significance of their isolation from the skin. Although essentially all group A streptococcal strains are beta hemolytic, not all streptococci producing beta hemolysis belong to group A. The Lancefield classification of streptococcal groups (A–T) is based on the C carbohydrate antigens of the cell wall. Since serologic grouping of streptococci is not generally available, a reasonably accurate presumptive test for group A streptococci is necessary. Bacitracin disk ("Taxos S") sensitivity has been widely used; group A organisms are, almost without exception, susceptible to the low concentration of bacitracin contained in the disk, whereas streptococci of other groups are often resistant.

The primary invasive streptococcal pyodermas are due almost exclusively to group A streptococci. The invasive potential of group A streptococci is usually considerably greater than that of other streptococci. Nonsuppurative postinfectious complications have been limited to those produced by group A organisms. Thus, group A streptococcal infections merit antibiotic treatment and eradication.

The presence of streptococci of other groups than A in skin lesions may represent either surface colonization or actual secondary infection in preexisting dermatoses. Group C and group G streptococci have occasionally been implicated in impetiginous lesions, secondarily infected dermatitis, wound infections with lymphangitis, and even in erysipelas and cellulitis. Streptococci of groups B and D have been isolated from infections of skin lesions secondary to ischemia or venous stasis, and have particularly involved the perineal area and operative wound sites. As with most secondary infections, those due to group B and group D streptococci are frequently mixed infections with enteric bacteria or *S. aureus*.

The hallmarks of group A streptococcal infection are profuse edema, rapid spread through tissue planes, and the relatively thin character of the exudative response. Infection may spread via the lymphatic or hematogenous routes and result in a fulminant clinical course.

Epidemiology of group A streptococcal infections. Group A streptococci are usually spread by transfer of organisms from an infected person or carrier through close personal contact. The major source of such spread is from patients with infections in the upper respiratory tract. A variety of skin lesions and puerperal sepsis also may be the source of intrahospital spread of infection. Group A streptococci introduced into the operating room in the form of a minor skin infection, or even through perianal carriage by a surgeon or anesthetist, may be responsible for an epidemic of streptococcal wound infections. In the past, milk- and food-borne epidemics occurred, but they no longer represent a major problem.

Although viable streptococci are found on a variety of articles in the immediate surroundings of a carrier or infected individual, the major factor in spread is not the articles in the contaminated environment but rather proximity to an individual disseminating the organisms. Since many patients with group A streptococcal skin infections harbor the same organism in their pharynxes, they are, for both reasons, potential sources for spread of infection in a hospital. Particular care must be taken to prevent spread of infection by isolating such patients until antibiotic therapy has rendered them noncontagious.

Despite the salutory effects of penicillin on morbidity and mortality, the overall incidence of streptococcal disease has probably not decreased. Localized epidemics have continued to appear periodically. During such outbreaks, the carrier and infection rates in the community increase. Carriers then may enter the hospital environment. In this way, streptococci can be introduced into surgical incisions and lacerations, and initiate infection. Operative infections, because of the rapidity with which they progress, may be more severe and dramatic than those caused by staphylococci.

After recovery (without antibiotic treatment) from streptococcal pharyngitis some individuals may carry the organism for prolonged periods. The carrier state may also occur in the absence of overt antecedent infection. Ten to forty percent of school children carry group A streptococci in the throat.

Delayed nonsuppurative sequelae. The incidence of invasive complications (lymphangitis, suppurative lymphadenitis, bacteremia) of streptococcal infections of the skin has decreased in the antibiotic era. Besides these pyogenic complications, a variety of nonsuppurative complications (acute rheumatic fever, acute glomerulonephritis, erythema nodosum) may follow group A streptococcal infections. Distinct differences exist between acute rheumatic fever and acute glomerulonephritis in the site of the antecedent infection, the length of the latent period, and the streptococcal serotypes involved [2,3]. Acute rheumatic fever may be a complication of group A streptococcal pharyngitis or tonsillitis, but it does not occur following streptococcal skin infections. In contrast, acute nephritis may follow infection of either the skin or the upper respiratory tract. The latent period between streptococcal pharyngitis and the onset of rheumatic fever is 2 to 3 weeks; whereas the latent period for pharyngitis-associated nephritis is about 10 days. A longer latent period, about 3 weeks, is characteristic of acute nephritis associated with streptococcal pyoderma. While there is as yet no strong evidence of an association between infection with any specific group A serotypes and the subsequent development of rheumatic fever, several serotypes (particularly type 5) have been implicated in a few outbreaks of streptococcal sore throat complicated by this sequela [4]. However, there is a clear relationship between infection with certain serotypes and the subsequent occurrence of nephritis—the so-called nephritogenic serotypes. Type 12 is the classic serotype responsible for pharyngitis-associated acute nephritis, but other serotypes such as 1, 4, 25, and 49 have been implicated. The pyoderma-associated nephritogenic strains generally belong to different serotypes: types 2, 49, 55, 57, and 60 [3,5]. The skin (rather than the pharynx) is the principal site of antecedent streptococcal infection causing nephritis, and impetigo is now the most common form of such predisposing skin infections. Major epidemics of pyoderma-associated nephritis have been observed in communities, and multiple cases of overt and subclinical nephritis have occurred within families. The frequency of acute glomerulonephritis following infection with a known nephritogenic strain is 10 to 15 percent; the frequency of rheumatic fever following an unrecognized or inadequately treated pharyngeal infection by any serotype of group A streptococcus is 2 to 3 percent or less. The distinction between nephritogenic strains of streptococci and other strains of streptococci that might be associated with rheumatic fever can be seen in studies from Trinidad, a hyperendemic area for pyoderma-associated nephritis. There, the streptococcal serotypes causing outbreaks of nephritis differed from the serotypes associated with sporadically occurring cases of acute rheumatic fever in the same population [4].

Antibody response and immunity. The immune response to group A streptococcal infection depends to a large measure on the site of infection. Following streptococcal pharyngitis, specific antibodies develop to many of the extracellular enzymes of the streptococci. Eighty-five percent of patients with acute rheumatic fever and a proven preceding streptococcal infection will have an elevated or increasing antistreptolysin O (ASO) titer. The serologic demonstration of an antecedent streptococcal infection in this situation can be increased to virtually 100 percent by the simultaneous testing for several other antibodies (antihyaluronidase, anti-DNase B). Antibodies to extracellular products, with the exception of antibody to the erythrogenic toxin of scarlet fever, appear to have no effect on the manifestations of illness. Streptococcal immunity is type-specific (but not group-specific), long-lasting, and depends on the production of bactericidal antibodies to the specific M proteins of the 63 different serotypes of group A organisms. Although recurrent pharyngeal infections due to the same serotype are most unusual, repeated clinical infections due to different types are not uncommon. Early treatment of streptococcal upper respiratory tract disease with antibiotics may suppress the appearance of type-specific antibody (and immunity) as well as the development of antibody to the extracellular products of the organism.

In contrast to pharyngeal infections, the ASO response with streptococcal skin infections or pyoderma-associated nephritis is feeble. To define the latter serologically, anti-DNase B (or antihyaluronidase) titers are much more reliable. Although pyoderma strains of streptococci produce M proteins and although type-specific antibody may develop in patients with pyoderma-associated nephritis, the frequency of production of such antibodies and their role in protection against reinfection are unclear. While pharyngeal reinfection with the same streptococcal serotype is probably unusual, some evidence suggests that the same serotype can be associated with repeated episodes of pyoderma.

Specific diseases due to group A (and other) streptococci

Superficial pyoderma. Streptococcal pyodermas include all types of superficial streptococcal skin infections except erysipelas, i.e., impetigo, ecthyma, and secondary infections of preexisting skin lesions (e.g., insect bites, abrasions, eczema).

Impetigo (contagiosa). DEFINITION. Impetigo is a primary, initially vesicular, later crusted superficial infection of the skin. It is commonly due to group A streptococci. *S. aureus* is the etiology of bullous impetigo (see "Staphylococcal Skin Infections" below).

EPIDEMIOLOGY AND BACTERIOLOGY. Impetigo is a highly communicable infection predominantly of preschool-age children. Its peak seasonal incidence is in the late summer and early fall. Group A streptococcus is the single most common isolate from impetigo in the United States [6]. Mixtures of streptococci and *S. aureus* are isolated from about half the patients with nonbullous impetigo, but the role of *S. aureus* here appears to be a subsidiary one. In nonbullous impetigo *S. aureus* alone is isolated from less than 10 percent of cases. In other parts of the world staphylococcal impetigo has been reported as more frequent [7]. Non-group A (groups B, C, and G) streptococci may be responsible for rare cases of impetigo; group B streptococci are associated with impetigo in the newborn. Whereas many different serotypes of group A streptococci may cause pharyngitis, a limited number of newly described types predominates in impetigo (types 49, 52, 53, 55-57, 59, and 61).

PATHOGENESIS AND PATHOLOGY. Group A streptococci appear on normal skin of children about 10 days prior to the development of impetigo and they are not recovered from the nose and throat of the same patients until 14 to 20 days after skin acquisition of the organism. Streptococci are recovered from the respiratory tract of about 30 percent of children with skin lesions but there is no clinical evidence of streptococcal pharyngitis. Thus, the sequence of spread in a given patient is from normal skin to lesions and eventually to respiratory tract [8]. In contrast, the sequence of spread of *S. aureus* (in cases of impetigo in which it is the only organism isolated) is from nose to normal skin (about 11 days later) to skin lesions (after another 11 days).

Following acquisition of a streptococcal strain on normal skin from another family member or close contact (whose skin was already colonized or contained a pyoderma), minor traumas (insect bites, abrasions) predispose to the appearance of infected lesions.

The inflammatory process of impetigo is superficial, with a unilocular vesicopustule located between the stratum corneum above and the stratum granulosum below. This is usually situated near the opening of a hair follicle. Organisms, as well as leukocytes and epithelial cell debris, fill the vesicle.

CLINICAL MANIFESTATIONS
History. Crowding, poor hygiene, and neglected minor skin trauma contribute to the spread of streptococcal impetigo in families. Minor outbreaks have also occurred among athletes involved in contact sports. Although the majority of cases occur in children, particularly of preschool age, young adults are also affected. Impetigo may complicate preexisting skin lesions such as scabies, varicella, or eczema. Systemic response is minimal unless complications occur.

Cutaneous lesions. Streptococcal impetigo begins as transient, thin-roofed, small vesicles, sometimes with a small inflammatory halo. Pustulation rapidly occurs. Vesicles and pustules easily rupture. The purulent discharge subsequently dries, forming a thick, soft, golden-yellow "stuck-on" crust (Figs. 176-1 to 176-3 and A1-24), the hallmark of impetigo. Removal reveals a red, weeping surface which rapidly becomes encrusted again. Exposed areas of the skin such as the extremities are most commonly involved, but, in infants particularly, the lesions may occur anywhere. Satellite lesions appear, spread by autoinoculation. The individual lesions rarely exceed 1 to 2 cm, but occasionally the crusted lesions may be large through coalescence of lesions. As the process progresses peripherally, central healing occurs, producing an appearance that sometimes mimics that of a superficial fungal infection (Fig. 176-4). The lesions are superficially located, do not ordinarily produce ulcerations or deep infiltration, and heal without scarring or atrophy. Regional lymphadenopathy is present in the majority of cases. Pruritus and burning may occur but the lesions are usually painless.

Classical staphylococcal impetigo (see below) is characterized by intact bullae that lack a surrounding zone of

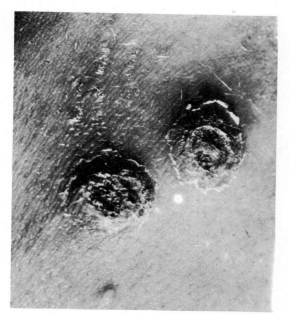

Fig. 176-1 Dried, crusted lesions of impetigo.

erythema or by ruptured bullae with thin, "varnishlike," light brown crusts.

LABORATORY FINDINGS. A slight leukocytosis is sometimes present, more commonly in those cases due to streptococci. A Gram-stained smear of early vesicle fluid reveals gram-positive cocci. Culture of the weeping area or of the area beneath an unroofed crust reveals group A streptococci, or a mixture of streptococci and *S. aureus* (particularly from older crusted lesions). The lesions of bullous impetigo are usually caused by *S. aureus* of phage group II.

DIAGNOSIS AND DIFFERENTIAL DIAGNOSIS. The diagnosis usually presents no difficulties when the lesions are seen at the stage of crusting. The initial vesicular lesion may resemble varicella, but the later crusted stage of varicella is readily distinguished by its hard, dark brown character. Occasionally, a fungal infection is suggested by the central clearing of a cluster of lesions. However, the vesicles in tinea circinata are usually very small and peripheral, and thick crusts are not formed. Herpes simplex may mimic impetigo, particularly as the contents of the vesicles become turbid. A drug eruption due to iodides and bromides may mimic a pyoderma, but it is usually not as superficial a process as impetigo and resembles a folliculitis.

COURSE AND PROGNOSIS. Untreated, the process may persist and new lesions may develop over a course of several weeks; thereafter the infection tends to resolve spontaneously unless there is some underlying cutaneous disorder such as eczema. Complicating deep cellulitis or bacteremia are most unusual. The major serious sequela is nephritis.

TREATMENT. Penicillin is the drug of choice in the treatment of streptococcal pyoderma, administered either as a single injection of long-acting benzathine penicillin (300,000 to 600,000 units for children; 1,200,000 for adults) or orally (25,000 to 100,000 units/kg per day in divided doses every 6 h for 10 days). Erythromycin (30 to 50 mg/kg per day by mouth in divided doses every 6 h for children; 250 to 500 mg by mouth every 6 h for adults administered for 10 days) is a suitable alternative drug in patients allergic to penicillin. Whether administration of penicillin is effective in reducing the incidence of pyoderma-associated nephritis remains a moot point. Although the latent period following impetigo is longer than that following pharyngeal infection, the mildness of the illness delays or negates the seeking of medical attention. Topical treatment (removal of dirt, crusts, and debris, by soaking with soap

Fig. 176-2 Impetigo. Yellow, dried "stuck-on" crusts on the face of a young woman.

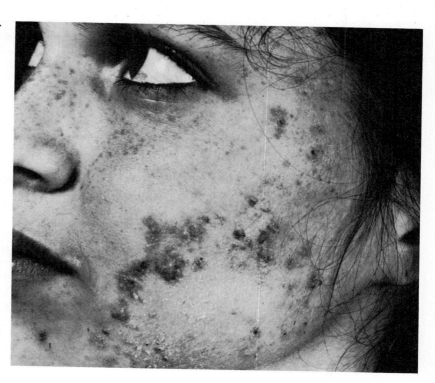

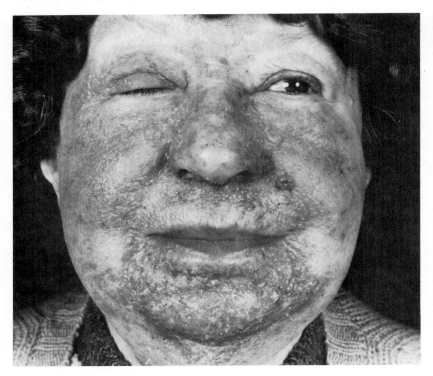

Fig. 176-3 Bullous impetigo. Extensive encrusted areas on the face containing many soft yellow crusts.

and water) is a valuable adjunct. Although penicillin treatment will clear the lesions of impetigo and prevent recurrence for a short time, streptococci can persist on or newly colonize normal skin in spite of this therapy.

Ecthyma. DEFINITION. This disease is very similar to the superficial vesiculopurulent pyoderma, impetigo. It begins

Fig. 176-4 Impetigo. In some of the lesions central healing has occurred.

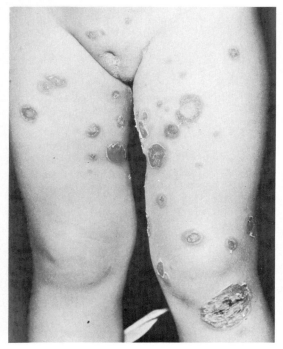

in the same fashion, but the process extends more deeply, penetrating through the epidermis to produce a shallow ulcer. Group A streptococci often initiate the disease or complicate preexisting superficial ulcers. However, lesions having the same ultimate appearance may be produced in the course of *Pseudomonas* septicemia (see Chap. 177).

CLINICAL MANIFESTATIONS. The lesions tend to occur most commonly on the lower extremities of children or neglected elderly patients following minor trauma such as insect bites or excoriations. Poor hygiene is an element in pathogenesis. Multiple ecthymatous ulcers on the ankle and dorsum of the foot were the most common pyodermas seen in the army in the rice paddies of Vietnam [9]. The initial lesion is a vesicle or vesicopustule with an erythematous base and surrounding halo. This enlarges over several days to a diameter of 0.5 to 3 cm and then crusts over. The ulcer has a "punched out" appearance when the dirty grayish yellow crust and purulent material are removed. The margin of the ulcer is indurated, raised, and violaceous (Fig. 176-5) and the granulating base extends deeply into the dermis. The lesions are slow to heal, requiring several weeks of antibiotic treatment for resolution. Problems of spread by autoinoculation, or by insect vectors, and of poststreptococcal sequela (glomerulonephritis) are the same as with impetigo.

Erysipelas. DEFINITION. Erysipelas is a characteristic type of superficial cellulitis of the skin with marked lymphatic-vessel involvement due to group A (or very uncommonly group C or G) streptococci. Group B streptococci may cause erysipelas in the newborn. Rarely, a similar clinical picture may be produced by infection with *S. aureus*.

CLINICAL MANIFESTATIONS

History. Erysipelas occurs most commonly in infants, very young children, and older adults; thus, not in the age groups most frequently involved in streptococcal respira-

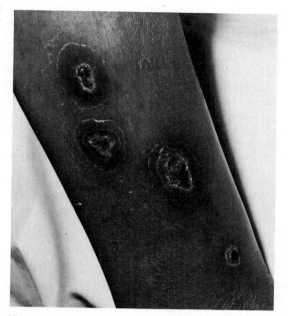

Fig. 176-5   Ecthyma with superficial ulcer in a raised margin.

tory tract infections. The process often begins in a small break in the skin, which is usually no longer evident by the time the infection has developed. The source of streptococci is commonly the upper respiratory tract, and a history of such an antecedent infection is obtained in one-third of patients. However, when the skin lesion is present, nose and throat cultures may no longer reveal streptococci. In cases of erysipelas developing after surgery or in wounds, organisms may have been transmitted from the nose, throat, or hands of attendants, the patient, or other patients. The skin of the face and head is most commonly involved, although in the neonate the lesion may take origin in an infection of the umbilical stump, spread rapidly over the anterior abdominal wall, and eventuate in bacteremia. In some neonates the omphalitis may be a more localized process persisting for weeks as an indolent infection at the umbilical stump. In adults, the portal of entry may be at the margin of an ulcer, at a site of chronic edema, in an area of devitalized skin, or about a dermatophytic lesion. Patients with nephrotic syndrome appear to be particularly susceptible to erysipelas. The initial lesion begins as a small area of redness which may be easily overlooked. The febrile onset of the disease may occur quite abruptly (even before the skin lesion is recognized) and may be associated with a frank rigor. The process evolves rapidly, and the patient appears quite ill with high fever.

Cutaneous lesions. The lesion has a characteristic brawny, edematous, indurated (peau d'orange) appearance and spreads peripherally. It is hot, shiny, and bright red, and has an advancing elevated margin that is sharply demarcated from the surrounding skin (Fig. A1-20). The involved area becomes painful only at this stage. The periphery of the lesion may appear irregular because of projections of the inflammatory process. As the lesion advances, no islands of normal skin are left behind. Small vesicles and occasionally large bullae may develop in the lesion, particularly in more severe infections. Petechiae

and even ecchymoses may appear during the active stage. With healing, local superficial desquamation of the skin occurs.

The most common form of erysipelas involves the bridge of the nose and one or both cheeks ("butterfly" distribution). The process usually halts at the hairline of the scalp or beard.

LABORATORY FINDINGS. A leukocytosis of 15,000 or greater occurs. Bacteriologic study is frequently of little help. Group A streptococci may be isolated from the throats of a few patients. Culture of the surface of the involved skin usually does not yield group A streptococci. Streptococci are only rarely cultured from aspirated tissue fluid from the advancing edge of the lesion.

PATHOLOGY. The histologic hallmarks of this disease are intense edema, marked vascular dilatation, and a profuse infiltration of tissue spaces and lymphatic channels with streptococci. The streptococci are not found in the blood vessels themselves, but their presence in the lymphatics produce an inflammatory reaction about these vessels. The dermis is markedly edematous, and there is infiltration with neutrophils and mononuclear cells. The epidermis is only secondarily involved.

DIAGNOSIS AND DIFFERENTIAL DIAGNOSIS. The diagnosis is made on clinical grounds. Unilateral facial erysipelas may be distinguished from early herpes zoster involving the maxillary division of the fifth cranial nerve by the presence of hyperesthesia and pain prior to the appearance of lesions in the latter. Osteomyelitis of the maxillary or frontal bones (secondary to paranasal sinusitis) producing erythema and edema of overlying tissues may suggest erysipelas. The lack of sharply defined borders and evidence of sinus disease on history and transillumination serve to differentiate between these processes.

Occasionally contact dermatitis, or angioneurotic edema may be mistaken for erysipelas, but the absence of fever is helpful in distinguishing these from erysipelas. An erysipelas-like skin lesion, apparently not due to infection, may occur recurrently in patients with familial Mediterranean fever. Diffuse inflammatory carcinoma of the breast may present a picture mimicking low-grade erysipelas.

Erysipelas should be differentiated from erysipeloid (see Chap. 178), which commonly occurs on the hand or finger of a person in contact with fish, shellfish, or animal products, and which is not associated with high fever or evidence of toxicity. Rarely, in immunosuppressed patients, skin lesions morphologically very similar to erysipelas have been produced by other organisms (e.g., coliform bacilli).

COURSE AND PROGNOSIS. Uncomplicated erysipelas remains confined primarily to the lymphatics and subcutaneous tissues. Even in the days prior to antibiotic therapy, it was often a self-limited process subsiding over 7 to 10 days. Occasionally, the organisms spread beyond the lymphatics, producing cellulitis and subcutaneous abscesses. This sequence may then be followed by bacteremia with metastatic infection in various organs. Antibiotic therapy produces improvement in the general condition of the patient in 24 to 48 h, but it takes several more days for subsidence of the local lesion to be clearly evident. Prompt treatment prevents both suppurative and nonsuppurative complications. However, in young infants and elderly debilitated patients and in individuals receiving corticosteroids, the disease may progress with devastating rapidity to a fatal outcome.

Erysipelas has a tendency to recur in the same area, perhaps due to the predisposing effects of chronic lymphatic obstruction, edema, and even elephantiasis caused by earlier infections. Such recurrent infections may produce persistent swelling of the lips (macrocheilia), cheeks (particularly the lax tissues beneath the eyes), or lower extremities. A bizarre, irregular, cutaneous overgrowth, designated *elephantiasis nostras verrucosa,* may be produced by chronic lymphedema secondary to recurrent erysipelas. Areas of lymphatic obstruction are predisposed to recurrent infections; for example, following radical mastectomy some patients are liable to recurrent episodes of what appears to be erysipelas in the area of lymphedema.

Acute cellulitis. DEFINITION. This is an acute, spreading inflammation of the skin involving particularly the deeper subcutaneous tissues. Group A streptococci and *S. aureus* are by far the most common etiologic agents, but occasionally other bacteria are implicated (e.g., group B streptococci in the newborn; rarely pneumococci; in patients with underlying diabetes mellitus or an immunosuppressive illness, a variety of atypical organisms such as gram-negative bacilli and even cryptococci can be the etiology as a result of local injury or blood-borne dissemination).

CLINICAL MANIFESTATIONS

History. Usually there is a history of an antecedent lesion (stasis ulcer, puncture wound), followed within a day or two by local erythema and tenderness. Systemic symptoms (malaise, fever, and chills) may then develop rapidly. Erythema at the site of infection rapidly intensifies and spreads. Local pain is often marked.

Cutaneous lesions. The involved area may be extensive, with a markedly red, hot, infiltrated edematous appearance. The borders of the lesion are not elevated or sharply defined. Tender regional lymphadenopathy is common, often with lymphangitis extending proximally. Superficial vesicles may form and rupture. Local abscesses may develop with necrosis of overlying skin.

A peculiar form of dissecting cellulitis may occur on the scalp, characterized by multiple small nodules and draining abscesses. The process is characteristically chronic, with a tendency toward burrowing. This disease usually occurs in young adults and is often associated with marked acne or hidradenitis suppurativa.

Streptococcal cellulitis may occur in unusual locations. Perianal cellulitis in children is a painful process with striking erythema about the anus [10]. The involved tissues have a boggy consistency. Group A streptococci can be readily isolated from the erythematous area. Antecedent or associated streptococcal pharyngitis or impetigo is often noted.

Streptococcal cellulitis as an operative wound infection is uncommon today in contrast to several decades ago. However, in the presence of streptococcal epidemics in the community, these organisms may be carried into the operating room and result in a particularly fulminating type of postoperative wound infection. Such sepsis may be manifest within 6 to 48 h of the surgery, more rapidly than that due to *S. aureus.* Hypotension (often due to bacteremia) may be the initial manifestation even before local erythema is evident. A thin serous discharge can be ex-

pressed from the wound area, and on Gram's stain shows myriads of gram-positive cocci in chains.

An unusual form of cellulitis may occur at the saphenous vein donor site of patients who have recently undergone coronary artery bypass [11]. Erythema and edema extend along the incision; tenderness is marked. In some patients the illness is quite acute with high fever, prostration, and tachycardia. In a few patients lymphangitic streaks are evident. The localized area of tenderness and erythema may suggest thrombophlebitis. Group A streptococci have been isolated from the skin lesions or blood of a few patients. The appearance of the lesions, the occasional associated lymphangitis, and the response to treatment with penicillin G suggest that this is most often a streptococcal process. The infection probably takes origin in a minor break in the skin in the interdigital web areas, usually secondary to tinea pedis. The lymphedema resulting from lymphatic interruption accompanying saphenous vein removal predisposes to development of cellulitis once organisms reach that area. Since streptococcal infection in an area of lymphedema begets further lymphedema, episodes of infection tend to recur. Topical treatment of the interdigital dermatophytosis with miconazole or clotrimazole cream is an important element in management and prophylaxis. Although the cellulitis responds well to penicillin, the response may be slower in patients with peripheral arterial disease. Also, it is important to recognize that the *rubor* of dependency in such a patient may exaggerate the appearance of cellulitis about the saphenous incision. Thus, it is advisable to examine the leg from day to day in the same (horizontal) position.

LABORATORY FINDINGS. There is almost always a brisk polymorphonuclear leukocytosis (15,000 to 40,000) with a marked shift to the left. Blood cultures should be performed, since the local process may be complicated by bacteremia.

DIAGNOSIS AND DIFFERENTIAL DIAGNOSIS. Like erysipelas, the diagnosis is based almost solely on the physical appearance of the lesion. The main point of differentiation between the two lesions centers on the nature of the margin of the lesion: raised, sharply demarcated from the uninvolved skin in erysipelas; indistinct and gradually blending with uninvolved adjacent areas in cellulitis.

COURSE AND PROGNOSIS. This process, because of its tendency to spread through lymphatics and bloodstream, is a serious disease if not treated early. In older patients, involvement of the lower extremities may be complicated by thrombophlebitis. In patients with chronic edema, the process may spread extremely rapidly and recovery may be slow, despite sterilization of the lesions by antibiotics. Occasionally, superinfection of necrotic areas, principally with gram-negative organisms, complicates recovery.

Acute lymphangitis. DEFINITION. Acute lymphangitis is an inflammatory process involving the subcutaneous lymphatic channels. It is due most often to group A streptococci but occasionally may be caused by *S. aureus;* rarely, soft tissue infections with other organisms, such as *Pasteurella multocida,* may be associated with acute lymphangitis.

CLINICAL MANIFESTATIONS

History. The portal of entry is commonly a wound on an extremity, an infected blister, or a paronychia. The systemic manifestations of infection may occur either before any evidences of infection are present at the site of inoculation, or after the initial lesion has subsided. The patient may notice pain over an area of redness proximal to the original break in the skin. Systemic symptoms are often more prominent than one might expect from the degree of local pain and erythema.

An unusual spread of streptococcal infection of the thumb (paronychia) or of the interdigital webs between the thumb and index finger may occur occasionally [10]. Lymphatic drainage from this area can bypass the lymph nodes at the elbow and drain into the axillary nodes, which in turn communicate with the subpectoral nodes and the pleural lymphatics. As a consequence, subpectoral abscesses and pleural effusion develop. The subpectoral infection may dissect downward and appear over the lower chest and upper abdomen as an area of cellulitis. This is a very serious illness. The clinical clues to the development of this sequence of events are provided by the location of the original infection on the thumb or medial surface of the index finger and the early occurrence of axillary pain.

Cutaneous lesions. Red linear streaks which may be a few millimeters to several centimeters in width extend from the local lesion toward the regional lymph nodes, which are usually enlarged and tender. The lymphangitic streaks are characteristically irregular and tender, and may be mistaken for linear excoriations. Occasionally, breakdown of overlying skin and ulceration will occur in the course of bacterial lymphangitis, but this is rare in the antibiotic era.

LABORATORY FINDINGS. The peripheral white blood cell count is elevated with a marked increase in polymorphonuclear cells. The offending organism cannot be cultured from the skin, since the infection is restricted to the lymphatic channels. However, the primary portal of entry or a suppurative lymph node, if overt infection is present, may reveal the etiologic agent.

DIAGNOSIS AND DIFFERENTIAL DIAGNOSIS. The combination of a peripheral lesion with proximal red linear streaks leading toward regional lymph nodes is diagnostic of lymphangitis. In the lower extremities, thrombophlebitis may produce somewhat similar linear areas of tender erythema. The absence of a portal of entry and of tender regional adenopathy is helpful in distinguishing this process from lymphangitis.

COURSE AND PROGNOSIS. The frequent development of bacteremia with metastatic infection in various organs makes this a potentially serious disease. The infection responds readily to penicillin therapy if instituted promptly.

Streptococcal gangrene. DEFINITION. Gangrene due to group A streptococci is a rare entity, with a high mortality rate, usually developing at the site of a laceration, needle puncture, or surgical wound, but sometimes occurring without any obvious portal of entry. It represents a cellulitis that has progressed rapidly to gangrene of the subcutaneous tissue, followed by necrosis of the overlying skin [12]. It is also known as *necrotizing fasciitis*. This nomenclature is confusing, because it is now recognized that the term necrotizing fasciitis includes not only group A streptococcal gangrene but also a similar-appearing entity due to other bacterial species (usually a mixture of anaerobic and facultative organisms). The latter process will be considered separately (see ''Necrotizing Fasciitis,'' below).

CLINICAL MANIFESTATIONS

History. Although cases have been reported in patients with underlying diseases (diabetes, myxedema), the majority of cases have occurred in otherwise healthy persons. Initially there are local redness, edema, heat, and pain in the involved area, typically on an extremity. Fever and other constitutional symptoms are prominent as the inflammatory process extends rapidly over the next 1 to 3 days.

Cutaneous lesions. From 36 to 72 h after onset of the cellulitis, the characteristic findings of streptococcal gangrene appear: the involved area becomes dusky blue in color; vesicles or bullae containing initially yellowish, then red-black fluid appear. The bullae rupture, and extensive, sharply demarcated cutaneous gangrene develops. At this point the area may be numb, and the black necrotic eschar with surrounding irregular border of erythema resembles a third-degree burn. This sloughs off by the end of a week or 10 days. Peripheral areas of involvement develop about the principal lesion, and metastatic lesions may occur as a consequence of bacteremia. Secondary thrombophlebitis is common, but lymphangitis and lymphadenitis are not.

LABORATORY FINDINGS. Organisms can usually be cultured from the yellow fluid in the bullous lesions. However, after these lesions rupture and undergo necrosis, a variety of other organisms not directly responsible for the lesion may be cultured from the area. Blood cultures usually contain streptococci.

PATHOLOGY. The prominent angiitis and focal dermal necrosis with spread along fascial planes suggest that the disease is fundamentally a gangrene of the subcutaneous tissues followed by necrosis of the overlying skin. Microscopically, fibrinoid necrosis is present in the media of many arteries and veins passing through the destroyed fascia. Fibrin thrombi are present. The epidermis, dermis, and skin appendages in the area of gangrene undergo coagulation necrosis. Numerous polymorphonuclear leukocytes and mononuclear cells infiltrate the lesion, and the upper layers of the dermis contain large numbers of gram-positive cocci.

DIAGNOSIS AND DIFFERENTIAL DIAGNOSIS. The gross appearance may suggest a third-degree burn or violent trauma, particularly if the patient is not able to provide a history and if the lesions have already reached the gangrenous phase.

COURSE AND PROGNOSIS. Prior to the availability of antibiotic therapy, the lesions commonly progressed and patients developed increasing toxemia and died from metastatic infection or shock. In rare cases, the process became sharply demarcated and self-limited. Even since the advent of antibiotics the mortality rate remains high.

TREATMENT. Surgical debridement and decompression with removal of the gray necrotic fascia is crucial in management, along with appropriate antibiotic therapy of the streptococcal infection. Because extensive undermining is often present, thorough exploration and filleting of involved tissues is necessary to control the spreading infection.

Necrotizing fasciitis. Necrotizing fasciitis other than that due to group A streptococci will be considered here. This is a mixed infection in which one or more anaerobes (e.g., *Peptostreptococcus, Bacteroides)* are involved along with at least one facultative species (non-group A streptococci;

members of the Enterobacteriaceae such as *Enterobacter, Proteus,* etc.) [13].

CLINICAL MANIFESTATIONS

History. Antecedent injury to soft tissues, abdominal surgery, perirectal abscess, decubitus ulcer, and intestinal perforation are common predisposing events. Diabetes mellitus, alcoholism, or parenteral drug abuse are additional contributing factors. The onset is usually acute and the course is rapidly progressive with high fever and prominent toxicity.

Cutaneous lesions. This infection most commonly occurs on the lower extremities, abdominal wall, perineum, and about operative wounds [14]. It is important to recognize that this infection may present in the thigh (dissection along the psoas muscle) or abdominal wall from an intestinal source (occult diverticulitis, rectosigmoid neoplasm). The involved area is swollen, red, warm, painful, and tender. The process is more extensive than the extent of the overlying skin changes would suggest. Within several days the skin color becomes purple, bullae develop, and frank cutaneous gangrene ensues. At this stage the involved area is no longer tender, and, in fact, has become anesthetic due to occlusion of small blood vessels and destruction of superficial nerves in the subcutaneous tissues. Crepitus is often present, particularly in patients with diabetes mellitus.

A special form of necrotizing fasciitis which occurs about the male genitalia is known as *Fournier's gangrene* (streptococcal scrotal gangrene, perineal phlegmon) [15]. It is caused by the same mixture of facultative and anaerobic organisms described above. In rare cases group A streptococci have been implicated. The process may be limited to the scrotum or spread to the penis, perineum, and abdominal wall. Pain, swelling, and crepitus in the scrotum are marked. Foul-smelling drainage occurs, and purplish discoloration of the scrotum progresses to frank gangrene. If the process invades the abdominal panniculus of an obese patient, especially one with diabetes mellitus, progression can be extraordinarily rapid.

Another variant of necrotizing fasciitis is known as *synergistic necrotizing cellulitis* (necrotizing cutaneous myositis, synergistic nonclostridial anaerobic myonecrosis). This process involves skin and muscle as well as fascia and subcutaneous tissue. The lower extremities, perineum, and abdominal wall are common sites [16]. The initial skin lesions may appear as skin sinuses (with surrounding areas of gangrene) draining foul-smelling brownish ("dishwater") pus. Between the draining tracks the skin appears uninvolved even though extensive necrosis of underlying fascia, muscle, and subcutaneous tissues has occurred. Crepitus is present in about 25 percent of cases.

LABORATORY FINDINGS. A leukocytosis is almost always present. Gram-stained smears of the exudate show a mixture of organisms (both gram-positive cocci and gram-negative bacilli of various sizes; occasionally, gram-positive bacilli consistent with *Clostridium* species are also present). Blood cultures are frequently positive for one or more bacterial species.

COURSE AND PROGNOSIS. This can be a rapidly progressive life-threatening infection if the diagnosis is not made promptly and appropriate surgical debridement is not carried out. This applies particularly when the process is secondary to a bowel perforation. Even with treatment the mortality rate is about 35 percent.

TREATMENT. The major cause of delay in instituting appropriate therapy is the failure to appreciate involvement of fascia and deep subcutaneous tissue, leading to the misdiagnosis of this infection as cellulitis. Prompt exploration of the involved area is of paramount importance. Easy passage of a hemostat along a plane just superficial to the deep fascia (not expected with early cellulitis) should make the diagnosis. A frozen-section soft tissue biopsy performed early in the course of the illness may provide a definitive diagnosis and expedite appropriate treatment [17]. Debridement should be carried out beyond the area of involvement until completely normal fascia is reached. All necrotic fascia and fat should be removed and the wound should be left open. If there is any question as to the adequacy of the initial debridement, a "second-look" procedure is indicated 24 to 48 h later. Prior to obtaining results from cultures, initial antimicrobial therapy should be based on knowledge of a prominent role of anaerobic bacteria in this infection and on the specific findings on Gram-stained smear of the exudate.

Progressive bacterial synergistic gangrene. DEFINITION. Progressive synergistic gangrene is a gangrenous ulceration of the skin due to a mixed bacterial infection in which microaerophilic streptococci together with *S. aureus* (or sometimes a gram-negative bacillus such as *Proteus*) are implicated. The lesion was designated synergistic gangrene because Brewer and Meleney [18] and Meleney [19] were able to reproduce the same type of lesion in dogs by injecting microaerophilic streptococci and *S. aureus* into the skin. Neither organism alone would produce such a lesion.

CLINICAL MANIFESTATIONS

History. This characteristic infection usually follows abdominal or thoracic infection (empyema) or trauma, and is frequently associated with the use of through-and-through stay sutures in surgery. It is sometimes seen in the area of a colostomy or ileostomy opening or in proximity to a chronic ulceration on an extremity.

Cutaneous lesions. The infection usually starts in the first or second postoperative week with local redness, tenderness, and swelling. A small, painful, superficial ulcer develops and gradually enlarges. The central shaggy ulcer is characteristically surrounded by a rim of gangrenous skin. The latter, in turn, is encircled by a zone of purple erythema which blends into a peripheral pink edematous area (Fig. 176-6).

LABORATORY FINDINGS. Anaerobic cultures from the advancing edematous margin of the lesion usually show microaerophilic or anaerobic streptococci, while *S. aureus* (rarely *Proteus* or several other gram-negative bacilli) is found in the central ulcerated area.

COURSE AND PROGNOSIS. If untreated, the process extends slowly but progressively, ultimately resulting in enormous ulcerations.

TREATMENT. This is usually a very difficult lesion to treat. Local bacitracin irrigations (about 50 units/mL) and systemic antibiotic therapy with large doses of penicillin or other antibiotic (based on antibiotic susceptibility tests) are sometimes helpful. However, most often the lesion can be controlled only by wide surgical excision combined with antibiotic therapy.

Scarlet fever. DEFINITION. Scarlet fever is a diffuse erythematous eruption resulting from the production and sub-

Fig. 176-6 Infant with progressive bacterial synergistic gangrene showing central ulceration around the anus and surrounded by a rim of gangrenous skin.

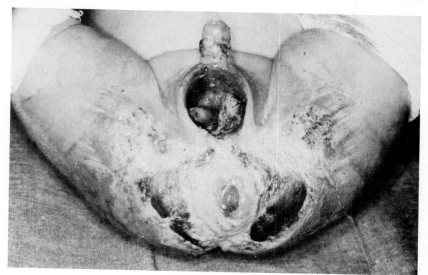

sequent circulation of erythrogenic toxin produced by group A streptococci usually located in a pharyngeal infection. The only difference between streptococcal tonsillopharyngitis and scarlet fever is the greater toxicity and the eruption in the latter.

BACTERIOLOGY AND PATHOGENESIS. Erythrogenic toxin is produced by most, but not all, strains of group A streptococci (a similar toxin is produced by certain strains of group C and group G streptococci) and is related to the presence of a lysogenic bacteriophage in the streptococcus. This relationship is very similar to that involving bacteriophage infection and toxin production in *Corynebacterium diphtheriae*. There appear to be three immunologically distinct erythrogenic toxins, but one type appears to be produced by 80 percent of strains of toxin-producing streptococci. It is possible to have repeated group A streptococcal infections, but an individual usually has scarlet fever only once because of the development of protective specific antitoxic antibody. The few patients with documented recurrent attacks of scarlet fever may represent cases in which the episodes have been due to either of the other two immunologically distinct toxins. The immune status of a patient will determine the response to exposure to a given erythrogenic toxin-producing strain of group A streptococcus; it consists of two parts—type-specific antibacterial immunity and antitoxic immunity. The responses fall into three patterns: (1) Patients with type-specific antibacterial immunity (± antitoxic immunity) to a given streptococcal type (e.g., type 12) will develop no clinical disease when exposed to that type. (2) Patients with no type-specific antibacterial immunity (but with antitoxic immunity) will develop streptococcal pharyngitis. (3) Patients with neither antibacterial nor antitoxic immunity will develop pharyngitis plus scarlet fever (unless treated early with appropriate antibiotics).

It has been suggested that the rash of scarlet fever requires both the presence of erythrogenic toxin and the existence of delayed-type skin reactivity to streptococcal products, the latter stemming from prior exposure to the organism. In support of this is the observation that although streptococcal infections are not uncommon in infants and very young children, scarlet fever is rarely seen in this age group, and these infants fail to react to intradermal injection of erythrogenic toxin (Dick test). This failure to react does not appear to be correlated with transfer of antibody from the mother. Similarly, infant guinea pigs are not susceptible to intradermal injection of erythrogenic toxin. Following immunization with the toxin in Freund's adjuvant, they become sensitized and the Dick test becomes positive.

CLINICAL MANIFESTATIONS

History. The disease occurs usually in children (the maximal incidence being in the 2- to 10-year age group) but only rarely in adults.

The clinical onset of the disease with the appearance of pharyngitis and fever is often abrupt after a 2- to 4-day incubation period. The temperature may be only slightly elevated in mild cases, but it often rises rapidly to 38.9 to 40°C. Nausea and vomiting, headache, malaise, diffuse abdominal pain, and chilly sensations are prominent initial constitutional manifestations. The fever reaches its peak by the second day, and the temperature gradually returns to normal in the average case in 5 to 6 days. The rash appears 24 to 48 h after the onset of pharyngeal symptoms. Although the streptococcal focus of most patients with scarlet fever is in the pharynx, occasional patients develop a form of the disease, surgical scarlet fever, as a consequence of operative or other wound (burn, etc.) infection.

The acute manifestations of scarlet fever consist of those symptoms and signs related to the invasive streptococcal process at the portal of entry and those findings produced by erythrogenic toxin (malaise, nausea, vomiting, headache, fever, generalized lymphadenopathy, rash).

The severity of scarlet fever has declined over the past three decades; this trend even antedates the advent of effective chemotherapy.

Cutaneous lesions. The major physical findings relate to the enanthem and exanthem.

1. *Enanthem.* The pharynx is beefy red in color, with edema involving the tonsillar area and extending anteriorly to include the soft palate and uvula (Fig. A3-2a and c). The tonsils are enlarged, reddened, and often covered with discrete patches of white or yellow exu-

date filling the tonsillar crypts. Occasionally, the exudate becomes confluent. Bilateral tender submandibular lymphadenopathy is present.

During the first several days of the illness, the tongue is white and furred, but the edges and tip remain reddened. The papillae soon become reddened and hypertrophied and project through the white coating, producing what has been called the "white-strawberry" tongue. By the fourth or fifth day, the white coating has disappeared and the tongue assumes a bright red color punctuated with very prominent papillae, the so-called red-strawberry tongue. Punctate erythema and scattered petechiae are often present over the soft palate.

2. *Exanthem.* The rash usually appears first on the neck, then rapidly encompasses the trunk, and finally spreads to the extremities (Fig. A3-2b). The involvement of the body is usually complete within 36 h, but the palms and soles are spared. The rash is a diffuse erythema, blanching on pressure, with numerous 1- to 2-mm punctate papular elevations, giving a rough sandpaper quality to the skin. There usually are no discrete lesions on the face but only a marked flushing of the cheeks and forehead, contrasting quite sharply with the circumoral pallor. On the body the rash is most marked in the skin folds of the inguinal, axillary, antecubital, and abdominal areas and about sites of pressure such as the buttocks and sacrum. The eruption often exhibits a linear petechial character in the antecubital fossae and axillary folds (Pastia's lines) (Fig. A3-2b). In those cases in which the eruption is intense, pinhead vesicular lesions (miliary sudamina), seen in a variety of prolonged febrile illnesses, may appear on the abdomen and chest. In mild cases the rash may be localized to the trunk and be seen as only a faint erythema. In the black patient the rash is often difficult to recognize but may be felt as punctate papular lesions resembling "gooseflesh" or sandpaper. At its peak the rash has a diffuse, bright scarlet appearance. Capillary fragility is increased in the severer cases, and the tourniquet test result is positive. Occasional patients may develop frank purpura, with or without thrombocytopenia.

The exanthem usually persists for 4 or 5 days but in mild cases may be very transient. One of the most characteristic features of the illness is the desquamation which begins as the rash starts to fade. It commences on the face, usually about the ears, and spreads to the trunk and extremities, involving the hands and feet last (between the second and third weeks of illness). The desquamation on the face and trunk has a brawny character, and frequently a punched-out appearance of the abdomen results from the peeling off of circular areas of skin. Skin on the hands and feet is frequently shed in large sheets. The desquamation is so prominent a feature that it may be helpful in making a retrospective diagnosis in a case in which the eruption was minimal. Similar changes in the nail bed produce a transverse groove in the nails.

Other physical findings. Generalized lymphadenopathy is a common finding, and splenomegaly is present occasionally.

LABORATORY FINDINGS. The blood picture in the early stages shows a polymorphonuclear leukocytosis, and later in the illness eosinophilia (5 to 10 percent) is a common finding. Throat culture reveals group A streptococci. If direct bacteriologic confirmation cannot be made during the early phases of the illness, determination of the antistreptolysin O titer may provide, retrospectively, evidence of a recent streptococcal infection. Slight microscopic hematuria is found not infrequently during the peak of the exanthem and does not represent acute glomerulonephritis. It is usually transient and may be related to a generalized effect of the erythrogenic toxin on capillaries.

PATHOLOGY. There is an outpouring of polymorphonuclear leukocytes and scattered red blood cells into the skin about small blood vessels. The punctiform lesions are represented by dilated small blood vessels and a focal accumulation of exudate. The suppurative and nonsuppurative sequelae are the same as are seen with any group A streptococcal infection.

DIAGNOSIS AND DIFFERENTIAL DIAGNOSIS. The diagnosis is usually made on the basis of clinical features—fever, vomiting, exudative pharyngitis, and an erythematous punctiform eruption going on to desquamation. Confirmatory evidence is provided by isolation of group A streptococci from the pharynx. Two other confirmatory tests that have been employed extensively in the past are no longer necessary:

1. *Dick test.* This is a test for the presence of antitoxic immunity and is performed by an intracutaneous inoculation of 0.1 mL of a standard diluted preparation of erythrogenic toxin. The appearance of a 1-cm or greater area of local erythema at 24 h is a positive test result and indicates a lack of antitoxic immunity (i.e., susceptibility to scarlet fever). A negative Dick test indicates immunity to the effects of erythrogenic toxin. A positive Dick test during the first several days of illness becoming negative 1 to 2 weeks later is highly suggestive of scarlet fever.
2. *Schultz-Charlton phenomenon.* Intradermal injection of 0.1 mL of antitoxin into an area of scarlet fever rash produces "blanching" at the site of injection within 12 to 24 h. The test must be performed during the very early phase of the eruption before exudation into the lesion makes the skin changes irreversible. The blanching test is not used now because of the danger of sensitization to horse serum, and because the use of antitoxin of human origin carries the risk of introducing viral hepatitis.

Although the total clinical picture is highly suggestive of scarlet fever (due to group A streptococci), scarlatiniform eruptions may occur in other conditions and cause confusion in diagnosis. Infection with toxin ("exfoliatin"), producing strains of *S. aureus* belonging to phage group II, may produce a rash resembling that of scarlet fever (see section on "Staphylococcal Skin Infections" below). Strains of *S. aureus* producing pyrogenic exotoxin C are responsible for the toxic shock syndrome, an acute febrile illness which also produces a generalized scarlatiniform eruption. In infants and young children particularly, exanthem subitum and rubella may be mistaken for scarlet fever, but the lack of a pharyngeal focus is important in distinguishing these conditions. Also, neither of these processes is followed by extensive desquamation. Patients with infectious mononucleosis may develop an erythematous eruption, and this, together with lymphadenopathy and membranous pharyngitis, may mimic scarlet fever. The typical blood picture and the heterophil agglutination test are helpful points in distinguishing between these diseases. Diffuse erythroderma as part of a drug-sensitivity reaction (sulfonamides, streptomycin, penicillin) may be mistaken for scarlet fever, as may the fever and cutaneous blush associated with atropine toxicity. Sunburn in a child with pharyngitis may be a cause of confusion, but the distribution of the lesions is the crucial distinguishing point.

COURSE AND PROGNOSIS. The acute febrile course of the untreated, uncomplicated case lasts about 4 to 5 days; desquamation may continue for several weeks thereafter. Many cases seen nowadays are mild and last only a few days. The course of the illness is dramatically altered by the administration of penicillin, which produces a prompt subsidence of fever and of constitutional symptoms. Adequate, early penicillin treatment eradicates the streptococci from the pharyngeal or other foci, interferes with the development of antistreptolysin O antibodies, and prevents the development of suppurative and nonsuppurative sequelae. The prognosis is excellent, and deaths today due to scarlet fever are extremely rare.

Cutaneous manifestations of subacute bacterial endocarditis. A variety of skin lesions has been described in subacute bacterial endocarditis (usually due to viridans streptococci). Although often ascribed to embolic phenomena, it appears that many of these lesions represent local areas of vasculitis.

PETECHIAE. These are the most common of the skin and mucous membrane lesions in bacterial endocarditis and are found in about half of patients with this disease. These small, reddish brown, flat lesions do not blanch on pressure. They occur particularly on the extremities and upper chest. Mucous membrane involvement (conjunctivae, palate) is common. The petechiae frequently occur in small crops. Rarely, the lesions may be extremely numerous and involve primarily the lower extremities. They usually deepen in color, last only a few days, and then fade away. It is important to distinguish capillary angiomas, which may be present on the chests of some patients, from petechiae. This can be done by applying pressure with a glass slide and demonstrating blanching of the angiomas.

The limited information on the histology of petechiae in subacute bacterial endocarditis does not suggest local bacterial multiplication or embolization as the basis for the lesions. The endothelial proliferation, hemorrhage, and round-cell infiltration found are consistent with small-vessel inflammation. Increased capillary fragility can be demonstrated in some patients.

SUBUNGUAL "SPLINTER HEMORRHAGES." These small, dark red streaks resembling splinters beneath the nail are suggestive of the diagnosis of subacute bacterial endocarditis (Fig. 176-7). Similar lesions may occur beneath the distal portion of the nail as a result of trauma (in dishwashers, carpenters, etc.) or poor hygiene. Splinter hemorrhages may occur as part of the clinical picture in trichinosis and vasculitis. Subungual hemorrages may occur in acute meningococcemia with extensive petechiae and purpura. "Splinters" located near the middle third of the nail are more suggestive of subacute bacterial endocarditis,

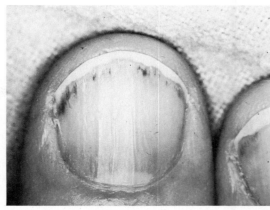

Fig. 176-7   Subungual "splinter" hemorrhages in subacute bacterial endocarditis.

since they are less likely to be of traumatic origin. True splinter lesions in subacute bacterial endocarditis will migrate distally as the nail grows out.

OSLER'S NODES. These are split-pea-sized, erythematous, painful, nodular lesions. They appear to be in the skin and in some ways resemble an urticarial wheal, often with a whitish center. The most common location of these swellings is on the pads of the fingers and toes, on the thenar and hypothenar eminences, and over the arms. They are quite transient, lasting 12 to 24 h or perhaps several days. They are not numerous and tend to occur in crops. They may desquamate but do not ulcerate. Currently, they are seen in about 5 percent of patients with bacterial endocarditis.

Histologic examination has not confirmed the suggested embolic nature of the Osler's nodes occurring in subacute bacterial endocarditis. Endothelial swelling and a perivascular inflammatory response have been found at the center of such lesions, but no bacteria or fibrin emboli were observed. Although at first suggested as pathognomonic findings in viridans streptococcal subacute bacterial endocarditis, Osler's nodes have been observed in subacute and acute endocarditis, due to a variety of organisms, including *S. aureus*. Histologic examination of Osler's nodes from several patients with acute endocarditis due to *S. aureus* and *Candida albicans* has revealed microemboli in dermal arterioles and adjacent microabscesses in the papillary dermis [20]. In these cases the responsible organism has been identified on Gram's stains or cultures of aspirates.

It appears that Osler's nodes in acute bacterial endocarditis may be caused by minute infective emboli; in subacute bacterial endocarditis they may be due to immunologic phenomena resulting in small-vessel arteritis of the skin.

JANEWAY LESIONS. These lesions, consisting of small erythematous macules or occasionally minimally nodular hemorrhages in the palms or soles, are seen in subacute bacterial endocarditis, but more frequently in acute endocarditis (often due to *S. aureus*). They may be rather numerous and, unlike Osler's nodes, are painless. Histologically, there is usually a polymorphonuclear infiltration of the walls of blood capillaries, some extravasation of red blood cells, and microabscess formation in the dermis.

Poststreptococcal (group A) nonsuppurative
cutaneous sequelae

Erythema nodosum. See Chap. 99.

**Erythema marginatum (cutaneous lesions of acute rheumatic
fever).** See Chap. 157.

Purpura fulminans (gangrenosa). DEFINITION. Purpura fulminans is an uncommon, acute, severe, usually fatal nonspecific hemorrhagic infarction and necrosis of the skin
that occurs in the course of, or immediately following, a
variety of infections, particularly those due to group A
streptococci. Marked depletion of multiple coagulation factors (disseminated intravascular coagulation) occurs in this
condition. Closely related, if not the identical process, is
the symmetric peripheral gangrene which sometimes is
seen (particularly in infants) during bacteremias.

EPIDEMIOLOGY. Purpura fulminans occurs most often in
children, but has been seen at all ages. The antecendent
or concomitant infections with which it has been associated
include those due to bacteria (scarlet fever; group A streptococcal, staphylococcal, and pneumococcal bacteremias,
and meningococcemia), and, less commonly, those of a
viral etiology (varicella). In patients with purpura fulminans after varicella, secondary streptococcal infection may
have been an important etiologic factor.

ETIOLOGY AND PATHOGENESIS. Purpura fulminans is one
of several cutaneous syndromes whose common feature is
a hemorrhagic tendency developing secondary to the acute
intravascular activation of the clotting mechanism. The
exact means of initiation of the consumption coagulopathy
is not yet fully understood. Rarely, a case appears to be
associated with drug allergy. A host of coagulation abnormalities has been noted at one time or another. This variability probably reflects the rapid changes that occur during
the evolution of the process and the effects of "secondary"
fibrinolysis. The abnormalities more commonly recorded
include thrombocytopenia; depression of prothrombin
(factor II), fibrinogen (factor I), proaccelerin (factor V),
and antihemophilic factor (factor VIII); and findings of
secondary fibrinolysis (i.e., increased plasminogen levels
or evidences of fibrinogen or fibrin breakdown products).
It is of interest that the coagulopathy and microscopic
pathology in purpura fulminans are very similar to those
found in rabbits with generalized Shwartzman reaction (see
Chap. 175).

CLINICAL MANIFESTATIONS

History. The eruption develops during, or on convalescence from, one of the infections noted earlier. Chills and
fever usually herald the onset of the hemorrhagic lesions,
and the patient appears acutely ill.

Cutaneous lesions. The lesions are localized, massive
ecchymoses, often with sharp, irregular ("geographic")
borders. They are usually symmetric and on the extremities, particularly in areas of pressure, but may involve the
lips, ears, nose, and trunk. There may be a narrow surrounding zone of erythema. Hemorrhagic blebs may develop in the ecchymotic areas associated with edema of
the areas. The peripheral ecchymotic lesions, especially of
the digits, may rapidly blacken and progress to gangrene.

Other physical findings. The other findings are those of
a systemically ill patient with high fever and tachycardia.

The disease often rapidly progresses over 48 to 72 h, with
peripheral vasoconstriction and shock supervening.

LABORATORY FINDINGS. There is usually a leukocytosis.
The number of platelets is markedly reduced and coagulation factors V, VII, VIII and prothrombin and fibrinogen
are decreased. As a result, the prothrombin time and the
partial thromboplastin time are prolonged. Split products
of fibrinogen and fibrin may be present.

PATHOLOGY. The involved areas show occlusion of arterioles with fibrin thrombi. A dense polymorphonuclear
reaction occurs in the dermis in the areas of infarction
necrosis. Bacteria are not seen in the lesions. Similar lesions may occur in the viscera, but often they are restricted
to the skin.

DIAGNOSIS AND DIFFERENTIAL DIAGNOSIS. All the causes
of gross purpura must be considered in the differential
diagnosis. The relationship of specific infections, the striking geographic nature of the lesions, and their location on
the extremities are suggestive of the diagnosis. Rarely,
morphologically similar lesions have been described as
complications of coumarin therapy.

TREATMENT. Treatment includes vigorous antibiotic
management of any associated infection. Only if bleeding
is significant during the course of diffuse intravascular coagulation in the patient with purpura fulminans is replacement of platelets and coagulation factors undertaken and
consideration given to the use of heparin (10 to 15 units/
kg/h as a continuous intravenous infusion) to inhibit the
intravascular clotting process.

COURSE AND PROGNOSIS. The mortality rate is extremely
high. In those patients who survive, amputation of extremities or extensive skin grafting may be necessary to deal
with the gangrenous areas.

**Other skin lesions accompanying or following group A strep-
tococcal infections.** ERYTHEMA MULTIFORME-LIKE LESIONS.
Round erythematous macules, up to 1.5 cm in diameter,
some developing bright borders and subsequently showing
clearing in the center, may occur during bacteremia due to
group A streptococci (or *S. aureus*) in infants and young
children.

Treatment of group A streptococcal skin infections

Antibiotic management. GENERAL PRINCIPLES. Penicillin G
is the drug of choice in the treatment of known group A
streptococcal skin infections. When the etiology is not
known immediately (e.g., in cellulitis) and when *S. aureus*
is also a distinct consideration, a semisynthetic penicillin
(nafcillin or oxacillin) should be employed initially. Penicillin treatment should be continued for at least 10 days to
insure eradication of the infection. Since as many as 40
percent of isolates of group A streptococci may be resistant
to the tetracyclines, this group of drugs should not be used
in the treatment of known streptococcal disease. Prophylactic penicillin therapy is indicated for close family contacts (particularly children) of patients with streptococcal
pharyngitis.

SPECIFIC TREATMENT. Mild infections such as impetigo,
scarlet fever, or certain cases of erysipelas and cellulitis
may be treated at home with intramuscular procaine penicillin (600,000 units once or twice daily), or with oral
penicillin V (250 to 500 mg 4 times daily). When staphy-

lococcal infection is suspected, oxacillin (0.5 to 1.0 g orally 4 times daily) should be substituted. In adults allergic to penicillin, erythromycin (0.25 to 0.5 g orally 4 times daily) is a reasonable alternative.

In more severe streptococcal skin infections (e.g., extensive erysipelas, cellulitis, or streptococcal gangrene), the above dosage of antibiotics is insufficient. Patients with such conditions should be hospitalized, and treatment with parenteral aqueous penicillin G (600,000 to 2,000,000 units every 4 to 6 h) should be begun. In the very ill patient in whom a staphylococcal etiology is suspected, one of the semisynthetic penicillins (e.g., nafcillin 1.0 to 1.5 g intravenously every 4 h) should be employed. In the patient with a questionable penicillin allergy, cephalothin (1.0 g intravenously every 3 to 4 h) may be substituted. If the patient has had an immediate type of reaction to penicillin (anaphylaxis or angioneurotic edema, etc.) then vancomycin (1.0 to 1.5 g intravenously daily) would be a reasonable alternative for treatment of a staphylococcal infection.

LOCAL AND OTHER MEASURES. Care of the local lesion of erysipelas and cellulitis includes immobilization and elevation of the involved area to reduce local edema. Cool, sterile saline dressings decrease the local pain and are particularly indicated in the presence of bullous lesions. The use of a footboard may protect the affected area from trauma. The application of moist heat may aid in the localization of a cellulitis, but it should not be used in a patient with arterial insufficiency in the involved extremity. Subsequent drainage may be necessary for areas of abscess formation; extensive debridement and grafting may be required for the necrotic areas of streptococcal gangrene.

Superficial lesions (such as ecthyma and secondarily infected dermatoses) benefit from sterile saline dressings. Bacitracin ointment may be of value in softening and removing crusted lesions.

Patients hospitalized with group A streptococcal infections should be isolated until the organisms have been eradicated by antibiotic treatment.

Staphylococcal skin infections

General features

Bacteriology and pathogenic aspects. S. aureus is the causative agent in some of the primary pyodermas and cellulitides as well as a colonizer or secondary invader on diseased dermatitic skin. The organisms are readily demonstrated on smear of pus as large gram-positive cocci in small clusters.

In contrast to the relative rarity of group A streptococci, S. aureus is frequently found distributed over the skin, particularly in nasal carriers. The presence of S. aureus often represents a carrier state or its passage as a transient [21]. The biologic attributes (cellular components, extracellular products) of S. aureus bearing on the disease-producing potential of the organism are not well understood, with the exception of the role of the exfoliating toxin in the staphylococcal scalded-skin syndrome and bullous impetigo and the role of pyrogenic exotoxin C (enterotoxin F) in the toxic shock syndrome. The production of coagulase, leukocidin, alpha toxin, etc., may be the same in strains isolated from staphylococcal cellulitis as in those

from the normal skin of the carrier. Thus, a variety of host factors (therapy with corticosteroids and immunosuppressive agents, etc.) appears to play an important, if not the major, role in the pathogenesis of staphylococcal infections. This is not to say that as yet unidentified virulence factors in certain staphylococcal isolates will not eventually explain the apparent heightened pathogenicity of particular strains. Preexisting tissue injury or inflammation (surgical wound, burn, trauma, exudative dermatitis, retained foreign body) is of major importance in the pathogenesis of staphylococcal disease. The production of coagulase, a factor capable of clotting plasma, remains, at present, the most widely employed in vitro criterion of the potential pathogenicity of a staphylococcal strain. Coagulase may play a role in the development of the staphylococcal abscess by producing local fibrin thrombi that protect organisms and concentrate toxic factors elaborated by these pathogens. The elaboration of surface slime, a substance facilitating adherence of coagulase-negative staphylococci to surfaces of foreign bodies, may contribute to the newly appreciated virulence of these organisms when they infect immunosuppressed individuals or patients with indwelling catheters or prostheses.

One of the major problems in dealing with staphylococcal infections has been the emergence of resistance to a variety of antibiotics. Although the presence of resistance, usually to penicillin G and other drugs, has been of paramount importance in the outcome of infection, there is no evidence that the intrinsic virulence of such strains is any greater than that of pencillin-sensitive organisms. The introduction of the pencillinase-resistant penicillins has altered considerably the picture for serious staphylococcal infections. S. aureus strains resistant to the semisynthetic penicillinase-resistant penicillins have emerged as a significant problem in the past five years in this country.

Epidemiology. The ubiquity of the staphylococcus and the difficulty in distinguishing among strains has, until recently, impeded an understanding of the epidemiology of infections due to this organism. Initially, the high frequency of staphylococcal colonization of the respiratory tract and the frequency of staphylococci in our immediate environment suggested that their spread from person to person occurred principally via respiratory transmission or fomites. Careful epidemiologic studies utilizing phage-typing techniques suggest that transfer of organisms to patients occurs predominantly via the hands of personnel rather than through the air. This appears to be particularly true in newborn nurseries, where this route is of importance in dissemination of the organisms from nasal carriers and also in transfer of staphylococci between babies. Individuals, whether infants or adults, with open staphylococcal lesions are particularly dangerous potential transmitters of infection. Good nursery technique, careful handling of patients, strict handwashing procedures, and isolation of patients with open draining staphylococcal infections are important in the reduction of transmission of staphylococci.

Immunity. The prevalence of staphylococci and staphylococcal infections is substantiated by the almost universal presence in adults of circulating antibody to one or more cell-wall antigens or extracellular toxins. The occurrence of staphylococcal infections in the presence of these antibodies suggests that they are not the primary determinants of resistance to such infections. Immunization of experimental animals with alpha toxin does not afford protection against staphylococcal disease following challenge. Hypersensitivity may play a role in recurrent staphylococcal skin infections in humans.

Superficial staphylococcal pyodermas

Impetigo. Two clinical types of impetigo occur. The first is a thick, yellow, crusted variety which is transiently vesicular in its early stage. Group A streptococci or a mixture of streptococci and *S. aureus* usually are isolated from these lesions. When both organisms are present, group A streptococci appear to be the primary pathogen and staphylococci are secondary invaders of the lesions (see earlier section on "Impetigo"). *S. aureus* alone is isolated from 5 to 10 percent of cases of this type of impetigo in the United States [5,22], but a higher percentage of cases in Europe [7]. Production of bacteriocins (highly bactericidal to group A streptococci) by certain *S. aureus* strains (phage group 71) may be responsible for the isolation of only *S. aureus* from some lesions due initially to streptococci. Overall, however, it would appear that in conventional impetigo with typical crusted lesions, the group A streptococcus is etiologically most frequent; *S. aureus* may be responsible for a minority of cases, and these tend to heal spontaneously, faster than those due to streptococci. The second type of impetigo is bullous impetigo, characterized by large bullae which rupture and form varnishlike crusts. This infection is specifically associated with *S. aureus* of phage group II (usually type 71).

Bullous impetigo. Three types of skin lesions can be produced by phage group II staphylococci: (1) bullous impetigo, (2) exfoliative disease (staphylococcal scalded-skin syndrome), (3) nonstreptococcal scarlatiniform eruption. All three represent varying cutaneous responses to an extracellular exfoliative toxin ("exfoliatin") produced by these staphylococci (for descriptions of the toxin and the latter two types of lesions see "Staphylococcal Scalded-Skin Syndrome" below).

CLINICAL MANIFESTATIONS. Bullous impetigo occurs mainly in the newborn and in older children, and is characterized by the rapid progression of vesicles to flaccid bullae. The latter arise on areas of grossly normal skin, and the Nikolsky sign is not present. The bullae contain initially clear yellow fluid which subsequently becomes dark yellow and turbid. There is no erythema surrounding the bullous lesions which are sharply demarcated. They soon rupture, collapse, and form thin, light brown crusts. *S. aureus* belonging to phage group II can be cultured from the contents of intact bullae. The uncommon bullous variant of varicella probably represents the occurrence of superinfection by *S. aureus* (phage group II) of varicella lesions. Pemphigus neonatorum (Ritter's disease) is an extensive form of bullous impetigo, often accompanied by fever, and represents the staphylococcal "scalded-skin syndrome" in the newborn (see Fig. A7-13). This type of infection, in the past, has spread in epidemics in infant nurseries.

Staphylococcal scalded-skin syndrome (see also Chap. 55).
DEFINITION. This is the most severe form of skin disease due to the exfoliative exotoxin produced by *S. aureus* of phage group II, and is characterized by generalized bulla formation and exfoliation. Unlike bullous impetigo, where the staphylococcal infection is in the skin at the site of the lesion, in the staphylococcal "scalded-skin syndrome" (SSSS) the infection often is at a distant site or not on the skin at all (bacteremia, localized abscesses, conjunctivitis).

A more general term, toxic epidermal necrolysis (TEN, Lyell's syndrome) (see Chap. 54 for illustrations), is often used to include both SSSS and a morphologically identical syndrome due to other etiologies (viral infections, drug reactions). However, since drug-induced TEN can be distinguished histologically from SSSS, it is reasonable to reserve the term TEN only for the drug-induced (and virus-related) syndrome and SSSS for the staphylococcal process.

BACTERIOLOGY AND PATHOGENESIS. Only staphylococci belonging to phage group II (types 3A, 3B, 3C, 55, 71) appear to be responsible for the staphylococcal scalded-skin syndrome. Exfoliative toxin (ET) is produced by these organisms in vivo or in vitro on enriched media with 10% CO_2. The toxins (there are probably four molecular species) are relatively heat-stable proteins with molecular weights of about 24,000. They are antigenic and distinct from the *a*-hemolysin of *S. aureus*. The genes for ET production in some strains of *S. aureus* are extrachromosomal; in other strains they are chromosomally determined.

Staphylococcal strains isolated from the skin lesions or other sites of infection in patients with the scalded-skin syndrome, when inoculated into neonatal mice, produce generalized exfoliation. Similar changes are produced by injection of ET into mice less than 5 days of age (prior to the appearance of hair) but not in older mice. Within 1 to 2 h of injection of ET, the Nikolsky sign can be elicited. Subsequent bulla formation and exfoliation develop whether the toxin is administered intraperitoneally or subcutaneously [23]. Intradermal injection of ET in humans produces similar cutaneous changes at the site of inoculation.

PATHOLOGY. The characteristic histologic changes in SSSS are the formation of a cleavage plane high in the epidermis, in the granular cell layer, and separation of the epidermal layer by edema fluid producing typical bullae. There is little associated inflammatory reaction in the dermis or epidermis [24]. In contrast, in drug-induced TEN the split in the skin is at the basal cell level.

CLINICAL MANIFESTATIONS. Staphylococcal scalded-skin syndrome usually occurs in either newborn infants (Ritter's disease) or in young children, but it may occur in older children or rarely in adults. It begins abruptly (sometimes several days following pharyngitis, rhinorrhea, conjunctivitis, or a discrete staphylococcal infection) with diffuse erythema resembling that of scarlet fever, marked skin tenderness, and fever. Within 12 to 14 h the Nikolsky sign is present. Large flaccid bullae filled with clear fluid develop and rupture almost immediately; these are not conventional bullae but represent passive fluid accumulation beneath detached epidermis. Large sheets of skin separate, wrinkle, and exfoliate, exposing a moist, bright red surface (see Figs. 55-2 and 55-3). Because of the extensive exfoliation, temperature regulation and fluid balance are particular problems in the newborn. Generally, with appropriate antibiotic and fluid therapy, patients recover and the skin is healed within 10 to 14 days of the onset of erythema, unless secondary infection has occurred.

STAPHYLOCOCCAL SCARLET FEVER. This is identical with the generalized scarlatiniform rash with skin tenderness observed in the initial stage of SSSS. As in streptococcal scarlet fever the skin is diffusely erythematous with a sandpaper roughness. Pastia's lines are present. Pharyngitis is not a feature usually, but patients are febrile for the first few days. The strawberry tongue and palatal enanthem are not seen. Bullae and exfoliation do not occur although Nikolsky's sign may be present in an occasional patient. After 2 to 5 days of erythema, desquamation begins, initially on the face, and extends to involve most of the body. Healing of the skin occurs within 10 days.

Staphylococci belonging to phage group II are recovered from sites of staphylococcal infection (conjunctivitis, abscesses, bacteremia, external otitis). Staphylococcal scarlet fever can be considered a forme fruste of SSSS.

Toxic shock syndrome. DEFINITION. The toxic shock syndrome (TSS) is an acute febrile illness due to certain toxin-producing strains of *S. aureus* and characterized by a generalized erythematous eruption. Additional elements making up the syndrome include (1) hypotension, (2) functional abnormalities in at least three organ systems, and (3) desquamation following the scarlatiniform eruption. Over 1600 cases occurred in a nationwide outbreak between 1979 and 1982 primarily, but not exclusively, in menstruating women [25].

BACTERIOLOGY AND PATHOGENESIS. *S. aureus* strains isolated from patients with TSS are usually penicillin-resistant and over 93 percent of them produce two exotoxins, pyrogenic exotoxin C and enterotoxin F. (In contrast, only 12 to 14 percent of *S. aureus* strains from patients with other types of staphylococcal infections make these toxins. It is likely that the two exotoxins represent different activities of the same protein. Since *S. aureus* bacteremia is rare in association with TSS and since the manifestations of this illness involve multiple organ systems, TSS is thought to be mediated by these (or other) exotoxins.

About 85 to 90 percent of cases of TSS have occurred in women at the time of menstruation; almost all have been tampon (particularly superabsorbent types) users. *S. aureus* has been isolated from vaginal cultures of more than 90 percent of menstruating women with TSS, but from only 10 percent of healthy menstruating women. Staphylococcal infections (soft tissue, bone, lung) in children, men, and nonmenstruating women have accounted for the remaining 10 to 15 percent of cases of TSS. Cervicovaginal ulcerations, possibly produced or aggravated by tampon use, may have provided the initiating infection and the portal for toxin absorption in menstruating women who developed TSS.

CLINICAL MANIFESTATIONS. Fever, hypotension (or shock) and an erythematous rash are the initial hallmarks of TSS. The rash may be indistinguishable from that of scarlet fever or may be less striking and suggest the flush associated with fever. Desquamation of palms and soles occurs one to two weeks later. Other early clinical features may include pharyngeal redness, strawberry tongue, conjunctival injection, diarrhea, and vomiting. Evidences of multiple other organ dysfunctions are seen in TSS: (1) *muscular system*—myalgias and rhabdomyolysis, (2) *central nervous system*—toxic encephalopathy, (3) *kidney*—azotemia, (4) *liver*—elevated levels of SGOT and serum bilirubin, (5) *blood*—thrombocytopenia.

LABORATORY FINDINGS. Leukocytosis and thrombocytopenia are usually present. Microscopic hematuria may be present. Elevated BUN and creatinine levels occur in the majority of patients, and abnormal liver function tests are frequent. Increased serum creatinine kinase levels reflect muscle injury, and myoglobinuria occurs in some patients. Hypocalcemia occurs in many patients but the basis is unclear.

DIAGNOSIS AND DIFFERENTIAL DIAGNOSIS. Diagnosis is made on the basis of the clinical constellation of findings in a patient who has a *S. aureus* infection or in a menstruating woman, particularly if a tampon user. The differential diagnosis includes scarlet fever (not usually associated with hypotension or shock), SSSS (in which bullae and a positive Nikolsky sign are expected), a febrile drug reaction (not usually associated with hypotension), Kawasaki's disease (usually in children and features prominent lymphadenopathy), and meningococcemia (in which rash is petechial rather than scarlatiniform).

TREATMENT. Staphylococcal impetigo responds quite promptly to appropriate treatment. In the adult oxacillin (or similar penicillinase-resistant semisynthetic penicillin) 0.5 g orally 4 times daily or erythromycin (in the penicillin-allergic patient) 0.25 g orally 4 times daily should be used if the process is extensive or bullous in character. Treatment should be continued for 5 to 7 days (10 days if streptococci are isolated). Local treatment with removal of crusts and maintenance of cleanliness, as in the management of streptococcal impetigo, is sufficient to cure many mild cases. However, the results are further improved, particularly in extensive cases, by the administration of antibiotics, as noted above. The frequency of isolation of group A streptococci makes systemic antibiotic therapy a reasonable approach in most patients with a significant degree of involvement.

Intravenous use of a penicillinase-resistant penicillin (nafcillin or oxacillin) is indicated in the initial treatment of *S. aureus* scalded-skin syndrome and of staphylococcal scarlet fever because of the relation of these processes to active staphylococcal infections of the skin or elsewhere and because of the rapid progression and potential seriousness of the illness. Nafcillin is administered at a dosage of 50 to 100 mg/kg per day in the newborn and at a dosage of 100 to 200 mg/kg per day (in divided doses every 4 to 6 h) for older children. The adult dose is 6 to 10 g daily, in divided doses every 4 to 6 h. Oxacillin is administered in similar dosage. A switch to oral therapy (e.g., cloxacillin 50 mg/kg per day in divided doses every 6 h) should not be made until there has been extensive clearing of the lesions or the initiating focus of staphylococcal infection has been controlled.

Systemic corticosteroids alone should not be used in the treatment of SSSS. Their use clinically has been associated with continued progression of the lesions and in hydrocor-

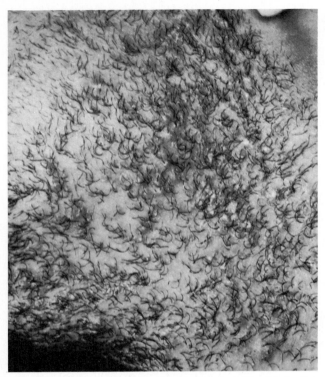

Fig. 176-8 Sycosis barbae. Deep chronic folliculitis in the bearded area.

tisone-treated experimental animals only 1/100 to 1/1000 of the usual infecting dose of *S. aureus* was needed to produce exfoliation [23]. Corticosteroid therapy may be indicated in the treatment of drug-induced TEN. In cases of TEN where it is unclear whether a staphylococcal etiology or drug sensitivity is responsible, consideration may be given to the use of combined antibiotic and corticosteroid therapy.

For topical management of the lesions of SSSS and TEN, cool saline compresses are used. Flurandrenolide ointment (0.025 to 0.05%) may be useful subsequently in selected cases where there is no direct infection of the skin.

Treatment of TSS involves (1) immediate institution of vigorous fluid replacement to combat the hypotension, (2) attention to focal staphylococcal infections (drainage of abscesses, removal of tampons), and systemic antimicrobial therapy aimed at penicillinase-producing *S. aureus* (nafcillin 1.0 to 1.5 g intravenously in the adult every 4 h).

Folliculitis. This is a pyoderma located within the hair follicle. There are two main subdivisions: superficial and deep. Follicular impetigo (Bockhart's impetigo) is a superficial folliculitis. It is a form of impetigo in which a small dome-shaped pustule occurs at the opening of a hair follicle, often on the scalps of children. There are several distinctive forms of deep folliculitis.

SYCOSIS BARBAE. This is a deep folliculitis with perifollicular inflammation occurring in the bearded areas of the face (Figs. 176-8 and A1-22). If uncared for, the lesions become deeper seated and chronic. Local treatment with warm saline compresses and local antibiotics (bacitracin) is sufficient to control the infection. More extensive cases

require systemic antibiotic therapy. The major condition to be considered in differential diagnosis is tinea barbae. In the latter fungal infection, the hairs are usually broken or loosened and there are suppurative nodules rather than discrete pustules.

LUPOID SYCOSIS. This is a deep, chronic, cicatricial form of sycosis barbae, usually occurring as a circinate lesion.

"CORAL REEF GRANULOMA." This rare disease begins as a staphylococcal folliculitis, usually on sun-exposed areas of the upper extremities, and spreads peripherally with ulcerations, erosions, and sinus tract formation [26]. There is profuse purulent drainage from multiple openings of burrowing lesions. The process continues for many months with active infection, scarring, and pseudoepitheliomatous hyperplasia progressing apace. Ultimately, the process burns itself out leaving an irregular "coral reef" scar.

Furuncles and carbuncles. DEFINITION. A furuncle, or boil, is a deep-seated inflammatory nodule which develops about a hair follicle, usually from a preceding, more superficial folliculitis. A carbuncle is a more extensive, deeper, infiltrated lesion which develops when suppuration occurs in thick inelastic skin.

CLINICAL MANIFESTATIONS

History. Furuncles occur only in areas where there are hair follicles, particularly in regions subject to friction and perspiration: neck, face, axillae, buttocks. They may complicate preexisting lesions such as scabies, pediculosis, or abrasions; but more often occur in the absence of any local predisposing causes. In addition, a variety of systemic host factors is associated with furunculosis. These include obesity, blood dyscrasias, defects in neutrophil function (defects in chemotaxis associated with eczema and high levels of IgE; defects in intracellular killing of organisms as in chronic granulomatous disease of childhood), treatment with corticosteroids and cytotoxic agents, and immune globulin deficiency states. Whether diabetes mellitus predisposes to furunculosis is still controversial; once established, however, the process is often more extensive in patients with diabetes. The majority of patients with problems of furunculosis appear to be otherwise healthy.

Cutaneous lesions. A furuncle starts as a hard, tender, red nodule which enlarges and becomes painful and fluctuant after several days (Fig. A1-23). Rupture occurs, with discharge of pus and often a core of necrotic material. The pain about the lesion then subsides, and the redness and edema diminish over several days to several weeks.

A *carbuncle* is a larger, more serious inflammatory lesion with a deeper base. It characteristically occurs as an extremely painful lesion at the nape of the neck, the back, or thighs. Fever and malaise often are present, and the patient may appear quite ill. The involved area is red, and indurated and multiple pustules soon appear on the surface, draining externally around multiple hair follicles. The lesion soon develops a yellow-gray irregular crater at the center which may then heal slowly by granulating, although the area may remain deeply violaceous for a prolonged period. The resulting permanent scar is often dense and readily evident.

LABORATORY FINDINGS. Extensive furunculosis or a carbuncle may be associated with a leukocytosis, particularly when there is a large amount of unliberated pus, surrounding cellulitis, or bacteremia. *S. aureus* is almost always the etiology of furuncles and carbuncles.

PATHOLOGY. A dense polymorphonuclear inflammatory process in the subcutaneous fat characterizes a carbuncle. Multiple abscesses, separated by connective tissue trabeculae, infiltrate the dermis and pass along the edges of the hair follicles, reaching the surface through openings in the undermined epidermis.

DIAGNOSIS AND DIFFERENTIAL DIAGNOSIS. The diagnosis is made on the basis of the clinical appearance. Simple folliculitis, due to *S. aureus* or *S. epidermidis,* is easily distinguished by the absence of significant redness and induration about the hair follicle.

COURSE AND PROGNOSIS. The major problems with furunculosis and carbuncles are bacteremic spread of infection and recurrence. Lesions about the lips and nose raise the specter of spread via the facial and angular emissary veins to the cavernous sinus. Invasion of the bloodstream may occur from furuncles or carbuncles at any time, in an unpredictable fashion, producing osteomyelitis, acute endocarditis, brain abscess, or other metastatic foci. *Squeezing such lesions is particularly dangerous and frequently produces spread of infection via the bloodstream.* Fortunately, these complications are not common.

Recurrent furunculosis is a troublesome process which may recur over many years. Most often these lesions are limited to the area of the follicles, but sometimes they extend to produce surrounding cellulitis or bacteremia. Individuals who perspire excessively or who have poor skin hygiene appear more disposed to recurrent furunculosis.

TREATMENT. *Simple furunculosis* may be treated by local application of moist heat, which relieves discomfort, aids in the localization of the infection, and promotes drainage. Such cases do not require the use of either local or systemic antibiotics. A *carbuncle* or a *furuncle* with surrounding cellulitis, or one associated with fever, should be treated with a systemic antibiotic. In view of the high frequency of penicillin-resistant *S. aureus,* a semisynthetic penicillin such as oxacillin (0.50 to 0.75 g orally every 4 to 6 h in the adult) should be used. In the penicillin-allergic adult, clindamycin (150 to 300 mg orally 4 times a day) or erythromycin (0.25 to 0.5 g orally 4 times daily) may be substituted. For severe infections or infections in a dangerous area, maximal antibiotic dosage should be employed by the parenteral route, the patient should be put to bed, and the involved area should be immobilized. Antibiotic treatment should be continued for at least 1 week.

When the lesions are large but localized, painful, and fluctuant, drainage (limited to the necrotic fluctuant area) is indicated. Antimicrobial therapy should be continued until evidences of inflammation have regressed. After adequate drainage (spontaneous or surgical) has occurred, moist dressings should not be applied because of the danger of local spread enhanced by tissue maceration. Application of a thin layer of bacitracin ointment (500 units/g) about the lesion protects the surrounding skin. Such draining lesions should be covered with a sterile dressing to prevent autoinoculation. Hands should be thoroughly washed after contact with the lesions.

The management of patients with *recurrent furunculosis* presents a special and frequently exasperating problem. There is no evidence that this disease is due to any specific

staphylococcal strains with special biologic properties. In addition to the treatment of acute lesions, as above, management involves steps in the prophylaxis of recurrent episodes:

1. Careful evaluation for underlying causes.
    a. Systemic processes: previously discussed.
    b. Specific localized predisposing factors: industrial exposure to chemicals, oils; poor hygiene; obesity; hyperhidrosis.
    c. Sources of staphylococcal contact: pyogenic infections in the family; contact sports such as wrestling; autoinoculation; nasal carriage.
2. General skin care. The aim of these measures is to reduce the numbers of *S. aureus* on the skin. General skin care of both hands and body with water and soap is important. The patient should avoid trauma to the skin, as well as potential skin irritants such as strong soaps and deodorants. A separate washcloth (and towel) should be used and carefully washed in *hot* water prior to reuse.
3. Care of clothing. Large numbers of staphylococci are frequently present on the sheets and underclothing of patients with furunculosis and may cause reinfection of the patient and infection of other members of the family. In problem cases it is not unreasonable to recommend that these items be carefully and separately washed in boiling water, and changed daily.
4. Care of dressings. Dressings should be changed frequently if purulent drainage collects. They should be carefully discarded into a paper bag that can be sealed and disposed of immediately.
5. General measures. Despite the above measures, some patients continue to have recurrent cycles of lesions. Sometimes the problem can be ameliorated or abolished by removing the patient from the regular routine of work. This is particularly pertinent in individuals under considerable emotional stress and physical fatigue. A vacation for several weeks, ideally in a cool, dry climate, may help considerably by providing rest and also the time needed for carrying out the program of careful skin care.
6. Measures of unproved worth.
    a. Staphylococcal vaccines of various types (autogenous, toxoid made from exotoxins, and bacteriophage-lysed preparations) have been used in attempts to protect against infection by inducing further humoral immunity. A controlled evaluation of the use of a staphylococcal bacteriophage-lysed vaccine showed that it had no significant effect on the course of recurrent furunculosis [27].
    b. Local use of antibiotic ointments (bacitracin) in the nasal vestibule has been suggested. It does reduce the nasal carriage of *S. aureus* and secondarily reduces the "shedding" of organisms on the skin. Such an approach may be justified in cases of recurrent furunculosis not responding to the measures outlined earlier. However, controlled studies of its use are lacking.
    c. Use of rifampin orally may be tried, when other measures have failed, to eradicate (at least temporarily) nasal carriage of *S. aureus* and thus, perhaps, minimize the possible role of nasal shedding in per-

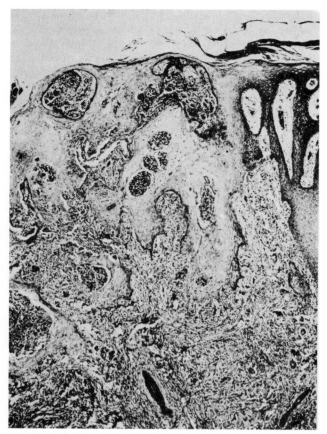

Fig. 176-9 Staphylococcal botryomycosis. This is not a fungal disease, but the photomicrograph is reproduced here because the microscopic pathologic change is easily confused with that of actinomycosis. X100. (AFIP 130847. Micrograph by Wallace H. Clark, Jr., M.D. Courtesy of Dr. Elson B. Helwig.)

petuation of this cycle. Rifampin, in a dose of 600 mg orally daily for 10 days, has eliminated the nasal carrier state in some healthy carriers [28]. To minimize the emergence of rifampin-resistant strains (particularly when carriage is of methicillin-resistant strains), use of the combination of rifampin plus trimethoprim has also been studied [29].

Hidradenitis suppurativa. (See also Chap. 70.) DEFINITION. This is an extremely troublesome, chronic, recurrent, suppurative infection of blocked aprocrine glands occurring in the axillary, perianal, and genital regions. The organisms initially found may be *S. aureus,* but subsequently the predominant organisms may be gram-negative bacilli such as *Proteus.*

CLINICAL MANIFESTATIONS. (Figs. 70-7 and 70-8). The initial lesions are tender, reddish purple nodules, appearing very much like furuncles. They subsequently become fluctuant, drain, and form irregular sinus tracts. Repeated crops of nodules with further burrowing constitute the usual sequence. Vegetative granular masses develop with deep boggy nodules, and there is marked hypertrophic scarring. The lesions occur in either men or women, but always after puberty. With extensive involvement, some patients exhibit constitutional symptoms such as fever and

weight loss. The chronic process may eventually become quiescent after destroying most of the apocrine glands of the body.

DIFFERENTIAL DIAGNOSIS. To be considered in the differential diagnosis are acne conglobata, multiple infected sebaceous cysts, and cutaneous blastomycosis. Predominant involvement about the inguinal and perianal areas may suggest lymphogranuloma venereum.

TREATMENT. Treatment is difficult because of the multiple, deep-seated sites of inflammation and infection not accessible to antibiotics. However, guided by Gram-stained samples and cultural evidence (as well as in vitro susceptibility tests), one can employ an appropriate systemic antibiotic. This will not cure the disease but will help to quiet the active acute process. Local moist heat may help to establish drainage, but surgical drainage of the frank abscesses is usually mandatory. Unfortunately, this does not prevent recurrent infection in many residual, blind-ended sinus tracts. In the very severe cases that are marked by chronicity and scarring and have resisted the above measures, radical surgical excision of most of the involved area, followed by skin grafting, may be the only avenue remaining. This is a very extensive and difficult surgical procedure requiring considerable skill and experience. Excision of isolated, resistant, infected apocrine glands is also sometimes effective therapy.

Actinophytosis (botryomycosis). This a very rare pyogenic disease in humans (Fig. 176-9). The lesions (usually solitary) can occur in skin, bone, liver, etc., and, on gross examination of the pus, pinhead-sized, whitish yellow granules are evident. When examined under the microscope, as on a fresh mount or in 20% potassium hydroxide (KOH), these granules appear coarsely lobulated and are seen to contain tightly packed clublike projections (resembling the ''sulfur granules'' of actinomycosis). Examination of Gram-stained preparations of crushed granules shows only masses of staphylococci, not the ray fungus appearance of actinomycosis. Cultures grow out typical *S. aureus.*

The cases of involvement of the skin in *botryomycosis* have usually had a solitary lesion or only a few lesions, often occurring in the genital area. The lesion has the gross appearance of an infected sebaceous cyst, with mild reddening of the skin over the circumscribed, slightly tender mass. In the majority of reported cases, a foreign body (fish bone, broom straw, etc.) has played a role in initiating or perpetuating the lesion. Surgical drainage will usually produce rapid resolution.

It appears that this rare lesion may be related in some way to a balance between numbers of organisms and host defenses. This condition should not be mistaken for granuloma pyogenicum (which has been given also the confusing designation botryomycosis hominis), a lesion that consists of small, pedunculated, raspberry-like vegetations of overgrowth of granulation tissue, particularly newly formed blood vessels, occurring at the site of trauma.

Skin lesions in *S. aureus* bacteremia and endocarditis. In acute bacteremia or endocarditis due to *S. aureus,* skin lesions can provide a clue to the nature of the infecting organism. These lesions include pustules, subcutaneous abscesses, and purulent purpura. The purulent purpura

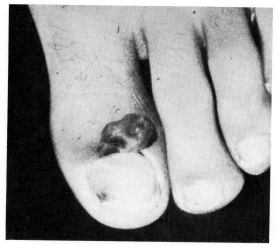

Fig. 176-10   A skin lesion of staphylococcal bacteremia.

consists of an area of purpura with a white purulent center (Fig. 176-10). Gram-stained smear of the aspirated contents of the center shows gram-positive cocci in clusters and polymorphonuclear inflammatory cells.

Rarely, a patient will develop multiple, tender, 2- to 4-cm nodules in the subcutaneous tissues as part of a systemic staphylococcal infection. The overlying skin is mildly erythematous. The nodules are firm and do not suppurate. The lesions are often found on the trunk and in this location suggest those of Weber-Christian disease (relapsing febrile nonsuppurative panniculitis). Low-grade fever is associated with these lesions, but the patients do not appear acutely ill. Blood cultures have only occasionally been positive, although the lesions probably represent metastatic infection in the subcutaneous tissue. Biopsy shows a nonspecific inflammatory response, and culture of the nodule shows *S. aureus*. The lesions promptly regress on antibiotic treatment.

Cutaneous manifestations of infections due to *Clostridium perfringens (C. welchii)*

Anaerobic cellulitis and gas gangrene (myonecrosis) are two forms of C. *perfringens* infection involving subcutaneous tissues and muscles, respectively. The etiologic agent is an obligate anaerobe that is normally found in the bowel. Cutaneous manifestations are evident in each process. It should be recalled, however, that gas-forming infections may sometimes be caused by *Escherichia coli, Klebsiella, Bacteroides,* or anaerobic streptococci (see Chap. 177).

Anaerobic cellulitis

This is a clostridial infection of devitalized tissue usually occurring in a dirty or inadequately debrided wound several days after injury. The onset is more gradual than in gas gangrene. The anaerobes are able to grow in the depths of the wound and extend rapidly through tissue planes, with attendant formation of large quantities of gas. A thin, dark gray-brown, foul, serous discharge is produced. Gram-stained smear of the drainage reveals short, plump, blunt-ended, gram-positive rods without spores and with a

variable number of polymorphonuclear leukocytes. Unlike clinical gas gangrene, there is relatively little local pain or edema, change in overlying skin, toxemia, or extension of the process to involve muscle. At operation the muscles appear normal, but gas may extend diffusely and is readily evident through the exudate. This type of infection must be distinguished from clostridial myositis (gas gangrene) to avoid needless mutilating surgery and amputations. Treatment consists of opening the wound, removing necrotic debris, and administering antibiotics (penicillin preferably, or a broad-spectrum antibiotic). Antitoxin administration is not necessary.

Anaerobic myositis (myonecrosis)

This is a rapidly progressing, toxemic, potentially lethal infection involving muscle but with secondary changes in the overlying skin. The infection may develop as a complication of a traumatic dirty wound with extensive muscle and soft-tissue damage. In addition, gas gangrene also may occur after surgery on the bowel or gallbladder.

The incubation period is often short (12 to 24 h) but may be delayed, and occasionally gas gangrene develops following anaerobic cellulitis. The first symptom is usually local pain, followed by edema. Gas formation is not prominent and may be completely obscured by local swelling of the subcutaneous tissues. The skin often takes on a dark yellow or bronze discoloration, with tense blebs or bullae containing dark brown fluid. A serosanguineous exudate can be expressed from the wound. Gram's stain of the exudate reveals plump gram-positive rods and only a few white blood cells. Subsequently, green-black patches of necrosis of the skin at the margin of the wound may develop. Evidences of toxemia are present: high fever, tachycardia, hypotension, and oliguria. Intravascular hemolysis does not usually occur in this type of process, in contrast to septic abortion with septicemia due to this organism.

Treatment consists of wide surgical debridement of all devitalized muscle and parenteral administration of penicillin in dosage of about 10,000,000 units daily. The use of hyperbaric oxygen "drenching," particularly in patients with far-advanced disease involving the trunk in whom surgical excision would be mutilating, appears to have a place in current therapy. Polyvalent gas gangrene antitoxin (40,000 to 60,000 units every 6 h for several doses) has been administered often in the past, but there has been no clear evidence of its efficacy. This antiserum is no longer commercially available.

Erythrasma

Definition

Erythrasma is a common superficial bacterial infection of the skin characterized by well-defined but irregular reddish brown patches occurring in the intertriginous areas.

Epidemiology

Erythrasma is widespread and has been found in about 20 percent of subjects randomly studied in a temperate climate. The generalized disease is much more common in the tropics. It is more common in men, where it may be present in an asymptomatic form in the genitocrural area. It does not appear to be significantly contagious [30].

Etiology

The causative agent has been shown to be not a dermatophyte or *Nocardia* species, as was formerly believed, but a *Corynebacterium* species. The organism is a short, gram-positive rod with subterminal granules. It is best cultivated on a medium containing 20% fetal bovine serum, 78% tissue culture medium No. 199 in 2% agar and 0.05% Tris, pH 6.8 to 7.2. Growth occurs as small, shiny, moist, whitish gray translucent colonies, which fluoresce orange to coral-red under Wood's lamp.

Clinical manifestations

History. The manifestations vary from a completely asymptomatic form, through a genitocrural form with considerable pruritus, to a generalized form with scaly lamellated plaques on the trunk and extremities.

Cutaneous lesions (Fig. A6-18). The lesions are reddish brown, rather superficial, finely scaly and finely wrinkled, and slowly spreading macular patches. Axillary and genitocrural areas are the principal sites of infection.

Pathology

Gram-stained imprints of the horny layer of the skin show rod-like, gram-positive organisms in large numbers. Bacilli have been demonstrated within cells of the horny layer on examination by electron microscope.

Diagnosis

The diagnosis is strongly suggested by the location and superficial character of the process. A characteristic "coral-red" fluorescence seen over the involved areas under Wood's lamp confirms the diagnosis. Cultivation of the specific *Corynebacterium* in abundance from the lesion corroborates the diagnosis. Tinea versicolor is distinguished from erythrasma by the lesions on the trunk seen in the former. Tinea cruris is more rapidly progressive and has a deeper, more inflammatory character.

Treatment

A 5- to 7-day course of erythromycin, 1.0 g orally daily, usually produces clearing of the lesions within several weeks. Topical antibiotics are not as effective.

Course and prognosis

The disease may remain asymptomatic for years or may undergo periodic exacerbations. Relapses occasionally occur even after successful antibiotic treatment.

References

1. Duma RH et al: Streptococcal infections. A bacteriologic and clinical study of streptococcal bacteremia. *Medicine (Baltimore)* **48**:87, 1969

2. Uhr JW (ed): *The Streptococcus, Rheumatic Fever, and Glomerulonephritis*. Baltimore, Williams & Wilkins, 1964

3. Wannamaker LW: Differences between streptococcal infections of the throat and of the skin. *N Engl J Med* **282**:23, 78, 1970

4. Bisno AL: Acute rheumatic fever: current concepts and controversies, in *Current Clinical Topics in Infectious Disease 5*, edited by JS Remington, MN Swartz. New York, McGraw-Hill, 1984, p 316

5. Dillon HC Jr: Impetigo contagiosa: suppurative and nonsuppurative complications. *Am J Dis Child* **115**:530, 1968

6. Dajani AS et al: Natural history of impetigo. II. Etiologic agents and bacterial interactions. *J Clin Invest* **51**:2863, 1972

7. Mobacken H et al: Epidemiologic aspects of impetigo contagiosa in western Sweden. *Scand J Infect Dis* **7**:39, 1975

8. Ferrieri P et al: Natural history of impetigo. I. Site sequence of acquisition and familial patterns of spread of cutaneous streptococci. *J Clin Invest* **51**:2851, 1972

9. Allen AM et al: Cutaneous streptococcal infections in Vietnam. *Arch Dermatol* **104**:271, 1971

10. Amren DP: Unusual forms of streptococcal disease, in *Streptococci and Streptococcal Diseases,* edited by LW Wannamaker, JM Matsen. New York, Academic Press, 1972, p 545

11. Baddour LM, Bisno AL: Recurrent cellulitis after saphenous venectomy for coronary bypass surgery. *Ann Intern Med* **97**:493, 1982

12. Meleney FL: Hemolytic streptococcus gangrene. *Arch Surg* **9**:317, 1924

13. Giuliano A et al: Bacteriology of necrotizing fasciitis. *Am J Surg* **134**:52, 1977

14. Casali RE et al: Postoperative necrotizing fasciitis of the abdominal wall. *Am J Surg* **140**:787, 1980

15. Finegold SM: *Anaerobic Bacteria in Human Disease.* New York, Academic Press, 1977, chap 13

16. Stone HH, Martin JJ Jr: Synergistic necrotizing cellulitis. *Ann Surg* **175**:702, 1972

17. Stamenkovic I, Lew PD: Early recognition of potentially fatal necrotizing faciitis. The use of frozen-section biopsy. *N Engl J Med* **310**:1689, 1984

18. Brewer GE, Meleney FL: Progressive gangrenous infection of the skin and subcutaneous tissues, following operation for acute perforative appendicitis. A study in symbiosis. *Ann Surg* **84**:438, 1926

19. Meleney FL: Bacterial synergism in disease processes with a confirmation of the synergistic bacterial etiology of a certain type of progressive gangrene of the abdominal wall. *Ann Surg* **94**:961, 1931

20. Alpert JS et al: Pathogenesis of Osler's nodes. *Ann Intern Med* **85**:471, 1976

21. Tuazon CU: Skin and skin structure infections in the patient at risk: carrier state of *Staphylococcus aureus. Am J Med* **76(5A)**:166, 1984

22. Dajani AS: The scalded-skin syndrome: relation to phage-group II staphylococci. *J Infect Dis* **125**:548, 1972

23. Melish ME et al: The staphylococcal epidermolytic toxin: its isolation, characterization, and site of action. *Ann NY Acad Sci* **236**:317, 1974

24. Elias PM et al: Staphylococcal scalded skin syndrome: clinical features, pathogenesis, and recent microbiological and biochemical developments. *Arch Dermatol* **113**:207, 1977

25. Institute of Medicine, National Academy of Science: Conference on the Toxic Shock Syndrome. *Ann Intern Med* **96**:835, 1982

26. Georgouras K: Coral reef granuloma. *Cutis* **3**:37, 1967

27. Bryant RE et al: Treatment of recurrent furunculosis with staphylococcal bacteriophage-lysed vaccine. *JAMA* **194**:123, 1965

28. Wheat LJ et al: Long-term studies of the effect of rifampin on nasal carriage of coagulase-positive staphylococci. *Rev Infect Dis* **5**:S459, 1983

29. Ward TT et al: Observations relating to an inter-hospital outbreak of methicillin-resistant *Staphylococcus aureus:* role of antimicrobial therapy in infection control. *Infect Control* **2**:453, 1981

30. Sarkany I et al: The etiology and treatment of erythrasma. *J Invest Dermatol* **37**:283, 1961

Bibliography

Bonventre PF et al: Production of staphylococcal enterotoxin F and pyrogenic enterotoxin C by *Staphylococcus aureus* isolates from toxic shock syndrome-associated sources. *Infect Immun* **40**:1023, 1983

Dillon HC: Streptococcal infections of the skin and their complications: impetigo and nephritis, in *Streptococci and Strepto-coccal Diseases,* edited by LW Wannamaker, JM Matsen. New York, Academic Press, 1972, p 571

Dillon HC et al: M-antigens common to pyoderma and acute glomerulonephritis. *J Infect Dis* **130**:257, 1974

Kapral FA, Miller MM: Product of *Staphylococcus aureus* responsible for the scalded-skin syndrome. *Infect Immun* **4**:541, 1971

Koblenzer PJ: Acute epidermal necrolysis (Ritter von Rittershain-Lyell). A clinicopathologic study. *Arch Dermatol* **95**:608, 1967

Lyell A: A review of toxic epidermal necrolysis in Britain. *Br J Dermatol* **79**:662, 1967

Rammelkamp CH Jr: Epidemiology of streptococcal infections. *Harvey Lect* **51**:113, 1957

Rudolph RI et al: Treatment of staphylococcal toxic epidermal necrolysis. *Arch Dermatol* **110**:559, 1974

Schievert PM: Staphylococcal scarlet fever: role of pyrogenic exotoxins. *Infect Immun* **31**:732, 1981

CHAPTER 177

GRAM-NEGATIVE COCCAL AND BACILLARY INFECTIONS

Arnold N. Weinberg and Morton N. Swartz

Many of the characteristic cutaneous manifestations of infection with gram-negative organisms are due to direct microbial invasion of the skin or subcutaneous tissues. In addition, platelet depression, the dermal or generalized Shwartzman reaction, disseminated intravascular coagulation, and effects of toxic products of these bacteria may produce varied hemorrhagic cutaneous manifestations. The typical skin lesions in meningococcal or *Pseudomonas* septicemia, often among the earliest indications of generalized infection, can provide immediate and important clues to early diagnosis.

Infections due to *Neisseria meningitidis* (meningococcus)

General features

Three clinical syndromes associated with cutaneous involvement occur in meningococcal disease: meningitis, acute meningococcemia, and chronic meningococcemia. Skin lesions are frequently the most dramatic manifestations and graphically add to the aura of fear attached to these infections.

Bacteriology and pathogenesis

The *Neisseria* are obligate, aerobic, gram-negative, kidney bean-shaped cocci that pair with their long axes in parallel. *N. meningitidis* grows well on blood-enriched media (chocolate agar), supplemented by an atmosphere containing 5 to 10 percent CO_2 and approximately 50 percent humidity. In potentially mixed bacterial exudates these organisms should be grown on a selective medium (e.g., Thayer-Martin); they can be distinguished from *N. gonorrhoeae* by their fermentation of both glucose and maltose rather than of glucose alone. Meningococci are separable into 13 serologic groups on the basis of capsular antigens. Agglutination and capsular swelling reactions identify groups A, B, C, Y, and W135 as the major pathogens involved in human disease today [1].

The presence of virulent strains colonizing the nasal mucous membranes of a nonimmune host precedes clinical disease. Initial colonization may be facilitated by pili that attach to specific receptors on mucosal epithelial cells [2,3] and by production of an IgA protease which neutralizes host secretory IgA [4]. Encapsulated organisms resist phagocytosis and with the onset of a viral respiratory infection they may multiply locally and invade the blood stream or be aspirated into the lower respiratory tract. Meningitis, meningococcemia, or pneumonitis can result. Predisposition to sporadic and occasionally recurrent meningococcal disease occurs in patients with congenital or acquired complement deficiencies, particularly late-acting components C5 to C8 [4a,4b].

The skin lesions associated with meningococcemia and meningococcal meningitis result from damage to small dermal blood vessels. By light and electron microscopy, bacteria are found within endothelial and polymorphonuclear cells [5]. Organisms can sometimes be seen when aspirates from involved areas of skin are Gram-stained. Local endothelial damage, thrombosis, and necrosis of the vessel walls occur. Immunoglobulins and complement are present, even in early vascular lesions [5]. Edema, infarction of overlying skin, and extravasation of red blood cells are responsible for the characteristic macular, papular, pete-chial, hemorrhagic, and bullous lesions. Similar vascular lesions occur in the meninges and in other tissues.

In addition to direct involvement of skin vessels by me-ningococci, many of the cutaneous hemorrhagic lesions may be due to the direct effects of endotoxin, or via the *dermal* Shwartzman reaction. Data supporting this view have been presented showing that purified meningococcal endotoxin, in contrast to endotoxin derived from *Esche-richia coli*, was uniquely potent in production of the dermal Shwartzman reaction in mice [6]. The frequency of hem-orrhagic cutaneous manifestations in meningococcal infec-tions, compared to infections with other gram-negative organisms, may be due to increased potency and/or unique properties of meningococcal endotoxins for the dermal re-action. On the other hand, lipopolysaccharide (LPS) en-dotoxins from meningococci and *E. coli* are equally potent producers of the *generalized* Shwartzman reaction and le-thality in mice [6].

The profound effects on small blood vessels, directly related to bacterial invasion or indirectly due to LPS en-dotoxin, may lead to diminished blood volume, lowered cardiac output, anoxia in vital organs, myocardial failure, hypotension, acidosis, and diffuse intravascular coagula-tion [7–9].

Meningococci can be isolated from the blood in chronic meningococcemia, usually during periodic fevers, rash, and joint manifestations. The pathogenesis of this form of disease is less well understood than that of the acute pro-cess. Recent observations have linked this chronic form of meningococcal infection to absence of terminal compo-nents of complement in several patients, an association that may provide new insights into pathogenic mechanisms in this unusual host-parasite interaction [9a]. The absence of bacteria, bacterial antigenic material, vascular damage, and granulocytic inflammation contrasts with the positive findings seen in acute infections. The chronic course of the disease, lack of endotoxin-like manifestations (even with demonstrated bacteremia), and the potentiality for meta-morphosis to meningitis or endocarditis suggest that an unusual host-parasite relationship is central to this persis-tent infection [10].

Epidemiology

Humans are the only known natural hosts and nasopha-ryngeal carrier rates vary from 5 to 15 percent ordinarily. In crowded conditions, like schools or military camps, or when a carrier of a new strain develops disease in a day-care nursery or family setting, carrier rates can increase dramatically, independent of clinical disease [11].

Asymptomatic exposure to a variety of encapsulated and nonencapsulated *N. meningitidis* strains can stimulate pro-tective bactericidal antibody [12]. In addition, a variety of nonmeningococcal microorganisms like *E. coli* K1 strains and *N. lactamica* stimulate production of cross-reacting protective antibodies to these potential pathogens [13]. Immunity to meningococci increases with age due to sub-clinical interactions with *N. meningitidis* or to other anti-genically related bacteria. As a result, protective bacteri-cidal antibodies, both IgG and IgM, are found in 70 to 95 percent of young adults [14]. Newborn infants are often resistant to meningococcal disease and this protection lasts

until approximately 3 to 6 months of age, by which time passively acquired maternal IgG antibody levels have markedly diminished [12,14]. Some young adults with acute meningococcal disease have circulating bactericidal antibody present at the outset. This paradoxical situation may be explained by the finding that such patients can have serum IgA antibody that blocks the bactericidal re-action [15]. Even though individuals acquire group-specific antibody from subclinical exposures in youth, the presence of other immune globulins may interfere with this protec-tive mechanism. Any endogenous microorganisms that stimulate IgA antibody, like *E. coli* K1 strains, could par-adoxically interfere with the protective effects of bacteri-cidal antibody [16].

In the military, sporadic cases often emerge in boot camp where young, susceptible recruits are brought together in situations of overwork, stress, and crowding. In civilian populations, adult family members probably introduce the organism into the household, but secondary cases are most frequently spread from children ages 1 through 14 to other family members in the same age group, especially under crowded conditions [17]. Household spread is 300 to 1000 times more frequent than secondary cases in the commu-nity at large [18]. An exception to this is the increased incidence of secondary cases in day-care centers where large numbers of susceptible children congregate [19].

Serogroup A isolates have most often been associated with epidemic disease, but recent experience has revealed that serogroups C and B are also identified in outbreaks as well as sporadic cases. Isolates belonging to groups Y and W135 have increased in frequency in the past decade [1]. Many of these have occurred in cases of respiratory dis-ease in older individuals. The disease occurs worldwide, including equatorial Africa ("meningitis belt") and Alaska. Most cases occur in early childhood (to age 4 years) and adolescence, but older individuals also become ill during epidemics. Absence of the spleen has been associated with severe meningococcal disease just as reported for other encapsulated organisms. *N. meningitidis* has been isolated from the genitourinary tract in individuals practicing oro-genital sex and in homosexuals [21].

Acute meningococcemia and meningitis

Clinical manifestations. HISTORY. The disease often follows a mild upper respiratory infection associated with head-ache, grippelike complaints, nausea and vomiting, and muscle soreness. These symptoms can be so brief that fever, obtundation, and other manifestations of meningitis are the initial findings. In fulminant meningococcemia, vomiting, stupor, hemorrhagic rash, and hypotension may be evident within a few hours of onset of symptoms. Milder cases, developing at a slower pace, also occur.

CUTANEOUS LESIONS. The skin findings associated with acute meningococcal infections are characteristically pe-techial, but transient urticarial, macular, or papular lesions, that can resemble viral exanthems, may be noted initially [22]. The petechiae are small and irregular, have a "smudged" appearance, and are often raised with pale grayish vesicular centers. While most commonly located on the extremities and trunk, lesions also can be found on the head, palms, soles, and mucous membranes. More extensive bullous and hemorrhagic lesions with central necrosis (suggillations) can develop (Fig. A3-17). Gangrenous hemorrhagic areas (indistinguishable from purpura fulminans) (see Chap. 176) can appear in patients with severe meningococcemia, often complicated by disseminated intravascular coagulation (DIC). Skin lesions and bacteremia are rarely seen with meningococcal pneumonia [23].

OTHER PHYSICAL FINDINGS. Patients with meningitis display signs of meningeal irritation and altered consciousness. Occasionally, agitated or maniacal behavior predominates. Cranial nerve palsies, long-tract signs, seizures, and alterations in vital signs associated with changes in intracranial pressure may be present.

Obtundation and hypotension without meningeal signs associated with the syndrome of DIC are characteristic features of acute fulminating meningococcemia [8]. Rarely, meningococcemia may result in septic foci in other areas: (1) *septic arthritis* with a pyogenic effusion in one or several joints: (2) *purulent pericarditis* with precordial pain, enlarging cardiac silhouette, and findings of cardiac tamponade; and (3) *bacterial endocarditis*. More commonly, a delayed immune complex-mediated syndrome can result in a sterile arthritis, pericarditis, or episcleritis.

Laboratory findings. A polymorphonuclear leukocytosis is present in the peripheral blood and cerebrospinal fluid (CSF). The CSF protein level is increased and the glucose value is commonly reduced. Characteristic organisms may be seen on Gram-stained smears of fluid and meningococci are usually isolated from CSF. *N. meningitidis* is isolated from the blood of approximately one-third of patients with meningitis and from almost 100 percent of patients with acute meningococcemia. Demonstration of organisms from cutaneous lesions has been variable. The most optimistic results include 27 positive smears and 35 cultured isolates in one series of 40 cases [24] and 70 percent positive petechial smears in another [25], but most modern reports indicate less success in finding organisms in skin lesions.

The development of rapid, accurate, and inexpensive procedures for detection of soluble antigens in CSF has been a major advance in laboratory methodology. The latex agglutination method is sensitive, and very specific, and is available as univalent or polyvalent reagents that will detect group A, B, C, Y, or W135 antigens in CSF and possibly in concentrates of urine [26].

Pathology. See "Bacteriology and Pathogenesis" above.

Differential diagnosis. Meningococcal infection should always be considered in a patient with fever and a petechial eruption, especially if meningitis is present. The differential diagnosis should include the following conditions:

1. *Acute bacteremias and endocarditis.* Petechial eruptions may be present, with or without changes in platelet numbers. In endocarditis, mucous membrane and conjunctival lesions as well as subungual "splinter" hemorrhages occur. In acute gonococcemia, the skin lesions are usually nodular, hemorrhagic, few in number, and usually located on the distal parts of the extremities (see Chap. 205).
2. *Acute "hypersensitivity" vasculitis.* The lesions are usually palpable, present in greatest profusion on the lower extremities, and are symmetric. Renal involvement and hypertension may be present. Pathologically, the major focus of inflammation is in precapillary arterioles (see Chap. 107).
3. *Enteroviral infections.* Fever, petechial eruptions, and aseptic meningitis are characteristic features of enteroviral disease. Echo (e.g., type 9) and Coxsackie viruses are most often implicated.
4. *Rocky Mountain spotted fever.* The history of exposure to ticks in an endemic area, absence of an antecedent respiratory infection, delay in appearance of the rash, and the location first on the distal parts of the extremities, including palms and soles, are helpful clues (see Chap. 183).
5. *Toxic shock syndrome* (see Chap. 176).

Course and prognosis. Untreated, the disease ends fatally with the exception of a rare case of meningitis. Occasionally the meningitis assumes an indolent course without therapy. The prognosis for treated meningitis or meningococcemia is excellent, with recovery in over 90 percent of patients.

In severe meningococcemia, especially with the rapid emergence of cutaneous hemorrhages, hypotension, and DIC, the entire course from onset to death can be measured in hours. These cases are often associated with massive adrenal hemorrhage (Waterhouse-Friderichsen syndrome). The mortality remains close to 100 percent, but gradations in severity of the illness make it difficult to assign an accurate prognosis in an individual case.

Chronic meningococcemia

Clinical manifestations. HISTORY. The manifestations of chronic meningococcemia are indefinite and vague at onset, but tend to establish a pattern over a period of weeks or months [27,28]. Initially, there may be an acute febrile illness, but this wanes and the patient is left with vague intermittent complaints of muscle aches and pains, joint soreness, mild headache, and anorexia with weight loss. The simultaneous emergence of a localized rash with several days of fever and joint soreness are characteristic symptoms. As the fever recedes, the rash usually fades too, and the patient may be totally free of overt skin manifestations for days at a time. This periodic fever and rash may recur over a period of a few weeks to as long as 6 to 8 months. The average duration of reported cases is 6 to 8 weeks. Untreated cases may eventually evolve into acute meningococcemia, meningitis, or endocarditis. Some recent case reports relate this syndrome to absence of a terminal component of complement, a finding also observed in some sporadic and recurrent acute meningococcal infections [9a].

CUTANEOUS LESIONS. Variability is the hallmark of the eruption associated with chronic meningococcemia. Several different types of skin lesions have been noted, usually distributed about one or more painful joints or on pressure areas. They may vary in appearance and in size (1 to 20 mm) from one crop of lesions to the next and include: (1) pale to rose-colored macular and papular lesions (the most common type), occurring in about 30 percent of cases; (2) slightly indurated and tender erythema nodosum-like nodules, mainly on the lower extremities; (3) petechiae of variable size; (4) petechiae with vesicular or pustular centers; (5) hemorrhage (minute) with an areola of paler erythema (very characteristic when it occurs); (6) gross hemorrhagic areas with pale blue-gray centers; or (7) hemorrhagic tender nodules which are located deep in the dermis.

OTHER PHYSICAL FINDINGS. Aside from the rash, the physical findings are minimal, except for occasional joint swelling and tenderness. If the disease progresses to an acute complication such as meningitis, the new findings will be those of the complicating process.

Pathology. Pathologically, the skin lesions in chronic meningococcemia differ from those in acute meningococcemia. Bacteria are absent and meningococcal antigens cannot be recognized using fluorescent antibody techniques. In addition to the absence of bacteria or their recognized products, thrombi do not occlude capillaries and venules, endothelial cell swelling is absent, and the perivascular infiltrate consists of round cells rather than the polymorphonuclear leukocytes seen in acute infections. An allergic basis for the skin lesions has been suggested in chronic meningococcemia, even though bacterial antigens are not identifiable [10].

Diagnosis and differential diagnosis. During the febrile periods, blood cultures are frequently positive and provide the specific means of diagnosis. Serologic tests have not proved helpful and there are no available data for the use of CIE or latex agglutination in chronic meningococcemia.

A number of diseases with periodic fever, skin lesions, and joint involvement resemble chronic meningococcemia, including:

1. *Subacute bacterial endocarditis.* A prolonged febrile course with a pleomorphic petechial rash, joint symptoms, and no overt focus make this an important consideration. A prominent heart murmur, evidence of renal impairment, and positive blood cultures help to establish the diagnosis.
2. *Acute rheumatic fever.* This diagnosis may be suggested when the fever is prolonged, joint findings are prominent, and macular and papular rashes appear (see Chap. 157).
3. *Henoch-Schönlein purpura.* The petechial hemorrhagic rash in association with symptoms of arthritis and fever suggests an illness not unlike chronic meningococcemia; the eruption is more often symmetric, usually on the lower extremities only, and does not have the periodicity of the rash of meningococcemia.
4. *Rat-bite fever.* This disease may be acute (mimicking acute meningococcemia) or chronic (resembling chronic meningococcemia). Intermittent fever, rash, and joint manifestations are hallmarks of an illness which follows a rodent bite or ingestion of contaminated milk (see Chap. 178).
5. *Erythema multiforme.* This diagnosis is suggested by the symmetric distribution of the eruption and the iris-type configuration of the lesions.
6. *Gonococcemia* (chronic) (Fig. A3-18). The cutaneous and joint manifestations may continue for many days or even weeks. The presence of tenosynovitis in gonococcemia, in contrast to its absence in meningococcemia, can be an important clue.

Course and prognosis. Some patients with chronic meningococcemia spontaneously recover without specific therapy, while others develop serious systemic complications, like endocarditis. The prognosis for treated infection is excellent; almost 100 percent of patients are cured with antibiotic therapy.

Treatment and prophylaxis

Chemotherapy. The therapy of meningococcal infections became complicated by the emergence of sulfonamide-resistant strains over 20 years ago. Initially, these strains belonged predominantly to serogroup B, but the majority of sulfonamide-resistant isolates in recent years have been from serogroups C or A [1]. These variations in sensitivity patterns have resulted in penicillin G supplanting the sulfonamides as the treatment of choice for acute meningococcal infections. The usual adult dosage is 2 million units intravenously every 2 h until approximately 7 days after the temperature has returned to normal. Treatment of chronic meningococcemia does not require "meningeal doses" of penicillin; 6 to 12 million units divided into 4 to 6 daily doses, intravenously or intramuscularly for 10 days, should be effective therapy. In the penicillin-allergic patient, chloramphenicol (1.0 g intravenously every 6 h) should be used. Sulfonamide-susceptible strains are ideally treated with sulfisoxazole (Gantrisin) intravenously and then orally, maintaining a blood level of 10 to 15 mg/dL for 1 week after the temperature has returned to normal.

Serotherapy. Preliminary results have been encouraging for the use of antiserum prepared in humans to a core lipopolysaccharide of the *E. coli* J5 mutant. This antibody for endotoxin appears to react with all gram-negative microorganisms and is clinically effective in preventing deaths in gram-negative infections, including *N. meningitidis* [29].

Supportive therapy. Efforts to prevent acute brain swelling are essential in patients with meningitis. These include prevention of overhydration, reduction of body temperature, and employment of agents like mannitol or dexamethasone (if evidences of rising intracranial pressure develop).

Although it has been postulated that hypotension in acute meningococcemia may be due to adrenal failure associated with the Waterhouse-Friderichsen syndrome (adrenal hemorrhage), blood cortisol levels and corticosteroid secretion rates have been found elevated in this syndrome. The modern treatment of shock in sepsis includes appropriate use of volume expanders, beta adrenergic-stimulating drugs like dopamine or isoproterenol, sodium bicarbonate infusions for severe acidosis, and, in selected patients, peripheral vasodilators and corticosteroids [30,31].

Severe meningococcal infections can be complicated by the syndrome of DIC. The diagnosis is usually made by a composite of associated hematologic abnormalities, including thrombopenia and hypofibrinogenemia, prolongation of the prothrombin time and partial thromboplastin time, and presence of fibrin split-products. If clinical bleeding occurs, fresh frozen plasma and heparin may be required. Each case must be individualized since therapy may be harmful and produce more problems than the DIC syndrome, especially if adult respiratory distress syndrome is present also [32].

Prophylaxis. Reliance on sulfonamide prophylaxis has been abandoned because of the presence of sulfonamide-resistant meningococcal strains, but the need for reliable chemoprophylaxis continues to exist. In civilian experiences, especially in association with day-care nursery exposures or crowded household contacts, secondary cases can emerge rapidly, often within 24 to 48 h of an index case [19]. Currently recommended prophylactic drug regimens in the adult favor rifampin, 600 mg orally twice daily for two days [33]; alternatively, minocycline 100 mg orally daily for five days can be used [34]. The effectiveness of these agents appears to be due to their presence in effective concentrations in upper respiratory and salivary secretions [35].

Immunization. Polysaccharide vaccines have been developed from groups A, C, Y, and W135 *N. meningitidis* and have proved to be safe and effective in preventing meningococcal disease in adults and in children over the age of 2 years [11,33]. The efficacy of the group C vaccine for younger children is uncertain for inadequate antibody levels are detected below age 2 years, and titers fall rapidly. Group C vaccine was routinely administered to all U.S. Army inductees and has essentially eliminated group C disease from recruit camps [11]. The development of an effective group B vaccine and improved methods of stimulating protective antibody in children (less than 2 years of age) are current goals of immunization research [36]. While chemotherapy prophylaxis provides immediate potential protection for exposure to all serogroups, immunization protection has a lag of 1 to 2 weeks and is available for serogroups A, C, Y, and W135 only, as individual vaccines or an effective quadrivalent preparation [33].

Infections due to *Pseudomonas aeruginosa*

General features

These ubiquitous gram-negative bacilli can cause serious infections, especially in individuals with altered defenses or receiving intense antibiotic therapy, or in hospitalized patients. Cutaneous manifestations of *Pseudomonas* infections are common and characteristic. They may represent the only overt findings in septicemias or be the localizing focus in serious infections of the ear. In addition, trivial cutaneous lesions involving nails, toe webs, skin, and the external auditory canal are produced by these organisms.

Bacteriology and pathogenesis

Pseudomonas aeruginosa is a nonfermentative, obligately aerobic, gram-negative bacillus. Some strains produce a blue pigment (pyocyanin) that is soluble in chloroform, or a yellow-green substance (fluorescein) which is water soluble. Using Wood's ultraviolet lamp, the presence of organisms in lesions of skin or nails and in the urine can be identified if fluorescein is produced by that particular strain. Either of the pigments, or their combination, impart a characteristic greenish color to the surrounding growth media or the tissue substrate involved in clinical disease

(e.g., "green nail" syndrome). In addition, growth of these microorganisms is often accompanied by an odor of grapes, characteristic of trimethylamine.

These organisms gain entry through breakdown of the skin or mucous membrane barriers at sites of trauma, foreign bodies (e.g., indwelling venous or urinary catheters), or via aspiration or aerosolization into the respiratory tract. Infections in otherwise healthy individuals are unusual; when they occur, the involved regions are often areas with increased moisture (toe webs, external auditory canal). Infection may begin in the base of the nail in persons having their hands in water frequently. This can progress to paronychia, followed by development of a green-blue discoloration of the nail due to local pigment production. Another example of the ability of this organism to infect healthy but moistened skin are the numerous reports of a diffuse rash on areas of skin of people immersed in public whirlpools, hot tubs, and swimming pools [37]. These organisms can sometimes be aggressive secondary invaders in open wounds, decubiti, and skin ulcerations, or in association with thermal burns. Rarely, a superficial pyoderma due solely to *Pseudomonas* is engrafted upon a generalized or localized dermatitis, such as tinea pedis or eczema, producing irregular pustular areas with macerated and eroded borders.

Serious invasive infections occur in debilitated patients; malnourished infants; individuals whose normal bacterial flora has been suppressed by antibiotics; patients with neoplastic diseases, granulocytopenias of various etiologies, or with impaired circulating or cellular immunity; and individuals requiring mechanical respiratory assistance. These organisms frequently colonize body surfaces and survive exposure to antibiotics. *Pseudomonas aeruginosa* can spread widely via the bloodstream, producing a disseminated infective vasculitis. Occasionally, features of the generalized Shwartzman reaction are found, but less frequently than in infections due to *N. meningitidis* or *Salmonella typhi*. Whole dead *Pseudomonas* cells injected into experimental animals produce little if any toxicity compared to the effects of live bacteria. This suggested to Liu and his associates that the pathogenicity of this organism might reside in an exotoxin rather than in the classic endotoxin of gram-negative bacteria. Studies during the past 15 years have confirmed the relevance of a number of toxic substances to pathogenesis. Among these, collagenase and elastase may be important determinants for the development of hemorrhagic lesions. A phospholipase similar to the alpha toxin of *Clostridium perfringens* may have a major role in the pathogenesis of respiratory infections through destruction of pulmonary surfactant [38]. Studies have led to the identification and characterization of a potent protein, exotoxin A. The mechanism of action of this toxin is identical to that of diphtheria cytotoxin, but it differs in its cellular specificities, molecular properties, and clinical expression. Exotoxin A and other *Pseudomonas* toxins have recently been reviewed [39]. An antitoxin can neutralize the effects of the toxin in vivo. Efforts to produce a toxoid are in progress. The importance of the contribution of this exotoxin to the pathogenesis of *Pseudomonas* infections has not been definitely established. There is evidence in experimental burn sepsis that synthesis of the exotoxin occurs in local lesions, and the toxin can be identified in the serum [40].

Epidemiology

Pseudomonas aeruginosa is found widely distributed in nature—in air, water, dust particles, and soil; thus, it is not surprising that it may occasionally contaminate plants, vegetables, and medicinal preparations such as procaine and fluorescein eye drops. In humans, the moist regions of skin folds and the external auditory canal are the most common sites of natural colonization (approximately 3 to 5 percent of individuals). *P. aeruginosa* is found in small numbers in the feces of 10 to 20 percent of the population, but in larger numbers in as many as 35 to 50 percent of hospitalized patients. Moist or weeping cutaneous lesions (e.g., thermal burns) encourage the growth of *Pseudomonas,* as well as of other gram-negative bacteria. Procedures which increase humidity in the environment are frequently associated with overgrowth of these organisms. Systemic infection with these indigenous gram-negative bacteria depends primarily on altered susceptibility of the host rather than on spread from individual to individual or on increased pathogenicity. However, there may be exceptions to this in newborn nurseries, respiratory care units, and, occasionally, urologic wards, where dissemination from a primary source may occur. In hospitalized patients who are immunocompromised, increasing numbers become colonized and a larger number suffer disease due to this organism.

Local and secondarily infected lesions

Pseudomonas produces a number of characteristic lesions. In addition, these organisms contaminate and complicate other skin diseases and open wounds [41].

Clinical manifestations. HISTORY. Painful paronychial lesions, with or without characteristic green or blue discoloration of the nails, occur most often in women with a history of chronic immersion of hands in water with soaps and detergents. People with toe web infection characteristically work or live in an atmosphere of high humidity and often have wet feet. Symptoms usually include slight persistent soreness and scaling of the web tissues. There are a large number of reports of therapeutic recreational whirlpool-, hot tub-, and swimming pool-associated skin rashes developing in healthy individuals within 1 to 5 days after use of public bathing facilities. In all instances, *P. aeruginosa* was isolated in large numbers from the pool water. The skin rash was self-limited, clearing without therapy within one week but often accompanied by fatigue, malaise, low-grade fever, external otitis, and mastitis [37].

CUTANEOUS LESIONS. In addition to a tender paronychial lesion, patients with "green nail" syndrome may have part or all of the associated nail colored green to blue. The color may be in horizontal bands, representing intermittent activity of the infection at the nail base. Individuals with toe web *Pseudomonas* infections have thick, macerated, scaling, slightly green discolored areas between the toes. External otitis due to any type of bacteria presents a characteristically swollen, macerated appearance in the local area, without any specific lesion involving the eardrum. Intense swelling and discoloration with excruciating pain on movement of the pinna, are characteristic of external otitis, often referred to as "swimmer's ear." If the skin is

traumatized naturally, or during a surgical procedure, local infection can spread to the pinna, producing a perichondritis and chondritis with intense tender swelling of the ear. Cartilagenous necrosis may result from pressure effects or inflammatory damage unless immediate drainage with through-and-through incisions and appropriate antibiotics are instituted. Organisms other than *P. aeruginosa* may be causal, including *S. aureus* and streptococci [42]. The most severe form of this infection, malignant external otitis, has a high mortality if therapy is delayed or inadequate [43].

This serious infection usually occurs in elderly diabetics with significant small-vessel disease. The onset and early progression are insidious. Swelling, erythema, moderate discharge, and pain are present without fever or constitutional symptoms. As the surface breaks down, invasion of the soft tissues occurs at the junction of cartilage and bone, and the process then advances to involve cartilage, mastoid, and temporal bone. Inflammation at the stylomastoid and jugular foramena can lead to 7th nerve and 9th to 11th nerve palsies, the 7th being the earliest objective neurologic defect seen. Diagnosis is made clinically and early if there is adequate visibility, and granulation tissue can be seen erupting at the cartilage–bone interface in the posterior inferior canal wall. The pinna is often swollen and intense pain is present [44].

Patients who develop folliculitis usually give a history of exposure to warm water in a whirlpool, a public bath like a hot tub, or some recreational spa for swimming or a water slide. The rash can be very local if a limb has been immersed in a whirlpool, or generalized in distribution in swim suit and intertriginous areas. The rash begins as papules, evolves to papulopustules, and eventually heals with fine desquamation. Pruritus and pain may accompany the lesions and localized areas of mastitis and external otitis [37].

In secondarily infected open skin areas, the presence of *Pseudomonas* is sometimes associated with a prominent greenish-blue color to the purulent exudate. Widespread, irregular, superficial pustular lesions may be superimposed on the underlying skin disease; the margins of these regions are usually sharply defined and irregular, and may exhibit the characteristic grapelike odor and pigmented exudate.

Diagnosis and differential diagnosis. Nail and skin lesions are recognized by the characteristic pigment and "fruity" odor of the exudate. The organisms can be identified as thin gram-negative rods, or a mixed infection (e.g., with *Candida*) may be observed. Identification of the organism isolated in routine culture is based on pigment production and fermentation reactions. Fluorescence, demonstrated with a Wood's lamp, can help to support the diagnostic impression. Occasionally *Aspergillus* infection of the nails produces a greenish color, but there is usually no associated paronychia, and bacteria are not found on careful study of nail clippings. A subungual hematoma may superficially resemble *Pseudomonas* nail infection.

Course and prognosis. Patients with minor *Pseudomonas* infections such as onychia and paronychia, toe web inflammation, whirlpool-associated skin rash, and external otitis usually improve rapidly with topical therapy and drying of the affected area. Malignant external otitis requires systemic antibiotics directed against *Pseudomonas,* utilizing an aminoglycoside and fourth-generation penicillin like ticarcillin. High doses and prolonged therapy are combined with surgical debridement to limit spread to bone, nervous system structures, and the meninges [44].

Septicemia and cutaneous involvement

Clinical manifestations. HISTORY. In individuals ill with *Pseudomonas* septicemia, the history is most frequently centered around the underlying problem and antecedent therapy. A premature infant may have required resuscitation and treatment of a nonspecific pneumonitis prior to developing high fever, obtundation, and macular or hemorrhagic vesicular skin lesions. Infants may present initially with omphalitis or severe diarrhea, followed by septicemia and skin lesions. Urinary tract infections complicating congenital lesions such as exstrophy of the bladder may predispose to bacteremia. In adults, there is usually a history of antibiotic therapy, treatment with corticosteroid hormones or antitumor agents, or the use of indwelling venous catheters. Frequently, the patient is granulopenic, has already had a significant febrile illness and may still be receiving antibiotics when one of the characteristic cutaneous manifestations develops. The local lesions are rarely painful, but in the authors' experience the patient is usually too sick to focus on the local problem. Occasionally, hemorrhagic manifestations may occur secondary to involvement of small vessels supplying the skin, to platelet reduction, or to DIC.

Pseudomonas involvement of the gastrointestinal tract, particularly in the tropics, may produce the picture of an acute enteric infection with headache, high fever, diarrhea, and ''rose spots''—a syndrome described as *Shanghai fever* and resembling typhoid fever [45].

CUTANEOUS LESIONS. The skin lesions, the most characteristic part of the physical findings in *Pseudomonas* septicemia, consist of four types [46]:

1. *Vesicles and bullae.* These occur singly or in clusters, spread in random fashion over the skin, frequently becoming hemorrhagic as they evolve (Fig. A3-19). Occasionally, in infants, they may be surrounded by large erythematous halos and may be mistaken for erythema multiforme.
2. *Ecthyma gangrenosa.* The lesion in this disorder consists of a round, indurated, ulcerated, painless area with central necrotic black or gray-black eschar and surrounding erythema. This lesion often evolves from a necrotic vesicle. Frequently, but not exclusively, the lesion is in the anogenital or axillary region.
3. *Gangrenous cellulitis.* This is a sharply demarcated, superficial, painless, necrotic lesion that may resemble a decubitus ulcer, but is located in a nonpressure area and may complicate a prior area of injury like a thermal burn.
4. *Macular or papular nodular lesions.* These are small, oval, and painless, located predominantly over the trunk, and resemble rose spots of typhoid fever (see above).

Another cutaneous manifestation of *Pseudomonas* septicemia, usually occurring after days or weeks, is nodular cellulitis. The lesions are red, warm, sometimes fluctuant, but often situated deeply enough to feel solid. Surgical incision reveals suppuration, and *P. aeruginosa* can be cultured from the lesions [47].

Other lesions that have been described include petechiae, ecchymoses, dermal Shwartzman-like reactions, and purpura fulminans. Occasionally, the cutaneous expression of *Pseudomonas* infection may take the form of a typical erythema multiforme reaction. Patients with extensive burns may develop lesions of the above types on areas of normal skin, as well as more florid diffuse growth secondarily infecting the burn surface.

OTHER PHYSICAL FINDINGS. Patients with *Pseudomonas* septicemia frequently exhibit physical findings associated with the underlying diseases: malnutrition, mucous membrane ulcerations, glossitis and stomatitis secondary to antibiotics and granulopenia, urinary tract infections, proctitis, adenopathy, hepatosplenomegaly, and hemorrhagic bronchopneumonia.

Laboratory findings. Routine hematologic examination may reveal leukocytosis or leukopenia, with modifications based on underlying illnesses (aleukemic leukemia, leukemia, etc.). Platelets may be diminished and fibrinogen and other clotting factors reduced in association with consumption coagulopathy, liver disease, or profound malnutrition.

Characteristically, in *Pseudomonas* septicemia, aspirated material from bullae, areas of cellulitis, and papular or nodular lesions reveals numerous organisms but few leukocytes. Cultures of these lesions and of blood are almost always positive.

Pathology. The distinctive finding in *Pseudomonas* lesions is a necrotizing vasculitis in which the walls of small arteries and veins are invaded by myriads of bacteria [48]. The internal elastic lamellae may be destroyed by microbial elastase [39], but the endothelial surface is rarely damaged and thrombosis is unusual. Extravasation occurs around the vessels, the perivascular and adventitial regions are extensively involved with edema and bland necrosis, and blood flow to the region supplied by the affected vessel is curtailed. This in turn leads to the formation of cutaneous lesions (bullae, hemorrhagic cellulitis, and gangrenous changes). Organisms tend to spread along the exterior surfaces of vessels and invade the skin. Lungs, liver, kidneys, and brain may be similarly involved by bacterial invasion of their respective blood vessel walls, with the production of characteristic discrete nodular necrotic lesions.

Diagnosis and differential diagnosis. The characteristic ecthyma gangrenosum skin lesions in an acutely ill patient suggests the diagnosis of *Pseudomonas* septicemia. The finding of abundant, thin, gram-negative rods with rare granulocytes in vesicle fluid or in association with gangrenous or hemorrhagic cellulitis constitutes further presumptive evidence.

The differential diagnosis of *Pseudomonas* septicemia includes other infections which can produce skin lesions through direct involvement of blood vessels (e.g., those caused by *N. meningitidis, Aeromonas hydrophilia, E. coli,* and fungi of the *Aspergillus* and *Rhyzopus* groups). In addition, other gram-negative bacteria may produce petechial, ecchymotic, and gangrenous skin lesions suggestive of the Shwartzman reaction.

Course and prognosis. *Pseudomonas* septicemia is frequently the terminal event in a complex illness involving a patient with malignant disease or altered cellular and humoral defense mechanisms. Therapy may be effective and recovery complete in some instances, especially when the septicemia occurs in patients with more favorable underlying problems like thermal burns, or in individuals with urinary tract foci of infection or in association with the use of percutaneous venous catheters.

Treatment. LOCAL INFECTIONS. Superficial skin and toe web infections and onychia usually respond to acetic acid, silver nitrate, or gentian violet compresses applied 2 to 3 times daily between long periods of drying. Paronychia is best treated by surgical drainage, nail trimming, and 4% thymol in chloroform. Acetic acid in 50% alchohol, polymixin (0.1%) in acetic acid, or corticosteroids with neomycin are effective for otitis externa. When acetic acid is used topically on chronic ulcers, a 5% solution is often effective. In addition, topical silver nitrate (0.5%), sulfamylon acetate, or silver sulfadiazine have been used to eradicate these organisms in burn patients (see Chap. 122).

SYSTEMIC INFECTIONS. *Pseudomonas* septicemia requires early and vigorous systemic bactericidal antibiotic therapy. Effective therapeutic agents include the aminoglycosides gentamicin, tobramycin, and amikacin. One of these drugs is usually combined with carbenicillin, ticarcillin, or piperacillin in patients who are acutely ill. Gentamicin or tobramycin should be given every 8 h in 1.5 mg/kg doses intramuscularly or intravenously. Ticarcillin is administered in doses of 2 to 3 g every 4 h. In the presence of hypotension or of any renal impairment, the dosage of aminoglycoside antibiotics must be drastically reduced; in such circumstances, therapy should be guided by determinations of "peak" and "trough" serum levels of the aminoglycoside drug employed.

In addition to parenteral administration of antibiotics, nodular and fluctuant lesions should be drained surgically. Leukocyte transfusions have been effective in granulopenic patients, and experimental use of human anticore lipopolysaccharide antiserum or specific *Pseudomonas* exotoxin A antibody preparations are under development and in early use [29,39,49].

PROPHYLAXIS. Infections caused by *P. aeruginosa* are difficult to treat because they often occur in altered hosts and the organisms are highly resistant to many antibiotics. There is no place for prophylactic antibiotics against *P. aeruginosa* because of drug toxicity and emergence of resistant strains. This reality has led to attempts to develop a polyvalent vaccine against the limited number of serotypes of *P. aeruginosa*. Preliminary clinical trials have been encouraging but variable in patients with thermal burns, cystic fibrosis, and in volunteers. Results are less favorable in seriously ill individuals with leukemia or other diseases with impaired host defenses [49,50]. A recent review of the clinical aspects of *Pseudomonas* disease includes a thoughtful discussion of passive and active immunization as well as antimicrobial therapy [51].

Skin infections due to *Hemophilus influenzae*

General features

The characteristic feature of infection of the skin with *H. influenzae* is a cellulitis that usually involves the face, neck, or upper extremities. Most cases occur in young children (6 to 24 months old), but examples in adults have been described in recent years.

Bacteriology and pathogenesis

Hemophilus influenzae is a small, coccobacillary pleomorphic gram-negative organism. It is nonmotile and has fastidious growth requirements, including heme (X factor) and nicotinamide nucleoside (V factor). In mixed cultures the presence of organisms like *S. aureus* can provide these growth factors and this allows *H. influenzae* colonies to grow well, as "satellites" of the feeding staphylococcus. There are rough and encapsulated forms, the latter divided into six serologic types (a through f) based on capsular polysaccharide antigens.

Most infections with *H. influenzae*, including meningitis, epiglottitis, and cellulitis, are caused by encapsulated type b strains (Hib). The ribosylribitol phosphate capsule inhibits phagocytosis in nonimmune individuals and allows a period of unchecked bacterial growth and invasiveness to occur. Rough, unencapsulated, nontypable, noninvasive species are commonly found in the upper part of the respiratory tract and are especially incriminated in surface infections like exacerbations of bronchitis in older individuals with chronic lung disease and in young children with otitis media.

The mechanism involved in the development of cellulitis is uncertain, but in the majority of cases is an antecedent upper respiratory infection (URI). The characteristic localization of the cellulitis to the upper part of the body argues for the sequence of URI, fallout onto or invasion of the skin locally and then bacteremia. This sequence is seen in adult as well as in pediatric cases. The association of otitis media with cellulitis has led to the hypothesis that the ear may serve as the primary focus in cases involving the face [52]. A primary bacteremic mechanism with secondary localization in the skin would be favored by a more random and widespread distribution of lesions than is seen. Localization of a subclinical bacteremia could follow trauma and has been suggested as a possible antecedent predisposing event [53]. The analogy to group A beta streptococcal erysipelas seems relevant, since the organisms are usually located in the upper respiratory tract, produce cellulitis locally, and bacteremia is a secondary complication, although less often seen than in Hib cellulitis.

Epidemiology

Humans are the only known natural host for *H. influenzae*. Carrier rates appear to be highest in young children between ages 1 and 5, especially in families and day-care groups with a recent case of Hib disease [54]. These potentially pathogenic bacteria are carried in the oropharynx and nasopharynx as part of the normal indigenous flora. Susceptibility to Hib disease appears to be greatest among certain ethnic groups and in socioeconomically disadvantaged populations. Genetic factors, prompt antibiotic treatment of Hib disease, congenital and acquired complement and antibody deficiency, and asplenia may also be responsible for increased susceptibility to disease and to recurrent episodes in traditional age groups as well as in adults. Spread is via droplet aerosol or close contact, and infection frequently occurs in association with a viral URI. Susceptibility to *H. influenzae* disease appears to be greatest between the ages of 3 months and 3 years. Although the early observations of Fothergill and Wright (1933) that this correlated with the absence of significant titers of bactericidal antibody has been questioned [55], there is general agreement that complement-dependent anticapsular and bactericidal antibodies increase with age and are protective [56]. Paradoxically, Hib disease may occur in individuals endowed with adequate levels of bactericidal antibody. It has been postulated that circulating IgA antibody may block the function of specific IgG [15], or that assay methodology provides false-positive results in vitro [57]. Although the mechanism of protection in the newborn period remains uncertain, it probably involves transplacental IgG transfer. The majority of adults beyond 15 years likewise have bactericidal and anticapsular antibody, and in this age group *H. influenzae* disease is unusual [58].

In addition to antibody induction by clinical or subclinical *H. influenzae* disease, protective anticapsular antibody may be formed in response to cross-reacting antigens from vegetables, like legumes, nonencapsulated *Hemophilus* species, other commensals, and enteric bacteria (e.g., *E. coli* K 100) [59].

Clinical manifestations

History. Typically, a young infant or child (under age 3) develops an area of swelling and discoloration on the face or arm following several days of coryza and abruptly rising temperature [60]. Rarely, a similar process occurs in adults as a complication of respiratory tract infection involving the upper airway [61].

Cutaneous lesions. The typical lesion is a single, circumscribed, indurated area, usually located on the face, neck, upper chest, or upper extremity. Although described in infants as characteristically blue-red to purple-red in color and surrounded by a zone of edema, the early lesion may be an area of pale edema [53]. The margins are indistinct, in contrast to the sharply defined borders of erysipelas. Regional adenopathy is rarely present.

Other physical findings. Associated infections of the upper respiratory tract including otitis media, sinusitis or epiglottitis, and pneumonia occur. The patient may appear lethargic and, occasionally, metastatic infections such as septic arthritis or meningitis may occur. Fever, in the range of 38.9° to 40°C is common.

Laboratory findings

The white blood cell count is invariably elevated, usually in the 20,000 range. Blood cultures are positive in greater than 80 percent of cases. Aspiration and culture of the margin of the cellulitis has been successful in about half the patients encountered, and Gram-stained smears should be studied [52]. Latex agglutination of soluble Hib capsule material has replaced CIE as the method of choice for antigen detection in CSF and other body fluids. It is more rapid, easier to perform, and more sensitive than CIE and can provide diagnostic information after antibiotic exposure [26].

Pathology

No information is available about the histologic changes associated with this lesion, but the inflammatory response is doubtless an acute pyogenic reaction.

Diagnosis and differential diagnosis

Hemophilus influenzae cellulitis should be suspected when a child, age 3 to 24 months, develops an acute facial cellulitis with high fever. There may be concomitant upper airway inflammation. Immediate confirmation of the diagnosis may be possible from inspection of Gram-stained smears of an aspirate of the lesion. While cellulitis caused by other microorganisms is more common in adults, Hib disease should be considered in patients with respiratory infections and upper body cellulitis.

Streptococcal (especially group A) or pneumococcal cellulitis may produce a similar discoloration of the skin. Erysipelas, which rarely occurs in infants, is usually homogeneously erythematous and margins of the plaquelike swelling are distinct compared with the indefinite borders of *H. influenzae* cellulitis. Occasionally, *Staphylococcus aureus* can produce a similar process, but the presence of pustules or boils is helpful in distinguishing this type of lesion.

Course and prognosis

Most patients do well with antibiotic therapy even though the disease is usually associated with bacteremia. The patient is often brought to a physician quickly since the abrupt onset of high fever and easily observed cellulitis indicates the urgency of the situation. Constant vigil must be maintained for suppurative complications in the upper airways, lungs, bones, joints, or other organs.

Treatment and prophylaxis

Ampicillin (150 to 250 mg/kg per day intravenously in four to six divided doses) has been effective treatment for most pediatric patients, but the emergence of plasmid-mediated (beta lactamase-producing), ampicillin-resistant strains has led to alternative recommendations [62]. Chloramphenicol (50 to 100 mg/kg daily in children above the age of 3 months) alone, or in combination with ampicillin, has become the initial treatment of choice for serious infections while awaiting the results of antibiotic susceptibility tests [62]. Cefamandole and the third-generation cephalosporins have activity against both ampicillin-sensitive and resistant strains. Additionally, the combination of trimethoprim and sulfamethoxazole is a potent alternative in serious Hib infections, and useful for selected patients.

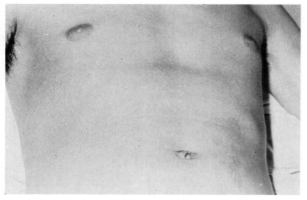

Fig. 177-1 Typhoid fever "rose spots." These lesions are not macular, but are 1- to 3-mm pink papules that blanch on pressure. The lesions last only 3 to 4 days, but others may develop over 2 to 3 weeks. (Courtesy of Dr. S. Yip, Hong Kong.)

Chemoprophylaxis has been studied in a variety of settings and rifampin appears to be effective in significantly lowering carrier rates in selected populations like households with an index case of Hib disease. Results are less impressive in other populations, such as day-care groups, and recurrent carrier rates increase more rapidly than has been the experience with *N. meningitidis* prophylaxis. At the present time rifampin is recommended for children and adults (reduced for infants) in doses of 20 mg/kg per day (up to 600 mg maximum) for four days, when an index case of Hib invasive disease occurs in a family where other children under age 4 reside [63].

Immunization with a vaccine prepared from Hib capsular polysaccharide (polyribosylribitol phosphate) has been successful in increasing circulating anticapsular antibody and protecting susceptible children. Unfortunately, the current material is not effective in infants and children below age 18 months, the most critical period for invasive Hib disease. A number of studies have confirmed the ease of administration, safety, and efficacy for older children, and work is in progress to enhance the immunogenicity of the vaccine for the age group most in need of protection. The vaccine is now available commercially. A two-dose schedule, commencing at age 18 months, has been recommended [64].

Cutaneous manifestations of *Salmonella* infection (enteric fever)

General features

Salmonella infections are usually manifest as gastroenteritis, enteric fever (typhoidlike illness), or septicemia. "Rose spots," the classical skin lesions of systemic *Salmonella* infection (Figs. 177-1 and A3-7), have been variably reported (10 to 60 percent) during the natural (untreated) evolution of typhoid fever, but less frequently in enteric fevers due to other *Salmonella* species.

Bacteriology and pathogenesis

Salmonellae are not fastidious organisms, but their isolation from stool is made difficult by the fact that, when present, they represent only a small part of the abundant fecal flora. Extragastrointestinal isolates (abscesses, blood, skin lesions) are easier to identify, since they usually are pure cultures of a given *Salmonella* species. Isolation of the organisms from stool specimens is aided by the use of selective inhibiting media (e.g., MacConkey SS agar) that decrease the growth of gram-positive organisms as well as many gram-negative species. Salmonellae are motile, gram-negative bacilli that do not ferment lactose. From a practical viewpoint, in stool bacteriology, initial selection of non-lactose-fermenting colonies is followed by biochemical and serologic (agglutination) procedures for identification and serotyping of the organism. There are three primary species: *Salmonella typhi* (1 serotype); *S. choleraesuis* (1 serotype); and *S. enteritidis* (over 1700 serotypes). By habit organisms are often referred to as *Salmonella* (plus serotype designation—e.g., *typhimurium*) but the correct nomenclature is *Salmonella enteritidis*, serotype *typhimurium*, etc.

There is a latent period of from 3 to as long as 50 days (usually 7 to 14) between ingestion of bacteria and the dramatic onset of clinical symptoms of enteric fever. Shorter latent periods often follow ingestion of larger numbers of organisms. When due to salmonellae other than *S. typhi*, symptoms tend to begin earlier and are milder. During the latent period, organisms multiply in the distal small bowel and invade and multiply in lymphoid tissues in the area of Peyer's patches in the terminal ileum. Invasion of the bloodstream from this focus heralds the onset of the clinical illness with chills and fever and other constitutional effects of circulating endotoxin. Manifestations of infection occur in many organs and often in a predictable sequence: respiratory and central nervous system symptoms during the first week; skin manifestations during the second week; diarrhea, usually following a period of constipation, during the second and third weeks. Bacterial invasion of the skin, liver, gallbladder, bones, and joints, as well as manifestations of endotoxemia usually occur during the bacteremic phase of the illness (first 10 days). Organisms are cleared by the reticuloendothelial system (RES), leading to hyperplasia of these elements in the liver, spleen, and other lymph nodes. Persistence of organisms in the gallbladder, biliary radicals, or the RES may lead to a chronic asymptomatic carrier state.

Epidemiology

S. typhi and other *Salmonella* species causing enteric fever are acquired by ingestion of contaminated water or food. Humans are the only hosts for *S. typhi* and the chronic carrier state that may follow clinical typhoid fever is almost always asymptomatic except for manifestations of gallbladder disease if cholelithiasis and active cholecystitis are present. Other *Salmonella*, serotypes of *S. enteritidis*, e.g., *typhimurium*, *schottmulleri*, and *hirshfeldii*, can produce an enteric fever syndrome similar to, but usually milder than, typhoid fever. Unlike *S. typhi*, these other *Salmonella* serotypes are ubiquitous in nature (occurring in animals, birds, reptiles, poultry products) and are difficult to control as sources of human infection.

A number of factors, exclusive of inoculum size, determine whether disease will occur after ingestion of *Salmonella*. Achlorhydria and previous gastric surgery allow organisms to escape destruction by the acid barrier of the stomach. Rapid transit of a smaller inoculum in a liquid vehicle may allow adequate numbers of viable bacteria to reach the distal small bowel. Underlying illnesses such as Hodgkin's disease which alters cellular immunity can interfere with the host defense mechanisms that normally eradicate these pathogens; hemoglobinopathies, such as sickle cell disease, appear to predispose to systemic *Salmonella* infections and osteomyelitis by saturating the protective RES with red cell fragments and occluding small blood vessels, leading to local chronic foci; and, finally, tumor immunosuppression therapy may be factors predisposing patients to salmonellosis. Infants and young children, as well as the very elderly, appear to be especially susceptible to serious disease as well as to gastroenteritis.

Clinical manifestations

History. Symptoms begin several days to several weeks after ingestion of contaminated water or food. Headache, fever, generalized aching, bronchitis, and constipation are often present. Delirium or mental torpor are not unusual, especially when there is a high fever. The pulse rate may be slower than expected for the magnitude of the fever. Symptoms increase in intensity, and the fever often reaches 39.5° to 40.5°C by the end of the first week. During the second week, rose spots may appear on the trunk and diffuse abdominal cramping becomes prominent, sometimes accompanied by diarrhea. In areas endemic for typhoid fever, the abdominal symptoms may be present from the onset, and diarrhea can be an early manifestation too [65].

Cutaneous lesions. After about 7 to 10 days of high fever, the characteristic rose spots may appear. These lesions are 2 to 3 mm in size, slightly raised, pink *papules,* which blanch on pressure (Fig. A3-7) and are nontender. They appear in crops of approximately 10 to 20 lesions and are usually located between the nipple area and the umbilicus on the anterior trunk, rarely on the back or extremities. Without therapy, the crops of spots usually become brownish as they fade and disappear in 3 to 4 days. New lesions emerge over the ensuing 2 to 3 weeks in untreated patients. Their presence in 63 percent of a group of 62 patients in a contemporary study should encourage careful observation for this subtle rash [66]. Antibiotic therapy instituted early in the course of the illness may be responsible for the decreasing incidence of rose spots [67]. The rash is less frequently reported in blacks, but this may be because of difficulty in detecting the small, scarce lesions on dark skin.

Rose spots occur infrequently in enteric fevers caused by other *Salmonella* species, but when they do appear, they may be present in greater numbers and in a more widespread distribution.

A variety of other skin changes have been described in enteric fever during the acute phase of illness. Erythema typhosum, an erythematous rash that is confluent and widely scattered, may occur during the first week of the disease. Erythema nodosum and urticarial lesions have been noted and ascribed to hypersensitivity phenomena. Transient loss of hair and changes in nails reflect the acute

catabolic stress. It is distinctly uncommon to observe herpes labialis in enteric fever.

Other physical findings. During the acute phase of the disease, at the time the cutaneous lesions are appearing, the patient may be disoriented and have signs of pneumonia. The abdomen is often distended, tympanitic, and diffusely tender with some localization to the right lower quadrant. The spleen is often enlarged, but may be difficult to palpate because of abdominal distension and guarding.

Laboratory findings

Leukopenia or low normal leukocyte counts are often present, but values range from 3,000 to 20,000 mm³. The percentage of mononuclear cells may be increased, and atypical lymphocytes can appear in small numbers, suggesting a viral illness. Thrombocytopenia may occur, and rarely hemolysis is observed. During the initial week of illness, blood cultures are usually positive. During the second week, or when diarrhea begins, stool cultures become positive and the white blood cell count may increase. In addition to blood and stool, the typical rose spots should be cultured, preferably using the technique of skin snips [66]. In addition to blood and fecal cultures, bone marrow and skin lesion material may be positive in approximately 65 to 95 percent of cases, even when routine blood cultures simultaneously done are negative or when antibiotics are being administered [66]. Antibodies to somatic ("O") antigens develop after about two weeks of illness and rise over the ensuing months. Unfortunately, the serologic tests (Widal agglutination) are positive in about half of patients studied, and antibodies are detected nonspecifically in a variety of other infectious diseases. A more specific and sensitive serologic test for systemic *Salmonella* infections merits development.

Pathology

The rose spot characteristically blanches on pressure, and examination of the lesion histologically reveals gross dilatation of capillaries, described by some pathologists as "capillary atony." Extravasation of blood is not observed, but there is considerable edema and an abundant pericapillary infiltration with macrophages; organisms may be present within these cells [68]. Rose spots have been produced experimentally by injecting purified *S. typhi* endotoxin intradermally [69].

Diagnosis and differential diagnosis

The diagnosis of *Salmonella* enteric fever may be difficult in a sporadic case, especially if the characteristic rash and gastrointestinal symptoms have not yet appeared and there is no history of travel in an endemic area. Headache, cough, and high fever are not very specific findings. However, when these symptoms are associated with delirium, relative bradycardia, and leukopenia with increased numbers of circulating mononuclear cells, the diagnosis of enteric fever should be considered. The diagnosis is usually made by obtaining blood cultures, which are positive in approximately 80 percent of untreated cases during the first week to 10 days. Serologic tests (Widal) are usually negative during the early phase of the illness, and may not be diagnostic later. Likewise, enteric fever due to other *Salmonella* species can usually be diagnosed by blood cultures. Other cultured material (marrow, rose spots) may be important, especially in patients who have had prior antibiotic therapy.

The differential diagnosis includes a wide range of diseases. Prominent cough and severe headache in the early phases may suggest a viral or atypical pneumonia (*Legionella pneumophila, Mycoplasma pneumoniae,* psittacosis, or Q fever). Typhus and Rocky Mountain spotted fever can usually be excluded by geographic and epidemiologic considerations, serologic studies, the characteristic petechial component to the rash, and, in the case of spotted fever, the distribution of the rash on the distal parts of the extremities. Miliary tuberculosis may begin as an acute febrile illness with similar symptoms, leukopenia, and splenomegaly. The diagnosis may be delayed until a secondary complication such as meningitis occurs, or until biopsy material (liver, lymph node) reveals granulomas, sometimes containing acid-fast organisms.

Among the viral diseases, the diagnosis of infectious mononucleosis is suggested by headache, cough, high fever, lymphadenopathy, splenomegaly, and a blood picture with leukopenia and atypical mononuclear cells.

Malaria and toxoplasmosis are two parasitic illnesses that deserve consideration. Epidemiologic information plus intermittency of symptoms usually suggest the diagnosis of malaria. In generalized toxoplasmosis, the symptoms may be very similar to those of early enteric fever: prominent cough, high fever, a rash that is located on the trunk, and a mononucleosis-like blood picture. The rash tends to be more florid than the crops of 10 to 20 lesions seen in enteric fever, and is macular with a petechial component, rather than papular. Diagnosis usually requires identification of *Toxoplasma gondii* in biopsy material or a rising antibody titer (19S fluorescent antibody or hemagglutination inhibition).

Course and prognosis

The response of patients with enteric fever to antibiotic therapy is usually prompt, although it may take 2 to 4 days for the temperature to return to normal. With prolonged treatment, the incidence of relapse has been reduced, but this will vary with the age, nutritional conditions, and general health of the patient. The major complications in the preantibiotic days were perforation and hemorrhage. Although rare, these complications still occur even with prompt, effective chemotherapy, and are responsible for approximately 75 percent of the mortality in enteric fever. Deaths have been reduced from approximately 10 percent to 1 to 2 percent with antibiotic therapy. Following typhoid fever, approximately 1 to 2 percent of patients continue to harbor organisms in the gallbladder and excrete them in the stools for an indefinite period, becoming a major potential source for infecting other individuals.

Treatment and prophylaxis. Chloramphenicol remains the preferred drug for the treatment of the enteric fever syndrome of salmonellosis, whether it is caused by *S. typhi* or by other *Salmonella* species. It is administered intravenously, 0.75 to 1.0 g every 6 h, and should be continued for approximately 3 weeks. Chloramphenicol can be given

by the oral route once clinical improvement is well established, but the intramuscular route is not effective. During treatment, the synthetic functions of the bone marrow should be watched carefully with leukocyte, reticulocyte, and differential blood counts, and the patient should be under close medical supervision.

In patients for whom chloramphenicol is not the drug of choice because of allergy, toxicity, or resistance of the *Salmonella* strain, ampicillin is the first alternative and may be equal to chloramphenicol in effectiveness. It should be given by the intravenous route in doses of 1.5 to 2.0 g every 4 h (in adults). The combination of trimethoprim-sulfamethoxazole (TSM) has also been extensively studied and found effective for most cases of enteric fever due to *S. typhi* or other *Salmonella* species. The dose of TSM is 160 mg trimethoprim plus 800 mg of sulfamethoxazole three times per day for approximately 3 weeks. It is mandatory to carry out sensitivity tests on all isolates from cases of enteric fever since some strains are resistant to chloramphenicol, ampicillin, trimethoprim-sulfamethoxazole, or to all three agents. The cephalosporins have been disappointing when used, even with favorable in vitro results.

Corticosteroid therapy for a period of several days has been advocated in addition to antibiotic treatment for severely toxic and febrile patients, but its efficacy is unproved. A recent report found that high doses of dexamethasone reduced mortality significantly [70]. Among the major complications, hemorrhage usually responds to conservative management, but perforation, often in the ileocecal region, requires immediate surgery.

Identification and eradication of the biliary carrier of *S. typhi* is an important preventive measure for controlling enteric fever. In the presence of stones, antibiotic therapy should be combined with cholecystectomy. In the absence of stones, a prolonged course of treatment with ampicillin or amoxicillin may eradicate the carrier site [71].

Individuals traveling to areas of the world endemic for *S. typhi* or *S. paratyphi* A should be instructed in commonsense methods of eating and drinking to avoid potentially contaminated materials. Immunization is available for *S. typhi* and is probably effective for all but massive exposures, but careful personal hygiene and avoidance of suspicious water or foods (e.g., leafy greens) will eliminate most encounters with *S. typhi* and other Salmonellae capable of causing enteric fever.

Cutaneous manifestations of infection with other gram-negative bacilli

General features

An acute cellulitis, with or without production of gas, may be caused by *Escherichia coli, Proteus* spp., *Klebsiella* spp., *Enterobacter* spp., *Serratia marcescens,* a variety of other facultative and nonfermenting bacilli, and members of the obligate anaerobic group of *Bacteroides*. These infections have often, but not exclusively, been described in the very elderly and in diabetic patients following trauma, surgery, or bowel or perineal inflammation. Drug addicts may develop mixed infections with these organisms when "skin popping," resulting in lesions like necrotizing fasciitis [72]. Prior exposure to broad-spectrum antibiotics and altered host defenses can predispose to this type of infection which is often nosocomial in origin. The finding of gas in the tissues frequently leads to an erroneous provisional diagnosis of clostridial cellulitis or gas gangrene.

Bacteriology and pathogenesis

The family Enterobacteriaceae is composed of a number of bacilli that grow readily on blood agar and selective media. By means of a number of biochemical reactions and growth characteristics, seven tribes of Enterobacteriaceae have been recognized [73]. *E. coli* is closely related to *Shigella; Salmonella* spp. to *Citrobacter; Klebsiella-Enterobacter-Serratia* make up a third tribe; *Proteus-Providence* comprise a fourth main division. There are a variety of facultative gram-negative bacilli that do not belong to this family, metabolize sugars variably, and can be recognized by utilizing other specialized biochemical tests. In addition, the obligate anaerobic *Bacteroides* spp. reside in the oral cavity, colon, and female vaginal region, and are identified by their anaerobic growth requirements as well as a variety of other characteristics [74].

Infection can result from contamination of skin or subcutaneous tissues in an area of injury, surgery, or ischemia. Bacteria can also invade the subcutaneous tissues via the circulation from a distinct source or by direct spread from contiguous structures like the colon. By dissection along fascial planes, cellulitis can erupt in areas removed from the initial focus. The process is often necrotizing, containing a mixture of facultative and anaerobic bacteria and, especially in diabetic individuals, can be associated with gas formation (mainly hydrogen). Edema, bleb formation, ischemia, and gangrene result from thrombosis of nutrient blood vessels. The underlying muscle is almost always spared [75]. Polymorphonuclear leukocytes are abundantly present compared to the relative scarcity of acute inflammatory cells in clostridial infections.

Epidemiology

Cellulitis usually follows contamination of adjacent tissues by bowel contents or a breakdown of skin. The conditions predisposing patients to this type of infection include: (1) bowel perforation (appendicitis, neoplasm, diverticulitis, rectal mucosal tear), (2) colon surgery, (3) chronic edema, (4) vascular insufficiency, (5) decubitus ulcers, (6) percutaneous lines, and (7) superficial perineal dermatitis, including diaper rash. The health of these patients is often further impaired by poorly controlled diabetes, alterations in host defense mechanisms (granulopenia, etc.), and poor nutrition. Crepitant (gas-containing) cellulitis results from infection with gas-forming strains of bacteria, especially in patients with poorly controlled diabetes, or when *Bacteroides* spp. or anaerobic streptococci are present too [76].

Clinical manifestations

History. Diabetes mellitus, malnutrition, chronic illness (e.g., paraplegia with decubitus ulcers), or several other conditions described under "Epidemiology" usually are present. The onset may be insidious over 4 to 5 days or abrupt, with high fever, shaking chills, hypotension, and pain in the area of cellulitis. Symptoms of gastrointestinal inflammation like appendicitis or diverticulitis may precede the cellulitis illness. Rectal or perineal pain can indicate a

local process that may be especially devastating in a patient deficient in granulocytes.

Cutaneous lesions. The areas of involvement have the typical findings of cellulitis with warmth and brawny edema. In the early stages, the skin is rarely discolored beyond a pink hue, and vesicles and blebs or bullae are almost never present. At this juncture, the process may easily be overlooked, especially if the infection is located in a less obvious area or the patient is obtunded. As the cellulitis progresses, edema and redness increase and areas of gangrene may appear. Palpable tenderness and crepitus, if present, can help define the anatomic extent of the process.

In addition to cellulitis, with or without gas formation, macular, papular, and ecthymatous lesions indistinguishable from those caused by *P. aeruginosa* occasionally occur.

SUPERFICIAL NASAL LESIONS. Several species of *Klebsiella* that infect the upper respiratory tract can produce unique superficial diseases. Ozena is a chronic productive rhinitis caused by infection with *Klebsiella ozaenae*. The process remains internal without any cutaneous manifestations except a profuse mucopurulent foul-smelling discharge [77]. *Klebsiella rhinoscleromatis* is the etiologic agent of a hypertrophic, granulomatous infection of the external nares which is known as scleroma. This disease often produces changes in the overlying nasal skin (Fig. 177-2) and the contiguous surfaces of the respiratory and posterior pharyngeal regions. Most cases have been described from very local areas of Eastern and Central Europe (where the disease is known as "Slavic leprosy"), from Africa, the Near East, and parts of Central and South America [78]. Dissemination of the organism is by prolonged close contact, often in family settings of crowding and poor sanitation. Infected individuals can shed organisms for years, with the result that hyperendemic areas are recognized. As seen in leprosy, the disease rarely becomes clinically apparent in children. Patients complain of chronic nasal and cutaneous discharge, obstructive symptoms, or cutaneous nasal masses. Diagnosis depends upon biopsy identification of characteristic vacuolated Mikulicz cells and isolation of the organism on routine cultures, with biochemical and serologic confirmation [79]. Both *K. ozaenae* and *K. rhinoscleromatis* are susceptible to streptomycin and the newer aminoglycosides, trimethoprim, sulfamethoxazole, tetracycline, and chloramphenicol. Prolonged (6 to 8 weeks) treatment of scleroma is important and results are favorable except for residual fibrotic and destructive changes.

Other physical findings. The clinical course often is dominated by systemic manifestations such as decreased mental alertness, hypotension, and dehydration. Abdominal distension and other manifestations of localized or generalized peritonitis may be present. Extreme tenderness of the rectum, with or without a mass, can indicate the local source of a perineal process.

Laboratory findings

The leukocyte count is usually elevated, in the range of 20,000 to 30,000 mm^3, but may be markedly diminished in the presence of gram-negative septicemia. Elevated blood glucose values and findings of ketoacidosis are not unusual.

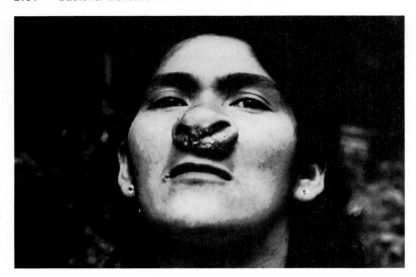

Fig. 177-2 Scleroma. Illustrated is the granuloma of the external nares in a patient from Honduras. *(Courtesy of Dr. Eric Kraus.)*

In the presence of crepitant cellulitis, roentgenograms of the soft tissue may show the depth and extent of the gas-forming process [76]. In the absence of palpable gas a soft tissue x-ray may indicate gas formation as part of the inflammatory process.

Pathology

Edema, necrosis, gangrene of overlying skin, and a thin exudate containing visible fat droplets and polymorphonuclear leukocytes is usually present. Gas may be seen in the subcutaneous tissues. Blood vessels are often involved in a necrotic, thrombotic inflammatory reaction. The underlying muscle is usually not involved unless there is septicemia associated with major vascular thrombosis.

Diagnosis and differential diagnosis

A specific etiologic diagnosis can be made by needle aspiration of the cellulitis or an overlying bleb. Several morphologic forms of gram-positive as well as gram-negative organisms may be present and when gas is present, anaerobic cocci and clostridia must also be considered. The presence of anaerobes in the exudate may be accompanied by a foul, fetid odor.

Course and prognosis

The process may be indolent and quickly respond to effective antibiotic therapy. Unfortunately, especially in obese diabetic patients with perineal lesions, progression may be astonishingly rapid, even with vigorous antibiotic and surgical therapy. When the process is located centrally, in the perineal-gluteal area, the mortality is often as high as 50 percent. Infection of an extremity is often treated by antibiotics and amputation, with more favorable results. The course is often prolonged and complex due to metabolic and nutritional complications.

Treatment

Immediate antibiotic therapy and surgical drainage are essential, guided by Gram-stained smears of the exudate and the extent of the process. Extensive debridement is usually unnecessary and hyperbaric oxygen is not indicated. Judgment and experience are vital in surgical decisions that include the question of amputation. The existence of a "feeding" source of contamination should be sought (e.g., from a ruptured appendix, diverticulum, or rectal tear). If a lower-bowel leak is found, a diverting colostomy should be performed in addition to a local drainage procedure. Decubitus ulcers must be carefully evaluated for undermining necrosis, abscess formation, and cellulitis [80].

Recent antibiotic usage, status of renal and hepatic function, and prior hospital exposure are factors that will help determine the choice of antibiotics. Single or multiple agents are used, depending on the above information and the results of Gram-stained smears of exudate. Hospitalized patients already exposed to antibiotics and acutely ill should be given an aminoglycoside, like gentamicin (1.5 mg/kg every 8 h parenterally). If the cellulitis is crepitant, then chloramphenicol (750 mg intravenously every 6 h) should be added since this may indicate coinfection with *Bacteroides fragilis*. Metronidazole (1 to 2 g daily in two to four doses), clindamycin (2.4 g in four divided doses intravenously), and selected second- and third-generation cephalosporins can substitute for chloramphenical. Tobramycin or amikacin may be preferred to gentamicin for certain hospital-acquired infections with *Pseudomonas, Klebsiella,* or *Serratia.* If gram-positive cocci are present on initial stained smears, penicillin or nafcillin should be added.

References

1. Band JD et al: Trends in meningococcal disease in the United States, 1975–1980. *J Infect Dis* **148:**754, 1983
2. Gibbons RJ, Van Houte J: Adherence in oral microbial ecology. *Annu Rev Microbiol* **29:**19, 1975
3. DeVoe IW, Gilchrist JE: Piliation and colonial morphology among laboratory strains of meningococci. *J Clin Microbiol* **7:**379, 1978
4. Kornfeld SF, Plaut AG: Secretory immunity and the bacterial IgA proteases. *Rev Infect Dis* **3:**521, 1981
4a. Heaney MR et al: Recurrent bacterial meningitis in patients with genetic disorders of terminal complement components. *Clin Exp Immol* **40:**16, 1980

4b. Ross SC, Densen P: Complement deficiency states and infection: epidemiology, pathogenesis and consequences of neisserial and other infections in an immune deficiency. *Medicine (Baltimore)* 63:243, 1984

5. Sotto MN et al: Pathogenesis of cutaneous lesions in acute meningococcemia in humans: light, immunofluorescent, and electron microscopic studies of skin biopsy specimens. *J Infect Dis* 133:506, 1976

6. Davis CE, Arnold K: Role of meningococcal endotoxin in meningococcal purpura. *J Exp Med* 140:159, 1974

7. DeVoe IW, Gilka F: Disseminated intravascular coagulation in rabbits: synergistic activity of meningococcal endotoxin and materials egested from leukocytes containing meningococci. *J Med Microbiol* 9:451, 1976

8. McGehee WG et al: Intravascular coagulation in fulminant meningococcemia. *Ann Intern Med* 67:250, 1967

9. DeVoe IW: The menigococcus and mechanisms of pathogenicity. *Microbiol Rev* 46:162, 1982

9a. Adams EM et al: Absence of the seventh component of complement in a patient with chronic meningococcemia presenting as vasculitis. *Ann Intern Med* 99:35, 1983

10. Fass RJ, Saslaw S: Chronic meningococcemia: possible pathogenic role of IgM deficiency. *Arch Intern Med* 130:943, 1972

11. Artenstein MC et al: Immunoprophylaxis of meningococcal infection. *Milit Med* 139:91, 1974

12. Goldschneider I et al: Human immunity to the meningococcus. II. Development of natural immunity. *J Exp Med* 129:1327, 1969

13. Robbins JB et al: Enteric bacteria cross-reactive with *Neisseria meningitidis* groups A and C and *Diplococcus pneumoniae* types I and III. *Infect Immun* 6:651, 1972

14. Goldschneider I et al: Human immunity to the meningococcus. I. The role of humoral antibodies. *J Exp Med* 129:1307, 1969

15. Griffiss JM, Bertram MA: Immunoepidemiology of meningococcal disease in military recruits. II. Blocking of serum bactericidal antibody by circulating IgA early in the course of invasive disease. *J Infect Dis* 136:733, 1977

16. Griffiss JM: Epidemic meningococcal disease: synthesis of a hypothetical immunoepidemiologic model. *Rev Infect Dis* 4:159, 1982

17. Munford RS et al: Spread of meningococcal infection within households. *Lancet* 2:1275, 1974

18. Meningococcal Disease Surveillance Group: Meningococcal disease. *JAMA* 235:261, 1976

19. Jacobson JA, Holloway JT: Meningococcal disease in day-care centers. *Pediatrics* 59:299, 1977

20. Gallaid EI et al: Meningococcal disease in New York City 1973–1978: recognition of groups Y and W135 as frequent pathogens. *JAMA* 244:2167, 1980

21. Salet IE et al: Seroepidemiologic aspects of *Neisseria meningitidis* in homosexual men. *Can Med Assoc J* 126:38, 1982

22. Feldman HA: Meningoccal infections. *Adv Intern Med* 18:177, 1972

23. Koppes GM et al: Group Y meningococcal disease in United States air force recruits. *Am J Med* 62:661, 1977

24. Bernhard WG, Jordan AC: Purpuric lesions in meningococci infections: diagnosis from smears and cultures of the purpuric lesions. *J Lab Clin Med* 29:273, 1944

25. Hoyne AL, Brown RH: Meningococcic cases, an analysis. *Ann Intern Med* 28:248, 1948

26. Tilton RC et al: Comparative evaluation of three commercial products and counterimmunoelectrophoresis for the detection of antigens in cerebrospinal fluid. *J Clin Microbiol* 20:231, 1984

27. Benoit FL: Chronic meningococcemia. *Am J Med* 35:103, 1963

28. Leibel RL et al: Chronic meningococcemia in childhood. *Am J Dis Child* 127:94, 1974

29. Ziegler EJ et al: Treatment of gram-negative bacteremia and shock with human antiserum to a mutant *Escherichia coli*. *N Engl J Med* 307:1225, 1982

30. Winslow EJ et al: Hemodynamic studies and results of therapy in 50 patients with bacteremic shock. *Am J Med* 54:421, 1973

31. Sprung CL et al: The effects of high-dose corticosteroids in patients with septic shock. *N Engl J Med* 311:1138, 1984

32. Corrigan JJ Jr: Heparin therapy in bacterial septicemia. *J Pediatr* 91:695, 1977

33. Meningococcal vaccines. *MMWR* 34:255, 1985

34. Devine LF et al: Selective minocycline and rifampin treatment of group C meningococcal carriers in a new naval recruit camp. *Am J Med Sci* 263:79, 1972

35. Hoeprich PD: Prediction of anti-meningococcal chemoprophylactic efficacy. *J Infect Dis* 123:125, 1971

36. Peltola H: Meningococcal disease: still with us. *Rev Infect Dis* 5:71, 1983

37. Gustafson TL et al: Pseudomonas folliculitis: an outbreak and review. *Rev Infect Dis* 5:1, 1983

38. Liu PV: Extracellular toxins of *Pseudomonas aeruginosa*. *J Infect Dis* 130 (suppl):S94, 1974

39. Woods DE, Iglewski BH: Toxins of *Pseudomonas aeruginosa*: new perspectives. *Rev Infect Dis* 5:S715, 1983

40. Saelinger CB et al: Experimental studies on the pathogenesis of infections due to *Pseudomonas aeruginosa*: direct evidence for toxin production during pseudomonas infection of burned skin tissues. *J Infect Dis* 136:555, 1957

41. Hall JH et al: *Pseudomonas aeruginosa* in dermatology. *Arch Dermatol* 97:312, 1968

42. Bassiouny A: Perichondritis of the auricle. *Laryngoscope* 91:422, 1981

43. Zaky DA et al: Malignant external otitis: a severe form of otitis in diabetic patients. *Am J Med* 61:298, 1976

44. Doroghazi RM et al: Invasive external otitis. Report of 21 cases and review of the literature. *Am J Med* 71:603, 1981

45. Stanley MM: *Bacillus pyrocyaneus* infections (2 parts). *Am J Med* 2:253, 1947

46. Forkner CE et al: Pseudomonas septicemia. *Am J Med* 25:877, 1958

47. Reed RK et al: Peripheral nodular lesions in *Pseudomonas* sepsis: the importance of incision and drainage. *J Pediatr* 88:977, 1976

48. Teplitz C: Pathogenesis of *Pseudomonas* vasculitis and septic lesions. *Arch Pathol* 80:297, 1965

49. Pollack M: Antibody activity against *Pseudomonas aeruginosa* in immune globulins prepared for intravenous use in humans. *J Infect Dis* 147:1090, 1983

50. Jones RJ et al: A new *Pseudomonas* vaccine: preliminary trial on human volunteers. *J Hyg (Camb)* 76:429, 1976

51. Bodey GP et al: Infection caused by *Pseudomonas aeruginosa*. *Rev Infect Dis* 5:279, 1983

52. Nelson JD, Ginsburg CM: An hypothesis on the pathogenesis of *Hemophilus influenzae* buccal cellulitis. *J Pediatr* 88:709, 1976

53. Dajani AS et al: Systemic *Haemophilus influenzae* disease: an overview. *J Pediatr* 94:355, 1979

54. Granoff DM, Ward JI: Current status of prophylaxis for *Haemophilus influenzae* infections. *Curr Top Infect Dis* 5:290, 1984

55. Shaw S et al: The paradox of *Hemophilus influenzae* type B bacteremia in the presence of serum bactericidal activity. *J Clin Invest* 58:1019, 1976

56. Robbins JB et al: *Haemophilus influenzae* type b: disease and immunity in humans. *Ann Intern Med* 78:259, 1973

57. O'Reilly RJ et al: Circulating polyribophosphate in *Haemophilus influenzae* type b meningitis. *J Clin Invest* 56:1012, 1975

58. Smith DH et al: Studies on the prevalence of antibodies to *Hemophilus influenzae*, type B, in *Hemophilus influenzae*, edited by S Sell. Nashville, Vanderbilt Univ Press, 1973

59. Schneerson R, Robbins JB: Induction of serum *Haemophilus*

influenzae type b capsular antibodies in adult volunteers fed cross-reacting *Escherichia coli* 075:K100:H5. *N Engl J Med* **292:**1093, 1975

60. Granoff DM, Nankervis GA: Cellulitis due to *Haemophilus influenzae* type b antigenemia and antibody responses. *Am J Dis Child* **130:**1211, 1976

61. Drapkin MS et al: Bacteremic *Hemophilus influenzae* type b cellulitis in the adult. *Am J Med* **63:**449, 1977

62. Katz S et al: Ampicillin-resistant strains of *Hemophilus influenzae* type b. *Pediatrics* **55:**145, 1975

63. Prevention of secondary cases of *Haemophilus influenzae* type b disease. *MMWR* **31:**672, 1982

64. Cochi SL et al: Immunization of US children with *Hemophilus influenzae* type b polysaccharide vaccine. *JAMA* **253:**521, 1985

65. Wicks ACB et al: Endemic typhoid fever: a diagnostic pitfall. *Q J Med [New Series XL]* **159:**341, 1971

66. Gilman RH et al: Relative efficacy of blood, urine, rectal swab, bone-marrow, and rose-spot cultures for recovery of *Salmonella typhi* in typhoid fever. *Lancet* **1:**1211, 1975

67. Gulati PD et al: Changing patterns of typhoid fever. *Am J Med* **45:**544, 1968

68. Litwack KD et al: Rose spots in typhoid fever. *Arch Dermatol* **105:**252, 1972

69. Hornick RB et al: Typhoid fever: pathogenesis and immunologic control. *N Engl J Med* **283:**739, 1970

70. Hoffman SL et al: Reduction of mortality in chloramphenicol-treated severe typhoid fever by high-dose dexamethasone. *N Engl J Med* **310:**82, 1984

71. Nolan CM, White PC: Treatment of typhoid carriers with amoxicillin. *JAMA* **239:**2352, 1978

72. Giuliano A et al: Bacteriology of necotizing faciitis. *Am J Surg* **134:**52, 1977

73. Brenner DJ et al: *Taxomonic and Nomenclature Changes in Enterobacteriaceae.* Atlanta, Centers for Disease Control, 1977

74. Moore WEC et al: Identification of anaerobes from clinical infections, in *Anaerobic Bacteria,* edited by A Balows et al. Springfield, IL, Charles C Thomas, 1974, p 51

75. Culbertson WR: Acute non-clostridial crepitant cellulitis. *Arch Surg* **77:**462, 1958

76. Bessman AN, Wagner W: Nonclostridial gas gangrene. *JAMA* **233:**958, 1975

77. Goldstein EJ et al: Infections caused by *Klebsiella ozaenae:* a changing disease spectrum. *J Clin Microbiol* **8:**413, 1978

78. Altmann G et al: Rhinoscleroma. *Isr J Med Sci* **13:**62, 1977

79. Malowany MS et al: Isolation and microbiologic differentiation of *Klebsiella rhinoscleromatis* and *Klebsiella ozaenae* in cases of chronic rhinitis. *Am J Clin Pathol* **58:**550, 1972

80. Galpin JE et al: Sepsis associated with decubitus ulcers. *Am J Med* **61:**346, 1976

CHAPTER 178

MISCELLANEOUS BACTERIAL INFECTIONS WITH CUTANEOUS MANIFESTATIONS

Morton N. Swartz and Arnold N. Weinberg

This chapter encompasses a group of "exotic" diseases rarely seen in urban practice in the United States. The thread of continuity that can be woven among this miscellaneous group involves epidemiologic considerations. If the occupation and travel history, the possibility of animal exposure, and the duration of the incubation periods are considered, the diagnosis can often be made expeditiously. Many of the illnesses described in this chapter, e.g., anthrax and rat-bite fever, are systemic infections having a major cutaneous component which helps to suggest the proper diagnosis.

Diseases related to intimate contact with animals, fish, fowl, or their products

Anthrax

Definition. The most common form of infection with *Bacillus anthracis* is an acute cutaneous lesion called "malignant pustule" [1]. Anthrax is primarily a disease of domestic and wild animals, but humans become accidentally involved through exposure to animals and their products.

Bacteriology and pathogenic aspects. BACTERIOLOGY. *Bacillus anthracis* is a large, gram-positive, square-ended rod that forms spores in the external environment and on culture, but not in tissues. Growth occurs readily on blood agar medium without a hemolytic reaction. This characteristic, plus pathogenicity for mice and lack of motility, helps to distinguish this organism from saprophytic *Bacillus* species.

PATHOGENIC ASPECTS. Cutaneous infection usually follows introduction of spores at the site of an abrasion. Following germination, the encapsulated organisms resist phagocytosis, and elaborate an exotoxin (composed of three distinct proteins: edema factor, lethal factor, and protective antigen) which probably is responsible for the characteristic gelatinous edema of the local lesion. Exotoxin may also be responsible for irreversible shock following bacteremia. Toxin production by virulent strains of *B. anthracis* is determined by plasmids which code for the toxin itself or for regulatory proteins. These plasmids are temperature-sensitive. Thus, it appears that Pasteur's original anthrax vaccine (strain of *B. anthracis* obtained by repeated subculture at increased temperature) against animal anthrax was attenuated through elimination of the plasmid genes for toxin production.

Epidemiology. Natural infection occurs in many domestic and wild animals. Highly resistant spores persist for many years in products of these animals and in pastures where they live. Vaccination and animal control programs have essentially eliminated reservoirs of infection in the United States, but imported animal products from the Middle and Near East, Africa, and South America introduce spores into a selected industrial environment. Infection in this country is almost entirely limited to persons working in animal product-associated industries, particularly individuals handling raw materials in wool factories. Shaving brushes, imported bongo drums, and piano keys (ivory) have been implicated in sporadic infections in persons not related to the above industries. In recent years, as regulations to safeguard employees in these plants have been strictly enforced, cases have become extremely rare. Most often infection occurs on an exposed part (face, neck, or arms) in an area of previous injury, since the organisms cannot penetrate the intact epidermis. In addition to direct inoculation through abrasions, inhalation of spores may rarely result in sinus or pulmonary infection ("woolsorter's disease"). Ingestion of spores may rarely be followed by intestinal anthrax.

Clinical manifestations. HISTORY. The patient almost invariably is employed in an animal product industry, usually handling wool, goat and other animal hair, hides, bones, etc. The initial symptoms, following a 1- to 3-day incubation period, are usually low-grade fever and malaise. A painless papular lesion is usually noted on an exposed area. Itching or burning may accompany the early lesion; progressive edema, discoloration, and enlargement then occur. The initial symptoms of inhalation anthrax are insidious, with fever, fatigue, and malaise, progressing to nonproductive cough, dyspnea, cyanosis, and collapse. In this form of the disease, as well as in septicemic anthrax, meningitis may develop and dominate the clinical picture.

CUTANEOUS LESION. The cutaneous lesion ("malignant pustule") is the classical primary infection in anthrax, occurring in greater than 95 percent of cases. It is most often located on an exposed area of the head, neck (Fig. 178-1), or upper extremity, beginning as a pimple or papule. The lesion enlarges and develops into a vesicle with surrounding brawny, gelatinous, nonpitting edema. During its evolution, the vesicle becomes hemorrhagic and then necrotic, and may be surrounded by small satellite vesicles. The area of nonpitting edema increases, an eschar forms, and the red discoloration becomes more intense, *but without pain*. Rarely, the area of necrosis extends over most of the edematous region, or edema may be present without any detectable primary lesion or necrosis. Regional lymph nodes may be slightly enlarged and tender, but there is no lymphangitis.

OTHER PHYSICAL FINDINGS. Systemic manifestations (high fever, tachycardia, hypotension) may accompany either extensive cutaneous involvement or dissemination from a skin site. In woolsorter's disease, tachypnea, stridor, and cyanosis may be prominent. A thick, gelatinous, hemorrhagic nasal discharge may accompany acute sinusitis due to *B. anthracis*.

Laboratory findings. The white blood cell count is usually elevated, with a preponderance of polymorphonuclear leukocytes. If meningitis is present, the cerebrospinal fluid is characteristically hemorrhagic and gram-positive bacilli may be seen.

Pathology. The prominent features are hemorrhagic edema, dilatation of lymphatics, and necrosis of the epidermis in the area of the eschar. Bacteria may be seen in the area of cellulitis.

Diagnosis and differential diagnosis. The diagnosis is usually suspected on the basis of the character of the lesion and the occupational history. Demonstration of large gram-positive rods in vesicle fluid or upon aspiration beneath the eschar supports the diagnosis. Definitive diagnosis requires culture of the organism and demonstration of its susceptibility to specific bacteriophage lysis. Identification of organisms in smears of exudate or in tissue specimens is possible utilizing a direct fluorescent antibody technique. Occasionally, the organism can be isolated from the blood during the acute cutaneous illness as well as in disseminated anthrax. Retrospective serodiagnosis is possible with the demonstration of a titer rise in an indirect microhemagglutination test.

Acute staphylococcal cellulitis with a central pustular lesion or a carbuncle with necrotic eschar may be confused with early anthrax. Pyogenic staphylococcal lesions are usually very painful and tender, and the etiologic agent is usually present on Gram-stain examination.

Treatment. Parenteral crystalline penicillin G (2 million units every 6 h) is the treatment of choice. In one study, smears and cultures from vesicles or from the necrotic tissue beneath the eschar became negative within 6 h of initiation of penicillin therapy [2]. For systemic infection (inhalation, gastrointestinal, meningeal), higher doses of penicillin (2 million units every 2 h for the adult) are indicated.

Treatment of cutaneous anthrax should continue until

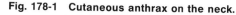
Fig. 178-1   Cutaneous anthrax on the neck.

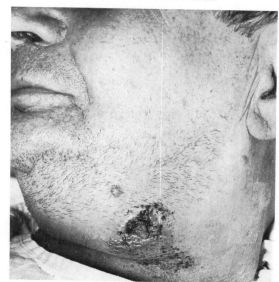

the local edema has disappeared or the lesion has dried up, i.e., for 7 to 14 days. When the edema has almost completely resolved, penicillin therapy may be switched to the oral route to complete the treatment course. In the penicillin-allergic individual, tetracycline (1.0 to 2.0 g daily intravenously in the adult), erythromycin, or chloramphenicol are alternatives.

Incision and debridement should be avoided in this disease, since this increases the opportunity for bacteremia. The disease does not appear to impart permanent immunity. A cell-free vaccine prepared from a nontoxigenic mutant strain suitable for human use is available for employees in high-risk industries [3].

Course and prognosis. Rapid defervescence and clinical improvement follow the institution of appropriate antibiotic therapy. In pulmonary, intestinal, septicemic, and meningeal anthrax the prognosis is exceedingly grave, especially if the disease is not recognized promptly.

Brucellosis

Definition. Brucellosis is an acute or chronic infection (due to any one of four species of the genus *Brucella*) transmitted to humans from contact with animals or animal products. Such infections may be acute with bacteremia, or chronic with a variety of symptoms and signs.

Bacteriology and pathogenic aspects. BACTERIOLOGY. The brucellae are nonmotile, coccobacillary gram-negative rods that require enriched media, and an atmosphere containing 8 to 10% CO_2 for optimal growth.

PATHOGENIC ASPECTS. Contact with infected animals or contaminated excretions allows organisms to enter through small skin abrasions. Another portal for these organisms is ingestion of contaminated unpasteurized milk or cheese. The organisms can multiply intracellularly in a variety of tissues and produce acute symptoms. They may persist within cells for prolonged periods, leading to chronic brucellosis. The effects of endotoxin as well as hypersensitivity to brucella antigens appear to contribute to the clinical manifestations.

Epidemiology. Domestic animals are the reservoir of brucella; humans are infected primarily by direct contact with animal material or by ingestion of raw milk or unpasteurized cheese. The majority of patients (75 percent) are males employed as abattoir workers in the meat-packing industry, engaged in livestock raising, or are veterinarians [4]. In the past most infections in the United States were due to *B. abortus* secondary to contact with infected cattle. More recently 70 percent of blood culture isolates from meat-processing-plant employees with brucellosis have been *B. suis.*

Another important group of patients with brucella infection are travellers who have become infected in endemic areas (countries of the Mediterranean littoral, the Middle East, Mexico) through ingestion of unpasteurized cow's or goat's milk or cheese. Unpasteurized cheese sent from abroad to friends or relatives in the United States may also be a source of infection. In recent years a brucella species, *B. canis,* that produces abortion or prostatitis and epididymitis in dogs, has been recognized as a cause of infection in individuals (pet owners, veterinarians) in contact with infected canines.

Clinical manifestations. HISTORY. In the majority of cases, contact with animals or their products is an essential feature of the history. The incubation period is usually 1 to 3 weeks, followed either by an acute febrile illness with headache (sometimes with involvement of local areas such as liver, joints, or meninges), or an indolent disease with weakness, anorexia, and low-grade fever which may persist for weeks or months. Brucella involvement of the spine in the form of vertebral body osteomyelitis is not infrequent. Rarer forms of infection include suppurative lymphadenitis and endocarditis.

CUTANEOUS LESIONS. There are no typical cutaneous lesions, although rashes have been reported in 5 to 9 percent of cases [5]. Erythematous, papular, urticarial, and vesicular lesions may appear during the course of the illness, and burning, itching, and desquamation also have been described following contact with infected animal products [6]. Rarely, subcutaneous abscesses or cutaneous sinus tracts may develop as a result of extension of suppuration from infected lymph nodes or sites of osteomyelitis, or following introduction of organisms through a skin abrasion. A severe hypersensitivity reaction to brucella antigen may occur among veterinarians and animal handlers exposed directly to infected material. This may be manifested by an acute febrile reaction and the appearance of discrete, elevated, red papules on the hands or arms that may progress to ulceration. Dramatic reactions of this type have occurred in veterinarians who have accidentally inoculated themselves with the attenuated strain of brucella used to immunize farm animals [7].

OTHER PHYSICAL FINDINGS. Among the characteristic findings may be lymphadenopathy, hepatosplenomegaly, suppurative arthritis, and evidence of osteomyelitis or spondylitis.

Laboratory findings. The white blood cell count is usually normal or depressed, and anemia is frequently present. Blood cultures may be positive during the acute illness.

Pathology. Lesions in the liver, spleen, and other organs frequently consist of small, noncaseating granulomas. Rarely larger areas with caseation necrosis and calcification occur in infections due to *B. suis.*

Diagnosis and differential diagnosis. The diagnosis of brucellosis is usually based upon epidemiologic information (animal contact), cultures (blood, bone marrow, organ granulomas), and *rising* serum agglutination titer. A titer of greater than 1:160 should raise the possibility of this disease, and warrant repetition of the test 7 to 14 days later. The presence of a prozone phenomenon and the development of "blocking antibody" may occasionally require modifications in the performance of the agglutination test. The antibody response to brucella infection is initially that of IgM followed by IgG antibodies. The IgM response may last for many months up to several years, but the IgG antibodies decrease rapidly following antimicrobial therapy. In patients with chronic symptomatology, the presence of IgG antibodies indicates continuing or recrudescent active infection. Skin testing with brucella antigen may lead to falsely positive serologic values and should not be performed. Cross reactions with *Francisella tularensis* occur uncommonly, and vaccination within the year for cholera may stimulate a brucella agglutinin titer.

The differential diagnosis includes other acute bacterial infections such as salmonellosis, listeriosis, tuberculosis, and endocarditis. Hodgkin's disease may mimic many of the findings of brucellosis. Vertebral osteomyelitis may sometimes be the primary or sole manifestation of brucellosis. Occasionally, a prolonged low-grade form of this illness is mistakenly considered as a psychoneurosis.

Treatment. For the adult, tetracycline 0.5 g orally, 4 times daily for 3 to 4 weeks, is given alone or combined with streptomycin (1 g daily intramuscularly for the first 7 to 14 days of treatment). Doxycycline has also been used successfully. Trimethoprim-sulfamethoxazole (480 mg trimethoprim-2400 mg sulfamethoxazole daily) for at least 4 weeks is a reasonable alternative in the patient whose infection has relapsed following combined tetracycline-streptomycin therapy or who cannot tolerate the latter antibiotics.

Course and prognosis. Early treatment results in rapid improvement. Brucellosis recurs in approximately 1 to 10 percent of treated patients. Chronicity, often in the form of osteomyelitis or joint infection, may lead to more permanent disability.

Erysipeloid

Definition. Erysipeloid is an acute infection of traumatized skin caused by a slender, gram-positive rod, *Erysipelothrix rhusiopathiae,* occurring in fishermen, butchers, and others handling raw fish, poultry, and meat products [8].

Bacteriology. *Erysipelothrix rhusiopathiae* is a thin, gram-positive, slightly curved bacillus which tends to form filaments in culture. Growth occurs best on media fortified with serum. The bacillus is microaerophilic and nonmotile, and is hardy enough to survive drying, putrefaction of tissue, and saltwater or freshwater exposure. There are certain morphologic and cultural similarities between *E. rhusiopathiae* and *Listeria monocytogenes.*

Epidemiology. *Erysipelothrix rhusiopathiae* is the cause of a cutaneous and systemic infection of swine, and is present also in the slime of saltwater fish, on crabs and other shellfish, or associated with poultry (especially turkeys), meats, and by-products such as hides and bones. Occurrence of the disease is limited almost exclusively to persons handling contaminated products. Most cases occur during summer months. Usually the organisms are inoculated through a break in the skin of the hands. There have been epidemics among crab fishermen ("crab dermatitis") and bone button makers. The disease does not seem to confer lasting immunity.

Clinical manifestations. HISTORY. Usually the patient is employed in fishing or animal product industries. Initially, there is burning pain at a site of injury. The incubation period is 2 to 7 days. A violaceous, raised area appears and enlarges. Lymphangitis and regional lymphadenopathy

occasionally occur. Constitutional symptoms include low-grade fever and malaise. Occasionally, an adjacent joint is involved. Rarely, bacteremia and even endocarditis may follow [9].

CUTANEOUS LESION. The distinctive lesion is usually on a finger or hand, is violet or purple-red in color, warm and tender, and has well-defined, raised margins (Fig. A1-21). As the process advances peripherally, the central region clears without desquamation or ulceration [10]. The lesion may enlarge considerably (Fig. 178-2). Rarely, dissemination occurs with multiple lesions distant from the original site of injury. Brownish discoloration develops as the lesion resolves [11].

OTHER PHYSICAL FINDINGS. Arthritis may be associated with the local lesion, and, rarely, distant joints are involved. Bronchitis may follow inhalation of organisms. Conjunctivitis also occurs. Typical peripheral stigmata as well as cardiac findings of endocarditis or septicemia have been reported [12,13]

Laboratory findings. There are no characteristic findings, and the organism is seldom seen on Gram's stain of material from the surface of the lesion or from aspirated material. Culture of a biopsy from the advancing edge of the lesion may reveal the organism.

Pathology. Dilatation of vessels in the papillary and subpapillary areas, and perivascular cellular infiltrates deep in the dermis are present. The depth of the process may explain why organisms rarely are seen or cultured from the lesion.

Diagnosis and differential diagnosis. The character of the local lesion in a person handling fresh meat or fish products suggests the diagnosis. Other forms of bacterial cellulitis

Fig. 178-2 Erysipeloid. The purple-red area is very slightly tender and warm, not hot, to touch.

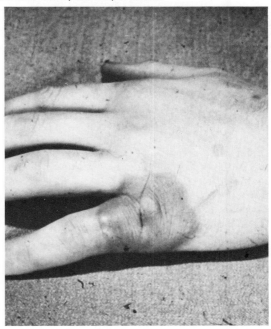

or erysipelas may be confused with erysipeloid. "Seal finger" may be mistaken for erysipeloid.

Treatment. Penicillin, in doses of *2 to 3 million units daily,* orally or intramuscularly, for 7 to 10 days, is the treatment for erysipeloid. Erythromycin is an alternative for a penicillin-allergic patient. If arthritis, septicemia, or endocarditis is present, the dose of penicillin should be raised to 2 to 4 million units every 4 h, administered intravenously (for 4 weeks in the case of endocarditis).

Course and prognosis. In the untreated patient, the lesion usually lasts for 2 to 3 weeks but may persist with cycles of improvement and worsening over several months. If penicillin is administered, the improvement is dramatic and recurrence is rare. In systemic infection, the course and prognosis depend on early and appropriate treatment.

Glanders

Definition. Glanders is an equine disease caused by the bacterium *Pseudomonas mallei.* This infection rarely is transmitted to humans. The clinical picture takes one of two forms: (1) an acute, febrile, disseminated, infectious process whose entire course may encompass only 10 to 30 days; (2) an indolent, relapsing, chronic infection, with multiple cutaneous and subcutaneous abscesses and draining sinuses. "Farcy," the name given to the disease in horses, refers to the nodular subcutaneous abscesses occurring along the course of lymphatics.

Bacteriology. *Pseudomonas mallei* is an aerobic, nonmotile, gram-negative bacillus, with bipolar staining. It can be cultured on ordinary nutrient media. Antigenically and biochemically it is distinct from *Pseudomonas pseudomallei,* the cause of melioidosis.

Epidemiology. Control measures have almost completely eradicated this previously common equine infection and essentially eliminated transmission to humans in the United States. Occasional cases still occur in Asia, Africa, and South America. Humans are infected by direct contact with horses. The organisms gain entry through abrasions in the skin, via the conjunctivae, or by inhalation or ingestion.

Clinical manifestations. HISTORY. In the acute fulminating form, the incubation period is usually 2 to 5 days. The onset is abrupt, with headache, malaise, chills, high fever, nausea, and vomiting. In the chronic form of glanders, the onset of malaise, headache, muscle pains, arthralgias, and low-grade fever is gradual. After many weeks, typical cutaneous and subcutaneous nodules, abscesses, and draining sinuses develop.

CUTANEOUS LESIONS. In acute glanders, a nodule or cellulitis appears at the site of inoculation. Local swelling and suppuration occur, and the lesion ulcerates. The ulcer is painful and has irregular edges with a gray-yellow base. Nodular sores rapidly develop along lymphatics draining the lesion; they become necrotic and ulcerated, and sinuses form. Regional lymphadenopathy is present. Widespread dissemination quickly follows, with multiple nodular necrotic abscesses in subcutaneous tissues and muscle. Lesions frequently coalesce into gangrenous areas. During this phase of bacteremic spread, a characteristic eruption appears which may be generalized or localized to the face and neck. The lesions (papules, bullae, and pustules) appear in crops. Involvement of the nasal mucosa, either initially or by secondary spread, is prominent. Mucopurulent, bloody nasal discharge is commonly noted. Infection may spread to the paranasal sinuses, pharynx, and lung.

In chronic glanders, cutaneous and subcutaneous nodules appear on the extremities and occasionally on the face. The lesions ulcerate, and draining sinuses develop. Repeated cycles of healing and breakdown of nodules may continue for weeks or months. Finally, conversion to the acute form of the disease can occur.

OTHER PHYSICAL FINDINGS. Bacteremic spread of infection may produce pneumonia, empyema, meningitis, septic arthritis, or osteomyelitis. Splenomegaly and hepatomegaly are sometimes present in both acute and chronic glanders. Pulmonary infiltrates and pneumonia occur, particularly after accidental (laboratory) inhalation.

Laboratory findings. A normal leukocyte count is usual, but a mild leukocytosis or leukopenia may occur.

Pathology. In acute glanders the pathologic picture is that of a suppurative, necrotic process, containing numerous intracellular and extracellular bacteria. In the chronic form of glanders, a granulomatous process (with few giant cells) suggesting tuberculosis is usually observed.

Diagnosis and differential diagnosis. The diagnosis is made on the basis of the epidemiologic background, examination of Gram-stained smears of pus, isolation of the organism from abscesses or blood, and serologic tests. Acute glanders may resemble miliary tuberculosis or typhoid fever during the initial stages. The multiple subcutaneous abscesses suggest staphylococcal or mycotic infections, or melioidosis. Lymphatic nodularity resembles the lesions of sporotrichosis.

Treatment. Experience with modern chemotherapy is limited. Sulfonamides (sulfadiazine 100 mg/kg daily in divided doses) have been used successfully, particularly in laboratory-acquired (pulmonary) infections. A combination of intramuscular streptomycin with tetracycline has recently been recommended. Patients should be isolated.

Course and prognosis. Without antibiotic therapy, acute glanders has a mortality rate of over 90 percent. Chronic glanders has a better prognosis, especially since the advent of chemotherapy.

Streptobacillus moniliformis infection ("rat-bite fever")

Definition. Rat-bite fever is an acute infection which is usually acquired from rodents and is characterized by fever, polyarthralgias or arthritis, and a rash [14].

Bacteriology. *Streptobacillus moniliformis* is a gram-negative, pleomorphic bacillus. Growth in culture occurs as chains of bacilli and filamentous forms, interspersed with swollen bodies that look like *Candida (Monilia)*, hence the name *moniliformis*. In blood cultures these microaerophilic organisms typically grow as small "puff balls" after prolonged incubation. On occasion, this organism may grow as an L form on initial culture.

Epidemiology. *Streptobacillus moniliformis* is found in the nasopharynx of approximately 50 percent of wild and laboratory rats. In recent years, the latter have been an increasing source of infection. Sporadic cases without contact with rats have been reported. Infection may occur also following ingestion of contaminated food. One such milk-borne outbreak occurred in Haverhill, Massachusetts, in 1926, and this illness was designated "Haverhill fever" (erythema arthriticum epidemicum) [15].

Clinical manifestations. HISTORY. The incubation period averages 1 to 5 days. The rat bite has often healed by the time the illness begins suddenly, with fever, chills, headache, and myalgias.

CUTANEOUS LESIONS. An erythematous macular or papular rash may develop within 2 to 3 days of the onset of symptoms. It is most marked on the extremities, (often involving palms and soles), particularly about joints, but may become generalized, resembling measles. Sometimes, the lesions are petechial.

OTHER PHYSICAL FINDINGS. Within a week of onset arthritis can develop involving larger joints such as the knee. Regional lymphadenopathy may be present.

Laboratory findings. Polymorphonuclear leukocytosis is common. *S. moniliformis* usually can be isolated from blood or joint fluid, or sometimes from an abscess developing at the bite site. Serologic diagnosis involves use of agglutination, fluorescent antibody, or complement fixation tests.

Diagnosis and differential diagnosis. The skin lesions are not specific. The diagnosis should be suspected in any febrile patient with a history of a recent rat bite. Blood cultures are the best way to establish the diagnosis. The other form of rat-bite fever (*Spirillum minus*) (sodoku) may cause a similar illness, but several features are helpful in distinguishing between the two conditions [14]:

1. *Streptobacillus moniliformis* infection has a shorter incubation period (usually less than 10 days).
2. The bite site usually has healed by the time of onset of fever in *S. moniliformis* infection.
3. The incidence of arthritis is low in *S. minus* infection.

The differential diagnosis should also include meningococcemia, gonococcemia, viral exanthems, and Rocky Mountain spotted fever.

Treatment. Penicillin, 600,000 units intramuscularly every 6 h for 10 to 12 days, is the drug of choice. Tetracycline or streptomycin are alternatives in the penicillin-allergic patient.

Course and prognosis. Untreated, the disease may last from a few days to several weeks. Rarely, it is complicated by endocarditis. Penicillin produces a prompt clinical response.

Diseases associated primarily with a specific geographic distribution

Bartonellosis (Carrión's disease)

Definition. *Bartonella bacilliformis* produces a disease exhibiting two characteristic stages: (1) a severe acute febrile illness with hemolytic anemia, known as Oroya fever; (2) a benign, nodular, cutaneous eruption, referred to as verruga peruana or Peruvian warts [16].

Bacteriology and pathogenic aspects. BACTERIOLOGY. Both phases of the disease are caused by the motile, gram-negative coccobacillus *B. bacilliformis*. This organism grows on media containing 10 percent fresh rabbit serum and hemoglobin. Growth characteristically is slow (8 to 10 days).

PATHOGENIC ASPECTS. Organisms are introduced into a susceptible individual by a bite from an infected sand fly. They subsequently are found in the cells of the reticuloendothelial system and attached to red blood cells, causing them to become fragile, and leading to the profound anemia of Oroya fever [17]. Cutaneous lesions represent late bacterial invasion of the blood vessels of the dermis, resulting in proliferating vascular nodules.

Epidemiology. The distribution of *B. bacilliformis* is confined to the valley regions of the Andes Mountains in South America, particularly in Colombia, Ecuador, and Peru. Humans are the only natural host, though monkeys and other animals have been experimentally infected. The sand fly (*Phlebotomus*) is the vector; its natural habitat is coextensive with the distribution of the disease (750 to 2800 meters elevation) in arid river valleys of the Andes.

Clinical manifestations. HISTORY. Characteristically, the patient lives in or has visited the endemic area, but may have no recollection of having been bitten by sand flies. Since the incubation period is 19 to 30 days, there is ample time for visitors to return to distant parts of the world before the onset of symptoms. Oroya fever is characterized by intermittent fever, myalgias, malaise, headache, gastrointestinal irritability, and, finally, symptoms due to increasingly severe hemolytic anemia. During convalescence from Oroya fever numerous discrete nodules may appear on the extremities, without recurrence of fever, malaise, or anemia. Occasionally, the cutaneous eruption occurs alone or precedes the systemic illness, and this is not accompanied by constitutional symptoms.

CUTANEOUS LESIONS. Oroya fever is not accompanied by skin lesions. The cutaneous lesions of the second stage of the disease (verruga peruana) usually appear during convalescence from Oroya fever. The incubation period is 30 to 60 days. The most common eruption consists of miliary lesions (erythematous macules and papules) on the face and extensor surfaces of the extremities (Fig. 178-3). The lesions bleed readily and may ulcerate. The eruption heals without scarring. Involvement of the conjunctivae and nose and throat may occur. The other type of lesions

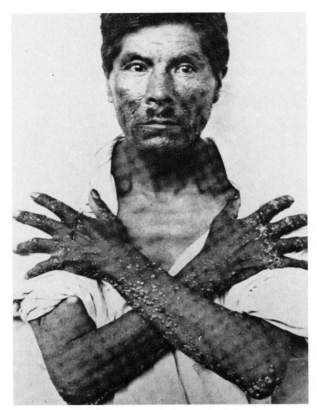

Fig. 178-3   Bartonellosis (verruga peruana). *[Courtesy of Dr. O. Canizares. From Canizares O (ed): Clinical Tropical Dermatology. Oxford, Blackwell, 1975, p 149.]*

are round, soft, hemangiomatous, subcutaneous nodules which may reach 1 to 2 cm in size. Sessile or pedunculated lesions also occur. They tend to occur in crops, are located on the extremities, spare the trunk, and may ulcerate and bleed.

OTHER PHYSICAL FINDINGS. Oroya fever is accompanied by marked pallor, mild icterus, and splenomegaly.

Laboratory findings. A profound (macrocytic) hemolytic anemia, with a reticulocytosis of up to 50 percent and erythroblasts and normoblasts in the peripheral blood, is not unusual [18]. On Giemsa-stained blood smears, numerous *B. bacilliformis* can be seen on or in red blood cells, and as many as 95 percent of cells may be parasitized. With the onset of convalescence from Oroya fever the *Bartonella* become less numerous and change from bacillary to coccoid forms. Bilirubinemia, predominantly of the unconjugated fraction, is present. Leukocytosis may occur but is usually due to a complicating infection.

Pathology. The skin nodules show capillary and endothelial cell proliferation resembling capillary hemangiomas. They appear neoplastic, with many mitotic figures. Phagocytized *Bartonella* can be seen in endothelial and histiocytic cells of verrugas [19].

Diagnosis and differential diagnosis. The diagnosis depends primarily on an appropriate geographic history and on characterization of the etiologic agent. In Oroya fever, the

organisms can be seen in red blood cells on stained smears, and blood cultures are almost always positive. In the cutaneous phase and even during convalescence, low-grade bacteremia may be present; also, organisms can be seen in and isolated from the nodular lesion.

Other rare forms of systemic (bacteremic) hemotrophic bacterial infections have been described [20]. The geographic confines of bartonellosis and the cultural characteristics of *B. bacilliformis* distinguish acute (Oroya fever) bartonellosis from these other hemotrophic infections; the distinctive skin lesions of verruga peruana are readily distinguished from the macules and petechiae that may be present in other hemotrophic bacterial infections.

Treatment. Penicillin, streptomycin, tetracycline, and chloramphenicol have all been used successfully. Chloramphenicol (0.5 g orally every 4 to 6 h) is preferred if there is any suspicion of an accompanying *Salmonella* bacteremia (see Chap. 177). A therapeutic response usually is evident within 48 h. Control of sand flies with insecticides is the most important preventive measure.

Course and prognosis. The mortality rate of untreated Oroya fever is approximately 40 percent, and is due to profound anemia and also to concurrent infections (malaria, amebiasis, tuberculosis, and salmonellosis). Salmonella septicemia has been reported in approximately 40 percent of affected individuals. The mechanism of this predisposition to secondary salmonella infection is unknown, but it may reflect a saturation of the reticuloendothelial system, with subsequent failure to clear these organisms.

In treated cases, the course is usually one of rapid improvement. The course and prognosis of the cutaneous syndrome are entirely favorable, in keeping with the concept that this represents a manifestation of developing immunity to the infection. Second attacks are extremely rare.

Melioidosis

Definition. Melioidosis is an infectious disease of animals and humans, endemic in Southeast Asia, but also occurring in Africa, South America, and the Middle East, between 20° north and south latitudes, and caused by the gram-negative bacillus *Pseudomonas pseudomallei* [21]. Apart from rare cases of laboratory-acquired infections, melioidosis has occurred in only those United States residents who have traveled abroad. During the recent war in Vietnam extensive exposure to this organism resulted in cases of melioidosis (some fatal) among American servicemen. Melioidosis is very similar to glanders clinically and pathologically, but is entirely different epidemiologically. The clinical manifestations of this disease take one of two principal forms: (1) acute melioidosis with suppurative skin infection, pneumonia, or septicemia; (2) chronic melioidosis, the most common form of the disease, which involves the lung (unresolved pneumonia or cavitary lesions), skin (subcutaneous abscesses and draining sinuses), bones, joints, liver, spleen, etc.

Bacteriology. The etiologic agent is a small, pleomorphic, gram-negative bacillus with bipolar staining that can be grown aerobically on common laboratory media.

Epidemiology. The etiologic agent of melioidosis can be isolated widely from soil, vegetables, and water in the rice-growing areas of Southeast Asia. Melioidosis appears to be transmitted by contamination of abraded skin with infected soil. The prominence of pulmonary findings in many patients, and of diarrhea in some, has suggested the possibility that it may be transmitted by inhalation or ingestion. Person-to-person transmission of melioidosis is rare [22].

Clinical manifestations. HISTORY. The incubation period is variable. It has been as short as 3 days and the disease has also remained latent for years. The acute pneumonic form may begin with a short prodrome (malaise, anorexia, and diarrhea), but more commonly its onset is abrupt, with chills, fever, cough, dyspnea, and chest pain. The acute septicemic form may start with an ulceration at the site of inoculation, lymphangitis, and regional lymphadenitis. Chronic melioidosis may follow the acute disease. More often it develops as an indolent pulmonary infection or as a low-grade febrile illness with multiple superficial abscesses. Recrudescence of a previous latent or clinical infection months or years after initial exposure to the organism may be precipitated by various illnesses (e.g., thermal burns, diabetic ketoacidosis, pneumonia) [23].

CUTANEOUS LESIONS. Cutaneous manifestations are not a specific or diagnostic feature of melioidosis. The acute septicemic form may complicate a superficial ulceration and cellulitis. In chronic melioidosis, subcutaneous abscesses and draining sinuses (from bone or lymph nodes) are common features and may occur even in the absence of fever.

OTHER PHYSICAL FINDINGS. In acute pulmonary melioidosis, the findings range from those of bronchitis to those of acute pneumonia or lung abscess. Septicemic spread of the disease leads to jaundice, hepatosplenomegaly, miliary pulmonary densities, myocarditis, and severe gastroenteritis. Chronic pulmonary melioidosis produces signs suggestive of fibrocavitary tuberculosis or lung abscess. The disseminated form of chronic disease may extend over many months with septic arthritis, osteomyelitis, suppurative lymphadenopathy, and visceral abscesses.

Laboratory findings. The peripheral white blood cell count is usually normal or only moderately elevated.

Pathology. Sharply circumscribed abscesses are found in many organs and in the subcutaneous tissues. There may be a surrounding granulomatous response.

Diagnosis and differential diagnosis. The various forms of melioidosis and the multiplicity of organs involved characterize this disease as a great imitator. Acute melioidosis may mimic typhoid fever, staphylococcal pneumonia, mycotic infections, or septicemia. In its chronic form, it must be differentiated from pulmonary tuberculosis, nocardiosis, fungal infections, and lung abscess. Chronic skin infections and draining sinuses in individuals from endemic areas should raise the possibility of melioidosis.

The diagnosis is suspected on epidemiologic grounds. Culture of the organism establishes the etiology. Hemagglutination, direct agglutination, and complement-fixation tests are helpful when a rise in titer is demonstrated.

Treatment. Antibiotic susceptibility must be determined on each isolate because of variations from strain to strain. In the adult with mild disease, chloramphenicol (3.0 g per 24 h) or tetracycline (2 g per 24 h) have been effective. Sulfisoxazole is an alternative. Trimethoprim-sulfamethoxazole has also been used successfully. For the severely ill patient the combination of tetracycline and chloramphenicol has been recommended in even higher dosage. Antibiotic therapy should be continued for at least 4 weeks and combined with surgical drainage of accessible abscesses.

Course and prognosis. Untreated, acute melioidosis is often fatal. Although antibiotic therapy has significantly improved the mortality rate in chronic melioidosis, it is still over 50 percent in the septicemic form.

Plague

Definition. Plague is a severe, acute, febrile infection in humans caused by *Yersinia pestis* [24]. Transmission between the natural reservoir of this disease (wild and commensal rodents) and human beings is effected by fleas. Infection occurs in three forms: (1) bubonic plague; (2) bubonic-septicemic plague (a more acute and severe form of bubonic plague with bacteremia and delirium); (3) pneumonic plague (fulminant form of infection resulting from respiratory spread of *Y. pestis*).

Bacteriology. *Yersinia pestis* is an aerobic gram-negative bacillus with "safety-pin" bipolar staining. It produces an intracellular toxin (plague toxin) which is plasmid encoded and an important virulence factor [25].

Epidemiology. Endemic (sylvatic) plague is firmly established among wild rodents in the western United States. In this country, human plague is almost always fleaborne and is usually of the bubonic type. Between 1956 and 1983, 231 cases of plague were reported in the United States. Most occurred during the warmer months and were transmitted by flea bites. "Off-season" (October to February) plague occurs during rabbit-hunting season in the western states and is associated with direct contact (skinning, dressing) with animal (rabbits, bobcats) carcasses [26]. In recent years, epizootics have occurred among prairie dogs in the Southwest, and sporadic human cases have been identified on several Indian reservations [27]. The disease is also endemic in Vietnam. Rarely, plague pneumonia secondary to bacteremia complicating bubonic plague may initiate respiratory spread to other persons.

Clinical manifestations. HISTORY. The incubation period is approximately 1 to 6 days, followed by the sudden onset of malaise, myalgias, backache, tachycardia, and high fever.

CUTANEOUS LESIONS. In bubonic plague, the initial skin manifestation is related to the flea bite. Usually, this cannot be seen, but occasionally a small papule or vesicopustule persists. Painful, tender, enlarged lymph nodes are present in the area draining the bite site. The nodes become matted (buboes) (Fig. 178-4), and there is extensive surrounding subcutaneous gelantinous edema. Bacteremia may supervene and lead to overwhelming systemic illness [28,29]. In this setting petechiae and ecchymosis often occur due to

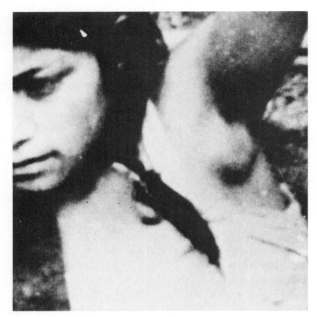

Fig. 178-4   Painful lymphadenitis in plague (bubo). Diagnosis is established by culture of the aspirate. [Courtesy of Drs. L. Leon and R. Leon, Quito, Equador. From Canizares O (ed): Clinical Tropical Dermatology. Oxford, Blackwell, 1975, p 344.]

the effects of plague toxin or to the development of a disseminated intravascular coagulopathy.

OTHER PHYSICAL FINDINGS. The onset of pneumonic plague is abrupt, with high fever, tachycardia, and tachypnea. Signs of consolidation may appear, and within 24 h of onset the patient is critically ill, raising bloody sputum loaded with *Y. pestis.* Meningitis may complicate all three forms of plague.

Laboratory findings. Leukocytosis occurs in all forms of the disease. In septicemic plague, bacilli can sometimes be seen on stained smears of venous blood (buffy coat).

Pathology. In the bubonic form, acute inflammatory changes are seen in the involved nodes.

Diagnosis and differential diagnosis. Bubonic plague should be distinguished from tularemia, lymphogranuloma venereum, cat-scratch disease, and suppurative lymphadentis. Plague pneumonia must be differentiated from other acute bacterial pneumonias. Epidemiologic considerations and the tempo of the illness are major points in the differential diagnosis. Even minimal epidemiologic information provides sufficient grounds to begin treatment, for delays may be fatal in this rapidly progressive infection. The diagnosis is firmly established by examination of Gram-stained or specific-fluorescent antibody-stained smears of infected material and by culture of the organism from blood, sputum, or aspirated buboes. Serologic methods can be used for retrospective diagnosis.

Treatment. Streptomycin is the drug of choice, administered intramuscularly (2 g daily in divided doses in the adult) for 10 days. Chloramphenicol or tetracycline are alternatives, or may be added initially since strains resistant to streptomycin have been recovered. The dosage of chloramphenicol in the adult is 4 g daily for 2 days, followed by 3 g per day; that of tetracycline, 2.0 g daily intravenously for 1 week, then 1.5 g daily for a second week. Preliminary results suggest that kanamycin may be as effective as streptomycin, and may be the most appropriate alternative should streptomycin-resistant strains increase. Strict isolation of pneumonia cases is essential to prevent spread via the respiratory route. Buboes should not be drained until the lesion is well localized and the patient has been treated with antibiotics.

Course and prognosis. Pneumonic and septicemic plague, if untreated, are almost invariably fatal. Untreated bubonic plague has a mortality rate of 30 to 70 percent. Early antibiotic therapy has reduced the mortality rate to 5 to 10 percent. Even the severest forms of the infection respond to antibiotic treatment, if instituted promptly.

Diseases associated with random animal contact independent of geographic or occupational considerations

Francisella tularensis infections (tularemia)

Definition. Tularemia is a disease of humans caused by *Francisella tularensis,* an organism that normally resides in a wide range of animal species. In human beings, most cases follow direct animal contact or transmission by insect vectors. The clinical manifestations fall into four major patterns: (1) ulceroglandular (most common form), (2) oculoglandular, (3) typhoidal, (4) pulmonary.

Bacteriology. *Francisella tularensis* is a pleomorphic, gram-negative coccobacillus which grows best on cysteine blood agar or in thioglycollate heart infusion medium. Intracellular parasitism of the reticuloendothelial system of humans and experimental animals is characteristic.

Epidemiology. Infection in humans, particularly among hunters, most commonly follows contact with infected rabbits, but may follow exposure to foxes, squirrels, skunks, and muskrats. Aquatic animals (voles, beavers) and mud and water from streams may also be a source of infection. The organisms are commonly introduced through a minimal abrasion or puncture wound. Bites of infected deerflies or ticks are also sources of infection in humans and are responsible for maintaining the disease in animals. Rarely, ingestion of meat or conjunctival contamination leads to infection.

Clinical manifestations. HISTORY. After an incubation period of 2 to 10 days, the onset of any of the four forms of disease is similar to that of most other acute infections: headache, malaise, myalgias, and high fever. A primary lesion then develops at the site of inoculation (usually on the hand), accompanied by regional adenopathy.

CUTANEOUS LESIONS. In ulceroglandular tularemia, a reddish, tender papule appears at a site of trauma or insect bite, usually on a finger or hand. A small vesicular pustule may develop, and the area rapidly enlarges and becomes necrotic. The lesion then evolves to an ulcer with raised margins, often covered by a black eschar, and appears

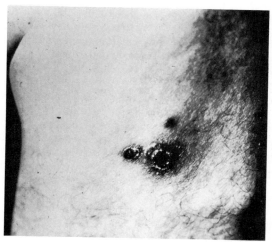

Fig. 178-5 Primary cutaneous lesions of tularemia. The black eschar is characteristic.

chancre-like (Fig. 178-5). Regional nodes are enlarged and tender. Systemic signs of toxicity may be marked and pneumonia may accompany dissemination of infection. A macular and papular or petechial exanthem on the trunk and extremities may occur in a minority of patients as the disease progresses.

In oculoglandular tularemia, the organism is directly introduced via the conjunctivae. The findings are those of a purulent conjunctivitis with marked pain, edema, and congestion. Small yellow nodules may appear on the conjunctivae and ulcerate. Corneal perforation may occur. Preauricular and submaxillary adenopathy is prominent.

OTHER PHYSICAL FINDINGS. Splenomegaly and generalized lymphadenopathy are relatively common, and hepatomegaly may occur. Ulcerative or exudative pharyngotonsillitis with cervical lymphadenopathy may follow ingestion of the organism which may also be associated with the "typhoidal" form of the disease. Tularemic pneumonia may occur occasionally following inhalation of organisms but is more often secondary to bacteremia. Pleural effusion and mediastinal node enlargement are sometimes evident.

Laboratory findings. The white blood cell count is normal or low, but a polymorphonuclear leukocytosis may be seen.

Pathology. Following inoculation, the organism progresses through lymphatic channels and nodes to the bloodstream. The organism survives intracellularly in phagocytes, and small granulomatous lesions develop in lymph nodes, liver, and spleen. Some of the lesions may caseate or progress to frank abscess formation.

Diagnosis and differential diagnosis. The primary lesion resembles a furuncle, paronychia, ecthyma, or the initial lesion of anthrax, *Pasteurella multocida* infection, or sporotrichosis. The prominent regional adenopathy suggests cat-scratch disease, plague, melioidosis or glanders, or lymphogranuloma venereum. Epidemiologic factors and systemic manifestations are points that suggest tularemia rather than other causes of a chancre-like lesion. A febrile

illness occurring after a tick bite might suggest Rocky Mountain spotted fever, but an exanthem is usually present in that condition. The skin lesion of Lyme disease, exanthem chronicum migrans, is a larger distinctive lesion that occurs after a tick bite in circumscribed geographic regions (Cape Cod, Long Island, Connecticut, Wisconsin, etc.). A febrile illness with hepatomegaly and granulomas (on liver biopsy) resembles tuberculosis, brucellosis, or other causes of granulomatous hepatitis. Isolation of *F. tularensis* from ulcer, blood, or bone marrow requires special media and is difficult to accomplish. The diagnosis is usually made by serologic (agglutination or microagglutination) tests showing a fourfold or greater rise in titer. Cross reactions occur in brucellosis. A skin test (delayed hypersensitivity), utilizing antigens from *F. tularensis,* becomes positive during the first week of disease, and may be helpful in diagnosis [30]. Unfortunately the skin test reagent is not commercially available.

Treatment. Streptomycin (1.0 to 2.0 g intramuscularly per day, in adults) is curative in all forms of tularemia if administered early. Clinical improvement is evident within 24 to 48 h, but treatment should be continued for at least 7 to 10 afebrile days. Tetracycline and chloramphenicol are alternative drugs, but clinical relapses are more frequent with these drugs particularly if given for less than 14 days. Gentamicin has been used successfully in a small number of cases. Lymph node drainage should be avoided until late in therapy.

Course and prognosis. Untreated, the course may be weeks. Prior to the use of antibiotics, the mortality rate was about 5 percent in ulceroglandular disease and about 30 percent in typhoidal and pulmonary forms. Recovery provides immunity to systemic tularemia, but reinfection may produce a recurrent primary ulcer.

Leptospirosis

Definition. Leptospirosis is an acute febrile illness caused by any one of the serovarieties (serovars) of the species *Leptospira interrogans.* Although specific serovars have been reported with specific syndromes (canicola fever, Weil's disease, pretibial fever), any serovar may be responsible for a variety of clinical pictures, and a given clinical picture may be produced by many different serovars [31].

Bacteriology. These organisms are spirochetes that can be cultured on special (Fletcher semisolid) media. More than 170 antigenically different types have been described. They are now defined as serovarieties of the species *Leptospira interrogans.* Thus, for example, a specific antigenic serotype would bear a designation such as *L. interrogans* serovar *canicola.* The most common serovars in the United States are *canicola, icterohaemorrhagiae, pomona, autumnalis,* and *grippotyphosa.*

Epidemiology. The reservoir of leptospira is in the animal population: farm animals (cattle, swine); domestic animals (dogs); wild animals (squirrels, rats). Infection in humans occurs as a result of direct contact with an animal (either a sick animal or an asymptomatic urinary "shedder"), or indirectly through contaminated water or soil. Organisms usually enter the body through a break in the skin, or less often through the mouth or conjunctiva. The disease is most prevalent among children (from playing in contaminated puddles or ponds), farmers, hunters, or abattoir workers.

Clinical manifestations. HISTORY. The incubation period is usually between 7 and 14 days, and the illness typically has a biphasic course. The onset is sudden, with headache, fever, chills, nausea, vomiting, abdominal pain, and myalgias. This initial nonspecific phase continues for about a week, when defervescence occurs. The patient is then relatively asymptomatic for several days. The second phase of illness begins with low-grade fever and often with meningeal symptoms, and persists for another 2 to 4 days, or even for several weeks. In the initial phase (leptospiremic), leptospiral organisms are present in the bloodstream, CSF, and other tissues. The second ("immune") phase coincides with the appearance of IgM antibodies. Clinically it is characterized by the onset of meningitis, rash, uveitis, and, in more severe cases, by hepatic and renal involvement.

CUTANEOUS LESIONS. Scleral conjunctival injection appears on the third or fourth day of illness. Skin lesions, usually on the trunk (consisting of macules, papules, urticaria, and petechiae), occur in less than half the cases. Peripheral desquamation and infarction of portions of the hands and feet have been observed in a few children with leptospirosis [32]. Weil's disease, often but not exclusively due to serovar *icterohaemorrhagiae,* is a form of the disease with prominent hepatic (jaundice) and renal (hematuria, azotemia) involvement. Hemorrhagic manifestations occur in a variety of organs, including the skin. Pretibial ("Fort Bragg") fever is a form of leptospirosis (serovar *autumnalis)* that has a rather distinctive rash occurring on the fourth or fifth day of illness and consisting of slightly raised, 1- to 5-cm, tender, erythematous lesions on the pretibial areas [33]. The rash subsides within 4 or 7 days. Erythema nodosum has occurred in association with infection due to *L. interrogans* [34].

OTHER PHYSICAL FINDINGS. These depend on the particular syndrome that is presented.

1. Pyrexia of unknown origin—localizing signs lacking
2. Aseptic meningitis—nuchal rigidity
3. Weil's disease—jaundice and hepatomegaly; interstitial nephritis; generalized hemorrhagic tendency with epistaxis, hematuria, and gastrointestinal bleeding
4. Pretibial fever—splenomegaly is common

In up to 20 percent of patients with leptospirosis, generalized lymphadenopathy (particularly involving cervical nodes) may be observed. Pulmonary involvement with cough and radiologically demonstrable infiltrates occurs rarely.

In children, curiously, acalculous cholecystitis has been observed occasionally, as a manifestation of leptospirosis. Rarely, myocarditis is a feature of leptospirosis.

Laboratory findings. The white blood cell count varies from a leukopenia to a mild leukocytosis. In Weil's disease white blood cell count may reach levels of 40,000 per cubic millimeter. A cerebrospinal fluid pleocytosis, with up to several hundred mononuclear cells, may be present. Abnormalities of liver function are common, even in patients lacking overt jaundice. Azotemia and hematuria occur in patients with renal involvement, and jaundice is usually present in these.

Diagnosis and differential diagnosis. Skin manifestations are not specific but may suggest leptospirosis in the context of jaundice and aseptic meningitis. Conjunctival suffusion may be a helpful clue. The differential diagnosis includes viral hepatitis, all the causes of a lymphocytic meningitis, nephritis, and the causes of a fever of unknown origin. The diagnosis is established most commonly by serologic means: a fourfold or greater rise in microagglutination titer (to ≥ 1:100), an indirect hemagglutination test, or an ELISA test. It can also be confirmed by isolation of the organism from blood, during the first 10 days of illness. In a recent series of cases of leptospirosis among military personnel in Panama, leptospires were isolated from blood cultures of 23 of 29 patients studied [35].

Treatment. In the past, studies of the effectiveness of antibiotics (tetracyclines, penicillin) in the treatment of leptospirosis have been inconclusive. Recently, in a controlled trial in anicteric leptospirosis, doxycycline therapy has proved effective, when administered early, in reducing the duration of illness and in preventing leptospiruria [35]. Doxycycline, administered orally on a once weekly basis, has been used successfully by the military as a prophylactic measure for short-term exposure in a hyperendemic area [36].

Course and prognosis. Recovery is the rule in anicteric cases. In the presence of jaundice, the mortality rate may be as high as 40 percent.

Pasteurella multocida infections

Definition. Infections produced by *Pasteurella multocida* follow one of several patterns: (1) local skin infection with adenitis following animal bites (the most common form of infection); (2) septic arthritis and osteomyelitis following an animal bite (usually of the hand); (3) respiratory tract infections or colonization; (4) systemic infections such as meningitis, bacteremia, spontaneous bacterial peritonitis [37].

Bacteriology. *Pasteurella multocida* is a small, ovoid, gram-negative rod. Its prominent bipolar staining may, from time to time, mistakenly suggest *Neisseria* or *Hemophilus influenzae.* It grows readily on nutrient blood agar and can be identified by biochemical tests and agglutination reactions.

Epidemiology. Although this organism is primarily a pathogen among animals, causing "hemorrhagic septicemia," it occasionally infects humans. *P. multocida* can be isolated from the upper respiratory tract of healthy cats, dogs, rats, and mice.

Clinical manifestations. HISTORY. Local pain and swelling occur within a few days of a cat or dog bite. There is little if any fever.

CUTANEOUS LESIONS. Redness, swelling, ulceration, and a small amount of seropurulent drainage develop at the bite site. Cellulitis may progress rapidly and extensively, with associated lymphangitis. Local necrosis and abscess formation may follow.

OTHER PHYSICAL FINDINGS. Regional adenopathy may be present. Complicating osteomyelitis may occur as a result of the introduction of organisms beneath the periosteum by the animal bite.

Laboratory findings. Mild leukocytosis is present. After several weeks, an x-ray of underlying bone may show osteomyelitis.

Pathology. This infection produces an acute pyogenic response.

Diagnosis and differential diagnosis. The diagnosis is suspected when a painful infection develops at the site of an animal bite. It must be distinguished from cat-scratch disease. Local ulceration and proximal lymphadenitis mimic ulceroglandular tularemia. The diagnosis is established by isolation of the organism.

Treatment. Most strains of *P. multocida* are susceptible to penicillin, the drug of choice. In patients with simple cellulitis, oral penicillin (penicillin VK at 500 to 750 mg orally four times daily for adults) may reasonably be used, but close follow-up is mandatory. If the prior animal bite is suspected to have penetrated deeply close to periosteum, parenteral penicillin (e.g., 2 to 4 million units intramuscularly daily) should be administered until the local lesion is well healed, to avert possible osteomyelitis. For the penicillin-allergic patient, tetracycline is a suitable alternative, but susceptibility testing must always be performed. Chloramphenicol may be effective therapy for the rare patient unable to tolerate either penicillin or tetracycline. Abscesses should be surgically drained.

Course and prognosis. The infection responds to local measures and antibiotic therapy.

Uncommon diseases in which animal contacts or geographic factors may occasionally be relevant

Listeria monocytogenes infections (listeriosis)

Definition. Infection with *Listeria monocytogenes* produces characteristic acute disease in infants (neonatal septicemia, meningitis, and septic granulomatosis) and in both healthy and immunosuppressed adults (septicemia, meningitis, vaginal infection, pneumonitis, and oculoglandular syndrome) [38].

Bacteriology. *Listeria monocytogenes* is a small, thin, gram-positive rod that often appears coccoid in infected tissues and body fluids. It may resemble a streptococcus or pneumococcus. On the other hand, its appearance mimics that of a diphtheroid, and this pathogen has occasionally been dismissed erroneously as a "contaminant." It is non-spore-forming, beta-hemolytic, and exhibits a characteristic tumbling motility when grown in broth at room temperature. This is the classical facultative intracellular

bacteria against which host resistance is mediated by thymus-derived lymphocytes (and macrophages).

Epidemiology. *L. monocytogenes* is found in the feces of many wild animals and birds and in soil and vegetation. One to four percent of humans (this is probably a minimal figure since it is difficult to isolate the organism from stool) appear to be fecal carriers of the organism. Higher rates of carriage have been observed in family contacts of patients with listeriosis. For undetermined reasons, pregnant women may acquire self-limited or asymptomatic genital infections. The highest incidence of infections is in the perinatal period, suggesting that the fetus either becomes infected in utero or on passing through the birth canal. Many but not all adult cases occur on a background of altered cellular immunity (Hodgkin's disease, immunosuppression for organ transplantation, etc.) or cirrhosis. Occasionally, veterinarians handling stillborn or ill newborn animals develop cutaneous infections.

Most cases in the United States occur in urban areas without obvious animal contact. The portal of infection for most cases is unknown but introduction through the intestinal tract seems likely. Food-borne (unpasteurized or improperly pasteurized milk; coleslaw made from cabbage grown on a farm where sheep manure had been used as fertilizer) outbreaks have been described [39].

Immunocompromised and pregnant patients (neonatal infection) are at particular risk [39,40].

Clinical manifestations. HISTORY. An acutely ill, moribund infant who was meconium-stained at birth, and who subsequently exhibits pustular, papular, or petechial skin lesions, suggests neonatal infection. *Listeria,* group B streptococci, *Herpes simplex,* etc., are etiologies to be considered. Listeriosis in the adult may present as a nonspecific acute febrile illness in which the findings of meningitis may predominate. Veterinarians may develop an acute febrile illness with headache, malaise, and rash 2 to 3 days after handling infected bovine fetuses.

CUTANEOUS LESIONS. In neonatal septicemia and infant granulomatosis, the skin rash consists of generalized erythematous papular or petechial lesions which may become pustular but only rarely vesicular. Veterinarians may develop tender, red papular lesions on the hands and arms, some of which evolve into pustules. Characteristic gram-positive rods can be demonstrated in these skin lesions. Tender axillary adenopathy is frequently present. In oculoglandular infection, there is acute conjunctivitis with preauricular adenitis.

OTHER PHYSICAL FINDINGS. In infants, meconium staining of the skin, hepatosplenomegaly, and lethargy are commonly present. Acute meningitis is accompanied by typical signs in infants and adults.

Laboratory findings. A significant monocytosis occurs only rarely. In adults with meningitis, the inflammatory reaction is usually a predominantly neutrophilic pleocytosis; in infants, the response in the cerebrospinal fluid is sometimes mononuclear.

Pathology. Skin lesions show focal necrosis and infiltration by polymorphonuclear leukocytes and monocytes about blood vessels. Abscesses are found in viscera and granuloma formation may also be evident.

Diagnosis and differential diagnosis. Listeriosis should be suspected in any newborn with meconium-stained skin who exhibits intrauterine growth retardation, fails to thrive, or develops a papular skin eruption. Gram's stain of meconium shows the characteristic gram-positive rods. The skin lesions, cerebrospinal fluid, or blood cultures reveal the etiologic agent.

The differential diagnosis includes other forms of in-utero neonatal infection such as toxoplasmosis, cytomegalovirus infection, rubella, disseminated *Herpes simplex* infection, and a variety of disseminated bacterial infections. The latter include those due to group B streptococci, *Escherichia coli, Salmonella,* and *Pseudomonas.*

Treatment. Penicillin (or ampicillin) is the antibiotic of choice, administered by the intravenous route in 2 or 3 divided doses. Care must be exercised in adjusting the dosage of penicillin in the newborn period to 50,000 to 250,000 units/kg per day; ampicillin is administered in a dosage of 100 to 200 mg/kg per day. Tetracycline (or erythromycin) is an alternative in the penicillin-allergic adult. In adults with meningitis or septicemia, the dosage of penicillin should be in the range of 1 to 2 million units intravenously every 2 h. If tetracycline is employed, then 1.0 to 1.5 g should be given daily by the intravenous route.

Course and prognosis. In neonatal septicemia and meningitis, the prognosis is extremely poor. In adult infections, treatment is effective and recovery is the rule, unless the underlying disease prevents this.

Diphtheria

Definition. Diphtheria is an acute febrile illness involving primarily the pharynx and mucous membranes of the upper respiratory tract. The major manifestations of this disease are due to (1) local membranous obstruction of the airway, and (2) the effects of a potent cytotoxin on the myocardium and peripheral nervous system. The hallmark of the local lesion is a gray, leathery membrane. Rarely, the primary lesion may be located on the skin, or the infection may complicate a preexisting wound. This is characteristically seen in tropical areas.

Bacteriology. The causative organism (*Corynebacterium diphtheriae*) is a gram-positive rod that exhibits metachromatic bipolar granules on staining with methylene blue. It grows well on ordinary media, but its presence may be obscured by other bacteria in the pharynx or on the cutaneous lesion. For this reason, it is necessary to use selective media such as Loeffler's or tellurite agar to inhibit other organisms.

Identification of toxigenic strains requires either an Elek plate (agar diffusion precipitin reaction) or demonstration of protection from dermonecrosis in guinea pigs by antitoxin neutralization of a suspension of the isolate of *Corynebacterium.*

Epidemiology. Humans are the only natural host for *C. diphtheriae.* The organism is carried in the pharynx of asymptomatic individuals. Infection occurs when a nonimmune person is infected by a toxigenic strain of *C. diphtheriae;* epidemics occur when such a strain becomes widespread in a population of nonimmune individuals. Most commonly, the site of primary infection is the nasopharynx or pharynx.

Cutaneous diphtheria and wound diphtheria occur in tropical areas ("jungle sore") and in association with poor hygiene. There has been an increase in skin diphtheria in the United States in the Pacific Northwest and in the South [41]. The contagiousness of cutaneous diphtheria may be greater than that of respiratory infection among school children [42].

Diphtheria is primarily a disease of young children, and in the United States most cases occur among poor, crowded, unimmunized individuals. Because of the widespread use and protective effect of toxoid immunization, the disease is rare in this country. It should be stressed, however, that this protection does not prevent the development of the carrier state and subsequent spread of organisms to susceptible individuals. In the past two decades, increasing numbers of cases have occurred in unimmunized migrant farm worker families, and in older alcoholics living in "skid row" situations.

In underdeveloped and overcrowded parts of the world, diphtheria remains an important health problem, with many carriers and susceptible individuals. The majority of cases of cutaneous and wound diphtheria occur in this setting and are associated with poor hygiene and skin trauma.

Clinical manifestations. HISTORY. Faucial diphtheria usually presents with pharyngitis and low-grade fever. Toxicity is out of proportion to the degree of fever and local findings. As the disease progresses, swelling and pain in the neck, symptoms of airway obstruction, or unilateral nasal discharge may develop. Cutaneous diphtheria occurs in the presence or absence of pharyngeal disease. However, 20 to 40 percent of patients with cutaneous diphtheria carry the identical strain of *C. diphtheriae* in their respiratory tract. The skin lesions are usually indolent but tender and on the extremities. Symptoms of cranial or peripheral neuritis or of myocarditis may complicate the course. The latter usually occurs 5 to 14 days after the onset of the illness, whereas the former may develop any time from 2 weeks to several months after the primary lesion. Myocarditis is extremely rare as a complication of cutaneous diphtheria. Neurologic symptoms such as blurred vision, diplopia, numbness of tongue, palatal paralysis, long-tract sensory and motor findings, and the Guillain-Barré syndrome have occurred in 3 to 5 percent of patients with ulcerated diphtheritic skin lesions.

CUTANEOUS LESIONS. There are basically three types of skin involvement [43]: (1) Wound diphtheria is a secondary infection of a preexisting wound, occurs in temperate as well as tropical climates, and may involve any part of the body. The lesion is usually partially covered with a membrane; a purulent exudate is present, and a zone of edema and erythema surrounds the area. (2) Primary cutaneous diphtheria begins acutely as a tender, pustular lesion which then breaks down and enlarges to form an oval punched-out ulcer with a gray membrane at the base. Later the membrane becomes dark brown. This ulcer does not extend below the fascia, has edematous, rolled, bluish margins, is usually located on a lower extremity, and is most often seen in the tropics. (3) Superinfection of eczematized skin lesions by C. *diphtheriae* evokes a more superficial, membranous, tender, edematous reaction.

Skin lesions with the appearance of impetigo, ecthyma, infected insect bites, etc., have been described as yielding C. *diphtheriae* on culture [41]. Whether these represent true infections with C. *diphtheriae* or are the cutaneous equivalent of the respiratory carrier state is unclear.

OTHER PHYSICAL FINDINGS. A membranous pharyngitis may accompany cutaneous diphtheria. Cranial or peripheral nerve palsies may be present.

Laboratory findings. The organism can be isolated on appropriate media from the skin ulcer or pharyngeal membrane.

Pathology. There is nothing characteristic about the pathologic picture of the diphtheritic lesion. The membrane is composed of coagulation necrosis and inflammatory cells.

Diagnosis and differential diagnosis. A presumptive diagnosis is usually based on the findings of membranous pharyngitis in faucial diphtheria, and of a shallow membrane-covered ulcer in cutaneous involvement. In methylene blue-stained smears of material from the edge of the membrane, the characteristic beaded metachromatically stained rods can be seen, but proof of the diagnosis must await culture results and demonstration of toxin production. However, the presence of a pharyngeal membrane, with or without typically appearing organisms, should be presumptive evidence of infection with C. *diphtheriae,* and treatment should be started immediately. Occasionally, membranous infectious mononucleosis can mimic the picture of faucial diphtheria, or be complicated by diphtheria.

Tropical ulcers may be confused with diphtheritic skin lesions, but the former usually occur in malnourished individuals and penetrate below the fascia, involving muscle and tendons. Bacterial infections in ulcerated wounds and following trauma usually are purulent and without membrane formation. Cutaneous mycotic infections are frequently more proliferative, and their margins are irregular, without surrounding reactive edema. Nonpathogenic (non-toxigenic) diphtheroids may be present in open skin lesions as superficial contaminants. Impetigo-like lesions and nondistinctive secondary pyodermas should be cultured in any contacts of a patient with diphtheria because of the contagiousness of cutaneous diphtheria.

Treatment. In faucial diphtheria, treatment consists of both specific equine antitoxin and penicillin. Treatment is initiated on the basis of clinical suspicion without awaiting cultural confirmation, since toxin elaborated in the intervening period could lead to irreversible myocardial damage.

In ulcerative cutaneous diphtheria, bed rest is essential for healing. Antitoxin in doses of 20,000 to 40,000 units is given by the intravenous route after careful testing for horse serum hypersensitivity. Injection of antitoxin into the subcutaneous area around the ulcer and also the surface application of antitoxin on the lesion have been suggested. Penicillin (2 to 4 million units intramuscularly daily) or erythromycin (2.0 g orally daily) is administered for 7 to 10 days. A few inducible erythromycin- and clindamycin-resistant strains of *Corynebacterium diphtheriae* have

been isolated recently from the lesions of cutaneous diphtheria. The lesion should be debrided and kept clean once antitoxin and antibiotics have been administered.

Course and prognosis. If treatment is begun early, the prognosis is excellent for full recovery. In untreated, unimmunized persons with cutaneous diphtheria, ulcers may persist for as long as 6 months. Neuritic symptoms and signs may occur as late as 5 months after the onset of illness. The neurologic defects are almost always completely reversible.

Infections due to *Vibrio* species

Definition. Infections caused by *Vibrio* species produce several different clinical syndromes: (1) gastroenteritis (the most common), (2) wound (and ear) infections, (3) septicemia (either "primary" or secondary to a wound infection) [44].

Bacteriology and pathogenic aspects. BACTERIOLOGY. Nine *Vibrio* species in addition to *Vibrio cholerae* have been associated with human disease. Four species are capable of producing wound infections: *V. parahaemolyticus, V. vulnificus, V. alginolyticus,* and *V. damsela.* Of these, *V. vulnificus* is capable of causing severe wound infections and a "primary septicemia" syndrome with a mortality rate of almost 50 percent. The *Vibrio* species grow in regular blood culture media and on blood agar. Selective media such as thiosulfate-citrate-bile salts-sucrose (TCBS) are necessary to isolate the organisms from stool cultures.

PATHOGENIC ASPECTS. Markers for pathogenicity have been described for some *Vibrio* species. Almost all *V. parahaemolyticus* strains associated with disease (diarrhea, wound infections) in humans produce a hemolysin (Kanagawa phenomenon). This organism also produces a toxin capable of causing intestinal fluid accumulation in suckling mice and, as well, is capable at times of invasiveness, producing a dysentery-like syndrome. *V. vulnificus* produces extracellular collagenolytic, proteolytic, and elastolytic activities which may be important in the tissue invasiveness of this pathogen. Among the *Vibrio* species, *V. vulnificus* exhibits a striking pathogenicity when introduced into animal models by either the gastrointestinal or parenteral routes.

Epidemiology. *V. parahaemolyticus* is commonly found in salt water, and in fish and shellfish. It has been implicated in 24 percent of reported cases of food-borne gastroenteritis in Japan; it also has been involved in shellfish-associated outbreaks of gastroenteritis in the United States. *V. parahaemolyticus* is responsible for occasional wound infections incurred following lacerations from shellfish or in sea water [45]. Wound infections with *V. vulnificus* typically follow cuts of the hand acquired while cleaning crabs or shrimp. Primary septicemia due to *V. vulnificus* is associated with the eating of raw oysters, and particularly in the setting of hepatic cirrhosis or hemochromatosis.

Clinical manifestations. HISTORY. Gastroenteritis is most commonly associated with *V. parahaemolyticus,* but wound infections and septicemia also occasionally occur. After an incubation period of 4 to 96 h, abdominal cramps, nausea, and vomiting occur in the majority of patients;

chills and fever occur in about 25 percent of patients. *V. vulnificus* may occasionally cause a similar gastroenteritis. More typically it is responsible for a wound infection occurring several days after a laceration sustained in sea water or brackish inland lakes. Primary septicemia with *V. vulnificus* may follow 24 to 48 h after consumption of raw oysters. This is more likely to occur in individuals with underlying chronic diseases such as cirrhosis, diabetes, leukemia, renal failure, or conditions requiring corticosteroid therapy. Fever, chills, nausea, vomiting, abdominal pain, and diarrhea are frequent symptoms in patients with primary septicemia, suggesting an initial gastrointestinal site of infection.

CUTANEOUS LESION. Traumatic wound infections due to *V. vulnificus* may consist of pustular lesions, lymphangitis and lymphadenitis, or cellulitis. These infections may be mild or develop into rapidly progressive cellulitis with myositis and extensive skin necrosis. Secondary bacteremia may ensue. Occasionally, cellulitis develops spontaneously without antecedent overt skin trauma but following exposure to sea water.

Skin lesions, in the form of large hemorrhagic bullae on the extremities or trunk, develop commonly in the course of primary *V. vulnificus* septicemia [46]. These progress to necrotic ulcers.

OTHER PHYSICAL FINDINGS. Systemic manifestations (high fever, tachycardia, hypotension) are common in *V. vulnificus* septicemia. One-third of patients are in shock on presentation or within the first 12 h of hospitalization.

Laboratory findings. Although *V. parahaemolyticus* usually produces a watery diarrhea, occasional patients will have a dysentery-like syndrome with leukocytes and blood present in the stool. In *V. vulnificus* primary septicemia, leukopenia is more frequent than leukocytosis. Thrombocytopenia is common, and may progress rapidly to disseminated intravascular coagulation. *V. parahaemolyticus*, *V. vulnificus,* and other *Vibrio* species can be grown on blood agar media and isolated from routine blood cultures. TCBS media is used for isolation of *Vibrio* species from stool.

Diagnosis and differential diagnosis. Infection with a pathogenic *Vibrio* species should be suspected when gastroenteritis occurs in the summer months when there is a history of recent ingestion of shellfish (particularly raw oysters or crabs) or exposure to sea water, especially along the Gulf Coast. The development of unexplained fever, shock, and bullous skin lesions in a patient with cirrhosis who has recently eaten raw oysters should alert the physician to the possible diagnosis of primary vibrio septicemia.

Differential diagnosis of the gastroenteritis syndrome includes other causes of watery diarrhea (*V. cholerae,* toxigenic *Escherichia coli*). Wound infections sustained in fresh water would suggest *Aeromonas hydrophila* rather than *Vibrio* species which are more typically involved in infected wounds sustained in a salt-water environment. Bullous lesions occurring in a hypotensive febrile patient might suggest the diagnosis of bacteremic *Pseudomonas aeruginosa* infection or even clostridial myonecrosis. The latter would be suggested by the presence of crepitus in the involved area and the presence of typical gram-positive blunt-ended bacilli in the contents of the bullae. *Pseudo-monas* bacteremia would be unlikely in a nonleukopenic nonhospitalized patient without a prior history of infection and antibiotic usage.

Treatment. *V. parahaemolyticus* gastroenteritis usually is a mild to moderately severe form of diarrheal disease that requires no treatment other than oral fluid replacement (e.g., glucose-electrolyte solution). Management of *V. vulnificus* septicemia involves the treatment of hypotension with fluid replacement and treatment of systemic infection with both tetracycline (or chloramphenicol) and an aminoglycoside. There is a role for antimicrobial therapy in infected traumatic wounds due to *V. vulnificus* (or other *Vibrio* species) in view of the potential invasiveness of these organisms. Debridement of necrotic lesions is indicated.

Course and prognosis. *V. parahaemolyticus* gastroenteritis is a self-limited disease. In contrast, the mortality rate for *V. vulnificus* primary septicemia is 50 to 60 percent, about three times as high as the mortality for wound infections due to the same organism. In view of the mortality associated with septicemic *V. vulnificus* infection, patients with cirrhosis and hemochromatosis should be advised against consuming raw shellfish.

Rhinoscleroma

Rhinoscleroma is a chronic granulomatous disease caused by *Klebsiella rhinoscleromatis*. The principal endemic foci are in Mexico and Central and South America, but cases have also been reported from central and eastern Europe, India, North Africa, and the United States. Most cases are found in areas with primitive living conditions and it is mildly contagious. The granulomas involve the nasal mucosa but may spread to the larynx, trachea, and bronchi. The diagnostic marker for the disease is the Mikulicz cell (a large histiocyte containing cytoplasmic bacilli). The clinical lesions consist of nodules that are painless, waxy, and red, often with ulceration (see Fig. 177-2). Treatment with streptomycin or tetracycline is often quite successful after two to three months in all but the patients with extensive disease.

References

1. Gold H: Anthrax: a report of 117 cases. *Arch Intern Med* **96:**387, 1955
2. Ronaghy HA et al: Penicillin therapy of human anthrax vaccine. *Curr Ther Res* **14:**721, 1972
3. Brachman PS et al: Field evaluation of human anthrax vaccine. *Am J Pub Health* **52:**632, 1962
4. Buchanan TM et al: Brucellosis in the United States, 1960–1972. *Medicine (Baltimore)* **53:**413, 1974
5. Young EJ: Human brucellosis. *Rev Infect Dis* **5:**821, 1983
6. Berger TG et al: Cutaneous lesions in brucellosis. *Arch Dermatol* **117:**40, 1981
7. Spink WW: The significance of bacterial hypersensitivity in human brucellosis: studies of infection due to strain 19 *Brucella abortus*. *Ann Intern Med* **47:**861, 1957
8. Woodbine M: *Erysipelothrix rhusiopathiae* bacteriology and chemotherapy. *Bacteriol Rev* **14:**161, 1950
9. Grieco MH, Sheldon C: *Erysipelothrix rhusiopathiae. Ann NY Acad Sci* **174:**523, 1970

10. Nelson E: Five hundred cases of erysipeloid. *Rocky Mountain Med J* **52**:40, 1955

11. Klauder JV et al: A distinctive and severe form of erysipeloid among fish handlers. *Arch Dermatol Syphilol* **14**:622, 1926

12. Park C et al: *Erysipelothrix* endocarditis with cutaneous lesion. *South Med J* **69**:1101, 1976

13. Simberkoff MS, Rahal J: Acute and subacute endocarditis due to *Erysipelothrix rhusiopathiae*. *Am J Med Sci* **266**:53, 1973

14. Brown TMcP, Nunemaker JC: Rat-bite fever. A review of the American cases with re-evaluation of etiology. *Bull Johns Hopkins Hosp* **70**:201. 1942

15. Place EH, Sutton LE: Erythema arthriticum epidemicum (Haverhill fever). *Arch Intern Med* **54**:659, 1934

16. Peters D, Wigand R: Bartonellaceae. *Bacteriol Rev* **19**:150, 1955

17. Herrer A: Bartonellosis, in *Tropical Medicine*, 5th ed, edited by GW Hunter et al. Philadelphia, WB Saunders, 1976, p 256

18. Reynafarje C, Ramos J: The hemolytic anemia of human bartonellosis. *Blood* **17**:562, 1961

19. Recavarren S, Lumbreras H: Pathogenesis of the verruga of Carrion's disease. *Am J Pathol* **66**:461, 1972

20. Archer GL et al: Human infection from an unidentified erythrocyte-associated bacterium. *N Engl J Med* **301**:897, 1979

21. Gilbert DN et al: Potential medical problems in personnel returning from Vietnam. *Ann Intern Med* **68**:662, 1968

22. McCormick JB et al: Human-to-human transmission of *Pseudomonas pseudomallei*. *Ann Intern Med* **83**:512, 1975

23. Sanford JP, Moore WL Jr: Recrudescent melioidosis: a Southeastern Asian legacy. *Am Rev Respir Dis* **104**:452, 1971

24. Davis DHS et al: Plague, in *Diseases Transmitted from Animals to Man*, 6th ed, edited by WT Hubbert et al. Springfield, IL, Charles C Thomas, 1975, p 147

25. Portnoy DA et al: Characterization of common virulence plasmids in *Yersinia* species and their role in the expression of outer membrane proteins. *Infect Immun* **43**:108, 1984

26. Centers for Disease Control: Winter plague—Colorado, Washington, Texas 1983–1984. *MMWR* **33**:145, 1984

27. Reed WB et al: Bubonic plague in Southwestern United States. *Medicine (Baltimore)* **49**:465, 1970

28. Mengis CL: Plague. *N Engl J Med* **267**:543, 1962

29. Cantey JR: Plague in Vietnam, clinical observations and treatment with kanamycin. *Arch Intern Med* **133**:280, 1974

30. Buchanan TM et al: The tularemia skin test—325 skin tests in 210 persons: serologic correlation and review of the literature. *Ann Intern Med* **74**:336, 1971

31. Heath CW Jr et al: Leptospirosis in the United States: analysis of 483 cases in man, 1949–1961. *N Engl J Med* **273**:857, 915, 1965

32. Wong ML et al: Leptospirosis: a childhood disease. *J Pediatr* **90**:532, 1977

33. Daniels WB, Grennan HA: Pretibial fever. *JAMA* **122**:361, 1943

34. Derham RLJ: Leptospirosis as a cause of erythema nodosum. *Br Med J* **2**:403, 1976

35. McClain JBL et al: Doxycycline therapy for leptospirosis. *Ann Intern Med* **100**:696, 1984

36. Takafuji ET et al: An efficacy trial of doxycycline chemoprophylaxis against leptospirosis. *N Engl J Med* **310**:497, 1984

37. Weber DJ et al: *Pasteurella multocida* infections. Report of 34 cases and review of the literature. *Medicine (Baltimore)* **63**:133, 1984

38. Gray ML, Killinger AH: *Listeria monocytogenes* and *Listeria* infections. *Bacteriol Rev* **30**:309, 1966

39. Sclech WF et al: Epidemic listeriosis—evidence for transmission by food. *N Engl J Med* **308**:203, 1983

40. Stamm AM et al: Listeriosis in renal transplant recipients: report of an outbreak and review of 102 cases. *Rev Infect Dis* **4**:665, 1982

41. Belsey MA et al: *Corynebacterium diphtheriae* skin infections in Alabama and Louisiana. A factor in the epidemiology of diphtheria. *N Engl J Med* **280**:135, 1969

42. Koopman JS, Campbell J: The role of cutaneous diphtheria infections in a diphtheria epidemic. *J Infect Dis* **131**:239, 1975

43. Flor-Henry P: Cutaneous diphtheria: brief historical review and discussion of recent literature, with presentation of two cases. *Med Serv J Canada* **17**:823, 1961

44. Morris JG, Black RE: Medical Progress. Cholera and other vibrioses in the United States. *N Engl J Med* **312**:343, 1985

45. Bonner JR et al: Spectrum of *Vibrio* infections in a Gulf Coast community. *Ann Intern Med* **99**:464, 1983

46. Tacket CO et al: Clinical features and an epidemiologic study of *Vibrio vulnificus* infections. *J Infect Dis* **149**:558, 1984

Bibliography

Berman SJ et al: Sporadic anicteric leptospirosis in South Vietnam. *Ann Intern Med* **79**:167, 1973

Buchner LH, Schneierson SS: Clinical and laboratory aspects of *Listeria monocytogenes* infections. *Am J Med* **45**:904, 1968

Gantz NM et al: Listeriosis in immunosuppressed patients. *Am J Med* **58**:637, 1975

Howe C, Miller WR: Human glanders: report of six cases. *Ann Intern Med* **26**:93, 1947

Kerdel-Vegas F: Rhinoscleroma, in *Clinical Tropical Dermatology*, edited by O. Conizares Oxford, Blackwell, 1975

Martone WJ, Kaufmann AF: Leptospirosis in humans in the United States, 1974–1978. *J Infect Dis* **140**:1020, 1979

Redfearn MS, Palleroni NJ: Glanders and melioidosis, in *Diseases Transmitted from Animals to Man*, 6th ed, edited by WT Hubbert et al. Springfield, IL, Charles C Thomas, 1975, p 110

Riddel GS: Cutaneous diphtheria: epidemiological and dermatological aspects of 365 cases amongst British prisoners of war in the Far East. *J R Army Med Corps* **95**:64, 1950

Roughgarden JW: Antimicrobial therapy of rat-bite fever. A review. *Arch Intern Med* **116**:39, 1965

Schmid GP et al: Clinically mild tularemia associated with tick-borne *Francisella tularensis*. *J Infect Dis* **148**:63, 1983

Young LS et al: Tularemia epidemic: Vermont, 1968. *N Engl J Med* **280**:1253, 1969

CHAPTER 179

MYCOBACTERIAL DISEASES: TUBERCULOSIS AND ATYPICAL MYCOBACTERIAL INFECTIONS

Klaus Wolff and Gert Tappeiner

While improved hygiene, living standards, and chemotherapy have greatly reduced the prevalence of tuberculosis in North America and Europe, infections due to mycobacteria are still very common in the developing countries. In addition, the so-called "atypical" mycobacteria are increasingly recognized as human pathogens and, especially in regions with a warm climate, some of them are common causes of skin disease. It has been estimated that the genus *Mycobacterium* probably causes more suffering for humans than all the other bacterial genera combined [1].

It is well documented that the immune and tissue response of the host plays a decisive role in determining the type and extent of disease produced by mycobacterial infection. This has been studied extensively in infections with *M. tuberculosis, M. bovis,* and *M. leprae* and, to a lesser degree, with *M. ulcerans.* Obligatory and facultatively pathogenic mycobacteria are distinguished. In contrast to the obligate mycobacterial pathogens, the environmental, facultatively pathogenic mycobacteria only rarely cause disease by person-to-person spread [2]. Infections due to the latter primarily depend on the occurrence and distribution of the organisms in the environment, the opportunities for contact with susceptible individuals, and the immunologic state of these individuals which makes them susceptible for infection [3–5]. There is evidence suggesting that previous contact with the nonpathogenic, environmental flora is of importance in determining the nature of the immune response to subsequently encountered pathogenic species [6].

The present chapter will first discuss *tuberculosis* of the skin—a spectrum of skin conditions due to infection with the obligatory mycobacterial pathogens *M. tuberculosis* and *M. bovis* (including the attenuated BCG organism). Subsequently we will deal with the *mycobacterioses,* diseases due to infection with mycobacteria previously designated as "atypical" or MOTT (mycobacteria other than tuberculosis). Although biologically different from *M. tuberculosis* and *M. bovis,* these facultatively pathogenic mycobacteria may cause disease patterns which are quite similar to those encountered in tuberculosis. Infection due to *M. leprae* will be discussed in Chap. 180.

Classification of mycobacteria

Mycobacteria are acid-fast, weakly gram-positive, nonsporulating and nonmotile rods. The family Mycobacteriaceae consists of only one genus, *Mycobacterium,* which includes the obligate human pathogens, *M. tuberculosis, M. africanum, M. bovis,* and *M. leprae* as well as a number

of facultatively pathogenic and nonpathogenic species, the so-called atypical mycobacteria. Between 1954 and 1959 Runyon developed the first useful classification of atypical mycobacteria [7] which groups them in a slow-growing and a fast-growing group; the former was subdivided according to pigment-forming properties in culture. Thus, three groups were distinguished among the slow growers: group I: photochromogens, capable of pigment formation upon exposure to light; group II: scotochromogens, capable of pigment production without light exposure; and group III, nonchromogens. Group IV includes all rapid growers.

Since that time much taxonomic work has been done [3,8,9] so that today the genus *Mycobacterium* stands among the best classified bacterial genera. Today 41 species of mycobacteria are recognized [10]. The main distinction made is between the slow growers and the rapid growers, as this seems to have occurred early in the development of the genus [1]. The old Runyon groups are still frequently used when referring to a slow-growing mycobacterium species.

For clinical purposes, the organisms may further be subdivided into obligate and facultative pathogens and nonpathogens; a classification scheme of the genus *Mycobacterium* is presented in Table 179-1. *M. leprae* has not been included as it has not been grown in culture and thus has not been available for biochemical testing. The listing of nonpathogens or animal pathogens is not exhaustive and some of them may still emerge as facultative pathogens. A complete list of the mycobacteria species recognized today can be found elsewhere [10].

Tuberculosis of the skin

Definition and classification

Tuberculosis of the skin is caused by *M. tuberculosis, M. bovis* and, under certain conditions, the bacillus Calmette-Guérin (BCG) which is an attenuated strain of *M. bovis;* the clinical manifestations comprise a considerable number of skin changes, usually subclassified into more or less distinct disease forms. Morphologic classification originated at a time when the pathogenesis of tuberculosis of the skin was not well understood, and the fact that clinically similar skin manifestations may originate in different ways and may vary in their histologic appearance was not appreciated. More recent classifications are based on the mode of infection or the immunologic state of the host but they, also, fail to satisfy completely because different routes of infection may sometimes lead to identical skin

Table 179-1 Classification of mycobacteria

	Runyon group
Slow-growing mycobacteria	
Obligate human pathogens:	
M. tuberculosis-bovis group including bacillus Calmette-Guérin (BCG) and M. africanum	
Facultative human pathogens:	
M. kansasii	I
M. marinum	I
M. simiae	I
M. scrofulaceum	II
M. szulgai	II
M. avium-intracellulare complex	III
M. haemophilum	III
M. ulcerans	III
M. xenopi	III
Nonpathogens:	
M. gordonae	II
M. flavescens	II
M. terrae complex	III
M. triviale	III
M. gastri	III
(others)	
Rapidly growing mycobacteria	IV
Facultative human pathogens:	
M. fortuitum complex (including M. fortuitum biovar and M chelonei biovar.)	
Nonpathogens:	
M. smegmatis	
M. phlei	
M. vaccae	
(others)	

Note: *M. leprae* is not included in this table.

Table 179-2 Classification of cutaneous tuberculosis

Exogeneous infection
  Primary inoculation tuberculosis
    (Infection of the nonimmune host)
  Tuberculosis verrucosa cutis
    (Infection of the immune host)
Endogeneous spread
  Lupus vulgaris
  Scrofuloderma
  Metastatic tuberculous abscess (tuberculous gumma)
  Acute miliary tuberculosis
  Orificial tuberculosis
Tuberculosis due to BCG vaccination
Tuberculids
  Tuberculids
    Lichen scrofulosorum
    Papulonecrotic tuberculid
  Facultative tuberculids
    Nodular vasculitis
    Erythema nodosum
Non-tuberculids*

* These conditions are not related to tuberculosis but for completeness are discussed in the text.

lesions and mycobacterial spread in comparable states of immunity may result in different forms of skin tuberculosis. The classification used in this chapter distinguishes between exogenous infection and endogenous spread of *M. tuberculosis/bovis*, conditions caused by vaccination with BCG, and a group of eruptions, the tuberculids, which are nosologically and pathogenically less well understood (Table 179-2). Some entities of nontuberculous nature which were previously thought to be related to tuberculosis and were thus also termed *tuberculids* will be briefly mentioned at the end of this section.

Historical aspects

Some forms of tuberculosis of the skin, especially lupus vulgaris, were described repeatedly in the seventeenth and eighteenth centuries, and the term *lupus* was used by some of the early authors. Bayle was the first to discover that tuberculosis was not confined to the lungs, but could affect the entire body. However, even after Villemin had proved that tuberculosis was infectious, tuberculous skin diseases continued to be mistaken for other dermatoses. Although tuberculosis was successfully transmitted to experimental animals and its histopathologic characteristics were described in detail by Rokitansky and Virchow, and although the great similarity of the histologic appearance of lupus vulgaris and tuberculosis of other organs was demonstrated

by Friedlaender, no absolute proof of the cause of the tuberculous skin lesions was available. Koch's [11] discovery of the tubercle bacillus and the confirmation of its role in the cause of tuberculosis of the skin finally provided this evidence.

Epidemiology and incidence

The worldwide incidence of infectious tuberculosis is estimated to be 15 to 20 million with the highest proportion in the developing countries [12]. Tuberculosis of the skin also has a worldwide distribution and, whereas in the past it was more prevalent in regions with a cold and humid climate and a few hours of daily sunlight, it is now appreciated that it occurs also in other geographic regions and in the tropics. Reports from southeast Asia and South Africa suggest that it is not uncommon at all in these regions [13–17]. In Western countries the incidence of skin tuberculosis has shown a steady decline over the past decades. This seems to be true for all countries and parallels the decreasing incidence of pulmonary tuberculosis. In times of crises, for instance after the two world wars, certain forms of skin tuberculosis occurred more frequently. Malnutrition coupled with breakdown in normal living conditions may well explain this temporary resurgence. Lower socioeconomic status seems to be associated with a higher incidence of cutaneous tuberculosis, especially lupus vulgaris. Urban or rural residence does not affect the incidence.

In the United States tuberculosis of the skin has always been a rare disease. In Europe it was quite common during the first quarter of this century but it now represents less than 0.5 percent of all cases seen. In the Federal Republic of Germany only 300 to 400 new cases are now estimated to occur every year [16]. The two most frequent forms are lupus vulgaris and scrofuloderma, but there are considerable differences in the incidence in different geographic regions [18]; in the tropics, for instance, lupus vulgaris is rare whereas scrofuloderma and verrucous lesions predominate [12].

Certain forms of skin tuberculosis affect one sex more than the other. For example, lupus vulgaris is more than twice as frequent in women as in men, while tuberculosis verrucosa cutis is most often found in male patients. As far as age distribution is concerned, generalized miliary tuberculosis is seen in infants (and adults with severe immunosuppression) and so is primary inoculation tuberculosis; scrofuloderma usually occurs in adolescents and the elderly while lupus vulgaris may affect all age groups.

Etiology and pathogenesis

Causative for all forms of skin tuberculosis are *M. tuberculosis*, *M. bovis* and, under certain conditions, the attenuated BCG organism. After having gained access to the host's tissues, the mycobacteria multiply intracellularly. The invasion by *M. tuberculosis* is characterized by the appearance of polymorphonuclear leukocytes, an influx of mononuclear cells, and, later on, the development of epithelioid cells and necrosis. Large amounts of mycobacteria are initially found in the tissue. The mere presence of mycobacteria in the skin, however, does not necessarily lead to clinical disease, and it is well to remember that infection with *M. tuberculosis* is not necessarily synonymous with tuberculosis.

The development of a certain type of skin tuberculosis depends on a number of independent and interrelated factors which, by interaction, determine its clinical manifestations, pathology, course, and prognosis. The three most important factors are the properties of the causative organism, the general condition and reactivity of the host, and the mode of introduction of the bacteria into the skin.

The mycobacteria. Different mammalian species vary in their susceptibility to infection with different mycobacteria. In humans, *M. tuberculosis* and *M. bovis* cause identical skin manifestations. The incidence of skin tuberculosis elicited by these two organisms varies and is determined by the probability of exposure to either human or bovine tuberculosis. On the other hand, the virulence and number of the bacteria are of importance, as they may be subject to considerable variation. In 50 to 90 percent of the cases of lupus vulgaris, the bacteria exhibit a reduced virulence [19,20] which may approach that of the attenuated BCG organism. In many forms of skin tuberculosis, the number of bacteria in the lesions is so small that it may be difficult to find them, whereas in the primary chancre or in acute miliary tuberculosis, large numbers of bacteria can be demonstrated in the affected tissue.

The host. The human species is quite susceptible to tuberculous infections, but differences exist among populations and individuals. Populations whose contact with tuberculosis spans many centuries are, in general, less susceptible than races that have come into contact with mycobacteria for the first time. The decline of tuberculosis has been ascribed, in part, to a gradually enlarging population partially immunized by natural infections with a variety of mycobacteria [20]. Heredity also plays a role, for the concordance of tuberculosis is higher in monozygotic twins than in dizygotes [21]. Age, state of health, and somatic type of the individual are of importance, as are the environmental factors. In blacks, tuberculosis frequently takes an unfavorable course, and it has been claimed that in this race tuberculin sensitivity is more intense than in whites [22], but this may also be the result of environmental factors.

After mycobacteria have invaded the tissue of the host, they may either multiply and lead to progressive disease, or their multiplication is checked or completely arrested. The balance between bacterial multiplication and destruction is determined not only by the properties of the invading organisms but also by the inherent or acquired power of the host to control such an infection. The skin of an individual previously infected with tuberculosis shows an altered response upon a second exposure to the organism. This changed reactivity was first demonstrated by Koch [23], who showed that if virulent mycobacteria were injected subcutaneously into a previously infected guinea pig, a massive inflammatory response and necrosis developed at the site of injection. Koch went on to show that an extract containing the specific protein of the mycobacteria (tuberculin) was able to elicit the same phenomenon. von Pirquet [24] interpreted the different and unduly severe reaction to the second infection as an "allergic" response, the term *allergy* denoting the altered reaction capacity of an individual to the same stimulus. Subsequently, the tuberculin reaction became a standard test in clinical tuberculosis.

The tuberculin reaction is due to delayed-type hypersensitivity, mediated by sensitized T lymphocytes which, when injected into a nonsensitized individual, transfer the hypersensitivity [25,26]. Patients with sarcoidosis, whose cell-mediated immunologic capacities are compromised, will transiently support local passive transfer with living cells [27]. Conversely, patients with hypogammaglobulinemia in whom the immunologic mechanisms mediated by circulating immunoglobulins are impaired show no reduction in their capacity to produce hypersensitivity to tuberculin [28].

Sensitization is induced either by the living mycobacterium (e.g., during primary infection with tuberculosis) or, under experimental conditions, with killed bacteria or with bacteria suspended in Freund's adjuvant. The substance which proved effective in the elicitation of hypersensitivity reaction in sensitized individuals was designated *tuberculin* by Robert Koch [23]. It was obtained originally from cultures of mycobacteria in glycerol broth which had been concentrated, sterilized by heat, and filtrated. This "old tuberculin" (OT) was widely used for skin testing, but now has been replaced by a purified derivative (purified protein derivative, PPD). This consists of the immunologically active tuberculoproteins from which some other constituents have been removed, and is preferable to OT as its potency and composition are more constant [29]. Still, even commercial, standardized PPD-tuberculins available today are subject to some variation in human sensitivity [30] and do not eliminate cross-reactions due to sensitization by other mycobacteria [31]. The different mycobacterial species contain antigens unique to themselves but also antigens shared by other mycobacteria [32]. The low specificity of PPD is also due to the procedures employed in the denaturation of the antigens and the avoidance of protein denaturation has recently yielded a class of tuberculins which are much richer in PPDs in species-specific antigens [33] and have been given the generic name *new tuberculins* [34].

If tuberculin is administered to a sensitized individual,

a reaction develops that may vary in expression, depending on the test dose employed and the route of administration. Local intradermal injection (the method most widely used) leads to the local tuberculin reaction, which usually reaches its maximal intensity after 48 h. It consists of a sharply circumscribed area of erythema and induration and, in highly hypersensitive recipients or after large doses, may eventually lead to a pallid central necrosis. Histologically, the earliest changes consist of an accumulation of mononuclear cells that form prominent cuffs around small veins [35,36], and in severe reactions the small venules are plugged with leukocytes, chiefly mononuclear cells, encased in a fibrinous coagulum [37].

Tuberculin sensitivity usually develops 2 to 10 weeks after infection with *M. tuberculosis* and tends to persist throughout life. It may diminish with age or if the infection is treated in its earliest stages. Its intensity may be reduced by conditions which nonspecifically diminish delayed hypersensitivity reactions such as acute viral infections or vaccination with live virus; immunosuppression by drugs and corticosteroids, disease, and malnutrition; and malignant disease, particularly lymphoma. In addition, about 5 percent of individuals with tuberculosis who have none of these conditions still do not react to ordinary intermediate strength doses of tuberculin for unknown reasons [30].

The state of sensitivity of an individual infected with *M. tuberculosis* is of considerable significance in the pathogenesis of tuberculous skin lesions. Obviously, a primary infection of the skin (tuberculous chancre) will result in clinical manifestations that are quite different from those occurring after inoculation of mycobacteria into the skin of a previously sensitized individual (tuberculosis verrucosa cutis). Similarly, the hematogenous spread of mycobacteria in individuals with low or greatly diminished sensitivity will evolve into a skin disease (for instance miliary tuberculosis of the skin) which is unlike that occurring in persons in whom sensitivity is high (lupus vulgaris).

The relationship between hypersensitivity and immunity in tuberculous disease is still not entirely clear but is now becoming better understood. At various times hypersensitivity had been held responsible for immunity, and it was formerly believed that the allergic reaction to mycobacteria played a part in the defense mechanisms of the body. Indeed, in animals inoculated with mycobacteria there is unrestricted bacterial multiplication before the onset of hypersensitivity; bacterial destruction begins at about the time hypersensitivity develops and is practically complete when the state of hypersensitivity has reached its maximal levels [25]. In patients with clinical tuberculosis an increase of skin sensitivity usually indicates a rather favorable prognosis, and in tuberculous skin disease with high levels of skin sensitivity the number of bacteria within the lesions is small. However, tuberculin sensitivity is not necessary for immunity against *M. tuberculosis,* and sensitivity and immunity do not always parallel each other [38]. Although both phenomena are cell-mediated and transferable by lymphocytes, there is now sufficient evidence that they are dissociable and that a high degree of tuberculin sensitivity may even be antagonistic to protection [4]. Strains of mice which become only weakly sensitive to tuberculin are relatively resistant to *M. tuberculosis* injected intravenously but are susceptible to intradermal inoculation. The opposite occurs in animals that develop high levels of tuberculin hypersensitivity [5]. Mycobacterial infection therefore seems to elicit at least two cell-mediated immune responses both of which produce positive tuberculin tests but vary in their protective efficacy, depending on the site of infection: one is the result of macrophage activation and is protective while the other is a necrotic Koch-type reaction which is usually irrelevant to, or antagonistic to, protection [30]. It is currently believed that delayed hypersensitivity and immunity are two separate processes involving separate T-lymphocyte populations and different lymphokines as mediators [4].

Any disturbance of the balance between the state of immunity on the one hand, and the degree of invasion and virulence of the bacteria on the other, has its bearing on the course of the disease. As in tuberculosis of other organs this is also true for tuberculosis of the skin. Infectious diseases, particularly measles, as well as diabetes, lymphomas, and the systemic administration of corticosteroids or cytostatic agents may upset this balance.

Route of infection. The mode of introduction of mycobacteria into the skin and the properties of the particular tissue components affected are also essential pathogenic factors. The infection may be exogenous (i.e., from an outside source), it may occur by autoinoculation, or it may be endogenous. Exogenous infection will lead to the tuberculous chancre or to tuberculosis verrucosa cutis, whereby the immunologic state of the host determines which of the clinical manifestations eventually develops. Lupus vulgaris at the site of BCG vaccination represents another example of exogenous infection, in this instance by attenuated mycobacteria (see below).

Endogenous spread of mycobacteria may occur by continuous extension of a tuberculous process underlying the skin (scrofuloderma), by way of the lymphatics (lupus vulgaris), or by hematogenous dissemination (acute miliary tuberculosis of the skin or lupus vulgaris).

Finally, the structure and vascular supply of the tissue invaded by mycobacteria also has to be taken into account. Lesions developing in the upper dermis assume a clinical appearance and course which may be quite different from those of tuberculous lesions developing in the subcutaneous tissues. Disturbances of vascular circulation have an important additive effect.

Tuberculosis of the skin due to *M. tuberculosis/bovis* infection

Primary inoculation tuberculosis (tuberculous chancre; tuberculous primary complex)

Definition. Primary inoculation tuberculosis results from the inoculation of mycobacteria into the skin of a host not previously infected with tuberculosis. The tuberculous chancre and the affected regional lymph nodes constitute the tuberculous primary complex of the skin.

Incidence. This entity has always been considered uncommon, and in 1930 it was estimated to constitute 0.14 percent of all primary tuberculous lesions [39]. However, it may be not quite as rare as generally believed, for in 1953 Miller [40] was able to observe some 30 cases within a five-year period in the northeast part of England; in some geographic regions, particularly in Asia, where the incidence of tuberculosis is still high and where living conditions and hygiene are poor, primary inoculation tuberculosis of the skin is not unusual.

Most patients are children, but the lesions may also occur in adolescents and young adults [41–43], particularly in people working in medically related professions [44–47]. All parts of the body may be affected, but predilection sites are the face and lower extremities, which are readily injured. Approximately one-third of the lesions are found on the mucous membranes of the conjunctiva and oral cavity [40].

Pathogenesis. Since tubercle bacilli cannot penetrate intact skin [48], they are introduced into the tissue at the site of minor abrasions or wounds. Organisms from the sputum of phthisic patients are transmitted to infants by kisses, and mycobacteria present in the dust of tuberculous households gain entry into the skin through lacerations or at the site of pyogenic infections. Primary inoculation tuberculosis used to be a common complication of ritual circumcision when performed by tuberculous rabbis [43,49], and a rare "venereal" inoculation tuberculosis occurred in healthy individuals who had had sexual contact with patients suffering from genitourinary tuberculosis [50,51]. Lesions in the mouth may be due to bovine bacilli from nonpasteurized milk and occur after mucosal trauma or tooth extraction [40]. Primary inoculation tuberculosis following mouth-to-mouth resuscitation has been reported [47].

After bacteria have gained entry into the tissue they remain at the site of infection, multiply, and after 2 to 4 weeks produce the skin lesion. They also pass on to the regional lymph nodes where they lead to tuberculous lymphadenitis. As sensitivity develops, the tuberculin test converts to positive, and with increasing acquired immunity the process is localized to the particular region involved.

Clinical manifestations. The tuberculous chancre initially presents as a small papule, scab, or wound with little tendency to heal. A painless ulcer develops which may be quite insignificant or may enlarge to attain a diameter of over 5 cm [52] (Fig. 179-1). It is shallow and exhibits a granular or hemorrhagic base which is often studded with miliary abscesses or covered by necrotic membranous deposits. The ragged edges are undermined and of a reddish-blue hue; as the lesions grow older they become more indurated, and thick adherent crusts develop.

Lacerations inoculated with tubercle bacteria may heal temporarily but break down eventually, giving rise to granulating ulcers. Lesions on the conjunctiva are characterized by shallow ulcers or fungating granulations [40]. In the mouth, painless ulcers occur on the gingiva or the palate. Primary inoculation tuberculosis of the finger may clinically manifest as painless paronychia [46], and accidental inoculations of mycobacteria by poorly sterilized needles have resulted in subcutaneous abscesses [53,54].

Regional lymphadenopathy develops 3 to 8 weeks after the infection and may rarely be the only clinical symptom. The lymph node glands enlarge slowly and harden but are usually painless and are the most common complaint for which the physician is consulted (Fig. 179-1). Usually a benign course results but after weeks or months the lymph nodes may soften and cold abscesses form which perforate to the surface of the overlying skin. Sinuses result, and

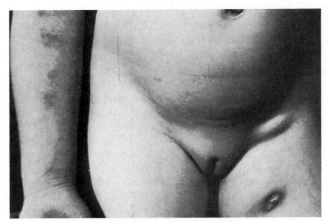

Fig. 179-1 Primary inoculation tuberculosis. Note tuberculous chancre on the thigh and regional lymphadenopathy.

the lymph nodes draining the primary glands may also be affected.

In about half the cases there are no systemic signs and symptoms. However, the temperature may be slightly raised and, occasionally, lymph node enlargement, abscess formation, and perforation take a more acute course. Fever, pain, and inflammatory swelling of the surrounding tissues may be concomitant features simulating a pyogenic infection [55].

Histopathology. In the early phases there is a banal acute inflammatory reaction with necrosis and ulceration, and mycobacteria are easily detected in sections stained for acid-fast organisms. After 3 to 6 weeks the infiltrate acquires a more tuberculoid appearance, exhibiting epithelioid cells, Langhans' giant cells, and lymphocytes. Typical caseation necrosis now becomes evident and mycobacteria are scarce. Similar changes occur in the regional lymph nodes which initially exhibit nonspecific inflammation and later develop tubercles with central caseation, densely packed epithelioid cells, and a peripheral rim of lymphocytes.

Diagnosis and differential diagnosis. Lack of awareness of the condition is probably the most common reason for an erroneous diagnosis. An ulcer with little or no tendency to heal and unilateral regional lymphadenopathy in a child should always arouse suspicion. Acid-fast organisms can be demonstrated in histologic sections or in smears obtained from the primary ulcer and draining glands in the initial stages of the disease but may be difficult to find in older lymph nodes. The diagnosis is verified by bacterial culture. The reaction to intradermal PPD is negative in the initial phases, but during the course of the disease it converts to positive. A previous tuberculous infection (such as a pulmonary Ghon focus) should be reasonably well excluded.

Differential diagnosis should consider other forms of skin tuberculosis, particularly tuberculosis verrucosa cutis and scrofuloderma. Primary inoculation tuberculosis has to be separated, both clinically and by laboratory procedures, from the primary complexes of syphilis, tularemia, cat-scratch fever, sporotrichosis, and from ulcerative lesions of other mycobacterioses.

Course. Without treatment, the condition may last up to 12 months. Skin and mucous membrane lesions heal by scarring, but in rare cases lupus vulgaris develops at the site of a healed tuberculous chancre. Scars also mark the previous sites of sinuses draining liquefied lymph nodes. In more than 50 percent of the cases calcium is deposited in the regional nodes [55].

Usually, the primary tuberculous complex procures satisfactory immunity and a state of high sensitivity, as shown by the tuberculin test. Calcification of the lymph nodes is not necessarily a sign for a favorable outcome, and reactivation of the disease may occur later. Hematogenous dissemination of bacteria from such latent foci may give rise to tuberculosis of other organs, particularly of the bones and joints [49,56]. Depending on the size of the inoculum, the age and resistance of the host, primary inoculation tuberculosis may also progress to acute miliary disease with fatal outcome [43]. Erythema nodosum is a feature in approximately 10 percent of the cases [55].

Tuberculosis verrucosa cutis (warty tuberculosis)

Definition. This is a verrucous form of skin tuberculosis in previously infected and sensitized individuals due to exogenous reinfection with *M. tuberculosis* or *M. bovis.*

Incidence. In Western countries tuberculosis verrucosa cutis is one of the rare forms of skin tuberculosis, but in certain regions it may be quite common; for instance, in Hong Kong it is the most frequently encountered form of tuberculous skin disease, accounting for more than 40 percent of the cases [15].

Pathogenesis. This is an inoculation tuberculosis occurring in persons who have had previous contact with *M. tuberculosis* and who have thus acquired a certain degree of immunity and sensitivity. Therefore, intradermal tests with PPD reveal a high degree of hypersensitivity and the regional lymph nodes are usually not involved. The inoculation of mycobacteria occurs at sites of minor wounds or abrasions, and their source is usually extraneous. Rarely, inoculation of mycobacteria may also occur by the patient's own sputum. In the past, certain professional groups were most liable to develop warty tuberculosis, particularly physicians, pathologists, medical students, and laboratory attendants, who were accidentally infected by tuberculous patients or by autopsy material (*verruca necrogenica, anatomist's wart, postmortem wart).* Farmers, butchers, and knackers contracted the disease from tuberculous cattle and in these cases *M. bovis* was responsible. In low socioeconomic environments, children become infected by playing and sitting on ground contaminated with tuberculous sputum [15,57].

Clinical manifestations. Tuberculosis verrucosa usually occurs on the hands, most often on the radial border of the dorsum, and on the fingers. In children the predilection sites are the lower extremities, which are most liable to be traumatized. The lesions are asymptomatic and start as a small papule or papulopustule with a purple inflammatory halo. The lesion becomes hyperkeratotic and warty and often is mistaken for a common wart. Slow growth and peripheral expansion lead to the development of a verru-

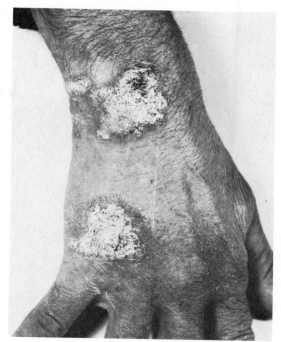

Fig. 179-2　Tuberculosis verrucosa cutis on the dorsum of the hand.

cous plaque with an irregular outline and a papillomatous horny surface (Fig. 179-2). Deep clefts and fissures extend into the underlying infiltrated base which is brownish red to purplish in color. The consistency is usually firm, but in the center it may be soft, and pus and keratinous material may be expressed from the fissures. As a rule, tuberculosis verrucosa is solitary, but multiple lesions may occur. The lymph nodes are usually not affected, but in some cases tuberculous involvement of the regional nodes has been described [57]. More commonly, however, enlargement of regional lymph nodes occurs after secondary bacterial infection.

Histopathology (Fig. 179-3). The most prominent features are pseudoepitheliomatous hyperplasia with marked hyperkeratosis and dense inflammatory infiltrates consisting of polymorphs and lymphocytes. Abscesses form in the superficial dermis, subepithelially, or within the pseudoepitheliomatous rete pegs. Epithelioid cells and giant cells are found in the midportions of the dermis and beneath the epidermis, but typical tubercles with characteristic caseation are not common. Mycobacteria can be demonstrated occasionally. At times, the dermal infiltrate may be nonspecific altogether [58].

Diagnosis and differential diagnosis. Early lesions resemble warts or keratoses. Hyperkeratotic lupus vulgaris exhibits "apple-jelly" nodules at the periphery and occurs in sites where tuberculosis verrucosa in rare. Blastomycosis, chromomycosis, and bromoderma may be similar clinically and histopathologically. Negative fungal cultures and small tuberculoid foci are diagnostic aids. Chronic vegetating pyoderma and hyperkeratotic lesions due to other, atypical mycobacteria may be difficult to exclude [59]. Hypertrophic lichen planus is pruritic, and usually other cuta-

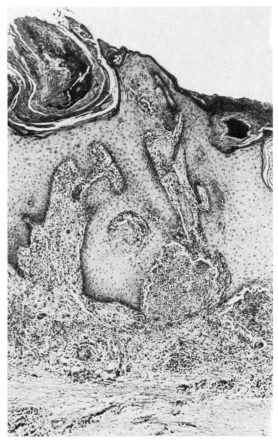

Fig. 179-3 Tuberculosis verrucosa cutis. There is pronounced epidermal hyperplasia, with hyperkeratotic masses on the surface of the epidermis. Abscesses are seen within and below the hyperplastic epithelium, and giant cells are present in the dermal infiltrate.

neous and mucosal lesions are found. Tertiary syphilis is not quite as verrucous and is accompanied by diagnostic serologic changes.

Course. The evolution of the lesions is slow and, without treatment, the course extends over many years. Secondary pyogenic infection may lead to temporary inflammatory changes of a more acute character, and lymphangitis and regional lymphadenitis ensue. Spontaneous involution does occur and usually results in sunken atrophic scars. Occasionally, ulcerative and sclerotic lesions or fungating granulomas are observed [57].

Lupus vulgaris

Definition. Lupus vulgaris is an extremely chronic and progressive form of tuberculosis of the skin occurring in individuals with a high degree of tuberculin sensitivity.

Incidence. Although the incidence of lupus vulgaris has steadily declined during the past decades, it was estimated in 1960 that some 50,000 new cases occurred throughout the world every year [60]. Early in this century it was so common that in some European countries special hospitals were available for the treatment of this condition alone. In 1938 the incidence in Germany was 430 per million [61],

and in the mid-1950s similar assessments in Denmark disclosed some 775 cases per million [60]. This contrasts sharply with present figures which estimate 300 to 400 new cases of all forms of skin tuberculosis in a population of 60 million in West Germany [16]. For the United States no exact figures are available, but lupus vulgaris has always been less common than in Europe. There is a greater prevalence of the disease in regions with a rather cool, humid climate, but the incidence is not influenced by rural or urban residence. Females appear to be affected about 2 to 3 times as often as males [60,61], but this may be in part because, for cosmetic reasons, women seek medical advice more frequently and earlier than men. Lupus vulgaris occurs at any age, and, in contrast to earlier estimates, the incidence is uniformly distributed among all age groups [62].

Pathogenesis. Lupus vulgaris is a postprimary form of skin tuberculosis arising in previously sensitized individuals. Immunity is only moderate in patients with lupus vulgaris, for the lesions progress steadily and, although spontaneous involution does occur, new lesions arise within old scars and, without therapy, complete healing is only rarely observed. Hypersensitivity to PPD is high, and only in early anergic stages of postexanthematic lupus it is reduced.

Lupus vulgaris originates from a tuberculous condition or a clinically inapparent tuberculous focus elsewhere in the body by hematogenous, lymphatic, or contiguous spread. Rarely it may follow primary inoculation tuberculosis or BCG vaccination [63] (see below); more frequently it develops from a tuberculous condition beneath the surface of the skin and in about 30 percent of the cases it is preceded by scrofuloderma; tuberculous involvement of the mucous membranes of the nose and throat is also a common source [61,64].

Most often lupus vulgaris develops after cervical adenitis or pulmonary tuberculosis. Hematogenous dissemination also has to be taken into account in those patients in whom there is no preceding tuberculous disease and in whom only an old pulmonary primary complex is found. It may be that mycobacteria disseminated into the skin reside there in a latent form to be activated by various stimuli [65].

Clinical manifestations. The lesions are usually solitary, but two or more sites may be involved simultaneously, and in patients with active pulmonary tuberculosis multiple foci may develop [66,67]. In about 90 percent of the patients the head and neck are involved [64]. Lupus vulgaris usually starts on the nose or cheek and by slow expansive growth extends onto adjacent areas. The earlobes are often affected, and solitary patches may be encountered on the scalp. Only a small percentage of the lesions occur on the extremities, and, except for cases with disseminated lupus vulgaris, involvement of the trunk is rare.

In general, lupus vulgaris is asymptomatic. The initial lesion is the lupus macule or papule, characterized by a brownish-red color and a soft consistency. Upon diascopy (i.e., the use of a thin piece of glass pressed against the skin), the infiltrate exhibits a diagnostic "apple-jelly" color, and if the lesion is probed, the instrument breaks through the overlying epidermis. Early lesions measure only a few millimeters in diameter; they are rather ill-

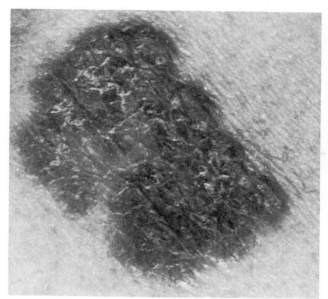

Fig. 179-4 Slightly raised, brownish plaque of lupus vulgaris.

defined, slightly raised or within the level of the skin, and may reveal a smooth surface or may be covered by a scale. Larger patches are formed by peripheral enlargement and coalescence of smaller papules, and further progression is characterized by an elevation of the lesions and an intensification of their brownish color (Fig. 179-4). Involution in one area and simultaneous expansion in another result in plaques with a gyrate outline. Since the course of this disease is marked by ulceration and scarring and since a number of complications ensue, the clinical manifestations of lupus vulgaris are diverse.

Plane forms manifest as flat plaques with a serpiginous or polycyclic configuration, a smooth surface or psoriasiform scaling (Fig. 179-5). *Hypertrophic forms* may present as tumorous growths of soft consistency that exhibit a nodular, knobby surface (Fig. 179-6) or show epithelial hyperplasia with the production of hyperkeratotic masses (Fig. 179-7). Edema, lymphatic stasis and recurrent erysip-

Fig. 179-5 Large plaque of lupus vulgaris of 10 years' duration involving the cheek, jaw, and ear.

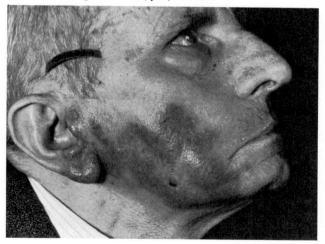

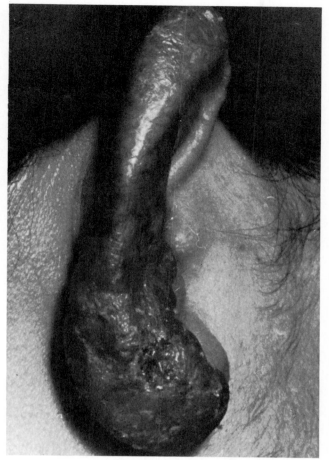

Fig. 179-6 Hypertrophic form of lupus vulgaris involving the ear. There is a tumorlike thickening of the earlobe; the lesion is brown and soft.

elas, elephantiasic thickening, and vascular dilatation accompany these tumorlike forms and may lead to gross deformity. In the *ulcerative forms* necrosis of the tissue predominates, and large progressive ulcers develop. The underlying tissue may be affected, and if the nasal or auricular cartilage is involved, extensive destruction takes place (Fig. 179-8). Granulations at the floor of the ulcers lead to vegetating papillomatous lesions.

Scarring is a prominent feature of lupus vulgaris. Atrophic scars occur subsequent to or independent of ulceration, and new "apple-jelly" nodules may develop within the cicatricial areas. Sometimes scarring is very pronounced and keloid-like fibrosis leads to contractures. The destruction of the tissues and cartilage and subsequent cicatricial changes are responsible for excessive deformities and mutilation.

LUPUS VULGARIS OF MUCOUS MEMBRANES. The buccal, nasal, or conjunctival mucosa either are primarily involved or are affected by extension of skin lesions. Small gray or pink papules of soft consistency ulcerate, and shallow mucosal defects develop which bleed easily. A dry rhinitis is often the only symptom of early nasal lupus, but progressive lesions destroy the cartilage of the nasal septum. Small transparent nodules, granulating masses, or ulcers characterize lupus vulgaris of the buccal mucosa, palate, gin-

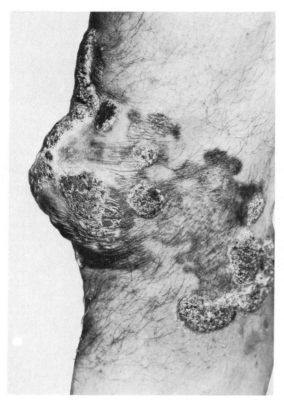

Fig. 179-7 Hyperkeratotic lupus on the knee.

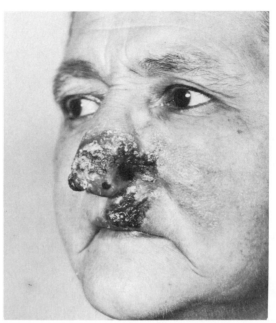

Fig. 179-8 Lupus vulgaris of long duration, having led to the destruction of the left nostril.

giva, larynx, and upper pharynx. Cicatricial deformities of the soft palate and stenosis of the larynx may result.

LUPUS POSTEXANTHEMATICUS. In rare cases, multiple disseminate lesions arise simultaneously in different regions of the body. The eruption is due to hematogenous spread from a latent tuberculous focus and follows a temporary reduction of immunity, particularly after measles. During and following the eruption a previously positive tuberculin test may become negative but will usually revert to positive as the general condition of the patient improves [68]. Clinically and histopathologically the lesions of postexanthematic lupus are typical for lupus vulgaris and this distinguishes the condition from acute miliary tuberculosis of the skin.

Histopathology (Fig. 179-9). The most prominent feature is the formation of typical tubercles with epithelioid cells, Langhans' giant cells, and a peripheral zone of lymphocytes. Caseation necrosis is sparse or may be absent, and acid-fast organisms are only rarely found in appropriately stained sections. More often than in other forms of cutaneous tuberculosis, secondary changes are superimposed: epidermal changes include thinning and atrophy or acanthosis with excessive hyperkeratosis and, occasionally, pseudoepitheliomatous hyperplasia. Necrosis and ulceration are usually accompanied by nonspecific inflammatory reactions which may partially conceal the tuberculous structures. Granulomatous reactions of the foreign-body type may develop. Long-standing quiescent lesions are composed chiefly of epithelioid cells, and it is impossible to distinguish them from sarcoidal infiltrates. During involution, small epithelioid foci are encased in fibrous connective tissue; they eventually disappear.

Diagnosis and differential diagnosis. Typical lupus vulgaris plaques do not present diagnostic problems; they have to be separated from lesions of sarcoidosis, lymphocytoma cutis, discoid lupus erythematosus, tertiary syphilis, leprosy, blastomycosis or other deep mycotic infections, lupoid leishmaniasis, and chronic vegetating pyodermas. Criteria helpful in the diagnosis are the softness of the lesions, the brownish-red color, and the slow evolution. The "apple-jelly" nodules revealed by diascopy are highly characteristic; finding them may be decisive, especially if the lesions are ulcerated, crusted, or hyperkeratotic. Histologic examination is mandatory and in some cases sparse acid-fast bacilli can be demonstrated. Bacterial culture verifies the diagnosis. The tuberculin test is strongly positive with the exception of early phases of postexanthematic lupus [68].

Course. This form of skin tuberculosis is extremely chronic, and without therapy its course usually extends over many years or even decades. This explains why in adults or older patients more extensive lesions are encountered than in children [69]. Although there are periods of relative inactivity, lupus vulgaris is incessantly progressive and leads to considerable impairment of function and to disfiguration. Contractions result in a reduction of joint mobility, and ulceration and destruction of the cartilaginous structures of the face lead to severe mutilation. Sequelae are cicatricial ectropion, with its complications, and microstomia with impairment of speech and food intake.

The most serious complication of long-standing lupus vulgaris is the development of carcinoma (Fig. 179-10). Early in this century this complication was not infrequent, having been estimated to be almost 10 percent [70]. Squamous cell carcinomas outnumber basal cell carcinomas by far, and the incidence of metastases is surprisingly high [71]. There is no causal relationship between previous x-ray treatment of the tuberculous lesions and the subsequent malignancy. Sarcomas following lupus vulgaris also have been described, but some of these tumors have actually represented highly dedifferentiated carcinomas.

The relation of lupus vulgaris to tuberculosis of other organs. In 40 percent of patients with lupus vulgaris there is associated tuberculous lymphadenitis or lupus of the mucous membranes; 10 to 20 percent have pulmonary tuberculosis or tuberculosis of the bones and joints [69]. The morbidity of lupus vulgaris patients from pulmonary tuberculosis is 4 to 10 times higher than in the general population, and in the majority of the cases the pulmonary disease represents postprimary phthisis [72].

In the past it was believed that pulmonary tuberculosis had a good prognosis if it was associated with lupus vulgaris of the skin, and a protective or immunizing effect was ascribed to the cutaneous condition [70,73]. This impression has not been substantiated. In all age groups more patients with lupus vulgaris die of tuberculosis than could be predicted from the mortality ratios in the general population [74]. In some cases lupus vulgaris may be regarded as a symptom of another tuberculous disease running a serious course. [69].

Scrofuloderma (tuberculosis colliquativa cutis)

Definition. This describes a subcutaneous process originating from tuberculosis beneath the skin and leading to cold abscess formation and a secondary breakdown of the overlying skin.

Incidence. In the past, tuberculosis colliquativa was a relatively frequent disorder, particularly in individuals with tuberculosis of the lymph nodes. It appears to be the most common form of skin tuberculosis in Mexico [75] and other tropical countries. In the United Kingdom it is more common in individuals of African or Asian origin [76].

Pathogenesis. Scrofuloderma results from contiguous involvement of the skin overlying another tuberculous process—most commonly tuberculous lymphadenitis, tuberculosis of bones and joints, or tuberculous epididymitis. It may affect all age groups although there is a higher prevalence among children, adolescents, and old individuals. Rarely, tuberculosis colliquativa may develop after accidental or intentional introduction of exogenous bacilli into the subcutaneous tissue by trauma or injection in individuals with previous latent or manifest tuberculosis [77].

Clinical manifestations (Fig. 179-11). Tuberculosis colliquativa most often occurs in the parotidal, submandibular, and supraclavicular regions as well as on the lateral aspects of the neck [78]; owing to the involvement of lymph nodes in these areas, the lesions are often bilateral. On the extremities or on the trunk the lesions accompany tuberculous disease of the phalangeal bones, joints, the sternum, and the ribs.

The skin lesions first present as firm, subcutaneous nodules or a well-defined, asymptomatic infiltrate, which initially is freely movable. As the infiltrate enlarges it becomes doughy, but it may take months before there is liquefaction with subsequent perforation. Ulcers and sinuses develop and discharge watery and purulent or caseous material. The ulcers are linear or serpiginous; their edges are undermined, inverted, and of bluish color; their

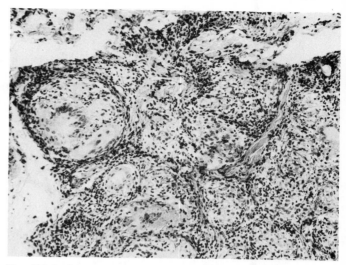

Fig. 179-9 Lupus vulgaris. Epithelioid cell tubercles with peripheral lymphocytes, but without caseation, are present. Giant cells are clearly visible.

floors are uneven, soft, and granulating. Sinusoidal tracts undermine the skin, and clefts and dissecting subcutaneous pockets alternate with soft gummatous nodules; cordlike scars develop and bridge ulcerative areas or even stretches of normal skin. Tuberculin sensitivity is usually pronounced.

Histopathology. Massive necrosis and abscess formation found in the center of the lesion are nonspecific. However, the periphery of the abscesses or the margins of the sinuses

Fig. 179-10 This patient had mutilating lupus vulgaris of the face, necessitating plastic surgery. Squamous cell carcinoma secondary to lupus vulgaris has developed below the left eye.

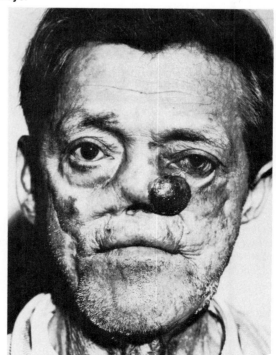

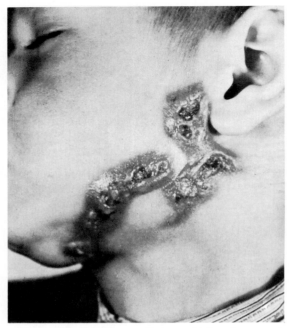

Fig. 179-11   Scrofuloderma. Note multiple ulcers and sinuses bridged by hypertrophic granulation tissue and incipient scar formation.

contain tuberculoid granulomas and true tubercles with caseation necrosis. *M. tuberculosis* can be demonstrated in the sections.

Diagnosis and differential diagnosis. If there is an underlying tuberculous lymphadenitis or bone and joint disease, the diagnosis usually presents no difficulty. Syphilitic gumma, deep fungal infections, particularly sporotrichosis, actinomycosis, severe forms of acne conglobata, and hidradenitis suppurativa have to be excluded. A confirmation of the clinical diagnosis is achieved by bacterial culture.

Course. Spontaneous healing does occur, but the course is very protracted, and it may take years before the inflammatory and ulcerative lesions have been completely replaced by scar tissue. The cordlike keloidal scars are characteristic enough to permit a correct diagnosis even after the process has become quiescent. Tuberculin sensitivity is pronounced, and not infrequently lupus vulgaris develops at the site or in the vicinity of scrofuloderma.

Metastatic tuberculous abscess (tuberculous gumma)

Definition and pathogenesis. The metastatic tuberculous abscess is due to hematogenous spread of mycobacteria from a primary focus during a period of lowered resistance or breakdown of immunity, resulting in singular or multiple subcutaneous-cutaneous lesions. It usually occurs in undernourished children of low socioeconomic status, in immunodeficiency, or in severely immunosuppressed patients.

Clinical manifestations. Subcutaneous abscesses, which are generally nontender and fluctuant, arise either singly or as multiples on the trunk, extremities, or head (Fig. 179-12). The lesions may coalesce with the overlying skin and break

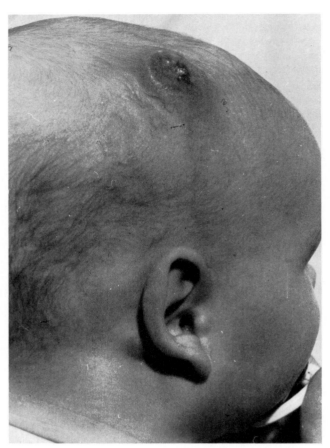

Fig. 179-12   Metastatic tuberculous abscess on the scalp in an infant with combined immunodeficiency.

down forming fistulas and ulcers. Metastatic tuberculous abscesses may occur with progressive organ tuberculosis [79] and in miliary tuberculosis [80] but also without any underlying tuberculous focus, suggesting silent bacillemia as the pathogenic mechanism [67,81]. Abscess formation may develop at sites of previous trauma, which suggests localization of blood-borne organisms in the injured tissue [81,82]. One patient presented with erythema nodosum-like lesions from which *M. tuberculosis* was cultured [67]. Tuberculin sensitivity is usually present but is lower than in other forms of skin tuberculosis and may be absent in severely ill patients.

Histopathology. As in scrofuloderma, massive necrosis and abscess formation are found. Acid-fast stains usually reveal copious amounts of mycobacteria.

Diagnosis and differentiated diagnosis. All forms of panniculitis, deep fungal infections, syphilitic gumma, and hidradenitis suppurativa have to be excluded. A confirmation of the clinical diagnosis is obtained by histopathology, acid-fast stains of the tissue and smears, and bacterial culture.

Orificial tuberculosis (tuberculosis ulcerosa cutis et mucosae)

Definition. This is a tuberculosis of the mucous membranes and skin of the orifices due to autoinoculation of mycobacteria from progressive tuberculosis of internal organs.

Incidence. The condition is rare; in one series it was found in only about 0.2 percent of patients with internal tuberculosis [83]. Males are more frequently affected than females, and although the disease may occur in practically all age groups, it is most common in middle-aged or older persons [84].

Pathogenesis. The underlying disease is far advanced, pulmonary, intestinal, or, rarely, genitourinary tuberculosis. Mycobacteria shed from these foci in massive numbers are inoculated into the mucous membranes of the orifices, usually after preceding trauma. Considering the frequency of positive sputums in patients with pulmonary involvement, it is surprising that oral tuberculosis is rare, but it seems that the constant bathing of the oral mucous membranes by salivary and mucous secretions and their constant motion render them rather resistant to tuberculous inoculation. However, histologic examinations at autopsy of patients with pulmonary tuberculosis have revealed a much higher incidence of oral lesions than was expected [85] and it may be that, clinically, many mucosal lesions go undiscovered. Most patients show a positive intradermal tuberculin reaction, but in terminal stages anergy develops.

Clinical manifestations. In orificial tuberculosis of the mouth, the tongue is most frequently affected, particularly the tip and the lateral margins, but the soft and hard palate are also common sites and, occasionally, a lesion develops in a tooth socket following extraction. In far advanced cases the lips are also involved [84,86–89] and the oral condition often represents an extension of ulcerative tuberculosis of the pharynx and larynx. In cases with intestinal tuberculosis, lesions develop on and around the anus and in females with active genitourinary disease the vulva is involved.

A small yellowish or reddish nodule appears on the mucosa and, by breaking down, forms a circular or irregular ulcer with a typical punched-out appearance and soft consistency (Fig. 179-13). The edges are undermined, and the surrounding mucosa is swollen, edematous, and inflamed. The floor of the ulcer is usually covered by pseudomembraneous material and often exhibits multiple yellowish tubercles and eroded vessels. Lesions may be single or multiple and are extremely painful. The tenderness is often out of proportion to the size of the ulcers and results in dysphagia and inability to eat.

Histopathology. There is a massive nonspecific inflammatory infiltrate and necrosis, but tubercles with caseation may be found deep in the dermis. Mycobacteria are easily demonstrated in acid-fast stained sections.

Diagnosis and differential diagnosis. Painful ulcers of the mouth in patients with pulmonary tuberculosis should arouse suspicion. Large numbers of acid-fast organisms can be detected in histologic sections, and bacterial culture confirms the diagnosis. Syphilitic lesions, aphthous ulcers, and carcinoma have to be excluded.

Course. The outcome depends on the course of the underlying disease. In general, individuals developing orificial tuberculosis run a downhill course, and as the internal condition progresses the orificial lesions enlarge and spread. Orificial tuberculosis is a symptom of advanced internal disease with a most unfavorable prognosis.

Acute miliary tuberculosis of the skin (tuberculosis cutis miliaris disseminata)

Definition and pathogenesis. Miliary tuberculosis of the skin, which most often occurs in babies or infants, is an extremely rare skin manifestation of fulminating miliary tuberculosis due to hematogenous dissemination of mycobacteria. The initial focus of infection is either meningeal or pulmonary and it may follow infections such as measles which reduce the immunologic defense mechanisms [90]. Two babies with typical skin lesions associated with congenital miliary tuberculosis have been reported but organisms have not been cultured from the lesions [91]. Although extremely rare, acute miliary tuberculosis does occur in adults [92]. Tuberculin sensitivity is usually absent.

Clinical manifestations. Disseminate lesions occur on all parts of the body, particularly on the trunk. They consist of minute erythematous macules or papules and or purpuric lesions. Sometimes vesicles or a central necrosis and crust develop. Removal of the crust discloses a minute umbilication.

Histopathology. In the acute phases the histologic changes are nonspecific; one finds necrosis and occasionally signs of vasculitis, extravasation of red blood cells, and nonspecific inflammatory infiltrates, which sometimes form small abscesses. Mycobacteria are present both intravascularly and in the perivascular tissue [93]. In later stages (if the patient develops immunity) lymphocytic cuffing of the vessels and even tubercles may be observed.

Diagnosis. The eruption occurs in individuals already gravely ill and, because of the severity of the underlying process, often goes unnoticed. A multitude of papular, macular, and purpuric rashes must be excluded, but the diagnosis is usually substantiated by the evidence of acute miliary disease of the internal organs.

Fig. 179-13 Orificial tuberculosis in far advanced cavitary pulmonary tuberculosis.

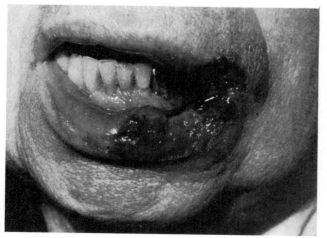

Course. Children usually run a downhill course, and the prognosis is poor. Cases with a favorable outcome after therapy have been described [94,95].

Tuberculosis of the skin due to BCG vaccination

While it is now generally accepted that vaccination with the attenuated bovine bacillus Calmette-Guérin (BCG) affords protection against tuberculosis [96–98], doubts about its effectiveness in developing countries have recently been revived [99]. However, a study from England published in 1984 has shown rather convincingly that neonatal BCG vaccination substantially reduces the incidence of childhood tuberculosis, the suggested level of protection being above 75% [100]. Untoward reactions are rare but it is important to be aware of these complications, particularly since BCG vaccination in adults has come into wide use as immunotherapy for cancer. BCG has immunopotentiating effects and macrophage-activating properties and is therefore undergoing extensive clinical trials.

The clinical course of a normal BCG vaccination is as follows [101]: approximately 2 weeks after vaccination an infiltrated papule develops which, after 6 to 12 weeks, attains a size of about 10 mm, ulcerates, and then slowly heals, leaving a scar. Vaccination may provoke an accelerated reaction if given to a subject previously infected but with a negative tuberculin test. The regional lymph nodes may enlarge but usually heal without breaking down. Tuberculin sensitivity appears 5 to 6 weeks after vaccination.

Nonspecific complications include keloid formation, epithelial cysts, granulomas, eczema, generalized hemorrhagic rashes, erythema nodosum, and other eruptions [101,102]. Specific complications comprise tuberculous processes caused by the BCG organism [103]. The large majority of these are lymphoglandular and skin reactions which mimic cutaneous responses to "natural" mycobacterial infection. Their true incidence is difficult to ascertain, but it is extremely low in comparison to the great number of vaccinations performed [96]. According to Horwitz and Meyer [103] nonfatal generalized complications occur in 1 or 2 persons per million; a perforating regional adenitis was seen in 2 percent of vaccinated children in Denmark, and the incidence of postvaccinal lupus vulgaris was estimated to be from 5 to 10 per million [103,104]. Usually the BCG reactions run a milder course than "spontaneous" tuberculosis of the skin and occur more often after revaccination [102,105].

Specific lesions originating from BCG vaccination include: (1) *Lupus vulgaris* may develop at or in the vicinity of the vaccination site after a latency period of several months or after 1 to 3 years (Fig. 179-14). Its clinical appearance, course, and response to treatment do not differ from "normal" lupus vulgaris. BCG organisms can be recovered from only one-fourth of the lesions [103]. In some cases lupus vulgaris has developed after vaccination with the Vole bacillus [106]. (2) Individuals previously sensitive to tuberculin may exhibit a type of *Koch's phenomenon.* Necrosis and ulceration occur as in normal nonsensitive individuals but are accelerated with time. Regional adenitis is common, and general symptoms may be present [103]. (3) Local *subcutaneous abscesses* may form if the vaccination material has been injected too deeply into the skin, and excessive ulceration may ensue [101]. (4) Severe

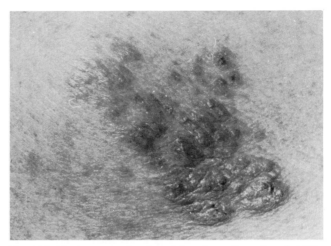

Fig. 179-14 Lupus vulgaris arising from the site of BCG vaccination in a patient undergoing immunotherapy for malignant melanoma.

regional adenitis is definitely the most common complication and occurs more often in the younger age groups. *Scrofuloderma* may develop and suppuration may persist for 6 to 12 months. (5) Generalized *tuberculid-like eruptions* have rarely been observed [101,102]. (6) *Generalized adenitis, osteitis,* and *tuberculous foci* in *distant organs* (e.g., the joints) have occurred occasionally [96]. After repeated vaccinations *fever, chills, arthralgia,* and *malaise* may occur. *Anaphylaxis* and a tuberculin shock-like syndrome may be fatal [107]; *hepatic dysfunction* and noncaseous granulomas containing the organisms have been noted. *Fatal disease* due to generalized BCG tuberculosis is rare—1 per 10 million vaccinated [96]—and occurs in immunologically compromised individuals [108]. In 1980 Rosenthal [109] collected 17 fatal disseminated cases, the majority of whom had immunodeficiencies.

The tuberculids

This term [110] is used to denote recurrent skin eruptions which are usually disseminate and show a tendency to spontaneous involution. It originally encompassed lichen scrofulosorum, erythema induratum, papulonecrotic tuberculids, lupus miliaris disseminatus faciei, and some eruptions with rather exotic designations. Tuberculids were originally considered to represent reactions to toxins of tubercle bacilli and were thus separated from the "true" cutaneous tuberculoses. More recent opinion holds that they result from a hematogenous dissemination of mycobacteria whereby the interplay of mycobacterial number and virulence as well as the resistance of the skin determine the clinical manifestations.

During the first half of this century tuberculids were eruptions quite familiar to dermatologists, but with the sharp decline of tuberculosis in the developed countries the tuberculids have also become rare. This does not appear to apply to geographic regions where tuberculosis is still not so uncommon [17], and with the recent resurgence of tuberculosis in some Western countries some tuberculids have also been observed again in these regions [111,112]. The pathogenesis of these conditions and their relation to tuberculosis are still poorly understood and, while there is no doubt that in some of these conditions such a relation exists, there are good reasons to doubt it in others. Therefore, before describing these entities it appears necessary to briefly discuss the evidence in favor of and against a causal relation between tuberculids and tuberculosis. Such evidence could rest on the demonstration of mycobacteria in the lesions, on the histopathology, the patient's sensitivity to mycobacterial antigens, the presence of proved concomitant tuberculosis elsewhere in the body, and the response to tuberculostatic therapy.

1. Mycobacteria. Early in this century several cases were described in which bacteria were recovered from the lesions [113–116]. Some of these conditions were atypical both clinically and histologically, and at that time the criteria for the identification of *M. tuberculosis* were not as stringent as today: during this period "mycobacteria" were even found in lesions of lupus erythematosus, granuloma annulare, and sarcoidosis. The results of a later study in which mycobacteria were detected in 2 out of 72 patients with erythema induratum [117] have not been confirmed [118] and it is accepted today that mycobacteria cannot be found in tuberculids. The failure to demonstrate mycobacteria in histologic sections, by bacterial culture, or by guinea pig inoculation has been ascribed, by the supporters of the tuberculid concept, to the small number of organisms or their rapid destruction [119].

2. Histology. Most tuberculids exhibit tuberculoid features histologically. However, tuberculoid granulomas are produced by a multitude of conditions, and, conversely, "tuberculids" have been described which lacked tuberculoid structures. Therefore, the histologic evidence is of questionable value.

3. Tuberculin sensitivity. The tuberculin reaction is moderate to strong in most patients, and in the past was considered positive evidence for the tuberculous nature of the lesions. However, a considerable number of the patients show only a low sensitivity, and the reactions may vary within wide limits [119]. Today, it is generally agreed that positive tuberculin reactions do not establish pathogenicity with respect to the lesions [118–120].

4. Previous and concomitant tuberculosis of other organs. In the older literature, patients with tuberculids often presented with a family or personal history of tuberculosis. Tuberculous disease was quite common in the first half of this century, and the chances of finding individuals with evidence of tuberculosis were rather high in the general population. However, in large series published in 1954 [121] and 1960 [122] active tuberculosis was found only in a small percentage of patients with tuberculids and was described to be just as common as, for instance, focal bacterial infections [122]. On the other hand, cases have only recently been published in whom active tuberculosis and concomitant eruptions satisfying the clinical criteria for tuberculids are documented [17,111,112,123]. The development of lupus vulgaris from lesions of papulonecrotic tuberculids certainly appears to be a strong argument in favor of a tuberculous etiology in these cases [17].

5. The therapeutic test. Tuberculostatics have been found beneficial in some cases and the involution of tuberculid lesions concomitant with the improvement of underlying tuberculosis has been described [17,112]. However, it should also be kept in mind that some tuberculids tend to involute spontaneously, that some cases do not respond to antituberculous treatment [119,124], and that many react equally well to other antibiotics or even to plain rest and nonspecific measures [118].

In summary then, the evidence supporting the tuberculous etiology of tuberculids is largely circumstantial and not necessarily convincing in all cases. One gets the impression that this term has been used too liberally in the past for conditions which are in fact unrelated to tuberculosis; it also is quite clear today that some tuberculids have a multifactorial etiology where *M. tuberculosis* or its products can, at best, be considered as one of several possible causes. On the other hand, positive evidence disproving the tuberculous nature of some of these eruptions is equally lacking and in some an etiopathogenetic link to tuberculosis cannot be denied.

The following discussion therefore employs a restrictive classification which acknowledges as tuberculids only those conditions for which a reasonable amount of evidence supporting a tuberculous etiopathogenesis exists (Table 179-3): *Tuberculids* therefore comprise only lichen scrofulosorum and papulonecrotic tuberculid. *Facultative tuberculids* are conditions in which *M. tuberculosis* or its antigens can be considered one of several possible causes: they comprise nodular vasculitis and erythema nodosum. Finally, *"non-tuberculids"* are all those conditions which were formerly regarded as tuberculids but can now be considered to be unrelated to tuberculosis.

Lichen scrofulosorum

Definition. Lichen scrofulosorum is a lichenoid eruption of minute papules occurring in children with tuberculosis.

Incidence and pathogenesis. The disorder was recognized by Hebra and was rather uncommon even in the past [125]. It usually occurred in children but was observed also in

---

Table 179-3   Tuberculids

Tuberculids (conditions in which *M. tuberculosis/bovis* appears to play a significant role)	1. Lichen scrofulosorum 2. Papulonecrotic tuberculid
Facultative tuberculids (conditions in which *M. tuberculosis/bovis* may be one of several etiopathogenic factors)	1. Nodular vasculitis (erythema induratum) 2. Erythema nodosum
Non-tuberculids (conditions formerly designated tuberculids; there is no relation to tuberculosis)	1. Lupus miliaris disseminatus faciei 2. Rosacea-like tuberculid 3. Lichenoid tuberculid

adolescents and adults [70]. Today this diagnosis is made only rarely, but a number of well-documented cases have recently been described [111,112]. Lichen scrofulosorum is usually associated with chronic tuberculous disease of the lymph nodes and bones, or with specific pleurisy, but is rare in phthisic patients [70]; it has been observed following BCG vaccination [101]. It is ascribed to a hematogenous spread of mycobacteria in an individual strongly sensitive to *M. tuberculosis* [70,111,112,125] and its pathogenesis has been considered to be analogous to that of postexanthematic lupus vulgaris [70]. The tuberculin reaction is positive.

Clinical manifestations. The eruption is asymptomatic and is usually confined to the trunk. The lesions consist of small, firm, follicular or parafollicular papules of a yellowish or pink color; they have a flat top or bear a minute horny spine or fine scales on their surface and, rarely, there may be superficial pustulation which is barely visible. Lichenoid grouping is pronounced and results in the formation of rough, discoid plaques which tend to coalesce. The lesions persist for months, but spontaneous involution eventually ensues. Antituberculous therapy results in complete resolution within a matter of weeks [111]. An association of lichen scrofulosorum and tuberculous dactylitis has been described [112].

Histopathology. Superficial tuberculoid granulomas develop around hair follicles but may also occur independent of the adnexae. They consist of epithelioid cells with some Langhans' giant cells and a narrow margin of lymphocytes [58]. Mycobacteria are not seen in the sections and cannot be cultured from biopsy material [111].

Diagnosis. Eczematoid eruptions, seborrheic and autosensitization dermatitis may be similar clinically. Lichen planus, lichen nitidus, lichenoid secondary syphilis, and micropapular forms of sarcoidosis should be excluded.

Papulonecrotic tuberculid

Definition. This is a symmetric eruption of necrotizing papules appearing in crops and healing with scar formation. The old names follicles and acnitis probably denoted variants of this disorder [70].

Incidence. Reports on papulonecrotic tuberculids were quite common in the older dermatologic and pediatric literature but have become rather rare. Today the condition still appears to be not so uncommon in populations with a high prevalence of tuberculosis—in 1974 Morrison and Fourie reported 91 cases seen in South Africa over a 17-year period [17]. It preferentially occurs in children or young adults.

Pathogenesis. As a rule, bacteria cannot be demonstrated in lesions, but a few authors are regularly cited who supposedly succeeded in recovering the organism [113–116,126]. However, these findings do not stand up to critical analysis. In most cases a single (!) acid-fast "rod" was found histologically and, with one exception [126], guinea pig inoculations were invariably negative. However, in a series of 91 cases published more recently [17], lupus vul-

garis was seen to evolve from papulonecrotic tuberculids in four patients and *M. tuberculosis* was cultured from two. This suggests that mycobacteria may have been present, in a covert form, in the papulonecrotic lesions but does not exclude the possibility that they may have lodged in these lesions secondarily.

In most cases the tuberculin test is positive [121] and in earlier writings the frequency of associated tuberculous lymph nodes of internal organs has been stressed [127]. In the series of Morrison and Fourie [17] a deep focus of tuberculosis, most commonly cervical adenopathy—some with scrofuloderma—was found in one-third of cases. A prompt response to antituberculous therapy—whether a tuberculous focus was known to exist or not—has been described [17]. Anticomplementary activity and in vivo conversion of C3 to C3c observed in five patients indicated the presence of immune complexes. Morrison and Fourie [17] believe that from a tuberculous focus bacilli periodically enter the circulation where they are opsonized with antibodies and complement and settle out preferentially in slow-flowing capillaries in the skin; they suggest that the papulonecrotic tuberculid represents an Arthus reaction followed by a delayed-hypersensitivity response to mycobacteria.

On the other hand, an association with discoid lupus erythematosus, arthritis, or erythema nodosum also has been observed in patients with papulonecrotic tuberculids [128] and concomitant focal bacterial infections are found frequently [122]; the antistreptolysin titer is increased in almost 65 percent of the cases [122] and a number of them respond to antibiotics other than tuberculostatic agents [120]. Some forms of papulonecrotic tuberculid may therefore be triggered by other antigens than those of *M. tuberculosis*.

Clinical manifestations. Predilection sites are the extensor aspects of the extremities, particularly the knees and elbows, buttocks, and lower trunk (Fig. 179-15). The distribution is usually symmetric, but localized papulonecrotic tuberculids have been reported, for instance, on the penis [129,130]. The lesions occur in crops, they are disseminate, and they present as dusky red, symptomless, pea-sized papules; they may show a central depression and an adherent crust and may develop necrosis in the center which, upon removal, results in a crater-like ulcer. If the lesions are seated more deeply, they may enlarge to a diameter of 1 cm and acquire a more livid color. There is spontaneous involution, and pitted scars result. Usually there are not systemic symptoms.

Histopathology. The most prominent feature of well-developed lesions is a wedge-shaped necrosis of the upper dermis extending to and involving the epidermis. The inflammatory infiltrate surrounding this necrotic area may be nonspecific but usually exhibits tuberculoid features. Epithelioid cells and occasionally Langhans' giant cells are present. Involvement of the blood vessels is a cardinal feature and consists of an obliterative and sometimes granulomatous vasculitis leading to thrombosis and complete occlusion of the vascular channels. Recanalization of the vessels may be observed. Early lesions have been described to mimic an Arthus type reaction with intraluminal collections of polymorphs and fibrin, vessel damage, extravasation of red blood cells, perivascular leukocytoclasia, and edema. In one case of papulonecrotic tuberculid the histopathology of one lesion was considered similar to Churg-Strauss vasculitis but an absence of eosinophils was noted [123].

Diagnosis and differential diagnosis. Although the clinical picture is characteristic, the histology should be consulted before the diagnosis is established. The exclusion of pityriasis lichenoides et varioliformis acuta may present difficulties. This condition is more widespread and involves also the trunk, palms, and soles; histologically it represents lymphocytic vasculitis [131,132]. Eruptions due to leukocytoclastic necrotizing vasculitis also have to be separated; the history, clinical appearance, and histology make the diagnosis. The distinction from lichen urticatus, prurigo, and secondary syphilis is easily established.

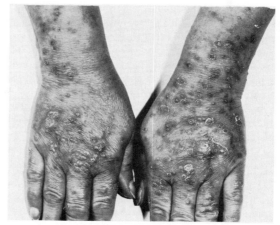

Fig. 179-15 Papulonecrotic tuberculid on the forearms and dorsa of the hands of a 62-year-old woman.

Nodular vasculitis (see also Chap. 99)

Definition. This term is used to describe a chronic recurring nodular and ulcerative disorder of the lower legs of women. Formerly the condition was considered to be the classical example of a tuberculid and was termed *erythema induratum of Bazin*.

Incidence. Nodular vasculitis is quite common, particularly in Europe. According to one report these cases comprise some 0.1 to 0.2 percent of all dermatologic patients seen at a University hospital [118]. The disease is found predominantly in women; men account for only 5 to 10 percent of the cases [117,118]. The age of onset varies from the early teens to old age, but there are two peaks of incidence: one in adolescence and one at about the time of menopause. There is a prevalence for certain seasons, particularly winter and early spring.

Pathogenesis. The elemental lesion is connected with the circulation, and most cases present erythrocyanotic changes of the lower extremities [133]. These women usually have heavy, column-like calves, the skin is thick and firm but not edematous, and follicular perniosis may be present. Cutis marmorata is common, and the pathogenic significance of the vasculature is clearly demonstrated by the histologic pattern which reveals features of vasculitis. The vessels of the patients react to changes of temperature in an abnormal manner, and the eruptions are usually associated with the action of cold [133].

It has long been contended that mycobacteria disseminated during transient bacteremia are caught up in areas of vascular stasis and that they or their decomposition products produce a reaction which is both induced by and superimposed upon the basic circulatory disorder [133]. However, active tuberculosis is found only rarely in these patients [118,121] and the fact that, very occasionally, tuberculous disease has developed subsequent to erythema induratum [117,121] does not establish pathogenicity with regard to skin disease. Similarly, the tuberculin test is of no pathogenic significance; many patients exhibit high sensitivity, but up to 60 percent do not react to a 1:10,000 dilution of OT [118].

The introductory comments on the relation of the tuberculids to tuberculosis are particularly relevant to the problem of "erythema induratum." Nodular vasculitis [117,133] today represents a multifactorial syndrome of lobular panniculitis in which tuberculosis may or may not be one of a multitude of etiologic components. Immune complexes play a pathogenic role in this condition in which both streptococcal and (in one study) mycobacterial antigens have been found in the lesions [134].

Today most authors accept a subdivision of the erythema induratum–nodular vasculitis complex into two groups: one with and one without tuberculous etiology [117,118]. At the same time, however, it is agreed that the term erythema induratum should be reserved for the first group, i.e., for those cases in which the tuberculous origin can be proved [117,135]. From the foregoing discussion on the validity of such proofs, the demonstration and culture of mycobacteria emerges as the only reliable criterion; if it is remembered that bacterial examinations of erythema induratum lesions have almost invariably yielded negative results, it becomes apparent that it may be impossible to pinpoint the alleged "tuberculous" cases.

Clinical manifestations. The clinical manifestations, histopathology, and course of nodular vasculitis are discussed in Chap. 99.

Erythema nodosum

Erythema nodosum is a cutaneous reaction pattern manifesting as septal panniculitis; it is associated with a variety of disease processes and results from immunologic reactions which may be triggered by a multitude of antigenic stimuli including, among others, viral, bacterial, and mycobacterial antigens.

For a detailed description of erythema nodosum see Chap. 99.

Non-tuberculids (conditions with nontuberculous etiology, previously considered tuberculids)

The older dermatologic literature abounds with entities that were considered tuberculous in nature. Great significance was attached to nomenclature, and the resulting confusion is still reflected in some more recent writings [136,137]. In none of these conditions has the tuberculous etiology been proved; they all exhibit tuberculoid features histologically; tuberculin sensitivity is low or inconstant; there is no associated visceral tuberculosis; and the incidence of past tuberculous disease among patients with these conditions does not exceed that of the general population. Mycobacteria cannot be recovered from the lesions.

In order to avoid a perpetuation of the terminologic jumble, many of the older designations are not mentioned in this text. Most of them are synonymous.

Lupus miliaris disseminatus faciei. This is a papular eruption of the face, running a chronic course and terminating with spontaneous involution. Originally it was considered a variant of lupus vulgaris or a tuberculid [136,138], but there is no evidence supporting a link to tuberculosis [139]. The histology exhibits tuberculoid features; the tuberculin test is inconstant and most often negative; the course is self-limited, leading to spontaneous involution; there is not concomitant tuberculosis [121]; mycobacteria cannot be recovered from the lesions; and there is no response to antituberculous drugs. The cause and pathogenesis of this condition are unknown and, therefore, the designation lupus miliaris disseminatus is not appropriate. Some cases may represent micropapular forms of sarcoidosis, but most represent a sarcoidal form of rosacea. An allergic etiology has been discussed [139].

The eruption is not uncommon and occurs in adults and adolescents of both sexes. It consists of multiple indolent papules, 1 to 3 mm in diameter, symmetrically distributed in the centrofacial regions. The lower portions of the forehead, the bridge of the nose, the cheeks, the nasolabial folds, and the perioral areas are preferentially involved (Fig. 179-16), but occasionally more widespread dissemination occurs [139]. The papules develop quite rapidly, may be follicular or nonfollicular, and are distributed at random. Their surface is smooth, their color brownish red; diascopy reveals an infiltrate similar to the "apple-jelly" nodules of lupus vulgaris. Their consistency is rather firm, but occasionally it may be soft, and in some cases pustulation has been observed.

Histopathology reveals well-defined globular masses of tuberculoid structures composed of epithelioid cells, giant cells, and an encircling rim of sparse lymphocytes in the upper dermis. In the center there may be frank necrosis, and thus the similarity to true tubercles may be striking (Fig. 179-17).

The condition runs a self-limited course. Individual papules regress, leaving pitted atrophic scars, and new crops of lesions arise. After a period of months or up to 2 years, the condition involutes spontaneously. Tetracyclines exert a beneficial effect.

Rosacea-like tuberculid. Originally described by Lewandowsky [140], this condition was separated from ordinary rosacea on the basis of its tuberculoid histopathology. This has caused much confusion; no uniform concept has ever emerged regarding its classification. Laymon and Michelson [136] found the term objectionable and replaced it with the designation "micro-nodular tuberculid," which did not help to clarify the situation. Today it is largely agreed that rosacea-like tuberculid represents a micropapular form of rosacea with pronounced tuberculoid features.

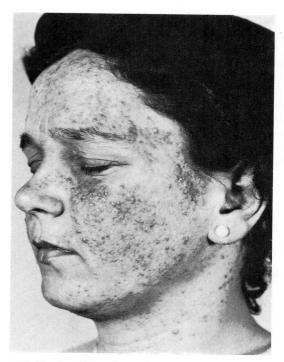

Fig. 179-16 Condition formerly termed lupus miliaris disseminatus faciei, with the characteristic distribution of small follicular and nonfollicular papules. This represents a sarcoidal form of rosacea.

Lichenoid tuberculid. This condition was described by Ockuly and Montgomery [141] in a study based on 15 patients and was thought to represent a hematogenous form of skin tuberculosis. Evidence to support this consisted of (1) the demonstration of "acid-fast bacilli" in one case (guinea pig inoculations were negative); (2) the eruptive onset; (3) the symmetric distribution; and (4) a tuberculoid histologic picture. However, the fact that most cases were tuberculin negative, that, histologically, epithelioid cells predominated, and that only 2 out of 15 cases had evidence of tuberculosis elsewhere in the body make it more probable that the eruptions represented sarcoidal reactions. Only a few additional cases have been described [142,143].

Clinically, there is a generalized eruption with sudden onset, symmetric distribution, and a preferential localization on the extremities. There may be extensive involvement of the entire cutaneous surface. The lesions are papular, of the size of a split pea, and of a brownish to violaceous color. Their surface may be capped by an adherent scale, and telangiectases are present. Grouping and coalescence are prominent, and annular lesions may be formed. Involution results in brownish macules, but there is no residual scarring.

Histopathologically, well-demarcated "tubercles" composed chiefly of epithelioid cells, are found in the superficial and midportions of the dermis. They show a tendency for perivascular arrangement, and central necrosis is quite common.

Therapy of skin tuberculosis

As in the management of tuberculosis of other organs, chemotherapy is the treatment of choice in cutaneous tu-

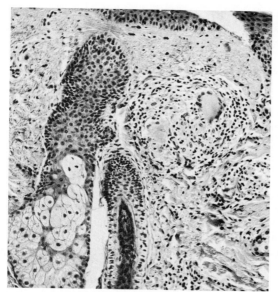

Fig. 179-17 Histopathology of what was formerly termed lupus miliaris disseminatus faciei. A small tuberculoid focus consisting of epithelioid cells, Langhans' giant cells, and peripheral lymphocytes in a perifollicular localization.

berculosis. The skin does, however, pose special problems, and ancillary measures may be required to provide the patient with the best care. The type of cutaneous involvement, the stage of the disease, the level of immunity, and the general condition of the patient are important factors to be considered. Early recognition of the disease and adequate follow-up are essential. Cutaneous tuberculosis associated with mycobacterial disease of internal organs requires a well-coordinated, multidisciplinary plan of therapy. Problems of drug resistance and possible side effects have to be taken into account. General measures, such as adequate nourishment, the control of intercurrent disease, the elimination of possible sources of reinfection, etc., are essential.

Chemotherapy. The aim of chemotherapy for tuberculosis is to cure the disease as rapidly as possible, to prevent the emergence of resistant strains and to reduce the rate of relapses. Chemotherapy should consist of at least two drugs to which *M. tuberculosis* is sensitive; it should be started as early as possible and should be continued at least for 12, preferably for 18 to 24, months. Short-course chemotherapy (6 to 9 months) is being evaluated and has shown promising results [144]. Phase I of chemotherapy is directed toward the rapid destruction of large populations of multiplying mycobacteria and therefore consists of initial, intensive chemotherapy [30]. Phase II is maintenance chemotherapy which aims at the elimination of remaining, "dormant" organisms: it relies on the effect of drugs on the spurts of metabolic activity of "dormant" bacilli which in a nonmetabolizing state are unaffected by chemotherapy [30].

A ranking of drugs currently employed in chemotherapy of tuberculosis—as evaluated by their sterilizing efficacy on tuberculous lesions—leads to the following list: rifampin, pyrazinamide, isoniazid, streptomycin, ethambutol, and thiacetazone [30]. In clinical practice, drug efficacy, side effects, development of resistance and, particularly in

developing countries, cost and patient compliance have to be taken into account when choosing an appropriate antituberculous treatment. First-line drugs which are highly effective and are used mainly in the initial treatment of susceptible organisms are isoniazid, rifampin, streptomycin, and ethambutol. Second-line drugs used mainly in the treatment of patients with drug-resistant mycobacteria are *p*-aminosalicyclic acid, pyrazinamide, ethionamide, viomycin, kanamycin, capreomycin, and cycloserine.

Isoniazid remains the mainstay of antituberculous therapy. It is both tuberculostatic and tuberculocidal in vitro. It penetrates into all body fluids and cells and also into sclerotic tissue so that it proves effective also in old fibrous lesions. The common daily dose of the drug is 5 mg/kg with a maximum of 300 mg. Bacterial resistance of isoniazid usually develops after prolonged treatment and since primary resistance of *M. tuberculosis* occurs (1 in 10^6 tubercle bacilli) it is not surprising that treatment with isoniazid alone will lead to selection of these bacteria [145]. Side effects seen in 5.4 percent of patients treated include fever (1.2 percent), skin eruptions (2 percent), peripheral neuritis (0.2 percent), and hematologic complications (agranulocytosis, eosinophilia, anemia, and thrombocytopenia) [146]. Vasculitis, antinuclear antibodies, and arthritic symptoms may occur and severe hepatic injury has been observed, particularly in older patients. Peripheral neuritis is the most common side effect of isoniazid and may occur in as many as 20 percent of patients receiving 6 mg/kg and no concurrent supportive therapy with pyridoxine. The latter should be given concurrently with isoniazid to forestall such reactions.

Ethambutol, primarily a bacteriostatic drug given in doses of 15 to 25 mg/kg, is always used in combination with other drugs, usually rifampin and isoniazid. It accumulates in patients with impaired renal function, which may necessitate adjustment of dosage. It should not be given to children under 13 years of age [145].

The incidence of side effects is low—these include diminished visual acuity, rashes, and drug fever [146]—and because of this and better patient acceptance, this drug has essentially replaced *p*-aminosalicylic acid in combined antituberculous regimens.

Rifampin, a semisynthetic derivative of an antibiotic produced by *Streptomyces mediterranei,* is one of the most effective drugs for the treatment of tuberculosis. It should not be used alone as mycobacteria rapidly develop resistance as a one-step process [145]. Although it produces a number of side effects, the incidence of these is low, seldom necessitating interruption of treatment [145]. Rifampin rapidly penetrates into tissues and cavities of the body and is rapidly bactericidal in vivo [30]; for sensitive organisms a combination of isoniazid and rifampin is probably as effective as regimens employing three or more drugs [147]. Rifampin is administered as a single oral dose of 600 mg per day and patients should be warned that the drug may impart an orange stain to bodily excretions, including saliva, tears, and sweat.

Streptomycin, a time-honored antibiotic in the treatment of tuberculosis, is bactericidal for *M. tuberculosis* in vitro but its activity in vivo is essentially suppressive [145]. It does not penetrate cell membranes (and can thus not kill intracellular organisms) and has been demonstrated to be more active in an alkaline medium. It is considered to be more effective against bacilli metabolizing in the extracellular fluid [144]. The toxicity of streptomycin prohibits continuous long-term therapy; nearly 75 percent of patients given 2 g of streptomycin daily for 60 to 120 days manifest vestibular disturbances, and impairment of hearing may also occur in an appreciable number of patients [145]. Other side effects include peripheral neuritis, dysfunction of the optic nerve, rashes, fever, exfoliative dermatitis, and blood dyscrasias, but there is less nephrotoxicity than with other aminoglycoside antibiotics [148]. Streptomycin is never used alone in the treatment of tuberculosis and since other drugs have become available its use has been sharply reduced. It is given in doses of 1 to 2 g per day; it is usually combined with two other drugs and is employed in the more serious forms of tuberculosis.

Drug combinations and regimens. In the recent past, clinical research on the treatment of tuberculosis has been directed mainly at identifying the best combination of drugs and the duration of treatment in phase I and phase II chemotherapy. In Western countries the majority of previously untreated tuberculosis is caused by mycobacteria that are sensitive to isoniazid, rifampin, ethambutol, and streptomycin. Since development of resistance to these agents frequently occurs, treatment must consist of at least two drugs to which the bacilli are sensitive. Isoniazid should be included in the regimen and rifampin should be used if isoniazid cannot be given [145]. A combination of rifampin and isoniazid is presently the most effective treatment available, to which a third drug should be added in life-threatening disease. Recommendations of the American Thoracic Society [149] for the treatment of tuberculosis are as follows: (1) isoniazid and ethambutol should be taken for 18 months; (2) large pulmonary cavitation, massive involvement of other organs and tissues, or prevalence of drug resistance in the particular geographic area require the addition of streptomycin; (3) substitution of PAS for ethambutol in children; (4) combination of isoniazid and ethambutol during pregnancy; and (5) use of second-line drugs in the case of drug resistance.

In Europe the combination of rifampin, ethambutol, and isoniazid is the most commonly used regimen in phase I (which will last up to 3 months); this is continued in phase II by a combination of two drugs, usually rifampin and isoniazid [147]. Changes in sensitivity pattern may necessitate a change of drugs used in the regimen which will be continued for at least one year.

In recent years there have been a number of trials employing short-course chemotherapy regimens, particularly in developing countries, because of compliance and economic problems [144,147,150,151]. These indicate that a 6- to 9-month regimen employing rifampin and isoniazid can be sufficient if a third drug (for instance, ethambutol) is added during the initial 2 months of treatment.

Intermittent therapy given twice weekly is also being evaluated. It provides the opportunity for direct administration and thus eliminates the problem of patient compliance and it is economical and reduces drug toxicity. When preceded by 2 months of intensive daily treatment and administered for an additional 16 months, it appears to be as effective as any other regimen [30].

Special considerations in the therapy of tuberculosis of the skin. Essentially, the treatment of tuberculosis of the skin

is that of tuberculosis in general. A full antituberculous regimen is administered even in localized forms of skin tuberculosis where a primary focus or evidence of an underlying organ tuberculosis or tuberculosis of lymph nodes exists. Special considerations may apply to warty tuberculosis and localized forms of lupus vulgaris without evidence of associated internal tuberculosis where isoniazid has been given alone with a high cure rate [152–156]. Prolonged treatment, extending up to 12 months, is necessary also in these forms of lupus vulgaris and total doses of 80 to 140 g may be required. As viable mycobacteria have been cultured from clinically healed lesions [153], treatment should be continued for at least 2 months after complete involution of the lesions [154]. If, however, there is concomitant internal tuberculosis or if drug resistance emerges, combination therapy is mandatory also in localized lupus vulgaris.

Careful observation and follow-up are essential. Surgical intervention is quite important in the treatment of scrofuloderma. It reduces morbidity and shortens the period necessary for chemotherapy. There is no rule as to when surgery should be performed: this has to be decided for each case on an individual basis. Small lesions of lupus vulgaris or tuberculosis verrucosa cutis are also best excised, but tuberculostatics should be given concomitantly. Plastic surgery is important as a corrective measure in long-standing lupus vulgaris with mutilation.

Caustics have lost their value in the treatment of localized lesions, and so has cryotherapy. However, in selected cases, residual lupus nodules within scarred areas may be conveniently destroyed by cryotherapy or electrocautery. Ultraviolet radiation therapy with the Finsen or Kromayer lamp, x-ray treatment, and vitamin D_2 are obsolete.

Other mycobacterial diseases

Historical aspects

Beside the overshadowing problem of infectious disease caused by *M. leprae* or *M. tuberculosis,* probably the largest single cause of infectious disease, the pathogenic potential of other slow-growing mycobacterial species, has been recognized only in the last four decades. The reason for this is in part that these infections usually closely mimic infections with *M. tuberculosis* or, in rare instances, with other organisms, and in part their strict and often unusual culture requirements.

M. ulcerans was identified as the cause of an ulcerating skin condition in Australia in 1948 [157] and in the Buruli district of Uganda (hence the name *Buruli ulcer)* in 1958 [158]. *M. marinum,* which has been known since 1926, was isolated from patients with swimming pool granuloma in 1954 [159]. Several other mycobacteria have since been identified as pathogens and further mycobacterial species may be found to cause disease in the future.

The rapid growers have been known as human pathogens since 1938 when Da Costa isolated an organism from a postinjection skin abscess which he named *M. fortuitum* [160]. It was later found to be identical with the known frog pathogen *M. ranae* [161], which name has since become obsolete [162].

The current classification of these mycobacteria is found in Table 179-1 and is discussed earlier in this chapter.

Table 179-4   Mycobacterial infections

Species	Organ involvement			
	Skin, subcutis	Lymph nodes	Lungs and other organs	Post operative
M. tuberculosis-bovis complex (incl. *M. africanum* and bacillus Calmette-Guérin)	+	+	+	−
M. marinum	+	−	−	−
M. ulcerans	+	−	−	−
M. kansasii	+	+	+	−
M. avium-intracellulare complex (including *M. scrofulaceum*)	+	+	+	
M. szulgai	+	−	+	−
M. simiae	−	−	+	−
M. xenopi	−	−	+	−
M. haemophilum	+	−	−	−
M. fortuitum complex (including *M. chelonei*)	+	−	+	+

Identification of mycobacteria

As in other infectious diseases, the diagnosis of mycobacterial infection depends on the characterization of the microorganism isolated from the host; various biologic fluids, scrapings, or biopsy specimens may be used for culture. Specimens should be sent to a special laboratory familiar with the culture requirements of mycobacteria as these vary somewhat from those of other microorganisms: other incubation temperatures, special media, prolonged times in culture, as well as proper identification procedures are needed. It should be noted that several species of mycobacteria are sensitive to sodium and therefore specimens should not be brought into contact with saline solutions as this may result in false-negative cultures.

Classification of mycobacteria is made on the basis of their rate of growth, pigment production, and enzymatic activities. Antigens for intradermal skin testing (PPDs) of many of the clinically relevant mycobacterial species have been prepared analogously to PPD from *M. tuberculosis* (PPD-S). Although a higher degree of reactivity with a particular PPD seems to correlate with that particular infection [163], cross-reactivities are frequent and, since the reagents are not generally available, many workers in the field feel that the use of these PPDs is limited to epidemiologic and clinical studies [164,165].

Pathology and pathogenesis

These infections tend to occur as sporadic cases, but certain types of exposures may lead to small community outbreaks. As in *M. tuberculosis* infection, any organ or organ system may be affected (Table 179-4) but there seems to be much less tendency to dissemination.

Pulmonary infections, which most frequently occur in patients with a ventilatory defect, e.g., after long-term silica exposure, are pathologically indistinguishable from tuberculosis; however, primary complexes have usually not been identified. Skin and lymph node lesions may be granulomatous, suppurative, or mixed. They can closely mimic tuberculosis, sporotrichosis, or other conditions. Only two organisms, *M. ulcerans* and *M. marinum* cause a disease with a distinct clinical picture.

In contrast to *M. tuberculosis,* atypical mycobacteria are usually not transmitted by person-to-person contact.

They are acquired from environmental sources (water, soil) and their occurrence reflects their natural distribution. These mycobacteria are widely distributed in different environments and usually are commensals or saprophytes rather than pathogens. In most instances it is not known what allows these microorganisms to become pathogenic. However, an immunosuppressed state of the host or damage to a particular organ (e.g., in *M. kansasii* infection of the lung) seems to be required for the development of some types of infection. In recent years, a number of patients have developed infections with fast-growing mycobacteria after minor or major surgical procedures.

Infections with atypical mycobacteria usually run a more benign and limited course than those with *M. tuberculosis*. They are, as a rule, much less responsive to antituberculous drugs, but may be sensitive to other chemotherapeutic agents. However, adequate studies of mycobacterial drug sensitivities are still scarce.

New mycobacterial pathogens are described from time to time, suggesting that we do not yet appreciate the full pathogenic potential of this genus. It seems desirable to develop a unifying concept of mycobacterial disease and its treatment, but at the present time, our knowledge of this area is not advanced enough to allow us to do so. Thus, mycobacterial skin infections are discussed here according to their causative organisms.

Skin infections with atypical mycobacteria

M. marinum

This *Mycobacterium* occurs in fresh and salt water including swimming pools (thus the older name *M. balnei*) and in fish tanks. It has been identified as the causative organism of a granulomatous eruption in swimmers since the early 1950s [159]. Depending on the source of infection, the disease occurs sporadically [166–168] or in small community outbreaks [159,169].

Clinical manifestations. The disease begins as a violaceous papule at the site of a trauma about 2 to 3 weeks after inoculation. Patients may present with an ulcerated plaque or a psoriasiform or verrucous lesion at the site of inoculation, usually the hands, feet, elbows, or knees (Fig. 179-18). As a rule, lesions are solitary but occasionally a

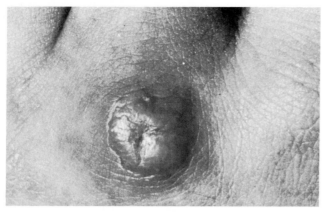

Fig. 179-18 *M. marinum* infection of the hand. Granulomatous nodular lesion with central ulceration at the site of inoculation. *(Courtesy of Dr. A. Kuhlwein.)*

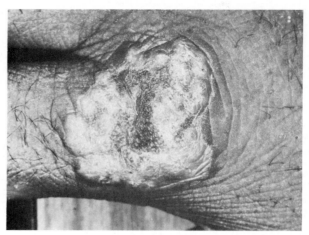

Fig. 179-20 *M. marinum:* residual scarring in granuloma that has undergone spontaneous involution.

centripetal spread reminiscent of sporotrichosis develops [67,169] (Fig. 179-19). These lesions frequently heal spontaneously with residual scarring within 1 to 2 years (Fig. 179-20). Sometimes penetration to underlying structures (bursae, joints) may occur [170] and, in endemic areas, skin lesions resembling those of cutaneous leishmaniasis may develop [171]. Regional lymph nodes are, as a rule, not involved, but in one patient with widespread skin lesions, lymph node involvement has been described. Occasionally the lesions are suppurative rather than granulomatous and may be multiple in normal [172] or immunosuppressed hosts [173].

It has been suggested that many of the cases thought to represent "inoculation lupus vulgaris" as well as "swimmer's lupus" have in fact been due to *M. marinum* infection [174].

Histopathology. There is a granulomatous inflammatory infiltrate in the dermis. Lymphocytes and epithelioid cells predominate and are arranged in tubercles. Infrequently, there may also be Langhans' giant cells and caseation

Fig. 179-19 *M. marinum:* sporotrichosis-like spread proximal to the inoculation site. *(Courtesy of Dr. D. W. Owens.)*

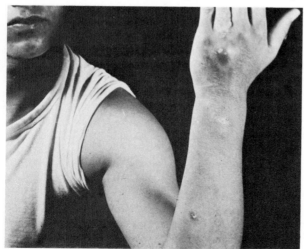

necrosis. Occasionally, the infiltrate also predominantly contains granulocytes, leading to abscess formation [172,173,175,176].

Diagnosis and differential diagnosis. As in all mycobacterial diseases, the diagnosis requires a high index of suspicion. An appropriate history (handling of fish, use of swimming pools) and the presence of a tuberculoid granuloma in the histopathology are suggestive. Proof of the diagnosis can only be obtained by the demonstration of *M. marinum* in culture from a minced biopsy specimen. Skin testing with PPD is generally not found to be helpful. Many other granulomatous infectious processes of the skin have to be considered in the differential diagnosis; depending on the geographical area other mycobacterial infections, blastomycosis, coccidioidomycosis, histoplasmosis, sporotrichosis, as well as nocardiosis, tertiary syphilis, and yaws have to be ruled out. The most frequent differential diagnoses are, however, verruca vulgaris and tuberculosis verrucosa cutis and certain cutaneous neoplasms.

Treatment. Like most atypical mycobacteria, *M. marinum* is poorly susceptible to antituberculous drugs. Therefore, in the past, treatment usually consisted of surgical excision of skin lesions or in destruction by cryosurgery or electrodesiccation with or without adjuvant antituberculous therapy. Recently, tetracycline, minocycline, and TMPS (trimathoprim and sulfamethoxazole) have been reported to be effective [177,178]; as spontaneous healing frequently occurs, this is as yet somewhat difficult to evaluate in the absence of controlled studies. It has been recommended to begin treatment with tetracycline, 2 g per day, or minocycline, 200 mg per day, for 1 to 2 months. If there is no regression of lesions, then rifampin 600 mg and ethambutol 15 mg per kg body weight daily should be given for 18 months [2].

M. ulcerans

This organism was first recognized in Australia in 1948 to cause a specific type of skin ulceration. Later a similar disease was observed in Central Africa, New Guinea, Mexico, and Bolivia. The natural habitat of *M. ulcerans* is still not known, and it has never been found outside the human

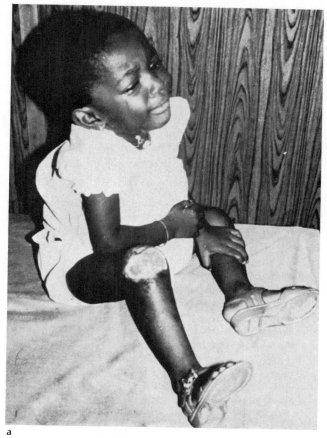

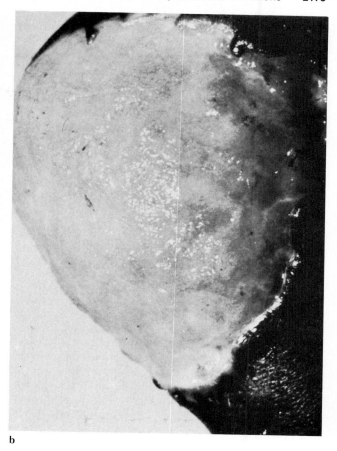

a

b

Fig. 179-21 (a) *M. ulcerans* infection on the knee of a child in Uganda. (b) Detail of lesion shows ulcer with infiltrated undermined margin and a base of necrotic adipose and connective tissue. *(Courtesy of Dr. M. Dietrich.)*

body, but the disease occurs in wet, marshy, or swampy areas [179]. It is possibly introduced into skin by microtrauma, probably by pricks or cuts from certain plants [180]. Person-to-person transmission does not seem to occur.

Clinical manifestations. The disease is found most often in children and young adults; there is a female prevalence. After an incubation period of about three months, a painless subcutaneous swelling develops [181]. The nodule gradually enlarges and eventually ulcerates; a blister may develop before ulceration. The ulcer is deeply undermined and necrotic fat is discharged (Fig. 179-21). The nodule as well as the ulcer is painless and the patient continues to feel well. The lesions may occur anywhere on the body but in adults tend to be limited to the extremities; they may be large, involving a whole limb. The ulceration may persist for months and years and then heal spontaneously. However, this may lead to an appreciable and sometimes disabling amount of scarring and to lymphedema.

No lymphadenopathy nor any constitutional signs appear at any time during the disease process if it is not complicated by bacterial superinfection.

Histopathology. Central necrosis originating in the interlobular septa of the subcutaneous fat is surrounded by gran-

ulation tissue with giant cells but no typical caseation necrosis or tubercles. Acid-fast organisms can always be demonstrated in tissue sections of the lesions.

Diagnosis and differential diagnosis. Diagnosis is made on the basis of histopathology and microbial culture from a subcutaneous node or an ulcer in an individual with a proper history. *M. ulcerans* can be isolated from diseased human tissue; its temperature requirements in culture are quite narrow (32° to 33°C). In culture, *M. ulcerans* produces a toxin which, when injected into the skin of guinea pigs, produces necrosis and ulceration that heals with scar formation after several weeks [182]. Skin testing with mycobacterial antigens is of no diagnostic value. While the lesions progress the patient is always nonreactive to an antigen prepared from *M. ulcerans* [183]. Healing of the lesions is always preceded by reversal of this anergic state. Unfortunately it is not yet known how this reversal is brought about; in fact, reactive and nonreactive areas may be found in the same patient within healing and progressing parts of the ulceration [1].

The differential diagnosis of *M. ulcerans* infection depends on the stage of the disease. The subcutaneous nodule or node must be distinguished from a variety of processes, such as foreign-body granuloma, phycomycosis, nodular fasciitis, panniculitis, nodular vasculitis, sebaceous cysts, or appendageal tumors. When the ulcerative stage is reached, necrotizing cellulitis, blastomycosis, and other deep fungal infections, pyoderma grangrenosum and suppurative panniculitis have to be considered.

Treatment. The treatment of choice is simple excision of the early lesion; when ulceration has developed, wide excision and skin grafting is necessary. Local heat therapy [184], hyperbaric oxygen [185], and chemotherapy with rifampin [186] and TMPS have been shown to be of some value as adjunctive measures. BCG vaccination of exposed populations seems to be of value, providing about the same amount of protection as to tuberculosis and to tuberculoid lepra [187]. Clofazimine has been shown to be ineffective [188].

M. kansasii

By lipid analysis this is the atypical mycobacterium most closely related to *M. tuberculosis* [189]. The organism is usually acquired from the environment; it has been found in tap water and in wild and domestic animals. However, its natural habitat remains obscure but it may have a source in the urban environment. The disease is endemic in Texas, Louisiana, the Chicago area, California, and Japan. Skin disease due to *M. kansasii* usually occurs in adults with or without an underlying condition, such as Hodgkin's disease or immunosuppression for renal transplantation [67,190]. The route of entry usually is through minor trauma such as a puncture wound [67].

Clinical manifestations. Clinically, *M. kansasii* infection may present in several forms: most frequently, a sporotrichoid condition develops [191,192]; sometimes, the subcutaneous tissues and deep structures are affected and this has resulted in a carpal tunnel syndrome [193] or in joint disease [67,194,195]; an ulcerated plaque may also develop as a metastatic lesion [196,197]; disseminated disease due to *M. kansasii* infection occurs in immunosuppressed patients [67,190] and such patients have cellulitis and abscesses rather than granulomatous lesions [197].

The most commonly affected organ is the lung, usually in patients with other pulmonary conditions (silicosis, emphysema) [198,199]. Like *M. tuberculosis, M. kansasii* present in nasopharyngeal secretions can lead to periorificial cutaneous infection [199]. Cervical lymphadenopathy may also be caused by *M. kansasii*.

M. kansasii infections usually progress slowly [200], although a chronic persistent lesion or even spontaneous regression may sometimes occur. Therefore, drug therapy should be initiated as soon as the diagnosis is made.

Histopathology. *M. kansasii* infection is histopathologically indistinguishable from tuberculosis.

Diagnosis and differential diagnosis. The diagnosis can be confirmed only by the demonstration of *M. kansasii* in bacterial culture. Histopathology is not useful in ruling out tuberculosis and skin testing is usually noncontributory. The differential diagnosis includes sporotrichosis, tuberculosis, *M. marinum, M. chelonei,* and other granulomatous infections of the skin.

Treatment. *M. kansasii* is more susceptible to antituberculous drugs than other atypical mycobacteria, particularly to streptomycin, rifampin, and ethambutol. Multiple-drug regimens have been of value, and the in vivo response does not always parallel in vitro sensitivities [2]. As in *M. marinum* infection, treatment with minocycline hydrochloride, 200 mg daily, has resulted in complete resolution of sporotrichoid *M. kansasii* infection in one case [201], but more extensive studies of this regimen are not yet available. In localized skin disease or in cervical lymphadenitis, surgical excision should also be performed.

M. scrofulaceum

This organism is widely distributed and has been isolated from tap water, soil, and other environmental sources. Infection probably occurs in children by accidental infestation or inhalation while playing.

Clinical manifestations. The usual manifestation of *M. scrofulaceum* infection is cervical lymphadenitis in young children, mainly between the ages of 1 and 3 years. Submandibular and submaxillary nodes are usually involved rather than the tonsillar and anterior cervical nodes characteristic for *M. tuberculosis* infection. The disease is frequently unilateral. There are no constitutional symptoms except mild pain in the neck, but nodes enlarging slowly over several weeks and eventually ulcerating and draining are seen. There is no evidence of lung or other organ involvement [202], and only in older individuals with preexisting lung disease pulmonary infection may rarely occur; very rarely, various internal organs may be affected, usually in patients with underlying malignant disease. Usually, however, the disease is benign and self-limited.

Histopathology. *M. scrofulaceum* lymphadenitis is histopathologically indistinguishable from tuberculous disease.

Diagnosis and differential diagnosis. Unilateral cervical lymphadenitis in a young child with a normal chest roentgenogram should make one think of this diagnosis. Skin testing with PPD-S is usually negative. The diagnosis needs confirmation by bacterial culture from a biopsy specimen. Differential diagnoses include all causes of cervical lymphadenitis, both infectious and neoplastic, which have to be ruled out by proper serologic, hematologic, and histopathologic investigations.

Treatment. *M. scrofulaceum* is not very sensitive to antituberculous drugs: the treatment of choice for cutaneous and lymph node disease is surgical excision. For more widespread disease, combinations of antituberculous drugs have to be tried until results from bacterial sensitivity testing are available.

M. avium-intracellulare

This species complex encompasses organisms with a wide variety of microbiologic and pathogenic properties. Well over 20 subtypes can be separated by immunologic techniques [203], although this is not necessary for clinical purposes.

They are usually grouped together with *M. scrofulaceum*

in the so-called MAIS (*M. avium-intracellulare-scrofulaceum*) complex but are separated here for clinical reasons. While *M. scrofulaceum* produces only a benign, self-limited lymphadenopathy with no organ involvement, *M. avium-intracellulare* usually causes lung disease, or less frequently, osteomyelitis. It may also cause a cervical lymphadenitis with sinus formation that is clinically indistinguishable from tuberculous scrofuloderma.

Clinical manifestations. Primary skin disease due to *M. avium-intracellulare* has been reported in rare instances. A chronic, slowly progressive skin condition of many years' duration has been described. In one case multiple lesions consisting of an erythematous border surrounding an ulcer with a yellow crusted base had spread to involve 20 percent of the body surface [204]; *M. intracellulare* was identified in culture. Another patient on steroid therapy developed a painless, scaling, yellow plaque on his right forearm which histopathologically resembled lepromatous leprosy but yielded *M. avium* on culture [205]. A third patient merely had a small ulcer with an erythematous border and a yellow "shaggy" base on the dorsum of his left foot [206]. Sometimes, skin involvement occurs secondary to disseminated infection with *M. avium-intracellulare* [5]. Skin lesions have included generalized cutaneous ulcerations, multiple cutaneous granulomas, infiltrated erythematous lesions on the extremities, pustular lesions, or soft-tissue swelling. Generalized lymphadenitis due to *M. avium-intracellulare* has developed in patients with the acquired immunodeficiency syndrome [207].

Histopathology. This shows noncaseating granulomas with epithelioid and giant cells; acid-fast bacilli can be found within giant cells and extracellularly.

Diagnosis and differential diagnosis. Demonstration of *M. avium-intracellulare* in bacterial culture is necessary to establish the diagnosis. The differential diagnosis includes all chronic granulomatous conditions of the skin.

Treatment. Where feasible, surgical treatment of *M. avium-intracellulare* infection is advisable as the organism seems to be poorly susceptible to chemotherapeutic agents. If dissemination of the disease does not allow curative surgery, combination therapy with multiple antituberculous drugs should be tried. In a recent report [208], a synergistic effect of several antituberculous drug combinations against *M. intracellulare* in vitro has been shown.

M. szulgai

The development of cervical lymphadenitis as well as cellulitis or draining nodules and plaques has been associated with *M. szulgai* [209]. The organism has also been found to cause bursitis and pneumonia; it is more susceptible to antituberculous drugs than are other atypical mycobacteria.

M. haemophilum

This is an organism requiring media supplemented with hemin or ferric ammonium citrate in culture [210]. Not much is yet known about its natural habitat. It was iden-

tified as the causative organism of a subcutaneous granulomatous eruption in several immunosuppressed patients in Sydney, Australia [211,212]. Histopathologically, there was a mixed polymorphonuclear and granulomatous inflammation, the so-called dimorphic inflammatory response, with no caseation necrosis, similar to that seen in *M. fortuitum* complex infection.

The organism may be sensitive to rifampin and *p*-aminosalicylic acid, but further observations of such infections are required.

M. fortuitum complex

This is the only species of rapid-growing mycobacteria that has so far been found to cause human disease. The species complex includes *M. chelonei*, which is the more common pathogen, and *M. fortuitum*. *M. chelonei* can be divided into two subspecies, *M. chelonei chelonei*, found predominantly in Europe, and *M. chelonei abscessus*, the more common variant in Africa and the United States. *M. fortuitum* occurs in the three biotypes, A, B, and C, of which A is the most important pathogen. These organisms seem to be widely distributed and can commonly be found in soil and in water supplies. Contamination of various material including surgical supplies occurs and does not always result in clinical disease [213].

Clinical manifestations. Infection usually follows a puncture wound or a surgical procedure. In a recent large series it was found that cutaneous disease accounted for 59 percent of 125 cases; of these, 54 percent were due to surgery and 46 percent to accidental inoculation [214]. When the skin and subcutaneous tissues are affected, the disease manifests itself as a painful, red, infiltrated area at the site of inoculation; there are no signs of dissemination and no constitutional symptoms. This type of infection has followed augmentation mammoplasty [215], median sternotomy [216,217], and a variety of other procedures usually involving percutaneous catheterization. Cold postinjection abscesses, especially when occurring in the tropics, may also be due to fast-growing mycobacteria. The source usually seems to be found in contaminated injection solutions. It has been suggested that so-called fixation abscesses, found in tuberculosis patients after intramuscular injections, have frequently also been due to inoculation *M. fortuitum* complex organisms [218].

Primary cutaneous inoculation through skin injuries is found in all age groups and without immunosuppression. The lesion presents as a dark red, infiltrated node, often with abscess formation and draining a clear liquid. Disseminated disease involving the skin also occurs, usually in immunologically compromised patients. The skin lesions consist of multiple recurrent episodes of abscesses on the extremities or as a generalized macular and papular eruption. Other manifestations of *M. fortuitum* complex infection include pneumonitis or osteomyelitis, lymphadenitis, and postsurgical endocarditis.

Histopathology. The lesions are characterized by the simultaneous occurrence of polymorphonuclear microabscesses and granuloma formation with foreign body-type giant cells, the so-called dimorphic inflammatory response.

There usually is necrosis but no caseation. Acid-fast bacilli may occasionally be demonstrated within microabscesses.

Diagnosis and treatment. Organisms of the *M. fortuitum* complex including *M. fortuitum* and *M. chelonei* with their subspecies may be identified by special laboratories. This is of more than epidemiologic interest as *M. fortuitum* is more susceptible to amicacin, doxycycline, and sufonamides than is *M. chelonei,* while subspecies of the latter have markedly different susceptibilities to cefoxitin, erythromycin, and tobramycin. Thus, a rational treatment has to await the results of identification of the organism and in vitro susceptibility testing.

References

1. Grange JM: Mycobacteria and the skin. *Int J Dermatol* **21**:497, 1982
2. Yaeger H Jr: Other mycobacterium species, in *Principles and Practice of Infectious Diseases,* edited by GL Mandell et al. Chichester, John Wiley & Sons, 1979, p 1953
3. Wolinsky E: Nontuberculous mycobacteria and associated disease. *Am Rev Respir Dis* **119**:107, 1979
4. Youmans GP: Relation between delayed hypersensitivity and immunity in tuberculosis. *Am Rev Respir Dis* **111**:109, 1975
5. Rook GAW, Stanford JL: The relevance to protection of three forms of delayed skin-test response evoked by *M. leprae* and other mycobacteria in mice. Correlation with the classical work in the guinea pig. *Parasite Immunol* **1**:111, 1979
6. Kardjito T, Grange JM: Immunological and clinical features of smear-positive pulmonary tuberculosis in East Java. *Tubercle* **61**:231, 1980
7. Runyon EH: Pathogenic mycobacteria. *Adv Tuberc Res* **14**:235, 1965
8. Runyon EH: Ten mycobacterial pathogens. *Tubercle* **55**:235, 1974
9. American Lung Association: *Diagnositc Standards and Classification of Tuberculosis and other Mycobacterial Diseases.* New York, American Lung Association/American Thoracic Society, 1974
10. Approved lists of bacterial names: Mycobacteria. *Int J System Bacteriol* **30**:324, 1980
11. Koch R: Die Ätiologie der Tuberculose. *Klin Wochenschr* **19**:221, 1882
12. Moschella SL: Mycobacterial infections of the skin, in *Dermatology Update, Reviews for Physicians,* edited by SL Moschella. New York, Elsevier, 1979, p 45
13. Pandhi RK et al: Cutaneous tuberculosis—a clinical and investigative study. *Indian J Dermatol* **22**:99, 1977
14. Sharma RC et al: Microbiology of cutaneous tuberculosis. *Tubercle* **56**:324, 1975
15. Wong KO et al: Tuberculosis of the skin in Hong Kong. (A review of 160 cases). *Br J Dermatol* **80**:424, 1968
16. Jung HD, Holzegel K: Klinik der Hauttuberkulose heute. *Dtsch Dermatol* **30**:365, 1982
17. Morrison JGL, Fourie ED: The papulonecrotic tuberculide. From Arthus reaction to lupus vulgaris. *Br J Dermatol* **91**:263, 1974
18. Spitzer R: Geographische Verteilung der Hautkrankheiten, in *Handbuch der Haut- und Geschlechtskrankheiten,* Ergänzungswerk, vol VIII, edited by J Jadassohn. Berlin, Springer-Verlag, 1967, p 1
19. Jensen KA, Frimodt-Möller J: Studies on the types of tubercle bacilli isolated from man. II. Strains with attenuated virulence. *Acta Tuberc Scand* **10**:83, 1936
20. Youmans GP: Natural resistance to tuberculous infection, in *Tuberculosis,* edited by GP Youmans, Philadelphia, WB Saunders, 1979, p 202
21. Simonds B: *Tuberculosis in Twins.* London, Pitman, 1963
22. Rich AR: *The Pathogenesis of Tuberculosis,* 2d ed. Springfield, IL, Charles C Thomas, 1951
23. Koch R: Weitere Mitteiling über das Tuberculin. *Dtsch Med Wochenschr* **17**:1189, 1891
24. Pirquet C von: Allergie. *Munch Med Wochenschr* **53**:1457, 1906
25. Arnason BG, Waksman BH: Tuberculin sensitivity: immunologic considerations. *Adv Tuberc Res* **13**:1, 1964
26. Turk JL: *Frontiers of Biology,* vol IV, *Delayed Hypersensitivity,* North-Holland Research Monographs, edited by A Neuberger, EL Tatum. Amsterdam, North-Holland, 1967
27. Urbach F et al: Passive transfer of tuberculin sensitivity to patients with sarcoidosis. *N Engl J Med* **247**:794, 1952
28. Good RA et al: Immunological deficiency diseases. Agammaglobulinemia, hypogammaglobulinemia, Hodgkin's disease, and sarcoidosis. *Prog Allergy* **6**:187, 1962
29. Seibert FB: Progress in the chemistry of tuberculin. *Adv Tuberc Res* **3**:1, 1950
30. Sbarraro JA: Tuberculosis. *Med Clin North Am* **64**:417, 1980
31. Edwards LB, Palmer CE: Epidemiological studies of tuberculin sensitivity. I. Preliminary results with purified derivatives prepared from atypical acid-fast organisms. *Am J Hyg* **68**:213, 1958
32. Stanford JL, Grange JM: The nature and structure of species as applied to mycobacteria. *Tubercle* **55**:143, 1974
33. Stanford JL, Rook GAW: Environmental mycobacteria and immunization with BCG, in *Medical Microbiology,* vol 2, edited by CS Easmon, J Jeljaszewicz. London/New York, Academic Press, 1983, p 43
34. Editorial: New tuberculosis. *Lancet* **1**:199, 1984
35. Dienes L, Mallory TB: Histological studies of hypersensitive reactions. I. The contrast between the histological responses in the tuberculin (allergic) type and the anaphylactic type of skin reactions. *Am J Pathol* **8**:689, 1932
36. Laporte R: Contribution à l'étude des bacilles paratuberculeux. II. Histo-cytologie des lésions paratuberculeuses. *Ann Inst Pasteur (Paris)* **65**:415, 1940
37. Gell PGH, Hinde IT: The histology of the tuberculin reaction and its modification by cortisone. *Br J Exp Pathol* **32**:516, 1951
38. Raffel S: The mechanism involved in acquired immunity to tuberculosis, in *Symposium on Experimental Tuberculosis: Bacillus and Host,* Ciba Foundation Symposium, edited by GEW Wolstenholme, MP Cameron. London, Churchill, 1955, p 261
39. Ghon A, Kudlich H: Die Eintrittspforten der Infektion vom Standpunkte der pathologischen Anatomie, in *Handbuch der Kindertuberkulose,* edited by S Engel, CV Pirquet. Leipzig, Georg Thieme Verlag, 1930, p 20
40. Miller FJW: Recognition of primary tuberculous infection of skin and mucosae. *Lancet* **1**:5, 1953
41. Fischer I, Orkin M: Primary tuberculosis of the skin. Primary complex. *JAMA* **195**:314, 1966
42. O'Leary PA, Harrison MW: Inoculation tuberculosis. *Arch Dermatol Syphilol* **44**:371, 1941
43. Holt LE: Tuberculosis acquired through ritual circumcision. *JAMA* **61**:99, 1913
44. Rytel MW et al: Primary cutaneous inoculation tuberculosis. *Am Rev Respir Dis* **102**:264, 1970
45. Sahn SA, Pierson DJ: Primary cutaneous inoculation drug-resistant tuberculosis. *Am J Med* **57**:676, 1974
46. Goette DK et al: Primary inoculation tuberculosis of the skin. Prosector's paronychia. *Arch Dermatol* **114**:567, 1978
47. Heilman KM, Muschenheim C: Primary cutaneous tuberculosis resulting from mouth to mouth respirations. *N Engl J Med* **273**:1035, 1965

48. Koch H: Die Tuberculose des Säuglingsalters. *Ergeb Inn Med Kinderheilk* **14**:99, 1915

49. Wolff E: Über Zirkumzisiontuberkulose. *Klin Wochenschr* **58**:1531, 1921

50. Strad S: Tubercular primary lesion on penis—cancer penis. Venereal tuberculosis. *Acta Derm Venereol (Stockh)* **26**:461, 1946

51. Bjørnstadt R: Tuberculosis primary infection of genitalia. *Acta Derm Venereol (Stockh)* **27**:106, 1947

52. Michelson HE: The primary complex of tuberculosis of the skin. *Arch Dermatol Syphilol* **32**:589, 1935

53. Heykock JB, Noble TC: Four cases of syringe transmitted tuberculosis. *Tubercle* **42**:25, 1961

54. Valledor T et al: Tuberculosis primaria de la piel en la infancia. *Rev Cutan Pediatria* **26**:147, 1954

55. Miller FJW, Cashman JM: The natural history of peripheral tuberculosis lymphadenitis associated with a visible primary focus. *Lancet* **1**:1286, 1955

56. Duken J: Über Verlaufsarten der extrapulmonalen Primärtuberkulose. *Z Kinderheilk* **55**:687, 1933

57. Mitchell PC: Tuberculosis verrucosa cutis among Chinese in Hong Kong. *Br J Dermatol* **66**:444, 1954

58. Montgomery H: Histopathology of various types of cutaneous tuberculosis. *Arch Dermatol Syphilol* **35**:698, 1937

59. Getzler NA et al: Atypical cutaneous tuberculosis. *Arch Dermatol* **84**:439, 1961

60. Horwitz O: Lupus vulgaris cutis in Denmark 1895–1954. Its relation to the epidemiology of other forms of tuberculosis. *Acta Tuberc Scand [Suppl]* **49**:1, 1960

61. Kalkoff KW: *Die Tuberkulose der Haut.* Stuttgart, Georg Thieme Verlag, 1950

62. Proppe A, Wagner G: Die Altersdisposition bei Lupus vulgaris. *Z Hautkr Geschlechtskr* **14**:376, 1953

63. Marcussen PV: Lupus vulgaris following BCG vaccination. *Br J Dermatol* **66**:121, 1954

64. Horwitz O: The localization of lupus vulgaris of the skin. *Acta Tuberc Scand [Suppl]* **47**:175, 1959

65. Ustvedt HJ, Ostensen IW: The relation between tuberculosis of the skin and primary infection. *Tubercle* **32**:36, 1951

66. Brown FS et al: Cutaneous tuberculosis. *J Am Acad Dermatol* **6**:101, 1982

67. Beyt BE et al: Cutaneous mycobacteriosis: analysis of 34 cases with a new classification of the disease. *Medicine (Baltimore)* **60**:95, 1980

68. Sundt H: A case of lupus disseminatus (postexanthematic miliary tuberculosis cutis). *Br J Dermatol* **37**:316, 1925

69. Horwitz O, Christensen S: Numerical estimates of the extent of the lesion in lupus vulgaris cutis and their significance for epidemiologic and clinical research. *Am Rev Respir Dis* **82**:862, 1960

70. Volk R: Tuberculose der Haut, in *Handbuch der Haut- und Geschlechtskrankheiten,* vol X/1, edited by J Jadassohn. Berlin, Springer, 1931, p 1

71. Hekele K, Seyss R: Die malignen Tumoren in Lupo vulgari. *Hautarzt* **2**:349, 1951

72. Clasen K, Horwitz O: The morbidity from pulmonary tuberculosis in patients suffering from extrapulmonary tuberculosis disease, lupus vulgaris cutis. *Adv Tuberc Res* **10**:237, 1960

73. Kutschera-Aichbergen H: Die Bekämpfung schwerer Lungentuberculose durch künstlich erzeugte Hauttuberculose. *Wien Klin Wochenschr* **50**:1544, 1937

74. Kalkoff KW: Die Lungentuberkulosesterblichkeit bei Lupuskranken im Vergleich zu Hautgesunden. Gleichzeitig ein Beitrag zum Altersaufbau und zum Durchschnittslebensalter der westfälishcen Lupuskranken. *Arch Dermatol Syphilogr* **186**:144, 1948

75. Amezquita R: Tuberculosis cutanea. Aspectos clinicos y epidémiológicos en Mexico. *Acta Leprologica* **16**:1, 1963

76. Editorial: Scrofula today. *Lancet* **1**:335, 1983

77. Chien JTT, Wiggins, ML: Self-inoculation with *M. tuberculosis* and *P. aeruginosa* by a diabetic woman. *Am Rev Tuberc* **69**:818, 1954

78. Michelson HE: Scrofuloderma gummosa (tuberculosis colliquativa). *Arch Dermatol Syphilol* **10**:565, 1924

79. Kleid JJ, Rosenberg RF: Pulmonary tuberculosis with noncommunicating chest wall abscess. *NY State J Med* **70**:2993, 1970

80. Munt PW: Miliary tuberculosis in the chemotherapy era: with a clinical review of 69 American adults. *Medicine (Baltimore)* **51**:139, 1971

81. Stead WW, Bates JH: Evidence of a "silent" bacillemia in primary tuberculosis. *Ann Intern Med* **74**:559, 1971

82. Glynn KP: Isolated subcutaneous abscesses caused by *Mycobacterium tuberculosis. Am Rev Respir Dis* **99**:86, 1969

83. Bryant JC: Oral tuberculosis. *Am Rev Tuberc* **39**:738, 1939

84. Sheingold MA, Sheingold H: Oral tuberculosis. *Oral Surg* **4**:239, 1951

85. Katz HL: Tuberculosis of the tongue. *Q Bull Seaview Hosp* **6**:239, 1941

86. Engleman WR, Putney FJ: Tuberculosis of the tongue. *Trans Am Acad Ophthalmol Otolaryngol* **76**:1384, 1972

87. Mc Andrew PG et al: Miliary tuberculosis presenting with multifocal oral lesions. *Br Med J* **1**:1320, 1976

88. Weaver RA: Tuberculosis of the tongue. *JAMA* **235**:2418, 1978

89. Fisher JR: Miliary tuberculosis with unusual cutaneous manifestation. *JAMA* **238**:241, 1977

90. Platou RV, Lennox RH: Tuberculous cutaneous complexes in children. *Am Rev Tuberc* **74**(2, part 11):160, 1956

91. McCray MK, Esterly NB: Cutaneous eruptions in congenital tuberculosis. *Arch Dermatol* **117**:460, 1981

92. Schermer DR et al: Tuberculosis cutis miliaris acuta generalisata. *Arch Dermatol* **99**:64, 1969

93. Leiner C, Spieler F: Über disseminierte Hauttuberulosen im Kindesalter. *Ergeb Inn Med Kinderheilkd* **7**:59, 1911

94. Lees AW, Munro ID: Skin lesions and deafness in disseminated tuberculosis. *Br Med J* **I**:496, 1954

95. Kurnedy C, Knowles GK: Miliary tuberculosis presenting with skin lesions. *Br Med J* **III**:356, 1975

96. Rouillon A, Waaler H: BCG vaccination and epidemiological situation. A decision making approach to the use of BCG. *Adv Tuberc Res* **19**:65, 1976

97. Ten Dam HG, Hitze KL: Does BCG vaccination protect the newborn and young infant? *Bull WHO* **58**:37, 1980

98. Anonymous: BCG vaccination in the newborn. *Br Med J* **281**:1445, 1980

99. Tuberculosis Prevention Trial. Trial of BCG vaccines in South India for tuberculosis prevention: first report. *Bull WHO* **57**:819, 1979

100. Curtis HM et al: Incidence of childhood tuberculosis after neonatal BCG vaccination. *Lancet* **1**:145, 1984

101. Dostrovsky A, Sagher F: Dermatological complications of BCG vaccination. *Br J Dermatol* **75**:181, 1963

102. Jörgensen BB, Horwitz O: Dermatological complications of BCG vaccination. *Acta Tuberc Scand* **32**:179, 1956

103. Horwitz O, Meyer J: The safety record of BCG vaccination and untoward reactions observed after vaccination. *Adv Tuberc Res* **8**:245, 1957

104. Waaler H, Rouillon A: BCG vaccination policies according to the epidemiological situation. *Bull Int Union Tuberc* **29**:166, 1974

105. Izumi AK, Matsunaga J: BCG vaccine-induced lupus vulgaris. *Arch Dermatol* **118**:171, 1982

106. Maguire A: Lupus murinus. The discovery, diagnosis and treatment of seventeen cases of lupus murinus. *Br J Dermatol* **80**:419, 1968

107. Aungst CW et al: Complications of BCG vaccination in neoplastic disease. *Ann Intern Med* **82**:666, 1975

108. Passwell J et al: Fatal disseminated BCG infection. An investigation of the immunodeficiency. *Am J Dis Child* **130**:433, 1976

109. Rosenthal SR: *BCG Vaccine: Tuberculosis-Cancer.* Dayton, OH, PSG Publishing Co, 1980

110. Darier MJ: Les "tuberculides" cutanées. *Ann Dermatol Syphiligr (Paris)* **7**:1431, 1896

111. Smith NP et al: Lichen scrofulosorum. A report of four cases. *Br J Dermatol* **94**:319, 1976

112. Graham Brown RAC, Sarkany I: Lichen scrofulosorum with tuberculous dactylitis. *Br J Dermatol* **103**:561, 1980

113. Philippson L. Über Phlebitis nodularis necrotisans. *Arch Dermatol Syphilogr* **55**:215, 1901

114. Whitfield A: A case of unusual papulonecrotic tuberculide. *Br J Dermatol* **25**:168, 1913

115. Tanimura C: Über papulonekrotische Tuberkulide und über den positiven Befund von Tuberkelbacillen. *Arch Dermatol Syphilogr* **146**:335, 1924

116. Dittrich O: Über den Tuberkelbazillennachweis bei Tuberkuliden. *Dermatol Wochenschr* **84**:734, 1927

117. Montgomery H et al: Nodular vascular diseases of the legs. *JAMA* **128**:335, 1945

118. Eberhartinger C: Das Problem des Erythema induratum Bazin. Ein Beitrag zur Kenntnis der rezidivierenden subakuten nodösen Gefäßprozesse am Unterschenkel. *Arch Klin Exp Dermatol* **217**:196, 1963

119. Miescher G: Über katamnestische Untersuchungen bei Fällen mit Tuberkulid. *Dermatologica* **110**:23, 1955

120. Flegel H: Die Stellung des Tuberculids im Rahmen der Tuberkulose. *Dermatol Wochenschr* **145**:609, 1962

121. Strauss H: Katamnestische Untersuchungen von Fällen mit Tuberkulid. *Arch Dermatol Syphilogr* **198**:417, 1954

122. Sonck CE: Focal infections and tuberculids. *Acta Derm Venereol (Stockh)* **2**:195, 1960

123. Iden DL et al: Papulonecrotic tuberculid secondary to *Mycobacterium bovis.* *Arch Dermatol* **114**:564, 1978

124. Formia FE et al: Isoniazid (nydrazid) in the treatment of cutaneous diseases: cutaneous tuberculosis, leprosy, sarcoidosis and miscellaneous dermatoses. *Arch Dermatol Syphilol* **68**:536, 1953

125. Rauschkolb JW: Tuberculosis of the skin. *Arch Dermatol Syphilol* **29**:398, 1934

126. Leiner C, Spieler F: Zum Nachweis der bazillären Ätiologie der Folliklis. *Arch Dermatol Syphilogr* **81**:221, 1906

127. Hempelmann TC: Frequency of tuberculides in infancy and childhood and their relation to prognosis. *Arch Pediatr* **34**:362, 1917

128. Irgang S: Superficial papulonecrotic tuberculid in the Negro. *Arch Dermatol Syphilol* **47**:627, 1943

129. Hellerström S: Papulo-nekrotische Tuberkulide mit Lokalisation an der Glans Penis. *Acta Derm Venereol (Stockh)* **23**:170, 1942

130. Stevanovic DV: Papulonecrotic tuberculids of glans penis. *Arch Dermatol* **78**:760, 1958

131. Szymanski JF: Pityriasis lichenoides et varioliformis acuta: histopathological evidence that it is an entity distinct from parapsoriasis. *Arch Dermatol* **79**:7, 1959

132. Montgomery H: *Dermatopathology.* New York, Harper & Row, 1967

133. Wilkinson DS: The vascular basis of some nodular eruptions of the legs. *Br J Dermatol* **66**:201, 1954

134. Parish WE: Microbial antigens in vasculitis, in *Vasculitis,* edited by K Wolff, RK Winkelmann. London, Lloyd and Luke Ltd, 1980, p 129

135. Michelson HE: Inflammatory nodose lesions of the lower leg. *Arch Dermatol Syphilol* **66**:327, 1952

136. Laymon CW, Michelson HE: The micropapular tuberculid. *Arch Dermatol Syphilol* **42**:625, 1940

137. Bologa EI: Betrachungen zur Nosologie, Pathogenese und Erkennung der rosacea-ähnlichen Tuberculide von Lewandowsky sowie deren Beziehungen zur Rosacea. *Hautarzt* **12**:508, 1961

138. Peck SM: Beitrag zur Lehre vom Lupus miliaris disseminatus faciei. *Arch Dermatol Syphilogr* **158**:545, 1929

139. Simon N: Ist der Lupus miliaris disseminatus tuberkulöser Ätiologie? *Hautarzt* **26**:625, 1975

140. Lewandowsky F: Über rosacea-ähnliche Tuberkulide des Gesichtes. *Korrespondenz-Blatt für Schweizer Ärzte* **47**:1280, 1917

141. Ockuly OE, Montgomery H: Lichenoid tuberculid. A clinical and histopathologic study. *J Invest Dermatol* **14**:415, 1950

142. Kowalenko W: Über ein lichenoides Exanthem unklarer Pathogenese. (Zur Kenntnis des "Lichenoid Tuberculid" von Montgomery). *Dermatol Wochenschr* **147**:13, 1963

143. Schuhmachers R: 2 Fälle eines lichenoiden Tuberculids (= Lichen scrophulosorum). *Hautarzt* **18**:81, 1967

144. Fox W, Mitchinson DA: Short course chemotherapy for pulmonary tuberculosis. *Am Rev Respir Dis* **111**:845, 1975

145. Mandell GL, Sande MA: Antimicrobial agents. Drugs used in the chemotherapy of tuberculosis and leprosy, in *The Pharmacological Basis of Therapeutics,* 6th ed, edited by A Goodman et al. New York, MacMillan, 1980, p 1200

146. Pitt FW: Tuberculosis prevention and therapy, in *Current Concepts of Infectious Diseases,* edited by EW Hook et al. New York, John Wiley & Sons, 1977, p 181

147. British Thoracic and Tuberculosis Association: Short-course chemotherapy in pulmonary tuberculosis. *Lancet* **1**:119, 1975

148. Sande MA, Mandell GL: Antimicrobial agents. The aminoglycosides, in *The Pharmacological Basis of Therapeutics,* 6th ed, edited by A Goodman et al. New York, MacMillan 1980, p 1162

149. American Thoracic Society: Treatment of mycobacterial disease. *Am Rev Respir Dis* **115**:185, 1977

150. East African/British Medical Research Councils: Controlled clinical trial of four short-course (6 months) regimens of chemotherapy for treatment of pulmonary tuberculosis. *Lancet* **2**:237, 1974

151. East African/British Medical Research Councils: Controlled clinical trial of four short-course (6 months) regimens of chemotherapy for treatment of pulmonary tuberculosis. *Lancet* **2**:1100, 1974

152. Hentschel V: Vorschläge für eine Standardtherapie der Haut-tuberkulose. *Dermatol Monatsschr* **160**:1009, 1974

153. Meyer-Rohn J, Schulz KH: Experimentelle und klinishe Erfahrungen bei der Isonicotinsäurehydrazid-Therapie der Hauttuberkulose. *Arch Dermatol Syphilogr* **197**:160, 1954

154. Krakauer R: Die Behandlung der Hauttuberkulose mit INH (Rimifon) in den Jahren 1952–1959 an der Züricher Dermatologischen Klinik. *Dermatologica* **120**:323, 1960

155. Brück D, Westbeck-Carlsson AM: Treatment of lupus vulgaris with INH exclusively. *Acta Derm Venerol (Stockh)* **44**:223, 1964

156. Ehring F: Die gegenwärtige Epidemiologie und Bakteriologie der Hauttuberkulose in der Bundesrepublik Deutschland, in *Proceedings of the 13th International Congress of Dermatology,* vol II, edited by W Jadassohn, CG Schirren. New York, Springer-Verlag, 1968, p 1308

157. MacCullum P et al: New mycobacterial infection in man: clinical aspects. *J Pathol Bacteriol* **60**:93, 1948

158. Clancey JK et al: Mycobacterial skin ulcers in Uganda. *Lancet* **2**:951, 1961

159. Linell F, Norden A: *Macrobacterium balnei.* A new acid-fast bacillus occurring in swimming pools and capable of producing skin lesions in humans. *Acta Tuberc Scand [Suppl]* **33**:1, 1954

160. Da Costa Cruz J: "*Mycobacterium fortuitum*," un novo bacilo acido resistente patogenico par o homem. *Acta Medica Rio de Janeiro* **1**:297, 1938

161. Kuster E: Über Kaltblütertuberkulose. *Munch Med Wochenschr* **52**:57, 1905

162. Runyon EH: Conservation of the specific epithet fortuitum in the name of the organism known as *Mycobacterium fortuitum* da Costa Cruz. *Int J System Bacteriol* **22**:50, 1972

163. Marmorstein BL, Scheinhorn DJ: The role of nontuberculous mycobacterial skin test antigens in the diagnosis of mycobacterial infections. *Chest* **67**:320, 1975

164. Fogan L: Atypical mycobacteria: their clinical, laboratory, and epidemiologic significance. *Medicine (Baltimore)* **49**:243, 1970

165. Hsu KHK: Diagnostic skin test for mycobacterial infections in man. *Chest* **64**:1, 1973

166. Brown J et al: Infection of the skin by *Mycobacterium marinum:* report of five cases. *Can Med Assoc J* **117**:912, 1977

167. Heineman HS et al: Fish tank granuloma: a hobby hazard. *Arch Intern Med* **130**:121, 1972

168. Jänner M et al: Infektion mit *Mycobacterium marinum* aus einem Aquarium. *Hautarzt* **34**:635, 1983

169. Philpott JA et al: Swimming pool granuloma. *Arch Dermatol* **88**:158, 1963

170. Jolly HW Jr, Seabury JK: Infections with *Mycobacterium marinum*. *Arch Dermatol* **106**:32, 1972

171. Even-Paz Z et al: *Mycobacterium marinum* skin infections mimicking cutaneous leishmaniasis. *Br J Dermatol* **94**:435, 1976

172. King AJ et al: Disseminated cutaneous *Mycobacterium marinum* infection. *Arch Dermatol* **119**:268, 1983

173. Gombert ME et al: Disseminated *Mycobacterium marinum* infection after renal transplantation. *Ann Intern Med* **94**:486, 1981

174. Hellerström S: Collected cases of inoculation lupus vulgaris. *Acta Derm Venereol (Stockh)* **31**:194, 1951

175. Schaefer WB, Bavis CL: A bacteriologic and histopathologic study of skin granulomas due to *Mycobacterium balnei*. *Am Rev Respir Dis* **84**:837, 1961

176. Marsch WC et al: The ultrastructure of *Mycobacterium marinum* granuloma in man. *Arch Dermatol Res* **262**:205, 1978

177. Wolinsky E et al: Sporotrichoid *M. marinum* infection treated with rifampin-ethambutol. *Am Rev Respir Dis* **105**:964, 1972

178. Izumi AK et al: *M. marinum* infections treated with tetracycline. *Arch Dermatol* **113**:1067, 1977

179. Barker DJ: Epidemiology of *Mycobacterium ulcerans* infection. *Trans R Soc Trop Med Hyg* **67**:43, 1972

180. Feldman RA: Primary mycobacterial skin infection: a summary. *Int J Dermatol* **13**:353, 1974

181. Uganda Buruli Group: Clinical features and treatment of pre-ulcerative Buruli lesions (*Mycobacterium ulcerans* infection) *Br Med J* **2**:390, 1970

182. Krieg RE et al: Toxin of *Mycobacterium ulcerans*. Production and effects in guinea pig skin. *Arch Dermatol* **110**:783, 1974

183. Stanford JL et al: The production and preliminary investigation of Burulin, a new skin test reagent for *Mycobacterium ulcerans* infection. *J Hyg (Camb)* **74**:7, 1975

184. Meyers WM et al: Heat treatment of *Mycobacterium ulcerans* infections without surgical excision. *Am J Trop Med Hyg* **23**:924, 1974

185. Krieg RE et al: Treatment of *Mycobacterium ulcerans* infection by hyperbaric oxygenation. *Aviat Space Environ Med* **46**:1241, 1975

186. Stanford, JL, Philipps I: Rifampicin in experimental *Mycobacterium ulcerans* infection. *J Med Microbiol* **5**:39, 1972

187. Uganda Buruli Group: BCG vaccination against *Mycobacterium ulcerans* infection (Buruli ulcer). *Lancet* **1**:111, 1969

188. Revill WD et al: A controlled trial of the treatment of *Mycobacterium ulcerans* infection with clofazimine. *Lancet* **2**:873, 1973

189. Chapman JS: *The Atypical Mycobacteria and Human Mycobacteriosis*. New York, Plenum Press, 1977

190. Hagmar B et al: Disseminated infection caused by *M kansasii*. Report of a case and brief review of the literature. *Acta Med Scand* **186**:93, 1969

191. Duncan WC: Cutaneous mycobacterial infections. *Tex Med* **64**:66, 1968

192. Owens DW, McBride ME: Sporotrichoid cutaneous infection with *Mycobacterium kansasii*. *Arch Dermatol* **100**:54, 1969

193. Kaplan H, Clayton M: Carpal tunnel syndrome secondary to *M. kansasii* infection. *JAMA* **208**:1186, 1969

194. Owen DS, Toone E: Soft tissue infection by group I atypical mycobacteria. *South Med J* **63**:116, 1970

195. Gunther SF, Elliot RC: *Mycobacterium kansasii* infection in the deep structures of the hand. *J Bone Joint Surg* **58A**:140, 1976

196. Hirsh FS, Saffold OE: *Mycobacterium kansasii* infection with dermatologic manifestations. *Arch Dermatol* **112**:706, 1976

197. Fraser DW et al: Disseminated *Mycobacterium kansasii* infection presenting as cellulitis in a recipient of a renal homograph. *Am Rev Respir Dis* **112**:125, 1975

198. Bailey WC et al: Silico-mycobacterial disease in sandblasters. *Am Rev Respir Dis* **110**:115, 1974

199. Ahn CH et al: Ventilatory defects in atypical mycobacteriosis. *Am Rev Respir Dis* **113**:273, 1976

200. Francis PB et al: The course of untreated *M. kansasii* disease. *Am Rev Respir Dis* **111**:477, 1975

201. Dore N et al: A sporotrichoid-like *Mycobacterium kansasii* infection of the skin treated with minocycline hydrochloride. *Br J Dermatol* **101**:75, 1979

202. Lincoln EM, Gilbert LA: Disease in children due to mycobacteria other than *M tuberculosis*. *Am Rev Respir Dis* **105**:683, 1972

203. Schaefer WB: Incidence of serotypes of *M. avium* and atypical mycobacteria in human and animal diseases. *Am Rev Respir Dis* **97**:18, 1968

204. Cox SK, Stransbough LJ: Chronic cutaneous infection caused by *Mycobacterium intracellulare*. *Arch Dermatol* **117**:794, 1981

205. Cole GW, Gebhard J: *Mycobacterium avium* infection of the skin resembling lepromatous leprosy. *Br J Dermatol* **101**:71, 1979

206. Schmidt JD et al: Cutaneous infection due to a Runyon group III atypical mycobacterium. *Ann Rev Respir Dis* **106**:469, 1972

207. Fainstein V et al: Disseminated infection due to *Mycobacterium avium-intracellulare* in a homosexual man with Kaposi's sarcoma. *J Infect Dis* **145**:586, 1982

208. Heifets LB: Synergistic effect of rifampin, streptomycin, ethionamide and ethambutol on *Mycobacterium intracelluare*. *Am Rev Respir Dis* **125**:43, 1982

209. Sybert A et al: Cutaneous infection due to *Mycobacterium szulgai*. *Am Rev Respir Dis* **115**:695, 1977

210. Dawson DJ, Jennis F: Mycobacteria with a growth requirement for ferric ammonium citrate, identified as *Mycobacterium haemophilum*. *J Clin Microbiol* **11**:190, 1980

211. Mezo A et al: Unusual mycobcteria in 5 cases of opportunistic infection. *Pathology* **11**:277, 1979

212. Walder BK et al: The skin and immunosuppression. *Aust J Dermatol* **17**:94, 1976

213. Centers for Disease Control: Follow up on mycobacterial contamination of porcine heart valve prothesis—United States. *MMWR* **27**:92, 1978

214. Wallace RJ et al: Spectrum of disease due to rapidly growing mycobacteria. *Rev Infect Dis* **5**:657, 1983

215. Centers for Disease Control: Mycobacterial infections associated with augmentation mammaplasty—Florida, North Carolina, Texas. *MMWR* **27**:513, 1978

216. Robicsek F et al: *Mycobacterium fortuitum* epidermis after openheart surgery. *J Thorac Cardiovasc Surg* **75**:91, 1978
217. Hoffman PC et al: Two outbreaks of sternal wound infections due to organisms of the *Mycobacterium fortuitum* complex. *J Infect Dis* **143**:533, 1981

218. Borghans JG, Stanford JR: *Mycobacterium chelonei* in abscesses after injection of diptheria-tetanus-polio vaccine. *Am Rev Respir Dis* **107**:1, 1973

CHAPTER 180

MYCOBACTERIAL DISEASES: LEPROSY

Stanley G. Browne*

Definition and classification (Table 180-1)

Leprosy is a chronic granulomatous disease caused by *Mycobacterium leprae*. Its principal clinical manifestations are determined more by the nature and vigor of the host's response to the infection than by the multiplication of the causative agent in the tissues. *M. leprae* has a predilection for the dermis, the mucosa of the upper respiratory tract, and the peripheral nerves.

Although leprosy was one of the earliest human diseases to be associated with a specific microorganism, it is among the last of the infections to yield its major secrets. Fascinating in its variegated clinical pattern, important because of its wide distribution in the world, and intriguing by reason of its accompanying peripheral neuropathy and unsolved pathologic and epidemiologic riddles, leprosy constitutes a continuing challenge to the physician and the research worker.

Recently acquired knowledge of immunology is making leprosy a better understood entity. The capacity of the exposed individual to mount a successful cell-mediated immune response through thymus-sensitized lymphocytes determines the outcome of the parasite-host confrontation and the characteristics of the lesions in target tissues, if leprosy develops.

Historical aspects

Notwithstanding popular beliefs that leprosy is one of the oldest diseases afflicting humanity, the earliest indubitable description of true leprosy dates from the sixth century B.C., and skeletal remains showing the specific changes due to leprosy (erosion of the anterior nasal spine and the alveolar process of the maxilla) are not known earlier than about 200 B.C. Bones from this period have recently been unearthed in an oasis in the Nile delta.

In the Western world, Aristotle may have referred to leprosy as "leontiasis" or "satyriasis." Leprosy seems to have appeared in Greece as a new disease shortly after the return of Alexander the Great's troops from the Indian campaign (327-326 B.C.). Alexandrian physicians in the

third century B.C. were calling it elephantiasis, whence it later became known as *elephantiasis Graecorum* (Galen, 133-201 A.D.). Years before, Nubian slaves may have carried leprosy into Egypt from the Sudan and further south. Pompey's troops returning from Egypt (62 B.C.) spread leprosy into Italy and the Mediterranean littoral; centuries later the Crusaders took leprosy from the Middle East to the countries of western Europe where it had already appeared.

Slaves from West Africa introduced leprosy to the Western hemisphere, and migrating Europeans from both Scandinavia and the Latin lands of southern Europe established foci of the disease in North, Central, and South America. In the Far East, Chinese (and, to a small extent, Japanese) have taken leprosy with them into the islands of the South Pacific and Australia.

References to leprosy in both the Old and New Testaments are imprecise and uncertain. The generic nonspecific Hebrew word *tsara'ath* (translated "leprosy") refers to a change in color of skin, cloth and leather, and damp walls of houses, with connotations of ceremonial defilement. The Greek *lepra*, used in the Septuagint and the New Testament, is a popular and all-inclusive term denoting scaliness; it had been used for scurf and summer prurigo and it probably included true leprosy, since the disease was present in the lands of the Mediterranean littoral in the first century A.D.. None of the pathognomonic signs or symptoms of true leprosy are mentioned in either the Old or the New Testament. No skeletal remains showing changes due to leprosy have been discovered in Palestine or Israel. While these considerations may not absolutely exclude leprosy, they make it unlikely that *tsara'ath* or *lepra* refers only or mainly to the disease we know today as leprosy. See Chap. 79 for an historical discussion of vitiligo and leprosy.

It was as recently as 1847 that Danielssen and Boeck differentiated leprosy clinically from other diseases, and in 1874 Hansen first described the "slender brown rods" now known as *Mycobacterium leprae* (hence, Hansen's disease as an eponymous alternative to leprosy).

Any scaly, ulcerating skin condition may engender fear and revulsion. Leprosy, by reason of its mysterious origin, capriciousness of attack, insidious onset, relentless prog-

---

* Deceased.

Table 180-1   Natural history and classification of leprosy

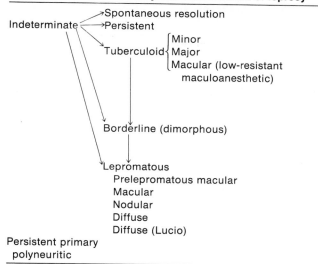

ress, destructive features, and resistance to treatment, has in the past been surrounded in many lands with an aura of superstition, dread, and taboo, and with social and religious sanctions. In this respect, it is a condition unique in medicine and civilization.

Epidemiology

Completely reliable figures of the worldwide prevalence of leprosy are not available. Recently available statistics from mainland China indicate that at present about 300,000 sufferers from leprosy are under treatment. It is claimed that the health service has reasonably complete records of all cases of leprosy in the country. No statistics are available from some countries where there is a high or very high prevalence of leprosy, and where the administrative machine is less able to collect accurate and full information. Data collected by the World Health Organization and incorporating the results of complete whole population surveys, sampling surveys, administrative estimates, and inspired guesses put the total number of leprosy sufferers at about 11 million. Thus, the figure of 15 million for the world would not be very wide of the mark. Past estimates have usually proved very much below the true prevalence. When facilities for treatment are provided, initial estimates of prevalence are seen to be too low; when the propaganda value of cured patients becomes apparent, the numbers increase again; and when rehabilitation services are provided, more patients come out of hiding.

The bulk of the victims of leprosy are to be found within the medicogeographical tropics—Africa (4.0 million), the subcontinent of India (4.0 million is the official estimate), and the whole of Southeast Asia. There are nearly 0.5 million in the Americas, including 3000 in the United States (mainly in the southern states). In Europe, the figure is around 30,000, including over 300 in the United Kingdom. Very few countries (e.g., Denmark, Switzerland, Chili) are thought to be completely spared.

The documented prevalence may reach as high as 50 percent in some villages in Central Africa and India, and the number of estimated and nonregistered patients may

comprise over 5 percent of the population in some countries of West and East Africa.

Until the causative organism can be both cultured on artificial media and easily and routinely inoculated successfully in an experimental animal with the production of progressive and generalized granulomatous disease, many epidemiologic questions must remain unanswered. Some outstanding fundamental issues of resistance or lack of it, of immunity, and of hereditarily transmitted genetic susceptibility to infection also await complete explanation.

Method of spread

Infection has been supposed to be by contagion, by "prolonged and intimate close (i.e., skin to skin) contact" between an infectious index case and a susceptible contact, but each of these concepts is challenged and disputed. Droplet infection from nasal mucus shed by a patient suffering from untreated multibacillary leprosy is probably the most common mode of contagion. A highly bacilliferous index case may harbor extremely few bacilli in the epidermal cells, and transepidermal shedding of viable organisms is unusual. Only a small proportion of leprosy patients will admit any close or intimate contact with a known case of leprosy. It may be that the infective contact was a chance meeting with someone with early or unsuspected lesions. While *M. leprae* has been regarded as an obligatory parasite of certain cells in human beings, it has been demonstrated that an organism resembling *M. leprae* in essential characteristics and causing a disease closely resembling human leprosy, has been found in feral armadillos in Louisiana, U.S.A., and in Mangabey monkeys in West Africa. The epidemiologic importance of these findings in the etiology of human disease has not yet been elucidated. When investigative methods permit, it is possible that *M. leprae* may be demonstrated and identified in other situations.

Age

No age is exempt from leprosy. While congenital infections have been recorded, they are exceedingly rare, and to all intents and purposes leprosy is not a hereditary disease in the true sense of the term. In most reported series, there is a preponderance of new infections among children, adolescents, and young adults, but this may indicate the opportunities and degrees of exposure rather than any specific susceptibility of younger age groups. Any form of leprosy, from the transient to the rapidly progressive, may occur at any age.

Sex

In most series, males are affected rather more than females, the proportion generally varying from 1:1 to 3:1. This, again, may be fortuitous, and express such factors as incomplete data, selected populations attending for diagnosis and treatment, seclusion of females, opportunities of contact between traveling and employed males, sex selection in school populations, etc. The main factors determining the prevalence of leprosy are the numbers of untreated bacilliferous index cases shedding viable bacilli and the opportunities for repeated exposure to massive bacillary challenge.

Genetic factors

Genetic factors determining resistance or susceptibility to leprosy infection have long been suspected, and recent experience showing concordance rates of 80 percent in monozygotic twins (for leprosy, and for the type of leprosy) are very suggestive. Investigation of genetic markers, however, has given equivocal results. Histocompatibility antigens in patients and their family contacts are at present the subject of study.

General health

The general health has no bearing on susceptibility to leprosy infection or the type of leprosy acquired. Prolonged undernourishment may predispose to infection, but the nutritional state does not noticeably affect the response to treatment.

Climate

Climate has no direct bearing on endemic leprosy, though leprosy is at present most common in hot and humid lands. A century ago leprosy was endemic in Scandinavia, and today some colder countries (e.g., Iceland, North Korea, Japan, North China) have a sizable leprosy problem. Leprosy lesions may first appear, suddenly multiply, or undergo acute exacerbation during the hotter and wetter months.

Hormonal state

The hormonal state has some definite though ill-understood effect on leprosy. Thus, the first lesion may appear at puberty, during pregnancy, or after parturition. At such times, existing skin lesions may become raised and succulent and new lesions may appear; the clinical state may deteriorate or evidence of hypersensitivity (i.e., erythema nodosum leprosum) may appear for the first time.

Race

As such, race plays no easily demonstrable part in leprosy infection, though the clinical pattern of leprosy does vary from one country to another. These variations may be associated with different strains of *M. leprae,* impossible at present to demonstrate, or with patterns of susceptibility to bacterial and viral infections. The further one goes from Central Africa, the more serious does leprosy seem to be: the ratio between the self-healing and the progressive forms decreases; the proportion of patients with severe multibacillary disease responding slowly to treatment increases; the incidence and severity and duration of episodes of acute exacerbation and of polyneuritis and iridocyclitis also increase.

The degree of cutaneous pigmentation may be fortuitously associated with these differences: the greater the pigment the less severe the disease. In the deeply pigmented African, susceptibility to contagion may be high, but the tuberculoid/lepromatous ratio may be 10:1 or even

12:1; whereas the light-skinned Caucasian or Mongoloid succumbs most frequently to multibacillary disease and is subject to severe, frequent, and prolonged reactional episodes.

Diet

Various articles of diet have in the past been suspected as predisposing to or actually causing leprosy infection (e.g., dried fish, various tubers, palm oil, manioc, etc.), but no evidence exists of any causal connection.

Transmission

Since it has been believed that *M. leprae* is found only in human tissues, transmission in theory must take place from a patient with "open" or bacilliferous lesions. These lesions are in the skin and nasal mucosa. The intact skin does not permit the entry or the exit of leprosy bacilli. Open ulcers of the lepromatous skin (as distinct from the neuropathic ulcerations of the extremities which but very rarely contain *M. leprae*) may discharge innumerable viable microorganisms. The only site showing leprosy bacilli on its surface is the perinasal skin contaminated by bacilli-laden nasal discharge. Infection may thus be transmitted by nasal droplets shed on foodstuffs, utensils, clothing, bedding, etc.

Various insects have been suspected from time to time of transmitting *M. leprae*, e.g., cockroaches, mosquitoes, fleas, lice. Acid-fast organisms may be found in the intestinal contents of insects, whether they feed on human beings or not, and biting insects may mechanically transmit *M. leprae* from one person to another. Viable leprosy bacilli have been demonstrated in the stomach, salivary glands, and biting parts of flies that have recently fed on untreated leprosy patients.

Some epidemiologic findings suggest that patients with tuberculoid leprosy may not be as innocent as sources of contagion as the rarity of bacilli in their tissues would imply. Their lesions may, of course, pass through phases of bacillary activity, or they may shed viable organisms that are not stainable by standard methods. In any case, since in any community there may be much more tuberculoid than lepromatous leprosy, the relative importance of the former in ensuring persistence of endemic leprosy should not be underestimated.

Etiology and pathogenesis

As seen in preparations from any tissue where it is present (skin, nasal mucosa, peripheral nerves, lymphatic nodes, deep organs, etc.), *M. leprae* is a slender rod, straight or slightly curved, about 3 μm long and 0.5 μm broad, acid-fast and alcohol-fast, and gram-positive. It is found either singly or in small clumps, or (and most characteristically) in masses of 40 to 60 (sometimes 200 to 300) called globi, enclosed within a glial membrane, or the ghostlike remains of the cytoplasm of a reticuloendothelial cell.

So far, since Koch's postulates have not been fulfilled to the satisfaction of all workers, *M. leprae* must strictly be referred to as the "suspected" cause of leprosy, but at present its etiologic role is unquestioned. It is present in uncountable numbers in the dermis in lepromatous leprosy, and can almost always be found on prolonged search in paucibacillary disease. It is not known to pass through a viral or submicroscopic phase, though some observations suggest that *M. leprae* may not always be disclosed by standard fixing and staining techniques. Aberrant forms, coccoid forms, long and club forms, mycoplasma-like bodies, diphtheroid, and L forms have all been demonstrated.

M. leprae in many respects seems to be the ultimate species in a series of related microorganisms with similar though varying culturable, inoculable, immunologic, and biochemical characteristics (mycobacterial contaminants such as *M. scrofulaceum* are frequently isolated from biopsy material). So far, and despite numerous claims over the years, it has not been successfully cultured in artificial media, though recent attempts appear promising. Thus, Eagle's medium, soft agar, and the addition of hyaluronic acid to special nutrient media have all been recently acclaimed. Confirmation of these claims is eagerly awaited, with the fulfillment of stringent criteria laid down by independent bodies. Growth characteristics in susceptible animal models, the long generation time, the dopa-oxidase test, scanning surface electron microscopy, and the presence of specific antigens are part of the screening process.

Localized and limited, though mathematically demonstrable, multiplication of *M. leprae* has been shown to occur in the mouse footpad and in the earlobes and testes of golden hamsters. It has recently been established that, when inoculated into thymectomized mice that have been subjected to high-dose (900 r) total-body irradiation, *M. leprae* will multiply in widely disseminated granulomata. Some success, also, is attending investigations with inoculation of slowly multiplying tissue cell strains with *M. leprae*. Its generation time appears to be about 12 to 13 days.

The nine-banded armadillo and some other species have been found to be susceptible to experimental inoculation with *M. leprae* derived from human sources. With their long lifespan, low body temperature, and immunologic configuration (similar in many respects to that of humans), the armadillo succumbs in 40 percent of cases to a progressive multibacillary leprosy infection. The wild female produces litters of four identical young. Leprosy bacilli are now available for biochemical and immunologic fractionation and for many kinds of investigation. Recently, wild armadillos in Louisiana have been found with a leprosy-like skin infection, caused by an organism closely resembling, if not identical with, *M. leprae*.

Work is proceeding on the ultramicroscopic structure of *M. leprae*, and on the antigenic pattern of its complex cell wall and cellular protoplasm. The morphology of *M. leprae* is indicative of its viability or nonviability. By an elegant investigative procedure, it is found that "solid-staining rods" of *M. leprae* are viable, whereas such changes as absence of central staining or diffuse or irregular polar staining are indicative of nonviability.

Although it is almost unknown for a child to be born with leprosy, and very rare for an infant to show signs of the disease, child household contacts of a lepromatous mother run a variable risk of contracting the disease, some reports suggesting a risk as high as 1 in 3. Where the household index case is suffering from paucibacillary leprosy and not apparently shedding any *M. leprae*, the risk of a child's contracting the disease is greater than in the general population. Where the prevalence of leprosy in a rural environment is greater than 1 percent, everybody must be considered to be a "contact."

Accidental inoculation of leprosy has been suspected to occur through the use of contaminated instruments in tattooing and smallpox vaccination, or in the course of a surgical operation. Recorded cases of inoculation of volunteers with material from leprosy patients do not bear scientific investigation. Where it is ascertainable, the shortest "silent period" between the supposed inoculation and the appearance of an overt lesion is between 2 and 3 years.

The majority of healthy persons exposed constantly to leprosy infection will, after several months, develop a subclinical infection which is shown only by heritable changes in the lymphocyte population; these can be demonstrated by special tests.

Clinical manifestations

Prodromal manifestations

The nonspecific and systemic symptoms formerly regarded as early signs of leprosy infections are mostly valueless for purposes of diagnosis.

It is now believed, on the basis of investigations using the Lymphocyte Transformation Test, that subclinical leprosy infection is very common, and that, in fact, the majority of persons who have been daily exposed for more than a few months in an environment in which live *M. leprae* are being disseminated, will demonstrate transmissible changes in their lymphocytes that give evidence of such exposure. No clinical signs of such infection are visible, or likely to become visible, unless the subject succumbs to a recognizable clinical infection with *M. leprae*, the nature of which will depend on his/her innate capacity to mount—or not to mount—a degree of cell-mediated immunity.

For a variable time, usually about 2 to 5 years, the patient passes through a silent or latent period, sometimes referred to as the incubation period. The length of this period is related both to the long generation time of *M. leprae* and to the indolent tissue response to the infection. Toward the end of this stage, the symptoms are those of irritation of nerve endings in the skin, and consist of persistent or recurrent paresthesiae and numbness localized to certain areas, with no accompanying visible alterations in the corresponding skin and no objectively demonstrable impairment of the peripheral nervous system. These symptoms are suggestive, without being pathognomonic. At this stage there may rarely occur transient macular skin rashes and perhaps occasional slight epistaxis, a reddish tingeing of the nasal mucus. The indicative value of these phenomena is best appreciated in retrospect. The onset of leprosy is thus insidious and painless, and its progress in the early stages is slow. Years may elapse before a diagnosis is made, and patients are frequently labeled "hysterics" until indubitable signs in skin and nerves make the true diagnosis obvious.

Before long, cutaneous lesions appear. These are so varied that their true nature is often missed, even by experienced dermatologists. If only the possibility of leprosy could be entertained whenever the clinician is confronted with a chronic nonirritating rash that is unusual or atypical,

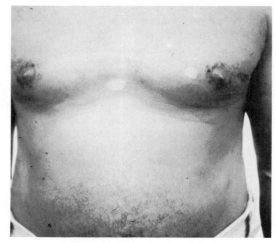

Fig. 180-1   Indeterminate leprosy, nearing tuberculoid.

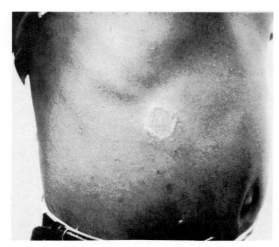

Fig. 180-2   Minor tuberculoid leprosy.

or is unresponsive to treatment, leprosy would be diagnosed earlier than it often is. Similarly, a patient with a positive geographical history who shows early signs of peripheral nerve disorder may have leprosy.

Cutaneous lesions (Figs. A6-1 to A6-8)

The bewildering varieties of skin manifestations of leprosy are reduced to recognizable order when the disease is regarded as the visible expression of a continuing process, sometimes constant, sometimes variable—the host response to the invasion of a parasite with rather special features. It is the tremendously wide variation in this response that leads to confusion. On the one hand, *M. leprae* may multiply in unrestrained fashion in the dermis and nasal mucosa: it may be seen by the thousand between the fibers of the main peripheral nerves; in these cases, the cellular reaction is minimal or negligible. On the other hand, *M. leprae* may be extremely scanty in the skin and nerves, but the vigor of the cell-mediated response and the subsequent fibrosis may itself cause widespread local damage and open the door to the severe muscle paralysis and neuropathic ulceration of the extremities habitually associated with leprosy among the laity and the profession. The descriptions that follow, representing a consensus of informed opinion from various countries, are conveniently based on the accepted classification. The clinical criteria run generally parallel with bacterioscopic findings, with the immunologic state (as shown in the lepromin test), and with the histopathologic picture.

Indeterminate leprosy

The skin lesions are the early manifestations of leprosy infection and consist of scattered, small, ill-defined macular areas numbering from 1 to 12 or more, slightly hypopigmented in dark skin, hypopigmented or pinkish in light skin (Fig. 180-1). At this early stage, there are no clinically demonstrable changes in tactile sensitivity, sweating, or hair appearance.

The slit-smear examination is usually negative; the lepromin test may be positive or negative; in the young child, it is frequently negative or doubtful. The histologic picture

is unconvincing and by no means pathognomonic; it consists of small collections of round cells scattered indiscriminately in the dermis. Prolonged examination of serial sections stained by the Fite-Faraco or Triff method may reveal isolated acid-fast organisms within the Schwann cells of the papillary layer and elsewhere.

These lesions may resolve spontaneously within a few months, remain stationary for a year or two before regressing, or develop unmistakable signs of one or other of the following "determined" or definite types of leprosy.

Tuberculoid leprosy

The skin lesions may be single or multiple, arising at once or in successive crops. From their earliest appearance, they may be typical, or they may arise from indeterminate lesions. The essence of the tuberculoid lesion is that it is a well-defined hypopigmented area in which the adnexa and the pigment-forming cells are subject to a greater or lesser degree of damage. The vigor of the cellular reaction to a paucibacillary infection determines the clinical appearances and the amount of consequential tissue destruction. The size of the individual lesions varies from a few millimeters in diameter to an area covering the whole trunk. The lesions may heal spontaneously in a few months or persist with very slow peripheral extension for a lifetime. They may heal centrally and extend peripherally. They are usually raised, especially around the edge, above the level of the surrounding skin, and a ring of papules set just within the advancing ameboid hypopigmented zone is very characteristic (Fig. 180-2). The height of the margin above the level of the surrounding skin, and hence the thickness of the granuloma, is the basis of the descriptive varieties of tuberculoid leprosy, "minor" and "major."

In addition to these raised lesions, there is a macular variety, referred to by Indian leprologists as maculoanesthetic. The lesions are completely flat, single or multiple, of uniform hypopigmentation; the surface may be micropapulate. These lesions are often indolent and repigment very slowly under treatment.

Except in the earliest stages, established tuberculoid lesions show the symptoms and signs of local nerve damage. Not only is the function of the pigment-forming cells interfered with (leading generally to hypopigmentation), but there is impairment of tactile sensation (shown by loss of tactile discrimination on examination with a wisp of cotton wool) and of thermal sensation (shown by confusion or inability to correctly identify test tubes containing hot and cold water). Sweating is impaired or in the last stages completely abolished, so that the surface of the lesion is dry and rough. The hair is lost when the follicles become fibrosed, and does not regenerate.

Nerve damage is characteristic of tuberculoid leprosy in all but the slightest forms. Locally, and in the neighborhood of a lesion, small cutaneous twigs may be grossly enlarged, especially near a joint (knee or elbow) and in the scapular region. Focally, and corresponding to the site of the skin lesion, the related peripheral nerve trunk at a site of predilection may be enlarged, hard, and tender. Generally, and even in patients with minimal cutaneous signs, many of the peripheral nerves of the extremities, at their sites of predilection, may be similarly affected. These sites are the ulnar, above the elbow; the external popliteal as it winds around the neck of the fibula; the posterior tibial, midway between the internal malleolus and the point of the heel. Not so frequently involved are the median (just above the wrist and in the antecubital fossa), the musculospiral in its groove, the great auricular leash as it lies over the sternocleidomastoid muscle, the facial over the malar bone, the supraorbital and supratrochlear, and the roots, trunks, and branches of the brachial plexus.

These symptoms and signs are transient if the granuloma is shallow and yields readily to treatment, and quasicomplete resolution and restoration of function may occur. When the granuloma, however, occupies the whole of the dermis from the basal layer of the epidermis to the deep fascia, the adnexa are permanently damaged.

The histopathologic picture is essentially that of an aggregation of tuberculoid foci, arranged primarily around the adnexa, i.e., there is a focalization of the granuloma. *M. leprae* are extremely scanty. Giant cells of the Langhans' type may be numerous, but caseation almost never occurs, except in nerve trunks and lymph nodes. A pathognomonic and differentiating feature is the infiltration with round cells of the nerve fibrils in the dermis, the cells being arranged cufflike and also between the fibers.

The lepromin test is positive in tuberculoid leprosy, and the degree of positivity in general corresponds to the vigor of the cellular response in the skin lesions and in the nerves.

Resolution may be spontaneous in the less severe and less extensive types of tuberculoid leprosy; this resolution may be accelerated by treatment. Nerve damage may be completely prevented by early treatment. Resolution may be characterized by true scarring or by repigmentation. Residual hypopigmentation, patchy dyschromia, or hyperpigmentation may mark the site of a healed tuberculoid lesion.

Lepromatous leprosy

This represents the completely anergic type in which there is an unrestrained multiplication of *M. leprae* in certain tissues, with late damage to the peripheral nerves. The lepromin reaction is consistently negative. There is a complete and permanent absence of cell-mediated immunity.

Several types are described, but the distinctions between these types are not clear-cut: one may precede another, and several may coexist. A common sequence is for lepromatous macules to precede by some years the appearance of discrete nodules, and for nodules to arise on skin that is the site of diffuse infiltration.

Prelepromatous macular leprosy or juvenile macular leprosy consists of numerous small and very slightly hypopigmented areas (in the dark skin), slightly pinkish or dull yellow (in the light skin). The best (and perhaps only) way of distinguishing these lesions is to examine attentively the tensed skin of the patient's back as he slowly turns around in a very good light: slight differences in skin coloring or shininess may be the only evidence of the condition. At this stage, no sensory disturbances can be detected, and the sweat glands function normally. Bacilli may not be demonstrable by the slit-smear method, and hence the diagnosis will be in doubt. However, with continued (and justifiable) temporizing and observation, the diagnosis will become obvious when innumerable *M. leprae* appear in material obtained by the slit-smear method. The earlier the diagnosis is made the better. Some patients diagnosed as having indeterminate leprosy are in reality suffering from prebacillary lepromatous macular leprosy.

Macular lepromatous leprosy. This may develop from prelepromatous lesions or from lesions called indeterminate. It usually shows itself by the appearance of numerous symptomless, small, ill-defined macules, slightly hypopigmented or erythematous. After some months or years, coalescent hypopigmented macules may occupy the entire body surface (except the inguinal and axillary regions notably), and so deceive even the expert. They may be seen first on the back, but may occur anywhere. Sweating may be slightly impaired, and very slight sensory loss is demonstrable on careful examination. After 3 or 4 years, the nerve trunks of the extremities become enlarged and tender. Bacterioscopic examination of the skin at this stage clinches the diagnosis. *M. leprae* are present singly and in globi in the lesions themselves, and also in the earlobes and in the mucosa covering the nasal septum. They may be shed in the nasal mucus.

Nodular lepromatous leprosy. This often follows macular leprosy after a lapse of some years, but it may arise de novo. The nodules appear on the face, the ears (lobes and helices), forehead, cheeks, nares, lips, and chin, and less frequently on the trunk and limbs (Fig. 180-3). They may be single or in groups or scattered diffusely over the whole body. As they increase in size, they may coalesce and form huge, raised, plaquelike masses of granulomatous tissue. The nodules are aggregations of *M. leprae* enclosed in masses of reticuloendothelial cells. All the peripheral nerve trunks are generally enlarged and tender.

Diffuse lepromatous leprosy. This may occur in the absence of macules or nodules, or it may coexist with both. It is characterized by a diffuse thickening of the dermis by a highly bacilliferous granuloma. The thickening leads to gross distortion and puckering of the skin, producing the classical leonine facies. The eyebrows and eyelashes are lost, as is the hair of the beard; the hairy scalp is but rarely

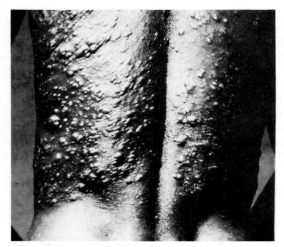

Fig. 180-3 Nodular leproma (back).

affected, except in Japan, where leprous alopecia is not uncommon.

Diffuse leprosy of Lucio. This is diffuse lepromatous infiltration of the skin with no obvious localized stigmata of leprosy. There is some atrophy of the epidermis, some wasting of the digital pulps, and (in Central America) loss of eyebrows. Despite the absence of local lesions in this "beautiful leprosy," *M. leprae* may be found in large numbers in the dermis anywhere in the body. This condition, virtually but not absolutely confined to Mexico and neighboring countries, is subject to acute multiple ulceration, with the appearance of polygonal necrotic areas.

Extremely numerous *M. leprae* are present within the major peripheral nerve trunks in all cases of lepromatous leprosy, but demonstrable damage occurs only when cellular infiltration makes its appearance, coinciding usually with the breakdown of some bacilli and characterized by local edema and ischemia. The essential pathology in all varieties of lepromatous leprosy is the development of a bacilliferous granuloma, with extremely numerous *M. leprae* massed in reticuloendothelial cells.

Borderline or dimorphous leprosy

This is the rather unsatisfactory designation of a wide variety of lesions occupying the broad and variable inter-

Fig. 180-4 Active borderline leprosy of cheek.

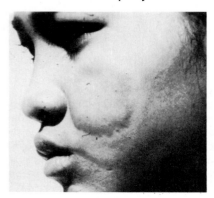

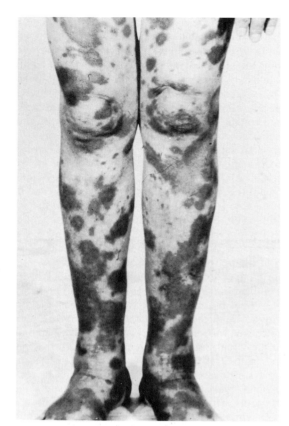

Fig. 180-5 Multiple dimorphous lesions involving the patient's legs in a generally symmetric fashion. *(Courtesy of U.S. Public Health Service Hospital, Carville, Louisiana.)*

mediate zone between the two "polar" types, tuberculoid and lepromatous.

The skin lesions are very diverse: some are near tuberculoid and others near lepromatous. The near-tuberculoid lesions are reasonably well-defined, and hypopigmented, and tend to be dome shaped (Figs. 180-4 and 180-5). The hypopigmentation is usually uniform, showing little or no tendency to spontaneous central healing (Fig. 180-6).

Fig. 180-6 Borderline leprosy with predominantly tuberculoid features.

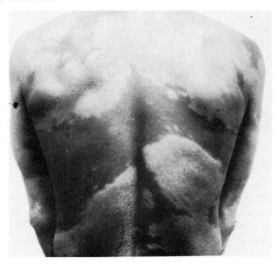

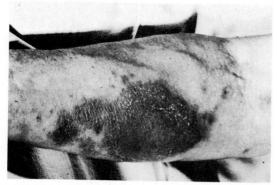

Fig. 180-7 A typical lesion of dimorphous leprosy showing a large erythematous plaque with a number of satellite lesions in the vicinity. *(Courtesy of U.S. Public Health Service Hospital, Carville, Louisiana.)*

Around the main lesion, small daughter lesions are frequently seen (Fig. 180-7). Such lesions tend to deteriorate toward the lepromatous—a downgrading reaction—often following repeated episodes of exacerbation. Sensory impairment and disturbances of sweating are marked within the lesion. Bacilli are scanty. The lesions are often larger and more numerous than in polar tuberculoid leprosy. Nerve damage is local, focal, and general; usually it appears earlier and is more widespread than in tuberculoid leprosy.

At the other extreme, the near-lepromatous lesions include a wide variety of raised or slightly raised elements of all sizes, from numerous, small, buttonlike elevations to large, slightly raised, and uniformly hypopigmented plaques occurring anywhere on the body. Small, discrete lenticulate nodules sometimes occur on the ears, the cheeks, and the chin. A very characteristic appearance in longstanding lesions is of a raised ring surrounding a central, flat "immune area."

The nerves are affected early and widely (Fig. 180-8); a generalized acute polyneuritis may be the presenting sign, or an early and obvious sign. Injudicious treatment may apparently precipitate a severe and widespread polyneuritis. Nerve damage is frequently symmetrical and rapidly progressive.

Fig. 180-8 Borderline leprosy with gross nerve involvement.

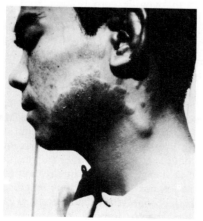

The histologic picture is variable; it may vary from one lesion to another, from the superficial to the deep aspect of the same lesion, from the border of the lesion to the center, and at different stages in the patient's history. There is often an admixture of diverse elements: numerous bacilli in lepra cells together with giant-cell systems; a diffuse bacilliferous granuloma together with focalization of round cells around the cutaneous adnexa.

The lepromin reaction corresponds to the presumed immunologic state: it varies with the individual, being most often doubtful or slightly positive. In the same patient, it may vary from time to time, generally becoming less positive in the course of a downgrading reaction.

In addition to these well-defined varieties of leprosy, all of which (except the indeterminate) may be accompanied or complicated by some degree of peripheral neuritis, *primary and persistent polyneuritis* may occur, in which no skin changes are apparent. This form must be distinguished from cases in which peripheral neuritis persists when the skin lesions are healed, and those where precocious polyneuritis precedes by a variable period the first cutaneous change due to leprosy. The affected nerves are usually enlarged, hard, and tender, and typical distal effects may develop.

Histologic examination of a superficial sensory nerve establishes the diagnosis of leprosy, and the kind of cellular infiltration indicates the type of leprosy concerned—usually borderline, sometimes tuberculoid. A small sliver of a cutaneous sensory nerve (such as the radial cutaneous or a twig coursing over the dorsum of the hand) may be removed for histopathologic examination.

Nerve damage

Enough has been said to show the overriding importance of peripheral nerve damage in leprosy. The neurologically distal results of transient or irreversible interruption of motor and sensory pathways in the mixed nerves of the extremities need no emphasis: atrophy of muscle, hypoasthesia, disturbance of sweating, pigmentation, changes in the caliber of blood vessels, etc. The secondary effects of nerve damage are seen in the so-called surgical complications of leprosy: the neuropathic ulceration of the extremities due, in the main, to repeated unappreciated traumata to insensitive tissues; the muscular wasting, following generally a predetermined pattern (in hands, feet, eyelids, face); the pareses and paralyses (claw hand, drop foot, everted foot, facial palsy); the neuropathic (Charcot's) joints, etc. For full consideration of these results of nerve damage in leprosy, standard works should be consulted.

Course of the disease

Leprosy may be a mere passing phase—a symptomless self-healing macule—or it may be a relentlessly progressive disease. The less severe the leprosy, the more likely is spontaneous regression to occur with no risk of nerve damage. Even extensive tuberculoid leprosy may eventually burn itself out, leaving the patient mutilated and sightless. Lepromatous leprosy very rarely heals without treatment. Borderline leprosy, untreated, usually tends to degenerate; it becomes more bacilliferous, the patient having the worst of both worlds.

Acute exacerbation—a neutral noncommittal term—covers the varied inflammatory phenomena that may occur in any form of leprosy (except the indeterminate). The precipitating cause may not be obvious or the onset may apparently be associated with some intercurrent infection (especially viral, or smallpox vaccination), or a change in the hormonal state consequent on pregnancy or parturition, or some acute mental stress. Or the phase may be ushered in by a reduction in the bacillary load after effective chemotherapy, or by pyrexia of diverse origin.

These reactions are conveniently classified as follows:

Type I reactions occur in nonlepromatous leprosy (tuberculoid, near-tuberculoid, and borderline tuberculoid). They are characterized by the more or less sudden appearance of hyperemia and edema in a single lesion or in all the lesions. In particular, the edges of the skin lesions become raised, red, and succulent; they may desquamate and ulcerate, and the patient may complain of itching or a burning sensation—rather unusual symptoms in leprosy. When the acute phase is over, either spontaneously or as the result of anti-inflammatory chemotherapy, the swelling subsides, the hyperemia disappears, and the fibrosis in the dermis leads to puckering of the skin.

The most important feature of this Type I reaction lies not in the skin, but in the peripheral nerves. Similar changes take place in subjacent nerves (as in the upper fibers of the facial nerve in association with a lesion on the cheek), or in the main peripheral nerve trunks at the sites of predilection. The consequent loss of sensory and/or motor modalities may be serious and permanent.

The broad intermediate borderline zone of essentially paucibacillary leprosy, ranging from the near-tuberculoid to the near-lepromatous, may show an increase in the level of cellular immunity that often follows successful chemotherapy: this is termed *reversal reaction*. Although the ultimate prognosis in the light of the infective process may be favorable, the accompanying changes in the peripheral nerves are frequently followed by fibrosis and destruction of nerve fibers, with unfortunate distal consequences.

A decrease in cell-mediated immunity is termed a *downgrading reaction*. These reactions tend to recur: new skin lesions appear, and existing lesions become red and edematous. Successive crops of lesions become less typically tuberculoid in appearance, and *M. leprae* become increasingly abundant in the lesions. In addition to severe pain in the nerves themselves, there may be systemic symptoms such as pyrexia, generalized malaise, and pain in the large muscle masses.

The clinical presentation of these two kinds of reaction—reversal and down-grading—may be difficult to distinguish on clinical grounds alone, but by recourse to the Lymphocyte Transformation Test and histology, it is possible to deduce the direction of the immunologic shift.

Type II reactions occur in patients suffering from multibacillary forms of leprosy, particularly the polar lepromatous form. They may arise spontaneously in patients who have never received treatment, but are more common nowadays in those receiving chemotherapy. The presenting feature of these reactions is erythema nodosum leprosum (ENL). ENL is seen in the established disease (unlike the erythema nodosum of tuberculosis). The individual lesions are situated superficially or deeply in the dermis, are tender to the touch, last for a few days, and arise in crops. Their distribution is quite unlike that of the erythema nodosum of tuberculosis, and the last place to look for ENL is the pretibial region. The lesions of ENL are most common on the extensor surfaces of thighs and forearms, the face, and the trunk. They leave a postinflammatory hypermelanotic imprint after they have faded. When large areas of dermis are affected, the overlying skin becomes hard and dark, and leathery to the touch. It may ulcerate in places and the discharge may be highly bacilliferous.

Common complications are: epistaxis, iridocyclitis, peripheral neuropathy, lymphadenitis, orchitis, fusiform dactylitis, and arthritis (perhaps with effusion). There are usually systemic signs and symptoms.

The essential histologic lesion is a diffuse panniculitis, with the blood vessels the target organs; hence, there is hyalin degeneration of the media of the smaller arterioles, vasculitis, thrombosis (and consequent localized gangrene of the skin area supplied), and a polymorphonuclear infiltration of the whole dermis. This type of cellular infiltrate may invade the peripheral nerves and the lymph nodes. This diffuse panniculitis may present localized areas of concentrated cellular infiltration with the formation of microabscesses that may erode the epidermis and lead to indolent ulcerations discharging bacilli-laden necrotic material.

The essential immunologic feature seems to be a complicated interplay of antigen, antibody, complement, and immune complexes, with the release of proteolytic enzymes that produce necrosis and acute tissue inflammation. The antigen is released from groups of degenerating *M. leprae* to initiate this complex sequence of events.

The mechanism of the changes that show themselves in polar lepromatous leprosy is dependent on an antigen-antibody reaction, accompanied by the deposit of immune complexes in target tissues and organs, particularly the skin, peripheral nerves, the uveal tract of the eye, and the kidney. The precipitating factors are those known to produce physical or mental stress, viral diseases, smallpox vaccination, pyrexia, hormonal changes, etc. The episode itself is frequently heralded by an attack of erythema nodosum leprosum, the lesions of which appear on arms, forearms, thighs, trunk, and face, and may be superficial or deep-seated in the pannus. It is accompanied by pyrexia, malaise, painful polyneuritis, polyarthritis (perhaps with effusion), lymphadenitis, and perhaps by iridocyclitis. Acute orchitis or acute mastitis may also occur. The first such episode may be slight and self-limited, and may not recur; or the condition may become chronic and intractable, gradually merging into progressive lepra reaction.

The lepromin test

The lepromin test consists of the intradermal inoculation of a small quantity of biologically standardized extract of lepromatous tissue, prepared according to one of the accepted methods. The early (Fernandez) reaction, read at 48 h, is in some respects comparable to the Mantoux reaction; the late (Mitsuda) reaction is a kind of delayed-hypersensitivity reaction and attains its maximum usually by the 21st day, and indicates potential reactivity of the tissues when challenged by the (impure) antigen. The reaction gives no indication of previous or present leprosy infection. The lepromin test is completely negative in the presence of lepromatous leprosy, and variably positive in

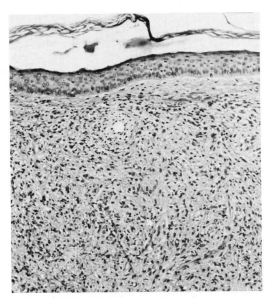

Fig. 180-9   Lepromatous leprosy. The clinical nodularity of this form of the disease is due to the presence of tumorlike accumulations of altered macrophages associated with innumerable acid-fast organisms. In this micrograph one sees such a large number of altered macrophages that the reticular dermis is virtually obliterated. The papillary dermis, however, is spared, in contrast to its common involvement in tuberculoid leprosy. ×100. (See Fig. 180-12.) *(Teaching Set No. 4, U.S. Public Health Service Hospital, Carville, Louisiana. Courtesy of Richard E. Mansfield, M.D. Micrograph by Wallace H. Clark, Jr., M.D.)*

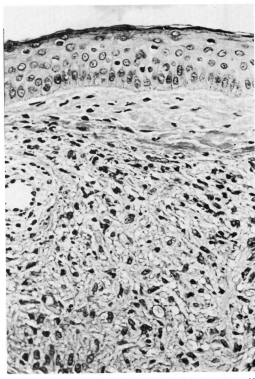

Fig. 180-10   Lepromatous leprosy. A higher-magnification view of a portion of Fig. 180-9. Note the sparing of the papillary dermis. ×256. *(Teaching Set No. 4, U.S. Public Health Service Hospital, Carville, Louisiana. Courtesy of Richard E. Mansfield, M.D. Micrograph by Wallace H. Clark, Jr., M.D.)*

tuberculoid and borderline leprosy, being highly positive in major tuberculoid leprosy.

There are no specific serologic tests for leprosy. The total protein in the serum is increased, the increase being largely in the globulin fractions.

Pathology

Biopsy

Small specimens of skin including the dermis are excised according to standard practice. After fixation in Zenker's or Ridley's solution, sections are cut and stained by the Fite-Faraco or Triff method to demonstrate acid-fast bacilli and to show the type of cellular response to the infection.

The salient features of the pathology have already been indicated in the section dealing with the clinical features of the disease, since an understanding of the pathologic basis for the symptoms and signs of this disease will provide a rational explanation of what would otherwise be complicated and confused (Figs. 180-9 through 180-13).

The earliest skin lesions of leprosy suggest that the Schwann cells provide the key. *M. leprae* seems to have a positive chemotaxis toward peripheral nerve tissue, while sparing the central nervous system. Thereafter, the cellular response to infection revolves around the neurovascular bundles, the pilosebaceous follicles, the hair follicles, and the pigment-forming cells.

In lepromatous leprosy the bacilli multiply, eventually producing a continuous sheet of lepra cells (Virchow, or "foamy") occupying the whole dermis, and separated generally from the basal layer by a well-marked subepithelial clear zone.

The virtual absence of toxemia in the presence of colossal numbers of *M. leprae* is as remarkable as the widespread involvement of the nerves of the extremities. In the latter, fibrosis follows edema and ischemia, and the nerve trunk is eventually reduced to a slender hard fibrous cord. Autolysis ("abscess formation") sometimes occurs in these nerve trunks at the same sites of predilection as those in which the earliest and most marked clinical changes occur, and the nerve may rarely calcify at these sites or in tubular fashion.

The advancing granuloma of lepromatous leprosy in the upper respiratory mucosa may eventually lead to death from asphyxia. Death is more often due to amyloid disease, kidney failure, pulmonary tuberculosis, dysentery, inanition, or toxemia from infection.

Reference has already been made to some immunologic aspects of leprosy. To reiterate, cellular immunity (that is, cell-mediated immunity) provides the important mechanism of defense against leprosy infection, preventing the establishment of the bacilli in the tissues, or preventing the appearance of overt lesions, or limiting the infection. The adequacy of the immune response may vary from the complete to the partial.

Humoral immunity also exists in leprosy, but apparently subserves no useful function. As a matter of fact, the albumin/globulin ratio is reversed in lepromatous leprosy, the gamma globulins are increased, and such moieties as

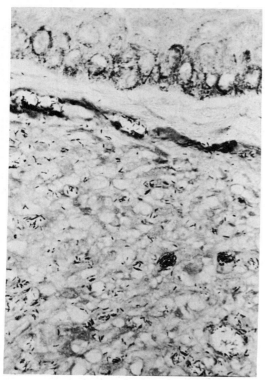

Fig. 180-11 Lepromatous leprosy, Fite stain. The upper part of the micrograph shows the basal region of the epidermis and the spared papillary body; the remainder of the picture shows numerous, dark lepra bacilli. Some are disposed in dense packets (globi), which appear as oval holes with a bit of amorphous material in hematoxylin and eosin sections. ×640. *(Teaching Set No. 4, U.S. Public Health Service Hospital, Carville, Louisiana. Courtesy of Richard E. Mansfield, M.D. Micrograph by Wallace H. Clark, Jr., M.D.)*

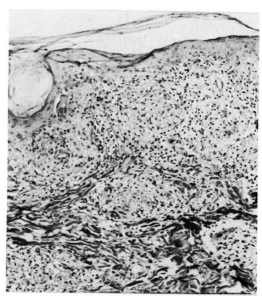

Fig. 180-12 **Tuberculoid leprosy. The histologic response is distinctly granulomatous with tubercle formation and is, therefore, more easily confused with tuberculosis and sarcoidosis than is lepromatous leprosy. Acid-fast organisms may be rare or absent in tuberculoid leprosy. Any granulomatous infiltrate such as that shown in this micrograph should be carefully searched for involvement of small nerves, for such involvement may suggest that the process is tuberculoid leprosy. ×100.** *(Teaching Set No. 37, U.S. Public Health Service Hospital, Carville, Louisiana. Courtesy of Richard E. Mansfield, M.D. Micrograph by Wallace H. Clark, Jr., M.D.)*

cryoglobulins, euglobulins, antithyroid factor, and antinuclear factor may be present. Despite this, a multibacillary infection establishes itself, with hematogenous dissemination of bacilli from ruptured endothelial cells lining the blood vessels.

During the episodes of acute inflammation occurring during the course of lepromatous leprosy—under treatment or arising spontaneously—the focal and systemic signs are apparently due to the deposit in the tissues of antigen, antibody, and immune complexes. When these substances are present in target tissues and target organs, such as the skin, the peripheral nerves, the uveal tract, or the glomeruli of the kidney, permanent damage to structure and function may result. In the kidney, deposits of amyloid may destroy the glomeruli. In the skin, the localized or diffuse polymorphonuclear panniculitis is characterized by local abscess formation, thrombosis in small vessels (with consequent localized gangrene in the area of skin supplied), and hyalin degeneration of the media of the small arterioles.

Demonstration of *M. leprae*

One means of examination is the slit-smear method. Cleanse with ether the skin over the most active part of the edge of the lesion and exsanguinate a skin fold by compressing it between thumb and forefinger of the left hand. With a sharp and sterile scalpel make an incision 5 mm long through the epidermis and into the dermis. Turn the scalpel through a right angle and scrape firmly the slightly gaping edge of the incision. Spread on a fresh microscopic slide the tissue juice collected on the tip of the scalpel. Fix by heat. Stain by Ziehl-Neelsen's method. Examine under the oil-immersion lens.

Material may be obtained by this technique from any site. Those recommended are, in order, the active edge of a lesion, the earlobe, the mucosa of the nasal septum, the anterior surface of the thigh, the finger, the buttocks, and apparently normal skin.

When standard techniques are used by a practiced technician, the numbers of bacilli present in the average microscopic field and the number of globi present may be estimated and expressed according to a standard notation: the average from the sites examined constitutes the bacterial index. Similarly, the average percentage of morphologically normal bacilli may be calculated, and expressed as the morphologic index.

Diagnosis and differential diagnosis

The positive diagnosis of leprosy is based on the clinical appearance, together with either the demonstration of impairment of tactile sensitivity in a skin lesion or the presence of *M. leprae*. Very strong presumptive evidence is furnished by the presence of enlarged, hard, and tender

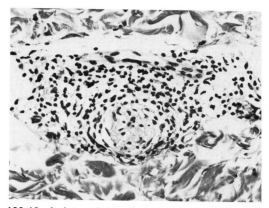

Fig. 180-13 Indeterminate leprosy, neural involvement. Lymphocytes are clustered about a small nerve branch. Though not diagnostic of leprosy, such a distribution of inflammatory cells is quite unusual in other inflammatory diseases of the skin. ×256. (Teaching Set, U.S. Public Health Service Hospital, Carville, Louisiana. Courtesy of Richard E. Mansfield, M.D. Micrograph by Wallace H. Clark, Jr., M.D.)

nerve trunks at the sites of predilection or near a hypopigmented area of skin.

The use of the eyes and a piece of cotton wool will provide convincing evidence of leprosy in the great majority of patients. Where the clinical findings are doubtful, little help can be expected from slit-smear and histologic examination (except in macular lepromatous leprosy) or from the lepromin test. The best basis for diagnosing leprosy is a knowledge of the diverse skin manifestations of the disease, and especially an acquaintance with the disease as it shows itself in the local people. General physicians and dermatologists may fail to diagnose leprosy because they do not consider the possibility, whereas leprologists are apt to see leprosy in any skin condition.

Differential diagnosis cannot be adequately dealt with in brief fashion since leprosy may be simulated by, or resemble in some way, literally hundreds of conditions, congenital and acquired, infective, parasitic, neoplastic, traumatic, etc. The only way to differentiate leprosy from these numerous other diseases is to bear leprosy in mind as a possible diagnosis and to search for suspicious or confirmatory positive signs. If the latter are not present, it is justifiable to temporize rather than saddle the patient with a wrong diagnosis, with all its adverse social and personal implications.

Each of the many typical lesions of leprosy—the macular, the nodular, the infiltrative, the polyneuritic—has its numerous imitators, but an accurate history and a painstaking physical examination will exclude most of them with relative ease. Slit-smear and histologic examination should exclude most of the rest. The only two conditions in which the nerves of the limbs are enlarged, hard, and tender and accompanied by signs of peripheral neuropathy are so rare as to be pathologic curiosities: hereditary familial hypertrophic neuropathy and chronic diffuse amyloidosis of nerves.

Treatment

In general, once the diagnosis of leprosy has been made, treatment should be started even though some patients

with self-healing disease may receive treatment unnecessarily. If the patient is suffering from an acute exacerbation, acute peripheral neuritis, or acute psychosis, it may be advisable to defer specific antileprosy treatment.

Most patients can with perfect safety be treated in their own homes; in fact, about 90 percent are so treated. In mass campaigns, competent medical auxiliaries undertake quite satisfactorily the treatment of the vast majority of patients. Central institutions are, however, necessary as bases for such campaigns, and hospital beds are required for patients undergoing acute exacerbation, suffering from such conditions as iridocyclitis or acute polyneuritis, sensitive or resistant to some antileprosy drug, awaiting stabilization of drug dosage, and for patients undergoing surgery or receiving physiotherapy or vocational training. Patients suffering from leprosy may be admitted to general hospital wards if the ordinary precautions of barrier nursing are observed in the care of those who are contagious.

Two factors now necessitate a radical reappraisal of the treatment of leprosy: first, the appearance of secondary dapsone-resistance in more than 25 countries where the drug has been used and of primary dapsone-resistance in several of them; wherever dapsone has been given for more than five years as the sole drug for the treatment of patients with multibacillary forms of leprosy, and especially where the drug has been taken irregularly and in low doses, relapse due to the emergence of dapsone-resistant organisms has been observed; second, the demonstration that leprosy bacilli may remain inactive but still alive in deep tissues (such as bone marrow, lymphatic nodes, muscle or nerve tissue, endothelial cells) for long periods and after apparently adequate chemotherapy. The bacilli do not multiply or spread. They are not metabolizing and hence do not absorb drugs present in inhibitory concentrations in their vicinity. When unknown conditions become propitious, they begin to multiply again; the patient suffers a relapse, and drug-sensitive bacilli reappear. Such "persister" bacilli have been found after 10 years of treatment with dapsone, five years with clofazimine, or two years with rifampicin. In view of these findings, it is now recommended that multidrug regimens should be followed by all newly diagnosed patients, as follows:

1. For patients with multibacillary forms of leprosy (that is, lepromatous, borderline lepromatous, borderline, and smear-positive indeterminate):

    Rifampicin 600 mg and clofazimine 300 mg once monthly, and should not be given unless supervised by a physician
    Clofazimine 50 mg and dapsone 100 mg daily
    This regimen should be followed for at least two years until bacterial negativity has been attained. In practice, the presence of acid-fast material in routine skin smears is held to be indicative of persistent activity, though it is probable that only "solid-staining rods" are evidence of infectivity.

2. For patients with paucibacillary forms of leprosy (that is, tuberculoid, borderline tuberculoid, smear-negative indeterminate):

    Rifampicin 600 mg monthly, and should not be given unless supervised by a physician
    Dapsone 100 mg daily
    To counter the argument that this regimen is in reality monotherapy with rifampicin if the infection is due to

dapsone-resistant organisms, it may be said that the mycobactericidal effect of rifampicin is such that, with the concurrence of the patient's own cell-mediated immunity, the infection will be overcome.

3. For patients with multibacillary forms of leprosy already undergoing treatment with dapsone alone, interventionist therapy should be used. These patients are probably already harboring potentially dapsone-resistant organisms (mutants). They should be given a six-month course of monthly rifampicin (600 mg) and clofazimine (300 mg), together with daily dapsone (100 mg).

The purpose of these recommendations is to minimize the risk of the emergence of dapsone-resistant organisms, and thereby reduce the bacterial load so that the numbers of drug-sensitive "persisters" will pose virtually no threat of relapse after treatment has been completed.

Notes on drugs used: Rifampicin is mycobactericidal, and kills 99.98 percent of leprosy bacilli within a few days. The monthly dose now advocated has proved as effective as daily doses, and is not followed by the side effects that complicate intermittent dosage. *Clofazimine* (Lamprene, Geigy; B 663) is an excellent second-line drug, which has mycobacteriostatic activity as well as anti-inflammatory properties when given daily in lepromatous leprosy. *Dapsone* (diaminodiphenylsulfone, DDS) is still a most useful drug in all varieties of leprosy. It is mycobacteriostatic when given in standard doses. It is relatively free from side effects, can be safely given by mouth for long periods, and is inexpensive. *Acedapsone* (DADDS, Hansolar), given by intramuscular injection every 75 days, releases into the bloodstream an amount of active sulfone equivalent to an oral dose of about 3 mg daily. Because of the low serum concentrations obtained, it is recommended that when acedapsone is given, it should be supplemented by daily oral dapsone.

The acute exacerbation of lepromatous leprosy (erythema nodosum leprosum and its accompanying or following complications) is treated by rest and sedation. If this simple regimen does not succeed, then the condition may yield to antimonials or antimalarials. For most physicians confronted with such a patient, the easiest line of treatment is to give corticosteroids at the outset, in adequate dosage, and to reduce the dose as rapidly as possible, keeping at bay the signs of the acute phenomena in skin, nerves, and eyes.

In the case of tuberculoid leprosy, especially when the risk of damage to neighboring underlying nerves is considerable (as in the facial nerve, in the presence of a skin lesion on the cheek), adequate doses of corticosteroids should be given.

It should be remembered that clofazimine is not only a mycobacteriostatic drug in leprosy, but also it has anti-inflammatory properties, preventing the appearance of erythema nodosum leprosum if given as a treatment for lepromatous leprosy. It is also useful when given as treatment for established acute exacerbation. It may be given in doses up to 300 mg daily, but this dose should not be given for more than one month.

Thalidomide has a proven action in controlling the clinical manifestations of the hypersensitive state in lepromatous leprosy; it has no antileprotic properties.

The surgical complications of untreated or neglected leprosy are now receiving much attention, but they cannot be considered here in detail. Orthopedic and plastic procedures may be indicated, including operations for drop and flail foot, tendon transfer in the hand, sling operations on the eyelids for lagophthalmos, relief of severe nerve pain by longitudinal incision of the fibrous sheath, as well as operations for deformed nose, gynecomastia, madarosis, sagging face, unsightly earlobes, wasted thumb webs, persistently enlarged and visible great auricular nerves, etc.

The question of shoes (molded microcellular rubber insoles, on a rigid sole) and appliances and artificial limbs is beyond the scope of this article.

Physiotherapy and vocational training are part and parcel of the modern treatment of leprosy.

The recognition and treatment of the psychological accompaniments of leprosy, the provision of sympathetic care and understanding, and the avoidance of social dislocation and the evils of institutionalization are as much part of the "treatment" of the leprosy patient as is the education of the laity about leprosy.

Course and prognosis

The typical course of the different kinds of leprosy having been summarily dealt with under the appropriate heads, it remains to underline the extremely wide variation in the course and prognosis of the disease. Between patients showing a tendency to self-healing, on the one hand, and those facing the prospect of relentless progress of the disease, on the other, is the mass of leprosy sufferers who could be cured through early diagnosis and proper treatment. Lepromatous leprosy may sometimes reduce a healthy young man to a sick, pain-racked skeleton in a few short years, but treatment entirely changes this grim outlook.

In the best conditions, a leprosy infection can be eradicated and neurologic complications completely prevented. Even when the treatment of a patient with lepromatous leprosy has been started too late to prevent nerve damage and resultant deformities, much may be recuperated. Surgery may restore usefulness and dignity to the most deformed and neglected patient.

Prophylaxis and prevention

For the medical attendant and those in constant close contact with "open" cases of leprosy, the ordinary standard precautions of washing the hands with soap and water several times during a morning's clinic, for instance, will suffice to prevent contagion. When operating on infected tissues or taking smears from the skin or nasal mucosa, the physician should wear gloves and mask. A protective coat is also indicated. No medicinal prophylactic is recommended.

The value of BCG vaccination as a prophylactic measure against leprosy is still in dispute, the evidence from well-conducted trials in Uganda, Burma, and Papua New Guinea being equivocal. However, since BCG vaccination is of value in protecting children from tuberculosis, it may have some nonspecific effect in enhancing potential cell-mediated immunity against leprosy challenge.

There is also evidence that regular administration of dapsone for some years to child contacts of "open" cases of leprosy will reduce, by a similar proportion of about three-quarters, the number of new cases.

Since both investigations are still proceeding, it is not yet possible to make a more definite statement or recommendation. Many theoretical questions still remain unanswered, and the whole subject bristles with immunologic and practical difficulties.

Under the guidance of the WHO, and especially its IMMLEP Committee, much work is proceeding through cooperating laboratories in several countries on the production of a specific and safe vaccine. Utilizing armadillo-derived leprosy bacilli and a variety of related mycobacteria, research workers hope to find a mixture of antigens that will stimulate (or even create) specific cell-mediated immunity against leprosy.

Bibliography

Shepard CC: The experimental disease that follows the injection of human leprosy bacilli into foot-pads of mice. *J Exp Med* **112**:445, 1960

World Health Organization Expert Committee on Leprosy: First report. *WHO Tech Rep Ser* **71**:1, 1953

World Health Organization Expert Committee on Leprosy: Second report. *WHO Tech Rep Ser* **189**:1, 1960

World Health Organization Expert Committee on Leprosy: Third report. *WHO Tech Rep Ser* **319**:1, 1966

World Health Organization Expert Committee on Leprosy: Fourth report. *WHO Tech Rep Ser* **459**:1, 1970

World Health Organization Expert Committee on Leprosy: Fifth report. *WHO Tech Rep Ser* **607**:1, 1977

World Health Organization Report of Study Group: Chemotherapy of leprosy for control programmes. *WHO Tech Rep Ser* **675**:1, 1982

Section 27

Fungal Diseases with Cutaneous Involvement

CHAPTER 181

MYCOLOGIC INFECTIONS

J. Blake Goslen and George S. Kobayashi

SUPERFICIAL DERMATOPHYTOSES

Mycology

Background

The dermatophytes are a group of taxonomically related fungi capable of colonizing keratinized tissues such as the stratum corneum of the epidermis, nails, hair, the horny tissues of various animals, and the feathers of birds. As a consequence of this predilection for keratin, these organisms are referred to frequently as the "keratinophilic fungi." Keratin, however, is not an essential metabolite for these fungi and the reasons for their selective colonization of tissues containing this protein are unknown.

While there is very early documentation that these organisms produce disease in humans, their systematic study began only about 150 years ago when Remak described the mycelial nature of the clinical disease favus. This observation was later supported by Schoenlein. Clearly, the most significant report to follow was that of Gruby, who in 1841 isolated the organism of favus in culture and experimentally produced disease in normal skin. From an historical point of view, Gruby's studies preceded by almost four decades the work of Koch and the formulation

of his criteria for assessing the etiology of infection. Despite this early start, the study of medical mycology did not witness the accelerated scientific advances seen in bacteriology and for the next 40 years the major activities were rather pedestrian. The scientific literature from this period was characterized by a series of disorganized and incomplete descriptions of fungi found in association with skin infections. At about the turn of the century, the systematic studies of the dermatophytes by Raymond Sabouraud began to appear. Sabouraud was credited with bringing order to the chaotic situation that existed with the taxonomy of the dermatophytes. He recognized four genera of dermatophytes based on cultural and microscopic features of the fungi along with clinical aspects of the diseases they produced. The culmination of this work was published in his classical treatise *Les Tiegnes* in 1910. Unfortunately, this period of time was again followed by a period during which numerous species of dermatophytes were described, based mostly on their trivial morphologic differences. In 1934 Emmons critically reviewed the taxonomic status of the dermatophytes. In summary he accepted only three genera, *Microsporum*, *Trichophyton*, and *Epidermophyton*, and defined each of them according to the systematic rules of nomenclature and taxonomy. Further developments occurred in 1957 when Georg reexamined the work of Emmons and supplemented them with studies on nutritional and physiologic characteristics of the dermatophytes.

Other studies have emphasized various epidemiologic and ecologic aspects of the dermatophytes. For example, of the various species of keratinophilic fungi that have been described, several have been found only in soil and, while the potential may exist, most of them have not been reported as causing diseases in humans or animals. From an ecologic viewpoint these fungi are referred to as geophilic species represented by such organisms as *M. gypseum*, *M. fulvum*, and *T. terrestre*. Several species are found frequently in association with domestic and wild animals; they are called zoophilic species and include *M. canis*, *M. equinum*, *M. gallinae*, *M. nanum*, *T. verruccosum*, and *T. mentagrophytes* var. *mentagrophytes*. A third group has been found only in association with human beings. These are called the anthropophilic species and include *M. audouinii*, *T. rubrum*, *T. mentagrophytes*, var. *interdigitale*, *T. schoenleinii*, *T. tonsurans*, *T. violaceum*, and *E. floccosum*.

A recent development in the study of these organisms has been the observation that many of them have a sexual phase of reproduction. While these findings have obvious genetic implications, there have been few studies in this regard. Of the more than 20 species in which sexual reproduction has been observed (Table 181-1), all have been classified in either of two genera, *Nannizzia* or *Arthoderma* of the family Gymnoascaceae in the subdivision Ascomycotina. Without exception, the teleomorphic state (sexual) of species in the genus *Microsporum* has been *Nannizzia* and for the species of *Trichophyton* has been *Arthoderma*. The sexual phase of *Epidermophyton* has not, as yet, been discovered.

Mycologic Procedures

The presumptive diagnosis of superficial or dermatophyte infection should be supported by direct microscopic examination of clinical material and confirmed by culture of the specimen on suitable mycologic media. Clinical specimens must be properly collected in order to ensure the success of revealing fungal elements if they are present.

Direct microscopic examination

1. *Hair*: When the lesions involve hairy areas of the body such as the scalp and beard, examination by ultraviolet light emitted at 365 nm (such as the Wood's lamp) will frequently reveal hairs infected with various species of *Microsporum*, e.g., *M. audouinii*, *M. canis*, and *M. ferrugineum*. These can be plucked with a pair of tweezers for microscopic examination and seeded onto fungal medium for culture. Suspected hairs are placed on clear microscope slides in a drop of clearing solution.* A

coverslip is placed over the preparation and the specimen is examined by low-power (10× objective) microscopy. Infected hairs will appear as:

  a. An ectothrix infection characterized by a mosaic of round arthrospores surrounding the hair shaft as a sheath (Fig. 181-1);
  b. An endothrix infection characterized by round arthospores in a mosaic pattern contained within the hair shaft proper (Fig. 181-2); or
  c. A "favic" infection which is characterized by the linear arrangement of hyphal fragments, usually vacuolated, in chains along the longitudinal axis of the hair shaft (Fig. 181-3).
  Table 181-2 summarizes the type of parasitized hair caused by the various dermatophytes.

2. *Skin and nails:* Specimens from skin and nails are taken from the active margins of the lesion by scraping with the dulled edge of a scalpel or clean glass slide and deposited onto a clear microscope slide.

  A coverslip is placed over the collected debris and a drop of clearing solution (10% KOH and ink) is carefully placed on the edge of the coverslip. The solution should flow evenly beneath the coverslip by surface tension. The alkaline clearing solution will digest the proteins, lipids, and most of the other epithelial debris that are present but the fungal elements resist this treatment because of their chitinous cell wall. The clearing process can be hastened by gently heating the slide. In a positive preparation fungi will appear as septate and branching hyphal elements (Fig. 181-4). This only denotes that fungal elements are present. In order to identify the specific agent the organism must be cultured on suitable medium and examined accordingly.

Culture procedures

Definitive identification of the etiology of dermatophyte infections rests solely on the macroscopic, microscopic, and, in some cases, the physiologic characteristics of the organism. For these reasons, clinical specimens must be cultured on media suitable for growth of these fungi. Sabouraud's dextrose agar† is the most commonly used medium in medical mycology and serves as the basis for most of the morphologic descriptions of these fungi. Unfortunately, saprophytes grow rapidly and well on this medium and since they frequently contaminate body surfaces from which clinical specimens are taken, they will overgrow any pathogens that may be present, thus making it difficult to isolate and identify pathogens. To circumvent this problem, chloramphenicol (0.05 g/L) and cyclohexamide (0.4 g/L) are usually incorporated into Sabouraud's dextrose agar to make the medium highly selective for the isolation of dermatophytes. The chloramphenicol inhibits bacterial growth and the cyclohexamide inhibits most saprophytic fungi. The medium is available commercially as Mycosel or Mycobiotic medium. Cultures should be maintained at

---

* The clearing solution consists of 10% KOH made up in Parker Super Quink permanent Blue Black Ink. (Swartz JH, Lamkins BE: *Arch Dermatol* **89**:149, 1964). When KOH is added to the ink, an amorphous precipitate forms. This can be removed by centrifugation (2000 rpm/10 min). The clear supernatant fluid should be stored in a plastic bottle to prevent formation of insoluble carbonates.

---

† Sabouraud's dextrose agar, formulation:
  Dextrose 40 g
  Peptone 10 g
  Agar 20 g
  Distilled water adjusted to pH 5.5 1000 ml

Fig. 181-1 Microscopic examination of ectothrix type hair involvement with arthrospores outside of hair shaft.

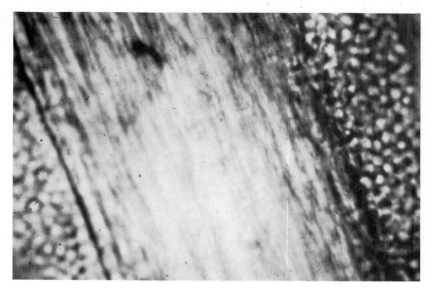

Fig. 181-2 Microscopic examination of endothrix type hair invasion.

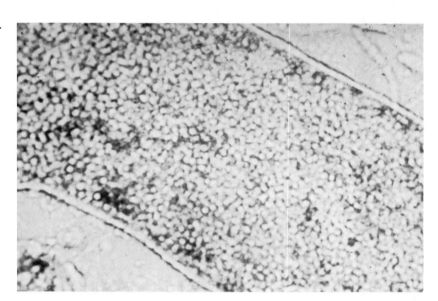

Fig. 181-3 Favic hair invasion due to _T. schoenleinii_.

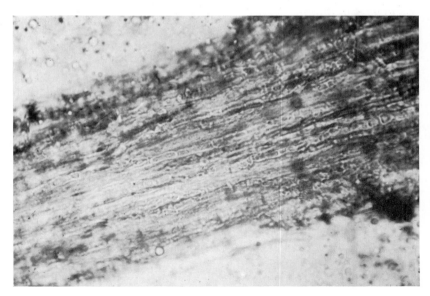

Table 181-1   Sexual state of dermatophytes*

Imperfect state (Deuteromycotina)	Perfect state (Ascomycotina)
Microsporum gypseum	*Nannizzia incurvata*
M. nanum	*N. obtusa*
M. gypseum	*N. gypsea*
M. fulvum	*N. fulva*
M. persicolor	*N. persicolor*
M. vanbreuseghemii	*N. grubyia*
M. canis	*N. otae*
M. cookei	*N. cajetani*
Trichophyton simii	*Anthroderma simii*
T. mentagrophytes	*A. benhamiae*
T. mentagrophytes	*A. vanbreuseghemii*
T. ajelloi	*A. uncinatum*
T. terrestre	*A. lenticularum*
T. gloriae	*A. gloriae*
T. georgiae	*A. ciferrii*

* Nomenclature of imperfect state (left column) and corresponding nomenclature of perfect state (right column).

Table 181-2   Parasitized hairs

Ectothrix	Endothrix	Favic
M. audouinii	*T. tonsurans*	*T. schoenleinii*
M. canis	*T. violaceum*	
M. ferrugineum		
M. gypseum		
M. nanum		
T. verrucosum		
T. mentagrophytes		

room temperature (26°C) for up to 4 weeks before they are discarded as showing no growth.

Identification and speciation of the dermatophytes require careful observation of gross colonial morphology and microscopic examination of properly prepared samples. The number of species of dermatophytes is large and for proper identification one should rely on a suitable reference source. An excellent treatise is the manual *Dermatophytes, Their Recognition and Identification*, Revised Edition, by Gerbert Rebell and David Taplin, University of Miami Press, Coral Gables, 1979.

The remainder of this chapter is a discussion of the various clinical disorders caused by the superficial fungi and the dermatophytes.

Tinea nigra

Definition

Tinea nigra is an asymptomatic superficial fungal infection of the stratum corneum caused by *Exophiala werneckii*. Lesions usually appear as brownish-black, nonscaly macules on the palm.

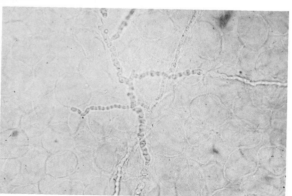

Fig. 181-4   Ten percent potassium hydroxide preparation showing septate, branching hyphae of typical dermatophyte infection.

History

Early reports of tinea nigra were probably erroneous descriptions of tinea versicolor [1]. The first authentic description was by Cerqueira in 1891. Horta isolated the organism and named it *Cladosporium werneckii* [2]. Subsequently, the name was changed to *Exophiala werneckii* (Horta) v. Arx [3].

Etiology

Although the causative organism is *E. werneckii* in the vast majority of cases, there is some evidence that other species of dematiaceous fungi (*Stenella araguata*) may produce the same clinical picture [1]. The dematiaceous fungi reside in soil, sewage, decaying vegetation, and on wood or shower stalls in very humid environments [1]. Person-to-person transmission has been suspected, but occurs only rarely [4]. Yet, inoculation onto the skin of volunteers has resulted in clinical disease; in one case the incubation period may have been 20 years [5].

The disease is most commonly seen in tropical or subtropical areas (Central and South America, Africa, Asia). About 75 cases have been reported from North America since 1950 [1]. Cases from Florida [6], Texas [7], and North Carolina [4] are well documented. With increasing awareness of the disease, more North American cases can be expected.

Clinical manifestations

The clinical lesion appears as a nonscaly, asymptomatic, mottled brownish or greenish-black macule on the palm or volar aspect of the fingers (Fig. 181-5). Bilateral plantar involvement [8] as well as concomitant palm and sole involvement have been reported [6]. The lesion gradually spreads centrifugally and may darken, especially at the border. The color resembles a silver nitrate stain.

Laboratory findings

Tinea nigra is readily diagnosed by a 10% KOH examination of a scraping from the lesion. On microscopic examination, brownish or olive-colored hyphae and budding cells are seen. The hyphae are septate and freely branching, ranging from 1.5 μm to 5 μm in diameter. Oval to spindle-shaped yeast cells, 3 × 10 μm in size, occur singly or paired, separated by a cross wall that is centrally located.

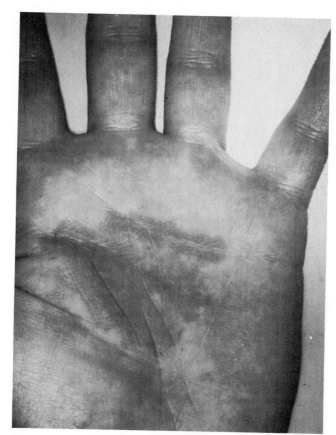

Fig. 181-5   Typical clinical presentation of tinea nigra palmaris showing an irregular, brownish-black macule on the palm.

Pathology

Skin biopsy shows hyperkeratosis without dermal inflammation. Hyphae are noted readily by H&E stain, but can be stained selectively with a Gomori methenamine silver preparation. Branched, brown hyphae are seen readily in the upper layers of the stratum corneum.

Diagnosis

Tinea nigra may sometimes be confused with melanocytic lesions (i.e., junctional nevi or melanoma). The importance of recognizing this differentiation is underscored by reports of unnecessary surgical removal of lesions in misdiagnosed cases of tinea nigra [9]. Other considerations in the differential diagnosis include pigmentation from Addison's disease, syphillis, pinta, or from a variety of chemicals or dyes. All of these entities are readily excluded by KOH examination.

Treatment and prognosis

Cure can be accomplished by the topical use of keratolytic and antifungal preparations such as Whitfield's ointment, topical 10% thiabendazole, tincture of iodine, or miconazole nitrate [1,10]. Griseofulvin is not effective. Treatment should be continued for 2 to 3 weeks to prevent recurrence [4].

Mycology

The organism can be isolated from clinical specimens on media containing chloramphenicol and cycloheximide where the growth is initially yeastlike and brownish to shiny black in color. Microscopic examination of these cultures reveals the typical two-celled, yeastlike morphology. As the culture ages, mycelial growth predominates. Aerial hyphae develop on the surface of the pigmented colonies giving the appearance of a fuzzy, grayish-black growth. Microscopic examination reveals deeply pigmented thick septate hyphal cells, 7 to 10 μm in diameter.

Tinea versicolor (pityriasis versicolor)

Definition

Tinea versicolor is a superficial, chronically recurring fungal infection of the stratum corneum characterized by scaly, hypo- and hyperpigmented, irregular macules usually located on the trunk and proximal extremities and caused by *Pityrosporum orbiculare* (*Malassezia furfur*).

History

In 1846, Eichstedt first recognized tinea versicolor as a fungal infection. In 1889, Baillon [11] originated the name *Mallassezia* to distinguish this yeastlike organism from the *Microsporum* species of dermatophytes. Gordon [12] first isolated the causative organism from lesional and normal-appearing skin. In 1961, Burke [13] produced clinical disease after inoculation of the organism on the skin of normal subjects. More recently, *M. furfur* and *P. orbiculare* have been found to be the same organism by immunologic and ultrastructural studies [14–16].

Etiology and pathogenesis

P. orbiculare is a dimorphic, lipophilic organism that grows in vitro only with the addition of a medium-chain fatty acid (C12–C24) source [17]. The organism is culturable from normal as well as lesional skin and, hence, can be a member of the normal skin flora [18]. Under appropriate conditions it converts from the saprophytic yeast to the pathogenic, mycelial phase. The latter is associated with clinical disease. Factors thought to be responsible for this transformation include a warm, humid environment, an inherited predisposition, endogenous or exogenous Cushing's disease, immunosuppression, or a malnourished state [13,19,20]. Tinea versicolor, therefore, represents an opportunistic infection. Experimentally, infection can be induced in rabbits and normal human volunteers by inoculation under occlusion. The associated rise in humidity, temperature, and CO_2 tension is responsible. When the occlusive state is terminated, self-healing occurs. The organism, however, is not eradicated from the skin and can be cultured from clinically resolved areas [21]. It may also colonize follicular structures. For these reasons, a high clinical recurrence rate is expected.

Although *P. orbiculare* is common in sebum-rich areas of skin and at an age when sebum production is high, no

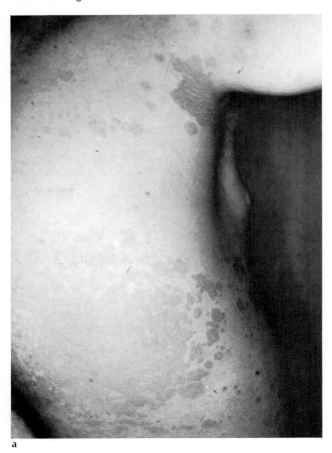

a

Fig. 181-6   Fawn-colored lesions of tinea versicolor in typical locations.

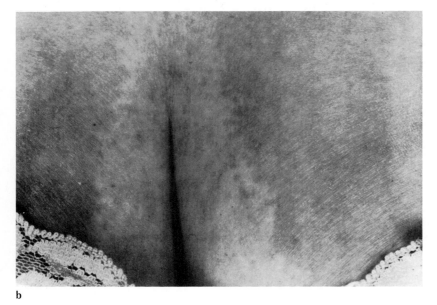

b

consistent differences in surface lipid composition between patients and controls have been found [22].

Clinical features

Clinical infection with *P. orbiculare* may take three forms: (1) papulosquamous lesions, (2) folliculitis, and (3) inverse tinea versicolor.

In the most common presentation, scaly hypo- or hy-perpigmented macules are observed in characteristic areas (e.g., chest, back, abdomen, and proximal extremities) (Figs. 181-6 and A1-34). Less common areas of involvement include the face, scalp, and genitalia. The characteristic scale is described as dustlike or furfuraceous. It can be produced by lightly scraping the fingernail over the involved area (the "fingernail sign") [23]. The color of the lesions varies from almost white to reddish brown or fawn-colored. The presenting complaint is usually a cosmetic

Fig. 181-7 Hypopigmented lesions of tinea versicolor.

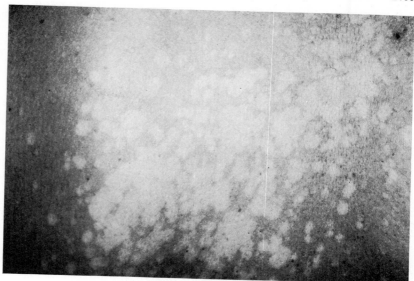

one as lesions often fail to tan with sun exposure. Pruritus is mild or absent.

The cause of the hypopigmentation is unclear (Fig. 181-7). Ultrastructural studies have shown an abnormality of melanosome number and packaging, with hypopigmented areas demonstrating a decreased number of individually dispersed melanosomes [24]. Also, extracts from *P. orbiculare* cultures have been found to contain C9-C11 dicarboxylic acids that may competitively inhibit tyrosinase [25]. In dark-complexioned children a severe, rapidly spreading variant may occur (achromia parasitica). Lesions usually begin in the diaper area and are markedly hypopigmented [19].

Pityrosporum folliculitis is a well-recognized and often misdiagnosed clinical entity [26]. Lesions typically appear on the back, chest, and sometimes on the extremities. Pruritus is more common than with typical tinea versicolor. The primary lesion is a perifollicular, erythematous, 2- to 3-mm papule or pustule. Only by appropriate culture and KOH examination can it be distinguished from a bacterial folliculitis. Frequently, biopsy with special stains for fungus is necessary. Diabetes mellitus, prior corticosteroid or antibiotic therapy can predispose one to this disorder [27]. Inverse tinea versicolor refers to clinical disease located predominantly in flexural areas [28]. In this location, lesions can be confused with seborrheic dermatitis, psoriasis, erythrasma, candidiasis, and dermatophyte infections.

Rarely, *P. orbiculare* can infect organs other than the skin. A premature infant on total parenteral nutrition with Intralipid supplementation has been reported who showed no skin lesions but had an extensive vasculitis of small pulmonary arteries and bronchopneumonia [29]. *P. orbiculare* organisms were seen microscopically in areas of lipid deposition. The organism has also been cultured from peritoneal dialysate and blood (also in a patient receiving parenteral Intralipid supplementation) [30]. Presumably, Intralipid provided an appropriate culture medium for the *Pityrosporum* organism.

All of the clinical variants have an equal sex distribution and tend to flare during warmer weather. Late adolescent and early adult age groups are predominantly affected. Small children and elderly patients are infected only in

unusual circumstances (e.g., prolonged occlusion or an immunosuppressed state) [28,31].

Immunology

Immunologic data are scarce in tinea versicolor. Elevated specific antibody titers are seen in patients and also in age-matched normal controls [32]. A defect in lymphokine production by patients with chronic tinea versicolor has been demonstrated [33]. Complement activation via the alternative pathway has been demonstrated in vitro with *P. orbiculare* but the significance of this finding remains unclear [34].

Laboratory findings

The organism is readily identified in 10% potassium hydroxide (KOH) preparations. Alternatively, cellophane tape can be used to pick up scale from the lesion. The tape is mounted on a glass slide with methylene blue, and the organism is selectively stained [35]. Microscopically, grapelike clusters of yeasts (4 to 6 μm) and short, septate hypae ("spaghetti and meatballs") are seen (Fig. 181-8). Culture is not necessary for diagnosis. A Wood's lamp examination may show yellowish fluorescence of involved skin.

Pathology

The organisms are seen in the stratum corneum. They may be observed with H&E stain alone. Periodic acid-Schiff staining is confirmatory. There is usually no dermal infiltrate. In *Pityrosporum* folliculitis organisms are noted in widened follicular ostia admixed with keratinous material. Rupture of the follicular wall can occur with a resulting mixed inflammatory cell and foreign-body giant cell response. Organisms can occasionally be identified in the perifollicular dermis.

Diagnosis

The clinical appearance of tinea versicolor is usually characteristic and KOH examination is confirmatory. Occa-

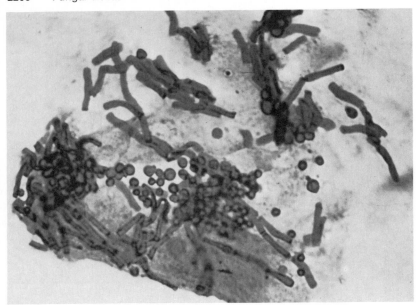

Fig. 181-8 "Spaghetti and meatballs" appearance of tinea versicolor on KOH examination.

sionally, pityriasis alba, confluent and reticulated papillomatosis of Gougerot and Carteaud, pityriasis rosea, seborrheic dermatitis, vitiligo, or secondary syphilis can enter into the differential diagnosis.

For the folliculitis variant, bacterial or candidal folliculitis should be considered. The skin lesions of disseminated candidiasis can sometimes be confused with *Pityrosporum* folliculitis [36].

Treatment

There are multiple topical products that are useful in treating tinea versicolor. The most widely used has been 2.5% selenium sulfide lotion. This can be applied on a variety of schedules. We prefer to apply it liberally over and beyond the affected areas. This is left on for 5 to 10 min and then washed off. The cycle is repeated every day for 2 weeks. Subsequently, we recommend applying the drug 1 or 2 times per month to prevent recurrence. Other topical agents that have been used include miconazole 2%, clotrimazole 1%, tolnaftate, 25% sodium thiosulfate, sulfur-salicylic acid soaps or shampoos (Sebulex) [37], or keratolytic agents such as 50% propylene glycol [38].

Griseofulvin is not helpful in this condition, but ketoconazole has been used successfully [39]. It is not necessary to give ketoconazole for the usual case of tinea versicolor. However, the drug may be useful prophylactically in a dose of 200 to 400 mg once or twice a month [40].

Course and prognosis

Tinea versicolor is often recurrent. Prophylactic measures as discussed above and fastidious cleanliness may lessen the risk of recurrence.

Mycology

Sabouraud's dextrose agar overlayed on the surface with olive oil or lanolin readily supports the growth of this lipophilic, yeastlike organism. Antibiotics such as penicillin, streptomycin, and cycloheximide are incorporated into this medium when primary clinical specimens are cultured to reduce growth of contaminating organisms. Microscopic examination reveals oval budding yeast cells ca. 2.5 × 3.5 μm in size (Fig. 181-8). In general, cultures are not necessary for diagnosis since the organism can be demonstrated with ease in skin scrapings treated with 10% potassium hydroxide.

Piedra

Definition

Piedra is an asymptomatic fungal infection of the hair shaft caused by *Piedraia hortae* (black piedra) and *Trichosporon beigelii* (white piedra).

History

The disease was reported initially by Beigel in 1865; however, he may have been describing an *Aspergillus* contaminant. The two diseases were distinguished by Horta in 1911.

Etiology

Black piedra is seen commonly in tropical areas of South America, the Far East, and the Pacific Islands. It is seen less frequently in Africa or Asia. For some cultures the infection is encouraged for social or religious reasons [41]. The scalp hair is the most commonly infected area.

White piedra is seen in temperate climates of South America, Europe, Asia, Japan, or the Southern United States [42]. Cases are more sporadic. Usually beard, mustache, or pubic hair is more commonly infected than is scalp hair [43].

In piedra the source of infection is unknown but related organisms can be found on animal hair, in soil, or in stagnant water [41].

Clinical manifestations

In black piedra, firmly attached, hard, brown-black nodules are present on the hair shaft. They vary in size from microscopic to a few millimeters and are gritty to feel. When the hair is combed a metallic sound may be heard [44].

In white piedra nodules are less firmly adherent and softer. They may vary in color from light brown to white.

Both forms of piedra may result in weakening of the hair shaft and subsequent breaks. Otherwise, the infections are asymptomatic.

There have been reports of disseminated infections with *T. beigelii* and other *Trichosporon* species [45–49]. These have occurred exclusively as opportunistic infections in an immunosuppressed host. Cutaneous manifestations of dissemination may include erythematous or purpuric papules or papulovesicles [50]. The responsible organism can be cultured from the skin lesions and seen in biopsy material [45].

Laboratory findings

When examined microscopically with 10% KOH, black piedra is characterized by nodules largely on the outside of the hair shaft. The periphery of the nodules shows aligned hyphae while the center consists of a packed, well-organized stroma of thick-walled cells (4 to 8 μm in diameter) that house the sexual (ascomycetous) phase of this organism. These are cemented together and the resultant structure has been termed "pseudoparenchyma" because of its resemblance to organized tissue [41,43].

The nodules of white piedra are soft in consistency, commonly intrapilar, and demonstrate less obvious external growth in comparison to black piedra. In contrast to *P. hortae*, *T. beiglii* grows in the asexual phase on infected hairs. The structure shows hyphae that are perpendicular to the hair surface and lack the organized appearance of black piedra [41–43]

Diagnosis

Microscopic examination readily distinguishes piedra from pediculosis, hair casts, monilethrix, trichorrhexis nodosa, and trichomycosis axillaris. In the latter case, smaller nodules (<1 μm) are seen, and the hairs may fluoresce under Wood's lamp examination.

Treatment

Shaving the infected hair is curative. Topical agents such as bichloride of mercury (1:2000), 3% sulfur ointment, and 2% formalin have also been advocated [41].

Mycology

P. hortae grows well on most laboratory media, but *T. beiglii* is inhibited by cycloheximide-containing media. Cultures of *P. hortae* grow slowly, have a dark brown to black pigmentation, and initially have a glaborous quality upon which develop aerial mycelia. Microscopic examination reveals septate hyphae, chlamydospores, and irregularly shaped hyphal elements. The asexual phase of this fungus is most frequently cultured from clinical material. The sexual (ascomycetous) phase which occurs on infected hairs, can be cultured only under various stringent culture conditions.

Clinical specimens of *T. beiglii* readily grow on Sabouraud's dextrose agar. The yeastlike growth is typically cream colored. As the colony ages, the surface growth develops furrows and convolutions that radiate out from the center. Microscopic examination reveals septate hyphae that readily fragment into arthroconidia, 3 to 7 μm in size. These cells rapidly take on an oval morphology and exhibit budding.

Dermatophytosis

Definition

Dermatophytosis represents a superficial infection of keratinized tissue caused by the dermatophytic fungi. In contrast, dermatomycosis refers to any fungal infection of the skin including the systemic or deep fungi that may have prominent cutaneous manifestations in addition to visceral disease.

History

The study of dermatophytosis has been aided by the superficial nature of its clinical manifestations. These infections have been described since the earliest historical accounts. "Tinea," a name which remains today, literally refers to an insect larva (clothes moth) that was felt by the Romans to be the cause of the infection [51].

In the 1800s, the work of a number of observers was culminated by the culture of the organism responsible for favus by Gruby [52] and the experimental production of disease by cutaneous inoculation of the mold.

In 1910 Sabouraud [53] published *Les Teignes* in which he classified the dermatophytes and made other clinical and therapeutic observations which remain accurate today. For this work, Sabouraud is justly considered the father of modern medical mycology.

In the 1920s, the scientific studies of the dermatophytes by Benham and Hopkins formed the foundations of modern-day medical mycology. Subsequent work by Emmons, Conant, Geary and others consolidated these efforts [51]. Finally, in 1959 the identification of the sexual stage of *T. ajelloi* led to taxonomic refinements that continue to assist in the scientific study of these organisms [54].

A major therapeutic advance in dermatophytosis occurred in 1958 with the development of griseofulvin [55]. The studies of Blank and colleagues solidified the role of griseofulvin in dermatologic therapeutics [56].

Epidemiology

The dermatophytes represent 39 closely related species in three imperfect genera: *Microsporum*, *Trichophyton*, and *Epidermophyton*. The perfect or sexual state has now been recognized for 21 of the dermatophytes. Cleistothecia, which are fruiting bodies or ascocarps, are formed through the conjugation of two compatible mating types and sexual spores or ascospores develop within these structures. The two perfect (sexual phase, telemorphic) genera are *Nan-*

Table 181-3 Ecology of dermatophytes

Geophilic	Zoophilic	Anthropophilic
(Microsporum boullardii)*	(M. amazonicum)	Epidermophyton
M. cookei	M. canis	floccosum
M. fulvum	M. distortum	M. audouinii
M. gypseum	M. equinum	M. ferrugineum
(M. magellanicum)	Trichophyton equinum	M. praecox
M. nanum	T. mentagrophytes	T. concentricum
	var. erinacei	
(M. racemosum)	(T. flavescens)	T. gourvilii
(M. ripariae)	T. gallinae	T. mentagrophytes
		var. interdigitale
M. vanbreuseghemii	T. mentagrophytes	T. megninii
T. ajelloi		T. rubrum
(T. georgiae)	T. mentagrophytes	T. schoenleinii
	var. quinckeanum	
(T. gloriae)		T. soudanense
(T. longifusum)	T. verrucosum	T. tonsurans
(T. phaseoliforme)		T. violaceum
T. simii		T. yaoundei
(T. terrestre)		
(T. vanbreuseghemii)		

* Organisms in parenthesis are not known to cause human disease.
Modified from Otcenasek [59].

nizzia and *Arthroderma* in the subdivision *Ascomycotina.* In general, *Nannizzia* corresponds to the *Microsporum* imperfect state and *Arthroderma* corresponds to *Trichophyton.* No perfect state has yet been found for the genus *Epidermophyton.* The existence of a perfect state for many of the dermatophytes has allowed a more precise classification and identification of these closely related fungi [57]. For example, mating studies have been used to clarify the origin of certain isolates of *T. mentagrophytes.* The inflammatory and often incapacitating *T. mentagrophytes* infection present in many U.S. soldiers in Vietnam [58] was of a single mating strain endemic in that area and not in the United States. Hence, the infections were acquired in Vietnam—a finding that provided valuable epidemiologic data [51]. As the dermatophytes evolve toward human parasitism, their ability to form a perfect state is diminished.

Although 39 species of dermatophytes have been identified, only a few are responsible for most human infections [51]. Many of the other species are soil-inhabiting keratinophiles with little tendency to infect humans. Thus, an important concept in understanding dermatophyte infections is a knowledge of their ecology, that is, whether the particular species in question resides predominantly in the soil (geophilic), on animals (zoophilic), or on humans (anthropophilic). This concept provides a useful classification of these organism (Table 181-3).

Geophilic organisms are adapted for soil habitation. These fungi sporadically infect humans and when they do, the resulting disease is usually inflammatory. *M. gypseum* is the most common geophile isolated in human infections. Although soil isolates of *M. gypseum* are of low virulence, strains cultured from humans are more virulent and account for epidemic spread of the infection under appropriate conditions [60–62].

Zoophilic species primarily infect higher animals but can be transmitted to humans sporadically. The zoophiles may have specific animal hosts largely because of a special affinity for the keratin of these hosts [59]. Infections often occur in rural areas where animal contact is likely. Do-

mestic animals and pets, however, are becoming an increasing source for these infections (i.e., *M. canis* in cats or dogs) in urban areas [63]. Transmission may occur through direct contact with a specific animal species (Table 181-4) or indirectly by infected animal hair carried on clothing or contaminated stalls, barns, or feed. Exposed areas of the body are favored sites of infection (i.e., scalp, beard, face, arms). Interestingly, although human infections with zoophiles are often suppurative, animal infection may be clinically silent. Under these conditions animals serve as asymptomatic carriers and, thereby, underscore the unique adaptation that these organisms have for their animal hosts [59–61].

Anthropophilic species have adapted away from soil or animal reservoirs and infect humans. Unlike the sporadic geophilic and zoophilic infections, anthropophilic infections are often epidemic in nature. They are transmitted from human to human either by direct contact or indirectly through fomites. In contrast to zoophilic infections, anthropophilic organisms may produce a relatively noninflammatory infection, often located on covered areas of the body (i.e., feet, groin). The chronic *T. rubrum* infections that occur in certain individuals are examples of the tolerance that can exist for this anthropophilic equilibrium with the host.

Yet, not all anthropophilic infections are noninflammatory [51,64,65]. Because of differences in susceptible hosts or strain virulence, markedly inflammatory reactions can occur. Kerion formation, suppuration or other manifestations of inflammatory tinea can facilitate early diagnoses in these cases. Noninflammatory disease, on the other hand, fosters the existence of a clinically silent "carrier" state that serves to delay the diagnosis and propagate the infection.

Host differences play a role in the epidemiology of anthropophilic infections. Not only are intercurrent diseases of the host important (e.g., dermatophytosis may be more severe or recalcitrant to therapy in patients with diabetes mellitus [66,67], lymphoid malignancies [68], immunologic

Table 181-4   Animal hosts for zoophilic dermatophytes

Organism	Animal hosts*
M. canis	Dog, cat, cattle, sheep, pigs, rodents, monkeys
M. distortum	Dog, cat, horses, monkeys
M. equinum	Horses
T. equinum	Horse, dog
T. mentagrophytes var. erinacei	Rodents (hedgehogs)
T. gallinae	Fowl, rodents, cat
T. mentagrophytes var. mentagrophytes	Cat, dog, cattle, sheep, pigs, horses, rodents, monkeys
T. verrucosum	Dog, cattle, sheep, pigs, horses

* Italics indicate the usual or preferred host.

compromise [69], or Cushing's syndrome [70]), but other factors including age, sex, race [64], habits, geographic location [71–73], and genetic background [74] should be addressed.

For example, children are the population at risk for anthropophilic tinea capitis [60,75–77]. In one study black male children appeared to be particularly susceptible [64]. In adults, however, tinea capitis due to anthropophilic organisms—especially T. tonsurans—is rare and when it occurs in the United States is largely confined to blacks or Hispanics. These differences hold true even after socioeconomic factors are considered. It is clear, at least for tinea capitis, that an age-dependent incidence applies [64]. When other dermatophytoses (tinea pedis, tinea unguium, or tinea cruris) are considered, however, the reverse prevails.

In a similar manner, sexual differences play a role in susceptibility to dermatophyte infections. Overall, there appear to be fewer overt anthropophilic infections in females [64]. This may be explained partially by their less frequent exposure to an environment conducive to the spread of the organism (i.e., athletic organizations, military service, etc.). When these factors are equalized, the incidence of tinea in women approaches that in men. Yet, even with this adjustment, tinea cruris remains predominantly a male dermatophytosis. Trichophyton tinea capitis, when occurring in adults, is far more common in women [78].

It is well known that the type of dermatophytosis present may vary depending on geographic location [71–73]. Multiple factors are responsible for this fact. Certain strains of dermatophytes are endemic to specific geographic areas (Table 181-5). Because of patterns of travel to and from these areas, resident dermatophytes may either remain restricted geographically or become more cosmopolitan. T. yaoundei, T. gourvillii, and T. soudanense, for example, are found only in Central and West Africa. T. concentricum—the causative organism of tinea imbricata—is found chiefly in the South Pacific [51]. Yet, with time these relationships may change. Earlier in this century, M. audouinii was the predominant cause of tinea capitis in the United States. In the last 10 to 15 years, T. tonsurans has assumed that role. The spread of this infection appears to correlate well with the ingress of Mexican and Puerto Rican immigrants to this country [75,77]. With the facility of world travel that is now possible, infections caused by geographically restricted dermatophytes may be seen more and more frequently in other areas of the world [79].

Furthermore, it appears that dermatophytes indigenous

to certain areas of the world have adapted themselves to their human hosts in these areas and vice versa. In Vietnam, U.S. combat personnel often acquired a disabling, inflammatory, zoophilic T. mentagrophytes infection. South Vietnamese soldiers, under similar environmental conditions, however, did not become infected with this organism. Presumably, adult Vietnamese had acquired a resistance to the infection [80]. Often infection seen in the resident population is chronic and noninflammatory while the same infection in virgin hosts is markedly inflammatory and self-limited.

The location of the dermatophytosis is partially dependent on climatic conditions of the area and the customs of the resident population. Tinea pedis, for example, is more common in areas where occlusive footwear is used [59]. In locations where the inhabitants wear sandals or go barefoot, the infection is markedly less common. In a similar fashion, tinea capitis is impeded in areas where the population uses hair oils [71,72]. The hair oil may, in fact, be inhibiting the initiation of the infection. In extremely hot, humid climates, tinea corporis may occur readily under occlusive garments [60,81,82].

Finally, there is some evidence to suggest that certain human populations may be genetically more susceptible to particular dermatophyte infections. T. concentricum is not transmitted readily to individuals of different races living with the susceptible population [51]. In fact, one study [83] has shown convincing evidence of an autosomal recessive inheritance for the susceptibility to this infection. Likewise, T. rubrum infections within a household favor relatives; conjugal pairs, in contrast, are less commonly infected even though environmental exposure to the organism is equivalent [74].

It is clear that the epidemiology of dermatophyte infections is dependent on many of the host factors discussed above. When the individual clinical infections are discussed later, these points will be expanded.

In addition to host and geographic factors, the virulence of the infecting organism must be considered. An important point is that strain to strain differences may exist for the same dermatophyte. The classic example is the difference between strains of T. mentagrophytes. T. mentagrophytes var. mentagrophytes is a zoophilic organism capable of producing a marked inflammatory infection in the human host. Its granular culture differs from the anthropophilic downy variant, T. mentagrophytes var. interdigitale. The latter variant produces a rather noninflammatory infection. Interestingly, the differences that exist between these two

Table 181-5 Geographically limited species

Organism	Endemic region
M. nanum	Cuba
T. concentricum	Pacific Islands, Far East, India, Ceylon; areas of North, Central, and South America
T. ferrugineum	Africa, India, Eastern Europe, Asia
T. megninii	Portugal, Sardinia
T. soudanense	Central and West Africa
T. yaoundei	Central and West Africa
T. gourvilii	Central and West Africa
M. distortum	New Zealand, United States
T. equinum	Western Europe, Canada, United States
T. ajelloi	Certain areas of North and Central America, Europe, Japan, Australia

Adapted from Ajello [72].

variants are alterable. Virulence may be enhanced by passage of the organism through a series of infections on guinea pigs. As the virulence is enhanced, the culture characteristics also are modified—to the granular pattern [61,84]. A similar phenomenon is postulated for different T. rubrum strains [61].

Pathogenesis

How a dermatophyte infection is initiated and maintained provides information that can be useful in understanding the clinical manifestations of these infections. Much of these data have come from experimentally induced infections [85]. It takes more than just a large inoculum of fungal organisms to initiate clinical disease. Studies of experimental tinea pedis by Baer and Rosenthal [86,87] demonstrate that volunteers who immersed a foot in water teeming with T. rubrum or T. mentagrophytes failed to get an active infection unless the foot was first traumatized. Hence, the presence of a suitable environment on host skin is of critical importance in the development of clinical dermatophytosis [88]. In addition to trauma, increased hydration of the skin with maceration is important. Occlusion with a nonporous material increases the temperature and hydration of the skin and interferes with the barrier function of the stratum corneum. Natural occlusion produced by wearing nonporous shoes definitely contributes to the development of tinea pedis [59,60]. In tropical climates, nonacclimatized subjects often develop lesions of tinea corporis, in part because of occlusive clothing [60,81,82].

If the host skin is inoculated under suitable conditions, there follow several stages through which the infection progresses. Although initially described for tinea capitis, these stages apply to most superficial dermatophyte infections [51,89,90]. The stages include a period of incubation and then enlargement followed by a refractory period and a stage of involution.

During the incubation period a dermatophyte grows in the stratum corneum, sometimes with minimal clinical signs of infection. A carrier state has been postulated when the presence of a dermatophyte is detected on seemingly normal skin by KOH examination or culture. Controversy exists in the literature regarding the importance of the carrier state [91–94]. In tinea capitis, for example, an asymptomatic carrier state has been found in 5 to 10 per-

cent of cultured scalps in a population of school children in an endemic area [95]. In another study, dermatophytes were cultured not only from clinically apparent areas of infection but also from normal-appearing skin up to 6 cm from the margin of the lesion [96]. These findings suggest that during the early (i.e., incubation) phase of dermatophyte infections, organisms are present but are clinically silent. This does not account for all the presumed "carriers," however, for only a limited number of these patients will develop clinical disease during a several-month follow-up period [95]. These individuals presumably represent true carriers.

Once infection is established in the stratum corneum, two factors are important in determining the size and duration of the lesion. These are the rate of growth of the organism and the epidermal turnover rate. The fungal growth rate must equal or exceed the epidermal turnover rate or the organism will be shed quickly [88].

Labeling indices done from various sites in an annular dermatophytic lesion revealed a fourfold increase in epidermal turnover at the inflammatory rim of the lesion [97]. In other areas of the lesion the labeling index was comparable to that of normal skin. It appears that the inflammatory response at the rim of the lesion stimulates an increased epidermal turnover in an effort to shed the organisms. However, lag periods undoubtedly exist between the initiation of the infection, the host inflammatory response, and the increased epidermal turnover. Therefore, probably only the organisms at the inflammatory rim are being shed while those just ahead maintain the infection. The annular appearance of most dermatophyte infections is compatible with these findings. The center of the lesion has relatively few organisms in contrast to the "battleground" of the peripheral rim. In chronic infections (i.e., chronic T. rubrum infections), inflammation is often minimal. Presumably, a suppressed delayed-hypersensitivity response by the host results in less inflammation which, in turn, leads to a lowered epidermal turnover rate in the lesion. A chronic area of infection would then result [88].

The affinity of dermatophytes for keratin is the sine qua non of their existence. Interestingly, different species of dermatophytes are attracted to different types of keratin. T. rubrum, for example, seldom attacks hair but frequently involves nails and glabrous skin. E. floccosum rarely involves nails and never infects hair [98]. Presumably, differences in the type of keratin and/or differences in the organism's ability to metabolize this material account for these findings.

Keratinases and other proteolytic enzymes are produced by dermatophytes [98,99]. The role of these enzymes in the pathogenesis of clinical infection is not totally understood. There is evidence that actual enzymatic digestion of keratin may be occurring [100,101]. In one study, such enzymes resulted in epidermal-dermal separation [102]. In Vietnam, U.S. soldiers developed a particularly inflammatory T. mentagrophytes infection. Many of these organisms produced elastase and there was a significant correlation between inflammation and elastase production [58]. The obvious conclusion of these studies is that not only the immunologic response but also enzymes or toxins produced by the organism account for some of the clinical findings in dermatophytoses [103].

On the other hand, there is evidence, at least in in vitro

studies, that keratin is not the ideal medium for supporting dermatophyte growth [97]. Furthermore, using a surface skin biopsy technique, certain investigators have found that dermatophytes prefer to spread between horn cells of the stratum corneum rather than through them as might be postulated in a keratin digestion process [104].

The pathogenesis of dermatophytosis is, therefore, not totally understood. Other factors are probably involved that have not yet been elucidated. The host's role in these infections is undoubtedly additive to the points made above and should be discussed separately.

Immunology

The immunology of dermatophyte infections has been studied thoroughly in recent years. Excellent reviews have been written by Emmons et al [105], Ahmed [106], and Grappel et al [107]. Nevertheless, our understanding of this area is still incomplete.

Resistance to dermatophyte infections may involve non-immunologic as well as immunologic mechanisms [108]. For example, a natural resistance to tinea capitis caused by *M. audouinii* exists after puberty. Rothman et al [109] have attributed this resistance to the increase in fungistatic and fungicidal long-chain, saturated fatty acids that occurs after puberty. In addition, a substance known as serum inhibitory factor (SIF) appears to limit the growth of dermatophytes, under most circumstances, to the stratum corneum [110–112]. This substance is not an antibody but is a dialyzable, heat-labile component of fresh sera [110]. Unsaturated transferrin is a likely SIF candidate [113]. Transferrin binds the iron that dermatophytes need for continued growth [114]. An α_2-macroglobulin keratinase inhibitor has also been identified in sera and may function to modify the growth of the organisms [115].

The importance of SIF is underscored by observations during the induction of experimental infections that skin traumatized mildly—not producing oozing or serous drainage—will support a subsequent fungal inoculation [85]. Yet, when trauma is overly zealous and weeping of tissue fluids occurs, the experimental inoculum fails to grow [89]. Furthermore, a patient described by Blank et al [116], who had a low titer of SIF, developed a widespread granulomatous *T. rubrum* infection—ostensibly due to the SIF deficiency.

The consensus of most investigators is that the humoral limb of the immune system has a minor role in the development of acquired resistance to dermatophyte infections [105–108]. Infection produces precipitating, hemagglutinating, and complement-fixing IgG, IgM, IgA, and IgE antibodies [117]. However, these antibodies are not species-specific and cross-react with other dermatophytes and saprophytic fungi including the airborne molds [107,118]. The antibodies have also been found to cross-react with the human blood group A isoantigen [119] and the intercellular substance of the epidermis [120,121]. Studies on the pathogenesis of chronic dermatophyte infections have cited these latter cross-reactions as evidence of how immunologic tolerance can occur in dermatophytosis [106]. Chronic *T. rubrum* infections and dermatophytids have been accompanied by complement-fixing and precipitating antibodies [108]. Their role in the pathogenesis of these disorders is not known. In fact, hyperglobulinemia E is probably contributory to chronic infections as will be discussed below [122].

The major immunologic defense mechanism in dermatophyte infections is the type IV delayed hypersensitivity response [105–108,123,124]. This is best illustrated during the course of human experimental infections [125]. When patients, who have not been previously infected with a dermatophyte, are experimentally infected with *T. mentagrophytes*, the initial response is one of slight inflammation and scaling. At this time the trichophyton skin test is negative. Between 10 and 35 days into the infection, the site abruptly becomes inflammatory and pruritic. Repeat trichophyton skin testing at this time is positive. After the development of cell-mediated immunity, the infected area becomes less inflammatory and eventually spontaneously involutes. If a second infection with the same organism is produced in the same subject at a later time, the site becomes inflammatory very early on and resolves relatively quickly. With the previous sensitization the recall of delayed hypersensitivity to trichophyton is brisk. Organisms are less often demonstrated in these secondary reactions [108].

A plausible mechanism by which the delayed hypersensitivity response may cause dermatophyte inhibition has been proposed by Jones et al [125] and others [126,127]. During the host's first exposure to the trichophyton cell wall [128,129] glycopeptide antigen [107,108], the antigen diffuses from the stratum corneum to stimulate sensitized lymphocytes. Inflammatory mediators and lymphokines are produced by these cells and probably act on the host cells rather than on the dermatophyte. Because of this response, the epidermal barrier is abrogated and SIF gains access to the otherwise privileged layers of the stratum corneum. SIF is fungistatic and so the cell-mediated immune response typically leads to inhibition but not complete destruction of the dermatophyte. Hence, the organism is still identified in cultures and KOH preparations of the infected area. The greater the inflammation, however, the fewer the number of organisms that can be found. In most circumstances, therefore, the cell-mediated immunity that exists is relative rather than absolute [125,126].

The use of the intradermal trichophyton skin test has identified two groups of patients based on the types of reactions ensuing from this test. Immediate (20 min) and delayed (48 h) reactions have been noted. The latter appears to correlate best with an active delayed-hypersensitivity response resulting from an acute infection with dermatophytes. On the other hand, patients showing immediate reactions often (75 percent) have chronic infections, most commonly with *T. rubrum* [106,107,130–132].

The entire question of chronic dermatophyte infections deserves special consideration. Chronic infections are characterized clinically by relatively long-standing, widespread disease, often with palmar and plantar involvement with little or no associated inflammatory response. There is often a negative delayed trichophyton skin test but a positive immediate one. The causative organism is usually *T. rubrum* typically resistant to therapy with griseofulvin [133,134]. When other organisms are found, there may be a higher incidence of serious underlying disease (i.e., diabetes, hypercortisolism, lymphoma, etc.) [133] (Table 181-6). As many as 50 percent of patients chronically infected with *T. rubrum* may have associated atopy

Table 181-6 Conditions associated with chronic dermatophytoses

	Reference
Atopy	[108,122]
Cushing's disease	[70]
Diabetes mellitus	[67]
Drugs (corticosteroids)	[133]
Immunodeficiency diseases	[108,135]
Familial endocrinopathies	[108]
Peripheral vascular disease	[133]
Disorders of keratinization	[108,133]
Collagen vascular disease	[133]
Tumors (lymphoma, thymoma, Kaposi's sarcoma)	[68,108,136]
Chronic mucocutaneous candidiasis	[133,137]

[106,122,130,131,138]. They usually have an elevated IgE serum level [124,139]. In vitro lymphocyte transformation studies in these patients often reveal a selective failure to respond to trichophyton antigen while mitogen responses remain intact [130,134,140,141].

There is evidence to suggest that patients with this "atopic-chronic-dermatophytosis syndrome" are capable of delayed-hypersensitivity skin test reactions, but these reactions are inhibited by the more sensitive, preceding type I response [122]. Evidence to support this conclusion stems from studies in which intradermal chlorpheniramine and trichophytin injected simultaneously are able to uncover an otherwise suppressed delayed skin test response [139]. In addition, other studies have demonstrated the antagonistic effects of histamine on the cell-mediated immune response [142–144]. This finding has important therapeutic relevance as the use of an H_2 histamine blocker (cimetidine) may prevent this antagonism and ultimately enhance the patient's own delayed-hypersensitivity reaction [145].

Dermatophytid reactions are an important part of the discussion of dermatophyte immunology. These are secondary inflammatory reactions of the skin at a site distant from the associated fungal infection. In contrast to material obtained from the dermatophytosis, cultures and KOH examinations of the "id" lesions are negative. Id reactions are usually accompanied by a reactive delayed trichophyton skin test. The mechanism responsible for the id response is unknown but may involve a local immunologic response to systemically absorbed fungal antigen [105–108,146].

Clinically, id reactions may take several forms [147] (Table 181-7). These reactions tend to occur at the height of the dermatophyte infection or slightly thereafter. They also may occur commonly just after initiation of systemic antifungal therapy [149]. The incidence of ids in an unselected patient population with dermatophytosis has been found to be 4 to 5 percent [64,107]. Disappearance of the dermatophytid reaction occurs when the dermatophyte infection is successfully treated. Occasionally, concomitant topical or systemic steroid therapy is warranted in addition to griseofulvin—especially if the dermatophytid is extremely widespread or inflammatory.

Clinical types

Tinea capitis. DEFINITION. Tinea capitis is a dermatophytosis of the scalp and associated hair that is caused by a variety of species of the genera *Microsporum* and *Trichophyton*. *Epidermophyton* species have not been associated with the disease.

EPIDEMIOLOGY. The true incidence of tinea capitis is unknown. Epidemics have occurred in the United States, but infection rates have ranged between only 5 to 20 percent of the population at risk [153]. The source of an infection depends on whether the causative organism is geophilic, zoophilic, or anthropophilic (see above). These factors also play a part in determining the degree of clinical inflammation. The anthropophilic organisms maintain their virulence in human-to-human transmission, thereby allowing epidemicity to be a prominent feature of these infections [60]. The specific organisms involved will be discussed below.

The patients most commonly affected are children between the ages of 4 and 14 years [60]. Adult infections are more unusual but do occur, especially when the causative organism is a species of *Trichophyton*.

Many studies have demonstrated a significant male predominance in infections caused by the *Microsporum* organisms. With *T. tonsurans* the male:female infection rate is equal in childhood [153–155], but favors females in adulthood [156–158].

In many cases, especially with inflammatory infections or in infections with *M. audouinii*, the disease is self-limited and seldom extends beyond puberty. *T. tonsurans* infections can also be self-limited [94]; however, they have been felt to extend into the adult population more commonly than *M. audouinii* [159].

In some series blacks and Hispanics have been found to have a higher incidence of tinea capitis, especially that caused by *T. tonsurans* [153,154]. Whites are affected more commonly with *Microsporum* species [154].

Some of these differences can be explained by the fact that transmission of certain forms of tinea capitis is fostered by the existence of overcrowding or poor personal hygiene. Low socioeconomic conditions and, in one report, protein malnutrition [160] have also been implicated. It is clear that organisms responsible for tinea capitis can be cultured from brushes, combs, caps, pillow cases, theater seats, and other inanimate objects. The disease can also be transmitted from child to child through exposure at schools or day care centers. Affected hairs can harbor infectious organisms for a year or more after they have been shed from the host [161,162]. As mentioned previously, overcrowding improves the chances for transmission. In several reports, the rate of the infection appeared to vary directly with the size of the family unit [60]. On the other hand, there are cases in which individuals are spared who have had ample exposure to the disease.

The existence of an asymptomatic carrier state in tinea capitis has been repeatedly documented. The finding has important epidemiologic implications, as silent sources of

Table 181-7 Types of dermatophytids

	Reference
Follicular papules	[148]
Erythema nodosum	[149]
Vesicular id of hands and feet	
Erysipelas-like	[150]
Erythema annulare centrifugum	[151]
Urticaria	[152]

Table 181-8   Classification of organisms causing tinea capitis

Species	Ecology	Geographic distribution
Ectothrix		
Microsporum:		
M. audouinii	Anthropophilic	Cosmopolitan
M. canis	Zoophilic	Cosmopolitan
M. gypseum	Geophilic	Cosmopolitan
M. fulvum	Geophilic	South America; rare in United States
M. ferrugineum	Anthropophilic	Africa, India, Asia, South America
Trichophyton:		
T. mentagrophytes	Zoophilic, anthropophilic	Cosmopolitan
T. rubrum	Anthropophilic	Cosmopolitan
T. verrucosum	Zoophilic	Cosmopolitan
T. megninii	Anthropophilic	Europe
Endothrix		
Trichophyton:		
T. tonsurans	Anthropophilic	Cosmopolitan
T. violaceum	Anthropophilic	Cosmopolitan
T. soudanense	Anthropophilic	Central and West Africa
T. gourvilli	Anthropophilic	Central and West Africa
T. yaoundei	Anthropophilic	Central and West Africa
T. schoenleinii	Anthropophilic	Europe, Near East, Mediterranean; rare in United States

infection are more difficult to detect and eradicate. In one report, school classes that had clinically affected members also had a 12 to 30 percent rate of asymptomatic carriers. In school classes without clinical disease the rate dropped to 1 to 5 percent [163].

ETIOLOGY AND PATHOGENESIS. Virtually any species of *Microsporum* or *Trichophyton* can cause tinea capitis. Exceptions are *T. concentricum* and *E. floccosum*. The causative organisms can be classified according to their host preference (i.e., anthropophilic, zoophilic, geophilic) and according to whether they produce arthrospores outside or just under the cuticle of the hair (ectothrix) or within the hair (endothrix). These features are summarized in Table 181-8.

As can be seen, most of the dermatophytes causing tinea capitis are ubiquitous in their geographic distribution. Others such as *M. ferrugineum* and the African species *T. yaoundei*, *T. gourvillii*, and *T. soudanense* cause disease in a relatively limited geographic area. It is important for the clinician to be cognizant of the prevalent organism or organisms responsible for each dermatophytosis in his geographic area. Although these trends are relatively stable, they are not absolutely so and may change with time. An example is the case of tinea capitis in the United States. In the 1940s the most common cause for epidemic tinea capitis in the United States was *M. audouinii*. In the late 1950s, however, *T. tonsurans* began to appear increasingly in the Southwest as the primary cause of this infection. Now it is the most common cause of tinea capitis in this country [77,154,157]. *M. audouinii*, on the other hand, has inexplicably dropped from view. Similarly, changes in the frequency of certain organisms can be expected to occur elsewhere, perhaps facilitated by the ease of world travel. Rarely, tinea capitis can be caused by a mixed infection of two or more dermatophytes, and this may serve to confuse the clinical picture [164–166].

The pathogenesis of tinea capitis has been studied by Kligman [89,90] and others. Hair appears to be susceptible to ectothrix dermatophytes during mid to late anagen. The infection usually begins in the perifollicular stratum corneum. Following a period of incubation, hyphae generally spread into and around the hair shaft. They descend the follicle and penetrate the midportion of the hair. Subsequently, hyphae descend within the intrapilary portion of the hair until they reach the border of the keratogenous zone. Here they continue to grow in delicate equilibrium with the keratinization process, so that they proceed no deeper than the upper limit of the keratogenous zone. The hyphae never enter the nucleated zone and, therefore, appear to discern the subtle differences between the partially keratinized and the fully keratinized hair. In this location the terminal tuft of hyphae is termed Adamson's fringe. Intrapilary hyphae proliferate and divide into arthrospores that reach the cortex of the hair and are transported upward on its surface. When the hair is plucked it breaks at its weakest point, just above Adamson's fringe. When the plucked hair is visualized microscopically, therefore, it is the numerous ectothrix spores that are seen rather than the intrapilar hyphae.

With endothrix infections (i.e., *T. tonsurans*), the same process occurs until the hair is penetrated. The arthrospores are formed rapidly and, with time, replace much of the intrapilary keratin while leaving the cortex intact. The hair is fragile, however, and with trauma breaks at its weakest point—the surface of the scalp where it loses the supporting follicular wall. When observed clinically the remaining hair in this infected follicle resembles a black dot and, hence, endothrix infections are often referred to as "black dot ringworm." A final important difference between endothrix and ectothrix infections is that endothrix infections may continue past the anagen phase of the hair cycle and into telogen. Therefore, these infections tend to be more chronic than those caused by the ectothrix organisms [65].

CLINICAL MANIFESTATIONS. The different organisms causing tinea capitis may present with several different clinical patterns [94,153–167] (Table 181-9):

Noninflammatory, human, or epidemic type. This clini-

Table 181-9   Organisms associated with clinical types of tinea capitis*

Inflammatory	Noninflammatory	"Black dot"	Favus
M. canis	M. audouinii	T. tonsurans	T. schoenleinii
M. gypseum	T. tonsurans	T. violaceum	T. violaceum
T. mentagrophytes	M. canis		M. gypseum
T. tonsurans	M. ferrugineum		
T. verrucosum			
T. schoenleinii			
M. audouinii			
M. nanum			

* Some organisms produce more than one clinical type.

cal pattern is produced most commonly by *M. audouinii* or *M. ferrugineum*. The lesion begins as a small erythematous papule surrounding a hair shaft. Subsequently, the lesion spreads centrifugally, involving all hairs in its path. Typically, there is scaling with minimal inflammation. One or more well-demarcated patches are seen usually on the occiput or posterior neck. Hairs in the infected area are gray and lusterless in appearance due to their coating of arthrospores ("gray patch" ringworm) (Fig. 181-9). They frequently break off just above the level of the scalp, rather than being shed entirely [167]. Occasionally, infections with *M. audouinii* may present with just a few scattered, infected hairs that cannot be detected without a Wood's lamp examination. Kerions may occur rarely (2 to 3 percent) and consist of an inflammatory, boggy mass studded with broken hairs and oozing purulent material from follicular orifices (Fig. 181-10) [168]. A kerion is the clinical manifestation of the host's cellular immune response to the organism.

Inflammatory type. In this form of tinea capitis there is significantly more inflammation present. These infections are caused most commonly by zoophilic organisms (e.g., *M. canis*) or geophilic dermatophytes (e.g., *M. gypseum*) [169]. Clinically, a spectrum of inflammatory changes may be seen ranging from a pustular folliculitis to kerion formation. These infections usually present with more subjective symptoms of pruritus, fever, and pain. There may

Fig. 181-9   Extensive infection and alopecia secondary to M. audouinii.

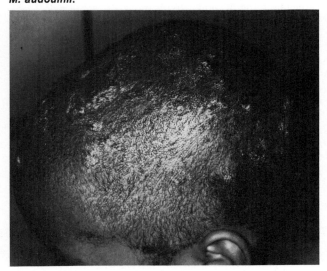

be associated regional lymphadenopathy. Occasionally, additional lesions are found on glabrous skin. Because of the degree of inflammation generated, scarring alopecia is often seen subsequently.

"Black dot" tinea capitis. This variety of tinea capitis is most often caused by endothrix organisms such as *T. tonsurans* or *T. violaceum*. Because of the location of the arthrospores, the hair shaft is extremely brittle and breaks at the level of the scalp. The remnant of hair left behind in the infected follicle appears as a black dot on clinical examination (Fig. 181-11). The appearance of this type of infection is variable [159]. There may be diffuse scaling with minimal hair loss or inflammation. In this circumstance, the infections can be readily confused with seborrheic dermatitis, atopic dermatitis, or psoriasis [170]. When hair loss occurs, the affected areas are characteristically multiple or polygonal in outline with indistinct, fingerlike margins [171,172]. This is in contrast to *M. audouinii* infections which usually appear as larger, solitary, annular patches. Within the areas of involvement, "black dot" infections commonly spare some hairs so that areas of alopecia are sprinkled with a few normal hairs. "Black dot" infections may also be quite inflammatory with changes ranging from a pustular folliculitis to furuncle-like lesions or obvious kerions [157]. Finally, "black dot" tinea capitis may present without obvious black dots, making a high index of suspicion for this infection imperative [75,170].

T. tonsurans also may infect glabrous skin or nails concurrently with scalp involvement [168]. In fact, these areas may be infected alone with complete sparing of the scalp [173].

LABORATORY FINDINGS. Laboratory confirmation of dermatophyte infections is imperative. Wood's lamp examination is valuable in infections caused by *M. audouinii*, *M. canis*, *M. ferrugineum*, or *M. distortum*. Here one typically sees a bright green band of fluorescence in the hair just above the level of the scalp. The examination can be positive only when a few hairs are infected. The fluorescence is thought to be produced by pteridines [174] generated as the fungus infects actively growing hairs [51]. Hairs infected in vitro do not appear to produce the substance. Rarely, Wood's lamp-negative variants of *M. audouinii* and *M. canis* are reported [168,175]. *T. tonsurans* infections typically do not fluoresce. In these instances, careful KOH examination and proper cultural techniques are crucial in making the correct diagnosis.

There are several methods of obtaining material suitable for culture or examination. One may scrape the infected scaly area with a #15 scalpel blade. In this maneuver

Fig. 181-10   Kerion on the occiput.

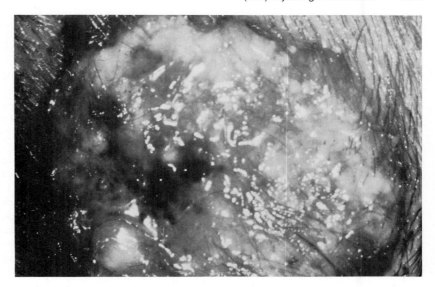

infected squames and portions of involved hair are recovered. In a similar manner, a sterile toothbrush may be used to recover infected material. The bristles of the toothbrush are then pressed directly into the appropriate culture medium. When large areas of scalp are involved—as in a seborrheic dermatitis-like presentation—a sterile plastic scalp massager can be used similarly [77,95,176]. In the case of the fluorescence-producing *Microsporum* species, the Wood's lamp may be helpful in locating individually infected hairs. These can then be plucked with epilating forceps and cultured directly. In "black dot" infections the remnant of infected hair should be extracted from the follicle, again with the use of epilating forceps or a Schamberg comedo extractor, and used for KOH examination and culture.

When examining infected hairs microscopically, 10% to 15% KOH is used. The architecture of the hair is maintained if the specimen is not heated. Hence, endothrix infections can be more easily identified. An examination technique described by Shelley and Wood [177] uses xylene as the mounting medium after the plucked hair(s) is

crushed. If the hairs are heavily pigmented, the melanin can be cleared partially by the use of 50% hydrogen peroxide.

Examination of the properly mounted specimen will demonstrate the type of hair parasitism involved. In ectothrix infections arthrospores are seen outside the hair shaft (Fig. 181-1); endothrix infections have intrapilar spores (Fig. 181-2). Hyphae can be seen within the hair in both types of infection.

Specimens obtained for culture should be inoculated on Sabouraud's dextrose agar with antibiotics and incubated at room temperature. The organism can be subsequently identified by colony characteristics and microscopic examination.

PATHOLOGY. In tinea capitis hyphae are identified both around and within the hair shaft. Special stains serve to emphasize their presence (i.e., PAS, methenamine silver). The dermis demonstrates a perifollicular mixed cell infiltrate with lymphocytes, histiocytes, plasma cells, and eosinophils. If follicular disruption has occurred, an adjacent foreign-body giant cell reaction is seen [178,179].

Fig. 181-11   "Black dot" ringworm secondary to *T. tonsurans.*

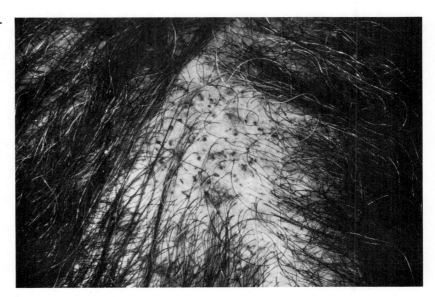

In the more inflammatory lesion (i.e., kerions), an intense dermal infiltrate is seen with polymorphonuclear leukoycytes forming abscesses in the dermis and within the follicle [153,179]. In these markedly inflammatory reactions fungal organisms are seen with difficulty. Immunofluorescence techniques, however, have demonstrated the presence of fungal antigens [180].

DIAGNOSIS. The differential diagnosis of tinea capitis includes seborrheic dermatitis, atopic dermatitis [170], and psoriasis when minimally inflammatory diffuse scaling is the major clinical presentation. When alopecia is more pronounced, diseases such as alopecia areata, trichotillomania, secondary syphilis, or pseudopelade can be entertained. Alopecia due to tinea capitis fails to produce the typical exclamation point hairs seen in alopecia areata or the artifactual-appearing areas with hairs of varying lengths seen in trichotillomania.

In inflammatory tinea capitis, bacterial pyodermas (furunculosis, impetigo) can be simulated. Folliculitis decalvans or perifolliculitis capitis abscedens et suffodiens can also enter into the differential diagnosis. After scarring has occurred, noninfectious processes such as discoid lupus erythematosus, lichen planopilaris, pseudopelade, or radiation dermatitis are often considered in the differential diagnosis.

THERAPY. Tinea capitis may resolve spontaneously. Rothman felt that *M. audouinii* infections cleared at puberty. However, more recent data indicate that these infections as well as many caused by *T. tonsurans* resolve within a year without therapy and with no relation to puberty. Inflammatory zoophilic and geophilic infections tend to resolve spontaneously in a period of time that varies inversely with the inflammation. Despite the data cited above, *T. tonsurans* and *T. violaceum* infections are more prone to be persistent into adulthood than are *M. audouinii* infections.

Tinea capitis should be treated with a systemic antifungal such as griseofulvin. The usual dose is 1.0 g/day of the microcrystalline variety or 0.5 g/day of the ultramicrosized drug. For children the dose is 10 to 12 mg/kg per day. Therapy should be continued until a clinical and cultural cure is obtained, usually 4 to 8 weeks. Although most griseofulvin therapy is conducted using daily doses, single megadose therapy has found support, particularly in economically deprived areas where access to physicians and medication is limited. In several reports, single doses of 3 to 5 g have yielded acceptable one-year cure rates for tinea capitis caused by *M. audouinii* [181,182]. Weekly treatment protocols have also been used successfully [183].

Occasionally, topical products are used in conjunction with systemic treatment. In one report the use of a selenium sulfide shampoo in conjunction with griseofulvin was curative while the griseofulvin alone was not [184]. Clearly, topical therapy alone is seldom successful.

In markedly inflammatory tinea capitis, oral corticosteroids may be helpful in reducing the incidence of scarring. The therapy is particularly helpful in the treatment of kerions. The usual dose of prednisone is 1 mg/kg per day given at one time in the morning.

When anthropophilic tinea capitis is identified, it is important to examine close contacts of the patient for evidence of disease. Segregation of infected children in school is not warranted if effective therapy is provided [153]. If zoophilic organisms are cultured, examination of pets (i.e., kittens, puppies) for evidence of dermatophytes is warranted. If infection is suspected, the pets should be treated.

Tinea favosa. DEFINITION. Tinea favosa or favus (L. honeycomb) is a chronic, mycotic infection of the scalp, glabrous skin, and/or nails characterized by the formation of yellowish crusts within the hair follicles (scutula) and eventuating in a cicatrizing alopecia.

EPIDEMIOLOGY. Favus is typically a chronic infection that begins early in life and commonly extends into adulthood [185]. The disease is seen predominantly in rural areas and often is associated with conditions of poor hygiene, malnutrition, and squalor. The infection is generally family-centered rather than school-centered as seen commonly with other tinea capitis-producing dermatophytes. A relatively intimate and prolonged contact is probably required for transmission [186].

Although favus is seen in families, generation after generation, attack rates within families can vary, suggesting that there may be an inherited susceptibility or resistance to the infection [167]. In addition, simple measures to improve personal hygiene in the at-risk population often result in markedly decreased transmission [187]. It is known that *T. schoenleinii* can survive for years on epilated hairs. For this reason, cleanliness with the removal of hairs or other sources of infection is an important factor in controlling the disease [161].

Although animal favus is known to occur, there is no evidence to substantiate the existence of an animal reservoir to explain human infections [187].

Sex differences do not seem to exist in the incidence of favus, except in those chronic infections extending into adulthood. Here, there is an increased number of females affected [168].

ETIOLOGY. The most common dermatophyte producing favus is *T. schoenleinii*. However, other organisms can produce a favus-like clinical picture (i.e., *T. violaceum*, *M. gypseum*). A variety of different organisms are known to produce animal favus [51].

Favus is commonly seen in certain geographic areas. In some of these locations it is the most common cause of tinea capitis [76]. The infection is endemic in the Middle East and Mediterranean basin area, Southeastern Europe, France, Southern Asia, and Greenland. In South Africa the disease is quite common and among the Bantu is referred to as "witkop" [51]. In the Americas endemic pockets of the disease exist. There are reports from areas of Quebec, the United States (Kentucky, West Virginia, Arkansas, New York) [153], Guatemala, and Brazil [51]. In many of these areas the infection can be traced to immigrants from endemic areas such as Russia or Poland. The disease is then passed on from generation to generation.

CLINICAL FEATURES. In the early stages of infection hyphae invade the hair follicle and gradually distend the follicular opening. Clinically, very little is seen within the first three weeks of infection except a slight amount of perifollicular scaling.

Scutula are found in most cases of favus. These concentrations of hyphae and keratinous debris take root at the opening of the hair follicle. Here, they gradually expand from a yellowish-red papule to form a yellowish, cup-shaped structure that may become 1 cm or more in diam-

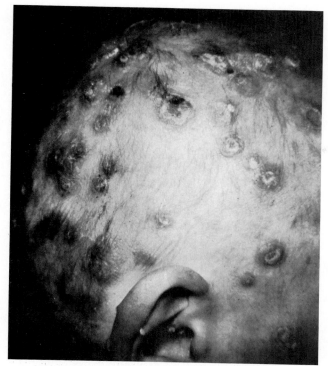

Fig. 181-12 Favus with scutula.

eter. The center of the scutulum is often pierced by a single, lusterless, dry hair (Fig. 181-12). The color is due to the invasion of the hair by multiple intrapilar hyphae. The hair is not as brittle as with *T. tonsurans* endothrix infections and, for that reason, hairs in favus may frequently attain a normal length. If the scutulum is removed from its attachment to the epidermis, an oozing, erythematous base is noted. Scutula may expand peripherally and, during the course of the infection, form large, adherent mats of scutula and hair. Hygienic conditions are particularly lacking in this stage of the disease and a characteristic "mousy" odor may be appreciated [51,57].

In the classic presentation, therefore, lesions appear in a patchy distribution on the scalp and with time coalesce. The borders of the infected lesions represent areas of advancing disease and are often polycyclic in shape [187]. The center of the infected area in time becomes extensively scarred and almost totally devoid of hair.

Besides scalp involvement, favus may involve glabrous skin and nails. The skin infections may be of various types (i.e., vesicular, papulosquamous, tinea circinata-like). Oftentimes true scutula are formed. Nail involvement occurs in 2 to 3 percent of infections [168] and is indistinguishable from onychomycosis due to other organisms [105].

In some cases, especially when personal hygiene is relatively good, favus lesions may be atypical in appearance [168,186]. For example, scutula may be small or absent and the disease may present with diffuse scaling of the scalp [168]. In these instances, the infection is difficult to distinguish from seborrheic dermatitis, psoriasis, or tinea amiantacea. In later stages of infection a cicatricial alopecia may be present. In this end stage presentation, the condition may be identical to that noted in cicatrizing alopecia after radiation or chemical injury or the scarring

alopecia seen in some cases of pseudopelade, folliculitis decalvans, lupus erythematosus, or lichen planopilaris.

LABORATORY FINDINGS. The laboratory diagnosis of favus requires the use of KOH examination and cultural techniques discussed previously. On microscopic examination an endothrix type of hair invasion is seen. The favus hair shows hyphae coursing lengthwise and no arthrospores [51,57]. Because of autolysis, vacant tunnels are formed within the hair and these may appear as air spaces microscopically [188] (Fig. 181-3).

With Wood's lamp examination a pale green fluorescence is seen along the entire length of the infected hair. The fluorescence may be subtle and can be difficult to appreciate, especially in patients with gray hair [57].

HISTOPATHOLOGY. Using histopathologic techniques, scutula show intermingled masses of mycelia, scale, and granular debris. The degenerating hyphae and necrotic material are seen most typically in the center of the scutulum while the viable organisms reside at the periphery. Under the scutulum there is an atrophic epithelium; acanthosis is noted at the lateral margins [178]. In the dermis an extensive chronic plasma cell or granulomatous perifollicular infiltrate is commonly seen and is particularly dense subjacent to the scutulum. No fungi are noted when the dermis is examined with special stains. Fragments of hair can be seen in the dermis, however, with polarized light. In the later stages of infection, the dermis may simply show fibrosis with a diminished inflammatory cell response.

THERAPY. Favus is effectively treated with griseofulvin in a dosage similar to that used in tinea capitis [189]. Nail infections require a longer course of therapy (6 to 12 months). It is important to examine and treat all affected family members simultaneously [51]. Improvement of hygienic conditions is also beneficial as are efforts to locally debride areas of extensive crusting.

Tinea barbae. DEFINITION. Tinea barbae (also known as tinea sycosis, "barber's itch") is a fungal infection limited to the coarse hair-bearing beard and moustache area of men. In women and prepuberal boys, infection in the facial areas (tinea faciale) is classified with the other glabrous skin infections [57].

EPIDEMIOLOGY. Tinea barbae is by definition seen only in males. Usually, the infection is contracted by exposure to animals, most commonly cattle and dogs. The infection is most often seen in a rural setting [51,57,190,194], oftentimes affecting dairy farmers or cattle ranchers. Prior to the introduction of modern-day antiseptic techniques, tinea barbae—then called barber's itch—was transmitted from person to person by contaminated barbers' razors or clippers [51].

ETIOLOGY AND PATHOGENEIS. Overall the most common dermatophytes causing tinea barbae are the zoophilic organisms—*T. mentagrophytes* and *T. verrucosum* [190,191]. *M. canis* is causative in a fewer number of cases [192]. Anthropophilic organisms (*T. rubrum*, *T. violaceum*, *T. schoenleinii*, and *T. megninii*) have been implicated in urban areas [193] or in areas where these fungi are endemic. In general, the infection caused by the anthropophiles is less inflammatory than that caused by the zoophilic dermatophytes.

The pathogenesis of tinea barbae, while not studied as carefully as tinea capitis, is thought to be similar to that of

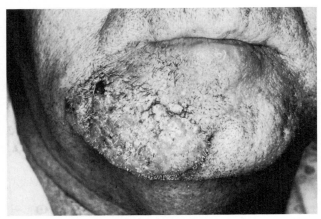

Fig. 181-13   A boggy, kerion-like *T. verrucosum* infection of the beard area.

the latter. Coarse hairs are uniquely susceptible; occasionally one may see concurrent involvement of the beard and scalp area [167].

CLINICAL MANIFESTATIONS. Three clinical types of tinea barbae have been recognized: (1) inflammatory or kerion-like; (2) superficial or sycosiform type [194]; and (3) the circinate, spreading type.

The inflammatory variety is analogous to kerion formation in tinea capitis (Fig. 181-13). In tinea barbae the lesions are usually unilateral; common areas of involvement are the chin, neck, maxillary and submaxillary areas. The upper lip is usually spared [51,195]. The inflammatory lesions are most often caused by *T. mentagrophytes* and *T. verrucosum*. Lesions are nodular and boggy; there is often an associated weeping of seropurulent material with subsequent crusting. Perifollicular pustulation is observed; coalescence of these inflammatory areas yields abscess-like collections of pus. The hairs within the infected areas are loose and easily epilated; commonly they are lusterless and brittle as well. Eventually, undermining and sinus tract formation can occur. Scarring and permanent alopecia is the ultimate outcome in severely affected areas.

The superficial type of tinea barbae more typically resembles a bacterial folliculitis. There is a diffuse erythema associated with perifollicular papules and pustules [194]. The organisms causing this clinical picture are the relatively noninflammatory anthropophiles. Hairs may be affected depending on the organism involved. For example, *T. violaceum* infections commonly result in brittle, lusterless hair due to endothrix invasion. Conversely, *T. rubrum* infections produce hair invasion less often.

The circinate tinea barbae is analogous to tinea circinata of glabrous skin. There is an active, spreading vesiculopustular border with central scaling. There may be a relative sparing of hair in this variant [194].

Atypical tinea barbae may also be seen, especially if the course of the disease is altered by corticosteroid or other therapy [168]. Infection caused by *M. canis* may demonstrate unusual clinical patterns. For example, in children, isolated involvement of the eyebrows may occur with this organism [51]. In addition, other authors have described infected granuloma annulare-like lesions or abscess-like tumors in patients infected with *M. canis* [196]. Finally, *E. floccosum* has been found to produce verrucous, granulo-

matous-appearing lesions on the face and body termed *verrucous epidermophyton* [195]. One must have a high index of suspicion for these dermatophyte infections so that atypical infections can be recognized.

LABORATORY FINDINGS. Epilated hairs or scale can be examined with 10% KOH as described for tinea capitis. Depending on the organisms involved, endothrix or ectothrix hair invasion can be seen as well as stratum corneum infections. Wood's lamp examination is useful only for infections by *M. canis* where a bright green fluorescence can be seen. Of course, cultures of the hair and infected squames should be done using Sabouraud's dextrose agar with antibiotics. In tinea barbae, epilated hairs may show a bulbous, white material surrounding the hair bulb; usually these hairs prove to be culture-positive.

PATHOLOGY. Histopathologic findings are similar to those seen in tinea capitis. Fungi are seen in the hair keratin and sometimes in the stratum corneum by using special stains. No organisms are seen in the surrounding dermis. Neutrophils may be seen within the hair follicle, but a chronic, sometimes granulomatous inflammatory response is noted perifollicularly. In extremely inflammatory lesions, fungi may be sparse or absent [179].

DIAGNOSIS. Tinea barbae should be differentiated from a bacterial folliculitis (sycosis vulgaris), perioral dermatitis, candidal infection, acneform dermatitis, pseudofolliculitis barbae, contact dermatitis, halogenoderma, or herpes simplex. A bacterial folliculitis is usually bilateral and may involve the upper lip. There can be more pain or fever in this instance than in tinea barbae [195]. The other entities mentioned can be differentiated by an accurate history and the use of such diagnostic procedures as patch testing, Tzanck smears, or viral cultures.

TREATMENT. As with tinea capitis, griseofulvin in a dose of 500 mg to 1 g per day (microsized) is used. Therapy is continued for 2 to 3 weeks after clinical resolution has occurred. Local measures such as topical antifungals, wet compresses, and debridement of crusted debris are additive. Occasionally, in severely inflammatory infections, a course of systemic corticosteroid therapy is helpful.

If no treatment is given, most inflammatory infections resolve spontaneously in a few weeks. Less inflammatory, superficial infections may, in contrast, persist for months [51,194].

Tinea corporis (tinea circinata). DEFINITION. Tinea corporis arbitrarily includes all dermatophyte infections of glabrous skin with the exclusion of certain specific locations (i.e., palms, soles, and groin).

ETIOLOGY. All species of dermatophytes belonging to the genera *Trichophyton*, *Microsporum*, or *Epidermophyton* are capable of producing tinea corporis. The three most common causative organisms are *T. rubrum*, *M. canis*, and *T. mentagrophytes*; however, variations may occur based on the existence of endemic species in specific geographic areas [63]. Oftentimes the prevalent organism causing tinea capitis in children in a certain geographic area is the organism producing tinea corporis in adults of the same region [51,167]. *T. concentricum* is the organism responsible for a variant of tinea corporis endemic in the Pacific Islands—tinea imbricata which is also known as Tokelau ringworm.

EPIDEMIOLOGY. The organism responsible for tinea corporis may be transmitted by direct contact with other infected individuals or by infected animals. It may also be transmitted from inanimate fomites such as clothing, furniture, etc. Although there is some controversy on this point, many authors feel that tinea corporis results from the transfer of infection from other involved sites on the same patient. Under appropriate environmental conditions (warmth, humidity) a reservoir of infection on the feet or elsewhere may be the source of tinea corporis [681,82]. Whether or not the infection originates in this manner, it is clear that a tropical or subtropical climate is associated with more frequent and severe tinea corporis.

Children appear to have an increased incidence of tinea corporis caused by zoophilic organisms. Many of these infections are with *M. canis* [195]. The organism is most likely transmitted by contact with pets (especially cats and dogs).

Tinea imbricata, caused by *T. concentricum*, has a unique epidemiology among the organisms causing tinea corporis. The organism is geographically limited to certain areas of the Far East, South Pacific, and South and Central America. Here a large proportion of the native population may be affected; interestingly non-natives may be spared even though they have resided in endemic areas for long periods. Like favus, tinea imbricata is probably contracted in early childhood and can persist for a lifetime [197]. There is some evidence that the susceptibility to tinea imbricata is hereditarily determined through an autosomal recessive trait [83].

PATHOGENESIS. The organisms responsible for tinea corporis generally reside in the stratum corneum (Fig. 181-14). Presumably, serum inhibitory factor is responsible for limiting the infection [110,111]. The pathogenic sequence of events has been outlined previously [51] (see "Dermatophytosis" above). The first step involves invasion of the stratum corneum, possibly with the help of warm, moist, occlusive conditions [198]. After a 1- to 3-week incubation period, centrifugal spread occurs. The active, advancing border of infection has an increased epidermal turnover rate [97]. Presumably, the host epidermis is attempting to shed the organism by increasing epidermal turnover to exceed the fungal growth rate. This defense mechanism is successful to a certain extent as there is relative clearing of infection in the center of the annular cutaneous lesion. Temporary resistance to reinfection occurs in this area for a variable time; however, second waves in infection are commonly seen later [51,57].

Most organisms causing tinea corporis are located superficially in the stratum corneum. Hair follicle involvement can occur—especially with *T. rubrum* or *T. verrucosum* [179]—and seems to be associated with increased inflammation [57]. Other correlates of increased inflammation are the type of organism (zoophilic or geophilic being more inflammatory) and the nature of the host response.

CLINICAL MANIFESTATIONS. Tinea corporis may be diverse in its clinical presentation [199–216]. Table 181-10 summarizes the clinical variants that can be seen along with distinguishing features of each. The most common presentation is the typical annular lesion with an active, erythematous and sometimes vesicular border (Fig. 181-15). Commonly, the center of the lesion shows clearing; yet, variations may occur (Fig. 181-16). The center often shows concentric rings in tinea imbricata and *T. rubrum* infections (Fig. 181-17). With *T. rubrum* large, confluent plaques of infection may occur [216] (Fig. 181-18). Polycyclic or psoriasiform lesions are also seen frequently. It is clear that a high index of suspicion should exist for tinea corporis. Any red, scaly rash deserves at least a thorough microscopic examination to exclude this entity.

Tinea corporis can occur on any area of the body. When the infection is due to a zoophilic organism, the lesions are commonly seen on exposed skin (head, neck, face, and arms). When such an infection occurs with *M. canis*, lesions may be unusually numerous for body ringworm. Tinea corporis due to anthropophilic organisms often occurs in occluded areas or in areas of trauma (i.e., perifolliculitis of the legs in women may be associated with leg shaving).

LABORATORY FINDINGS. Because clinical signs are variable in many cases of tinea corporis, the clinician must often rely on laboratory findings for the correct diagnosis.

In the usual lesion of tinea corporis—the spreading ring-

Fig. 181-14 Stratum corneum parasitism by a dermatophyte (PAS stain).

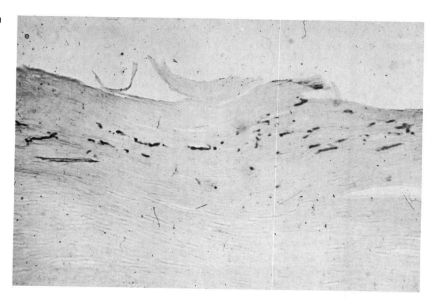

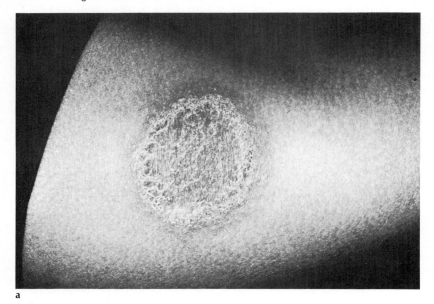

a

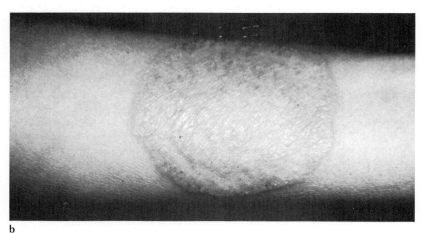

b

Fig. 181-15 Tinea corporis with typical ringworm-like lesions.

worm with the active, erythematous border—specimens for KOH examination should be obtained from the actively spreading border of the lesion. Here organisms are more numerous, and the chances of a positive examination are higher. One sees septate, branching hyphae in the stratum corneum (Fig. 181-4). If bullous lesions are present, the greatest numbers of organisms are found by examining the roof of the blister. Finally, if dermal granulomatous lesions occur, the greatest positivity on culture is obtained by using biopsy material as the inoculum [202].

It is important not to rely on KOH examination alone to prove or disprove the existence of a dermatophyte infection, particularly if the index of suspicion is high. In some reports the KOH examination is positive in only one-third of patients with tinea corporis [217]. Fungal culture is, therefore, imperative. Infected material should be inoculated on Sabouraud's dextrose agar with antibiotics even when direct KOH examination is negative. Four weeks of incubation at room temperature is required before the culture plates are discarded.

PATHOLOGY. Histopathologically, fungal organisms can be seen in the stratum corneum in the usual case of tinea circinata. With hematoxylin and eosin, they appear basophilic; with PAS, the fungal elements stain red; with silver methenamine, they stain black [179].

If organisms are not found, the histopathology is nonspecific and may resemble an acute or chronic dermatitis. If vesiculation is present, it is often seen histologically as a spongiotic vesicle. In the nodular perifolliculitis variant caused by *T. rubrum*, there is a perifollicular granulomatous reaction, often associated with central necrosis and suppuration. Organisms are seen in the hairs as well as in the dermis. Here, spores may be large (6 μm) and located within multinucleated giant cells [179].

DIAGNOSIS. The differential diagnosis of tinea corporis is variable because the clinical findings are, themselves, variable. In the usual annular ringworm infection, entities such as erythema annulare centrifugum (EAC), nummular eczema, and granuloma annulare (GA) should be considered. EAC generally shows scaling at the trailing edge of the advancing border; whereas, tinea corporis shows scaling over the entire advancing edge. In nummular eczema, lesions show eczematous change or crusting throughout the entire lesion; no central clearing is seen. Furthermore,

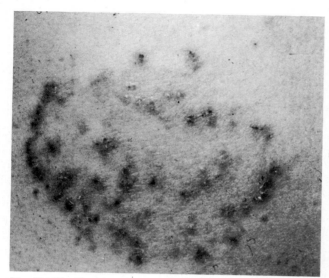

Fig. 181-16 Variant of tinea corporis showing spotty areas of vesiculation and crusting not limited to the peripheral rim of the lesion.

lesions tend to be more numerous and symmetrical than in tinea corporis. In GA, intradermal papules without significant epidermal change make up the border of the lesions.

If the clinical lesion is more papulosquamous in appearance, other typically papulosquamous entities can be considered (i.e., psoriasis, lichen planus, secondary syphilis, seborrheic dermatitis, pityriasis rosea, or pityriasis rubra pilaris). Most of the above conditions are readily distinguished by their characteristic clinical features as well as by biopsy.

For the inflammatory variants of tinea corporis, bacterial, candidal, or deep fungal infections enter the differential diagnosis. Verrucous and granulomatous lesions may mimic acid-fast infections or North American blastomy-

cosis. Deeper lesions may resemble bacterial abscesses, panniculitis, or nodular vasculitis.

Tinea faciale may resemble lupus erythematosus or dermatomyositis. The history of photoexacerbation in tinea faciale as well as the absence of a distinct raised scaly border are misleading [210]. Most tinea faciale lesions lack follicular plugging and the true poikiloderma of connective tissue diseases. Other entities to be considered include photodermatoses such as polymorphous light eruption, contact dermatitis, or acne rosacea.

TREATMENT. For isolated lesions of tinea corporis, topical agents such as miconazole nitrate 1%, clotrimazole 2%, and other topical imidazoles or ciclopirox olamine 1% are the most effective.

For widespread or more inflammatory lesion, griseofulvin is used in a dose equivalent to 500 mg to 1 g per day of the micronized drug. For serious infections not responding to griseofulvin, ketoconazole may be helpful (see "Therapy of Superficial Fungal Infections").

Tinea cruris. DEFINITION. Tinea cruris is a dermatophytosis involving the groin area and includes infections of the genitalia, pubic area, perineal and perianal skin [218–220].

EPIDEMIOLOGY. Tinea cruris is almost exclusively a male dermatophytosis [78]. The reasons for this preference may depend on several factors: (1) men wear more occlusive clothing than do women; (2) because of the scrotum, skin in the groin area of men may be subject to a greater area of occlusion; (3) in general, men are more physically active than women, and the groin may remain warm and moist for longer periods; (4) finally, there may be a greater incidence of other sites of dermatophyte infection in men (i.e., tinea pedis), which may function as a reservoir for new cases of tinea cruris [51,57]. Close direct or indirect physical contact does not appear to equalize the differences cited above. For example, in the examination of multiple infections within a single household, conjugal transmission is rare despite ample exposure to infectious material [74].

Fig. 181-17 Polycyclic pattern of tinea corporis.

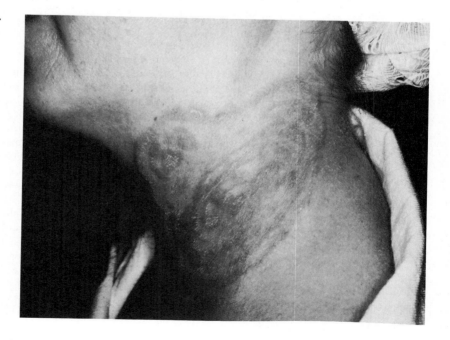

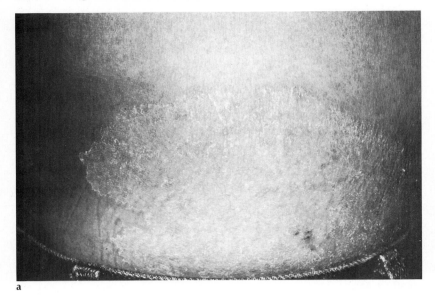

a

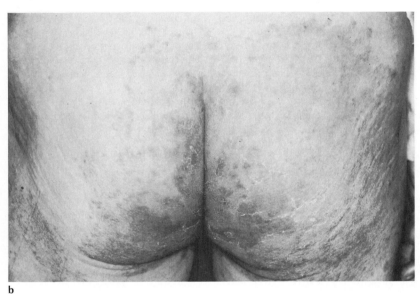

b

Fig. 181-18 Diffuse, confluent involvement characteristic of *T. rubrum* infections.

The transmission of tinea cruris may occur by several mechanism. Direct contact, between infected and noninfected individuals, may serve to transmit the disease in some cases. The role that trauma plays in colonization of uninvolved areas is implied but not fully appreciated. More commonly, however, indirect transmission can occur through contact with nonliving objects that carry infected scales. Cultures from items such as bed linens, towels, articles of clothing, and even bedpans and urinals have been positive for dermatophytes in situations where epidemic spread of tinea cruris is occurring [60,221]. The causative dermatophytes (especially *E. floccosum*) have been found to survive for long periods on shed squames [51]. These infected scales provide a difficult-to-eradicate source for future infections.

Environmental factors are important in the initiation and propagation of tinea cruris. It is well known that these infections occur more commonly in the summer months or in tropical climates where ambient warmth and humidity are highest. If occlusion from clothing or wet bathing apparel is added, an optimal environment for the initiation or recrudescence of this infection exists [51,57].

A final important epidemiologic consideration is the role played by dermatophytoses elsewhere on the body in providing a reservoir for autoinfection in tinea cruris. Other sites of infection may coexist with tinea cruris. The most common association is the tinea pedis and cruris caused by *T. rubrum* [222]. Many investigators feel that the feet are a likely source of the infecting organism in nascent cases of tinea cruris [51,218]. Others have implicated the scrotum in this reservoir role. Although clinical signs of scrotal infection in tinea cruris are minimal, organisms have been detected by microscopic examination and by culture in a surprisingly high percentage of scrotal specimens [223–225].

ETIOLOGY. The most common organisms causing tinea

Table 181-10   Variants of tinea corporis

Name	Causative organism(s)	Clinical description
Noninflammatory:		
Tinea circinata	Any dermatophyte (commonly *T. rubrum*, *T. mentagrophytes*, *M. canis*)	Annular lesions with central clearing and an active, spreading border
Bullous tinea corporis [199–201]	Usually *T. rubrum*	Spongiotic or subcorneal vesicles/pustules; may be herpetiform
Tinea imbricata	*T. concentricum*	Widespread; multiple concentric, polycyclic scaly lesions with minimal inflammation; there may be an increased immediate hypersensitivity and decreased cell-mediated immunity to trichophytin antigen [197]
Inflammatory:		
Kerion of glabrous skin [202]	Zoophilic organisms (usually *T. verrucosum* or *T. mentagrophytes*)	Similar to kerion of scalp
Majocchi's granuloma [203,204]	*T. rubrum, T. violaceum, T. tonsurans, T. mentagrophytes*	In Majocchi's original description the lesions were perifollicular, granulomatous nodules seen mostly on the scalps of children. They were often painless without pustulation, and often associated with underlying disease
Nodular granulomatous [203,204] perifolliculitis of the legs (Fig. 181-19)	*T. rubrum*	This variant of Majocchi's disease is characterized by lesions occurring in women on the lower two-thirds of the legs; the disease is often unilateral; *T. rubrum* is usually present elsewhere (nails, feet)
Agminate folliculitis [57]	Zoophilic organism	Well-defined, erythematous plaques studded with perifollicular pustules
Subcutaneous abscess (tinea profunda)	*T. mentagrophytes* [205], *T. violaceum* [206], *T. crateriforme, (tonsurans)* [207], *T. rubrum* [116], *M. audouinii* [208]	Deep subcutaneous nodules are present; there is rarely lymph node involvement [208] and associated hematogenous spread [209]
Mycetoma [208]	*M. audouinii, T. verrucosum, T. mentagrophytes, T. violaceum, T. tonsurans, M. ferrugineum, M. canis*	Subcutaneous masses
Either inflammatory or noninflammatory:		
Tinea faciale [209–212] (Fig. 181-20)	Usually *Trichophyton* species; occasionally *M. canis*	This disease represents 3 to 4% of tinea corporis; erythematous, scaly plaques with or without active borders are present; telangiectasia, atrophy, and photoexacerbation may mimic lupus erythematosus
Tinea incognito [57,213,214]	Any dermatophyte infection modified by corticosteroid treatment	Lesions are often atypical appearing; inflammation, scaling, and symptoms may be absent, or kerion-like lesions may occur; there are usually dermal nodules present.
Verrucous epidermophyton [135,215]	*E. floccosum*	Verrucous-like lesions are present on the head, neck, and buttocks; cutaneous anergy may be present
Miscellaneous and widespread infections	*T. rubrum* [122,131–133]	There is often atrophy and a selective CMI defect to trichophytin
	M. audouinii [69]	There may be an associated depressed CMI and a deficient plasma factor needed for lymphocytic blastogenesis

cruris are *E. floccosum*, *T. rubrum*, and *T. mentagrophytes*. Differences in the number of infections caused by each organism exist and depend on the prevalence of that organism in the population being surveyed. Interestingly, the groin is by far the most common site for infections caused by *E. floccosum*. The epidemics of tinea cruris reported in some series are caused predominantly by this dermato-

phyte [218,219]. Infections with other dermatophytes, such as species of *Microsporum*, have been reported but they are extremely rare [220].

CLINICAL MANIFESTATIONS. Pruritus is a common symptom; pain may be present if the involved area is macerated or secondarily infected. In classic tinea cruris, one sees bilateral but often asymmetrical involvement of the geni-

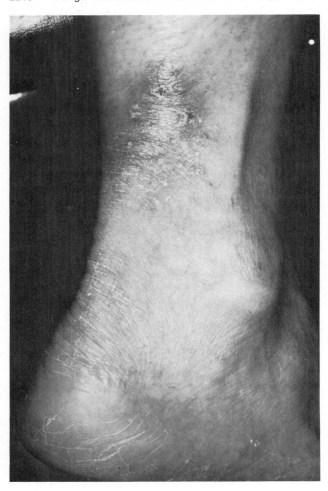

Fig. 181-19   Nodular granulomatous folliculitis of the leg caused by *T. rubrum*.

Fig. 181-20   Tinea faciale due to *M. canis*.

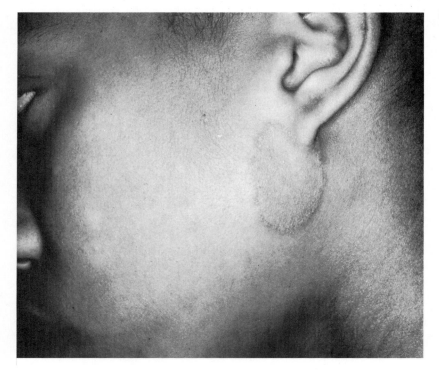

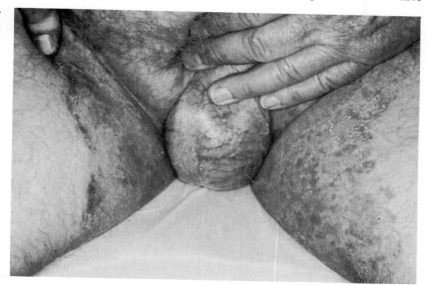

Fig. 181-21 Tineacruris. Note the more extensive involvement of the left medial thigh.

tocrural area and medial upper thigh (Fig. 181-21). Often the left thigh adjacent to the scrotum is the first site involved.

The clinical lesion (Fig. A1-17) is characterized by a well-marginated, raised border that may be composed of multiple erythematous papulovesicles. Rarely pustules may be seen at the border, but the satellite pustules typical of candidal infections are unusual (Fig. 181-22). The scrotum may appear completely normal or only minimally involved, even though microscopic examination and culture show the presence of organisms [224]. Candida, in contrast, often presents with obvious clinical disease on the scrotum or penis.

The two most common organisms causing tinea cruris may have differences in their clinical lesions. *E. floccosum* typically presents as described above with an active, spreading papulovesicular border and central clearing. The lesions seldom extend beyond the genitocrural crease and medial upper thigh. *T. rubrum* lesions, however, often coalesce and spread to involve wider areas of adjacent skin in the pubic, lower abdominal, buttock, and perianal areas (Fig. 181-18a) [51,57].

Secondary changes may complicate the clinical picture of tinea cruris. Chronic scratching may cause lichenification and present a lichen simplex chronicus-like picture. Secondary bacterial infection may obscure a more chronic tinea cruris. Weeping, maceration, and areas of pustulation may exist. Finally, a secondary allergic or irritant contact dermatitis may be present if sensitizing or irritating topical products have been used in treatment.

LABORATORY FINDINGS. As noted previously, infected scales examined by a 10% to 15% potassium hydroxide preparation show septate hyphae coursing through infected squames. Cultures inoculated onto Sabouraud's media with antibiotics and incubated at room temperature will grow the responsible organism within two weeks.

PATHOLOGY. The histologic findings are identical to those described with tinea corporis.

DIAGNOSIS. The diagnosis is made by the presence of a typical clinical picture associated with positive micro-

scopic or cultural evidence. Other dermatoses presenting a similar clinical picture in the crural area are psoriasis, seborrheic dermatitis, a therapeutic dermatitis, candidiasis, erythrasma, lichen simplex chronicus, or even Darier's disease and benign familial chronic pemphigus (Hailey-Hailey).

Candidiasis is distinguished by a greater incidence of obvious scrotal involvement and by the presence of satellite pustules peripheral to brightly erythematous plaques (Fig. 181-22). Erythrasma can be distinguished by examining the suspected lesion under the Wood's lamp. The involved skin in erythrasma shows a coral red fluorescence; lesions of tinea cruris do not. Biopsy may be necessary to totally exclude some of the other diagnoses mentioned.

TREATMENT. Efforts to decrease occlusion and moisture in the involved area are helpful. This can be accomplished by lighter and better-ventilated clothing as well as by the judicious use of absorbent powder.

Fig. 181-22 *Candida* infection with satellite pustules.

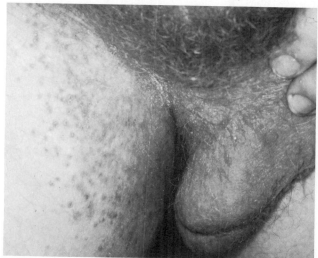

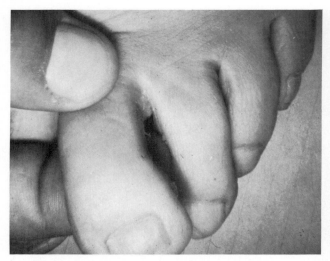

Fig. 181-23 Tinea pedis with interdigital involvement.

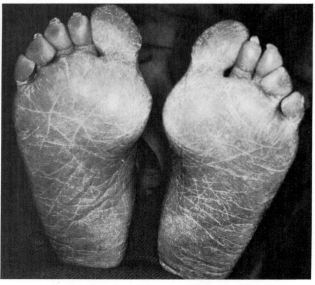

Fig. 181-25 Mocassin-like tinea pedis due to *T. rubrum*.

In most cases tinea cruris can be managed by local topical measures. A variety of agents have been used including haloprogin, tolnaftate, and the topical imidazoles (miconazole, clotrimazole, or econazole). A powder or minimally occlusive cream base for these products is recommended.

For more widespread or inflammatory infections, treatment with griseofulvin (500 to 1000 mg/day of the micro-sized preparation) is indicated.

Tinea pedis and tinea manuum. DEFINITION. Tinea pedis is a dermatophyte infection of the feet. Tinea manum is a dermatophyte infection of the palmar and interdigital areas of the hand.

Fig. 181-24 Tinea pedis with plantar involvement.

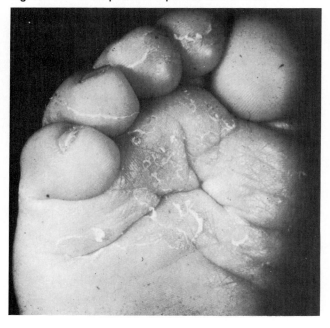

HISTORY. Tinea pedis represents a dermatophytosis of relatively recent onset. It probably was not common until humans began wearing occlusive footwear [51,60]. Tinea manuum was first described by Fox in 1870 [226], but tinea pedis was not reported until 1888 [227]. At present both infections are common worldwide; in fact, they represent the most common forms of dermatophyte infections.

EPIDEMIOLOGY. The epidemiology of tinea pedis has been extensively studied [60,61]. The infection is common during the summer months or in tropical or semitropical climates. Footwear is an important variable, and the incidence of tinea pedis is definitely higher in any population that wears occlusive shoes. In general, the patients infected are from civilized, urban areas; primitive populations, in which individuals rarely wear shoes, are spared.

The infection rate is increased in individuals using communal baths or pools [228,229]. The number of infections can be related to the frequency in which these facilities are utilized. Cultures from swimming pool or washroom floors as well as items of clothing in contact with infected areas [230,231] are often positive for the responsible organism. It is generally accepted, therefore, that tinea pedis is an exogenously transmitted infection in which cross-infection among susceptible individuals readily occurs [232]. Previous theories have postulated that dermatophytes frequently populated normal interdigital areas [236,233], and that under appropriate conditions (heat, humidity, trauma), a symptomatic infection could arise from the patient's endogenous flora. In fact, these workers found that infections were difficult to produce experimentally using exogenous inocula alone [86,87,234].

The sex or age of the host is not a direct risk factor in this disease as infection rates are comparable if the nature and degree of exposure are equivalent [61]. The increasing incidence of this infection with age is probably a function of an increased opportunity for exposure. Approximately 10 percent of the total population can be expected to have a dermatophytic foot infection at any given time [57]. If only closed communities of individuals (athletic teams,

Fig. 181-26 Bilateral, chronic tinea manuum due to *T. rubrum*.

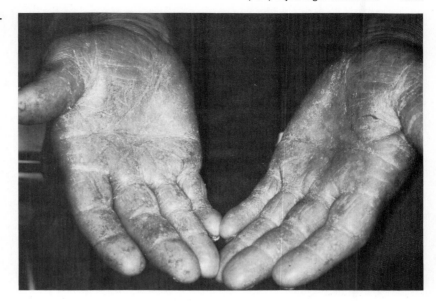

military organizations, boarding schools) are considered, the rate of infection is much higher.

ETIOLOGY. Tinea pedis is caused most commonly by *T. rubrum*, *T. mentagrophytes*, or *E. floccosum*. In rare instances sporadic infections with *T. violaceum*, *T. megninii*, *M. persicolor*, and *M. canis* have been described. Although slight differences may exist in relative frequency, the common causative organisms are the same worldwide. In the United Kingdom [57] *T. rubrum* accounts for 60 percent of the cases, while *T. mentagrophytes* is seen in 25 percent. *E. floccosum* is found in 10 percent of the cases in the United Kingdom and 20 percent of the cases in the United States [51]. A 3 to 5 percent incidence of mixed infections has been noted in some series [57].

T. rubrum commonly produces a dry, hyperkeratotic, mocassin-like involvement of the feet and/or hands; *T. mentagrophytes* often produces a vesicular pattern; and *E. floccosum* may produce either of the two patterns described above. Toenail involvement, however, is less common with *E. floccosum*.

CLINICAL MANIFESTATIONS. Tinea pedis may present as one of four clinically accepted variants or as an overlap of one or more of these types. The chronic, intertriginous type is the most common and is characterized by fissuring, scaling, or maceration in the interdigital or subdigital areas (Fig. 181-23). The lateral (i.e., 4th to 5th or 3rd to 4th) toe webs are the most common sites of infection (Fig. A1-14). From here infection may spread to the sole or instep of the foot but it seldom involves the dorsum (Fig. 181-24). A common aggravating feature in this type of infection is warmth and humidity. Hyperhidrosis may be an underlying problem for a number of these patients and should be treated along with the dermatophytosis.

Interesting studies on the microbial ecology of interdigital foot infections have been done by Leyden and Kligman [235,236]. It is clear that the disease we know as "athlete's foot" is not caused solely by dermatophytes. Normal-appearing toe webs have a skin flora consisting of Micrococcaceae (usually *Staphylococcus*), aerobic coryneforms, and small numbers of gram-negative organisms. Dermatophytes can also colonize normal toe webs frequently [233,234]. When toe web interspaces clinically demonstrated scaling or peeling without maceration or symptoms, the bacterial flora was unchanged from that of normal interspaces. Dermatophytes were isolated, however, in about 85 percent of these cases.

On the other hand, if an interspace showed maceration, white hyperkeratosis or erosions with increasing patient symptomatology, an overgrowth of the bacterial flora including gram-negatives was noted. Using clever manipulations of the interspace microflora in different patient groups, it was found that the clinical picture of symptomatic "athlete's foot" results from the interaction of bacteria and dermatophytes. Overgrowth of bacteria alone or the presence of dermatophytes alone produced a relatively mild clinical picture that was short-lived and relatively asymptomatic [235,236].

Another variant of tinea pedis is the chronic, papulosquamous pattern. This is usually bilateral and is characterized by minimal inflammation and a patchy or diffuse mocassin-like scaling over the soles (Figs. 181-25 and A1-16). *T. rubrum* and occasionally *T. mentagrophytes* are the usual causative organisms. In addition to the feet, the hands may be involved as well as multiple toenails (Fig. 181-26). A common but puzzling presentation is the "one hand, two feet" presentation observed frequently with *T. rubrum* infections (Fig. 181-27).

The third variant is the vesicular or vesiculobullous type. This is usually caused by *T. mentagrophytes* var. *interdigitale*. Small vesicles or vesicopustules are seen near the instep and on the midanterior plantar surface (Fig. 181-28). There usually is associated scaling in these areas as well as in the toe webs. Larger bullae are more unusual but can be seen. This type of infection may become clinically quiescent during the cooler months of the year only to become symptomatic again in the summer.

The fourth pattern is the acute ulcerative variant which is commonly associated with maceration, weeping denu-

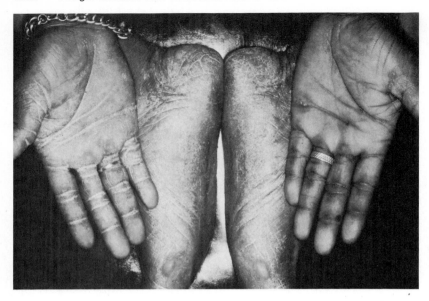

Fig. 181-27 The "one hand, two feet" presentation of *T. rubrum.*

dation, and ulceration of sizable areas of the sole of the foot. Obvious white hyperkeratosis and a pungent odor are characteristically present. This infection is often complicated by a secondary bacterial (often gram-negative) overgrowth.

The final two variants are commonly seen in conjunction with a vesicular "id" reaction either as a dyshidrotic-like distribution on the hands or on the lateral foot or toe area

Fig. 181-28 Vesicular tinea pedis in a common location on the foot.

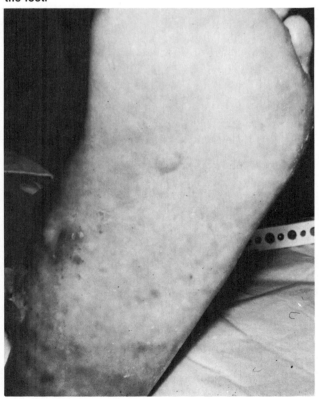

(Fig. 181-29). Cultures of these blisters are by definition sterile.

LABORATORY FINDINGS. KOH examination of scales is positive for septate, branching hyphae in tinea pedis. If vesiculobullous lesions are present, examination of a portion of the blister roof yields the highest rate of positivity. Cultures should be done using Sabouraud's media with cycloheximide and chloramphenicol added.

PATHOLOGY. Histologic examination reveals different patterns depending on the clinical variant involved. The hyperkeratotic, scaling variety shows acanthosis, hyperkeratosis, and a sparse, chronic superficial perivascular infiltrate in the dermis. On occasion, foci of neutrophils may be seen in the stratum corneum. In the vesicular variant, there is spongiosis, parakeratosis and subcorneal or spongiotic intraepithelial blisters. Neutrophils are likewise seen in the stratum corneum. In both histologic patterns special stains (PAS or methenamine silver) show organisms in the horny layer.

DIAGNOSIS. With a compatible clinical picture and a positive KOH preparation and/or culture, the diagnosis of tinea pedis can be made comfortably. If these findings are negative, however, a sizable differential diagnosis is possible. Interdigital scaling, fissuring, or maceration can be seen with bacterial secondary infection. The more severe the signs and symptoms, the greater is the probability of isolating gram-negative organisms (i.e., *Pseudomonas* or *Proteus* spp. in particular). Even if dermatophytes are present they are more difficult to isolate under these circumstances [235,236]. Other disorders to consider in evaluating an interdigital dermatosis are candidiasis, erythrasma (commonly has a coral red fluorescence with Wood's lamp examination), or soft corns.

In the scaly, hyperkeratotic variety of tinea pedis, confusion can occur with diseases such as psoriasis, hereditary or acquired keratodermas of the palms and soles, pityriasis rubra pilaris, or Reiter's syndrome. In contact dermatitis from shoes, lesions are seen on the dorsum of the foot more commonly than with tinea pedis. In children, peridigital dermatitis or atopic dermatitis is more common than

Fig. 181-29 Dermatophytid reaction associated with an inflammatory *T. mentagrophytes* infection of the feet.

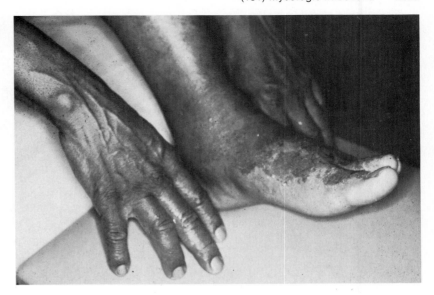

tinea pedis. In the vesicular or vesiculopustular presentation, tinea pedis can be confused with pustular psoriasis, pustulosis palmaris et plantaris, or bacterial pyodermas. In many cases careful examination of the nails can reveal convincing signs of dermatophytosis that are not seen with many of the above diagnoses.

PREVENTION AND TREATMENT. Tinea pedis can be transmitted by contact with infected scales on bath or pool floors as well as on clothing. Laundering of clothing is not always effective in removing infectious material, and it is impossible to prevent most infected individuals from using communal baths or swimming facilities [230]. Control of concomitant hyperhidrosis is important in preventing tinea pedis. Talcum powder or antifungal powders (undecylenic acid or tolnaftate powders) can be used along with absorbent socks and nonocclusive shoes. On occasion the use of 20% to 25% aluminum chloride hexahydrate topically will help to curb excessive moisture [237].

In overt tinea pedis, griseofulvin, ultramicrosized 0.5 g per day for 3 months is optimal. The prolonged treatment time is because of the increased turnover period of the thickened stratum corneum on the hands or feet. Cure rates with this treatment regimen are 90 percent. In intertriginous tinea pedis, griseofulvin and a topical imidazole are recommended for a 3-month course [238].

When there is maceration, erythema, or denudation of skin associated with pain, a secondary bacterial infection must be ruled out with cultures and Gram stains. Appropriate systemic antibiotics based on sensitivity studies should be started if bacterial infection is documented. Gram-negative organisms as well as *Staphylococcus aureus* are frequent pathogens in this area. Adjunctive topical measures such as using antibacterial soaks (e.g., ¼% acetic acid for *Pseudomonas* overgrowth) are helpful. Colorless Castellani's paint (phenolated resorcinol) is also used frequently.

Tinea unguium and onychomycosis. DEFINITION. Tinea unguium is clinically defined as a dermatophyte infection of the nail plate. Onychomycosis, on the other hand, includes all infection of the nail caused by any fungus, including nondermatophytes and yeasts.

EPIDEMIOLOGY. Onychomycosis is a common infection and accounts for 20 percent of all nail disease [51]. Approximately 30 percent of patients with dermatophytic infections on other parts of their body also have tinea unguium. Fungal nail infections are almost exclusively an adult malady. Children can be affected during household epidemics [57,239], but the faster nail growth in children appears to make infection more difficult [240]. Mold infections usually affect the elderly where underlying nail diseases allow room for these secondary invaders [241].

Although the overall susceptibility to dermatophyte nail infections is higher in men than in women, the number of cases affecting the toenails is increased in women. This may reflect differences in footwear in the female population where narrow-toed shoes allow increasing crowding of and trauma to the toenails. Paronychial infections caused by *Candida* spp. are also much more commonly seen in the fingernails of women. This most likely reflects the greater burden of wet work performed by females [240].

The epidemiologic considerations discussed in the section on tinea pedis apply also to tinea unguium. Yet, because fungal nail infections are more chronic and recalcitrant to therapy, these infections provide an endogenous source for reinfection of the feet. This is especially true if a nidus of infection is combined with the environmental conditions of warmth and humidity provided by the climate or by occlusive footwear [240].

ETIOLOGY AND PATHOGENESIS. Onychomycosis can be caused not only by dermatophytes but also by certain yeasts and nondermatophytic molds [241]. The most common dermatophytes causing tinea unguium worldwide are *T. rubrum*, *T. mentagrophytes* var. *interdigitale*, and *E. floccosum*. Yet, if a dermatophyte is endemic to a certain geographic area, it is often the cause of nail infections as well as other dermatophytoses in that areas. As noted in Table 181-11, *Microsporum* nail infections are extremely rare [243]. Table 181-12 groups the causative dermatophytes according to other anatomic areas that are often concurrently affected. Clearly *T. rubrum* is the most common cause of fingernail infections, but toenails can be infected by many of the different organisms cited.

Many nondermatophytic fungi have been associated with

Table 181-11   Dermatophyte fungi reported to produce tinea unguium

Organism	Geographic area
T. rubrum	Cosmopolitan
T. mentagrophytes	Cosmopolitan
T. violaceum	Europe, Africa, Near East,
T. schoenleinii	Eastern Europe, North Africa, Near East; rarely in the Americas
T. tonsurans	Cosmpolitan
T. megninii	Spain, Portugal, Sardinia
T. concentricum	South Pacific, portions of South and Central America
T. soudanense	Central and West Africa
T. gourvilli	Central and West Africa
E. floccosum	Cosmopolitan
M. gypseum	Cosmopolitan
M. audouinii	Cosmopolitan
M. canis	Cosmopolitan

Modified from Zaias N [242].

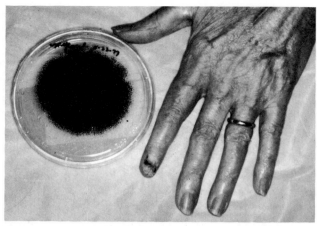

Fig. 181-30   Onychomycosis can be due to nondermatophytic fungi including *Aspergillus niger*.

nail infections [244]. Among the yeasts, *Candida albicans* is found to invade the nail only in chronic mucocutaneous candidiasis. Other species of *Candida* such as *C. parapsilosis* have been isolated from toenails [240,242]. The nondermatophytic molds have also been cultured frequently from nails clinically felt to be onychomycotic (Fig. 181-30). Strict criteria are necessary, however, to implicate these organisms as primary pathogens as they are often considered to be contaminants when routine cultures are examined [245]. English has outlined these criteria as follows [246]: (1) if a dermatophyte is isolated on culture, it is considered to be pathogen; (2) if a mold or yeast is cultured, it is considered significant only if hyphae, spores, or yeast cells are seen on microscopic examination; (3) confirmation of an infection by a nondermatophyte requires isolation of the organism on at least 5 out of 20 inocula without concurrent isolation of a dermatophyte. In general, it appears that nondermatophytic onychomycosis favors antecedently diseased nails or aged nails [241]. Toenails are the usual site of involvement [247].

Zaias [242,247] has divided onychomycosis into four clinical types: (1) distal subungual onychomycosis (DSO), (2) proximal subungual onychomycosis (PSO), (3) white superficial onychomycosis (WSO), and (4) candidal ony-

Table 181-12   Causative organisms according to anatomic site of infection

Tinea unguium + tinea pedis and/or tinea manuum
   T. rubrum
   T. mentagrophytes var. interdigitale
   E. floccosum
Tinea unguium + tinea corporis + tinea pedis
   T. rubrum
   T. mentagrophytes var. interdigitale
   E. floccosum
Tinea unguium + tinea capitis or favus
   T. tonsurans
   T. violaceum
   T. megninii
   T. schoenleinii
Tinea unguium + tinea imbricata
   T. concentricum

chomycosis. Characteristically, infected nails coexist with normal-appearing nails (Figs. 181-31 and A1-15).

Distal subungual onychomycosis is the most common type and starts by invasion of the stratum corneum of the hyponychium and distal nail bed. Subsequently, the infection moves proximally in the nail bed and invades the ventral surface of the nail plate. Subungual hyperkeratosis results from a hyperproliferative reaction of the nail bed in response to the infection [240]. As the process continues, invasion of the nail plate results in a progressively dystrophic nail unit.

Proximal subungual onychomycosis is the least common variant of onychomycosis. It starts by fungal invasion of the stratum corneum of the proximal nail fold and subsequently the nail plate.

White superficial onychomycosis differs from the other variants by primarily invading the dorsal surface of the nail plate. Interestingly, the morphology of the fungus in WSO is typically that of a saprophyte. There are "eroding fronds" or "perforating organs" as seen with in vitro hard keratin invasion [242,248].

Candidal onychomycosis is seen in patients with chronic mucocutaneous candidiasis. It may affect toenails and fingernails by invasion of the nail plate via the hyponychial epithelium. The entire thickness of the nail plate is commonly affected [242]. The dystrophic nails seen with candidal paronychia do not result from direct fungal invasion and should not be confused with true onychomycosis.

Table 181-13 summarizes the common causative organisms for the different variants of onychomycosis.

The mechanism and relative facility of nail invasion has been studied previously.. Zaias [247] found, by using [^{14}C]cystine-labeled keratin during in vitro invasion studies, that *T. mentagrophytes* was a more active destroyer of the nail than was *T. rubrum*. This may correlate with the clinical findings of slow, chronic infections caused by *T. rubrum*. The mechanism of nail destruction is unclear. Some authors have postulated a mechanical separation of nail laminae rather than true keratinolysis [251]. Other authors using ultramicroscopic data have seen evidence of corneocyte penetration and obvious keratinolysis [252]. Probably both mechanisms are operative depending on the specific organisms involved.

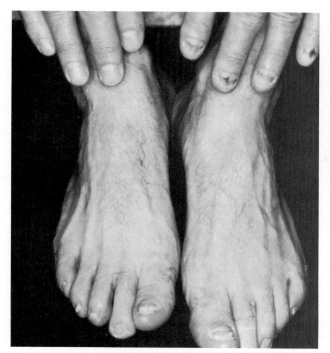

Fig. 181-31   Tinea unguium with sparing of certain nails.

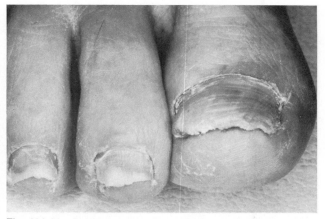

Fig. 181-32   Distal subungual onychomycosis (DSO).

CLINICAL MANIFESTATIONS. The different clinical types of onychomycosis have been described previously. Each type has a rather characteristic clinical picture.

Distal subungual onychomycosis begins as a whitish or brownish-yellow discoloration at the free edge of the nail or near the lateral nail fold. As the infection progresses, subungual hyperkeratosis may lead to a separation of nail plate and nail bed (Fig. 181-32). Fungi invade the nail plate from the ventral surface, and in time the entire nail may become friable and discolored. The subungual debris also provides a site for opportunistic secondary infection by bacteria or other molds and yeasts. Hence, a wide spectrum of clinical changes can occur when the infection is advanced.

White superficial onychomycosis [248] appears as white, sharply outlined areas on the surface of the toenails (Fig. 181-33). The fingernails are not affected. Any area of the nail can be affected initially and with time much of the nail surface can be involved. The surface of the nail is usually rough and friable as the "eroding fronds" of the organisms remain quite superficial. As discussed previously, *T. mentagrophytes* is the most common organism producing WSO. Recently, *T. rubrum* has been reported as an infrequent cause [253].

Proximal subungual onychomycosis is the least common variant of onychomycosis. The first clinical sign of this type of infection is a whitish to whitish-brown area on the proximal part of the nail plate. This area may gradually enlarge to affect the entire nail. Like DSO the organisms invade the ventral surface of the nail plate from the proximal nail fold.

Candida onychomycosis (Fig. A1-18) is seen in patients with chronic mucocutaneous candidiasis. Both toenails and

Table 181-13   Common causative organisms for variants of onychomycosis

Distal subungual onychomycosis (DSO)
 Toenails
  Dermatophytes: *T. rubrum, T. mentagrophytes, E. floccosum*
  Molds: *Scopulariopsis brevicaulis, Aspergillus, Fusarium, Cephalosporium*
  Yeasts: *C. albicans, C. parapsilosis, C. tropicalis, Geotrichum candidum, Hendersonula toruloidea*
 Fingernails
  Dermatophytes: *T. rubrum*
  Yeasts and molds: *C. albicans*
Proximal subungual onychomycosis (PSO)
 Toenails
  T. rubrum, T. megninii, T. schoenleinii, T. tonsurans, T. mentagrophytes
  Molds and yeasts: not documented
 Fingernails:
  Dermatophytes: *T. rubrum, T. megninii*
  Molds and yeasts: not documented
White superficial onychomycosis (WSO)
 Toenails
  Dermatophytes: *T. mentagrophytes,* rarely *T. rubrum*
  Molds: *Aspergillus, Cephalosporium, Fusarium*
 Fingernails: WSO does not occur on fingernails

Modified from Norton [249] and Baron [250].

Fig. 181-33   White superficial onychomycosis (WSO).

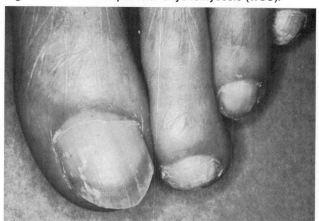

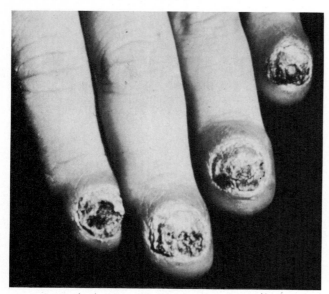

Fig. 181-34 Candidal onychomycosis in chronic mucocutaneous candidiasis.

fingernails are affected. Clinically, the appearance of these nails resembles DSO with thickening of the nail bed and nail plate. Unlike DSO, the entire nail plate is invaded by the organisms. The surface of the nail becomes opaque, rough, and furrowed. It is usually discolored and may be brownish or brownish-yellow in color. Oftentimes a surrounding paronychial inflammatory response is present, and the digit tip may become bulbous (Fig. 181-34).

LABORATORY FINDINGS. Attempts to document fungal infections of the nail involve the use of KOH preparations and fungal cultures. Unfortunately, microscopy may frequently be negative in nails that clinically appear to be infected. Furthermore, nails that are positive by microscopic examination often yield negative cultures [240,244,254,255]. A reason for this discrepancy is that fungi seen on KOH examination may not be viable and hence do not grow as expected. Since the most commonly sampled area of the nail is the distal tip with its associated subungual debris, we must reevaluate whether better results could be obtained by devising better sampling methods.

Samman recommends soaking full-thickness clippings of the affected nail in 5% KOH for 24 h prior to examination [256]. English [246] and others [244,257] have used a dental drill with a suction apparatus attached to obtain nail dust from affected areas. By doing this the rate of culture positivity has been increased to 88 percent from the usual 50 to 75 percent.

Another method of sampling the nail has been described by Shelley and Wood [258]. Here one selects sites of early, active infection. These appear as whitish areas of discoloration with a normal overlying nail. A razor blade is used to trim away the normal nail and reach the powdery white area of infection. This material is then mounted with xylene and examined microscopically.

Cultures are done on Sabouraud's dextrose agar with and without added chloramphenicol and cycloheximide. Cycloheximide will suppress the growth of nondermatophytic organisms and should not be used if these fungi are suspected.

PATHOLOGY. Histologically, hyphae are seen lying between the laminae of nail parallel to the surface. The ventral nail and the stratum corneum of the nail bed are preferentially affected [259]. The epidermis may show spongiosis and focal parakeratosis. The inflammatory response in the dermis is minimal.

DIAGNOSIS. Onychomycosis can be confused with a variety of nail disorders. The diagnosis is further complicated by the high incidence of false-negative KOH examinations and cultures.

Psoriasis can closely mimic onychomycosis; however, the pitting seen in psoriasis is infrequent in fungal nail infections. The dystrophic nails seen in conjunction with hand eczema usually are transversely ridged and eczematous changes are apparent in the surrounding skin. Other entities that can be confused with onychomycosis are the nails of Reiter's syndrome, Darier's disease, lichen planus, exfoliative dermatitis, pachyonychia congenita, and Norwegian scabies. Usually these disorders are separated from onychomycosis by history or evidence of characteristic skin lesions or biopsy findings.

White superficial onychomycosis must be distinguished from acquired or congenital leukonychias. Among these leukonychias, those due to trauma are the most common.

TREATMENT. Therapy of onychomycoses is often a challenging endeavor for the clinician. Topical agents are usually of little benefit. Systemic therapy with griseofulvin is usually effective for fingernails if given for 4 to 6 months [260]. Toenails may require 12 to 18 months to clear and are associated with a high relapse rate. Ketoconazole may be more helpful with organisms such as *T. rubrum*, but even with this drug there is a high relapse rate.

Some authors have advised chemical removal of nail using 40% urea compounds [261] or surgical avulsion of the nail combined with topical agents and oral griseofulvin [247,256]. This regimen may increase the cure rate for dermatophyte infections. Of course, avulsion or chemical destruction of the nail in nondermatophytic fungal infections is the only therapy that is effective [247].

Therapy of superficial fungal infections

The therapy of specific superficial fungal infections has been outlined in previous sections. Here, we describe characteristics of the therapeutic agents used in many of these infections.

Unfortunately, the wide variety of antibiotics used in the treatment of bacterial infections is not equalled by antimycotic drugs. In part this is due to the similarity between host and fungal cells—both are eukaryotic. It has been difficult to find antimycotic drugs that are efficacious and, at the same time, relatively nontoxic [51,262]. Among the agents that have been found, we will discuss the polyenes, griseofulvin, the imidazoles including ketoconazole, and a variety of older topical agents that still have a place in therapy.

Polyene antibiotics

Nystatin, a polyene antibiotic, was the first specific antifungal agent [51]. Subsequently, a number of polyenes have been developed. Unfortunately, problems with solubility, stability, absorption, and toxicity have limited their use.

The polyenes are characterized by a macrolide ring of

Fig. 181-35 Chemical structure of amphotericin B.

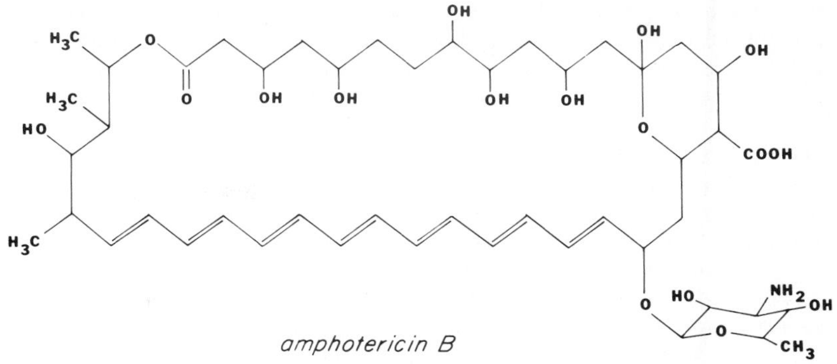

amphotericin B

carbon atoms closed by the formation of an internal ester or lactone. A conjugated double-bond system is maintained within the lactone (Fig. 181-35). The polyenes appear to act by binding to membrane sterols (i.e., ergosterol) and, in so doing, alter the permeability characteristics of the membrane. Subsequently, a loss of intracellular cations (particularly K^+) occurs, and cell death follows. The preferential effect of the polyenes on fungal cell membranes is explained by the more avid binding of the antibiotic to ergosterol than to cholesterol (the principal sterol in mammalian cells [263,264].

Of the polyenes available, nystatin and amphotericin B are the only drugs used clinically. The other drugs (pimaricin, filipin, candicidin, etc.) are considered too toxic. Nystatin is insoluble in water and is not absorbed when given orally. The drug is derived from an actinomycete, *Streptomyces noursei*. Nystatin is too toxic for parenteral use but has been useful as a topical product and for oral use to clear gastrointestinal candidiasis. Topically, it is used for the therapy of cutaneous and mucous membrane candidal infections. The drug is unstable with excessive heat, light, moisture, and air. Aqueous suspensions are stable for only 10 days under refrigeration [265].

Amphotericin B is rarely used for superficial cutaneous fungal infections. It is, however, extremely effective for many systemic fungal infections. Amphotericin B is a heptaene lactone linked with mycosamine. It is the least toxic polyene for systemic use [266]. Recent reviews have adequately outlined the pharmacology of amphotericin B [263,264,267]. It is interesting that in addition to binding

membrane sterols, amphotericin B may also act as an immunoadjuvant [264].

Griseofulvin

Griseofulvin, 7-chloro-2',4,6-trimethoxy-6'-methylspiro-[benzofuran-2(3H),1'-(2)cyclohexene]-3,4'-dione (Fig. 181-36), is a metabolic product of certain *Penicillium* species. It was discovered in 1939 [268], and its chemical structure ($C_{17}H_{17}ClO_6$) was characterized in 1947. The drug was first used medically in 1958 [55,56]. Since then it has been an extremely safe and effective agent for cutaneous dermatophyte infections.

The properties of griseofulvin were described initially by Brian and his colleagues [269]. The drug was termed "curling factor" due to its ability to induce stunted and abnormal growth of certain test organisms. The precise mechanism of action of griseofulvin is unclear. The drug is fungistatic, however, and interferes with cell wall, protein, and nucleic acid synthesis of actively growing organisms. It appears that griseofulvin affects the microtubular system and interferes with the mitotic spindle as well as the cytoplasmic microtubules [262,270,271]. The molecular action of griseofulvin is thought to be different from other compounds (i.e., colchicine, vinca alkaloids) that bind to receptors on tubulin and inactivate the free subunits of microtubules [265,262]. If griseofulvin does interfere with cytoplasmic microtubules, the role of these structures in transporting secretory material to the periphery of the cell would be interrupted. Faulty processing of synthesized cell

Fig. 181-36 Structures of commonly used antifungals.

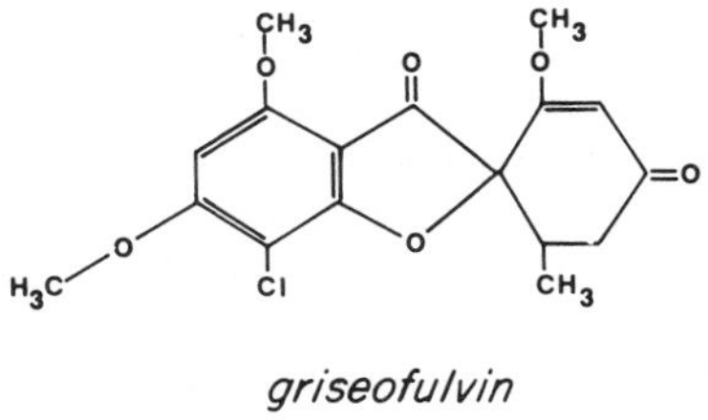

griseofulvin

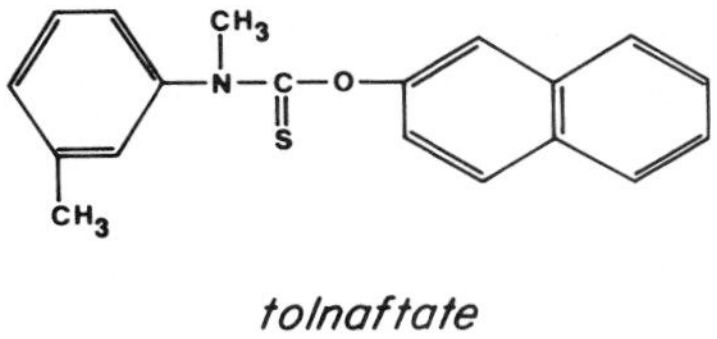

tolnaftate

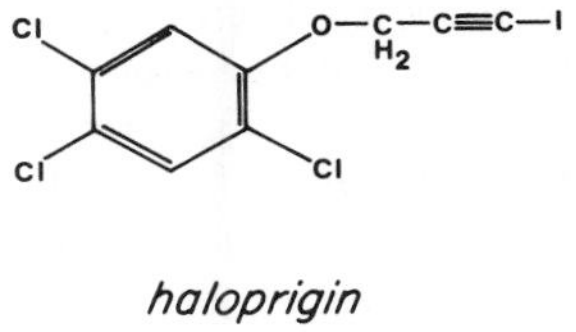

haloprigin

wall material for growing hyphae would then result [271]. In addition to the antimitotic properties of the drug, griseofulvin has also been found to be anti-inflammatory [272] and antichemotactic for polymorphonuclear leukocytes [271].

Griseofulvin is effective in the treatment of most dermatophyte infections in a serum concentration of <1 μg/ml [51,266]. In vitro resistance to the drug can be induced by growing certain dermatophyte strains with increasing concentrations of the drug [273]. In addition, natural resistance to the drug can occur. A mean inhibitory concentration (MIC) of >3 μg/ml is considered indicative of relative griseofulvin resistance. Recently, T. rubrum was found to be the most common isolate in griseofulvin-resistant dermatophyte infections [274]. Griseofulvin has no activity against yeast or bacterial infections.

After oral administration of 0.5 g, a peak plasma level of 1 μg/ml is seen at about 4 h [275]. Because of poor water solubility, absorption of the drug is erratic [276]. Absorption can be enhanced by reduction of particle size (i.e., microsized, ultramicrosized) or by administering a supersaturated solution of the drug in polyethylene glycol [266]. The absorption of griseofulvin is more rapid if taken with a fatty meal [277], but the total absorption in 24 h is unchanged [278]. The drug has a plasma half-life of about 1 day and need only be given once daily.

After absorption from the gastrointestinal (GI) tract, the drug is detectable and selectively concentrated in the stratum corneum within 4 to 8 h. Similarly, there is a rapid disappearance of the drug from the stratum corneum within 48 to 72 h after an oral dose [279]. Griseofulvin does not fix to keratin-producing cells and move outward with them as previous studies suggested [280]. Sweat also serves to concentrate the drug in the stratum corneum by a "wick effect" [279].

Remarkably few adverse effects have been attributed to griseofulvin. Fifty-five percent of patients may complain of headaches at the onset of therapy. This is usually a transient symptom that commonly disappears with continued therapy. Other side effects include nausea, vomiting, diarrhea, and other symptoms of GI distress or neurologic symptoms such as confusion, lethargy, or peripheral neuritis. A drug eruption can occur and is usually urticarial. Occasionally, a phototoxic reaction is seen. Hematologic abnormalities such as leukopenia have been reported but fortunately are infrequent [57,281]. Finally, renal abnormalities such as proteinuria or cylinduria are described.

Griseofulvin can precipitate or aggravate systemic lupus erythematosus [281] and acute intermittent porphyria [282]. Simultaneous administration of barbituates and griseofulvin results in lowered blood levels of griseofulvin. This is due to an interference by the barbituate with the absorption of griseofulvin [283]. Griseofulvin diminishes the anticoagulant effect of warfarin through induction of hepatic microsomal enzymes. Finally, reduced alcohol tolerance has been reported in a few patients taking griseofulvin [57].

The effectiveness of griseofulvin for dermatophyte infections has been well documented in the literature. Griseofulvin has been found to have the following cure rates: tinea capitis, 93.1 percent; tinea of glabrous skin, 64.8 percent; tinea of the palms and soles, 53.3 percent; tinea of the fingernails, 56.9 percent; and tinea of the toenails,

16.7 percent [284]. Reasons for failure of the drug are variable. Recently, studies demonstrating in vitro griseofulvin-resistant organisms have appeared [274]. In deciding whether or not to use long-term griseofulvin, particularly with chronic T. rubrum infections, a determination of griseofulvin sensitivities may be helpful.

The dose of griseofulvin depends on the preparation used. In general, microcrystalline preparations are given in a dose of 500 to 1000 mg/day depending on body weight. In children, a dose of 10 mg/kg per day is generally used. With the ultramicronized preparations, dosages may range between one-half and two-thirds of the microsized variety.

The imidazoles

With the exception of ketoconazole, the imidazoles are used topically in the treatment of superficial fungal infections. A number of substituted imidazole derivatives are now available, including thiabendazole [285], miconazole, clotrimazole, econazole [286], and sulconazole (Fig. 181-37). These agents are particularly useful because they are effective against a wide range of fungi, including *Candida* and dermatophytes, as well as certain bacteria.

The imidazoles, including ketoconazole, appear to function by inhibiting ergosterol synthesis in fungi by blocking C-14 demethylation. This results in a decrease in ergosterol and an accumulation of C-14 methyl sterol intermediates, such as lanosterol. This alteration in membrane sterols results in cell membrane permeability changes or structural defects that lead to growth inhibition or cell death [287].

Applied topically in the treatment of uncomplicated dermatophytic or *Candida* infections, a representative imidazole, miconazole, has achieved a 95 percent cure rate [266]. Adverse reactions from these agents are rare, but irritant and allergic contact dermatitis have been reported [288]. The development of resistance to these agents by fungal organisms is unusual.

Ketoconazole is a dibasic piperazine imidazole (Fig. 181-37) that is effective orally in the treatment of several deep and superficial fungal infections. At present the drug is approved by the Food and Drug Administration of the United States for the treatment of candidiasis, coccidioidomycosis, histoplasmosis, chromomycosis, and paracoccidioidomycosis. It is also effective in dermatophyte infections.

The mode of action of ketoconazole is similar to that of the other imidazoles. It inhibits ergosterol synthesis in fungal cell membranes, resulting in an accumulation of lanosterol. In addition, ketoconazole may inhibit the uptake of RNA and DNA precursors by the organism as well as interfere with the synthesis of oxidative or peroxidative enzymes. Ketoconazole also appears to have a synergistic effect with host defense mechanisms [287]. The drug, however, is fungistatic and is not able to sterilize tissues in the presence of defective cell-mediated immunity [289].

Ketoconazole is water-soluble and is well absorbed from the gastrointestinal tract. Peak serum concentrations are obtained 1 to 4 h after a 200-mg dose. Absorption may be enhanced by administering the drug with 4 ml 0.2 N HCl and drinking it through a plastic straw to protect the teeth followed by a glass of water. Achlorhydria or the simultaneous administration of antacids, anticholinergics, or the H_2 blockers, cimetidine or ranitidine, impair absorption.

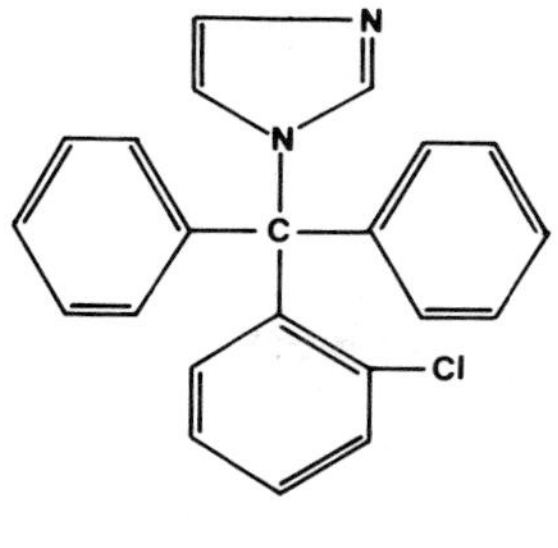

clotrimazole

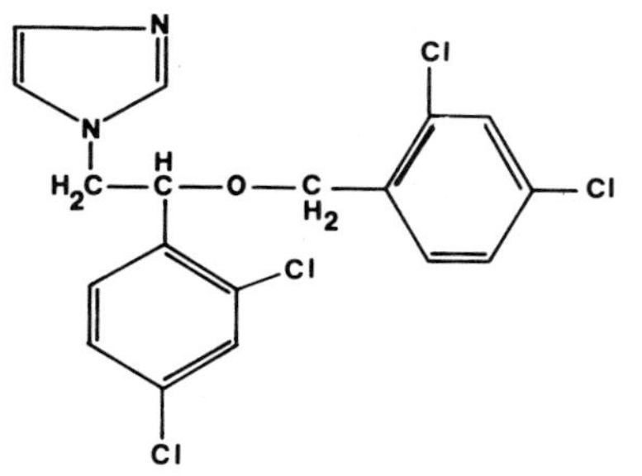

miconazole

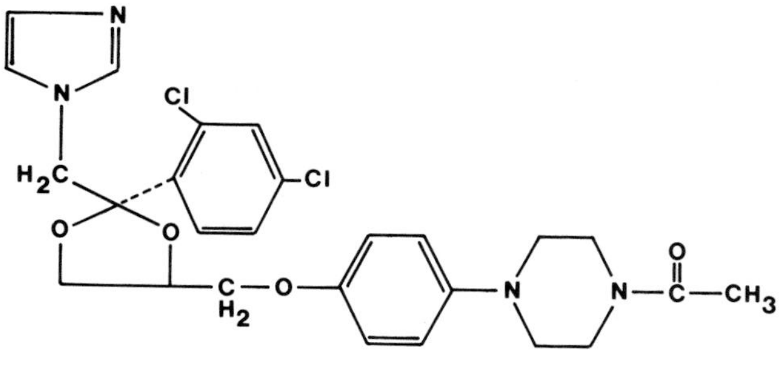

ketoconazole

Fig. 181-37 Structures of commonly used imidazole antifungals.

The drug is metabolized by the liver and excreted in an inactive form via the bile. The renal excretion is minimal, and alterations of drug dosage due to renal failure are unnecessary [290].

Ketoconazole has been particularly useful in the management of chronic mucocutaneous candidiasis [267,291]. Unfortunately, resistant *C. albicans* organisms have been identified and have recently been correlated with a poor clinical response to the drug [292].

The drug has also been effective in dermatophyte infections and tinea versicolor. Recalcitrant, griseofulvin-resistant *T. rubrum* infections usually respond to the drug but may relapse after therapy is stopped [293–296]. As expected, palmar/plantar or nail infections responded more slowly and commonly relapsed after discontinuation of therapy [293,294,297,298].

The usual dosage of ketoconazole is 200 to 400 mg/day. Side effects commonly include nausea and vomiting in 3 to 10 percent of patients. Abdominal pain, pruritus, headache, fever and chills, and photophobia are seen in fewer

than 1 percent of patients [291]. Interestingly, gynecomastia may occur possibly due to an inhibition of testosterone synthesis [299]. Likewise, a block in adrenal steroid synthesis, in the absence of clinical hypoadrenalism, has been found [300].

The most disturbing adverse effect has been the occurrence of an idiosyncratic hepatotoxic reaction to the drug [299–302]. More commonly, transient mild liver enzyme rises have been noted which resolve with continued therapy. Symptomatic hepatic reactions have been estimated to occur in 1 in 10,000 patients treated. The reaction is usually noted early in the course of therapy and does not seem to be related to daily or cumulative dosage of the drug [303–305]. Fortunately, most of these reactions subside after the drug is discontinued.

Other topical agents

A wide variety of older but still efficacious topical products are available for the treatment of superficial fungal infections.

Whitfield's ointment is a combination of benzoic (12%) acid and salicylic (6%) acid. It has keratolytic and antifungal properties and is used commonly for tinea nigra.

Colorless Castellani's paint has local anesthetic, antibacterial and antifungal properties. It is particularly useful for intertriginous infections. Excessive dryness or irritation may occur, however.

Short-chain organic fatty acid and fatty acid salts have long been recognized to have antifungal properties [306]. A preparation containing 5% undecylenic acid and 20% zinc undecylenate (Desenex) is sold over-the-counter relatively inexpensively. The powder is particularly useful as a prophylactic measure for tinea pedis.

Tolnaftate (*m*,N-dimethylthiocarbanilic acid O-2 naphthyl ester) (Fig. 181-36) is a safe, odorless and nonstaining topical preparation that is effective against dermatophytes and tinea versicolor. It is not effective, however, against *C. albicans*. Its mode of action has not been determined.

Haloprogin (3-iodo-2-propynyl-2,4,5-trichlorphenyl ether) (Fig. 181-36) is effective against dermatophytes, *Candida*, and some gram-positive bacteria. The drug may work by disrupting cell membrane function. Skin irritation and contact allergy are occasional side effects [51,266,269].

Ciclopirox olamine is a relatively new topical agent that has antibacterial, antiyeast, and antidermatophyte properties [266]. It is a pyridone ethanolamine salt and is available as a 1% cream. The drug appears to act by blocking the uptake of macromolecular precursors by the organism [307]. Preliminary controlled double-blind studies have shown equal to higher cure rates when ciclopirox was compared to clotrimazole. Because the drug penetrates highly cornified tissue well, it may be more useful than previously discussed drugs in the therapy of palmar/plantar or nail infections [308,309].

CANDIDIASIS

Definition

Candidiasis (or candidosis) is an infection, with protean clinical manifestations caused by *Candida albicans* or, on occasion, by other yeasts of the genus *Candida*. The in-

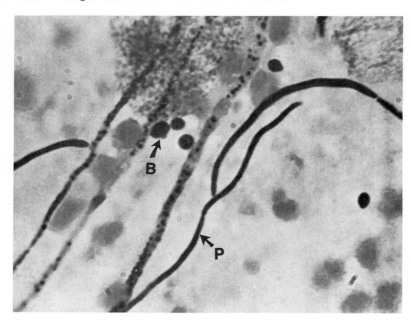

Fig. 181-38 Gram stain of *C. albicans* illustrating blastospores (B) and pseudohyphae (P). X1000. *(Photograph courtesy of B. H. Cooper.)*

fections are usually confined to the skin, nails, mucous membranes, and gastrointestinal tract but can be systemic and infect multiple internal organs.

History

The clinical manifestations of candidiasis have been recognized since ancient times and were discussed in the writings of Hippocrates, Galen, and Pepys. In 1839, Langenbeck discovered the organism in a lesion of thrush. Berg in 1841 and Bennett in 1844 supported this finding and demonstrated that the fungus was indeed the etiologic agent of thrush. Thereafter, and until the genus *Candida* was constructed by Berkhout in 1923, a confusing taxonomy ensued. Initially classified as a *Sporotrichum* by Gruby, it was placed in the genus *Oidium (Oidium albicans)* by Robin in 1847. Later it was confused with another fungus isolated from rotting vegetation *(Monilia candida)* and was renamed *Monilia albicans* by Zopf in 1890. The name *Monilia* was stubbornly defended by Castellani and probably accounts for the term moniliasis being used as a synonym for candidiasis even in the relatively modern literature. Of course, the term *Monilia* is a misnomer and actually refers to the imperfect stage of certain ascomycetes and has no relationship whatsoever to the genus *Candida.*

In 1877 further progress was made when Grawitz described the dimorphic nature of the organism. In the late 1800s and 1900s the protean clinical manifestations of candidiasis were unraveled. In 1853 Robin first described the occurrence of systemic candidiasis. Interestingly, cutaneous candidiasis and chronic mucocutaneous candidiasis were described relatively late, in 1907 and 1909, respectively. Diaper dermatitis was not described formally until 1911. Finally after the genus *Candida* was established in 1923, efforts toward speciating yeasts placed in this genus were forged by Martin in 1937. The importance of candidiasis as an opportunistic infection was first appreciated in the postantibiotic era of the 1940s when an increase in the number of candidal infections was noted.

Controversy over nomenclature persists, and while candidiasis is the accepted term for this infection in the United States, candidosis is preferred in Canada, the United Kingdom, France, and Italy.

Etiology

From a taxonomic viewpoint the genera *Candida* and *Torulopsis* accomodate a heterogeneous collection of yeast species which do not produce ascospores or teliospores and do not possess morphologic or biochemical characteristics which would classify them in the more homogeneous genera of imperfect yeasts. At the present time, the morphologic feature that separates these two genera are based on the capacity of the yeast to form pseudomyecelia (Fig. 181-38). In the genus *Candida,* pseudomycelia are well developed whereas in the genus *Torulopsis* they are absent or poorly developed. There is presently a controversy concerning the separation of these two genera and since the criteria for defining various genera of imperfect fungi are arbitrary, some authors have suggested they be classified in one single artificial genus *(Candida).* Since this would require the renaming of a great number of species and invariably lead to confusion and disagreement among mycologists and clinicians, this chapter will recognize *Candida* and *Torulopsis* as two separate genera. Of the various species in the genus *Candida, C. albicans,* is the most common cause of superficial and systemic candidiasis. Several of the more than 80 other species classified in this genus can also be responsible for clinical disease under certain circumstances (e.g., host immunosuppression, indwelling catheters, intravenous drug delivery, etc). Most of these infections are systemic but can be localized (Table 181-14). Together *C. albicans* and *C. tropicalis* account for about 80 percent of the species isolated from medical specimens [310,311]. The species of *Candida* have been graded by descending degree of pathogenicity as follows: *C. albicans, C. stellatoidea, C. tropicalis, C. parapsilosis, C. pseudotropicalis, C. guilliermondii,* and *C. krusei.*

Table 181-14 Regular isolates other than *C. albicans* in certain types of candidiasis

Causative organism	Clinical disease
C. parapsilosis	Paronychia, endocarditis, otitis externa
C. tropicalis	Vaginitis, intestinal, bronchopulmonary, and systemic infections, onychomycosis, bone and joint CNS
C. stellatoidea	Vaginitis, systemic, bone, and joint
C. guilliermondii	Endocarditis, cutaneous candidiasis, onychomycosis, bone and joint
C. pseudotropicalis	Vaginitis, urethritis
C. (Torulopsis) glabrata	Esophagitis, vaginitis, endocarditis
C. krusei	Endocarditis, vaginitis
C. zeylanoides	Onychomycosis
C. viswanathi	CNS
C. lusitaniae	Systemic

Pathogenesis

C. albicans is frequently found as a saprophyte and colonizes certain mucous membrane surfaces of warm-blooded animals. As many as 80 percent of normal individuals may show such colonization of the oropharynx, gastrointestinal tract, and vagina [312]. In contrast, the organism is rarely isolated from normal human skin except sporadically from certain intertriginous areas. Likewise the organism is seldom isolated from soil, vegetation, or air samples.

The development of disease due to *Candida* species is dependent on the complex interaction that exists between the innate pathogenicity of the organism and the defense mechanisms of the host. *Candida* infections, therefore, are largely opportunistic ones made possible by diminished host defenses. Certain predisposing factors have been classically associated with an increased incidence of colonization and infection by these yeasts (Table 181-15).

Various factors regarding the intrinsic pathogenicity of *Candida* species as they relate to skin and mucous membrane infections are important to consider. The species of *Candida* differ in their ability to initiate cutaneous infection in an experimental animal model [313]. Using the staphylococcal toxin epidermolysin to cleave the epidermis selectively below the granular layer, Ray et al [314] demonstrated that only *C. albicans* and *C. stellatoidea* inoculated into this cleft were capable of invading the stratum corneum and eliciting inflammation. Other species were excluded even under occlusive experimental conditions. These findings were supported by Maibach and Kligman in experimental human cutaneous candidiasis, clearly demonstrating differences in virulence among the species of *Candida* [315].

Other important factors in the initiation of candidal infections include adherence of the organism to epithelial cells and subsequent invasion [312,316]. The mechanism of invasion is unclear but may involve elaboration of keratinolytic enzymes, phospholipases, or strain-specific proteolytic enzymes [317–319]. Ultrastructurally, pseudo-hyphae can be seen penetrating intracellularly into corneocytes in clinical lesions of candidiasis. A prominent clear space is usually seen around the organisms, suggesting an ongoing process of epithelial tissue lysis [320,321]. It appears that mycelial growth predominates in invasive disease states, while the blastospore growth phase predominates in saprophytic states.

The induction of cutaneous candidiasis in humans under experimental conditions pointed the way to important subsequent data examining the pathogenesis of the inflammatory response in the disease. Maibach and Kligman noted that the epicutaneous inoculation of *C. albicans* could produce cutaneous disease only if the site of inoculation was occluded [315]. Within 36 to 72 h typical erythematous, pustular lesions developed. The severity of the infection was proportional to the size of the inoculum [322]. Biopsy of these pustules showed them to be subcorneal in location. Using special stains, organisms were not seen within the pustules but were only in the stratum corneum. Cutaneous lesions were similarly produced using a sterile extract of disintegrated candidal cells and a sediment of killed ruptured cells. The authors postulated the existence

Table 181-15 Factors predisposing to *Candida* infections

Mechanical factors:
  Trauma (burns, abrasions, etc.)
  Local occlusion, moisture and/or maceration (dentures, occlusive dressings or garments, obesity)
Nutritional factors:
  Avitaminosis
  Iron deficiency (chronic mucocutaneous candidiasis)
  Generalized malnutrition
Physiologic alterations:
  Extremes of age
  Pregnancy
  Menses
Systemic illnesses:
  Down's syndrome
  Acrodermatitis enteropathica
  Diabetes mellitus and certain other endocrinopathies (Cushing's, hypoadrenalism, hypothyroidism, hypoparathryoidism)
  Uremia
  Malignancy (especially hematologic, thyoma)
  Intrinsic immunodeficiency states (DiGeorge's syndrome, Nezelof's syndrome, severe combined immunodeficiency syndrome, myeloperoxidase deficiency, Chédiak-Higashi syndrome, hyperimmunoglobulinemia E syndrome, chronic granulomatous disease, AIDS)
Iatrogenic causes:
  Barrier-weak factors (indwelling catheters, i.v. drug abusers)
  X-irradiation
  Medications:
  Corticosteroids and other immunosuppressive agents
  Antibiotics (especially broad-spectrum, metronidazole)
  Tranquilizers
  Oral contraceptives (especially estrogen-dominant)
  Colchicine
  Phenylbutazone

of an endotoxin-like substance that mediated the pustular response [315]. Subsequently, Ray et al [323] demonstrated that a purified mannan cell wall polysaccharide from *C. albicans* is capable of activating complement via the alternative pathway, thereby generating products such as C5a that induce neutrophil chemotaxis. This material also exhibits in vitro endotoxin-like activity. In this way, highly antigenic or toxic products of candidal organisms are able to induce vigorous host response mechanisms that, at the same time, both limit infection and produce the typical cutaneous manifestations of the disease. Such a mechanism may explain certain findings in systemic candidiasis. For example, circulating mannan has been demonstrated in systemic invasive candidal infections. By alternative pathway complement activation in this setting, the leukopenia and early neutrophilic tissue response associated with disseminated candidal infections may be partially explained. Furthermore, *Candida* antigen, immunoglobulin, and complement have been found in the nephritic kidney of a patient with *Candida* endocrinopathy syndrome [324]. In contrast, other cell wall ''toxic'' products of candidal organisms have been found to interfere with host neutrophil chemotaxis and phagocytosis [325]. Furthermore, cell wall polysaccharide products may interfere with T lymphocyte-mediated defenses [312,326,327]. The mechanisms of host defense operative during *Candida* infections are complex and still not completely understood. The broad categories include nonimmune and immune factors [328,329].

The nonimmune factors include the following: (1) interaction with other members of the microbial flora, (2) the functional integrity of the stratum corneum, (3) the desquamation process induced by inflammation-induced epidermal proliferation, (4) opsonization and phagocytosis, and (5) other serum factors. The host microbial flora are protective in that they compete with *Candida* for nutrients and epithelial adherence sites and produce by-products toxic to the yeast. Likewise, normal intact skin with its constant sloughing and regeneration provides an effective barrier against *Candida*. Skin surface lipids are partially inhibitory as well [312]. Abrogation of this barrier by mechanical means or occlusion facilitates infection. As with cutaneous dermatophyte infections, the skin increases its turnover rate significantly during the early stages of infection, and this increased desquamation helps shed the organism [330].

The process of phagocytosis and killing of candidal organisms is accomplished primarily by polymorphonuclear leukocytes (PMN) and macrophages. The PMN is probably the most important in this regard [331]; patients with neutropenia or diseases affecting PMN function (Table 181-15) are particularly susceptible to candidal infections. As noted previously, the PMN is the predominant early inflammatory cell seen histologically in candidal infections. It is recruited in part by mannan activation of the alternative complement pathway and the ensuing generation of potent chemotactic factors [323]. The importance of this process to host defense against *Candida* is emphasized in experimental studies on complement-depleted (using cobra venom factor) rodents or hereditary C5-deficient animals. In this setting experimental candidal infections do not elicit a PMN response. In addition, the organism invades much more rapidly and extensively than in normal animals

[313,332]. Likewise, macrophages participate in opsonization, phagocytosis, and killing of yeasts. PMN and macrophages have C3b surface receptors, and the deposition of C3b opsonins on *Candida* organisms may therefore facilitate phagocytosis [333,334]. PMN and macrophages accomplish intracellular killing by both oxidative (myeloperoxidase-hydrogen peroxide-halide system) and nonoxidative means. This mechanism is not absolute, however, and some organisms, while phagocytosed, are not killed while larger hyphae may not be phagocytosed at all. Neutrophils, however, appear to be able to recognize these hyphae and attach to them. While not phagocytizing the yeasts, they do inflict damage by extracellular oxidative antimicrobial mechanisms [329,335].

Serum factors that may be important in containing candidal infections include the controversial serum ''clumping'' factor described by Louria and Brayton [336]. Although initially thought to be important in fungistasis, this clumping phenomenon may simply reflect the entanglement of hyphal elements grown in serum [337]. Transferrin, by binding iron necessary for fungal growth, may inhibit candidal proliferation [338], and lactoferrin, a neutrophil-derived iron-binding substance, may function similarly as well as contribute to neutrophil adherence and other functions [329,339].

The immune mechanisms responsible for protection against *Candida* infections include both humoral and cell-mediated responses. The latter are considered to be more important in this regard. Proof for this assertion comes from experience with chronic mucocutaneous candidiasis, where a defect in cell-mediated immunity leads to extensive superficial candidiasis despite normal, or even exaggerated, humoral defenses. Serum antibody production to the principal cell wall glycoprotein antigens of *Candida* occurs in low titers in normal individuals. The protective role of these antibodies, however, is controversial and may reflect a response to colonization of the gastrointestinal tract early in life. There is evidence in certain experimental situations, such as using passive transfer of serum, that a degree of protection may be provided [340,341]. Yet, in the clinical setting, it is clear that patients with primarily B-cell deficiency states are not at high risk for candidal infections [328]. There is also conflicting evidence for the role of secretory IgA in limiting mucosal infections [328,342]. It is probable that the various innate, nonimmune factors in conjunction with cell-mediated immunity and complement activation contribute more to host defense against candidal infections than does humoral immunity [312].

Clinical manifestions

The cutaneous and mucosal manifestations of candidiasis are varied but in most cases characteristic. They may be categorized broadly as shown in Table 181-16.

Oral candidiasis (see also Chap. 101)

The recognized clinical syndromes of oral candidiasis have been categorized as in Table 181-16.

Acute pseudomembranous candidiasis or *thrush* may present early in life as candidal organisms, presumably originating from the maternal birth canal, colonize the

Table 181-16 Classification of cutaneous syndromes of candidiasis

I. Mucous membrane involvement
  A. Oral
    1. Acute pseudomembranous candidiasis (thrush)
    2. Acute atrophic candidiasis
    3. Chronic atrophic candidiasis
    4. Cheilosis (perlèche angular cheilosis)
    5. Chronic hyperplastic candidiasis (leukoplakia)
    6. Other: black hairy tongue, median rhomboid glossitis
  B. Vulvovaginitis
  C. Balanitis
II. Cutaneous involvement
  A. Localized
    1. Intertrigo
    2. Folliculitis
    3. Paronychia and onychomycosis
    4. Perioral dermatitis
    5. External otitis
    6. Suppurative peripheral thrombophlebitis
    7. Skin abscesses
    8. Cellulitis
  B. Generalized
    1. Congenital and neonatal candidiasis
    2. Disseminated candidiasis with cutaneous manifestations
III. Chronic mucocutaneous candidiasis (CMCC)
IV. Candidids

mouth of the neonate. A very few organisms may produce clinical disease in this setting [310]. Thrush is the most common form of oral candidiasis and may affect up to 5 percent of newborns and 10 percent of debilitated, hospitalized, elderly patients [343]. Concomitant illnesses such as diabetes mellitus [344], malignancies, and immune deficiency states may also be predisposing factors (Table 181-15). Oral candidiasis may be the primary presenting manifestation in some patients with acquired immunodeficiency syndrome (AIDS) [345]. Clinically there are discrete white patches that may become confluent on the buccal mucosa, tongue, palate, or gingiva (Fig. 181-39). This friable pseudomembrane resembles milk curds and consists of desquamated epithelial cells, fungal elements, inflammatory cells and food debris. When scraped off, a raw, brightly erythematous surface is exposed. Microscopic examination of this material reveals masses of tangled pseudohyphae and blastospores. Severe cases may show ulcerations and necrosis of the mucosal surface.

Acute atrophic candidiasis (antibiotic candidasis) may occur de novo or after sloughing of the pseudomembrane of thrush [343]. It is commonly associated with broad-spectrum antibiotic administration but can be seen with the use of topical, inhaled, or systemic corticosteroids [329,346]. The most common location is on the dorsal surface of the tongue where there are patchy depapillated areas with minimal pseudomembrane formation.

Chronic atrophic candidiasis (denture stomatitis) is a very common form of oral candidiasis among denture wearers. In one study it was found in 24 percent of surveyed denture wearers [347] and in 60 percent of those older than 65 years of age [348]. Female patients are affected more commonly than males. The condition is characterized by chronic erythema and edema of the palatal mucosa that contacts the dentures. Angular cheilitis is commonly present as well. It is often not symptomatic or only mildly so. *C. albicans* is recovered more commonly from the surface of the denture material than from the mucosal surface [349]. Presumably, the chronic low-grade trauma and occlusion provided by dentures predisposes to candidal colonization and subsequent infection.

Candida cheilosis or *perlèche* is characterized by erythema, fissuring, maceration and soreness at the angles of the mouth (Fig. 181-40) from which the organism *C. albicans* can be isolated. It occurs in habitual lip lickers or in those elderly patients with sagging skin at the oral commissures. Loss of vertical dimension in the lower one-third of the face due to loss of dentition or poorly fitting dentures and malocclusion may also be predisposing factors [350].

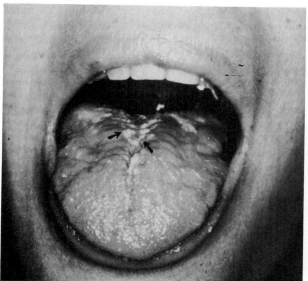

Fig. 181-39 Clinical features of acute pseudomembranous candidiasis or thrush. Note the characteristic white patches on the surface of the tongue (arrows) which consist of yeasts and pseudohyphae.

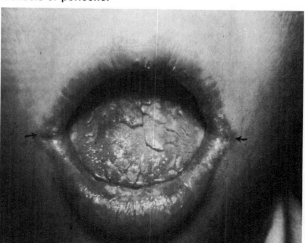

Fig. 181-40 Erythema and fissuring at the corners of the mouth (arrows) characterize the clinical features of *Candida* cheilosis or perlèche.

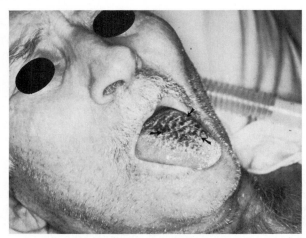

Fig. 181-41 The condition of black hairy tongue is characterized by pigmented hypertrophied filiform papillae of the dorsum of the tongue (arrows). This condition is usually associated with oral antibiotic therapy.

It is often associated with chronic atrophic candidiasis due to denture wear. A true candidal cheilitis has been described where chronic erosive or granular changes appear on the lower lips of compulsive lip lickers. Satellite lesions may spread beyond the vermilion in this case [351].

Chronic hyperplastic candidiasis or candidal leukoplakia is characterized by adherent (unlike thrush), firm, raised areas on the buccal mucosa or tongue that are translucent to white in color with surrounding erythema and from which *C. albicans* can frequently be isolated.

Median rhomboid glossitis is a central papillary atrophic condition of the dorsal surface of the tongue. Some consider it to be a developmental anomaly [352], but others point to histologic and microbiologic evidence suggesting that it represents a true candidal infection [353].

Black hairy tongue has been associated etiologically with *C. albicans*. However, the organism probably is a secondary invader of hypertrophied filiform papillae on the dorsum of the tongue (Fig. 181-41) that characterizes the condition [310].

Vaginal and vulvovaginal candidiasis

C. albicans may be isolated from vaginal cultures in roughly 8 percent of normal women. This percentage increases to 25 percent in patients with symptoms of vaginitis [354]. Factors thought to predispose to an increasing incidence of candidal vaginitis include pregnancy, diabetes mellitus, oral contraceptives and antibiotic administration, and occlusive tight-fitting garments such as pantyhose and leotards. Patients present with a thick vaginal discharge associated with burning or itching and sometimes dysuria. Examination shows whitish plaques on the vaginal wall with underlying erythema and surrounding edema. Areas of involvement may spread to the labiae and perineal area. Recurrent and chronic candidal vulvovaginitis is a particularly difficult problem for certain patients. The pathogenesis of such recurrent vaginitis is unclear and controversial but has been thought to reflect intestinal or urethral colonization or penile colonization in the male partners of affected women [355,356]. In some cases, concomitant poly-

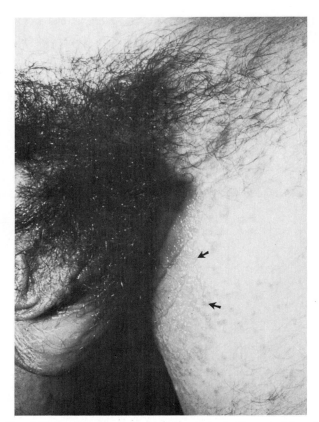

Fig. 181-42 Genitocrural candidiasis typically consists of pruritic, erythematous, macerated areas of skin with satellite vesicopustules (arrows).

microbial infections may explain poor responses to therapy and frequent relapses [357].

Balanitis or balanoposthitis

Balanitis due to *C. albicans* may present as small papules or fragile papulopustules on the glans or in the coronal sulcus. These break to leave superficial erythematous erosions with a collarette of whitish scale. A thrushlike membrane may form in some cases. Infection may spread to the scrotum and inguinal areas. In diabetics or immunosuppressed patients, a severe edematous, ulcerative balanitis may occur [358]. Occasionally, patients may present with a transient erythema and burning occuring shortly after intercourse with partners having candidal vaginitis. This presentation had been felt to represent a hypersensitivity response to the organism [359]. Factors predisposing to balanitis include candidal vaginal infection in sexual partners, diabetes mellitus, and an uncircumcised state.

Cutaneous candidiasis

C. albicans has a predilection for colonizing moist, macerated folds of skin. For that reason intertrigo in its various forms is the most common clinical presentation of candidiasis on glabrous skin. Common locations for the infection include the genitocrural (Fig. 181-42), subaxillary, gluteal (Fig. 181-43), interdigital (Fig. 181-44), submam-

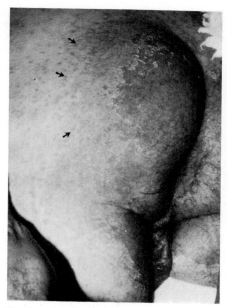

Fig. 181-43 Candidiasis of the gluteal area with satellite lesions (arrows) studding the area of intense erythema. The disease sometimes spreads to involve the perianal region.

mary (Fig. 181-45) areas, and between the folds of skin of the abdominal wall. Predisposing conditions include obesity, occlusive clothing, diabetes mellitus, and occupations favoring excessive exposure to moist occlusive conditions. The clinical appearance is typical and consists of pruritic, erythematous, macerated areas of skin in intertriginous areas with satellite vesicopustules. These pustules are fragile and break, leaving a red macular base with a collarette of easily detachable necrotic epidermis (Fig. A1-19). Several varieties of intertrigo caused by *Candida* deserve special mention. *Diaper dermatitis* in infants can be of multiple etiologies. *Candida*, however, can colonize this area from the gastrointestinal tract of these children [360]. The chronic occlusive state provided by diaper wear propagates the infection. Lesions appear first in the perianal area and spread to the perineum and inguinal creases with pronounced erythema in the latter area. Concomitant thrush or candidal involvement of other intertriginous areas may

be present in severe cases. *Erosio interdigitalis blastomycetica* refers to interdigital candidal infection of the hands and usually affects the area between the third and fourth fingers (Fig. 181-44). *Candida miliaria* affects the back in bedridden patients, particularly those who are febrile and sweating profusely. Lesions start as isolated vesicopustules that are positive for fungal forms. *Candida* can also colonize and infect the skin around wounds that are being dressed occlusively, especially if broad-spectrum topical antibiotics are being used.

An *erythematous pustular folliculitis* has been described due to *C. albicans*. Although the lesions are perifollicular in location, true hair shaft invasion is usually not observed [361]. A common location for these lesions is in the perioral area [329]. Typical perioral dermatitis presenting as erythematous papulopustules has been described secondary to *C. albicans* as has a more severe pyoderma faciale-like eruption in the perioral area [362,363].

Candida paronychia is extremely common in individuals whose hands are chronically involved in wet work (e.g., housewives, bakers, fishermen, bartenders, etc.). At times the clinical presentation may be complicated by a concomitant bacterial infection. Typically there is redness, swelling, and tenderness of the paronychial area with prominent retraction of the cuticle toward the proximal nail fold (Fig. 181-46). Occasionally, pus can be expressed from beneath this area. Secondary nail changes can occur and include onycholysis and transverse ridging of the nail plate with a brownish or green discoloration along the lateral borders (Fig. A1-18). True *Candida* invasion of the nail plate occurs in chronic mucocutaneous candidiasis; in this case the entire thickness of the nail plate is involved [364].

A more generalized cutaneous involvement can occur due to *C. albicans*. The rare syndrome of *congenital candidiasis* usually presents at birth or shortly thereafter (within 12 hours of life) and is due to infection acquired in utero. The disease has been reported after amniocentesis [365]. Lesions occur diffusely over the trunk, extremities, head, and neck and spare the mouth and diaper area. They appear as red macules that progress to papulovesicles or pustules which later desquamate and resolve spontaneously. Fever and other constitutional symptoms are lacking, and patients usually have a benign course. Fatal dissemination, however, has been described, especially in

Fig. 181-44 Interdigital candidiasis sometimes referred to as erosio interdigitalis blastomycetica is characterized by macerated, desquamated lesions occurring between the fingers (arrows).

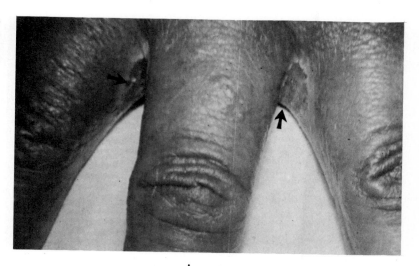

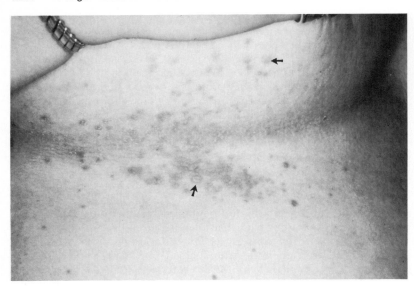

Fig. 181-45 Candidiasis of the submammary area, as with other forms of *Candida* intertrigo, commonly presents as an acute or chronic pruritic rash. Vesicles often occur but they rupture quickly leaving characteristic macules (arrows).

infants with low birth weights or concomitant respiratory distress [366].

The incidence of *disseminated candidiasis* is steadily rising as more patients with serious hematologic malignancies are treated aggressively with potent immunosuppressive drugs, and more and more patients undergo bone marrow and other organ transplants [367]. Other factors that may predispose one to disseminated candidal infection are listed in Table 181-15. The organisms responsible for such infections include *C. albicans, C. tropicalis, C. pseudotropicalis, C. krusei,* and *C. parapsilosis* [368]. These organisms may gain hematogenous access from the oropharynx or gastrointestinal tract, when the mucosal barrier function is compromised (e.g., mucositis secondary to chemotherapy), or through contaminated intravenous catheters. Organs most commonly involved include the lungs, spleen, kidneys, liver, heart, and brain [369]. The eye findings include an endophthalmitis that correlates well with multiple organ involvement [370]. Skin lesions may occur in 10 to 13 percent of patients with disseminated infection [371]. The recognition of such lesions may be important in early diagnosis as antemortem blood cultures are negative

in a high percentage of patients with autopsy-proved systemic candidiasis [372].

The characteristic skin lesions are 0.5 to 1.0 cm erythematous papulonodules that tend to become hemorrhagic particularly in patients with associated thrombocytopenia (Fig. 181-47). They are usually located on the trunk and extremities and may be numerous of few [373]. Associated findings may include fever and myalgias [374,375]. Necrotic cutaneous lesions resembling ecthyma gangrenosum (due to *Pseudomonas aeruginosa*) have also been described due to candidiasis [376,377]. A distinctive syndrome in intravenous heroin abusers has been described where macronodular and folliculitis-like skin lesions occurred in the scalp and other terminal hair-bearing areas. Infiltration of the hair follicules with candidal organisms has been observed histologically [378].

Chronic mucocutaneous candidiasis

Chronic mucocutaneous candidiasis (CMC) is a term used to describe a heterogeneous group of clinical syndromes characterized by chronic, treatment-resistant, superficial

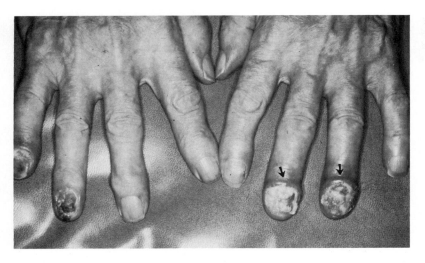

Fig. 181-46 *Candida* paronychia is a chronic inflammatory infection of the nail folds (arrows). This condition may also involve the nail (onychomycosis).

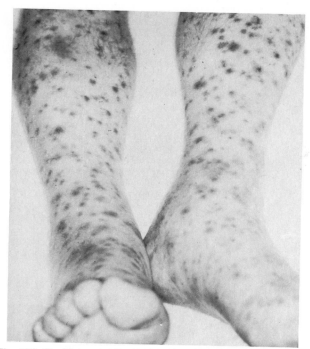

Fig. 181-47 The cutaneous manifestations of disseminated candidiasis are usually a late manifestation of disease and appear as an erythematous, papular exanthema.

candidal infections of the skin, nails, and oropharynx. There is virtually no propensity for disseminated, visceral candidiasis. In many cases there are narrow but specific abnormalities in cell-mediated immunity. In others the defects are more global. The clinical findings and immunologic defects have been extensively reviewed [379].

Clinical syndromes. A suitable clinical classification of the major subtypes of CMC was described by Lehner [380] and Wells et al [381]. Table 181-17 provides an updated categorization of these syndromes and a summary of their distinguishing features. In general, the various syndromes may be familial or sporadic in nature. When presenting in childhood, lesions are usually detected before the age of 3 years. Usually oral lesions or a papular diaper dermatitis appear first followed by angular cheilitis or perlèche, lip fissures, nail and paronychial involvement, vulvovaginitis, and cutaneous involvement. In some cases of CMC, markedly hyperkeratotic, hornlike, or granulomatous lesions may appear (*Candida* granuloma). These heavily crusted lesions may appear on the face, eyelid, scalp, lips, or acral areas (Fig. 181-48). On the scalp they may resemble the lesions of favus and can lead to alopecia. Other cutaneous lesions may appear atypical for candidiasis and can have erythematous, serpiginous borders [382] or areas of brownish desquamation on a background of mild erythema [383] (Fig. 181-49). Concomitant dermatophyte infection of skin may appear commonly and confuse the clinical presentation.

Nail involvement is characterized by markedly thickened and dystrophic nail plates which are invaded through their entire thickness by *Candida*. The paronychial areas are red and edematous, and the digital tips are often bulbous in appearance.

Conditions that have been associated with CMC include: *Candida* esophagitis or laryngitis [384,385], endocrinopathies (usually hypoparathyroidism, hypoadrenalism, hypothyroidism) [386], circulating autoimmune antibodies [387], diabetes mellitus, vitiligo with antibodies to melanocytes [388], iron deficiency [389], chronic active hepatitis, pernicious anemia, malabsorption, alopecia totalis, dental enamel dysplasia, keratoconjunctivitis, pulmonary fibrosis, KID syndrome (keratitis, ichthyosis, and deafness) [390], and recurrent pyogenic [379], viral [391], or other fungal infections [392]. When CMC first appears in adulthood, it is often associated with a thymoma and the other conditions listed in Table 181-17 [393]. Some of these associations are found in only certain clinical subtypes of CMC (e.g., endocrinopathies); others are observed more broadly (e.g., esophagitis/laryngitis, dermatophytosis, etc.).

Immunology. In CMC numerous inmunologic defects have been described. These usually involve abnormalities in cell-mediated immunity (CMI) while humoral immunity is largely intact. In up to 25 to 30 percent of patients with CMC, however, no immunologic defect has been found [394]. In many cases the CMI defects may reflect a selective deficiency in the recognition and processing of *Candida* while handling of other antigens is intact. The following is a listing of some of the commonly described immunologic abnormalities [391,394,395]:

1. There may be complete anergy to a battery of common skin test antigens or selective nonresponsiveness to *C. albicans* antigen. This group can be further divided based on in vitro lymphocyte transformation and lymphokine production studies to *Candida*. In most cases, lymphocyte response to mitogens such as phytohemagglutinin are normal in CMC.
   A. Lymphocyte transformation negative and lymphokine production positive
   B. Lymphocyte transformation positive and lymphokine production negative
   C. Both lymphocyte transformation and lymphokine production negative
2. Selective IgA deficiency
3. Plasma inhibitor to lymphocyte transformation by *C. albicans* [327]
4. Serum inhibitor to polymorphonuclear leukocyte chemotaxis [396] and killing of *C. albicans* [397]
5. Abnormal monocyte chemotactic [398] and killing responses [399]
6. Combined abnormality of monocyte mobility and phagocytosis-killing [400]
7. Abnormal complement function [401]
8. Abnormal macrophage function
9. Hyperimmunoglobulinemia E and impaired granulocyte chemotaxis [402]
10. Defective suppressor T-cell function [403]
11. Defective mannan handling by monocytes [404]
12. Impaired generation of helper T cells [405]

In some cases the observed immunologic defect is reversed after successful antifungal therapy. This suggests that a massive antigenic load (particularly mannan) may interfere with CMI—perhaps by the generation of specific T suppressor cells [328].

Table 181-17 Classification of chronic mucocutaneous candidiasis (CMC)

Clinical syndrome	Inheritance	Age of onset	Distrubution of lesions	Endocrinology	Associated findings	Notes
Chronic oral candidiasis	Sporadic	Any	Mucosa of tongue, lips, buccal cavity; perlèche; no skin or nail involvement	None	Esophagitis	Denture stomatitis is a variant
Chronic candidiasis with endocrinopathy	Autosomal recessive	Childhood	Mucous membranes, skin, and/or nails	Frequent (hypoadrenalism, hypothyroidism, hypoparathyroidism, or polyendocrinopathy)	Alopecia totalis, thyroiditis, vitiligo, chronic hepatitis, pernicious anemia, gonadal failure, malabsorption, diabetes mellitus	Endocrinopathy may be delayed in onset
Chronic candidiasis without endocrinopathy	Autosomal recessive	Childhood	Mucous membrane, perlèche, and nail involvement; less common skin involvement	None	Blepharitis, esophagitis, laryngitis	
	Autosomal dominant	Childhood		None	Dermatophytosis, loss of teeth, recurrent viral infections	
Chronic localized mucocutaneous candidiasis	Sporadic	Childhood	Mucous membrane, skin, and/or nails	Occasionally	Pulmonary infections, esophagitis	Hyperkeratotic lesions (*Candida*), granuloma
Chronic diffuse candidiasis	Autosomal recessive	Childhood	Widespread mucous membrane, skin, and nail involvement	None		Erythematous, serpiginous skin lesions
		Adolescence	Widespread mucous membrane, skin, and nail involvement	None	History of frequent courses of antibiotics	
Chronic candidiasis with thymoma	Sporadic	Adulthood (after 3rd decade)	Mucous membranes, nails, and skin	None	Thymoma, myasthenia gravis, aplastic anemia, neutropenia, hypogammaglobulinemia	CMC often precedes diagnosis of thmoma

Cutaneous candidids

There is controversy in the literature as to the existence to allergic cutaneous reactions (id reactions) to localized infections with *C. albicans*. Certain recalcitrant cases of erythema annulare centrifugum, chronic urticaria, and groin or hand dermatitis have been attributed to this phenomenon and have cleared with successful therapy of the underlying candidal infection.

Laboratory findings

Of the more than 80 species of yeast that have been classified in the genus *Candida* only about 10 have been identified as capable of producing or contributing to disease of humans and animals. Because of the ubiquity of these unicellular organisms in nature and the fact that they are often found as transient colonizers of the skin and appendages of humans, the clinical diagnosis of candidiasis should be confirmed by laboratory tests for identification of the species of yeast involved. In addition to the clinical evaluation of the patient, direct microscopic examination of specimens for the presence of yeast and isolation of yeast in culture are needed for definitive proof of infection. In superficial candidal infections, the diagnosis can be made by performing an examination of skin scrapings and observing typical budding yeasts with hyphae or pseudohyphae. *C. albicans* grows readily on bacterial media, but Sabouraud's agar with added antibiotics is usually recommended for isolation. Whitish, mucoid colonies grow within 2 to 5 days. Of all superficial infections, chronic paronychiae may have the lowest yield of positive cultures.

In systemic candidiasis with skin lesions, the diagnosis usually can be made from histopathologic examination and culture of appropriate skin biopsy specimens. Blood cultures may frequently be negative in this setting [406]. Serologic studies using immunodiffusion, counterimmunoelectrophoresis, and latex agglutination methods may be somewhat helpful in the diagnosis of systemic candidiasis. However, false-negative and false-positive reactions are rather frequent. More promising are techniques to detect circulating candidal antigens (e.g., mannan) or metabolic

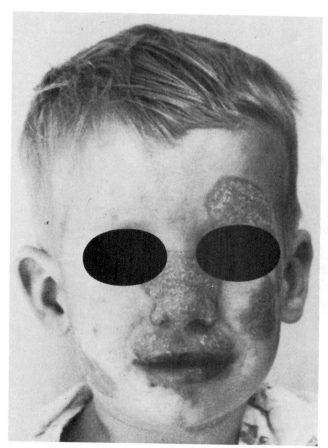

Fig. 181-48 Well-demarcated granulomatous lesions of chronic mucocutaneous candidiasis.

products (e.g., arabinitol) [407]. Occasionally, muscle biopsy of symptomatic muscle groups may show organisms histologically [375].

Microscopic studies

Since the clinical manifestations of infections caused by species of *Candida* are protean, the types of specimens taken from patients for laboratory examination will vary from body fluids to surgical biopsy. Direct microcopic examination of these specimens for the presence of yeast forms provides rapid evidence in support of the presumptive clinical diagnosis. Body fluids such as urine and cerebrospinal fluid should be centrifuged and the sediment examined. This procedure increases the probability of finding yeasts. Sputum and other viscous secretions along with surgical biopsies and tissue scrapings must be treated with a clearing agent such as 10% potassium hydroxide and ink before the material is examined (see "Superficial Dermatophytoses" above). Yeast forms in the genus *Candida* will appear as oval budding cells, elongated filamentous cells connected in a sausage-like manner (pseudohyphae), or as truly septate hyphae (Fig. 181-38). The presence of such forms in clinical material does not permit species identification but does provide evidence that fungi consistent with the morphology of *Candida* are present. Species identification relies on isolation of the yeast in pure culture and biochemical and physiologic tests.

Culture methods

All clinical specimens should be freshly taken and cultured onto suitable media as rapidly as possible. Sediment from centrifuged body fluids, tissue from biopsies, and scrapings should be inoculated onto Sabouraud's dextrose agar containing antibacterial antibiotics. Cultures are incubated at room temperature (ca. 25° to 27°C) and examined periodically for growth of yeast. Negative cultures are discarded after 4 weeks. All colonies of yeast must be subcultured and tested further for identifying morphologic and biochemical characteristics before they can be speciated. Several reference sources are available for speciating yeasts in the genus *Candida*. One excellent procedure is described by Cooper and Silva-Hutner in the *Manual of Clinical Microbiology* [408].

Pathology

Superficial candidiasis is characterized by subcorneal pustules. Organisms are seldom seen within the pustule but can be visualized with the aid of a periodic acid-Schiff (PAS) stain in the stratum corneum. The histology of a candidal granuloma shows marked papillomatosis, hyperkeratosis and a dense dermal infiltrate consisting of lymphocytes, granulocytes, plasma cells, and multinucleated giant cells. Again, organisms are usually seen only within the stratum corneum.

In systemic candidal infections with skin involvement, biopsies show focal areas in the dermis and within blood vessels where organisms can be identified using PAS or methenamine silver stains. Hematoxylin and eosin staining alone is insufficient. There may be a surrounding bland mononuclear cell infiltrate [371], leukocytoclastic vasculitis, or microabscess formation. It may be necessary to do multiple sections through the biopsy material in order to identify the areas of involvement.

Diagnosis

The diagnosis of most superficial cutaneous candidal infections can be made by the typical appearance of the clinical lesions and the presence of satellite vesicopustules. This can be confirmed by KOH examination and culture of skin scrapings. Nevertheless, intertriginous candidiasis can be confused occasionally with tinea infections, eczema, seborrheic dermatitis, intertriginous psoriasis, erythrasma, bacterial intertrigo, familial benign pemphigus, Leiner's disease, glucagonoma, or flexural Darier's disease.

Chronic paronychiae can be seen due to bacterial infections or with hypoparathyroidism, celiac disease, acrodermatitis enteropathica, Reiter's syndrome, acrokeratosis paraneoplastica, or retinoid therapy.

Typical oral thrush is characteristic, but the atrophic or ulcerative forms of oral candidiasis can be confused with mucositis due to chemotherapeutic drugs, herpetic infections, erythema multiforme, blistering disorders such as pemphigus, lichen planus, histoplasmosis, leukoplakia, secondary syphilis, or an aspirin burn. Perlèche-like lesions may be seen in secondary syphilis, avitaminosis (e.g., riboflavin), glucagonoma syndrome, or iron-deficiency states.

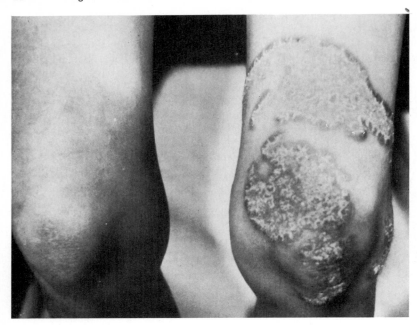

Fig. 181-49 Heavily crusted lesions of chronic mucocutaneous candidiasis with well-demarcated serpiginous borders.

The lesions of chronic mucocutaneous candidiasis (CMC) should be differentiated from those of tinea (e.g., favus), bacterial pyoderma, acrodermatitis enteropathica, or halogenoderma. The immunodeficiency states listed in Table 181-15 should be remembered in evaluating patients with widespread CMC.

Papular cutaneous lesions similar to those seen in systemic candidiasis can be observed with *Pityrosporum* folliculitis [409], bacterial sepsis (e.g., gonococcal, meningococcal, pseudomonal, staphylococcal), or other disseminated fungal infections (e.g., mucormycosis, aspergillosis, etc.). Necrotic cutaneous lesions due to *Candida* may appear identical to *Pseudomonas* ecthyma, or deep fungal infections (e.g., cryptococcosis, torulopsosis, or sporotrichosis).

Therapy

An important aspect of the treatment of all forms of candidiasis is the correction, if possible, of any of the predisposing factors listed in Table 181-15. For example, efforts to prevent chronic occlusion and maceration in cases of candidal intertrigo are particularly important. In systemic candidiasis, removal of potentially colonized intravenous or Foley catheters is the first step in successful management.

Fortunately, there are a number of antimicrobial agents effective against *Candida*. For oral infections, the most commonly used drugs include nystatin suspension (400,000 to 600,000 units qid) held in the mouth and then swallowed, clotrimazole troches (10 mg dissolved in the mouth five times per day), 1% to 2% gentian violet, or amphotericin B (80 mg/ml) rinses. There is some evidence that the clotrimazole troche regimen is most effective in therapy as well as prophylaxis of oral candidiasis [410–412]. For infants clotrimazole 100 mg suppositories can be inserted tightly into the tip of a slit pacifier and the child allowed to suck on this qid [413]. At times sytemic therapy of strictly oral candidiasis is indicated, and ketoconazole 200 to 400 mg per day orally is the drug of choice.

Candidal vulvovaginitis is usually treated by one of the topical imidazole creams or tablets (e.g., miconazole, or clotrimazole). The duration of therapy is controversial, but there is evidence to suggest that high-dose, shorter courses of therapy (two 100-mg clotrimazole tablets inserted intravaginally nightly for three days) are as effective as the standard 7-day course [414,415]. Ketoconazole, 400 mg orally per day for three days, has also been used successfully [416]. For chronically recurrent vaginitis, treatment of concomitant intestinal *Candida* may be helpful (nystatin oral tablets 500,000 units qid for 10 to 14 days) [361,417]. Treatment of sexual partner(s) may also be beneficial [355,356].

Intertriginous and many of the other forms of cutaneous candidiasis (with the exception of CMC) can be treated topically with creams or ointments containing nystatin, amphotericin B, or the imidazoles (miconazole, clotrimazole, econazole, or sulconazole). Powder preparations containing nystatin may be useful in moist, intertriginous areas. The long-held theory that cornstarch application exacerbates candidiasis by providing nutrient support for the organism is probably erroneous [418].

Chronic paronychial infections due to *C. albicans* are more resistant to therapy. All wet work should be minimized. Topical therapy should be applied to the nail folds and allowed to drain under the proximal nail fold if possible. Occlusion using a finger cot may allow better drug penetration. Of the agents available, haloprogin, clotrimazole, or miconazole solutions are the most helpful. Four percent thymol in chloroform or absolute alcohol has anticandidal activity and is drying. Oral ketoconazole or even surgical marsupialization of the proximal nail fold area have been recommended in resistant cases.

Congenital cutaneous candidiasis, although usually resolving spontaneously, can be treated with any of the topical anticandidal agents listed above. Some authors favor treatment of all such cases in order to prevent subsequent disseminated disease [419].

Chronic mucocutaneous candidiasis, in the past, has been notoriously resistant to therapy. However, with the recent addition of ketoconazole to the treatment armamentarium, dramatic improvement is obtainable [420–422]. The usual adult oral dosage is 200 to 400 mg per day. It is essential to perform liver function tests before treatment and at monthly or more frequent intervals during treatment, especially in patients who will be on prolonged therapy. Oral lesions usually clear early followed by cutaneous lesions; nail infections require several months of therapy. Relapse may occur after the drug is discontinued. Other systemic antifungals that have been used in CMC include 5-fluorocytosine [423], amphotericin B, miconazole, or clotrimazole. Other patients have improved with parenteral iron administration [424]. Immunomodulating drugs used in the past include transfer factor, thymosin, cimetidine [425], and levamisole [394,424].

Systemic candidal infections require the use of parenteral amphotericin B.

References

1. Rippon JW: Superficial infections: tinea nigra, in *Medical Mycology: The Pathogenic Fungi and the Pathogenic Actinomycetes*. Philadelphia, WB Saunders, 1982, p 145
2. Horta P: Sobre un caso de tinha preta e un novo cogumelo (*Cladosporium werneckii*). *Rev Med Cirug Brazil* **21**:269,1921
3. McGinnis MR: Taxonomy of *Exophiala werneckii* and its relations to *Microsporum mansonii*. *Sabouraudia* **17**:145, 1979
4. Van Velsor H, Singletary H: Tinea nigra palmaris: a report of 15 cases from coastal North Carolina. *Arch Dermatol* **90**:59, 1964
5. Blank H: Tinea nigra: a twenty-year incubation period? *J Am Acad Dermatol* **1**:49, 1979
6. Helfman RJ: Tinea nigra palmaris et plantaris. *Cutis* **28**:81,1981
7. Spiller WF et al: Tinea nigra. *J Invest Dermatol* **27**:187,1956
8. Isaacs F, Reiss-Levy E: Tinea nigra plantaris: a case report. *Australas J Dermatol* **21**:13, 1980
9. Vaffee AS: Tinea nigra palmaris resembling malignant melanoma. *N Engl J Med* **283**:1112, 1970
10. Carr JF, Lewis CW: Tinea nigra palmaris: treatment with thiabendazole topically. *Arch Dermatol* **111**:904, 1975
11. Baillon H: *Traite de Botanique Medical Cryptoganique*. Paris, Octave Doin Editeur, 1889, p 234
12. Gordon M: Lipophilic yeast-like organisms associated with tinea versicolor. *J Invest Dermatol* **17**:267, 1951
13. Burke RC: Tinea versicolor: susceptibility factors and experimental infection in human beings. *J Invest Dermatol* **36**:389, 1961
14. Tanaka M, Imamura S: Immunological studies on *Pityrosporum* genus and *Malassezia furfur*. *J Invest Dermatol* **73**:321, 1979
15. Faergemann J et al: Antigenic similarities and differences in genus *Pityrosporum*. *J Invest Dermatol* **78**:28, 1982
16. Barnes WG et al: Scanning electron microscopy of tinea versicolor organisms. *Arch Dermatol* **107**:392, 1973
17. Porro MN et al: Growth requirements and lipid metabolism of *Pityrosporum orbiculare*. *J Invest Dermatol* **66**:178,1976
18. Roberts SOB: *Pityrosporum orbiculare*: incidence and distribution on clinically normal skin. *Br J Dermatol* **81**:264, 1969
19. Rippon JW: Superficial infections: pityriasis versicolor, in *Medical Mycology: The Pathogenic Fungi and the Pathogenic Actinomycetes*. Philadelphia, WB Saunders, 1982, p 140
20. Roberts SOB: Pityriasis versicolor: a clinical and mycological investigation. *Br J Dermatol* **81**:315, 1969
21. Faergemann J: Experimental tinea versicolor in rabbits and humans with *Pityrosporum orbiculare*. *J Invest Dermatol* **72**:326, 1979
22. Catterall MB: Tinea versicolor: a reappraisal. *Int J Dermatol* **19**:84, 1980
23. Dahl MV: *Common Office Dermatology*. New York, Grune & Stratton, 1983, p 35
24. Karaoui R et al: Tinea versicolor: ultrastructural studies on hypopigmented and hyperpigmented skin. *Dermatologica* **162**:69, 1981
25. Nazzaro-Porro M, Passi S: Identification of tyrosinase inhibitors in cultures of *Pityrosporum*. *J Invest Dermatol* **71**:205, 1978
26. Potter BS et al: *Pityrosporum* folliculitis: report of seven cases and review of the *Pityrosporum* organism relative to cutaneous disease. *Arch Dermatol* **107**:388, 1973
27. Berretty PJM et al: *Pityrosporum* folliculitis: is it a real entity? *Br J Dermatol* **103**:565, 1980
28. Burkhart CG et al: An unusual case of tinea versicolor in an immunosuppressed patient. *Cutis* **27**:56, 1981
29. Redline RW, Dahms BB: *Malassezia* pulmonary vasculitis in an infant on long-term Intralipid therapy. *N Engl J Med* **305**:1395, 1981
30. Wallace M et al: Isolation of lipophilic yeast in "sterile" peritonitis. *Lancet* **2**:956, 1979
31. Wyre HV, Johnson WT: Neonatal pityriasis versicolor. *Arch Dermatol* **117**:752, 1981
32. DaMert GJ et al: Comparison of antibody responses in chronic mucocutaneous candidiasis and tinea versicolor. *Int Arch Allergy Appl Immunol* **63**:97, 1980
33. Sohnle RG, Collins-Lech C: Cell-mediated immunology to *Pityrosporum orbiculare* in tinea versicolor. *J Clin Invest* **62**:45, 1978
34. Sohnle RG, Collins-Lech C: Activation of complement by *Pityrosporum orbiculare*. *J Invest Dermatol* **80**:93, 1983
35. Popkess FG: A practical office method for the diagnosis of tinea versicolor. *Ann Allergy* **22**:42, 1964
36. Klotz SA et al: *Pityrosporum* folliculitis: its potential for confusion with skin lesions of systemic candidiasis. *Arch Intern Med* **142**:2126, 1982
37. Bamford JTM: Treatment of tinea versicolor with sulfur-salicylic shampoo. *J Am Acad Dermatol* **8**:211, 1983
38. Faergemann J, Fredricksson T: Propylene glycol in the treatment of tinea versicolor. *Acta Derm Venereol (Stockh)* **60**:92, 1980
39. Urcuyo FG, Zaias N: The successful treatment of pityriasis versicolor by systemic ketoconazole. *J Am Acad Dermatol* **6**:24, 1982
40. Borelli D: Treatment of pityriasis versicolor with ketoconazole. *Rev Infect Dis* **2**:592, 1980
41. Rippon JW: superficial infections: piedra, in *Medical Mycology: The Pathogenic Fungi and the Pathogenic Actinomycetes*. Philadelphia, WB Saunders, 1982, p 148
42. Lassus A et al: White piedra: report of a case evaluated by scanning electron microscopy. *Arch Dermatol* **118**:208, 1982
43. Emmons EW et al (eds): Black piedra, white piedra and trichomycosis axillaris, in *Medical Mycology*. Philadelphia, Lea & Febiger, 1977, p 181
44. Conant NF: Piedra, in *Manual of Clinical Mycology*, 3rd ed. Philadelphia, WB Saunders, 1971, p 632
45. Manzella JP et al: *Trichosporon beigelii* fungemia and cutaneous dissemination. *Arch Dermatol* **118**:343, 1982
46. Winston DJ et al: Disseminated *Trichosporon capitatum* infection in an immunosuppressed host. *Arch Intern Med* **137**:1192, 1977
47. Rivera R, Cangir A: *Trichosporon* sepsis and leukemia. *Cancer* **36**:1106, 1975
48. Watson KC, Kallinchurum S: Brain abscess due to *Trichosporon cutaneum*. *J Med Microbiol* **3**:191, 1970
49. Kirmani N et al: Disseminated *Trichosporon* infection: occurrence in an immunosuppressed patient with chronic active hepatitis. *Arch Intern Med* **140**:277, 1980
50. Evans HL et al: systemic mycosis due to *Trichosporon cutaneum*. *Cancer* **58**:591, 1980
51. Rippon JW: Dermatophytosis and dermatomycosis, in *Medi-*

cal Mycology: The Pathogenic Fungi and the Pathogenic Actinomycetes. Philadelphia, WB Saunders, 1982, p 154

52. Gruby D: Sur les mycodermes que constituent la teigne faveuse. *C R Acad Sci (Paris)* **13**:309, 1841

53. Sabouraud R: *Les Teignes.* Paris, Masson et Cie, 1910

54. Dawson CO, Gentles JC: The perfect stage of *Keratinomyces ajelloi. Nature* **183**:1345, 1959

55. Gentles JC: Experimental ringworm in guinea pigs: oral treatment with griseofulvin. *Nature* **182**:476, 1958

56. Blank H, Roth FJ: The treatment of dermatomycoses with orally administered griseofulvin. *Arch Dermatol* **79**:259, 1959

57. Roberts SOB, Mackenzie DWR: Mycology, in *Textbook of Dermatology,* edited by A Rook et al. London, Blackwell, 1979, p 767

58. Blank H et al: Cutaneous *Trichophyton mentagrophytes* infections in Vietnam. *Arch Dermatol* **99**:135, 1969

59. Otcenasek M: Ecology of the dermatophytes. *Mycopathologica* **65**:67, 1978

60. Philpot CM: Some aspects of the epidemiology of tinea. *Mycopathologica* **62**:3, 1977

61. Georg LK: Epidemiology of the dermatophytoses: sources of infection, modes of transmission and epidemicity. *Ann NY Acad Sci* **89**:69, 1960

62. Whittle CH: A small epidemic of *M. gypseum* ringworm in a plant nursery. *Br J Dermatol* **66**:353, 1954

63. Caprilli F et al: Etiology of ringworm of the scalp, beard, and body in Rome, Italy. *Sabouraudia* **18**:129, 1980

64. Blank F et al: Distribution of dermatophytosis according to age, ethnic group and sex. *Sabouraudia* **12**:352, 1974

65. Hernandez AD: An approach to the diagnosis and therapy of dermatophytosis. *Int J Dermatol* **19**:540, 1980

66. Mandel EH: Diagnosis: tinea circinata and onychomycosis (*Trichophyton purpureum*): resistance to griseofulvin during uncontrolled diabetes. *Arch Dermatol* **82**:1027, 1960

67. Jolly HW, Carpenter CL: Oral glucose tolerance studies in recurrent *Trichophyton rubrum* infections. *Arch Dermatol* **100**:26, 1969

68. Lewis GM et al: Generalized *Trichophyton rubrum* infection associated with systemic lymphoblastoma. *Arch Dermatol* **67**:247, 1953

69. Allen DE et al: Generalized *Microsporum audouinii* infection and depressed cellular immunity associated with a missing plasma factor required for lymphocyte blastogenesis. *Am J Med* **63**:991, 1977

70. Nelson LM, McNiece KJ: Recurrent Cushing's syndrome with *Trichophyton rubrum* infection. *Arch Dermatol* **80**:700, 1959

71. Philpot CM: Geographical distribution of the dermatophytes: a review. *J Hyg (Lond)* **80**:301, 1978

72. Ajello L: Geographic distribution and prevalence of the dermatophytes. *Ann NY Acad Sci* **89**:30, 1960

73. Binazzi M et al: Skin mycoses—geographic distribution and present-day pathomorphosis. *Int J Dermatol* **22**:92, 1983

74. Many H et al: *Trichophyton rubrum:* exposure and infection within household groups. *Arch Dermatol* **82**:226, 1960

75. Saferstein HL et al: Endothrix ringworm: a new public health problem in Philadelphia. *JAMA* **190**:115, 1964

76. Malhotra YK et al: A study of tinea capitis in Libya (Benghazi). *Sabouraudia* **17**:181, 1979

77. Georg LK: *Trichophyton tonsurans* ringworm—a new public health problem. *Public Health Rep* **67**:53, 1952

78. Blank F, Mann SJ: *Trichophyton rubrum* infections according to age, anatomical distribution and sex. *Br J Dermatol* **2**:171, 1975

79. Rippon JW et al: *Trichophyton simii* infection in the United States. *Arch Dermatol* **98**:615, 1968

80. Allen AM, Taplin D: Epidemic *Trichophyton mentagrophytes* infections in servicemen: source of infection, role of environment, host factors, and susceptibility. *JAMA* **226**:864, 1973

81. Sanderson PH, Sloper JC: Skin disease in the British army in S.E. Asia III: The relationship between mycotic infections of the body and of the feet. *Br J Dermatol* **65**:362, 1953

82. Taplin D et al: Environmental influences on the microbiology of the skin. *Arch Environ Health* **11**:546, 1965

83. Ravine D et al: Genetic inheritance of susceptibility to tinea imbricata. *J Med Genet* **17**:342, 1980

84. Georg LK: The relationship between the downy and granular forms of *Trichophyton mentagrophytes. J Invest Dermatol* **23**:123, 1954

85. Knight AG: A review of experimental human fungus infections. *J Invest Dermatol* **59**:354, 1972

86. Baer RL et al: Newer studies on the epidemiology of fungous infections of the feet. *Am J Public Health* **45**:784, 1955

87. Baer RL, Rosenthal SA: The biology of fungous infections of the feet. *JAMA* **197**:1017, 1966

88. Hernandez AD: An approach to the diagnosis and therapy of dermatophytosis. *Int J Dermatol* **19**:540, 1980

89. Kligman AM: The pathogenesis of tinea capitis due to *Microsporum audouini* and *Microsporum canis:* I. Gross observations following the inoculation of humans. *J Invest Dermatol* **18**:231, 1952

90. Kligman AM: Tinea capitis due to *M. audouini* and *M. canis:* II. Dynamics of the host-parasite relationship. *Arch Dermatol* **71**:313, 1955

91. English MP, Gibson MD: Studies in the epidemiology of tinea pedis. I. Tinea pedis in school children. *Br Med J* **1**:1442, 1959

92. Davis CM et al: Dermatophytes in military recruits. *Arch Dermatol* **105**:558, 1972

93. Raubitchek F: Infectivity and family incidence of black-dot tinea capitis. *Arch Dermatol* **79**:477, 1959

94. Friedman L et al: The course of untreated tinea capitis in Negro children. *J Invest Dermatol* **42**:237, 1964

95. Ive FA: The carrier stage of tinea capitis in Nigeria. *Br J Dermatol* **78**:219, 1966

96. Knudsen FA: The areal extent of dermatophyte infection. *Br J Dermatol* **92**:413, 1975

97. Berk SH et al: Epidermal activity in annular dermatophytosis. *Arch Dermatol* **112**:485, 1976

98. Yu RJ et al: Two cell-bound keratinases of *Trichophyton mentagrophytes. J Invest Dermatol* **56**:27, 1971

99. Meevootisom V, Niederpruem DJ: Control of exocellular proteases in dermatophytes and especially *Trichophyton rubrum. Sabouraudia* **17**:91, 1979

100. Mercer EH, Verma BS: Hair digested by *Trichophyton mentagrophytes. Arch Dermatol* **87**:357, 1963

101. Verma BS: The use of fluorescence microscopy in the study of *in vitro* hair penetration by ringworm fungi. *Br J Dermatol* **78**:222, 1966

102. Cruickshank CND, Trotter MD: Separation of epidermis from dermis by filtrates of *Trichophyton mentagrophytes. Nature* **177**:1085, 1956

103. Kligman AM: Pathophysiology of ringworm infections in animals with skin cycles. *J Invest Dermatol* **27**:171, 1956

104. Marks R, Dawber RPR: *In situ* microbiology of the stratum corneum: an application of skin surface biopsy. *Arch Dermatol* **105**:216, 1972

105. Emmons CW et al (eds): Dermatophytoses, in *Medical Mycology.* Philadelphia, Lea & Febiger, 1977, p 117

106. Ahmed AR: Immunology of human dermatophyte infections. *Arch Dermatol* **118**:521, 1983

107. Grappel SF et al: Immunology of dermatophytes and dermatophytosis. *Bacteriol Rev* **38**:222, 1974

108. Dahl MV: Host defense: fungus, in *Clinical Immunodermatology.* Chicago, Year Book Medical Publishers, 1981, p 127

109. Rothman S et al: The spontaneous cure of tinea capitis in puberty. *J Invest Dermatol* **8**:81, 1947

110. Lorincz AL et al: Evidence for a humoral mechanism which

prevents growth of dermatophytes. *J Invest Dermatol* **31:**15, 1958

111. Roth FJ et al: An evaluation of the fungistatic activity of serum. *J Invest Dermatol* **32:**549, 1959

112. Memmesheimer AR et al: Studies of fungistatic activity in normal human blood serum. *Sabouraudia* **2:**1, 1962

113. King RD et al: Transferrin, iron, and dermatophytes. I. Serum dermatophyte inhibitory component definitely identified as unsaturated transferrin. *J Lab Clin Med* **86:**204, 1975

114. Mosher WA et al: Nutritional requirements of the pathogenic mold: *T. interdigitale. Plant Physiol* **11:**795, 1936

115. Yu RJ et al: Inhibition of keratinases by alpha-2-macroglobulin. *Experientia* **28:**886, 1972

116. Blank HD et al: Widespread *Trichophyton rubrum* granulomas treated with griseofulvin. *Arch Dermatol* **81:**779, 1960

117. Grappel SF et al: Circulating antibodies in dermatophytosis. *Dermatologica* **144:**1, 1972

118. Jones HE et al: Apparent cross-reactivity of airborne molds and the dermatophytic fungi. *J Allergy Clin Immunol* **52:**346, 1973

119. Young E, Roth FJ: Immunological cross-reactivity between a glycoprotein isolated from *Trichophyton mentagrophytes* and human isoantigen A. *J Invest Dermatol* **72:**46, 1979

120. Peck SM et al: Intercellular antibodies: presence in a *Trichophyton rubrum* infection. *J Invest Dermatol* **58:**133, 1972

121. Hopfer RL et al: Antibodies with affinity for epithelial tissue in chronic dermatophytosis. *Dermatologica* **151:**135, 1975

122. Jones HE: The atopic-chronic-dermatophytosis syndrome. *Acta Derm Venereol [Suppl] (Stockh)* **92:**81, 1980

123. Conant NF et al: Immunology of the dermatomycoses, in *Manual of Clinical Mycology,* 3rd ed. Philadelphia, WB Saunders, 1971, p 587

124. Brahmi Z et al: Depressed cell-mediated immunity in chronic dermatophytic infections. *Ann Immunol (Paris)* **131C:**143, 1980

125. Jones HE et al: Acquired immunity to dermatophytes. *Arch Dermatol* **109:**840, 1974

126. Delamater ED, Benham RW: Experimental studies with the dermatophytes. I. Primary disease in laboratory animals. *J Invest Dermatol* **1:**451, 1938

127. Delamater ED, Benham RW: Experimental studies with the dermatophytes. II. Immunity and hypersensitivity in laboratory animals. *J Invest Dermatol* **1:**451, 1938

128. Holden CA et al: A method for identification of dermatophyte antigens *in situ* by an immunoperoxidase technique and electron microscopy. *Clin Exp Dermatol* **6:**311, 1981

129. Holden CA et al: The antigenicity of *Trichophyton rubrum: in situ* studies by an immunoperoxidase technique in light and electron microscopy. *Acta Derm Venereol (Stockh)* **61:**207, 1981

130. Hanifin JM et al: Immunological reactivity in dermatophytosis. *Br J Dermatol* **90:**1, 1974

131. Hay RJ, Brostoff J: Immune responses in patients with chronic *Trichophyton rubrum* infections. *Clin Exp Dermatol* **2:**373, 1977

132. Kaaman T: The clinical significance of cutaneous reactions to *Trichophyton* in dermatophytosis. *Acta Derm Venereol (Stockh)* **58:**139, 1978

133. Hay RJ: Chronic dermatophyte infections. I. Clinical and mycological features. *Br J Dermatol* **106:**1, 1982

134. Hay RJ, Shennan G: Chronic dermatophyte infections. II. Antibody and cell-mediated immune responses. *Br J Dermatol* **106:**191, 1982

135. Marmor MF, Barrett EV: Cutaneous anergy without systemic disease: a syndrome associated with mucocutaneous fungal infection. *Am J Med* **44:**979, 1968

136. Alteras I et al: The high incidence of tinea pedis and unguium in patients with Kaposi's sarcoma. *Mycopathologica* **74:**177, 1981

137. Shama SK, Kirkpatrick CH: Dermatophytosis in patients with chronic mucocutaneous candidiasis. *J Am Acad Dermatol* **2:**285, 1980

138. Jones HE et al: A clinical, mycological, and immunological survey for dermatophytosis. *Arch Dermatol* **108:**61, 1973

139. Jones HE et al: Immunologic susceptibility to chronic dermatophytosis. *Arch Dermatol* **110:**213, 1974

140. Helander I: Lymphocyte transformation test in dermatophytes. *Mykosen* **21:**71, 1978

141. Hunziker N, Brun R: Lack of delayed reaction in presence of cell-mediated immunity in *Trichophyton* hypersensitivity. *Arch Dermatol* **116:**1266, 1980

142. Wang SR, Zweiman B: Histamine suppression of human lymphocyte responses to mitogens. *Cell Immunol* **36:**28, 1978

143. Rocklin RE: Modulation of cellular-immune responses *in vivo* and *in vitro* by histamine receptor-bearing lymphocytes. *J Clin Immunol* **57:**1051, 1976

144. Rocklin RE: Histamine-induced suppressor factor (HSF): effect on migration inhibitory factor (MIF) production and proliferation. *J Immunol* **118:**1734, 1977

145. Presser SE, Blank H: Cimetidine: adjunct in treatment of tinea capitis. *Lancet* **1:**108, 1981

146. Jillson OF: Immunology of dermatophytosis: lack of immunity and hyperimmunity. *Cutis* **30:**159, 1982

147. Jillson OF: Dermatophytids and candidids. *Semin Dermatol* **2:**60, 1983

148. Jadassohn J: *Korblatt Schweiz Aerzte* **42:**22, 1912

149. Martinez-Roig A et al: Erythema nodosum and kerion of the scalp. *Am J Dis Child* **136:**440, 1982

150. Waisman M: Recurrent, fixed erysipelas-like dermatophytid. *Arch Dermatol* **53:**10, 1946

151. Jillson OF: Allergic confirmation that some cases of erythema annulare centrifugum are dermatophytids. *Arch Dermatol* **70:**355, 1954

152. Weary PE, Guerrant JL: Chronic urticaria in association with dermatophytosis: response to the administration of griseofulvin. *Arch Dermatol* **95:**400, 1967

153. Rudolph AH et al: Tinea capitis, in *Clinical Dermatology,* edited by DJ Demis et al. Philadelphia, Harper & Row, 1978

154. Prevost E: Nonfluorescent tinea capitis in Charleston, SC: A diagnostic problem. *JAMA* **242:**1765, 1979

155. Laude TA et al: Tinea capitis in Brooklyn. *Am J Dis Child* **136:**1047, 1982

156. Ridley CM: Tinea capitis in an elderly woman. *Clin Exp Dermatol* **4:**247, 1979

157. Bronson DM et al: An epidemic of infection with *Trichophyton tonsurans* revealed in a 20-year survey of fungal infections in Chicago. *J Am Acad Dermatol* **8:**322, 1983

158. Seale ER, Richardson JB: *Trichophyton tonsurans:* a follow-up of treated and untreated cases. *Arch Dermatol* **8:**125, 1960

159. Pipkin JL: Tinea capitis in the adult and adolescent. *Arch Dermatol* **66:**9, 1952

160. Vanbreuseghem R: Tinea capitis in the Belgian Congo and Ruanda Urundi. *Trop Geogr Med* **10:**103, 1958

161. Guirges SY: Viability of *Trichophyton schoenleinii* in epilated hairs. *Sabouraudia* **19:**155, 1981

162. Rosenthal SA, Vanbreuseghem R: Viability of dermatophytes in epilated hairs. *Arch Dermatol* **85:**143, 1962

163. Clayton YM, Midgely G: New approach to the investigation of scalp ringworm in London school children. *J Clin Pathol* **21:**791, 1968

164. Crozier WJ, Searls S: "Double" or "mixed" fungal infections: significant, or not? *Australas J Dermatol* **20:**43, 1979

165. Grigoriu D, Delacretaz J: Mixed dermatophytical infection of the scalp. *Dermatologica* **164:**407, 1982

166. Varadi DP, Rippon JW: Scalp infection of triple etiology. *Arch Dermatol* **95:**299, 1967

167. Wilson JW, Plunkett OA: Dermatophytosis, in *The Fungous*

Diseases of Man. Berkeley, Univ of California Press, 1965, p 213

168. Rook A, Dawber R: Infections and infestations, in *Diseases of the Hair and Scalp.* Oxford, Blackwell, 1982, p 367

169. Feuerman EJ et al: Kerion-like tinea capitis and barbae caused by *Microsporum gypseum* in Israel. *Mycopathologica* **58:**165, 1976

170. Honig PJ, Smith LR: Tinea capitis masquerading as atopic or seborrheic dermatitis. *J Pediatr* **94:**604, 1979

171. Howell JB et al: Tinea capitis caused by *Trichophyton tonsurans* (sulfureum or crateriforme). *Arch Dermatol* **65:**194, 1952

172. Rudolph AH: The clinical recognition of tinea capitis from *Trichophyton tonsurans. JAMA* **242:**1770, 1979

173. Foged EK, Sylvest B: Occurrence of *Trichophyton tonsurans* infections in the Danish island of Funen. *Acta Derm Venereol (Stockh)* **62:**159, 1982

174. Wolf FT et al: Fluorescent pigment of *Microsporum. Nature* **182:**475, 1958

175. Beare M, Walker J: Non-fluorescent *Microsporum audouini* and *canis* infections of the scalp. *Br J Dermatol* **67:**101, 1955

176. Mackenzie DWR: "Hairbrush diagnosis" in detection and eradication of non-fluorescent scalp ringworm. *Br Med J* **2:**363, 1963

177. Shelley WB, Wood MG: New technic for instant visualization of fungi in hair. *J Am Acad Dermatol* **2:**69, 1980

178. Graham JH, Barroso-Tobila C: Dermal pathology of superficial fungus infections, in *Human Infection with Fungi, Actinomycetes, and Algae,* edited by RD Baker et al. New York, Springer-Verlag, 1971, p 211

179. Lever WF, Schaumburg-Lever G: Fungal diseases, in *Histopathology of the Skin,* 6th ed. Philadelphia, JB Lippincott, 1983, p 328

180. Imamura S et al: Use of immunofluorescence staining in kerion. *Arch Dermatol* **111:**906, 1975

181. Friedman L et al: The control of tinea capitis among indigent populations. *Am J Public Health* **54:**1588, 1964

182. Vanbreuseghem R et al: Mass treatment of scalp ringworm by a single dose of griseofulvin. *Int J Dermatol* **9:**59, 1970

183. Oskui J: Intermittent use of griseofulvin in tinea capitis. *Cutis* **21:**689, 1978

184. Allen HB et al: Selenium sulfide: adjunctive therapy for tinea capitis. *Pediatrics* **69:**81, 1982

185. Khan KA, Anwar AA: Study of 73 cases of tinea capitis and tinea favosa in adults and adolescents. *J Invest Dermatol* **51:**474, 1968

186. Joly J et al: Favus: twenty indigenous cases in the province of Quebec. *Arch Dermatol* **114:**1647, 1978

187. Hakendorf AJ et al: Favus. *Australas J Dermatol* **8:**22, 1965

188. Dvoretzky I et al: Favus. *Int J Dermatol* **19:**89, 1980

189. Sams WM: Favus treated with griseofulvin. *Arch Dermatol* **81:**802, 1960

190. Nierman MM, Landay ME: *Trichophyton verrucosum* in Indiana: infection in two cases. *Cutis* **26:**591, 1980

191. Hall FR: Ringworm contracted from cattle in western New York state. *Arch Dermatol* **94:**35, 1966

192. Loewenthal K: Tinea barbae due to *Microsporum canis. Arch Dermatol* **91:**60, 1965

193. McAleer R: Fungal infection as a cause of skin disease in Western Australia. III. Tinea barbae. *Australas J Dermatol* **21:**40, 1980

194. Jansen GT et al: Tinea barbae, in *Clinical Dermatology,* edited by DJ Demis et al. Philadelphia, Harper & Row, 1978

195. Domonkos AN et al: Diseases due to fungi, in *Andrews' Diseases of the Skin,* 7th ed. Philadelphia WB Saunders, 1982, p 341

196. Alteras I, Feuerman EJ: Atypical cases of *Microsporum canis* infection in the adult. *Mycopathologica* **74:**181, 1981

197. Hay RJ et al: Immune responses of patients with tinea imbricata. *Br J Dermatol* **108:**581, 1983

198. Gill KA et al: Fungus infections occurring under occlusive dressings. *Arch Dermatol* **88:**348, 1963

199. Cullen SI, Ioannides G: Bullous dermatophyte infections. *Cutis* **6:**661, 1970

200. Costello MJ: Vesicular *Trichophyton rubrum (purpureum)* infection simulating dermatitis herpetiformis. *Arch Dermatol* **66:**653, 1952

201. Tolmach JA, Schweig J: Generalized *Trichophyton purpureum* infection simulating dermatitis herpetiformis. *Arch Dermatol* **41:**732, 1940

202. Powell FC, Muller SA: Kerion of glabrous skin. *J Am Acad Dermatol* **7:**490, 1982

203. Wilson JW et al: Nodular granulomatosus perifolliculitis of the legs caused by *Trichophyton rubrum. Arch Dermatol* **69:**258, 1954

204. Schreiber MM: *Trichophyton rubrum* perifollicular granuloma of legs. *Cutis* **3:**1083, 1967

205. Smith EB, Head ES: Subcutaneous abscess due to *Trichophyton mentagrophytes. Int J Dermatol* **21:**338, 1982

206. Swart E, Smit FJA: *Trichophyton violaceum* abscesses. *Br J Dermatol* **101:**177, 1979

207. Araviysky AN et al: Deep generalized trichophytosis (endothrix in tissues of different origin). *Mycopathologica* **56:**47, 1975

208. McAleer R: Fungal infection as a cause of skin disease in Western Australia. I. Tinea corporis. *Australas J Dermatol* **21:**25, 1980

209. West BC, Kwon-Chung KJ: Mycetoma caused by *Microsporum audouinii. Am J Clin Pathol* **73:**447, 1980

210. Shanon J, Raubitschek F: Tinea faciei simulating chronic discoid lupus erythematosus. *Arch Dermatol* **82:**268, 1960

211. Gilgor RS et al: Lupus-erythematosus-like tinea of the face (tinea faciale). *JAMA* **215:**2091, 1971

212. Rist TE et al: Tinea faciale: an often misdiagnosed clinical entity. *South Med J* **67:**331, 1974

213. Shapiro L, Cohen JH: Tinea faciei simulating other dermatoses. *JAMA* **215:**2106, 1971

214. Ive FA, Marks R: Tinea incognito. *Br Med J* **3:**149, 1968

215. Burkhart CG: Tinea incognito. *Arch Dermatol* **117:**606, 1981

216. Fisher BK et al: Verrucous epidermophytosis, its response and resistance to griseofulvin. *Arch Dermatol* **84:**375, 1961

217. Emtestam L, Kaaman T: The changing clinical picture of *Microsporum canis* infections in Sweden. *Acta Derm Venereol (Stockh)* **62:**539, 1982

218. McAleer R: Fungal infection as a cause of skin disease in Western Australia. II. Tinea cruris. *Australas J Dermatol* **21:**33, 1980

219. Blank F, Prichard H: Epidemic ringworm of the groin. *Arch Dermatol* **85:**410, 1962

220. Gip L: Isolation of *Trichophyton gallinae* from 2 patients with tinea cruris. *Acta Derm Venereol (Stockh)* **44:**251, 1964

221. Neves H, Xavier NC: The transmission of tinea cruris. *Br J Dermatol* **76:**429, 1964

222. Rosman N: Infections with *Trichophyton rubrum. Br J Dermatol* **78:**208, 1966

223. Hopkins JG et al: Dermatophytosis at an infantry post. *J Invest Dermatol* **8:**291, 1947

224. LaTouche CJ: Scrotal dermatophytosis: an insufficiently documented aspect of tinea cruris. *Br J Dermatol* **79:**339, 1967

225. Davis CM et al: Dermatophytes in military recruits. *Arch Dermatol* **105:**558, 1972

226. Fox T: Tinea circinata of the hand. *Br Med J* **1:**116, 1870

227. Pellizari C: Recherche sur *Trychophyton tonsurans. Giornale Italiano Della Malattie Veneree* **29:**8, 1888

228. Gentles JC, Holmes JG: Foot ringworm in coal-miners. *Br J Ind Med* **14:**22, 1959

229. English MP et al: Studies in the epidemiology of tinea pedis. *Br Med J* **1:**1083, 1961

230. Broughton RH: Reinfection from socks and shoes in tinea pedis. *Br J Dermatol* **67**:249, 1955

231. Ajello L, Getz ME: Recovery of dermatophytes from shoes and shower stalls. *J Invest Dermatol* **22**:17, 1954

232. Munro-Ashman D, Clayton Y: Tinea pedis in adolescence. *Proc R Soc Med* **55**:551, 1962

233. Ajello L et al: Observations in the incidence of tinea pedis in a group of men entering military life. *Johns Hopkins Med Bull* **77**:440, 1945

234. Strauss JS, Kligman AM: An experimental study of tinea pedis and onychomycosis of the foot. *Arch Dermatol* **76**:70, 1957

235. Leyden JJ: Microbial ecology in interdigital "athlete's" foot infection. *Semin Dermatol* **1**:149, 1982

236. Leyden JJ, Kligman AM: Interdigital athlete's foot. *Arch Dermatol* **114**:1466, 1978

237. Leyden JJ, Kligman AM: Aluminum chloride in the treatment of symptomatic athlete's foot. *Arch Dermatol* **111**:1004, 1975

238. Arndt KA: *Manual of Dermatologic Therapeutics*, 3d ed. Boston, Little, Brown, 1983, p 82

239. Jewell EW: *Trichophyton rubrum* onychomycosis in a four month old infant. *Cutis* **6**:1121, 1970

240. Ramesh V et al: Onychomycosis. *Int J Dermatol* **22**:148, 1983

241. English MP, Atkinson R: Onychomycosis in elderly chiropody patients. *Br J Dermatol* **91**:67, 1974

242. Zaias N: Onychomycosis. *Arch Dermatol* **105**:263, 1972

243. Tuzun Y: *Microsporum* infections of the nails. *Arch Dermatol* **116**:620, 1980

244. Zaias N: Fungi in toe nails. *J Invest Dermatol* **53**:140, 1969

245. Onsberg P: The fungal flora of normal and diseased nails. *Curr Ther Res* **22**:20, 1977

246. English MP: Nails and fungi. *Br J Dermatol* **94**:697, 1976

247. Zaias N: Onychomycosis, in *The Nail: In Health and Disease*. New York, SP Medical & Scientific Books, 1980, p 91

248. Zaias N: Superficial white onychomycosis. *Sabouraudia* **5**:99, 1966

249. Norton LA: Nail disorders: a review. *J Am Acad Dermatol* **2**:451, 1980

250. Baron R: Onychia and paronychia of mycotic, microbial and parasitic origin, in *The Nail*, edited by M Pierre. New York, Churchill Livingstone, 1981, p 39

251. Raubitschek F, Maoz R: Invasion of nails in vitro by certain dermatophytes. *J Invest Dermatol* **28**:261, 1957

252. Meyer JC et al: Onychomycosis (*Trichophyton mentagrophytes*): a scanning electron microscopic observation. *J Clin Pathol* **8**:342, 1981

253. Reiss F: Leukonychia trichophytica caused by *Trichophyton rubrum*. *Cutis* **20**:223, 1977

254. Gentles JC: Laboratory investigations of dermatophyte infections of nails. *Sabouraudia* **9**:149, 1971

255. Davies RR: Mycological tests and onychomycosis. *J Clin Pathol* **21**:729, 1968

256. Samman PD: Fungous infection, in *The Nails in Disease*, 3d ed. London, Heinemann Medical Books, 1978, p 40

257. Epstein S: Examination of nails for fungi. *Arch Dermatol* **51**:209, 1945

258. Shelley WB, Wood MG: The white spot target for microscopic examination of nails for fungi. *J Am Acad Dermatol* **6**:92, 1982

259. Scher RK, Ackerman AB: Subtle clues to diagnosis from biopsies of nails. *Am J Dermatopathol* **2**:255, 1980

260. Blank H et al: Griseofulvin for systemic treatment of dermatomycoses. *JAMA* **171**:2168, 1959

261. White MI, Clayton YM: The treatment of fungus and yeast infections of nails by the method of "chemical removal." *Clin Exp Dermatol* **7**:273, 1982

262. Kobayashi GS, Medoff G: Antifungal agents: recent developments. *Annu Rev Microbiol* **31**:291, 1977

263. Medoff G, Kobayashi GS: Strategies in the treatment of systemic fungal infections. *N Engl J Med* **302**:145, 1980

264. Medoff G et al: Antifungal agents useful in therapy of systemic fungal infections. *Annu Rev Pharmacol Toxicol* **23**:303, 1983

265. Arndt KA: *Manual of Dermatologic Therapeutics*, 3d ed. Boston, Little, Brown, 1983, p 258

266. D'Arcy PF, Scott EM: Antifungal agents. *Prog Drug Res* **22**:93, 1978

267. Graybill JR, Craven PC: Antifungal agents used in systemic mycoses: activity and therapeutic use. *Drugs* **25**:41, 1983

268. Oxford AE et al: Studies in the biochemistry of microorganisms: LX. Griseofulvin, $C_{17}H_{19}O_6Cl$, a metabolic product of penicillium griseofulvum. *Biochem J* **33**:240, 1939

269. Brian PW et al: Biological assay, production and isolation of "curling factor." *Trans Br Mycol Soc* **29**:173, 1946

270. Borgers M, Van den Bossche H: The mode of action of antifungal drugs, in *Ketoconazole in the Management of Fungal Disease*, edited by HB Levine. New York, Adis Press, 1982, p 25

271. Borgers M: Mechanism of action of antifungal drugs, with special reference to the imidazole derivatives. *Rev Infect Dis* **2**:520, 1980

272. D'arcy PF et al: The anti-inflammatory action of griseofulvin in experimental animals. *J Pharm Pharmacol* **12**:659, 1960

273. Lenhart K: Griseofulvin resistant mutants in dermatophytes. *Mykosen* **13**:139, 1970

274. Artis WM et al: Griseofulvin-resistant dermatophytosis correlates with *in vitro* resistance. *Arch Dermatol* **117**:16, 1981

275. Sande MA, Mandell GL: Antimicrobial agents, in *The Pharmacological Basis of Therapeutics*, 6th ed, edited by AG Goodman et al. New York, Macmillan, 1980, p 1232

276. Ginsburg CM et al: Effect of feeding on bioavailability of griseofulvin in children. *J Pediatr* **102**:309, 1983

277. Crounse RG: Human pharmacology of griseofulvin: the effect of fat intake on gastrointestinal absorption. *J Invest Dermatol* **37**:529, 1961

278. Epstein WL et al: Dermatopharmacology of griseofulvin. *Cutis* **15**:271, 1975

279. Epstein WL et al: Griseofulvin levels in stratum corneum: study after oral administration in man. *Arch Dermatol* **106**:344, 1972

280. Scott A: Behaviour of radioactive griseofulvin in skin. *Nature* **187**:705, 1960

281. Blank H: Commentary: Treatment of dermatomycoses with griseofulvin. *Arch Dermatol* **118**:835, 1982

282. Berman A, Franklin RL: Precipitation of acute intermittent porphyria by griseofulvin therapy. *JAMA* **192**:1005, 1965

283. Riegelman S et al: Griseofulvin-phenobarbital interaction in man. *JAMA* **213**:426, 1970

284. Anderson DW: Griseofulvin: biology and clinical usefulness. A review. *Ann Allergy* **23**:103, 1965

285. Battistini F et al: Clinical antifungal activity of thiabendazole. *Arch Dermatol* **109**:695, 1974

286. MacKie RM: Topical econazole in cutaneous fungal infections. *Practitioner* **224**:1311, 1980

287. Borgers M et al: The mechanism of action of the new antimycotic ketoconazole. *Am J Med (suppl)* **74**:2B, 1983

288. Samsoen M, Jelen G: Allergy to daktarin gel. *Contact Dermatitis* **3**:351, 1977

289. Graybill JR, Drutz DJ: Ketoconazole: a major innovation for treatment of fungal disease. *Ann Intern Med* **93**:921, 1980

290. Ketoconazole (Nizoral^R): a new antifungal agent. *Med Lett Drugs Ther* **23**:85, 1981

291. Hume AL, Kerkering TM: Ketoconazole. *Drug Intelligence and Clinical Pharmacy* **17**:169, 1983

292. Horsburgh CR, Kirkpatrick CH: Long-term therapy of chronic mucocutaneous candidiasis with ketoconazole: experience with twenty-one patients. *Am J Med (suppl)* **74**:23, 1983

293. Cox FW et al: Oral ketoconazole for dermatophyte infections. *J Am Acad Dermatol* **6**:455, 1982

294. Robertson MH et al: Ketoconazole in griseofulvin-resistant dermatophytosis. *J Am Acad Dermatol* **6**:224, 1982

295. Hay RJ, Clayton YM: Treatment of chronic dermatophyte infections: the use of ketoconazole in griseofulvin treatment failures. *Clin Exp Dermatol* **7**:611, 1982

296. Jones HE et al: Oral ketoconazole: an effective and safe treatment for dermatophytosis. *Arch Dermatol* **117**:129, 1981

297. Welsh O, Rodriquez M: Treatment of dermatomycoses with ketoconazole. *Rev Infect Dis* **2**:582, 1980

298. Galimberti R et al: The activity of ketoconazole in the treatment of onychomycosis. *Rev Infect Dis* **2**:596, 1980

299. Pont A et al: Ketoconazole blocks testosterone synthesis. *Arch Intern Med* **142**:2137, 1982

300. Pont A et al: Ketoconazole blocks adrenal steroid synthesis. *Ann Intern Med* **97**:370, 1982

301. Tkach JR, Rinaldi MG: Severe hepatitis associated with ketoconazole therapy for chronic mucocutaneous candidiasis. *Cutis* **29**:482, 1982

302. Heiberg JK, Svejgaard E: Toxic hepatitis during ketoconazole treatment. *Br Med J* **283**:825, 1981

303. Jones HE: Ketoconazole. *Arch Dermatol* **118**:217, 1982

304. Janssen PAJ, Symoens JE: Hepatic reactions during ketoconazole treatment. *Am J Med (suppl)* **74**:80, 1983

305. Graybill Jr: Summary: Potential and problems with ketoconazole. *Am J Med (suppl)* **74**:86, 1983

306. Lyddon FE et al: Short chain fatty acids in the treatment of dermatophytoses. *Int J Dermatol* **19**:24, 1980

307. Sakurai K et al: Mode of action of 6-cyclohexyl-1-hydroxy-4-methyl-2(1H)-pyridone ethanolamine salt (HOE 296). *Chemotherapy* **24**:68, 1978

308. Dittmar W: Penetration and antimycotic efficacy of ciclopirox olamine in keratinized body tissue. *Arzneimittelforsch/Drug Res* **31**:1353, 1981

309. Qadripur SA et al: On the local efficacy of ciclopirox olamine in onychomycosis. *Arzneimittelforsch/Drug Res* **31**:1369, 1981

310. Rippon JW: Candidiasis and the pathogenic yeasts, in *Medical Mycology: The Pathogenic Fungi and the Pathogenic Actinomycetes*. Philadelphia, WB Saunders, 1982, p 484

311. Hopfer RL: Mycology of *Candida* infections, in *Candidiasis*, edited by GP Bodey, V Fainstein. New York, Raven Press, 1985, p 1

312. Smith CB: Candidiasis: pathogenesis, host resistance, and predisposing factors, in *Candidiasis*, edited by GP Bodey, V Fainstein. New York, Raven Press, 1985, p 53

313. Ray TL, Wuepper KD: Recent advances in cutaneous candidiasis. *Int J Dermatol* **17**:683, 1978

314. Ray TL et al: Experimental cutaneous candidiasis: role of the stratum corneum. *Clin Res* **24**:495A, 1976

315. Maibach HI, Kligman AM: The biology of experimental human cutaneous moniliasis (*Candida albicans*). *Arch Dermatol* **85**:233, 1962

316. King RD et al: Adherence of *Candida albicans* and other *Candida* species to mucosal epithelial cells. *Infect Immun* **27**:667, 1980

317. Kapica L, Blank F: Growth of *Candida albicans* on keratin as sole source of nitrogen. *Dermatologica* **115**:81, 1957

318. Pugh D, Cawson RA: The cytochemical localization of phospholipase A and lysophospholipase in *Candida albicans*. *Sabouraudia* **13**:110, 1975

319. Staib F: Proteolysis and pathogenicity of *Candida albicans* strains. *Mycopathologia* **37**:345, 1969

320. Scherwitz C: Ultrastructure of human cutaneous candidosis. *J Invest Dermatol* **78**:200, 1982

321. Montes LF, Wilborn WH: Fungus-host relationship in candidiasis: a brief review. *Arch Dermatol* **121**:119, 1985

322. Rebora A et al: Experimental infection with *Candida albicans*. *Arch Dermatol* **108**:69, 1973

323. Ray TL et al: Purification of a mannan from *Candida albicans* which activates serum complement. *J Invest Dermatol* **73**:269, 1979

324. Chesney RW et al: *Candida* endocrinopathy syndrome with membranoproliferative glomerulonephritis: demonstration of glomerular *Candida* antigen. *Clin Nephrol* **5**:232, 1976

325. Diamond RD et al: Properties of a product of *Candida albicans* hyphae and pseudohyphae that inhibits contact between the fungi and human neutrophils in vitro. *J Immunol* **125**:2797, 1980

326. Piccolella E et al: Generation of suppressor cells in the response of human lymphocytes to a polysacchride from *Candida albicans*. *J Immunol* **126**:2151, 1981

327. Fischer A et al: Specific inhibition of in vitro *Candida* induced lymphocyte proliferation by polysaccharidic antigens present in the serum of patients with chronic mucocutaneous candidiasis. *J Clin Invest* **62**:1005, 1978

328. Rogers TJ, Balish E: Immunity to *Candida albicans*. *Microbiol Rev* **44**:660, 1980

329. Ray TL: Candidosis, in *Dermatologic Immunology and Allergy*, edited by J Stone. St Louis, CV Mosby, 1985, p 511

330. Sohnle PG, Kirkpatrick CH: Epidermal proliferation in the defense against experimental cutaneous candidiasis. *J Invest Dermatol* **70**:130, 1978

331. Louria DB: *Candida* infections in experimental animals, in *Candidiasis*, edited by GP Bodey, V. Fainstein, New York, Raven Press 1985, p 29

332. Ray TL, Wuepper KD: Experimental cutaneous candidiasis in rodents. II. Role of the stratum corneum barrier and serum complement as a mediator of a protective inflammatory response. *Arch Dermatol* **114**:539, 1978

333. Solomkin JS et al: Phagocytosis of *Candida albicans* by human leukocytes: opsonic requirements. *J Infect Dis* **137**:30, 1978

334. Wilton JMA et al: The role of F_c and $C3_b$ receptors in phagocytosis by inflammatory polymorphonuclear leukocytes in man. *Immunology* **32**:955, 1977

335. Diamond RD et al: Damage to pseudohyphae forms of *Candida albicans* by neutrophils in the absence of serum in vitro. *J Clin Invest* **61**:349, 1978

336. Louria DB, Brayton RG: A substance in blood lethal for *Candida albicans*. *Nature* **201**:309, 1964

337. Lehrer RT, Cline MJ: Interaction of *Candida albicans* with human leukocytes and serum. *J Bacteriol* **98**:996, 1969

338. Caroline L et al: Reversal of serum fungistasis by addition of iron. *J Invest Dermatol* **42**:415, 1964

339. Boxer LA et al: Lactoferrin deficiency associated with altered granulocyte function. *N Engl J Med* **307**:404, 1982

340. Pearsall N et al: Immunologic responses to *Candida albicans*. III. Effects of passive transfer of lymphoid cells or serums on murine candidiasis. *J Immunol* **120**:1176, 1978

341. Mourad S, Friedman L: Passive immunization of mice against *Candida albicans*. *Sabouraudia* **6**:103, 1968

342. Epstein JB et al: Oral candidiasis: pathogenesis and host defenst. *Rev Infect Dis* **6**:96, 1984

343. Dreizen S: Oral candidiasis. *Am J Med* **77(4D)**:28, 1984

344. Tapper-Jones LM et al: Candidal infections and populations of *Candida albicans* in mouths of diabetics. *J Clin Pathol* **34**:706, 1981

345. Klein RS et al: Oral candidiasis in high-risk patients as the initial manifestation of the acquired immunodeficiency syndrome. *N Engl J Med* **311**:354, 1984

346. Pingleton WW: Oropharyngeal candidiasis in patients treated with triamcinolone acetonide aerosol. *J Allergy Clin Immunol* **60**:254, 1977

347. Nyquist G: A study of denture sore mouth: an investigation of traumatic, allergic and toxic lesions of the oral mucosa arising from the use of full dentures. *Acta Odontol Scand* **10 (suppl 9)**:11, 1952

348. Budtz-Jorgensen E et al: An epidermologic study of yeasts

in elderly denture wearers. *Community Dent Oral Epidemiol* **3:**115, 1975

349. Odds FC: Candidiasis of the oropharynx, in *Candida and Candidosis*. Baltimore, University Park Press, 1979, p 83
350. Chernosky ME: Relationship between vertical facial dimension and perlèche. *Arch Dermatol* **93:**332, 1966
351. Jansen GT et al: *Candida* cheilitis. *Arch Dermatol* **88:**325, 1963
352. McCarthy PL, Shklar G: *Diseases of the Oral Mucosa*. Philadelphia, Lea & Febiger, 1980, p 88
353. Coohe BED: Median rhombaid glossitis: candidiasis and not a developmental anomaly. *Br J Dermatol* **93:**399, 1975
354. Odds FC: Ecology and epidemiology of *Candida*, in *Candida and Candidosis*. Baltimore, University Park Press, 1979, p 50
355. Sobel JD: Vulvovaginal candidiasis—what we do and do not know. *Ann Interern Med* **101:**390, 1984
356. Odds FC: Genital candidosis. *Clin Exp Dermatol* **7:**345, 1982
357. Meech RJ et al: Pathogenic mechanisms in recurrent genital candidosis in women. *N Z Med J* **98:**1, 1985
358. Waugh MA: Clinical presentation of candidal balanitis—its differential diagnosis and treatment. *Chemotherapy* **28 (suppl 1):**56, 1982
359. Catterall RD: *Candida albicans* and the contraceptive pill. *Lancet* **2:**830, 1966
360. Rebora A, Leyden JJ: Napkin (diaper) dermatitis and gastrointestinal carriage of *Candida albicans*. *Br J Dermatol* **105:**551, 1981
361. Jorizzo JL: The spectrum of mucosal and cutaneous candidosis. *Dermatologic Clinics* **2:**19, 1984
362. Bradford LG, Montes LF: Perioal dermatitis and *Candida albicans*. *Arch Dermatol* **105:**892, 1972
363. Brandrup F et al: Perioral pustular eruption caused by *Candida albicans*. *Br J Dermatol* **105:**327, 1981
364. Zaias N: Onychomycosis. *Dermatologic Clinics* **3:**445, 1985
365. Delaplane D et al: Congenital mucocutaneous candidiasis following diagnostic amniocentesis. *Am J Obstet Gynecol* **147:**342, 1983
366. Chapel TA et al: Congenital cutaneous candidiasis. *J Am Acad Dermatol* **6:**926, 1982
367. Bodey GP: Candidiasis in cancer patients. *Am J Med* **77(4D):**13, 1984
368. Bodey GP, Fainstein V: Systemic candidiasis, in *Candidiasis*, edited by GP Bodey, V Fainstein. New York, Raven Press, 1985, p 135
369. Hughes WT: Systemic candidiasis: a study of 109 fatal cases. *Pediatr Infect Dis* **1:**11, 1982
370. Edwards JE et al: Ocular manifestations of *Candida* septicemia: review of seventy-six cases of hematogenous *Candida* endophthalmitis. **53:**47, 1974
371. Bodey GP, Luna M: Skin lesions associated with disseminated candidiasis. *JAMA* **229:**1466, 1974
372. Bodey GP: Fungal infections complicating acute leukemia. *J Chronic Dis* **19:**667, 1966
373. Grossman ME et al: Cutaneous manifestations of disseminated candidiasis. *J Am Acad Dermatol* **2:**111, 1980
374. Jarowski CI et al: Fever, rash, and muscle tenderness: a distinctive clinical presentation of disseminated candidiasis. *Arch Intern Med* **138:**544, 1978
375. Kressel B et al: Early clinical recognition of disseminated candidiasis by muscle and skin biopsy. *Arch Intern Med* **138:**429, 1978
376. File TM et al: Necrotic skin lesions associated with disseminated candidiasis. *Arch Dermatol* **115:**214, 1979
377. Fine JD et al: Cutaneous lesions in disseminated candidiasis mimicking ecthyma gangrenosum. *Am J Med* **70:**1133, 1981
378. Collingnon PJ, Sorrell TC: Disseminated candidiasis: evidence of a distinctive syndrome in heroin abusers. *Br Med J* **287:**861, 1983
379. Kirkpatrick CH, Sohnle PG: Chronic mucocutaneous can-

didiasis, in *Immunodermatology*, edited by B Safai, RA Good. New York, Plenum Press, 1981, p 495
380. Lehner T: Classification and clinico-pathological features of candida infections of the mouth, in *Symposium on Candida Infections*, edited by HI Winner, R Hurley. Baltimore, Williams & Wilkins, 1966, p 119
381. Wells RS et al: Familial chronic muco-cutaneous candidiasis. *J Med Genet* **9:**302, 1972
382. Kirkpatrick CH: Host factors in defense against fungal infections. *Am J Med* **77(4D):**1, 1984
383. Odds FC: Chronic mucocutaneous candidosis, in *Candida and Candidosis*. Baltimore, University Park Press, 1979, p 121
384. Dudley JP et al: *Candida* laryngitis in chronic mucocutaneous candidiasis: its association with *Candida* esophagitis. *Ann Otol Rhinol Laryngol* **89:**574, 1980
385. Kobayashi RH et al: *Candida* esophagitis and laryngitis in chronic mucocutaneous candidiasis. *Pediatrics* **66:**380, 1980
386. Price ML, MacDonald DM: *Candida* endocrinopathy syndrome. *Clin Exp Dermatol* **9:**105, 1984
387. Zouali M et al: Evaluation of auto-antibodies in chronic mucocutaneous candidiasis without endocrinopathy. *Mycopathologia* **84:**87, 1983/1984
388. Howanitz N et al: Antibodies to melanocytes: occurrence in patients with vitilgo and chronic mucocutaneous candidiasis. *Arch Dermatol* **117:**705, 1981
389. Higgs JM, Wells RS: Chronic mucocutaneous candidiasis: associated abnormalities of iron metabolism. *Br J Dermatol* **86 (suppl 8):**88, 1972
390. Harms M et al: KID syndrome (keratitis, ichthyosis, and deafness) and chronic mucocutaneous candidiasis: case report and review of the literature. *Pediatr Dermatol* **2:**1, 1984
391. Sams WM et al: Chronic mucocutaneous candidiasis: immunologic studies of three generations of a single family. *Am J Med* **67:**948, 1979
392. Chipps BE et al: Non-candidal infections in children with chronic mucocutaneous candidiasis. *Johns Hopkins Med J* **144:**179, 1979
393. Kirkpatrick CH, Windhorst DB: Mucocutaneous candidiasis and thymoma. *Am J Med* **66:**939, 1979
394. Jorizzo JL: Chronic mucocutaneous candidosis: an update. *Arch Dermatol* **118:**963, 1982
395. Valdimarsson H et al: Immune abnormalities associated with chronic mucocutaneous candidiasis. *Cell Immunol* **6:**348, 1973
396. Cates KL et al: Cell-directed inhibition of polymorphonuclear leukocyte chemotaxis in a patient with mucocutaneous candidiasis. *J Allergy Clin Immunol* **65:**431, 1980
397. Walker SM, Urbaniak SJ: A serum-dependent defect of neutrophil function in chronic mucocutaneous candidiasis. *J Clin Pathol* **33:**370, 1980
398. Synderman R et al: Defective mononuclear leukocyte chemotaxis: a previously unrecognized immune dysfunction. *Ann Intern Med* **78:**509, 1973
399. Bortolussi R et al: Phagocytosis of *Candidia albicans* in chronic mucocutaneous candidiasis. *Pediatr Res* **15:**1287, 1981
400. Yamazaki M et al: A monocyte disorder in siblings with chronic candidiasis. *Am J Dis Child* **138:**192, 1984
401. Drew JH: Chronic mucocutaneous candidiasis with abnormal function of serum complement. *Med J Aust* **2:**77, 1973
402. Van Scoy RE et al: Familial neutrophil chemotaxis defect, recurrent bacterial infections, mucocutaneous candidiasis, and hyperimmunoglobulinemia E. *Ann Intern Med* **82:**766, 1975
403. Arulanantham K et al: Evidence for defective immunoregulation in the syndrome of familial candidiasis endocrinopathy. *N Engl J Med* **300:**164, 1979
404. Fischer A et al: Defective handling of mannan by monocytes in patients with chronic mucucutaneous candidiasis resulting

in a specific cellular unresponsiveness. *Clin Exp Immunol* **47**:653, 1982

405. Ruiz-Arguelles A et al: Impaired generation of helper T cells in a patient with chronic mucucutaneous candidiasis and malignant thymoma. *J Clin Lab Immunol* **10**:165, 1983

406. Myerowitz RL et al: Disseminated candidiasis: changes in incidence, underlying diseases, and pathology. *Am J Clin Pathol* **68**:29, 1977

407. Penn RL et al: Invasive fungal infections: the use of serologic tests in diagnosis and management. *Arch Intern Med* **143**:1215, 1983

408. Cooper BH, Silva-Hutner M: Yeasts of medical importance, in *Manual of Clinical Microbiology*, 4th ed, edited by EH Lennette et al. Washington, DC, American Society for Microbiology, 1985, chap 49, p 526

409. Klotz SA et al: *Pityrosporum* folliculitis: its potential for confusion with skin lesions of systemic candidiasis. *Arch Intern Med* **142**:2126, 1982

410. DeGregorio MW et al: *Candida* infections in patients with acute leukemia: ineffectiveness of nystatin prophylaxis and relationship between oropharyngeal and systemic candidiasis. *Cancer* **50**:2780, 1982

411. Quintiliani R et al: Treatment and prevention of oropharyngeal candidiasis. *Am J Med* **77(40)**:44, 1984

412. Owens NJ et al: Prophylaxis of oral candidiasis with clotrimazole troches. *Arch Intern Med* **144**:290, 1984

413. Mansour A, Gelfand EW: A new approach to the use of antifungal agents in infants with persistent oral candidiasis. *Pediatrics* **98**:161, 1981

414. Robertson WH: A concentrated therapeutic regimen for vulvovaginal candidiasis. *JAMA* **244**:2549, 1980

415. Masterton G et al: Three-day clotrimazole treatment in candidal vulvovaginitis. *Br J Vener Dis* **53**:126, 1977

416. Fregoso-Duenas F: Ketoconazole in vulvovaginal candidosis. *Rev Infect Dis* **2**:620, 1980

417. Miles MR et al: Recurrent vaginal candidiasis: importance of an intestinal reservoir. *JAMA* **238**:1836, 1977

418. Leyden JJ: Corn starch, *Candida albicans*, and diaper rash. *Pediatr Dermatol* **1**:322, 1984

419. Johnson DE et al: Congenital candidiasis. *Am J Dis Child* **135**:273, 1981

420. Drouhet E, Dupont B: Chronic mucocutaneous candidosis and other superficial and systemic mycoses successfully treated with ketoconazole. *Rev Infect Dis* **2**:606, 1980

421. Petersen EA et al: Treatment of chronic mucocutaneous candidiasis with ketoconazole: a controlled clinical trial. *Ann Intern Med* **93**:791, 1980

422. Hay RJ et al: Treatment of chronic mucocutaneous candidosis with ketoconazole: a study of 12 cases. *Rev Infect Dis* **2**:600, 1980

423. Lin C-Y: Treatment of chronic mucocutaneous candidiasis with 5-fluorocytosine. *Ann Allergy* **49**:298, 1982

424. Hay RJ: Management of chronic mucocutaneous candidosis. *Clin Exp Dermatol* **6**:515, 1981

425. Jorizzo JL et al: Cimetidine as an immunomodulator: chronic mucocutaneous candidiasis as a model. *Ann Intern Med* **92**:192, 1980

CHAPTER 182

DEEP FUNGAL INFECTIONS

John P. Utz and H. Jean Shadomy

The skin lesions seen in the systemic mycoses are, with the exception of mycetoma and perhaps sporotrichosis and paracoccidioidal granuloma, acquired by the hematogenous route, rather than from direct implantation. The portal of entry is generally the respiratory tract, and a focus of infection is established in the lung. This infection is accompanied by a spectrum of disease which ranges from inapparent infection to severe, fulminant, and inexorably fatal illness. The factors responsible for the severity are known in part and include the amount of inoculum, e.g., histoplasmosis, and such important predisposing factors as diabetes mellitus, Hodgkin's disease, and corticosteroid or immunosuppressive therapy. The spread of disease, characteristically hematogenous, from the focus of infection in the lung is to remote organs in patterns that are distinctive for each disease. Skin involvement is most common in blastomycosis, and this disease is readily suspected from inspection of the lesions. Somewhat less characteristic lesions are important features in coccidioidomycosis, cryptococcosis, and in some cases of actinomycosis. Contagious spread from person to person or from patient to hospital staff is not known to occur. At the present time,

several systemic antifungal agents are available for virtually all these diseases.

Actinomycosis

Definition

Actinomycosis is a chronic infectious disease of the cervicofacial area, thorax, or abdomen, caused by the anaerobic, gram-positive bacterium *Actinomyces israelii,* a commensal of humans, and characterized pathologically by a suppurative, fibrosing inflammation which spreads directly to contiguous tissue. Lumpy jaw, a similar infection occurring in cattle, is caused by a related organism, *A. bovis.*

Historical aspects

In 1877, Bollinger [1] described the disease in cattle, and in 1878 Israel [2] reported infection in humans. In 1891 Wolff and Israel cultured the microorganism. Lord, in 1910, established that *A. israelii* is present in carious teeth and tonsils of otherwise normal persons. In 1938, Cope

[3], in an excellent review, summarized 1330 reported cases. Successful treatment of the disease with penicillin dates to 1943 and the report of Nichols and Harrell in 1947 [4].

Epidemiology

Actinomycosis is worldwide in distribution. In the United States it is more common in males. The incidence of disease is difficult to determine, since it is not reportable and there is no skin test material for population surveys. A widespread current clinical impression is that the disease, once the most common of the systemic fungal diseases, is now one of the rarest.

Etiology and pathogenesis

Although the species are almost indistinguishable, human disease usually is caused by *A. israelii* and rarely by *A. bovis*, *A. naeslundii*, or *A. viscosus*.

Since *A. israelii* is present in various studies in approximately 50 percent of excised tonsils and is a normal commensal of humans [5], the disease is regarded as being acquired endogenously by direct extension to contiguous tissues, probably as a result of minor local trauma. Predisposing factors, other than this assumed one, are not known.

Clinical manifestations

There are three major forms of the disease: cervicofacial, thoracic, and abdominal. In earlier studies, approximately 60 percent of disease was cervicofacial, 20 percent thoracic, and 15 percent abdominal. More recently, 60 percent has been abdominal, 25 percent cervicofacial, and 15 percent thoracic. In rare instances, infection appears to spread via the bloodstream to such other sites as the meninges or endocardium.

The cervicofacial form begins as a swelling over the lower part of the face or neck with formation of an irregular, woody, indurated lesion which drains and heals at various sites. Regional lymph node involvement is characteristically absent. Invasion and destruction of bone occur early, with periostitis and osteomyelitis.

In thoracic actinomycosis, the cutaneous lesion is generally a draining sinus tract or subcutaneous abscess, occasionally with local induration and discoloration. Cough productive of sputum, and pleuritic chest pain are pulmonary symptoms. The chest roentgenogram characteristically shows a dense infiltrate with signs of pleural thickening and occasionally mediastinitis.

Abdominal actinomycosis presents in cutaneous form, again as a draining sinus tract or subcutaneous abscess. An abdominal mass is usually present, and occasionally a psoas abscess occurs. Signs of incomplete intestinal obstruction in the form of vomiting or cramping pain occasionally occur. On x-ray examination, a sinus tract can sometimes be visualized. In other instances, there is evidence of partial obstruction or an extraintestinal mass. Ten to twenty new patients are reported annually now with pelvic disease from intrauterine contraceptive devices (IUD). From 2 to 5 percent of IUD users are infected as determined by direct immunofluorescent study of Papanicolaou smears of the cervix [6].

In all forms of the disease, there may be such constitutional symptoms as fever, shaking chills, drenching night sweats, anorexia, weight loss, and marked easy fatigability.

A normocytic, normochromic anemia is frequent, but leukocytosis is mild and occasionally absent. The erythrocyte sedimentation rate is usually elevated [7].

Pathology

The gross pathologic picture is that of a chronic infection localized to a particular site. There are multiple, small and occasionally larger, coalescent abscesses with communicating sinuses. Tissues are frequently yellow, indurated and firm. The "sulfur" granules occasionally can be recognized. These are sandlike particles composed of tangled hyphal forms of *A. israelii*. On microscopic examination (Fig. 182-1), one finds chronic inflammation with granulation tissue, occasionally giant cells, and frequently large numbers of macrophages.

Diagnosis and differential diagnosis

The diagnosis is established by the isolation and identification of the causative microorganism in cultures of tissue or exudate from characteristic lesions.

The diagnosis is virtually certain if "sulfur" granules are seen in pus, exudate, or tissue sections.

Laboratory diagnosis. DIRECT EXAMINATION. Sputum, bronchial aspirates, pleural, joint, and pericardial fluids, pus, and biopsy material should be examined for "sulfur" granules. All granules should be studied both in a wet preparation (water, never potassium hydroxide) and by Gram's stain.

Specimens initially are removed to a drop of water on a slide, covered with a coverslip, and examined under reduced light. A characteristic feature consists of "clubs," inflammatory tissue reactions surrounding the hypal tips. Granules are then prepared for staining by removing the coverslip and crushing the specimen between two slides. After the material dries, the slides are fixed by heat and stained with Gram's stain. *A. israelii* produces gram-positive, small (1.0 μm or less in diameter), beaded hyphae, which may branch or break up into diphtheroid elements.

The absence of granules in a specimen does not rule out

Fig. 182-1 Actinomycosis. The distinctive sulfur granule forms the center of an area of suppuration and is surrounded by neutrophils. ×100. (AFIP 71607; courtesy of Dr. Elson B. Helwig. Micrograph by Wallace H. Clark, Jr., M.D.)

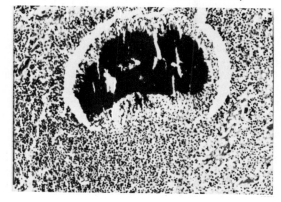

actinomycosis, nor does their presence establish the diagnosis. They may be present in other lesions (or infections) due to *Nocardia* spp., other fungi that cause mycetoma, and bacteria (*Staphylococcus aureus*).

CULTURE. Granules must be well washed before inoculation to reduce chances of bacterial contamination. One may do this in either drops or small tubes of sterile saline solution, taking the granules through a series of at least 10 washings until adherent pus or debris is gone. A ''cleaned'' granule is placed in a drop of sterile saline solution, crushed, and spread on brain-heart infusion agar plates, with and without 10 percent rabbit blood, on Garrod's starch agar plates with 10 percent rabbit blood, and in several fresh tubes of glucose-thioglycollate broth. Use of a cold catalyst anaerobic jar in conjunction with ''Gaspak'' (Baltimore Biological Laboratories, product No. 06-112) provides a simple method for anaerobiosis and appears to be nontoxic for *Actinomyces* spp.

Specimens other than granules are homogenized or centrifuged when appropriate (e.g., biopsy material, cerebrospinal fluid) and planted as above.

Media are generally incubated at 37°C, although *Actinomyces* spp. will grow at temperatures from 30 to 37°C. Anaerobic conditions are essential. The actinomycetes are susceptible to antibacterial agents; these, therefore, are not used in culture media.

On agar plates, colonies of *A. israelii* at 48 h are long, branching, and filamentous or spider-like. After a week to 10 days the colonies become white, glistening, irregular, or lobulated. They remain small and may penetrate the agar. In glucose-thioglycollate broth, *A. israelii* produces granular colonies without turbidity.

In contrast, *A. bovis,* usually isolated from cattle and swine, produces on agar at 48 h pinhead size ''dewdrop'' colonies which enlarge by a week to 10 days, becoming similar to *A. israelii* colonies, but possessing an entire border. In glucose-thioglycollate broth, the hyphae of *A. bovis* break up early, producing turbidity and a dense sediment.

Actinomyces spp. and anaerobic diphtheroids, which they closely resemble culturally, can be differentiated by the positive catalase activity of the diphtheroids; species other than *A. viscosus* are uniformly catalase-negative. This test is performed on a microscopic slide with a drop of fresh hydrogen peroxide and a portion of colony growth mixed in it. The formation of gas bubbles, seen microscopically, indicates a catalase-positive reaction. Species other than *A. naeslundii* are urea negative.

ANIMAL INOCULATION

Pathogenicity test. This study is best done in 3- to 4-week-old male golden hamsters. Seven- to 10-day-old broth cultures are centrifuged, and the sediment is washed several times in sterile saline solution and crushed with a glass rod. One milliliter of a 2% concentration (v/v) is then injected intraperitoneally into each of several hamsters. At 4 weeks they are killed, and peritoneal abscess material is removed for Gram's stain and cultural procedures, as described.

Isolation. Animal inoculation is not employed in the primary isolation of *Actinomyces* spp. from clinical specimens.

Differential diagnosis. Cervical facial actinomycosis must be distinguished from chronic infections due to *Mycobac-*

terium tuberculosis, Staphylococcus aureus, Nocardia asteroides, or other systemic mycoses. The abdominal form resembles other chronic infectious diseases (tuberculosis) and, occasionally, regional enteritis and malignancy. The thoracic form must be distinguished from tuberculosis, other fungal infections, and malignancy.

Treatment

Treatment of actinomycosis is twofold: surgical (incision and drainage of abscesses and excision of chronic, fibrotic, avascular tissue) and chemotherapeutic (penicillin notably).

Chemotherapy must be prolonged usually for at least 3 months. Customary dosage early in the course is from 10 to 20 million units daily of penicillin G, administered intravenously for approximately a 4-week period. Following this, oral phenoxymethyl penicillin in daily dosage of from 4 to 6 g should be continued. Therapy should not be stopped until lesions have cleared completely, or until they have been stable for 6 weeks. In patients who are allergic to penicillin, therapy may be with tetracycline, erythromycin, or chloramphenicol, each of which has been reported successful in patients.

Course and prognosis

The course of the disease is characteristically prolonged, indolent, and marked by the closure of one sinus tract and the opening of another.

With specific chemotherapy most patients can be cured, although therapy must be prolonged and patients may be left with chronic residual local scarring, respiratory embarrassment from lung tissue destruction, or mild gastrointestinal obstructive phenomena.

Nocardiosis

Definition

Nocardiosis is an acute or subacute infectious disease, acquired by the respiratory route, with a focus of infection in the lungs, with frequent hematogenous dissemination, characteristically to the brain, and caused by an organism, *Nocardia asteroides,* intermediate between true fungi and bacteria.

Historical aspects

Nocard, in 1888, described an illness characterized by lymphatic swelling in cattle and caused by an aerobic, partially acid-fast actinomycete [8]. The first description of the disease in humans was that of Eppinger [9], who reported a patient with a brain abscess and caseous disease of the lungs and pleura.

Epidemiology

Nocardiosis is worldwide in distribution and occurs more frequently in men and after middle age.

Unlike *A. israelii, N. asteroides* is not a commensal of humans. It has been isolated from soil and, because of its resistance to higher temperature, from composting vegetation. Despite this, the disease is not recognized to be more common in farmers and gardeners.

Etiology and pathogenesis

Factors predisposing to nocardiosis are not known. The infection generally occurs as an "opportunist."

Clinical manifestations

Skin lesions due to *N. asteroides* are limited to sinus tracts from abscesses or rarely to primary cutaneous lesions [10]. The pulmonary symptoms in nocardiosis are commonly cough, occasionally blood-tinged sputum, chest pain, and dyspnea. On x-ray examination a dense infiltrate is usually seen unilaterally, sometimes with cavitation of either the honeycomb or the large variety, and frequently with markedly thickened pleurae.

It is a peculiarity of this disease that there is a strikingly increased frequency of hematogenous dissemination to the brain with abscess formation. Findings on neurologic examination depend on the location of the lesion, but headache and signs of increased intracranial pressure are the most common. Less frequently there are abscesses in the kidney, spleen, or liver.

With all manifestations of the disease there are usually fever, chills, night sweats, malaise, anorexia, and weight loss. Such manifestations of infection as leukocytosis, anemia, elevated sedimentation rate, and elevated serum globulin levels also usually are present.

Pathology

Tissue reaction to *N. asteroides* is characteristically pyogenic, with the formation of multiple, but occasionally confluent, abscesses. There tends to be less induration, fibrotic tissue formation, and sinus tract formation than in actinomycosis, the disease it resembles.

The organism, *N. asteroides,* is readily seen with Gram's stain of tissues. Hyphae are beaded and vary in size from 0.5 to 1.0 μm in diameter and 10 to 40 μm in length. Branching is seen frequently.

Diagnosis and differential diagnosis

The diagnosis of nocardiosis is established by the isolation and identification of *N. asteroides* in culture. Typical organisms seen on microscopic examination of tissues suggest the diagnosis, although there is always some uncertainty, as *Mycobacterium tuberculosis* is also acid-fast and *Actinomyces israelii* is similarly branching.

Laboratory diagnosis. DIRECT EXAMINATION. Sputum and bronchial aspirates, pleural, joint, and pericardial fluids, pus, cerebrospinal fluid, and biopsy material should all be studied microscopically by Gram's and modified acid-fast stain procedures. Small, cream- to white-colored granules may be produced by *N. asteroides,* and occasionally "clubs" may be present. The granules should be studied as described for actinomycosis. When granules are not present, the organism is seen as freely branching filaments which are gram-positive and acid-fast. To perform the latter staining procedure, the preparation is destained with 0.5% aqueous sulfuric acid instead of with acid alcohol.

CULTURE. Colony formation is identical at 30 and 37°C. *N. asteroides* is sensitive to antibacterial agents, and these are not used in isolation media. The microorganism will grow on media for *Mycobacterium* isolation and may be mistaken for rapidly growing members of this genus (group IV).

Clinical material is inoculated onto brain-heart infusion or Sabouraud's agar and incubated at 30°C, or more often at 37°C. Growth develops in approximately 1 week at 30°C, and within 3 or 4 days at 37°C. Colonies vary from chalky-white to yellow and orange and are raised, folded, and cerebriform. Colonies must be differentiated from *Mycobacteria* spp. by structure and from *Streptomyces* spp. by acid-fast studies, biochemical reactions, and pathogenicity tests.

Morphology. Slide cultures demonstrate the ability, generally, of *N. asteroides* to produce aerial hyphae, whereas *Mycobacteria* spp. do not.

Acid-fast stain. *N. asteroides* is acid-fast with beaded hyphae when the modified acid-fast stain is used. *Streptomyces* spp. are not acid-fast.

Biochemical reaction. *N. asteroides* does not hydrolyze casein and will not grow on gelatin medium. *N. brasiliensis* hydrolyzes casein and grows well on gelatin medium. *Streptomyces* spp. hydrolyze casein but grow poorly in gelatin medium, producing a flaky or stringy type of growth.

ANIMAL INOCULATION

Culture confirmation. Determination of pathogenicity of isolates from clinical specimens frequently is required [11,12] and is most easily performed in the laboratory. Four Sabouraud's agar slants are inoculated and incubated at either 30 or 37°C until heavy growth covers at least half of each slant (1 to 2 weeks). The growth is removed to a mortar and ground with an equal quantity of gastric mucin. One milliliter is injected intraperitoneally into each of two guinea pigs. At death they are examined for acid-fast hyphae in lesions. If death does not occur, one guinea pig is killed at 2 weeks, the other at 4 weeks postinoculation, and they are examined. Pathogenicity is demonstrated by the presence of lesions and acid-fast hyphae.

Isolation. This procedure is not done with clinical material.

Differential diagnosis. It is of historical interest that the first reported patient had been thought to have tuberculosis. For many years nocardiosis was not well distinguished from actinomycosis. Nocardiosis clinically also may resemble more chronic lung and brain abscesses due to such organisms as anaerobic *Streptococcus,* occasionally *Staphylococcus aureus,* or *Klebsiella pneumoniae.* It may mimic other fungal infections such as histoplasmosis, blastomycosis, and coccidioidomycosis [13].

Treatment

As shown by studies in animals and experience in humans, members of the sulfonamide group, notably sulfadiazine, have been the most active chemotherapeutic agents. Chemotherapy must be combined with drainage of abscesses, but despite such therapy, treatment has been unsuccessful in so many patients that it has been customary to use another agent such as tetracycline, chloramphenicol, or large doses of penicillin (though this agent is less active in animal infections). Impressive in vitro and in vivo studies of amikacin have been confirmed by successful use in a renal transplant recipient after failure on multiple other regimens [14].

Prognosis

Even today with such therapy, case fatality rates in nocardiosis are approximately 50 percent. This high rate appears to be a function of disseminated disease and abscess formation at such vital sites as the brain when the illness is first recognized and diagnosed, as well as the impaired immunity from the underlying disease or treatment.

Mycetoma (madura foot, maduromycosis)

Definition

Mycetoma is a chronic infectious disease of the subcutaneous tissues, skin, and bone, characteristically of the foot but occasionally of the hand, back, or shoulder following implantation, at the site, of one of a variety of *Actinomyces* spp. or true fungi, notably *Nocardia brasiliensis, Streptomyces madurae, Pseudallescheria boydii, Madurella mycetomi, Madurella grisea,* and *Phialophora jeanselmei.*

Historical aspects

The synonym for the disease is derived from the area in India from which the earliest cases were reported, primarily by Vandyke Carter in 1860.

Epidemiology

In addition to India, other sites where the disease is seen frequently include the Sudan area in Africa, southern Asia, and tropical areas of Central and South America. The disease is relatively rare in the United States, although one of the causative fungi, *Pseudallescheria boydii,* has been isolated frequently from soil in this country. The disease is seen more commonly in blacks, but this seems to be more a reflection of population in the geographic location of the fungi and the prevalence there of the practice of walking without shoes. The disease is more common in young adults and in workers in rural areas exposed frequently to accidental injury to the bare foot.

Etiology and pathogenesis

Four species of actinomycetes and 13 of true fungi have been associated with mycetomas.

It seems clear that humans acquire the disease through accidental traumatic or occasionally subclinical implantation by thorns or splinters contaminated by one of the causative fungi. The most common site for such implantation is the foot or leg, though occasionally the lesions are seen on the upper part of the back because of irritation by contaminated sacks used to carry sugar cane [15].

Clinical manifestations (Fig. A6-21)

The hallmark of the disease is swelling with marked distortion of the normal anatomy, draining sinus tracts, and bloody or purulent drainage, with only mild impairment of

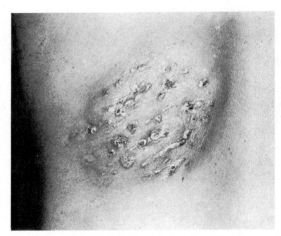

Fig. 182-2   Nocardiosis: multiple fistulas. *(Courtesy of Dr. Jan Schwarz, Cincinnati, Ohio.)*

mobility and relatively little pain (Figs. 182-2 to 182-4). Radiologic examination of the affected extremity shows soft-tissue swelling and areas of rarefaction and fibrosis characteristic of osteomyelitis in contiguous bone.

Pathology (Fig. 182-5)

The gross appearance of the lesion is as described above.

A characteristic finding in material draining from the

Fig. 182-3 *Nocardia* **infection resulting in marked distortion of the tissues, draining sinuses, and verrucous tumors.** *(Courtesy of Dr. Jan Schwarz, Cincinnati, Ohio.)*

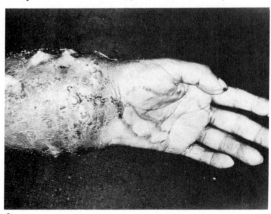

a

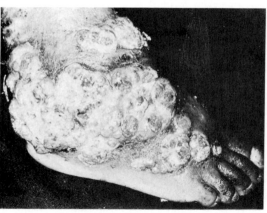

b

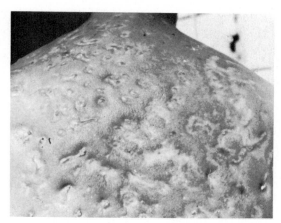

Fig. 182-4   Severe atrophic scarring resulting from *Nocardia* infection. *(Courtesy of Dr. Jan Schwarz, Cincinnati, Ohio.)*

sinus tracts is that of granules visible to the naked eye, which on microscopic examination are seen to be colonies of fungal hyphae with a shell or crust of fibrin derived from the host tissues. They vary in color from pink to yellow, white, brown, or black. Tissues at the site of these granules characteristically show suppuration with, in addition, epithelioid and multinucleated giant cells. Fibrosis is prominent in areas between the abscesses.

Diagnosis and differential diagnosis

The diagnosis is established by the clinical appearance of the lesion and the presence of characteristic granules; cultural studies of pus and tissue usually show one of the implicated fungi, but, in addition, bacteria such as *Staphylococcus aureus*. Gram's stain showing branching, filamentous microorganisms, aerobic and anaerobic cultures, and special stains, such as periodic acid-Schiff's and Gomori's methenamine silver or Gridley's may be helpful in demonstrating the causative microorganisms.

Laboratory diagnosis. DIRECT EXAMINATION. Biopsy material and pus from draining sinuses should be examined for granules. Processing for microscopic study and culture is outlined under "Actinomycosis," earlier in this chapter. If granules cannot be found in biopsy tissue, it should be teased apart and reexamined. Granules are studied for consistency of the granule, pigmentation, hyphal size and septation, morphologic characteristics, and manner of fragmentation.

CULTURE. Colony production may be best at 30 or 37°C, depending on the causative agent. Therefore, cultures should be made by cleansing the granules (see "Actinomycosis"), crushing and culturing them on Sabouraud's dextrose agar, and incubating at both temperatures.

To avoid contaminated material, biopsy specimens for culture should be of deep tissue.

The various organisms most often seen in mycetoma are identified in Table 182-1.

ANIMAL INOCULATION. Most of the causative fungi are not pathogenic for animals, and animal studies are not done [16].

Differential diagnosis. Mycetoma must be distinguished from osteomyelitis due to *Staphylococcus aureus* (which is usually more acute, accompanied by more pain but by less distortion of tissues) or to *Mycobacterium tuberculosis*.

Treatment

Treatment of mycetomas has been notoriously unsatisfactory with a few exceptions. Those infections due to *Actinomyces* spp. have responded partially to therapy with penicillin, sulfonamides, or tetracycline. Some strains of *M. mycetomi* have been shown sensitive to levels of amphotericin B which can be achieved in the serum. However, there are no extensive data on the use of this agent in these infections.

Some attempts have been made, without notable suc-

Fig. 182-5   Mycetoma. Large, dark-staining granule, formed by fungal colony, in an abscess with a thick fibrous capsule (seen in part at lower left). Bar=100 μm. *(From D. M. Dixon and H. J. Shadomy, Department of Microbiology, Virginia Commonwealth University, Richmond, with permission.)*

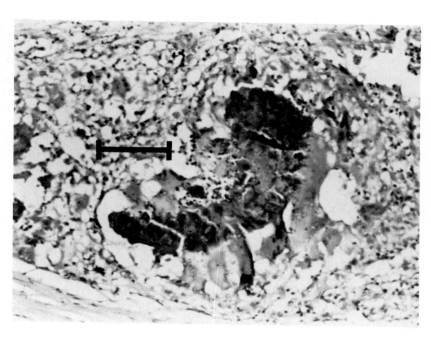

Table 182-1   Organisms most often seen in mycetoma

Organism	Presentation	Culture on Sabouraud's dextrose agar	Microscopic appearance
Actinomycetes: *Nocardia brasiliensis*	Granules soft, irregularly spherical, white to yellow, with or without "clubs."	Small, wrinkled, heaped colony, tan to yellow or orange. May have chalky surface because of short aerial hyphae. Some strains produce browning of the medium.	Short, irregular rods, long branched hyphae in liquid culture. Partially acid-fast, often beaded hyphae. Proteolytic activity −; amylase activity −.
Streptomyces madurae	Granules large, irregular to serpiginous, white to yellow or slightly pink, "clubs" numerous, long, tapered, and sometimes branching.	Cream-colored, glabrous colony with a firm, hard surface. Some stains produce powdery, white aerial hyphae.	Delicate branched hyphae; not acid-fast; conidia in chains. Proteolytic activity +; amylase activity +.
Higher fungi: *Pseudallescheria boydii*	Granules soft, round or lobulated, white to yellow, no "clubs" but instead surrounded by chlamydospore-like terminal cells.	Fluffy colonies, at first white but later gray to nearly black.	*Monosporium apiospermum* stage: hyaline hyphae with pale brown, oval to clavate conidia, on simple or branched conidiophores. Many strains also produce cleistothecia (sexual fruiting body of the *Pseudallescheria boydii* stage), particularly at the edge of the colony. Proteolytic activity +; amylase activity +.
Madurella mycetomi	Granules hard, brittle, round or lobed, black, no "clubs," but instead chlamydospores produced at the periphery. Brown pigment particles in hyphae and chlamydospores.	Flat, membranous or fluffy colonies, tan to yellow-brown or olivaceous. Brown, diffusible pigment produced.	Chlamydoconidia. Some strains produce conidia from small phialides; black sclerotia. Proteolytic activity +; amylase activity +.
Madurella grisea	Granules soft at first, hardening with age, round or lobed, black with hyaline hyphae at the unpigmented center, dark brown hyphae at periphery. No brown pigment particles in the hyphae.	Slow-growing, tan to gray or olivaceous, velvety colony with both hyaline cylindric hyphae and chains of dark, budding cells. Chlamydospores rare.	Chlamydoconidia rare. No micro-, sclerotia, or hyphal inclusions. Proteolytic activity +; amylase activity +.
Exophiala jeanselmei	Granules soft, irregular, black, made up mostly of dark brown chlamydospores, rare brown hyphae.	Slow-growing, black colony, at first membranous, later grayish and velvety.	Begins as chains of budding cells; later hyphae develop. Conidia produced from tapering annelides. Proteolytic activity +; amylase activity +.

cess, to treat the disease by surgical resection of tissue. Amputation is frequently necessary.

Course and prognosis

The course of disease is prolonged. In the areas where it occurs, other infections, and amyloidosis are the usual causes of death.

Cryptococcosis (torulosis, European blastomycosis)

Definition

Systemic cryptococcosis, a disease caused by the yeast *Cryptococcus neoformans* (perfect state: *Filobasidiella neoformans* [17]), is a chronic infectious process acquired by the respiratory route, with the primary focus of infec-

tion in the lungs, and with occasional hematogenous dissemination, characteristically to the meninges, occasionally to the kidneys, and to the skin.

Historical aspects

Although San Felice, in 1894 [18], reported the presence of an encapsulated yeast in peach juice, and thus probably described for the first time what is known as *C. neoformans,* it was Busse and Buschke in 1895 who first reported disease in humans due to this agent. In 1905 Hansemann observed the yeast in a patient who had died of meningitis, and Verse, in 1914, recognized the disease antemortem. An important advance in 1951 was a report by Emmons of the isolation of *C. neoformans* from soil and later from pigeon excreta, nests, and other sources associated with this bird [19].

Epidemiology

The disease is worldwide in distribution. It is more common in males than in females, by a ratio of approximately 2:1. The disease is relatively rare in children and more common in patients over the age of 40. The important evidence of association with pigeon excreta has been extended to show that the microorganism has been discovered in almost every area where pigeons have been congregating. Cases of cryptococcosis have also been noted in patients exposed to air conditioners contaminated with pigeon excreta. Pigeon breeders have been shown to have higher levels of antibody to *C. neoformans* antigen than persons without such contact. The organism has been isolated from various species of animals such as cow, cat, dog, horse, gazelle, mink, koala, and wallaby.

Etiology and pathogenesis

The causative microorganism is *C. neoformans*. It seems highly probable that the disease is acquired by inhalation of microorganisms from dust, since the fungus is so ubiquitous. However, defective host defenses are probably equally as important in disease induction. Such defects appear to be present in such diseases as diabetes mellitus, lymphoma, Hodgkin's disease, and sarcoidosis. A focus of infection is established in the lung, from which site the microorganism disseminates hematogenously.

Clinical manifestations

Approximately 10 to 15 percent of patients with cryptococcosis have skin lesions. These usually occur as a result of hematogenous spread from the lungs. In most instances they are papules or nodules with surrounding erythema. They occasionally break down and exude a liquid, mucinous material. Other lesions less frequently noted are ulcers, acneform pustules, granulomas, and purple plaques (Fig. 182-6).

Pulmonary disease as the sole manifestation of infection is being recognized with increasing frequency. Most patients with this condition are free of pulmonary complaints, and the lesion is discovered on a routine chest roentgenogram. A few, however, have a productive cough and, rarely, hemoptysis. The chest roentgenograms show a variety of lesions, including multiple fluffy infiltrates, extensive miliary lesions, "coin" lesions, dense pneumonic infiltrates, or loculated pleural effusions. Abscesses and cavities occur in about 15 percent [20].

Approximately a third of patients with systemic cryptococcosis have renal involvement, as attested to by the culture of *C. neoformans* from urine. Except for an occasional case of pyelonephritis or perinephritic abscess, the renal form of disease has not been well characterized.

Cryptococcosis, unlike blastomycosis, histoplasmosis, or coccidioidomycosis, involves the bones and joints in less than 5 percent of cases.

The most commonly observed form of the disease is meningitis, with headache the chief complaint in approximately 80 percent of patients. Mental confusion or impaired vision is seen in about 40 percent of patients. Onset is generally gradual, sometimes with symptoms going back 2 or 3 months, or more. In 15 percent meningitis occurs

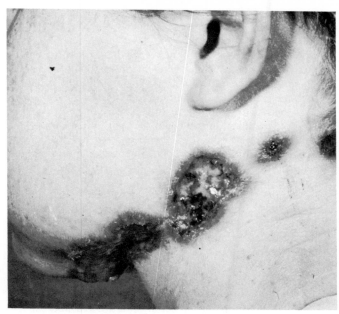

Fig. 182-6   Cryptococcosis.

without symptoms referable to the central nervous system. Examination of cerebrospinal fluid usually reveals a leukocytosis, predominately lymphocytic, an elevated protein level, and in approximately 50 percent of patients, a depressed glucose value [21].

Other than the above findings in the cerebrospinal fluid, consistently abnormal laboratory values are not encountered.

Infection is seen as part of the usually fatal acquired immunodeficiency syndrome (AIDS) [22].

Pathology

One of the hallmarks of *C. neoformans* infections is an absence of, or only a minimal, inflammatory response. With proper stains the organism can be seen in tissue with relatively little round cell or polymorphonucler response. In the brain, there are lytic lesions, with multiple organisms in the resulting cysts. Occasionally histiocytic granulomas are present. Rarely, giant cells which contain one or more fungal cells are seen. In pulmonary lesions there may be conspicuous fibrosis.

Diagnosis and differential diagnosis

The diagnosis is established by the isolation and identification of the causative microorganism in culture from skin lesions, pus, sputum, and urine, but especially from the cerebrospinal fluid. The diagnosis is virtually established if budding yeast forms with a capsule are seen with an india ink preparation.

In the rare instance when material for culture is not available, the diagnosis may rest on finding the characteristic fungal cells after microscopic examination of specially stained tissue sections. The organism may be confused with *Blastomyces dermatitidis* or (though this is less likely) with *Histoplasma capsulatum*.

Detection of antigen by agglutination or enzyme-linked

immunosorbent assay (ELISA) techniques may also be helpful [23].

Laboratory diagnosis. DIRECT EXAMINATION. Lumbar or ventricular cerebrospinal fluid or urine should be centrifuged and studied by a wet mount preparation, preferably with an agent such as india ink, to delineate the capsule of *C. neoformans*. The organism may vary in size from 4 to 20 μm depending on the age of the cell. The mucopolysaccharide capsule may vary from large to nearly indistinguishable (rarely), and is visible in a negative fashion with reduced light intensity as a halo between the cell and the india ink particles (Fig. 182-7).

The capsule of *C. neoformans* is not visibly affected by 10% to 20% potassium hydroxide. When sputum or pus is mixed with this mounting agent, the organism and capsule may be demonstrated in outline by the cellular debris present in the specimen.

In brain tissue, crushed between a slide and coverslip to a thin layer, the organism and its capsule are readily demonstrated.

Other specimens are generally not studied microscopically in fresh preparations. They may be cultured, and appropriate specimens may be prepared for histopathologic procedures.

CULTURE. Culturally, *C. neoformans* is identical at 30 and 37°C and grows well on all standard mycologic media containing no cycloheximide, which inhibits it. Colonies are at first whitish gray, pasty with either a dull or shiny surface, and sticky and stringy because of the presence of capsular material. After about 2 weeks, the color becomes tan but the colony retains it stickiness.

The individual organisms are spherical, colorless, yeast-like budding cells producing rare pseudohyphae and, under standard conditions, no hyphae.

C. neoformans differs from other related organisms in having a polysaccharide capsule and a narrow pore between mother and daughter cell, in producing urease and utilizing some sugars but fermenting none, in growing as a yeast at both 30 and 37°C, and in being pathogenic for and producing hydrocephalus in mice. The latter feature differentiates *C. neoformans* from the nonpathogenic cryptococci.

ANIMAL INOCULATION

Cultural confirmation. Mice are generally used for animal studies of *C. neoformans*. Several routes of inoculation may be used. A saline suspension of 24- to 48-h culture grown on yeast malt extract agar is prepared to contain approximately 10^6 organisms per milliliter. Six adult mice should be inoculated intraperitoneally with 0.5 mL or intravenously with 0.2 mL. Intracerebral inoculation of young mice should not exceed 0.02 to 0.04 mL of approximately 10^5 per milliliter.

On autopsy of animals at weekly intervals from 2 to 4 weeks after inoculation, heart blood, viscera, lungs, and brain are removed for culture. Small portions of the brain should be crushed between microscope slides and coverslips, and direct microscopic examination for the budding encapsulated yeasts performed.

Isolation. From the numbers of microorganisms required to infect mice as indicated above, it is obvious that direct inoculation of mice with patients' specimens is not generally performed.

Differential diagnosis. Cryptococcosis of the skin must be distinguished from pyoderma and other bacterial or fungal skin lesions. The pulmonary form must be distinguished from tuberculosis, malignancy, other fungal infections, and from more chronic bacterial disease. Cerebrospinal fluid findings typical of *C. neoformans* meningitis may be seen in tuberculosis, other fungal infections, sarcoidosis, meningeal carcinomatosis, and, rarely, such viral diseases as mumps and lymphocytic choriomengitis.

Treatment

Chemotherapy is the most critical factor in the management of disease, and there are at least four options. If the isolate is sensitive to the drug, 5-flucytosine is the first. If such data cannot be obtained, or treatment must begin immediately, amphotericin B must be used. In patients with meningitis both drugs should be used.

5-Flucytosine is administered by the oral route in a daily dose of 150 mg/kg per day in four equally divided doses. Intervals between doses must be increased according to serum creatinine values or to creatinine clearances.

Amphotericin B is administered intravenously (see under "Blastomycosis" later in this chapter). Optimal total dose should be, according to one schedule, approximately 1 to 2 g or, by a second schedule, a 10-week course at 20 mg per day.

If both drugs are used, a 6-week course of therapy is customary, with a daily dose of 5-flucytosine of 150 mg/kg, and of amphotericin B of 20 mg.

When such therapy is unsuccessful in meningitis patients, intrathecal administration of amphotericin B is justified. The dose should not exceed 1.0 mg, at 2- to 3-day intervals. Amphotericin B should be diluted in the syringe with approximately 5.0 mL of cerebrospinal fluid.

If other options are unsuccessful miconazole intravenously may be useful [24].

Fig. 182-7   India ink preparation showing the capsule of *C. neoformans*.

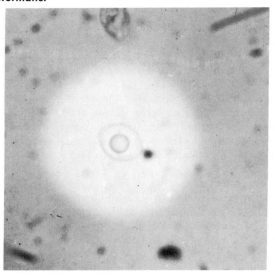

Course and prognosis

Once meningitis appears, the disease is considered inexorably fatal, unless treated as described above. Pulmonary forms of disease have a more variable course, and some appear to persist for long periods without worsening or disseminating. The skin forms of disease as well as the bone forms have a chronic, slowly progressive course.

Histoplasmosis

Definition

Histoplasmosis is a chronic infectious disease, acquired by the respiratory route, with a primary focus of infection in the lungs, with occasional hematogenous dissemination (characteristically to such reticuloendothelial organs as liver, bone marrow, and spleen), and caused by a dimorphic fungus. *Histoplasma capsulatum* (perfect state: *Emmonsiella capsulata* [25]).

Historical aspects

In 1906, Darling [26] reported his studies of a fatal illness in three patients in whom he found a great many microorganisms that he suspected of being protozoa, but which seem clearly to have been fungal. In 1934, DeMonbreum [27], in a beautiful series of experiments, demonstrated the causative agent to be indeed a fungus.

A second form of the disease, acute primary histoplasmosis, was delineated as a result of observations of localized outbreaks for the most part, by Christie, Peterson, Palmer, and Furcolow during the mid-1940s.

Furcolow is also to be credited with the description of the third form of disease, chronic cavitary histoplasmosis, which he identified in tuberculosis sanatorium patients who had a disease closely resembling tuberculosis but who had negative tuberculin skin tests [28].

A notable contribution to the knowledge of the epidemiology of histoplasmosis was the recognition by Emmons, in 1949 [19], of the presence of the causative organism in soil, particularly where there has been a deposit of bird and chicken excreta [29].

Epidemiology

Although the disease has been reported from 30 widely scattered countries, it is recognized most commonly in eastern and central United States. In these areas, as high a proportion as 80 percent of the adult population will have skin test evidence of prior infection. There is a marked preponderance of disease in patients above the age of 60 and (uniquely among the systemic mycoses) in infants and children below the age of 10 years. In adults the disease is far more common in males. The largest outbreak, in Indianapolis, affected 100,000 residents [30].

H. capsulatum can be recovered, occasionally in abundance, from soil naturally enriched by chicken or bird excreta. The causative fungus has been isolated from a large number of wild and domestic animals, including notably the dog, skunk, raccoon, woodchuck, cow, horse, and sheep. Animal-to-human or human-to-human spread does not occur, however.

Etiology and pathogenesis

Since *H. capsulatum* is ubiquitous in nature, and infection is widespread in certain areas, as indicated by delayed hypersensitivity skin reactions to histoplasmin, it appears certain that important factors other than exposure to the fungus are necessary for production of disease. One of these is probably the size of the inoculum. Decreased host resistance (as seen in lymphoma and Hodgkin's disease) and impaired antibody response probably play a role, although most likely a lesser one than in other fungal infections, e.g., those due to *Candida* spp., *C. neoformans*, and the Phycomyces.

Clinical manifestations (Fig. A6-22)

Glabrous skin involvement in histoplasmosis is highly unusual, other than by the hypersensitivity phenomenon of erythema nodosum. Mucous membrane lesions due to invasion of the mouth, pharynx, and larynx by the fungus may be commonly noted in progressive disseminated histoplasmosis.

Acute primary histoplasmosis has been characterized chiefly from observations of illnesses occurring in localized outbreaks of disease. Constitutional symptoms are commonly malaise, fever, chills, sweats, and lethargy. Pulmonary symptoms are generally those of cough (61 percent), chest pain (55 percent), and hemoptysis (6 percent). On the chest roentgenogram infiltrates, hilar or mediastinal lymphadenopathy or both occur in 85 percent of patients. Lesions may appear or heal with diffuse calcification, suggesting a miliary process.

In progressive disseminated histoplasmosis, the aforementioned constitutional symptoms are present frequently. The organ most often involved is the liver, and approximately 80 percent of patients have either abnormal function or cultural evidence of disease. An important additional lesion is ulceration of the soft palate, oropharynx, epiglottis, or stomach and intestine, resulting in pain, dysphagia, and weight loss (Fig. 182-8). Overt Addison's disease or lesser manifestations of adrenal involvement may be present in the form of decreased serum cortisol levels.

The chronic cavitary form is recognized from the characteristic upper-lobe pulmonary disease. A productive cough, dyspnea on exertion, and progressive respiratory embarrassment are the common findings.

The usual laboratory findings in the progressive disseminated form are those of impaired liver function. Anemia and leukocytosis are present only in a minority of patients. Laboratory tests in the two other forms of disease are not especially helpful.

Pathology

Darling [26], in his original description of histoplasmosis, reported "an intense invasion of large endothelial-like cells." The presence of *H. capsulatum* in histiocytes and macrophages is the hallmark of the histopathologic change of this disease. Lesions are seen most commonly in lymph nodes, liver, and spleen, which are a part of the reticuloendothelial system.

In nonfatal histoplasmosis, the characteristic histologic lesion is an epithelioid cell granuloma, usually with Lan-

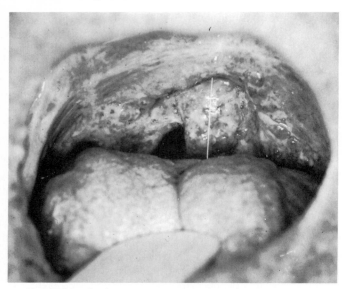

Fig. 182-8 Oral mucous membrane lesions in histoplasmosis.

ghans' giant cells. Such lesions may be seen in pulmonary tissue, biopsies of oral or gastrointestinal ulcers, or in the liver. Gomori's methenamine silver or the periodic acid-Schiff (PAS) stains are particularly helpful in rapid screening examinations of tissues for the presence of typically staining fungal cells (Fig. 182-9).

Diagnosis and differential diagnosis

The diagnosis is established by the isolation and identification of the causative fungus in culture from oral lesions, bone marrow, sputum, blood, urine, lymph node, or liver biopsy.

The diagnosis is virtually established if on microscopic examination of tissue, organisms are seen that are typical of *H. capsulatum* in size and staining. These must be distinguished from the endospores of *Coccidioides immitis*

(in lesions of which spherules can usually be seen), from *C. neoformans* (in which typical capsules can be recognized with the use of Mayer's mucicarmine stain), from small intracellular forms of *Blastomyces dermatitidis* (in which the fungal cells are usually multinuclear), from *Toxoplasma gondii* (which are smaller and characteristically not in histiocytes), and from *Leishmania donvani* (in which the kinetoplast can easily be seen).

Skin and seriologic tests are rarely helpful and virtually never diagnostic in active disease [31].

Laboratory diagnosis. DIRECT EXAMINATION. Slide preparations may be made from specimens such as sputum, bronchial aspirates, urine, peripheral blood, or bone marrow, cerebrospinal fluid, lymph nodes, and pus or material from ulcers. The preparation is fixed with methyl alcohol for 10 min and then stained with either Giemsa's or Wright's stain. The yeasts are found extracellularly, or intracellularly in monocytes or macrophages, as 2- to 3-μm by 3- to 4-μm cells composed of deeply stained, cup-shaped protoplasm at one end of the cell, and, usually, a large vacuole.

CULTURE

37°C incubation. This temperature is not used for primary isolation. The organism may not grow, and when it does, neither the small budding cells, which resemble many other yeastlike forms, nor the soft, white, creamy colony formed is characteristic. When inoculated with the mycelial form, a relatively unstable yeastlike growth is produced only with difficulty.

30°C incubation. Mycosel (Difco) or Sabouraud's agar with added chloramphenicol is most often used for primary isolation of the fungus from clinical material. Colonies develop slowly (10 days to more than 3 weeks after inoculation), producing, initially, white cottony aerial hyphae which darken with age from buff to light brown. Microscopically, two types of conidia are found: smooth-walled, oval or pyriform microconidia (2 to 4 μm) borne on short lateral stalks (conidiophores), and round to pyriform macroconidia (7 to 18 μm) on short or long conidiophores and

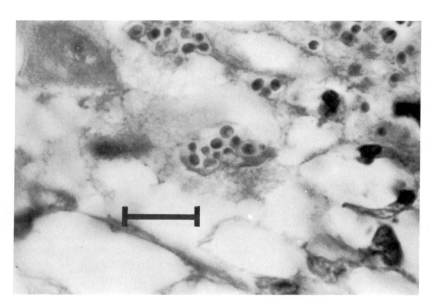

Fig. 182-9 *Histoplasma capsulatum* intracellularly in macrophages and extracellularly in a bone marrow specimen. H&E, bar = 10 μm.

characterized by tuberculate appendages formed from condensed cell-wall material covering the entire spore.

ANIMAL INOCULATION

Cultural confirmation. Certain saprophytic fungi closely related to *H. capsulatum* have macroconidia resembling those of this organism. Therefore, other verification of cultural findings may be necessary.

Isolation. Mice are susceptible to *H. capsulatum:* intraperitoneal inoculation of a patient's specimen or a saline spore suspension from cultural growth at 30°C leads to infection and usually death of the animals. At weekly intervals 2 to 6 weeks after inoculation, animals are killed, and impression smears made aseptically of liver and spleen. In these smears, after Wright's or Giemsa's stain, the characteristic tissue yeast phase of the fungus may be seen. Liver and spleen are then homogenized and inoculated onto Mycosel agar. When the inoculum is incubated at 30°C, colonies develop on this medium as described above.

Differential diagnosis. The acute primary form of histoplasmosis usually cannot be distinguished from a flulike, acute viral illness of the upper part of the respiratory tract, or atypical pneumonia, unless microbiologic studies are performed. The progressive disseminated form most closely resembles a lymphoma, such as Hodgkin's disease, or hematogenous tuberculosis. The chronic cavitary form is distinguishable from the similar form of tuberculosis only by laboratory diagnostic tests.

Treatment

Antifungal chemotherapy is essential in those patients with more severe acute primary illness, in all patients with a progressive disseminated form of disease, and in most patients with the chronic cavitary form. Amphotericin B is presently the therapeutic agent confirmed by 25 years' experience. The details of treatment are given under "Blastomycosis," below.

Members of the sulfonamide group, notably sufadiazine, have been shown, under specific controlled conditions in experimental infections in mice, to have chemotherapeutic effect. Because it has minimal activity, however, the use of this drug should be reserved for mild infections, e.g., when the laboratory reports the culture of *H. capsulatum* some time after an acute illness from which the patient seems to be recovering spontaneously.

Ketoconazole, in dosage of 400 to 600 mg daily, orally has been useful in preliminary studies [32].

In some patients with chronic cavitary histoplasmosis, surgical resection of irreversibly diseased pulmonary tissue is sometimes advisable.

Course and prognosis

The acute primary form is usually a mild disease, although fatalities have been reported in patients massively infected. In the progressive disseminated form, spontaneous recovery is rare and 80 percent of patients die within 1 year of the diagnosis. The chronic cavitary form is less often fatal, although most patients have progressive respiratory and ventilatory impairment.

Blastomycosis

Definition

Blastomycosis is a chronic infectious disease acquired by the respiratory route, with a primary focus of infection in the lungs, and with occasional hematogenous dissemination (characteristically to the skin, bone, and genital part of the genitourinary tract); it is caused by a dimorphic fungus, *Blastomyces dermatitidis* (perfect state: *Ajellomyces dermatitidis* [33]).

Historical aspects

The disease in its cutaneous form was first described by Gilchrist and Stokes at a meeting of the Baltimore and Washington Dermatologic Association in 1894. In 1898 the same authors named the causative organism *Blastomyces dermatitidis* [34]. In 1964, Emmons et al reported, for the first time, culturally authenticated cases originating outside the North American continent, in Africa [35].

Epidemiology

This disease occurs in the Americas and Africa. It is encountered with the greatest frequency in the southeastern United States. It is at least 6 times as common in males as in females, and occurs more often in farmers and laborers. The majority of illnesses are seen in patients of 50 years and older. The disease occurs not infrequently in dogs and has been reported once in a horse and a sea lion. The natural habitat of the fungus has yet to be unequivocally demonstrated, but wood has been implicated.

Disease in dogs continues to be encountered, occasionally as harbingers of disease in humans [36].

Etiology and pathogenesis

Since *B. dermatitidis* does not appear to be ubiquitous in nature, and because there is no skin test survey evidence of widespread infection (as in histoplasmosis and coccidioidomycosis), disease may represent rare instances of infection. It appears to occur with increased frequency in persons who have diabetes mellitus and tuberculosis, but opportunistic infection continues to be rare.

Although once thought to be due to cutaneous implantation, blastomycosis has been considered, since the work of Schwarz and Baum [37], a disease acquired by inhalation, with a primary focus in the lungs.

Clinical manifestations

When infection disseminates from the lung, a number of cutaneous forms of the disease are seen. The most characteristic is an elevated, verrucous, crusted, varicolored lesion which has a sharply slanting serpiginous border and a tendency toward central healing, with a thin depigmented atrophic scar. The peripheral border extends on one side only, resembling a one-half to three-quarter moon (Fig.

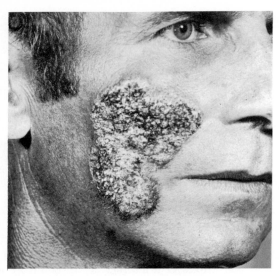

Fig. 182-10   Verrucous plaque of blastomycosis.

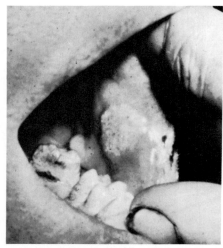

Fig. 182-12   Blastomycosis. Mucosal plaque in a patient with pulmonary, laryngeal, and cutaneous foci. *(Courtesy of Dr. Jan Schwarz, Cincinnati, Ohio.)*

182-10). These lesions are most commonly seen on the exposed surfaces of the body: face, hands, and arms. When one of the crusts is lifted, pus exudes. In approximately half the patients, the lesions are multiple. Another form of cutaneous disease is that of small superficial ulcerative lesions (Fig. 182-11). A third form of the disease consists of a raised, firm, subcutaneous nodule, containing occasionally many small pustules over its surface. In extraordinarily rare instances of accidental inoculation into the skin, e.g, in a laboratory worker, the disease has been quite different, characterized by a chancre with a reddened area of induration, by lymphangitis and lymphadenopathy, and by the absence of hematogenous spread. Erythema nodosum may be seen as a sign in blastomycosis, but is more common as a manifestation of coccidioidomycosis and histoplasmosis.

Pulmonary involvement occurs in virtually all patients but is clinically important (i.e., with lesion on chest roentgenogram or positive sputum culture) in only one-half of them. Approximately a quarter of all patients have a mul-

Fig. 182-11   Superficial ulcerative lesion of blastomycosis. *(Courtesy of Dr. Jan Schwarz, Cincinnati, Ohio.)*

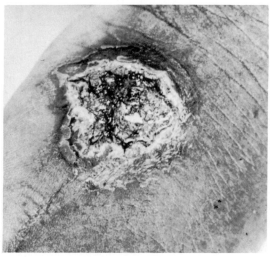

tiple lobe involvement. Miliary and cavitary lesions occasionally are seen. Pleural disease or pulmonary calcification is rare [38].

Bone lesions in the form of osteomyelitis are seen in approximately a third of the patients. The most common sites are the thoracic and lumbar vertebrae, pelvis, sacrum, skull, ribs, and long bones of the extremities. In some of these patients, extension to subcutaneous areas, with a large abscess, especially in the psoas area, may be the first manifestation of this type of disease. The most common symptoms from bone involvement are pain and tenderness at the site [39].

Disease of the genital tract occurs in approximately a third of the male patients. The prostate, seminal vesicles, and testes are affected; the kidney is virtually never involved. Symptoms and findings are characteristically pain, often described as "heaviness" in the perineum, or swelling of the scrotal contents [40].

Approximately a quarter of the patients have oral or nasal mucous membrane lesions (Fig. 182-12). Of this fraction, only one-half are from a contiguous cutaneous lesion.

Rarely, the disease may be manifest by meningoencephalitis, cerebral abscess, endocarditis, or involvement of the liver, adrenals, spleen, or gastrointestinal tract.

Constitutional symptoms such as chills, fever, night sweats, anorexia, weight loss, malaise, and lassitude are seen in only 50 percent of patients.

Leukocytosis and anemia in one-quarter of patients, increased erythrocyte sedimentation rate in two-thirds, and hyperglobulinemia in approximately three-quarters are the most common laboratory findings [39].

Pathology

The histologic pattern of blastomycosis is a characteristic combination of suppurative and granulomatous changes (Fig. 182-13). In these inflammatory areas, especially within giant cells, the budding fungus can be seen, even with hematoxylin and eosin stain (Fig. 182-14). The Gridley fungus stain is especially helpful in finding the fungus in screening examinations of tissue.

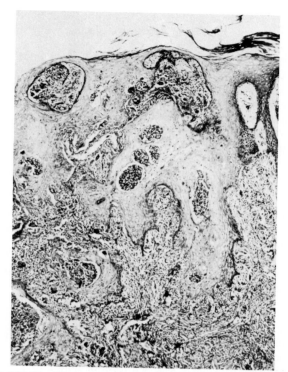

Fig. 182-13 Blastomycosis. The cutaneous reaction is characterized by pseudoepitheliomatous hyperplasia associated with intraepithelial neutrophilic abscesses and underlying granulomatous inflammation. Many deep fungi produce pseudoepitheliomatous hyperplasia. ×40. (AFIP 923367; courtesy of Dr. Elson B. Helwig. Micrograph by Wallace H. Clark, Jr., M.D.)

In skin lesions, pseudoepitheliomatous hyperplasia is characteristically seen.

Diagnosis and differential diagnosis

The diagnosis is established by the isolation and identification of the causative fungus in culture from skin lesions,

pus, sputum, urine, or rarely, cerebrospinal fluid, blood, or bone marrow.

The diagnosis is almost as certainly, and more quickly, established by finding characteristic budding cells with thick walls on direct microscopic examination of the above-mentioned specimens. This tentative diagnosis should, however, be confirmed by cultural procedure.

In the rare instances when material for culture is not available, the diagnosis rests on finding characteristic cells on direct microscopic examination of stained tissue sections. These cells may be confused with *C. immitis*, *H. capsulatum*, *H. duboisii*, and *C. neoformans*. The mucicarmine stain is helpful in distinguishing *B. dermatitidis* from the last-named fungus; *B. dermatitidis* does not stain well with mucicarmine, whereas *C. neoformans* does.

Skin and serologic tests usually are not helpful and virtually never diagnostic of active disease.

Laboratory diagnosis. DIRECT EXAMINATION. Pus or material from a swab from the periphery of an ulcerated lesion, mixed with a drop of 10% or 20% potassium hydroxide, is examined microscopically. Under reduced light intensity the fungus may be seen as large (8 to 15 μm), usually single, budding cells with a thick "double-contoured" wall and a wide pore of attachment (Fig. 182-15). It is more difficult to differentiate the microorganism from artifacts in sputum, cerebrospinal fluid, and pleural exudates, and direct examination should always be followed by confirmatory cultural procedures.

CULTURE

37°C incubation. Material planted on blood agar continues to produce the yeastlike phase with single and multiple budding similar to that seen in tissue, as well as with pseudohyphal development. The colony is a light buff-to-brown color with a dry, wrinkled surface often described as mealy.

30°C incubation. On either Sabouraud's or Mycosel (Difco) agar planted with suitable material, *B. dermatitidis* forms the same yeastlike growth initially as at 37°C, but hyphae will develop rapidly, and a white fluffy colony is formed. In some stains, the colony becomes brown with

Fig. 182-14 *Blastomyces dermatitidis* forms in patients with disseminated disease. (Cytoplasm contracted in fixation artifactually, but thickness of wall notable.) Bar = 10 μm. (From D. M. Dixon and H. J. Shadomy, Department of Microbiology, Virginia Commonwealth University, Richmond, with permission.)

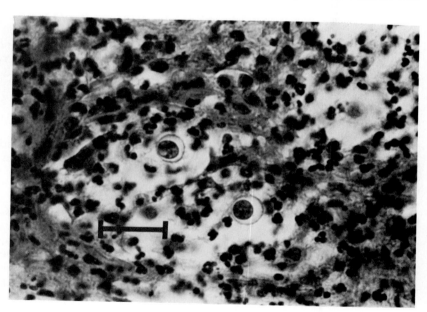

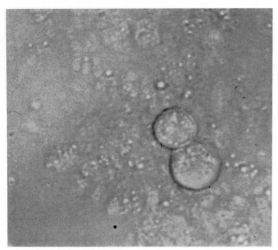

Fig. 182-15 Fresh preparation demonstrating budding cells of *Blastomyces dermatitidis*.

age and may produce a dark diffusible pigment. The hyphae are relatively fine (2 to 3 μm in diameter) and septate. After 2 to 3 weeks, short lateral conidiophores are formed bearing single hyaline, smooth-walled conidia (2 to 10 μm in diameter). Although the spores are usually spherical or slightly oval, occasional strains of *B. dermatitidis* produce pyriform conidia. With the development of large numbers of these conidia, the surface of the colony flattens and may become powdery or granular.

Transfer of the 37°C yeastlike culture to 30°C leads to the development of the characteristic mold colony by which *B. dermatitidis* may be identified.

ANIMAL INOCULATION

Cultural confirmation. In some cases it is not possible to obtain typical growth of *B. dermatitidis* at both 30 and 37° C. If the true identity of the fungus is questioned, the virulent nature of the organism may be tested by the intraperitoneal inoculation of a saline suspension of spores into white Swiss mice. Disease may not be fatal, but autopsy of the animals at weekly intervals 3 to 6 weeks after inoculation should demonstrate lesions in lungs, the peritoneal cavity, liver, spleen, and often on the diaphragm.

Isolation. Use of mice for initial isolation of *B. dermatitidis* from clinical material is usually less helpful than proper cultural techniques.

Differential diagnosis. The skin lesions of blastomycosis must be distinguished from squamous cell carcinoma or chronic skin lesions due to tuberculosis, tertiary syphilis, leprosy, staphylococcal infection, and bromism. The pulmonary lesions must be differentiated from carcinoma with atelectasis and pneumonia, tuberculosis, other fungal infection, or, rarely, more chronic bacterial infections such as those due to *Klebsiella pneumoniae*. The bone and genitourinary lesions resemble those due to tuberculosis.

Treatment

Chemotherapy is indicated in all patients, and surgical drainage of abscesses or resection of chronically diseased tissue occasionally is essential. A number of chemotherapeutic agents have been demonstrated clearly in the past to be efficacious.

The first chemotherapeutic agent proved effective was 2-hydroxystilbamidine. It is administered intravenously in a daily dose of 225 mg, for a total dose of 8 g. This drug is well tolerated but is relatively contraindicated in patients with hepatic disease, since it is stored in the liver.

Amphotericin B is a more effective agent. It is administered intravenously with an initial dose of 1 mg. The drug is suspended in 5% glucose solution (the drug precipitates in sodium or potassium salt solution, in a concentration not greater than 1 mg per 10 mL), and infused over a period of 2 to 4 h. The use of a smaller-gauge (No. 23 or 24) needle and heparin may be helpful in preventing phlebitis. The dosage should be increased thereafter by daily increments of 5 to 10 mg.

There are two opinions as to optimal daily dosage, total amount of drug, and duration of therapy. One recommends an optimal daily or alternate daily dose of 1 mg/kg [not to exceed 50 mg and meant to achieve a serum level approximately 10 times the minimal inhibitory concentration (MIC)], a total amount of approximately 1 to 2 g, and duration sufficient to achieve that (usually 4 to 6 weeks). A second opinion is that a lower optimal dosage 15 to 30 mg (meant to achieve a serum level of only 2 to 3 times the MIC) is given, a total amount of less importance, and a duration of 10 weeks. The toxicity of the drug is usually less with the second regimen.

Amphotericin B produces fever, chills, nausea, vomiting, anorexia, headache, and, in most patients, irreversible renal damage of at least mild degree. Anemia and hypokalemia also are occasionally encountered. Fifty milligrams of the succinate salt of hydrocortisone injected into the bottle or tubing at the onset of infusion is the most effective means of preventing vomiting, chills, fever, and malaise.

Preliminary data suggest ketoconazole may also be effective in doses of 200 to 600 mg daily, orally [41].

Course and prognosis

It was formerly thought that the disease was inexorably fatal, but more recent studies suggest that at least in some patients it is only mildly progressive or even self-limited. Progressive disease and death occur, however, so that the illness is considered by some to be serious and deserving of treatment.

Paracoccidioidal granuloma (South American blastomycosis, Lutz-Splendore-Almeida disease)

Definition

Paracoccidioidal granuloma is a chronic infectious disease, beginning characteristically on the skin or mucosa about the mouth or nose, or occasionally in the lungs, with subsequent involvement of regional lymph nodes, and occasional dissemination hematogenously (characteristically to the spleen, or to other organs); it is caused by the fungus

Paracoccidioides brasiliensis, thought to be a saprophyte of soil or decaying vegetation.

Historical aspects

Lutz, in 1908, described a patient and the fungus causing his disease. A more complete description of the clinical illness and of the causative organism was published subsequently by Splendore. In a series of reports, Almeida [42] distinguished this illness from others with which it had been confused in the literature.

Epidemiology

Paracoccidioidal granuloma is an important disease in Brazil and it has been reported from virtually all countries in South America, and from Costa Rica and Mexico as well. The disease is 5 times more common in whites than blacks, and approximately 10 times more common in males than in females. It is more frequent in the 20- to 30-year age group. It seems to occur more frequently in rural areas, especially in farmers.

Etiology and pathogenesis

After many years of doubt and controversy it now seems well established from the work of Londero [43] that infection is acquired by the respiratory route, no matter what organ is affected, and that such involvement is secondary to hematogenous dissemination. Recent confirmation of this stems from demonstration of the fungus in the lung of a woman, mummified about 290 A.D., near the village of Auk, Chile [44].

Clinical manifestations

The vast majority of patients present with painful ulcerative lesions of the mouth or because of ulcerative or verrucous lesions of the skin (Fig. 182-16). These latter are most commonly seen about the face and are usually multiple. Less frequently there is a solitary pustular lesion or subcutaneous abscess and draining sinus tract.

Involvement of the regional lymphatics is characteristic of the disease, and occasionally swelling or drainage of a lymph node, especially those of the cervical region, is the first sign noted by the patient.

Occasionally disease begins with cough, chest pain, and a pulmonary infiltrate on the chest roentgenogram.

From the above lesions disease may disseminate to such organs as bone, adrenal glands, central nervous system, and, in virtually all patients, the spleen.

Pathology

The histopathologic findings are characteristically both granulomatous and suppurative. In skin lesions there is usually pseudoepitheliomatous hyperplasia, with both the Langhans' type of granuloma and such pyogenic inflammatory cells as neutrophils, lymphocytes, and plasma cells. In these respects, as well as in the appearance of the fungus in giant cells or tissue, the pathologic change closely resembles that of blastomycosis. Although the character-

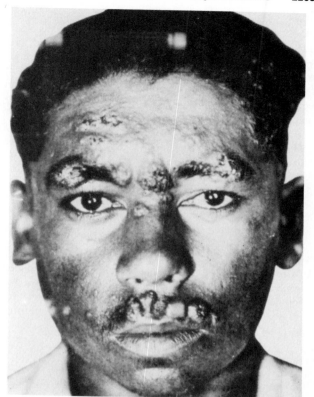

Fig. 182-16   South American blastomycosis. [*Courtesy of Dr. A. Rothberg, Brazil, and Dr. Orlando Canizares. Canizares O (ed): Clinical Tropical Dermatology. Oxford, Blackwell, 1975, p 31.*]

istic budding fungal cells stain with hematoxylin and eosin, the special fungal stains demonstrate them more strikingly.

Diagnosis and differential diagnosis

The diagnosis is established by the isolation and identification of the causative fungus, *P. brasiliensis,* in culture. Skin test material and serologic procedures are not generally available.

Laboratory diagnosis. DIRECT EXAMINATION. Sputum or other body fluids, crusts of ulcers, and pus (particularly from draining lymph nodes) may be examined microscopically by potassium hydroxide preparation. The large (10 to 60 μm in diameter) spherical to oval cells are easily visualized. The cell wall is as thick as in *B. dermatitidis* and is differentiated from the latter by the single to multiple buds. Buds are usually not larger than 2 to 10 μm in diameter. Chains of multiple budding cells frequently are seen.

CULTURE

37°C incubation. Material planted on blood agar will maintain the budding tissue form of the fungus. Growth is cream- to tan-colored, and either smooth and soft in consistency or verrucose and waxy.

30°C incubation. P. brasiliensis is probably the slowest growing of the systemic fungi: a small heaped colony may appear in from 2 to 3 weeks, but occasionally 2 months or more may be required. On standard mycologic media (preferably neutral or alkaline in pH) the colony, usually small even at maturity, is white, compact, flat or wrinkled, and velvety. Occasionally glabrous, irregularly folded colonies may develop. Microscopically, the colony is made up of fine septate hyphae and chlamydospores. Some pyriform conidia attached either directly to hyphae or on short sterigmata have been described [45].

ANIMAL INOCULATION

Cultural confirmation. The budding tissue forms are most easily obtained on blood agar at 37°C, but occasionally animals may be used to obtain this characteristic phase. The intratesticular inoculation of male guinea pigs with a heavy suspension of the yeast phase of the fungus leads to orchitis, with draining sinuses and abscesses in which the characteristic budding tissue forms may be seen.

Isolation. Not done.

Differential diagnosis. The disease must be distinguished from blastomycosis (in which mucosal lesions are rare and regional lymphadenopathy is characteristically absent), tuberculosis (especially scrofula), yaws, syphilis, sporotrichosis, and leishmaniasis.

Treatment

For many years the sulfonamides have been known to suppress but not cure the infection.

Amphotericin B administered intravenously in total dosage ranging from 1 to 8 g has been shown to be effective in patients now numbering in excess of 100. In view of the known renal toxicity and the response in some patients to lower doses of drug, it would seem advisable to limit the total dose to less than 3 g. At daily doses of 1 mg/kg, approximately 4 to 8 weeks are necessary for such therapy.

Preliminary data suggest that ketoconazole at doses of 200 to 600 mg daily is at least as effective as amphotericin B and has the advantage of the oral route of administration [41].

Course and prognosis

Disease was formerly invariably fatal, although its course has occasionally been prolonged. The chronicity of the process is markedly increased by sulfonamides, and the case fatality rate has been markedly reduced by amphotericin B and ketoconazole.

Coccidioidomycosis

Definition

Coccidioidomycosis is an acute or chronic infectious disease acquired by the respiratory route, with a primary focus of infection in the lungs, with occasional hematogenous dissemination (characteristically to subcutaneous tissues, bone, skin, or meninges), and caused by the dimorphic fungus *Coccidioides immitis*.

Historical aspects

Posadas and Wernicke, in 1891, described the first reported patient, a soldier in Argentina with coccidioidomycosis of the disseminated form, involving especially the skin of the face. They, as well as Rixford and Gilchrist [46], who reported the next case, from the San Joaquin Valley of California, believed that the causative microorganism was a protozoon, for which the name *C. immitis* was suggested. In 1900, Ophuls and Moffitt described an additional case, and correctly identified and characterized the causative agent as a fungus. In a series of papers beginning in 1915, Dickson described and identified the illness, respiratory in origin, that constitutes the primary acute form of the disease. Gifford [47] is credited with the definition of the syndrome, known as "San Joaquin Valley fever," and marked by fever, pleurisy, erythema nodosum, and occasionally, joint pains or rheumatism.

Epidemiology

In a long series of beautifully conducted studies, Smith [48] and colleagues succeeded in defining the epidemiology of the infection in the endemic areas of Southern California.

Coccidioidomycosis is sharply and dramatically limited in geographic occurrence to the areas of southern California, Arizona, New Mexico, southwestern Texas, northern Mexico, and areas of northern Argentina and Paraguay. Cases reported from other areas represent, without much question, infection by fomites or previous residence in endemic areas, e.g., cases in freight and cargo handlers in eastern United States, and in Italians previously quartered as prisoners of World War II in California. It has been estimated that approximately 50,000 persons are newly infected annually with *C. immitis* and, of these, approximately one-half have a clinical illness. Infection appears to occur equally in all ages, both sexes, and all races. However, blacks are 14 times, and Filipinos 175 times, more likely than Caucasians to have severe and disseminated disease. It is interesting that Mexicans, although darker-skinned, appear to be only about 3 times more susceptible to severe illness than light-skinned persons.

C. immitis has been found frequently in the soil from endemic sites; persistence of the fungus is favored by a dry climate, alkaline soil, infrequently severe frost, an annual rainfall of about 12 to 50 cm, and a season of several months' duration with mean temperatures between 26 and 32°C. The fungus remains viable during the hot summer months in rodent burrows at depths of from 6 to 8 in. Infection has been reported in a large variety of domestic and wild animals, including the dog, cat, cow, coyote, monkey, and gorilla.

Etiology and pathogenesis

Since this fungus is so ubiquitous in certain geographic areas, and since in these areas infection occurs in 80 to 90 percent of the inhabitants (as judged by delayed-hypersensitivity skin reactions to coccidioidin), it seems likely that certain factors are important in the induction and in the severity of the disease. Among these is race, as previously mentioned. Pregnancy also predisposes towards more severe disease. In contrast to other systemic mycoses, such diseases as lymphoma, leukemia, and diabetes mellitus do not appear to be predisposing factors.

Clinical manifestations

Erythema nodosum is a characteristic but nonspecific feature of the primary infection, valley fever. Erythema multiforme is less frequently seen. In the disseminated disease there are characteristic draining sinus tracts to the skin. Granulomas, verrucous and nodular lesions are commonly seen; ulcerative lesions are less frequently noted (Fig. 182-17) [49].

Acute primary coccidioidomycosis, which has an incubation period of from 10 to 18 days, is usually an influenza- or grippelike illness, characterized by fever, chills, aching, malaise, pleuritic chest pain, and cough occasionally productive of blood-streaked sputum. Anorexia is common, and weight loss from 4.5 to 9 kg may occur during the illness.

Disseminated coccidioidomycosis results from hematogenous spread of the fungus. There are characteristically subcutaneous cellulitis, abscess formation, and multiple draining sinus tracts, some of which heal spontaneously, only to be replaced by new tracts at other sites. Bone is commonly involved, and the osteomyelitis may be the presenting illness. The psoas area is frequently involved, with drainage posteriorly or anteriorly below the inguinal ligament. Meningitis, also a common manifestation of dissemination, is characterized by headache and stiff neck. In most patients with severe disseminated disease, such constitutional symptoms as fever and chills, weight loss, malaise, sweats, and lassitude and anorexia are present.

Chronic residual coccidioidomycosis is the term for such continuing lesions in the lung as cavities (characteristically thin-walled), pulmonary fibrosis, and possibly, bronchiectasis [50].

Pathology

In pulmonary disease the early lesion of pulmonary coccidioidomycosis is a pyogenic reaction, with leukocytes

Fig. 182-17   Cutaneous lesions of coccidioidomycosis.

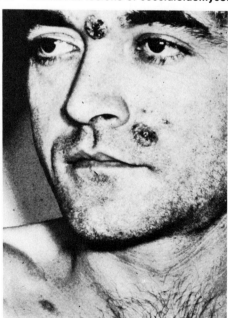

about the released sporangiospores. The inflammatory response to the larger sporangia (spherules) is characteristically granulomatous, with histiocytes, foreign-body giant cells, and lymphocytes. It has been recognized recently that there may be hyphal forms of the arthroconidia type in tissues in as many as 75 percent of resected lesions. When disease disseminates from the lung, characteristic lesions may be seen in skin, subcutaneous tissue, bone, meninges, lymph nodes, spleen, liver, and kidney. Again suppuration or granuloma may predominate.

Diagnosis and differential diagnosis

The diagnosis is established by the isolation and identification of the causative fungus in culture from sputum, sinus tract drainage, blood, urine, lymph node, or cerebrospinal fluid. Frequently on direct microscopic examination of these specimens, sporangia can be seen.

For information on histopathologic aids see "Blastomycosis" earlier in this chapter.

Laboratory diagnosis. DIRECT EXAMINATION. Sputum, pus, aspirates, and biopsy specimens are all best studied microscopically in potassium hydroxide preparations. The sediment of centrifuged cerebrospinal fluid may be examined directly with no mounting agent. Care must be taken, however, to dispose of the latter slide in disinfectant immediately after study, as *C. immitis* is capable of germination with production of the hyphal forms under these conditions.

Since the sporangia in these specimens are large (30 to 60 μm), they may be readily visualized under the microscope with reduced light. However, the smaller, single sporangiospores (endospores) may be difficult to differentiate from debris and artifacts.

CULTURE *37°C incubation.* Cultural procedures to produce the tissue phase are complex and not performed in routine laboratories. Standard media inoculated and incubated at 37°C produce the same type of growth as that seen at 30°C.

30°C incubation. C. immitis grows well on standard mycologic media. Cultures should be made in cotton-plugged tubes and incubated at 25 to 30°C. This fungus is the most rapid growing of all the systemic fungi. Within 2 to 4 days a gray-white floccose colony (which darkens with age) develops, covering the entire surface. The first characteristic-shaped arthroconidia appear on side branches of the vegetative hyphae in from 1 to 2 weeks after the colony is first seen. They are produced along the hyphal branches alternately with smaller empty cells and they vary somewhat in size from 2.5 to 4 by 3 to 6 μm. At maturity these empty cells rupture, freeing the infective arthroconidia. This phenomenon occurs rapidly after maturation of the culture. Therefore, all suspected colonies should be transferred within 1 week after initial observation of growth to containers appropriate for preventing infection to personnel. If the culture has any aerial hyphae, it is advisable to flood the surface with saline solution before obtaining material either for subculture or for microscopic examination.

ANIMAL INOCULATION *Cultural confirmation.* A sterile suspension of saline solution is flooded over the surface of a culture, and the arthroconidia are dislodged mechanically with a sterile inoculating needle. The suspension of spores is then removed to a sterile serum bottle and sealed with a rubber diaphragm. This material is used for animal inoculation studies. Mice and guinea pigs are susceptible to *C. immitis.*

In the guinea pig, intratesticular inoculation of 0.1 mL of the spore suspension produces orchitis, usually within a week to 10 days. With a sterile syringe, fluid is then withdrawn from the testes and examined for characteristic sporangia and sporangiospores produced in the tissue phase. If pus is present, a potassium hydroxide preparation will also demonstrate sporangia.

In the mouse, 0.5 to 1.0 mL of the spore suspension should be inoculated intraperitoneally. Mice are killed at weekly intervals from 2 to 4 weeks, and lungs, spleen, and liver are removed. Exudates from these organs, examined microscopically after potassium hydroxide preparation, show sporangia and sporangiospores.

Presence of the sporangia with sporangiospores confirms identifications of a culture as *C. immitis.*

Isolation. Animals may be inoculated directly with clinical material. Specimens must be held for 1 h at room temperature in concentrations of 10,000 units penicillin G and 1 mg of streptomycin or of 0.05 mg chloramphenicol per milliliter prior to animal inoculation to reduce the probability of bacterial infection. Animals should be autopsied and organs examined as previously described.

The diagnosis is virtually established if microorganisms typical in size of sporangia or sporangiospores are seen in properly stained tissues.

Precipitin and complement-fixation tests are helpful, though rarely diagnostic. Skin tests with coccidioidin or spherulin are not helpful [51].

Differential diagnosis. The acute primary form usually cannot be distinguished from influenza or severe infection of the upper part of the respiratory tract without cultural studies, unless it has the classical hallmarks of valley fever. The severe disseminated form most closely resembles hematogenous tuberculosis (though the latter disease is usually more acute and severe), other fungal disease such as blastomycosis or actinomycosis, or, less closely, a pyogenic infection due to *S. aureus.* Meningitis must be distinguished from that due to *C. neoformans* or *M. tuberculosis.* Erythema nodosum and erythema multiforme are nondiagnostic, and the underlying cause must be determined. The cutaneous granulomas of systemic coccidioidomycosis must be distinguished from cutaneous blastomycosis, tuberculosis, tertiary syphilis, cryptococcosis, and disease from bacterial causes.

Treatment

Antifungal chemotherapy is essential to the treatment of all patients with the severe disseminated form of disease. There is less certainty as to whether chemotherapy is necessary for patients with chronic cavities, who may need pulmonary resection, or for patients with more severe forms of acute primary disease.

Amphotericin B is not as effective in this disease as it is in cryptococcosis, histoplasmosis, or blastomycosis. More experienced workers in California believe that 3 g of drug should be the limit by the intravenous route. They also recommend for meningitis, intrathecal therapy at the

cisternal site 2 to 3 times weekly for prolonged periods, e.g., at least 2 to 3 years. For greater details of the administration of amphotericin B, see the treatment sections under "Blastomycosis" and "Cryptococcosis," both earlier in this chapter.

Ketoconazole in high doses (600 to 1200 mg daily) has been recommended, though recently discovered side effects have dampened enthusiasm for this drug [52,53].

Course and prognosis

In the majority of infected residents of endemic areas, disease does not occur or is mild, heals spontaneously, and is not distinguishable clinically. However, the disseminated form is serious, and patients must be studied intensely and treated as early as possible. A continuing negative delayed-hypersensitivity skin reaction to coccidioidin or aspirin and a high or rising titer of serologic antibodies may indicate early or impending dissemination. Some doubt exists even today as to whether any patient with meningitis has been cured. However, there is unquestionable evidence that many patients have improved and have sustained remissions with continuing therapy [50].

Aspergillosis

Definition

Aspergillosis comprises a group of clinical conditions unified only by sensitization to, saprophytic colonization of, or actual tissue invasion of, a number of species of the genus *Aspergillus.*

Historical aspects

Aspergillus fumigatus was described first by Fresenius in 1850. One of the earliest identifiable illnesses in humans was reported by Virchow in 1856. Much of the interest in the disease in Europe, sustained even to today, stems from Renon's classic paper of 1897 [54].

Epidemiology

It is difficult to say whether the preoccupation in Europe with this disease is a result of the early work of Renon, or whether it is due to an actual prevalence of illnesses ascribed to this fungus on that continent. However, the disease is probably worldwide in distribution. It is more common in men.

A great variety of *Aspergillus* spp. grow abundantly as saprophytes in nature. They are thermophilic and can be found frequently in such decaying vegetation as compost heaps.

A. fumigatus is an important cause of severe disease and death in young birds and in penguins in zoos. Animal-to-human spread, however, is not considered important.

Etiology and pathogenesis

Because of the ubiquity of these species in nature, humans are exposed repeatedly and probably continuously to the large variety of *Aspergillus* spp. Principally the respiratory tract and also the skin, cornea, external auditory canal, gastrointestinal tract, nasopharynx, vagina, and urethra have been primary sites of infection. There are at least four important mechanisms of production of disease. The most important and serious of these is hematogenous dissemination of *A. fumigatus* in patients who have impaired immune responses from a variety of causes. The second is by the production of a "fungus ball" in a part of the body such as the bronchus. Third, various *Aspergillus* spp. are allergenic and produce asthma in sensitive persons. Fourth, *Aspergillus* spp. produce episodic bronchial obstruction, transient infiltrates, and other findings (allergic bronchopulmonary aspergillosis) or a chronic necrotizing pneumonia.

Clinical manifestations

Except for an occasional association with otitis externa, *Aspergillus* spp. are usually not considered factors in cutaneous disease.

Some patients with bronchial asthma or asthmatic bronchitis show immediate-type cutaneous hypersensitivity to extracts of *Aspergillus* spp. Occasionally during attacks these species can be cultured from bronchial secretions. For these reasons it has been customary to consider them as allergens, and thus they may be related to such symptoms as wheezing, shortness of breath, agitation, and cyanosis occurring with asthma.

One of the most characteristic and striking manifestations of aspergillosis is the fungus ball. This is composed of colonies of *Aspergillus* spp., inflammatory exudate, cells, and fibrin in the form of a sphere measuring from 1 to 5 cm in diameter. This appears on the chest roentgenogram as a ball covered by a thin meniscus of air. The sphere acts as a ball valve, trapping air during expiration and resulting in increased intracavitary pressure. This pressure tends to expand the cavity, and the fungus ball grows to fill this expanding space. Most patients with a fungus ball are asymptomatic, although occasionally it induces hemoptysis, which has been fatal.

In some patients, especially those with lymphoma or malignancy and those who are receiving corticosteroids or other immunosuppressive drug treatment, *A. fumigatus* is capable of invading tissues directly and of disseminating hematogenously, characteristically to the brain and kidney. In most such patients the clinical picture is that of the predominating underlying disease, with such general symptoms of infection as fever, chills, inanition, shock, altered consciousness, and anorexia. Occasionally there are pulmonary symptoms, and an infiltrate is seen on the chest roentgenogram. In some instances, endocarditis and symptoms typical of it have been encountered.

A more recently defined form, chronic necrotizing aspergillosis, is characterized by fever, productive cough, weight loss, progressive parenchymal destruction, and extensive pleural reaction in patients with a mean age of 60 years [55].

Pathology

In the characteristic pulmonary lesion, fungus ball, there is a mass of *Aspergillus* spp. hyphae, typically without invasion or marked inflammatory response in the contiguous tissue.

In the invasive form of the disease, the *Aspergillus* spp. hyphae are surrounded by acute inflammatory cells and a pyogenic reaction. Rarely, there may be giant cells and granulomas.

Such special stains as the Gridley, Gomori methenamine silver, or the periodic acid-Schiff may be necessary to demonstrate the fungi. With these stains hyphae are generally seen to be 3 to 4 µm in diameter and branching, characteristically at an angle of less than 45°, to produce the forked-stick appearance.

Diagnosis and differential diagnosis

The ubiquitous nature of *Aspergillus* spp. leads to difficulty in interpreting reports of the culture of this genus from sputum, skin, or pus. Furthermore, in the clinically characteristic form, the fungus ball, *A. fumigatus* may be cultured only with difficulty from the sputum. Even when there is hematogenous dissemination or endocarditis, the fungus cannot usually be cultured from the blood. Last, the diagnosis of disseminated disease is made by seeing hyphae or culturing *A. fumigatus* from the tissues only at autopsy or rarely at biopsy, usually too late to benefit the patient.

Laboratory diagnosis. DIRECT EXAMINATION. Potassium hydroxide preparations may be made from specimens such as bronchial washings, sputum, and biopsy material; wet mounts may be made with ear canal scrapings.

SIGNIFICANCE AND CULTURE. *Aspergillus* spp. are ubiquitous in nature and are frequently contaminants in the laboratory. Therefore, as with the phycomycetes, the same *Aspergillus* spp. must be isolated repeatedly from clinical specimens, and characteristic hyphal fragments must be demonstrated in tissue sections, before a disease can be called aspergillosis. When histologic specimens are not available, hyphal fragments or microconidia and the repeated culture of a single *Aspergillus* spp., in the absence of any other pathogen, are presumptive evidence of aspergillosis.

Media are usually incubated at room temperature, although *A. fumigatus* is capable of growing at temperatures of up to 45°C. Temperatures above 37°C favor development of this species and inhibit growth of many contaminants.

Standard mycologic media (e.g., Sabouraud's agar), which do not incorporate cycloheximide, may be used for clinical specimens. Growth is rapid, and the characteristic structures are produced early in colonial development.

The genus *Aspergillus* characteristically produces, along the hyphae, septate or nonseptate stalks (conidiophores) which broaden at the apex to form a vesicle. Finger-like projections, phialides, are produced, covering approximately one-third to all the outside of the vesicle, depending on the species. Certain *Aspergillus* spp. produce secondary phialides. Conidia are produced by a budding at the tip of the phialides and, in young cultures, are held together in short or long chains. Conidia vary in color, shape, and smoothness of cell wall, and these are several of the characteristics used in their identification.

The species most often encountered as a human pathogen, *A. fumigatus,* is identified as follows: colony color—gray-green; gradual widening of the conidiophore into a vesicle; production of a single row of phialides covering the upper half to two-thirds of the vesicle; bending upwards of the lower phialides to approximate a parallel attitude with the upper ones; columnar masses of gray-green conidia.

A. niger is seen frequently as a laboratory contaminant, but it is also associated with otomycosis and fungus ball. The colony at first has a white floccose color, becoming yellowish and finally black within 4 to 5 days. There is widening of the long, smooth conidiophores to a spherical vesicle, as well as phialides borne in a single row radially over the entire surface of the vesicle, with chains of brown to black, spherical rough conidia.

Young cultures are preferable for species identification; *The Genus Aspergillus* [56] is suggested for identification of the many *Aspergillus* species.

ANIMAL INOCULATION. Not done.

Differential diagnosis. Otomycosis must be differentiated from chronic otitis externa of other causes, i.e., swimmer's ear, seborrheic dermatitis, psoriasis, etc. The fungus ball is generally classic in its appearance, although other fungi have now been implicated. The allergic bronchopulmonary and chronic necrotizing forms mimic other fungal pneumonias, tuberculosis, and more chronic bacterial diseases, e.g., actinomycosis, nocardiosis. The disseminated form of disease must be distinguished from other severe, terminal illnesses, including bacterial sepsis, candidiasis, tuberculosis, or infection with *Pneumocystis carinii*.

Treatment

The otomycosis is best treated topically, not necessarily with an antifungal agent.

The allergic manifestations are best controlled by measures for a hypersensitivity state.

The saprophytic colonization of bronchi by *Aspergillus* spp. does not by itself warrant therapy. The fungus ball does not generally respond to chemotherapy but may need to be removed surgically if hemoptysis is severe. Intravascular (bronchial artery) coagulotherapy is in an investigative stage.

The disseminated form is generally of such short duration that chemotherapy cannot be instituted in time. Furthermore, the minimal inhibitory concentrations of available antifungal drugs against most strains of *A. fumigatus* are generally greater than levels that can be obtained in the patient's serum. Despite this, however, chemotherapeutic activity of amphotericin B has been demonstrated in experimental infections in laboratory animals, and there are isolated reports of recoveries in patients who received this drug intravenously. Rather less drug is necessary than in other systemic mycoses, since the infection tends to be of shorter duration, and if the patient is living 5 to 10 days after the diagnosis has been made, amphotericin B therapy can usually be discontinued. For details, see treatment section under "Blastomycosis," earlier in this chapter.

Ketoconazole has been disappointing in preliminary studies.

Course and prognosis

The otitis externa, allergic manifestations, and saprophytic colonization are virtually never disabling or fatal forms of *Aspergillus* infection. A number of patients have now died of fatal exsanguination from a fungus ball. The chronic necrotizing form may produce ventilatory compromise, but is not usually fatal. The invasive, systemic form of aspergillosis is generally a terminal, fatal disease.

Phycomycosis (mucormycosis, zygomycosis) (see also Chap. 181)

Definition

Mucormycosis is an acute or fulminant infectious disease, arising usually in the eye, nose, or sinus, with characteristic early invasion of blood vessels and with dissemination to the brain or other organs, caused by a variety of the members of the class Phycomycetes.

Under the term *phycomycosis*, another form of disease is characterized by inflammatory subcutaneous swellings, involving fat, muscle, and fascia, that spreads widely over the upper part of the chest, neck, or arms, heals spontaneously, and is caused by a member of the Phycomycetes class, notably *Basidiobolus ranarun*.

Historical aspects

Although Paltauf is credited with the first known report of mucormycosis, the disease was so rarely recognized that in 1957 Baker could title a paper, "Mucormycosis: A New Disease."

Lie, in 1956, first described the characteristic subcutaneous mycosis in Indonesia caused by the strain of *B. ranarun*. Workers in that area and Emmons in the United States have contributed most to the knowledge of this form of disease.

Epidemiology

The pulmonary and upper respiratory forms of mucormycosis are worldwide in distribution. Infections with *B. ranarun* have been reported from Indonesia and Africa.

The causative fungi, *Absidia corymbifera*, *Mucor* and *Rhizopus* spp., and *B. ranarun*, are ubiquitous fungi present on decaying vegetation, fruits, bread, or other vegetable material containing sugar.

Etiology and pathogenesis

A striking feature in the pathogenesis of at least a third of the patients with this disease has been concomitant diabetic ketoacidosis. In the remainder of the patients, some other disease has almost invariably been present; among these have been leukemia, bone marrow hypoplasia, malignancy, or treatment with corticosteroids, irradiation, antimetabolite, or immunosuppressive drugs.

Clinical manifestations

The orbital, nasal, sinus, or oropharyngeal form of disease begins with pain, reddish and then gangrenous skin, or mucosal change with purulent drainage (Fig. 181-18). Induration and swelling appear, so that there is often marked and disfiguring tumescence, including proptosis. There are usually fever and leukocytosis. Disease may begin in the

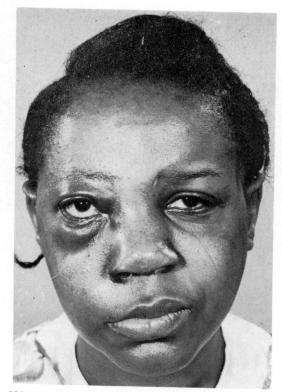

Fig. 182-18 Marked swelling caused by mucormycosis.

Laboratory diagnosis. DIRECT EXAMINATION. Owing to the fulminant nature of phycomycosis, fresh materials for direct examination are usually not submitted. Direct laboratory examination may be performed, if specimens are obtained. Fungi of this group may sometimes be identified in biopsy specimens of the nasal sinuses. They are visualized by adding a piece of tissue to a drop of potassium hydroxide and teasing it apart. Large, broad, nonseptate, branching hyphae are characteristic of the Phycomycetes.

Pus and sputum examined in a potassium hydroxide preparation may demonstrate the same characteristic large hyphae.

CULTURE. The significance is the same as was discussed for *Aspergillus* spp. Cultures are grown at 30°C. Strains of some species are inhibited by cyclohexhimide, and therefore material should be cultured on media without this additive. The genera encountered in phycomycosis are *Mucor, Rhizopus, Absidia, Mortierella,* and *Basidiobolus.* They are differentiated culturally by their morphologic characteristics.

1. *Mucor.* The colony grows rapidly, is at first white, but darkens to gray or brown with age. Hyphae are coenocytic i.e., nonseptate; sporangiophores arise singly from hyphae and may be profusely branched to unbranched; rhizoids (rootlike structures) are not formed. Columellae are present at the tip of the conidiophore and extend with the sporangium.
2. *Rhizopus.* The colony grows rapidly, is at first white, but darkens to gray-black or yellow-brown with age. Hyphae are coenocytic; several nonbranched sporangiophores arise on the hyphae at a node opposite the rhizoids. Columellae are present at the tip of the conidiophore and extend within the sporangium.
3. *Absidia.* The colony is as in *Rhizopus,* but with branched sporangiophores arising on stolons between two nodes, never opposite the rhizoids.
4. *Mortierella.* The colony grows rapidly, is at first white, then later gray or yellowish. Hyphae are submerged or adherent to agar, usually with little aerial hyphae. Sporangiophores are simple or branched, with no columellae present.
5. *Basidiobolus.* The colony grows rapidly as a thin, flat, glabrous sheet of mycelium on the surface of agar, is at first gray or yellowish, and later may develop short, white aerial hyphae. Hyphae are sinuous, with occasional septums. Sporangia are borne on sporangiophores with a bulb-shaped tip, from which they bud. Many chlamydoconidia are present.

ANIMAL INOCULATION. Not done.

Differential diagnosis. The disease of the upper part of the respiratory tract is probably most closely mimicked by midline lethal or Wegener's granuloma. Acute orbital cellulitis, nasal sinusitis, or oral pharyngitis due to pyogenic organisms, such as *Staph. aureus* or *Streptococcus pyogenes,* may similarly resemble mucormycosis.

The subcutaneous form is so bizarre that only lymphoma or tumor, such as Burkitt's, would be suggested.

Treatment

Successful treatment of the pulmonary form has usually been with amphotericin B. For the rhinocerebral form,

lung, with pleuritic chest pain, cough, and fever. Early invasion of blood vessels is a characteristic feature, resulting in central nervous system meningitis and abscess formation [57].

The subcutaneous form appears usually over the upper part of the chest, back, neck, and arms and is marked by disfiguring swelling and boardlike induration, but entails little pain and few systemic signs and symptoms.

Pathology

The reaction to the Phycomycetes is marked by early invasion of blood vessels, vascular occlusion, infarction, and ischemia or hemorrhage. Rarely are there giant cells or other manifestations of a more chronic process. In contrast to many other fungi, Phycomycetes take hematoxylin stain readily. The hyphae are characteristically larger (10 to 15 µm in diameter) and rarely septate, and these distinguishing features in tissues have been the basis for diagnosis of most instances of disease [58].

Diagnosis and differential diagnosis

Because of the ubiquity of these fungi, care must be taken in ascribing disease to one of the Phycomycetes. In the past and for practical purposes at present, tissue invasion of the fungi is virtually essential to the diagnosis. Because of the fulminant course of the pulmonary form and that in the upper part of the respiratory tract, the diagnosis must usually be presumptive: many patients have died before biopsy tissue sections could be studied or cultural results obtained.

surgical debridement has been necessary almost always. In a recent summary of reported cases [59] overall survival has increased to 70 (from 50) percent, is better when other disease is not present, is least likely when diabetes mellitus is present, is improved to 79 percent with amphotericin B, and to 89 percent with accompanying surgery.

Course and prognosis

As previously mentioned, the disease in the pulmonary form and in the upper part of the respiratory tract is usually fulminant and fatal. In the subcutaneous form, spontaneous recovery without therapy seems to occur.

Chromoblastomycosis (chromomycosis, verrucous dermatitis)

Definition

Chromoblastomycosis is a chronic cutaneous and subcutaneous infection of the skin, caused by species of *Phialophora*, *Cladosporium*, and *Fonsecaea* which form wart-like lesions on the skin (Fig. 182-19). It is most common in the tropics and subtropics but occasionally is seen in the United States.

Clinical features (Fig. A6-20)

Chromomycosis occurs mainly in rural tropical areas, following trauma to the legs. It usually begins with a nodule that ulcerates and gradually spreads, forming a large mass on the skin surface. It is a persistent infection, lasting many years, and heals with scarring and keloid formation. It is not systemic. The disease is seen more frequently in males, and in rural workers. These differences are produced by environment, i.e., workers without shoes or protective clothing on their lower extremities are more likely to suffer trauma on the feet and legs (Fig. 182-20), into which the fungus may be introduced. Lesions may also occur less frequently on the hands, arms, or on the trunk. Transmission does not occur from human to human or from animals to humans.

Fig. 182-19 Verrucous lesions of chromoblastomycosis. (Courtesy of Dr. Jan Schwarz, Cincinnati, Ohio.)

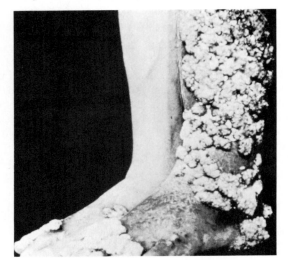

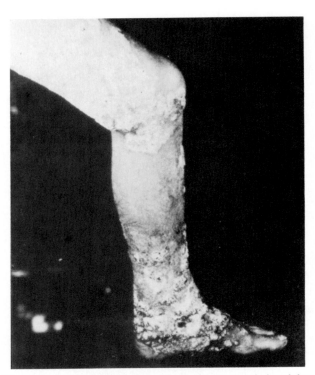

Fig. 182-20   Disseminated form of chromomycosis involving a lower extremity. [Courtesy of Dr. P. Lavalle, Mexico. Canizares O (ed): Clinical Tropical Dermatology. Oxford, Blackwell, 1975, p 39.]

Historical aspects

Rudolph first reported a case of chromomycosis from Brazil in 1914. Lane and Medlar in 1915 reported the first case from the United States, and Thaxter named the causative agent *Phialophora verrucosa*. Owing to the variations seen in the cultures, the true relationship between *P. verrucosa* and the other fungi viz., *Fonsecaea compactum*, *F. pedrosoi*, and *Cladosporium carrionii*, is not yet known. They have been identified as sufficiently different from one another culturally to create new species, while exhibiting many similar features and some identical ones.

In tissue and exudate, all species produce the same type of dark brown cells which are septate (Medlar bodies) and occur in pairs or small clusters.

On culture, all species produce similar heaped-up dark colonies with short aerial hyphae, producing a gray, green, or brown velvety surface resembling a mouse pelt. The various causal agents are differentiated microscopically, a task for only the most experienced mycologists.

Microscopically the species are differentiated as follows:

P. verrucosa produces almost exclusively the phialophora type of sporulation.

F. pedrosoi produces predominantly acrogenous (spores developing at the tip of a conidiophore) or pleurogenous (spores borne on the sides of a conidiophore or hypha) conidia. The conidia may bud, forming short, branching chains of spores. Phialides identical to those seen in *P. verrucosa* may also be formed by this species.

F. compactum produces colonies which resemble those of *F. pedrosoi* but which develop slowly. Conidia are formed in compact heads with short chains which are not readily dissociated. Spores are separated from one another by thick septums appearing as black lines under the microscope. Under certain conditions (when *F. compactum* is grown on cornmeal agar) phialides may be produced.

Wangiella dermatitidis has been isolated a few times. It originates as a black, slimy, moist colony which produces conidia in a manner similar to that of *Aureobasidium pullulans*. As the colony continues to grow, aerial hyphae develop and conidial production decreases. Occasional conidiophores of the *A. pullulans* type may be found.

C. carrionii is the only known etiologic agent of chromomycosis in Australia. It has been isolated in South Africa and Venezuela. Cultural growth is slow at 22°C and is almost inhibited at 37°C. Long-branching chains of small conidia resembling the saprophytic strains of *Cladosporium* are the only spores seen.

Treatment

The treatment of choice is with amphotericin B. Reports of successful treatment with potassium iodide either orally or intravenously are not convincing.

Amphotericin B may be given intravenously until a dose of 2 to 3 g is reached. It may also be injected into the skin lesions locally (for details, see "Blastomycosis" earlier in this chapter).

Sporotrichosis

Definition

Sporotrichosis is a chronic disease that usually follows accidental implantation of the fungus, *Sporothrix schenckii,* into the skin, from which site it may spread via the lymphatics. A second form is pulmonary, and a third is other organ involvement, presumptively from hematogenous dissemination.

Historical aspects

The first description of sporotrichosis was made in the United States by Schenck in 1898; in the same year he isolated the causative agent, *S. schenckii.*

Until the early 1920s it was most frequently seen in France. It is rarely found there today. By far the greatest number of cases was reported from Witwatersrand, South Africa [61], in 3000 mine workers who developed the disease within a period of approximately 2 years by contact with mine timbers on which *S. schenckii* was growing. In all cases studied, the infection was of the cutaneous lymphatic type and none disseminated. The epidemic was halted by use of antifungal agents on the timbers.

Epidemiology

Sporotrichosis is seen in all age groups. Although white, adult males are most often infected, occupation and exposure are probably more important than are race, sex, or age. The usual reservoir in nature is vegetation on which *S. schenckii* grows saprophytically.

Infection usually occurs after traumatic or inapparent implantation of the fungus by thorns, splinters, or other vegetal objects. Barberry, rose bushes, sphagnum moss,

soil, and contaminated mine timbers have been the usual source. Sporotrichosis is seen in horses and occasionally in other animals such as dogs, cats, and rats.

Etiology

The single species *S. schenckii* is diphasic with a tissue and a hyphal phase. The tissue phase is difficult to demonstrate on direct microscopic examination of exudate or skin scrapings stained with Gram's or fungal stains, or even in specially stained sections of histopathologic material.

Clinical description

Primary cutaneous sporotrichosis presents a variety of clinical lesions, but central lymphatic spread from a single lesion on the dorsum of the hand is the most characteristic form of this disease. The initial lesion begins as a papule, pustule, or nodule which ulcerates, with subsequent associated multiple, cutaneous nodules spreading in linear fashion in the lymphatics (Fig. 182-21). The initial lesion is indurated and ulcerative and has a ragged undermined border; it slightly resembles the primary lesion of syphilis. It is painless except when secondary bacterial infection is present.

The pulmonary form is that of a chronic pneumonia.

The disseminated form spreads from a primary lesion of often undetermined site, to lymph nodes, bone, muscle, joints, viscera, and central nervous system.

Differential diagnosis

Cutaneous lymphatic sporotrichosis is differentiated from tularemia and staphylococcal lymphangitis primarily by the

Fig. 182-21 Multiple lymphatic nodules of sporotrichosis.

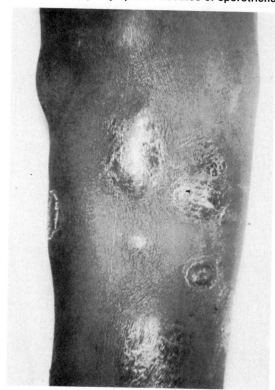

afebrile nature of the former, and by culture from a my-cobacterial infection. The pulmonary form must also be distinguished from tuberculosis and other fungal infection. The disseminated form, as a single or multiple organ infection, resembles other chronic infections, as in septic arthritis.

Pathology

Sporotrichosis is difficult to diagnose by histopathologic techniques, since the fungus usually cannot be seen in lesions even with special stains. In inoculated laboratory animals or rarely in human disease, *S. schenckii* appears as basophilic, small, either ovoid or cigar-shaped budding cells, occurring singly or in clumps. Local tissue reaction is one of suppuration and granuloma.

Diagnosis and differential diagnosis

In a patient with an ulcer at the tip of a finger and a chain of swollen nodules along the lymphatics extending up the arm, the diagnosis is frequently either sporotrichosis or infection due to atypical mycobacteria. In this, the pulmonary, and in disseminated disease, the diagnosis is established by culture of *S. schenckii*.

Laboratory diagnosis. DIRECT EXAMINATION. Because the organisms are so few in lesions or infected tissue, this is not generally done.

CULTURE. On Sabouraud's dextrose agar with or without antibiotics, at room temperature, the fungus first appears as a moist, cream-colored colony, which darkens to brown, and later to nearly black, and becomes leathery in most cases. Rarely the colony remains cream-colored or tan, and pigment production may be lost on subculture.

Microscopically, extensive, branched, septate, fine (1 to 2 μm in diameter) hyphae are seen, with comparatively large conidia produced along the hyphae or in clumps (rosettes) on short stalks. The conidia may be round, oval, or pyriform and are from 2 to 5 μm in length. The conidia are attached to the hyphae by fine short phialides, which are seen only on careful focusing with the microscope.

Occasionally, animal inoculation may be required for definitive identification. Rats, mice, and hamsters are susceptible. An inoculation intratesticularly or intraperitoneally of 0.2 mL of a dense suspension of the mycelial culture produces orchitis and, with appropriate stains, the cigar-shaped budding forms may be found in the infected sites on direct examination or in mounts from cultures grown on special media at 37°C.

Treatment

The treatment is a saturated solution of potassium iodide, 10 drops 3 times a day after meals, until lesions have cleared; it may be necessary, in some cases, to increase the dose to maximum tolerance. When iodides are not tolerated or are ineffective, amphotericin B should be given intravenously (see "Blastomycosis" earlier in this chapter). In preliminary studies ketoconazole has been helpful in a few cases [41]. Griseofulvin has been used but is not of proved value. Topical therapy is worthless.

Laboratory techniques for superficial and deep mycoses

In dealing with dermatophytic problems there is a tendency to minimize the necessity for cultural confirmation. The general impression appears to be that modern antifungal agents negate such requirements. However, Emmons et al [62] state: "Clinical variations of dermatophytosis are so great and the resemblance of some other skin diseases are so close that a clinical diagnosis needs to be supported by a laboratory diagnosis." Certainly in a percentage of patients this is an accurate evaluation.

Collecting the appropriate specimen, handling, processing, and culturing them correctly are skills acquired through practice.

Collection and cultures for patient specimens

Cultures should be examined daily. If saprophytic fungi appear, subcultures should be made of any colonies suspected of being dermatophytes or systemic fungi. All inoculated media must be held for at least 4 weeks before being considered negative.

In general, inoculated media should be incubated at 22°C and 37°C in an attempt to isolate the tissue phase of diphasic fungi, to aid in the differentiation of *C. neoformans* from other *Cryptococcus* spp., and in the special instances as indicated in the various diseases.

Dermatophytes. INFECTED HAIRS. Since several of the dermatophytes that infect hairs fluoresce under appropriate conditions, an ultraviolet light with a Wood's filter (360 nm) may be used both to collect infected hairs and to separate fluorescing from nonfluorescing types of infection. Many other materials may also fluoresce, and the technique should be used only when the skin or scalp is clean and free from ointments. Hairs may be individually epilated with sterile forceps, or adhesive tape may be placed on the lesion surface and pulled off rapidly, removing damaged and infected hairs. Sufficiently infected or questionably infected hairs should always be epilated both for cultural purposes and for direct potassium hydroxide mount study; at least 10 to 15 hairs should be obtained. Hairs suspected of being infected should be placed on Sabouraud's dextrose agar and on medium containing chloramphenicol and cycloheximide (Mycosel agar, Baltimore Biological Co., or Mycobiotic agar, Difco Co.). Care should be taken to ensure maximum contact of the hairs with the surface of the agar.

SKIN SCRAPINGS. The skin should be adequately cleansed, preferably with 70% alcohol. Application should be brisk, and a few minutes' contact time allowed for the alcohol to control the surface contaminants. Alcohol should never be applied with cotton balls because they leave fibers which make a potassium hydroxide mount difficult to interpret. The roof of unopened vesicles may be removed with sterile scissors for culture. However, suppurated or macerated areas are generally heavily contaminated with bacteria, and should be avoided. One should always obtain a sample that is good in both quality and quantity. Too little material causes useless discomfort to the patient and is usually culturally negative. The best approach is to obtain sufficient material by scraping deep into the tissue, causing it to weep. *Scrapings must be collected from the margins of the lesions, where the fungus will be actively growing.* This area is the most productive for both culture and potassium hydroxide mount. Skin scales are placed on the surface of Sabouraud's dextrose agar medium containing chloramphenicol and cycloheximide; the antibiotics are omitted in cases where the suspected fungus might be sensitive to either one or the other. The scales should be spread out and flattened on the surface. Scales that have excessive portions extending into the air rarely produce growth on culture media.

NAIL SCRAPINGS. The nail must be cleansed by scraping off all debris and then applying 70% alcohol, again making sure not to use cotton balls. Debris under the nail is poor material for culture. Rather, scrapings taken at the union of apparently healthy and infected nail should be used for both potassium hydroxide mount and culture. All thick pieces of nail should first be sliced into smaller ones before further manipulation. After being cut into small pieces, this material should be cultured as above. If a *Candida* spp. rather than a dermatophyte is the suspected causal organism, exudate from the inflamed, swollen paronychial tissue, if collected on sterile swabs, may be used for both cultural purposes and for microscopic study. However, material from the eroded nail at the lateral fold is best for direct microscopic examination and for culture.

Specimens for other than dermatophytes. SPUTUM. Specimens collected before breakfast and after rinsing the mouth are preferable. Purulent or bloody portions of the specimen should be inoculated directly onto Sabouraud's dextrose agar medium containing chloramphenicol and cycloheximide, and onto blood agar plates with added chloramphenicol and cycloheximide. The latter should be incubated at both 22°C and 37°C. (If systemic infection caused by diphasic fungus is suspected, media containing chloramphenicol and cycloheximide should be kept at 22°C only, since the yeast phases of the systemic fungi are sensitive to these antibiotics at 37°C.)

URINE. A well-mixed, representative sample of fresh, preferably first voided morning urine should be centrifuged for 15 min at 2500 rpm. The supernatant is discarded, leaving only several milliliters, and the sediment is resuspended. Portions of this material should be inoculated onto Sabouraud's dextrose agar and incubated at 22°C and 37°C, and onto one tube of Sabouraud's dextrose agar containing chloramphenicol and cycloheximide, at 22°C. The material should be spread to cover the entire surface.

CEREBROSPINAL FLUID. The entire specimen should be centrifuged for 15 min at 2500 rpm. The supernatant may be discarded, or used for chemical evaluations, or frozen and kept for serologic or other studies. Inoculation is made onto Sabouraud's dextrose agar and blood agar or chocolate agar, with incubation at both 22°C and 37°C.

GRANULES. See "Actinomycosis."

BLOOD. Place 5 mL or more directly into 50-mL bottles of brain-heart infusion or trypticase soy broth with sodium citrate and 5 to 8 mL Sabouraud's agar added. At least two bottles should be inoculated from the same blood specimen.

BIOPSY. Inoculate pus or caseous material directly onto desired media and prepare two smears for Gram's and PAS stains. *Mince the tissue with sterile scissors, grind with*

sterile Sabouraud's broth, and add 0.2 to 0.5 mL of the homogenate to appropriate media.

BONE MARROW. Inoculate appropriate media and streak it across the entire surface with a loop. If the specimen is obtained in a syringe, draw up several milliliters of broth into the syringe and discharge it into 20 mL of Sabouraud's broth.

Collection and direct examination for patient specimens*

Dermatologic specimens. HAIR. Epilated hairs should be studied immediately. Several hairs are placed on a slide, 10 to 20% potassium hydroxide and a coverslip are added, and the slide is warmed without boiling. After sitting for 15 to 30 min, the slide may be examined for the presence of fungi. For this and most other microscopic examinations, the substage or condenser diaphragm should be closed to approximately one-half its normal opening area and the condenser lowered until best contrast with the specimen is obtained.

All *Microsporum* species produce small spores (2 to 3 μm) around the outside of the hair shaft (ectothrix) in a mosaic fashion. *M. gypseum,* however, produces larger spores (5 to 8 μm). *Trichophyton* species produce generally larger spores, which may be either outside (ectothrix) or within (endothrix) the hair in chains. Several species sometimes produce both ectothrix and endothrix infection. Spores may become dislodged in heavily damaged hairs, and then only the mycotic nature of the infection, not the genus, may be determined.

For *T. schoenleinii,* the yellowish scales, crusts, or hairs are the best material for direct microscopic examination. The microscopic field shows spores of varying size and shape. Particularly typical is the sausage-shaped spore. [JH Swartz, *Elements of Medical Mycology,* 2d ed. New York, Grune & Stratton, 1949, Fig. 63 (p 107) and Fig. 64 (p 108)]. Hyphae are septate and rather coarse. In some fields, the organism may be missing but vestigial traces containing air bubbles are present.

SKIN SCRAPINGS. Several pieces of the scrapings should be placed on a glass slide without overlapping. Potassium hydroxide (10 to 20%) and a coverslip are added; the specimen is gently heated and then allowed to stand for about 10 min. The specimen may then be studied for hyphae, arthrospores, or, occasionally, budding cells (Fig. 182-22). One cannot identify specific organisms, usually, but only note their presence or absence.

NAIL SCRAPINGS. Several thin pieces of the specimen should be placed on a glass slide without overlapping. A few drops of potassium hydroxide (10 to 20%) and a coverslip are added. The slide is gently heated to near-boiling and then allowed to sit for approximately ½ h. Avoid boiling, which produces bubbles that both disrupt the fungus

---

* A rapid clearing and staining method for fungi in skin scales, nail scrapings, and hairs was developed by Swartz and Lamkins in 1963 (JH Swartz, BE Lamkins, *Arch Dermatol* 89:89, 1964). In addition to staining the fungi, this method has significant advantages over the widely used potassium hydroxide technique; e.g., it produces fewer artifacts and causes no damage to the microscope. The stain is also useful for preparing culture mounts.

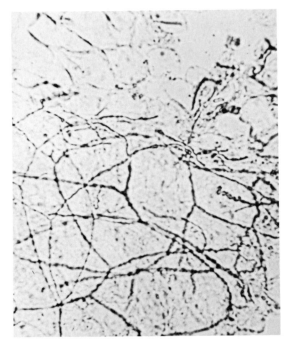

Fig. 182-22 Direct microscopic examination of infected skin scales, showing septate branching mycelium. × 250. Stained with the method described by Swartz and Lamkins. *(From Swartz JH, Lamkins BE, Arch Dermatol 89:89, 1964. Used by permission.)*

and produce artifacts. The specimen may then be studied for hyphae and budding cells.

BIOPSIED TISSUE. This material is handled by the same general procedure as are skin scrapings. However, the tissue must first be ground or minced into minute pieces before placement on a microscope slide or culture.

Specimens for other than dermatophytes. SPUTUM. Fresh sputum, not saliva, should be collected in a sterile container. A loopful of the material is mixed with a drop of potassium hydroxide (10 to 20%) on a microscope slide, a coverslip is placed on top, and the specimen is studied microscopically. Clearing by gently heating may occasionally be necessary. *Candida* spp., *B. dermatitidis, Cryptococcus* spp., *C. immitis* spherules, and hyphal strands of either saprophytic or opportunistic fungi (e.g., *Aspergillus, Mucor*) may be visualized in this manner. The cells of *H. capsulatum* are too small to be seen in a potassium hydroxide preparation, although sputum smears, dried and stained with Giemsa's stain, may at times be useful for elucidating this organism when it is examined under oil immersion.

URINE. Following centrifugation of the specimen, a drop of the sediment is placed on a slide and covered with a coverslip; under reduced light, hyphae and budding cells such as those produced by *B. dermatitidis* may be visualized. Gram's stain may demonstrate hyphae and yeast cells compatible with *Candida* spp.

CEREBROSPINAL FLUID. An India ink preparation is mandatory if *C. neoformans* is suspected or if yeast cells are seen in the specimen.

GRANULES. See "Actinomycosis."

BONE MARROW. A small portion should be placed be-

tween two slides, smeared, and dried. Gram's and PAS stains are then performed.

Other specimens for culture generally require special laboratory preparation or culture media. The laboratory to which the specimen will be sent should be notified first, to ensure that the most appropriate specimen will be collected, and to alert the laboratory to anticipate the specimen.

References

1. Bollinger O: Über eine neure Pilzkrankheit beim Rinde. *Zbl Med Wiss* **15:**481, 1877
2. Israel J: Neue Beobachtungen auf dem Gebiete der Mykosen des Menschen. *Virchows Arch [Pathol Anat]* **74:**15, 1878
3. Cope VZ: *Actinomycosis*. London, Oxford Univ Press, 1938, 246 pp
4. Nichols DR, Harrell WE: Penicillin in the treatment of actinomycosis (abstr). *J Lab Clin Med* **32:**1405, 1947
5. Emmons CW: The isolation of *Actinomyces bovis* from tonsillar granules. *Public Health Rep* **53:**1967, 1938
6. Valicenti JF et al: Detection and prevalence of IUD associated Actinomyces colonization and related morbidity. A prospective study of 69,925 cervical smears. *JAMA* **247:**1175, 1982
7. Slack JM, Genescser MA: *Actinomyces, Filamentous Bacteria*. Minneapolis, Burgess, 1975
8. Nocard ME: Note sur la maladie des boeufs de la Guadeloupe connue sous le nom de farçin. *Ann Inst Pasteur (Paris)* **2:**293, 1888
9. Eppinger H: Über eine neue Pathogene Cladothrix und eine durch sie hervorgerufene Pseudotuberculosis. *Wien Klin Wochenschr* **3:**321, 1890
10. Satterwhite TK, Wallace RJ Jr: Primary cutaneous nocardiosis. *JAMA* **242:**333, 1979
11. Frazier AR et al: Nocardiosis, a review of 25 cases occurring during 24 months. *Mayo Clin Proc* **50:**657, 1975
12. Folb PI et al: *Nocardia asteroides* and *Nocardia brasiliensis* infections in mice. *Infect Immun* **13:**1490, 1976
13. Curry WA: Human nocardiosis. A clinical review with selected case reports. *Arch Intern Med* **140:**818, 1980
14. Yoger R et al: Successful treatment of *Nocardia asteroides* infection with amikacin. *J Pediatr* **96:**771, 1980
15. Mackinnon JE: Mycetomas as opportunistic wound infections. *Lab Invest* **11:**1124, 1962
16. Mariat F: *Les Principaux Actinomycetes Aerobes Responsables de Mycetomes*. Paris, Mycologie Médicale l'Expansion Scientifique Française, 1958
17. Kwon-Chung KJ: A new genus, *Filobasidiella*, the perfect state of *Cryptococcus neoformans*. *Mycologia* **67:**1197, 1975
18. San Felice F: Contributo alla morfologia e biologica dei blastomiceti che si sviluppano nei succhi di alcuni frutti. *Ann Hygiene Sperimentale* **4:**463, 1894
19. Emmons CW: Isolation of *Cryptococcus neoformans* from soil. *J Bacteriol* **62:**685, 1951
20. Kerkering TM et al: The evolution of pulmonary cryptococcosis. Clinical implications from a study of 41 patients with and without compromising host factors. *Ann Intern Med* **94:**611, 1981
21. De Wyte CN et al: Cryptococcal meningitis: a review of 32 years' experience. *J Neurol Sci* **53:**283, 1982
22. Godwin JD et al: Fatal pneumocystis pneumonia, cryptococcosis, and Kaposi's sarcoma in a homosexual man. *AJR* **138:**580, 1982
23. Scott EN et al: Enzyme linked immunosorbent assays in murine cryptococcosis. *Sabouraudia* **19:**275, 1982
24. Bennett JE, Remington JS: Miconazole in cryptococcosis and systemic candidiasis: a word of caution. *Ann Intern Med* **94:**708, 1981

25. Kwon-Chung KJ: *Emmonsiella capsulata*: perfect state of *Histoplasma capsulatum*. *Science* **177**:368, 1972

26. Darling ST: A protozoon general infection producing pseudotubercles in the lungs and focal necrosis in the liver, spleen, and lymph nodes. *JAMA* **46**:1283, 1906

27. DeMonbreun WA: The cultivation and cultural characteristics of Darling's *Histoplasma capsulatum*. *Am J Trop Med* **14**:93, 1934

28. Furcolow ML, Brasher CA: Chronic progressive (cavitary) histoplasmosis as a problem in tuberculosis sanatoriums. *Am Rev Tuberc* **73**:609, 1956

29. Schwartz J, Baum GL: The history of histoplasmosis, 1906–1956. *N Engl J Med* **256**:253, 1957

30. Wheat LJ et al: A large urban outbreak of histoplasmosis: clinical features. *Ann Intern Med* **94**:331, 1982

31. Jacobson ES, Strauss SE: Reevaluation of diagnostic histoplasma serology. *Am J Med Sci* **281**:143, 1981

32. Hawkins SS et al: Progressive disseminated histoplasmosis: favorable response to ketoconazole. *Ann Intern Med* **95**:446, 1981

33. McDonough ES, Lewis AL: The ascigerous stage of *Blastomyces dermatitidis*. *Mycologia* **60**:76, 1968

34. Gilchrist TC, Stokes WR: A case of pseudo-lupus vulgaris caused by a blastomyces. *J Exp Med* **3**:53, 1898

35. Emmons CW et al: North American blastomycosis: two autochthonous cases from Africa. *Sabouraudia* **3**:306, 1964

36. Legendre AM et al: Canine blastomycosis: a review of 47 clinical cases. *J Am Vet Med Assoc* **178**:1163, 1981

37. Schwarz J, Baum GL: Blastomycosis. *Am J Clin Pathol* **21**:999, 1951

38. Sarosi GA, Davies SF: Blastomycosis. *Am Rev Resp Dis* **120**:911, 1979

39. Witorsch P, Utz JP: North American blastomycosis: a study of 40 patients. *Medicine (Baltimore)* **47**:169, 1968

40. Schwarz J: Mycotic prostitis. *Urology* **19**:1, 1982

41. Restrepo A et al (eds): First International Symposium on Ketoconazole. *Rev Infect Dis* **2**:519, 1980

42. Almeida F: Consideraçoes sôbre a blastomicose sulamericana em sua forma queloideana. *Rev Inst Adolfo Lutz* **10**:31, 1951

43. Londero AT: The gamut of progressive pulmonary paracoccidioidomycosis. *Mycopathologia* **75**:65, 1981

44. Allison MJ et al: Paracoccidioidomycosis in a Northern Chilean mummy. *Bull NY Acad Med* **55**:670, 1979

45. Neves JA, Bogliolo L: Researches on the etiological agents of the American blastomycosis. I. Morphology and systemic of the Lutz's disease agent. *Mycopathologia* **5**:133, 1951

46. Rixford E, Gilchrist TC: Two cases of protozoan (coccidioidal) infection of the skin and other organs. *Johns Hopkins Hosp Rep* **1**:209, 1896

47. Gifford MA: Coccidioidomycosis in Kern County, California. *Proc Pacific Sci* **5**:791, 1942

48. Smith CE: Epidemiology of acute coccidioidomycosis with erythema nodosum ("San Joaquin" or "Valley fever"). *Am J Public Health* **30**:600, 1940

49. Schwartz RA, Lamberts RJ: Isolated nodular cutaneous coccidioidomycosis: initial manifestation of disseminated disease. *J Am Acad Dermatol* **4**:38, 1981

50. Stevens DA: *Coccidioidomycosis*. New York, Plenum Press, 1980

51. Gifford J, Catanzaro A: A comparison of coccidioidin and spherulin in the diagnosis of coccidioidomycosis. *Am Rev Resp Dis* **124**:440, 1981

52. Graybill JR et al: Ketoconazole therapy for systemic fungal infections. Inadequacy of standard dosage regimens. *Am Rev Resp Dis* **126**:171, 1982

53. Grosso DS et al: Ketoconazole inhibition of testicular secretion of testosterone and displacement of steroid hormones from serum transport proteins. *Antimicrob Agents Chemother* **23**:207, 1983

54. Renon L: Étude sur L'Aspergillose chez les Animaux et chez l'Homme. Paris, Masson, 1897

55. Binder RE et al: Chronic necrotizing pulmonary aspergillosis: a discrete clinical entity. *Medicine (Baltimore)* **61**:109, 1982

56. Raper KB, Fennel DI: *The Genus Aspergillus*. Baltimore, Williams & Wilkins, 1965

57. Lehrer RI et al: Mucormycosis. *Ann Intern Med* **93**:93, 1980

58. Symmer WStC: Histopathologic aspects of the pathogenesis of some opportunistic fungal infections, as exemplified in the pathology of aspergillosis and the phycomycetoses. *Lab Invest* **11**:1073, 1962

59. Blitzer A et al: Patient survival factors in paranasal sinus mucormycosis. *Laryngoscope* **90**:635, 1980

60. Costello MJ et al: Chromoblastomycosis treated with local infiltration of amphotericin B solution. *Arch Dermatol* **79**:184, 1959

61. Helm MAF, Bermann C: Sporotrichosis infection in mines of the Witwatersrand: a symposium, in *Proceedings of the Transvaal Mine Medical Officers Association*. Johannesburg, Transvaal Chamber of Mines, 1947

62. Emmons CW et al: *Medical Mycology*. Philadelphia, Lea & Febiger, 1963

Bibliography

Glimp RA, Bayer AS: Fungal pneumonias. Part 3, Allergic bronchopulmonary aspergillosis. *Chest* **80**:85, 1981

Louria DL: Fungal infections in the compromised host. *Diseases of the Mouth* **27**:1, 1981

Massa MC, Doyle JA: Cutaneous cryptococcosis simulating pyoderma gangrenosum. *J Am Acad Dermatol* **5**:32, 1981

McDonough ES, Kuzma JF: Epidemiological studies on blastomycosis in the state of Wisconsin. *Sabouraudia* **18**:173, 1980

Ozols II, Wheat LJ: Erythema nodosum in an epidemic of histoplasmosis in Indianapolis. *Arch Dermatol* **117**:709, 1981

Section 28

Rickettsial and viral diseases with cutaneous involvement

CHAPTER 183

THE RICKETTSIOSES

William Schaffner

Rickettsiae are pleomorphic coccobacillary obligate intracellular parasites with characteristics of both bacteria and viruses. Transmitted to humans by arthropods, they produce acute systemic infections of varying severity (Table 183-1).

The most frequent rickettsial infection in the United States is Rocky Mountain spotted fever; reported cases have increased annually since 1960, predominantly in the southeastern states. Because the dermatologic characteristics of the rickettsioses provide the basis for clinical differential diagnosis and the initiation of proper therapy, they will be emphasized in the discussion that follows.

Historical aspects

Classical louse-borne epidemic typhus has been one of the major scourges of civilization, particularly during periods of famine or war. As Zinsser has dramatically described, typhus—not strategy—has determined the outcome of many military campaigns, thus exerting a direct influence on history. In the epidemics of typhus that swept through Russia and eastern Europe from 1918 to 1922, it is estimated that 30 million persons became ill, and 3 million died.

In the 1890s, Wood and Maxcy described an unusual disease of high mortality in Idaho which was later named Rocky Mountain spotted fever. In the early 1900s Howard Taylor Ricketts established the tick as the vector of Rocky Mountain spotted fever. The rickettsiae were named for this investigator, who died of typhus while studying that disease in Mexico. In 1910 Brill described a series of patients in New York City who had a disease similar to, but distinct from, typhoid fever. Subsequently, Zinsser correctly postulated that this illness represented a recurrent form of epidemic typhus appearing in patients who had previously had the classical disease. In 1915 two Polish investigators, Weil and Felix, discovered that patients re-

Table 183-1   The rickettsial diseases

Group	Disease	Rickettsial species	Arthropod vector	Reservoir	Weil-Felix reaction
Spotted fever	Rocky Mountain spotted fever	R. rickettsii	Tick	Small mammals, ticks	Positive
	Boutonneuse fever South African tick-bite fever (see Fig. 183-5) Kenya tick typhus Indian tick typhus	R. conorii	Tick	Dogs, rodents	Positive
	Siberian tick typhus	R. sibiricus	Tick	Rodents	Positive
	Queensland tick typhus	R. australis	Tick	Marsupials, rodents	Positive
Typhus	Rickettsialpox	R. akari	Mite of house mouse	House mouse	Negative
	Endemic	R. typhi (R. mooseri)	Rat flea	Rat	Positive
	Epidemic	R. prowazekii	Human body louse	Humans, flying squirrel	Positive
	Brill's disease	R. prowazekii	Unknown	Recurrence of dormant epidemic typhus	Low or negative
	Scrub	R. tsutsugamushi	Mite	Rodents, mites	
Trench fever Q fever	Trench fever Q fever	R. quintana R. burnetii	Louse Inhalation of dried tick feces	Humans Cattle, sheep, goats	Negative Negative

covering from rickettsial infection had an agglutinin in their serums for certain otherwise unrelated *Proteus* bacteria. The Weil-Felix test is still used as a nonspecific but rapid method of screening for certain rickettsial diseases. In the 1920s and 1930s the work of Maxcy, Dyer, and others established the existence of another form of typhus transmitted not only by the body louse, but by the rat flea, thereby explaining the many cases of mild typhus unassociated with lousiness which had so long puzzled investigators.

Pathogenesis

Infected arthropods transmit rickettsiae to humans in two ways: ticks and mites (vectors of spotted fevers and scrub typhus) inoculate rickettsiae directly at the time of the bite, and lice and fleas (carriers of epidemic and endemic typhus) defecate feces containing rickettsiae while biting. Rickettsiae are introduced into the wound by scratching the irritated site. Rarely, epidemic typhus may be acquired via the airborne route when the garments of a patient are shaken, thus dispersing an aerosol of infected louse feces.

After inoculation it is postulated that initial rickettsial multiplication occurs at the site of introduction, and significant skin lesions at the site of the arthropod bite are the rule in rickettsialpox, scrub typhus, and fievre boutonneuse.

Rickettsia rickettsii, the agent causing Rocky Mountain spotted fever, may be considered the rickettsial prototype. It produces the most marked pathologic changes and the most severe disease. The size of the microorganisms (0.2 by 1.0 μm) and their staining characteristics (purple with Giemsa's stain or red with Macchiavello's stain) enable

them to be visualized with the light microscope if they are carefully sought in tissue sections. The members of the spotted fever group of rickettsiae multiply in both the nucleus and the cytoplasm of infected cells. Rickettsiae of the typhus group grow only in the cytoplasm.

Diffuse vasculitis is the pathologic hallmark of rickettsial disease. During the incubation period it is surmised that rickettsemia occurs, seeding the endothelial cells of capillaries, arterioles, and venules. With rickettsial multiplication the endothelial cells proliferate, swell, and degenerate, resulting in partial or complete thrombosis of the vascular lumen. In Rocky Mountain spotted fever the rickettsiae also invade the smooth-muscle wall of arterioles, producing further vascular damage, with resultant microinfarction and extravasation. Accumulations of polymorphonuclear and mononuclear inflammatory cells surround such areas of vascular injury. These changes occur at intervals along the vessels, leaving normal vascular architecture in intervening areas. In severe cases, thrombosis involves larger vessels, and microinfarction of the affected tissue is extensive (Fig. 183-1).

The vascular lesions described account for most of the observed clinical findings, the location of the lesion determining its clinical expression. The skin most directly reflects vascular damage, the rash coinciding with the point and extent of vascular injury. In the brain the glial nodule is its counterpart; in the heart an interstitial myocarditis and microinfarctions are produced. A patchy interstitial rickettsial pneumonitis may occur.

The pathologic changes produced by the rickettsiae causing the typhus fevers closely resemble those described for Rocky Mountain spotted fever, but their extent and severity are usually more limited, there is less tendency to

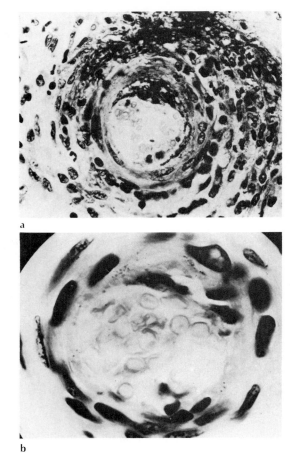

Fig. 183-1 **(a) The vascular lesion of Rocky Mountain spotted fever as seen in an arteriole in the epididymis. An early thrombus is present. (b) Rickettsiae are seen in endothelial cells in a biopsy from scrotal skin.** *(From the collection of the late Prof. S. Burt Wolbach, with permission of Arthur T. Hertig, M.D., Dept. of Pathology, Harvard University.)*

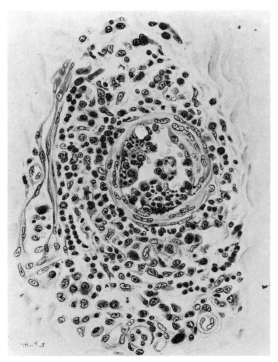

Fig. 183-2 **The vascular lesion of typhus as depicted in an artist's representation of a skin biopsy taken on the eighth day of the eruption.** *(From the Wolbach collection, with permission of Arthur T. Hertig, M.D.)*

thrombosis, and invasion of the arteriolar smooth muscle almost never occurs (Figs. 183-2 and 183-3).

The cause of the toxic and febrile state produced by rickettsial infection remains obscure. Rickettsial toxins (lethal for mice) have been described, but their role in the pathogenesis of disease is uncertain. There is no explanation for the fact that the rash of Rocky Mountain spotted fever begins peripherally and spreads centrally while that of typhus erupts first on the trunk and later appears on the extremities.

Rocky Mountain spotted fever

Rocky Mountain spotted fever, caused by *R. rickettsii,* transmitted via tick bite, is the most severe of the rickettsial infections. The illness ranges from a virtually asymptomatic form to a fulminant disease with fatality rates ranging from 20 to 80 percent in untreated cases.

The infection is seasonal, the early summer peak of the disease corresponding to the increased seasonal activity of ticks and increased human contact with them. The reservoir of the disease is thought to be in small mammals, but ticks can infect their offspring transovarially, thus also serving as a reservoir. In the western United States the

wood tick, *Dermacentor andersoni,* is the vector of the disease; in the eastern United States, however, the dog tick, *D. variabilis* is the principal vector. Possibly this explains the high incidence in children in the eastern United States and the high incidence in men in the mountain woods of Montana and other western states.

Clinical manifestations (Fig. A3-9)

The incubation period ranges from 3 to 12 days, with a mean of 7 days. The onset is generally abrupt, with the sudden appearance of fever, chills, severe headache, myalgia, and arthralgia. The rash, the most characteristic aspect of the disease, generally appears on the fourth day of fever (range, 2 to 6 days). *It goes through a very regular and unique progression, first erupting on the wrists, ankles, and forearms.* It is pink and *macular,* fades on pressure, and is accentuated by warm compresses or a rise in the patient's temperature. After 6 to 18 h the rash involves the *palms* and *soles* and then extends centrally to the arms, thighs, trunk, and face. After 1 to 3 days the rash becomes *macular and papular* and a deeper red (Fig. 183-4). After 2 to 4 days petechiae appear in the rash and the lesions no longer fade on pressure. Pressure from a sphygmomanometer may induce an additional shower of petechiae (Rumpel-Leede test, indicating capillary fragility), and the lesions coalesce and form ecchymoses. Small areas of gangrene may appear over the toes, fingers, earlobes, nose, scrotum, or vulva. Involvement of the scrotum or vulva often serves as a diagnostic clue. The more severe the infection, the more extensive the rash and the more rapid the progression. The rash may not be noticed in black patients.

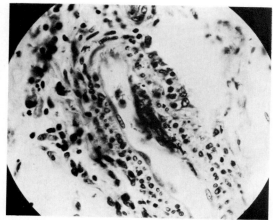

Fig. 183-3 Thrombosis in a cutaneous arteriole from a patient with typhus. *(From the Wolbach collection, with permission of Arthur T. Hertig, M.D.)*

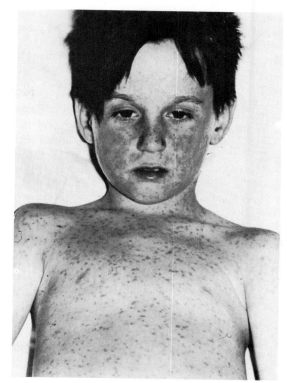

Fig. 183-4 Rocky Mountain spotted fever.

The diffuse vasculitis of the severe cases results in transudation of plasma, diminishing intravascular volume, falling blood pressure, and rising pulse, and patients appear profoundly ill. These changes are accentuated by the diffuse myocarditis and by the lowered serum albumin level, thought to be a consequence of liver involvement. Such patients, especially children, may appear quite edematous. Impaired circulatory dynamics further leads to diminished renal function.

A firm spleen is palpable in half the cases. Abdominal distension and muscular tenderness may combine to mimic appendicitis or other intraabdominal disease. Severely ill patients may be comatose. Further evidence of neurologic damage, such as seizures or hemiplegia, is associated with a very poor prognosis.

On recovery, the areas involved by the rash develop secondary pigmentation which may persist for some time.

Laboratory diagnosis

The usual laboratory determinations do not aid in diagnosis. A normochromic, normocytic anemia may develop during the second week of the disease. The white blood cell count is generally within the normal range, although leukopenia or a mild leukocytosis may be observed. Cerebrospinal fluid examination generally reveals only a few red blood cells and lymphocytes. Thrombocytopenia and various derangements of the blood clotting mechanisms often accompany the moderate and severe forms of the disease as a consequence of diffuse intravascular coagulation. Elevated blood urea nitrogen values usually reflect a prerenal azotemia, and liver function studies show degrees of impairment, especially diminished serum albumin concentrations.

The Weil-Felix test, with OX-K, OX-19, and OX-2 strains of *Proteus vulgaris,* is used extensively to help in narrowing diagnostic possibilities to rickettsial disease. A titer of less than 1:320 is not definitely diagnostic, and demonstration of a rising titer in acute and convalescent serum specimens is desirable. The Weil-Felix test will *not* distinguish between the spotted and typhus fevers. It is thus important to have specific complement fixation or indirect fluorescent antibody studies performed with acute and convalescent serums. These tests are available through state health departments and the Centers for Disease Control in Atlanta, Georgia. Antibiotic therapy, if started early in illness, may delay the appearance of both Weil-Felix and more specific antibodies. Biopsy of skin lesions which can be processed within 8 h is helpful in establishing the diagnosis; the microorganisms are found by immunofluorescent staining in the walls of the small blood vessels of the skin.

Isolation of the microorganism is difficult and dangerous. Unless a laboratory specially equipped to work with rickettsiae is available, serologic methods should be relied upon to establish the diagnosis.

Differential diagnosis

A history of tick bite in a person who has been in an endemic area is helpful but is frequently not available. The two other diseases most frequently considered are meningococcemia and measles. Meningococcemia is the most important as it, too, may kill rapidly. The rash may be entirely similar, ranging from macular to macular and papular to petechial and ecchymotic. In meningococcemia, the rash appears earlier in the course of the illness and does not have the characteristic progression of Rocky Mountain spotted fever rash. A coverslip touch preparation of a lightly scraped meningococcal lesion may reveal the microorganisms on Gram's stain. Cultures will reveal the meningococci in petechiae, blood, and cerebrospinal fluid if meningitis is present. In practice these diseases often cannot be differentiated with certainty. Thus therapy for *both* diseases often must be instituted and subsequently modified when further information becomes available.

Coryza, conjunctivitis, cough, and Koplik's spots help

to distinguish measles, in which the rash usually starts on the face and only rarely becomes petechial. The presence of edema (a parent's history of a child's puffy eyes, for example) can be very helpful in suggesting Rocky Mountain spotted fever rather than measles. So-called atypical measles (see Chap. 186) may also mimic Rocky Mountain spotted fever.

The rose spots (papules) of typhoid fever are a delicate pink, are usually few in number, and are found on the abdomen and lower part of the thorax. They do not become petechial.

Some of the enteroviruses produce summer febrile illnesses with a rash. Usually appearing in epidemics, sometimes associated with diarrhea, the illness is short and mild and the rash only rarely becomes petechial.

Treatment

Tetracycline and chloramphenicol are extremely effective in the treatment of Rocky Mountain spotted fever when administered early in the disease. The dose of either drug is 50 to 100 mg/kg per day (no more than 2 g per day for children or 4 g per day for adults). Because of the hematologic involvement of Rocky Mountain spotted fever, tetracycline is preferred. Therapy is continued for about 4 days after the patient has become afebrile, to prevent relapse.

When initial therapy should also be directed against the meningococcus, 20 million units of intravenous penicillin G daily should be added to the regimen. Under *no* circumstances should the sulfonamides be employed, as they appear to *enhance* rickettsial infection.

Supportive measures, including intravenous administration of albumin, plasma, plasma expanders, or whole blood, may be of use in the severely ill patient. Corticosteroids have been employed to reduce fever and toxicity more rapidly, but whether they alter prognosis is unknown. Heparin has been administered to patients with associated disseminated intravascular coagulation, but no definite recommendation can yet be made.

Spotted fever groups: boutonneuse fever, South African tick-bite fever, Siberian tick typhus, and Queensland tick typhus

The rickettsiae producing the mild diseases making up this group are closely related to one another and to *R. rickettsii,* the agent of Rocky Mountain spotted fever. The diseases are transmitted by ticks and occur in various parts of the Eastern Hemisphere. Boutonneuse fever, caused by *R. conorii,* is the prototype of the group.

Clinical manifestations

After a 5- to 7-day incubation period the illness begins with fever and headache. A primary lesion, the *tache noir,* at the site of the tick bite is characteristic of all the Eastern Hemisphere rickettsioses. It consists of a small ulcer with a black center surrounded by a red halo. It is associated with regional lymphadenopathy. A generalized, red, macular and papular rash erupts on the fourth day (Fig. 183-5). It involves the palms and soles and rarely becomes hemorrhagic. The disease is milder than Rocky Mountain spotted fever, and those who succumb usually have un-

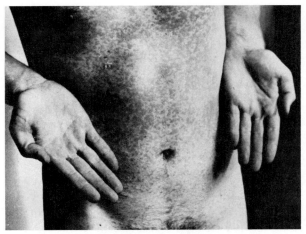

Fig. 183-5   South African tick-bite fever. (Courtesy of Dr. Evelyn Wallace, Monterey, California.)

derlying disease. Imported cases occurring in travelers have been described.

The Weil-Felix reaction becomes positive in convalescence and specific antibodies develop.

Treatment

Therapy with tetracycline or chloramphenicol is effective.

Rickettsialpox

Rickettsialpox, a mild disease caused by *R. akari,* was first identified in New York City in 1946. It is transmitted by the mite of the house mouse. It has been recognized in urban locations along the eastern seaboard of the United States, and in Russia. It is unique among rickettsial diseases in that its eruption is vesicular.

Clinical manifestations

A local lesion at the site of the mite bite appears 1 to 2 days after the bite and precedes the febrile illness. The lesion is a red papule which becomes quite large (1 to 1.5 cm in diameter). A vesicle forms in the center, leaving an erythematous halo. The vesicle dries and a black eschar results which is present when the patient develops systemic symptoms (Fig. 183-6). The febrile illness lasts about a week, during which period the rash appears. It is a generalized macular-papular-vesicular eruption, which is often sparse. Usually on the face, trunk, and extremities, it may involve the palms, soles, and oral mucosa. The lesions develop a scale but no permanent scars. Therapy with tetracycline or chloramphenicol shortens the course.

The Weil-Felix test *remains negative* after this disease, but specific complement-fixing or indirect fluorescent antibodies do develop.

Differential diagnosis

Now that smallpox has been eradicated, the major differential diagnosis is with chickenpox. Chickenpox generally occurs in children and has no initial lesion. Its rash appears with the fever, and the whole papule is transformed into a vesicle. In rickettsialpox, fever generally precedes the

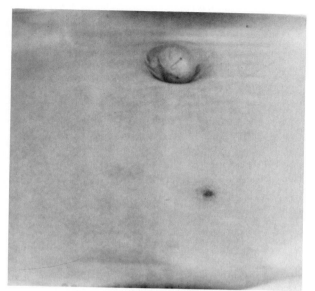

Fig. 183-6 Rickettsialpox. Initial lesion depicting the black eschar resulting from rupture of vesicle. (Courtesy of Dr. F. Daniels, Jr.)

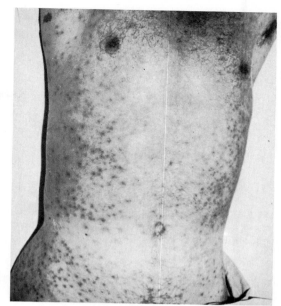

Fig. 183-7 The diffuse macular-petechial eruption of epidemic typhus. The distribution is primarily trunkal. (From the personal collection of Dr. Theodore E. Woodward.)

rash, and the papular base is always discernible under and around the vesicle.

Typhus group

Endemic typhus

Endemic or murine typhus is caused by *R. typhi* (formerly *R. mooseri*) which is transmitted to humans by the rat flea. It is most prevalent about harbors and granaries where humans are likely to have contact with rats, the reservoir for the disease.

Clinical manifestations. After an incubation period of 8 to 16 days, the onset of illness is heralded by chills, fever, severe headache, malaise, nausea, and vomiting. The rash generally appears on the fifth day. It is initially macular, becoming macular and papular. It is not petechial. The distribution of the rash helps to differentiate this disease from Rocky Mountain spotted fever. The lesions are located primarily over the trunk, with limited involvement of the face, extremities, palms, and soles, as opposed to the distal distribution of spotted fever lesions. The rash may be very evanescent and is absent in 10 percent of cases.

Typhus is generally milder than Rocky Mountain spotted fever, and it has a low mortality rate. One-fourth of patients have a palpable spleen.

The Weil-Felix test becomes positive in convalescence, and type-specific, complement-fixing and indirect fluorescent antibodies appear.

Treatment is as for the other rickettsial diseases.

Epidemic typhus

Classical typhus is caused by *R. prowazekii* and is transmitted by the human body louse. Hence, the disease is easily spread from person to person. The reservoir for the disease is thought to be humans, lice becoming infected

from patients with recrudescent typhus (Brill's disease). Sporadic cases of classical typhus recently have been reported in this country, primarily from rural or suburban areas of the eastern United States. The majority of cases have occurred during the cold months of December, January, and February. Most of the patients have had contact with flying squirrels or their nests. This animal now has been shown to be a sylvatic reservoir of *R. prowazekii*, but the mode of transmission to humans is unknown.

Clinical manifestations. The incubation period is about 7 days. As in other rickettsial diseases, the onset is characterized by fever, chills, headache, malaise, and weakness. On the fifth febrile day the rash appears, first in the axillae, then over the trunk, and later on the extremities. The rash initially consists of pink macules, which may become petechial and confluent (Fig. 183-7). The rash does not become papular.

Epidemic typhus is generally at an intermediate level of severity between murine typhus and Rocky Mountain spotted fever. In severe cases of louse-borne typhus, the clinical manifestations detailed for spotted fever, including widespread vascular thrombosis, are also observed (Fig. 183-8). Treatment is as for Rocky Mountain spotted fever.

In convalescence, Weil-Felix agglutinins and specific complement-fixing and indirect fluorescent antibodies develop.

Brill's disease

For unknown reasons, some patients who have had classical louse-borne typhus in the distant past develop a recurrence of the disease. The clinical manifestations are in all ways similar to those of a mild episode of typhus, and therapy is the same.

Interestingly, the Weil-Felix test is frequently negative

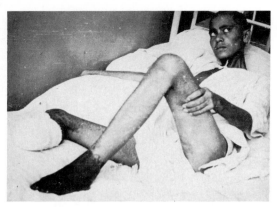

Fig. 183-8 Epidemic typhus. Thrombosis of large vessels may result in significant gangrene. *(From the collection of Dr. Theodore E. Woodward.)*

or, at best, weakly positive, while specific antibodies rise rapidly to high titers in an anamnestic-like response.

Scrub typhus

Rickettsia tsutsugamushi, transmitted by the bite of a mite, causes scrub typhus in India, Southeast Asia, and Australia. There is marked strain variation in virulence, and mortality rates have varied from 0 to 60 percent.

Clinical manifestations. After an incubation period of 6 to 18 days, illness begins suddenly with fever, chills, and headache. The primary lesion, a vesicle or black eschar on an erythematous papular base, can usually be found, associated with local and moderate generalized lymphadenopathy (Fig. 183-9). On the fifth day of fever the red macular and papular rash develops, primarily over the trunk. Unlike the other rickettsial eruptions, it fades within a few days.

The disease resembles the other typhus fevers with two exceptions: early in the disease there is a bradycardia relative to the elevated temperature, and pneumonitis is more frequent.

Agglutinins to the OX-K strain of *Proteus* appear in convalescence. The OX-19 and OX-2 *Proteus* agglutinins remain negative. Repeated attacks of scrub typhus are not unusual, as there is considerable antigenic variation in strains.

Therapy is the same as described for the other rickettsial diseases, scrub typhus responding more rapidly than any of the other rickettsial diseases.

Trench fever

Rickettsia quintana, a louse-transmitted microorganism, produces a mild, though sometimes prolonged, illness in humans, characterized by fever, chills, headaches, and a very characteristic myalgia, especially in the lower part of the back and in the legs. The rash consists of red macules confined to the trunk; the extremities and face are infre-

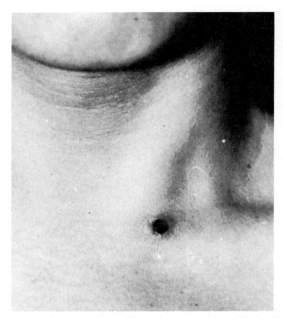

Fig. 183-9 Scrub typhus. The primary lesion with its black eschar ("cigarette burn") is associated with regional lymphadenopathy. *(From the collection of Dr. Theodore E. Woodward.)*

quently involved. The rash appears during the first day of illness and then waxes and wanes with the height of the fever. The spleen is usually palpable and quite firm. As the disease has been seen only in association with the two world wars, data on the efficacy of therapy are lacking.

Q fever

R. burnetii, the agent of Q fever, produces an acute self-limited pneumonitis and hepatitis in humans. It is the only rickettsial pathogen that does not produce cutaneous manifestations.

Bibliography

Barrett-Conner E, Ginsberg MM: Imported South African tick typhus. *West J Med* **138:**264, 1983

Brettman LR et al: Rickettsialpox: report of an outbreak and a contemporary review. *Medicine (Baltimore)* **60:**363, 1981

Burnett JW: Rickettsioses: a review for the dermatologist. *J Am Acad Dermatol* **2:**359, 1980

Duma RJ et al: Epidemic typhus in the United States associated with flying squirrels. *JAMA* **245:**2318, 1981

Hattwick MAW et al: Rocky Mountain spotted fever: epidemiology of an increasing problem. *Ann Intern Med* **84:**732, 1976

Schaffner W et al: Thrombocytopenic Rocky Mountain spotted fever: case study of husband and wife. *Arch Intern Med* **116:**857, 1965

Torres J et al: Rocky Mountain spotted fever in the mid-south. *Arch Intern Med* **132:**340, 1973

Walker DH et al: Laboratory diagnosis of Rocky Mountain spotted fever. *South Med J* **73:**1443, 1980

Zinsser H: *Rats, Lice and History.* Boston, Little, Brown, 1935

CHAPTER 184

VIRAL DISEASES: GENERAL CONSIDERATIONS

Douglas R. Lowy

Skin manifestations are a prominent feature of many viral diseases. In some instances, cutaneous lesions may suggest a particular viral illness whose diagnosis can be quickly established by appropriate procedures. At other times, the physician may be confronted with a patient whose differential diagnosis includes several viral as well as nonviral illnesses. The latter situation presents both a challenge and a source of frustration to the clinician because establishing the correct diagnosis may involve diagnostic procedures that are costly, specialized, time consuming, and are not definitive. Nonetheless, achieving the correct diagnosis is not only intellectually satisfying but may also be critical for both the patient and the community in the surveillance and control of infectious disease. The availability of chemotherapeutic agents that are useful in treating certain viral illnesses provides an additional incentive for the specific diagnosis of viral infections.

Definition of viruses

Viruses form a diverse group of infectious agents that share a distinctive composition and a unique mode of replication. Viruses are not cellular organisms. Although certain viruses encode a small number of enzymes, viruses do not possess functional ribosomes or other cellular organelles. These agents therefore lack much of the machinery required for their own multiplication. They multiply only inside cells, where they make use of the cellular synthetic apparatus to produce the components of the virus. It is because of their dependence on the cell for their replication that viruses are often referred to as "obligate intracellular parasites."

The most important element of a virus is its genetic information (the viral *genome*), which may be either deoxyribonucleic acid (DNA) or ribonucleic acid (RNA), depending on the type of virus. The life cycle of a virus may be divided into two parts. One is as a particle or *virion,* where the viral genetic information is surrounded by a highly organized protein coat that can be readily visualized in the electron microscope. The virus exists in this form outside of cells. The virion serves to transmit the viral genetic information, functionally intact, to a susceptible host. The second portion of the viral life cycle is that period when the viral genetic information is present inside a cell, where it is usually found in a nonparticulate form. Certain pathogenetic aspects of virus infection occur during the nonparticulate portion of the virus life cycle.

Classification of viruses

No single virus is capable of infecting all classes of cells. Each virus is broadly classified as a bacterial, plant, or animal virus on the basis of the type of cell it can infect. The animal viruses have been divided into several large families according to the size, shape, and structure of the virion and the type of viral nucleic acid within it, as shown in Table 184-1. Viruses of a given family can be identified by physical methods, such as the size and shape of their virions in the electron microscope, by antigenic cross-reactivity, or by nucleic acid homology.

As noted above, the virion is composed of the viral genetic core surrounded by a protective protein coat called the *capsid*. The capsids in certain virus families (such as herpesviruses) are located inside a virion *envelope* (composed of lipid, protein, and carbohydrate) which is required for infectivity. In the virion, the viral genome consists of only a single type of nucleic acid, either DNA or RNA. Although viruses have been grouped principally by virion morphology and nucleic acid composition, many functional, genetic, biochemical, and immunologic features are shared by viruses within the same family. Viruses within a given family may be further classified according to their relatedness at the nucleic acid level, their antigenic cross-reactivity, or the host cells that they infect.

Examples of virions from the three families of viruses (papovaviruses [papillomaviruses], herpesviruses, and poxviruses) which frequently multiply in the epidermis are shown in Figure 184-1. The viral genome of these three families is composed of DNA. Papillomaviruses possess naked (nonenveloped) capsids, and herpesviruses have enveloped virions. Poxvirus virions are large, have a very complex structure, and are enveloped, but their envelope is not required for their virions to be infectious.

Viral replication

Viruses replicate inside cells by synthesizing their various structural components separately and then assembling them into multiple virions, in contrast to cells, which multiply by binary fission (the production of two progeny cells from a single parental cell). As noted earlier, viruses utilize the host cell machinery to synthesize and assemble new virions, since these agents do not contain the apparatus required for their own replication.

It is important to recognize that viral genomes encode two different functional classes of proteins. Some virus-encoded proteins form virions; these proteins are called structural or virion proteins. Viral genomes also encode nonvirion proteins; as their name implies, these proteins are not incorporated into virions, although their production may be essential to the replication of the virus. The antimetabolite acyclovir inhibits herpesvirus replication because the drug is activated by virus-encoded nonvirion enzymes (proteins) that promote DNA synthesis.

Table 184-1   Major groups of animal viruses

Group	Size, nm	Shape	Symmetry	Envelope	Nucleic acid	Site of replication*	Examples of viruses
Parvovirus	20	Spherical	Icosahedral	No	DNA	N	Erythema infectiosum
Papovavirus	45–55	Spherical	Icosahedral	No	DNA	N	Wart, JC, BK, polyoma, SV-40
Adenovirus	70–80	Spherical	Icosahedral	No	DNA	N	32 human serotypes
Herpesvirus	150	Spherical	Icosahedral	Yes	DNA	N	Herpes simplex (types 1 and 2), varicella-zoster, cytomegalo, EB
Poxvirus	100–300	Brick	Complex	No†	DNA	C	Vaccinia, cowpox, variola, orf, milker's nodules, molluscum contagiosum
Unclassified	42	Spherical	Icosahedral	No	DNA	N	Hepatitis B (4 serotypes)
Picornavirus	20–30	Spherical	Icosahedral	No	RNA	C	Rhino (more than 90 serotypes), entero (3 polio, 33 echo, 30 Coxsackie serotypes)
Togavirus	40–60	Spherical	Icosahedral	Yes	RNA	C	Some arboviruses, rubella
Bunyavirus	90–100	Spherical	Helical	Yes	RNA	C	Some arboviruses
Arenavirus	85–120	Spherical	Helical?	Yes	RNA	C	Lassa fever
Coronavirus	80–120	Spherical	Helical	Yes	RNA	C	3 human serotypes
Retrovirus	100–120	Spherical	Helical	Yes	RNA	N + C	Rous sarcoma virus, murine leukemia virus, HTLV
Orthomyxovirus	80–120	Spherical and filamentous	Helical	Yes	RNA	C	Influenza types A + B + C (many subtypes)
Paramyxovirus	100–200	Spherical and filamentous	Helical	Yes	RNA	C	Mumps, parainfluenza, measles?
Rhabdovirus	70–180	Bullet	Helical	Yes	RNA	C	Rabies
Reovirus	50–80	Spherical	Icosahedral	No	RNA	C	Infantile diarrhea

* N = Nucleus; C = cytoplasm.

† Envelopes sometimes surround poxvirus virions, but are not necessary for infectivity.

Nonvirion proteins of certain viruses may redirect the cell to synthesize the proteins required by the virus at the expense of those required for normal function of the cell. Many tumor viruses, including papillomaviruses, encode nonvirion proteins that enhance cell growth and lead to inappropriate control of cell division (see Chap. 73). The intracellular pathogenicity of a virus may therefore result in part from effects of nonvirion proteins.

The viral replication cycle, which has been studied in detail in tissue culture, involves several more or less sequential steps: attachment (adsorption), penetration, uncoating, biosynthesis, virion assembly, and release. Attachment of virions to cells involves a specific interaction between the viral capsid or envelope (for those viruses that possess enveloped virions) and receptors on the cell surface. Cells that lack the appropriate cell surface receptors for a particular virus will therefore not be infected by that virus. Following penetration of the virion into the cell, cellular enzymes degrade the envelope and capsid (uncoating), which begins that nonparticulate phase of the virus life cycle.

Viruses vary in their size and complexity. The genome of poliovirus, which is a small virus with a simple virion structure, encodes a single precursor protein which is cleaved to give rise to the structural and nonstructural viral proteins. By contrast, poxviruses, whose virions are more than 10 times larger than poliovirus virions and are much more complex structurally, encode dozens of structural and nonstructural proteins.

During biosynthesis, the viral genome instructs the cells to produce the proteins encoded by the viral genes. The virions of most viruses, including papillomaviruses, herpesviruses, and poxviruses, are assembled inside the cell and then released following cell death and lysis. However, enveloped viruses whose virions are assembled at the cell surface (such as paramyxoviruses and retroviruses) are released by budding from intact cells; with these viruses, productive infection and release of virions may not always be accompanied by toxic effects on the infected cell. Each virus has its characteristic site of replication within the cell. Papillomaviruses and herpesviruses are assembled in the nucleus (Figs. 184-2 and 184-3). Poxviruses, which are the only DNA viruses that replicate in the cytoplasm, synthesize their virions in organized cytoplasmic "viral factories" containing "viroplasm" (Fig. 184-4).

Typically, hundreds or thousands of new virions are produced from each infected cell, and they in turn infect previously uninfected cells. One cycle of virus replication may last 3 to 36 h, depending on the virus and cell involved. Interruption of any step will prevent the development of new infectious virions.

Each virus can infect and replicate in only a limited number of cell types. The spectrum of susceptible cells depends on the virus. Human papillomaviruses (HPV) can infect a very narrow range of cells, namely certain differentiating human epidermal cells. Other viruses can infect a much broader range of cells; herpes simplex viruses can replicate in many different human and nonhuman cell types.

Even within a given tissue, a virus may be infectious

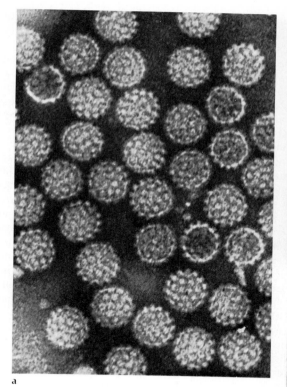

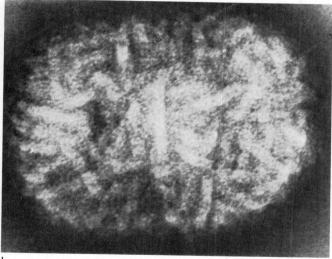

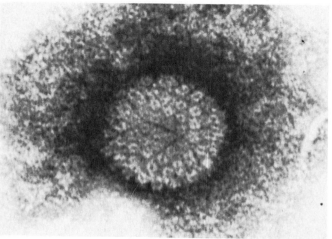

Fig. 184-1 Electron micrographs of negatively stained virions (X200,000). (a) Papovavirus: multiple nonenveloped human papillomavirus (wart) virions showing capsid subunits (capsomeres). (b) Poxvirus: single molluscum contagiosum virus virions, showing complex tubular structures. (c) Herpes virus: single varicella-zoster virus virion showing capsid inside envelope. *(Parts (a) and (b) courtesy of A. F. Howatson, J. D. Almeida, and M. G. Williams. Part (c) by permission of Almeida JD et al, Virology 16:353, 1962.)*

only for cells with a specific degree of differentiation. The important role of the differentiated state of the cell in determining whether or not a virus will undergo replication is seen in the skin lesions of molluscum contagiosum. Since molluscum contagiosum virus (MCV) particles are sometimes found in cells of the upper dermis, the virus is capable of attachment and penetration in these cells. MCV does not, however, replicate in dermal cells, indicating that an intracellular block to MCV synthesis exists in these dermal cells. MCV particles are also found in the basal layer of epidermal cells, but synthesis of new viral components does not begin until the cells reach the suprabasal layers. This observation implies that MCV replication can take place only in partially differentiated epidermal cells.

Cellular consequences of viral infection

Typically, infected cells develop gross and often characteristic cytopathic changes and eventually die. Infections of this type are termed *cytocidal* or *lytic*. However, some viruses can replicate without causing irreversible damage to the host cell. Noncytocidal infection of this type may occur in tissue culture with measles virus and many other enveloped RNA viruses, leading to a chronically infected culture.

Two other types of noncytocidal infection are neoplastic transformation and viral latency. Tumor viruses, when they transform cells, alter the normal control of cellular proliferation. In general, tumor viruses (such as the papovavirus SV-40) do not synthesize new virions in neoplastically transformed cells, although such transformation requires the continued expression of a portion of the viral genome. It is interesting to note that SV-40 is exclusively cytocidal for some cell types (permissive infection), induces transformation exclusively in other cells (nonpermissive infection), and induces both types of infection in still other cell types (semipermissive infection), again underlining the importance of the host cell in affecting the outcome of infection. Epidermal cells are semipermissive for papillomavirus infection. Virus-induced neoplasia is discussed in greater detail in Chap. 73.

Viral latency, which occurs commonly with herpes viruses, papillomaviruses, and retroviruses, represents the other type of noncytocidal infection. Latently infected cells probably either produce very small numbers of new virions so that spread to uninfected cells is minimal, or they syn-

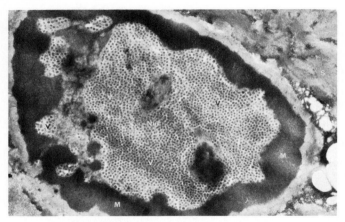

Fig. 184-2 Papillomavirus (a papovavirus). Electron micrograph (X20,000). Nucleus (Nuc) of a stratum corneum cell, filled with papillomavirus virions (V); chromatin is marginated (M). Mature keratin can be seen in an adjacent cell (S).

thesize no new virus but retain an intact and potentially activatable viral genome.

Pathogenesis of viral infections in the skin

Virus infections may affect the skin by three different routes: direct inoculation, systemic infection, or local spread from an internal focus. In warts, herpes simplex, chickenpox, herpes zoster, molluscum contagiosum, and smallpox, the shedding of virus from human skin lesions represents an important source in the transmission of virus to other people. Skin lesions may be produced by the direct effect of virus replication on infected cells, the host response to the virus, or the interaction of these two phenomena. Relatively little is currently known about the role of the immune response in the pathogenesis of skin lesions induced by viruses.

The viruses of warts, molluscum contagiosum, vaccinia, orf, milker's nodules, and (primary) herpes simplex, all of

Fig. 184-3 Varicella-zoster virus (a herpesvirus). Electron micrograph (X24,000). Portion of cell of the stratum spinosum. The nucleus (Nuc) contains varicella-zoster virions (V). Chromatin is marginated at (M). Virions (V) and tonofilaments (T) are shown in the cytoplasm (Cyt).

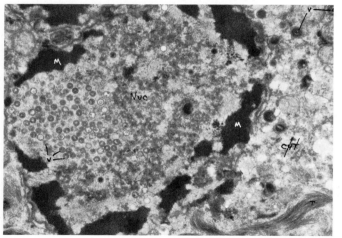

which infect the skin by direct inoculation, replicate in the epidermis. Their viral cytopathic effects account for the appearance of early lesions. The contribution of the immune response to the evolution of these lesions remains conjectural. The incubation period is generally short because the lesions develop at the site of inoculation. The incubation period for warts is longer presumably because the virus replicates slowly or cell-to-cell spread of virus occurs to only a limited extent. Latent papillomavirus infection has also been demonstrated in clinically normal laryngeal tissue of patients with a history of laryngeal papillomas, suggesting that host-specific factors may also play a significant role in some papillomavirus-induced lesions.

In systemic infections, the skin is infected during viremia, so that the dermis is generally infected earlier than the epidermis. It is not known how the distribution of viral exanthems is determined. In chickenpox and smallpox, the damage from cytocidal infection of the skin is a prime cause of the lesions. On the other hand, there is suggestive evidence from patients with impaired cellular immunity that the lesions of rubella and measles result in part from cell-mediated immune response to the virus. The basis of most exanthems associated with enteroviral infections remains to be established; there is significant cytocidal viral replication in the skin in hand-foot-and-mouth disease.

Recurrent herpes simplex and herpes zoster represent the local spread of virus to the skin following reactivation of the latent viral infection present in peripheral nerves. Cytocidal infection clearly plays an important role in these lesions, although lesions often contain less virus than during primary infection, presumably because of immunity.

Host response

The severity of illness induced by a particular virus varies considerably from person to person. While the size of the viral inoculum and the portal of entry play some role, it is believed that host factors usually account for most of this variation. Both immunologic and nonimmunologic responses appear to be important.

Antibody responses to viral infection represent the major host defense against reinfection by the same virus; the prophylactic administration of type-specific antibodies can prevent or modify primary illness even in patients with impaired cellular immunity. Humoral immunity is not thought, however, to contribute to the recovery from most primary viral infections, as viral infection of patients with isolated deficiencies of humoral immunity usually follows a normal course. There are several mechanisms by which antibodies may inhibit the spread of virus. These include neutralization of virus through prevention of viral attachment to target cells (which may be increased by complement), enhancement of viral uptake by phagocytic cells which then inactivate the virus, and (complement-mediated) immune lysis of infected cells.

Specific cell-mediated immunity (CMI) is also elicited during viral infections and apparently influences the course of many viral infections. While CMI sometimes increases the degree of cellular pathology (as in the eruption of measles), it is usually protective. Patients with impaired CMI often have difficulty handling primary or recurrent viral infection. Such patients are at risk of developing severe primary virus infections, as well as warts, chronic herpes simplex virus infections, and disseminated herpes zoster. The antiviral mechanism of CMI has not yet been established. Sensitized T cells are known to be capable of lysing infected cells and of liberating lymphokines which attract phagocytic cells.

Inflammatory cells may produce some of their antiviral effects via the production of interferons, a unique family of closely related cell-encoded proteins which are active against viruses. Interferon, which can be induced by foreign RNA or DNA (including viral nucleic acids), is secreted into the extracellular fluid. Resistance to virus infection is induced in those cells that come in contact with the interferon. Virtually all viruses are capable of inducing interferon and are susceptible to its action, but viruses differ greatly in their efficiency of interferon induction and in their sensitivity to its action. The presence of interferon correlates with the recovery phase of several viral infections. Genetic factors may also play a role in determining the outcome of viral infections. In animal models, genes can determine the susceptibility to viral infection at several levels, including virion attachment to cells, viral replication, and viral-induced immune responses.

Diagnosis of viral infections

Four major approaches are used in the laboratory to diagnose viral infection: serology, virus isolation, microscopy, and viral antigen detection. Sensitive techniques to identify viral nucleic acids have also been developed, but these procedures are still too complex for routine application. As with all laboratory tests, the results must be interpreted in the context of the clinical setting. Fortuitous infection with a virus unrelated to the illness should always be considered. Serologic studies are very important for epidemiologic purposes, but the information is rarely helpful in patient management because the results are not available for several weeks. Virus isolation is expensive and may also be time consuming. Since microscopic techniques involve the direct examination of clinical material, they may be accomplished rapidly. Unfortunately, microscopy alone may not be definitive. The development of sensitive specific immunologic assays for viral antigen in clinical material represents a significant advance in the rapid diagnosis of viral infection.

In the determination of serum antibody levels, both acute and convalescent sera are needed. The acute specimen should be taken as early in the illness as possible, and the convalescent specimen 2 to 4 weeks later. Serum should be separated immediately from the coagulated blood and refrigerated or preferably frozen at $-20°C$ until antibody tests can be run simultaneously on both specimens. A fourfold or greater rise in antibody titer between first and second specimen generally indicates recent infection. A variety of assays are used to measure antibody levels, each detecting a certain type of antigen–antibody reaction. For each type of assay, serial dilutions of the test sera are reacted with a constant amount of antigen or whole virus. The antibody titer of a given serum is defined as the reciprocal of the highest dilution that gives a positive reaction. Some commonly used tests include:

1. Complement fixation. Sensitized sheep red blood cells fail to be lysed because antigen–antibody complexes have bound the complement.
2. Virus neutralization. Virus–antibody complexes inhibit infection.

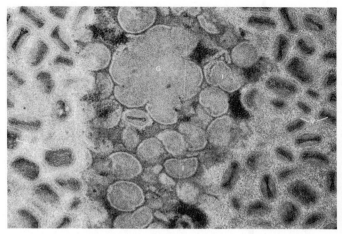

Fig. 184-4 Molluscum contagiosum (a poxvirus). Electron micrograph (X45,000). Cytoplasm of a spinosum cell filled with mature molluscum contagiosum virions (V), immature virus forms (I), and viroplasm in a gyrate pattern (G).

3. Immunodiffusion. Soluble antigens and antibody diffuse toward each other in agar, forming precipitin lines.
4. Hemagglutination inhibition. Viral-mediated hemagglutination is prevented by antibodies coating the virus.
5. Radioimmunoassay. Radioactively labeled antigen is bound to antibody from the test serum and precipitated (direct assay), or radioactively labeled antibody is prevented from binding to unlabeled antigen because the antigen is bound to antibody present in the test serum (competition assay).
6. Enzyme-linked immunosorbent assay (ELISA). Viral antigen, bound to a solid surface, binds viral antibody in the test serum. The bound antibody is detected by a colorimetric change induced by addition of an enzyme linked to a second antibody that binds to the serum antibody.
7. Immunoelectron microscopy. Antibody aggregates virions into clumps.

If virus isolation is attempted, specimens should be obtained as early in the disease as possible. Fluid from an early vesicle is often a good source of virus. Lesional specimens are less likely to be positive with nonvesicular exanthems. Specimens should also be obtained from other sites as indicated. Each specimen should be placed in a sterile tube with 2 to 5 mL of a buffered isotonic balanced salt solution containing penicillin and streptomycin. Preferably, it should be transported on ice immediately to the laboratory. If this is not practical, the specimen should be frozen (at $-70°C$, if possible). The suspected pathogen(s) should be indicated, since it may determine the type of cell culture or test animal to be inoculated.

For those lesions that contain large numbers of viral particles, electron microscopy of a lesion or its extract may provide morphologic identification of the virus. The light microscopic appearance of lesions may also be diagnostic. For example, Tzanck smears of the base of a blister may indicate the presence of an infection with a virus of the herpes group.

The positive identification of specific viral antigen in clinical material through use of immunologic techniques permits a more specific diagnosis than direct microscopy.

For example, these techniques will distinguish between herpes simplex and varicella-zoster. Radioimmunoassay, ELISA, immunoelectron microscopy, fluorescent antibody, or immunoperoxidase techniques identify viral antigen by the use of viral-specific antibody.

Therapy and prevention (see also Chap. 222)

Prophylaxis of viral infection has thus far proved more successful than the specific treatment of established infection. Vaccines have been extremely useful in the prevention of a variety of viral illnesses. In addition to vaccines that induce active immunity, the passive administration of type-specific antibody soon after exposure can prevent chickenpox in compromised hosts. Sensitive procedures for the detection of hepatitis B antigen in potential blood donors can drastically reduce the incidence of transfusion-mediated hepatitis.

Because viruses are adapted to the cells they infect and make use of cellular machinery, many chemotherapeutic agents that have been considered as potential antiviral agents affect cells to about the same extent as they affect viruses. 5'-Iododeoxyuridine, adenine arabinoside, and acyclovir are antimetabolites that have been approved for use in selected herpesvirus infections. Acyclovir, which is preferentially activated by herpesvirus-infected cells through its affinity for two herpesvirus enzymes involved in DNA synthesis, appears to have the best therapeutic index. Its mode of action makes it unlikely that acyclovir will be active against nonherpesviruses. As in the case of vaccines, acyclovir is much more effective in the prevention of clinical disease than in the treatment of an established self-limited infection. Although the drug can effectively inhibit viral replication in recurrent herpes simplex virus infection, its administration during active recurrent herpes labialis or progenitalis has little effect in this setting on healing time. In primary or chronic herpes simplex infections, which have a longer duration of active disease, the drug can decrease healing time.

Interferon is a potentially potent antiviral agent that inhibits most viruses and at low dosages is relatively nontoxic to cells. Biologically active interferon can now be produced in large quantities, and trials are currently in progress for various diseases. Its greatest therapeutic effects have thus far been in the treatment of some papillomavirus infections. It has been found to eliminate several types of cutaneous warts and to suppress laryngeal papillomas in children. Further studies are required to determine whether the promise of these preliminary studies will be fulfilled.

Bibliography

Brinton MA, Nathanson N: Genetic determinants of virus susceptibility: epidemiologic implications of murine models. *Epidemiol Rev* **3**:115, 1981

Burns WH, Allison AC: Virus infections and the immune responses they elicit, in *The Antigens,* vol 3, edited by M Sela. New York, Academic Press, 1975, p 479

David BD et al: *Microbiology,* 3d ed. Hagerstown, MD, Harper & Row, 1980

Fenner FJ, White DO: *Medical Virology,* 2d ed. New York, Academic Press, 1976

Field AM: Diagnostic virology using electron microscopic techniques. *Adv Virus Res* **27**:2, 1982

Goldstein LC et al: Monoclonal antibodies to herpes simplex viruses: use in antigenic typing and rapid diagnosis. *J Infect Dis* **147**:829, 1983

Haglund S et al: Interferon therapy in juvenile laryngeal papillomatosis. *Arch Otolaryngol* **107**:327, 1981

Hirsch RL: The complement system: its importance in the host response to viral infection. *Microbiol Rev* **46**:71, 1982

Hsiung GD: *Diagnostic Virology,* 3d ed. New Haven, Yale Univ Press, 1982

Joklik WK et al: *Zinsser Microbiology,* 18th ed. Norwalk, CT, Appleton-Century-Crofts, 1984

Melnick JL: Taxonomy and nomenclature of viruses, 1982. *Prog Med Virol* **28**:208, 1982

Moller G (ed): MHC restriction of anti-viral immunity. *Immunol Rev* **58**:1, 1981

Nilsen AE et al: Efficacy of oral acyclovir in the treatment of initial and recurrent genital herpes. *Lancet* **2**:571, 1982

Peterson LR, Balfour HH: Advances in clinical virology. *Prog Clin Pathol* **8**:239, 1981

Schonfeld A et al: Intramuscular human interferon-beta injections in treatment of condylomata acuminata. *Lancet* **1**:1038, 1984

Solomon A et al: The Tzanck smear in the diagnosis of cutaneous herpes simplex. *JAMA* **251**:633, 1984

Steinberg BM et al: Laryngeal papillomavirus infection during clinical remission. *N Engl J Med* **308**:1261, 1983

Straus SE et al: Suppression of frequently recurring genital herpes. A placebo-controlled double-blind trial of oral acyclovir. *N Engl J Med* **310**:1545, 1984

Yolken RH: Enzyme immunoassays for the detection of infectious agents in body fluids: current limitations and future prospects. *Rev Infect Dis* **4**:35, 1982

RUBELLA (GERMAN MEASLES)

Stephen E. Gellis and Sydney S. Gellis

Rubella (German measles) is a common communicable infection of children and young adults, characterized by a short prodromal period, enlargement of cervical, suboccipital, and postauricular glands, and a rash of approximately 2 to 3 days' duration. The disease has rare sequelae, and were it not for its devastating effect on the fetus, would be of relatively little significance in terms of morbidity or complications.

Epidemiology

Epidemics of rubella have been noted at 5- to 7-year intervals. The disease is worldwide in its distribution and tends to occur most frequently during the spring months in North America. It is rare in young infants and is most common in school-age children, adolescents, and young adults. It is spread via the respiratory route, and the period of infectivity extends from the end of the incubation period to the disappearance of the rash. A single attack confers lifelong immunity in most individuals, although subclinical reinfections can be demonstrated by laboratory tests in some "immune" individuals who are subsequently exposed to the wild virus. Two attacks of rubella with rash are most unlikely to be encountered; in such instances, one of the episodes is usually not rubella but is due to another virus infection.

The virus of rubella may be recovered from the pharynx as early as 7 days before and up to 14 days after the onset of the rash. Viremia is rarely demonstrated after the onset of the rash [1].

Clinical manifestations (Table 185-1)

The incubation period ranges between 14 and 21 days and is usually 16 to 18 days. Prodromal signs and symptoms are rare in young children, and the rash usually appears without prior complaint. In older children, adolescents, and adults, low-grade fever, headache, conjunctivitis, sore throat, rhinitis, cough, and lymphadenopathy may precede the rash by 1 to 4 days and disappear rapidly after the rash appears. In some adults, however, these symptoms and signs may persist longer and be more severe, and the infection under such circumstances may be difficult to distinguish from rubeola (measles) unless Koplik's spots characteristic of measles are observed. The rash of rubella is first noted on the face (Fig. A3-5) and rapidly spreads to the neck, arms, trunk, and legs. It consists of pink-red macules and papules which are discrete and remain so on the extremities, coalescing on the trunk to give a uniform red blush.

The rash, which usually disappears by the end of 2 or 3 days, clearing first from the face, may occasionally be followed by fine desquamation. This rapid disappearance is in contrast to measles (rubeola) which persists for longer periods. An enanthem is often seen at the end of the prodromal period or beginning of the rash, consisting of red spots, pinhead in size, scattered over the soft palate. The lymphadenopathy of rubella is striking; it involves all lymph nodes, but enlargement and tenderness are most common in the suboccipital, postauricular, and anterior and posterior cervical nodes. In older children and adults lymphadenopathy may be noted several days before the rash but in both children and adults the enlargement and tenderness are most striking on the first day of the rash. Enlargement of glands may persist for days to weeks but tenderness rapidly subsides. Splenomegaly may occasionally be detected. The fever of rubella is usually low-grade and seldom lasts beyond the first day or two of the eruption except in individuals who have joint involvement and in whom fever may persist. Arthritis due to rubella occurs much more frequently in adults than in children and is usually first noted as the rash fades. Small and large joints may become painful, with or without swelling, and may simulate rheumatic fever or rheumatoid arthritis. In one epidemic, joint involvement was seen in 25 percent of children under the age of 11 years and in 52 percent of patients 11 years of age or older [2]. Striking effusions into joints have been reported. The arthritis of rubella usually lasts 1 to 2 weeks but occasionally may persist for longer periods or may be recurrent.

Complications

Rubella is essentially a benign disease. Rarely, it may produce an encephalitis which tends to be mild and is usually followed by complete recovery and with no effect on intellectual function. Thrombocytopenic purpura which may result from rubella may be accompanied by epistaxis, petechiae, ecchymoses, intestinal hemorrhage, and hematuria. These manifestations frequently clear within a month of onset but occasionally may persist for longer periods. Rarely, a peripheral neuritis may follow rubella.

Laboratory findings

The white blood count is usually low but may be normal. Increased numbers of atypical lymphocytes may be noted, and in some cases increased numbers of plasma cells have been reported. In cases with meningoencephalitis, varying numbers of lymphocytes may be found in the cerebrospinal fluid.

Congenital rubella (Table 185-2)

Gregg in 1941 [3] was the first to record the devastating effects of rubella infection in the fetus and to describe the

Table 185-1 Some distinctive features of the rashes of rubella, measles, and scarlet fever

	Rubella	Rubeola (measles)	Scarlet fever
Prodromata	1–2 days of mild fever and respiratory symptoms	2–4 days of fever with moderate-to-severe respiratory symptoms	1–2 days of fever and sore throat
Duration of rash	Average 1–2 days	Average 3–5 days	Varies with treatment
Color	Pink-red	Purple-red to brown before fading	Yellow-red (may blanch on pressure)
Distribution	Scattered to generalized	Generalized (variable in modified measles) Koplik's spots (early)	Generalized (altered by treatment) Circumoral pallor "Strawberry" tongue
Nature	Macular to macular and papular	Macular to macular and papular	Punctate lesions on erythematous skin
	Discrete with minimal coalescence about thorax	Discrete with marked coalescence about face and thorax	Pinhead-sized lesions imparting sandpaper-like texture to skin Accentuation in flexor creases
Postexanthem desquamation	Occasional and branny	Common and branny	Typical and severe, often occurring on the hands and feet

congenital rubella syndrome. Approximately 50 percent of infants who acquire rubella during the first trimester of intrauterine life will show clinical signs of damage from the virus. The earlier the infection, the more severe is fetal damage. In such infants multiple congenital defects include low birth weight, microcephaly with mental retardation, cataracts, nerve deafness, and congenital heart disease (usually patent ductus arteriosus or ventricular septal defect). Following completion of organ development in the fetus, infection with rubella may produce a variable clinical picture which may include hepatitis, splenomegaly, pneumonitis, myocarditis, encephalitis, and osteomyelitis. When the bone marrow is affected, the infant may be born with thrombocytopenia and bleeding into the skin, producing a striking picture of petechiae and ecchymoses given the colorful term of "blueberry muffin baby." In congenital rubella a retinopathy is commonly found, consisting of a diffuse deposit of black pigmentation.

Diagnosis

Infants with congenital rubella may be chronically infected for many months. Virus can be cultured from the nasopharynx, urine, cerebrospinal fluid, and even from the lens of infants with congenital cataract. As time passes, the amount of virus shed in the nasopharynx and urine gradually declines and disappears. Approximately 85 percent of infants infected in utero will excrete virus in the first month of life; 1 to 3 percent continue to excrete virus in the second year of life. The large amounts of virus from congenitally infected infants are very hazardous to pregnant women working with such infants and who may be susceptible to infection. The infant with congenital infection will usually have elevation of IgM due to antibody produced by the infant itself, together with elevated IgG caused by passive transfer of antibodies in the maternal blood. IgG traverses the placenta in contrast to IgM which does not. The IgG antibodies disappear over the first few months of life. Passively acquired IgG by the fetus from an immune mother may explain the rarity of acquired rubella in early infancy. The antibodies against rubella consist of neutralizing, complement-fixing, and hemagglutination-inhibition antibodies. Neutralizing and hemag-

glutination-inhibition antibodies usually persist for life. The hemagglutination-inhibition antibodies are easily and quickly measured and serve to determine whether a recent infection can be attributed to rubella by an increase in titer in the convalescent period over the titer in the acute stage. A fourfold increase or more is considered diagnostic of the

Table 185-2 Some manifestations of the congenital rubella syndrome

Teratogenic findings—congenital malformations:
  1. Heart*
     a. Patent ductus arteriosus
     b. Coarctation of pulmonary vessels
     c. Ventricular septal defects
     d. Combination of above
     e. Others
  2. Eye*
     a. Cataracts
     b. Microphthalmia
     c. Retinopathy
     d. Glaucoma
     e. Cloudy cornea
  3. Hearing defects*
  4. Central nervous system*
     a. Microcephaly
     b. Hydrocephaly
  5. Bone;* disturbances of growth of skull
  6. Abnormal dermatoglyphics
  7. Agammaglobulinemia
  8. Other organ systems
Other findings:
  1. Intra- and extrauterine growth retardation*
  2. Prematurity*
  3. Meningoencephalitis
  4. Pneumonitis
  5. Hepatitis*
  6. Cardiac tissue injury
  7. Rarefaction bone*
  8. Thrombocytopenia with or without purpura*
  9. Anemia
  10. Rubelliform skin rash
  11. Generalized adenopathy

* More commonly encountered.
Source: Adapted from papers in Rubella Symposium, *Am J Dis Child 110:*345, 1965.

infection. Testing for these antibodies also enables the physician to determine whether a woman of childbearing age is immune or susceptible to German measles.

Differential diagnosis

See Atlas 3 and Table 185-1.

Immunity and immunization

Lifelong immunity usually follows an attack of rubella. Reinfection can occur but it is usually not accompanied by clinical signs and symptoms. A rise in antibody level can occur; viremia from subclinical reinfection is very rare. Thus, congenital rubella is very unlikely in an infant whose mother has had an attack of rubella in the past and acquires a reinfection during pregnancy. The availability of rubella vaccine [4,5] and its widespread use has reduced markedly the frequency of congenital infection, although in some areas of Canada the congenital rubella syndrome is increasing due to failure to immunize susceptible women [6].

In the United States rubella vaccine is usually given together with mumps and measles vaccines in a single injection after the age of 15 months [7]. In the United Kingdom rubella vaccine is administered to girls just before adolescence to ensure that antibody titers will be at their highest during the early childbearing period. The child or adult to whom rubella vaccine is administered does not shed sufficient virus to infect susceptible individuals in close contact. As a result, it is safe to immunize children in a family in which the mother is pregnant. If a woman of childbearing age is to be immunized, it is important to obtain her rubella hemagglutination-inhibition titer since she may be immune as a result of an unrecognized or subclinical infection in the past and will therefore not require immunization. If she is susceptible and therefore is to be immunized, she must understand that pregnancy must be avoided for the following 3 months, a period during which attenuated virus from the vaccine may persist in her tissues. If a woman shown to be susceptible to rubella because of the absence of antibody is inadvertently given vaccine when she is pregnant, abortion is no longer recommended. Although rubella vaccine virus has been demonstrated in the fetal membranes and amniotic fluid, there has been no risk of the congenital rubella syndrome [8]. Because of the risk to the fetus from proved rubella infection in the pregnant woman, abortion is recommended.

References

1. Cooper LZ, Krugman S: Clinical manifestations of postnatal and congenital rubella. *Arch Ophthalmol* **77**:434, 1967
2. Jedelsohn RG, Wyll SA: Rubella in Bermuda; termination of an epidemic by mass vaccination. *JAMA* **223**:401, 1973
3. Gregg NM: Congenital cataract following German measles in the mother. *Trans Ophthalmol Soc Aust* **3**:35, 1941
4. Meyer HM Jr et al: Attenuated rubella virus. II. Production of an experimental live-virus vaccine and clinical trial. *N Engl J Med* **275**:575, 1966
5. Meyer HM Jr, Parkman PD: Rubella vaccination: a review of practical experience. *JAMA* **215**:613, 1971
6. Middleton PJ et al: Guide to the management of rubella problems. *Can Med Assoc J* **116**:484, 1977
7. Preblud SR et al: Assessment of susceptibility to measles and rubella. *JAMA* **247**:1134, 1982
8. Anonymous: Rubella and congenital rubella—United States, 1983. *Morbidity and Mortality Weekly Report* **33**:237, 247, 1984

Bibliography

Krugman S et al: *Infectious Diseases of Children*, 6th ed. St. Louis, CV Mosby, 1977
Feigin RD, Cherry JD: *Textbook of Pediatric Infectious Diseases*. Philadelphia, WB Saunders, 1981

CHAPTER 186

MEASLES

Louis Z. Cooper

Definition

Measles is an almost universal, highly contagious, acute viral disease of childhood. It is characterized by high fever, cough, coryza, conjunctivitis, and Koplik's spots which precede the appearance of a florid, generalized macular and papular rash.

Historical aspects

The term *measles* is thought to come from the Latin *misellus* or *misella*, a diminutive of the Latin *miser*, meaning miserable, which described the inmate of a medieval leper house. *Morbilli,* the diminutive of *morbus,* was introduced to distinguish minor rash disease from bubonic plague, *morbus,* the major disease. Morbilliform is a synonym for measles-like which is still in common use.

No accurate information is available on the early history of measles. The tenth-century Arabian physician Rhazes has generally been credited with distinguishing measles from smallpox, although he cited El Yehudi, a Hebrew physician from the first century, as first describing the disease. However, it was probably not until the severe epidemics of measles during the seventeenth century that these diseases were clearly separated; e.g., the astute clinical and epidemiologic observations by Thomas Sydenham were completed at this time [1].

In more recent times, transmission of measles to monkeys was first reported by Josias [2], and other investigators [3,4] demonstrated that monkeys could be infected with blood or nasopharyngeal secretions obtained from patients.

The isolation of measles virus in tissue culture by Enders and Peebles [5] provided the essential techniques for definitive characterization of the virus excretion and antibody response in this disease and for its ultimate control. In 1958, Enders and his coworkers successfully attenuated measles virus [6], and after extensive field trials, a live measles virus vaccine was licensed for general use in the United States in 1963. Since that time, the administration of approximately 150 million doses of vaccine has significantly decreased the incidence of this infection in this country.

Epidemiology

Measles is a universal illness, worldwide in distribution, which occurs primarily in children. However, the age incidence varies according to the environmental setting. In congested urban areas, the highest attack rate occurs in infancy and early childhood. In rural and less-crowded areas, the attack rate is highest in the early school years, ages 5 to 10 years. When measles has been introduced into isolated communities, the attack rate has approached 100 percent among the susceptible population of all ages. Very young infants, under 4 months of age, are usually protected by the persistence of transplacentally acquired maternal measles antibody.

Neither race nor sex affects the attack rate of measles, but the general state of health and nutrition clearly affect morbidity and mortality rates. Measles is primarily a disease of winter and spring in temperate climates, with the peak incidence of infection usually occurring in March or April.

The epidemiology of measles in the United States has changed dramatically because of the impact of massive immunization programs for eradication of this disease. The reported incidence of measles has declined since license of live attenuated measles virus vaccine in 1963, and elimination of indigenous measles has become a realistic national goal.

Etiology and pathogenesis

Measles virus has been classified as a paramyxovirus. Its structure and many of its biologic properties are similar to those of the larger members of the myxovirus group, i.e., mumps, Newcastle disease virus (NDV), and parainfluenza viruses. It is a heat-labile virus, with an RNA core and an outer envelope of protein and lipoprotein. The virus is stable at low temperatures (especially in the presence of protein) but is rapidly inactivated by ultraviolent radiation, ether, trypsin, acetone, and β-propiolactone. Complement fixation, hemagglutination, and hemolysis are properties of the virus which have been utilized for laboratory diagnosis (see "Diagnosis," below). Initial isolation in tissue culture

is most readily accomplished in primary cultures of human or simian renal or human amnion cells, but the virus has been adapted by serial passage to grow well in numerous continuous cell lines.

At the time of the initial isolation of measles virus in tissue culture, certain characteristic cytopathic effects were noted which were strikingly similar to previously well recognized pathologic changes occurring during natural infection in humans. These included formation of syncytia, or multinucleated giant cells with intranuclear and intracytoplasmic eosinophilic inclusions.

Measles virus is antigenically stable and distinct from mumps virus and the other larger myxoviruses. There is some degree of cross-reactivity with the agents of canine distemper and bovine rinderpest, but these cause no difficulty in serodiagnosis in humans.

The natural route of infection is by droplet spread of infectious secretions from an infected patient to the respiratory tract of a person who is susceptible. It is suspected that after local multiplication at this site of entry there may be an early viremia, but this has not been documented. During the prodromal period, virus can be detected in nasopharyngeal secretions, lymphatic tissue, blood, and urine [7], and virus may persist in the urine for 4 days after onset of the rash [8]. However, viremia and pharyngeal shedding of virus cease by the second day of rash, a time when measles antibody reaches detectable levels in the serum.

The mechanism of the rash has not been established; rash may be a direct effect of viral invasion on epithelial and vascular endothelial cells, or it may result from the damaging effects of a virus–antibody complex. In support of the latter theory is the temporal relationship between onset of rash and appearance of antibody (the same is true in rubella, another exanthem caused by a virus possibly in the myxovirus group), and the absence of rash in the few rare children, usually those with leukemia, who have developed chronic measles infection without rash or antibody production but with fatal giant cell pneumonia [9]. The experience of these children is in sharp contrast to that of children with classical (Bruton type) agammaglobulinemia, who respond to measles infection in a normal fashion [10]. Delayed allergy (tuberculin-type skin sensitivity) is intact in these children, and they may make small quantities of humoral antibody as well. Similarly, two complications of measles, encephalitis and thrombocytopenia purpura, are suspected of having an allergic basis, but direct evidence is not available to clarify these points.

Clinical manifestations

The course of measles may be divided into three distinct phases: (1) an essentially asymptomatic incubation period of 10 or 11 days following exposure; (2) a prodromal phase characterized by fever, malaise, and increasing severe coryza, conjunctivitis, and cough which persists for 3 or 4 days before (3) onset of the rash, which usually reaches its maximum within several days and rarely persists longer than 5 to 6 days. The pathognomonic Koplik's spots usually appear in the mouth 24 to 48 h before onset of the rash and may remain discrete for 2 or 3 days. A typical clinical course is illustrated in Fig. 186-1.

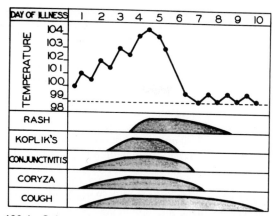

Fig. 186-1 Schematic diagram illustrating clinical course of typical measles. *(From Krugman S, Ward R: Infectious Diseases of Children, 3d ed. St. Louis, CV Mosby, 1964.)*

Prodromal symptoms

The coryza, conjunctivitis, cough, and fever which characterize the measles prodrome increase in severity until the rash has reached its peak. The coryza is similar to that in a severe common cold. The conjunctivitis is most strikingly palpebral, extending to the lid margin so that the eyes appear to be red-rimmed. Lacrimation, lid edema, and photophobia accompany the conjunctivitis. A brassy or barking cough, due to the diffuse involvement of the tracheobronchial tree, may be quite severe even in the absence of a complicating pneumonia, and may persist for a week after the coryza. The temperature frequently reaches 40 to 40.5°C at the peak of the rash but falls promptly to normal in the absence of complications. Generalized adenopathy is common in measles.

Rash (Fig. A3-4b and c)

After a prodromal period of 1 to 7 days, an erythematous, discrete, macular and papular rash appears behind the ears and over the forehead. It spreads down over the neck and trunk and then distally over the upper and lower extremities. The hands and feet are involved. This progression is usually complete, and the rash most intense, within 3 days, which coincides with the peak of the other major clinical signs of fever, cough, and conjunctivitis. Those areas in which the rash appears first tend to be most heavily involved, and confluence of lesions on the face and upper neck is common. Lesions on the legs usually remain discrete and macular and papular. The exanthem begins to fade in the order of its appearance; sometimes clearing of the face begins on the third day while the eruption is still discrete and fresh on the legs. Although the early erythematous rash blanches on pressure, the fading rash consists of a brown staining (inflammatory melanosis with old hemorrhage) which does not blanch [11]. Variable degrees of fine, branny desquamation may be present as the rash clears. In the United States, the desquamation is never as extensive as that which may occur in severe scarlet fever, but desquamation has been described as quite marked in certain areas of the world such as Nigeria [12].

The severe hemorrhagic measles (black measles) associated with extreme toxicity, respiratory tract and gastrointestinal bleeding, hyperpyrexia, and significant mortality rate is now rare and should not be confused with the purpuric lesions that may be seen in fair-skinned children during the course of ordinary measles.

Oral lesions

The earliest oral lesions, according to Weinstein [11], are a "series of pin-point elevations connected by a network of minute vessels on the soft palate." These red dots then coalesce as the entire pharynx becomes reddened. Herrman spots, bluish gray or white areas on the tonsils, also may be present. Neither of these lesions is pathognomonic of measles. The pathognomonic lesions of measles described by Henry Koplik [13], a New York pediatrician, begin as small, irregular, bright red spots, which usually precede onset of the rash by 24 to 48 h. In the center of each red spot is a minute bluish white speck. These Koplik's spots are most heavily clustered on the buccal mucosa opposite the second molars (Fig. A3-4a), but occasionally are on the conjunctivae at the inner canthus, and at autopsy in the large intestine [14]. During the first day of rash, the Koplik's spots usually are easy to see as a cluster of fine grains of sand on a red background. They usually become less distinct as the rash progresses.

Complications

The complications of measles fall into two categories: those that are due to the measles infection alone and/or the patient's response to the infection, and those due to superinfection with pathogenic bacteria. Encephalitis, which occurs in approximately 1 out of every 800 cases, is the most dreaded and unpredictable complication of measles. Although most children recover completely, death or permanent brain damage occurs in a significant minority of children who develop measles encephalitis. Purpura, usually associated with thrombocytopenia, may be severe. These complications may be due to a direct effect of measles virus on the target tissues, or there may be an immunologic component. Common bacterial complications are otitis media and pneumonia caused by the pneumococcus, group A hemolytic streptococcus, *Hemophilus influenzae*, or, occasionally, *Staphylococcus aureus*. The onset of these complications is frequently accompanied by a secondary fever spike or prolongation of fever at a time when defervescence would ordinarily be expected.

Measles may aggravate or exacerbate tuberculosis. The reasons for this and for the transient anergy it produces are unknown. Both measles and measles vaccine may depress the tuberculin skin test reaction for 2 or 3 weeks.

A complication, new since the "vaccine era," has been described in children who received killed measles virus vaccine and subsequently were exposed to and infected with natural measles [15]. Some of these children have developed atypical infection characterized by urticarial, vesicular, and petechial rashes, swollen hands and feet, severe pneumonia, high fever, and extreme prostration. Although children may be quite sick with this syndrome, the illness appears to be self-limited. Similarly, administration of the live attenuated measles virus vaccine after prior immunization with the killed vaccine may produce erythema, edema, and even vesiculation at the injection site with or without fever for several days.

Another late-developing complication of measles is subacute sclerosing panencephalitis (SSPE). Patients with this progressive and usually fatal disease recover uneventfully after acute measles. Months or years later, mental and motor deterioration, often with myoclonic seizures, are associated with a characteristic spike and wave pattern of the electroencephalogram, remarkably elevated serum and cerebrospinal fluid (CSF) measles antibody titers, and elevated total CSF IgG. In brain tissue, measles virus antigen has been demonstrated by immunofluorescence, measles-like nucleocapsids have been seen on electron microscopy, and infectious virus with the characteristics of measles has been isolated in tissue culture by meticulous techniques of cocultivation and serial passage. Fortunately, this rare complication (estimated at 5 to 10 cases per million cases of measles) appears to be even less common among children protected by attenuated measles vaccines (1 case per million doses of vaccine).

Laboratory findings

In uncomplicated measles, routine laboratory tests are unremarkable and not particularly helpful. There is a mild leukopenia, and the chest roentgenogram frequently reveals an increase in bronchovascular markings. Cytologic examination of nasal secretion and sputum may demonstrate characteristic multinucleated giant cells.

Isolation of measles virus from blood, urine, or pharyngeal secretions during the prodromal and early rash period (see "Etiology and Pathogenesis," above) requires virus laboratory facilities which are available in only a limited number of research and reference institutions.

Serologic tests for measles include measurements of neutralizing, complement-fixing (CF), and hemagglutination-inhibiting (HI) antibodies. Paired serums taken shortly after onset of rash and 2 weeks later will show diagnostic (fourfold or greater) rises in measles antibody measured by each of these tests. Neutralizing and HI antibody persist at detectable levels for many years after natural infection (probably for life in most instances), but CF antibody persistence is not so predictable [16]. The most sensitive and convenient of these serologic tests are the HI technique [17] and the enzyme-linked immunosorbent assay (ELISA) [18]. These tests, which are specific for measles, can be most helpful in clarifying the cause of the unusual case of atypical measles. Bacterial superinfections and measles encephalitis are usually associated with a polymorphonuclear leukocytosis.

Pathology

The measles exanthem begins with hyaline necrosis of epidermal cells, followed by exudation of serum around the superficial vessels in the dermis and by proliferation of endothelial cells [19]. The epithelial cells become necrotic. Intranuclear inclusions may be seen. In the later stages, there are leukocytic infiltration of the dermis and lymphocytic cuffing of vessels. In uncomplicated measles, the invariable presence of multinucleated giant cells in the respiratory tract and lymphoid tissues (Warthin-Finkeldey cells) throughout the body has been accepted as evidence of measles virus invasion of these tissues (see "Etiology and Pathogenesis," above). Tracheobronchitis is as much a part of measles as the exanthem. Rarely, a fatal pneumonia, characterized by the presence of giant cells in the lungs, occurs in children with underlying disease such as leukemia. The histopathologic characteristics of measles encephalitis are similar to those observed in other postviral encephalitides. Early lesions include lymphocytic infiltration of the walls of small veins in gray and white matter, measured cellular infiltration, degeneration of ganglion cells, and microglial proliferation. Perivascular demyelinization follows these initial changes. Adams et al [20] described intranuclear and intracytoplasmic inclusions and small giant cells in brain tissue obtained from fatal cases of measles encephalitis. Confirmation of these observations by others would add indirect support to the concept that direct invasion of the central nervous system by measles virus is of pathogenic significance in measles encephalitis.

Diagnosis

The clinical course of full-blown measles is so characteristic that diagnosis should represent no problem. The 3- to 4-day prodrome of cough, conjunctivitis, coryza, with appearance of Koplik's spots, then a macular and papular rash, is unambiguous. Laboratory confirmation is usually not necessary. (For differential diagnosis of febrile exanthems, including rubella, see Atlas 3.) However, when measles has been modified by prophylactic administration of human immunoglobulin at the time of exposure (see "Treatment," below), the disease may be significantly attenuated; it may consist of various combinations of brief fever, cough, and rash, or it may be subclinical.

The unusual clinical picture seen in patients who develop measles despite prior immunization with inactivated (killed) measles vaccine may be diagnosed on the basis of a prior history of such immunization and recent measles exposure (see "Complications," above).

Treatment

As in other systemic viral infections, there is no specific therapy for measles. Supportive therapy, consisting of rest, diet, hydration, aspirin, a vaporizer, and mild antitussive agents appropriate for the febrile child with tracheobronchitis, is frequently helpful in management of the self-limited disease. The prophylactic administration of antibiotics is unwarranted, since it does not prevent bacterial complications and, in fact, may predispose the patient to superinfection with a treatment-resistant organism [21]. Antibiotic therapy should be instituted promptly, however, if bacterial complications develop (see "Complications," above). Therapy for measles encephalitis is also supportive.

Prevention

Measles is preventable. Immunization with a single injection of live attenuated measles virus vaccine produces long-lasting, perhaps lifetime, protection. Vaccination should be deferred until the age of 15 months so that persistence of maternal measles antibody does not interfere with a "take." In part because of this interference of maternal antibody, measles has remained a major cause of morbidity and mortality among young infants in developing countries. Recently, Sabin et al demonstrated in a small trial that children age 4 to 6 months and older could be immunized successfully by live measles virus vaccine administered as an aerosol by a nebulizer and face mask [22]. The practical value of this approach cannot be determined until larger-scale studies are completed. Because of the evidence that use of the inactivated (killed) type of measles vaccine may be followed by severe, atypical measles when the vaccine is subsequently exposed to natural ("virulent") measles, this type of vaccine is no longer licensed in this country.

Immune serum globulin (ISG) may be used to modify or prevent measles in susceptible persons if given within six days of exposure. The recommended dose is 0.25 mL/kg of body weight (maximum dose 15 mL). ISG may be especially useful for infants under age one year and older immunosuppressed individuals, for whom live virus vaccine is contraindicated.

Course and prognosis

Uncomplicated measles runs a self-limited course, lasting about 10 days, with no sequelae. However, the prognosis varies greatly with the age of the patient and the nutritional and general health status. In recent years, just prior to widespread measles immunization, in the United States approximately 500 deaths were attributed to measles each year. The mortality rate is highest in infants under 1 year of age—approximately 30 per 100,000 cases [23]. In less well developed countries, the morbidity and mortality rates associated with measles establish this disease as a major problem of child health. For example, an estimated 84,500 children died from measles in India in 1959; this represents a case fatality rate 153 times greater than that in the United States [24]. In one Nigerian hospital, measles and its complications accounted for 16 percent of pediatric admissions and represented the most frequent cause of death (22 percent) [12]. These morbidity and mortality figures provide ample justification for the present efforts to eradicate measles by extensive immunization programs in many areas of the world.

References

1. Katz SL, Enders JF: Measles virus, in *Viral and Rickettsial Infections of Man,* 4th ed, edited by FL Horsfall Jr, I Tamm. Philadelphia, JB Lippincott, 1965, p 784
2. Josias A: Récherches expérimentales sur la transmissibilité de la rugeole aux animaux. *Med Mod* **9**:158, 1898
3. Anderson JF, Goldberger J: Experimental measles in a monkey; a preliminary note. *Public Health Rep* **26**:847, 1911
4. Blake FG, Trask JD Jr: Studies on measles. I. Susceptibility of monkeys to the virus of measles. *J Exp Med* **33**:385, 1921
5. Enders JF, Peebles TC: Propagation in tissue cultures of cytopathogenic agents from patients with measles. *Proc Soc Exp Biol Med* **86**:277, 1954
6. Enders JF et al: Studies on an attenuated measles-virus vaccine. I. Development and preparation of the vaccine: technics for assay of effects of vaccination. *N Engl J Med* **263**:153, 1960
7. Enders JF: Measles virus: historical review, isolation and behavior in various systems. *Am J Dis Child* **103**:282, 1962
8. Gresser I, Katz SL: Isolation of measles virus from urine. *N Engl J Med* **263**:452, 1960
9. Mitus A et al: Persistence of measles virus and depression of antibody formation in patients with giant cell pneumonia after measles. *N Engl J Med* **261**:882, 1959
10. Janeway CA, Gitlin D: The gamma globulins. *Adv Pediatr* **9**:65, 1957
11. Weinstein L: *The Practice of Infectious Disease.* New York, McGraw-Hill, 1958
12. Morley DC: Measles in Nigeria. *Am J Dis Child* **103**:230, 1962
13. Koplik H: The diagnosis of the invasion of measles from a study of the exanthema as it appears on the buccal mucous membrane. *Arch Pediatr* **13**:918, 1896
14. Corbett EU: The visceral lesions in measles. *Am J Pathol* **21**:905, 1945
15. Rauh LW, Schmidt R: Measles immunization with killed virus vaccine: serum antibody titers and experience with exposure to measles epidemic. *Am J Dis Child* **109**:232, 1965
16. Krugman S et al: Studies on immunity to measles. *J Pediatr* **66**:471, 1965
17. Rosen L: Hemagglutination and hemagglutination-inhibition with measles virus. *Virology* **13**:139, 1961
18. Parker JC et al: Sensitivity of enzyme-linked immunosorbent assay, complement fixation, and hemagglutination inhibition serological tests for detection of Sendai virus antibody in laboratory mice. *J Clin Microbiol* **9**:444, 1979
19. Robbins FC: Measles: clinical features. *Am J Dis Child* **103**:266, 1962
20. Adams JM et al: Inclusion bodies in measles encephalitis. *JAMA* **195**:290, 1966
21. Weinstein L: Failure of chemotherapy to prevent the bacterial complications of measles. *N Engl J Med* **253**:679, 1955
22. Sabin AB et al: Successful immunization of children with and without maternal antibody by aerosol measles vaccine. *JAMA* **249**:2651, 1983
23. Langmuir AD: Medical importance of measles. *Am J Dis Child* **103**:224, 1962
24. Taneja PN et al: Importance of measles to India. *Am J Dis Child* **103**:226, 1962

Bibliography

Editorial: Reactions following measles vaccination. *N Engl J Med* **277**:265, 1967
Katz SL et al (eds): International Symposium on Measles Immunization. *Rev Infect Dis* **5**:389, 1983
Krugman S: Present status of measles and rubella immunization in the United States. A medical progress report. *J Pediatr* **90**:1, 1977

CHAPTER 187

EXANTHEM SUBITUM (ROSEOLA INFANTUM)

Philip A. Brunell

Definition

Exanthem subitum is a disease of infants that is characterized by the onset of rash following 3 to 5 days of high fever. Symptoms other than fever are usually absent during the preeruptive phase.

Historical aspects

Zahorsky [1] provided the first description of this disease which clearly set it apart from the toxic or infectious erythemas of childhood. The name *exanthem subitum,* which means "sudden rash," was subsequently suggested as a more appropriate designation for this illness than roseola infantum [2].

Epidemiology

Good epidemiologic data are not available for exanthem subitum, since the disease is not reportable and is frequently misdiagnosed. The available data, however, indicate that the clinical illness (1) probably occurs less commonly than other childhood exanthems, e.g., chickenpox or measles, (2) occurs sporadically during the late fall or spring months [3–5], (3) rarely causes secondary cases in families [1,2], and (4) is seen most frequently in infants between the ages of 6 months and 2 years [1,3]. Exanthem subitum is commonly seen in children up to age 4, and, in rare instances, cases have been reported in children as old as 9 and 14 years of age [1]. Exanthem subitum is rarely seen in infants under 6 months of age. Young infants do not get the disease, either because they are protected by maternal antibodies or because they have limited exposure to a relatively noncontagious illness.

The infrequent occurrence of secondary cases in families and the low incidence as compared with other childhood exanthems indicate that the disease either is only slightly contagious or has a high subclinical attack rate.

The incubation period of exanthem subitum has been estimated, from outbreaks in orphanages, to be from 5 to 15 days [6]. Secondary cases are not commonly seen following admission of children with exanthem subitum to hospital wards.

Etiology and pathogenesis

Although many attempts have been made to isolate the etiologic agent, none has been successful. The disease has been produced in an infant by inoculation of serum from a patient with exanthem subitum. Monkeys inoculated with serum or throat washings from an affected child develop fever and a decrease in white blood cell count [7].

Clinical manifestations

The preeruptive phase is characterized by the sudden onset of fever. Temperatures are in the range of 38.9 to 40.5°C. Fever is fairly constant; it ordinarily lasts 3 to 5 days, then usually decreases by crisis.

Children appear remarkably well in spite of their high temperature. Their appetite is unimpaired. A slight injection of the pharynx and fauces is usually found. An exanthem has been described on the soft palate [3]. Swelling of the eyelids has also been observed prior to the onset of rash [8]. Suboccipital lymphadenopathy appears during the febrile period and persists during the eruption [5].

Convulsions may occur at the onset of the preeruptive phase. It is not clear whether this is because of the rapid rise in fever or because of an encephalitic component of the illness.

The onset of rash coincides with the disappearance of fever. Skin lesions are commonly found on the trunk. When there is extensive involvement, the rash may also be present to a lesser extent on the proximal extremities, neck, and face. The lesions are discrete and small, 3- to 5-mm pink macules. Some are papular with a clear halo. The rash is ordinarily present for about 24 h but may last only a few hours or as long as 2 days. The rash does not, as a rule, desquamate or become pigmented.

Leukopenia is usually found during the course. White blood cell counts in the range of 3000 to 5000 per mm^3 are common. A relative lymphocytosis occurs, and atypical leukocytes may be seen. Nucleogeminy has been observed in cells from urine sediment obtained from patients [9]. There are no specific serologic tests for this disease.

Diagnosis

During the preeruptive phase, it is difficult, if not impossible, to make a diagnosis since there is a paucity of physical signs. The children may receive medications which produce rashes and further confuse the picture.

With the appearance of rash, several diagnoses are suggested. A history of exposure to rubella, scarlet fever, or measles should always be determined. If it can be ascertained that the child is immune to measles or rubella because of previous infection or immunization, these infections can usually be ruled out.

Although measles also has a febrile prodrome, cough, conjunctivitis, and coryza are usually marked. The rash in measles tends to be confluent and appears first on the face and back of the ears. Specific laboratory tests are available to confirm the diagnosis of measles.

Fever is not usually as high in rubella as in exanthem subitum. In rubella, prominent postauricular and suboccipital nodes can be palpated, while the lymph nodes are unremarkable in exanthem subitum. In rubella, the rash is ordinarily prominent on the face. Specific laboratory tests are available to confirm the diagnosis of rubella.

Scarlet fever is accompanied by obvious signs of pharyngitis. The rash is confluent and has a characteristic distribution and appearance that distinguish this disease from exanthem subitum. Laboratory evidence of streptococcal infection can usually be obtained.

Erythema infectiosum (fifth disease) and rashes due to certain enteroviruses, e.g., echo 9 or echo 16, must be considered in the differential diagnosis.

Treatment

There is no specific therapy.

Course and prognosis

Children have remarkably little disability despite their high temperatures. With the appearance of rash, there is a return of well-being. Except for rare neurologic complications, there are no sequelae [10].

References

1. Zahorsky J: Roseola infantum. *JAMA* **61**:1446, 1913
2. Veeder BS, Hempelmann TC: Febrile exanthem occurring in childhood (exanthem subitum). *JAMA* **77**:1787, 1921
3. Clemens HH: Exanthem subitum (roseola infantum): report of 80 cases. *J Pediatr* **26**:66, 1945
4. Berenberg W et al: Roseola infantum (exanthem subitum). *N Engl J Med* **241**:253, 1949
5. McEnery JT: Postoccipital lymphadenopathy as a diagnostic sign in roseola infantum (exanthem subitum). *Clin Pediatr (Phila)* **9**:512, 1970
6. Barenberg LH, Greenspan L: Exanthema subitum (roseola infantum). *Am J Dis Child* **58**:983, 1939
7. Kempe CH et al: Studies on etiology of exanthema subitum (roseola infantum). *J Pediatr* **37**:561, 1950
8. Berliner BC: A physical sign useful in diagnosis of roseola infantum before the rash. *Pediatrics* **25**:1034, 1960
9. Gittes RF: Observation of nucleogeminy in urinary-sediment cells in roseola-infantum syndrome. *N Engl J Med* **269**:446, 1963
10. Burstine RC, Paine RS: Residual encephalopathy following roseola infantum. *Am J Dis Child* **98**:144, 1959

CHAPTER 188

HAND-FOOT-AND-MOUTH DISEASE

Antoinette F. Hood and Martin C. Mihm, Jr.

Hand-foot-and-mouth disease (HFMD), a distinctive clinical syndrome caused by an enterovirus, is clinically manifested by characteristic lesions in the mouth and on the extremities. In 1958 Robinson et al [1] described an epidemic of vesicular stomatitis with an exanthem on the hands and feet from which Coxsackie virus type A_{16} was isolated. A second epidemic, in England, was described by Alsop et al [2] who coined the term *hand-foot-and-mouth disease*. Subsequently epidemics and individual cases have been reported from around the world. The epidemic disease is usually associated with Coxsackie A_{16} virus or enterovirus 71 [3,4]. Sporadic cases have been reported in association with Coxsackie A_5 [5], A_9 [6], A_{10} [7,8], B_2 and B_5 [9]. HFMD usually affects children under the age of 10, although in one series 10 of 11 patients were 15 years of age [10].

Pathogenesis

Infections due to an enterovirus, a member of the picornavirus group, typically develop according to a basic pathogenic mechanism [11]. Initial viral implantation in the buccal mucosa and ileum is followed within 24 h by extension to regional lymph nodes. At 72 h, a viremia occurs followed by the seeding of viruses to the sites of secondary infection, which, in HFMD, are the oral mucosa and the skin of the hands and feet. By the seventh day there is a rise in serum antibodies, and the virus disappears from the blood and other sites of implantation.

Epidemiology

The incubation period in HFMD is short, from 3 to 6 days. The disease is highly contagious and the spread of virus from person to person occurs by the oral–oral and fecal–oral routes.

During epidemics of HFMD, there is spread from child to child (horizontal spread) and then to adults (vertical spread) in various family groups. In one study 44 percent of asymptomatic family contacts had laboratory evidence of infection; 53 percent of infected asymptomatic individuals were adults [12]. In temperate climates there is usually a seasonal pattern for the occurrence of the clinical syndromes caused by enterovirus, as well as for the isolation of the virus from the sewage and fecal samples taken from populations where epidemics occur. Epidemic outbreaks of HFMD tend to occur in the warmer months between June and October; however, one winter-month episode occurred in England in 1965–1966 [13].

Clinical manifestations

The typical signs and symptoms of HFMD may be preceded by a brief prodrome of 12 to 24 h characterized by

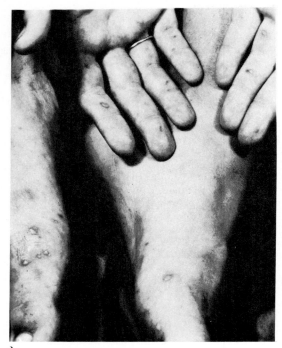

a

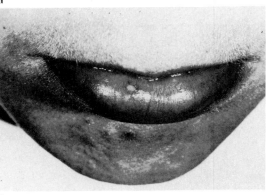

b

Fig. 188-1   (a) Small vesicular and papular lesions distributed on the hands and feet are characteristic of hand-foot-and-mouth syndrome. (b) Vesicles on the lips may accompany mucosal ulcerations as part of the oral manifestation of Coxsackie virus A$_{16}$ infection.

low-grade fever, malaise, and abdominal pain. The most frequent finding of the disease is ulcerative oral lesions. In one series, sore mouth and refusal to eat were the presenting complaints in over 80 percent of laboratory-confirmed cases; oral lesions were present in 100 percent [12]. The number of oral lesions averages between 5 and 10. Although the lesions may be found anywhere within the oral cavity, they appear most frequently on the tongue, hard palate, and buccal mucosa [12]. The oral lesions begin as erythematous papules 2 to 8 mm in diameter, then progress to form gray, thin-walled vesicles surrounded by a zone of erythema. The vesicular stage is short and rarely seen since the vesicles progress to form shallow, yellow to gray ulcerations with an erythematous halo. Small lesions may coalesce to form larger ones. These lesions are usually painful and may interfere with eating; however, they usually resolve in 5 to 10 days without treatment.

The cutaneous lesions appear together with or shortly after the oral lesions. They may vary in number from a few to over 100. The dorsal surfaces and sides of the fingers, hands, toes, and feet are more often involved than the palms and soles. Each lesion begins as an erythematous macule or papule, 2 to 10 mm in size, in the center of which arises a gray, round to oval vesicle [13]. The lesions often run in or parallel to the skin lines (Figs. A3-6c and d). The vesicles are often surrounded by a red areola (Fig. 188-1); they may be asymptomatic or tender. They crust after a few days and gradually disappear over the course of 7 to 10 days.

Macular and papular erythematous lesions have also been described in association with the more typical lesions of HFMD in infants. This eruption occurs principally on the buttocks, but is occasionally generalized [13–17].

Patients may present with either enanthem or exanthem, but most patients manifest both aspects of the disease. In general, the disease is accompanied by minimal or mild signs and symptoms, such as low-grade fever, vague malaise, and sore mouth. Some patients, however, are afflicted with high fever, marked malaise, diarrhea, and occasionally even joint pains [16]. In Japan, epidemics of HFMD caused by enterovirus 71 have been associated with an 8 to 24 percent incidence of neurologic signs and symptoms such as headache, nuchal rigidity, hyperreflexia, tremor, ataxia, myoclonus, and CSF pleocytosis [3]. Most commonly, however, the entire disease runs its course in 7 to 10 days without the patient's awareness of debility. A few cases of prolonged or recurrent HFMD have been observed [14,17]. Serious sequelae rarely occur; however, Coxsackie virus has been implicated as the etiologic agent in cases of myocarditis [18,19], meningoencephalitis [18], aseptic meningitis [18,20], paralytic disease [21], and a systemic illness resembling rubeola [22]. Infection acquired during the first trimester of pregnancy may result in spontaneous abortion [23].

Diagnostic procedures

The causative viral agent may be isolated from an affected subject by inoculation of suckling mice and appropriate tissue culture with fluid from vesicles, throat washings, and stool specimens. More than one technique is suggested for virus isolation because the various strains of these viruses possess different characteristics and differ in their ease of isolation.

Serum-neutralizing antibody against these viruses appears early in the illness and often rapidly disappears; therefore, serologic examination performed during the course of the illness may demonstrate antibody only during the acute, and not during the convalescent, phase of the disease.

Significantly elevated titers of complement-fixing antibody may be detected in serum drawn from a patient during the convalescent stage of the illness. These antibodies, however, are usually group specific, rather than type specific.

Histopathology

The characteristic cutaneous lesion is an intraepidermal vesicle containing neutrophils, mononuclear cells, and pro-

Fig. 188-2 (a) An intraepidermal bulla with focal loss of the epidermis at the base. The blister cavity is filled with neutrophils and mononuclear cells. H&E; X140. **(b)** Higher magnification of blister roof showing numerous dyskeratotic epidermal cells and exocytosis of mononuclear cells. H&E; X400.

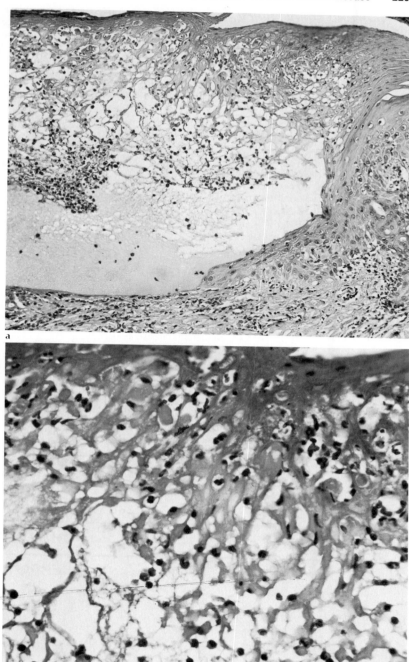

teinaceous eosinophilic material. As the lesion ages, there may be focal loss of the basal cell layer resulting in a subepidermal bulla. The roof of the blister is often necrotic with discrete eosinophilic dyskeratotic and acantholytic epidermal cells. The epidermis immediately adjacent to the vesicle exhibits intercellular and intracellular edema or so-called reticular degeneration (Fig. 188-2). Eosinophilic intranuclear inclusions have been described [24]. The dermis beneath a vesicle is edematous and contains a perivascular polymorphous infiltrate composed of lymphocytes and neutrophils.

Intracytoplasmic particles in a crystalline array charac-teristic of Coxsackie virus have been observed with electron microscopy [24].

Material obtained by scraping the base of a vesicle, smeared on a glass slide, and stained with Giemsa's stain reveal no multinucleated giant cells or inclusion bodies [10,25].

Treatment

There is no specific treatment for HFMD. Topical application of dyclonine HCl solution (Dyclone) or lidocaine

(Xylocaine, ointment or viscous) may reduce the discomfort accompanying the oral ulcerations.

References

1. Robinson CR et al: Report on an outbreak of febrile illness with pharyngeal lesions and exanthem. Toronto, Summer 1957—isolation of group A Coxsackie virus. *Can Med Assoc J* **79**:615, 1958
2. Alsop J et al: "Hand-foot-and-mouth disease" in Birmingham in 1959. *Br Med J* **2**:1708, 1960
3. Ishimaru Y et al: Outbreaks of hand, foot, and mouth disease by enterovirus 71. *Arch Dis Child* **55**:583, 1980
4. Tagaya I et al: A large-scale epidemic of hand, foot and mouth disease associated with enterovirus 71 infection in Japan in 1978. *Jpn J Med Sci* **34**:191, 1981
5. Flewett TH et al: "Hand, foot, and mouth disease" associated with Coxsackie A_5 virus. *J Clin Pathol* **16**:53, 1963
6. Hughes RP, Roberts C: Hand, foot, and mouth disease associated with Coxsackie A_9 virus. *Lancet* **2**:751, 1972
7. Clarke SKR et al: Hand, foot, and mouth disease (letter). *Br Med J* **1**:58, 1964
8. Duff MF: Hand-foot-and-mouth syndrome in humans: Coxsackie A_{10} infection in New Zealand. *Br Med J* **2**:661, 1968
9. Lindenbaum JE et al: Hand, foot, and mouth disease associated with Coxsackie virus group B. *Scand J Infect Dis* **7**:161, 1975
10. Miller GD, Tindall JP: Hand, foot, and mouth disease. *JAMA* **203**:827, 1968
11. Cherry JD, Nelson DB: Enterovirus infections: their epidemiology and pathogenesis. *Clin Pediatr* **5**:659, 1966
12. Adler JL et al: Epidemiologic investigation of hand, foot, and mouth disease. Infection caused by Coxsackie A_{16} in Baltimore, June through September 1968. *Am J Dis Child* **120**:309, 1970
13. Higgins PG, Warin RP: Hand, foot, and mouth disease: a clinically recognizable virus infection seen mainly in children. *Clin Pediatr* **6**:373, 1967
14. Evans AD, Waddington E: Hand, foot and mouth disease in South Wales, 1964. *Br J Dermatol* **79**:309, 1967
15. Meadow SR: Hand, foot, and mouth disease. *Arch Dis Child* **40**:560, 1965
16. Fields JP et al: Hand, foot, and mouth disease. *Arch Dermatol* **99**:243, 1969
17. Mihm MC Jr et al: A clinical, epidemiologic, and virologic study of hand, foot, and mouth syndrome. *Proceedings of the Third Joint Meeting of the Clinical Society and Commissioned Officers Association of the United States Public Health Service, March 25–29, 1968, San Francisco, California,* p 64
18. Wright HT et al: Fatal infection in an infant associated with Coxsackie virus group A, type 16. *N Engl J Med* **268**:1041, 1963
19. Baker DA, Phillips CA: Fatal hand-foot-and-mouth disease in an infant caused by Coxsackie virus A_7. *JAMA* **242**:1065, 1979
20. Froeschie JE et al: Hand, foot, and mouth disease (Coxsackie A_{16}) in Atlanta. *Am J Dis Child* **114**:278, 1967
21. Magoffin RL, Lenette EH: Nonpolioviruses and paralytic disease. *Calif Med* **97**:1, 1962
22. Gohd RS, Faigel HC: Hand-foot-and-mouth disease resembling measles. A life-threatening disease: case report. *Pediatrics* **37**:644, 1966
23. Ogilvie MM, Tearne CF: Spontaneous abortion after hand-foot-and-mouth disease caused by Coxsackie virus A_{16}. *Br Med J* **281**:1527, 1980
24. Kimura A et al: Light and electron microscopic study of skin lesions of patients with the hand, foot and mouth disease. *Tohoku J Med* **122**:237, 1977
25. Cherry JD, Jahn CL: Hand, foot, and mouth syndrome. Report of six cases due to Coxsackie virus, group A, type 16. *Pediatrics* **37**:637, 1966

CHAPTER 189

HERPANGINA

Robert H. Parrott

Definition [1–4]

Herpangina is a specific infectious disease in which, characteristically, peculiar lesions appear on the mucous membrane around the soft palate, tonsillar pillars, and fauces. In temperate climates it appears almost exclusively in the summertime and early fall, and it affects children primarily. The etiologic agent has been established as any of six or seven different group A Coxsackie virus types, although some authorities have suggested that herpangina may also occur as part of a larger clinical syndrome in response to other enteroviruses.

Historical aspects [1]

Zahorsky first described herpangina as a specific entity in 1920. Outbreaks of an illness similar to what he called herpangina were reported in summer camps and nursery schools in 1939 and 1941. Later, Huebner and his associates recovered viruses of the Coxsackie group A from throat washings and feces of a group of patients with herpangina. This was the first suggestion that specific viruses caused the disease. The clinical association has been confirmed in many reports since that time.

Epidemiology [3]

The viruses that are responsible for herpangina may also result in subclinical infection or febrile illness without typical oropharyngeal lesions. These viruses also may be isolated from as many as 1.5 to 7.5 percent of persons who are not ill during the summer in a temperate climate. The group A Coxsackie viruses may spread readily in a family or neighborhood group, and, in fact, from patient to patient in hospitals. Virus may persist in the feces for up to 47 days after acute infection. Fecal material is a common source of isolation of virus, although in herpangina the agent may be recovered from saliva, nasal secretions, the oropharynx, and stomach washings. Undoubtedly the major method of spread early in illness is from oropharyngeal secretions. Herpangina and the group A Coxsackie agents which cause it have been reported from many parts of the world; the disease is presumably worldwide in distribution.

Etiology and pathogenesis [3,4]

The clinical association of group A Coxsackie viruses with herpangina has occurred much more often than would be expected by chance. In most studies the virus types recovered have been the same—A_2, A_4, A_5, A_6, A_8, and A_{10}. Type 3 was found in cases of herpangina in one locale during one season. Whether the oropharyngeal lesions sometimes seen during infection with other Coxsackie viruses or echo viruses should be considered herpangina is a matter of definition. The herpangina strains of group A Coxsackie virus can cause febrile illness without visible oropharyngeal lesions, and this situation should be strongly suspected when one finds fever and pharyngitis in siblings of a patient who has clinically distinct herpangina.

There is no sex difference and no known difference by race or national origin in the occurrence of the disease. In Washington, D.C., 50 percent of cases occur in July, 35 percent in August, 5 percent in June, and 10 percent in September. The incubation period is approximately 4 days. Permanent immunity occurs to the type-specific agent. However, since there are several group A Coxsackie viruses which can cause the disease, the clinical syndrome may recur.

Clinical manifestations [2]

The child affected with herpangina is usually in good health until a sudden onset of fever. In Zahorsky's description: "The child feels tired and often complains of pain in the back and extremities. Headache and pains in the back of the neck are frequently marked symptoms and lead one to expect poliomyelitis at times. This impression is often accentuated by the tenderness of the extremities on movement."

In 68 cases studied at Children's Hospital in Washington, D.C., temperature ranging from 38.3 to 40.5° C was found in 89 percent of the patients and lasted for 1 to 4 days. Five percent had convulsions with the onset of fever. Seventy percent complained of anorexia, dysphagia, or sore throat. There was vomiting in 38 percent, abdominal pain in 21 percent, and headache in 16 percent.

The characteristic feature of the disease is the presence of gray-white papulovesicular lesions, about 1 to 2 mm in diameter (Fig. 189-1), which progress to slightly larger ulcers. A zone of erythema surrounds the lesion usually. The lesions are distributed, in order of frequency, on the anterior pillars of the tonsillar fauces, the soft palate, the uvula, and the tonsils themselves. The lesions may persist for 4 to 6 days. During the illness there is usually a diffuse pharyngeal hyperemia. Occasionally there is nonpurulent conjunctivitis, and rarely a rash. Similar lesions have been reported occurring in the vagina in the course of what was otherwise typical herpangina. In a Washington, D.C. se-

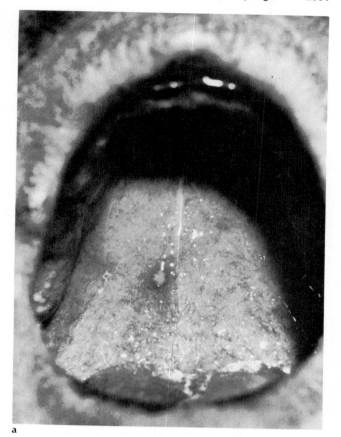

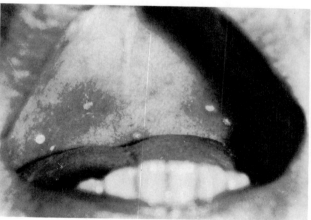

Fig. 189-1 The typical feature of herpangina is the presence of gray-white papulovesicular lesions on the palate, as illustrated. These progress to slightly larger ulcers. A zone of erythema surrounds the lesions. *(Courtesy of K. Wolff, M.D.)*

ries, total peripheral white blood cell counts were under 10,000 per cubic millimeter in 53 percent of the cases; 20 percent ranged from 10,000 to 15,000; and 27 percent were over 15,000.

Pathology

The only visible lesions occurring in the course of this disease are the oropharyngeal lesions already described and the diffuse pharyngeal hyperemia. Specific histologic studies of these lesions have not been reported.

Diagnosis and differential diagnosis [3,5]

The diagnosis is primarily clinical. It can be confirmed in the laboratory either by obtaining material from the oropharyngeal lesions or an anal swab for recovery of group A Coxsackie viruses or by type-specific serologic study with blood specimens obtained early in the illness and during convalescence. The group A Coxsackie viruses induce flaccid paralysis and marked muscle degeneration but no significant central nervous system lesions in suckling mice and cause no apparent disease in adult mice. Most of the herpangina strains of Coxsackie virus can be recovered only in suckling mice and not as readily in tissue culture as most of the other Coxsackie viruses.

The clinical conditions that may be confused with herpangina are infectious gingivostomatitis due to herpes simplex virus, acute lymphonodular pharyngitis (also due to a group A Coxsackie virus), or possibly the other oropharyngeal lesions sometimes described in the course of enteroviral infections. Infectious gingivostomatitis is also a common childhood illness. There is fever, with vesicles or ulcers in the oral cavity, occasionally in the pharnyx. It occurs throughout the year. The onset is more gradual than that of herpangina. The major symptoms include fever, dysphagia, sore mouth with a very fetid odor to the breath, and bleeding gums. There are cervical lymphadenopathy and hyperemia, hypertrophy, and hemorrhage of the gums, none of which occurs in herpangina. The vesicles and ulcers are on the gums, tongue, lips, and buccal mucous membrane, as well as occasionally in the location of herpangina lesions. Fever lasts longer, and the oropharyngeal lesions persist for 8 to 14 days. The child with gingivostomatitis is much more severely ill than the one with herpangina.

Acute lymphonodular pharyngitis is an illness that also primarily affects children and is due to Coxsackie A_{10} virus, as reported by Steigman et al [5]. There are headache, malaise, and anorexia with fever. Lesions located on the uvula, palate, anterior pillars, and posterior pharynx, as in herpangina, are described as raised, discrete, white-to-yellow nodules, surrounded by erythema. These lesions do not ulcerate. Symptoms and lesions persist somewhat longer than in herpangina.

Various authors have described vesicles, ulcers, and other types of lesions in the faucial and soft-palate area in the course of infection with Coxsackie viruses B_1 through B_5, with Coxsackie A_7 and A_9, and with echo 9 and 16. In these cases the clinical picture is not that described by Zahorsky and others. These cases suggest that various enteroviruses may produce lesions in this particular location. Some authors have, therefore, suggested that the term *herpangina* be used as a description of oropharyngeal lesions rather than as a description of a specific disease.

In the differential diagnosis of herpangina one must also exclude occasional cases of oral moniliasis; infectious mononucleosis; the enanthems of measles, varicella, scarlatina, and diphtheria; certain heavy-metal poisonings; and deficiency diseases and hematologic disorders. Aphthae which occur as a result of trauma, allergy, or psychogenic factors are not usually accompanied by fever. (For differential diagnosis, see Chap. 101.)

Treatment

The major importance of herpangina for the physician is that making the diagnosis relieves the fear which accompanies sudden fever in children. No specific treatment is available or necessary. Antipyretic or anticonvulsant treatment might be indicated in individual cases.

Course and prognosis

The fever of herpangina rarely lasts more than 4 days, and the lesions rarely more than a week. With the exception of the occasional child who suffers a convulsion, the prognosis is good and the course benign.

References

1. Cole RM et al: Studies of Coxsackie viruses: observations on epidemiological aspects of group A viruses. *Am J Public Health* **41**:1342, 1951
2. Parrott RH, Cramblett HG: Nonbacterial infections affecting nasopharynx. *Pediatr Clin North Am* **4**:115, 1957
3. Parrott RH: Clinical importance of group A Coxsackie viruses. *Ann NY Acad Sci* **67**:230, 1957
4. Cherry JD, Jahn CL: Herpangina: etiologic spectrum. *Pediatrics* **36**:632, 1965
5. Steigman AJ et al: Acute lymphonodular pharyngitis: newly described condition due to Coxsackie A virus. *J Pediatr* **61**:331, 1962

CHAPTER 190

HERPES SIMPLEX

Clyde S. Crumpacker

The human herpes simplex virus consists of two closely related viruses designated herpes simplex virus type 1 (HSV-1) and herpes simplex virus type 2 (HSV-2) (Fig. 190-1). The viruses cause a wide variety of mucocutaneous infections and produce both primary and recurrent infections. The primary infection by herpes simplex virus is more severe and has a different natural history than recurrent disease. Following a primary infection, the virus establishes a latent or dormant state and recurrent disease is caused by reactivation of this dormant virus; then travels

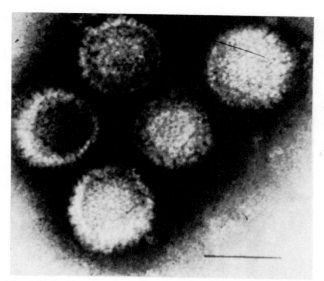

Fig. 190-1   Herpes simplex virion.

down the nerve fiber to establish skin infection. Recurrent facial-oral herpes simplex infection, known as "fever blisters" or "cold sores," afflicts between 25 to 40 percent of people in the United States, and it is the most common manifestation of infection with herpes simplex virus. Facial-oral herpes simplex infection is usually a self-limited infection with mainly cosmetic consequences, but in immunocompromised patients, severe lesions can occur which encompass a large surface area, and produce painful ulcers in the mouth and esophagus.

Genital infection with herpes simplex virus has increased markedly during the past two decades. Data obtained from patient consultations with private physicians indicate that patient consultation for genital herpes increased 3.4 per 100,000 in 1960, to 29.7 per 100,000 in 1979. In the United Kingdom, genital herpes simplex virus infection is increasing at the rate of 11 percent per year [1]. These figures support the estimates that genital herpes infections also occur in primary and recurrent forms and the large majority of genital herpes infections are sexually transmitted. In the college-educated middle-class populations, genital herpes is the most frequently occurring sexually transmitted disease. The natural history and transmission of these viral infections pose a significant health problem. Effective antiviral therapy for these diseases remains an important medical goal. In this chapter, the clinical presentations, diagnosis, and treatment of herpes simplex infections will be discussed.

The viruses

Herpes simplex virus types 1 and 2 contain a double-stranded linear DNA genome of molecular weight 160×10^6 surrounded by a protein coat and lipid envelope. The genomes of HSV-1 and HSV-2 have about 50 percent of the nucleotide sequence in common and 50 percent variable. The viral genomes encode for about 50 viral-specific proteins. These include 5 to 6 viral-specific glycoproteins which are present on the viral surfaces and on the surface of viral-infected cells. These glycoproteins are important for induction of neutralizing antibodies to the virus and

regulate cell fusion exhibited by these viruses. Only one of these surface glycoproteins, gC for HSV-1 and gG for HSV-2, appears to be type specific. There is significant cross-reactivity of antibodies raised against the other glycoproteins between HSV-1 and HSV-2.

The major glycoproteins which induce neutralizing antibodies, the gD glycoprotein of HSV-1 and HSV-2, share 80 percent of the amino acids in common and neutralizing antibodies raised against HSV-1 readily neutralize HSV-2. The viral core proteins and structural proteins comprise 20 viral-specific proteins. The viral protein coat consists of protein arranged in 162 capsomeres around the viral nucleic acid.

The herpes simplex virus genome encodes a number of nonstructural proteins which are important for viral DNA replication. These include a viral thymidine kinase, DNA polymerase, ribonucleotide reductase, and alkaline DNAse. These enzymes have all been mapped to precise locations on the viral genome and mutants of herpes simplex virus have been isolated which contain mutations in the genes encoding these viral enzymes. These viral enzymes, which differ in significant ways from cellular enzymes, can be selectively inhibited by antiviral drugs. The development of antiviral drugs which selectively inhibit viral-specific enzyme targets, such as viral DNA polymerase, has progressed rapidly and permitted the successful application of antiviral chemotherapy for the treatment of herpes simplex infections. The use of rapid techniques of viral diagnosis to make an early diagnosis of herpes simplex infection and begin therapy with drugs, such as acyclovir, has made it possible to effectively treat many forms of mucocutaneous infection with herpes simplex virus.

Primary infection

A hallmark of infections caused by herpes simplex virus is that they occur initially in mucocutaneous locations and then remain dormant in neuronal cells located in ganglia before recurring as outbreaks of mucocutaneous infection. The natural histories of primary and recurrent infections differ, the response to treatment may differ, and they need to be considered separately. Primary infection with herpes simplex occurs primarily by direct exposure through mucocutaneous contact with another infected individual. Primary infection is defined as the first infection with herpes simplex virus in a seronegative patient. There are no reliable well-documented examples of herpes simplex virus being transmitted by the respiratory route. Even though some experimental studies have shown that the virus can persist on surfaces like towels, toilet seats, or counter tops for as long as 30 min, there is no case of a herpes simplex infection being acquired by contact with such a surface. The virus may persist in water or on a wet surface for a short period of time also, but the presence of any halogenated compound in the water inactivates the virus infectivity immediately. There is no evidence that herpes simplex infection can be acquired through water transmission.

For primary facial-oral herpes infection, exposure to herpes simplex in a mother's vaginal secretions during the process of delivery can result in a primary neonatal infection in about 50 percent of the infants exposed to the virus. This usually is first noted at day 4 to 7 of life by the development of characteristic herpetic skin lesions (Fig.

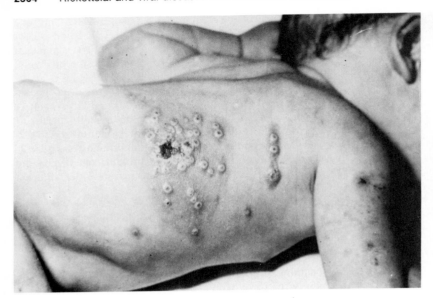

Fig. 190-2 Disseminated herpes simplex in a newborn infant.

190-2). The skin infection commonly occurs in areas of trauma on the body and may begin in areas where scalp electrodes were placed to facilitate fetal monitoring during labor. Neonatal infection with herpes simplex virus may also occur in the absence of skin lesions and directly involve the CNS and visceral organs such as the liver. In the absence of skin lesions, primary neonatal herpes simplex infection is very difficult to diagnose and remains an important challenge for the pediatric clinician. Primary herpes simplex infection in the neonate is a devastating life-threatening infection which must be diagnosed and treated promptly with antiviral drugs.

Primary facial-oral herpes infection usually occurs as an acute gingivostomatitis and ulcers may occur throughout the buccal mucosa (Fig. 190-3). Many cases of herpes gingivostomatitis occur early in life and are probably not diagnosed. It is estimated that a great majority (90 to 95 percent) of an American or British urban population has evidence of herpes simplex facial-oral infection by age 15, whereas only about 30 percent of middle-class college-age American students have antibody to herpes simplex infection [2,3].

Primary genital herpes infection occurs following sexual exposure in perhaps 95 percent of cases. The usual time period of an outbreak of genital herpes is overt between 3 to 14 days following sexual relations with a person with active genital lesions.

Recurrent infection

A characteristic feature of all the herpes viruses is that after primary infection occurs, the virus has the ability to establish latent or dormant infection and then to reactivate to produce recurrent disease (Fig. 190-4). The recurrent disease is usually milder and of shorter duration than the primary infection. In the facial-oral herpes simplex infection, the virus is almost always HSV type 1 and, following the primary episode of stomatitis, the virus migrates to the trigeminal ganglion. In the ganglion of the nerve, the viral genome remains in a suppressed state primarily as a circular episome of viral DNA with very few of the viral genes being expressed. Certain triggering events such as

exposure to sunlight, severe stress, or neurosurgical manipulation of the ganglia will cause the latent virus to reactivate and express its genome to make intact viral particles. The viral particles move down the nerve, probably by axonal flow, and replicate in the epithelial cells of the skin to produce an outbreak of cold sores (Fig. 190-4). Between episodes there is no evidence of viral particles, viral proteins, or viral nucleic acids in the skin at the affected site. These general principles apply to recurrent episodes of herpes infections in all common sites, especially facial-oral herpes, genital herpes, herpes whitlow, and herpes keratitis. In recurrent herpes infections, patients possess antibody to the virus, and immunologically active mononuclear cells and lymphocytes contribute to the pathogenesis and healing of the recurrent outbreak.

Clinical manifestations

Primary gingivostomatitis

Primary herpetic infection of the mouth and pharynx is a disease of children and young adults. The peak years of

Fig. 190-3 Primary facial-oral infection with herpes simplex virus involving the buccal mucosa.

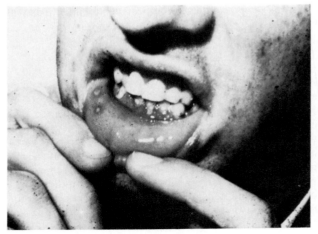

Fig. 190-4 Recurrent facial-oral herpes infection of the lip—"cold sore."

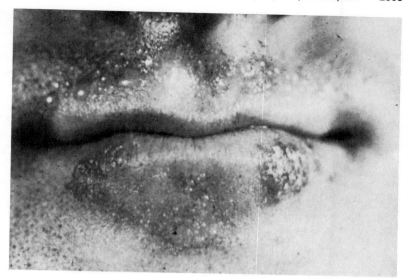

incidence usually occur between age 1 to 5. A study at a large university health service estimated that primary herpes simplex virus infection was a significant cause of sore throats in college students [3]. The infection may be mild and inapparent to severe with high fever. The usual onset is with fever, sore throat and painful vesicles, and ulcerative erosions on the tongue, palate, gingiva, buccal mucosa, and lips. The vesicles on the mucous membranes coalesce to form plaques covered with a gray membrane. Severe oral lesions are associated with drooling, bad breath, enlarged lymph nodes, inability to eat, fever, and generalized complaints. The time from exposure to onset of symptoms is from 5 to 10 days. The diagnosis is suggested by the early onset of lesions in discrete clusters before they spread to extensively involve the entire buccal mucosa. Diagnosis is confirmed by culturing herpes simplex virus from the lesions, or identifying herpes simplex antigens with the use of monoclonal antibodies and immunofluorescent analysis.

The differential diagnosis of primary herpetic gingivostomatitis includes streptococcal pharyngitis, diphtheria, Coxsackie virus infection, aphthous ulcers, infectious mononucleosis, severe candidiasis, pemphigus vulgaris, Behçet's disease, and erythema multiforme.

Recurrent facial-oral herpes simplex

After a primary infection with herpes simplex virus, patients develop antibody to the virus. In population studies in the United States and Great Britain, neutralizing antibody has been found in 40 to 90 percent of a study population. In a study of university students, however, only 30 percent had neutralizing antibody to HSV-1, suggesting that a majority of children from middle-income families reach adulthood without antibody. It is estimated that about one-third of the population of the United States experiences recurrent episodes of facial-oral infection with HSV, known as recurrent herpes labialis or cold sores. The incidence of recurrences is variable in different populations but 15 percent of young adults surveyed had recurrences of at least one lesion per year and in a series of over 1000 young adults, 20 percent have recurrent episodes. The usual number of recurrences is 3 to 4 per year [4,5].

The onset of a cold sore is heralded by itching and burning at the vermilion border of the lip. This may be associated with an erythematous papule which rapidly goes on to become vesicular and to then ulcerate to produce a sore. The open sore crusts over in about 4 days, the scab falls off, and complete healing occurs in 8 to 9 days. Virus can be isolated from cold sores for about 3.5 days and the virus is overwhelmingly HSV-1. Neutralizing antibodies do not prevent recurrent episodes and most patients with recurrent herpes labialis have high levels of neutralizing antibody at the time of recurrence. The most common triggering events to bring on recurrent cold sores are sun exposure, trauma to the lips, emotional stress, and fatigue [6].

Recurrent herpes labialis must be distinguished from other ulcerative lesions such as aphthous ulcers, erythema multiforme, impetigo, and vaccinia infection. The usual location for recurrent herpes labialis is at the skin–lip junction. Recurrent erosive ulcers inside the mouth are most commonly due to aphthous ulcers or erythema multiforme rather than herpes simplex infection. An important distinguishing feature of herpes in the mouth from aphthous ulcers (canker sores) is that herpes begins as a few clustered lesions on one part of the buccal mucosa whereas aphthous ulcers begin as sores on widely separated parts of the buccal mucosa.

Primary genital herpes

In industrial countries, herpes simplex virus is the most common cause of genital ulcerations and accounts for 20 to 50 percent of ulcerative lesions in patients attending sexually transmitted disease clinics. It is estimated that 95 percent of episodes of primary genital herpes occur following sexual exposure to a sexual partner with active lesions. The usual time period between sexual exposure to a person with active genital herpes and development of an acute episode is between 3 to 14 days. The outbreak begins with small grouped vesicles (Fig. 190-5) which break and progress to ulcerative lesions in 2 to 4 days. Most patients present to the physician with ulcerative lesions. The first episode of genital herpes usually has multiple lesions which are present bilaterally and coalesce to involve a larger

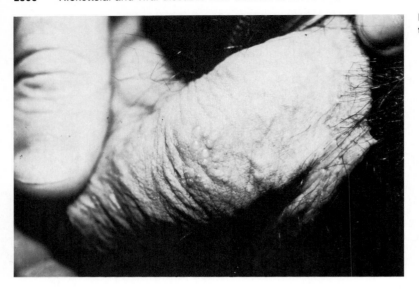

Fig. 190-5 Herpes simplex-induced vesicle on the shaft of a penis.

surface (Fig. 190-6). Recurrent genital herpes frequently presents as a single ulcer. Painful enlarged inguinal lymph nodes are common and the nodes are usually tender on palpation, nonfixed, and slightly firm. About 35 percent of women and 13 percent of men with primary genital herpes will have an aseptic meningitis with fever, stiff neck, headache, photophobia, and pleocytosis in the spinal fluid [7]. The spinal fluid protein may be elevated to near 100 mg/dL and the glucose may fall below 40 mg. Cells are mainly lymphocytes (200 to 1000 per mm³). It is also clear that approximately 20 percent of patients with primary genital herpes will have painful difficulty on urination which may require catheterization of the urinary tract for relief. This is essentially never present in recurrent genital herpes. The dominant local symptoms of primary genital herpes are pain, itching, dysuria, and vaginal and urethral discharge. The severity of these symptoms increases over the first 6 to 7 days of the illness, and peaks at day 8 to 10. New

Fig. 190-6 Primary herpetic vulvovaginitis causing intense edema, pain, and urinary retention.

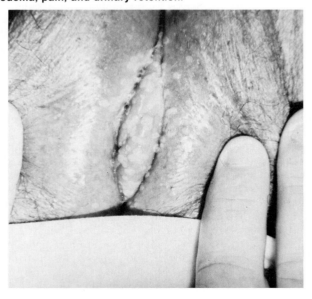

lesions continue to form during the first week of illness in about 75 percent of patients. Both HSV-1 and HSV-2 cause primary genital herpes with 80 percent being associated with isolation of HSV-2 from lesions. Both produce an identical clinical picture, but HSV-1-induced primary disease is associated with many fewer recurrences than when HSV-2 is isolated from the primary episode. Herpes simplex virus has been isolated from the pharynx of 11 percent of patients with primary genital herpes and in only 1 percent of those with recurrent disease [7]. Clinical signs of herpes simplex virus pharyngitis may be mild erythema or diffuse ulcerative and exudative pharyngitis of the posterior pharynx. This may be associated with tender anterior cervical adenopathy and may mimic streptococcal pharyngitis.

The course of primary genital herpes may last 18 to 21 days and virus shedding is present for about 11 days; this correlates with the time from onset of symptoms to the development of crusting. The differential diagnosis of other infections which cause genital ulcers and inguinal lymphadenopathy includes syphilis, chancroid, lymphogranuloma venereum, and granuloma inguinale.

Herpes simplex virus cervicitis

During primary herpes genital infection, virus can be isolated from the cervix in 88 percent of women with primary HSV-2 infection and in 80 percent of women with primary HSV-1 infection. Virus is isolated in 65 percent of women with non-primary first episodes of genital HSV-2 infection. Herpes virus is isolated from the cervix in only 12 percent of women who present with recurrent genital lesions. The cervix appears abnormal in approximately 90 percent of women from whom herpes simplex virus is isolated during the primary episode. The most common abnormality is diffuse friability, but extensive ulcerative or severe necrotic cervicitis has been found. Symptomatic and asymptomatic excretion of herpes simplex virus is found during first episodes of genital infection. It has been suggested that acute herpetic cervicitis may be the only manifestation of first-episode genital herpes simplex infection [8], and about 8 percent of women attending a sexually transmitted disease clinic had herpes simplex virus isolated with mucopurulent cervicitis without evidence of external genital lesions [7]. In the first episode of genital herpes, ulcers occur on both the endocervical and stratified squamous cells of the exocervix. When shedding of herpes simplex virus from the cervix in the absence of genital symptoms has occurred, it has been very infrequent, occurring in 1.6 to 8 percent of women attending sexually transmitted disease clinics and in 0.25 to 1.5 percent of patients seen in private gynecologic practice [9]. Duration of asymptomatic shedding has been short and the virus has been present in much lower titer than in those women with symptomatic cervicitis.

Recurrent genital herpes

It is estimated by the Centers for Disease Control that recurrent genital herpes infection affects about 30 million adults in the United States. Following the primary infection, about 50 percent of men will have a recurrence in 4 months, whereas 50 percent of women will not have a recurrence until 8 months after the initial outbreak. While recurrent episodes may be more common in men following the initial episode, the recurrent episodes appear to be more painful in women. The average number of recurrences is 3 or 4 per year whereas perhaps 15 percent of patients with recurrent disease have 8 or more recurrences per year. The severity of symptoms, duration of symptoms, and duration of viral shedding are all much shorter in recurrent episodes than in primary disease. Virus can be cultured for 3 to 4 days, mean time for crusting is 4 to 5 days, and time to complete healing is 9 to 10 days in recurrent genital herpes. The mean lesion area is much smaller in recurrent disease and new lesion formation is much less. New lesions occur for only 1 to 2 days in recurrent disease as compared to 5 to 6 days in primary disease. Symptoms of fever, aseptic meningitis, and headache are also much less frequent in recurrent disease. With recurrent disease, 40 to 50 percent of episodes have a prodrome consisting of tingling, burning, or dysesthesias which may occur 1 or 2 days to a few hours before the appearance of vesicles. This prodrome may be associated with buttock pain or pain radiating down the back of the thigh and mimicking sciatic pain. In patients with recurrent genital herpes, HSV-1 is isolated much less frequently than in primary episodes. The recurrence rate is definitely much greater with genital herpes associated with HSV-2.

A major cause of morbidity with recurrent genital herpes is the frequency of recurrences and the fear of transmission of disease to infants or to sexual partners. Patients should be instructed to avoid sexual intercourse when prodromal symptoms or lesions occur and to resume sexual activity only when lesions completely reepithelialize. Herpes can be isolated from lesions rarely at the crust stage of disease.

Herpes infection in the immunocompromised patient

Herpes simplex virus infections are a major cause of infectious problems in patients who are immunosuppressed, and represent a most important group of virus infections in these patients. Immunocompromised patients infected with herpes simplex develop progressive, deep ulcers in the facial (Fig. 190-7), oral (Fig. 190-8), and anogenital

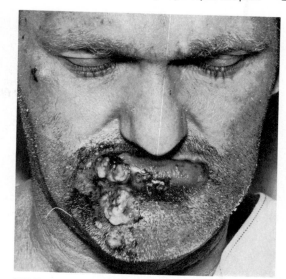

Fig. 190-7   Herpes simplex infection of the face of a patient with severe immunodeficiency due to lymphoma. *(Courtesy of Skin and Cancer Hospital, Philadelphia.)*

regions. The lesions coalesce and are much larger than in patients with normal immune defenses. Herpes virus can be isolated for long periods in these patients, even up to several months. Herpes simplex infections, usually HSV-1, in the mouth and buccal mucosa can produce a painful stomatitis which leads to herpes esophagitis and herpes pneumonitis. Immunocompromised patients with recurrent genital herpes or facial-oral herpes may develop disseminated infection with herpes viremia and herpes hepatitis. A bone marrow transplant patient developed herpes pneumonia and had HSV-2 isolated from lung parenchyma [10]. Early antiviral therapy can be dramatically effective in reducing morbidity in these patients and in prophylaxis. The differential diagnosis of mouth ulcers in immunocompromised patients must include herpes simplex, candidiasis, and drug-induced neutropenia.

Fig. 190-8   Primary herpetic gingivostomatitis in a child.

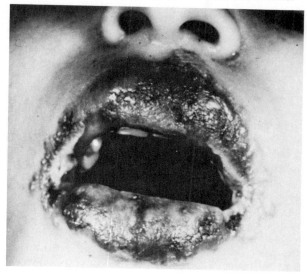

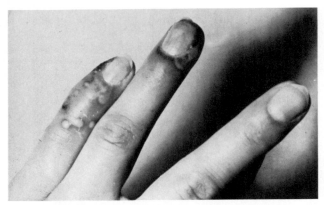

Fig. 190-9   Herpetic whitlow on the finger of a dental technician.

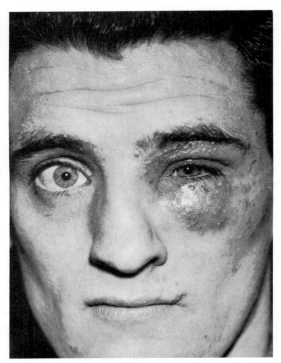

Fig. 190-10   Herpetic vesicles of the eyelids may be associated with herpetic keratitis. *(Courtesy of Skin and Cancer Hospital, Philadelphia.)*

Herpes whitlow

The term herpetic whitlow applies to a primary or recurrent herpes simplex infection of the fingers (Fig. 190-9) and hands. The disease is a common occupational hazard in members of the medical and dental professions. In the study of natural history or recurrent facial-oral herpes simplex infection, HSV was detected in the saliva in 8 percent of the episodes and the amount of virus was high in cultures taken early in the episode. Members of the normal adult population may have herpes virus in the saliva periodically; therefore, doctors, nurses, dentists, or dental technicians who work in and around the mouth of patients may become inoculated in the fingers or hands with virus, particularly in areas where there is an abrasion or break in the skin. Following inoculation, a primary infection lasting 2 to 6 weeks may follow. This is characterized by vesicles and swelling on the finger. The area of the finger tip may become erythematous and edematous and a streak of erythema may extend up to the forearm and up the arm. It is not uncommon for the axillary lymph nodes to become enlarged and tender. In many aspects the process may mimic bacterial cellulitis. The appearance of vesicles at the margin of infected skin is an important clinical finding that represents herpetic whitlow. The presence of a positive culture of multinucleate giant cells in the lesion on direct examination will also establish this diagnosis. Herpetic whitlow can recur in a periodic manner and the recurrences can be severe with significant swelling of the hand and forearm. It is not clearly established that the course of herpetic whitlow benefits from antiviral therapy.

Herpetic keratoconjunctivitis

Herpes simplex virus infection of the eye can cause recurrent erosions of the conjunctiva and cornea (Fig. 190-10). The initial phase of the ophthalmologic disease is a superficial corneal ulcer. This is usually specifically diagnosed by a slit-lamp examination. With repeated recurrences, deeper ulcers develop and stromal keratitis occurs. With each episode stromal scarring may progress and blindness may develop. Herpes simplex keratitis is now regarded as the leading cause of infectious blindness in the United States. The differential diagnosis of herpetic keratoconjunctivitis includes herpes zoster, adenovirus infection, vaccinia, and chlamydial conjunctivitis. Early treatment with topical antiviral drugs such as Vidarabine or trifluorothymidine can enhance healing and minimize stromal scarring.

Recurrent lumbosacral herpes simplex

Recurrent cutaneous herpetic lesions on the low back and buttocks can occur in the absence of actual genital lesions. Recurrent outbreaks of "buttock herpes" usually occur in men and women over the age of 40 and comprise a small percentage—usually only 10 percent of herpes outbreaks in the pelvic and genital area. The lesions are frequently triggered by stress, fatigue, or the onset of the menstrual cycle. The lesions usually occur on one side of the buttocks or another, begin as clusters on an erythematous base (Fig. 190-11), and heal with hyperpigmentation and minimal scarring. Recurrences can develop on a periodic basis and go on for several years. A central feature of recurrent lumbosacral herpes simplex is the prodrome associated with deep pelvic aching for 1 to 3 days before the cutaneous lesions appear. Some patients may experience pain going down the back of the leg and mimicking "sciatic pain." Patients have even undergone myelograms in evaluation of this pain. The differential diagnosis of lumbosacral herpes simplex infection must include low back strain, herniated lumbosacral disk, impetigo, and herpes zoster.

Recurrent herpes simplex and erythema multiforme

In a small subset of patients the development of recurrent facial-oral herpes simplex infection may be followed in 7 to 10 days by development of erythema multiforme (Fig.

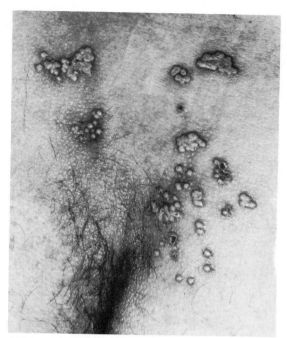

Fig. 190-11 Recurrent lumbosacral herpes simplex.

190-12). This probably represents a hypersensitivity reaction to herpes virus antigens. It may be present only as painful intraoral lesions or may develop into a typical erythema multiforme picture with target lesions present on the extremities. Recurrent bullous erythema multiforme may occur with painful erosions in the mouth and on the skin. In preliminary trials erythema multiforme may respond to treatment with acyclovir. In terms of pathogenesis, this provides evidence that herpes simplex antigens are playing a crucial role in the development of lesions.

Eczema herpeticum

Patients with preexisting skin disorders such as atopic dermatitis and Darier's disease may develop widespread cutaneous infections with herpes simplex virus. Eczema herpeticum (Fig. 190-13) begins as clusters of umbilicated vesicles in areas where the skin has been previously abnormal. The eruption spreads widely over a period of 7 to 10 days and may be associated with fever, malaise, and lymphadenopathy. The vesicular lesions coalesce into large erosions which frequently become secondarily infected with bacteria. The primary episode of eczema herpeticum will run its usual course and heal in 2 to 6 weeks. Patients with chronic skin damage may have recurrent episodes which are milder and not associated with systemic symptoms. The differential diagnosis of eczema herpeticum includes widespread impetigo and a Kaposi's varicelliform eruption caused by vaccinia virus.

Herpes simplex encephalitis

Herpes simplex encephalitis is a highly fatal sporadic encephalitis which usually produces a hemorrhagic necrosis of the temporal-parietal lobes. A prior history of facial-oral or genital herpes simplex is of no clinical relevance concerning the likelihood of developing herpes encephali-

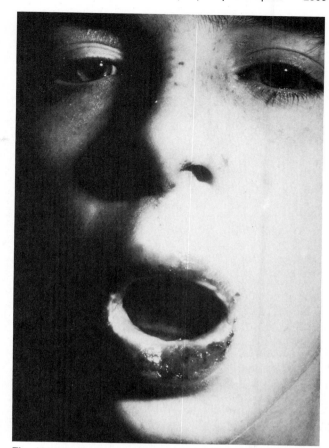

Fig. 190-12 Erythema multiforme associated with recurrent facial-oral herpes simplex.

tis. The disease can occur in young healthy adults and children with no previous evidence of herpes simplex infection, but 70 percent of cases occur in patients who possess neutralizing antibody for herpes simplex [11]. The onset is frequently characterized by recent memory loss, confusion, and temporal lobe signs such as experiencing peculiar smells and odors. The diagnosis is suggested by abnormal EEG tracings or brain scan and arteriogram localized to the temporal lobe. An abnormal head CT scan is useful to follow the course of the disease.

A brain biopsy is still the most definitive way to make the diagnosis and a carefully done brain biopsy has only minimal complications. The virus will grow from infected brain tissue within 5 days in 95 percent of cases. Spinal fluid culture is usually negative for herpes simplex virus even when brain biopsy specimens are positive. Spinal fluid culture has little role in making a precise diagnosis. Other methods of making a diagnosis such as immunofluorescence of brain tissue or electron microscopic pictures of brain tissue for viral particles are not as effective as growing the virus in tissue culture. Antiviral therapy has dramatically altered the course of herpes encephalitis.

Diagnosis

Viral culture

The most reliable way to make a precise diagnosis of herpes simplex infection is to grow the virus from skin

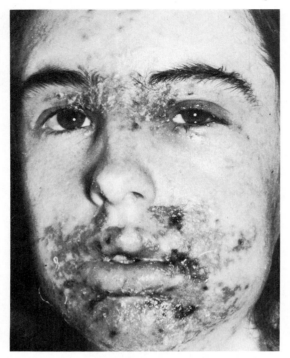

Fig. 190-13   Eczema herpeticum in atopic dermatitis.

lesions. The virus obtained from skin lesions can be quantitated by plaque titration, typed, and its sensitivity to antiviral agents determined. When compatible skin lesions are present and viral culture obtained from skin lesions yields herpes simplex virus, this essentially establishes the diagnosis. In the setting of characteristic lesions on the lip–skin junction which progress from papule to vesicle to erosion or ulcer to crusting state, no other virus or pathogen except HSV has ever been isolated. In our clinical trials, lesions which appear to be due to herpes will produce positive virus on culture about 85 to 90 percent of the time [6]. The percent of positive viral cultures obtained from clinical lesions is quite variable but in most large series this has varied between 60 and 90 percent. All other current methods of making a specific viral diagnosis of herpes simplex-induced skin lesions are less sensitive than viral culture.

Tzanck preparation

A valuable clinical approach to making a rapid diagnosis of HSV relies on taking a smear of cells from the base of the skin lesion, spreading the cells on a glass slide, and staining with Wright's or Giemsa's stain to look for multinucleated giant cells in a Tzanck preparation. With experience, a clinician can reliably distinguish multinucleated giant cells from cellular debris, crushed cells, and artifacts. In the case of genital herpes, multinucleated giant cells can also be identified on cytologic examination of Papanicolaou smears. A comparison of the yield of positive cultures for HSV with the appearance of multinucleated giant cells obtained from clinical specimens of genital herpes in women revealed that about 60 percent of specimens that grew HSV also possessed multinucleated giant cells on cytologic examination. In another study of biopsy-proved HSV encephalitis, examination of brain tissue by histo-

pathology, immunofluorescence, and electron microscopy demonstrated evidence of HSV infection in 56, 70, and 45 percent, respectively, of cases where herpes simplex virus was cultured from brain tissue [11]. This study also indicated that false-positive results were obtained in 14, 9, and 2 percent of HSV-negative specimens of brain biopsies by histopathology, immunofluorescence, and electron microscopy, respectively. Taken together, these studies document the importance of obtaining a positive culture for HSV in establishing a precise diagnosis.

Monoclonal antibodies

The use of specific monoclonal antibodies directed against HSV-1 and HSV-2 proteins is currently being evaluated in the laboratory as a means of making a rapid and precise viral diagnosis of facial-oral herpes simplex virus infection and genital herpes simplex. In a study employing monoclonal antibodies to confirm HSV in tissue cultures by immunofluorescence, the monoclonal antibodies for HSV-1 and HSV-2 have proved to be sensitive and specific [12] with an 88 percent correlation with tissue culture results. The use of monoclonal antibodies has considerable potential for the future in making rapid precise viral diagnosis of herpes infections.

Nucleic acid hybridization

The development of nucleic acid probes derived from the HSV genome for use in DNA-DNA hybridization assays to detect viral nucleic acids in infected tissue is also progressing. The clinical usefulness of all of these new rapid diagnostic approaches, however, will be judged by comparison with the viral culture, the method which remains the most sensitive and specific.

Treatment of herpes simplex infection

Acyclovir (9-[2-hydroxyethoxy-methyl]-guanine) is the prototype of a class of antiviral drugs that employ the viral-specific thymidine kinase enzyme to add a phosphate group to the guanosine analogue. The guanosine analog, acyclovir, utilizes the viral thymidine kinase enzyme to form the acyclovir monophosphate. Cellular guanyldylate kinase and guanosine diphosphate kinase then form acyclovir triphosphate, a potent inhibitor of viral DNA polymerase. Acyclovir triphosphate is incorporated as the terminal base in an elongating strand of DNA and functions as a chain terminator to inhibit chain elongation [13]. Acyclovir triphosphate also appears to form an irreversible bond between elongating DNA and viral DNA polymerase, leading to inactivation of the DNA polymerase [14]. This has been described as an example of how acyclovir triphosphate also acts as a competitive inhibitor of guanosine triphosphate on viral DNA polymerase function. In addition to requiring viral thymidine kinase for activation and inhibition of viral DNA polymerase at a 30-fold less concentration of acyclovir triphosphate than is required to inhibit cellular polymerase functions, acyclovir is taken up preferentially in cells that express a viral TK activity. This third area of specificity, decreased uptake of acyclovir by uninfected cells, probably accounts for the remarkable lack of toxicity associated with high doses of acyclovir.

In carefully randomized placebo-controlled trials, acyclovir is the only drug that has been effective in the treatment of mucocutaneous herpes simplex infections.

Treatment of facial-oral herpes

Therapy of recurrent facial-oral herpes simplex infection with a topical 5% ointment of acyclovir polyethylene glycol in normal patients has revealed that the early application of the ointment would result in a significant antiviral effect with the virus being eradicated more rapidly from the skin of patients treated in the first 8 h of clinical occurrence of facial-oral HSV [15]. This antiviral effect was not associated with any clinical benefit and treated cold sores did not heal more quickly, nor did pain and discomfort resolve more rapidly. Recurrence rate of facial-oral herpes was not affected by acyclovir treatment. In another study in fewer patients employing acyclovir 5% ointment in modified aqueous cream, an increased rate of healing of cold sores was noted in patients treated with acyclovir [16].

Treatment of genital herpes

In primary genital herpes, however, topical acyclovir or oral acyclovir therapy is associated with an antiviral effect and also more rapid healing. Topical acyclovir in a 5% ointment was applied 4 times a day for 7 days. Topical acyclovir reduced viral shedding from 7.0 days to 4.1 days, and time to complete crusting was reduced from 10.5 to 7.1 days [17]. Intravenous and oral acyclovir treatment of primary and initial genital herpes shortened median healing time by about 50 percent. Treatment with oral acyclovir, 200 mg, 5 times daily for 10 days, decreased median duration of viral shedding from 9 to 2 days, time for healing from 16 to 12 days, duration of pain from 7 to 5 days, and the number of patients forming new lesions after 48 h in therapy was decreased from 62 to 18 percent [18]. Other studies with patients having true primary disease had similar results. In nonprimary initial disease, the symptoms are intermediate in severity between primary and recurrent disease. Oral acyclovir is probably effective in treatment of nonprimary disease, but sufficient numbers of these patients have not been studied to document efficacy. In all of the studies employing oral acyclovir therapy for 10 days, there was no effect noted in the proportion of patients who developed recurrent disease episodes nor in the frequency of these episodes. When patients with severe initial cases of genital herpes have an inability to urinate and require urinary catheterization or have severe meningitis with systemic symptoms, they may require hospitalization and treatment with intravenous acyclovir. Oral acyclovir will be the therapy of choice, however, for most patients with initial disease. Oral acyclovir will replace the less effective topical acyclovir therapy for this indication.

Suppression of recurrent disease

In a large double-blind trial comprising 143 patients with a mean number of 1.07 recurrences of genital herpes per month, placebo was compared with oral acyclovir (200 mg) five times daily and oral acyclovir twice daily [19]. Patients received the therapy for 4 months and 94 percent of the placebo patients experienced recurrences during this period compared to 29 percent of those treated with acyclovir five times daily and 35 percent of those treated with acy-

clovir twice daily. The recurrences while patients were taking acyclovir were less frequent and of a shorter duration than among placebo recipients but recurrence rates returned to pretreatment rates once medication was discontinued. In another study, patients taking 3 or 4 capsules daily experienced a similar improvement [20]. In the study by Straus et al, 3 patients who developed recurrences while taking acyclovir had acyclovir-resistant HSV isolated from episodes that developed while they were taking the drug [20]. These episodes were described as "breakthrough recurrences" and were attributed to development of resistance while taking acyclovir for suppression. No serious toxicity was observed in any patient who was taking the drug for up to 6 months. Trials evaluating the effectiveness and safety of acyclovir when taken for 12 months or longer are in progress. The current recommendation of the FDA suggests limiting acyclovir suppressive therapy to 6 months in patients with 8 or more recurrences per year.

Treatment of recurrent genital herpes

The treatment of recurrent genital herpes with acyclovir in any form has been only marginally successful. Topical acyclovir treatment did not facilitate healing in women with recurrent disease but slight beneficial effects were observed in pain reduction and healing in men. Shortened time of virus shedding was observed with topical acyclovir therapy. Due to the slight clinical benefit of acyclovir therapy in recurrent genital herpes, topical treatment of recurrent genital herpes is not justified. In a large multicenter controlled trial, oral acyclovir treatment of recurrent genital herpes was evaluated by comparing patient-initiated therapy with therapy initiated by a physician or placebo [21]. Oral acyclovir capsules (200 mg) were taken five times daily, for 5 days. When patients had acyclovir at home and initiated therapy at the onset of a prodrome or at the first sign of lesions, therapy was more effective than when it was initiated by a physician within 48 h of the onset of symptoms. The patient-initiated treatment reduced viral shedding from 3.9 days in placebo-treated cases, to 2.1 days. Time to healing was reduced from 6.5 days in placebo-treated cases, to 5.5 days with patient-initiated treatment. The percent of patients forming new lesions was 22 percent with placebo treatment, and this was reduced to 7 percent in the patient-initiated treatment. When patients went to a physician and initiated therapy within 48 h of the onset of lesions, new lesion formation was reduced from 22 to 16 percent. The treatment of recurrent episodes with oral acyclovir offers marginal clinical benefit but the benefit is superior to that obtained with topical acyclovir. Patients with severe recurrent episodes who initiate therapy at the first sign of a recurrence will derive the greatest benefit. Treatment with acyclovir has no effect on subsequent recurrence rate.

Treatment of herpes infections in the immunosuppressed patient

In immunocompromised patients with severe herpes simplex infections, the need for effective antiviral therapy is greatest. In these immunocompromised patients acyclovir therapy for mucocutaneous herpes simplex infection can be lifesaving or dramatically successful. In these patients, healing of mucocutaneous herpes simplex infection occurs more quickly in those treated with acyclovir because inhibition of HSV replication reduces tissue destruction. In a randomized double-blind trial of intravenous acyclovir, in culture-proved herpes simplex infection that followed bone marrow transplantation, 13 of 17 patients who received acyclovir (750 mg per square meter per day) for seven days had a therapeutic response [22]. Only 2 of 17 placebo-treated patients improved. Intravenous acyclovir produced a shorter duration of positive cultures, shortened duration of pain, and hastened healing. These controlled trials have been performed in heart transplant patients and in other immunosuppressed patients. The accumulated data on intravenous acyclovir in immunocompromised patients with mucocutaneous herpes simplex infection indicate that acyclovir shortens the period of viral shedding, shortening the time interval to scabbing and healing, and shortens the duration of pain. On termination of acyclovir, reactivation of herpes simplex infection usually occurs. Intravenous and oral acyclovir are useful in preventing mucocutaneous herpes simplex infection in immunocompromised patients. A double-blind placebo-controlled trial of intravenous acyclovir in bone marrow transplant recipients indicated that 10 patients who were seropositive for antiherpes antibody and who received acyclovir in a dose of 250 mg per square meter every 8 h for 18 days starting at 3 days before transplantation did not develop herpes infection [23]. Virus-positive lesions developed in 7 of 10 patients who received placebo treatment. When acyclovir treatment was discontinued, however, herpes infection did develop. Oral acyclovir treatment has been found to be effective in preventing reactivation of HSV infections following bone marrow transplantation and in other immunosuppressed patients. Topical acyclovir therapy, however, has not been effective in suppressing recurrence in normal or immunosuppressed patients. In immunocompromised patients, oral acyclovir is more effective than topical acyclovir in treatment of mucocutaneous herpes infections, but severe or life-threatening infections caused by HSV should be treated with intravenous acyclovir. A comparison of the effects of ara-A and acyclovir in the treatment of a severe mucocutaneous infections caused by HSV in the immunocompromised patient indicates that ara-A was not very successful. Acyclovir is also much more soluble than ara-A and less fluid volume is required for treatment. Ara-A is also more inhibitory for proliferating granulocytes and bone marrow cells than is acyclovir. At doses of 30 mg/kg per day, adenine-arabinoside therapy will produce a megaloblastic anemia in patients. From the standpoint of efficacy and safety, acyclovir is the preferred therapy for mucocutaneous herpes simplex infections in immunocompromised patients.

Treatment of herpes simplex encephalitis

Herpes simplex virus is the most common cause of sporadic nonepidemic encephalitis. The disease commonly involves the temporoparietal lobes in a hemorrhagic necrosis, and without treatment has a mortality of greater than 70 percent. In a double-blind placebo-controlled trial in 1977, treatment of biopsy-proved herpes encephalitis with adenine arabinoside reduced the mortality from 70 percent in the placebo group to 44 percent survival at 6 months after treatment [24]. In a follow-up study, the mortality

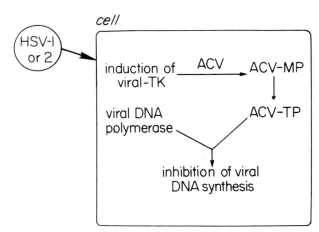

Fig. 190-14   Postulated mechanism of acyclovir.

was reduced to 39 percent and one-third of patients who survived had a return to normal function. The level of consciousness and age had the greatest impact on outcome. Patients under 30 years of age, and only lethargic at the beginning of therapy, had the highest recovery.

A comparison of acyclovir at 30 mg/kg per day and ara-A (15 mg/kg per day) for 10 days as treatment for biopsy-proved herpes encephalitis was carried out by the NIAID (National Institute of Allergy and Infectious Disease) collaborative antiviral study group of the National Institutes of Health and acyclovir was clearly superior. The mortality of the acyclovir-treated group was 28 percent compared with 54 percent for ara-A-treated patients. At 6 months after treatment, 38 percent of acyclovir patients were functioning normally and only 14 percent of ara-A-treated patients were normal [25]. This study concluded that acyclovir is the preferred treatment for biopsy-proved herpes encephalitis. In another study on 53 patients where there was not uniformity of diagnosis for herpes simplex encephalitis, adenine arabinosine therapy was associated with a mortality of 50 percent and acyclovir mortality at 6 months was 19 percent [26].

Over two-thirds of the acyclovir survivors returned to normal function. Both of these studies had remarkably similar outcomes in favor of acyclovir as the preferred treatment for herpes encephalitis.

Resistance of herpes simplex to acyclovir and its clinical importance

The postulated mechanism for the anti-HSV action of acyclovir is illustrated in Fig. 190-14. There are three known mechanisms to explain how resistance of HSV to acyclovir develops in vitro. Selection of TK⁻ mutants in a population is by far the most common mechanism, and accounts for all but one example of resistant cases seen with the clinical use of acyclovir. Selection is emphasized because of evidence that in any wild-type population of herpes there are TK⁻ mutants, viruses with an altered TK, and perhaps even viruses with an altered DNA polymerase; the use of acyclovir allows these to grow out and become dominant in the viral population [27]. There is no evidence to support the hypothesis that a genetic mutation occurs with the use of the drug; rather, mutants already present in nonsignificant amounts become dominant. In any wild-type population, between 0.4 and perhaps up to 4 percent of the total virions will be TK⁻ to begin with.

A second mechanism is selection of a mutant with an altered TK that will phosphorylate thymidine but not acyclovir. This has been shown by Darby, Field, and Salsbury [28] to occur by passing herpes simplex virus in resting cells that do not express a cellular TK, and replication of HSV in these cells in the presence of acyclovir permits selection of a mutant that will phosphorylate thymidine normally but not acyclovir.

The third mechanism of resistance is selection of mutants with an altered DNA polymerase activity. Evidence for this has not been found, however, either in animal or human clinical use of acyclovir. The demonstration of these mechanisms and their clinical relevance are discussed next.

The clinical importance of acyclovir resistance focuses on three points. First, if resistance develops, will it impede healing in the clinical use of the drug? Second, would resistant mutants that develop have altered pathogenicity, perhaps causing serious disease in ways that are as yet unknown? Third, will resistant virus be transmitted to other people? Transmission is not as great a problem with herpes simplex viruses as it is with influenza or other viruses spread by respiratory contact, but a major problem would be transmission of resistant viruses between sexual partners or between mother and infant. Although currently speculative, these possibilities should be closely watched for as our knowledge of acyclovir increases.

The occurrence of resistance of HSV to acyclovir in immunocompromised patients is well documented [29,30], but only one report [20] in the literature describes resistance occurring in normal patients taking acyclovir. This was in a patient with frequently recurrent genital herpes who was taking oral acyclovir in order to suppress recurrences of genital herpes.

In the cases of resistance noted to date in humans, the presence of an acyclovir-resistant mutant exhibiting diminished thymidine kinase activity has been associated with prolonged virus shedding. With the early courses of acyclovir, the herpes lesions healed dramatically, but subsequent courses of therapy in two children with combined immunodeficiency syndrome were characterized by low-grade chronic lesions that healed slowly. One of these acyclovir-resistant herpes simplex isolates obtained from a child with severe combined immunodeficiency and exhibiting diminished thymidine kinase activity was tested for pathogenicity in mice [30]. Intracerebral inoculation of mice with the resistant isolates was associated with a 1000-fold decrease for neurovirulence and death due to encephalitis. Cutaneous lesions produced by the resistant isolate (BW-R) were slow to heal, and a chronic infection resulted. The authors noted that some lesions eventually healed while others tended to persist for prolonged periods with ultimate death of the mouse. They also noted that this resistant isolate in the patient was present in the CSF, but in the absence of meningeal inflammation and perivascular infiltration in the brain. The claim that the development of acyclovir resistance of HSV-1 was associated with attenuated virulence may be true for neurovirulence leading to death, but this does not mean that these acyclovir-resistant mutants are truly less virulent in all circumstances. The presence of prolonged virus-positive lesions that are slow to heal or the persistence of HSV in the CSF is probably best described as an example of altered, rather than diminished, virulence.

Thymidine kinase-deficient mutants are capable of establishing latent infection, however, even at a decreased frequency, and the possibility exists that the TK-deficient mutant can revert to the wild-type strain that again produces large amounts of TK and reestablishes neurovirulence. There does not seem to be any evidence yet to indicate that this kind of virus will disseminate and produce disease elsewhere.

References

1. Sexually Transmitted Disease Surveillance, 1979. *Br Med J* **282:**155, 1981
2. Smith IW et al: The incidence of *Herpesvirus hominis* antibody in the population. *J Hyg (Camb)* **63:**395, 1967
3. Glezen WP et al: Acute respiratory disease of university students with special reference to the etiologic role of *Herpesvirus hominis*. *Am J Epidemiol* **101:**111, 1975
4. Embil JA et al: Prevalence of recurrent herpes labialis and aphthous ulcers among young adults on six continents. *Can Med Assoc J* **113:**627, 1975
5. Young SK et al: A clinical study for the control of facial mucocutaneous herpes virus infections. I. Characterization of natural history in a professional school population. *Oral Surg* **41:**498, 1976
6. Bader C et al: The natural history of recurrent facial-oral infection with herpes simplex virus. *J Infect Dis* **138:**897, 1978
7. Corey L et al: Genital herpes simplex virus infections: clinical manifestations, course and complications. *Ann Intern Med* **98:**958, 1983
8. Josey WE et al: Genital herpes simplex infection in the female. *Am J Obstet Gynecol* **96:**493, 1966
9. Jeansson SS, Molin L: On the occurrence of genital herpes simplex virus infection: clinical and virological findings and relation to gonorrhea. *Acta Derm Venereol (Stockh)* **54:**79, 1974
10. Ramsey PG et al: Herpes simplex virus pneumonia: clinical, virologic and pathologic features in 20 patients. *Ann Intern Med* **97:**813, 1982
11. Nahmias AJ et al and the Collaborative Antiviral Study Group: Herpes simplex virus encephalitis: laboratory evaluations and their diagnostic significance. *J Infect Dis* **145:**829, 1982
12. Goldstein LC et al: Monoclonal antibodies to herpes simplex viruses: use in antigenic typing and rapid diagnosis. *J Infect Dis* **147:**829, 1983
13. Elion GB et al: Selectivity of action of an antiherpes agent 9-(2-hydroxyethoxymethyl)-guanine. *Proc Natl Acad Sci USA* **74:**5716, 1978
14. Furman PA et al: Acyclovir triphosphate is a suicide inactivator of herpes simplex virus DNA polymerase. *J Biol Chem* **259:**9575, 1984
15. Spruance SL et al: Treatment of herpes simplex labialis with topical acyclovir in polyethylene glocol. *J Infect Dis* **146:**85, 1982
16. Fiddian AP et al: Successful treatment of facial-oral herpes with topical acyclovir. *Br Med J* **286:**1699, 1983
17. Corey L et al: A trial of topical acyclovir genital herpes simplex virus infections. *N Engl J Med* **306:**1313, 1982
18. Bryson Y et al: Treatment of first episode of genital herpes simplex infection with oral acyclovir, a randomized double-blind controlled trial in normal subjects. *N Engl J Med* **308:**916, 1982
19. Douglas JM et al: A double-blind study of oral acyclovir for

suppression of recurrences of genital herpes simplex virus infection. *N Engl J Med* **310:**1551, 1984

20. Straus SE et al: Suppression of frequently recurring genital herpes. *N Engl J Med* **310:**1545, 1984
21. Reichman RC et al: Treatment of recurrent genital herpes simplex infections with oral acyclovir. *JAMA* **251:**2103, 1984
22. Wade JC et al: Intravenous acyclovir to treat mucocutaneous herpes simplex infection after marrow transplantation: a double blind trial. *Ann Intern Med* **96:**265, 1982
23. Saral R et al: Acyclovir prophylaxis of herpes-simplex virus infections: a randomized double-blind controlled trial in bone marrow transplant recipients. *N Engl J Med* **305:**63, 1981
24. Whitley RJ et al: Adenine arabinoside therapy of biopsy proved herpes simplex encephalitis. *N Engl J Med* **297:**289, 1977
25. Whitley RJ et al: NIAID Collaborative Antiviral Study Group. Herpes simplex encephalitis: adenine arabinoside vs acyclovir therapy. *N Engl J Med,* in press
26. Skoldenberg B et al: Acyclovir versus vidarabine in herpes simplex encephalitis. Randomized multicenter study in consecutive Swedish patients. *Lancet* **8405:**707, 1984
27. Schnipper LE, Crumpacker CS: Resistance of herpes simplex virus to acycloguanosine: role of viral thymidine kinase and DNA polymerase loci. *Proc Natl Acad Sci USA* **77:**2270, 1980
28. Darby G et al: Altered substrate specificity of herpes simplex virus: thymidine kinase confers acyclovir resistance. *Nature* **289:**81, 1981
29. Crumpacker CS et al: Resistance to antiviral drugs of herpes simplex virus isolated from a patient treated with acyclovir. *N Engl J Med* **306:**343, 1982
30. Sibrack CD et al: Pathogenicity of acyclovir-resistant herpes simplex virus type 1 from an immunodeficient child. *J Infect Dis* **146:**673, 1982

CHAPTER 191

VARICELLA AND HERPES ZOSTER

Michael N. Oxman

Definition

Varicella (chickenpox) and herpes zoster (shingles, zoster) are distinct clinical entities caused by a single member of the herpesvirus family, varicella-zoster virus (VZV). The differences between these two diseases are due to differences in the host and in the circumstances of infection, and not to differences in their etiologic agent.

Varicella, an acute, highly contagious exanthematous disease that occurs most often in childhood, is the result of primary infection of a susceptible individual. It is characterized by a short or absent prodromal period and a generalized pruritic rash consisting of successive crops of lesions that progress rapidly from macules and papules to vesicles, pustules, and crusts. In normal children, systemic symptoms are usually mild and serious complications are extremely rare. In adults and in immunologically compromised individuals of any age, varicella is more likely to be associated with an extensive eruption, high fever, severe constitutional symptoms, pneumonia, and other life-threatening complications.

Herpes zoster is a localized disease characterized by unilateral radicular pain and a vesicular eruption limited to the dermatome innervated by a single spinal or cranial sensory ganglion. It occurs most frequently in elderly people. In contrast to varicella, which follows primary exogenous VZV infection, herpes zoster appears to represent reactivation of an endogenous infection that has persisted in latent form following an earlier attack of varicella.

Historical aspects

Herpes zoster, though sometimes confused with herpes simplex and other cutaneous eruptions, has been recognized as a distinct clinical entity since ancient times. Varicella, on the other hand, was confused with smallpox well into the nineteenth century. Herberden (1767) is credited with first differentiating varicella from smallpox, but more than a century later such authorities as Osler (1892) deemed it necessary to emphasize that the two diseases were indeed etiologically distinct [1–3]. The name "chickenpox" is probably derived from the Old English *gican,* to itch [4]. The infectious nature of varicella was demonstrated by Steiner in 1875 [5] who transmitted the disease to volunteers by the inoculation of vesicle fluid from patients with varicella. Tyzzer described the histopathology of the skin lesions of varicella in 1906 and called attention to the characteristic multinucleated giant cells and intranuclear inclusion bodies [6]. However, it was not until 1952 that Weller and Stoddard succeeded in isolating and propagating the virus from varicella vesicle fluid in vitro [7].

The relationship of herpes zoster to varicella was first noted by von Bokay in 1888, who observed that susceptible children acquired varicella after contact with individuals with herpes zoster [1,2,8]. It was further supported by Lipschutz [9] who noted that the skin lesions of herpes zoster were histologically identical to those of varicella previously described by Tyzzer.

Kundratitz (in 1922) and Bruusgaard (in 1925) inoculated

children with vesicle fluid from patients with herpes zoster and demonstrated that the same agent was responsible for both diseases [8]. Some recipients developed varicella-like lesions at the site of inoculation; others developed, in addition, a generalized exanthem which resembled varicella in every respect. Uninoculated children in contact with affected recipients developed typical varicella after a normal incubation period and transmitted the disease to other contacts. Children who had previously had varicella did not develop the disease when inoculated with vesicle fluid from patients with herpes zoster or when exposed to children who had developed a varicella-like exanthem following such inoculation. Vesicles from the site of inoculation and the generalized exanthem were histologically identical to those of ordinary varicella and herpes zoster. Early serologic studies [10] demonstrated that antigens derived from the vesicles and crusts of both varicella and herpes zoster reacted equally well in complement fixation tests with convalescent sera from patients with either disease. However, it was only with the isolation and propagation in vitro of the agents of varicella and herpes zoster that the common etiology of the two diseases was proved. Weller and his colleagues found that the viruses recovered from patients with varicella and herpes zoster were identical with respect to their physical, biologic, and immunologic attributes [11,12]. This identity has subsequently been confirmed in numerous studies [2,10,13].

The neurologic implications of the segmental distribution of the lesions of herpes zoster were recognized as long ago as 1831 by Richard Bright, and the inflammatory changes in the corresponding sensory ganglion and spinal nerve were first described by von Barensprung in 1862 [14–16]. The definitive work is that of Head and Campbell (1900) who published detailed postmortem examinations of 21 persons with herpes zoster, together with clinical observations on 450 individuals with the disease [14]. All of the gross and microscopic pathology is described and illustrated, including the acute lymphocytic inflammation, focal hemorrhage and neuronal destruction in sensory ganglia, the degeneration of sensory nerve fibers linking the affected neurons peripherally to the involved skin and centrally to the spinal cord and brain, and the later fibrosis of severely involved ganglia and nerves. Correlation of their detailed pathologic and clinical observations enabled Head and Campbell to map the area of skin (dermatome) innervated by each of the sensory ganglia. Their findings have been confirmed repeatedly by a number of subsequent studies [16–23], some of which employed newer techniques, such as electron microscopy and fluorescent antibody staining, to demonstrate virus particles and viral antigens within neurons and satellite cells in the sensory ganglia and within peripheral sensory nerves early in the disease. Together, these observations indicate that in herpes zoster, active infection of sensory neurons precedes involvement of the skin.

Epidemiology

Epidemiology of varicella

Varicella is worldwide in distribution, with no evidence of differing racial or sexual susceptibility. Humans are the only known reservoir, and there is no indication that arthropod vectors play any role in transmission. In metropolitan communities in temperate climates, varicella is endemic, with a regularly recurring seasonal prevalence in winter and spring, and periodic epidemics dependent upon the accumulation of susceptible persons. In urban areas of the United States, varicella is primarily a disease of childhood; 90 percent of cases occur in children less than 10 years of age and fewer than 5 percent in individuals over the age of 15 [1,2]. In tropical and semitropical countries, infection is delayed and varicella is seen more often in adults. In a serologic survey of parturient women in New York City, only 4.5 percent of those born in the United States lacked antibody to VZV, whereas 16 percent of those from Latin America were seronegative [24]. The proportion of susceptible adults is even higher in Asia, Africa, and the Middle East [2,13]. This can be an important consideration in delivering health care to immigrant populations and in controlling nosocomial varicella in hospitals with patients and staff from these areas.

Despite the lability of the virus, varicella is highly contagious. Attack rates of 87 percent among susceptible siblings in households, and nearly 70 percent among susceptible patients on hospital wards have been reported [1,25]. Most cases of varicella are clinically apparent, although on occasion the exanthem may be so sparse and transient that it is unnoticed. A typical patient is probably infectious for 1 to 2 days (rarely, 3 to 4 days) before the exanthem appears, and for 4 or 5 days thereafter, i.e., until the last crop of vesicles has crusted. The immunocompromised patient, who may experience successive crops of lesions for a week or more, is infectious for a longer period of time. The average incubation period of varicella is 14 or 15 days, with a range of 10 to 23 days [1,25]. The incubation period is often prolonged in patients who develop varicella after passive immunization with zoster-immune globulin (ZIG) or plasma (ZIP) [26–28]. The major route by which varicella is acquired and transmitted is thought to be the respiratory tract. Airborne droplets constitute an important mechanism of transmission [29,30] but infection is also spread by direct contact and, less frequently, by indirect contact. Unlike smallpox, varicella crusts are not infectious and the duration of infectivity of droplets containing the labile VZV must be relatively limited. The mechanism by which VZV is shed is unclear. Viremia occurs during the prodromal stage, when varicella can be transmitted to the fetus in utero and by blood transfusion from a donor incubating the infection. Lesions are not confined to the skin, but occur also in the respiratory, genitourinary, and gastrointestinal tracts. Though the infectiousness of patients with varicella is thought to depend largely upon virus shed from the mucous membranes of the upper respiratory tract, VZV has only rarely been isolated from pharyngeal secretions, whereas it can regularly be recovered from vesicle fluid [2,13].

One attack of varicella confers lasting immunity to the disease. Most of the rarely reported second attacks are probably examples of cutaneous dissemination in patients with herpes zoster (see below).

Epidemiology of herpes zoster

Herpes zoster occurs sporadically throughout the year without seasonal prevalence. It affects both sexes and all races with equal frequency. As expected with a disease that reflects the reactivation of latent endogenous infection, the occurrence of herpes zoster is independent of the prevalence of varicella, and there is no convincing evidence that herpes zoster can be acquired by contact with persons with varicella or herpes zoster [15,31,32]. Rather, the incidence of herpes zoster is determined by factors which influence the host–parasite relationship. One of these is age. The rate of occurrence is in the range of 1.3 to 5 per 1000 persons per year, and although the disease may be seen in any age group, including children, more than two-thirds of reported cases occur in individuals over 50 years of age and less than 10 percent of cases occur under the age of 20 years [1,15,31–37]. Hope-Simpson's tabulation of data from 192 cases occurring over a 16-year period in a population of 3500 individuals showed that the annual incidence per thousand rises from 0.74 in children under 10 years of age to a plateau of approximately 2.5 between ages 20 and 50, and thereafter increases to reach a level of over 10 in octogenarians. The incidence of herpes zoster among those who have already had an attack appears to be at least as high as that of first attacks in individuals of comparable age. Second attacks comprise 4 to 5 percent of reported series, and third attacks are not unheard of. Hope-Simpson estimated that if a cohort of 1000 people were to live to be 85 years old, half would have had an attack of herpes zoster and 10 would have had two attacks. However, patients suffering multiple episodes of zoster-like disease, especially involving the same anatomic location, are far more likely to be suffering recurrent zosteriform herpes simplex virus infections. The incidence of herpes zoster in immunosuppressed patients is increased 20 to 100 times, and the severity of the disease is also increased. The increased incidence and severity of herpes zoster in older individuals, as well as in individuals of any age who are immunosuppressed, is associated with deficient cell-mediated immune responses to VZV antigens (see below).

Herpes zoster is rare during the first few years of life. When it occurs in infants, there is usually no history of postnatal varicella, but there is almost always a history of maternal varicella during gestation [38]. Presumably, primary VZV infection and the establishment of neuronal latency occurred in utero.

Patients with herpes zoster are infectious. Virus can be isolated from vesicles in uncomplicated herpes zoster for up to seven days after the appearance of the rash, and for much longer periods in immunocompromised individuals. However, herpes zoster is less contagious than varicella; the infection rate in susceptible household contacts appears to be only about one-third that of varicella [1,8,15,31].

The increased incidence of herpes zoster in immunocompromised patients with cancer has led many physicians to assume that the occurrence of herpes zoster in an otherwise normal individual may be an indication of underlying malignancy. Consequently, many apparently normal patients with herpes zoster are subjected to aggressive and expensive workups for occult cancer. A recent prospective study of 590 patients with herpes zoster indicates that such workups are unnecessary because the incidence of cancer during the first year and the first five years after the diagnosis of herpes zoster is the same as the incidence of cancer in the general population [39].

Etiology

Varicella-zoster virus is a member of the herpesvirus family. Other members pathogenic for humans include herpes simplex virus type 1 (HSV-1) and type 2 (HSV-2), cytomegalovirus (CMV), and the Epstein-Barr virus (EBV) of infectious mononucleosis [40]. All of these herpesviruses are morphologically indistinguishable and share a number of properties, including a remarkable propensity for establishing latent infections that persist for the life of the host. VZV consists of an icosahedral capsid 100 nm in diameter that encloses the viral genome, a linear molecule of double-stranded DNA with a molecular weight of about 90 million. The capsid is composed of 162 protein subunits (capsomers), which resemble elongated hexagonal or pentagonal prisms with axial holes (Fig. 191-1b). The genome and capsid (the nucleocapsid) are surrounded by one or two additional layers of protein and, finally, by a loose lipoprotein envelope derived from the nuclear membrane of the host cell and containing radially oriented viral glycoproteins on its surface (Fig. 191-1a). The complete virion is roughly spherical with a diameter of 150 to 200 nm [41]. Only enveloped virions are infectious, and this accounts for the lability of VZV; infectivity is rapidly destroyed by organic solvents, detergents, proteolytic enzymes, heat, and extremes of pH. More than 30 virus-specific proteins and glycoproteins have been identified in purified virions and in VZV-infected cells. [13]. In addition to structural components of the virion, certain enzymes essential for virus replication, including a virus-specific DNA polymerase and a virus-specific deoxypyridine (thymidine) kinase, are synthesized in infected cells. Because these viral enzymes differ in substrate specificity from the corresponding host cell enzymes, they are important targets for specific antiviral chemotherapy.

There is only one VZV serotype. A number of antigens are present in the virion and produced in infected cells, but these are identical in viruses isolated from patients with varicella and herpes zoster throughout the world [2,10,11,13]. However, some VZV antigens cross-react with antigens of other members of the herpesvirus family and this limits the usefulness of certain serologic tests [2,10,11,13,42].

The DNA of viruses isolated from cases of varicella and herpes zoster throughout the world is basically similar, but minor variations in nucleotide sequence give the genomes of different clinical isolates of VZV slightly different restriction endonuclease cleavage patterns (i.e., each isolate has a unique pattern or "fingerprint"). More substantial differences distinguish the OKA live attenuated VZV vaccine (see below) from wild-type VZV isolates, and there is little resemblance between the restriction endonuclease cleavage pattern of VZV and those of the other human herpesviruses (HSV-1, HSV-2, CMV, and EBV). These differences are useful epidemiologically, in that isolates from common source outbreaks will have identical restriction endonuclease cleavage patterns, and when illness occurs in vaccinees or their contacts the responsible agent, vaccine virus or wild-type VZV, can be determined [13,44].

Studies of the molecular biology and pathogenesis of VZV infection have been hampered by difficulty in obtaining adequate quantities of cell-free virus and by the absence of suitable animal models. Some progress has been made in preparing cell-free virus, and the application of

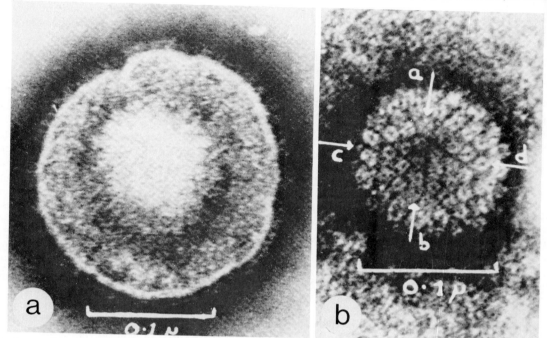

Fig. 191-1 Varicella-zoster virus stained with phospho-tungstic acid. (a) Intact particle showing envelope with radially oriented glycoproteins on its surface. (b) Rupture of the envelope reveals the nucleocapsid within. *(From Almeida et al [41], with permission.)*

molecular cloning procedures has facilitated the physical mapping of the VZV genome. VZV has now been propagated in guinea pig cells, and a guinea pig model of VZV infection and transmission has been established [13,45].

Pathogenesis

Pathogenesis of varicella

Our present concept of the pathogenesis of varicella is based primarily on circumstantial evidence, analogy with experimental models of other exanthematous diseases, and postmortem examination of fatal cases. Entry of the virus is probably through the mucosa of the upper respiratory tract and oropharynx. Initial multiplication at this portal of entry results in dissemination of small amounts of virus via the blood and lymphatics (the primary viremia). This virus is removed by cells of the reticuloendothelial system, which probably constitutes the major site of virus replication during the remainder of the incubation period.

The incubating infection is partially contained by nonspecific host defenses (e.g., interferon) and by developing immune responses. In most individuals, virus replication eventually overwhelms these defenses, so that about two weeks after infection a much larger viremia (the secondary viremia) occurs [46,47]. This causes fever and malaise, and disseminates virus throughout the body, especially to the skin and mucous membranes, where foci of infection are initiated by the infection of capillary endothelial cells [6,8,48–50]. The skin lesions appear in successive crops, reflecting a cyclic viremia which, in the normal host, is terminated after about three days by VZV-specific humoral and cellular immune responses. Virus in the blood is cell-associated; it appears to circulate and replicate in monocytes [51,52]. The frequent observations of abnormal electroencephalograms and elevated serum levels of hepatocellular enzymes in the acute stage of uncomplicated varicella [53–56] suggest the regular occurrence of asymptomatic viremic infection of many organs, including the central nervous system.

In addition to terminating the viremia, host immune responses play a critical role in limiting the progression of the focal lesions in the skin and other organs. Varicella pneumonia and most other complications of varicella reflect a failure to halt virus replication and dissemination, and to limit the progression of viseral and cutaneous foci of infection [48–50,57–59]. Their frequency in newborns and in patients with congenital, acquired, or iatrogenic immunodeficiencies is almost certainly due, in large part, to depressed cellular immunity. The pathogenic basis for the greater severity of varicella in normal adults than in children, however, is totally unknown.

IgG, IgM, and IgA antibodies to VZV are detectable within 2 to 5 days after the onset of clinical varicella and reach maximum titers during the second or third week. Thereafter, IgG antibodies decline slowly and persist at low levels for life. IgM and IgA antibodies decline more rapidly and are generally undetectable a year after infection [13,57,60–63]. Cell-mediated immunity to VZV also develops during the course of varicella and persists for many years [64,65]. The assays most frequently employed measure the capacity of peripheral blood leukocytes to synthesize DNA and proliferate in vitro in response to VZV antigens, but cell-mediated immunity to VZV has also been demonstrated by other techniques, including a skin test that correlates well with the results of antibody assays and efficiently identifies susceptible individuals [13,66].

The relative importance of humoral and cellular immunity in recovery from varicella is not clear. The disease is not particularly severe in children with agammaglobulinemia [67], and there is no obvious correlation between the endogenous antibody response and the severity of varicella [57,58,60]. Cellular immune responses, and perhaps interferon, appear more important in limiting the extent and duration of VZV infection; it is patients with congenital, acquired, or iatrogenic defects in cell-mediated immunity who suffer severe and life-threatening varicella [58,60,68–70]. However, passive immunization of these immunocompromised patients with antibody to VZV can protect them from severe or fatal varicella [26–28,71]. Clearly, control of primary VZV infection must involve a number of host defenses, and augmenting one (e.g., by administering antibody to VZV) may compensate for deficiencies in another.

Immunity to VZV is complex. In immunocompetent persons, one attack of varicella confers lasting immunity to varicella (i.e., to clinically apparent exogenous reinfection) but it does not prevent herpes zoster, a disease caused by the same virus. Serum antibody to VZV is an important factor in varicella immunity. People with detectable serum antibody do not usually become ill after exogenous exposure, whereas those devoid of serum antibody to VZV develop varicella [72,73]. Moreover, passive immunization can prevent varicella in susceptible immunocompetent individuals exposed to exogenous VZV [25,26,74]. However, the development and application of sensitive assays for humoral and cell-mediated immunity to VZV has revealed the dynamic nature of the VZV–host interaction. Subclinical reinfection, evidenced by a boost in the titer of IgG antibody to VZV, by the reappearance of IgM and IgA antibodies, and by an increase in the in vitro lymphoproliferative response to VZV antigens, is a frequent occurrence in normal immune individuals following household exposure to varicella [60,75,76]. This implies limited replication of VZV, at least at the portal of entry. Repeated exposures of this sort may help adults to maintain a high level of immunity to VZV [15]. Infants with transplacentally acquired maternal antibody regularly develop mild varicella after exposure [77], as do immunocompromised children passively immunized with varicella-zoster immune globulin (VZIG) [71]. It would thus appear that the presence of antibody to VZV in a normal host, with or without VZV-specific cellular immune responses induced by previous varicella, will prevent the development of disease but not the local replication of exogenous VZV at the portal of entry. The failure of the same antibody preparations to prevent disease in immunosuppressed patients implies the need for some nonspecific, presumably cellular, component(s) that may interact with antibody—perhaps cells capable of mediating antibody-dependent cytotoxicity.

It also appears that immunity in persons who develop modified varicella (e.g., because they are infected as infants in the presence of transplacentally acquired maternal antibody) is less durable than that which follows unmodified infection; such individuals may later respond to exogenous reinfection by developing mild varicella [77,78]. Similarly, while immunologically normal recipients of live attenuated VZV vaccines (see below) have had a greatly reduced incidence of varicella after subsequent exposures, a few have developed mild varicella in spite of having vaccine-induced antibody to VZV [79,80].

Taken together, these observations suggest that antibody alone will not guarantee total immunity to varicella, unless it is the result of a previous unmodified natural infection.

Pathogenesis of herpes zoster

The pathogenesis of herpes zoster is not fully understood, but clinical, epidemiologic, and pathologic data, as well as analogy with recurrent herpes simplex virus infections [81] support the following model [15]. During the course of varicella, VZV passes from lesions in the skin and mucosal surfaces into the contiguous endings of sensory nerves and is transported centripetally up the sensory fibers to the sensory ganglia. In the ganglia a latent infection is established in the sensory neurons, and the virus then persists silently and harmlessly; it is no longer infectious and does not multiply, but it retains the capacity to revert to full infectiousness. Although VZV might also reach the sensory ganglia via the blood stream during the course of the primary or secondary viremia of varicella, only the neural route can easily explain the selection of sensory rather than motor neurons as the site of latency and the coincidence of the anatomic pattern of the incidence of zoster in later life with the distribution of the rash in varicella. Herpes zoster occurs with the highest frequency in those dermatomes in which the rash of varicella achieves the greatest density [15,17], presumably because areas of skin with a denser rash during varicella transmit larger amounts of virus to the corresponding sensory ganglia and thus establish latent infection in a larger number of sensory neurons. If subsequent reactivation occurs at random, zoster should occur most frequently in areas of skin innervated by ganglia with the largest number of latently infected neurons.

Although the latent virus in the ganglia retains its potential for full infectivity, reversions are sporadic and infrequent. The mechanisms involved in the activation of latent VZV are unclear, but a number of conditions have been associated with the occurrence and localization of herpes zoster. These include immunosuppression in Hodgkin's disease and other malignancies; administration of immunosuppressive drugs and corticosteroids; irradiation of the spinal column; tumor involvement of the cord, dorsal root ganglion, or adjacent structures; local trauma; surgical manipulation of the spine; heavy metal poisoning or therapy; and frontal sinusitis, as a precipitant of ophthalmic zoster [14,15,82–86].

Even when latent virus does revert, usually nothing perceptible happens. The minute dose of infectious virus that results is immediately neutralized by circulating antibody or destroyed by cellular immune responses before it can infect other cells and multiply enough to cause perceptible damage. The small quantity of viral antigen released into the bloodstream during such "contained reversions" stimulates host immune responses [15,87,88], and this raises the level of host resistance (Fig. 191-2). A similar boost in the level of host resistance frequently follows contact with a patient with varicella (Fig. 191-2), reflecting subclinical exogenous reinfection [60,75,76,89]. When host resistance falls below a critical level, reactivated virus can no longer be contained and the next reversion is "successful." Virus multiplies and spreads within the ganglion, causing neuronal necrosis and intense inflammation, a process that is usually accompanied by severe neuralgia. Infectious VZV

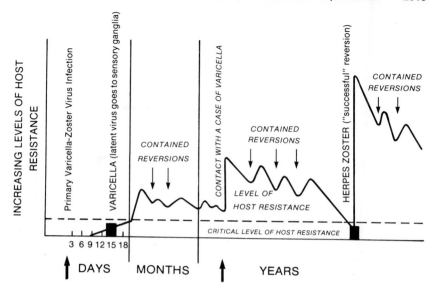

Fig. 191-2 Pathogenesis of herpes zoster. Heavy arrows = exogenous exposure to VZV; solid boxes = clinically apparent disease; dashed lines = critical level of host resistance. (Modified from Hope-Simpson [15].)

then spreads antidromically down the sensory nerve, causing intense neuritis, and is released around the sensory nerve endings in the skin where it produces the characteristic cluster of zoster vesicles. The frequent occurrence of neuralgia several days before the rash appears, and the presence of degenerative changes in cutaneous nerve fibrils on the first day of the eruption [19] provide additional evidence that infection in the sensory ganglion precedes involvement of the skin. Spread of the ganglionic infection proximally along the posterior nerve root to the meninges and cord results in local leptomeningitis, cerebrospinal fluid pleocytosis, and segmental myelitis. Infection of motor neurons in the anterior horn and inflammation of the anterior nerve root account for the local palsies that occasionally accompany the cutaneous eruption, and extension of infection within the central nervous system may result in ascending myelitis or meningoencephalitis, rare complications of herpes zoster [90,91].

During each successful reversion, hematogenous dissemination of virus from the affected ganglion [92] often produces aberrant vesicles at a distance from the primary dermatome, even in uncomplicated herpes zoster [34], and stimulates an anamnestic immune response that terminates the infectious process. Sometimes this response is sufficiently rapid to neutralize virus released into the skin and thus prevent the development of cutaneous lesions; the result is an episode of radicular pain without eruption (zoster sine herpete) and a coincident rise in antibody to VZV. The occurrence of this syndrome has now been well documented [83,87,93], as have completely asymptomatic rises in antibody to VZV that presumably reflect "contained reversions" [76,87,89]. If the anamnestic host response is delayed or deficient, as it appears to be in many immunosuppressed patients, the duration and severity of the local infection is increased and the hematogenous dissemination of VZV is more prolonged and extensive [82–86,92,94–97].

Hope-Simpson considered the level of antibody to be the critical determinant of the host's capacity to contain VZV reversions [15]. However, it now appears that cellular immunity is a more important factor in host resistance to

these recurrent VZV infections of endogenous origin [35,57,60,68–70,84–86,98–101].

A selective decline in cellular immune responses to VZV has been documented in elderly individuals, and this may explain the increased incidence and severity of herpes zoster observed in older people [102–104].

Clinical manifestations

Clinical manifestations of varicella

Prodrome of varicella. In young children, prodromal symptoms are infrequent and the illness usually begins, after an incubation period of 14 or 15 days, with the onset of the rash. The rash may be accompanied by a low-grade fever and malaise. In older children and adults, the rash is often preceded by 2 to 3 days of fever, chills, malaise, headache, anorexia, severe backache, and, in some patients, sore throat and dry cough. A fleeting scarlatiniform rash is sometimes observed just before or coincident with the vesicular eruption.

Rash of varicella. The rash begins on the face and scalp, and spreads rapidly to the trunk with relative sparing of the extremities. New lesions appear in successive crops, but their distribution remains central. The rash tends to be more profuse in hollows and protected parts of the body than on prominent and exposed parts. Thus it is denser in the hollow of the small of the back and between the shoulder blades than on the scapulae and buttocks, and more profuse on the medial than on the lateral aspects of the limbs. It is not uncommon to have a few lesions on the palms and soles. Vesicles often appear earlier and in larger numbers in areas of inflammation, such as diaper rash, sunburn, or eczema.

The most striking feature of the lesions of varicella is their rapid progression from rose-colored macules to papules to vesicles to pustules to crusts. The entire transition may take only 8 to 12 h. The typical vesicle of varicella is superficial and thin-walled, so that it looks like a drop of water lying on, rather than in, the skin. It is usually 2 to

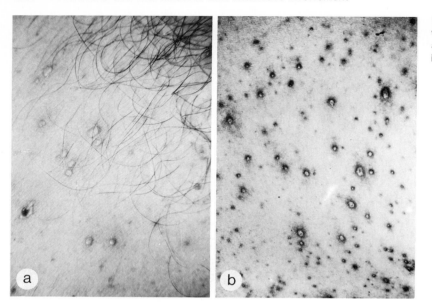

Fig. 191-3   Varicella. (a) Superficial thin-walled elliptical vesicles with their long axes parallel to the skin folds. (b) Lesions in all stages of evolution.

3 mm in diameter and elliptical, with its long axis parallel to the folds of the skin (Fig. 191-3a). The early vesicle is surrounded by an irregular area of erythema which gives the lesions the appearance of a "dewdrop on a rose petal" [105]. The vesicle fluid soon becomes cloudy with the influx of inflammatory cells which convert the vesicle to a pustule. The lesion then dries, beginning in the center, first producing an umbilicated pustule and then a crust. Crusts fall off in 1 to 3 weeks, depending upon the depth of the skin involvement, leaving shallow pink depressions that gradually disappear. Scarring is rare in uncomplicated varicella.

Vesicles also develop in the mucous membranes of the mouth, occurring most commonly over the palate. Mucosal vesicles rupture so rapidly that the vesicular stage may be missed. Instead, one sees shallow ulcers 2 to 3 mm in diameter. Vesicles may also appear on other mucous membranes, including those of the nose, pharynx, larynx, trachea, gastrointestinal tract, urinary tract, and vagina, as well as on the conjunctivae.

A distinctive feature of varicella is the simultaneous presence, in any one area of the skin, of lesions in all stages of development (Fig. 191-3b). This is due to the rapid evolution of individual lesions and the appearance of successive crops involving the same anatomic areas. In a typical case, three crops of lesions appear over a 3-day period, but there is wide variation, ranging from a single crop of a few scattered lesions to a series of five or more crops developing over a period of a week, with innumerable lesions covering the entire body. In general, the mildest cases are seen most frequently in infants and the most severe in adults (Fig. 191-4). Inapparent infections occur, but are rare [25].

Fever usually persists as long as new lesions continue to appear and its height is generally proportional to the severity of the rash. In typical cases it rarely exceeds 39°C (102°F); it may be absent in mild cases and rise to 40.5°C (105°F) in severe cases with extensive rash. Prolonged fever or recurrence of fever after defervescence may be seen with secondary bacterial infection or other complications. Headache, malaise, myalgia, and anorexia generally accompany the fever and are more severe in older children and adults. However, the most distressing symptom is usually pruritus, which is present throughout the vesicular stage.

Complications of varicella. In the normal child, varicella is a benign disease rarely attended by serious complications. The most frequent complication is the secondary bacterial infection of skin lesions, usually by staphylococci or streptococci, which may produce impetigo, furuncles, cellulitis, erysipelas and, rarely, gangrene. These local infections often lead to scarring and, very rarely, to septicemia with metastatic infection of other organs [106–109]. Bullous lesions may be produced when vesicles are infected with staphylococci that elaborate exfoliative toxin [110]. Secondary bacterial pneumonia is a rare complication that occurs mainly in children under 7 years of age and responds to appropriate antibiotic therapy, as do otitis media and suppurative meningitis [106,111,112]. In contrast to the situation in the normal host, bacterial superinfection is frequent and life-threatening in leukopenic patients, especially children with leukemia.

Other complications that appear to reflect some defect in the capacity of the host to limit VZV multiplication and dissemination account for the increased morbidity and mortality of varicella in adults, in newborns, and in immunocompromised patients of any age [48,58,83,107, 109,111–116].

Varicella, like many other viral infections, is generally more severe in adults than in children. Fever and constitutional symptoms are more prominent and prolonged. The rash is more profuse and complications more frequent. Primary varicella pneumonia is the major complication of adult varicella. It is rarely observed in normal children, and adults account for more than 90 percent of reported cases [106,107,111,113].

The incidence of primary varicella pneumonia depends upon the population of patients studied and upon the diagnostic criteria employed. Roentgenographic evidence of

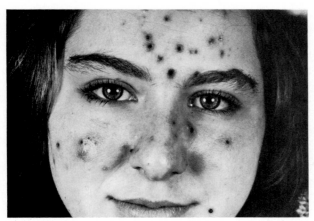

Fig. 191-4 Varicella. Facial involvement in an adult. This may lead to scarring.

pneumonia was found in 16 percent of healthy male military recruits with varicella, but clinical signs of pneumonia were present in only 4 percent [117]. The incidence and severity of varicella pneumonia are substantially higher in older patients and in the subset of adults with varicella admitted to hospitals [111,113]. Pneumonia generally appears 1 to 6 days after the onset of the rash, and the degree of pulmonary involvement correlates best with the severity of the cutaneous eruption. Some patients are virtually asymptomatic, but others develop severe respiratory embarrassment, with cough, dyspnea, tachypnea, high fever, pleuritic chest pain, cyanosis, and hemoptysis. The severity of the symptoms is usually out of proportion to the physical findings in the chest, but the roentgenogram typically reveals diffuse nodular densities throughout both lung fields, often peribronchial in distribution, with a tendency to concentrate in the perihilar regions and at the bases. Roentgenographic abnormalities disappear more slowly than the symptoms of pneumonia and, occasionally, the pulmonary lesions calcify and persist for years [107,113,118]. The mortality in adults with varicella pneumonia has been estimated to be between 10 and 30 percent, but it is probably closer to 10 percent if immunocompromised patients are excluded [107,113,116]. It is clear from postmortem examination of fatal cases that the pneumonia is but one manifestation of widespread hematogenous dissemination, with evidence of varicella infection in virtually every organ examined [113,119,120].

Varicella during pregnancy is a threat to both mother and fetus. Disseminated infection and varicella pneumonia may result in maternal death, but it is not clear that either the incidence or the severity of varicella pneumonia is greater when varicella occurs during pregnancy than when it occurs in the normal nonpregnant adult [121,122]. The fetus may sometimes die as a consequence of premature labor or maternal death in severe varicella pneumonia, but varicella during pregnancy has not increased the background level of fetal morbidity, mortality, or congenital malformations [121,122]. Nevertheless, even in uncomplicated varicella, maternal viremia may result in intrauterine (congenital) VZV infection.

When congenital VZV infection occurs early in gestation, the spectrum of disease ranges from severe congenital malformations to asymptomatic latency. A characteristic

syndrome of developmental abnormalities (including hypoplasia of an extremity, cicatricial skin scarring, cortical atrophy, ocular abnormalities, and low birth weight) has been observed in infants born to women who had varicella between the seventh and twentieth weeks of gestation [121–123]. This is a rare occurrence, with fewer than 30 cases reported worldwide. However, maternal varicella at any stage of pregnancy can cause a fetal infection that resolves before parturition without obvious sequelae. These infants are born without visible evidence of infection, but frequently develop herpes zoster at an early age without any history of previous varicella [38,121,122].

Congenital varicella (i.e., varicella occurring within 10 days of birth) appears to be more serious than varicella in infants infected postnatally, and the severity varies markedly depending upon the proximity of maternal disease to delivery. When an infant acquires VZV infection in utero but is born before the transplacental passage of sufficient maternal antibody to modify the infection during its incubation period (i.e., when the rash of varicella occurs in the mother less than 5 days before or within 2 days after delivery, or begins in an infant between 5 and 10 days of age), the result is often severe disseminated varicella, and the mortality is about 30 percent. When the onset of rash in the mother is 5 days or more before delivery (onset of rash in the infant at 0 to 4 days of age) sufficient maternal antibody has crossed the placenta to modify the infection, and all such infected infants can be expected to survive. These observations imply that immature perinatal defenses cannot, by themselves, restrain VZV replication and dissemination [121,122].

The morbidity and mortality of varicella are markedly increased in immunocompromised patients, including patients with leukemia and other malignancies who are receiving corticosteroids, chemotherapeutic agents, or radiotherapy at the time of infection; patients receiving corticosteroids for diseases such as nephrotic syndrome and rheumatic fever; and patients with congenital immunologic deficiencies [48,58,114,115,124–130]. In these patients, continued virus replication and dissemination result in a prolonged high-level viremia [51,59], a more extensive rash and a longer period of new vesicle formation, and frequent involvement of the lungs, liver, central nervous system, and other organs throughout the body. In one series, 19 of 60 children with leukemia who were receiving chemotherapy at the time of infection had visceral dissemination, and 4 died [58]. There was varicella pneumonia in all four fatal cases and fulminant encephalitis in two. Varicella hepatitis was also frequently present, but was not fatal in the absence of pneumonia. Disseminated varicella occurred more fequently in children with absolute lymphopenia (less than 500 lymphocytes per cubic millimeter). Immunosuppressed and corticosteroid-treated patients may also develop hemorrhagic complications of varicella that range in severity from mild febrile purpura to severe and often fatal purpura fulminans and malignant varicella with purpura [83,131–135]. The etiology of these hemorrhagic complications is complex and probably not the same in every case. In some, thrombocytopenia may be associated with the underlying disease, its therapy, the direct effect of VZV infection on the bone marrow, or immune-mediated platelet destruction [83,132,136]. In others, particularly those with malignant varicella and purpura fulminans, the primary factor may be infection of vascular endothelial cells, with endothelial damage initiating disseminated intravascular coagulation and thrombotic purpura.

Central nervous system (CNS) complications of varicella, which occur in fewer than 1 in 1000 cases, include several distinct syndromes [91]: (1) Reye's syndrome, (2) acute cerebellar ataxia, (3) encephalitis or meningoencephalitis, (4) acute ascending or transverse myelitis, and (5) Guillain-Barré syndrome. Varicella-associated Reye's syndrome (acute encephalopathy with fatty degeneration of the viscera), which typically occurs 2 to 7 days after the appearance of the rash, is not discernibly different from Reye's syndrome associated with influenza A, influenza B, or other viral infections. Although its pathogenesis is not understood, there is no inflammatory response in the CNS, and pathologic and virologic studies have essentially ruled out direct virus infection of the liver or brain. Instead, Reye's syndrome may be caused by some circulating toxin, perhaps a component of the virus or a substance elaborated by virus-infected cells [137]. From 15 to 40 percent of all cases of Reye's syndrome occur in association with varicella [138,139], and the mortality may be as high as 40 percent [109]. Reexamination of older reports of the CNS complications of varicella suggests that many of the cases described as "varicella encephalitis" in immunologically normal children were probably Reye's syndrome. Furthermore, Reye's syndrome appears to account for most of the fatalities in normal children that were attributed to varicella encephalitis. Two recent series [109,140] support this conclusion. In Takashima and Becker's review of 32 fatal cases of varicella in children, all 12 that occurred in otherwise normal children had clinical and pathologic findings compatible with Reye's syndrome. Of the remaining 20, 18 occurred in children with underlying diseases (12 of whom were receiving corticosteroids) and 2 were cases of neonatal varicella. Although typical inclusions were demonstrated in the brains of only 2, all 20 of these children had evidence of widespread VZV dissemination with inclusions in many internal organs. In a series of 96 patients hospitalized with varicella [109], there were 17 cases of Reye's syndrome in 81 immunologically normal children, and these accounted for 7 of the 10 fatalities recorded. Another of the deaths occurred in an infant who developed varicella 7 days after delivery; CNS involvement in this case was part of a widely disseminated VZV infection.

Varicella-associated Guillain-Barré syndrome is extremely rare, and many of the cases reported are almost certainly examples of varicella myelitis. Apart from the temporal association in the few cases recorded, there is no evidence directly implicating VZV in the pathogenesis of Guillain-Barré syndrome.

In acute cerebellar ataxia the onset of neurologic symptoms has ranged from 11 days before to 20 days after the appearance of the rash. Recovery without sequelae is the rule, and no pathologic data are available. However, its occurrence as early as 11 days before the onset of rash, i.e., during the primary viremia [141] and the detection of VZV antigens in the cerebrospinal fluid of two patients with this complication [142] suggest that acute cerebellar ataxia may reflect direct invasion of the CNS, presumably as a consequence of viremia and infection of vascular endothelial cells.

The pathogenesis of varicella encephalitis (meningoencephalitis) and myelitis remains obscure. Although many observers favor a postinfectious (autoimmune) demyelinating process like that observed in measles encephalomyelitis [143], there is increasing evidence that these complications of varicella result from direct VZV infection of the CNS. The therapeutic implications of this distinction are obvious (see below). Many cases of varicella meningoencephalitis and myelitis (and most cases that have come to postmortem examination) have occurred in patients with prolonged high-grade viremia and infection of many organs in addition to the skin and mucous membranes—a setting in which direct infection of the CNS is to be expected [51,58,90,120,140,144,145]. Furthermore, whereas characteristic intranuclear inclusions in the CNS have been reported in only a few cases [140,146], many others have shown pathologic features more consistent with direct VZV infection than with postinfectious (autoimmune) encephalomyelitis [147]. These have included perivascular infiltrates in the cortex and brain stem, scattered foci of necrosis, often hemorrhagic and often associated with swelling of endothelial cells and injury to vessel walls, and inflammatory infiltration of the leptomeninges. Moreover, because isolation of VZV from skin vesicles after more than 4 days of rash is uncommon [57] and because characteristic intranuclear inclusion bodies are not always observed in infected tissues, the failure to isolate VZV or demonstrate inclusion bodies is not compelling evidence against direct CNS infection. Finally, the infectious nature of varicella encephalitis and myelitis is further supported by the recent demonstration of antibody to VZV (presumably locally produced within the CNS) in the cerebrospinal fluid of patients with varicella encephalitis and transverse myelitis, and by the direct isolation of VZV from the cerebrospinal fluid of a patient with varicella encephalitis [148].

Other rare complications of varicella include myocarditis, glomerulonephritis, orchitis, appendicitis, pancreatitis, arthritis, Henoch-Schönlein vasculitis, optic neuritis, keratitis, and iritis. The pathogenesis of these complications has not been delineated, but direct parenchymal infection or vasculitis induced by VZV infection of endothelial cells appears to be responsible in many instances.

Although chemical evidence of mild hepatitis is common in uncomplicated varicella [54–56], clinical hepatitis is rare, except as a complication of progressive varicella.

Clinical manifestations of herpes zoster

Prodrome of herpes zoster. The first symptom of herpes zoster is usually pain and paresthesia in the involved dermatome. This generally precedes the eruption by several days and varies from superficial itching, tingling or burning, to severe, deep, boring or lancinating pain. It may be constant or intermittent, and it is often accompanied by tenderness and hyperesthesia of the skin in the involved dermatome. The preeruptive pain of herpes zoster may simulate pleurisy, myocardial infarction, duodenal ulcer, cholecystitis, biliary or renal colic, appendicitis, prolapsed intervertebral disk, or early glaucoma, and it may thus lead to serious misdiagnosis. Constitutional symptoms, including headache, malaise, and fever, occur in about 5 percent of patients, usually in children, and may precede the rash by 1 to 2 days [32,36,83].

A few patients experience acute segmental neuralgia

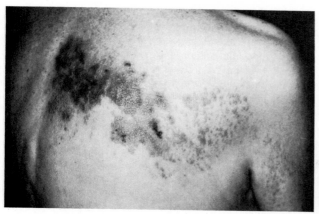

Fig. 191-5 Herpes zoster in the right second thoracic dermatome. *(Courtesy of Dr. D. A. Lopez.)*

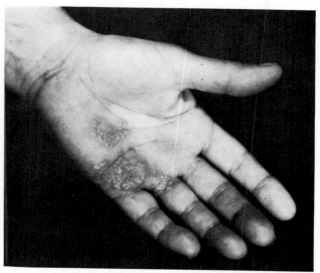

Fig. 191-6 Herpes zoster involving the C8 dermatome. Note closely grouped vesicles on an erythematous base. This may be difficult to distinguish from zosteriform herpes simplex; definitive diagnosis requires virus isolation or the direct detection and identification of VZV antigens or nucleic acids in the lesions.

without ever developing a cutaneous eruption, a syndrome called *zoster sine herpete* [83,87,93,133,149]. A concurrent rise in antibodies to VZV has now been demonstrated in a number of such episodes, providing evidence that they are, indeed, manifestations of herpes zoster [83,87,93]. However, while zoster sine herpete may explain some cases of trigeminal neuralgia, most patients with this syndrome do not have serologic evidence of herpes zoster. Similarly, although facial palsy frequently complicates cephalic herpes zoster, VZV infection does not appear to be responsible for most cases of "idiopathic" facial (Bell's) palsy [150].

Rash of herpes zoster. The most distinctive feature of herpes zoster is the localization of the rash, which is nearly always unilateral, does not cross the midline, and is usually limited to the area of skin innervated by a single sensory ganglion (Figs. 191-5 and A1-27). Individual sensory ganglia are not attacked at random; herpes zoster occurs with greatest frequency in those areas in which the rash of varicella is most abundant [15,17]. The area supplied by the trigeminal nerve, particularly the ophthalmic division, and the trunk from T3 to L2 are most frequently affected; the thoracic region alone accounts for more than one-half of reported cases (Figs. 191-5 and A1-27) and lesions rarely occur below the elbows or knees [14,15,32,37,83,151]. Regional lymphadenopathy occurs in the majority of cases, and the cerebrospinal fluid frequently shows a mild pleocytosis, predominantly lymphocytic, and an elevated protein content. Although the individual lesions of herpes zoster and varicella are usually indistinguishable, those of herpes zoster tend to evolve more slowly, and they often consist of closely grouped vesicles on an erythematous base rather than the discrete, randomly distributed vesicles of varicella (Fig. 191-6). The lesions begin as erythematous maculopapules that often first appear where superficial branches of the affected sensory nerve are given off, e.g., the posterior primary division and the lateral and anterior branches of the anterior primary division of spinal nerves [10,14,17,133]. Vesicles form within 12 to 24 h and evolve into pustules by the third day. These dry up and crust in 7 to 10 days. Crusts generally persist for 2 to 3 weeks. In normal individuals, new lesions continue to appear for 1 to 4 days (occasionally for as long as 7 days) and virus may be recovered from lesions for as long as a week after the appearance of the rash. The rash is most severe and

lasts longest in older people, and is least severe and of shortest duration in children [32,33,83,151]. Segmental pain, a prominent feature of herpes zoster in older individuals, generally remits as the crusts fall off. Pain is seldom a significant symptom of herpes zoster in children [152,153].

Ten to fifteen percent of reported cases of herpes zoster involve the ophthalmic division of the trigeminal nerve (Figs. 191-7 and A1-26). The rash of ophthalmic zoster may extend from the level of the eye to the vertex of the skull, but it does not cross the midline of the forehead. When only the supratrochlear and supraorbital branches are involved, the eye is usually spared. Involvement of the nasociliary branch, as evidenced by a herpetic rash on the tip and side of the nose (Fig. 191-7), occurs in about one-third of patients and is usually accompanied by conjunctivitis and occasionally by keratitis, scleritis, iridocyclitis, extraocular-muscle palsies, ptosis, and mydriasis. Thus, when ophthalmic zoster involves the side of the nose, careful attention must be given to the condition of the eye. VZV is not, however, as pathogenic for the eye as is herpes simplex virus.

Herpes zoster affecting the second and third divisions of the trigeminal nerve and other cranial nerves is uncommon, but when it occurs it may produce symptoms and lesions in the mouth, ears, pharynx, or larynx [16,133,154,155]. The so-called Ramsay Hunt's syndrome, which consists of facial palsy in combination with herpes zoster of the external ear or tympanic membrane, with or without tinnitus, vertigo, and deafness, results from involvement of the facial and auditory nerves [16].

Complications of herpes zoster. Postherpetic neuralgia (pain persisting after all crusts have fallen off) occurs in 10 to 15 percent of patients with herpes zoster [37,156]. It is uncommon in patients under 40 years of age, but occurs in more than one-third of patients 60 years old or older, especially those with ophthalmic zoster [32,33,83,156].

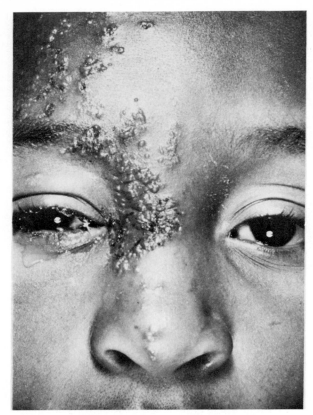

Fig. 191-7 Herpes zoster of the ophthalmic division of the 5th cranial nerve. Involvement of the nasociliary branch results in lesions on the tip and side of the nose and unilateral conjunctivitis. *(Courtesy of Dr. D. A. Lopez.)*

Anesthesia in the involved dermatome is another common sequela, and is particularly troublesome when it occurs in the area innervated by the ophthalmic nerve [83,157,158]. Postherpetic neuralgia is refractory to treatment, but usually remits spontaneously in 1 to 6 months.

When the rash is particularly severe, there may be superficial gangrene with delayed healing and subsequent scarring. As in varicella, secondary bacterial infection may also delay healing and cause scarring.

Ophthalmic zoster has a relatively high complication rate, especially when involvement of the nasociliary branches provides VZV with direct access to intraocular structures [37,157,158]. The eye is involved in 20 to 70 percent of patients with ophthalmic zoster. Complications include cicatricial lid retraction, paralytic ptosis, acute epithelial keratitis, scleritis, uveitis, secondary glaucoma, oculomotor palsies, chorioretinitis, and optic neuritis. Corneal sensation is almost always impaired, and when the impairment is severe it may lead to neurotrophic keratitis and chronic ulceration. Rarely, secondary bacterial infection may result in panophthalmitis requiring enucleation. Granulomatous cerebral angiitis with contralateral hemiplegia (see below) was observed in 4 of 86 patients with ophthalmic zoster seen at the Mayo Clinic between 1975 and 1980 [158].

Most other complications of herpes zoster appear to be associated with spread of virus from the involved ganglion, either via the bloodstream or by direct neural extension. When patients with herpes zoster are carefully examined,

17 to 35 percent are found to have at least a few vesicles in areas remote from the involved dermatome; this is due presumably to hematogenous dissemination of virus from the affected ganglion, nerve, or skin [10,34,83]. The disseminated lesions usually appear within a week of onset of the segmental eruption and, if few in number, are easily overlooked. More extensive dissemination, producing a varicella-like eruption (generalized herpes zoster), occurs in 2 to 10 percent of unselected patients with localized zoster, most of whom have immunologic defects due to underlying malignancy (particularly lymphomas) or immunosuppressive therapy [31–36,94].

On rare occasions, most often in children, infection disseminates widely from a small, painless area of zoster [36]. In such cases, the herpes zoster may go unnoticed and the disseminated eruption be mistaken for varicella. This probably explains some reported second attacks of varicella, as well as some of the cases of "atypical generalized zoster" (a disseminated varicella-like eruption without an accompanying dermatomal rash in a person with a history of varicella) reported primarily in immunocompromised patients [85]. However, symptomatic reinfections do occur, especially in immunocompromised patients and in people whose initial infection was modified by passively acquired antibody to VZV [13,80] (see above). These patients may have a prolonged incubation period, and they probably account for the majority of the cases of "atypical generalized zoster" observed in immunocompromised and apparently normal patients [85,159].

Motor paralysis is reported in 1 to 5 percent of patients with herpes zoster. It results from the direct extension of infection from the sensory ganglion to adjacent parts of the nervous system [14,16,83,133,160,161]. Mild motor deficits are often missed in thoracolumbar zoster, but when zoster involves the cranial nerves or the extremities the incidence of recognized motor involvement is 10 to 20 percent [91].

Paralysis usually begins within two weeks of the onset of the rash and almost always involves muscle groups with innervation that is contiguous with that of the affected dermatome; oculomotor and facial palsies are seen with cephalic zoster, unilateral diaphragmatic paralysis with homolateral cervical zoster, paralysis of the trunk and limbs with zoster involving corresponding dermatomes, and dysfunction of the bladder and anus with sacral zoster [14,83,133,161–165]. Rare cases in which the involved myotome and dermatome are widely separated may represent the result of more extensive myelitis [161,166]. Total or functional recovery occurs in most cases.

Posterior nerve roots contain sensory fibers originating in the viscera as well as the skin, which explains the occasional occurrence of visceral lesions in patients with herpes zoster. The affected viscera usually have innervation corresponding to the infected dermatome. Thus, vesicular lesions in the gastric mucosa have been observed in patients with thoracic herpes zoster [167], and herpes zoster hemicystitis has frequently been observed in association with sacral herpes zoster [168,169].

Although a lymphocytic pleocytosis, with or without an increase in the concentration of protein in the cerebrospinal fluid, is a regular feature of uncomplicated herpes zoster, the incidence of acute symptomatic meningoencephalitis and myelitis is low (0.2 to 0.5 percent). When these complications do occur, their onset usually follows that of herpes zoster by 7 to 10 days, but it may precede the rash by a week or more, or follow it by up to 2 months [91,170–174]. Clinical manifestations include fever, altered sensorium (frequently with delirium and hallucinations), headache, meningismus, and cranial or extracranial nerve palsies, often at a cord level corresponding to the rash. There is a lymphocytic cerebrospinal fluid pleocytosis, which usually ranges from 10 to 500 cells/mm³, a moderate elevation in protein concentration, and a normal glucose concentration. However, the cell count occasionally exceeds 1000/mm³, there may be 30 to 40 percent neutrophils, and the sugar concentration may be low. The incidence of meningoencephalitis appears to be increased in cranial zoster and in immunocompromised patients, and most cases occur in association with VZV dissemination [90,174]. Most patients recover and return to their pre-encephalitis cognitive status, but many are left with postherpetic neuralgia, chronic ophthalmologic infections, and motor palsies. Most cases probably represent actual VZV infection, with virus reaching the CNS by the hematogenous route in the course of disseminated herpes zoster, or by direct extension from the involved sensory ganglion [90,91,170,174; author's unpublished observations].

Another complication of herpes zoster, which is being recognized with increasing frequency, is granulomatous angiitis of cerebral arteries, which is responsible for a syndrome of ophthalmic zoster and delayed contralateral hemiplegia [175–177]. It usually occurs weeks to months after the episode of ophthalmic zoster (average interval about 8 weeks), and may present as an isolated cerebral infarction, multiple cerebral infarctions, stroke-in-evolution or transient ischemic attacks. Since the clinical manifestations are similar to hypertensive strokes and the delayed onset may obscure the relationship to herpes zoster, the syndrome is probably underdiagnosed. Cerebral arteriograms usually reveal segmental narrowing or occlusion of cerebral arteries ipsilateral to the ophthalmic zoster. Although multiple strokes may occur for several weeks, later recurrences are rare and the disease appears to be self-limited. The mortality in reported cases is about 15 percent.

Herpes zoster in the immunocompromised host. Certain types of malignancy, especially Hodgkin's disease and lymphocytic leukemia, and the administration of immunosuppressive therapy (e.g., radiation, antimetabolites, antilymphocyte serum, and corticosteroids) to patients with malignant and nonmalignant diseases markedly increase the incidence and severity of herpes zoster [82–86,90,94–97]. In fact, serious complications of herpes zoster occur almost exclusively in such immunocompromised patients. Twenty to 50 percent of patients with Hodgkin's disease develop herpes zoster, with the highest incidence in patients with far-advanced disease and those receiving radiation and combination chemotherapy [82–86,95–97]. The severity of the disease is also increased; necrosis of skin and scarring are fairly common, as is postherpetic neuralgia, and the incidence of cutaneous dissemination is 25 to 50 percent. Approximately 10 percent of patients with disseminated cutaneous lesions develop widespread, frequently fatal, visceral infection, particularly of the lungs, liver, and brain [18,21,94,129,130,170,178]. The incidence and severity of herpes zoster is also markedly increased in immunosuppressed renal, cardiac, and bone marrow transplant recipients [87,98,100,101,179].

A syndrome resembling progressive multifocal leukoencephalopathy (PML) has recently been reported following herpes zoster in two immunocompromised patients [180]. Both patients exhibited steadily progressive, asymmetric, multifocal neurologic deficits, including impaired mental function and focal seizures, and died after several months. At autopsy, there were multifocal lesions, primarily at the gray-white cortical junction, with demyelination, necrosis, and eosinophilic Cowdry type A intranuclear inclusion bodies in oligodendrocytes, neurons, and astrocytes. Herpesvirus-like particles and VZV antigens were detected in these cells. A remarkable feature of these two cases was the long interval (9 to 20 months) between their episode of herpes zoster and the onset of neurologic symptoms. This, as well as the long interval between ophthalmic zoster and the onset of symptoms in patients with granulomatous angiitis, suggests that in addition to latent infections, VZV can produce prolonged "smoldering" subclinical infections, especially in patients lacking the normal defenses that eliminate virus-infected cells and prevent cell-to-cell spread of VZV infection.

The presence or absence of a normal humoral response to VZV does not appear to be a major determinant of the response of these patients to herpes zoster. Rather, cellular immunity, as measured by lymphocyte blastogenesis and interferon production following exposure to VZV antigens, appears to be a major correlate of the host's capacity to limit VZV replication and dissemination [35,57,60,64,67–70,86,98–101].

Pathology

The cutaneous lesions of varicella and herpes zoster are histologically indistinguishable, and are similar to those produced by herpes simplex virus. The characteristic changes in infected cells, which can be observed in tissue culture as well as in vivo, are "ballooning degeneration," with the formation of intranuclear inclusion bodies and mutinucleated giant cells [10]. Individual infected cells become greatly enlarged with pale vacuolated cytoplasm. The nuclei exhibit margination of chromatin and contain inclusion bodies. Early in infection, the inclusion bodies may be homogeneous and moderately basophilic, and they often fill the nucleus. However, they rapidly evolve into sharply demarcated acidophilic inclusion bodies that are separated from the deeply basophilic ring of marginated chromatin at the nuclear membrane by a clear zone or halo. Multinucleated giant cells are formed primarily by the fusion of adjacent infected cells [49]. Cell fusion, which is mediated by viral glycoproteins that appear on cell membranes early in the VZV replication cycle, facilitates cell-to-cell spread of infection, even in the presence of antibody capable of neutralizing extracellular virus. Neither multinucleated giant cells nor intranuclear inclusion bodies are found in the vesicular lesions caused by poxviruses (smallpox, vaccinia) or enteroviruses (echo viruses, Coxsackie viruses).

Pathology of varicella

The initial event in the formation of the cutaneous lesions of varicella is probably infection of capillary endothelial cells in the papillary dermis, with subsequent spread of virus to epithelial cells in the epidermis, hair follicles, and sebaceous glands [6,8–10,48,49,181]. In early papular le-

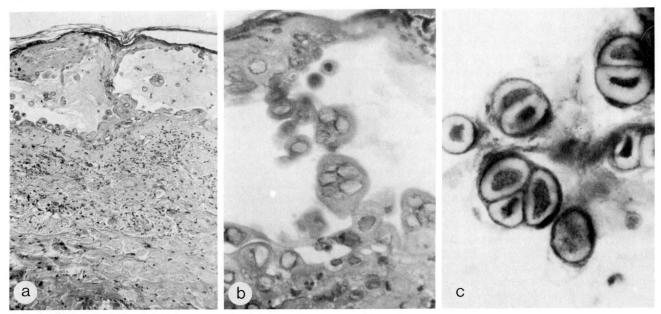

Fig. 191-8   Varicella zoster, early vesicle. (a) Intraepidermal vesicle. Infected epithelial cells show acantholysis, "ballooning degeneration," intranuclear inclusions, and multinucleated giant cell formation. Underlying dermis shows edema and mononuclear cell infiltration. H&E stain; ×100. (b) Multinucleated giant cells in walls and base of vesicle. H&E stain; × 400. (c) Tzanck smear from base of vesicle showing multinucleated giant cells with intranuclear inclusion bodies. H&E stain; ×1000. *[Parts (a) and (b) courtesy of Dr. R. J Barr.]*

sions the epithelium is slightly elevated due to swelling of the infected epithelial cells and to edema and vascular congestion of the underlying dermis. In the superficial dermis, capillary endothelial cells are swollen, and their nuclei frequently contain intranuclear inclusion bodies. Similar inclusion bodies may be seen in the nuclei of fibroblasts in the surrounding connective tissue, which is edematous and infiltrated by small numbers of mononuclear cells. Superficial lymphatics are dilated, and cells lining these structures are also swollen and may contain intranuclear inclusion bodies. In the epidermis, the cells initially involved are those of the germinal layer and the deeper portion of the stratum spinosum. These cells show ballooning degeneration with loss of intercellular bridges, and they are soon separated by intercellular edema (acantholysis). A few small multinucleated giant cells, containing three to eight nuclei, are usually seen at the base and periphery of these early epithelial lesions. The papular lesions rapidly evolve into intraepidermal vesicles as a result of the infection and degeneration of increasing numbers of epithelial cells, the fusion of adjacent areas of microscopic degeneration, and the continuing influx of edema fluid which elevates the uninvolved stratum corneum to form a delicate clear vesicle (Fig. 191-8a). At this stage, the vesicle fluid contains fibrin, degenerating and "ballooned" epithelial cells, and abundant cell-free infectious VZV. Multinucleated giant cells with eosinophilic intranuclear inclusion bodies are readily found in the walls and base of the vesicle (Fig. 191-8b). As the lesions progress, polymorphonuclear leukocytes and a small number of macrophages invade from the underlying dermis, and the vesicle fluid becomes cloudy; this transforms the vesicle into a pustule. The fluid is then absorbed, with the formation of a flat adherent crust that is eventually detached by the regrowth of subjacent

epithelial cells. The evolution from papule to early crusting can occur over a period of 8 to 12 h. Lesions of uncomplicated varicella usually heal without scarring. Lesions in mucous membranes develop in the same way, but the thin roof of the vesicle breaks down quickly, producing a shallow ulcer that heals rapidly.

In fatal varicella, focal lesions have been found in the mucous membranes of the respiratory, gastrointestinal, and genitourinary tracts, in the serosa of the pleural and peritoneal cavities, and in the parenchyma of virtually every organ, the lungs being the most frequent site of severe involvement [10,48–50,107,119,120,133,182–184]. There is widespread vascular damage, with characteristic acidophilic intranuclear inclusion bodies in the endothelial cells lining small blood vessels and lymphatics; capillaries within individual lesions are often destroyed, resulting in thrombosis and hemorrhage. In varicella pneumonia, the pleura are studded with hemorrhagic nodules and the lungs show widely disseminated interstitial pneumonia with numerous foci of hemorrhagic necrosis. Alveoli are filled with red cells, fibrin, inclusion-bearing mononuclear cells, and occasional multinucleated giant cells. Hyalin membranes are frequently seen. Typical acidophilic inclusion bodies are also seen within hyperplastic alveolar septal cells, swollen capillary endothelial cells, fibroblasts, and bronchiolar and tracheobronchial epithelial cells. Similar areas of vascular damage and focal necrosis are found in the parenchyma of the liver, spleen, and other organs throughout the body. In some cases, characteristic intranuclear inclusion bodies may be nearly or totally absent, in spite of unmistakable clinical and pathologic evidence of extensive VZV infection and the isolation of VZV from the liver, lungs, brain, and other tissues [120,183,184; author's unpublished observations].

There is now increasing evidence that (except for Reye's syndrome) the central nervous system complications of varicella and herpes zoster (see below) are caused by direct VZV infection, rather than autoimmune demyelination, as previously thought by many observers [91,147].

Pathology of herpes zoster

Although the histopathology of the skin lesions of herpes zoster and varicella is the same, herpes zoster is accompanied by acute inflammation of the corresponding sensory nerve and ganglion. The ganglion shows intense lymphocytic infiltration, necrosis of nerve cells and fibers, endothelial cell proliferation and lymphocytic cuffing of small vessels, focal hemorrhage, and inflammation of the ganglion sheath [14,16]. Satellite cells and neurons contain characteristic acidophilic intranuclear inclusion bodies, virus particles visible by electron microscopy, and VZV antigens demonstrable by immunofluorescence [10,18,20–23,83]. Some degree of neuronal degeneration and lymphocytic infiltration is also generally present in adjacent ganglia on the same side. The periperal nerve shows diffuse lymphocytic infiltration and focal hemorrhage, with axonal degeneration and demyelination of sensory fibers. Virus particles and VZV antigens are present in Schwann and perineural cells. These inflammatory and degenerative changes can be traced distally to branches innervating the affected skin [19]. The inflammatory reaction in the ganglion also extends proximally to the posterior nerve root and into adjacent regions of the cord or brainstem, producing a segmental myelitis that is predominantly unilateral and involves the posterior more than the anterior horns. There is degeneration of nerve fibers in the posterior columns and inflammatory changes in the gray matter of the posterior and anterior horns, with perivenous lymphocytic infiltration, scattered neuronal necrosis, and neuronophagia. These changes may extend two or more segments from the one corresponding to the cutaneous eruption. A mild lymphocytic leptomeningitis is generally present, and is most intense over the involved segments and nerve roots. Marked inflammation and degeneration of the anterior nerve root within the meninges and in the portion contiguous to the involved sensory ganglion may also be present, producing a true motor radiculitis [16]. When extensive, the acute inflammatory response is followed by fibrosis of the ganglion and nerve [14]. These observations, as well as the isolation of VZV from the sensory ganglion [22,23,185], cerebrospinal fluid [86,171,186,187], and CNS tissue [170,180,188; author's unpublished observations] indicate that the pathologic changes in herpes zoster are the direct result of VZV infection.

Herpes zoster is occasionally complicated by meningoencephalitis or myelitis, in which CNS involvement is not restricted to segments corresponding to the involved dermatome [91]. The pathologic findings in herpes zoster meningoencephalitis vary from focal mononuclear cell infiltration of the leptomeninges [83,173] to acute necrotizing encephalitis with perivenous encephalomalacia, myelin and axonal degeneration, macrophage infiltration, and typical intranuclear inclusion bodies and virus particles in oligodendrocytes, neurons, and astrocytes [170]. The presence of VZV in the involved brain tissue has been documented by virus isolation or immunoperoxidase staining in

several of these patients [170,180; author's unpublished observations]. Herpes zoster myelitis is rarely fatal, but in two patients who died of pulmonary embolism 12 days and 12 weeks, respectively, after the onset of herpes zoster, autopsy revealed extensive inflammatory necrosis of the spinal cord, which was maximal at the level of the dermatomal rash and extended above and below in a continuous but irregular pattern that did not correspond to any vascular topography [166,188]. In areas of most recent extension where necrosis was less complete, intranuclear inclusion bodies were present in glial nuclei [188]. VZV has also been isolated from the cerebrospinal fluid of a number of patients with herpes zoster meningoencephalitis and myelitis [86,148,171,174,186,187]. In herpes zoster myelitis, it seems clear that VZV reaches the spinal cord by direct extension from the infected dorsal root ganglion. The pathogenesis of herpes zoster encephalitis (or meningoencephalitis) is more obscure. The presence of perivascular mononuclear cell infiltrates and demyelination, and the lack of direct evidence of VZV infection in autopsied cases, has led many observers to favor a postinfectious (autoimmune) encephalomyelitis [91] like that observed in measles encephalomyelitis [143]. However, there is now much evidence that most or all of the CNS complications of herpes zoster are the direct result of VZV infection of the tissues involved, and that the demyelination observed in herpes zoster encephalitis can be accounted for by VZV infection of oligodendrocytes [180]. The frequent occurrence of herpes zoster encephalitis or meningoencephalitis in association with disseminated herpes zoster suggests that virus often reaches the brain as a result of viremia [90,91,174]. However, it may also reach the brain along neural routes, especially when meningoencephalitis occurs in association with herpes zoster of cranial dermatomes [174,180,189].

The contralateral hemiplegia that sometimes develops in patients with ophthalmic herpes zoster appears to be caused by segmental granulomatous angiitis involving ipsilateral cerebral arteries [175–177,190]. The temporal association with herpes zoster and the electron microscopic observation of herpesvirus-like particles in the walls of involved vessels and in adjacent glial cells [189,191,192] suggest that the angiitis is due to VZV infection of arterial walls. The virus may reach the vessels by direct spread from the trigeminal ganglion or along branches of the ophthalmic nerve that supply the meninges and most of the intracranial arteries that have been involved [193].

Lesions of the skin, lungs, and other organs in fatal cases of disseminated herpes zoster are identical to those observed in fatal cases of varicella [18,48–50,94,107,119, 120,178,182,184]. They result from the viremic spread of VZV in both diseases [46,51,57,59,92].

Clinical and laboratory diagnoses

Clinical diagnosis of varicella

Varicella can usually be diagnosed clinically on the basis of the character and evolution of the rash, particularly when there is a history of exposure within the preceding 2 to 3 weeks [105,107,133]. Characteristic diagnostic features include (1) the development, after a brief and mild (or absent) prodrome, of a papulovesicular eruption accompanied by fever and mild constitutional symptoms; (2) the appearance of lesions in crops, with a predominantly central distribution including the scalp; (3) the rapid evolution of individual lesions from macules to papules to delicate thin-walled vesicles to pustules and, finally, to crusts; (4) the presence of lesions in all stages of development in any one anatomic area throughout the acute disease; and (5) the presence of lesions in the mucous membranes of the mouth.

Severe varicella, especially in immunosuppressed patients, may resemble smallpox or generalized vaccinia. Conversely, mild variola, especially when modified by vaccination, may be indistinguishable from varicella. Generalized vaccinia, especially in patients with immunologic defects or eczema, may also be confused with varicella. Since the distinction between varicella and these poxvirus infections cannot be made with certainty on clinical grounds, prompt laboratory diagnosis is required. However, the eradication of smallpox and the consequent cessation of smallpox vaccination should eliminate this diagnostic problem.

Disseminated herpes simplex may occasionally resemble varicella, especially in the neonate, in immunosuppressed patients, and in patients with eczema. However, the distribution of lesions is rarely typical of varicella, and there is often an obvious concentration of lesions at the site of the primary or recurrent infection (e.g., the mouth or external genitalia). Marked toxicity and encephalitis are more common in neonatal herpes simplex than in neonatal varicella. The histopathology of lesions caused by herpes simplex virus (HSV) and VZV is indistinguishable. Thus differentiation of the two requires virus isolation or the detection and identification of viral antigens or nucleic acids in the lesions.

Other diseases that may be confused with varicella include impetigo, the vesicular exanthems of Coxsackie virus and echo virus infections (e.g., hand-foot-and-mouth disease syndrome), rickettsialpox, insect bites, papular urticaria, scabies, contact dermatitis, dermatitis herpetiformis, drug eruptions, secondary syphilis, and erythema multiforme. The character, distribution, and evolution of the lesions, together with a careful epidemiologic history, usually differentiate these diseases from varicella [107,133]. When any doubt exists, the clinical impression should receive laboratory confirmation.

Clinical diagnosis of herpes zoster

In the preeruptive stage, herpes zoster is easily confused with other causes of pain such as pleurisy, myocardial infarction, cholecystitis, appendicitis, renal colic, or collapsed intervertebral disk. Sometimes the early appearance of regional lymphadenopathy and localized cutaneous sensory abnormalities (e.g., hyperesthesia, dysesthesia) provide a clue to the diagnosis. When the eruption appears, the diagnosis is almost always obvious.

Zosteriform herpes simplex is often impossible to distinguish from herpes zoster on clinical grounds. A history of multiple recurrences at the same site is common in herpes simplex but exceedingly rare in herpes zoster. Virus isolation or the identification of VZV (or HSV) antigens or nucleic acids in material obtained from the lesions is the only reliable means of differentiating these entities.

Contact dermatitis, burns, vaccinia autoinoculation, and localized bacterial skin infections may occasionally resemble herpes zoster, but a careful history and examination of the lesions (including a Tzanck smear with the identification of multinucleated giant cells and intranuclear inclusion bodies) will eliminate any confusion.

Disseminated herpes zoster may be mistaken for varicella when there is widespread dissemination of VZV from a small painless area of zoster or from the affected sensory ganglion in the absence of an obvious dermatomal eruption [36,85,179].

Laboratory diagnosis

Routine laboratory determinations are not helpful in the diagnosis of either varicella or herpes zoster.

The presence of multinucleated giant cells and epithelial cells containing acidophilic intranuclear inclusion bodies distinguishes the cutaneous lesions produced by VZV from all other skin lesions except those produced by herpes simplex virus (Fig. 191-8). These cells can be demonstrated in Tzanck smears prepared at the bedside; material is scraped from the base of an early vesicle and stained with hematoxylin-eosin, Giemsa's, Papanicolaou's, or Paragon Multiple stain [194,195] (Fig. 191-8c). Every physician should become familiar with this simple diagnostic procedure and employ it in the initial evaluation of any patient with a vesicular eruption. Punch biopsies provide more reliable material for histologic examination and also facilitate diagnosis in the prevesicular stage [181]. Sputum from patients with varicella pneumonia may contain desquamated respiratory epithelial cells with acidophilic intranuclear inclusion bodies, but such cells are also found in patients with pneumonia caused by measles virus and in patients with respiratory tract infections caused by HSV. The identification of herpesvirus particles in vesicle fluid or biopsy material by electron microscopy provides another means of diagnosis. However, neither electron microscopy nor Tzanck smears can distinguish VZV from HSV infections.

The definitive diagnosis of VZV infection, as well as the differentiation of VZV from HSV, can be made by isolating VZV from vesicle fluid inoculated into suitable tissue cultures [42,196] or by direct identification of VZV antigens or nucleic acids in material from skin lesions or infected tissues [181,196,197].

VZV can be isolated and propagated in vitro in monolayer cultures of a variety of human (and certain simian) cells [10,42,196]. The cytopathic effect in such cell cultures is characterized by the formation of acidophilic intranuclear inclusion bodies and multinucleated giant cells similar to those seen in the cutaneous lesions of the disease. These changes are indistinguishable from those produced by HSV, but whereas HSV is released into the medium by initially infected cells and rapidly spreads to infect the remaining cells in the culture, the cytopathic effect of VZV remains focal. This is because infectious VZV remains cell-associated and is not released into the medium by the initially infected cells; infection proceeds from cell to cell only by direct contact, and the initial foci of infection gradually enlarge. Serial passage of VZV in tissue culture requires the transfer of infected cells. Cytopathic effects of VZV are generally not apparent until several days after specimen inoculation.

A rapid and specific diagnosis can be achieved by identifying VZV antigens or nucleic acids in vesicle fluid, cells scraped or swabbed from the base of vesicles or ulcers, crusts, or tissue obtained by biopsy. Viral antigens can be demonstrated in vesicle fluid or extracts of crusts by countercurrent immunoelectrophoresis (CIE) using antiserum to VZV [198]. Immunofluorescence or immunoperoxidase staining of cellular material from fresh vesicles or prevesicular lesions is a useful diagnostic technique in experienced hands; it can identify individual infected cells and structures, and can detect VZV antigens relatively late in the disease when cultures are no longer positive [20,23,42,181,196,199]. Enzyme immunoassays provide another rapid and sensitive method for antigen detection [197,200]. Monoclonal antibodies can improve the specificity of these techniques, but it is always important to examine aliquots of each specimen with antisera to VZV, HSV-1, HSV-2, and control antigen in parallel, together with positive and negative virus-infected tissue controls. Nucleic acid hybridization with radiolabeled or biotinylated probes can detect viral nucleic acids in clinical specimens [197] and this offers another sensitive and specific means for rapid diagnosis.

The lesions of varicella and herpes zoster are indistinguishable by histopathology. Both contain VZV virions, VZV antigens, and VZV nucleic acids.

Serologic tests can provide a retrospective diagnosis of varicella and herpes zoster when acute and convalescent sera are available for comparison, and they can also identify susceptible individuals who may be candidates for isolation or prophylaxis. The widely available complement-fixation (CF) test suffers from two disadvantages: (1) a rise in CF titer to VZV or HSV is not diagnostic if antibody to both viruses increases, because infection by either virus can induce a heterologous anamnestic response, and (2) the CF antibody titer drops within months after varicella infection and may reach undetectable levels. Thus, many adults who are immune to varicella may be CF antibody-negative. Consequently, the CF test is not useful for distinguishing between immune and susceptible adults [2,13,42,196]. Indirect fluorescent antibody tests have problems of specificity similar to those of the CF test [42,196]. VZV neutralization tests are both sensitive and specific, but they are time consuming and technically demanding, and are available only in research laboratories. A number of new and more sensitive techniques have been developed to measure humoral responses to VZV [13,42,196]. These include an immunofluorescence assay for antibody to VZV-induced membrane antigens (FAMA) [72,73,201] that distinguishes immune from susceptible adults; an immune adherence hemagglutination assay (IAHA), which is slightly less sensitive than the FAMA assay [202]; a rapid ^{125}I-labeled staphylococcal protein A radioimmunoassay, which is more sensitive and easier to perform than the FAMA assay [203]; enzyme-linked immunosorbent assays (ELISA), which are comparable to the FAMA assay in their ability to distinguish immune from susceptible adults, but which are more sensitive and simpler to perform [75,204]; and a solid-phase radioimmunoassay (RIA) for measuring VZV-specific IgG, IgM, and IgA responses [61,76]. In addition, measurement of the in vitro proliferative response of peripheral blood lymphocytes to VZV antigens [65,76] correlates well with immunity as measured by FAMA, RIA, and ELISA, and a VZV skin test has been widely and successfully used in Japan

to distinguish between immune and susceptible individuals [66,205,206]. With all of these assays, adequate controls are required to deal with the problem of heterotypic responses to infections by other herpesviruses [2,13,42,63,196].

Seroconversion to VZV is indicative of varicella. However, if the "acute" serum is obtained late it may already contain detectable antibody to VZV, and it may then only be possible to demonstrate an increase ($\geq$ fourfold) in antibody titer.

Most immunocompetent patients with herpes zoster show an anamnestic increase in humoral and cell-mediated immunity to VZV [61,76,80,87–89], but this may fail to occur in immunocompromised patients. Antibody to VZV appears in the cerebrospinal fluid of most patients with herpes zoster meningoencephalitis, presumably as a result of intrathecal synthesis [148]. As in the case of herpes simplex encephalitis, this may provide a useful means for retrospective diagnosis.

The presence of VZV-specific IgM antibody is indicative of recent active infection, but it can be induced by exogenous reexposure or by asymptomatic "contained reversions" of latent VZV (Fig. 191-2), as well as by symptomatic varicella and herpes zoster [61,63,76,89].

Treatment

Treatment of varicella

In normal children, varicella is generally benign and self-limited. Cool compresses or calamine lotion locally, and antihistamines orally, may help control the intense pruritis of the rash. Tepid baths with baking soda ($\frac{1}{4}$ cup per tub of water) may also relieve itching. Creams or lotions containing corticosteroids and occlusive ointments should not be used. Antipyretics are rarely indicated, and it has been recommended that salicylates be avoided because of their possible association with Reye's syndrome [138,207]. Fingernails should be kept short and clean to minimize secondary skin infections and the scarring that may result from scratching.

Complications are most frequently due to bacterial superinfection. Bacterial infections of local lesions are treated with warm soaks. Systemic antimicrobial drugs are indicated for bacterial cellulitis, otitis media, sepsis, bacterial meningitis, osteomyelitis, septic arthritis, and bacterial pneumonia. The prominence of *Staphylococcus aureus* and group A β-hemolytic *Streptococcus* as causes of these complications should be recognized, but therapy should be guided by the results of Gram-stained smears and cultures. Antibiotics are useless in varicella pneumonia unless there is bacterial superinfection.

Varicella pneumonia is rare in normal children, but more common in adults. Although it usually responds to supportive measures, including positive-pressure ventilation, antiviral chemotherapy should be used early to inhibit VZV replication. Antibiotics are indicated only when bacterial superinfection develops. There is no evidence that corticosteroids are beneficial, and their use is not recommended.

Reye's syndrome must be considered when a child with otherwise uncomplicated varicella develops lethargy, persistent vomiting, and confusion. Early diagnosis with supportive care and aggressive control of increased intracranial pressure and hypoglycemia should reduce the mortality and morbidity of this mysterious complication.

The most common neurologic complication of varicella in normal children is cerebellar ataxia, which is usually self-limited. However, recent evidence that it may be associated with VZV infection of the CNS (see above) suggests that the use of antiviral chemotherapy is warranted. Varicella encephalitis, meningoencephalitis, and myelitis are very rare complications in normal children. However, the evidence that they are the result of CNS VZV infection, rather than of some postinfectious autoimmune mechanism (see above), makes it reasonable to treat them with an antiviral agent.

Hemorrhagic complications should be treated on the basis of the results of coagulation studies and bone marrow examination. It is always important to rule out bacterial sepsis. Because of the possible involvement of VZV-induced endothelial damage in purpura fulminans, especially if this complication occurs when new vesicles are continuing to appear, these patients should receive antiviral chemotherapy.

In contrast to varicella in normal children, varicella in immunocompromised children and adults may be severe and life-threatening. Thus every effort should be made to prevent its occurrence (see "Prevention and Control" below). When this fails, antiviral therapy should be initiated as early in the illness as possible, and certainly before there is any clinical evidence of disseminated disease. Patients at risk include those with leukemia, lymphoproliferative disorders, metastatic malignancies, and congenital or acquired immunodeficiency diseases, as well as newborns and patients receiving cytotoxic drugs, corticosteroids, radiotherapy or antithymocyte globulin because of organ allografts, nephrotic syndrome, collagen-vascular diseases, etc. The risk is low in patients receiving low-dose alternate-day steroid therapy, but it is substantial in those receiving higher doses (e.g., 1 to 2 mg/kg per day of prednisone). If possible, cancer chemotherapy should be temporarily interrupted; however, treatment of malignancy should take precedence during induction therapy or therapy for disease in relapse. When treatment is stopped, it should be resumed 21 days after exposure or 7 days after complete crusting of all lesions. Steroids should be tapered during the incubation period and cytotoxic therapy stopped if possible. However, patients who have received prolonged courses of corticosteroids should continue to receive replacement therapy.

Two antiviral chemotherapeutic agents, acyclovir (9-[2-hydroxyethoxymethyl]guanine, acycloguanosine) and vidarabine (9-β-D-arabinofuranosyladenine, adenine arabinoside), as well as human interferon, have shown efficacy in VZV infections [208–211]. Acyclovir, a guanosine analog, is selectively phosphorylated by HSV and VZV thymidine kinases (it is a poor substrate for cellular thymidine kinase) and is thus concentrated in infected cells. Cellular enzymes then convert acyclovir monophosphate to acyclovir triphosphate, which interferes with viral DNA synthesis by inhibiting viral DNA polymerase [212]. At therapeutic concentrations, acyclovir is remarkably nontoxic, with no observed effects on hematopoietic precursor cells or the immune system [208–211]. Vidarabine, a purine nucleoside analog, is phosphorylated by cellular kinases to vidarabine triphosphate, which appears to inhibit herpesvirus DNA

polymerases to a greater extent than cellular DNA polymerases [208–211,213]. Despite its clinical efficacy, vidarabine has drawbacks. It is not a selective inhibitor of virus replication (vidarabine triphosphate also inhibits cellular DNA polymerases) and thus it is potentially cytotoxic. Its low solubility requires that it be administered in large volumes of fluid [208–211].

In placebo-controlled therapeutic trials, intravenous acyclovir (500 mg/m² each 8 h for 7 days), intravenous vidarabine (10 mg/kg per day over 12 h for 5 days), and parenteral human interferon alpha (3.5 × 10⁵ units/kg per day for 2 days, then 1.75 × 10⁵ units/kg per day for 3 days) have all been shown to markedly decrease the incidence of life-threatening visceral complications when administered within 72 h of onset to immunosuppressed patients with varicella [129,214,215]. These results, as well as experience gained in open protocols [216–218], suggest that acyclovir is at least as effective as vidarabine in patients with VZV infections but is free of vidarabine's toxicity and problems of fluid overload. Thus, until the results of studies directly comparing these agents are available, this author prefers to use intravenous acyclovir (500 mg/m² each 8 h for 7 days) because of its lower toxicity and ease of administration. Treatment must be initiated early in the disease to be effective, and the dosage must be reduced in patients with renal insufficiency [210].

Except for Reye's syndrome and bacterial superinfection, complications of varicella in both immunocompromised and normal patients appear to be associated with continuing VZV replication and dissemination. Thus, although efficacy has not yet been established, it seems reasonable to treat these complications with intravenous acyclovir (500 mg/m² each 8 h for 5 to 10 days).

Oral formulations of acyclovir are being tested in patients with VZV infections [219] and a number of new selective antiviral chemotherapeutic agents are beginning to be evaluated in clinical trials [209]. Treatment with systemic cytosine arabinoside (ara-C) or iododeoxyuridine (IUdR) should *not* be considered in patients with varicella or its complications. These compounds are toxic and are likely to adversely affect the outcome of the disease, especially in immunosuppressed patients.

Treatment of herpes zoster

During the acute phase of herpes zoster, analgesics and the application of cool compresses, calamine lotion, cornstarch, or baking soda may help to alleviate local symptoms and hasten the drying of vesicular lesions. Occlusive ointments should be avoided, and creams or lotions containing corticosteroids should not be used. After the acute phase, a bland ointment or olive oil dressings may help to soften and separate adherent crusts. Bacterial superinfection of local lesions is uncommon and should be treated with warm soaks; bacterial cellulitis requires systemic antibiotic therapy.

The major goals of therapy in patients with herpes zoster are to: (1) limit the extent, duration, and severity of disease in the primary dermatome; (2) prevent disease elsewhere; and (3) prevent postherpetic neuralgia. Since the pathology in the primary dermatome, as well as that responsible for the visceral and CNS complications of herpes zoster, appears to be the consequence of VZV replication, the first two goals can be achieved by limiting VZV replication and spread. If immunity is intact, herpes zoster is usually self-limited and there is rarely significant spread outside of the initially involved dermatome. In contrast, immunocompromised individuals, particularly those with deficiencies in cell-mediated immunity, have more severe and prolonged local disease and a much higher incidence of visceral and CNS complications. Obviously, it is these patients who have the most to gain from effective antiviral therapy.

Nucleoside analogs capable of inhibiting VZV replication have been administered parenterally in attempts to control the multiplication and dissemination of VZV in immunocompromised patients with herpes zoster. Cytosine arabinoside (ara-C) and iododeoxyuridine (IUdR) have proved ineffective and toxic when administered systemically.

The efficacy of vidarabine in immunocompromised patients with acute herpes zoster was established in a double-blind placebo-controlled crossover study [220] and, more recently, in a randomized double-blind placebo-controlled study [130]. When administered within 72 h of the onset of rash, vidarabine (10 mg/kg intravenously over 12 h each day for 5 days) shortened the period of new vesicle formation, accelerated healing, and reduced the spread of rash over the primary dermatome. Vidarabine also markedly reduced the incidence of cutaneous dissemination and of visceral and CNS complications. Patients with lymphoproliferative malignancies and those older than 38 years of age had the greatest risk of complications and thus benefited most from therapy. Vidarabine did not reduce the incidence of postherpetic neuralgia (45 percent in patients older than 38 years of age) but appeared to reduce its duration, and to reduce the duration of acute pain. Vidarabine toxicity, consisting mainly of nausea, vomiting, subclinical abnormalities in liver enzymes, jitteriness and hallucinations, was self-limited and did not necessitate cessation of therapy. Analysis of placebo recipients revealed that concomitant administration of corticosteroids did not reduce the frequency of postherpetic neuralgia, but did delay healing and prolong new vesicle formation.

Acyclovir has also proved effective. A randomized double-blind placebo-controlled study in immunocompromised patients with acute herpes zoster demonstrated that acyclovir (500 mg/m^2 intravenously each 8 h for 7 days) halted progression of herpes zoster, both in patients with localized disease and in patients with cutaneous dissemination before treatment [221]. Acyclovir accelerated the rate of clearance of virus from vesicles and markedly reduced the incidence of visceral and progressive cutaneous dissemination. Pain subsided faster in acyclovir recipients, and fewer reported postherpetic neuralgia, but these differences were not statistically significant. No acyclovir toxicity was observed.

Human interferon alpha (1.7 or 5.1 × 10^5 units/kg per day intramuscularly for 7 days) has also been shown to reduce new vesicle formation, cutaneous and visceral dissemination, and visceral and CNS complications [222,223]. Interferon also appeared to reduce the incidence of postherpetic neuralgia. Although reasonably well tolerated in these trials, interferon appears to be somewhat more toxic than vidarabine [208–211].

These results, as well as experience gained in open protocols and in treating varicella, suggest that acyclovir is at least as effective as vidarabine in immunocompromised patients with VZV infections. Clinical trials directly comparing the two drugs are now in progress.

Immunocompromised patients with herpes zoster who have a deficient or delayed antibody response to VZV have an increased incidence of severe disease and dissemination [35,224,225]. This led Stevens and Merigan [226] to conduct a double-blind controlled therapeutic trial of zoster immune globulin (ZIG) in immunocompromised patients with herpes zoster. Despite a much higher titer of antibody to VZV, ZIG did not appear superior to the normal immune serum globulin control in preventing dissemination or diminishing postherpetic neuralgia.

The efficacy of intravenous acyclovir in normal adults with herpes zoster has been evaluated in three small double-blind placebo-controlled trials [227–229]. Acyclovir (5 mg/kg or 500 mg/m^2 each 8 h for 5 days) shortened the period of virus shedding and of new vesicle formation, accelerated healing, and shortened the duration of pain during the acute phase of the disease. However, there was no effect upon the incidence of postherpetic neuralgia. The greatest effect of acyclovir treatment was observed in patients older than 67 years of age and those with fever (i.e., patients in whom the disease is more severe and prolonged without therapy) and in patients treated early [227]. No toxicity was observed in acyclovir recipients.

It is clear that in immunocompromised patients, parenterally administered acyclovir, vidarabine, or interferon can shorten the course of acute herpes zoster and markedly reduce the incidence of serious complications. However, parenteral antiviral therapy has only a small effect upon the course of herpes zoster in immunocompetent individuals (because normal host defenses alone are effective in limiting VZV replication and spread) and it does not appear to alter the incidence or severity of postherpetic neuralgia, which is the major cause of morbidity in immunologically normal patients with herpes zoster. While antiviral therapy may well prevent complications, such as motor paresis and meningoencephalitis, the potential benefits for most immunologically normal individuals do not appear to outweigh the expense and inconvenience of hospitalization for intravenous therapy. What is needed is an effective outpatient regimen, and progress is being made in this direction; studies are under way to determine the therapeutic potential of orally administered acyclovir, other antiviral chemotherapeutic agents [209], and intramuscularly administered human interferons in immunologically normal individuals with herpes zoster. Oral acyclovir has already been proved effective in patients with genital herpes, but treatment of VZV, which is less sensitive to acyclovir than HSV, will require larger doses than those used to treat genital herpes.

In view of the early and extensive involvement of the sensory ganglion and nerve, and the importance of contiguous rather than viremic spread in the genesis of CNS complications of herpes zoster in immunocompetent individuals, it seems unlikely that topical therapy applied to the skin will reduce the incidence or severity of most complications of herpes zoster (including postherpetic neuralgia) in immunologically normal persons. Moreover, while many forms of topical therapy have been advocated, few have been subjected to well-controlled clinical evaluation. An exception is iododeoxyuridine (IUdR) in dimethylsulfoxide (DMSO). Well-controlled studies have demonstrated that topical application of 5 to 40% IUdR in 100% DMSO, beginning early in the course of uncomplicated herpes zoster, shortens the vesicular phase and accelerates healing, and may also reduce the duration of pain [83,230]. However, these effects are small, the treatment protocol is inconvenient, and IUdR is not effective in more convenient ointment formulations. The IUdR-DMSO preparation is not licensed for use in the United States, and the cost and potential long-term toxicity of such high concentrations of drug and solvent should discourage its use elsewhere. Other forms of topical therapy, including topical and intralesional corticosteroids, should be avoided until their safety and efficacy are demonstrated by means of well-designed double-blind placebo-controlled clinical trials.

Postherpetic neuralgia, once established, is often refractory to therapy. Fortunately, it resolves spontaneously in most patients—within 3 months in about 50 percent and within a year in 75 percent or more. Nevertheless, a number of patients are left with persistent, often disabling, pain. Conventional analgesics should be tried, but they often fail, as do narcotics, which also carry a risk of addiction. A wide range of therapies have been advocated, including epidural injection of local anesthetic and corticosteroid, acupuncture, biofeedback, subcutaneous injections of triamcinolone, and systemic administration of a variety of compounds, but most have not been validated by controlled trials. Though of unproved benefit, an initial trial of cutaneous stimulation, either by frequent rubbing with a dry towel or with a cutaneous electrical stimulator, is advocated by many experts [231]. This should be continued for several weeks before being abandoned. The typical dull persistent aching pain of postherpetic neuralgia will often respond to tricyclic antidepressants [231]. In a controlled trial, amitriptyline provided excellent pain relief in about two-thirds of patients with postherpetic neuralgia. Carbamazepine may also be effective, especially for the lancinating pain that develops in some patients [231].

The possibility that postherpetic neuralgia may be caused by inflammation, necrosis, and subsequent scarring of the sensory ganglion and contiguous neural structures has provided the rationale for the use of corticosteroids during the acute phase of herpes zoster in an attempt to prevent this complication. However, the host defenses that cause tissue injury appear to be identical to those that terminate dermatomal VZV infection and prevent dissemination, and patients who develop herpes zoster while being treated with corticosteroids have an increased risk of dissemination and visceral complications. Nevertheless, two small controlled trials have suggested that the oral administration of 48 mg of triamcinolone or 40 mg of prednisolone per day, beginning during the early eruptive phase of the disease, may reduce the duration of postherpetic neuralgia in otherwise healthy patients over 60 years of age [232,233]. No complications of corticosteroid therapy were observed in either study. In view of the possibility that such large doses of corticosteroid may induce VZV dissemination, and the reported failure of corticosteroid therapy to reduce the incidence of postherpetic neuralgia in immunocompromised patients in a large, placebo-controlled vidarabine treatment study [130], these results

should be confirmed by means of a larger double-blind placebo-controlled trial before this form of therapy is accepted for general use. If the capacity of corticosteroid to reduce the incidence and severity of postherpetic neuralgia can be confirmed, any associated increase in VZV replication and dissemination might be prevented by the simultaneous administration of an antiviral agent. The NIAID Collaborative Antiviral Study Group has initiated a double-blind randomized study in which immunocompetent persons older than 50 years of age with herpes zoster will be treated orally with prednisone, acyclovir, prednisone plus acyclovir, or placebo. This trial should resolve the questions of the safety and efficacy of corticosteroid therapy and, in addition, determine the therapeutic potential of oral acyclovir alone and in combination with corticosteroid.

The eye is involved in 20 to 50 percent of patients with ophthalmic zoster, and the advice of an ophthalmologist should be sought in treating these patients. Therapy of ocular VZV infections is controversial. Mydriatics are used to prevent synechiae, and topical corticosteroids are frequently recommended for keratitis and uveitis, although their efficacy is unproved [157]. Topical antiviral drugs (IUdR, vidarabine, trifluorothymidine) are also frequently recommended and should be included whenever corticosteroids are used.

The following recommendations reflect the author's views and current state of knowledge. Progress in antiviral therapy is rapid, and these recommendations are certain to be altered by the results of studies now under way.

Herpes zoster in immunologically normal persons less than 50 years of age is generally benign and self-limited, and is very rarely complicated by postherpetic neuralgia. Thus antiviral therapy is not recommended, and the use of corticosteroids, even if it should be proven effective in preventing postherpetic neuralgia, is not warranted.

In immunologically normal older persons (over 50 years of age) the major complication of herpes zoster is postherpetic neuralgia, which can be expected to develop in 20 percent or more of these patients. Until a regimen of antiviral drug, corticosteroid, or both is clearly demonstrated to reduce the incidence or severity of this complication, neither is recommended for routine use. However, the high incidence of ocular and CNS complications observed in patients with ophthalmic zoster, including the syndrome of delayed contralateral hemiplegia [37,158,175–177] warrants consideration of antiviral therapy. The cost and inconvenience of intravenous therapy would certainly be justified if there were unequivocal evidence that the early initiation of antiviral therapy prevented the development of these complications. Until such evidence is available, therapeutic decisions should be made on a case-by-case basis, recognizing that the frequency and severity of complications increases with age. When a safe and effective oral regimen is available, its use will probably be warranted in all patients with herpes zoster who are more than 50 years of age.

Immunocompetent patients of any age who develop significant cutaneous dissemination (e.g., 20 or more vesicles at a distance from the primary dermatome) should be carefully evaluated, and those with evidence of visceral or CNS involvement should receive antiviral therapy. Pending the availability of the results of comparative studies, the author prefers to use acyclovir (500 mg/m² or 10 mg/kg intravenously every 8 h for 5 days) because of its ease of administration and lower toxicity.

In immunocompromised patients of any age with herpes zoster, the major objective is to prevent local, visceral and CNS complications, which are the direct consequence of VZV replication and spread. Accordingly, such patients are prime candidates for antiviral therapy. The only significant deterrent is the cost and inconvenience of intravenous administration. The development of safe and effective oral regimens will make it practical to treat most or all of these patients early in the course of their disease, when infection is localized to the primary dermatome. Early initiation of therapy is important because of the close temporal proximity of the onset of cutaneous dissemination to the onset of visceral and CNS complications; one would rather not wait for the occurrence of cutaneous dissemination to initiate antiviral therapy. Until an effective outpatient regimen is available, it would seem reasonable to treat herpes zoster in more severely immunocompromised patients (e.g., those with lymphoproliferative malignancies, advanced Hodgkin's disease, and organ allografts) with intravenous acyclovir (500 mg/m² or 10 mg/kg each 8 h for 7 days). Older patients with lesser degrees of immunosuppression, and all immunocompromised patients with ophthalmic zoster should probably also be treated. Treatment should be continued for 7 days or more, or until there is no longer evidence of continuing VZV replication. Untreated immunocompromised patients who develop cutaneous dissemination or evidence of visceral or CNS involvement should be treated with intravenous acyclovir at this dosage for 7 to 10 days or until there is no longer evidence of VZV replication. Patients with CNS involvement should probably be treated longer, and their physician should be alert for relapse. Both acyclovir and vidarabine require dose reduction in patients with renal insufficiency [210].

Prevention and control

Prevention and control of varicella

Varicella is almost always a benign disease in normal children. Since infection results in lifelong immunity, its acquisition in childhood eliminates the problem of varicella in the adult years. Therefore, no preventive measures are recommended for a normal child who has been exposed to varicella.

On the other hand, varicella is potentially fatal in susceptible patients undergoing immunosuppressive therapy, patients with an immunosuppressive malignancy such as Hodgkin's disease, susceptible newborn infants, and even normal adults. Thus it is desirable to prevent or modify varicella in these high-risk individuals. Potential approaches include passive immunization, active immunization, chemoprophylaxis, and prevention of exposure.

Passive immunization with large doses (0.6 to 1.2 mL/kg) of standard human immune serum globulin (ISG) administered within three days of exposure was shown to attenuate but not prevent varicella in normal children [25]. Passive immunization with zoster immune globulin (ZIG), prepared from the plasma of donors recovering from herpes zoster and containing a high titer of antibody to

VZV, has been shown to prevent varicella in susceptible normal children when administered within three days of exposure [74] and to modify the disease in immunosuppressed children [26,28]. One-third of the immunosuppressed recipients developed subclinical infection, and the disease was mild in most of the others. Similarly, zoster immune plasma (ZIP) obtained from otherwise healthy individuals during convalescence from varicella or herpes zoster has been shown to modify or prevent varicella in susceptible high-risk children when it is administered within five days of exposure [27,234]. In contrast to the favorable outcome in these passively immunized, high-risk children is the 32 percent mortality reported in a group of 106 leukemic children with unmodified varicella [127]. In order to overcome the relative shortage of zoster convalescent plasma and ZIG for the growing population of immunosuppressed patients, Zaia et al [235] screened outdated blood from blood banks and used those units with high levels of antibody to VZV to prepare batches of immune globulin (VZIG) with antibody levels equivalent to those in ZIG. In a randomized double-blind trial of their capacity to protect immunosuppressed children from severe varicella, ZIG and VZIG were comparable [71]. Clinical infection occurred in 44 percent of VZIG recipients and 37 percent of ZIG recipients, with no significant difference in severity in the two groups. Subclinical infections occurred in 16 percent of VZIG and 31 percent of ZIG recipients. It was also observed that 28 percent of patients with a negative history of previous varicella, but with FAMA antibody to VZV detectable in preimmunization serum, developed mild clinical illness. This suggests that in patients receiving blood and blood products who lack a history of varicella or herpes zoster, low levels of antibody to VZV may not indicate immunity to varicella. Such patients remain at risk of serious infection. When exposed to VZV they should receive passive immunization and they require isolation procedures to prevent nosocomial varicella. The incubation period is prolonged in ZIG, ZIP, and VZIG recipients who develop clinical disease.

VZIG has now been licensed for use by the FDA and can be purchased from a number of regional distribution centers [236]. Recommended criteria for the use of VZIG are listed in Table 191-1.

The availability of new serologic tests that permit the rapid identification of susceptible individuals, and the increased availability of VZIG, now make it possible to identify and passively immunize *susceptible* pregnant and nonpregnant adults with recognized exposure to varicella.

Unfortunately, protection afforded by VZIG is transient, whereas most susceptible people will experience repeated exposures to VZV. Furthermore, exposure to VZV is often unrecognized, and thus large numbers of immunocompromised patients will continue to develop unmodified varicella in spite of the availability of VZIG. Continuous prophylaxis by administration of VZIG on a monthly or bimonthly schedule is impractical; what is needed is a safe means of inducing long-lasting immunity to VZV in immunocompromised patients and susceptible adults.

A decade ago Dr. M. Takahashi and his colleagues announced the development of a live attenuated VZV vaccine (OKA strain) prepared by serial passage in human and guinea pig cell cultures of a strain of VZV isolated from a varicella vesicle [237]. Despite concerns about its degree

Table 191-1   Criteria for the use of varicella-zoster immune globulin (VZIG) for the prophylaxis of varicella*

1. Susceptible to varicella:
   a. Children <15 years of age with no or unknown history of varicella or herpes zoster
   b. Bone marrow transplant recipients regardless of pre-transplantation history of varicella or herpes zoster
   c. Immunocompromised adolescents and adults (≥15 years of age) with no or unknown history of varicella or herpes zoster
   d. Normal adolescents and adults (≥15 years of age) with no or unknown history of varicella or herpes zoster who lack antibody to VZV†.
2. One of the following underlying illnesses or conditions:
   a. Leukemia or lymphoma
   b. Congenital or acquired immunodeficiency
   c. Bone marrow transplant recipient *regardless of pretransplantation history of varicella or herpes zoster*
   d. Immunosuppressive treatment (including corticosteroids)
   e. Newborn of mother who had onset of varicella within 5 days before delivery or within 48 h after delivery
   f. Premature infant (≤28 weeks gestation, or ≤1000 g) regardless of maternal history of varicella or herpes zoster
   g. Premature infant (≥28 weeks gestation) whose mother lacks a history of varicella or herpes zoster
   h. Any infant ≤14 days of age whose mother lacks a history of varicella or herpes zoster
   i. Susceptible pregnant or nonpregnant adult†
3. One of the following types of exposure to person or persons with varicella or herpes zoster:
   a. Continuous household contact
   b. Playmate contact (generally >1 h play indoors)
   c. Hospital contact (in same 2-bed to 4-bed room *or* adjacent beds in a large ward *or* prolonged face-to-face contact with an infectious staff member or patient)
   d. Intrauterine contact (newborn of mother with onset of varicella 5 days or less before delivery or within 48 h after delivery)
4. Time elapsed after exposure is such that VZIG can be administered within 96 h of exposure (but preferably sooner)

* Patients should fulfill all 4 criteria.
† New serologic tests that permit the rapid identification of susceptible individuals, and the increased availability of VZIG, now make it possible to passively immunize *susceptible* pregnant and nonpregnant adults with recognized exposure to varicella. Immunologically normal adults with no history of varicella or herpes zoster are generally considered immune unless it is demonstrated that they lack serum antibody to VZV [236].

of attenuation, capacity to induce latent infections, and safety in immunocompromised patients, it has been extensively evaluated in Japan and, more recently, in the United States [78,79,237–241]. Administered to normal children and adults, it induces a mild papular or papulovesicular rash and slight fever in a small minority. Antibody to VZV, VZV-specific lymphoproliferative responses, and VZV-specific skin test reactivity are induced in almost all normal recipients and are generally long-lasting. Virus is rarely isolated from the rash in normal recipients, and there is no apparent transmission to contacts. However, in contrast to natural varicella, a few of these immunized normal persons have developed very mild varicella on subsequent exposure to VZV; the virus isolated from such patients is wild-type VZV. Herpes zoster has developed in less than 0.3 percent of normal recipients of the vaccine. Interestingly, the vaccine can prevent varicella in normal children if administered within 3 days of exposure. When children with leukemia in remission and off chemotherapy are vaccinated, fewer than 10 percent develop a papular or papulovesicular rash, and most develop antibody and cell-mediated immunity to VZV. When children on chemotherapy have it stopped for one week before and one week after vaccination, up to 40 percent develop rash. When the rash is vesicular, vaccine virus can be isolated and transmitted to susceptible normal siblings (who develop mild varicella). However, when vaccinated leukemic children are exposed to VZV, most are protected; only 10 to 20 percent develop clinical varicella, which is generally mild. Leukemic vaccinees develop herpes zoster (caused by the vaccine virus) at a rate comparable to that in similar patients with a history of natural varicella. These observations indicate that the OKA VZV vaccine can be safely administered to susceptible immunosuppressed children and will protect them from the morbidity and mortality that would otherwise result from subsequent exposures to varicella. However, even in normal individuals, the immunity induced by the vaccine is not as solid as that induced by wild-type VZV infection. Furthermore, vaccine virus can be transmitted from vaccinated patients to susceptible normal contacts who develop mild varicella, and it appears that a single passage in humans may result in increased virulence. Although the attenuated OKA VZV vaccine represents a tremendous advance in our ability to cope with the problem of varicella in immunocompromised patients, and may also be useful for the prevention of varicella in susceptible normal adults, questions of long-term safety and efficacy are still likely to preclude its use in normal children.

Chemoprophylaxis has not been developed for VZV. Exposure of susceptible patients to VZV warrants reduction in the dosage of corticosteroids to physiologic levels and the elimination or reduction of immunosuppressive drugs until their varicella has resolved or until it is clear that they have escaped infection. Such patients should receive VZIG immediately after exposure.

There is no need to prevent exposure of susceptible normal children; patients with varicella need only be kept at home until all vesicles have crusted [2,107]. On the other hand, rigid isolation should be enforced to prevent infection of susceptible immunocompromised patients and newborn infants. Contact with patients with varicella and herpes zoster, and with persons who may be incubating varicella, must be avoided. Hospital personnel without a clear history of varicella or herpes zoster should be tested for antibody to VZV. Hospitals should develop and implement effective procedures to prevent nosocomial varicella [2,29,107,242]. If such exposure occurs or is suspected, susceptible immunocompromised patients and newborn infants should receive prophylaxis with VZIG.

Prevention and control of herpes zoster

Herpes zoster is a sporadic disease that results from reactivation of latent endogenous VZV, rather than from exogenous infection. Thus, attempts at prophylaxis must be aimed at preventing the reactivation of endogenous VZV or inhibiting its subsequent replication and spread. It appears that natural resistance to herpes zoster is maintained by periodic antigenic stimulation, which results from subclinical episodes of exogenous reinfection and endogenous reactivation (see Fig. 191-2). The increased incidence and severity of herpes zoster observed in elderly persons appears to be associated with depressed immunity to VZV, primarily depressed cell-mediated immunity [102–104]. Depressed cell-mediated immunity also appears to be responsible for the increased incidence and severity of herpes zoster in immunocompromised patients. Accordingly, one approach to the prevention of herpes zoster is the stimulation of immunity to VZV in elderly and other high-risk individuals. The development of live attenuated VZV vaccine provides an opportunity to test this approach to prophylaxis in immunologically normal elderly individuals. The use of live attenuated vaccines is generally to be avoided in immunocompromised individuals, but the current VZV vaccine has proved to be relatively safe and effective in immunocompromised children with leukemia and other malignancies (see above). Berger et al [243] have recently administered attenuated VZV vaccine to 33 elderly adults with a history of varicella and antibody to VZV, but with a negative in vitro lymphoproliferative response to VZV antigen (stimulation index less than 3). Seventeen (52 percent) of the vaccine recipients subsequently developed a positive lymphoproliferative response to VZV antigen (stimulation index greater than 5) and an additional 11 (33 percent) became weakly positive (stimulation index of 3 to 5). It remains to be seen whether immunization of such elderly individuals will also result in a reduction in the incidence and severity of herpes zoster. Experimental vaccines consisting of purified VZV envelope glycoproteins and free of VZV DNA will provide another means of stimulating immunity that is more suitable for use in immunocompromised patients.

Patients with herpes zoster are infectious and may transmit varicella to susceptible individuals. Thus, susceptible high-risk patients should be protected from contact with individuals with herpes zoster.

Course and prognosis

Course and prognosis of varicella

In the normal child, varicella is a benign disease rarely attended by serious complications or sequelae. New skin lesions continue to appear for about 3 days and are all crusted by day 5; the rash persists for about a week. Fever is mild and persists as long as new lesions continue to appear. The disease is often trivial in young children but tends to be more severe in older children and adults. Except for Reye's syndrome (which occurs in immunocompetent children) serious complications of varicella occur almost exclusively in neonates, adults, and immunocompromised patients (see above), and these account for most of the morbidity associated with the disease. Mortality in the United States is less than 4 per 100,000, with most deaths occurring in patients with underlying diseases (e.g., leukemia) or Reye's syndrome.

Course and prognosis of herpes zoster

In the normal host, herpes zoster is a self-limited disease with little direct mortality. The rash is usually preceded by 1 to 3 days of neuralgic pain in the involved dermatome. New lesions continue to appear for 2 to 4 days (occasionally for as long as a week) and resolve somewhat more slowly than those of varicella; lesions generally crust in 7 to 10 days and the crusts fall off after about 2 weeks. The most frequent complication is postherpetic neuralgia, which is uncommon in normal persons under 40 years of age, but occurs in more than one-third of patients over 60 years of age. Postherpetic neuralgia is especially common in patients with ophthalmic zoster and in immunocompromised patients. Mortality in herpes zoster is associated with failure of the host to limit virus replication and dissemination; it occurs almost exclusively in immunocompromised patients.

References

1. Gordon JE: Chickenpox: an epidemiological review. *Am J Med Sci* **244**:362, 1962
2. Weller TH: Varicella-herpes zoster virus, in *Viral Infections of Humans, Epidemiology and Control*, 2d ed, edited by AS Evans. New York, Plenum Press, 1982, p 569
3. Osler W: *The Principles and Practice of Medicine*. New York, Appleton, 1892, p 65
4. Scott-Wilson JH: Why "chicken" pox? *Lancet* **1**:1152, 1978
5. Steiner: Zur Inokulation der Varicellen, *Wien Med Wochenschr* **25**:306, 1875
6. Tyzzer EE: The histology of the skin lesions in varicella. *Philipp J Sci* **1**:349, 1906
7. Weller TH, Stoddard MB: Intranuclear inclusion bodies in cultures in human tissue inoculated with varicella vesicle fluid. *J Immunol* **68**:311, 1952
8. Bruusgaard E: The mutual relation between zoster and varicella. *Br J Dermatol Syphilol* **44**:1, 1932
9. Lipschutz B: Untersuchungen uber die Atiologie der Krankheiten der Herpesgruppe (Herpes zoster, Herpes genitalis, Herpes febrilis). *Arch Derm Syph* **136**:428, 1921
10. Taylor-Robinson D, Caunt AE: *Varicella Virus*. Vienna, Springer-Verlag, 1972
11. Weller TH, Witton HM: The etiologic agents of varicella and herpes zoster: serologic studies with the viruses as propagated *in vitro*. *J Exp Med* **108**:869, 1958
12. Weller TH et al: The etiologic agents of varicella and herpes zoster: isolation, propagation, and cultural characteristics *in vitro*. *J Exp Med* **108**:843, 1958
13. Weller TH: Varicella and herpes zoster. Changing concepts of the natural history, control, and importance of a not-so-benign virus. *N Engl J Med* **309**:1362, 1434, 1983
14. Head H, Campbell AW: The pathology of herpes zoster and its bearing on sensory localization. *Brain* **23**:353, 1900
15. Hope-Simpson RE: The nature of herpes zoster: a long-term study and a new hypothesis. *Proc R Soc Med* **58**:9, 1965
16. Denny-Brown D et al: Pathologic features of herpes zoster: a note on "geniculate herpes." *Arch Neurol Psychiatr* **51**:216, 1944
17. Stern ES: The mechanism of herpes zoster and its relation to chicken-pox. *Br J Dermatol Syphilol* **49**:263, 1937
18. Cheatham WJ: The relation of heretofore unreported lesions to pathogenesis of herpes zoster. *Am J Pathol* **29**:401, 1953
19. Muller SA, Winkelmann RK: Cutaneous nerve changes in zoster. *J Invest Dermatol* **52**:71, 1969
20. Esiri MM, Tomlinson AH: Herpes zoster: demonstration of virus in trigeminal nerve and ganglion by immunofluorescence and electron microscopy. *J Neurol Sci* **15**:35, 1972
21. Ghatak NR, Zimmerman HM: Spinal ganglion in herpes zoster. *Arch Pathol* **95**:411, 1973

22. Bastian FO et al: Herpesvirus varicellae: isolated from human dorsal root ganglia. *Arch Pathol* **97**:331, 1974

23. Aoyama Y et al: Demonstration of viral antigens in herpes simplex and varicella-zoster infection. *Recent Advances in RES Research* **14**:90, 1974

24. Gershon AA et al: Antibody to varicella-zoster virus in parturient women and their offspring during the first year of life. *Pediatrics* **58**:692, 1976

25. Ross AH: Modification of chicken pox in family contacts by administration of gamma globulin. *N Engl J Med* **267**:369, 1962

26. Gershon AA et al: Zoster immune globulin: a further assessment. *N Engl J Med* **290**:243, 1974

27. Balfour HH Jr et al: Prevention or modification of varicella using zoster immune plasma. *Am J Dis Child* **131**:693, 1977

28. Orenstein W et al: Prophylaxis of varicella in high-risk children. Dose-response effect of zoster immune globulin. *J Pediatr* **98**:368, 1981

29. Leclair JM et al: Airborne transmission of chickenpox in a hospital. *N Engl J Med* **302**:450, 1980

30. Gustafson TL et al: An outbreak of airborne nosocomial varicella. *Pediatrics* **70**:550–556, 1982

31. Seiler HE: A study of herpes zoster particularly in its relationship to chickenpox. *J Hyg (Camb)* **47**:253, 1949

32. Burgoon CF et al: The natural history of herpes zoster. *JAMA* **164**:265, 1957

33. de Moragas JM, Kierland RR: The outcome of patients with herpes zoster. *Arch Dermatol* **75**:193, 1957

34. Oberg G, Svedmyr A: Varicelliform eruptions in herpes zoster—some clinical and serological observations. *Scand J Infect Dis* **1**:47, 1969

35. Miller LH, Brunell PA: Zoster: reinfection or activation of latent virus? *Am J Med* **49**:480, 1970

36. Rogers RS, Tindall JP: Herpes zoster in children. *Arch Dermatol* **106**:204, 1972

37. Ragozzino MW et al: Population-based study of herpes zoster and its sequelae. *Medicine (Baltimore)* **61**:310, 1982

38. Brunell PA, Kotchmar GS: Zoster in infancy: failure to maintain virus latency following intrauterine infection. *J Pediatr* **98**:71, 1981

39. Ragozzino MW et al: Risk of cancer after herpes zoster. A population-based study. *N Engl J Med* **307**:393, 1982

40. Roizman B, Batterson W: Herpesviruses and their replication, in *Virology,* edited by BN Fields et al. New York, Raven Press, 1985, p 497

41. Almeida JD et al: Morphology of varicella (chickenpox) virus. *Virology* **16**:353, 1962

42. Schmidt NJ: Varicella-zoster virus, in *Manual of Clinical Microbiology,* 4th ed, edited by EH Lennette et al. Washington, DC, American Society for Microbiology, 1985, p 720

43. Martin JH et al: Restriction endonuclease analysis of varicella-zoster vaccine virus and wild-type DNAs. *J Med Virol* **9**:69, 1982

44. Straus SE et al: Genome differences among varicella-zoster virus isolates. *J Gen Virol* **64**:1031, 1983

45. Myers MG et al: Experimental infection of guinea pigs with varicella-zoster virus. *J Infect Dis* **142**:414, 1980

46. Feldman S, Epp E: Detection of viremia during incubation of varicella. *J Pediatr* **94**:746, 1979

47. Asano Y et al: Viremia is present in incubation period in nonimmunocompromised children with varicella. *J Pediatr* **106**:69, 1985

48. Cheatham WJ et al: Varicella: report of two fatal cases with necropsy, virus isolation, and serologic studies. *Am J Pathol* **32**:1015, 1956

49. Johnson HN: Visceral lesions associated with varicella. *Arch Pathol* **30**:292, 1940

50. Eisenbud M: Chickenpox with visceral involvement. *Am J Med* **12**:740, 1952

51. Myers MG: Viremia caused by varicella-zoster virus: association with malignant progressive varicella. *J Infect Dis* **140**:229, 1979

52. Arbeit RD et al: Infection of human peripheral blood mononuclear cells by varicella-zoster virus. *Intervirology* **18**:56, 1982

53. Gibbs FA et al: Electroencephalographic abnormality in "uncomplicated" childhood diseases. *JAMA* **171**:1050, 1959

54. Pitel BA et al: Subclinical hepatic changes in varicella infection. *Pediatrics* **65**:631, 1980

55. Myers MG: Hepatic cellular injury during varicella. *Arch Dis Child* **57**:317, 1982

56. Ey JL et al: Varicella hepatitis without neurologic symptoms or findings. *Pediatrics* **67**:285, 1981

57. Gold E: Serologic and virus-isolation studies of patients with varicella or herpes-zoster infection. *N Engl J Med* **274**:181, 1966

58. Feldman S et al: Varicella in children with cancer: seventy-seven cases. *Pediatrics* **56**:388, 1975

59. Feldman S, Epp E: Isolation of varicella-zoster virus from blood. *J Pediatr* **88**:265, 1976

60. Brunell PA et al: Varicella-zoster immunoglobulins during varicella, latency, and zoster. *J Infect Dis* **132**:49, 1975

61. Arvin AM, Koropchak CM: Immunoglobulins M and G to varicella-zoster virus measured by solid-phase radioimmunoassay: antibody responses to varicella and herpes zoster infections. *J Clin Microbiol* **12**:367, 1980

62. Wittek AE et al: Serum immunoglobulin A antibody to varicella-zoster virus in subjects with primary varicella and herpes zoster infections and in immune subjects. *J Clin Microbiol* **18**:1146, 1983

63. Schmidt NJ, Gallo D: Class-specific antibody responses to early and late antigens of varicella and herpes simplex viruses. *J Med Virol* **13**:1, 1984

64. Jordan GW, Merigan TC: Cell-mediated immunity to varicella-zoster virus: in vitro lymphocyte responses. *J Infect Dis* **130**:495, 1974

65. Zaia JA et al: Specificity of the blastogenic response of human mononuclear cells to herpesvirus antigens. *Infect Immun* **20**:646, 1978

66. Asano Y et al: Soluble skin test antigen of varicella-zoster virus prepared from the fluid of infected cultures. *J Infect Dis* **143**:684, 1981

67. Good RA, Zak SJ: Disturbances in gamma globulin synthesis as "experiments of nature." *Pediatrics* **18**:109, 1956

68. Armstrong RW et al: Cutaneous interferon production in patients with Hodgkin's disease and other cancers infected with varicella or vaccinia. *N Engl J Med* **283**:1182, 1970

69. Ruckdeschel JC et al: Herpes zoster and impaired cell-associated immunity to the varicella-zoster virus in patients with Hodgkin's disease. *Am J Med* **62**:77, 1977

70. Patel PA et al: Cell-mediated immunity to varicella-zoster virus infection in subjects with lymphoma or leukemia. *J Pediatr* **94**:223, 1979

71. Zaia JA et al: Evaluation of varicella-zoster immune globulin: protection of immunosuppressed children after exposure to varicella. *J Infect Dis* **147**:737, 1983

72. Gershon AA, Krugman S: Seroepidemiologic survey of varicella: value of specific fluorescent antibody test. *Pediatrics* **56**:1005, 1975

73. Zaia JA, Oxman MN: Antibody to varicella-zoster virus-induced membrane antigen: immunofluorescence assay using monodisperse glutaraldehyde-fixed target cells. *J Infect Dis* **136**:519, 1977

74. Brunell PA et al: Prevention of varicella by zoster immune globulin. *N Engl J Med* **280**:1191, 1969

75. Iltis JP et al: Comparison of the Raji cell line fluorescent antibody to membrane antigen test and the enzyme-linked

immunosorbent assay for determination of immunity to varicella-zoster virus. *J Clin Microbiol* **16**:878, 1982

76. Arvin AM et al: Immunologic evidence of reinfection with varicella-zoster virus. *J Infect Dis* **148**:200, 1983

77. Baba K et al: Immunologic and epidemiologic aspects of varicella infection acquired during infancy and early childhood. *J Pediatr* **100**:881, 1982

78. Gershon AA et al: Live attenuated varicella vaccine: efficacy for children with leukemia in remission. *JAMA* **252**:355, 1984

79. Arbeter AM et al: Varicella vaccine trials in healthy children. *Am J Dis Child* **138**:434, 1984

80. Gershon AA et al: Clinical reinfection with varicella-zoster virus. *J Infect Dis* **149**:137, 1984

81. Stevens JG: Latent herpes simplex virus and the nervous system. *Curr Top Microbiol Immunol* **70**:31, 1975

82. Shanbrom E et al: Herpes zoster in hematologic neoplasias: some unusual manifestations. *Ann Intern Med* **53**:523, 1960

83. Juel-Hensen BE, MacCallum FO: *Herpes Simplex, Varicella and Zoster.* Philadelphia, JB Lippincott, 1972

84. Sokal JE, Firat D: Varicella-zoster infection in Hodgkin's disease. *Am J Med* **39**:452, 1965

85. Schimpff S et al: Varicella-zoster infection in patients with cancer. *Ann Intern Med* **76**:241, 1972

86. Feldman S et al: Herpes zoster in children with cancer. *Am J Dis Child* **126**:178, 1973

87. Luby JP et al: A longitudinal study of varicella-zoster virus infections in renal transplant recipients. *J Infect Dis* **135**:659, 1977

88. Weigle KA, Grose C: Molecular dissection of the humoral immune response to individual varicella-zoster viral proteins during chickenpox, quiescence, reinfection, and reactivation. *J Infect Dis* **149**:741, 1984

89. Gershon AA et al: IgM to varicella-zoster virus: demonstration in patients with and without clinical zoster. *Pediatr Infect Dis* **1**:164, 1982

90. Dolin R et al: Herpes zoster-varicella infections in immunosuppressed patients. *Ann Intern Med* **89**:375, 1978

91. McKendall RR, Klawans HL: Nervous system complications of varicella-zoster virus. In *Handbook of Clinical Neurology,* vol 34, edited by PJ Vinken, GW Bruyn. Amsterdam, North-Holland, 1978, p 161

92. Feldman S et al: A viremic phase for herpes zoster in children with cancer. *Pediatrics* **91**:597, 1977

93. Easton HG: Zoster sine herpete causing trigeminal neuralgia. *Lancet* **2**:1065, 1970

94. Merselis JG Jr et al: Disseminated herpes zoster. *Arch Intern Med* **113**:679, 1964

95. Goffinet DR et al: Herpes zoster-varicella infections and lymphoma. *Ann Intern Med* **76**:235, 1972

96. Goodman R et al: Herpes zoster in children with stage I–III Hodgkin's disease. *Radiology* **118**:429, 1976

97. Reboul F et al: Herpes zoster and varicella infections in children with Hodgkin's disease. *Cancer* **41**:95, 1978

98. Rand KH et al: Cellular immunity and herpesvirus infections in cardiac-transplant patients. *N Engl J Med* **296**:1372, 1977

99. Stevens DA et al: Cellular events in zoster vesicles: relation to clinical course and immune parameters. *J Infect Dis* **131**:509, 1975

100. Pollard RB et al: Specific cell-mediated immunity and infections with herpesviruses in cardiac transplant recipients. *Am J Med* **73**:679, 1982

101. Meyers JD et al: Cell-mediated immunity to varicella-zoster virus after allogenic marrow transplant. *J Infect Dis* **141**:479, 1980

102. Miller AE: Selective decline in cellular immune response to varicella-zoster in the elderly. *Neurology* **30**:582, 1980

103. Berger R et al: Decrease of the lymphoproliferative response to varicella zoster virus antigen in the aged. *Infect Immun* **32**:24, 1981

104. Burke BL et al: Immune response to varicella-zoster in the aged. *Arch Intern Med* **142**:291, 1982

105. Wesselhoeft C: The differential diagnosis of chicken pox and smallpox. *N Engl J Med* **230**:15, 1944

106. Bullowa JGM et al: Complications of varicella I. Their occurrence among 2,534 patients. *Am J Dis Child* **49**:923, 1935

107. Krugman S et al: Varicella-zoster infections, in *Infectious Diseases of Children,* 8th ed. St Louis, CV Mosby, 1985, p 433

108. Smith EW et al: Varicella gangrenosa due to group A-hemolytic streptococcus. *Pediatrics* **57**:306, 1976

109. Fleisher G et al: Life-threatening complications of varicella. *Am J Dis Child* **135**:896, 1981

110. Melish ME: Bullous varicella: its association with the staphylococcal scalded skin syndrome. *J Pediatr* **83**:1019, 1973

111. Weinstein L, Meade RH: Respiratory manifestations of chicken pox. *Arch Intern Med* **98**:91, 1956

112. Singer J: Postvaricella suppurative meningitis. Case reports and review of the literature. *Am J Dis Child* **133**:934, 1979

113. Triebwasser JH et al: Varicella pneumonia in adults. *Medicine (Baltimore)* **46**:409, 1967

114. Haggerty RJ, Eley RC: Varicella and cortisone. *Pediatrics* **18**:160, 1956

115. Gershon A et al: Steroid therapy and varicella. *J Pediatr* **81**:1034, 1972

116. Boughton CR: Varicella-zoster in Sydney: I. Varicella and its complications. *Med J Aust* **53(II)**:392, 1966

117. Weber DM, Pellecchia JA: Varicella pneumonia: study of prevalence in adult men. *JAMA* **192**:527, 1965

118. Mackay JB, Cairney P: Pulmonary calcification following varicella. *NZ Med J* **59**:453, 1960

119. Sargent EN et al: Varicella pneumonia. A report of 20 cases, with postmortem examination in six. *Calif Med* **107**:141, 1967

120. Waring JJ et al: Severe forms of chickenpox in adults. *Arch Intern Med* **69**:384, 1942

121. Oxman MN et al: Management at delivery of mother and infant when herpes simplex, varicella-zoster, hepatitis or tuberculosis have occurred during pregnancy, in *Current Topics in Infectious Diseases,* vol 4, edited by JS Remington, MN Swartz. New York, McGraw-Hill, 1983, p 224

122. Young NA, Gershon AA: Chickenpox, measles and mumps, in *Infectious Diseases of the Fetus and Newborn Infant,* 2d ed, edited by JS Remington, JO Klein. Philadelphia, WB Saunders, 1983, p 375

123. Williamson AP: The varicella-zoster virus in the etiology of severe congenital defects. *Clin Pediatr* **14**:553, 1975

124. Finkel KC: Mortality from varicella in children receiving adrenocorticosteroids and adrenocorticotropin. *Pediatrics* **28**:436, 1971

125. Scheinman, JI, Stamler FW: Cyclophosphamide and fatal varicella. *J Pediatr* **74**:117, 1969

126. Lux SE et al: Chronic neutropenia and abnormal cellular immunity in cartilage-hair hypoplasia. *N Engl J Med* **282**:231, 1970

127. Hattori A et al: Use of live varicella vaccine in children with acute leukaemia or other malignancies. *Lancet* **2**:210, 1976

128. Feldhoff CM et al: Varicella in children with renal transplants. *J Pediatr* **98**:25, 1981

129. Whitley R J et al: Vidarabine therapy of varicella in immunosuppressed patients. *J Pediatr* **101**:125, 1982

130. Whitley RJ et al: Early vidarabine therapy to control the complications of herpes zoster in immunosuppressed patients. *N Engl J Med* **307**:971, 1982

131. Smith H: Purpura fulminans complicating varicella: recovery with low molecular weight dextran and steroids. *Med J Aust* **54(II)**:685, 1967

132. Feusner JH et al: Mechanisms of thrombocytopenia in varicella. *Am J Hematol* **7**:255, 1979

133. Christie AB: Chickenpox (varicella); Herpes zoster, in *In-*

fectious Diseases: Epidemiology and Clinical Practice, 3d ed. Edinburgh, Churchill Livingstone, 1980, pp 262, 278

134. Charkes ND: Purpuric chickenpox: report of a case, review of the literature, and classification by clinical features. *Ann Intern Med* **54**:745, 1961

135. Yeager AM, Zinkham WH: Varicella-associated thrombocytopenia: clues to the etiology of childhood idiopathic thrombocytopenic purpura. *Johns Hopkins Med J* **146**:270, 1980

136. Espinoza C, Kuhn C: Viral infection of megakaryocytes in varicella with purpura. *Am J Clin Pathol* **61**:203, 1974

137. Ladisch S et al: Extrapulmonary manifestations of adenovirus type 7 pneumonia simulating Reye syndrome and the possible role of an adenovirus toxin. *J Pediatr* **95**:348, 1979

138. Centers for Disease Control: Reye syndrome—United States, 1984. *MMWR* **34**:13, 1985

139. Lichtenstein PK et al: Grade I Reye's syndrome. A frequent cause of vomiting and liver dysfunction after varicella and upper-respiratory-tract infection. *N Engl J Med* **309**:133, 1983

140. Takashima S, Becker LE: Neuropathology of fatal varicella. *Arch Pathol Lab Med* **103**:209, 1979

141. Goldston AS et al: Cerebellar ataxia with preeruptive varicella. *Am J Dis Child* **106**:197, 1963

142. Peters ACB et al: Varicella and acute cerebellar ataxia. *Arch Neurol* **35**:769, 1978

143. Johnson RT et al: Measles encephalomyelitis—clinical and immunological studies. *N Engl J Med* **310**:137, 1984

144. Applebaum E et al: Varicella encephalitis. *Am J Med* **15**:223, 1953

145. Boughton CR: Varicella-zoster in Sydney: II. Neurological complications of varicella. *Med J Aust* **53(II)**:444, 1966

146. Nicholaides NJ: Fatal systemic varicella. A report of 3 cases. *Med J Aust* **44(II)**:88, 1957

147. Griffith JF et al: The nervous system diseases associated with varicella. *Acta Neurol Scand* **46**:279, 1970

148. Gershon AA et al: Varicella-zoster-associated encephalitis: detection of specific antibody in cerebrospinal fluid. *J Clin Microbiol* **12**:764, 1980

149. Lewis GW: Zoster sine herpete. *Br Med J* **2**:418, 1958

150. Adour KK: Current Concepts in Neurology: diagnosis and management of facial paralysis. *N Engl J Med* **307**:348, 1982

151. Brown GR: Herpes zoster: correlation of age, sex, distribution, neuralgia, and associated disorders. *South Med J* **59**:576, 1976

152. Winkelmann RK, Perry HO: Herpes zoster in children. *JAMA* **171**:112, 1959

153. Brunell PA et al: Zoster in children. *Am J Dis Child* **115**:432, 1968

154. Eisenberg E: Intraoral isolated herpes zoster. *Oral Surg* **45**:214, 1978

155. Clark J: Herpes zoster of right glossopharyngeal nerve. *Lancet* **1**:38, 1979

156. Hope-Simpson RE: Postherpetic neuralgia. *J R Coll Gen Pract* **25**:571, 1975

157. Pavan-Langston D: Ocular viral infections. *Med Clin North Am* **67**:973, 1983

158. Womack LW, Liesegang TJ: Complications of herpes zoster ophthalmicus. *Arch Ophthalmol* **101**:42, 1983

159. Patterson SD et al: Atypical generalized zoster with lymphadenitis mimicking lymphoma. *N Engl J Med* **302**:848, 1980

160. Grant BD, Rowe CR: Motor paralysis of the extremities in herpes zoster. *J Bone Joint Surg* **43A**:885, 1961

161. Thomas JE, Howard FM: Segmental zoster paresis—a disease profile. *Neurology* **22**:459, 1972

162. Kendall D: Motor complications of herpes zoster. *Br Med J* **1**:616, 1957

163. Brostoff J: Diaphragmatic paralysis after herpes zoster. *Br Med J* **2**:1571, 1966

164. Jellinek EH, Tulloch WS: Herpes zoster with dysfunction of bladder and anus. *Lancet* **2**:1219, 1976

165. Izumi AK, Edwards J: Herpes zoster and neurogenic bladder dysfunction. *JAMA* **224**:1748, 1973

166. Rose FC et al: Zoster encephalomyelitis. *Arch Neurol* **11**:155, 1964

167. Wisloff F et al: Herpes zoster of the stomach. *Lancet* **2**:953, 1979

168. Gibbon NOK: A case of herpes zoster with involvement of the urinary bladder. *Br J Urol* **28**:417, 1956

169. Richmond W: The genitourinary manifestations of herpes zoster. *Br J Urol* **46**:193, 1974

170. McCormick WF et al: Varicella-zoster encephalomyelitis. *Arch Neurol* **21**:559, 1969

171. Gold E, Robbins FC: Isolation of herpes zoster virus from spinal fluid of a patient. *Virology* **6**:293, 1958

172. Applebaum E et al: Herpes zoster encephalitis. *Am J Med* **32**:25, 1962

173. Norris FH et al: Herpes-zoster meningoencephalitis. *J Infect Dis* **122**:335, 1970

174. Jemsek J et al: Herpes zoster-associated encephalitis: clinicopathologic report of 12 cases and review of the literature. *Medicine (Baltimore)* **62**:81, 1983

175. Reshef E et al: Herpes zoster ophthalmicus followed by contralateral hemiparesis: report of two cases and review of literature. *J Neurol Neurosurg Psychiatry* **48**:122, 1985

176. Bourdette, DN et al: Herpes zoster ophthalmicus and delayed ipsilateral cerebral infarction. *Neurology* **33**:1428, 1983

177. Hilt DC et al: Herpes zoster ophthalmicus and delayed contralateral hemiparesis caused by cerebral angiitis: diagnosis and management approaches. *Ann Neurol* **14**:543, 1983

178. Pek S, Gikas PW: Pneumonia due to herpes zoster: report of a case and review of the literature. *Ann Intern Med* **62**:350, 1965

179. Atkinson K et al: Varicella-zoster virus infection after marrow transplantation for aplastic anemia or leukemia. *Transplantation* **29**:47, 1980

180. Horten B et al: Multifocal varicella-zoster virus leukoencephalitis temporally remote from herpes zoster. *Ann Neurol* **9**:251, 1981

181. Olding-Stenkvist E, Grandien M: Early diagnosis of virus-caused vesicular rashes by immunofluorescence on skin biopsies. *Scand J Infect Dis* **8**:27, 1976

182. Frank L: Varicella pneumonitis: report of a case with autopsy observations. *Arch Pathol* **50**:450, 1950

183. Rotter R, Collins JD: Fatal disseminated varicella in adults; report of a case and review of the literature. *Wis Med J* **60**:325, 1961

184. Sander J et al: Fatal varicella pneumonia. *Scand J Infect Dis* **2**:231, 1970

185. Shibuta H et al: Varicella virus isolation from spinal ganglion. *Archiv fur die gesamte Virusforshung* **45**:382, 1974

186. O'Donnell PP et al: Recurrent herpes zoster encephalitis. *Arch Neurol* **38**:49, 1981

187. Andiman WA et al: Zoster encephalitis. Isolation of virus and measurement of varicella-zoster-specific antibodies in cerebrospinal fluid. *Am J Med* **73**:769, 1982

188. Hogan EL, Krigman MR: Herpes zoster myelitis. *Arch Neurol* **29**:309, 1973

189. Doyle PW et al: Herpes zoster ophthalmicus with contralateral hemiplegia: identification of cause. *Am J Clin Pathol* **14**:84, 1983

190. Rosenblum WL, Hadfield MG: Granulomatous angiitis of the nervous system in cases of herpes zoster and lymphosarcoma. *Neurology* **22**:348, 1972

191. Reyes MG et al: Viruslike particles in granulomatous angiitis of the central nervous system. *Neurology* **26**:797, 1976

192. Linnenmann CC, Alvira MM: Pathogenesis of varicella-zoster angiitis in the CNS. *Arch Neurol* **37**:329, 1980

193. Mayberg MR et al: Trigeminal projections to supratentorial pial and dural blood vessels in cats demonstrated by horseradish peroxidase histochemistry. *J Comp Neurol* **223**:46, 1984

194. Blank H et al: Cytologic smears in diagnosis of herpes simplex, herpes zoster, and varicella. *JAMA* **146**:1410, 1951

195. Barr RJ et al: Rapid method for Tzanck preparations. *JAMA* **237**:1119, 1977

196. Weller TH: Varicella and herpes zoster, in *Diagnostic Procedures for Viral, Rickettsial and Chlamydial Infections*, 5th ed, edited by EH Lenette, NJ Schmidt. Washington, DC, American Public Health Association, 1979, p 375

197. Richman DD et al: Rapid viral diagnosis. *J Infect Dis* **149**:298, 1984

198. Frey HM, Steinberg SP: Rapid diagnosis of varicella-zoster virus infections by countercurrent immunoelectrophoresis. *J Infect Dis* **143**:274, 1981

199. Schmidt NJ et al: Direct immunofluorescence staining for detection of herpes simplex and varicella-zoster virus antigens in vesicular lesions and certain tissue specimens. *J Clin Microbiol* **12**:651, 1980

200. Cleveland PH et al: An enzyme immunofiltration technique for the rapid diagnosis of herpes simplex virus eye infections. *J Clin Microbiol* **16**:676, 1982

201. Williams V et al: Serologic response to varicella-zoster membrane antigens measured by indirect immunofluorescence. *J Infect Dis* **130**:669, 1974

202. Kalter ZG et al: Immune adherence hemagglutination: further observations on demonstration of antibody to varicella-zoster virus. *J Infect Dis* **135**:1010, 1977

203. Richman DD et al: A rapid radioimmunoassay using ^{125}I-staphylococcal protein A for antibody to varicella-zoster virus. *J Infect Dis* **143**:693, 1981

204. Shanley J et al: Enzyme-linked immunosorbent assay for detection of antibody to varicella-zoster virus. *J Clin Microbiol* **15**:208, 1982

205. Kamiya H et al: Diagnostic skin test reaction with varicella virus antigen and clinical application of the test. *J Infect Dis* **136**:784, 1977

206. Steele RW et al: Varicella zoster in hospital personnel: skin test reactivity to monitor susceptibility. *Pediatrics* **70**:604, 1982

207. Fulginiti VA et al: Aspirin and Reye syndrome. *Pediatrics* **69**:810, 1982

208. Hirsch MS, Schooley RT: Treatment of herpesvirus infections. *N Engl J Med* **309**:963, 1034, 1983

209. Dolin R: Antiviral chemotherapy and chemoprophylaxis. *Science* **227**:1296, 1985

210. Savoia M, Oxman MN: Guidelines for antiviral therapy, in *Current Therapy in Infectious Disease: 1985–1986*, edited by EH Kass, R Platt. Toronto/Philadelphia, BC Decker, 1986, p 1

211. Nicholson, KG: Antiviral therapy. Varicella-zoster virus infections, herpes labialis and mucocutaneous herpes, and cytomegalovirus infections. *Lancet* **2**:677, 1984

212. Elion GB: Mechanism of action and selectivity of acyclovir. *Am J Med* **73**:7, 1982

213. Schwartz PM et al: Antiviral activity of arabinosyladenine and arabinosylhypoxanthine in herpes simplex virus-infected KB cells. Selective inhibition of viral deoxyribonucleic acid synthesis in the presence of an adenosine deaminase inhibitor. *Antimicrob Agents Chemother* **10**:64, 1976

214. Prober CG et al: Acyclovir therapy of chickenpox in immunosuppressed children—a collaborative study. *J Pediatr* **101**:622, 1982

215. Arvin AM et al: Human leukocyte interferon in the treatment of varicella in children with cancer. *N Engl J Med* **306**:761, 1982

216. Serota FT et al: Acyclovir treatment of herpes zoster infections. *JAMA* **247**:2132, 1982

217. Balfour HH Jr: Intravenous acyclovir therapy for varicella in immunocompromised children. *J Pediatr* **104**:134, 1984

218. Shulman ST: Acyclovir treatment of disseminated varicella in childhood malignant neoplasms. *Am J Dis Child* **139**:137, 1985

219. Novelli VM et al: Acyclovir administered perorally in immunocompromised children with varicella-zoster infections. *J Infect Dis* **149**:478, 1984

220. Whitley RJ et al: Adenine arabinoside therapy of herpes zoster in the immunosuppressed. *N Engl J Med* **294**:1193, 1976

221. Balfour HH Jr et al: Acyclovir halts progression of herpes zoster in immunocompromised patients. *N Engl J Med* **308**:1448, 1983

222. Merigan TC et al: Human leukocyte interferon for the treatment of herpes zoster in patients with cancer. *N Engl J Med* **298**:981, 1978

223. Merigan TC et al: Short-course human leukocyte interferon in treatment of herpes zoster in patients with cancer. *Antimicrob Agents Chemother* **19**:193, 1981

224. Rifkind D: The activation of varicella-zoster virus infections by immunosuppressive therapy. *J Lab Clin Med* **68**:463, 1966

225. Mazur MH et al: Serum antibody levels as risk factors in the dissemination of herpes zoster. *Arch Intern Med* **139**:1341, 1979

226. Stevens DA, Merigan TC: Zoster immune globulin prophylaxis of disseminated zoster in compromised hosts. *Arch Intern Med* **140**:52, 1980

227. Peterslund NA et al: Acyclovir in herpes zoster. *Lancet* **2**:827, 1981

228. Bean B et al: Acyclovir therapy for acute herpes zoster. *Lancet* **2**:118, 1982

229. McGill J et al: A review of acyclovir treatment of ocular herpes zoster and skin infections. *J Antimicrob Chemother* **12**:45, 1983

230. Wildenhoff KE et al: Treatment of herpes zoster with idoxuridine ointment, including a multivariate analysis of symptoms and signs. *Scand J Infect Dis* **11**:1, 1979

231. Price RW: Herpes zoster. An approach to systemic therapy. *Med Clin North Am* **66**:1105, 1982

232. Eaglstein WH et al: The effects of early corticosteroid therapy on the skin eruption and pain of herpes zoster. *JAMA* **211**:1681, 1970

233. Keczkes K, Basheer AM: Do corticosteroids prevent postherpetic neuralgia? *Br J Dermatol* **102**:551, 1980

234. Geiser CF et al: Prophylaxis of varicella in children with neoplastic disease: comparative results with zoster immune plasma and gamma globulin. *Cancer* **35**:1027, 1975

235. Zaia JA et al: A practical method for preparation of varicella-zoster immune globulin. *J Infect Dis* **137**:601, 1978

236. Centers for Disease Control: Varicella-zoster immune globulin for the prevention of chickenpox. *Ann Intern Med* **100**:859, 1984

237. Takahashi M et al: Live vaccine used to prevent the spread of varicella in children in hospital. *Lancet* **2**:1288, 1974

238. Brunell PA et al: Administration of live varicella vaccine to children with leukemia. *Lancet* **2**:1069, 1982

239. Asano Y et al: Five-year follow-up study of recipients of live varicella vaccine using enhanced neutralization and fluorescent antibody membrane antigen assays. *Pediatrics* **72**:291, 1983

240. Asano Y et al: Long-term protective immunity of recipients of the OKA strain of live varicella vaccine. *Pediatrics* **75**:667, 1985

241. Weibel RE et al: Live attenuated varicella virus, vaccine.

Efficacy trial in healthy children. *N Engl J Med* **310:**1410, 1984
242. Myers MG et al: Hospital infection control for varicella zoster infection. *Pediatrics* **70:**199, 1982

243. Berger R et al: Enhancement of varicella-zoster-specific immune responses in the elderly by boosting with varicella vaccine. *J Infect Dis* **149:**647, 1984

CHAPTER 192

SMALLPOX AND COMPLICATIONS OF SMALLPOX VACCINATION

Vincent A. Fulginiti

Smallpox (variola)

Definition

Smallpox is an acute exanthematous disease caused by infection with poxvirus variolae. The significant clinical features include a 3-day prodromal illness and a generalized centrifugal rash with rapidly successive papules, vesicles, pustules, umbilication, and crusting within 14 days.

Historical aspects

The first clinical description of smallpox was by Rhazes, an Arabian physician, in the tenth century A.D. Many curious beliefs concerning the cause and pathogenesis of the disease are recorded in the writings of the early physicians. Frequently smallpox was confused with chickenpox, syphilis, and measles. It is of interest that smallpox was known in China 11 centuries before the birth of Christ, and that inoculation to prevent the disease was described in the sixth century B.C. using dried crusts introduced into the nose. It is likely that smallpox was introduced into the Western world in the early centuries after Christ by the migrations of invading armies. Subsequent spread of smallpox in Europe and England is intertwined with the history of these areas. As one reads the various accounts of epidemics of this disease in the fifteenth and sixteenth centuries, and later in the United States, it becomes apparent that smallpox represented a major force in life, often affecting dynasties, determining the outcome of military conflicts, as well as influencing daily life. Until the advent of Jennerian vaccination, its widespread application, and the ultimate eradication of smallpox from most of the Western world, this disease continued to be a major threat, with widespread attack rates, persistent infection within a community, and a high mortality rate.

Epidemiology

In the last decade a remarkable event has occurred in public health. As of this writing the efforts of many coun-

tries coordinated by the World Health Organization have resulted in intensive case finding and application of smallpox vaccination across large populations. This has resulted in the eradication of smallpox from many countries, such as the entire Indian subcontinent, the Middle East, all of South America, and Africa. There have been no cases since October 1977 anywhere in the world.

Etiology and pathogenesis

Smallpox is caused by infection with poxvirus variola. It is believed that infection occurs strictly following contact with another infected human being. Evidence is accumulating that suggests a respiratory transmission, and the epidemiologic pattern supports this concept. Skin inoculation and fomite spread also may play a role in some instances.

Following contact, an asymptomatic period of 12 to 13 days follows. Despite the lack of symptoms, viral replication is massive. The pathogenic events that occur in the human being are suggested by analogy with Jenner's experimental mousepox infection. The virus, following introduction via the respiratory tract, undergoes local multiplication in the respiratory mucosa and regional lymphoid tissue. Primary viremia occurs, which spreads the virus widely throughout the reticuloendothelial system, where a massive multiplication occurs. A secondary viremia heralds the onset of the prodromal illness, resulting in spread to many organs and tissues, with primary manifestations in the skin. It has been postulated that serum antibody is not the significant factor in recovery from initial episodes of smallpox, and it appears likely that both delayed hypersensitivity and interferon production play some role in such recovery. Hemorrhagic forms of the disease are of interest in that a profound coagulation disorder is associated with a decrease in the number of serum platelets. Recent evidence indicates that depression of platelet formation occurs routinely in smallpox infection and that the hemorrhagic forms of the disease bear some similarity to disseminated intravascular coagulation, which results in reduction in coagulation factors, extensive hemorrhage, and death.

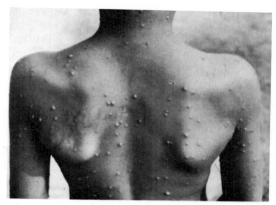

Fig. 192-1 Pustular smallpox: tense, clouded vesicles which maintain firm feel.

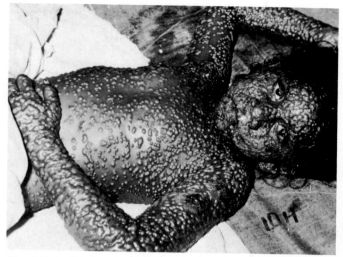

Fig. 192-3 Confluent smallpox. Note massive numbers of lesions, all in same stage of development, and confluency of many.

Clinical manifestations

History. An influenzal illness shortly after contact has been described ("illness of contact"). In nonendemic areas a history of contact is essential. Prior vaccination history and interval to symptoms are important, as the disease pattern may be altered. Prior to the onset of the typical cutaneous lesions, a prodromal period of 3 days' duration occurs, characterized by apprehension, sudden prostrating fever, severe headache, back pain, and vomiting. A prodromal rash is not uncommon; it is macular and papular or petechial, and when it occurs in the characteristic "swimming-trunk" distribution, it is felt to be pathognomonic.

Cutaneous lesions. The disease may take various courses. In the nonvaccinated, a discrete pox eruption is the most frequent form of illness. Severe forms of the disease are associated with confluent eruptions and/or cutaneous hemorrhage. Infrequently variola may occur without eruption, or with just a few pocks. A flat erythematous macular rash may precede the appearance of tense, deep-seated papules which rapidly vesiculate. These lesions are firm and more deep-seated than those of chickenpox. The rash may be very sparse, or individual vesicles may become confluent to form large patches. As the lesions mature, the classical "pustule" occurs (Fig. 192-1). These lesions do not contain bacteria, and the cloudiness represents accumulated white

blood cells, debris, and protein. Central umbilication is characteristic (Figs. 192-2 and 192-3), and eventually the lesion crusts over and heals, with scar formation. Although this is the classical evolution of smallpox, many variants are encountered, especially in individuals previously vaccinated. Lesions may present a flat disklike appearance or may undergo resolution without passing through the vesiculopustular stage.

There are two recognized hemorrhagic forms of the disease; one in which hemorrhage occurs in association with prodromal symptoms but death supervenes before any of the characteristic skin lesions can occur; and a second, characterized by hemorrhage into preexisting skin lesions. Both have almost universally fatal outcomes, the first within a week and the second after 8 to 12 days. Bacterial infection of smallpox lesions occurs, and localized abscesses, cellulitis, etc., may result.

Other physical findings. Secondary viremia with spread to many organs may result in clinically apparent illness. Particularly common are ulceration of the cornea, laryngeal lesions with symptoms of obstruction in the upper part of the airway, central nervous system involvement with encephalitis or acute psychotic behavior, and, less commonly, osteomyelitis, pneumonia, and orchitis.

Laboratory findings. Usual diagnostic laboratory measurements are of little value in smallpox. The white blood cell count may be elevated early in the disease, but this is not of diagnostic significance.

Virus is present in the blood of patients during the prodrome and occasionally thereafter. Virus is uniformly found in the skin lesions; the early papules and vesicles provide the richest source. In hemorrhagic forms of the disease, severe thrombocytopenia occurs; in addition, marked decrease in the level of accelerator globulin (factor V), moderate decreases in the amount of prothrombin and proconvertin, and a circulating antithrombin are noted in early hemorrhagic smallpox. The late hemorrhagic form of

Fig. 192-2 Pustular smallpox. Note tendency to confluence and beginning central umbilication in some lesions.

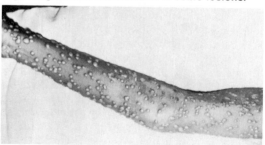

the disease is associated with a decrease in platelets without other coagulation disturbances.

Pathology

In the papular stage of the eruption, capillary dilatation and edema of the papillary layer of the dermis are observed. Perivascular inflammatory changes occur, with lymphocytic and histiocytic infiltration. Thickening and vacuolization in the epithelium result in vesicle formation. The vesicle is deep and, because of the destruction of cells, becomes separate. Leukocyte infiltration results in the "pustule formation," which resolves by epithelial migration and crusting. Typical cytoplasmic eosinophilic inclusion bodies have been described (Guarnieri's bodies). Histopathologic changes in the mucosa are similar, with added ulceration.

Diagnosis and differential diagnosis

Typical smallpox in endemic areas usually can be diagnosed clinically, and ancillary virologic laboratory aids are usually unnecessary. However, in the United States, as well as in most of the Western world, smallpox is sufficiently uncommon that it may be confused with severe chickenpox or not suspected at all. For this reason virologic diagnosis is *essential,* with confirmation of variola having public health implications, in countries free of the disease. Rapid means of laboratory diagnosis include (1) light microscopic identification of elementary bodies with appropriate stains, (2) electron microscopic identification of virus in vesicular fluid or scrapings from the base of a papule or early vesicle, and (3) fluorescent antibody staining of the virus from the same material. All these tests yield rapid, presumptive results in the hands of experienced workers, but definite diagnosis can be achieved only by isolation of the virus in the embryonated egg or in appropriate tissue culture systems and specific identification of the virus by neutralization with variola or vaccinal antiserum. Indirect but rapid methods utilize vesicular fluid as a hemagglutinin, complement-fixing, or precipitating antigen with specific variola vaccinia antiserum. Retrospective diagnosis can be afforded by evaluation of serum antibody rises in a 2- to 3-week interval, utilizing paired sera collected during the acute and convalescent phases of the illness.

In summary, the diagnosis of smallpox is primarily clinical and based upon obtaining an adequate history of exposure, the observation of an approximately 2-week incubation period followed by a severe 3-day prodrome, ultimately terminating in a typical rash with centrifugal distribution and all lesions in the same stage of development. One cannot rely on the presence of Guarnieri's bodies to establish the diagnosis, although they may be suggestive.

In the preeruptive phase of smallpox, distinction must be made from dengue, enterovirus infections, and other febrile illnesses. The prodromal rash may be confused with that of measles. History of contact and the appropriate incubation interval should serve to make one suspect smallpox.

Hemorrhagic smallpox, especially in nonendemic areas, may be confused with meningococcal septicemia, coagulation disorders, typhus, and other acute hemorrhagic exanthems. Eruptive smallpox is most frequently mistaken for chickenpox. The lack of prodromal symptoms, the successive appearance of crops of superficial vesicles, the centripetal distribution, and the varying stages of development of chickenpox lesions all serve to distinguish this disease from variola.

Treatment

This disease can be effectively prevented by Jennerian vaccination. No effective specific treatment is known, however. Thiosemicarbazone and antivariola or antivaccinia serum and immune globulin have thus far failed in the therapy of established smallpox.

Good nursing care with attention to the prevention of secondary bacterial infection is critical in treatment. Appropriate antimicrobial therapy for bacterial complications should be employed, and attention should be paid to the nutritional, fluid, and electrolyte needs of patients.

Course and prognosis

The overall mortality rate of smallpox approximates 25 percent, with confluent disease representing a greater risk than discrete eruptions. Fulminant smallpox is universally fatal, as are the hemorrhagic forms of illness.

Complications of smallpox vaccination (vaccinia)

Definition and classification

Vaccination against smallpox consists of the introduction of vaccinia virus into the outer layers of the intact skin. Local multiplication of virus occurs, and in some instances regional lymphadenopathy and systemic symptoms ensue. The infection is a localized one which heals by scarring and is limited by host response. A complicated vaccination is one in which any of the above components is altered. Complications may be classified as indicated in Table 192-1.

Historical aspects

With the reduction of smallpox in the world, the routine application of infant vaccination has been greatly diminished. As a result, complications of vaccinations are seen infrequently in most countries and not at all in many.

Epidemiology

Most complications may occur at any age, but they are usually seen among young infants and children. Primovaccination is most often administered to this age group, and almost all the significant complications occur most frequently, if not exclusively, after first vaccination. In addition, the infectious complications tend to occur in the immunologically deficient child, which also contributes to the clustering in early childhood. Bacterial superinfection in some instances is related to warm weather, with the opportunity for maceration of skin and with increased exposure of the vaccination site.

Complications are reported more commonly in the West-

Table 192-1   Classification of complications of vaccination

Major category	Specific syndromes	Comment
Noninfectious rashes	Erythema multiforme	Differentiate from
	Macular—toxic eruption	generalized
	Macular and papular	
	Vesicular	
	Urticarial	
Bacterial superinfection	Streptococcal	Often hyperkeratotic
	Staphylococcal	
	Mixed	
	Tetanus	
	Syphilis	Of historical interest in U.S.
Accidental inoculation (may occur in vaccinated individual)	Normal skin	
	Abnormal skin	
	Burns	
	Pyoderma	
	Exanthem	Examples: varicella, herpes
	Eczema	
	Other dermatides:	
	Mucosal	Usually oral or conjunctival
	Corneal	Vaccinal keratitis
Congenital vaccinia		
Generalized vaccinia	Benign becoming malignant with progression	
Progressive vaccinia (vaccinia gangrenosa, vaccinia necrosum)	In immunologically normal persons	
	In hypogamma-globulinemia:	
	Congenital sex-linked	
	Thymic alymphoplasia	
	In dysgammaglobulinemia	
	With malignancies:	
	Chronic lymphatic leukemia	
	Hodgkin's disease	
	Lymphoma	
Encephalitis	Postvaccinal	
Miscellaneous	Hemolytic anemia	
	Arthritis	
	Osteomyelitis	
	Laboratory infections	
	Pericarditis and myocarditis	

ern world, despite the prevalence of vaccination in the East. This undoubtedly represents reporting differences, not a true geographic or racial relationship. The incidence of postvaccinal encephalitis appears to be higher in the Netherlands. Whether this represents a true racial difference or simply reflects the fact of primovaccination in the adults is not clear.

Etiology and pathogenesis

The basic mechanisms of the complications of vaccination may be divided into three categories: (1) bacterial super-infection, (2) abnormal viral replication, and (3) altered reactivity, or "allergy," to some viral component.

Bacteria can invade the vaccination site; indeed, not all vaccine is bacteriologically sterile. That superinfection is not more common is remarkable. Apparently more than contamination is necessary; those factors of greatest importance are concurrent streptococcal infection elsewhere, and excessive trauma, maceration, and manipulation of the vaccination site.

Usually the virus remains localized at the site of implantation, but occasionally infection may be transposed to healthy or unhealthy skin elsewhere on the body, or even to another person. Etiologic factors include excessive manipulation, abnormal skin (burns, eczema, etc.), inflammatory lesions (blepharitis, herpes), and abnormal immune mechanisms. Any of these may contribute to spread of the virus away from the intended localized vaccination site.

Among the host factors that are responsible for limitation of viral spread and recovery from vaccination are development of serum antibody, delayed hypersensitivity, and interferon production. Serum antibody and delayed hypersensitivity are specific and are induced soon after infection; antibody would appear to be less important in recovery than delayed hypersensitivity. Interferon is nonspecific and has been found in the skin of animals recovering from vaccinia infection who have been rendered deficient in

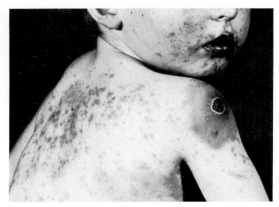

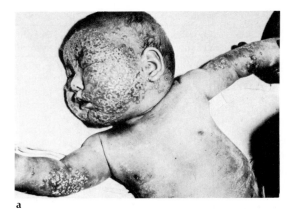

Fig. 192-4 Erythema multiforme following a smallpox vaccination. Note normal vaccination site, surrounding erythema, and a macular, papular, and vesicular eruption.

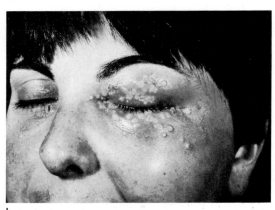

antibodies and in delayed hypersensitivity. It has also been found in human vaccination crusts. Individuals who lack antibody-synthesizing capacity may develop progressive and widespread vaccinal lesions. However, even these patients, if they retain delayed-hypersensitivity responsiveness, may undergo perfectly normal vaccinations. In addition, patients with normal antibody levels, but with absent delayed-hypersensitivity responsiveness, are susceptible to the progressive form of the disease. As indicated, interferon is also important and may account for recovery of animals in the absence of the other two functions. However, data for human beings are lacking, and the importance of this mechanism of resistance is not known.

Allergy, or presumed altered reactivity, to viral components appears to be responsible for the erythema multiforme type of skin rash observed in some individuals after primovaccination. This mechanism has also been implicated in the pathogenesis of postvaccinal encephalitis; it is assumed the virus or a virus–central nervous system complex invokes an immune response directed against brain antigens, which then results in an antigen–antibody inflammatory reaction and the clinical picture of encephalitis.

Fig. 192-5 Accidental inoculation in a pediatrician who was giving smallpox immunization.

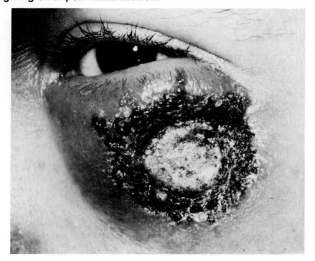

Fig. 192-6 Eczema vaccinatum. Lesions are in areas of active eczema. Note typical vaccinal character of individual lesions.

Clinical manifestations

Erythema multiforme-like eruptions. An intensely erythematous macular rash may follow smallpox vaccination. This rash has the characteristics of erythema multiforme in that iris or bull's eye lesions appear and tend to coalesce (Fig. 192-4). The rash is often symmetrical and florid, involving a large portion of the body. This is a totally benign manifestation representing an allergic reaction.

Bacterial superinfection. Purulent complications of smallpox vaccination today involve principally impetiginous infection with *Staphylococcus aureus* or group A beta-hemolytic streptococci. If poultices are employed, tetanus may be introduced by the soil or dung elements incorporated in such primitive techniques.

Accidental inoculation. Vaccinia virus can be implanted from the site of vaccination onto the skin or mucous membrane anywhere on the individual's body. They can also be transferred to another individual. Each of the lesions is characteristic of a primary smallpox vaccination with the exception that they do not tend to scar (Fig. 192-5). Certain implantations may be more hazardous than the occasional single-site inoculation. These include implantation onto large areas of abnormal skin (burns or other dermatoses), into the eye (vaccinal keratitis may result), extensive mucosal lesions, and implantation around various body

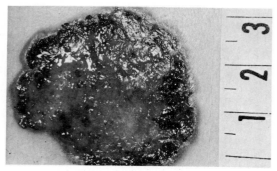

Fig. 192-7 Progressive vaccinia: large, nonhealing vaccination site with "soft, rubbery" border, high virus content, and lack of surrounding inflammatory response; present 4 months in 10-month-old male with variant of thymic alymphoplasia.

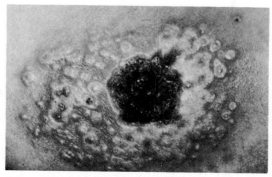

Fig. 192-8 Progressive vaccinia. Note necrotic center, extensive satellite lesions, and advancing border.

orifices which may impede certain bodily functions (Fig. 192-6).

Congenital vaccinia. Vaccination of the pregnant woman may result in disseminated disease fatal to the fetus. Congenital vaccination may also occur following exposure to a vaccinated individual. The infant may be stillborn or may develop lesions shortly after birth.

Generalized vaccinia. Generalized vaccinia as used in this classification refers to a benign generalized eruption, each lesion of which is identical to its primary smallpox vaccination. Although little is known of the immunology surrounding such a defect, it is clear that some children with isolated IgM deficiency are liable to this complication. This is not generally a lethal disease.

Progressive vaccinia (vaccinia gangrenosa, vaccinia necrosum). If a smallpox vaccination shows no evidence of normal resolution within 2 weeks of inoculation, a presumptive diagnosis of progressive vaccinia should be made. In this disease, the normal immunologic response to vaccination is impaired. This may occur in an otherwise normal individual or in persons with generalized defects in immunologic capacities.

In its complete form, the site of vaccination fails to heal and continues to enlarge, often for months. Usually, no systemic signs of illness are present and, in the absence of some other disease, physical findings are limited to the vaccination. These lesions differ from the normal in that little inflammatory response is observed. The vaccination initially has a soft, rubbery appearance with little scabbing (Fig. 192-7). As the lesion progresses in size, considerable central necrosis becomes evident, and thick, dark eschars form (hence the synonym, vaccinia necrosum). The initial lesion may become huge, with the entire upper arm and shoulder involved. In many cases secondary lesions are evident; in some, satellite vaccinations occur close to the primary one, and, in addition, viremic lesions may appear at distant sites (Fig. 192-8). Each of the secondary lesions progresses in the same fashion as the primary one (Fig. 192-9). Variations are observed in that the primary lesion may become ulcerative or may have a piled-up appearance, but the progression is characteristic.

Untreated disease or illness failing to respond to treatment may be of long duration, during which extensive tissue destruction, secondary bacterial infection and septicemia, mucosal lesions, pneumonia, and other complications may occur. The course is progressively downhill, although the patient may not manifest correspondingly severe constitutional symptoms until relatively late in the disease.

Encephalitis. A meningoencephalitis syndrome occurs rarely as a complication of smallpox vaccination. The sudden onset of headache and vomiting in the second week after vaccination may herald this illness. Convulsions, lethargy, coma, paralysis, signs of cerebral edema, increased intracranial pressure, and focal neurologic findings may occur. In other instances the disease may resemble aseptic meningitis or myelitis.

Laboratory findings

Virologic. Specimens from suspected vaccinal lesions can be inoculated into a variety of tissue culture systems or the embryonated hen's egg. Identification is by typical pock formation or by classical cytopathogenic effect with subsequent neutralization by antisera. Additionally, specific vaccinia antigen can be detected by a variety of an-

Fig. 192-9 Secondary, viremic lesions in progressive vaccinia. Two lesions on arm, which demonstrate variability, both positive for vaccinia virus, occurred in elderly female with chronic lymphatic leukemia; complete clearing with thiosemicarbazone therapy.

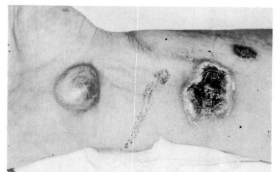

tibody methods, either from the original specimen obtained from the patient or from the infected cell cultures or egg fluids.

Immunologic and hematologic. Response to vaccinia virus may be critical in determining host susceptibility. Vaccinia-neutralizing antibody can be measured, as can a delayed-hypersensitivity reaction to inactivated vaccinia antigen.

In certain clinical states, total immunologic capacity may need to be surveyed as the vaccinal infection is simply an indicator or a more comprehensive immunologic defect. Assays for immunoglobulin antibody capacity and for cell-mediated immune function may need to be employed.

Treatment

Complications of vaccination can be reduced by recognizing those predisposing conditions which lead to each of the separate types of complication. Thus, individuals who have eczema or other skin lesions should not be vaccinated or exposed to an individual who is vaccinated. Individuals with immunologic deficiency, receiving immunosuppressive therapy, or suffering from diseases such as lymphatic malignancies which heighten susceptibility should avoid contact with vaccinia virus, and should not be vaccinated. If such individuals are exposed, use of either vaccinia immune globulin by injection or methisone (isatin thiosemicarbazone) can be expected to reduce the risk.

In the past, administration of vaccinia immune globulin (VIG) for complications of vaccination has been facilitated by its ready availability. Currently this product is no longer produced and is in limited supply. As a result, its use should be more stringent than in the past and it should be reserved for those severe complications in which a beneficial effect has been either demonstrated or suspected. Children with erythema multiforme or simple autoinoculation disease and vaccinal encephalitis should not receive this preparation as it is of no benefit. On the other hand, those with extensive intradermal involvement such as eczema vaccinatum or burns should be treated with either VIG or methisone. VIG should be used in conjunction with methisone and immunologic therapy in those severe complications such as progressive vaccinia.

Course and prognosis

As indicated in the separate sections, prognosis is variable. Most complications are self-limited or respond to simple measures; a few require extraordinary forms of therapy, and even with such treatment a small group remains who are unresponsive.

Bibliography

Smallpox (variola)
Bauer DJ et al: The chemotherapy of variola major infection. *Bull WHO* **26**:727, 1962
Bauer DJ et al: Prophylactic treatment of smallpox contacts with *N*-methylisatin β-thiosemicarbazone. *Lancet* **2**:494, 1963
Bremen JG, Arita I: The confirmation and maintenance of smallpox eradication. *N Engl J Med* **303**:1263, 1980
Dixon CW: *Smallpox*. London, Churchill, 1962
Downie AW: Smallpox, in *Medical History of the Second World War*, edited by Z Cope. London, HM Stationery Office, 1952
Downie AW, MacDonald A: Smallpox and related virus infections in man. *Br Med Bull* **9**:191, 1953
Downie AW et al: Studies on the virus content of mouth washings in the acute phase of smallpox. *Bull WHO* **25**:49, 1961
Fenner F: Global eradication of smallpox. *Rev Infect Dis* **4**:916, 1982
Kempe CH: Smallpox, in *The Biologic Basis of Pediatric Practice*, edited by R Cooke. New York, McGraw-Hill, 1965
Kempe CH, St Vincent L: Variola and vaccinia, in *Diagnostic Procedures in Viral and Rickettsial Infections*, edited by E Lennette. New York, American Public Health Association, 1964
Kempe CH et al: The use of vaccinia hyperimmune gamma globulin in the prophylaxis of smallpox. *Bull WHO* **25**:41, 1961
Rao AR et al: A study of 1,000 cases of smallpox. *J Indian Med Assoc* **35**:296, 1960
Wehrle P: A reality in our time—certification of the global eradication of smallpox. *J Infect Dis* **242**:636, 1980
WHO Expert Committee on Smallpox: *WHO Technical Report Series* **283**:1, 1964

Complications of smallpox vaccination (vaccinia)
Adels BR, Oppe TE: Treatment of eczema vaccinatum with *N*-methylisatin beta-thiosemicarbazone. *Lancet* **1**:18, 1966
Barbero GT et al: Vaccinia gangrenosa treated with hyperimmune vaccinal gamma globulin. *Pediatrics* **16**:609, 1955
Daly JJ, Jackson E: Vaccinia gangrenosa treated with *N*-methylisatin β-thiosemicarbazone. *Br Med J* **2**:1300, 1962
Davidson E, Hayhoe FG: Prolonged generalized vaccinia complicating acute leukemia. *Br Med J* **2**:1298, 1962
Dimson SB: Eczema vaccinatum. *Lancet* **2**:73, 1962
Ellis PP, Wenograd L: Ocular vaccinia. *Arch Ophthalmol* **68**:600, 1962
Erichson RB, McNamara MJ: Vaccinia gangrenosa: report of a case and review of the literature. *Ann Intern Med* **55**:491, 1961
Fekety FR Jr et al: Vaccinia gangrenosa in chronic lymphatic leukemia. *Arch Intern Med* **109**:205, 1962
Flewitt TH, Ker FL: A case of vaccinia necrosum (progressive vaccinia) with severe hypogammaglobulinemia, treated with *N*-methylisatin β-thiosemicarbazone (33T57). *J Clin Pathol* **16**:271, 1963
Fulginiti VA, Kempe CH: Poxvirus diseases, in *Brennemann's Practice of Pediatrics*, vol II, part 1, edited by V Kelley. Hagerstown, MD, Harper & Row, 1937, p 1
Fulginiti VA et al: Therapy of experimental vaccinal keratitis. *Arch Ophthalmol* **74**:539, 1965
Greenberg M: Complications of vaccination against smallpox. *Am J Dis Child* **76**:492, 1948
Kaufman H et al: A cure of vaccinia infection by 5-iodo-2'-deoxyuridine. *Virology* **18**:567, 1962
Kempe CH: Studies on smallpox and complications of smallpox vaccination. *Pediatrics* **26**:176, 1960
Kempe CH, Benenson AS: Smallpox immunization in the United States. *JAMA* **194**:161, 1965
Kempe CH et al: Hyperimmune vaccinal gamma globulin. *Pediatrics* **18**:177, 1956
Naidoo P, Hirsch H: Prenatal vaccinia. *Lancet* **1**:196, 1963
Nanning W: Prophylactic effect of antivaccinia gamma globulin against postvaccinal encephalitis. *Bull WHO* **27**:317, 1962
Neff JM: Smallpox vaccination: minimal complication rates, United States, 1963. Presentation at Annual Epidemiologic Intelligence Service, Communicable Disease Center, April 1965
O'Connel CJ et al: Progressive vaccinia with normal antibodies: a case possibly due to deficient cellular immunity. *Ann Intern Med* **60**:282, 1964

Sathe PV et al: Prevention of postvaccinal tetanus. *Indian J Pediatr* **31**:306, 1965

Spillane JD, Wells CEC: The neurology of Jennerian vaccination: a clinical account of the neurological complications which occurred during the smallpox epidemic in South Wales in 1962. *Brain* **87**:1, 1964

Sussman S, Grossman M: Complications of smallpox vaccination. Effects of vaccinia immune globulin therapy. *J Pediatr* **67**:1168, 1965

Wielenga G et al: Prenatal infection with vaccinia virus. *Lancet* **1**:258, 1961

CHAPTER 193

ORF

Ullin W. Leavell, Jr.

Definition

Orf is a viral disease endemic among sheep and goats. It can be transmitted to humans. Synonyms include ecthyma contagiosum, scabby mouth, sore mouth, bovine pustular dermatitis, and infectious pustular dermatitis. The disease usually develops in the vicinity of the mouth and nose of lambs, manifesting itself as a weeping erythematous eruption. In humans, it generally manifests itself as nodules on exposed areas. The lesions are similar in humans and lambs, and heal in about 35 days. Orf is classified as a near-neoplasm, since it stimulates pseudoepitheliomatous hyperplasia and exhibits a finger-like downward proliferation of the epidermis.

Historical aspects

Early writers who suggested that the disease was transmitted from animals to humans include Brandenberg, Newsom and Cross, and Peterkin.

Epidemiology

The disease is commonplace among sheepherders in all parts of the world, although many do not seek medical advice. Veterinarians, individuals on immunosuppressive drugs, and patients with eczema may develp the disease. It has been reported exclusively in the white race. Age is not a factor. Orf has been diagnosed in patients as young as 10 and as old as 72 years of age. Those acquiring it are engaged either in farming or work with infected animals. The closer the contact with infected animals, the more likely is infection. Individuals feeding milk from a bottle to infected, orphaned lambs frequently come in contact with the lamb's sore mouth and may contract the disease. Orf is more prevalent in the spring when newborn lambs, lacking immunity, fall prey to the disease. The infection may be acquired indirectly from virus on knives, barbed wire, barn doors, towels, and vehicles used in transportation of the animals.

Etiology

The virus is sturdy, surviving the winter months on barn doors, feeding troughs, and fences. Susceptible lambs become infected from contact with virus-containing objects.

The virus grows on primary human amnion and on other cell cultures, producing cells with pyknotic nuclei and vacuolated cytoplasm. Later, holes develop in the amnion sheet and are surrounded by clumps of granular cells. Electron microscopy of sheep tissue reveals partially and/or totally encapsulated viroplasm, viroplasm and nucleoid, and mature oval particles with a riblike outer structure. Elongated virions with central narrowing and bending of the elementary bodies may be present. The virus has been seen in the nucleus and cytoplasm of epidermal cells. A spiral has been demonstrated in the virus. The orf virus is a member of the poxvirus group.

Clinical manifestations

The cutaneous lesions average 1.6 cm in diameter. Usually, only one lesion is present, although as many as 10 have been reported. The lesion is most commonly located on the dorsal aspect of the right index finger. Regional lymphadenopathy is common; lymphangitis and fever may occur. Fever disappears within 3 to 4 days, lymphangitis within 3 to 4 weeks. Toxic erythema, erythema multiforme, and a widespread papulovesicular eruption of the skin and mucosae may occur. Amputation of a finger was necessary in a patient on immunosuppressive drugs for lymphoma.

Orf advances through six stages, healing uneventfully in about 35 days. Each stage lasts approximately 6 days. The papular phase is denoted by a red, elevated lesion (Fig. 193-1). The target stage has a nodule with a red center, a

Fig. 193-1 Orf tumor measuring 2 cm in diameter, located on left temple. Note red, weeping surface.

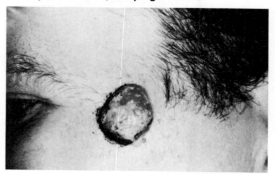

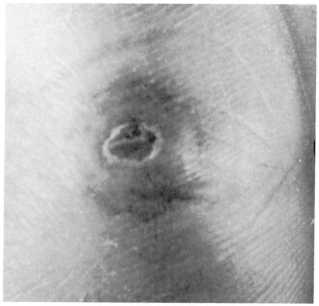

Fig. 193-2 The target stage in orf has a nodule with a red center, a white middle ring, and a red periphery.

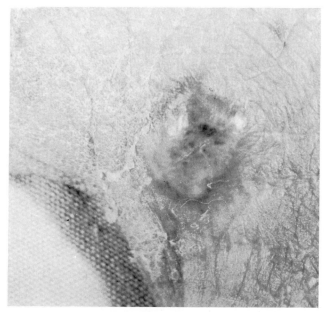

Fig. 193-3 Orf. A nodule with black dots over the surface is seen in the regenerative stage.

white middle ring, and a red periphery (Fig. 193-2). A red, weeping surface is present during the acute stage. In the regenerative stage (Fig. 193-3), a thin, dry crust through which black dots may be seen, covers the surface of the nodule. Small papillomas appear over the surface of the lesion during the papillomatous stage. In the regressive stage, a thick crust develops over the surface of the lesion, and a reduction in the size of the papillomas and in the elevation of the lesion occurs.

Pathology

The papular stage of orf has not been studied in humans. In the target stage, intranuclear and intracytoplasmic inclusions are present in superficial, vacuolated epidermal cells in areas corresponding to the white ring (Fig. 193-4).

Intracytoplasmic and intranuclear inclusions may also be seen in endothelial cells of papillary blood vessels. The dermis discloses a dense infiltrate of plasma cells, macrophages, histiocytes, and lymphocytes. The acute stage is distinguished by loss of epidermis over the central part of the lesion. Peripherally, there is reticular degeneration. Microvesicles are present. There are distension and loss of the epidermal cells of hair follicles. There is regeneration of the epidermis. The black dots observed clinically correspond to the accumulation of cellular breakdown products in the follicles. Many papillary elevations of the epidermis are seen in the papillomatous stage. In the regressive stage, the papillomas are reduced in size, and histiocytes, macrophages, lymphocytes, and plasma cells are decreased in number.

Those features that suggest neoplasia are acanthosis

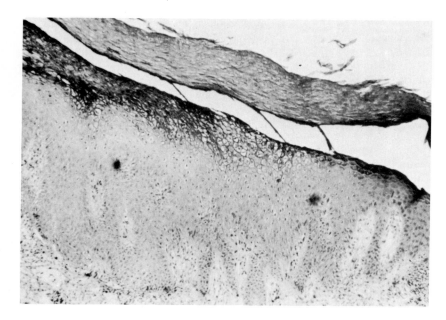

Fig. 193-4 Orf. The target stage with vacuolated epidermal cells, a trail of dead epidermal cells, and acanthosis. X100.

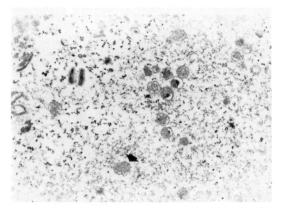

Fig. 193-5 Orf. Electron photomicrograph primarily showing immature particles. Arrow points to particles forming from viroplasm. Three of the immature particles exhibit a dense staining nucleoid. Note two mature particles at upper left. X52,500. *(By permission of Dr. Albert J. Dalton, National Institutes of Health, Bethesda, Maryland.)*

within the first week, followed by a finger-like downward proliferation of the epidermis. Papillomatosis and acanthosis occur within the papillomas. The infiltrate in the dermis contributes to the elevation of the lesion, giving it the appearance of a rapidly growing tumor.

The pathology of human regional lymph nodes has not been studied. In sheep, however, there is a progressive increase in the size of the lymph nodes and in the amount of infiltrate of plasma cells over a 14-day period.

Diagnosis

The diagnosis of orf is established by a history of contact with infected sheep or goats, the appearance of the lesions, passage of the virus to sheep, cell cultures, fluorescent antibody tests, and electron microscopy (Fig. 193-5). Complement-fixing antigen has been advanced as the most sensitive diagnostic technique for diagnosing contagious ecthyma. T-cell function, phytohemagglutinin and K-cell activity have been normal.

Treatment

Treatment is not specific. Compresses and antibiotics are of value when secondary bacterial infection ensues. Bacterial culture and antibiotic sensitivity is indicated when secondary bacterial infection is suspected. Following excision and cautery, lesions heal uneventfully within 2 to 3 weeks. Corticosteroids and immunosuppressive drugs should be avoided, inasmuch as acanthosis and pseudo-epitheliomatous hyperplasia may appear earlier and be more extensive as a result of their administration. No underlying disease has been found to predispose to orf, nor has residual pathologic change been reported. The prognosis is excellent.

Bibliography

Brandenberg TO: Lip and leg ulceration in sheep with report of two cases in man. *J Am Vet Assoc* **8:**818, 1932

Carr RW: A case of orf contracted by a human from a wild Alaskan mountain goat. *Alaska Med* **10:**75, 1968

Cutler TP: Orf: report of a case. *Clin Exp Dermatol* **6:**205, 1981

Dupre A et al: Orf and atopic dermatitis. *Br J Dermatol* **105:**103, 1981

Erickson GA et al: Generalized contagious ecthyma in a sheep rancher: diagnostic considerations. *J Am Vet Med Assoc* **166:**262, 1974

Guss SB: Contagious ecthyma (sore mouth, orf). *Mod Vet Pract* **61:**335, 1980

Leavell UW Jr: Ecthyma contagiosum. *J Ky Med Assoc* **58:**42, 1960

Leavell UW Jr et al: Ecthyma contagiosum (orf). *South Med J* **58:**238, 1965

Leavell UW Jr et al: Orf: report of 19 human cases with clinical and pathological observations. *JAMA* **204:**657, 1968

Nagington J et al: The structure of the orf virus. *Virology* **23:**461, 1964

Newsom IE, Cross F: Sore mouth transmissible to man. *J Am Vet Med Assoc* **84:**799, 1934

Peterkin GAG: The occurrence in humans of contagious pustular dermatitis of sheep ("orf"). *Br J Dermatol* **49:**492, 1937

Wilkinson JD: Orf: a family with unusual complications. *Br J Dermatol* **97:**447, 1977

Yeh HP, Soltani K: Ultrastructural studies in human orf. *Arch Dermatol* **109:**390, 1974

MILKER'S NODULES, MOLLUSCUM CONTAGIOSUM

Douglas R. Lowy

Milker's nodules

Definition

Milker's nodule is a benign viral skin disease which generally consists of one or a few nodules on the hand or forearm. The virus is usually transmitted to cattle handlers from infected cows.

Etiology

The disease is induced by paravaccinia virus, a poxvirus that is endemic to many cattle herds [1]. Lesions in cows, which may be chronic and recurrent, appear mainly on the teats, although other areas may be affected. In cows the condition is called *pseudocowpox*. There is no cross-immunity with the cowpox, vaccinia, or variola group of poxviruses. *Bovine papular stomatitis* is a closely related poxvirus infection of cattle characterized by lesions around the mouth [2]; because it induces lesions in humans that are identical to milker's nodules, some investigators believe that the two viruses may be identical [3].

Paravaccinia virus can be propagated in bovine or human cells in tissue culture [4,5]. It resembles the virus of orf (ecthyma contagiosum) morphologically and serologically [6,7]. As is true of other poxviruses, paravaccinia is a large (150 by 300 nm) brick-shaped deoxyribonucleic acid (DNA) virus that replicates in foci in the cytoplasm of infected cells. Infection often induces a mild degree of hyperplasia. The disease has been transmitted experimentally from human to human and from human to cow [8].

Epidemiology

Milker's nodule has a worldwide distribution, occurring where cattle are found. Most cases are sporadic, but small epidemics have been reported. Since the disease is usually transmitted to humans by direct contact with infected cattle, milkers are most at risk. Cases also occur among stockyard and slaughterhouse workers. Most cases occur among persons who have recently become milkers, and infection in humans usually induces lasting immunity. Indirect transmission from virus-contaminated material to patients with burned skin has been reported [9]. The incidence of subclinical infection is not known. Although infectious virus is found in human lesions, person-to-person transmission under natural conditions has not been documented.

Clinical manifestations

The typical case consists of a single asymptomatic or slightly painful 1-cm nodule on a finger (Fig. 194-1) [10,11].

There are usually no more than four lesions, and they are generally confined to the hand and forearm. Rarely, other areas of the skin may be involved, or numerous lesions may be present. Lymphadenopathy is uncommon.

The incubation period is usually 4 to 7 days, but may be as long as 2 weeks. In the absence of secondary bacterial infection, each lesion usually heals spontaneously in 4 to 6 weeks without scar formation. Leavell and Phillips [11] have described six clinical stages, each lasting about a week. Initially, the lesion begins as an erythematous macule, which soon becomes papular. The target stage is next: the lesion, which is papulovesicular, has a red center, surrounded by a white ring and a red halo. This stage is followed by a period of weeping and erosion. The lesion then becomes a firm, crusted nodule. Next, small papillomatous elevations develop on the nodule. Finally, during the regressive stage, the lesion darkens and sloughs.

Pathology

Pathologic changes are present in both epidermis and dermis; the precise histologic appearance depends on the clinical stage [11]. Epidermal changes include hyperkeratosis, parakeratosis, acanthosis, and striking elongation of the rete ridges. These alterations increase progressively as the lesion develops. In early lesions the upper portion of the malpighian layer may contain balloon cells and cells with many intracytoplasmic and some intranuclear inclusions. Later, reticular degeneration, multilocular vesicles, spongiosis, and intracellular edema may be the prominent findings. The dermis contains a marked increase in the number of capillaries and a nonspecific inflammatory infiltate that is most intense during the acute weeping stage. Electron micrographic examination of the superficial portion of a lesion usually reveals the characteristic cytoplasmic viral particles.

Diagnosis and differential diagnosis

The diagnosis is generally based on the history, clinical appearance, and biopsy. It can be established more definitively by the electron microscopic demonstration of viral particles or by propagation of the virus in tissue culture. Orf and bovine papular stomatitis must be excluded by history.

Milker's nodule must also be differentiated from a large number of other conditions, including true cowpox, herpetic whitlow, pyoderma, anthrax, tularemia, primary inoculation tuberculosis, atypical mycobacterial infection, syphilitic chancre, sporotrichosis, and pyogenic granuloma.

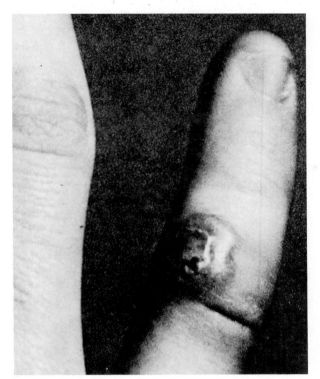

Fig. 194-1 Milker's nodule. (Courtesy of Dermatology Service, Walter Reed Army Medical Center.)

Course, prognosis, treatment, and prevention

Since the disease is self-limited, only symptomatic therapy is generally indicated. Prevention is limited to the isolation of infected animals.

Molluscum contagiosum

Definition

Molluscum contagiosum is a common, benign, viral disease of the skin and mucous membranes which generally affects children. In adults, the condition may be transmitted sexually. The fully developed lesion is an umbilicated papule, and most patients have multiple lesions.

Etiology

Molluscum contagiosum virus (MCV) is a poxvirus that is distinct morphologically and pathologically from other poxviruses [12,13]. It is a large (200 by 300 nm) DNA virus which replicates in the cytoplasm of infected cells and induces hyperplasia, as do other poxviruses. Serologically, MCV is distinct from the poxviruses vaccinia, cowpox, and fowlpox. Unlike most other poxviruses, MCV has not been reproducibly propagated in tissue culture. A report of the successful tissue culture growth of MCV [14] has not been confirmed [15]. It is not known whether only one or several MCV strains exist. Using viral particles extracted from lesions, researchers have noted minor differences in viral polypeptides [16] and in restriction endonuclease cleavage patterns in viral DNA [17], findings suggesting that distinct strains of MCV may exist.

Experimental transmission to humans has been achieved, with a reported incubation period of 2 to 7 weeks [12]. Attempts to induce the disease experimentally in other species have been unsuccessful. MCV infection has been thought to be confined to humans, but lesions that are clinically and histologically identical to those in human disease have been reported in the chimpanzee and kangaroo in captivity [18,19].

Epidemiology

The disease occurs throughout the world, but its frequency varies considerably [12]. On some Pacific islands, 5 percent of children under 10 years may be affected. The prevalence rate in the United States is much lower. Although the disease may develop at any age, the vast majority of cases are found in children, with boys being affected more frequently than girls. Multiple familial cases are uncommon.

The mode of person-to-person spread is unknown. Outbreaks have been reported among children attending swimming pools, and genital lesions in adults may be transmitted sexually [20,21]. The incidence of subclinical infection is not clear, nor is the role of immunity in recovery from infection or in the prevention of reinfection [22]. The results of experimental studies suggest that many adults are resistant to infection, and widespread lesions have been reported in adults with impaired immunity [23,24].

Clinical manifestations

The lesions, which begin as minute papules, are usually 3 to 6 mm, although rarely they may be as large as 3 cm in diameter. The individual lesions are discrete, smooth, pearly to flesh-colored, dome-shaped papules, often with central umbilication and a mildly erythematous base. Beneath the umbilication lies a white curdlike core which may be easily expressed [25].

Lesions may be located on any area of the skin and mucous membranes. They are usually grouped (Fig. 194-2) in one or two areas but may be widely disseminated. Most patients have fewer than 20 lesions, although some may have several hundred. In temperate climates, the head, eyelids, trunk, and genitalia are affected most often. In the tropics, lesions occur most commonly on the extremities.

Although lesions are usually asymptomatic, pruritus may be present, and an eczematous reaction may develop around some lesions. Conjunctivitis and keratitis may complicate lesions around the eyelid. Patients with atopic dermatitis may develop widespread lesions, and secondary bacterial infection also occurs.

Pathogenesis and pathology

The rate of cell division in the basal layer of lesional skin is twice that of normal skin. Viral growth is confined to the epidermis; virus particles are synthesized in cytoplasmic foci of cells in the malpighian and granular layers [22,26,27]. The infected cells, which are interspersed with uninfected cells, move more quickly than uninfected cells through the epidermis. Viral antigen is present in infected cells, and 90 percent of patients possess circulating antibody to this antigen.

The histologic appearance of the hypertrophied and hyperplastic epidermis is characteristic (Fig. 194-3) [25,28]. Above the normal-appearing basal layer are lobules of en-

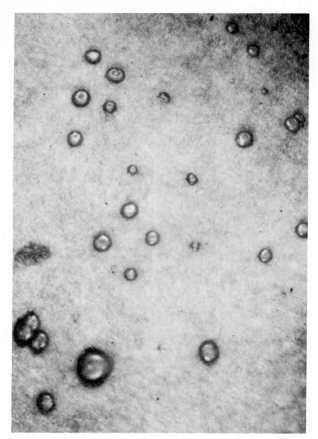

Fig. 194-2 Molluscum contagiosum. *(Courtesy of Dermatology Service, Walter Reed Army Medical Center.)*

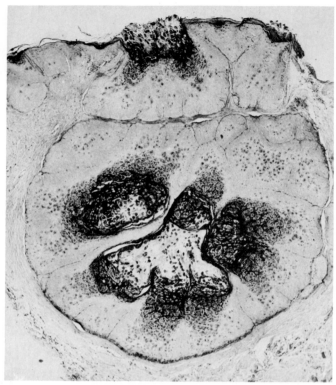

Fig. 194-3 Molluscum contagiosum. Extensive downgrowth of infected cells bearing the large, eosinophilic cytoplasmic inclusion bodies × 40. *(Micrograph by Wallace H. Clark, Jr., M.D.)*

Course and prognosis

Individual lesions may last 2 to 4 months, but the development of new lesions by autoinoculation is common. Most cases resolve spontaneously in 6 to 9 months, but some may persist for 3 years or longer.

References

Milker's nodules

1. Moscovici C et al: Isolation of a viral agent from pseudocowpox disease. *Science* **141**:915, 1963
2. Bowman KF et al: Cutaneous form of bovine papular stomatitis in man. *JAMA* **246**:2813, 1981
3. Rossi CR et al: A paravaccinia virus isolated from cattle. *Cornell Vet* **67**:72, 1977
4. Friedman-Kien AE et al: Milker's nodules: isolation of a poxvirus from a human case. *Science* **140**:1335, 1963
5. Thomas V: Biochemical and electron microscopic studies of the replication and composition of milker's node virus. *J Virol* **34**:244, 1980
6. Nagington J et al: Milker's nodule virus infections and their similarity to orf. *Nature* **208**:505, 1965
7. Leavell UW et al: Orf: report of 19 human cases with clinical and pathological observations. *JAMA* **204**:657, 1968
8. Sonck CE, Penttinen K: Milker's nodules: transmission from man to man. *Acta Derm Venereol (Stockh)* **34**:420, 1954
9. Schuler G et al: The syndrome of milker's nodules in burn injury: evidence for indirect transmission. *J Am Acad Dermatol* **6**:334, 1982
10. Wheeler CE, Cawley EP: The etiology of milker's nodules. *Arch Dermatol* **75**:249, 1957

larged epidermal cells which contain multiple Feulgen-positive intracytoplasmic inclusion bodies (*molluscum bodies* or *Henderson-Paterson bodies*). These inclusion bodies, which contain the viral particles, increase in size as the infected cell moves toward the surface. In the horny layer, the molluscum bodies are enmeshed in a fibrous network that dissolves in the center of the lesions, forming the central core which is composed primarily of molluscum bodies.

Diagnosis and differential diagnosis

The diagnosis is easily made by the distinctive clinical appearance of the lesions, by stained smears of the expressed core, and by biopsy. Molluscum contagiosum must be differentiated from warts, varicella, pyoderma, papillomas, epitheliomas, and lichen planus.

Treatment

Since the condition is usually self-limited and lesions heal without scarring in the absence of secondary bacterial infection, treatment is not always mandatory. Removal of lesions with a sharp curette or liquid nitrogen is simple, relatively painless, and usually effective. More than one treatment session is often necessary, either because of recurrence or the development of new lesions.

11. Leavell UW Jr, Phillips IA: Milker's nodules: pathogenesis, tissue culture, electron microscopy, and calf inoculation. *Arch Dermatol* **111**:1307, 1975

Molluscum contagiosum

12. Postlethwaite R: Molluscum contagiosum: a review. *Arch Environ Health* **21**:432, 1970
13. Brown ST et al: Molluscum contagiosum. *Am Vener Dis Assoc* **8**:227, 1981
14. Francis RD, Bradford HB Jr: Some biological and physical properties of molluscum contagiosum virus propagated in tissue culture. *J Virol* **19**:382, 1976
15. McFadden G et al: Biogenesis of poxviruses: transitory expression of molluscum contagiosum early functions. *Virology* **94**:297, 1979
16. Oda H et al: Structural polypeptides of molluscum contagiosum virus: their variability in various isolates and location within the virion. *J Med Virol* **9**:19, 1982
17. Parr RP et al: Structural characterization of the molluscum contagiosum virus genome. *Virology* **81**:247, 1977
18. Dagnall BG, Witson GR: Molluscum contagiosum in red kangaroo. *Australas J Dermatol* **15**:115, 1974
19. Douglas JD et al: Molluscum contagiosum in the chimpanzee. *J Am Vet Med Assoc* **151**:901, 1967
20. Brown ST et al: Molluscum contagiosum: sexually transmitted disease in 17 cases. *J Am Vener Dis Assoc* **1**:35, 1974
21. Wilkin JK: Molluscum contagiosum venereum in a women's outpatient clinic: a venereally transmitted disease. *Am J Obstet Gynecol* **128**:531, 1977
22. Shirodaria PV, Matthews RS: Observations on the antibody responses in molluscum contagiosum. *Br J Dermatol* **96**:29, 1977
23. Solomon LM, Telner P: Eruptive molluscum contagiosum in atopic dermatitis. *Can Med Assoc J* **95**:978, 1966
24. Peachy RDG: Severe molluscum contagiosum infection with T-cell deficiency. *Br J Dermatol* **97(suppl)**:49, 1977
25. Uehara M, Danno K: Cental pitting of molluscum contagiosum. *J Cutan Pathol* **7**:149, 1980
26. Epstein WL et al: Viral antigens in human epidermal tumors: localization of an antigen to molluscum contagiosum. *J Invest Dermatol* **40**:51, 1963
27. Epstein WL, Fukuyama K: Maturation of molluscum contagiosum virus (MCV) in vivo: quantitative electron microscopic autoradiography. *J Invest Dermatol* **60**:73, 1973
28. Kwittken J: Molluscum contagiosum: some new histologic observations. *Mt Sinai J Med (NY)* **47**:583, 1980

CHAPTER 195

CAT-SCRATCH DISEASE

Steven M. Passman and Irwin M. Freedberg

Definition and synonyms

Cat-scratch disease (CSD) is a benign, self-limited disease, most likely of infectious etiology, characterized in most cases by a history of cat contact and enlarged, localized lymph nodes which may suppurate. Synonyms include: cat-scratch fever, nonbacterial lymphadenitis, nonbacterial regional lymphadenitis, benign lymphoreticulosis, benign inoculation lymphoreticulosis, and subacute granulomatous lymphadenitis.

Epidemiology [1–4]

The disease occurs in all ages, although approximately 50 to 80 percent of patients are less than 20 years of age. There does not appear to be any sexual, racial, or geographic predilection. Although epidemic outbreaks have been reported, CSD usually occurs throughout the year in an endemic fashion, with most cases reported in the midwinter months. The vector animal most frequently has been a cat or kitten that shows no evidence of disease and has a negative CSD skin test. Clinical evidence of scratches is present in half the reported cases, and in 90 percent there is a history of both cat contact and scratches. CSD has also been reported after contact with dogs, monkeys, and chickens. In general, only one household member is affected at a time, although others may be similarly scratched. Multiple cases in the same household have been reported, usually with exposure to the same cat, but these occur months or years apart. No specific etiologic agent has been identified in any feline tissue (including nails, nodes, and saliva). Studies of the patients for bacteria (including *Chlamydia*), fungi, viral agents, and protozoan species, aimed at elucidating a specific agent, also have been unproductive until recently. Wear and his colleagues have reported the presence of delicate, small pleomorphic, gram-negative bacteria in the capillaries of the lymph node of patients with cat-scratch disease. The organisms have not been cultured and Koch's postulates have not been fulfilled.

Clinical manifestations [5–7]

Cat-scratch disease is most commonly benign and self-limited. The incubation period ranges from a few days to 2 weeks from the scratch to the onset of the primary lesion. One-third of the patients have only asymptomatic regional lymphadenopathy. Fever, occurring in 25 to 75 percent of cases, is usually low-grade. Common symptoms include malaise, headache, generalized myalgias and arthralgias, lassitude, and chills. These symptoms tend to increase as the nodes enlarge. The objective signs are the cat scratch itself, the primary lesion, and the lymphadenopathy. The primary lesion occurs in approximately 50 percent of the

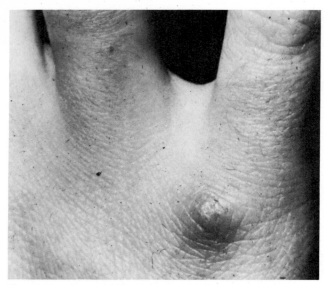

Fig. 195-1   Cat-scratch disease, illustrating the primary lesion, which is a nodule that has undergone necrosis with the development of a tiny ulcer. (Courtesy of Dr. Anne Baker.)

patients and is a 0.5- to 1-cm lichenoid papule, pustule, nodule (Fig. 195-1), or cluster of tiny nodules. In about 50 percent of the cases in which a primary lesion occurs, it is located on the arm or hand. The lesion persists for less than a month in two-thirds of the cases and up to 2 months in a third. Approximately 4 percent of patients have a viral-like, nonpruritic, macular and papular eruption which lasts several days. Erythema nodosum, erythema multiforme, figurate erythemas, and thrombocytopenic purpura have been observed.

The most alarming manifestation of the disease is the encephalopathy which is reported infrequently. This is characterized by a sudden onset of fever and coma progressing to convulsions and lasting only a few days. Deaths have been reported. The cerebrospinal fluid is usually normal, although there may be an increase in the protein or cell count.

Lymphadenopathy is the hallmark of the disease. The nodes are usually unilateral, regional, and primarily cervical. However, other lymph nodes, including the axillary, epitrochlear, submandibular, inguinal, and preauricular, may be involved. Nodes are single in about half the cases or multiple in single sites in the other half. Lymphadenopathy begins within 1 to 3 weeks after the appearance of the primary papule and is proximal to the primary lesion. The nodes are initially red and tender and gradually increase in size to become fluctuant and occasionally suppurative. They usually regress within 6 weeks, but many have lasted as long as 2 years.

Laboratory findings

Routine laboratory tests are not helpful except to exclude other causes of lymphadenopathy. The white blood count is normal or only slightly increased with occasional eosinophilia. Sedimentation rate is commonly increased to 40 to 50 mm/h.

Cat-scratch skin test [8]

The CSD skin test is a crude test at best, in which the nature of the antigen and any other components are poorly understood. Although there have been no reports of hepatitis or other diseases transmitted through the test, it is unlikely that this biologic product will ever be commercially available. The source of the antigen, much like the Kveim antigen in sarcoidosis, consists of aspirated purulent lymph node material from patients with the disease. This pus is diluted in saline and heated to kill infectious agents. Extensive sterilization tests are carried out prior to use. The final solution is injected intradermally in a volume of 0.1 mL and the test is read at 24 to 96 h. Areas of less than 5 mm of induration are considered negative, and 5 to 10 mm of induration is considered doubtful. Greater than 10 mm of induration is accepted as positive. Antigen potency varies among patient sources, and all new batches of antigen must be evaluated for their degree of antigenicity among known reactors prior to their being used for diagnostic purposes. Manipulation of the antigen to assure sterility reduces its potency as an indicator of CSD. Such variation in antigenicity may account for negative tests in settings of classical clinical disease. Skin-test reactivity persists indefinitely. If appropriately performed, the sensitivity of the test is good and approaches 98 percent positive reactions in patients who have a consistent clinical picture. Positive tests occur in 12 to 29 percent of veterinarians and in 18 to 20 percent of relatives of infected patients. These may reflect subclinical infections. In the general population, positive reactions range between 4 and 8 percent.

Histopathology [9,10]

The primary lesion is middermal and shows small areas of frank necrosis surrounded by necrobiosis. Surrounding the necrobiosis is a multilayered mantle of histiocytes in which the inner layer may be palisaded. Surrounding the histiocytes is a zone of lymphocytes of variable thickness and density. Multinucleated giant cells are seen in the lesion and eosinophils can be seen in the adjacent stroma. Epidermal changes are generally varied and nonspecific, showing parakeratosis, epidermal edema, or exocytosis of inflammatory cells through the epidermis.

Microscopic changes in lymph nodes are nonspecific, but may be helpful in making a diagnosis of CSD when the clinical picture is not typical. Initially, there is a reticular cell hyperplasia which progresses to an intermediate stage of caseating granulomas simulating tuberculosis. The centers are acellular and necrotic and are surrounded by histiocytes and peripheral lymphocytes reminiscent of the morphology found in the primary skin lesion. Late stages show multiple abscesses.

About 14 days after skin testing, a nodule can be palpated in the subcutaneous tissue. This is not a specific response since 4 to 8 percent of normal controls, as well as some patients with sarcoid and tuberculosis, also develop nodules. The histopathology of skin-test sites has recently been studied, and, like the lymph node, the skin-test sites mimic the granulomatous appearance of the primary lesion. Biopsy of the CSD skin test is not recommended in all cases, but, again, it may be helpful in some.

Diagnosis and differential diagnosis

The approach to the child or young adult with suspected CSD is the same as the approach to the patient with regional lymphadenopathy or generalized lymphadenopathy with regional accentuation [10,11].

A diagnosis of cat-scratch disease in a typical case must include three of the following criteria, and all four in an atypical case [12]: (1) regional lymphadenopathy; (2) a history of cat contact, cat scratch, or a consistent primary lesion; (3) a positive cat-scratch skin test; and (4) failure to demonstrate other possible causes. Some investigators have stressed lymph node biopsy for diagnosis because of the characteristic histopathologic findings. A negative cat-scratch skin response to two different antigen sources would indicate need for lymph node biopsy.

Treatment

CSD usually subsides spontaneously within a period of 1 to 2 months. Second attacks are not reported and sequelae from typical cases do not occur. Thus, treatment should be conservative, consisting of reassurance and analgesics. In some cases, spontaneous or therapeutic lymph node drainage is effective in relieving local pain and systemic symptoms. Antimicrobial agents have been singularly ineffective in shortening or ameliorating the course.

References

1. Brooksaler FS, Sulkin SE: Cat-scratch disease. *Postgrad Med* **36**:366, 1964
2. Warwick WJ: The cat-scratch syndrome, many diseases or one disease? *Prog Med Virol* **9**:256, 1967
3. Emmons RW et al: Continuing search for the etiology of cat-scratch disease. *J Clin Microbiol* **4**:112, 1976
4. Wear DJ et al: Cat-scratch disease: a bacterial infection. *Science* **221**:1403, 1983
5. Spaulding WB, Hennessy JN: Cat-scratch disease (a study of eighty-three cases). *Am J Med* **28**:504, 1960
6. Carithers HA et al: Cat-scratch disease (its natural history). *JAMA* **207**:312, 1969
7. Pickerill RG, Milder JE: Transverse myelitis associated with cat-scratch disease in an adult. *JAMA* **24**:2840, 1981
8. Carithers HA: Cat-scratch skin test antigen: purification by heating. *Pediatrics* **60**:928, 1977
9. Johnson WT, Helwig EB: Cat-scratch disease (histopathologic changes in the skin). *Arch Dermatol* **100**:148, 1969
10. Czarnetzki BM et al: Cat-scratch disease skin test (studies of specificity and histopathologic features). *Arch Dermol* **111**:736, 1975
11. Zitelli BJ: Neck masses in children: adenopathy and malignant disease. *Pediatr Clin North Am* **4**:813, 1981
12. Margileth AM: Cat-scratch disease: nonbacterial regional lymphadenitis (study of 145 patients and a review of the literature). *Pediatrics* **42**:803, 1968

CHAPTER 196

WARTS

Douglas R. Lowy and Elliot J. Androphy

Definition

Verrucae, or warts, are benign tumors that commonly involve skin and less frequently affect other epithelial tissues. These lesions are induced by *papillomaviruses* (PVs), which are deoxyribonucleic acid (DNA)-containing viruses. As sensitive techniques to detect PVs have been developed, these viruses have been recognized in an increasing number of clinical conditions [1].

Historical aspects

Warts have been recognized for millenia. The term *verruca,* meaning "a steep place," was used because warts resembled "small hills" on the skin [2]. The ancient Greeks and Romans noted that anogenital warts were sexually transmitted, but until the nineteenth century anogenital warts were considered to be a form of syphilis or gonorrhea. The infectious nature of warts was experimentally confirmed within the last century, when several investigators demonstrated that human skin inoculated with wart extracts induced new warts [3]. A viral etiology was proposed since warts developed at sites inoculated with wart filtrates that were free of cells and bacteria. Moreover, since inoculation of extracts from common, anogenital, or laryngeal papillomas could, at low frequency, induce verrucae when injected into a different site, it was postulated that all warts were caused by a single agent. Although all PVs are morphologically similar, recent studies have indicated a multiplicity of human (H) PV types; some are already known to possess a distinct regional predilection, biology, and histopathology [1,4].

Despite these advances, PVs have not been reproducibly propagated in culture. In addition to preventing fulfillment of all Koch's postulates to establish an etiologic relation between PV infection and warts, the inability to culture PVs has greatly hampered research into the biology and genetics of PVs. Recent applications of recombinant DNA technology have, however, partially circumvented this obstacle and have provided new insights into PVs.

Etiologic agent

PVs are small double-stranded DNA viruses; they form one group of the Papovavirus family [5]. The spherically shaped viral particle (virion) consists of an outer protein shell (the capsid) approximately 55 nm in diameter surrounding a single, covalently closed supercoiled circle of double-stranded DNA with a molecular weight of 5 million (about 8000 nucleotide base pairs). Unlike the herpes viruses, PV viruses do not possess a lipoprotein envelope surrounding the capsid.

Virions can remain infectious for months to years when warts are stored in glycerol at room temperature [3]. Treating virions with formalin, detergents, or 55°C temperature can block viral infectivity, but the virus is resistant to freezing or desiccation. Since it has no lipid envelope, the virion is not inactivated by dehyrating agents such as ether.

PV infection occurs commonly in many species, including humans, rabbits, cows, and deer [5]. All PVs are highly host-specific; PVs from one species have not been able to induce papillomas in heterologous species. Recent molecular studies have established that PVs are more closely related to each other than to other viruses, including other members of the Papovavirus family. The complete nucleotide sequence has been determined for several human and animal PVs [6]. These studies suggest that all PVs have a similar genetic organization.

Epidemiology

HPV infection occurs commonly in humans, although the prevalence of clinical lesions in the general population is unknown. Warts are most frequent in children and young adults, in whom it has been estimated that the incidence may approach 10 percent [3]. In 1982 there were an estimated 4 million patient visits for nonvenereal warts to private physicians; 50 percent of these were to dermatologists [7]. Seventy percent of these patients were between 10 and 39 years old. Since 1966, there has been a sixfold increase in the number of visits for anogenital warts [8]. There were approximately 1 million consultations to office-based physicians for anogenital warts in 1982 (15 percent to dermatologists) [7], more than three times the number of consultations for genital herpes [8]. Patients with impaired cell-mediated immunity (CMI) are particularly susceptible to HPV infection. Warts may develop in more than 40 percent of renal transplant patients on immunosuppressive therapy [9].

Papillomavirus types

The recent finding of multiple HPV types represents an important advance. HPVs are classified according to their immunologic (structural viral antigens) or genetic (DNA sequence) relatedness. Sera made by immunization with intact virions generate type-specific antibodies, and sera made with detergent-treated virions detect antigenic determinants shared by all PVs (but not by other viruses) [10]. These antibodies can be used for typing HPVs, as well as for in situ immunohistochemical visualization of PV antigen in fixed tissue (Fig. 196-1). This technique is at least as sensitive as electron microscopy and more specific. Since these antibodies recognize structural proteins, they cannot identify cells that contain PV DNA but are not synthesizing virion antigens, such as those in bowenoid papulosis and certain other PV-associated lesions that produce few or no virions.

PVs can also be detected and typed by molecular hy-

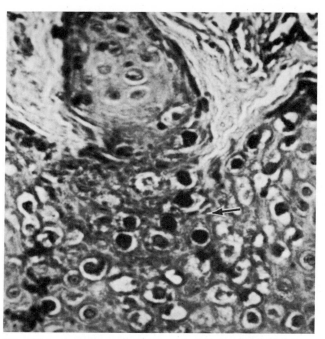

Fig. 196-1   Immunoperoxidase assay of a verruca in which the darkly stained nuclei (arrow) represent cells that contain PV virion structural antigens. The positive nuclei are found in some, but are not limited to, koilocytotic cells.

bridization, which is more sensitive but also more cumbersome than immunochemistry. These techniques, which can be performed on fixed tissue sections or on nucleic acids extracted from lesional skin, can detect PV DNA by determining whether the material will specifically bind (hybridize) to a known PV DNA. The complementarity of double-stranded DNA permits this specific binding if PV DNA is present in the lesion.

A new HPV type is defined when its DNA hybridizes by less than 50 percent to all other HPV types under stringent hybridization conditions [11]. However, 50 percent hybridization conditions imply close to 90 percent identity at the DNA sequence level. Some HPV types are actually quite closely related to each other and tend to induce similar lesions (see the following discussion).

The recent molecular cloning of many HPV DNA genomes has provided unlimited amounts of viral DNA for nucleic acid homology studies. The only source of viral antigen has thus far been wart tissue, but molecular cloning technology could in theory permit the production of any PV-encoded protein in vitro.

Many different HPV types have been described since 1975, with significant clinicopathologic correlations already noted for some types (see Table 196-1). In addition to those types listed in Table 196-1, several other unpublished HPV types are being characterized. Some of the listed HPV types have been isolated only rarely, although other types, such as HPV-1 through HPV-4, are found commonly throughout the world. Many rare HPV types have been identified predominantly in patients with epidermodysplasia verruciformis, a disease of unique susceptibility to chronic HPV infection (see Chap. 197).

Specific HPV types are commonly associated with infection of a defined body region or epithelial type, although

Table 196-1 Clinical associations of HPV types*

HPV type	Most common clinical lesions	Less common or rare lesions	Potential oncogenicity
1	Deep, painful plantar/palmar warts	Common warts	—
2	Common warts	Plantar, palmar, mosaic, oral, and anogenital warts	—
3,10	Flat warts	Flat warts in EV	HPV-10 rare in cervical and vulval carcinomas
4	Common warts	Plantar, palmar, mosaic, oral, and anogenital warts	—
5,8,9, 12,14,15 17,19–24	Macular warts in EV	Immunosuppressed patients	HPV-5, -8, -9 isolated from SCCs
6,11	Anogenital, laryngeal warts, cervical condylomata	Bowenoid papulosis, common warts	HPV-6, -11 in penile, vulval, cervical, and other urogenital tumors, including verrucous carcinoma
7	Butcher's warts	—	—
13	Oral focal epithelial hyperplasia	—	—
16,18	Bowenoid papulosis, cervical condylomata	Anogenital warts	HPV-16, -18 common in cervical dysplasias and carcinomas, urogenital Bowen's disease, and carcinomas

* *Note:* Abbreviations: HPV (human papillomavirus), EV (epidermodysplasia verruciformis), SCC (squamous cell carcinoma). For references see text.

this correlation is not rigorous [1,4]. For example, HPV-1 is typically isolated from deep plantar and palmar warts, but it may be found in common warts as well. Plantar warts may also be infected with HPV-2 or -4, although more often in mosaic warts than in deep, painful plantar types. HPV-3 and -10 are closely related by DNA hybridization, as are HPV-6 and -11; this homology extends to their pattern of clinical disease [12,13]. HPV-3 and -10 are found frequently in flat warts, and HPV-6 and -11 are both identified in anogenital and laryngeal papillomas.

Pathogenesis

Relatively little is known from experimental data about the pathogenesis of PV lesions. Humans are presumed to represent the only natural reservoir for HPV. Although PVs may usually be transmitted to uninfected individuals by close contact with an infected person, the marked stability of the virus suggests that transmission via desquamated epidermal cells can also occur.

It is thought that exogenously acquired PV is inoculated into the viable epidermis through breaks in the skin. Maceration of the skin may be an important predisposing factor, as suggested by the increased incidence of plantar warts in swimmers who frequent public pools [14]. Anogenital warts are usually transmitted by sexual contact, probably via microscopic abrasions to the epidermis.

Once an individual has been infected, new warts may develop over a small area or in distant sites. Each new lesion is thought to result from autoinoculation with virus rather than from blood-borne infection. Apposed lesions, which probably arise from autoinoculation, commonly appear on adjacent digits (Fig. 196-2) or in the anogenital region.

The contagion of PVs, which is highly variable, probably depends on many factors, including the location of lesions,

quantity of virus in them, degree and type of exposure, and general and PV-specific immunologic states of the exposed individuals. For example, in one study two-thirds of the sexual contacts of individuals with anogenital warts developed similar lesions, whereas sexual contacts of patients with nonvenereal warts did not have an increased incidence of genital warts [15].

The roles of immunity and genetic susceptibility to PV infection are poorly understood [1,9,16]. CMI, possibly in conjunction with humoral immunity, is believed to be critical in the host's defenses against PV infection, since individuals with defective CMI are particularly susceptible to PV infection [17]. The immune system may also play a significant role in wart regression [16]. Warts in patients with defective CMI are notoriously resistant to treatment. Conversely, treatment of one or a few warts may lead to resolution of many or all warts in nonimmunosuppressed patients. Flat warts commonly regress simultaneously in association with a mononuclear cell infiltrate. Other host factors may also be important in limiting PV infection. Although an individual may have several verrucae, widespread dissemination of the cutaneous infection is very rare.

In experimental PV inoculation, developing a clinically detectable verruca usually requires 2 to 6 months [3]. This result implies a relatively long period of subclinical infection, which could represent an unrecognized source of infection to others. Latent HPV infection also occurs; HPV DNA has been detected in normal-appearing areas in the larynx of patients with a history of laryngeal papillomatosis who were in clinical remission [18].

Certain aspects of viral replication are known, but the interactions between virus and host cell have not been well characterized. PV-associated lesions share several common features. The epidermis is acanthotic because of hyperplasia of a proliferative basal cell population and reten-

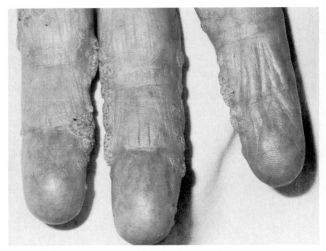

Fig. 196-2 Scaly, rough, keratotic papules typical of common warts, confluent on adjacent surfaces of the fingers (also known as "kissing" warts).

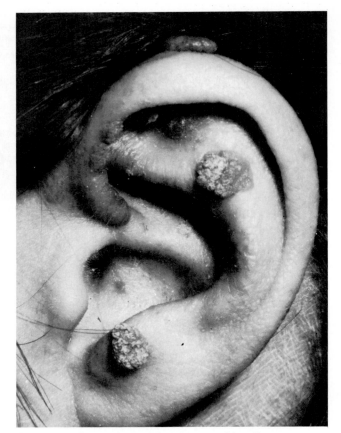

Fig. 196-4 Common warts in an unusual location.

tion of the upper stratifying keratinocytes. Although unproved, the assumption is that the virus infects the basal cells and stimulates them to divide. The viral DNA would then be carried in the nuclei of the daughter cells migrating upward through the differentiating epidermis. Viral DNA, virion antigens, and mature virions have been detected only in keratinocytes at or above the granular layer. Viral DNA replication and virion assembly take place in the nuclei of these cells. Since virus has not yet been detected in the lower epidermis, it is believed that virion antigen production is linked to the state of differentiation of the infected epidermal cell and that basal cells contain at most a few copies of viral DNA. The continued inability to propagate PVs in vitro is thought to be due to a failure to reproduce the milieu required for physiologic epidermal differentiation.

The relative abundance of virus particles in a verruca varies with the clinical setting and the HPV type [19]. Newer lesions tend to contain more virions than do older verrucae. Plantar warts containing HPV-1 have a high number of virions, whereas anogenital verrucae typically have small amounts of mature virus particles, and common

Fig. 196-3 Plantar warts.

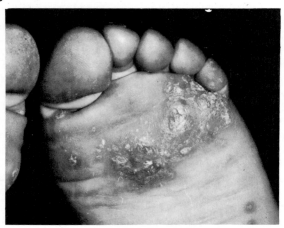

warts usually have intermediate numbers. The quantity and proportion of viral DNA that is not encapsidated into infectious virus also vary in these verrucae [19]. Nonencapsidated viral DNA remains in the form of free closed circles (episomes), i.e., self-replicating DNA that usually remains independent of the host cell's chromosomal DNA.

The production of virus particles and virion antigens also varies with the state of epithelial differentiation in the lesion. Virions are usually detected in cervical condylomas, but as lesions progress to an increasing degree of dysplasia, virion antigen and particle production decreases concomitantly [20]. Virion proteins are almost never observed in frank malignancies, although PV DNA may be detected.

Evidence from nonhuman PVs suggests that these viruses encode genes that directly alter cell proliferation, as do other tumor viruses. Bovine (BPV) and certain other animal PVs can induce tumorigenic transformation of certain nonepithelial cell lines in vitro [21]. This transformation causes the cells, which are normally contact-inhibited, to continue to divide and pile up with loss of contact inhibition upon infection. When injected into susceptible animals, these cells are able to form tumors. The transformed cells contain multiple copies of nonchromosomal PV DNA and do not produce PV virions, since they do not express the genes that encode the virion antigens. They do, however, express viral genes that encode nonvirion proteins. In BPV, at least two different nonvirion proteins encoded by the virus are involved in this transformation (unpublished data).

Fig. 196-5 The large, scaly, and horny warts contain HPV-2. The smaller, flatter, less scaly papules are warts that contain HPV-3.

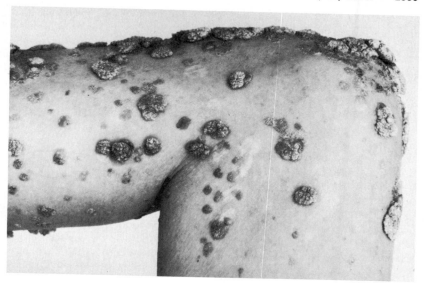

Clinical manifestations

Lesions are commonly classified by their clinical location or morphology as cutaneous and extracutaneous PV infections.

Cutaneous infections (Figs. 196-2 through 196-7)

Common warts (*verruca vulgaris*) are slightly scaly, rough papules or nodules, single or grouped, that may be found on any skin surface. They occur most often on the hands. Flat warts (*verruca plana*) are small, usually 2 to 4 mm, slightly elevated flattopped papules which may have no or minimal scale. These are usually multiple and frequent on the face and hands of children. Plantar and palmar warts are thick, endophytic, and hyperkeratotic lesions which may be painful with pressure. *Punctate black dots* ("seeds"), most evident after shaving away the outer keratinous surface, represent thrombosed capillaries in the papilloma. *Mosaic warts* result from the coalescence of planter or palmar warts into large plaques. *Butcher's warts* are verrucous papules, usually multiple, on the dorsal, palmar, or periungual hands and fingers of meat cutters [22]. Verrucae may also be filiform or appear as cutaneous horns. Epidermodysplasia verruciformis is discussed in Chap. 197.

Anogenital warts (also known as *condylomata acuminata, genital warts,* or *venereal warts*) consist of epidermal and dermal tumors on the perineum, genitalia, crural folds, and anus. They vary in size and can form large, exophytic ("cauliflowerlike") masses, especially in the moist environment of the perineum. Discrete, 1- to 3-mm sessile warts may occur on the penile shaft. Lesions that resemble common warts also occur in this region, but they are unusual. Anogenital warts may extend internally into the vagina, urethra, and rectum.

Bowenoid papulosis is a recently described clinicopathologic entity in which HPVs have been identified [23,24]. These are small 2- to 3-mm papules, often multiple, of the male and female genitalia [25]. Histologically, there is cellular atypia mimicking Bowen's disease, but clear evidence of transition to frank malignancy has not been demonstrated. DNA related to HPV-6 or -16 has been found in most lesions, but virion antigens have been detected less frequently [26].

Extracutaneous infections

Verrucous, horny papillomas, often of the palate, may have the appearance of common warts in the oral cavity [27]. Mucosal lesions of the oropharynx, termed *focal epithelial hyperplasia,* have also been demonstrated to contain HPVs [28]. These oral warts are small, slightly elevated, soft, often pink or white papules that may be found on buccal, gingival, or labial mucosa or hard palate. In *oral florid papillomatosis,* which is thought also to be caused by a PV, multiple large verrucae appear within the oral cavity. Progression to verrucous carcinoma (see the discussion that follows) may occur. *Oral condylomata acuminata* have been reported and may be considered uncommon sexually transmitted entities.

Laryngeal papillomatosis is characterized by the presence of many benign, noninvasive tumors that usually involve the larynx but may extend to the oropharynx and bronchopulmonary epithelia. Presenting symptoms are most commonly hoarseness and stridor. Most cases occur in infants, but the condition may develop at any age. These PV-associated papillomas may spontaneously remit, especially at puberty, but recurrences are frequent, perhaps because of the persistence of viral DNA despite clinical remission [18]. Since the HPV isolated from these lesions is frequently of the same type as that of anogenital warts, laryngeal papillomatosis in infants is believed to result from seeding of the larynx during parturition by virus from a mother with condyloma acuminatum or PV infection of the uterine cervix (see the following discussion). Several studies have confirmed the correlation of condylomata in mothers of infants with this disease [29]. Condylomata are common in the child-bearing age bracket, whereas laryngeal papillomatosis of infants is rare; it is therefore not clear whether cesarean section should be routinely performed in mothers with condylomata.

Warts may also occur about the meatus and in the urethra. They may rarely develop in the urinary bladder or in the lungs.

It has recently been recognized that many clinical lesions of the uterine cervix contain HPVs [30]. These lesions are usually termed *cervical warts* or *atypical condylomata*. They are usually flat and may require colposcopy and treatment of the cervix with acetic acid, whereupon they appear as white patches (Fig. 196-8). Atypical condylomata may mimic cervical dysplasia or carcinoma in situ histologically, with nuclear atypia and disorganized differentiation. Cells with a central nucleus and a surrounding clear halo (*koilocytotic cells*) may be seen histologically in these lesions as well as in common verrucae. The natural history of these cervical warts is not known, but progression to cervical dysplasia and carcinoma in situ has been reported [30–33]. PV virion antigens can be detected in fixed biopsies and atypical Papanicolaou's stains from cases of cer-

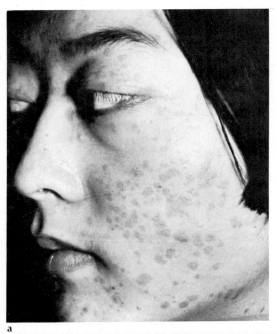

a

vical warts and dysplasias. Since HPV DNA has recently been found in a majority of cervical cancers (discussed in a later section), a possible role of the HPV in development of this malignancy has been speculated. The precise epidemiologic relation between anogenital warts and cervical warts is not yet known. Recent studies have shown that cervical cancers most frequently contain HPV-16 and -18, whereas the PVs found in anogenital warts are usually HPV-6 and -11 [13,34].

Relation of papillomaviruses and malignancy

Although most PVs are associated with biologically benign lesions only, increasing evidence suggests that certain PV types may have oncogenic potential. In humans, the association with infection by certain HPV types has been studied in greatest detail in patients with epidermodysplasia verruciformis (see Chap. 197). PVs do not appear to induce malignant tumors directly; it is more likely that potentially oncogenic PVs act by predisposing the infected cell to become malignant.

The benign epidermal hyperplasia induced in rabbits by the (Shope) cottontail rabbit PV can spontaneously convert to invasive squamous cell carcinoma. Small doses of chemical carcinogens induce a high rate of malignant conversion in these lesions [5]. In cattle, esophageal papillomas induced by BPV-4 become malignant if the infected animals graze on bracken fern, which contains a potential carcinogen.

Epithelial malignancy associated with PV infection may also develop in humans. Progression of the verrucae in laryngeal papillomatosis to invasive squamous cell carcinoma has been recognized to develop after x-irradiation. An immunosuppressed renal allograft patient developed a cutaneous squamous cell carcinoma containing HPV-5 DNA [35].

Epidemiologic evidence has linked penile, vulvar, and anal carcinoma with condylomata acuminata. The verrucous carcinoma is a low-grade, well-differentiated squamous cell carcinoma that is locally invasive but rarely metastasizes. This tumor, as well as some other epithelial urogenital tumors, has recently been found in some in-

Fig. 196-6   Flat warts are seen as small, flattopped papules with minimal or no scale.

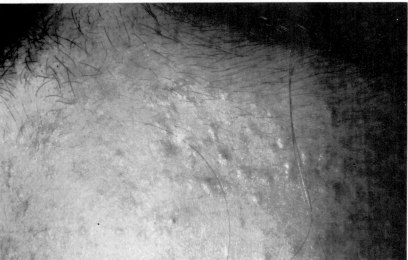

b

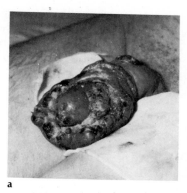

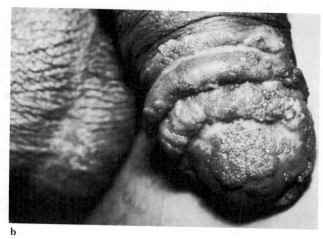

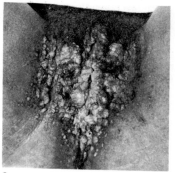

Fig. 196-7 Numerous nonscaly papules typical of anogenital warts in these locations.

stances to contain HPV DNA [23]. The giant condyloma acuminatum, also called the *Buschke-Loewenstein tumor,* and the squamous cell carcinoma that may arise from oral florid papillomatosis are forms of the verrucous carcinoma. *Epithelioma cuniculatum,* another rare type of verrucous carcinoma, is found on the sole and is thought to arise from a plantar wart.

The epidemiologic relation between cervical carcinoma and sexually transmitted diseases such as gonorrhea and herpes simplex has long been recognized. Anogenital and cervical warts represent another sexually transmitted disease associated with cervical cancer. New data support a possible role for HPV in this malignancy. Immunohistochemical techniques have detected HPV structural antigens in approximately 50 percent of cervical dysplasias (see preceding discussion). Using HPV-16 and -18 DNA as probes, identification of these or similar PV DNAs has been achieved in up to 80 percent of cervical carcinomas by highly sensitive hybridization techniques [34].

In summary, HPVs usually induce benign verrucae, but specific HPV types may be involved in development of malignant epithelial tumors.

Histopathology (Fig. 196-9)

Verrucae consist of an acanthotic epidermis with papillomatosis, hyperkeratosis, and parakeratosis [36]. The elongated rete ridges often point toward the center of the wart. The dermal capillary vessels are prominent and may be thrombosed. A mononuclear infiltrate may be present. Large keratinocytes with an eccentric, pyknotic nucleus surrounded by a perinuclear halo, termed *koilocytotic cells*

or *koilocytes,* are characteristic of PV-associated papillomas. Koilocytes do not usually contain keratohyaline granules, although they occur in the malpighian layer. They may, however, have small, eosinophilic granules; the origin of these granules is unknown, but they do not represent conglomerates of virus particles. Adjacent keratinocytes in this layer of the epidermis may contain dense clumps of basophilic keratohyaline granules. Flat warts have less acanthosis and hyperkeratosis and do not have parakeratosis or papillomatosis. Koilocytotic cells are usually abundant, indicating the viral origin of the lesion. Anogenital warts may possess slight to extensive acanthosis and parakeratosis; they lack a granular layer, since they are located on or adjacent to a mucosal surface. The rete ridges often form thick bands extending extensively into the underlying, highly vascular dermis. Koilocytes are often observed in these viral papillomas.

Diagnosis

The diagnosis of viral wart is usually made by the clinical appearance but can also be suggested by histologic examination. Immunohistochemical detection of PV structural proteins may confirm the presence of virus in a lesion. DNA hybridization techniques are currently limited to research laboratories.

Cutaneous warts are common in children and young adults, but they also occur in patients over 40 years of age. Multiple warts that do not spontaneously resolve or that recur after treatment, persist for years, or have an unusual morphology, especially if familial, suggest epidermodysplasia verruciformis. Immunocompromised patients, such

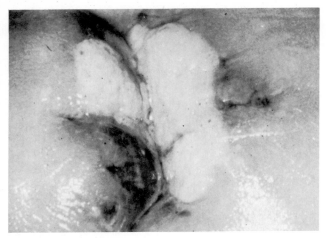

Fig. 196-8 Colposcopic view of cervical condylomata after treatment with acetic acid for visualization as white, elevated patch.

as those with lymphoproliferative disorders or on chemotherapeutic drugs, may have multiple warts.

Differential diagnosis

Papules of lichen planus may resemble flat warts; they may be differentiated by the presence of Wickham's striae and buccal involvement. Acrokeratosis verruciformis and epidermolytic hyperkeratosis are characterized by verrucous papules on the extremities. Common lesions such as seborrheic keratoses, acrocordons, clavi, and squamous cell carcinomas may resemble verrucae. Syphilitic condylomata need to be differentiated from venereal warts.

Treatment

The approach to management of warts depends on the age of the patient, the extent and duration of lesions, the patient's immunologic status, and the patient's desire for therapy. Children with common warts may not require therapy. Studies of spontaneous regression of warts in children suggest that two-thirds will remit within 2 years, with remaining verrucae continuing to resolve at this rate [37]. However, new warts may appear while others are regressing.

Current treatments for verrucae involve physical destruction of the infected cells; none is specifically antiviral. The existence of multiple treatment modalities reflects the fact that none is uniformly effective. Choice of treatment modality depends on the location, size, and type of wart, as well as the age and cooperation of the patient. Pain, inconvenience, risk of scarring, and experience of the physician are considerations to evaluate prior to treatment. In patients with anogenital warts, sexual partners should be examined and treated if necessary.

Cryotherapy utilizing liquid nitrogen or dry ice is a common and effective treatment for many types of warts [2,38]. Caustics and acids, such as salicylic acid, lactic acid, or trichloroacetic acid, peel off infected skin. Retinoic acid has been used topically to treat flat warts and probably has a similar mechanism of action. Induction of allergic contact dermatitis to topical dinitrochlorobenzene (DNCB) allows localization of inflammation to warts on which DNCB is painted; it has been speculated that this treatment stimulates local immunity. Uncontrolled studies have found DNCB to be effective, but since DNCB is positive in the Ames bacterial test of mutagenicity and squaric acid dibutyl ester is negative in this assay, the latter immunogen may be a suitable substitute [39]. Cantharidin is an extract of the green blister beetle which leads to blistering and focal destruction of epidermis.

A variety of chemotherapeutic agents are also widely employed. Topical podophyllin resin is a common treatment, particularly for anogenital warts, but is contraindicated during pregnancy [40]. Application of 5-fluorouracil has been reported to be effective in some cases of flat warts and condylomata acuminata [41]. Direct instillation has been used for urethral warts. Intralesional bleomycin may eradicate verrucae but must be used cautiously because of the possibility of extensive tissue necrosis [42].

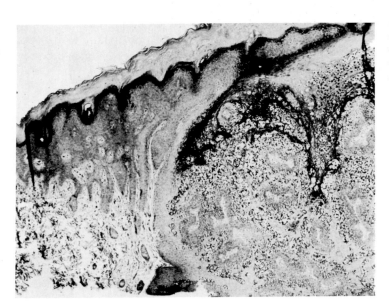

Fig. 196-9 Verruca vulgaris. The process is one of extensive hyperplasia, and the hyperplastic cells contain both intranuclear and intracytoplasmic inclusion bodies. ×40 (Micrograph by Wallace H Clark, Jr., M.D.)

Warts may be curetted or excised surgically, particularly large anogenital warts resistant to topical treatments. Electrodesiccation of condylomata acuminata requires local anesthesia but is effective. The advent of the CO_2 and argon lasers has potential utility for treating resistant warts. Microscopically controlled (Mohs) surgery has been particularly useful in the treatment of verrucous carcinomas [43].

Therapy for bowenoid papulosis is controversial, for lesions may spontaneously remit. However, since they frequently contain HPV-16, it is most prudent to treat these lesions with standard techniques such as cryotherapy, electrodesiccation, or excision. Examination of sexual partners, and particularly of the uterine cervix, is indicated.

Interferon has been effective in short-term studies in reducing warts in laryngeal papillomatosis and epidermodysplasia verruciformis, as well as common, plantar, and anogenital warts [44–46]. This therapeutic modality is currently under active investigation. X-irradiation of verrucae is probably contraindicated because of its association with the development of malignancy in laryngeal papillomatosis. In uncontrolled studies, vaccination with autogenous wart extracts has been reported to be highly effective in prevention of condyloma acuminatum recurrence [16].

References

1. Symposium on human papillomaviruses in *Clinics in Dermatology*, edited by S Jablonska, G Orth. Philadelphia, Lippincott, in press
2. Bunney MH: *Viral Warts: Their Biology and Treatment.* Oxford, Oxford Univ Press, 1982, p 1
*3. Rowson, KEK, Mahy BWJ: Human papova (wart) virus. *Bacteriological Reviews* **31**:110, 1967
4. Lutzner MA: The human papillomaviruses. *Arch Dermatol* **119**:631, 1983
*5. Lancaster WD, Olson C: Animal papillomaviruses. *Microbiol Rev* **46**:191, 1982
6. Danos O et al: Comparative analysis of the human type la and bovine type 1 papillomavirus genomes. *J Virol* **46**:557, 1983
7. *National Disease and Therapeutic Index, 1982.* Ambler, PA, IMS America.
8. Condyloma acuminatum—United States, 1966–1981. MMWR **32**:306, 1983
*9. Briggaman RA, Wheeler CE Jr: Immunology of human warts. *J Am Acad Dermatol* **1**:297, 1979
10. Jenson AB et al: Immunological relatedness of papillomaviruses from different species. *JNCI* **64**:495, 1980
11. Coggin J Jr, Zur Hausen H: Workshop in papillomaviruses and cancer. *Cancer Res* **39**:545, 1979
12. Green M et al: Isolation of a human papillomavirus from a patient with epidermodysplasia verruciformis: presence of related viral DNA genomes in human urogenital tumors. *Proc Natl Acad Sci USA* **79**:4437, 1982
13. Gissman L et al: Human papillomavirus types 6 and 11 DNA sequences in genital and laryngeal papillomas and in some cervical cancers. *Proc Natl Acad Sci USA* **80**:560, 1983
14. Gentles JC, Evans EGV: Foot infections in swimming baths. *Br Med J* **2**:260, 1973
15. Oriel JD: Natural history of genital warts. *Br J Vener Dis* **47**:1, 1971
16. Adler A, Safai B: Immunity in wart resolution. *J Am Acad Dermatol* **1**:305, 1979
17. Morison W: Viral warts, herpes simplex, and herpes zoster in patients with secondary immune deficiencies and neoplasms. *Br J Dermatol* **92**:625, 1975
18. Steinberg BM et al: Laryngeal papillomavirus infection during clinical remission. *N Engl J Med* **308**:1261, 1983
19. Grussendorf-Cohen E-I et al: Correlation between content of viral DNA and evidence of mature virus particles in HPV-1, HPV-4, and HPV-6 induced virus acanthomata. *J Invest Dermatol* **81**:511, 1983
20. Morin C et al: Confirmation of the papillomavirus etiology of condylomatous cervix lesions by the peroxidase-antiperoxidase technique. *JNCI* **66**:831, 1981
21. Nakabayashi Y et al: In vitro transformation by bovine papillomavirus. *J Invest Dermatol* **83 (suppl)**:12s, 1984
22. Orth G et al: Identification of papillomaviruses in butcher's warts. *J Invest Dermatol* **76**:97, 1981
23. Zachow KR et al: Detection of human papillomavirus DNA in anogenital neoplasias. *Nature* **300**:771, 1982
24. Ikenberg H et al: Human papillomavirus type-16 related DNA in genital Bowen's disease and in bowenoid papulosis. *Int J Cancer* **32**:563, 1983
25. Wade TR et al: Bowenoid papulosis of the genitalia. *Arch Dermatol* **115**:306, 1979
26. Guillet GY et al: Bowenoid papulosis: demonstration of human papillomavirus (HPV) with anti-HPV immune serum. *Arch Dermatol* **120**:514, 1984
27. Lutzner MA et al: Different papillomaviruses as the causes of oral warts. *Arch Dermatol* **118**:393, 1982
28. Pfister H et al: Characterization of human papillomavirus type 13 from focal epithelial hyperplasia Heck lesions. *J Virol* **47**:363, 1983
29. Quick CA et al: Relationship between condylomata and laryngeal papillomata. *Ann Otol* **89**:467, 1981
30. Meisels A et al: Human papillomavirus infection of the cervix: the atypical condyloma. *Acta Cytol (Baltimore)* **25**:7, 1981
31. Crum CP et al: Human papillomavirus type 16 and early cervical neoplasia. *N Engl J Med* **310**:880, 1984
32. Reid R et al: Genital warts and cervical cancer: I. Evidence of an association between subclinical papillomavirus infection and cervical malignancy. *Cancer* **50**:377, 1982
33. Welker PG et al: Natural history of cervical epithelial abnormalities in patients with vulval warts. *Br J Vener Dis* **59**:327, 1983
34. Durst M et al: A papillomavirus DNA from a cervical carcinoma and its prevalence in cancer biopsy samples from different geographic regions. *Proc Natl Acad Sci USA* **80**:3812, 1983
35. Lutzner MA et al: Detection of human papillomavirus type 5 DNA in skin cancers of an immunosuppressed renal allograft recipient. *Lancet* **2**:422, 1983
36. Gross G et al: Correlation between human papillomavirus (HPV) type and histology of warts. *J Invest Dermatol* **78**:160, 1982
37. Messing AM, Epstein WL: Natural history of warts: a two year study. *Arch Dermatol* **87**:306, 1963
38. Bunney MH et al: An assessment of methods of treating viral warts by comparative treatment trials based on a standard design. *Br J Dermatol* **94**:667, 1976
39. Dunagin WG, Millikan LE: Dinitrochlorobenzene immunotherapy for verrucae resistant to standard treatment modalities. *J Am Acad Dermatol* **6**:40, 1982
40. Guidelines for sexually transmitted diseases. *J Am Acad Dermatol* **8**:589, 1983
*41. Goette DK: Topical chemotherapy with 5-fluorouracil. *J Am Acad Dermatol* **6**:633, 1981
42. Shumer SM, O'Keefe EJ: Bleomycin in the treatment of recalcitrant warts. *J Am Acad Dermatol* **9**:91, 1983
*43. Swanson NA: Mohs surgery. *Arch Dermatol* **119**:761, 1983
44. Haglund S et al: Interferon therapy in juvenile laryngeal papillomatosis. *Arch Otolaryngol* **107**:327, 1982

* Reviews

45. Uyeno K, Ohtsu A: Interferon treatment of viral warts and some skin diseases, in *The Clinical Potential of Interferon,* edited by R Kono, J Vilcek. Tokyo, Univ of Tokyo Press, 1982, p 149

46. Androphy EJ et al: Response of warts in epidermodysplasia verruciformis to treatment with systemic and intralesional alpha interferon. *J Am Acad Dermatol* **11**:197, 1984

CHAPTER 197

EPIDERMODYSPLASIA VERRUCIFORMIS (LEWANDOWSKY-LUTZ SYNDROME)

Marvin A. Lutzner and Claudine Blanchet-Bardon

Definition

Epidermodysplasia verruciformis (EV) is a rare familial disease characterized by long-lasting, widespread papillomavirus-induced macules and papules, usually appearing in childhood. Within two to three decades, lesions in sun-exposed skin may degenerate into bowenoid carcinomas in situ, and then further progress to squamous cell carcinomas [1].

Historical aspects

Epidermodysplasia verrucciformis was first described by Lewandowsky and Lutz in 1922 [2]. These authors observed a patient in her third decade with a forehead cancer, who had suffered with multiple, flat, wartlike lesions since early infancy. Since this patient was the product of a consanguineous marriage, the authors concluded that EV was a familial disease which rendered the patient susceptible to warts and skin cancer.

Epidemiology

Incidence and geographic location

Since the original description of EV, over 200 cases have been reported (see reviews [1,3]). The disease appears to

have no geographic restrictions or racial preferences, but occurs more commonly in regions where the consanguinity rate is highest [1].

Age and sex

The average age of onset of benign macular and papular lesions is six, although onset may vary from early infancy to the second or third decade [1]. Skin cancers usually are first seen in the late twenties or early thirties, but the range of onset as reported in the literature is from age 10 to 50 [1]. Since transformation from benign to malignant lesions appears proportional to the amount of sun exposure [1], those with outdoor occupations in sunny climates are probably at greater risk.

Etiology

Genetic

Evidence for the genetic nature of EV rests on the observations that about 10% of EV patients are the product of

Table 197-1   Human papillomavirus types* found in benign EV lesions and arrangement into groups†

Group	Types
1	HPV 3, 10
2	HPV 5, 8, 12, 14, 19–23
3	HPV 9, 15, 17
4	HPV 24

* A human papillomavirus (HPV) can be categorized as a separate type if it exhibits less than 50 percent cross-hybridization with other known HPVs under stringent conditions in the Southern blot test [15].

† An HPV type found in an EV lesion which shows no cross-hybridization with other EV HPVs is placed in another group. HPVs in the same group show some cross-hybridization with each other, but less than 50 percent.

Source: From Kremsdorf et al [10] and G Orth et al, in preparation.

Fig. 197-1   Histology of a benign EV macular lesion. The stratum corneum is hyperkeratotic and exhibits parakeratosis. Large nests of pale-staining clear cells fill the epidermis down to the midstratum spinosum. Paraffin-embedded, H&E stained.

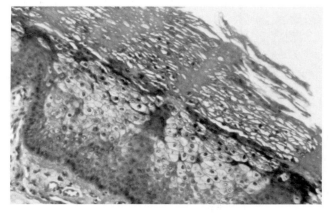

Fig. 197-2 Higher-magnification light micrograph of a macular EV lesion embedded in plastic. The enlarged, pale-staining clear cells fill the field. Nuclei are empty except for nuclear viral inclusions. Cytoplasm is filled with pale-staining homogenous material and rounded keratohyaline-like granules. Plastic-embedded, methylene blue stained.

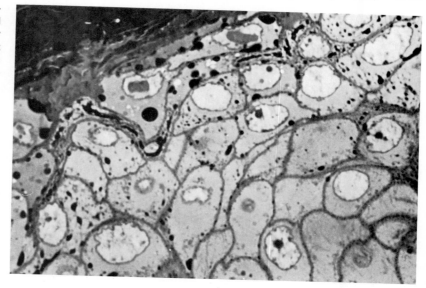

consanguineous marriages, and that about 10% of EV families have more than one sibling involved with the disease, suggesting an abnormal recessive gene [1–4]. It is to be anticipated that as in other hereditary diseases phenocopies may occur.

Viral

Reports of successful auto- and heteroinoculation studies established the infectious nature of EV [5,6], and visualization by electron microscopy of papillomavirus-like particles in EV benign lesions [7–9] as the probable role of a wart virus. Search for such particles in EV skin cancers with rare exception proved negative [8,9].

Recently, with the use of newly developed techniques,

Fig. 197-3 Macular-papular lesion from an immunosuppressed renal allogaft recipient infected with both HPV 3 and HPV 5 as determined by immunofluorescence. Cells to the left are pale-staining clear cells with rounded keratohyaline-like granules infected with HPV 5, typical for EV; to the right are smaller cells infected with HPV 3, typical for flat warts. The cytoplasm of these cells is empty and tonofilaments are clustered at the cell periphery. Plastic-embedded, methylene blue stained.

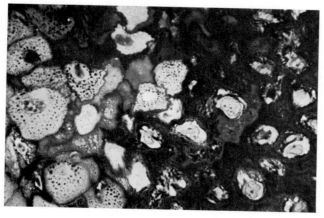

it was discovered that rather than a single papillomavirus, there were instead many, now numbering in the twenties [10,11] (see Chap. 184). Further it has been discovered that at least 15 of these human papillomavirus (HPV) types occur almost exclusively in benign lesions of EV patients [10–14] (Table 197-1). HPVs 3 and 10 are most commonly found in flat warts in non-EV patients; the other 13 EV HPVs are found almost exclusively in EV patients, HPV 5 being the most common [11,14]. EV patients are often infected with multiple HPVs [10–14,16]. Full virus particles are not usually seen in EV skin cancers by electron microscopy [8,9], nor has viral capsid protein been found in these cancers by immunofluorescence microscopy [11,14]. However, using the method of Southern blot hybridization, which can identify small amounts of viral DNA, HPV 5 and 8 genome copies have been found in a number of EV skin cancers, establishing these as probable oncogenic viruses [14,16–18]. Genome copies of the viral DNA remain episomic, rather than inserting into host cell DNA [19], and some information about a subgenomic transforming portion of an oncogenic papillomavirus is known [20]. Capsid protein does not appear to be produced in these cancers [14]. Some of the HPV DNAs have been sequenced [21,22], information which will hopefully lead to understanding both the infectious and transforming properties of these viruses.

Pathogenesis

The relatively long period of time between the onset of benign lesions and the onset of cancer in EV patients suggests a multifactorial process of HPV-induced oncogenesis.

Virus

In all papillomavirus-induced naturally occurring lesions to date, virus particles can be found only in cells of the upper strata of the epidermis within cells that have undergone differentiation, most commonly in cells of the gran-

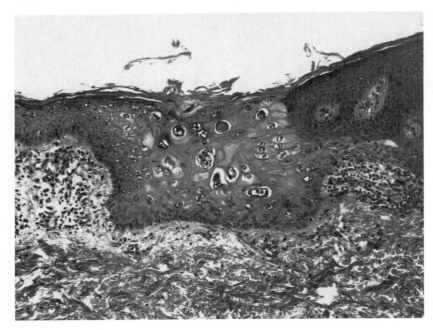

Fig. 197-4   A bowenoid carcinoma in situ lesion from an EV patient. The involved area is acanthotic and exhibits dyskeratotic cells with bizarre, hyperchromatic nuclei. Cells have lost their polarity. No abnormal cells have penetrated into the dermis. Paraffin-embedded, H&E stained.

ular layer [1,11,14]. The role of the virus in the production of benign EV lesions is well established by inoculation studies [5,6] and visualization of virus particles by electron microscopy [3,7–9]. However in EV cancers only a small number of genome copies of the viral DNA remain in the nuclei [12,14,18]. This transformation from permissive keratinocytes producing full virus particles to malignant keratinocytes which contain only small amounts of viral DNA

is not yet understood, but cofactors are likely involved in this conversion.

Genetics

The presence of an abnormal recessive gene renders EV patients in some unknown fashion susceptible to chronic infection with the specific EV HPVs shown in Table 197-1. In general, these patients are not more susceptible to infection with non-EV papillomaviruses [1,17], nor are they unduly susceptible to infections with other microorganisms.

Immunity

Ninety percent of EV patients have depressed cell-mediated immunity, although their humoral immunity remains intact [1,23]. This altered immunity may be secondary to generalized, chronic infection with papillomaviruses which may compromise the immune system [24], or the immune defect may be primary, perhaps a result of an abnormal gene, leading to specific susceptibility to infection by the EV HPVs, and perhaps susceptibility to oncogenic transformation by certain of these viruses. Further support for a role of the immune system in EV is the observation that immunosuppressed renal allograft recipients have a high incidence of warts and skin cancer, and the findings that the potentially oncogenic EV HPV type 5 is present in benign macular lesions in some of these patients [25], and genome copies are present in some skin cancers of a renal allograft recipient with an EV-like syndrome [26].

Sunlight

There is much circumstantial evidence that supports the role of sunlight as a cofactor in the production of skin cancers in EV patients: (1) Cancers develop most commonly in sun-exposed skin, especially the forehead of EV patients. (2) Blacks with EV seldom develop skin cancers;

Fig. 197-5   An invasive squamous cell carcinoma showing nests of epithelial malignant cells in the dermis. Nuclei are hyperchromatic, and cytoplasm is pale-staining in some cells in the invading nests. Paraffin-embedded, H&E stained.

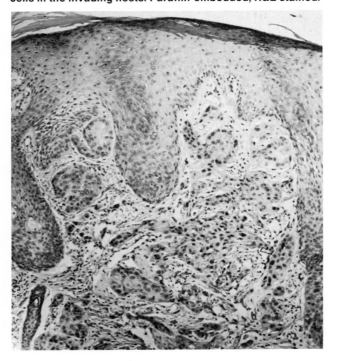

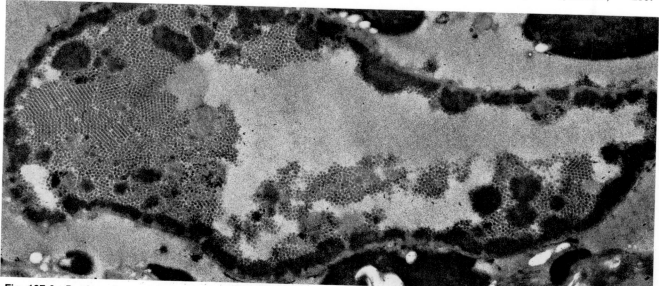

Fig. 197-6 Portion of a cell from an EV macular lesion infected with an EV HPV as visualized by electron microscopy. Clusters of papillomavirus-like particles can be seen in the nucleus. Masses of electron-dense chromatin can be seen. The rest of the nucleus is electron-lucid and filled with a finely granular or fibrillar material, which can be seen also in the cytoplasm immediately surrounding the nucleus. Electron-dense bodies in the cytoplasm are keratohyaline granules. Epon-embedded, lead and uranyl stained.

they are apparently protected by their skin pigment [27]. (3) Skin cancers in renal allograft recipients have a frequency directly proportional to the duration and intensity of sun exposure [28]. (4) Ocular cancers associated with papillomaviruses occur in cattle exposed to excessive sunlight [29]. (5) Sheep develop skin cancers associated with papillomaviruses in sun-exposed skin unprotected by hair or pigment [30]. (6) Human actinic (solar) keratoses have been found to be associated with papillomaviruses as well as sunlight exposure [31]. (7) Sunlight theoretically could reinforce the role of immunodeficiency in EV through the known effect of ultraviolet radiation which is capable of suppressing cell-mediated immunity [32,33].

Pathology

Benign lesions [1,3,11]

A benign EV lesion can be diagnosed in routine histologic sections by its characteristic picture. Nests of large pale-staining clear cells are seen in the upper spinous and granular layers (Fig. 197-1). Basal cells appear normal. The cytoplasm of the clear cells appears to contain only rounded keratohyaline granules. Nuclei have clear spaces and occasionally inclusion bodies can be seen, especially in plastic-embedded sections (Fig. 197-2). Macular lesions are not acanthotic; flat wartlike lesions show moderate acanthosis. True flat warts infected with HPV 3 and HPV 10 have a different picture (Fig. 197-3). Affected cells of the spinous and granular layer have empty cytoplasm except for a ring at the periphery composed of keratohyaline

Fig. 197-8 Pityriasis (tinia) versicolor-iike lesions on the trunk of an EV patient, showing the widespread scaly macular lesions. *(Courtesy of R. Caputo.)*

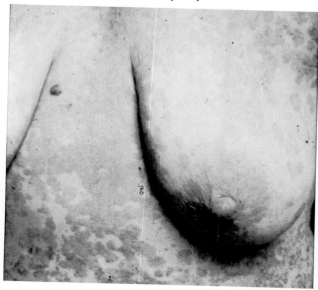

Fig. 197-7 Electron micrograph of negatively stained papillomavirus particles showing multiple capsomeres comprising the virus capsid. Phosphotungstic acid stained.

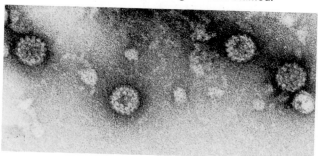

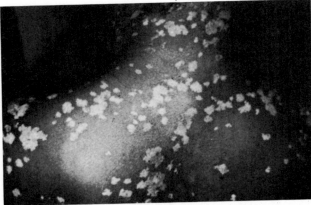

Fig. 197-9 Depigmented macular lesions on the trunk of a black EV patient.

granules and tonofilament bundles. The stratum corneum often shows a basket-weave pattern.

Bowen's carcinoma in situ

The histology of EV Bowen's lesions is no different from that of ordinary Bowen's disease lesions (Fig. 197-4). There is acanthosis, loss of cell polarity, dyskeratotic cells, and hyperchromatic and bizarre nuclei, which are often bi- or multinucleated [1,3,11].

Invasive squamous cell carcinoma

The histology of EV squamous cell carcinomas is similar to that of other squamous cell carcinomas, except that occasionally features characteristic of atypical cells in Bowen's lesions predominate. Nests of epidermal cells or single epidermal cells are present in the dermis and may be seen invading underlying structures (Fig. 197-5) [1,3,11,25].

Electron microscopy

Paracrystalline arrays of papillomavirus-like particles can be easily found in keratinocytes of benign lesions, especially those of the granular layer (Fig. 197-6). Nuclear clear spaces are evident. The cytoplasm contains only rounded

Fig. 197-10 Flat wartlike papular lesions on the dorsum of the hand of an EV patient.

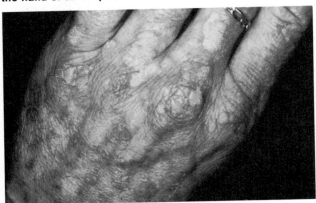

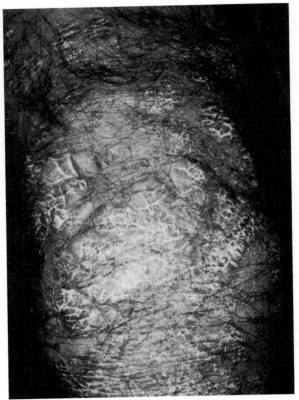

Fig. 197-11 Psoriasis-like lesions on the knees of an EV patient.

keratohyalin-like bodies. The clear areas within the cyto-plasmic and nuclear compartments are filled with very fine filaments. No virus particles can be found in cancer lesions [1,3,7–9,34]. Negative staining studies show the papillo-maviruses to be approximately 50 nm in diameter, spheri-cal, and to have 72 capsomeres comprising their capsid. All papillomavirus types have the same appearance with this technique (Fig. 197-7).

Clinical manifestations

Benign lesions

Macular scaly lesions begin to appear ordinarily in child-hood. They are often widespread and are most commonly seen first on the trunk and upper extremities, although they may occur anywhere on the skin (Fig. 197-8). The lesions range in color from tan to red, or may be depigmented or dark brown to black in EV patients with darkly pigmented skin (Fig. 197-9). Macules tend to become confluent and may have polycyclic borders. The eruption at times resem-bles pityriasis (tinia) versicolor, thus the name pityriasis versicolor-like or PV-like lesions. Lesions on the dorsa of the hands tend to be papular (Fig. 197-10) and are termed flat wartlike lesions. Lesions on the elbows and knees may resemble psoriasis (Fig. 197-11).

Bowenoid carcinomas in situ

These lesions most commonly occur in sun-exposed skin, especially the face and most often the forehead (Fig.

Fig. 197-12 An EV patient showing macular lesions on his back, bowenoid carcinomas in situ on his temple and forehead, and an invasive squamous cell carcinoma on his forehead.

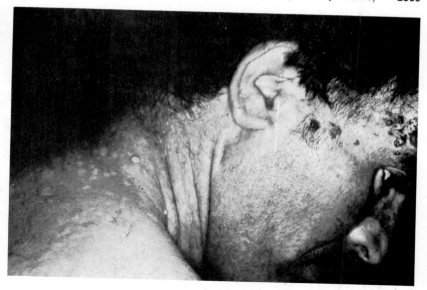

197-12). They are raised plaques that may be red or pigmented from tan to black. Lesions may ulcerate and crust, events which should evoke suspicion of early squamous cell carcinoma.

Invasion and metastases

Epidermodysplasia verruciformis cancers may metastasize to local lymph nodes, but this appears to occur less frequently than with non-EV squamous cell carcinomas, unless the EV cancers have been treated with x-irradiation after which, paradoxically, they tend to become more malignant in nature; radiation perhaps plays a further cofactor role in oncogenesis. Local invasion is not uncommon and vital organs or structures such as the orbit, sinuses, or brain may be penetrated and destroyed (Figs. 197-12 to 197-14) [1,3,14,17,18,26]. Cancers may be seen to develop in sites of benign lesions (Fig. 197-14).

Mental retardation

About 10 percent of EV patients have been reported to be mentally retarded at birth [1,3]. Others seem to have psychological disturbances [1]. Most are of normal intelligence and present normal behavior. Nothing is known of the mechanisms involved in the brain. Since mental retardation of various types is not uncommon among children born to consanguineous parents, the relationship of these mental aberrations to EV is not yet established.

Laboratory findings

Identification and typing of EV papillomaviruses

A clinically suspected diagnosis of EV can be partially confirmed by histologic findings as described above. Determination of the presence of a papillomavirus can be made by visualization of the virus by electron microscopy and by screening for papillomavirus "group" antigen by immunoperoxidase microscopy performed on routine paraffin sections using an antibody raised against any disrupted papillomavirus particles [11,35]. It is possible to type papillomaviruses by immunofluorescence on cryostat sections of lesions using antibody prepared against purified viruses of known types, each of which has its own specific capsid antigen [14,36] (Fig. 197-15). However, because it is not yet possible to culture papillomaviruses and since lesions contain ordinarily so little virus, such antibodies

Fig. 197-13 Hand of an EV patient showing macular pigmented lesions on the fingers and palm, a small squamous cell carcinoma at the base of the fourth finger, and a large fungating squamous cell carcinoma at the base of the thumb. The latter lesion had penetrated to the bone and required amputation of the thumb.

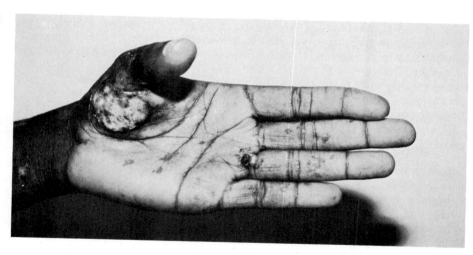

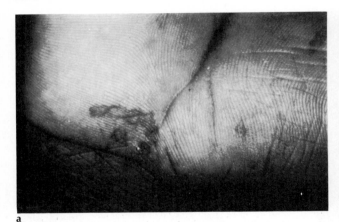

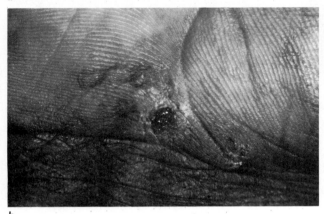

Fig. 197-14   (a) Portion of the palm of the other hand of the patient shown in Fig. 197-13, exhibiting a number of macular benign EV lesions. (b) The same area photographed 18 months later, showing that one of the macular lesions has degenerated into a nodular ulcerating lesion, which proved to be an invasive squamous cell carcinoma.

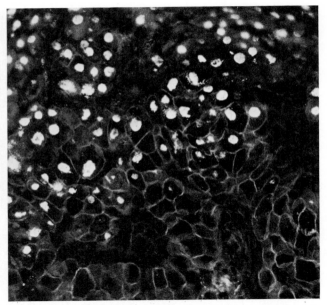

Fig. 197-15   Immunofluorescence microscopy using an antiserum raised against pooled EV HPVs. Positive nuclei indicate the presence of papillomavirus capsid protein in this macular lesion from a renal allograft recipient.

are available for only a few of the papillomaviruses and are not yet commercially feasible, although efforts are being made through genetic engineering and monoclonal antibody techniques to provide such reagents. At present, type identification of HPVs is a laborious task performed only in a small number of research laboratories. Methodology involves the extraction of viral DNA identification of papillomavirus DNA by its migration patterns on agarose gels and identification of DNA fragment patterns following restriction endonuclease digestions. If cloned type-specific DNA is available, final recognition can be made on Southern blots [10,12–14,16,18,19,26] (Fig. 197-16). Wider distribution of these cloned probes and simplified methodologies for papillomavirus typing will hopefully be accomplished in the future.

Immunologic testing

Since it is known that most EV patients have an impairment in cell-mediated immunity, delayed hypersensitivity skin testing using a battery of antigens, especially DNCB, is helpful in supporting the diagnosis [23]. Unfortunately, there are not at present any serologic tests available for diagnosing EV [23].

Differential diagnosis

The macular eruption of EV might be mistaken for pityriasis (tinia) versicolor because of the truncal and upper extremity distribution and the varied color of the lesions. However the persistence of the lesions and their resistance to the usual treatment of tinia versicolor should alert the physician to the diagnosis, which can be confirmed by biopsy examination. Papular lesions on the dorsa of the hands can be mistaken for ordinary flat warts, but here biopsy examination and virus typing help in the diagnosis. Confluent scaly lesions on the elbows and knees can resemble psoriasis; isolated papules on the extremities could be confused with lichen planus. Rarely EV macules may exhibit atrophy and may be mistaken for porokeratosis. The most difficult imitator of EV is the patient with widespread flat warts caused by HPVs 3 and 10, who may also be immunodepressed. Sometimes in these patients the final diagnosis can be made histologically or by virus typing, but the physician must be alert to watch such patients for the possible development of Bowen's and squamous cell carcinomas, especially if the patient is the product of a consanguineous marriage.

Treatment

There is no effective treatment for EV. Most important is early recognition of the disease and frequent examination for skin cancers so that they may be surgically removed. Patients should avoid excessive exposure to sunlight and should not receive treatment by x-rays. Intralesional alpha interferon injections appear successful in treating early Bowen's lesions, but this treatment is still in its experimental phases [37]. Oral retinoids such as etretinate seem to reduce the number of virus particles in benign lesions. Although use of this medication ordinarily results in the

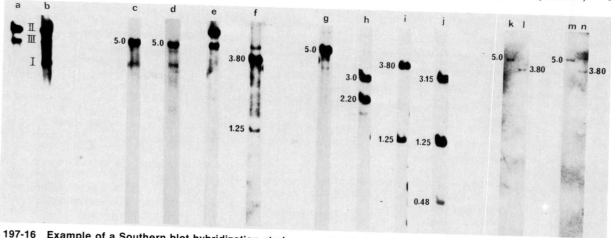

Fig. 197-16 Example of a Southern blot hybridization study using HPV 5 as a radioactive probe and a variety of restriction endonucleases. Lanes a and c–f contain DNA from benign lesions of a renal allograft recipient with an EV-like syndrome; whereas lanes b and g–j contain DNA from an EV patient's benign lesions known to be infected with HPV 5. Lanes k–n contain DNA from the renal allograft recipient's two cancers. The banding pattern of these lanes indicates the presence of HPV 5 DNA in both patients. For more details see [26].

flattening of papular lesions, and the reduction in scaling and abnormal pigmentation in macular lesions [38], lesions regress when the retinoids are stopped. Whether or not persistent use of retinoids over a period of years might prevent or reduce the number of skin cancers remains to be proved. Antiviral drugs effective against papillomaviruses might be developed, as well as a vaccine which, when given in childhood, would prevent papillomavirus infection.

Genetic counseling is useful for families who already have a child with EV, but prenatal diagnosis is not yet possible.

The cessation of immunosuppressive drugs in renal allograft recipients with multiple warts and cancers reduces the cancer incidence although loss of the allograft may occur [25,26].

Prognosis

If the diagnosis is made soon after the onset of benign lesions, cancer treatment is more effective because of close surveillance and early surgery. The development of skin cancers varies in incidence probably according to cofactor effects. The avoidance of sunlight, x-ray treatment, and immunosuppressive drugs is imperative. The darker the natural skin color, the better is the prognosis. Cancers appear to be slow to metastasize, however deaths have occurred from invasion of vital organs or metastases [1,17].

References

1. Lutzner MA: Epidermodysplasia verruciformis. An autosomal recessive disease characterized by viral warts and skin cancer. A model for viral carcinogenesis. *Bull Cancer (Paris)* **65:**169, 1978

2. Lewandowsky F, Lutz W: Eis Fall einer bisher nicht beschrieben Hauterkrankung (Epidermodysplasia verruciformis). *Arch Dermatol Syphilol (Berlin)* **141:**193, 1922

3. Rueda LA, Rodriguez G: Verrugas humanas por virus papova. Correlaçion clinica, histologica y ultrastructural. *Med Cutan Iber Lat Am* **2:**113, 1976

4. Rajogopalan K et al: Familial epidermodysplasia verruciformis of Lewandowsky and Lutz. *Arch Dermatol* **105:**73, 1972

5. Lutz W: A propos de l'epidermodysplasie verruciforme. *Dermatologica* **92:**30, 1946

6. Jablonska S, Formas I: Weitere positive Ergebnisse mit Auto und der Heteroinokulation bei Epidermodysplasia verruciformis. *Dermatologica* **118:**86, 1959

7. Ruiter M, Van Mullem J: Demonstration by electron microscopy of an intranuclear virus in epidermodysplasia verruciformis. *J Invest Dermatol* **47:**247, 1966

8. Aaronson CM, Lutzner MA: Epidermodysplasia verruciformis and epidermoid carcinoma. Electron microscopic observations. *JAMA* **201:**775, 1967

9. Jablonska S et al: On the viral etiology of epidermodysplasia verruciformis Lewandowsky Lutz. Electron microscopic studies. *Dermatologica* **137:**113, 1968

10. Kremsdorf D et al: Molecular cloning and characterization of the genomes of nine newly recognized human papillomavirus types associated with eipdermodysplasia verruciformis. *J Virol* **52:**1013, 1984

11. Lutzner MA: Papillomaviruses. A review. *Arch Dermatol* **119:**631, 1983

12. Kremsdorf D et al: Biochemical characterization of two types of human papillomaviruses associated with epidermodysplasia verruciformis. *J Virol* **43:**436, 1982

13. Pfister H et al: Characterization of a human papilloma virus from epidermodysplasia verruciformis lesions of a patient from Upper Volta. *Int J Cancer* **27:**645, 1981

14. Orth G et al: Epidermodysplasia verruciformis. A model for the role of papillomaviruses in human cancer, in *Cold Spring Harbor Conferences on Cell Proliferation,* vol 7, *Viruses in Naturally Occurring Cancers,* edited by M Essex et al. Cold Spring Harbor, NY, Cold Spring Harbor Laboratories, 1980, p 259

15. Coggin JR zur Hausen H: Workshop on papillomaviruses and cancer. *Cancer Res* **39:**545, 1979

16. Pfister H et al: HPV-5 DNA in a carcinoma of an epidermodysplasia verruciformis patient infected with various human papillomavirus types. *Cancer Res* **43:**1436, 1983

17. Lutzner MA et al: Clinical observations, viral studies and treatment trials in patients with epidermodysplasia verruciformis, a disease induced by specific human papillomaviruses. *J Invest Dermatol* **83 (suppl):**18s, 1984

18. Ostrow RS et al: Human papillomavirus DNA in cutaneous primary and metastasized squamous cell carcinomas from pa-

tients with epidermodysplasia verruciformis. *Proc Natl Acad Sci USA* **79**:1634, 1982

19. Howley P et al: Molecular characterization of papillomavirus genome, in *Cold Spring Harbor Conferences on Cell Proliferation*, vol 7, *Viruses in Naturally Occurring Cancers*, edited by M Essex et al. Cold Spring Harbor, NY, Cold Spring Harbor Laboratories, 1980, p 233

20. Lowy DR et al: In vitro tumorogenic transformation by a defined subgenomic fragment of bovine papillomavirus DNA. *Nature* **287**:72, 1980

21. Chen EY et al: The primary structure and genetic organization of the bovine papillomavirus type 1 genome. *Nature* **299**:529, 1982

22. Danos O, Yaniv M: Structure and function of papillomavirus genome, in *Advances in Viral Oncology*, vol 3, edited by G Klein. New York, Raven Press, 1983, p 59

23. Jablonska S et al: Immunopathology of papillomavirus-induced tumors in different tissues. *Springer Semin Immunopathol* **5**:33, 1980. Addendum: Lutzner MA: Immunopathology of papillomavirus-induced warts and skin cancers in immunodepressed and immunosuppressed patients.

24. Reid TMS et al: Generalized warts and immune deficiency. *Br J Dermatol* **95**:559, 1976

25. Lutzner MA et al: A potentially oncogenic human papillomavirus (HPV-5) found in two renal allograft recipients. *J Invest Dermatol* **75**:353, 1980

26. Lutzner MA et al: Detection of human papillomavirus type 5 DNA in skin cancers of an immunosuppressed renal allograft recipient. *Lancet* **2**:422, 1983

27. Jacyk JK, Subbuswamy SG: Epidermodysplasia in Nigerians. *Dermatologica* **159**:256, 1979

28. Hardie IR et al: Skin cancer in Caucasian renal allograft recipients living in a subtropical climate. *Surgery* **87**:177, 1980

29. Ford JN et al: Evidence for papillomaviruses in ocular lesions in cattle. *Res Vet Sci* **32**:257, 1982

30. Vanselow BA, Spradbrow PB: Papillomaviruses, papillomas and squamous cell carcinomas in sheep. *Vet Res* **110**:561, 1982

31. Spradbrow PB et al: Virions resembling papillomaviruses in hyperkeratotic lesions from sun-damaged skin. *Lancet* **1**:189, 1983

32. Fischer MS, Kripke ML: Systemic alteration induced in mice by ultraviolet carcinogenesis. *Proc Natl Acad Sci USA* **74**:1688, 1977

33. Hersey P et al: Immunological effects of solarium exposure. *Lancet* **1**:545, 1983

34. Lutzner MA: Electron microscopy in virus diseases of the skin and mucosa, particularly the human papillomavirus-induced diseases, in *Electron Microscopy in Skin Diseases*, edited by K Hashimoto, vol 3, *Electron Microscopy in Human Medicine*, edited by JV Johannessen. New York, McGraw-Hill, in press

35. Jenson AB et al: Immunological relatedness of papillomaviruses from different species. *JNCI* **64**:495, 1980

36. Orth G et al: Evidence for antigenic determinants shared by the structural polypeptides of (Shope) rabbit papillomavirus and human papillomavirus type 1. *Virology* **91**:243, 1978

37. Blanchet-Bardon C et al: Interferon treatment of skin cancer in patients with epidermodysplasia verruciformis. *Lancet* **1**:274, 1981

38. Lutzner MA, Blanchet-Bardon C: Oral retinoid treatment of human papillomavirus type-5 induced epidermodysplasia verruciformis. *N Engl J Med* **302**:1091, 1980

CHAPTER 198

INFECTIOUS MONONUCLEOSIS

Ben Z. Katz and Warren A. Andiman

Definition

Infectious mononucleosis (IM) is an acute, self-limited disease caused by the Epstein-Barr virus (EBV). Occasionally a similar syndrome may be caused by other agents, such as cytomegalovirus or *Toxoplasma gondii*. It is most frequently recognized as a clinical entity in adolescents and young adults in whom the disease is characterized by fever, generalized lymphadenopathy, pharyngitis, and lymphocytosis with atypical lymphocytes. These findings are often accompanied by mild hepatitis, dermatitis, and, less frequently, dysfunction of other organ systems. The presence of heterophile antibodies with a characteristic absorption pattern is specific for the disease, but 10 to 15 percent of patients with clinical illness are heterophile antibody negative. Some of these patients are infected with other agents, but most have EBV infections that require the application of virus-specific serologic tests for definitive diagnosis. This chapter will concern itself with IM caused by EBV.

Historical aspects

The recent recorded history of IM as a distinct nosologic entity originated with a description of a syndrome called "glandular fever" by Emil Pfeiffer in 1889. The disease consisted of fever, lymphadenopathy, pharyngitis, and, in severe cases, hepatosplenomegaly [1]. In 1920, Sprunt and Evans accurately described the disorder in young adults as we know it, reported the presence of atypical lymphocytes, and renamed the disease *infectious mononucleosis* [2]. A major development occurred in 1932 when Paul and Bunnell discovered agglutinating antibodies to sheep red blood cells (heterophile antibodies) in the serum of IM patients [3]. Three years later Davidsohn and Walker showed that the specificity of this agglutination reaction could be improved considerably by using guinea pig kidney and beef red blood cell antigens to absorb serum specimens prior to their reaction with sheep erythrocytes [4].

EBV was first seen by electron microscopy in 1964 in cells cultured from African Burkitt lymphoma tissue [5].

The causal relationship between EBV and IM was first observed in 1968. A previously seronegative technician working with the virus developed IM and, in its wake, antibodies to EBV-associated antigens that were present in cultured lymphoma cells [6]. Subsequent seroepidemiologic studies showed that heterophile-positive IM was invariably associated with the development of antibodies to EBV and that IM occurred only in individuals who previously lacked EBV antibodies [7].

Epidemiology

One must distinguish between the epidemiology of most EBV infections and that of IM. EBV is a ubiquitous agent. The clinical manifestations associated with infection are usually related to the age at which primary exposure occurs. Thus, in developing countries and in lower socioeconomic groups in industrialized nations, up to 90 percent of children develop antibodies to EBV by age six. In young children EBV infections are either mild or subclinical. In contrast, in higher socioeconomic groups, only 40 to 50 percent of adolescents have experienced infection previously and it is among the seronegatives that IM generally occurs. Among older adolescents 10 to 20 percent of susceptibles become infected every year, and the ratio of apparent to inapparent infection is between 1:1 and 1:3.

EBV is shed in oropharyngeal secretions during IM and intermittently or persistently thereafter. These secretions appear to be the major source of infectious virus. Therefore, IM is likely to be transmitted through close interpersonal contact such as kissing, mothers fondling their children, and toddlers sharing toys. However, infection is only modestly communicable, probably due to the lower titer of virus present in saliva even during acute infection. Hence, secondary attack rates are low. The virus is shed intermittently in the majority of seropositive individuals; at any one time 10 to 20 percent of such persons may be shedding virus, thereby serving as the principal reservoir of infection. Rarely, parenteral transmission of heterophile-positive IM has been documented following blood transfusions [8].

Etiology

EBV, a herpesvirus, was discovered by Epstein, Achong, and Barr during electron microscopic studies of cell lines derived from African Burkitt lymphoma tissue [5]. The mature, infectious particles measure approximately 180 nm in diameter and are composed of nucleic acid (double-stranded DNA), a capsid, and a lipid-containing outer coat. The viral capsid has icosahedral symmetry and is composed of 162 capsomeres. The virus itself, like other herpesviruses, is relatively large and fragile, easily degraded and inactivated [8].

EBV is tropic for B lymphocytes, and thus far, can only be cultured in vitro in the lymphocytes of humans and certain other primates. Its growth can also be supported by epithelial cells of the mouth and, perhaps, by certain cells of the salivary glands [9,10]. The virus confers upon infected lymphocytes the ability to grow continuously in cell culture, a process that has been termed *transformation* or *immortalization* [11].

Pathogenesis of infection

Epidemiologic studies suggest that EBV enters the oropharynx through salivary transfer. It multiplies locally, presumably in epithelial cells of the buccal mucosa or those of the salivary glands. This initial cycle of replication leads to the death of infected cells in the oropharynx and may contribute to the sore throat and exudative pharyngitis of IM. The local lymphatics are probably next invaded, and it is in these lymphoid tissues (Waldeyer's ring) that B lymphocytes are infected. The virus then spreads through the bloodstream to the liver, spleen, and other organs. A variety of lymphocytes is involved in limiting the continuous proliferation of infected B cells, such as suppressor T cells and natural killer cells. A detailed description of the immunology of IM is beyond the scope of this chapter; a good treatise on this subject can be found in the review by Sullivan [12].

Clinical manifestations

In the toddler and young child, primary infection with EBV is either asymptomatic or characterized by minor episodes of upper respiratory infection, diarrhea, pharyngitis, low-grade fever, otitis media, rash, adenopathy, and hepatosplenomegaly. In the adolescent and young adult, the more classical illness may be seen. The incubation period is usually 30 to 50 days. A prodrome of 3 to 5 days' duration may occur and is characterized by mild headache, malaise, and fatigue. Sore throat occurs in the first week of illness in about 85 percent of cases. Pharyngitis, uvular edema, palatal petechiae, and tonsillitis with an accompanying gray exudate may be seen. High fever sometimes lasts for as long as 10 days, followed by gradual lysis over a period of 7 to 10 days. Occasionally low-grade fever will persist for weeks. Generalized lymphadenopathy of gradual onset is the hallmark of IM. Cervical lymph nodes are the most commonly involved, but enlargement of almost any group is possible. The nodes are usually single, firm and tender, 2 to 4 cm in diameter, and not matted. Splenomegaly is seen in about 50 percent of patients in the second to third week of illness. Hepatomegaly and hepatic tenderness are seen in about 10 percent of patients, while overt jaundice is seen in less than 5 percent. Central nervous system (CNS) syndromes such as aseptic meningitis, encephalitis, acute psychosis, coma, transverse myelitis, acute cerebellar syndrome, Bell's palsy, infectious polyneuritis, and the Guillain-Barré syndrome have been described. Complications of a hematologic nature include hemolytic anemia and thrombocytopenia [8].

Rash

In cases of IM that are well documented clinically and serologically, the incidence of dermatitis is 3 to 19 percent [13–17]. The rash, when present, is usually located on the trunk and arms; rarely it may present solely as a palmar dermatitis [18]. It appears during the first few days of illness, lasts 1 to 6 days, and is described as being erythematous, macular, and papular, or morbilliform. Sometimes urticarial or scarlatiniform eruptions are seen [16,17,19]. Occasionally, cold-induced urticaria [20,21] and acrocyanosis [22] may be associated with IM. Rarely the rash may be petechial, vesicular, or hemorrhagic, but other more common and more serious causes of such rashes should be sought before they are ascribed to IM.

In 1967, Pullen, Wright and Murdoch [23] and Patel [24] nearly simultaneously observed an increased incidence of skin rashes in IM patients given ampicillin. The copper-colored rash begins 5 to 10 days after the drug is begun, mainly over the trunk. It then develops into an extensive, generalized (including the palms and soles) macular and papular pruritic eruption. It can last up to a week, with desquamation persisting for several more days. At its peak, the rash is confluent over exposed areas and pressure points and more marked over extensor surfaces. A faint macular rash is sometimes seen on the palatal and buccal mucosae. The incidence of this rash is greater than that of either nonantibiotic-associated dermatitis in IM or hypersensitivity to ampicillin. This rash may also be seen with ampicillin derivatives, such as amoxicillin [25–27] and other penicillins, such as methicillin [28]. Fortunately this rash does not represent a long-lasting hypersensitivity to ampicillin; the drug may be used again once the IM has subsided [29].

In 1982, Konno et al [30] described an association between infantile papular acrodermatitis (IPS) and EBV infection. The rash of IPS is distinctive and consists of firm 2- to 4-mm bright red papules distributed symmetrically over the face, limbs, and buttocks, lasting 20 days or more. Although IPS is usually associated with primary hepatitis B infection, confirmatory reports of IPS caused by EBV have appeared subsequently, but are based on serologic evidence only [31].

Eyelid edema

Eyelid edema may be seen in as many as 50 percent of all IM patients early in the disease. It may be difficult to appreciate unless the examiner is familiar with the patient's normal appearance, or it is pointed out by the patient or his family [17].

Oral lesions

Petechiae appear on the palate between the fifth and seventeenth days of illness in 2 to 25 percent of IM patients [13,15,17]. Six to 20 lesions are usually seen, grouped for the most part at the juncture of the hard and soft palate. They usually become brownish in color within 2 days of their appearance and then fade.

Laboratory findings

Hematologic changes

During the first week of illness the leukocyte count may be normal or decreased. By the second week, however, leukocytosis is commonplace and is accompanied by an absolute lymphocytosis, usually with greater than 10 percent atypical lymphocytes. Occasionally, thrombocytopenia and hemolytic anemia may be seen in the early weeks of illness [8].

Antibody responses

The heterophile antibodies were the first serologic markers discovered that could reasonably confirm the diagnosis of

Table 198-1   Heterophile antibody reactions in normal and IM sera

In the presence of:	Agglutination of sheep red blood cells after absorption with:	
	Guinea pig kidney cells	Beef red blood cells
Some normal human sera	−	+
Most IM sera	+	−

IM. Heterophile antibody tests are still used more frequently than any of the virus-specific assays. Most sera of patients with IM will cause sheep red blood cells to agglutinate after they have been absorbed with guinea pig kidney antigens, but not after absorption with beef red blood cells. The reverse is often true of normal sera (see Table 198-1). The heterophile antibody responsible for this differential absorption in IM patients has been shown to be principally of the IgM class, appears during the first or second week of illness, and disappears gradually over 3 to 6 months. The mechanism by which these antibodies develop is unknown. Several slide or spot tests have been developed which employ variations on the heterophile antibody detection technique for testing sera.

Specific antibodies to several EBV antigens appear during the acute disease or in convalescence in a specific sequence. Both IgM and IgG antibodies to the viral capsid antigen (VCA) are present at the onset of systemic illness and peak after 2 to 3 weeks; the VCA IgG antibodies persist for life. Antibodies to the EBV early antigens, which appear to be a complex of viral polymerases and other enzymes associated with viral replication, are present in 80 percent of recently infected persons and wane over a period of 2 to 6 months. Antibodies to the nuclear antigen of EBV (EBNA) begin to appear in a minority of patients in the third or fourth week of illness; virtually all late convalescent sera contain antibodies to EBNA. The diagnosis of acute IM or primary EBV infections is often based on the presence of both IgM and IgG antibody to VCA and the absence of antibody to EBNA [8].

Miscellaneous

Other laboratory findings frequently associated with IM include elevated liver enzymes and increased levels of IgM and IgG. The presence of cold agglutinins, cryoglobulins, and rheumatoid factor may be associated with the cold-induced urticaria and acrocyanosis that are occasionally seen in the disease. A false-positive biologic test for syphilis may also be observed [8].

Pathology

Because IM is generally a benign illness, pathologic studies have usually been limited to biopsy specimens, generally of lymph nodes or liver. Only rarely has autopsy material been available. Most of the pathologic changes consist of hyperplasia of lymphoid tissue. In some cases of IM the architectural patterns of the lymph nodes and liver are so distorted by the infiltrating lymphocytes that the pattern resembles that seen in leukemia or lymphoma. Occasionally the skin, heart, lungs, and digestive, genitourinary, and central nervous systems may be involved similarly. The lungs may show either a consolidated or an interstitial infiltrate. The histology of all other affected organs reveals infiltrates consisting mainly of both normal-appearing and atypical lymphocytes [32].

Diagnosis

The diagnosis of IM is usually based on the clinical picture and a characteristic heterophile agglutination pattern. However, 10 to 15 percent of patients with classic IM who develop specific EBV antibodies during the course of their illness are heterophile antibody negative; in such cases, viral-specific serologic testing may be necessary. Invasive diagnostic procedures such as lymph node, liver, or bone marrow biopsies are only necessary to rule out a malignancy if the clinical findings suggest such a process [8].

Treatment

As yet there is no specific treatment for IM. None of the antiviral chemotherapeutic agents, such as adenine arabinoside or acyclovir, which are effective against a limited number of other herpesvirus infections, have been shown to be useful for routine infections due to EBV. Therefore, treatment is entirely symptomatic. Aspirin, saline gargles, and codeine can provide short-term relief for the severe tonsillitis and cervical adenitis that are seen. Short courses of steroids have been used when the tonsillar enlargement is severe and respiratory embarrassment is imminent. They have also been recommended by some to treat other complications of the disease such as hemolytic anemia, thrombocytopenia, and those involving the CNS.

The amount of physical activity permitted should be determined on an individual basis. Contact sports must be prohibited in the face of splenic enlargement. Ampicillin should be avoided whenever possible because of the rash it may precipitate. Pharyngitis should be treated with antibiotics only if the throat culture is positive for group A beta-hemolytic streptococci [8].

Course and prognosis

The prognosis of IM is generally excellent, even in cases where the malaise persists for weeks. Rarely, splenic rupture, infectious polyneuritis and other neurologic symptoms, laryngeal edema, myocarditis, or hemorrhage may complicate the course. In patients with the X-linked lymphoproliferative syndrome and others in whom the immunologic response to EBV is blunted or aberrant, IM can be fatal [8,12].

References

1. Pfeiffer E: Drüsenfieber. *Jahrb Kinderheilkd* **29**:257, 1889
2. Sprunt TP, Evans FA: Mononuclear leukocytosis in reaction to acute infections (in infectious mononucleosis). *Bull Johns Hopkins Hosp* **31**:410, 1920
3. Paul JR, Bunnell WW: The presence of heterophile antibodies in infectious mononucleosis. *Am J Med Sci* **183**:91, 1932
4. Davidsohn I, Walker PH: The nature of heterophile antibodies in infectious mononucleosis. *Am J Clin Pathol* **5**:455, 1935
5. Epstein MA et al: Virus particles in cultured lymphoblasts from Burkitt's lymphoma. *Lancet* **1**:702, 1964
6. Henle G et al: Relation of Burkitt's tumor-associated herpes-type virus to infectious mononucleosis. *Proc Natl Acad Sci USA* **59**:94, 1968
7. Niederman JC et al: Infectious mononucleosis: clinical manifestations in relation to EB virus antibodies. *JAMA* **203**:205, 1968
8. Schooley RT, Dolin R: Epstein-Barr virus (infectious mononucleosis), in *Principles and Practice of Infectious Diseases,* edited by GL Mandell et al. New York, John Wiley & Sons, 1979, pp 1324–1341, and references therein
9. Lemon SM et al: Replication of EBV in epithelial cells during infectious mononucleosis. *Nature* **268**:268, 1977
10. Sixbey JW et al: Epstein-Barr virus replication in oropharyngeal epithelial cells. *N Engl J Med* **310**:1255, 1984
11. Gerber P et al: Transformation and chromosome changes induced by Epstein-Barr virus in normal human leukocyte cultures. *Proc Natl Acad Sci USA* **63**:740, 1969
12. Sullivan JC: Epstein-Barr virus and the X-linked lymphoproliferative syndrome, in *Advances in Pediatrics,* edited by LA Barness. Chicago, Year Book Medical Publishers, 1984, p 365
13. Paul JR: Infectious mononucleosis. *Bull NY Acad Med* **15**:43, 1939
14. Contratto AN: Infectious mononucleosis: a study of one hundred and ninety-six cases. *Arch Intern Med* **73**:449, 1944
15. Milne J: Infectious mononucleosis. *N Engl J Med* **233**:727, 1945
16. Press JH et al: Infectious mononucleosis: a study of 96 cases. *Ann Intern Med* **22**:546, 1945
17. McCarthy JT, Hoagland RJ: Cutaneous manifestations of infectious mononucleosis. *JAMA* **187**:153, 1964
18. Petrozzi JW: Infectious mononucleosis manifesting as a palmar dermatitis. *Arch Dermatol* **104**:207, 1971
19. Cowdrey SC, Reynolds JS: Acute urticaria in infectious mononucleosis. *Ann Allergy* **27**:182, 1969
20. Tyson CJ, Czarny D: Cold-induced urticaria in infectious mononucleosis. *Med J Aust* **1**:33, 1981
21. Barth JH: Infectious mononucleosis (glandular fever) complicated by cold agglutinins, cold urticaria and leg ulceration. *Acta Derm Venereal (Stockh)* **61**:451, 1981
22. Dickerman JD et al: Infectious mononucleosis initially seen as cold-induced acrocyanosis: association with auto-anti-M and anti-I antibodies. *Am J Dis Child* **134**:159, 1980
23. Pullen H et al: Hypersensitivity reactions to antimicrobial drugs in infectious mononucleosis. *Lancet* **2**:1176, 1967
24. Patel BM: Skin rash with infectious mononucleosis and ampicillin. *Pediatrics* **40**:910, 1967
25. Mulroy R: Amoxycillin rash in infectious mononucleosis (letter). *Br Med J* **1**:554, 1973
26. Glennie HR: Pivampicillin (ampicillin) and infectious mononucleosis (letter). *NZ Med J* **78**:222, 1973
27. Morris J: Infectious-mononucleosis rash after Talampicillin (letter). *Lancet* **1**:423, 1976
28. Fields DA: Methicillin rash in infectious mononucleosis (letter). *West J Med* **133**:521, 1980
29. Nazareth I et al: Ampicillin sensitivity in infectious mononucleosis—temporary or permanent? *Scand J Infect Dis* **4**:229, 1972
30. Konno M et al: A possible association between hepatitis-B antigen-negative infantile papular acrodermatitis and Epstein-Barr virus infection. *J Pediatr* **101**:222, 1982
31. Iosub S et al: Papular acrodermatitis with Epstein-Barr virus infection. *Clin Pediatr (Phila)* **23**:33, 1984
32. Custer R, Smith EB: The pathology of infectious mononucleosis. *Blood* **3**:830, 1948

Bibliography

Evans AS: *Viral Infections of Humans,* 2d ed. New York, Plenum, 1982

Mandell GR et al: *Principles and Practice of Infectious Diseases.* New York, John Wiley & Sons, 1979

CHAPTER 199

KAWASAKI DISEASE

Richard H. Meade III

Mucocutaneous lymph node syndrome, a descriptive phrase still in use, was the first name for the disorder now called Kawasaki disease or Kawasaki syndrome. It is named for Dr. Kawasaki who was the first to write about it, and whether it should be called a disease or a syndrome is debated. The fact that there is no known cause has led members of the Centers for Disease Control to recommend use of the word syndrome. Because it can be lethal and can produce quite severe and disabling manifestations, it seems appropriate to this author to call it a disease and this word will be used in the discussion that follows.

It was first reported in 1967 [1]; a total of 50 cases had been seen and it was believed to be a new disease. Over 20,000 cases have been seen in Japan since then. During the years that followed the first report it was seen in Hawaii [2], in Canada [3], and in Greece [4] in 1975. The first report from the continental United States was in 1976 [5] but was about cases seen in 1972 that had not at first been recognized. While at first it appeared that this was a new disease, there is now evidence that it may not be. One report dates back to 1870 and concerns a child who died of what was thought to be scarlet fever complicated by pneumonia and meningitis. At autopsy three aneurysms involving his coronary arteries were seen, ranging in size from 4 mm to 1.5 cm [6].

The cause is unknown but a number of possible causes have been discussed. An early suggestion was leptospirosis because antibody was present in one patient [7]. Others have searched unsuccessfully for this antibody [8]. In another study a fourfold rise in *Coxiella burnetii* antibody in a 9-month-old girl suggested Q fever [9]. The child had no antibodies to *Mycoplasma,* psittacosis, adenovirus, respiratory syncytial virus, influenza a, b, and c, parainfluenza virus 1 and 2, measles, mumps, herpes zoster, herpes simplex, cytomegalovirus, or EB virus. The list of negative results is long but the evidence for Q fever is only an antibody elevation in a patient with another disease. The authors point out that others have looked unsuccessfully for this antibody. They also cite another paper referring to the presence of rickettsia-like particles in children with the disease [10]. A child treated at Johns Hopkins Hospital had Rocky Mountain spotted fever antibody in association with Kawasaki disease but the authors did not attempt to show that the *Rickettsia* was responsible [11].

Of interest is the recent report of an association between exposure to rugs being cleaned and the development of Kawasaki disease. In one study 48 percent of the children had such an exposure, which was far larger than in a control population. The fact that over half were not exposed should make the relationship dubious [12]. Related to rugs, and possibly more significant, is the observation of mite-associated particles in children with the disease.

The possibility of a genetic predisposition has been considered and reports of different HLA antigens in patients have appeared. In a Japanese study HLA Bw22 was found

to be more common in patients than in controls [13]. In an American study one HLA B5 was found in patients and not in controls [14]. The antigen was found in 30 percent of patients and in only 4.9 percent of controls. The difference is significant but the number is not very large. Efforts to relate the disease to immunologic reactions have been published, showing that immune complexes were found in significantly greater abundance in patients than in controls [15].

Because the cause of Kawasaki disease is unknown, a list of criteria has been used to establish the diagnosis. There are six altogether, and it is considered necessary to have five of the different manifestations to allow the diagnosis to be made. The criteria are as follows:

1. *Fever.* Fever must be present for at least 5 days. There is no specified height. Some feel that antibiotic use should have been attempted to show that there was no response. Most patients get treated since in the beginning there may be only fever, or fever and enlarged cervical nodes.
2. *Conjunctival injection* (Fig. 199-1). Almost all patients have this and may have only a few dilated conjunctival vessels visible or there may be a great many. There is no exudate and the lids are not swollen. Uveitis occurs in up to 70 percent of children [16].
3. *Changes involving the lips and oral cavity.* The most common finding is reddening of the lips; there may be fissuring. The tongue may be swollen, reddened, and the papillae hypertrophied. A white coat is sometimes present (Fig. 199-2). the pharynx may be quite red and sometimes there are buccal mucosal ulcerations.
4. *Changes in the hands and feet* (Fig. 199-3). The palms and soles are often bright red early in the disease. A little later there can be swelling of the fingers and toes, often with a bluish tint to the skin. The entire hand or foot can be swollen and painful to use. During the second stage of the disease peeling of the fingertips or toes occurs. The rash need not have involved either hands or feet nor need it have been prolonged. Peeling can be confined to the tips of toes or fingers, but can involve the entire sole of the foot (Fig. 199-4). Peeling from other areas of the body occurs less often. After two or three months a transverse groove will appear crossing toenails or fingernails. There is only one per nail and it remains until the nail grows out.
5. *Polymorphous exanthema of the skin* (Figs. 199-5 to 199-9). A variable rash appears in almost every patient. It can be transient, lasting no more than a few days. It can be variable, looking like one type of eruption on one day and quite another on a later day.
6. *Lymph node enlargement* (Fig. 199-10). This is usually confined to nodes in the neck although others may be enlarged. The nodes can be large enough to be visible, but are often only palpably enlarged.

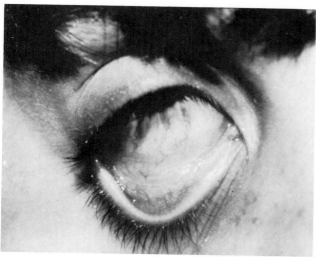

Fig. 199-1   Kawasaki disease. Severe conjunctivitis in a 15-year-old boy.

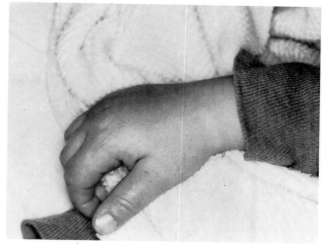

Fig. 199-3   Swollen, reddened hands in Kawasaki disease.

The disease is divided into two stages. In the first stage there is fever and all the manifestations of the disease appear. During the second stage fever begins to subside and the different visible abnormalities begin to subside as well. The rash fades, the eyes lose the conjunctival injection, the lips become normal, and the swelling of hands and feet disappears. The second stage can last for as long as a week and even longer as fever which had been sustained during the first phase begins to go down, but unevenly.

Clinical manifestations

The disease begins with fever in almost every case. There have been patients with other signs visible in whom fever was not high or even detected by a parent. In most cases, however, fever is the first abnormality seen. It is usually high and in the range of 40°C (104°F). There are no chills nor are there sweats. With the elevated temperature chil-

dren under the age of 4 become irritable. To be considered compatible with Kawasaki disease, fever must last for at least 5 days. It lasts no longer in a small number of cases but usually lasts for 10 to 14 days. In some, fever can be present for 8 weeks before it finally goes. Fever does not respond to antipyretic treatment. Confusion is created when a child is hospitalized, given aspirin, and found to be afebrile the next day. It is only when other children are seen whose fevers last for several weeks in spite of aspirin that it becomes clear that the temperature elevation is not responsive. Fever may be sustained at one level during much of the day, but can also fluctuate between nearly normal values and high levels during the course of the day. As the patient enters the second stage, fever often goes to normal for a day or two only to return and remain for another day before dropping once more. This up-and-down pattern can be repeated over the course of a week or 10 days.

Often with the onset of fever the doctor examining the child finds that the eardrum is red and presumes that otitis media is present. The drum is red, but it retains normal motility. It will not respond to antibiotic treatment, but

Fig. 199-2   Kawasaki disease. Strawberry tongue in second attack.

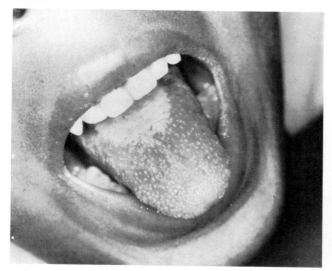

Fig. 199-4   Peeling in Kawasaki disease.

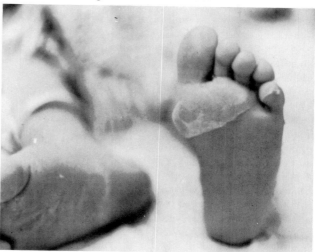

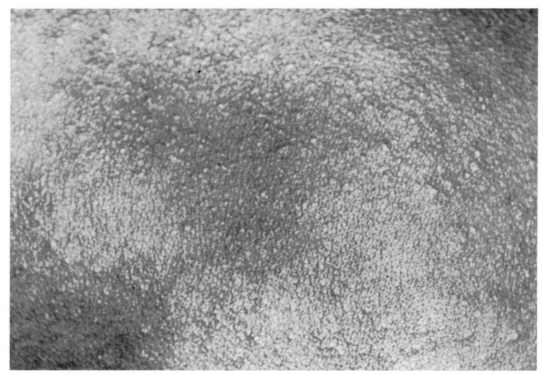

Fig. 199-5   Scarlatiniform rash in Kawasaki disease.

appears to improve when aspirin is given. The lesion is a myringitis, with inflammation similar to that of the eyes. Other children will have diarrhea which, with fever, leads to a diagnosis of gastroenteritis, a diagnosis that cannot be refuted by any means until other signs of Kawasaki disease appear. A third manifestation that can be present early in the course of the illness is a cough. This can be quite pronounced, and when a chest x-ray is obtained peribronchial cuffing is visible.

Following fever any of the following may appear. No one symptom is more likely to be first. Each manifestation is described separately but is not presented in order of occurrence.

Conjunctival injection is present in almost every patient. In some it is hardly visible since the vessels are not particularly prominent. It is often only because other signs are present and the diagnosis of Kawasaki disease under consideration that attention is given to this symptom. In others the injection is considerably more prominent. Vessels of both the bulbar and palpebral surfaces can be prominently inflamed. In a few there are perivascular hemorrhages.

Uveitis has been seen in up to 70 percent of patients [17]. There may be little visible and its presence is determinable only with a slit lamp. There can be considerable pain on exposure to light. A case was reported in which a retinal cotton-wool exudate was seen that, over the space of several months, enlarged so that it covered the optic disc [18]. Treatment with steroids was provided at this stage in the disease with no effect.

Mouth involvement is variable. The most common sign is reddening of the lips. This is easily seen in white-skinned children but is not so apparent in black, Hispanic, or Ori-

ental children. When the lips become fissured the change is obvious regardless of the color of the skin. Inside the mouth there may be a very red palate or pharynx. The tongue may be enlarged with hypertrophy of the papillae and a white coat on its surface. This looks exactly like the tongue in scarlet fever, and, as in that disease, the white coat disappears by receding posteriorly from the tip over the space of four days. What is left behind is a red tongue with enlarged papillae which has the appearance of the strawberry tongue of scarlet fever. The tongue does not become completely smooth as it does in scarlet fever. All that happens is that it returns to normal size and color and the papillae shrink back to their normal size. Small ulcerations can be seen on the inside of the cheek in some children. The mouth can be very obviously involved in many children but not all. Some have no visible abnormality of the lips, tongue, or throat.

The fourth manifestation involves changes in the hands and feet. In the very beginning the palms and soles can turn bright red. Their appearance is very striking. This change in color may occur with fever as the only accompanying sign and has often been the clue that made the diagnosis of Kawasaki disease seem likely. After a few days the fingers and toes are often swollen and occasionally they take on a bluish coloration. Sometimes, if the baby is small and plump, it is hard for the physician to see that swelling is present. The mother knows because shoes that fit the day before can no longer be put on. Children old enough to walk may complain of pain in the feet and usually if under two will refuse to walk. Older children continue walking but acknowledge discomfort. The hands and feet remain swollen during the first phase of the illness but resume normal size as the temperature begins to come

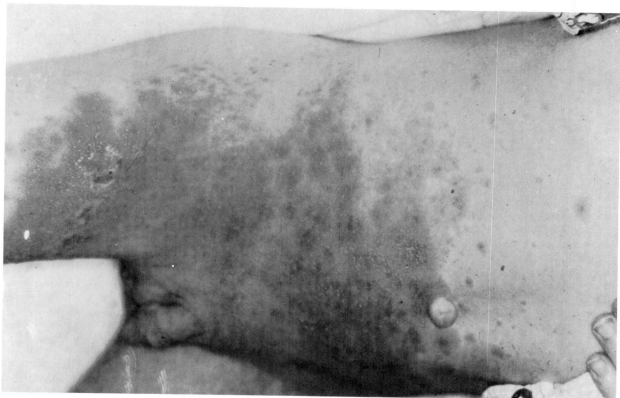

Fig. 199-6   Diaper area dermatitis in Kawasaki disease.

down. After the temperature has begun to decline, peeling appears. This is often confined to the finger and toe tips, and may be only on the feet. It may be considerably more extensive than the loss of only a few millimeters of skin and can involve the entire sole of the foot with a dense peel coming off in one piece from the heels to the toes. Peeling can occur elsewhere and has been seen on the face and on the trunk. Children with a diaper type skin eruption will often peel at the margins of the rash. Peeling is ordinarily superficial enough to produce no discomfort but may be deep enough in some children to leave a very uncomfortable denuded fingertip or palm. Various oily preparations with mineral oil, lanolin, or petrolatum are useful in relieving discomfort. Two or three months later the last

Fig. 199-7   Erythema multiforme-like eruption in Kawasaki disease.

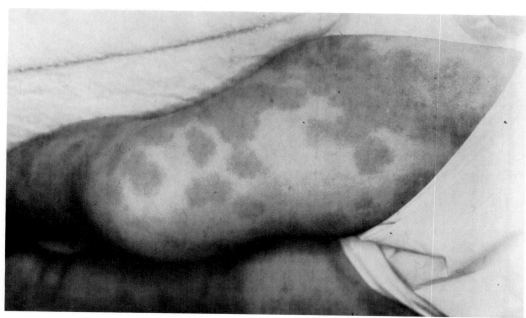

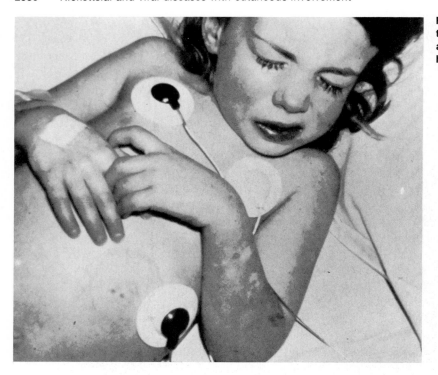

Fig. 199-8 Kawasaki disease. Typical eruption involving extremities and sparing trunk and also showing red lips and swollen hands.

event, the appearance of a transverse groove crossing the fingernail or toenail, occurs. Not all nails are involved; there may be only one, there are often two or three. The groove is narrow and less than a millimeter deep. There is no more than one and it goes as soon as the nail grows out.

The fifth manifestation is the skin eruption, of which there are many types. One type of eruption is a rash con-

fined to the diaper area. It is bright red and confluent. There are often lesions consisting of red papular spots on the knees or on the thighs. In one boy the lesions in the groin were accompanied by a very painful urethral inflammation. It was enough to make it hard for him to urinate. In one there were pustules superimposed on the red diaper area eruption. Both children developed peeling at the margins of the lesion. A second type of eruption seen during

Fig. 199-9   Pastia's lines in Kawasaki disease.

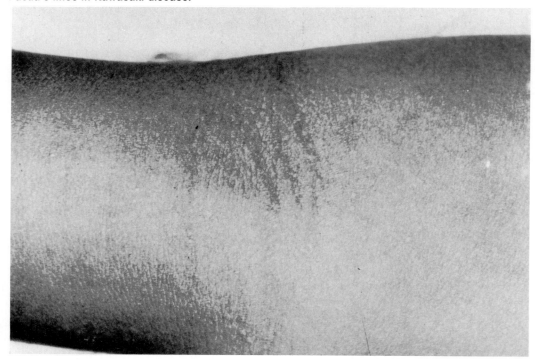

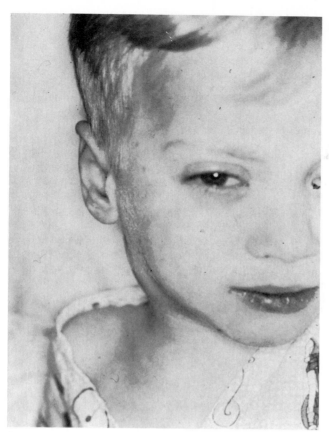

Fig. 199-10 Kawasaki disease. Cervical lymphadenitis causing bulge in the neck.

another season was one that looked like scarlet fever (Fig. 199-5). The rash was bright red with small follicles that could be palpated and produced a sensation of sandpaper. The creases of the antecubital fossa of the axilla and groin were purpuric as in Pastia's lines (Fig. 199-9). The face was not involved. What made it clear that the rash was not that of scarlet fever was the presence of conjunctival injection. But the rash in company with a strawberry tongue was identical with scarlet fever. A third eruption consists of the presence of large, rounded, brownish lesions that have been said to resemble the lesions of erythema multiforme (Fig. 199-7). To this author's eye the lesions are browner than those associated with erythema multiforme. In one child this eruption developed after she had presented with a red papular collection of lesions that resembled a viral exanthem. The child was sent home only to return a few days later with an almost ecchymotic eruption covering the trunk and involving the face as well. The lesions did not blanch on pressure and were densely scattered over the entire trunk. Another child had more circular lesions, some that had clear centers and central target spots. Peeling in both cases involved only the fingertips. The fourth eruption (Fig. 199-8) consists of broad red areas sharply demarcated from normal skin by a curving line. The lesions tend to be most prominent on the extremities. A fifth eruption is pustular. Lesions can be anywhere from the face to the trunk. The pustules are 3 to 4 mm in size and when opened and smeared they are seen to contain polymorphonuclear leukocytes. They do not drain nor do

they crust, although the overlying skin can dry and peel off.

The sixth manifestation can, like the discoloration of the palms and soles, appear early in the disease along with fever. This is cervical adenitis. It was seen in only half of Japanese children but was seen in 75 percent of children at a Boston hospital. The nodes are usually large enough to feel with ease and commonly can be so large they are seen to bulge out from the side of the neck (Fig. 199-10). Glands in other parts of the body are sometimes involved. Enlarged supraclavicular and axillary nodes are seen in some children, although this is not common. The node can be tender and when associated only with fever suggests the diagnosis of suppurative adenitis.

Visceral manifestations

A great deal more than the signs and symptoms of the six components of the diagnostic criteria are in progress in the patient with Kawasaki disease. Children under the age of four are irritable and unconsolable. Babies cry on what seems a continuous basis and sleep little and parents are rapidly exhausted. Occasionally babies sleep more than they normally do. Either type of behavior is a change from normal. Older children are not so affected and can be cheerful. About 25 percent of children have a stiff neck in association with irritability and when a lumbar puncture is done most will have evidence of an aseptic meningitis [19]. While the number of cells in the spinal fluid is greater than normal it is not very high. Counts ranging from 8 to 40 were seen in one series [19]. When there were no more than 8 cells the presence of 4 polymorphonculear leukocytes made the count abnormal. The sugar is normal and the protein is not elevated. Some children have combative behavior, suggesting encephalitis. Two of 25 children had a unilateral seventh cranial nerve palsy [19]. It lasted for only a week and no evidence of other cranial nerve involvement appeared.

Approximately 25 percent of children have a cough as part of the early symptoms of the disease. It may appear before much else is visible and is one of the reasons that Kawasaki disease has been attributed to a preceding viral disease. When an x-ray of the chest is taken, peribronchial cuffing is visible.

Abdominal symptoms are numerous. Ten to fifteen percent of children have right upper quadrant pain. There is tenderness to palpation which is the result of an enlarged gallbladder. Hydrops of the gallbladder develops in these children [20] and can be identified by ultrasound [21]. What is seen is an echo-free mass below the liver. In one case surgery was carried out and the cystic duct was found to be compressed by an enlarged node. In most other cases surgery is not required and the gallbladder returns to normal size within the space of a few days. While enlarged it can be associated with biliary obstruction, and jaundice has been seen in such children. Right upper quadrant pain can also be associated with hepatitis in which the liver is enlarged, tender, and accompanied by jaundice and elevated liver enzymes. Some patients have been admitted because of the jaundice and the impression was that they had hepatitis. Midepigastric pain is seen in a small number of children who have evidence of pancreatitis provided by an elevated amylase. A final intraabdominal disorder is paralytic ileus. This is a cause of abdominal distension and severe pain that can persist for as long as 5 or 6 days. The child is unable to eat and is in a great deal of pain that can be difficult to relieve except with narcotic agents.

Renal involvement is not accepted by all writers. It was pointed out in one study that when children with abnormal urinary sediment were catheterized, specimens of urine were obtained that contained no white or red cells [22]. The authors presumed from this that the abnormality seen was a result of urethritis. In this author's own experience changes were found that could not be explained on the basis of urethral inflammation [19]. Red cell casts were seen in some and in two children there was elevation of the BUN and creatine. The most likely explanation is a renal cortical vasculitis.

Most troublesome of all is the cardiovascular disease associated with Kawasaki disease. In this author's experience with patients seen during an outbreak, 66 percent of the children had one lesion or another as determined by electrocardiography or two-dimensional echocardiography. The lesions were not all serious and most were asymptomatic and only transiently present. Coronary artery involvement was seen in three (12 percent) and consisted of aneurysm formation in two and arterial occlusion in one. Myocarditis was present in the remainder with pericardial effusion in six (24 percent). Evidence for myocarditis was in the form of inverted T waves on electrocardiography and evidence of impaired ventricular motion by echocardiography. Arrhythmias were present in six patients with myocarditis. In seven there was ventricular hypertrophy. One patient with coronary aneurysm formation had only one artery involved. Another patient had three arteries with extensive aneurysms which involved most of each vessel. In this child aneurysms of the iliac and femoral arteries were present as well. In other patients aneurysms have been found in such other arteries as the hepatic artery; in one patient [23] the artery ruptured with extensive but not fatal intrahepatic bleeding. In an infant with coronary occlusion there were both clinical and laboratory signs of infarction. The child was 2 years old and arrived in the hospital clutching his chest much the way an adult would at the time of severe angina. His EKG showed deep Q waves, and he had a markedly elevated CPK. Unlike adults with a myocardial infarction the child was in pain for no more than a day and after 5 days had a normal electrocardiogram. Dilatation of the coronary arteries also occurs and is generally regarded as a benign effect. In one such patient, however, dilatation preceded aneurysm formation.

Autopsy studies of the heart show a vascular inflammatory lesion consisting of an infiltrate of polymorphonuclear cells plus lymphocytes extending from the perivascular space into the adventitia [24,25]. In addition to the infiltration of inflammatory cells there is edema. These changes are present in both the coronary arteries and in the myocardium as well. Endocarditis of the mitral and tricuspid valves has been described [26]. Most patients with coronary artery aneurysms recover and redevelop what appears to be a normal vascular channel. This is the result of intimal proliferation with filling in of the cavity produced by aneurysmal swelling. The vessel is now greatly thickened but within its walls a normal vascular channel has been reproduced [25]. While the muscularis remains damaged, the danger of rupture has been reduced.

Laboratory abnormalities associated with Kawasaki disease

While a number of abnormalities have been described as being present in patients with Kawasaki disease, they are neither diagnostic nor proof of the presence or absence of the disease. Patients with full-blown disease satisfying every criterion for clinical diagnosis have had normal blood values for white count and sedimentation rate and platelet count. In most cases, however, the laboratory findings are helpful in confirming doubtful cases in which the clinical findings are not so clear that diagnosis is easily established. The rash, for example, may be present only briefly, the fever may be present for no more than 5 days, and changes in the mouth and eyes are not very definite. In these cases a platelet count of a million, a white count of 20,000 with a shift to the left, and a sedimentation rate of 75 are helpful in making a diagnosis. One child had only a brief rash, mild but definite conjunctival injection, and prolonged fever. There were no other signs. She developed a platelet count of over a million, peeled from the fingertips, and had a pericardial effusion. She did not have enough criteria to support the diagnosis, but had other findings including laboratory abnormalities that confirmed it. Most of the time the white count is over 18,000 [19] and most patients have an elevated number of polymorphonuclear leukocytes, an elevated sedimentation rate, and an elevated platelet count. This last is usually elevated a little above normal when the child arrives in the hospital and over the course of the next 10 to 14 days it rises. This author has seen levels of 1,600,000 and has read of far higher numbers. It was pointed out at one time that elevated levels of IgE were present and this was regarded as a valuable laboratory tool in making the diagnosis. IgE is not always elevated and is normal in children even in the presence of coronary vasculitis. Elevated liver enzymes are present in a number of patients but not in all, and bilirubin values have been found to be elevated in some. Neither of these findings helps make the diagnosis of Kawasaki disease; they help only in defining the presence of liver involvement. A laboratory test that has been of value is the determination of the serum albumin content [19]. In all patients observed in one hospital, when the serum albumin was at a level of 3.2 g% or less there was evidence of carditis. Cardiac abnormalities were present in a few patients with normal values, but in all those with low serum albumins evidence of carditis was present. In a number of cases the low serum albumin was observed before echocardiographic abnormalities occurred.

The most intriguing laboratory abnormalities were demonstrated by Drs. Geha and Leung [27]. Abnormalities in both B- and T-cell lymphocyte function were documented. The number of helper T cells was increased, the number of suppressor T cells was decreased below the number found in control subjects. B lymphocytes when cultured were found to be secreting both IgG and IgM antibodies without stimulation. T cells were found to be cytotoxic to human fibroblasts. It was found that the supernatant fluid taken from suspensions of lymphocytes contained a substance that stimulated even normal B cells to form antibody.

It has been emphasized that there should be no evidence of other infection in patients with Kawasaki disease since a number of bacteria or viruses could be considered to be the cause of the rash or other signs of Kawasaki disease. Since the rash can resemble that of scarlet fever it would be important to have no streptococci on culture of the throat and to have no antibody in the serum. It is, however, possible to have two diseases concurrently or sequentially. Patients with Kawasaki disease will, in some cases, have elevated E-B virus antibody titers, or elevated ASLO antibody titers but have no evidence either of infectious mononucleosis or of streptococcal infection.

Unusual forms of Kawasaki disease

A number of patients have been seen with unusual manifestations of Kawasaki disease. Four of them will be described to indicate how varied the disease can be.

A 15-month-old girl had been sick for a month before she arrived in the hospital. She had had fever and attacks of what had been thought of as otitis media and bronchitis. Recurrent fever, rash, lymph node enlargement, and unusual appearance led the mother to seek additional help. The baby was unusual in appearance because of edema involving not only the hands and feet but also the arms and legs and the face as well. She was febrile, had a rash, conjunctivitis, and red lips. She had a right facial palsy, and when the lumbar puncture was done it was found that there were 40 cells in her spinal fluid. Over the course of the next several weeks it was found that she had a pericardial effusion, aneurysms of all her coronary arteries and of the femoral and iliac arteries as well. She became hypertensive and required propranolol treatment for control. It took four weeks in the hospital before her temperature began to remain in a normal range, for her serum albumin, which had fallen to 2.3 g, to begin to rise, for edema to begin to recede, and the platelet count of 1,600,000 to begin to return to normal. Finally the echocardiogram showed stabilization of the coronary artery aneurysms and after several more weeks she was allowed to go home. Over the course of 4 months the aneurysms began to heal and in time there was no remainder.

A girl of 34 months was sent to the hospital with the diagnosis of hemolytic uremic syndrome. She had fever and severe diarrhea. She was found to have a low platelet count and, on smear of her blood, schistocytes were seen. Both creatinine and BUN values were elevated. On arrival she was found to have a platelet count of 54,000. X-ray showed "fingerprinting" of the bowel mucosa. Schistocytes and helmet cells were seen on stained smear of her peripheral blood and, in the urine, red and white cells were present with granular casts. She was disoriented and combative and a spinal fluid analysis showed 12 white cells (3 polys, 9 lymphocytes) and her EEG was abnormal. The impression she gave to everyone when she arrived was of hemolytic uremic syndrome. Over the next several days she developed a petechial skin eruption, enlarged cervical nodes, conjunctivitis, and red lips. The diagnosis of Kawasaki disease was based on these findings plus the fact that her finger peeled a week later and her platelet count rose to over 600,000. While she had many features of hemolytic uremic syndrome, they cleared far more rapidly than in other children and it seems more likely that she had only Kawasaki disease.

A boy of 10 years was hospitalized because of what was thought to be resistant suppurative cervical lymphadenitis. Lymph node swelling and fever had not responded to an-

tibiotics given before admission. When he arrived he had an erythema multiforme type of skin eruption consisting of brown, circular lesions covering the trunk, many with central clearing and target spots. He had conjunctival injection with multiple perivascular circular hemorrhages. His systolic blood pressure was 70 and he had an S3 gallop rhythm. His heart was enlarged. His laboratory work showed a BUN of 37, creatinine of 1.7 mg%, and a platelet count of only 87,000. His serum albumin was 2.4 g and he had shifting pleural effusions as seen on chest x-ray. Treatment with dopamine, furosemide, and digoxin was provided during the first day with rapid improvement over the course of 24 h. His platelet count went to 623,000 during the course of an uneventful recovery. He was the second case to be seen with a low platelet count at the time of arrival.

The fourth patient was a $5\frac{1}{2}$-year-old boy who had had Kawasaki disease 2 years before. He was admitted with what was thought to be scarlet fever that had not responded to oral penicillin. He had a classical rash, with Pastia's lines, a strawberry tongue (Figs. 199-2 and 199-9) and large cervical nodes. Intravenous penicillin was given and soon after arrival he began to peel in what was thought to be a classic way for scarlet fever. Fever persisted and was accompanied by abdominal pain and distension due to paralytic ileus and hydrops of the gallbladder. Kawasaki disease was recognized as the cause of his disease a second time when a coronary aneurysm was found by echocardiography.

Treatment

No specific form of treatment is available. What is done for the patient is to provide what is hoped will be protection against coronary occlusion caused by platelet aggregation. Aspirin in a dose of 30 mg/kg of body weight is used in 4 daily doses. It is used during the first and second stages of the disease and is later reduced to one baby (85-mg) aspirin tablet daily. The similarity between this disease and polyarteritis nodosa led initially to the employment of steroids. In one study 1.5 mg/kg of prednisolone was administered to 17 patients, 11 of whom (64.7 percent) developed coronary aneurysms [28]. Aspirin in a dose of 30 mg/kg was given to 36 patients, 4 of whom (11 percent) developed aneurysms. Antibiotics were given to 20, of whom 5 developed aneurysms. The antibiotic was cephalexin and the incidence of aneurysms was not statistically larger than in the aspirin group. Both groups were associated with aneurysms significantly less often than were those given prednisone. The effect of aspirin on symptoms is minor. It does not reduce fever and has only modest effect on irritability. Fever lasts a variable time and one can be confused by seeing the temperature fall the day after aspirin is begun. Seeing other patients maintain fever for several weeks despite aspirin, however, makes its lack of effect clear. It is useful for the relief of joint pain.

Kawasaki disease has been regarded as a disease of children for a number of years, but an increasing number of adults are being seen [29,30]. This author has seen a young man of 22 with the disease and has spoken to a 45-year-old physician who was convinced he had the disease. It seems likely that as the number of cases seen increases so too will the number of adults. It is probable that Kawasaki disease is a lot more common than is now believed because there must be patients with the disease who do not satisfy all the diagnostic criteria. When the cause is found and a method for diagnosis established it is likely that it will be found to be more common than is now suspected.

References

1. Kawasaki T: MCLS—clinical observation of 50 cases. *Jpn J Allergy* **16**:178, 1967
2. Kawasaki T et al: A new infantile acute febrile mucocutaneous lymph node syndrome (MLNS) prevailing in Japan. *Pediatrics* **54**:271, 1974
3. Wentworth P, Silver MD: Fatal mucocutaneous lymph node syndrome in Canada. *Can Med Assoc J* **115**:299, 1976
4. Valaes T: Mucocutaneous lymph node syndrome in Athens, Greece (letter). *Pediatrics* **55**:295, 1975
5. Brown JJ et al: Mucocutaneous lymph node syndrome in the continental United States. *Pediatrics* **88**:81, 1976
6. Aterman K: A possible early example of mucocutaneous lymph node syndrome. *Pediatrics* **92**:1027, 1978
7. Humphrey T et al: Leptosporosis mimicking MLNS. *J Pediatr* **91**:853, 1977
8. Ohtaki C et al: Leptos viral antibody and MLNS. *J Pediatr* **93**:896, 1978
9. Swaby ED et al: Is Kawasaki disease a variant of Q fever? *Lancet* **1**:146, 1980
10. Hamashima Y et al: Rickettsia-like bodies in infantile acute, febrile mucocutaneous lymph node syndrome. *Lancet* **2**:42, 1973
11. Headings DL, Santosham M: Kawasaki disease associated with serologic evidence of Rocky Mountain spotted fever. *Johns Hopkins Med J* **149**:220, 1981
12. Patriarca PA et al: Kawasaki syndrome: association with the application of rug shampoo. *Lancet* **2**:578, 1982
13. Kato S et al: HLA antigen in Kawasaki disease. *Pediatrics* **61**:252, 1978
14. Krensky AM et al: HLA antigens in mucocutaneous lymph node syndrome in New England. *Pediatrics* **67**:741, 1981
15. Weindling AM et al: Circulating immune complexes in mucocutaneous lymph node syndrome (Kawasaki disease). *Arch Dis Child* **54**:241, 1979
16. Ohno S et al: Ocular manifestations of Kawasaki disease (mucocutaneous lymph node syndrome). *Am J Ophthalmol* **93**:713, 1982
17. Germain BF et al: Anterior uveitis in Kawasaki disease. *Pediatrics* **97**:780, 1980
18. Verghote M et al: An uncommon sign in mucocutaneous lymph node syndrome. *Acta Paediatr Scand* **70**:591, 1981
19. Meade RH III, Brandt L: Manifestations of Kawasaki disease in New England outbreak of 1980. *J Pediatr* **100**:558, 1982
20. Mofenson HC et al: Gallbladder hydrops. *NY State J Med* **80**:249, 1980
21. Magilavy DB et al: Mucocutaneous lymph node syndrome: report of two cases complicated by gallbladder hydrops and diagnosed by ultrasound. *Pediatrics* **61**:699, 1978
22. Dean AG et al: An epidemic of Kawasaki syndrome in Hawaii. *J Pediatr* **100**:552, 1982
23. Lipson MH et al: Ruptured hepatic artery aneurysm and coronary artery aneurysms with myocardial infarction in a 14 year old boy: new manifestations of mucocutaneous lymph node syndrome. *Pediatrics* **98**:936, 1981
24. Fujiwara H, Hamashima Y: Pathology of the heart in Kawasaki disease. *Pediatrics* **61**:100, 1978
25. Sasaguri Y, Kato H: Regression of aneurysms in Kawasaki disease: a pathological study. *Pediatrics* **100**:225, 1982
26. Kusakawa S, Heiner DC: Elevated serum IgE in acute febrile mucocutaneous lymph node syndrome. *Clin Res* **24**:180, 1976
27. Leung DYM et al: Immunoregulatory abnormalities in mucocutaneous syndrome. *Clin Immunol Immunopathol* **23**:100, 1982
28. Kato H et al: Kawasaki disease: effect of treatment on coronary artery involvement. *Pediatrics* **63**:175, 1979
29. Milgrom H et al: Kawasaki disease in a healthy young adult. *Ann Intern Med* **92**:467, 1980
30. Melish ME et al: Mucocutaneous lymph node syndrome in the United States. *Am J Dis Child* **130**:599, 1976

Section 29

Sexually transmitted diseases

CHAPTER 200

SEXUALLY TRANSMITTED DISEASES—AN OVERVIEW

Ernesto Gonzalez and Arthur R. Rhodes

Definition

The sexually transmitted diseases (STDs) comprise a large group of infections produced by different microorganisms including spirochetes, chlamydia, bacteria, mycoplasma, protozoa, fungi, parasites, and viruses (see Table 200-1) The traditional separation between major venereal diseases (such as syphilis, gonorrhea, chancroid, lymphogranuloma venereum, and granuloma inguinale) and the minor ones has become archaic since the sociocultural and economic impacts of some of the latter diseases have increased in recent years. The most common STD in England, for example, is a nonspecific urethritis produced by different organisms that can precipitate severe complications such as salpingitis, ectopic pregnancy, and sterility in females, and prostatitis, epididimitis, and even Reiter's disease in males [1]. Whereas the incidence of congenital and tertiary syphilis has diminished dramatically in recent years, the new generation of STDs has steadily increased not only in incidence, but also in severe complications, such as chlamydial pelvic inflammatory disease in females and pneumonia in newborns. Furthermore, response to drug therapy in many of the "minor" diseases has not been as predictable as in the "major" diseases.

Epidemiology

Of the 10 million cases of STD that occur annually in the United States, gonorrhea and nongonococcal urethritis, genital herpes, and syphilis are among the most common [2]. Although the number of reported cases of gonorrhea has decreased steadily since 1975, 960,633 new cases were reported in 1982 [3]. Syphilis continues to be the second most common reportable STD in the United States and the number of cases reported has increased each year since 1977 with primary and secondary cases totaling 33,613 in 1982 compared to 24,000 in 1976 [3]. Nongonococcal urethritis and genital herpes are nonreportable STDs in the United States and available data have to be extracted from other countries where these diseases are registered. In the United Kingdom, for example, the number of new cases of nongonococcal urethritis has increased from 105,210 in 1977 to 142,066 in 1982, an increase of 35 percent during this period (see Table 200-2) [4].

In the Genito-Infectious Disease Unit of the Massachusetts General Hospital, syphilis and gonorrhea accounted for 46 percent of all cases seen in 1982, while minor STDs accounted for 54 percent (see Table 200-3). The British surveillance system, on the other hand, showed that syphilis and gonorrhea accounted for only 22 percent of all notifiable STDs, while minor STDs comprised 50 percent (see Table 200-2) [4].

A strong case can be made for a comprehensive approach to the patient with a genitourinary complaint in view of the diversity of problems encountered in one venereal disease clinic setting [5]. Of 174 patients with minor STDs, dermatologic disease accounted for 70 percent of all problems; gonococcal balanitis, prostatitis, epididymitis, and pharyngitis also occurred with great frequency. Only 6.1 percent of patients had general medical problems, but these included potentially serious diseases—thyrotoxicosis, labial carcinoma, hepatitis, and sinusitis. In the same series, 13 percent of patients with suspected syphilis had gonococcal infections, and 4.6 percent (44) of patients with gonococcal infection had a second venereal disease—syphilis (21), trichomoniasis (12), moniliasis (7), and warts (4). About 37 percent of patients had either minor or nonvenereal disease. Of 56 men who sought care for a penile lesion, only 22 (39.2 percent) had syphilis.

A physician may feel comfortable in adequately treating

Table 200-1   Disorders and infectious agents associated with sexual transmission

Disorders caused by infectious agents:
  Nongonococcal urethritis
  Candidiasis
  Genital warts (condylomata acuminata)
  Trichomoniasis
  Genital herpes
  Molluscum contagiosum
  Cytomegalovirus infection
  Viral hepatitis type B
  Pubic lice
  Scabies
  Reiter's syndrome

Infectious agents causing various disorders:
  Corynebacterium vaginale
  Neisseria meningitides
  Protozoa and helminths: *Entamoeba histolytica,*
    Enterovirus vermicularis, Dientamoeba fragilis, Giardia
    lambia, Endolimax nana, Lobomoeba butschlii,
    Trypanosoma gambiense
  Other bacteria: *Salmonella* (typhoid fever), *Shigella,*
    Pseudomonas pseudomallei, Leptospira (leptospirosis)

a patient's gonorrhea or syphilis but may inadvertently allow a second "minor" disease to go untreated. On the other hand, the presence of a minor STD is important because its mode of acquisition increases the likelihood of coincidental syphilis and/or gonococcal infection. Blood tests for syphilis and appropriate cultures for gonorrhea are advisable for any individual with an STD. It should be recalled that social as well as sexual contact may allow

dissemination of minor STDs, and it may be impossible to predict the mode of transmission without a contact history and suspicion according to disease and age group.

The two most important events in the 1980s that focused attention on STDs were the recognition of a new disease called the acquired immunodeficiency syndrome (AIDS) and the linking of herpes progenitalis with cancer of the cervix. The impact that both events have had in the scientific community and the public compares with the mass hysteria produced by syphilis and leprosy during the biblical period. The effect has permeated epidemiologic reporting and precaution procedures in facilities providing care for AIDS patients; record keeping measures have had to be instituted in order to protect AIDS patients from being chastised and stigmatized. In addition, sexual and social practices have been altered drastically. In a Boston clinic caring for STD patients, with a prominent homosexual population, a 50 percent drop in attendance was recorded in the year that followed the widely publicized AIDS epidemic. The drop in attendance was presumably due to the reduction in sexual activity by this group, as well as the stigma generated by these new developments. Although the immediate aftermath of this medicosocial storm has died down with vigorous research and educational activities, for AIDS in particular, the effect of exposing such a vulnerable window in our sociocultural behavior will not be known for years to come.

Minor sexually transmitted diseases

Nongonococcal urethritis

The minor STDs have attained major prominence in the past 15 years. Nongonococcal urethritis (NGU), for example, has become the leading cause of urethritis among males in most developed countries. In STD clinics, it is estimated that up to 62 percent of urethritis cases in men have been identified as NGU [6]; in university student populations, NGU is 10 times more common than gonorrhea [7]. In England, where NGU is reportable, there were 2.4 cases of NGU in 1982 for each case of gonorrhea (see Table 200-2) [4]. In 1982, at the Massachusetts General

Table 200-2   Sexually transmitted diseases: reported new cases in 1977, 1980, 1982 in the United Kingdom*

Diagnosis	1977	1980	1982
Syphilis	4,780	4,443	3,929
Gonorrhea	65,963	60,850	58,782
Chancroid	49	65	137
Lymphogranuloma venereum	43	34	38
Granuloma inguinale	56	20	20
Nonspecific genital infection	105,210	125,476	142,066
Trichomoniasis	22,145	22,285	21,515
Candidiasis	41,144	48,060	56,126
Scabies	2,562	2,599	2,307
Pubic lice	6,769	8,928	10,900
Herpes simplex	8,399	10,780	14,836
Warts	26,063	31,780	37,334
Molluscum contagiosum	1,019	1,228	1,467
Other treponemal diseases	1,117	934	843
Other conditions requiring treatment	48,461	65,991	85,307
Other conditions not requiring treatment	104,539	117,070	127,234
Total new cases	438,319	500,543	562,841

* Modified from [4] (prepared by the Public Health Laboratory Service Communicable Disease Surveillance Centre and Communicable Disease [Scotland] Unit, with the assistance of the Academic Department of Genitourinary Medicine, Middlesex Hospital Medical School)

Table 200-3   Sexually transmitted diseases: reported new cases in 1977, 1980, 1982 in the Genito-Infectious Disease Unit of the Massachusetts General Hospital

Diagnosis	1977	1980	1982
Syphilis	125	83	79
Gonorrhea	1101	1085	976
Chancroid	1	—	—
Lymphogranuloma venereum	1	—	—
Granuloma inguinale	1	—	—
Nonspecific genital infection	934	1370	1481
Trichomoniasis	51	59	17
Candidiasis	239	340	236
Scabies	37	28	41
Pubic lice	83	100	101
Herpes simplex	213	151	223
Warts	159	139	111
Molluscum contagiosum	32	36	25
Total new cases	2977	3391	2290

Source: Pam Miles, R.N., Head Nurse GID Unit, Massachusetts General Hospital, Boston, MA.

Hospital Genito-Infectious Disease Unit, NGU accounted for 45 percent of clinic visits.

Nongonococcal urethritis may be viewed as a heterogeneous "group" of sexually transmitted infections primarily affecting males, for which no specific etiology was identified in 90 percent of cases prior to 1970. Since then, however, *Chlamydia trachomatis,* an obligate intracellular bacterium, has been established as the etiology in approximately 40 to 50 percent of cases [6,8]. The role of other etiologic agents in NGU is controversial, although studies using quantitative cultures and the response to antimicrobial agents with different activities against *Ureaplasma urealyticum* and *Chlamydia trachomatis* suggest that most cases of nonchlamydial nongonococcal urethritis are due to *U. urealyticum* [8]. In 10 to 20 percent of cases, however, the above organism cannot be identified, and the etiology remains unknown. Organisms that cause NGU infrequently, if ever, include *Corynebacterium vaginale, Trichomonas vaginalis, Candida* spp., *Herpes simplex,* cytomegalovirus, and certain commensal bacteria [9].

Concomitant infection with *Chlamydia trachomatis* is not infrequent among patients with gonococcal urethritis. This persistent urethritis following therapy for gonococcal urethritis is called *postgonococcal urethritis* (PGU), since the inflammation remains after treatment of gonococcal disease with penicillin, ampicillin, or spectinomycin. Between 19 and 29 percent of patients with gonococcal urethritis may have a double infection, and require treatment with a drug such as tetracyline, which covers both bacteria [6,10].

Evidence for sexual transmission of *Chlamydia* is provided by Holmes et al [6], who demonstrated a high yield of *Chlamydia* culture-positive female partners of patients with *Chlamydia*-positive NGU (14:21) compared with a low yield in female partners of *Chlamydia*-negative NGU (2:24, $p < 0.0001$). Compared to gonorrhea, NGU occurs more frequently in whites than in blacks, in men who have attained higher socioeconomic levels, and in men who have fewer sexual partners. NGU is also common in exclusively homosexual men [11].

The counterpart of NGU in females is referred to in England and Scandinavian countries as *nonspecific genital infection* (NSGI). The isolation rate of *Chlamydia trachomatis* in women attending venereal disease clinics in Sweden, for example, has varied from 16 to 38 percent while in women who were sexual contacts of men with known *Chlamydia* infection, *Chlamydia trachomatis* was isolated in 47 to 66 percent [10]. Conversely, Persson et al [12] demonstrated *Chlamydia trachomatis* in 5 percent of women consulting for general medical reasons and in 8 percent of women consulting for contraceptive advice.

The notoriety attained by NGU and NSGI in recent years is not due solely to an increasing incidence. Complications associated with *Chlamydia trachomatis* include formation of urethral strictures and acute epididymitis in men over 35 years of age [13,14], as well as endocarditis [15]; in females, complications include salpingitis and pelvic inflammatory disease. In Sweden, for example, it is estimated that 60 percent of cases of salpingitis may be due to *Chlamydia trachomatis* [16]. Transmission of *Chlamydia trachomatis* from an infected mother to the neonate may also occur during vaginal delivery, resulting in conjunctivitis [17]. Pneumonia has been reported in about 30 percent of children under six months of age infected with *Chlamydia trachomatis* during vaginal delivery.

Candidiasis

Vaginal candidiasis remains one of the most common gynecologic diseases in Europe and North America. In England, where this disease is notifiable, vaginal candidiasis is the third most common STD after nongonococcal urethritis and gonorrhea (see Table 200-2) [4]. Meanwhile, the frequency of candidiasis of the penis is about one-tenth that of the vagina [18].

The major epidemiologic and pathophysiologic factors involved in this infection are still not clear. *Candida* is commonly cultured from the vagina of asymptomatic women. Osborne cultured yeasts, mostly *C. albicans,* in vaginal specimens from 22 percent of asymptomatic college women [19]. The prevalence of *C. albicans* in genital sites in asymptomatic carriers is less than its prevalence in the mouth or rectum, suggesting that the gastrointestinal tract is the reservoir, and from there it spreads to the genitalia. About 48 to 75 percent of women with positive vaginal cultures also have positive stool cultures. With the introduction of methods for differentiation of individual *C. albicans* strains, it became evident that, in most of the cases, similar strains can be isolated from the mouth, anus, feces, and vagina, suggesting an endogenous source for *C. albicans.*

Candida may be transmitted sexually. Thin et al [20] demonstrated sexual transmission in 30 to 40 percent of cases of genital candidiasis. Ten percent of male contacts of females with vaginal yeast infections were noted to have *Candida* balanoposthitis [21], and the organism has been cultured from the semen in male partners of females with recurrent candidiasis [22]. Davidson [23] demonstrated that 80 percent of female contacts of yeast-positive males (from glans and foreskin) had yeast infection in contrast to 32 percent of contacts of yeast-negative males.

The fact that similar strains of *C. albicans* can be isolated from the genitalia of symptomatic and asymptomatic carriers and that *C. albicans* can be isolated from the vagina of asymptomatic carriers for up to four weeks [24] suggests that the change from commensal to pathogen is dependent on the host interaction with the yeast. So far, no one local or systemic factor has been identified to account for the change in the host–parasite interaction. However, several factors have been demonstrated to be important: high vaginal glycogen levels, low vaginal pH, and local occlusion with nylon underwear [18]. Pregnancy, and therapy with antibiotics, metronidazole, and systemic corticosteroids increase the risk for *Candida* infection. Metabolic, endocrinologic, and immunologic disorders, such as diabetes mellitus, obesity, hypoparathyroidism, hypothyroidism, pancreatitis, Addison's disease, and immune deficiency are often cited as underlying predisposing factors. The role of oral contraceptives in the predisposition to vaginal candidiasis has been controversial, and at this time there is no convincing evidence for a direct relationship [18]. The effect of iron metabolism in predisposing to vaginal candidiasis has been discounted [25].

Treatment of genital candidiasis is empirical and not always successful. With available topical and systemic imidazoles, mycologic cure is obtained in about 90 percent

Table 200-4   Human papillomavirus types

Predominant virus	Types of lesions
HPV-1	Plantar wart
HPV-2	Verruca vulgaris
HPV-3	Verruca plana
HPV-4	Plantar wart and verruca vulgaris
HPV-5*	Epidermodysplasia verruciformis
HPV-6	Genital warts
HPV-7	Meat-handler warts
HPV-8*	Epidermodysplasia verruciformis
HPV-9	Epidermodysplasia verruciformis
HPV-10	Verruca plana
HPV-11*	Genital warts, flat warts of the cervix, laryngeal papillomas
HPV-12*	Epidermodysplasia verruciformis
HPV-13	Focal epithelial hyperplasia Heck
HPV-16*	Flat warts of cervix, carcinoma of cervix
HPV-18*	Flat warts of cervix, carcinoma of cervix

* Types associated with malignancy.
Source: Modified from Bennett-Jenson et al [30].

of patients, but relapses are frequent [18]. Although it is presumed that eradicating *Candida* from the gut wall will reduce vaginal infection, no beneficial effect was demonstrated when an oral agent was combined with topical therapy in a double-blind study [26]. Sexual transmission may be more important in recurrent infection than endogenous seeding, and sexual partners should be treated with consideration to reservoirs of infection, including the oral cavity, nails, perianal region, and urethra. It is likely that the treatment of vaginal candidiasis may be simplified in the future. Recent evidence shows that the total dose of an imidazole preparation, such as miconazole, inhibits fungal growth for at least 48 h [27].

Genital warts

Condylomata acuminata are defined as fleshy, nonkeratinized growths occurring in moist areas of the body at the junction of squamous epithelium and mucous membrane, to be distinguished from common warts which also may occur in the genital area. There appear to be no morphologic differences between the virus of ordinary skin warts and that causing genital warts when studied by routine electron microscopy. This observation and the fact that human papillomaviruses (HPV) have not been propagated in cell culture have made the study of HPV difficult. Antigenic differences between genital and skin wart viruses were first demonstrated by one-way cross reactivity using immune electron microscopy [28]. More recently, multiple strains of HPV have been identified using DNA hybridization techniques and restriction enzyme analysis [29]. Several different types of viruses (HPV-1 to HPV-18) can be distinguished serologically and/or by molecular hybridization techniques. Current evidence suggests that the type of HPV determines, in part, the clinical and pathologic appearance, location, and natural fate of cutaneous warts and, perhaps, mucosal papillomas [30].

Table 200-4 illustrates the predominant types of HPV identified in these papillomas although, in some instances, more than one type of virus has been characterized. The

HPV that infect the genital tract, for example, include types 6, 11, 16, and 18 [31]. Types 6 and 11 are commonly found in acuminate warts but seldom found in invasive squamous cell cancer. On the other hand, types 16 and 18 are found almost exclusively in high-grade cervical intraepithelial neoplasia and invasive cancer [32]. Specifically, type 16 has been incriminated in the cervical "flat" warts which are inconspicuous, nonexophytic lesions visualized only by colposcopic examination and implicated as a precursor of cervical cancer [33].

Evidence for sexual transmission of HPV is provided by Oriel [34], who studied 332 men and women with genital warts and found that 64 percent of sex contacts developed genital warts with incubation periods as long as two years, averaging two months. In this same series, ordinary skin warts were no more common in those with genital warts than in controls, although skin warts of the penis could appear in patients with warts elsewhere, suggesting that in these cases, manifestations in the two sites are caused by the same virus, possibly autoinoculated to the genital area. About 10 percent of men and 20 percent of women with genital warts subsequently developed anal warts; the vast majority of these patients admit to anal intercourse [35].

Condylomata of the anus and genitalia, although rising in incidence for adults, are extremely rare in persons below age 10 years, approaching 2 per 100,000 population between 1950 and 1978 in Rochester, Minnesota [36]. Lesions appearing before age 12 months could be related to inoculations through an infected birth canal and they can be manifested as laryngeal papillomata [37], as well as genital warts [38]. Anal/genital warts appearing after age 18 months, however, should suggest the possibility of inappropriate sexual inoculation and possible sexual abuse, and mandates the need for a careful evaluation [39]. Sexual abuse may be very difficult to detect because children are often reluctant to incriminate close family contacts (the most frequent source of the problem) [40]. Warts on the oral mucosa in children may have the same implications as anal/genital warts, given the epidemiologic features of this phenomenon [41].

Other genital infections are common in patients with genital warts, including NGU, candidiasis, and trichomoniasis. Furthermore, young female children born to women with vulvar warts have been noted to develop vulvar warts and laryngeal papillomas [42–44].

The potential for malignant transformation of genital warts and the possible oncogenicity of HPV have been intensively studied in the past several years. Besides flat warts of the cervix, the extensive form of condyloma acuminatum of anorectum, penis, and vulva (Buschke-Lowenstein) may be difficult to distinguish from carcinoma. Despite extensive surgery and other modes of treatment, patients may die from this disorder and its complications [45]. A new variety of "genital wart," bowenoid papulosis, has been described; its similarity to multicentric pigmented Bowen's disease has been stressed [46]. Both the Buschke-Lowenstein tumor and bowenoid papulosis are suspected of having some relationship to HPV or condyloma acuminatum [47,48]. The viral features of these entities have not been well characterized to determine whether the type of HPV is one of the oncogenic viruses or whether they are induced by multiple HPV types, as in condyloma acuminatum. Recently, 50 women with vulvar condylomata acuminata attending a clinic for STDs were found to have a high prevalence of HPV infection of the cervix; changes of cervical intraepithelial neoplasia were detected, suggesting that there might be an association between vulvar condylomata and abnormalities of the uterine cervix [49]. Since it appears that there is an association between condylomata and genital malignant neoplasms, it is recommended that a Papanicolaou smear in women and close follow-up for both men and women be provided when genital condylomata are diagnosed [50].

Although other therapeutic modalities, such as Co_2 laser [51]. have been increasingly used to treat genital warts, podophyllum and cryotherapy are most frequently used. Besides being relatively ineffective (less than 50 percent of patients are cured after 1 to 2 applications [52]), podophyllum should be used with caution because it is potentially toxic. Podophyllum should not be used during pregnancy, not only because of its antimitotic properties and teratogenic potential, but also because of rare fetal and maternal complications due to systemic absorption after topical use, including stillbirth of the infant, and respiratory distress, cyanosis, and profound muscular weakness of the mother [53,54].

Trichomoniasis

In patients with vaginitis presenting to an STD clinic in the United States, 32 percent of cases were due to *Trichomonas vaginalis* [55]. The study evaluated simultaneously the sensitivity and specificity of clinical observations, wet-mount preparations, and two trichomonal culture systems. Although 56 percent of women infected with *T. vaginalis* described a discharge and 18 percent had dysuria, symptoms may not be helpful in diagnosing the infection because they may be equally common in women without trichomoniasis. Frothy, purulent discharge, for example, was found in only 12 percent of women with *T. vaginalis* and in 29 percent of women who did not have trichomoniasis. Conversely, 44 percent of women who grew *T. vaginalis* from the vagina did not complain of a discharge, and 19 percent did not show evidence of leukorrhea on vaginal inspection. While the wet-mount remains highly specific, cultures of *T. vaginalis* will detect twice as many trichomonal infections.

Although trichomoniasis may cause asymptomatic infection in males, this organism may be responsible for 5.6 percent of cases of nongonococcal urethritis [56]. In sex partners of males with trichomoniasis, most have evidence of infection. Most of the male consorts of infected women show evidence of infection when prostatic secretion and semen ejaculates are examined. The incubation period is often difficult to determine, but experimental inoculation of the vagina in women may establish infection in 4 to 20 days. Complications of trichomoniasis include neonatal infection, a rare syndrome of multiple penile ulcerations with urethritis and adenitis, and a high prevalence of concurrent infection with gonorrhea and candidiasis [56].

Metronidazole, the recommended treatment for trichomoniasis for many years, has recently come under scrutiny [57,58] because of reports linking it [59] and its human urine products [60] to mutagenicity in bacteria and carcinogenicity in mice fed daily doses of the drug for life [61]. However, there is no evidence that the drug is carcinogenic in humans, and there is considerable debate among clinicians over the bacterial and animal data cited. Treatment of the female without treating her steady sexual contacts is associated with more than double the reinfection rate [62]. There are no good alternatives to metronidazole for trichomoniasis. It is recommended, therefore, that only symptomatic males and females and their steady sexual partners be treated with a single oral dose of 2 g of metronidazole, avoiding this drug (where possible) in pregnant and nursing women. (This drug is secreted in human milk and is not approved for pregnant or nursing women in the United States.)

Genital herpes simplex

Genital herpes has become the malady of the last decade and, except for AIDS, it has attracted more attention from the scientific and lay communities than any other STD in recent years. Several factors have contributed to this phenomenon: (1) its incidence has continued to rise; (2) morbidity and rate of recurrence is higher than its counterpart, herpes labialis; (3) occurrence during pregnancy may endanger the fetus or newborn; (4) there has been an association with cervical carcinoma; and (5) a new antiviral drug, acyclovir, which seems to be safer and more effective than previous drugs, has been developed. The availability of antiviral therapy has attracted many investigators to study drugs in collaborative, well-controlled trials which have produced reproducible results and conclusions. The relationship between herpes simplex and carcinoma of the cervix has created an unprecedented hysteria, second only to AIDS, where the media have played an important role in diffusing information about the disease. Both AIDS and herpes genitalis have become the stigmata of the 1980s, influencing the sexual and social behavior of a large segment of the population.

Since HSV infections are not reportable in the United States, estimates of incidence are based on regional reports. Most epidemiologic studies demonstrate that the incidence of genital herpes has been rising dramatically. At the student health clinic of a large southwestern university, for example, herpes genitalis was 10 times more common than gonorrhea [63]. A study in another university student health service showed a first diagnosis of genital herpes in 5.9 per 1000 students during a one-month span [64], and a 15-year population-based epidemiologic study conducted in Rochester, Minnesota, showed a continuous increase in incidence peaking in 1979 at 128 cases per 100,000 population [65]. Recent estimates from the Centers for Disease Control suggest that visits to private physicians for genital herpes have increased from 29,500 in 1966 to 260,000 in 1979 [66]. In England, where the disease is reportable, there has been an increase of about 57 percent in the incidence of genital herpes from 1977 to 1982 (see Table 200-2) [4].

Viral types I (HSV-I) and II (HSV-II) may be isolated from symptomatic local genital infections: 89 percent HSV-II and 11 percent HSV-I for female genital herpes, and 97 percent HSV-II and 3 percent HSV-I for male genital herpes [67]. Biologic differences between type I and type II viruses are major factors in determining clinical manifestations and the natural course of recurrent disease. HSV type I produces a milder infection, and, while recurrences occur in 14 percent of patients infected with HSV-I, 60 percent of patients will have a recurrent episode during the first year if infected with HSV-II [68]. The difference in recurrence rate might be explained experimentally by mouse inoculation studies, which showed that type II strains establish latent infection in the dorsal root ganglia more readily than do type I strains [69]. Although reinfection is postulated to occur via reactivation of persisting virus from sacral and cranial nerve ganglia, local infection has been induced in persons with a history of recurrent herpes labialis or genitalis by inoculating virus into normal skin. This observation suggests that skin, eye, and cervix may not be protected by serum antibodies against exogenous infection [70]. Nahmias and Storr [67] claim an attack rate in sexual contacts of about 75 percent for genital herpes, but data are limited.

The increased prevalence of genital HSV infection in the United States may be responsible for a concomitant increase in neonatal HSV infection. While in Britain the incidence of neonatal HSV is very low (1 in 30,000 births) [71], the HSV infection rate at term in the United States is estimated at 1:300 to 1:1000, with clinically apparent infection in about 1 of 7500 deliveries [72]. The incidence of neonatal HSV infection in King County, Washington, increased progressively from a rate of 2.6 per 100,000 live births in the period between 1966 and 1969 to 11.9 per 100,000 live births from 1978 to 1981 [73]. Most of these neonatal infections are due to HSV type II virus. Early intrauterine infection during the first 8 weeks of gestation may result in spontaneous abortion, while late intrauterine infection may result in microcephaly, psychomotor retardation, encephalitis, chorioretinitis, and recurrent skin disease during infancy [74]. Neonatal infection may result in widely disseminated disease, with or without involvement of the central nervous system, eyes, skin, and oral cavity. A 50 percent mortality rate in neonatal disseminated disease, and significant neurologic and ocular sequelae in at least a third of survivors, has been described [75]. Approximately 50 percent of neonates showing HSV skin infection may have evidence of disseminated disease [76].

Asymptomatic shedding of infectious HSV without clinically detectable lesions is of major epidemiologic interest, particularly at parturition, since asymptomatic infection may cause neonatal infection. In a recent study of 56 women who delivered HSV-infected newborns, 70 percent had neither signs nor symptoms of genital HSV infection and only one-third of these women were considered high-risk mothers because of a previous history of herpes genitalis in them or their sexual partners [77]. Unfortunately, cesarean section cannot be used prophylactically in the above situation since there are no available predictable tests to identify those at high risk of neonatal infection. High-risk mothers, however, should be followed with cervical and vaginal HSV cultures weekly during the last month of pregnancy. If genital HSV infection is clinically apparent at the time of delivery or if cultures are positive for HSV within two weeks before delivery, a cesarean section should be performed if the fetal membranes have been ruptured for less than 4 h [78]. Otherwise, the risk of neonatal infection is 54 percent if the child is delivered vaginally. If a cesarean section is performed more than 4 h after the membrane is ruptured, the incidence of neonatal infection is 94 percent [79].

The evidence that genital HSV plays a role in the production of cervical carcinoma, although still circumstantial, is growing. This evidence has contributed significantly to the awareness by the public who consider infection and carcinoma synonymous. Herpes simplex-induced DNA-binding proteins, for example, are present in tissue taken from sites of cervical dysplasia and carcinoma [80]. In situ hybridization techniques show HSV-specific RNA in cervical intraepithelial neoplasia and in overt squamous cervical carcinoma [81]. The fact that a high proportion of women with HSV-II infections do not develop carcinoma of the cervix suggests that other factors must be implicated. The public should be made aware that cervical cancer is neither a certain consequence of infection nor an imminent danger. The problem should be approached rationally with periodic gynecologic examinations and Papanicolaou smears, rather than a fatalistic attitude.

An important factor that adds a sense of desperation to the sufferer of genital herpes simplex is the lack of adequate treatment to eradicate the virus. The advent of acyclovir, a guanosine analog that inhibits HSV replication by interfering with the action of viral DNA polymerase, has provided some optimism to these patients and rekindled enthusiasm among investigators that safe antiviral agents might be developed. Topical acyclovir may reduce virus shedding and shorten the clinical course of primary HSV infection, but there is no appreciable effect on the course of the recurrent infection [82]. More recently, oral acyclovir has become the subject of extensive cooperative trials which show that the drug is effective not only in reducing virus shedding, but also shortens significantly the clinical course of both primary and recurrent genital herpes if treatment is instituted early [83–86]. The effectiveness of oral acyclovir in immunocompromised patients has also been studied, and preliminary studies show that the therapeutic benefits are comparable to intravenous administration of the drug [87]. Furthermore, prophylactic therapy with lower doses can prevent recurrences in this high-risk population. Unfortunately, the drug does not prevent recurrences once it is discontinued. Because of the possibility of inducing resistant strains of the virus with prolonged therapy, most investigators recommend against prophylactic treatment except in exceptional high-risk situations. One major advantage of acyclovir over previous antiviral drugs is the relative lack of toxicity when administered intravenously for short periods of time, and topically or orally for up to six months [87]. Recently, oral acyclovir has been used successfully in a case of Kaposi's varicelliform eruption (eczema herpeticum), suggesting that the intravenous route may not be necessary [88].

Molluscum contagiosum

Molluscum contagiosum, a DNA virus resembling vaccinia and the largest of the poxvirus group, is difficult to grow and difficult to transmit to humans with experimental inoculation. Social transmission of this virus is suggested by an epidemic described in Alaskan children who lived in close quarters [89]. Circumstantial evidence implicates a venereal mode of transmission since infection often follows intercourse, and the site of infection is often confined to the genital area in sexually active males [90]. The incubation period is 3 weeks to 3 months after exposure. The natural course of the disease lasts a few years, with individual lesions persisting for an average of 2 months [91].

Complications are rare, but include giant molluscum, pruritus, secondary eczematous dermatitis, and the occurrence of foreign-body "abcess" when the molluscum body ruptures in the dermis.

Cytomegalovirus infection

Cytomegalovirus (CMV), a herpes virus which can cause both symptomatic and clinically inapparent infection, has been incriminated as the cause of severe brain damage in 400 infants born yearly in England and Wales. Since 1 to 3 percent of asymptomatic pregnant women excrete the virus in urine [92], and 1 percent of all pregnancies are associated with primary infection and the risk of fetal infection in such a pregnancy is 50 percent [93], it is relevant to consider the evidence suggesting that the disease may be transmitted sexually in adults: (1) the rate of cervical isolation of CMV is about 3.2 percent of women attending veneral disease clinics, compared with 0.7 percent of private antenatal patients [94]; (2) high titers of CMV have been demonstrated in the semen of symptomatic or asymptomatic males, persisting sometimes for months [95]; (3) in women with active infection, virus may be recovered from the throat, urine, and cervix [96]; (4) in women attending venereal disease clinics, there is a significant correlation between the presence of CMV antibody and gonococcal infection [97].

Positive cultures for CMV have been recovered from placenta, amniotic fluid, liver, and brain of a fetus aborted at 4 months in a woman who had clinical infection and positive urine and blood cultures for CMV during pregnancy [98]. In utero infection has been associated with cerebral and cerebellar atrophy, microcephalus, deafness, blindness due to optic atrophy and chorioretinitis, as well as multiple congenital anomalies. Where primary infection in utero can be documented, therapeutic abortion should be considered because of the likelihood of severe fetal damage. However, a prospective study was conducted on 147 neonates with positive cultures to determine whether perinatal CMV infection produced characteristic clinical symptoms or signs, or influenced their general morbidity. None of the manifestations that characterize this infection in utero or later on in life was present among these children, suggesting that contracting the disease after delivery is much more benign than when contracted in utero [99].

Hepatitis type B virus infection

Infection with hepatitis type B virus (HBV) is not restricted to the parenteral mode of transmission; at least half of those infected with HBV have no history of parenteral exposure. Studies by Krugman and Giles [100] demonstrated oral exposure as an important mode of transmission, and subsequent studies have shown the presence of hepatitis B-associated antigen (HBsAg) in saliva, sneeze droplets, vaginal secretions, tears, urine, blood, feces, and semen [101]. Evidence for sexual transmission of infection comes from studies showing that the risk of contagion was confined to spouses and sexual partners when household contacts of patients with HBV infection were followed closely for 12 months [102]. There is a suggestion that swallowing semen [103], involvement in predominantly anal intercourse, and large numbers of sexual partners [104] are factors responsible for the nine- to tenfold greater

prevalence of present or past HBV infection in homosexual males vs. heterosexual males in England and the United States [103,105,106].

The incubation period for "sexually" acquired HBV is not specifically known, but early experimental work in children suggests a time lag of 98 days after oral exposure compared to an average of 65 days after parenteral exposure to "serum hepatitis" antigen [100].

Phthirus pubis infestation

Although sexual transmission of pubic lice has not been carefully studied, it has been accepted that skin-to-skin transfer of organisms is common. Infection is reported to be largely confined to whites. About 38 percent of individuals with pubic lice have one or more other STDs [107].

Lice have a life expectancy of about 1 month, with eggs requiring 7 to 8 days to hatch and 3 to 4 weeks of evolution before adulthood and sexual reproduction. The period of incubation is about 30 days, but may be shorter. About 49 percent of individuals will show no reaction to the bite of the pubic louse, which remains attached to the skin, feeding on blood intermittently, and dying in 2 days without a blood meal. Urticaria, vesicles, and macular blue pigmentation may develop after bites [108].

Scabies

Experimental inoculation of adult scabies mites into previously uninfected human volunteers results in symptoms 4 to 5 weeks later, despite the appearance long before of burrows and invading organisms in the absence of inflammation. Reinfection of previously infected persons results in an immediate reaction, with itching at the site of invasion. Moreover, reinfection experiments are unsuccessful in 60 percent of cases, suggesting a host-immune response [109].

Close physical contact appears to be more pertinent to the spread of scabies than the sharing of bedding or clothing: in experiments where volunteers were exposed to the bedding and underwear of infected persons, only 2 of 38 persons so exposed developed infection, with the symptoms appearing more than a month after (primary) exposure. The rate of infection by exposure to clothing and other fomites was found to be directly related to the number of organisms present on an infected "source" individual [109]. The organism does not usually survive "dryness" for more than 48 h away from its "moist" host; organisms may survive for as long as a week or more in an artificial moist environment such as mineral oil papers.

Sexual transmission of scabies probably accounts for most infections occurring outside of household or institutional settings. Complications of this infection include severe itching, skin reactivity due to sensitization (urticarial and papular rash), pyoderma, glomerulonephritis [110], and coincidental occurrence of other STDs.

Reiter's syndrome

The etiology of Reiter's syndrome and the role played by veneral and dysenteric agents have been moot issues since the original suggestion by Reiter [111]. *Mycoplasma* [112] and *Chlamydia* [113] have been particularly incriminated, but evidence remains circumstantial and inconclusive.

Factors of genetic disposition [114,115] and immunologic responsiveness to a variety of infectious organisms [116,117] may be more relevant to the pathogenesis of the varied manifestations of this disease than a single infectious agent. The incidence of nonspecific genital infection with arthritis in British genitourinary clinics was less than 1 percent per 100,000 population in the first half of 1975, having shown a decreasing trend since 1971.

Corynebacterium vaginale infection

It is accepted that *Corynebacterium vaginale (Hemophilus vaginalis)* is a principal cause of bacterial vaginitis but only rarely a cause of nongonococcal urethritis. Its ability to produce vaginitis within 7 to 14 days when a pure culture of the organism is inoculated into disease-free vaginas has been well documented [118]. A venereal mode of transmission is suggested by the demonstration of urethral colonization in the majority of men whose wives are infected, the rare occurrence of the organism in premenarchial girls, and high association with other STDs (especially trichomoniasis) [119]. The overall prevalence of infection with *C. vaginale* appears to be less frequent than either gonorrhea or trichomonas and may reflect the low virulence of the organism or difficulty in making the diagnosis.

There have been reports of serious disease related to *C. vaginale*, including puerperal pyrexia, septic abortion, and maternal and neonatal infections [120]. Isolation of the organism requires specialized techniques, and no reliable serologic test is available. Direct visualization of epithelial cells with associated small gram-negative or variable rods (''clue cells'') has been considered characteristic, but not absolutely diagnostic. Pus cells are usually not present. Tetracycline, intravaginally or systemically, is effective therapy. Steady sexual partners should be advised to seek treatment in order to prevent reinfection.

Neisseria meningitidis infection

N. meningitidis, not a normal inhabitant of either genital or anal areas, is being recognized as a serious source of septic complications, with probable spread via oral–genital and oral–anal contact. In a report describing isolation of the organism from the urethra and anal canal from both sexes, most of the males were homosexuals and had no symptoms. Females frequently had vaginitis, cervicitis, and generalized disease, including sepsis, arthritis, endometritis, and salpingitis [121]. Further study is required to determine the importance of sexual transmission, host-immune factors, and incidence of infection.

Helminths and protozoa infestation

Parasites reported to cause sexually transmitted infection are those not requiring an intermediate host or long interval outside the host, and those surviving after ingestion, usually depending on oral–anal route of transmission. The following organisms have been occasionally associated with sexual transmission: *Iodamoeba butschlii, Endolimax nana, Giardia lamblia, Dientamoeba fragilis, Enterobius vermicularis,* and *Entamoeba histolytica.* Amebic vaginitis, cutaneous amebiasis of the prepuce and glans penis of the sexual partner, and urethritis due to *Entamoeba his-*

tolytica in males following rectal intercourse with infected partners, are notable examples [122,123].

Miscellaneous bacterial infections

Occasional reports in the literature suggest sexually transmitted leptospirosis [124], typhoid fever [125], shigellosis [123,126], *Pseudomonas pseudomallei* [127], and group A beta-hemolytic streptococci [128].

References

1. Catterall RD: Infections of the genital tract—recent trends. *Clin Exp Dermatol* **7**:369, 1982
2. *Health and Prevention Profile—US 1983.* Washington, DC, US Dept of Health and Human Services, 1983, p 253
3. Centers for Disease Control: Annual summary 1982: reported morbidity and mortality in the United States. *MMWR* **31**:29, 1983
4. Sexually transmitted disease surveillance in Britain: 1982. *Br Med J* **289**:99, 1984
5. Armstrong JH, Weisner PJ: The need for problem-oriented venereal disease clinics. *J Am Vener Dis Assoc* **1**:23, 1974
6. Holmes KK et al: Etiology of nongonococcal urethritis. *N Engl J Med* **292**:1199, 1975
7. Handsfield HH: Nongonococcal urethritis. *Cutis* **27**:269, 1981
8. Bowie WR et al: Etiology of nongonococcal urethritis: evidence for *Chlamydia trachomatis* and *Ureaplasma urealyticum. J Clin Invest* **59**:735, 1977
9. Bowie WR et al: Bacteriology of the urethra in normal men and men with nongonococcal urethritis. *J Clin Microbiol* **6**:482, 1977
10. Johannisson G: Studies on *Chlamydia trachomatis* as a cause of lower urogenital tract infection. *Acta Derm Venereol (Stockh)* **61 (suppl)**:93, 1981
11. Handsfield HH: Gonorrhea and nongonococcal urethritis: recent advances. *Med Clin North Am* **62**:925, 1978
12. Persson K et al: Prevalence of nine different microorganisms in the female genital tract. *Br J Vener Dis* **55**:429, 1979
13. Felman UM, Nikitas JA: Nongonococcal urethritis. *JAMA* **245**:381, 1982
14. Berger RE et al: *Chlamydia trachomatis* as a cause of acute ''idiopathic epididymitis.'' *N Engl J Med* **298**:302, 1978
15. Van der Bel-Kahn JM et al: *Chlamydia trachomatis* endocarditis. *Am Heart J* **95**:627, 1978
16. Holmes KK: The *Chlamydia* epidemic. *JAMA* **245**:1718, 1981
17. Harrison HR et al: *Chlamydia trachomatis* infant pneumonia. *N Engl J Med* **298**:702, 1978
18. Odds FC: Genital candidosis. *Clin Exp Dermatol* **7**:345, 1982
19. Osborne NG et al: Vaginitis in sexually active women: relationship to nine sexually transmitted organisms. *Am J Obstet Gynecol* **142**:962, 1982
20. Thin RW et al: How often is genital yeast infection sexually transmitted? *Br Med J* **2**:93, 1977
21. Oriel JD et al: Genital yeast infections. *Br Med J* **4**:761, 1972
22. Gilpin CA: Resistant monilial vaginitis—the male aspect. *J Fla Med Assoc* **54**:337, 1967
23. Davidson F: Yeasts and circumcision in the male. *Br J Vener Dis* **53**:121, 1977
24. Sautter RL, Brown WJ: Sequential vaginal cultures from normal young women. *J Clin Microbiol* **11**:479, 1980
25. Davidson F et al: Recurrent genital candidiasis and iron metabolism. *Br J Vener Dis* **53**:123, 1977
26. Milne JD, Warnock DW: Effect of simultaneous oral and vaginal treatment on the rate of cure and relapse in vaginal candidosis. *Br J Vener Dis* **55**:362, 1979

27. Odds FC, MacDonald F: Persistence of miconazole in vaginal secretions—implications for the treatment of vaginal candidosis. *Br J Vener Dis* **57**:400, 1982

28. Almeida JD et al: Characterization of the virus found in human genital warts. *Microbios* **3**:225, 1969

29. Coggin J, Zur Hausen H: Workshop on papilloma virus and cancer. *Cancer Res* **39**:545, 1979

30. Bennett-Jenson A et al: Human papilloma virus—frequency and distribution in plantar and common warts. *Lab Invest* **47**:491, 1982

31. Gissman L et al: Human papilloma virus types 6 and 11 DNA sequences in genital and laryngeal papillomas and in some cervical cancers. *Proc Natl Acad Sci USA* **80**:560, 1983

32. Durst M et al: A papillomavirus DNA from a cervical carcinoma and its prevalence in cancer biopsy samples from different geographic regions. *Proc Natl Acad Sci USA* **80**:3812, 1983

33. Crum CP et al: Human papillomavirus type 16 and early cervical neoplasia. *N Engl J Med* **310**:880, 1984

34. Oriel JD: Natural history of genital warts. *Br J Vener Dis* **47**:1, 1971

35. Oriel JD: Anal warts and anal coitus. *Br J Vener Dis* **47**:373, 1971

36. Chuang T-Y et al: Condyloma acuminatum in Rochester, Minn. 1950–1978: I. Epidemiology and clinical features. *Arch Dermatol* **120**:469, 1984

37. Felman Y, Nikitas JA: Condyloma acuminata. *NY State J Med* **11**:1747, 1979

38. Eftaiha M et al: Condyloma acuminata in an infant and mother. *Dis Colon Rectum* **21**:369, 1978

39. American Academy of Dermatology Task Force on Pediatric Dermatology: Genital warts and sexual abuse in children. *J Am Acad Dermatol* **11**:529, 1984

40. Sgroi SM: Pediatric gonorrhea and child sexual abuse: the venereal disease connection. *Sex Transm Dis* **9**:154, 1984

41. Fiumara NJ: The management of warts of the oral cavity. *Sex Transm Dis* **11**:267, 1984

42. Patel R, Groff DB: Condyloma acuminata in childhood. *Pediatrics* **50**:153, 1972

43. Cook TA et al: Laryngeal papilloma: etiologic and therapeutic considerations. *Ann Ontol Rhinol Laryngol* **82**:649, 1973

44. Storrs FJ: Spread of condyloma acuminata to infants and children. *Arch Dermatol* **113**:1294, 1977

45. Shah IC, Hertz RE: Giant condyloma acuminatum of the anorectum: report of two cases. *Dis Colon Rectum* **15**:207, 1972

46. Lupulescu A et al: Venereal warts vs. Bowen's disease: a histologic and ultrastructural study of five cases. *JAMA* **237**:2520, 1977

47. Kimura S et al: So-called multicentric pigmented Bowen's disease: report of a case and possible etiologic role of human papillomavirus. *Dermatologica* **157**:229, 1978

48. Guillet GY et al: Bowenoid papulosis—demonstration of human papillomavirus (HPV) with anti-HPV immune serum. *Arch Dermatol* **120**:514, 1984

49. Walker PG et al: Abnormalities of the uterine cervix in women with vulvar warts: preliminary communication. *Br J Vener Dis* **59**:120, 1983

50. Chuang TY et al: Condyloma acuminatum in Rochester, Minn, 1950–1978. II. Anaplasias and unfavorable outcomes. *Arch Dermatol* **120**:476, 1984

51. Ferenczy A: Using the laser to treat vulvar condyloma acuminata and intradermal neoplasia. *Can Med Assoc J* **128**:135, 1983

52. Von Krogh G: Topical treatment of penile condylomata acuminata with podophyllin, podophyllotoxin and cochicine. *Acta Derm Venereol (Stockh)* **58**:163, 1979

53. Chamberlain MJ et al: Toxic effect of podophyllin application in pregnancy. *Br Med J* **3**:391, 1972

54. Oriel JD: Genital warts—recent advances. *Clin Exp. Dermatol* **7**:361, 1982

55. Fouts AC, Kraus SJ: Trichomoniasis vaginalis: reevaluation of its clinical presentation and laboratory diagnosis. *J Infect Dis* **141**:137, 1980

56. Morton RS: Epidemiologic and social aspects (of trichomoniasis), in *Recent Advances in Sexually Transmitted Diseases,* edited by RS Morton, JR Harris. Edinburgh, Churchill Livingston, 1975, p 203

57. Is Flagyl dangerous? *Med Lett* **17**:53, 1975

58. Komaroff A et al: Alternatives to metronidazole. *JAMA* **235**:2081, 1976

59. Voogd CE et al: The mutagenic action of nitroimidazoles. 1. Metronidazole, nimorazole, dimetridazole and ronidazole. *Mutat Res* **26**:483, 1974

60. Speck WT et al: Mutagenicity of metronidazole: presence of several active metabolites in human urine. *J Natl Cancer Inst* **56**:283, 1976

61. Rustia M, Shubik P: Induction of lung tumors and malignant lymphomas in mice by metronidazole. *J Natl Cancer Inst* **48**:721, 1972

62. Gardner JL, Dukes CD: Clinical and laboratory effects of metronidazole. *Am J Obstet Gynecol* **89**:990, 1964

63. Sumaya CV et al: Genital infections with herpes simplex virus in a university student population. *Sex Transm Dis* **7**:16, 1980

64. Delva MD, McSherry JA: Herpes genitalis in a student population. *J Fam Pract* **18**:397, 1984

65. Chuang T-Y et al: Incidence and trend of herpes progenitalis: a 15 year population study. *Mayo Clin Proc* **58**:436, 1983

66. Genital herpes infection—United States 1966–1979. *MMWR* **31**:137, 1982

67. Nahmias AJ, Storr SE: Infections caused by herpes simplex viruses, in *Infectious Diseases,* 2d ed, edited by PD Hoeprich. Hagerstown, MD, Harper & Row, 1977, p 726

68. Reeves WC et al: Risk of recurrence after first episode of genital herpes: relation to HSV type and antibody response. *N Engl J Med* **303**:315, 1981

69. Nishiura J et al: Experimental studies on genital herpetic infections in mice. *Biken J* **23**:169, 1980

70. Blank H, Haines HG: Experimental human infection with herpes simplex virus. *J Invest Dermatol* **61**:223, 1975

71. Joel-Jensen B: Genital herpes. *Clin Exp Dermatol* **7**:355, 1982

72. Marshall WC, Peckham CS: The management of herpes simplex in pregnant women and neonates. *J Infect Dis* **6 (suppl)**:23, 1983

73. Sullivan-Bolyai J et al: Neonatal herpes simplex virus infection in King County, Washington. Increasing incidence and epidemiologic correlates. *JAMA* **250**:3059, 1983

74. Komorous JM et al: Intrauterine herpes simplex infections. *Arch Dermatol* **113**:918, 1977

75. Nahmias AJ et al: Cesarean section and genital herpes. *N Engl J Med* **296**:359, 1977

76. Nahmias AJ, Vinistine AM: Herpes simplex, in *Infectious Diseases of the Fetus and Newborn Infant,* edited by JS Remington, JO Klein. Philadelphia, WB Saunders, 1976, p 156

77. Whitley RJ et al: The natural history of herpes simplex virus infection of mother and newborn. *Pediatrics* **66**:489, 1980

78. Jarratt M: Herpes simplex infection (editorial). *Arch Dermatol* **119**:99, 1983

79. Nahmias AJ et al: Genital herpes infection—the old and the new, in *Sexually Transmitted Diseases,* edited by RD Catterall, CS Nicol. London, Academic Press, 1976, p 135

80. Dreesman GR et al: Expression of herpes virus-induced antigens in human cervical cancer. *Nature* **283**:591, 1980

81. Eglin RP et al: Detection of RNA complementary to herpes

simplex virus DNA in human cervical squamous cell neoplasms. *Cancer Res* **41**:3597, 1981

82. Corey L et al: A trial of topical acyclovir in genital herpes simplex virus infection. *N Engl J Med* **306**:1313, 1982

83. Nilsen AE et al: Efficacy of oral acyclovir in the treatment of initial and recurrent genital herpes. *Lancet* **2**:571, 1982

84. Bryson YJ et al: Treatment of first episodes of genital herpes simplex virus infection with oral acyclovir. *N Engl J Med* **308**:916, 1983

85. Reichman RC et al: Treatment of recurrent genital herpes simplex infections with oral acyclovir. *JAMA* **251**:2103, 1984

86. Mertz GJ et al: Double-blind placebo-controlled trial of acyclovir in first episode genital herpes simplex virus. *JAMA* **252**:1147, 1984

87. Straus SE et al: Oral acyclovir to suppress recurring herpes simplex virus infections in immunodeficient patients. *Ann Intern Med* **100**:522, 1984

88. Woolfson H: Oral acyclovir in eczema herpeticum. *Br Med J* **288**:531, 1984

89. Overfield TM, Brody JA: An epidemiologic study of molluscum contagiosum in Anchorage, Alaska. *J Pediatr* **69**:640, 1966

90. Jacobs PH: Molluscum contagiosum. *Aerospace Med* **41**:1196, 1970

91. Hawley TG: The natural history of molluscum contagiosum in Fiijian children. *J Hyg (Camb)* **68**:631, 1970

92. Numazaki Y et al: Primary infection with human cytomegalovirus: virus isolation from healthy infants and pregnant women. *Am J Epidemiol* **91**:410, 1970

93. Editorial: Congenital cytomegalovirus infection—more problems. *Lancet* **1**:845, 1974

94. Harris JRW: Cytomegalovirus infection, in *Recent Advances in Sexually Transmitted Diseases,* edited by RS Morton, JR Harris. Edinburgh, Churchill Livingstone, 1975, p 361

95. Lang DJ, Kummer JF: Cytomegalovirus in semen: observations in selected populations. *J Infect Dis* **132**:472, 1975

96. Diosi P et al: Cytomegalovirus infection associated with pregnancy. *Lancet* **1**:1063, 1967

97. Jordan MC et al: Association of cervical cytomegalovirus with venereal disease. *N Engl J Med* **288**:932, 1973

98. French MLV et al: Cytomegalovirus viremia with transmission from mother to fetus. *Ann Intern Med* **86**:748, 1977

99. Granstrom ML, Leinikki P: Illness during the first two years of life and their association with perinatal cytomegalovirus infection. *Scand J Infect Dis* **10**:251, 1978

100. Krugman S, Giles JPL: Viral hepatitis—new light on an old disease. *JAMA* **212**:1019, 1970

101. Gitnick GL et al: The liver and antigens of hepatitis B. *Ann Intern Med* **85**:488, 1976

102. Koff RS et al: Contagiousness of acute hepatitis B. *Gastroenterology* **72**:297, 1977

103. Lim KS et al: Australian antigen-positive hepatitis as a sexually transmitted disease, in *Sexually Transmitted Diseases,* edited by RD Catterall, CS Nicol. London, Academic Press, 1976, p 197

104. Szmuness W et al: On the role of sexual behavior in the spread of hepatitis B infection. *Ann Intern Med* **83**:489, 1975

105. Coleman C et al: Hepatitis B antigen and antibody in a male homosexual population. *Br J Vener Dis* **53**:132, 1977

106. Dietzman DE et al: Hepatitis B surface antigen (HBsAg) and antibody to HBsAg: prevalence in homosexual and heterosexual men. *JAMA* **238**:2625, 1977

107. Fisher I, Morton RS: *Phthirius pubis* infection. *Br J Vener Dis* **46**:326, 1970

108. Kraus JS, Glassman LH: The crab louse—review of physiology and the study of anatomy as seen by scanning electron microscopy. *J Am Vener Dis Assoc* **2**:12, 1976

109. Mellanby K: Scabies in 1976. *R Soc Health J* **97**:32, 1977

110. Svartman M et al: Epidemic scabies and glomerulonephritis in Trinidad. *Lancet* **1**:249, 1972

111. Reiter H: Über eine bisher Unerannte Spirochateninfektion (Spirochaetosis arthritica). *Dtsch Med Wochenschr* **42**:1535, 1916

112. Bartholomew LE: Isolation and characterization of mycoplasmas (PPLO) from patients with rheumatoid arthritis, systemic lupus erythematosus and Reiter's syndrome. *Arthritis Rheum* **8**:376, 1965

113. Gordon FB et al: Chlamydial isolates from Reiter's syndrome. *Br J Vener Dis* **49**:376, 1973

114. Arnett FC et al: Incomplete Reiter's syndrome: discriminating features and HL-A W27 in diagnosis. *Ann Intern Med* **84**:8, 1976

115. Lawrence JS: Family survey of Reiter's disease. *Br J Vener Dis* **50**:140, 1974

116. Sharp JT: Reiter's syndrome, a review of current status and hypothesis regarding its pathogenesis. *Curr Probl Dermatol* **5**:157, 1973

117. Urman JD et al: Reiter's syndrome associated with Campylobacter fetus infection. *Ann Intern Med* **86**:444, 1977

118. Criswell BD et al: *Haemophilus vaginalis* vaginitis by inoculation from culture. *Obstet Gynecol* **33**:195, 1969

119. Josey WE, Lambe DW: Epidemiologic characteristics of women infected with *Corynebacterium vaginale (Haemophilus vaginalis). J Am Vener Dis Assoc* **3**:9, 1976

120. Harris JRW: *Corynebacterium vaginale* infection, in *Recent Advances in Sexually Transmitted Diseases,* edited by SE Morton, JRW Harris. Edinburgh, Churchill Livingstone, 1975, p 354

121. Givan KF et al: Isolation of *Neisseria meningitidis* from the urethra, cervix and anal canal: further observations. *Br J Vener Dis* **53**:109, 1977

122. Harris JRW: Sexually transmitted protozoa and helminths, in *Recent Advances in Sexually Transmitted Diseases,* edited by SE Morton, JRW Harris. Edinburgh, Churchill Livingstone, 1975, p 365

123. Dritz SK: Patterns of sexually transmitted enteric diseases in a city. *Lancet* **2**:3, 1977

124. Turner HL: Leptospirosis. *Br J Med* **1**:537, 1973

125. Dritz SK, Braff EH: Sexually transmitted typhoid fever. *N Engl J Med* **296**:1359, 1977

126. Dritz SK, Back A: Shigella enteritis venerally transmitted. *N Engl J Med* **291**:1194, 1974

127. McCormick JB et al: Human to human transmission of *Pseudomonas pseudomallei. Ann Intern Med* **83**:512, 1975

128. Brosseau JD, Mazza JJ: Group A streptococcal sepsis and arthritis—origin from an intrauterine device. *JAMA* **238**:2178, 1977

CHAPTER 201

SYPHILIS AND OTHER TREPONEMATOSES

Arthur R. Rhodes and Anton F. H. Luger

Syphillis

Definition

Venereal syphilis (synonyms: lues, lues venerea) is a communicable disease caused by *Treponema pallidum*. In the early stages, transmission occurs most often via sexual contact, but nonvenereal transmission may also occur. The early stages of disease are systemic from the outset and are usually manifested by mucocutaneous lesions that tend to ulcerate. Years of asymptomatic latency may follow the infectious stages, to be succeeded in a minority of cases by late symptomatic disease. Transplacental infection is common in the early phases; any organ may be involved during the course of infection; and life-threatening consequences may occur in the cardiovascular and central nervous systems.

History

It has often been proposed that syphilis was imported to Europe from Hispaniola (Haiti) by the crews of Christopher Columbus (Columbian theory); these "infected" persons later joined the army of Charles VIII of France and presumably became the source of an epidemic ("great pox") which spread throughout Europe after the surrender of Naples on February 22, 1495, at 4:00 p.m. ("natal hour of syphilis"). This theory has been challenged by Hackett [1], who demonstrated syphilitic bone changes in skeletons of Australian, African, and Middle American aborigines. In addition, historical writings allude to the presence of syphilis in ancient Chinese, biblical, and Roman times, often masquerading under the guise of "venereal" leprosy (pre-Columbian theory). These findings and the existence of a treponemal infection in rabbits and some primates [2] support the theory that the disease may originally have been a less serious infection of humans and animals which differentiated into venereal and nonvenereal treponematoses between 15,000 and 3,000 B.C. Although no traces of syphilis have so far been uncovered in the pre-Columbian skeletons of Europe, it is considered probable that nonvenereal syphilis was once widespread on the Continent. It is postulated that as social conditions improved and crowding was reduced, nonvenereal transmission among children may have decreased and the venereal form of disease emerged. Foci of nonvenereal syphilis were present in Europe in Bosnia, Yugoslavia even after World War II, but have since been eradicated by mass campaigns. Because of crowded conditions in urban settings, small-scale reversals from venereal to nonvenereal syphilis have occurred in developed countries during the penicillin era [3].

The end of the fifteenth century saw the introduction of mercury into syphilotherapy, and the sixteenth century saw a more complete understanding of the clinical characteristics of syphilis. A complete description of clinical syphilis was given in 1530 by an Italian pathologist, Girolamo Fracastoro, in a poem entitled "Syphilis sive Morbus Gallicus," in which a mythical shepherd named Syphilus was afflicted with a sexually transmitted disease as punishment for blasphemy to the sun god. Jean Fernel (1506–1558) called the same disease "lues venerea" (*lues* is derived from the Latin, meaning plague, or pestilence) in one of his poems. By the end of the sixteenth century, clinicians were aware of the oral, cutaneous, joint and bone, and visceral lesions of syphilis, the communicable nature through sexual and nonsexual contact, and treatment with agents such as mercury, inorganic arsenic, guaiac wood, and sulfur baths.

The modern era of syphilis research began with the experimental transmission of the disease by Metchnikoff and Roux in 1903 from men to anthropoid apes. Subsequent advances include: the discovery by Schaudinn and Hoffmann in 1905 of the causative agent in the exudate of a syphilitic papule; the detection by Wasserman, Neisser, and Bruck in 1906 of lipoidal antibodies in the serum of infected individuals; the cultivation by Noguchi of a nonvirulent *T. pallidum;* the development of arsphenamine by Ehrlich and Hata (1909–1910); and fever therapy by Wagner-Juaregg (1917). Other notable events in the annals of syphilology were contributions in serologic standardization by Kolmer; the methods for synthesis and mass production of arsphenamine by Raiziss, Schamberg, and Kolmer; the codification of existing knowledge about syphilis in John H. Stoke's *Modern Clinical Syphilology;* and intensive intravenous chemotherapy using mapharsen (arsenoxide) by Chargin, Leifer, and Hyman in 1933. These efforts, however, were completely overshadowed in 1944 when Mahoney, Arnold, and Harris demonstrated that penicillin was effective therapy for early syphilis in the rabbit and man. World War II was partly responsible for the accelerated research and development of penicillin syphilotherapy in the United States; syphilis had become an urgent public health problem for the armed forces at home and abroad.

There is a suggestion by students of syphilis that the disease has changed over the course of recorded history. The pandemic of syphilis-like disease occurring at the end of the fifteenth century was associated with severe and often fatal systemic manifestations. Skin lesions were frequently extensive, destructive, and disfiguring. Syphilis of such severity is rarely seen in the twentieth century. Exuberant secondary lesions of skin and mucous membranes, ulcerative skin lesions, gummata, secondary infectious relapse, cardiovascular and neurosyphilis, and early prenatal syphilis are also rarely seen in the modern era. On the other hand, reinfections with syphilis, once seldom seen, are now common: in 1976, of 165 patients with early infectious syphilis seen in a London hospital, 22 (13.3 percent) had experienced 26 earlier attacks of the disease [3]. Multiple chancres, anorectal chancres, and atypical chancres as well as the classic Hunterian chancre are common presentations in modern syphilis; there is a suggestion that the disease has evolved from its original virulent presentation into a more stable and predictable course. Alternatively, clinicians may be diagnosing the more subtle manifestations of the disease in all its phases, aided by a more educated public reporting disease earlier in its course. The blanket of penicillin covering the past 30 years may also have altered the "natural course" of syphilitic infection [4].

Epidemiology [5]

Venereal syphilis occurs in all parts of the world and respects no social class, in contrast to nonvenereal syphilis, yaws, and pinta. The exact incidence or prevalence of syphilis can only be studied from areas of the world with reliable reporting systems; trends in developing countries can only be inferred.

In the United States and the United Kingdom, early syphilis (primary and secondary disease) is most common in the sexually active years, the most frequent age groups affected (in decreasing order) being 20 to 24 years, 25 to 29 years, 30 to 39 years, 15 to 19 years, and 40 to 49 years. Teenagers account for a minority of cases. Males outnumber females 2 to 6:1 [6,7], and may reflect inapparent syphilis in the female as well as a rising number of male patients who admit to acquiring disease from homosexual exposure. Approximately 46 percent of all males with syphilis in the United States in 1976 had sexual contact with other males, 12 percent occasionally, and 34 percent exclusively. In England, outside of London, 25 percent of acquired infections with primary and secondary syphilis occurred in male homosexuals, while in sections of London this figure approached 73 percent [3]. Homosexuality involves about 4 percent of adult males, and a moderately active homosexual male may have contact with 1000 partners in his lifetime. The total number of partners may not be as important as the fact that so many contacts are anonymous, making it nearly impossible to interrupt disease transmission in the gay male [8].

In the United States there had been a steady increase of all stages of syphilis during World War I and the postwar years, peaking during the years from 1935 to 1947. A decreasing trend in the reported cases of primary and secondary syphilis began in the mid-1940s (see Fig 201-1), with fluctuations in early syphilis incidence (primary and secondary) from World War II to the early 1980s (see Fig. 201-2). Control programs and the widespread use of penicillin accounted for a nadir in 1957, a subsequent rise and another slowdown in 1962 with renewed control efforts, another slight upward trend in 1969, and a 34 percent increase in new cases from 1969 to 1973. From 1973, there was a downward trend in reported new cases, possibly related to better control efforts [9]. However, the reported cases of primary and secondary syphilis in the United States increased by 43 percent between 1978 and 1981 [6,10]. These fluctuations in reported rates may also reflect erratic funding for the case-finding and treatment programs. Unfortunately, a decrease in syphilis incidence is accompanied by a proportionate lack of concern by the medical community, government, and public. These trends contrast sharply with the incidence curve for gonorrhea, which until 1975 had demonstrated a steady upward trend since the early 1960s despite extensive control efforts (see Fig. 201-1). Although there were 31,266 new cases of reported primary and secondary syphilis in 1981 [6], it is estimated that closer to 100,000 new cases occurred, since private physicians treat 83 percent of all syphilis but only 12 percent of all cases are reported to federal agencies.

Prenatal syphilis has shown a progressive decline over the past 20 years, from 4085 total cases (all types) reported in 1962 to 287 in 1981 [6]. This fall in cases reflects the incidence of acquired syphilis in the general population since mothers with early acquired syphilis are at greatest risk for having an infant with prenatal syphilis. The number of reported cases of prenatal syphilis in infants younger than 1 year of age fell progressively from 422 in 1971 to a low of 104 in 1978; 123 cases were reported in 1979, 107 in 1980, and 160 in 1981. During the same period, the number of reported cases of primary and secondary syphilis in females per 100,000 population rose from 4.8 for 1978 to 5.0 for 1979, 5.5 for 1980, and 6.6 for 1981 [6,11] (Fig. 201-3). The number of cases of prenatal syphilis in newborn infants reported per 100 cases of acquired infectious syphilis in the United States remained essentially

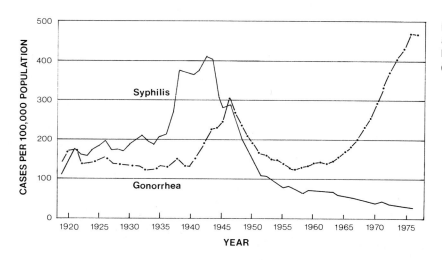

Fig. 201-1 Reported cases of gonorrhea and syphilis (all stages) per 100,000 population by year, United States, 1919–1976. *(From Centers for Disease Control [9].)*

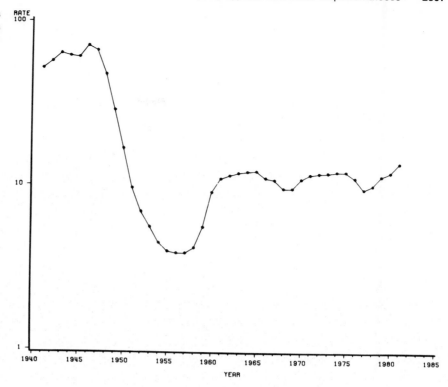

Fig. 201-2 Reported cases of syphilis (primary and secondary) in civilians per 100,000 population by year, United States, calendar years 1941–1981. (From Centers for Disease Control [6].)

constant during the period from 1978 through 1981 (2.0, 2.3, 1.7, and 2.0, respectively). This may indicate that the proportion of undetected pregnant women with syphilis remains relatively constant [6].

There is a suggestion that infectious venereal syphilis is increasing in most developing countries, but statistics are not reliable. High incidence rates exist in El Salvador, Chile, Johannesburg, New Guinea, and Addis Ababa. Even a rich developing country such as Singapore has an estimated incidence rate of 72:100,000 per year, at least 5 times the rate in the United States (10.8 to 12.1:100,000) and 30 times that in the United Kingdom [5].

In the United States, there has been a steady decline in the death rate due to syphilis, from 2193 deaths in 1966 to 272 deaths in 1975. This observation can be interpreted as the barometer of earlier case detection, earlier treatment, and prevention of late systemic complications. A change in the virulence of *T. pallidum* is also possible but less likely. Nonetheless, a reservoir of untreated syphilis, numbering more than 400,000 cases and detectable only by a blood test, is a constant reminder that case detection through serologic screening may be the only means of preventing life-threatening sequelae in a small but definite proportion of persons with latent syphilis.

The reasons for the worldwide occurrence of sexually transmitted diseases, and syphilis in particular, have been attributed to a change in sexual mores and the availability of contraception and medical abortion. Sex and venereal disease education, however, have probably not kept pace with this sexual "revolution." Also, available measures for syphilis control are too often inadequate for a mobile society. Sources of infection may be more frequently concealed or impossible to trace, and self-treatment with ineffective doses of antibiotics is more common today than in past years. The medical community and lay society is

barely able to keep up with the current endemic of syphilis and may have to be content keeping the incidence of disease at a low level. There is no indication that syphilis will be eradicated in this generation without further advances in the basic biology of the organism and the immune response of the human host.

Etiology

The causative agent in syphilis, *T. pallidum,* was identified in 1905 when Schaudinn and Hoffmann demonstrated its presence in the primary lesion and in the adjacent lymph glands of syphilitic patients. The organisms were subsequently found by Noguchi and Moore in the cerebral cortex of patients dying with general paresis.

T. pallidum belongs to the class of prokaryotic microorganisms: a nuclear membrane is not present, DNA is not subdivided into chromosomes, multiplication occurs by cross-fission, and the cell wall contains a mureine-macromolecule [12]. *T. pallidum* is in the same family as *Borrelia* and *Leptospira,* all in the order Spirochaetales. In addition, the order Spirochaetales comprises two genera nonpathogenic for humans (*Spirochaeta* and *Cristispira*) and found predominantly in sewage and contaminated mud and water, and in the intestines of mollusks in the case of *Cristispira.* Other organisms in the *Treponema* genus include the human pathogens (*T. pertenue, T. carateum,* causing yaws and pinta, respectively, and *T. pallidum,* the agent causing venereal and nonvenereal syphilis), the animal pathogens (*T. cuniculi,* the agent causing rabbit syphilis, and *T. Fribourg-Blanc,* monkey syphilis in endemic yaws areas) [3], and human or animal saprophytes (*T. microdentium* and *T. macrodentium,* which occur in the oral cavity about the gum margins and about the anus in fecal material of humans). Other nonpathogenic saprophytic strains in the *Tre-*

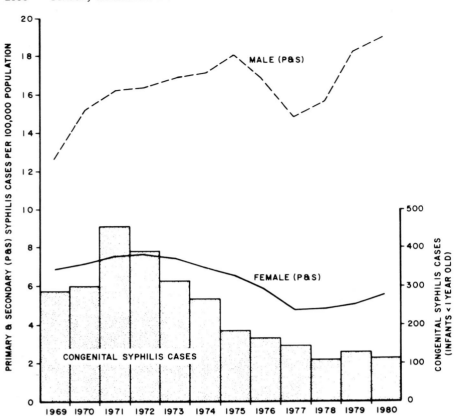

ponema genus include *T. refringens* (normal flora about male and female genitalia), *T. denticola* (oral cavity of humans and chimpanzees), *T. orale* (gingival crevice of humans), and *T. scoliodentium* and *T. vincentii* (oral cavity of humans). The saprophytic strains can be cultivated on artificial media and are antigenically distinguishable from the human pathogenic strains.

T. pallidum is a fine spiral organism measuring 5 to 20 μm in length and 0.1 to 0.2 μm in thickness, with 4 to 14 regular spirals. Three main elements are evident from ultramicroscopic studies: the protoplasmic cylinder (protoplast), axial filament, and outer envelope (cell wall). The protoplast is enclosed by a frail cytoplasmic membrane which functions as an osmotic barrier and is thus essential for cell metabolism, especially absorption and excretion. The axial filament consists of 6 to 8 elastic fibrils which are twisted around the protoplast in one or two bundles and may be responsible for the helicoid form. The outer envelope is composed of three layers: the middle layer is predominantly lipid and is radiolucent by electron microscopy, while the other two layers are osmophilic, consist of proteins and polysaccharides, and appear electron dense. An inner layer contains the heteropolymer peptidoglycan macromolecule—the mureine sacculus—which is formed by main strands of alternating sequences of *N*-acetyl muramic acid and *N*-acetyl-glucosamine, forming cross-links among tetrapeptide side chains. The peptidoglycan lattice functions as a strong skeleton for the organism, preserves its form, protects the fragile cytoplasm against physical insult, and functions as an inert filter for larger molecules [13,14]. An extracellular slime layer demonstrated by ruthenium red staining on *T. pallidum* occurring in vivo in

syphilitic rabbit testes, may protect the organism against phagocytosis [15].

Replication of the organism occurs via fission, with an interval of 30 to 33 h between divisions (most bacteria multiply every 20 to 40 min). *T. pallidum* has been previously thought to be an obligatory anaerobe, with oxygen having a negative effect on growth [16], despite its ability to live in the human host where oxygen tension is quite high. In vitro cultures have also not been possible in the past. Observations of in vitro growth of *T. pallidum* in baby hamster kidney cultured tissue cells in the presence of 7 percent CO_2 in air [17] and the maintenance of the organism in aerobic in vitro fibroblast cell cultures for several weeks using special medium have challenged all traditional views [18]. Moreover, it has been shown that *T. pallidum* requires molecular oxygen for survival and anabolic activity in cell-free and tissue culture systems [19–21]. Routine maintenance of virulent strains of *T. pallidum* may be performed by inoculation of infected material into rabbit testicles. An orchitis develops, and organisms may be reliably recovered between the sixth and tenth day after inoculation. Chimpanzees infected with *T. pallidum* exhibit clinical lesions and show signs of an immune response that is somewhat comparable to the course of early syphilis in humans. Rabbits develop similar reactions but the infection heals spontaneously after some time. *T. cuniculi* is morphologically indistinguishable from *T. pallidum* and causes a treponematosis that can be transmitted by copulation in free-living rabbits. Antibodies against *T. cuniculi* cannot be differentiated from immunoglobulins against *T. pallidum* in rabbit serum, and partial cross-immunity exists. Hamsters are susceptible to infection with *T. pallidum* but develop atypical lesions, while the same organism remains an inoffensive saprophyte in rats and mice.

Immunology

Because of technical difficulties, the nature of the immune response to syphilitic infection in humans remains poorly understood [22–24]. Visualization of the organism requires dark-field microscopy in vivo and silver impregnation or indirect immunofluorescence in vitro. The organism has only recently been maintained in vitro, and immunologic studies are limited by available animal models.

It is well known that experimental infection with *T. pallidum* promotes the development of immunity to reinfection, but only if disease is allowed to persist. In clinical studies carried out on previously infected human volunteers at Sing-Sing prison after World War II [25], it became clear that the reaction of the host to reinoculation was related to the stage of disease. Most patients who had been treated for early syphilis developed typical chancres containing *T. pallidum,* while patients with latent syphilis who never received treatment were refractory to reinoculation. Many patients with late latent or prenatal syphilis did not develop lesions or a change in the nontreponemal serologic titer, a significant proportion developed dark-field-negative lesions and a rise in the VDRL, and a few developed gummata at the inoculation site. These studies illustrate that late syphilitic infection resists rechallenge with *T. pallidum,* while patients treated for early disease are more susceptible to reinfection—a contradiction of the observation that *T. pallidum* in human and rabbit tissue persists years after ''adequate'' antibiotic therapy for late latent disease [26,27] (see ''Treatment Guidelines'').

In early disease, a humoral antibody response is evident with minimal delayed hypersensitivity response, whereas in later disease the delayed hypersensitivity response appears to account for the nature of clinical manifestations. A partial inhibition of the cell-mediated response in early disease may account for the failure to eradicate live organisms from infectious lesions. Alternatively, survival of *T. pallidum* may be related to site-specific poor access to immune products (aorta, brain, eye) and prevention of immune attack by accumulation of blocking antibody or slime coat around organisms in vivo, in the face of a brisk host immune response [28]. Both humoral and cell-mediated phenomena are active in syphilis infection and each must be examined to appreciate a poorly understood and complex interaction between the two.

Evidence that humoral immunity plays a role in syphilis infection is demonstrated by the following:

1. Nontreponemal and treponemal antibodies are regularly present in patients who have syphilis.
2. As syphilis progresses to latent and tertiary disease, immobilizing and inactivating antibodies to *T. pallidum* increase. The mechanism for such antibody action is unknown. There is some correlation between titer of immobilizing antibody and immunity but no correlation for antilipoidal antibodies, since their titer is often high in early infection when resistance is not fully developed, and low or negative in late disease when levels of immunity to reinfection are high. Antilipoidal antibodies reflect activity of the disease and tissue response to infection.
3. Although passive transfer of serum from syphilis-immune animals will confer partial immunity to rabbits, repeated immunization with killed treponemes will not offer protection despite the development of antibodies [29,30]. Hyperimmune serum has been shown to retard the course of experimental syphilis in rabbits [31,32].

Evidence for cell-mediated immunity in syphilis is provided by the following:

1. Delayed hypersensitivity to treponemal antigens is regularly present in latent and tertiary syphilis but is usually absent in early syphilis and normal controls.
2. In the nonimmune animal, treponemes rapidly spread from the site of inoculation to the regional lymph nodes, but in the immune host they remain localized [24].
3. In vitro studies have shown that rabbit peritoneal macrophages can incorporate *T. pallidum* [22].
4. Tertiary syphilis has a granulomatous histologic appearance.
5. Infection of neonatal rabbits with *T. pallidum* has resulted in a progressive runting syndrome leading to death with depletion of lymphocytes in spleen and thymus [33].
6. Immunization of rabbits with killed *T. pallidum* is usually unsuccessful in the induction of immunity, while organisms attenuated with irradiation given as a vaccine protect against rechallenge with the virulent organism [34]. A labile immunogenic fraction capable of inducing protection may only be found in living organisms.
7. Although the in vitro blastogenic response to phytohemagglutinin, pokeweed mitogen, and streptolysin is identical in syphilis patients and normal controls, the response to treponemal antigens and several fungal antigens is suppressed in patients with untreated early syphilis [22]. Following treatment for early syphilis, responsiveness returns to normal. Plasma from patients with primary and secondary syphilis was found to change the in vitro reactivity of normal lymphocytes when stimulated with different mitogens. Other studies suggest suppression of leukocyte migration late in disease and stimulation in early disease. The mechanism of suppressed lymphocyte reactivity, which has also been observed in cryptococcosis, tuberculosis, histoplasmosis, and leprosy is unknown but may be related to antigen load or the ratio of circulating T and B lymphocytes.

An absolute and relative T-lymphocytopenia has been observed in patients with primary and secondary syphilis [35,36]. In primary syphilis, T-helper lymphocytes (T cells with Fc receptors for IgM) may be responsible for the reduced number of T lymphocytes; in secondary syphilis, a reduced concentration of T-suppressor cells (T cells with Fc receptors for IgG) may be responsible [35]. In studies of patients with primary, secondary, and latent syphilis, the natural killer cell activity has been negatively associated with the presence of circulating lipoidal antibodies [37]. The sera of patients with primary, secondary, and latent syphilis contain immunoglobulin factors that depress the natural killer cell activity of healthy controls [38]. The lymphocytes of individuals with secondary syphilis respond poorly to in vitro stimulation with mitogens and treponemal antigens, lymphocyte responses are poorer in autologous syphilitic serum than in normal human serum, lymphocyte responsiveness to mitogen and antigen improve after therapy, and circulating immune complexes that are increased in amount before therapy decrease (but not in all cases) in amount after therapy [39]. The proportion of T-lymphocyte antibodies may be reduced in vitro by incubation with syphilitic sera, but antilymphocyte antibodies are not demonstrated [40]. Immune complexes in serum may play a central role in modulating the immune response in syphilis [39,41].

Another important but confusing aspect of immunity in syphilis is the relation between *T. pallidum* and the other human treponemal infections. The organisms causing venereal syphilis, nonvenereal syphilis, yaws, and pinta are indistinguishable morphologically, although subtle graded differences exist in infectivity, antibody response, host tissue response, and cross-protectivity of one to another. For instance, patients with pinta (*T. carateum*) cannot easily be infected with *T. pallidum* or *T. pertenue* (yaws), while yaws and syphilis patients are easily infected with *T. carateum*. Patients who have yaws are protected against developing syphilis, but the reverse is not certain. *T. pertenue* can be inoculated into monkeys, rabbits, and hamsters, although similar attempts have been successful for *T. carateum* only in the chimpanzee. Prenatal transmission and late complications of the cardiovascular and neurovascular systems are said not to occur with yaws and pinta, and only rarely with nonvenereal syphilis [42]. This view has been challenged in observations by Smith et al who demonstrated neuroophthalmologic abnormalities in late yaws and interstitial keratitis in pinta [43]. Hollander [44] argues that venereal syphilis, endemic syphilis, yaws, and pinta are explainable as different infection patterns (based on temperature) of a single pathogenic organism.

There is no way of formulating a unipartite concept in venereal syphilis from the above observations that explains the delay in cellular immune response and chronic course of disease in many cases [45]. Both cellular and humoral responses are stimulated, with cellular delayed hypersensitivity occurring only in latent and late syphilis, and immobilizing antibodies occurring early as well as late in the progression of disease. True immunity to reinfection in humans exists only in late syphilis. The waxing and waning of symptoms in early disease may be explained by suppression of lymphocyte reactivity due to *T. pallidum* itself, since the mucoid evelope is thought to render it resistant to phagocytosis [15,33,46], allowing antigen overload to proceed due to unchecked proliferation of organisms. The mucoid envelope may also act as a barrier against treponemicidal antibody. Another explanation for suppressed delayed hypersensitivity is that humoral antibody produced in response to early infection may coat *T. pallidum* and further delay the processing of antigen [47]. Such a privileged state of events, which allows prolonged antigenemia in the presence of antibody, provides conditions suitable for immune complex disease. In fact, immune complex glomerulonephritis presenting as the nephrotic syndrome has been reported in secondary and prenatal syphilis in humans [48,49]. A similar set of events could not be produced experimentally in rabbits [50], possibly because, in this host, relapses do not occur and infection is short-lived, probably related to the exquisite temperature sensitivity of *T. pallidum* and the higher body temperature in the rabbit.

Prolonged suppression of cellular immune responsiveness, directly related to properties of *T. pallidum*, may allow unchecked proliferation and destruction, until the host finally responds with a proper cellular response. The fact that the majority of syphilis infections in humans are self-healing suggests a heterogeneity of host responsiveness to infection. Such a situation is analogous to other diseases occurring in humans, including mycobacterial, fungal, and viral infections.

Clinical manifestations

Classification of clinical disease [51–57]. The natural history of syphilis may be described by using a combination of an older clinical plus a more recent epidemiologic terminology. The older classification is based on clinical manifestations of disease and includes the primary stage (chancre), secondary stage (mucocutaneous lesions with lymphadenopathy and other organ system involvement), the latent stage (a reactive serologic test for syphilis in the absence of signs or symptoms of disease), and the tertiary stage (cardiovascular, central nervous system, skin, and visceral involvement). The *epidemiologic* classification is based on the duration of infection and communicability, and is divided into an *early* and *late* stage. Although 4 years was previously the dividing line between early and late disease, 2 years is now the generally accepted span, since early symptomatic syphilis is continually infectious and early latent disease intermittently so, providing a high yield of serologic positives on sexual contact tracing. Late latent syphilis, on the other hand, is infectious to the newborn only exceptionally, and epidemiologic investigation of sexual contacts beyond the immediate family is generally not worthwhile.

For treatment purposes, there is yet another classification, where the duration of disease is the determining factor. Syphilis of more than 1 year's duration may more likely lead to progressive involvement of the central nervous system than disease of less than 1 year's duration. Syphilis of more than 1 year's duration, as well as indeterminate syphilis, is therefore treated the same way as neurosyphilis (see "Treatment Guidelines"). The following is a convenient classification of acquired syphilis, combining the clinical, epidemiologic, and treatment factors:

1. Early syphilis includes primary and secondary disease, as well as clinical relapses due to inadequate therapy, and usually lasts less than 1 year for treatment purposes.
2. Latent disease is subdivided into early (less than 2 years) and late (2 years or more) stages for contact tracing, and less than or more than 1 year for treatment purposes.
3. Late syphilis, usually more than 1 year, includes manifest disease: late benign (gumma), cardiovascular, and central nervous system involvement.

Transmission. Transmission of syphilis occurs through direct lesion contact, blood transfusion [58], and oral ingestion of menstrual blood and vaginal secretions in *acquired syphilis*, or via transplacental transfer from mother to fetus in *prenatal syphilis*. In acquired syphilis, the organism is ideally suited for sexual transmission since it requires moisture and tissue medium for survival; fomites are only a theoretical means of transfer and probably account for very few infections. Prosectors, blood handlers, and laboratory technicians remain at risk for accidental inoculation from infected material.

Progression of disease. Infection with syphilis begins almost immediately after contact. The spirochetes multiply locally and enter the lymphatics and bloodstream, where they continue to proliferate. At the site of inoculation, a chancre develops after an asymptomatic incubation period ranging from 10 to 90 days, with an average of 21 days. Variability of the incubation period may relate to the number of spirochetes in the inoculum, as illustrated by experimental infection in rabbits: the incubation period preceding the development of the chancre varied linearly with the size of the inoculum over a range of 2 to 200,000 treponemes with an average increment of 4 days for each tenfold decrease in the number of treponemes inoculated. Ten treponemes or more were required to infect rabbits [57].

Chancres, which may go unnoticed in 15 to 30 percent of infected individuals, may last from 1 to 5 weeks. Dark-field examination is positive during this early stage, while the nontreponemal serologic tests are usually negative until 1 week after the appearance of the chancre and usually positive by 4 weeks after the early lesion. Secondary skin lesions appear 6 to 12 weeks after the onset of the chancre and develop before or after the chancre disappears. The nontreponemal tests are positive during the secondary stage; dark-field examinations of secondary lesions are positive, although the yield of spirochetes in dry lesions is one-tenth the number obtained from moist lesions. Secondary lesions recede in 4 to 12 weeks, but relapses occur in 25 percent of untreated patients [59]. Usually, however, an untreated patient becomes noninfectious as early as 6 months after the disease has been contracted [57]. In 95 percent of cases, immunologic changes prevent the appearance of skin and mucous membrane lesions after this time, but not progression of the organisms to other tissues. Although there is less danger of direct transmission after 4 to 5 years of established infection, inoculation from gummata has occasionally been noted [57]. Latent disease follows secondary syphilis and may persist for life in an asymptomatic form in 60 to 70 percent of patients or progress to neurosyphilis (6.5 percent), cardiovascular disease (9.6 percent), or late benign gummata (16 percent) [60].

Primary syphilis. CLINICAL MANIFESTATIONS. The primary lesion of acquired syphilis is the chancre (Figs. 201-4 and 201-5), developing at the site of inoculation and classically described as single and painless, having a smooth, clean base with raised, indurated borders, associated with a scanty, serous exudate when gentle pressure is applied, and teeming with spirochetes. The chancre is initially an inflammatory papule, followed later by erosion and the formation of a grayish, slightly hemorrhagic crust, with the depth of the lesion varying between superficial and deep, occasionally assuming an ecthymatous appearance. The surrounding tissue shows little or no inflammatory signs. In the male, the chancre commonly appears at the inner part of the prepuce, near the frenulum, in the corona sulcus, and occasionally on the shaft or base of the penis. In the female, common locations for the chancre include the cervix, vagina, vulva, and around areas of the clitoris, urethral orifice, and the posterior labial commissure.

Nowadays, the classic Hunterian chancre is less often seen than the atypical form. In the literature since about 1950, an increase in the occurrence of "atypical" primary syphilis has been noted. In a study of 87 patients with primary syphilis in Rotterdam in 1972 [61], multiple ulcers or erosions were noted in 23 percent of patients, multiple lesions (Fig. 201-4a) with inflammatory edema or phimosis in 8 percent, erosive balanitis in 4.5 percent, multiple lesions with lymphangitis or thrombophlebitis of the dorsal vein in 1.1 percent, and an ulcer in the urethral orifice in 3.4 percent (Fig. 201-4c), for a total of 40 percent with atypical lesions. Atypical chancres have been described in circumcision and vasectomy surgical wounds, and "kissing" chancres on the labia minora are not uncommon. A chancre at the urethral orifice may present as nongonococcal urethritis, or, if left untreated, may occasionally cause an inflammatory phimosis resulting in gangrene of the penis. A dorsal incision of the preputium may be necessary to confirm syphilis infection in the uncircumcised male. Other studies of primary syphilis reveal atypical lesions in 40 to 50 percent of cases. Previous antibiotic treatment does not appear to explain the atypical presentation which may be accounted for by coincidental infection with primary herpes simplex or chancroid. Atypical primary syphilis occasionally may be mistaken for neoplastic disease, especially in the presence of marked adenopathy or systemic signs [62].

Chancres may occur in areas other than the genitalia, and only a high index of suspicion will lead to the correct diagnosis. Extragenital chancres may occur anywhere, but have been most commonly observed in the anus or rectum (Fig. 201-6), with or without proctitis and inguinal adenopathy, and occasionally mimicking polyps or tumor masses; mouth, lips, tongue, and tonsils; fingers [63], toes, and axillary areas; umbilicus, breasts, and eyelids (Fig. 201-7). Inoculation from an infant with prenatal syphilis, or varieties of sexual foreplay may often account for unusual locations. Extragenital chancres may be single or multiple, but are said to be more painful and have a more chronic clinical course. Chancres occurring on the genitalia may occasionally be slightly painful, especially when superinfected with other bacteria, but are rarely as painful as chancroid or herpes simplex, unless occurring together coincidentally. A careful speculum examination may be the only means of detecting cervical chancres. Healing of the chancre takes place over 3 to 6 weeks even without treatment, and leaves a thin atrophic scar; with treatment, there is progressive healing by 10 to 14 days.

DIFFERENTIAL DIAGNOSIS. Typical vesiculoulcerative lesions of genital herpes infection offer little difficulty in differential diagnosis, but once the vesicles rupture and coalesce, diagnosis may be more difficult. Coalescence of lesions to produce solitary ulcers has been reported in 6 percent of patients with genital herpes [64]. In one study, chancroid, which has multiple painful ulcerations, was suspected 3 times more than the causative agent, *Hemophilus ducrei,* and could be identified by smear or culture; clinical appearance of chancroid was more often caused by *T. pallidum* and *H. hominis* [65]. Genital ulcerations resembling chancroid may also be related to microaerophilic streptococci isolated by culture [66]. Infection with other pathogens, opportunistic infection of traumatic lesions, trauma alone, and changes induced by self-administered therapy may confuse the differential diagnosis of primary

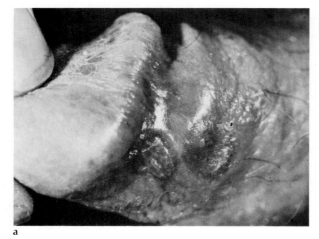

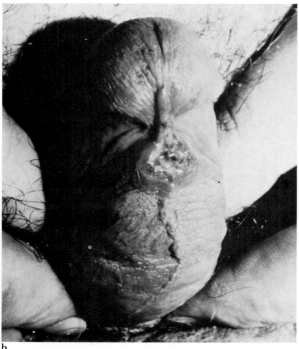

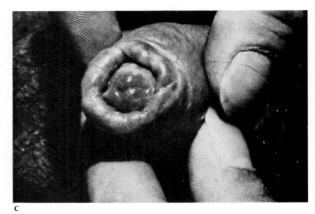

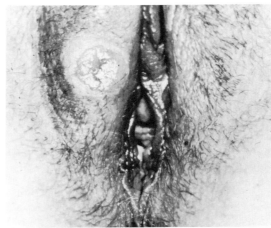

Fig. 201-4 Primary syphilis. Multiple chancres of penile shaft (a), chancre involving frenulum of penus (b), chancre of urethral meatus (c), and chancre of labia majorum (d).

syphilis. In lymphogranuloma venereum, nondiscrete tender adenopathy clinically overshadows skin lesions, which are transient and usually not present at the time of presentation for enlarged lymph nodes. Granuloma inguinale is more granulomatous and true lymph node enlargement is not evident. Other lesions in the differential diagnosis include erosive balanitis or vulvitis, squamous cell carcinoma of the penis or vulva, Behçet's syndrome, fixed drug eruption, lichen planus, psoriasis, Reiter's syndrome, superficial or deep mycotic infection, ulcus vulvae acutum, and pseudolues papulosa of the female genitalia. The diagnostic accuracy and index of suspicion are highest in the presence of a single ulceration on the genitalia, but both are reduced when there are multiple, inflamed, or tender lesions or when coincident infection with other pathogens is present [65].

DIAGNOSIS. In the absence of a definite diagnosis, repeat dark-field and serologic examinations for syphilis are re-

quired for all patients who have genital ulcerations. Patients who have self-administered antitreponemal drugs in inadequate doses require an even closer and more prolonged follow-up examination in order to detect serologic changes which make possible a legitimate retrospective diagnosis of syphilis, the completion of adequate therapy, and a thorough investigation of sexual contacts. Epidemiologic treatment (see "Treatment Guidelines") with syphilis therapy for "nonspecific" ulcerations may be indicated in some clinical circumstances, especially when patient follow-up is not assured. A highly suspect, undiagnosed lesion should be examined on 2 or 3 successive days; application of saline compresses is permitted, but soaps, disinfectants, or local antibiotics should be avoided. Secondary infection may be treated with sulfisoxazole, 1 g orally 4 times per day, without influencing syphilitic infection or serologic tests.

A tenable retrospective diagnosis of syphilis, in the presence of a dark-field-negative lesion, is possible when there are characteristic skin changes, regional nontender adenopathy, and a rising nontreponemal serologic titer. Nontreponemal serologic tests should be positive in an untreated chancre at the end of 4 weeks, although treatment with antitreponemal drugs in inadequate doses may prolong the "incubation period." Serologic testing should be

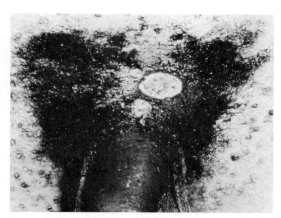

Fig. 201-5   Primary chancre at base of penis. Lesions in this location are commonly associated with the use of a condom.

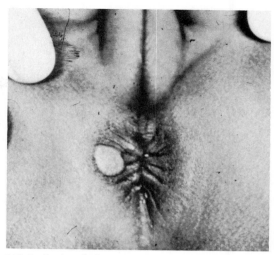

Fig. 201-6   Perianal chancre.

extended for 3 months to reliably exclude syphilis. Although in primary syphilis the FTA-ABS test is usually positive earlier than the nontreponemal tests (see "Serology of Syphilis"), it is not recommended as a screening test, since false positives will occur, especially in populations with a low prevalence of syphilis.

Primary syphilis is usually accompanied by painless regional adenopathy. The nodes are characteristically discrete, firm, nonsuppurative, movable, and without changes on the overlying skin. The lymphadenopathy may be unilateral, bilateral, or undetectable if the lesion occurs in an area where lymph nodes are not palpable (cervix, rectum). Occasionally the lymph nodes are tender, markedly enlarged, and may even be mistaken for malignancy. Suppurative inguinal lymphadenopathy may occasionally accompany atypical primary chancres [67], and superinfection of primary lesions with pyogenic organisms (including fusospirochetal organisms) may pose additional diagnostic difficulties [68]. Chancres of the urethral meatus and oral cavity may require aspiration of the regional lymph node to confirm the diagnosis by dark-field examination, since these mucosal sites are colonized by spirochetes difficult to differentiate morphologically from *T. pallidum*.

A diagnosis of primary syphilis may be made by detecting *T. pallidum* in lesions of early disease (primary, secondary, early prenatal). Serum from moist lesions or intentionally abraded dry lesions, needle aspiration of enlarged regional lymph nodes, and nasal secretions from infants with "snuffles" may be used to identify *T. pallidum*. Characteristic movements of *T. pallidum* in dark-field microscopy include a corkscrew rotation, a graceful bending like a bamboo pole, and a spiral spring stretching and shortening.

One method of identification of *T. pallidum* relies on direct immunofluorescence examination of dry secretions on glass slides. Such a method compares favorably with dark-field examination of fresh lesions and may be useful in settings where dark-field microscopy is unavailable, where syphilis has a low incidence, aboard ship (allowing retrospective diagnosis), and where the postal service is reliable. The seronegative oral primary lesion lends itself to this technique, since the direct fluorescence method is specific for *T. pallidum* [69].

HISTOPATHOLOGY OF PRIMARY SYPHILIS [70]. Vascular changes, characterized by endarteritis and periarteritis, are the most prominent histologic features of the human response to *T. pallidum*. Capillary dilatation with enodothelial cell swelling and proliferation leads to vessel lumen narrowing in an endarteritis, while proliferation of adventitial cells and a surrounding inflammatory infiltrate which includes lymphocytes, monocytes, and plasma cells, characterize the periarteritis (Fig. 201-8). Fibrosis and scar formation often occur with healing. Histopathology of the chancre reveals acanthosis at the lesion margins and absence of the epidermis toward the center. The changes in the dermis show a dense lymphocytic and plasma cell infiltrate at the center of the lesion and a loose perivascular array at the periphery. The endothelial cells show proliferation and swelling, and many treponemes demonstrated with silver stains (Levaditi's, Warthin–Starry) are found in the dermis around the walls of capillaries. Spirochetes are found predominantly in the perivascular areas, within phagolysosomes of endothelial cells, macrophages, neutrophils, and plasma cells; to a lesser extent in the intercellular spaces of the epidermis; and occasionally within epidermal cells. Fluorescent antibody staining methods are more specific in detecting spirochetes in tissue, since reticulin fibers take up silver stains and cause confusion. Specific antitreponemal antibodies may also be identified in the lymphoplasmocytic infiltrates of skin lesions using a modified direct immunofluorescence procedure [71].

In regional lymph nodes of primary syphilis, there is a chronic inflammatory infiltrate composed of many plasma cells in addition to endothelial proliferation, follicular hyperplasia, and, in some instances, noncaseating granulomas resembling sarcoidosis. Spirochetes can be identified using the Warthin–Starry silver stains or immunofluorescence techniques.

Secondary syphilis. The signs and symptoms of secondary syphilis may develop 2 to 6 months after infection, occasionally longer, and usually 6 to 8 weeks after appearance of the primary chancre. The primary chancre may still be present when the secondary lesions appear. Generalized clinical manifestations occur during this stage and may affect almost any organ system of the body. Nontrepone-

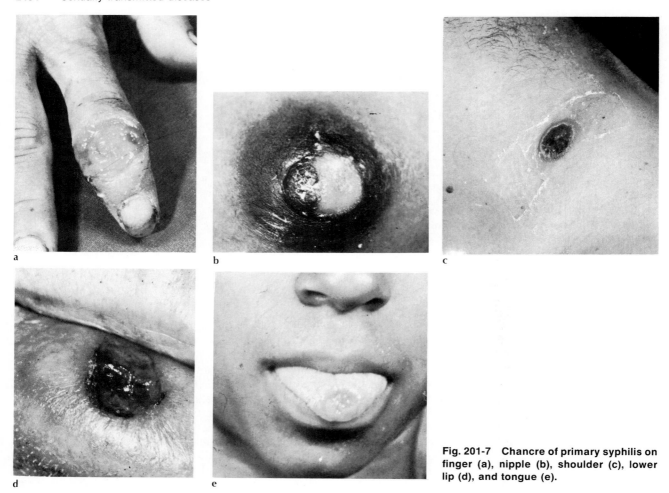

Fig. 201-7 Chancre of primary syphilis on finger (a), nipple (b), shoulder (c), lower lip (d), and tongue (e).

Fig. 201-8 Primary syphilis, the chancre. The process is characterized by a dense infiltrate of inflammatory cells, including lymphocytes, histiocytes, and plasma cells. Vascular spaces are frequently difficult to identify due to endothelial swelling. ×100. (Micrograph by Wallace H. Clark, Jr., M.D.)

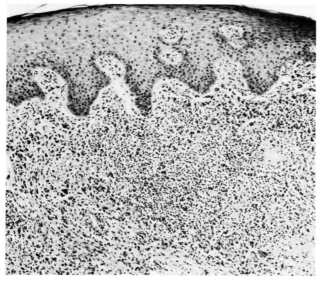

mal serologic tests (VDRL, ART, RPR) are always positive, and a negative serology requires a reconsideration of the clinical diagnosis or a reexamination for a prozone phenomenon (see "Serology of Syphilis"). Malignant syphilis may also occur with a negative serology.

The lesions of secondary syphilis represent a tissue reaction to *T. pallidum*, that is carried to the site by the blood and lymphatics. Lesions contain large numbers of motile treponemes, although gentle abrasion may be required in order to obtain serous fluid in dry lesions for dark-field examination. As a rule, the secondary lesions heal without scar formation in 2 to 10 weeks, with or without treatment, although atypical presentations are not uncommon (see below). Systemic signs, symptoms, and mucocutaneous manifestations may be subtle, transient, and easily overlooked; or obvious, indolent, and occasionally destructive. Clinical relapse of secondary manifestations, although stated by Thomas [57] to represent a failure of antibiotic therapy, probably represents natural progression of disease. In their follow-up of patients with untreated syphilis, Clark and Danbolt noted that approximately 25 percent of subjects experienced clinical secondary relapse, and of these, one-quarter had multiple episodes. More than two-thirds of the relapsers had relapsed by the end of 6 months, 90 percent by the end of 1 year, 95 percent by the end of 2 years, and 100 percent by the end of 5 years [59]. Moreover, progressive lesions in the untreated state represent not relapse but persistence of secondary syphilis and progression of one syphilitic eruption to another. Progressive serologic or clinical infection and communicability may exist even in the absence of clinical lesions. Serologic relapse may occur in the treated state and signify inadequate therapy, even with "effective" antibiotics. Longterm follow-up after treatment for early syphilis is therefore required (see "Treatment Guidelines"). A serologic rise occurring more than 2 years after adequate treatment probably represents reinfection rather than relapse.

CLINICAL MANIFESTATIONS. Skin and mucous membrane lesions of secondary syphilis are marked by a panoply of clinical patterns that bear a semblance of symmetry in early disease and asymmetry in later stages. Macular, papular, papulosquamous, follicular, pustular, or nodular varieties occur, with many forms often appearing simultaneously. Vesiculobullous lesions, although common in prenatal syphilis, are not found in adults. According to classic teachings, pruritus is generally not present, but recent reports indicate that as many as 8 to 42 percent of patients with secondary syphilis have pruritus [72,73], with a possibly higher rate among blacks, especially those with lichenoid or follicular varieties of skin lesions [74]. There is also a suggestion that secondary syphilis in the modern era is less polymorphous, more predictable, and less destructive than disease reported in older writings, although atypical forms still occur [75].

Macular lesions (macular syphilides, roseola syphilitica) are the earliest of the secondary skin manifestations, beginning 7 to 10 weeks after infection and 3 to 6 weeks after the chancre, remaining only a few days, and often overlooked, especially in blacks. The lesions are present as nonpruritic, nonscaling oval spots beginning on the torso and involving any area, including palms and soles. Progression and dissemination may occur, and take an annular shape around earlier lesions (annular syphilide) or simply increase in size (larger macular syphilide). Macules may undergo proliferative changes and coexist with papules and pustules.

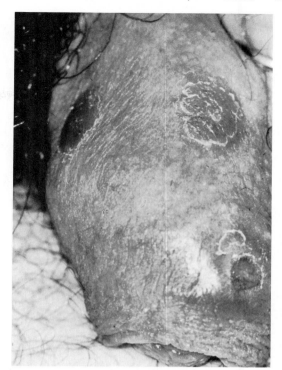

Fig. 201-10   Scaling lesions of secondary syphilis.

Fig. 201-11   Annular lesions of secondary syphilis on the face (a) and shoulder (b).

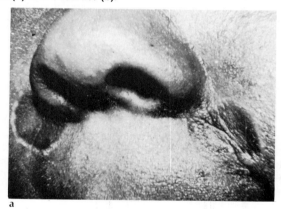

a

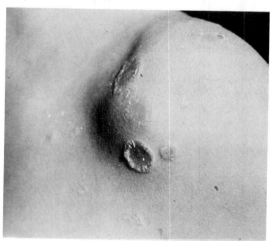

b

Fig. 201-9   Papular lesions of secondary syphilis.

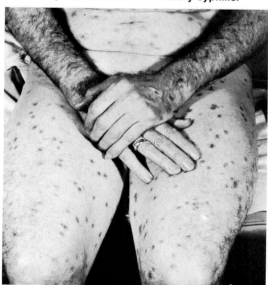

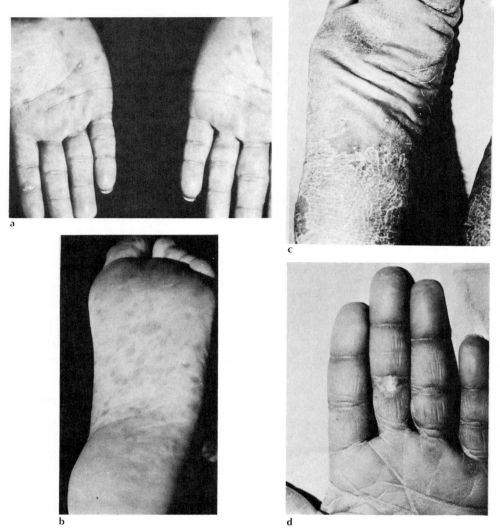

Fig. 201-12 Palm and sole lesions in secondary syphilis may present subtle manifestations of the generalized eruption. Papulosquamous (a) and papular (b) lesions are characteristic, while diffuse (c) or localized (d) hyperkeratosis may be mistaken for tinea pedis or simple callus (syphilitic "corn"). Parts (c and d) represent the same patient, whose palm and sole lesions cleared by 3 weeks after 2 doses of benzathine penicillin, 2.4 million units intramuscularly, separated by 1 week.

Papular lesions (papular syphilides) are the most frequent lesions encountered in secondary syphilis and are subdivided into several morphologic variants which include the following:

Follicular lesions (miliary papular syphilides) are pinhead to pinpoint in size, acuminate or rounded, erythematous, and develop in crops on the torso and extremities. Some lesions may be pustular (see below). These lesions tend to be pruritic, especially in blacks.

Lenticular papular lesions are pinhead to bean size or larger, brown to red in color, with a smooth or finely scaling surface. Predilection appears to be for the forehead and face, especially the buccal commissures, nasolabial folds, and genitalia. Pustulation may occur, but lesions do not coalesce in this variety.

Papulosquamous lesions (Figs. 201-9, 201-10, and A3-8a and b) are raised, with flat surfaces, discoid and scaling, red and indurated, and may assume a psoriasiform appearance. An annular (Fig. 201-11), serpiginous, concentric (cockade syphilide), or arcuate configuration is often seen. Head, neck, and palmar and plantar surfaces are common sites (Fig. 201-12). A pruritic lichenoid variety, clinically and histologically similar to lichen planus, has been reported in the penicillin as well as prepenicillin era [76]. On the palms and soles, diffuse hyperkeratosis may simulate dermatophytosis (Fig. 201-12c); localized hyperkeratosis may be confused with a simple callus (syphilis cornée, clavi syphilitici) (Fig. 201-12d).

Moist papular lesions (condylomata lata, Fig. 201-13) occur on the genital, anal, and umbilical regions, axillae, buccal commissures, interdigital webs, opposing surfaces of toes, and submammary folds. Lesions begin as papules but become flattened, macerated, and covered with a thick mucoid exudate. Papillomatosis, vegetations, and foul odor

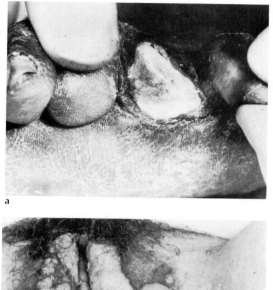

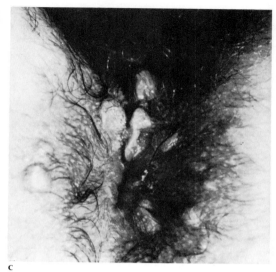

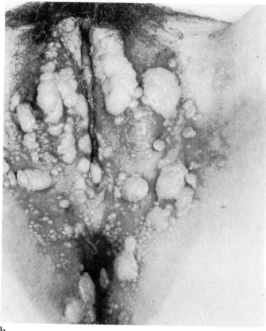

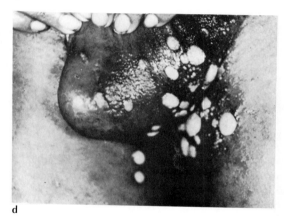

Fig. 201-13 Condylomata lata in toe web (a), female ano-genital region (b), perianal region (c), and scrotal area (d). The term *lata* (Latin adjective meaning "broad" or "flat") distinguishes these lesions from condylomata acuminata (Latin adjective *acuminata,* "pointed" or "sharp").

may result. These lesions are teeming with spirochetes; they are quite infectious whereas dry lesions are less so. Eroded lesions on the intertriginous parts of the body (Fig. 201-14) may proliferate and form large, elevated, brown-red, velvetlike lesions, or grow to hypertrophic nodular masses (framboesiform syphilide) [77,78]. Papules may be located on seborrheic areas of the face or trunk, may assume an annular configuration (Fig. 201-11) that may be confused with annular sarcoid and granuloma annulare, or may be placed in a ring along the edge of the hair ("corona veneris"). Concentric rings of papules, simulating tinea imbrication, rarely occur in secondary syphilis [79].

Corymbose syphilide (bombshell syphilide) is another variant of the papular morphology, with a large central papule surrounded by small satellite papules, usually occurring in the late secondary stage and rarely before 6 to 8 months of infection [80].

Pustular secondary syphilis may appear in several vari-eties, and include a small acuminate pustular syphilide (miliary pustular syphilide) often occurring with papular lesions and leaving depressed hyperpigmented areas when healed; a large acuminate pustular syphilide (acneform, varioliform, or obtuse syphiloderm) consisting of discrete perifollicular pustules with a firm base and often showing polymorphism [81]; a flat pustular syphiloderm (impetigi-noid or echthymiform syphilide), which often becomes confluent, forming a large crust called a carapace. A rare follicular papulopustular variant has been associated par-ticularly with abnormal CSF findings [82], while yet an-other variant is distinguished for its severely destructive behavior—malignant syphilis (rupial syphilide, lues ma-ligna, pustuloulcerative syphilide)—frequently seen in the seventeenth century ("la grand vérole"), but only rarely seen in the modern ear [83,84].

The skin lesions of *malignant syphilis,* which are often widespread yet reversible with adequate antibiotic treat-

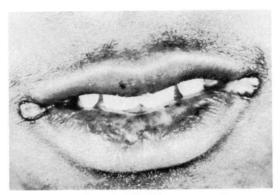

Fig. 201-14   Split papules of secondary syphilis.

ment, are preceded by a prodrome of fever, headache, and muscle pain. Lesions begin as papulopustules which soon become necrotic and result in sharply marginated ulcers covered by thick, dirty crusts found in layers resembling oyster shells (''rupioid''). The face and scalp are most commonly involved and lesions are associated with pain, toxicity, arthralgias, and occasionally hepatitis [85]. Oral ulcerations as well as mucous patches are not uncommonly associated with malignant syphilis.

Although malignant syphilis has been associated with a debilitated state as a predisposing factor, recent cases argue against such a mechanism. In cases where epidemiology can be traced, most have been contracted from patients with ordinary varieties of the disease, although one report describes three cases apparently infected from the same source [86]. Also, there is no evidence that there are *T. pallidum* organisms of different virulence causing different degrees of severity. Alternatively, an immunologic mechanism for the destructive process is postulated that is related to host responsiveness, with a syphilitic obliterative vasculitis of medium-sized vessels at the dermal-subcutaneous junction resulting in thrombosis of vessels and necrosis of overlying skin. Further studies of this process are needed. Active lesions respond dramatically to penicillin (see Fig. 201-18d and e) (see ''Treatment Guidelines'').

Nodular lesions of secondary syphilis are being reported with increasing frequency in the modern antibiotic era. Such manifestations are being mistaken for lymphoma or a granulomatous process due to foreign body or other infectious organisms [87-90].

Changes in pigmentation often accompany the skin lesions of secondary syphilis. Hyperpigmentation commonly occurs with healing, and in early secondary syphilis hypopigmentation may occur in the form of macular pigment loss on a darker, often hyperpigmented reticulated background on the sides of the neck (leukoderma colli syphiliticum, necklace of Venus), penis, or other sites [91,92]. Disseminated leukoderma masquerading as vitiligo was reported to have occurred with secondary syphilis in India, and the pigment changes resolved after two months following treatment for syphilis [93]. Atrophy may follow the healing of secondary skin lesions, possibly related to destruction of elastic tissue in the sites of previous inflammation (secondary anetoderma). Electron microscopic studies of the leukoderma of secondary syphilis reveals a normal or slightly reduced number of melanocytes, with partial inhibition of melanogenesis [94].

Nail changes with paronychia and secondary changes of the plate are said to occur sometimes in the secondary stage, but the appearance is not specific [95].

Hair loss can occur as a diffuse telogen effluvium [93] 3 to 5 months after infection begins, or as patchy ''moth-eaten'' thinning occurring in small, scattered and irregular areas (Fig. 201-15), predominantly on the posterior scalp and occasionally involving the eyebrows, beard, or other body sites, such as the legs [96]. Scarring is not present during this stage and regrowth occurs with or without treatment. Scarring of the scalp may occur with tertiary syphilis.

Mucous membrane lesions of secondary syphilis are similar to those on the surface of the skin, modified by influences peculiar to the oral, labial, anal, and vulvar mucosae. Stratum corneum is lacking in these locations, so lesions are easily abraded. Papules are characteristically rounded, flat, gray, superficially ulcerated, and teeming with spirochetes. These mucous patches (Fig. A3-8c) of gray-white color have a tendency to ulceration, and are seen on the tonsils, the inner surface of the lips and cheeks, and in the larynx where papules appear on the epiglottis and aryepiglottic folds and cause a characteristic hoarseness. On the surface of the tongue they appear as sharply defined, round or oval plaques (''plaques fouchées'') in which the papillae of the tongue are flattened and the mucous membrane is denuded.

Constitutional signs and symptoms may accompany or precede skin and mucous membrane lesions. Malaise, appetite loss, hoarseness, mild weight loss, headache, myalgias, arthralgias, and low-grade fever may be so mild as to go unnoticed, or florid enough to require hospitalization and consideration of other disease states (acute rheumatic fever, collagen vascular disease, tuberculosis, malignancy, etc.).

Lymph node involvement is almost always present in secondary syphilis, though not always appreciated; and is marked by nontender, firm, discrete adenopathy on palpation. Cervical (anterior and posterior), suboccipital, inguinal, epitrochlear, and axillary nodes are regularly involved. Spleen enlargement is common. Occasionally, painful lymphadenopathy has required biopsy for presumed reticuloendothelial disease or carcinomatosis, only to reveal secondary syphilis [97]; painful lymph nodes following alcohol ingestion, similar to Hodgkin's disease, have been described [98].

Abnormalities are found in other organ systems in secondary syphilis. Anemia, leukocytosis, a relative lympho-

Fig. 201-15   Moth-eaten alopecia of secondary syphilis.

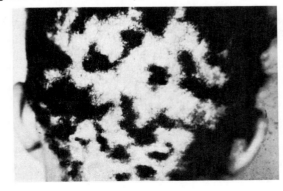

cytosis, and an elevated sedimentation rate are regularly observed. Both antinuclear antibodies and rheumatoid factors have been detected in patients with secondary syphilis [99]. Acute membranous glomerulonephritis manifested by the nephrotic syndrome, reversible after appropriate antibiotic therapy and resembling the glomerulopathy of prenatal syphilis, has been associated with the deposition of treponemal antigen–antitreponemal antibody complexes and C3 in the subepithelial basement membrane zone, as demonstrated by histologic, electron microscopic, and histochemical studies [100].

Hepatitis, manifested by a tender enlarged liver or simply an asymptomatic elevation of alkaline phosphatase, but rarely clinical jaundice, has been documented in 17 of 175 cases of early syphilis. An abnormal biopsy in most patients sampled, as well as treponemes present in the liver, and reduction in biopsy abnormalities and disappearance of treponemes from the liver 2 months after penicillin therapy suggest that syphilitic hepatitis may be more common than has been clinically suspected in the past [99,101,102].

Gastric lesions, interpreted as ulcerative or polypoidal by endoscopy, and manifested as clinical gastritis with epigastric pain and postprandial vomiting, have been attributed to secondary syphilis in rare instances. The lesions responded to antibiotic therapy for syphilis [103]. Painless swelling of the parotid gland may also be a rare manifestation of secondary syphilis [104].

Bone and joint changes, including skull and limb pain, backache, arthralgias, and arthritis may occur in as high as 4 percent of patients with secondary syphilis [105]. Headache, often thought to be due to early syphilitic meningitis with elevated CSF pressure and pleocytosis [55], may more likely be related to ostitic lesions of the skull, found in 7 of 80 patients with secondary syphilis [106]. A proliferative periostitis, osteomyelitis, tumefaction, severe pain at involved sites that is usually worse at night, and demonstration of spirochetes, bone necrosis, and intense plasma cell infiltration on biopsy characterize the bony lesions of secondary syphilis [107–110].

Periostitis, not always evident on x-ray and appearing as localized bone pain as the earliest and most common osseous manifestation, occurs in tibia, sternum, skull, and ribs, in decreasing order of frequency. Destructive lesions (osteitis and osteomyelitis) are rare and occur most frequently in the skull and sternoclavicular joint. The destructive bone lesions of secondary syphilis cannot be distinguished clinically from bacterial tuberculosis or neoplastic causes, and bone biopsy may be necessary for diagnosis, especially if appropriate antisyphilitic therapy does not rapidly improve symptoms within 48 h. X-ray changes may take 3 to 11 months for complete resolution [109]. Articular involvement, including symmetric or asymmetric arthritis, tenosynovitis, and bursitis, or back pain simulating early ankylosing spondylitis may be mild or severe, lasting weeks to months [105]. Joint complaints of secondary syphilis may even simulate acute rheumatic fever or rheumatoid arthritis.

Generalized myalgias are common in the secondary stage, but muscle weakness may occasionally present as inflammatory myopathy and respond to appropriate therapy. Contracture of the biceps muscle may rarely occur in early syphilis, with gummata in skeletal muscles presenting as a woody myositis affecting the proximal limbs and tongue may occur in the tertiary stage. Muscle weakness

is more usually the result of spinal cord or root involvement in the later stages of syphilis [111].

Eye involvement in the form of uveitis, iridocyclitis, choroidoretinitis, and, rarely, combined occlusion of the central retinal vein and artery due to vasculitis may occasionally occur in secondary syphilis. Symptoms include photophobia, lacrimation, and red and painful eyes. Inappropriate steroid administration may lead to deterioration, while appropriate antibiotic therapy will usually halt progression or result in rapid resolution of disease [112,113].

Central nervous system involvement, manifested by transient CSF pleocytosis or elevated protein and usually reactive VDRL tests, occurs in 30 to 70 percent of patients in the early stages of syphilis infection. About 20 percent of these affected patients, representing 7 to 9 percent of all untreated patients with early syphilis, will develop late symptomatic neurosyphilis 7 to 30 years after infection [114,115]. Other investigators have found a lower prevalence of abnormalities, and question the value of CSF examination in secondary syphilis unless CNS symptoms are present [103], since adequate treatment of the secondary stage will usually prevent progression to neurosyphilis (see ''Treatment Guidelines''). On the other hand, *acute syphilitic meningitis* can rarely occur in patients at this stage of disease, with manifestations of headache, vertigo, fever, and rarely convulsions, with accompanying abnormal spinal fluid protein, pleocytosis, elevated pressure, and a positive CSF and blood nontreponemal serology [116]. Transverse myelitis or thrombosis of cerebrospinal arteries may occur, and the occasional presence of papilledema may confuse this process for a mass lesion or focal cerebral damage [117]. The meningitis is usually basilar in location, with optic neuritis and asymmetric involvement of multiple cranial nerves, and the vast majority of cases occurs within the first year of infection and in about 10 percent is coincident with the skin rash of secondary disease. Response to appropriate antibiotic therapy is usually successful because the inflamed meninges enhance penetration of penicillin. Permanent neurologic damage may occur in untreated cases, although the natural process runs a relatively benign course with rare fatalities.

Perceptive deafness, with residual VIIIth nerve damage occurring despite adequate antibiotic therapy, will rarely complicate secondary syphilis. Vestibular symptoms, including persistent vertigo, may also occur. Signs of acute meningitis and abnormalities of the CSF commonly accompany these findings and emphasize the necessity for routine CSF examination in patients with sudden hearing loss [118]. Prednisone has been recommended for treatment of inner ear and auditory nerve involvement in secondary syphilis in order to prevent the worsening of symptoms occasionally occurring with the Jarisch–Herxheimer reaction (see ''Treatment Guidelines'').

Other rare manifestations of secondary syphilis include lesions in the lung [119] and cardiac conduction abnormalities [120].

DIFFERENTIAL DIAGNOSIS. The skin and mucous membrane lesions of secondary syphilis may be confused with many disease states. The initial macular rash (roseola) may be confused with drug eruptions, rubella, rubeola, viral exanthemata, and pityriasis rosea, to name a few (see Atlas 3). Papular syphilides may be difficult to differentiate from psoriasis, lichen planus, acne, or scabies; eroded papules may resemble impetigo, fungal infection (dermatophyte,

deep fungal), condylomata acuminata, ulcerated hemorrhoids, balanitis, psoriasis, and herpes simplex. Papules
on the palms and soles may be confused with psoriasis,
Reiter's syndrome, dermatophytosis, hyperkeratotic
eczema, clavi, or plantar warts. Papules in the mouth can
mimic aphthosis, herpangina, diphtheria, infectious mononucleosis, and perlèche. Ulcerative syphilides can be distinguished from ecthyma by dark-field examination and
serology; leukoderma syphiliticum may be similar to pityriasis versicolor except for a positive serology in the
former and a positive scraping for hyphae in the latter.
Alopecia areata can be distinguished from the moth-eaten
alopecia of secondary syphilis by the presence of excla-
mation-point hairs in the midst of bald spots in the former,
and ragged thinning of hair density and a positive serology
in the latter.

DIAGNOSIS. The diagnosis of secondary syphilis requires
a high index of clinical suspicion, given the variety of
manifestations and presentations. Nontreponemal serologic tests are usually positive in high titer ($> 1{:}16$), the
only exception being the prozone phenomenon (see "Serology of Syphilis"). Dark-field examination of moist or
intentionally abraded dry lesions, and histologic examination of tissue (lymph nodes, liver, skin, mucous membrane)
using silver stains or immunofluorescence for the detection
of spirochetes or specific antitreponemal antibodies may
be helpful to confirm the diagnosis.

HISTOPATHOLOGY OF SECONDARY SYPHILIS [70]. The histopathology of skin lesions in secondary syphilis (Fig.
201-16) is dependent on the clinical presentation. The number of spirochetes in tissue sections stained with silver
varies with the type of lesion, their number being few in
macular lesions, but present in great enough quantity to
be detected in the dermis around blood vessels of the
superficial plexus and in the epidermis in papular lesions
and condylomata lata (Fig. 201-17). The histology of macular lesions is not diagnostic; there is endothelial swelling
of superficial capillaries, surrounded by a meager infiltrate
of lymphocytes and plasma cells. Papular lesions show
superficial and deep vessel involvement with perivascular

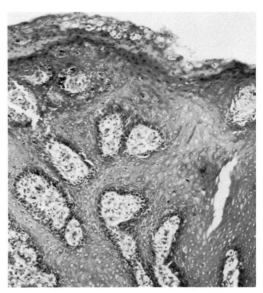

**Fig. 201-17   Condyloma latum. There is extensive epidermal
hyperplasia with a dense inflammatory infiltrate of the
stroma. ×100. (AFIP 138609. Micrograph by Wallace H. Clark,
Jr., M.D. Courtesy of Dr. Elson B. Helwig.)**

cuffing in the lower dermis and a diffuse scattering of cells,
in addition to perivascular infiltrates in the upper dermis.
Plasma cells are common in the infiltrate, and granulomas
often appear even in early secondary syphilis. Condylomata lata show acanthosis and edema between and within
cells of the epidermis, with elongation and broadening of
the rete ridges. Psoriasiform lesions resemble psoriasis
except for the dermal infiltrate, which is similar to that
found in papular lesions of secondary syphilis. Follicular
papulopustular lesions show granulomas consisting of epithelioid and giant cells in the perifollicular region, in addition to the perivascular coat-sleeve infiltrate of papular
lesions. Ulcerating lesions of malignant syphilis are distinctive in that they show accumulation of fibrinoid material within many vessels, which causes partial or complete
occlusion of the lumen and results in infarction of the upper
dermis and epidermis. The lesions of syphilis cornée show
the typical dermal changes of papular lesions, but, in addition, show a keratotic and in part parakeratotic plug
invaginating the epidermis.

Although the aforementioned pathologic changes are
considered typical in the lesions of secondary syphilis, the
absence or inconspicuous nature of the "classic" histologic findings has been stressed in a clinicopathologic review of 57 patients [121]: (1) in nearly one-quarter of the
biopsies, plasma cell infiltration was either absent or very
sparse; (2) vascular damage was seen in fewer than half,
and, where present, the vessel changes were almost entirely confined to swelling of the endothelial cells, while
endothelial cell proliferation was uncommon. On the other
hand, epidermal changes suggestive of eczematous dermatitis were frequently apparent and included exocytosis,
spongiosis, parakeratosis, and, most commonly, acanthosis. Occasionally Munro abscesses and spongiform pustulation occurred, simulating psoriasis.

Syphilis is as much an "imitator" for the pathologist as
for the clinician.

**Fig. 201-16   Secondary syphilis. Some lesions of secondary
syphilis show a sparse, quite nonspecific inflammatory response. Others, such as the one illustrated here, show a
dense infiltrate in the papillary dermis with some obscura-
tion of the dermal-epidermal interface. The presence of
plasma cells and endothelial swelling suggests that the
changes are due to syphilis, but the histologic diagnosis may
be difficult. ×100. (Micrograph by Wallace H. Clark, Jr. M.D.)**

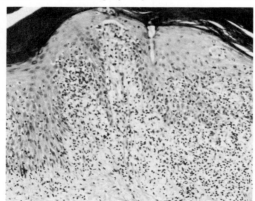

Latent syphilis. Latent syphilis is defined in an individual who has a repeatedly reactive nontreponemal serologic test for syphilis that is confirmed by a specific treponemal test in the absence of signs and symptoms of disease. The diagnosis is usually uncovered by serologic screening, the birth of a syphilitic child, or a history of syphilis exposure or of former skin lesions. Prenatal syphilis may be difficult to exclude in the absence of maternal history, physical findings suggesting prenatally acquired disease, or previous blood tests for syphilis. When the results of previous blood tests are known (marriage, military service, employment), a more exact timing of disease duration can be made. More commonly, however, the clinician must settle for a diagnosis of ''indeterminate'' latent syphilis because of a lack of information. Latency, or inactivity of disease, however, may not be diagnosed until a complete physical and neurologic examination, in addition to a sampling of CSF and an x-ray of the heart and aorta, are found to be normal. Abnormal spinal fluid findings will change the diagnosis to asymptomatic neurosyphilis, which requires treatment quite different from latent disease (see ''Treatment Guidelines'').

Latent syphilis begins with the disappearance of skin lesions of secondary syphilis and continues as such for life unless symptomatic disease occurs. Thomas estimates that approximately 25 percent of patients with latent disease will subsequently develop signs of late disease [57]. Of those patients with late latent disease left untreated in the Tuskegee study, the primary cause of death in one-third of patients was syphilitic involvement of the cardiovascular and central nervous systems; of those whose disease was allowed to progress more than 10 years and studied at autopsy, an estimated 50 percent showed cardiovascular system involvement (see ''Treatment Guidelines'').

Late benign syphilis [52–57,59,115]. CLASSIFICATION AND BACKGROUND. In Clark and Danbolt's follow-up of 1404 original patients with untreated early syphilis, initially studied by Boeck of Norway, late benign syphilis occurred in 14.4 percent of males and 16.7 percent of females. Approximately one-quarter of the males and one-third of the females had from 2 to 7 episodes of late benign lesions, which included skin (70 percent), skeletal (9.6 percent), and mucous membrane involvement (10.3 percent). Solitary (single structure) lesions were more common (90 percent) than multiple structure involvement (10 percent), and of the multiple structure lesions, the skin was one of the structures in more than half the patients. Gummata affected almost any organ of the body, including the liver and cardiovascular system. The majority of lesions developed by the end of the fifteenth year after healing of the secondary manifestations, with a range from 1 to 46 years. Spontaneous healing of a gumma did not usually occur [59,60].

The exact incidence of late benign syphilis in the last decade is not known but seems to be distinctly rare. The incidence of late syphilis (all ages, all types) from 1976 to 1980 in the United Kingdom varied from 1.81 to 4.56 (depending on sex, higher in males than females) new cases per 100,000 population per year [7]. Only a few cases of late benign syphilis of the skin have been seen at major university dermatology departments in Boston and Vienna in the past decade.

LATE BENIGN SYPHILIS OF THE SKIN. Cutaneous manifestations may develop any time after the secondary stage resolves, with ''precocious'' lesions noted within the first 2 years, and the late syphilides as late as 2 to 30 years, but in general most occur within 3 to 7 years. Isolated examples of gummata may appear as long as 60 years after infection and are generally associated with neurosyphilis. The longer the time between early disease and the appearance of the late benign skin lesions, the more solitary and destructive the process.

Skin lesions are manifest as nodules or plaques (Fig. 201-18), representing an inflammatory tissue response to the presence of rare organisms in tissue in patients chronically sensitized to *T. pallidum*. At this stage, delayed skin tests to *T. pallidum* are markedly positive, in contrast to early disease. In addition, persons previously sensitized chronically with *T. pallidum* may occasionally respond to new exogenous infection with the manifestation of benign late syphilis of the skin. Gummata are rarely infectious, although there has been documented transfer of infection from such lesions [57]. Patients with malignant syphilis are more likely to develop gummata, which suggests a unique host responsiveness to *T. pallidum* in this rare variant of secondary syphilis.

Serologic tests for syphilis are usually reactive and of high titer in active benign syphilis, although reports of gummata with nonreactive nontreponemal tests for syphilis do exist. Healed gummata following adequate treatment may be associated with a negative STS as well.

There is a tendency to partial healing of late benign syphilis of the skin even without therapy, but new lesions occur on the periphery and spontaneous complete healing is unusual without adequate treatment. Scarring is notable for its noncontractile and atrophic quality. Active lesions respond dramatically to penicillin (see ''Treatment Guidelines'').

The classification of skin lesions in late benign syphilis includes precocious syphilides and the late syphilides. Late syphilides include nodular and noduloulcerative lesions, pseudochancre redux, and gummata. The nodular syphilide is superficial, while the gummatous syphilide is deep. Transitional forms occur.

Precocious tertiary syphilides were not uncommon during the era of heavy metal therapy and were observed more frequently in inadequately treated rather than untreated patients. Lesions usually occurred during the first 4 years of infection, but occasionally appeared within weeks in a particularly malignant precocious form. Skin manifestations had characteristics that bordered between secondary and late cutaneous lesions, and consisted of papules in a grouped configuration, localized or generalized in distribution, with some degree of ulceration and reminiscent of nodular late syphilides. *T. pallidum* can rarely be demonstrated, and the lesions heal with little or no scarring.

Nodular and noduloulcerative lesions (tubercular syphilides) are superficial, firm, nodular gummata of the skin, several millimeters in size and brownish red in color. The nodules occur in a grouped configuration, rapidly extending peripherally in an unequal manner and healing in the center over weeks or months (simultaneous healing and progression), resulting in serpiginous plaques with arciform and scalloped borders (Fig. 201-18a, b, and d). Occasionally, waxy scales may impart a psoriasiform character, and

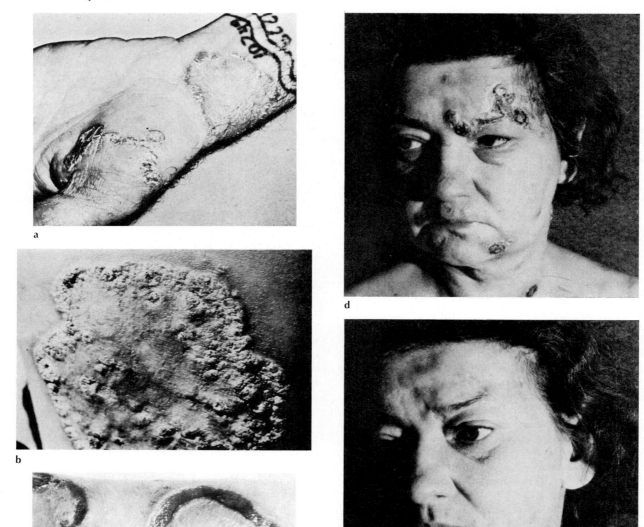

Fig. 201-18 Late benign syphilis, showing annular nodular syphilide of the wrist and hand (a), noduloulcerative syphilide of the femoral region (b), gumma of the leg (c), and early ulcerative syphilide of the face before (d) and 8 weeks after (e) treatment with 4.8 million units of benzathine penicillin.

lesions may closely resemble granuloma annulare or sarcoidosis. Crusts will cover the ulcerated forms that have slight pus formation and elevated borders. The lesions are without symptoms and occur on the extensor arms, back, and face. Atrophy, hyper- and hypopigmentation characterize the healing process. *Pseudochancre redux* is a term describing a solitary gumma of the penis. The *gumma* (Fig. 201-18c) is a deep granulomatous process involving epidermis secondarily, beginning as one or several painless subcutaneous tumors anywhere on the body but more regularly on the scalp, face, chest, and calf. Trauma may also affect the localization of lesions. The lesion has a tendency

to necrosis, with the formation of a stringy mass (of "gum")—hence its name *gumma*. As it increases in size and involves more superficial layers of the dermis, the skin appears red and eventually breaks down to form a punched-out ulcer, indistinguishable from other ulcers. The gumma may even begin in bone and eventually involve the dermis and skin surface. When the lesions spread laterally with small ulcerations and abscesses, they may be indistinguishable from noduloulcerative syphilides. Large gummata may have several skin perforations, with skin necrosis destroying intervening bridges of skin and the lesions assuming various geometric shapes (Fig. 201-18c). When lesions heal, new lesions form on the periphery, forming scalloped borders. The scars are indistinguishable from those caused by burns or other trauma, while retraction of the skin may be the only residual manifestation if ulceration has not occurred.

Differential diagnosis of late benign disease of skin includes cutaneous tuberculosis, psoriasis, deep and superficial fugal disease, ecthyma, ulceration due to vascular or hematologic disease, seborrheic dermatitis, Hansen's disease, mycosis fungoides, granuloma annulare, sarcoidosis, and occasionally squamous cell and basal cell carcinoma.

MUCOUS MEMBRANE LESIONS OF LATE BENIGN SYPHILIS. The tongue may be involved by a solitary elastic painless tumor which undergoes necrosis and ulceration, or a diffuse gummatous infiltration which often develops into a *chronic interstitial glossitis* with superficial atrophic changes or deep fissuring and lobulation. Patients with chronic interstitial or superficial changes must be periodically observed, since these lesions represent a precancerous condition even after adequate therapy for syphilis [122].

Other areas of involvement in the mucous membranes include the hard and soft palates (Fig. 201-19c) and the bony and cartilaginous structures of the nose (Fig. 201-19a and b). These areas are susceptible to ulceration and destruction (saddle nose); chronic perforations remain even after healing. Gummata, nodules, and diffuse ulcerative inflammation covered by a gray slough may involve the tonsils and pharynx. Gummata of the lips and buccal membranes are rare. Differential diagnosis of mucous membrane lesions includes leukoplakia, lichen planus, malignant tumor, and other forms of glossitis.

Gummata of the larynx may produce hoarseness or aphonia, while involvement of the trachea and bronchi is rare. Late syphilis of the lung may be manifested by chronic pulmonary infection resembling tuberculosis, with miliary lesions, a mass, or pleural effusion.

LATE SYPHILIS OF BONE AND JOINTS. Changes in bone occurred as commonly as in skin in 601 patients with late benign syphilis seen by Kampmeier from 1925 to 1943 [123], and may be classed as gummatous osteitis, periostitis, and sclerosing osteitis. Sites most commonly involved include the tibia, clavicle, skull, fibula, femur, and humerus, but almost any bone may be affected. The chief symptoms are nocturnal pain and swelling, and the most common sign is tenderness. X-ray examinations are rarely helpful unless signs or symptoms of bone disease are present. *Gummatous osteitis* is a destructive or osteomyelitic lesion associated with periosteal and/or osteal changes, with varying degrees of sclerosis occurring in neighboring bone. Swelling and sinus tract formation of surrounding soft tissues are commonly observed. Localized osteoporosis, frequently confused with tuberculosis or tumor of bone, often occurs at the diaphysis of long bones and rarely at the shaft. A common site is the sternal end of the clavicle. *Periostitis* is characterized by periosteal thickening and localized increased density, similar to cortical bone, often as laminations or as a diffuse thickening that may or may not be accompanied by destruction of bone. *Sclerosing osteitis,* in which a gumma may be small or obscure, represents a lesion in which the bone shows increased density and is usually accompanied by a periosteal reaction. Obliteration of the marrow cavity (ivory bone)

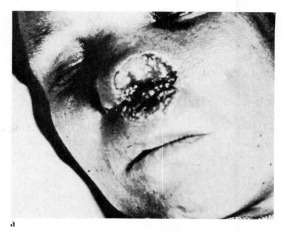

a

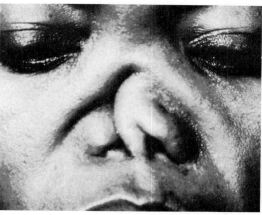

b

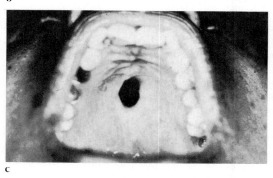

c

Fig. 201-19   Destructive effects of late syphilis. (a) Gumma involving the nose. (b) Destruction of vomer and nasal septum. (c) Perforation of the hard palate.

may occur and be confused with tuberculosis or tumor. Localized lesions of the lamina externa of the skull (caries sicca) are usually a reliable sign of late benign syphilis. Although antisyphilitic therapy will halt symptoms and progression of disease, bone lesions heal slowly.

Late syphilis of the joints may be manifested by arthralgias, synovitis, or arthritis due to adjacent periostitis or gummatous infiltration from bone or skin lesions. Bilateral syphilitic bursitis (of Verneuil) may occasionally ulcerate and expose the gelatinoid content of bursa. *Juxtaarticular nodes,* or fibroid gummata, are multilobed, firm lesions occurring beneath the skin in the region of joints, evolving slowly, occasionally ulcerating, and responding to adequate antibiotic therapy [52].

LATE BENIGN SYPHILIS OF OTHER ORGAN SYSTEMS. Late syphilis of the gastrointestinal tract is characterized by occasional involvement of the parotid glands (parotitis and gumma), esophagus (obstruction, by gumma), stomach (gumma presenting as peptic ulcer or scirrhous carcinoma), and liver (hepar lobatum caused by multiple gummata).

Although rarely clinically enlarged in late syphilis, the spleen may be found to contain gummata in rare instances at autopsy. Gummata may also involve pancreas, kidneys, heart, brain, bladder, uterine cervix, breasts, thyroid, and adrenal glands. Late syphilis of the eye is rare and appears in the form of a chronic iritis, chorioretinitis, interstitial keratitis, and atrophy of the optic nerve. The testicles may be involved with a painless, fibrosing interstitial orchitis that may result in atrophy. Almost any visceral organ may be involved by late benign syphilis.

DIAGNOSIS OF LATE BENIGN SYPHILIS. Diagnosis of this stage of syphilis may result from a combination of characteristic organ involvement, consistent histologic picture, positive nontreponemal and treponemal serologic tests, and healing in response to adequate antibiotic therapy (see "Treatment Guidelines"). *T. pallidum* may be demonstrated by indirect immunofluorescence microscopy, but not by dark-field microscopy illumination or silver stains [124]. Animal inoculation of involved tissue may be informative but is cumbersome and usually impractical.

HISTOPATHOLOGY OF LATE BENIGN SYPHILIS. The histopathology of late benign syphilis [70] is remarkable for a cellular infiltrate that is massive in the center and tends to have a perivascular arrangement at the periphery. The infiltrate is composed of lymphoid and plasma cells, histiocytes, fibroblasts, and granulomas containing epithelioid and giant cells. Vascular changes are notable for thickening of the wall, cellular infiltration, endothelial proliferation, and luminal narrowing. Caseation necrosis is prominent. In noduloulcerative syphilides, the granulomatous process is limited to the dermis, and caseation necrosis is absent, slight, or extensive (leading to ulceration). In the gumma, the granulomatous process is more extensive than in the nodular form and involves the subcutaneous tissue as well as the dermis. Caseation necrosis is extensive, and the large vessels of the subcutaneous layer are markedly involved. Histopathologic differentiation from lupus vulgaris, erythema induratum (Bazin), and sarcoidosis in cases where caseation is absent is sometimes difficult or impossible. Organisms are usually sparse and difficult to demonstrate except by using indirect immunofluorescence [124].

Cardiovascular syphilis [52–57,59,123]. The first scientific paper attempting to prove that syphilis was the cause of aortic aneurysm appeared in 1875 written by Welch, and was protested and deemed unacceptable to prominent English physicians. It was not until Reuter described the organism in the wall of the aorta in active aortitis in 1905 that a syphilitic origin to this cardiovascular lesion was generally accepted.

Although diffuse myocarditis and myocardial gummata may occur as manifestations of late syphilis, the common cardiovascular lesion is aortitis and includes uncomplicated aortitis, aortic insufficiency, and aneurysm. Cardiovascular syphilis is only rarely associated with prenatal syphilis [125,126] and occurs predominantly in acquired syphilis, and only in individuals who are infected after the age of 14 [59]. The incidence is more common in men and is 3 times higher in blacks than whites. Aneurysm alone occurs 6 times more frequently in males than females. In patients followed for untreated early syphilis by Boeck in Norway [59,115], about 10 percent developed cardiovascular syphilis; aortic insufficiency developed in 5.3 percent, saccular aneurysm in 2.5 percent, ostial stenosis in 0.5 percent, and uncomplicated aortitis was found at death in 0.3 percent. In the United States, aneurysms have occurred with one-quarter the frequency of syphilitic aortic regurgitation [123]. In patients with uncomplicated aortitis, aortic insufficiency or aneurysm is said to develop within 3 to 5 years, but follows initial infection by 15 to 30 years. Only about 7 percent of cases with cardiovascular syphilis will develop clinical disease within 5 years of infection. Abnormalities in the spinal fluid will be detected in 49 percent of patients with uncomplicated aortitis, 62 percent in those with aortic regurgitation, and 31 percent with saccular aneurysm. In general, neurosyphilis has been associated with cardiovascular syphilis in about one-third of patients.

The diagnosis of uncomplicated aortitis is difficult at best, and early diagnosis rests on the combined evaluation of relatively insignificant signs and symptoms and expert radiographic study. The ECG is unrevealing in early disease, and clinical manifestations do not occur until damage is severe. The wall of the aorta becomes severely scarred and weakened after a period of chronic obliterating endarteritis of the vasa vasorum, infiltration by lymphocytes and plasma cells, and necrosis and fragmentation of the elastic tissue in the media, accompanied by lymphocytic infiltrate and often miliary gummata of the adventitia. The clinicopathologic lesions of chronic syphilitic aortitis are thin, uneven, serpiginous scars, analogous to healed lesions of the skin. Focal weakening of the wall will produce a saccular aneurysm, while diffuse weakening may produce fusiform involvement of the descending and transverse aorta with subsequent dilatation of the aortic ring. Aneurysms of the abdominal aorta, arising above the renal artery, occur about one-tenth as often as thoracic lesions, but pressure symptoms may result in back pain (vertebral erosion) or disturbance of gastrointestinal function (mass lesion). A palpable pulsating tumor may be present in 60 percent of abdominal aneurysms due to late syphilis. Separation, sagging, and even inflammatory involvement of the aortic wall may also cause deformity and narrowing of the coronary ostia, impairing coronary circulation.

Thoracic aortic saccular dilation may cause pressure symptoms; common structures involved are the trachea, major bronchi and lungs, pulmonary arteries, esophagus, vertebrae, and vagus, sympathetic, and recurrent laryngeal nerves. Aortic incompetence will cause left ventricular hypertrophy and eventual decompensated congestive heart failure. Coronary ostial involvement may produce angina pectoris, myocardial infarction, or congestive cardiomyopathy. In necropsy series of patients with syphilitic aortitis, 25 to 51 percent of patients had coronary ostial stenosis. The right coronary ostium was found to be stenosed 8 times more commonly than the left, but isolated left coronary ostial occlusion due to syphilitic aortitis presenting as congestive myopathy and myocardial fibrosis without angina or aortic incompetence has been well documented [127]. Most patients with coronary ostial stenosis experience cardiac pain, but the absence of angina does not exclude the presence of such stenosis. In a young person with angina pectoris alone or disproportionate to the degree of associated aortic incompetence, or congestive myopathy with or without associated aortic incompetence, syphilitic ostial stenosis needs to be considered. Such a lesion is amenable to surgical therapy, with reasonable expectations of symptom relief if permanent damage has not occurred [128,129].

In aortic insufficiency due to syphilis, the average length of time between the appearance of the heart murmur and the initial manifestations of heart failure is estimated to be less than 6 months. Progressive heart failure will occur within 6 weeks for most patients, and death within another 18 months [130]. The absence of angina or congestive heart failure before treatment in the presence of uncomplicated aortitis has been associated with a more favorable prognosis. Established aortic regurgitation is not affected by penicillin therapy (see ''Treatment Guidelines''). The prognosis in untreated aortic aneurysm is gloomy, death occurring within months after the development of symptoms. Occasionally, a calcified aneurysm will self-heal.

While most patients with cardiovascular syphilis have reactive nontreponemal blood tests, as many as one-quarter of patients with specific anatomic lesions of cardiovascular syphilis in an autopsy study of 380 syphilitic patients had a nonreactive reaginic test for syphilis [131]. In patients with established aortic insufficiency due to syphilis, 10 to 15 percent were nonreactive to reaginic tests used prior to the VDRL. False-negative results may occur with the VDRL as well, but there are no recent studies to determine the rate [123].

Neurosyphilis [52–54,57,116]. CLASSIFICATION. Infection of the nervous system by *T. pallidum* results in clinical syndromes dependent upon the extent of involvement in the parenchyma, blood vessels, and meninges. Neurosyphilis may be divided into three groups, although this classification is not ideal: (1) asymptomatic, (2) meningeal and vascular, and (3) parenchymatous. The first group includes cases having abnormalities in the spinal fluid with no neurologic signs or symptoms of damage to the nervous system. The second group, meningeal and vascular involvement, includes acute and chronic meningitis, gummata of the brain (focal cerebral meningeal neurosyphilis), cerebral vascular syndromes similar to stroke caused by arteriosclerotic disease, and meningeal or vascular syphilis of the spinal cord. The third group, parenchymatous syphilis, includes tabes dorsalis (progressive locomotor ataxia) and dementia paralytica (general paresis of the insane). Combinations of vascular, meningeal, and parenchymatous involvement may exist, so any one patient does not necessarily fall neatly into the second or third groups.

In the Oslo study of untreated syphilis, approximately 8 percent of patients developed neurosyphilis; it is of interest that CNS disease had developed among those infected under the age of 15, while acquired infection after age 40 was rarely associated with the development of neurosyphilis [60]. Symptoms usually did not appear until after 5 to 35 years of infection. The distribution of disease in

676 cases of neurosyphilis studied by Merritt, Adams, and Solomon was as follows: asymptomatic, 31 percent; tabetic, 30 percent; paretic, 12 percent; taboparetic, 3 percent; vascular, 10 percent; meningeal, 6 percent; optic neuritis and spinal cord, 3 percent each; VIIIth nerve, 1 percent; and miscellaneous, 1 percent [116].

In the prepenicillin era, the proportion of patients with symptomatic neurosyphilis among all cases of syphilis after the secondary stage approached 29 percent, with a higher rate of involvement in males than females (4:1), and in whites than blacks (2:1). Although there has been a decrease in all forms of neurosyphilis in the past 30 years, there has recently been a reported increase of late neurosyphilis in England [132], Denmark [133,134], Switzerland [114], the German Federal Republic [135,136], and Italy [137]. The classic forms of neurosyphilis are becoming rare today and are being replaced by atypical forms [138]. Most patients are not brought to the hospital with the classical picture of tabes dorsalis, general paresis of the insane, or meningovascular syphilis. On the contrary, patients may present with a new seizure disorder, ophthalmic symptoms, stroke or confusion, dizziness, and personality changes, or, not uncommonly, neurosyphilis is discovered as an incidental finding during the course of a medical evaluation. For example, 43.2 percent of 241 patients with neurosyphilis studied from 1965 to 1970 were found to have the disease during the course of a general medical evaluation for unrelated problems, 24 percent presented with a seizure disorder, 12 percent with ophthalmic symptoms, 11 percent with stroke or confusion, 8 percent with dizziness, and 2 percent with personality changes [139].

The diagnosis of symptomatic neurosyphilis must be clinical, confirmed by appropriate serologic tests. However, nontreponemal serologic tests are not sensitive enough to detect all cases—in as high as 39 percent of cases of neurosyphilis these tests may be negative [140]. Treponemal tests are more sensitive, with the FTA-ABS test positive in 95 percent of the cases [141]. In Hooshmand's series of 241 patients with neurosyphilis, 48.5 percent had a reactive serum STS, 100 percent had a positive CSF STS. No case was found to have a reactive FTA-ABS in the CSF that was nonreactive in the blood [139]. The CSF FTA-ABS is a more sensitive indicator of neurosyphilis than the VDRL and may become more informative as experience using the test increases [142]. Other good indicators of active neurosyphilis are positive activity to the solid phase hemabsorption test for CSF-IgM (CSF-IgM-SPHA test) and a *T. pallidum* hemagglutination assay (TPHA) index above 100 [143] (see ''Serology of Syphilis'').

ASYMPTOMATIC NEUROSYPHILIS. Patients who have asymptomatic neurosyphilis usually present with a positive blood test for syphilis; a positive STS in the CSF is found during the course of evaluation. Although CSF abnormalities are occasionally manifested during early syphilis (see above), the prevalence in the modern era of a positive CSF serology in latent or indeterminate syphilis approaches 16 percent: of 92 patients evaluated for indeterminate syphilis, 15 had CSF VDRL-positive specimens, with pleocytosis noted in all, and one-quarter of the affected patients were totally asymptomatic [144]. In another series of asymptomatic patients with latent syphilis of indeterminate duration, 7 of 18 had CSF abnormalities sufficient to diagnose asymptomatic neurosyphilis [145]. In 26 consecutive patients with secondary or early latent syphilis, all with normal neurologic findings, 14 had one or more pathologic abnormalities in CSF [146]. The course of untreated asymptomatic neurosyphilis is spontaneous resolution, or progression to symptomatic neurosyphilis in 5 to 10 percent of untreated cases. Progression is usually prevented by adequate antibiotic therapy in the asymptomatic state [147]. Clinical evidence of syphilis elsewhere in the body, especially cardiovascular syphilis, is present in about 10 percent of the cases of asymptomatic neurosyphilis.

MENINGEAL AND VASCULAR NEUROSYPHILIS. Early symptomatic neurosyphilis may present as *acute syphilitic meningitis,* which may arise during the first 12 months of infection and be associated with the secondary rash in about 10 percent of cases (see "Secondary Syphilis"). Syphilitic meningitis is rarely fatal, but permanent cranial nerve palsies or focal cerebral damage is not uncommon in untreated cases. Although acute syphilitic meningitis was common 40 to 50 years ago when early syphilis was at its height, it is a distinct rarity today. *Chronic syphilitic meningitis* usually presents later but for the most part within 5 years of infection, and produces syndromes localized to the vertex or base of the brain, the optic nerve area, and the posterior fossa. Serologic tests are reactive and the CSF is abnormal.

Gummata of the brain, or focal cerebral meningeal neurosyphilis, commonly evolve from the pia mater and compress and invade the brain substance, producing signs and symptoms of an intracranial tumor. A diagnosis of cerebral gumma can only be made by biopsy, and given its rarity and lack of response to antibiotic therapy, surgical removal is the best solution [116]. The results of nontreponemal tests may be nonreactive in the serum and CSF. Treponemal tests are usually reactive, but exceptions occur.

Cerebral vascular syphilis describes those cases of neurosyphilis characterized pathologically by endarteritis and encephalomalacia, and clinically by the appearance of focal neurologic signs, such as aphasia and hemiplegia, similar to stroke caused by arteriosclerotic disease. Meningitis or meningoencephalitis is usually associated with cerebral vascular syphilis. The average time from initial infection to symptoms is about 7 years, and males are affected 3 times more frequently than females. In the present era, syphilis is rarely the cause of thrombosis of a major cerebral vessel or its branches, even in the setting of syphilitic neurovascular disease.

Meningeal or *vascular syphilis of the spinal cord* is rare, occurring in 1 percent of patients with untreated syphilis and one-tenth as frequently as tabes dorsalis. Damage to the cord or its roots via meningeal or vascular involvement produces meningomyelitis (pains, paresthesias, spastic weakness of the legs, muscular atrophy, sensory loss, sphincter disturbance), a spinal vascular syndrome (complete or incomplete transverse myelitis), gumma (rapidly growing intraspinal tumor), and spinal pachymeningitis (atrophy and weakness of muscles at the level of involvement, usually the cervical region). Symptoms usually occur 5 to 30 years after initial infection, and males are affected 4 times as frequently as females. Serologic tests for syphilis are commonly reactive in blood and CSF. Prognosis will be determined by the severity of pathologic damage prior to treatment.

PARENCHYMATOUS NEUROSYPHILIS. Invasion by *T. pallidum* into the parenchyma of the posterior columns and posterior roots of the spinal cord will result in *tabes dorsalis* (progressive locomotor ataxia), while involvement of the cerebral cortex will result in *dementia paralytica* (general paresis of the insane, syphilitic meningoencephalitis, paretic neurosyphilis). Symptoms may be psychiatric, neurologic, or both, and reflect the anatomic damage to the areas involved.

Tabes dorsalis. Degenerative changes take place in the posterior roots and posterior funiculi of the spinal cord, and the brainstem. The optic or other cranial nerves are shrunken where involved. Pathogenesis of tabes dorsalis is debated: one theory considers changes in the spinal cord secondary to degenerative changes in the posterior roots; a second theory postulates that changes in the posterior roots are a result of retrograde degeneration. Males are affected 4 to 6 times as often as females, and whites more commonly than blacks. While tabes is a rarity in the modern era, in the older literature it developed in 3 to 9 percent of untreated syphilis. Symptoms commonly appeared 10 to 25 years after infection, with a range of 5 to 50 years. Tabes dorsalis may also complicate prenatal syphilis and may occur before the age of 10 years.

The major symptoms in tabes dorsalis include lancinating pains, ataxia, bladder disturbance, paresthesias, gastric or visceral crises, visual loss, rectal incontinence, deafness, and impotence. Signs include pupillary abnormalities (including Argyle–Robertson pupils), loss of reflexes in large joints and muscles, Romberg's sign, impaired sensation (vibration, position, touch, and deep sensation), optic atrophy, ocular palsy, and Charcot's joints (see below). The pains of tabes dorsalis are present in over 90 percent of cases, described as "jabs of lightning" and "sticks of a sharp needle" and characterized as fleeting and recurrent. Visceral crises occur in 15 percent, usually in the right upper quadrant, and are accompanied by pain, nausea, and vomiting in various combinations. The ataxia of tabes dorsalis is related to loss of position sense, is compensated for by vision and decompensated in the dark (Romberg's sign). An uncertain and slapping gait, incoordination of leg movements, and an insecure equilibrium are common; locomotion may become impossible with severe involvement. A pupillary abnormality is found in over 90 percent of cases, with an Argyle–Robertson pupil found in over 50 percent—miosis, complete absence of response to light, normal reaction to accommodation–convergence, and impairment to sympathetic stimulation. Commonly involved cranial nerves include the optic, oculomotor, and auditory. In severe cases of optic atrophy, blindness may result. Paralysis of ocular muscles may be transient or permanent. Eighth nerve involvement is found in approximately 25 percent of patients with tabes dorsalis and will affect the auditory more than the vestibular portion of the nerve.

Trophic disorders, due to loss of proprioception and chronic repeated trauma, include an arthropathy of lower extremity joints and spine called *Charcot's joints* (Fig. 201-20a) (painless enlargement of joint with or without effusion, hypermotility, and deformity resulting from fractures, dislocations, erosions, and bony repair) and perforating ulcers known as *mal perforant* (Fig. 201-20b) (circular, indolent, painless sores on the plantar surface of the foot, usually at the base of the great toe and most often

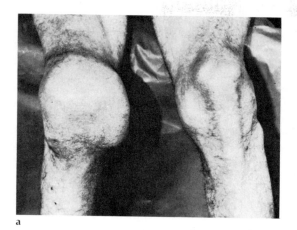

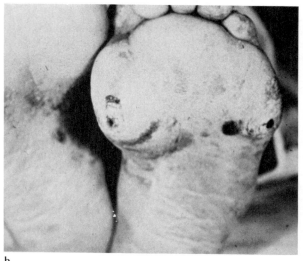

Fig. 201-20 Neurotrophic manifestations of tabes dorsalis, due to loss of proprioception and chronic repeated trauma, include Charcot's joint (a) and mal perforant (b).

associated with an arthropathy of the underlying tarso-metatarsal joint). Surgical treatment of the affected joint by removal of osteophytes may be required for the healing of these sores. Similar trophic changes may be found in other diseases, such as diabetes, leprosy, and syringomyelia. Hypotonicity of the extensor muscles may lead to an overextension of joints (genu recurvatum).

In early tabes dorsalis, blood and CSF nontreponemal and treponemal tests are positive, while in "burnt-out" cases the blood and CSF nontreponemal tests may be normal (see "Serology of Syphilis").

Tabes dorsalis is rarely fatal in itself, although complications may result from urinary and bladder disturbances, severe ataxia, or blindness. Untreated tabes may undergo spontaneous arrest, and progression may be halted with early treatment (see "Treatment Guidelines").

Dementia paralytica. The major pathology in paresis is a chronic meningoencephalitis which destroys or severely disturbs cerebral–cortical function. In the Oslo study of untreated syphilis, general paresis developed in 2.5 percent of males and 1.4 percent of females. At one time this disease accounted for 5 to 10 percent of first admissions to hospitals for mental disease, while today it is a rarity.

Disease does not generally become manifest before 10 to 20 years, and it only rarely occurs before the age of 10 in patients with prenatal syphilis.

The pathologic findings of paresis account for the varied clinical presentations. The brain is grossly atrophic, especially the anterior portion of the frontal and temporal lobes; granulations are present in the ventricles and hydrocephalus may result; the leptomeninges are thickened and adherent to the underlying cortex; and the cerebral sulci are widened. Spirochetes may be found throughout the nervous system, but predominantly in the gray matter of the frontal lobes, the meninges, in the walls of blood vessels, and in microglial cells. Nerve cells, their axons, and myelin sheaths are destroyed in the inflammatory process.

Clinical manifestations of paresis occur in three phases. The onset is usually incipient, but occasionally sudden. Irritability, personality changes, and forgetfulness are common findings. A cerebral vascular accident or convulsive seizure followed by neurologic deficit may also herald the onset of paresis. A period of full-blown psychosis follows, with simple deterioration being most common; memory defect, judgment impairment, or excessive mood lability progresses to imbecility. Grandiose ideation occurs in about 20 percent of cases, and delusions of grandeur contrast with a dilapidated appearance. Full-blown psychosis is followed by a period of decline and a terminal stage, characterized by epileptiform seizures and incontinence of urine and feces. Neurologic signs are variable and include pupillary abnormalities, paralytic facies, speech and handwriting disorders, and alterations in the reflexes.

Serologic tests for syphilis are reactive in the blood, and the CSF shows abnormalities in practically all cases, including a CSF-reactive VDRL, a moderate pleocytosis, an increased protein content, and an abnormal colloidal gold test, usually of the first zone type. Abnormal encephalography may be found in more than half the patients. Untreated cases will progress to death within months to 5 or more years, with an average of $2\frac{1}{2}$ years. Spontaneous remissions of months to a year's duration occur in 5 to 10 percent of cases. Progression may be halted in about 80 percent of cases with adequate antibiotic therapy, but in paresis, unlike other forms of neurosyphilis, disease may continue to worsen despite adequate treatment. Deterioration despite adequate treatment may be related immediately to a rapid change of affected tissue during the course of antibiotic therapy (therapeutic paradox), or subsequently due to contracting scars in the brain parenchyma or progression to normal-pressure hydrocephalus (caused by inhibition of CSF resorption after meningeal or ependymal inflammation [137].

Prenatal syphilis (congenital syphilis) [11,52–57]. DEFINITION AND CLASSIFICATION. Prenatal syphilis is defined as syphilis transmitted by the mother to the fetus in utero. *Congenital,* meaning existing at or from birth, is a less accurate term than *prenatal,* since syphilis acquired in utero may result in death before or after delivery as well as disease during infancy and childhood.

The time of appearance of clinical disease in prenatal syphilis very much depends on the time of infection, since spirochetemia may lead to fetal wastage, neonatal death, or nonlethal reversible and irreversible manifestations in infancy, childhood, and even adulthood. Thomas estimates that in untreated syphilis, about 25 percent of fetuses infected in utero die before birth as a result of infection; 25 to 30 percent of infected fetuses will die shortly after birth; and of those infected fetuses who survive infancy, about 40 percent of untreated cases will develop symptomatic syphilis [57]. Infection at the time of delivery via contact with infectious lesions in the birth canal (acquired syphilis) may lead to the development of a primary chancre in the newborn; nonsexual contact in infancy and early childhood (nonvenereal, or endemic, syphilis) may lead to a disease course quite different from prenatal or venereally acquired syphilis [see "Nonvenereal ('Endemic') Syphilis"].

Although the occasional demonstration of spirochetes in early abortuses suggests that infection may take place earlier, the clinical manifestations of prenatal syphilis rarely take place before the sixteenth week of gestation, at a time when the Langhans' layer of the chorion is said to atrophy and no longer function as an effective barrier to *T. pallidum*. This view is challenged by the electron microscopic demonstration of the layer in question throughout pregnancy [148,149], and the fact that spirochetes may cross the placenta as early as 8 to 9 weeks' gestation [150]. An alternative explanation for the lack of tissue changes of prenatal syphilis before the fifth month of development is the immunologic immaturity of the early fetus and its inability to mount an immune response to *T. pallidum* [151]. Whatever the explanation, generally accepted observations hold true: adequate therapy before the fourth month will almost always prevent infection in the newborn, while treatment after 18 weeks will usually bring about in utero cure but may not prevent bone or joint involvement, neural deafness, or interstitial keratitis in the newborn. It seems clear, then, that prenatal syphilis is a preventable disease. Since 80 percent of cases are not diagnosed until 1 year of age, an intensive program of serologic screening during the first trimester and at term would lead to earlier detection and treatment. First trimester serologic screening for syphilis was found to be economically advantageous when weighing the cost of such a screening program vs. the cost of manifest prenatal disease in an individual [152].

According to Thomas [57], the outcome of a pregnancy will be determined by the duration of syphilitic infection in the mother: the longer the duration of untreated syphilis in the mother before pregnancy occurs, the less the risk to the unborn fetus, especially if the mother has had infection for more than 2 years. An affected infant of a mother with late prenatal syphilis may be due to newly acquired sexually transmitted syphilitic infection [153,154].

If the mother acquires infection during pregnancy, the manifestations in the infant are dependent on *when* during pregnancy the mother became infected. Maternal infection occurring late during pregnancy may result in a normal-appearing mother and infant at delivery; manifestations of infection (clinical and serologic) may not appear for weeks or months later. On the other hand, infection of the fetus during early gestation may result in spontaneous abortion or a severely affected infant at birth. Infection during pregnancy, therefore, may result in spontaneous abortion (usually after 12 to 16 weeks' gestation), fetal death in utero, manifestations at birth or later in infancy, a normal-appearing infant with a persistent positive serology who develops late manifestations or heals spontaneously, or a

normal unaffected child, especially in mothers with disease of more than 2 years' duration. Successive pregnancies in a syphilitic mother may result in stillbirth for the first child, prenatal syphilis for the second, and healthy children thereafter.

The clinical manifestations of prenatal syphilis are arbitrarily divided into early prenatal syphilis (before age 2), late prenatal syphilis (after age 2), and stigmata. Early prenatal syphilis is analogous to secondary syphilis and rarely occurs before the second to sixth week of life, while late disease is analogous to the adult late form, developing after 2 years of age but seldom past 30 years. Prenatal syphilis can simulate any of the features of acquired syphilis, excluding cardiovascular manifestations. Some of the lesions of prenatal syphilis produce scars which persist indefinitely as stigmata of the disease, and these will be described separately.

EARLY PRENATAL SYPHILIS. Since spirochetemia is the source of infection from mother to fetus in utero, the "primary" stage of acquired syphilis is bypassed. Dead, macerated fetuses of spontaneous abortions and stillbirths, as well as babies dying soon after birth due to early severe disease, are remarkable for enormous numbers of *T. pallidum* in most of the tissues. In addition, spinal fluid tests of syphilitic infants show evidence of CNS involvement in a much higher proportion of cases than in patients with acquired secondary syphilis. Early prenatal syphilis, therefore, behaves in a more "malignant" manner than acquired secondary syphilis. Lesions may or may not be clinically evident, as in acquired secondary disease, and the time of appearance of disease depends on the time of maternal–fetal spirochetemia.

Early prenatal syphilis, appearing before age 2, may be subdivided into disease with active signs and symptoms at birth, and disease appearing after a delay of weeks to months or even longer. When disease is obvious at birth, the prognosis is usually poor, with a mortality rate approaching 50 percent. Although severe infection present at birth has been associated with a "classic" picture of marasmus, pot belly, withered skin, old man facies, and pseudoparalysis of Parrot (see below), other presentations may be more common. In a series of 10 consecutive cases of early prenatal syphilis in Singapore [155], all infants were small for dates or premature; the placentas were larger and heavier than expected; hepatosplenomegaly was a constant feature and accounted for a distended abdomen; and 4 infants presented with pallor, bloated abdomen, and edema—features of hydrops fetalis—which distracted attention from the diagnosis of prenatal syphilis. A striking finding in half of these cases was the presence of blistering, oozing, and raw areas on the ears and extremities. X-ray examination revealed osseous lesions in 9 infants, ranging from submetaphaseal radiolucent bands to severe osteomyelitis and periostitis of long bones. Anemia, reticulocytosis, normoblastemia, thrombocytopenia, and leukocytosis were present in the majority. Five infants died within the first week, and autopsy revealed gross hepatosplenomegaly, ascites in those with hydrops, and increased hematopoietic foci in the liver and spleen. Treponemata were demonstrated in lungs and pancreas, and interstitial fibrosis was noted in these same organs [155]. Congenital syphilis pneumonia may predispose to chronic lung disease later in childhood [156]. Among Bantu babies, the most common cause of thrombocytopenia and bleeding during the first few weeks of life is prenatal syphilis. A leukoerythroblastic anemia and macroglobulinemia associated with a coagulation disturbance are associated findings during this early stage of disease [103].

Usually there are no clinical signs at birth of prenatal syphilis, merely a positive STS in mother and child (see "Serology of Syphilis"), with the titer often higher in the child than in the mother. From 2 to 6 weeks after birth, the first manifestations may be coryzal symptoms often accompanied by rhinitis and hoarse breathing. Mucous patches and condylomata lata may be present in the first few months and often develop prior to the general exanthem. Cutaneous lesions are present in 52 percent of patients under 6 months and most often include macules and papules of copper-red hue, appearing most often on palms, soles, and diaper area.

Although rare, bullous lesions of early syphilis (syphilitic pemphigus) are characteristic for the disease. Blebs vary in size from 1 to 5 cm in diameter, are partially distended with eroded bases, appearing in a generalized fashion but more commonly localized to palms and soles, and usually intermixed with macules, papules, and pustules. Bullae and pustular lesions may signify a severe prognosis. Fissures of the lips, angles of the mouth, and anus are present in 75 percent of cases and produce permanent scarring in later life (rhagades). Syphilitic rhinitis (Fig. 201-21), producing a bright red, bloody nasal discharge (snuffles) is highly infectious, and may result in ulceration of the nasal septum with flattening of the nasal bridge, producing the characteristic saddle nose. Gummata and noduloulcerative lesions are not present in the early stage.

The most common early findings in early prenatal syphilis are related to bone and joints. The long bones are usually involved, and the most common lesion is osteochondritis, with the characteristic "sawtooth" metaphysis seen on x-ray. Pathologic fracture of involved bones may be an occasional presenting sign of early prenatal syphilis (personal observation, A.R.R.). Osteochondritis at the ends of long bones (epiphysitis) may cause local tenderness, swelling, and pain, so that the child will not move a limb (pseudoparalysis of Parrot). X-ray changes of epiphysitis have usually disappeared by the eighth month. Periostitis, which causes pain when acute and is commonly observed in the latter half of the first year, may lead to blunting of the scapular spines and anterior tibial margins in later life. A form of osteitis of the phalanges is rarely seen and may lead to syphilitic dactylitis during the first 2 years.

An infant with early prenatal syphilis is often restless and cries feebly but frequently. Central nervous system involvement occurs in 40 to 50 percent of affected infants and may be asymptomatic or symptomatic with meningitic or meningoencephalitic changes presenting as convulsions, bulging fontanelle, neck stiffness, "meningeal cry," and hydrocephalus. Lymphadenopathy may be present but is not a constant feature, while enlargement of liver and spleen is present in 64 percent of patients with early prenatal syphilis, with or without jaundice.

Renal disease may complicate early prenatal syphilis and includes the nephrotic syndrome and acute glomerulonephritis, with infants usually having features of both processes. Microscopic hematuria, marked hypertension,

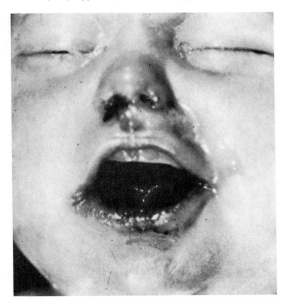

Fig. 201-21 Prenatal syphilis: snuffles and rhagades.

edema, proteinuria, and depressed serum protein may reflect immunologic involvement of the glomeruli. Coarse granular deposition of IgG and C3 on the glomerular basement membrane, subepithelial and intramembranous electron-dense deposits on electron microscopic examination, and resolution of clinical, laboratory, and histologic abnormalities on repeat biopsy after appropriate antibiotic therapy identify the lesion as an immune glomerulopathy. The renal lesion associated with prenatal syphilis is curable if patients are treated before irreversible renal damage occurs [157,158].

Other manifestations of early prenatal syphilis include a mild paronychia along the nail margin with secondary nail changes, peritonitis, iritis, and choroiditis.

LATE PRENATAL SYPHILIS (LATE SYPHILIS AFTER PRENATAL INFECTION, SYPHILIS CONGENITA TARDA) [11,57,159,160]. The course of prenatal syphilis after infancy is similar to acquired late syphilis, with lesions developing after age 2 and rarely past age 30. A possible exception is involvement of the cardiovascular system. Thomas stated he had never seen cardiovascular involvement in a patient with prenatal syphilis and therefore postulated a peculiar resistance to syphilitic infection of the infant aorta. A report of 15 cases of prenatal syphilis in which aortic and vascular lesions were present, however, questions the sparing effect during this stage of disease, although there is general agreement that such findings are rare [125]. Late prenatal syphilis may be in a latent form in 60 percent of cases of prenatal syphilis, and a diagnosis is made with serologic tests for syphilis. It may be impossible to distinguish between the acquired and prenatal forms of latent syphilis except by an examination of mother and siblings and an accurate history. In a series of 271 patients with late prenatal syphilis, the average age at first diagnosis was 29.3 years [159].

Interstitial keratitis (Figs. 201-22 and A4-24) has been observed in prenatal syphilis from 9 to 31 years of age, although it may be seen at any time after infancy. It was seen in 8.8 percent of 271 patients with late prenatal syphilis and the average age at onset was 13.5 years for men

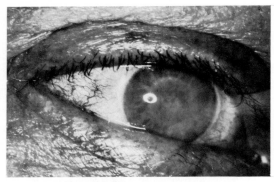

Fig. 201-22 Prenatal syphilis: interstitial keratitis.

and 27.1 years for women. The predominant symptoms are those of an acute iritis and include tearing and photophobia followed by clouding of the cornea and invasion of its surface and stroma by blood vessels. Unlike other manifestations of prenatal syphilis, invasion of the eye by *T. pallidum* does not explain all the findings. The keratitis, which is unresponsive to penicillin therapy but does *not* occur if early prenatal syphilis is adequately treated, presumably reflects an antigen–antibody reaction in a tissue sensitized by transient spirochetal invasion in fetal life. Histologic findings reveal necrosis of the stroma and a massive lymphocytic response, occurring early, and deep vascularization manifest during healing. Both eyes are affected, one after the other, and ulceration is rare. Interstitial keratitis is suppressed by topical corticosteroids, with reasonable expectation of fair visual acuity after treatment. There is little or no corneal scarring, and, if present (in the event of inadequate treatment), corneal transplantation may be used to restore vision, with at least a 50 percent chance that the grafts will remain clear. Glaucoma may be a late finding in patients with treated interstitial keratitis, so continual surveillance is indicated. Iritis and iridocyclitis may also occur, but are usually early in the course of interstitial keratitis.

Neurosyphilis occurs in one-third to one-half of patients with late prenatal syphilis, is usually asymptomatic, and is discovered only by examining the CSF. Mononuclear pleocytosis, elevated protein and depressed or normal glucose, and a positive CSF serology are common findings. Disease usually occurs after age 5 and is commonly established during the teen years, with whites more commonly affected than blacks (4:1). Many of the clinical syndromes described for acquired neurosyphilis may occur. In children, there is rarely sharply defined tabes or paresis; fewer than 1 percent will develop paresis. Adequate treatment in asymptomatic neurosyphilis will halt progression.

Eighth nerve deafness was seen in 3.3 to 38 percent of patients with late prenatal syphilis, usually during the teen years and only rarely beginning in adulthood. The lesion is considered primarily a labyrinthitis, the onset of disease heralded by vertigo, followed by a loss of hearing for higher frequencies and later for conversational tones, first in one ear and then the other. The prognosis is poor in untreated cases, and even with adequate antibiotic therapy deafness is progressive. Rarely is VIIIth nerve involvement the only sign of late prenatal syphilis. Spinal fluid examination is normal, and a biopsy of the endochondral bone of the labyrinthine capsule may reveal spirochetes. Some patients

respond to at least 4 weeks of combined systemic corticosteroid and antibiotic therapy [161,162].

Skin manifestations are essentially the same for acquired late benign syphilis and include gummata and gummatous inflammation, occurring at any time after age 2 and having an incidence similar to the acquired variety.

Bilateral hydroarthrosis (Clutton's joints), described in 1886, and usually occurring between ages 8 and 15 years, is a unique syphilitic synovitis especially of the knees, without involvement of bone or cartilage. The condition begins acutely or subacutely and is accompanied by fever, redness, warmth, and occasionally pain, contrary to the original description. The synovitis usually resolves spontaneously within several months without residual joint damage, responding to corticosteroids but not penicillin or salicylates.

Bone involvement in late prenatal syphilis may take the form of gummata in the palatine bones and vomer, leading to ulceration and perforation of the palate and the nasal septum (Fig. 201-19). A true arthritis may also occur in late prenatal syphilis [163] and take the form of either a perisynovitis or an epiphysitis which eventually involves the structure of the joint. The rare von Gies joint is a chondroosteoarthritis, which may lead to ankylosis. An early diagnosis and treatment with adequate antibiotic therapy may prevent permanent damage. Periostitis, producing new bone formation, commonly involves the tibia and rarely the fibula, radius, ulna, and clavicle. The affected bones show fusiform swelling (saber shins of the tibia, Higoumenakis sign of the sternoclavicular joint), and x-ray examination shows periosteal thickening.

Paroxysmal cold hemoglobinuria may occur with prenatal syphilis, and is associated with muscular cramping, headache, hyperpyrexia, and hemoglobinuria that clears within 24 h. Urticaria, acrocyanosis, and transient splenomegaly and jaundice may also occur. Episodes are precipitated by exposure to the cold, are decreased or eliminated by adequate antibiotic treatment, and are associated with a biphasic hemolysin of variable thermolability [164]. This disorder may also be unrelated to syphilis.

STIGMATA OF PRENATAL SYPHILIS. Inflammation of anatomic structures during prenatal syphilis may result in scarring and developmental changes that persist as characteristic features of the disease. Only a few of these stigmata are diagnostic for syphilis, but all may eventually be helpful in the diagnosis of late prenatal syphilis if present in a patient with a positive serologic test for syphilis.

In a review of 271 patients with late prenatal syphilis, Fiumara and Lessell made a careful analysis of the frequency of stigmata found on examination [159]:

Saddle nose, with or without nasal perforation, was present in 73.4 percent and is the end result of syphilitic rhinitis. Saddle nose may also be the result of infection or trauma and is not a diagnostic finding.

Frontal bossae (of Parrot) were present in 86.7 percent, appearing as lens-shaped bony prominences on exostoses representing sequelae of localized periostitis of the frontal and parietal bones. Rickets may produce identical findings.

Short maxillae, resulting from the local effect of syphilitic rhinitis on the development of adjacent structures, was present in 83.3 percent and appears as a shallow dish configuration. It is not diagnostic for syphilis.

Relative protuberance of the mandible (bulldog jaw) occurred in 25.8 percent, and is itself of normal size and shape, but appears proportionately longer and bigger because the maxilla is small. It is not diagnostic.

A *high arched palate,* appearing for the same reasons as the short maxillae, occurred in 76.4 percent and of itself is not diagnostic.

Higoumenakis sign, a unilateral irregular enlargement of the sternoclavicular portion of the clavicle as an end result of periostitis, occurred in 39.4 percent, usually on the right side of right-handed individuals. Fractures, rickets, and infection may result in the same appearance.

Rhagades (Fig. 201-21), linear scars like the spokes of a wheel radiating from the angle of the eyes, nose, mouth, chin, anus, and areas of moisture, are the end result of linear fissures or ulcers of early prenatal disease. Rhagades are not frequently seen (7.6 percent of patients), but when present are suggestive (though not diagnostic) of prenatal syphilis.

Saber shin (Fig. 201-23), observed in 4.1 percent, is a result of periostitis of the anterior and middle portion of the tibia, with a resultant thickening and bowing. Saber shin may also be seen as a sequela of rickets (lower two-thirds of tibia), fractures, tumors, and infection.

Scaphoid scapulae, manifested by a concavity of the vertebral border of the scapulae, were observed in only 0.7 percent.

Hutchinson's teeth (see Fig. 101-11), noted in 63.1 percent of the group, refers to an abnormality of the upper central incisors of the permanent dentition, appearing at age 6 or older. They are widely spaced, shorter than the lateral incisors, barrel or peg shaped, wider at the gingival margin than at the biting surface, thick in their anteroposterior diameter and laterally. A notch is present in the biting surface as a result of defective enamel formation. Teeth with the above appearance are diagnostic of prenatal syphilis.

Hutchinson's triad, described by Sir Jonathan Hutchinson in 1858 and considered pathognomonic of late prenatal syphilis, consists of the following stigmata: Hutchinson's teeth, interstitial keratitis, and VIIIth nerve deafness. One of these findings was detected in 204 of the 207 patients with late prenatal syphilis studied by Fiumara and Lessell [159]. Another diagnostic sign is *mulberry molars* (Moon's molars, Fournier's molars) (Fig. 201-24), observed in 64.9 percent of the group and usu-

Fig. 201-23   Saber shin. The anterior bowing of the tibia is a result of syphilitic periostitis.

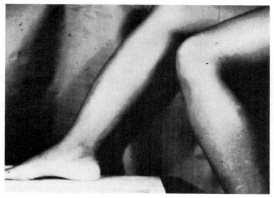

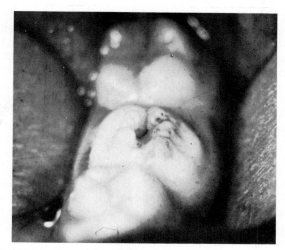

Fig. 201-24   Prenatal syphilis: mulberry molar.

ally accompanied by other findings. All of the molars may be affected, but the diagnostic one is the first lower molar, a sixth-year molar developing at the same time as the upper central incisors. It is dome shaped (the gingival margin is wider than the grinding surface) with poorly developed, more numerous cusps than the usual four well-formed cusps. The enamel is poorly formed, predisposing to cavities, so the molar has often been extracted at the time of examination.

DIAGNOSIS OF PRENATAL SYPHILIS. A dark-field examination of the umbilical vein at delivery will be positive in more than half the cases of early prenatal syphilis [11]. An attempt, moreover, should be made to visualize spirochetes in skin lesions and nasal secretions in an infant with physical signs of disease. In the absence of clinical signs in an infant born of a syphilitic mother, there must be reliance on serologic tests, although a negative result to lipoidal antigen assays in a neonate does not exclude prenatal syphilis if a fetus is infected late in gestation; a positive test does not prove infection, since passive transfer of IgG antibody to the fetus occurs even after adequate treatment of the mother during gestation. A seropositive mother should be investigated with specific treponemal tests to exclude a biologic false-positive reaction and, if positive, selective IgM assays to assess activity of disease; after birth, an asymptomatic child with positive serologic tests for syphilis should be investigated with specific IgM tests or be followed with serial quantitative tests for 6 months, to exclude active infection if treatment is withheld. Since the half-life of passively transferred reagin is about 32 days, there should be a 50 percent reduction in quantitative titers 32 days after birth. At 3 months postpartum, passively transferred *reagin* should not be detectable; at 6 months postpartum, passively transferred specific treponemal antibody should be undetectable as well. IgG reactivity to the TPHA test may persist for 9 months and even longer (see "Serology of Syphilis").

In an infant delivered to a mother adequately treated for syphilis during pregnancy, a positive serologic reaginic test probably represents maternal transfer. This issue can be clarified by detecting serum antitreponemal IgM antibodies using the IgM-SPHA or FTA-ABS (IgM) test (see "Serology of Syphilis"). Immunoglobulins of the IgM class do not pass the placental barrier, and their presence in serum in an infant suggests active infection. Occasional false positives [165], possibly related to degenerative changes in the placenta during pregnancy, and false negatives related to prenatal infection occurring late in gestation, should be kept in mind. In settings where the FTA-ABS (IgM) test is not readily available, passive maternal antibody transfer is suggested by a quantitative reaginic test titer in an infant that is identical to or lower than that in the mother; a repeat test will be lower still 1 week later and negative by age 3 months. If an infant has a reaginic test titer significantly higher than that of the mother, with no decreasing trend 1 to 3 weeks later, then prenatal infection is highly likely, and the infant should be treated. Adequate treatment must also be considered for neonates if active syphilis infection cannot be excluded, or if continuity of follow-up care for mother and infant cannot be assured (see "Treatment Guidelines").

Underdiagnosis of prenatal syphilis may be a problem, since up to 80 percent of cases may not be diagnosed until after 12 months of age. Unfortunately, *overdiagnosis* of early prenatal syphilis may also be a problem, since at least one-third of such cases are inaccurate or in doubt [166]. Thus, many infants with true infection are not discovered until later during the course of disease, and many infants are labeled as having infection even though adequate therapy has been given during pregnancy and/or criteria for active infection cannot be documented. Specific IgM tests may be helpful in this situation. Active disease in a mother or infant is likely in the presence of reactivity to IgM-SPHA and/or FTA-ABS (IgM) tests [167–173].

Aside from technical advances in the diagnosis and management of individual infants with prenatal syphilis, the single most important factor in the prevention of prenatal syphilis is the provision of adequate prenatal care. A serologic test for syphilis performed in the first trimester and at term in all pregnant women would in effect detect almost all cases of prenatal syphilis.

Serology of syphilis [174–178]

Classification. Invasion of humans by *T. pallidum* may induce the production of multiple antibodies of two basic types.

Nonspecific antibodies (reagins) are directed against lipoidal antigens of *T. pallidum,* as well as against mitochondrial and nuclear membranes of human cells (autoantibodies). *T. pallidum* appears to contain a phospholipid which is similar to structures in human mitochondrial membranes, and thus stimulates the production of two different types of antibodies [179,180]. One of these antibodies reacts with lipoidal antigens, which result from the interaction of human tissues and *T. pallidum*. These antibodies are measured by tests that employ cardiolipin-lecithin antigens, and are called nontreponemal antigen tests, or serologic tests for syphilis (STS). Lipoidal antigens are present in normal tissues, but are particularly evident in conditions that destroy cell nuclei. Those conditions giving rise to autoantibodies often produce false-positive reactions to nontreponemal tests.

Specific antitreponemal antibodies are directed against *T. pallidum,* and are measured using assays that require the whole organism or its components as the antigen. An-

tibodies in this category are of two types: (1) group-specific antibodies directed against commensal spirochetes, and (2) type-specific antibodies directed against *T. pallidum*. Various techniques are used to eliminate group-specific antibodies directed against commensal spirochetes in the performance of specific antitreponemal tests.

Identification of nonspecific reagins or specific treponemal antigens by observing in vitro antigen–antibody reactions is the basis of syphilis serology. Differences in serologic tests are determined by the antigen used and, therefore, the type of antibody detected. Table 201-1 lists most of the serologic assays; many of them are outdated (see below).

Antibodies of both the IgM and IgG classes, directed against lipoidal and treponemal antigens, are reactive in syphilis infection. IgM directed against both antigens is the first detectable sign of humoral immune response, and is detected by specific serum IgM assays by the end of the second week after *T. pallidum* infection. The IgM antibody has a molecular weight of one million, and is called 19S-IgM based on the fraction detected by ultracentrifugation. IgM antibodies directed against *T. pallidum* are not produced as an anemnestic response, so their presence in the sera of untreated individuals usually indicates active disease [181]. The large size of the IgM molecule prevents its permeation through intact placenta and the blood/brain barrier. IgM production decreases when IgG synthesis commences; IgM becomes undetectable about 3 months after adequate therapy for early syphilis, and within 12 months after adequate therapy for late syphilis [167,169,171–173,182–184]. The IgG antibody has a molecular weight of 150,000, and the sedimentation coefficient in the ultracentrifuge is 7 (hence the designation 7S-IgG). The synthesis of IgG antibodies in syphilis begins around the second week after infection, and their detection is possible by the fourth and fifth weeks after infection. In response to *T. pallidum* infection, IgG production far exceeds that of IgM, and high levels are attained within 2 to 4 weeks after infection. IgG synthesis decreases over time, but antilipoidal and antitreponemal activity may persist for years or indefinitely, even after "cure" by effective therapy [181]. Sera from patients with late syphilis show persistent concentrations of antilipoidal IgM and IgG and of antitreponemal IgG, but not antitreponemal IgM. The significance of IgA antibodies in the serology of syphilis, particularly its role in neurosyphilis [185], is not clear.

Table 201-1   Serologic tests for syphilis

Tests using lipoidal antigens	Tests using *Treponema pallidum* antigens
Complement fixation:	*T. pallidum* immobilization test (TPI)
Kolmer	
Wassermann	Fluorescent *T. pallidum* absorption test (FTA-ABS)
Flocculation:	
Kahn	*T. pallidum* hemagglutination assay (TPHA)
Kline	
Mazzini	
Hinton	Enzyme-linked immunosorbent assay (ELISA)
Slide assays—VDRL, RPR (PCT, USR, RPR teardrop, RPR circle, ART)	

Nontreponemal tests. Nontreponemal tests employ a purified cardiolipin–cholesterol (lipoidal) antigen to which lecithin has been added to produce standard reactivity. Syphilitic reagin, the antibody measured by these tests, is primarily of the IgM and IgG class and should not be confused with IgE or skin-sensitizing antibody. Reaginic antibodies may occur in normal individuals [186]; patients with syphilis, yaws, bejel, and pinta; or in nonsyphilitic persons as a response to nontreponemal disease, both acute and chronic. Nontreponemal tests are of two types—complement-fixation tests and flocculation tests. Both can be done as qualitative (antibody present or absent) or quantitative (the highest dilution of serum-containing antibody) procedures. Except for the VDRL and RPR, most of the other lipoidal antigens are not in use. None of the other lipoidal antigen assays offers an advantage over the VDRL or RPR [167], which are well standardized, simpler, and cheaper to perform (see Table 201-1).

Bordet in 1898 first described the use of complement-mediated serum hemolysis in the test tube, and at the turn of the century, Wassermann described the complement-fixation test. The complement-fixation tests (Kolmer, Wassermann), requiring multiple reagents and at least 24 h to complete, depend on the formation of an antigen–antibody complex between the cardiolipin–lecithin–cholesterol antigen and reagin which in turn binds complement, thereby preventing a trigger mechanism to the complement cascade and thus inhibiting hemolysis of sensitized erythrocytes in the indicator system. These tests, because they are so laborious, are no longer used in medically developed countries and will therefore not be discussed further.

In 1931, Kahn introduced a flocculation test that required no complement and only a few hours to read. A standardized purified antigen remained a problem in modifications of all of these tests until Panghorn successfully isolated pure cardiolipin and lecithin from beef heart in 1942, which made standardized and reproducible test results possible. The purified antigens led in turn to the development of microflocculation tests (read under the microscope) and the means for mass testing of sera for screening.

FLOCCULATION TESTS. Flocculation tests depend on the formation of physical aggregates of reaginic antibody contained in serum and a cardiolipin–lecithin–cholesterol antigen. The antigen–antibody combination is viewed directly and may be performed on slides, special cards, tubes, or an autoanalyzer. The most widely used nontreponemal test is the Venereal Disease Research Laboratory (VDRL) test, which is easily standardized and easily adapted to quantitative testing. The VDRL test requires inactivated serum plus antigen, while a modification of the test—the rapid plasma reagin (RPR) test—does not require heat inactivation of serum and may be carried out on disposable cards. Coal particles in the RPR test allow better distinction of reactive results, and specificity and reactivity are practically the same or slightly better than the VDRL. A modified VDRL antigen suspension is made more sensitive in the RPR test by adding choline chloride. Modifications of the original RPR test include the plasmacrit (PCT), the untreated serum reagin (USR), the RPR teardrop card test, the RPR circle card test, and the automated reagin test (ART). The ART offers the advantage of automation with the autoanalyzer continuous flow system in which a modified RPR card test antigen suspension containing charcoal and unheated serum or plasma are mixed and then deposited automatically on a moving strip of filter paper. The use of dilutions of serum before introduction into the autoanalyzer allows for a quantitative as well as a qualitative test [187]; prozones are uncommon with this technique, in contrast to most flocculation tests.

In clinical use, the PCT, USR, and RPR teardrop card tests should be regarded as screening procedures only with a high degree of sensitivity but low specificity (the *sensitivity* of a test in the diagnosis of a given disease is a measure of its ability to be positive in persons having the disease; *specificity* is a measure of the ability of the test to be negative in persons not having the disease). Specimens showing any degree of reactivity to these tests should be subjected to further testing with more specific procedures such as the VDRL slide test and the treponemal tests. The RPR circle card and the ART are as accurate in diagnosis as the VDRL slide test and compare favorably in sensitivity and specificity, both quantitatively and qualitatively. There is disagreement on final titers, however, which prevents equation of the ART, RPR circle card, and the VDRL; the titer response of the ART and RPR circle card test have not been fully evaluated in persons treated for syphilis or in persons previously treated who are experiencing relapse or reinfection. Quantitative testing is currently performed with the VDRL slide test (i.e., to follow titers after treatment) until more information is available on the other lipoidal antigen tests.

In the lipoidal test, a quantitative is more informative than a qualitative result, since it provides a standard from which change or lack of change can be measured. Active disease will show a rise in titer, treated active disease will show a fall in titer, and inactive "serofast" disease will not show a change in titer on subsequent testing. The last dilution to produce a reactive result is the titer of the test—a titer of 1:16 means the serum is reactive at 1:16 dilution but nonreactive at 1:32. Titers may be negative, low, or occasionally high (1:32 or higher) in primary syphilis, commonly high in secondary syphilis (1:32 or higher), and are variable in later stages. False-positive reactors (see below) have VDRL titers of 1:8 or below, although higher titers are found rarely [188]. A fourfold or greater change in titer is necessary to demonstrate a noteworthy change in the level of serum reaginic antibody, since twofold changes in titer are commonly related to technical error. Undiluted serum specimens with very high titers of reagin antibody will occasionally give a negative reaction. An estimated 1 percent of patients with secondary syphilis will have a negative result if undiluted serum is used in the test procedure, which on further dilution of the serum will become positive (the "prozone phenomenon"). Every physician ordering reaginic serologic tests for syphilis should be aware of procedures used since all laboratories do not routinely dilute serum [189].

A weakly reactive VDRL may be due to a technical error by the laboratory. Such a result, however, must *not* be disregarded until serum is retested with specific treponemal tests, since one study demonstrated that weakly reactive sera commonly indicate syphilitic infection—of 519 weakly reactive VDRL tests, 189 were reactive with more specific testing [190].

The antibody type detected by the VDRL is predominantly a 19S IgM immunoglobulin in early infection, and a

7S IgG immunoglobulin as disease progresses. Investigation in recent years suggests that another immunoglobulin reacting with lipoidal antigens is an autoantibody against substances of the mitochondrial membrane (usually 19S IgM) and may be of significance in biologic false-positive results. This *cardiolipin F* antibody was found frequently in early syphilis but not in late syphilis, was usually low in titer, disappeared rapidly after treatment, and is thought to differ from reagin antibody although it can be removed from sera by absorption with cardiolipin antigen [191]. There is also an increased production of other antibodies in patients with syphilis, including rheumatoid factors and cryoglobulins, their prevalence correlating with high-titer reagin antibody and duration of infection [175].

BIOLOGIC FALSE-POSITIVE REACTIONS WITH NONTREPONEMAL TESTS. Biologic false-positive (BFP) reactors for the reaginic tests are defined as patients in whom one or more of these tests (VDRL, Kahn, Wassermann, RPR, etc.) are repeatedly positive, but in whom tests for antitreponemal antibody (i.e., FTA and/or TPHA test) are negative. Acute reactors are arbitrarily defined as those in whom reagin positivity reverts to negative within 6 months of the first positive finding, and chronic reactors as those in whom positivity persists for 6 months or longer. False positivity rates for the flocculation tests run as high as 8 to 20 percent of reactive samples [192–194]. The rate of false positivity, however, is population dependent, with a markedly lower false positivity rate in groups where syphilis is more common, i.e., 3 percent of nonwhite compared to 28 percent of white patients, and 15 percent of clinic vs. 30 percent of private patients. Most of the false-positive tests had a titer of 1:1 to 1:4 but were occasionally 1:32 or higher. Of all biologic false-positive tests, 61 percent were acute reactors, and 39 percent chronic reactors. Of the chronic reactors, up to one-half were subsequently diagnosed as definite syphilis, and 50 percent were true biologic false positives often manifesting serious underlying disease [195].

Causes of transient (Table 201-2) biologic false-positive reactions have included smallpox vaccination (1 to 2 percent), [196,197], atypical pneumonia (2 percent), and enterovirus infection [198]. Accurate data on the frequency of acute false-positive tests in other diseases are not readily available in the literature. Immunization procedures other than the smallpox are unlikely to produce BFP reactions. Infectious mononucleosis was once attributed a false positivity rate of 20 percent [199], but more recent studies have reduced this figure to less than 1 percent [200,201].

Pregnancy has often been listed as a common cause of biologic false positivity in the reaginic tests—as high as one-third in several large series [195,202,203]; other studies dispute these findings and report a BFP rate of less than 1 in 2000 in a survey of more than 141,000 serum specimens obtained during pregnancy [204]. The differences in rates of false biologic positives may be population specific, with a lower false biologic positivity rate in a higher-risk population. The estimated rate of BFP in the general population is 1:4000 [205]. If an asymptomatic pregnant woman is found to have a confirmed positive VDRL, an attempt should be made to substantiate a diagnosis of syphilis with more specific treponemal tests. If specific tests are not available, treatment with recommended therapy should be administered in order to minimize the risk of infection in

Table 201-2 False-positive reactions to the nontreponemal tests

Transient reactors (less than 6 months' duration)	Chronic reactors (6 months or longer)
Technical error (low titer)	Leprosy
Smallpox vaccination	Elderly population
Mycoplasma pneumonia	Systemic lupus
Enterovirus infections	erythematosus
Infectious mononucleosis	Hashimoto's thyroiditis
Pregnancy	Rheumatoid arthritis
Narcotic abuse	Rheumatic heart disease
Other causes commonly	Other connective tissue
listed:	disorders
Advanced tuberculosis	Hepatic cirrhosis
Scarlet fever	Polyarteritis nodosa
Viral pneumonia	Narcotic abuse
"Pneumonia"	Malignant tumors
Brucellosis	Familial false positives
Rate-bite fever	Idiopathic
Relapsing fever	
Leptospirosis	
Measles	
Mumps	
Lymphogranuloma	
venereum	
Malaria	
Trypanosomiasis	
Protein deficiency	

the unborn fetus. A careful clinical and serologic follow-up of the infant should be performed in order to exclude active infection (see above).

Narcotic addicts exhibit a high rate of reactivity to a number of reaginic tests for syphilis—5 to 8 percent for women and 8 to 13 percent for men [206,207]. In drug addicts with reactive tests, false positivity varies from 33 to 95 percent [206,208,209]. In these studies there appeared to be no false reactors to treponemal tests, and no evident correlation of false reactivity and type B hepatitis, duration of heroin use, or last use of heroin. False-positive reagin reactions may persist in ex-addicts after 14 months abstinence from heroin, but may recede during methadone use [210].

Other commonly listed causes of acute biologic false positives are less well documented and include advanced tuberculosis, scarlet fever, pneumonia, brucellosis, rat-bite fever, relapsing fever, leptospirosis, viral pneumonia, measles, mumps, lymphogranuloma venereum, malaria, trypanosomiasis, and protein deficiency [211]. One study showed that the duration of reactivity in acute reactors was less than 10 weeks in 60 percent and most were below the age of 30. In contrast, most chronic reactors were over the age of 30; in the majority the duration of reactivity was more than 1 year. False biologic reactions were also more common with the complement-fixation type of reagin tests than with the flocculation type. There seemed to be no association of BFP with ABO blood group typing in acute or chronic reactors. Excluding pregnancy, overt disease that could have accounted for the false positivity was noted in 21 of 109 (20 percent) acute and 26 of 110 (25 percent) chronic reactors [212].

The causes of chronic BFP reaginic tests are multiple, but eventually include syphilis in 50 percent of the total group; careful follow-up studies and treponemal tests must be performed on all reactors [195]. Leprosy has been associated with chronic BFP, with rates varying between 8 and 28 percent of those with positive reaginic tests [202,213] and an even higher association in lepromatous leprosy [214]. Aging alone is reported as a common cause of chronic BFP, with a false-positive rate of 1.7 percent for persons 55 to 60 years of age and 9 to 10 percent for those 70 to 80 years of age [215–217]. The positive tests in the elderly group are associated with increased total globulins, antinuclear antibodies, and rheumatoid factor. Not all studies show such a high false positivity rate in the elderly population [218].

Patients with chronic BFP who are followed for a long period are more likely to develop systemic lupus erythematosus (SLE) [219], Hashimoto's thyroiditis [220], and other connective tissue disorders [212]. In 130 patients (94 women and 36 men) with chronic BFP followed for 1 to 12 years, the largest single illness represented was lupus erythematosus, in 10 women. Seventy-four patients had no diagnosis, and the remainder had a variety of chronic diseases including rheumatoid arthritis, rheumatic heart disease, possible connective tissue disease, hepatic cirrhosis, polyarteritis nodosa, Hashimoto's thyroiditis, and heroin addiction [221]. In addition, there was a high prevalence of antinuclear antibody, rheumatoid factor, elevated total gamma globulins, antithyroid antibodies, and cryoglobulins in the group of chronic reactors [195,222,223]. A chronic BFP may be present for several years before clinical SLE develops. The prevalence of BFP in patients with SLE may be as high as 11 percent, and 5 percent in patients with Hashimoto's thyroiditis [219]. Other unusual causes of chronic BFP reactions include an occasional instance of lymphoma [224], Waldenström's macroglobulinemia, and plasma cell dyscrasia [225].

A genetic basis for chronic BFP is suggested by findings in several families in which multiple relatives had chronic BFP and an increased frequency of elevated total gamma globulins, positive tests for antinuclear antibodies, and rheumatoid factor [219,226]. The predominant types of antibody found in the biologic false-positive reactor is of the 19S (IgM) fraction, 19S and 7S together, and only occasionally 7S alone. Patients with acquired syphilis, on the other hand, demonstrate specific reactivity in both the 19S and 7S fractions [227]. Addition of 2-mercaptoethanol, which specifically splits the IgM molecule, rendered 29 of 43 false positives but none of 107 syphilitic sera negative in the VDRL test [228]. This procedure may be applicable for determining true or false positives in patients with SLE, and positive reaginic and treponemal tests.

Treponemal tests. Treponemal antigen tests may be divided into five main groups depending on how the antigen–antibody complex is detected: (1) immobilization, in which the antigen is live *T. pallidum;* (2) complement-fixation, in which the antigen usually is an extract of the Reiter treponeme; (3) immunofluorescence, in which the antigen is fixed *T. pallidum;* (4) hemagglutination, in which red blood cells are coated with cell components of *T. pallidum;* and (5) enzyme-linked immunosorbent assay (ELISA), in which protein fractions of *T. pallidum* are used as antigens. These tests are more sensitive and specific than lipoidal antigen tests but some are technically difficult and expensive to perform.

TREPONEMA PALLIDUM IMMOBILIZATION (TPI). The *T. pallidum* immobilization test, first introduced in 1949 by Nelson and Mayer [229], requires live organisms obtained from experimentally infected rabbit orchitis. The test is technically difficult to perform, and the results are influenced by several sources of error [175,230]. The TPI test, which is available in only a few research laboratories, has been replaced by other treponemal tests that are easier to perform and appear to be just as reliable. In fact, one study claims that the TPI test adds no further diagnostic information once the result of the FTA-ABS test is known (see below) [231].

Treponemal tests based on complement-fixation—the Reiter protein complement-fixation (RPCF) and the one-fifth volume Kolmer with Reiter protein antigen (KRP)—are no longer routinely performed in the United States and have been replaced by the FTA-ABS test because of variance in batches of the Reiter protein and false positives with aging of the antigen.

FLUORESCENT TREPONEMAL ANTIBODY-ABSORPTION (FTA-ABS) TEST. The standard treponemal test in the United States is the manual fluorescent treponemal antibody-absorption (FTA-ABS) test, which is based on indirect immunofluorescence testing techniques and helps to demonstrate treponemal antibody by visualizing its combination with a Nichols strain of *T. pallidum* affixed to glass slides. The test serum of the patient is first mixed with a sorbent containing an extract from a Reiter strain of treponemes in order to absorb nonspecific group antigens. The absorbed serum is then added to the *T. pallidum* affixed to glass slides. Human globulins specific for syphilis infection adhere to the surface of the treponemes, and the globulins are detected using an indirect fluorescence technique with rabbit antihuman globulin conjugated with fluorescein. Results are dependent on the intensity of fluorescence and are noted as nonreactive, marginal (borderline), and reactive (1+ to 4+). Quantitative evaluation of test results are being performed in experimental studies only and are not yet useful clinically. The FTA-ABS shows reactivity with 19S IgM, 7S IgG, and IgA antibodies directed against *T. pallidum.*

At present, the FTA is the most sensitive serologic test in all stages of syphilis [232], rivaled only by the TPHA [170,233]. The automated version of the FTA-ABS test shows good agreement with the manual method [234], but the manual FTA-ABS may be less specific [235]. The false reactivity of the manual FTA-ABS test is usually related to the use of inefficient reagents (e.g., lyophilized treponemes, inadequate sorbent), failures in the emission spectrum of the ultraviolet lamp used for reading tests, and technician error. Occasionally, positive FTA-ABS reactions occur in healthy adults with no other evidence of syphilis and with negative lipoidal tests, and many positives will revert to negative within a year [236]. Most of these false-positive FTA-ABS tests are related to the presence of autoantibodies, such as rheumatoid factors [171]. False-positive FTA-ABS tests (Table 201-3) have also occurred in patients with genital herpes [237,238] (an estimated 1 percent false positive and 5 percent borderline FTA-ABS reactor rates), in pregnant women [239,240], in patients with systemic lupus erythematosus [241], alcoholic cirrhosis, scleroderma, and mixed connective tissue disease [242,243]. Positive FTA-ABS tests in the afore-

Table 201-3   False-positive reactions to the FTA-ABS test

Technical error
Inefficient sorbents
Healthy individuals without syphilis
Genital herpes simplex
Pregnancy
Lupus erythematosus (systemic or skin only)
Alcoholic cirrhosis
Scleroderma
Mixed connective tissue disease

mentioned disease states have occurred usually with the beaded or borderline pattern, but also rarely in a uniform pattern. Patients selected on the basis of an elevated ANA ($\geq$ 1:32) or rheumatic factor ($\geq$ 1:640), 12 and 20 percent of sera, respectively, showed some degree of reactivity; patients with borderline, 1+ homogeneous, and beaded patterns of fluorescence did not have syphilis. On the other hand, of 39 patients with discoid lupus erythematosus (DLE) and systemic lupus erythematosus (SLE) but without evidence of syphilis and a negative TPI, 41 percent of the patients were reactive or borderline to one or more serologic test for syphilis: 10 patients (26 percent) had homogeneous reactions in the FTA-ABS test (7 borderline, 3 reactive), 11 patients (28 percent) had reactive VDRL tests, 5 patients (13 percent) had reactive RPR tests, and 4 patients (10 percent) had reactive MHA-TP tests. None of these patients had beaded reactions in the FTA-ABS test, and reactive results in the VDRL, RPR, and MHA-TP tests were low in titer in all patients examined [244].

The beaded pattern of fluorescence has occurred at a prevalence rate of 0.04 percent of 9800 sera submitted for VDRL testing and 2.1 percent of "problem" sera (positive VDRL or evidence of syphilis). In certain patients with SLE, anti-DNA antibodies are responsible for the beading pattern and are inhibited when serum is preincubated with calf thymus DNA. Other sera with the beading phenomenon are not related to anti-DNA antibodies and the phenomenon may simply disappear with a decrease of IgM by serum aging. Occasionally, the beading phenomenon has occurred in patients with documented histories of syphilis [241]. Studies suggest that the beaded fluorescence pattern of the FTA-ABS test is not dependent on the presence of antinuclear antibody, but rather on the substrate (*T. pallidum*) and the method of preparation. The original test used a sonicated Reiter treponeme as the absorbing agent for group-specific antitreponemal antibodies, but for practical reasons a heat-stable sorbent is used in commercial preparations. The beaded phenomenon and false-positive reactivity in the FTA-ABS test using heat-stable sorbent could be abolished when fresh sonicated Reiter treponemes were used as the absorbing agent [243,245]. It is also not clear what role the antihuman globulin conjugate has in false reactivity in the FTA-ABS test. At present, a polyvalent conjugate containing antisera to all the components of the human globulin fraction is used. Monospecific conjugates may help the specificity of the test, but further studies are necessary.

Low false-positive rates to the FTA-ABS test have occurred in other studies of normal patients without syphilis—3 of 383 normals studied by Deacon et al [246] and 3 of 250 nuns studied by Goldman and Lantz [232]. These

"false positives" in the FTA-ABS test and 1 of 75 normal blood donors studied by Pien et al [241] should be distinguished from the BFP reactions using the lipoidal tests. False positivity for one specified treponemal serologic test does not always correlate with positivity for the other serologic tests: of 8 patients with SLE or LE with a borderline or reactive FTA-ABS test, 5 had a reactive VDRL, 3 had a reactive RPR, and 3 had a reactive MHA-TP test [244]. A variation of the manual FTA-ABS test, called the FTA blocking test, uses a rabbit anti-Reiter serum instead of the sorbing agent in order to reduce false-positive reactions [247]. Borderline reactions in the FTA-ABS test usually do not correlate well with the diagnosis of syphilis.

The FTA-ABS test is predominantly used for confirmation of positive results in other assays and in cases with discrepant test results [167].

TREPONEMA PALLIDUM HEMAGGLUTINATION ASSAY (TPHA). Passive hemagglutination of erythrocytes coated with antigen is a sensitive method for the detection of antibody. This method is the basis for a reliable test to detect antibodies against *T. pallidum* [248]. In the original report by Rathlev [249], the antigen was formalinized tanned sheep erythrocytes coated with ultrasonicated material from the Nichols strain of *T. pallidum;* treponemal antibody was indicated by macrohemagglutination when "positive" sera were added to the test suspension.

Experience with the microvariant of the TPHA test, the microhemagglutination assay with *T. pallidum* (MHA-TP), and its automated version (AMHA-TP), does not differ significantly from the TPHA [169,173,250–252]. The use of chemically stable polyurea microcapsules with red dye inside, instead of tanned sheep erythrocytes, may provide some advantage over the standard TPHA [253]. The automated version of the original test [254] using microvolume technique has provided the technical basis for an inexpensive, easy method for detecting specific treponemal antibodies, requiring much less technical skill and equipment than the FTA-ABS test. The TPHA test is being used as a screening or confirmatory assay for syphilis in many laboratories throughout the United States and Europe.

The usefulness of the TPHA is dependent on the quality of reagents, which may vary from kit to kit of the same producer [167]. The test is less sensitive in primary syphilis than either the FTA-ABS or the VDRL due primarily to the variable IgM-binding capacity of the reagents [167], is superior in sensitivity to both the FTA-ABS test and VDRL in secondary syphilis, and is at least as sensitive as the FTA-ABS test (and more sensitive than the VDRL) for latent and late latent syphilis. In treated syphilis, both early and late disease, the TPHA demonstrates seroreversal less frequently than does either the VDRL or the FTA-ABS test [255].

The specificity and sensitivity of the TPHA are high, i.e., each greater than 99.9 percent [133]. In studies of patients with false-positive tests for syphilis, the TPHA was reactive in 2 to 5 percent of cases, or less. Some of the false reactors detected by the TPHA may in fact have syphilis, confirmed by further studies [194]. False-positive or inconclusive tests in the TPHA have been reported in patients with infectious mononucleosis, pregnancy, narcotic addiction, autoimmune diseases, and leprosy. In the autoimmune disease category, false-positive results to the TPHA may be caused by autoantibodies [171,223]. Like other treponemal tests, the TPHA is not able to distinguish between infection due to *T. pallidum* and that due to other treponematoses. The usefulness of the TPHA in prenatal syphilis has not been fully investigated because of the small number of cases available for evaluation. However, passively transferred IgG antibodies to *T. pallidum* have been detected by the TPHA as long as 9 months after birth in noninfected children of previously infected mothers.

The TPHA is not useful in the evaluation of response to treatment, since the titer falls slowly if at all. In addition, there is no relationship to activity of disease or the clinical stage of syphilis using a quantitative TPHA. The TPHA, particularly its microvariants (the MHA-TP and AMHA-TP), may be used to screen normal populations for latent or late disease since the test is cheaper than the FTA-ABS and more sensitive than the VDRL at this stage of syphilis. It may also be used for retrospective confirmation of syphilitic infection, since the duration of reactivity after treatment for the TPHA is longer than the VDRL or FTA-ABS.

The TPHA should not be used as the sole treponemal test. Its simplicity, sensitivity, and low cost make it an attractive screening test. However, a positive reaction to the TPHA should be confirmed using the FTA-ABS test [16].

THE ENZYME-LINKED IMMUNOSORBENT ASSAY (ELISA) FOR SYPHILIS. The antigen for this assay utilizes an ultrasonicate of *T. pallidum;* protein fractions of the organism obtained by ultracentrifugation, extraction, or gel filtration [256–260]; or flagella of Reiter treponemes [261]. The antigen is fixed to wells of microtemplates, and is incubated with serum. Enzyme-linked antihuman globulin is added in a second incubation, and will bind serum antibodies to *T. pallidum* (if present). Peroxidase or alkaline phosphatase is used as the enzyme. A color change after addition of respective enzyme substrate (*o*-phenylenediamine or *p*-nitrophenoyl phosphate) indicates a positive reaction. The assay can be performed automatically, and photometric readings of the color change permit semiquantitation. The sensitivity and specificity of this new assay indicate comparable or superior results when compared to other tests for specific *T. pallidum* antibodies [260].

ASSAYS FOR THE DETECTION OF SPECIFIC ANTITREPONEMAL IGM ANTIBODIES. The significance of serum 19S IgM antibodies directed against *T. pallidum* has already been stressed (see above), particularly in the diagnosis of prenatal infection [168]. The reaginic tests for the diagnosis of syphilis are dependent upon reactions involving IgG, IgM, and IgA antibodies. Serum IgG in a newborn infant may be passively acquired transplacentally. Therefore, a positive reaginic test in the neonatal period could indicate either active infection in the infant or passively acquired antibodies from an infected mother.

In 1968, Scotti and Logan [262] reported a modification of the standard FTA-ABS test, using indirect fluorescence to detect IgM specific for *T. pallidum*. Since maternal IgM does not cross the placenta, it was postulated that the presence in an infant of IgM specific for *T. pallidum* represents a true host response to infection (and not placental transfer of antibody) [263]. Although this concept is theoretically sound and initial reports were enthusiastic, practical application of the IgM-FTA-ABS test indicates the need for cautious interpretation.

False-negative reactions to the IgM-FTA-ABS test have

occurred, probably due to competitive inhibition of IgM by IgG; the IgM receptors on the surface of treponemes appear to be "hidden" by high titers of IgG [171]. False-positive reactions to the IgM-FTA-ABS test have been caused by autoantibodies of the IgM class, i.e., rheumatoid factors, or even IgM directed against antitreponemal IgG [171,173]. According to an analysis of pooled results of the IgM-FTA-ABS test from several studies [264], there were no false-positive reactions in normal neonates (virtually 100 percent specific). In infants with positive reaginic tests due to maternal infection, but no neonatal syphilis infection, specificity was noted to be about 94 percent. Sensitivity of the IgM-FTA-ABS test correlates with the onset of disease: immediate onset (signs and symptoms within 4 weeks of birth) and delayed onset of disease (presence of signs or symptoms more than 4 weeks after birth) have been associated with sensitivities of 88 and 65 percent, respectively [264]. Higher sensitivity and specificity of the test have been reported [265], related possibly to the source and dilution of the conjugate used for the test. Leakage of maternal serum into the fetal circulation could theoretically create false positivity in the reaginic tests, as well as the IgM-FTA-ABS test. If this is suspected, the serum ceruloplasmin concentration may be useful; pregnant women have a concentration of ceruloplasmin 4 to 6 times that in nonpregnant adults, and the concentration in infants is only half that in adults [103].

The IgM-FTA-ABS test has been improved to reduce false-positive results by separating the 19S fraction of serum (to eliminate IgG) by gel filtration, and then applying the purified serum product using the same reagents for the IgM-FTA-ABS test. The various techniques for obtaining purified 19S IgM have been described [266,267]. Application of high-pressure liquid chromatography with electronic surveillance [266] requires 10 min for one separation, renders an absolutely pure 19S IgM fraction, and costs $10 per serum. The low cost for routine use of this new test will require examination of not fewer than 8,000 to 10,000 sera per month, i.e., 2000 to 3000 reactive samples per year [267]. Results are highly specific and sensitive; reactivity is detectable around the second week of infection, and is undetectable about 3 months after adequate therapy for early syphilis and within 12 months after effective therapy for late disease. Of all sera showing reactivity to the test, 3.4 percent are false positive and 3.6 percent are false negative [267]. The reliability in prenatal syphilis is 99 percent [168]. The microenzyme-linked immunosorbent assay for the detection of specific IgM antibodies in syphilis may eventually be a suitable alternative to the more technically complicated 19S(IgM)-FTA-ABS test [268].

THE IGM-SOLID PHASE HEMABSORPTION (IGM-SPHA) TEST [269]. In this test, a μ-chain-specific anti-IgM reagent is fixed to the wells of polystyrol microtemplates and incubated with test serum. IgM molecules in test serum bind to the wells and react in a second step with TPHA reagents. The test is as easy and inexpensive as the MHA-TP or the AMHA-TP, and an automated version can be used for mass examinations. Quantitative assessments of positive tests are performed routinely. A titer of 1:4 is considered borderline, 1:2 or below negative, and 1:8 or above positive. During the first weeks of infection, the sensitivity of the test is lower than the 19S IgM-FTA-ABS test, but is comparable to the MHA-TP [170,173,259,270–272]. False-negative results occur maximally in 8 percent of reactive sera, particularly at the onset of infection, due to low IgM-binding capacity of reagents [259,267,270,271]. False-positive findings are seen in less than 1 percent of all reactive samples. Therefore, a positive IgM-SPHA test very likely indicates active infection in untreated patients, particularly in children with prenatal syphilis, and in individuals with reinfection, cardiovascular syphilis, and neurosyphilis. A negative IgM-SPHA test does not always exclude active syphilis infection; reliability of the test is highly dependent on the quality of reagents, proper preparation of the test plates, and careful performance of the assay.

Comparative sensitivity of VDRL, TPI, FTA-ABS, and TPHA tests [194,246,248]. The tests commonly in use for the detection of untreated and treated syphilis infection have widely differing sensitivities in early, latent, and late disease. In primary untreated syphilis up to 6 weeks after infection, the FTA-ABS test is the most sensitive test with 91 percent reactive, compared to about 72 percent for the TPHA and 88 percent for the VDRL. For untreated secondary disease, the VDRL is 100 percent reactive, the FTA-ABS 99.2 percent, and the TPHA 100 percent, provided proper reagents are used [133,194,273]. For latent or indeterminate untreated syphilis, the VDRL is least sensitive (39 to 70 percent reactive) [194,246,274], while the FTA-ABS test is 81 to 100 percent reactive [193,246,274], and the TPHA is at least as sensitive as the FTA-ABS test. In untreated late disease (cardiovascular, CNS, or congenital), both the FTA-ABS and TPHA approach a sensitivity of 100 percent, while the VDRL is 61 to 70 percent reactive [246,274]; the TPHA is much more sensitive than the VDRL, and at least as sensitive as the FTA-ABS test, in late disease [142].

It is clear from these comparative reactivities that reliance on serologic tests must be correlated with the clinical stage of disease (Table 201-4). For instance, in primary syphilis, a definite early diagnosis may be made only with a dark-field examination of lesions. In secondary disease, the VDRL is usually positive, while in latent or late disease the VDRL is often negative and reliance must be placed on the FTA-ABS or TPHA.

Onset of reactivity of serologic tests for syphilis is marked first by the production of antitreponemal 19S IgM antibody and reactivity of the FTA-ABS (IgM) test by the end of the second week after infection. The FTA-ABS, using polyvalent antihuman globulin, becomes reactive during the third week, followed at close intervals by the TPHA (third week) and the VDRL (3 to 4 weeks after infection). Sometimes, reactivity to the TPHA or VDRL appears before the FTA-ABS, but only infrequently. The

IgM-FTA-ABS test, which is more often positive and higher in titer in untreated early syphilis when compared with untreated late latent disease, may eventually assist in distinguishing between these two stages [275] (Table 201-4).

Cerebrospinal fluid examination for syphilis infection [57,276,277]

The proper evaluation of cerebrospinal fluid requires three major determinations: (1) a nontreponemal serologic test; (2) a cell count; and (3) total protein determination. The colloidal gold test is not considered diagnostic and is of little value in the management of neurosyphilis.

Nontreponemal serologic test on spinal fluid. The most useful nonspecific test on the CSF is the VDRL slide test, reported as reactive or nonreactive. Quantitative tests on "reactive" spinal fluids provide a baseline of activity from which response to treatment or activity of disease can be assessed, although the response is less predictable than serum quantitative tests. A reactive VDRL will not distinguish between active or inactive disease, and such a determination can be more reliably made by examining CSF protein level and cell counts. Following successful treatment, the CSF cell count should return to normal, followed by the cerebrospinal fluid protein concentration, and finally the CSF VDRL. It may take many years for the CSF VDRL to become negative, depending on the duration of disease: 6 to 15 months after disease of less than 2 years' duration, and persisting in low titer for as long as 7 years in disease of more than 5 years' duration [57]. The CSF VDRL titer should drop progressively over time.

Unlike the serum nontreponemal tests, a false-positive VDRL in the spinal fluid is very rare, reported only in isolated cases of tuberculous meningitis, benign lymphocytic meningitis, meningococcal meningitis, subarachnoid hemorrhage, infectious mononucleosis, cerebral malaria, lymphoma, trypanosomiasis, poliomyelitis, collagen vascular disorders, and spinal cord tumor [276,278]. One of the authors (A.R.R.) is aware of a patient with false-positive CSF VDRL, ART, and FTA-ABS tests associated with a cranial glioblastoma multiforme, obstructive hydrocephalus, and elevated CSF protein (600 mg/100 mL); the CSF tests became nonreactive when the hydrocephalus and elevated protein were corrected, and at no time were blood tests for syphilis reactive. Meningeal carcinomatosis secondary to metastatic lung carcinoma has been reported to give a false-positive VDRL and FTA in the CSF [279]. Authentic false-positive spinal fluid Wassermann reactions have also been reported to occur in rare cases of intracranial tumor, encephalomalacia, and cranial trauma [280]. The prozone phenomenon was not detected for the CSF VDRL when more than 7000 CSF specimens were studied, and further dilution of more than 50 positive CSF VDRL specimens did not give stronger reactivity (W. P. Corbett, personal communication). However, the prozone phenomenon has been reported in CSF [281]. Contamination of a CSF specimen with blood in a syphilitic patient with a serum VDRL reactive at 1:256 or below and a strongly reactive serum FTA-ABS will produce a false-positive CSF VDRL test only if the CSF is grossly bloody, or a false-positive CSF FTA-ABS test if there are more than 1000

Table 201-4   Present-day application of serologic tests for syphilis

Serum screening	Confirmation of diagnosis	Assessment of activity of disease or efficacy of treatment
MHA-TP	FTA-ABS	VDRL quantitative
VDRL		IgM-SPHA quantitative
ART		19S IgM-FTA-ABS qualitative
RPR		

Source: WHO report [167]

red blood cells per cubic millimeter [276]. Contamination of CSF with acetic acid may also cause flocculation of the VDRL. Despite these rare exceptions, a reactive VDRL test on the CSF should be considered as indicative of syphilitic central nervous system infection, either active or inactive.

Although the specificity of a positive VDRL in the spinal fluid is almost always unquestioned, the sensitivity is less secure. A nonreactive VDRL in the CSF does not necessarily disprove CNS infection, since autopsy-proved neurosyphilis is occasionally reported with a negative CSF VDRL [282]. Other studies reveal that the CSF VDRL can be negative in 30 to 43 percent of patients with untreated neurosyphilis [142,179,283]. Signs and symptoms of infection and meningeal irritation may be present in primary and secondary syphilis as indicated by an increased CSF protein level and cell count in 3 to 5 percent of patients with primary syphilis and 3 to 15 percent of patients with secondary syphilis. The CSF VDRL is only rarely positive (< 5 percent) in early syphilis, except for acute symptomatic syphilitic meningitis in which the reaginic test for syphilis is usually positive [57,116]. On the other hand, it is not uncommon to find entirely normal spinal fluid findings in "burnt-out" cases of tabes dorsalis [116].

Cell count. The most sensitive indicator of activity of disease in the central nervous system is an increased CSF cell count. Counts of greater than 10 cells per cubic millimeter are unquestionably abnormal, 5 to 10 cells per cubic millimeter usually considered abnormal, and 2 to 5 cells per cubic millimeter considered borderline. Students of CNS syphilis do not always agree on what constitutes a normal cell count.

Total protein determination. A precipitating agent, such as trichloroacetic acid, and the degree of turbidity produced, detected by a colorimeter or spectrophotometer, are usually used to determine total protein in the CSF. Normal values in a given laboratory, which depend on the methods used, must be taken into account when assessing a given value. In general, a CSF protein greater than 40 mg per 100 mL is considered abnormal.

Tests for treponemal antibody in CSF. Soon after its introduction, the FTA test was applied to spinal fluid; it soon became evident that the FTA test was more sensitive than the nontreponemal tests. In particular, it became clear that the CSF-FTA (undiluted CSF, not absorbed with Reiter protein) was more sensitive than the CSF-FTA-ABS (spinal fluid diluted 1:5 with sorbent) and was associated with a 4.5 percent false-positivity rate [284]. In a review of the CSF-FTA test [285], 1 in 177 nonsyphilitic patients examined had a positive test when the CSF was used undiluted and unabsorbed, and the "false" positivity was abolished when the CSF was diluted in saline or sorbent. Blood containing a high-titer VDRL and contaminating the CSF did not account for false positives since the CSF would not produce a false-positive CSF-FTA unless there were more than 1000 red blood cells per cubic millimeter. In patients with latent syphilis and a negative CSF-VDRL test, there were false-positive results when the CSF-FTA test was used, and fewer false positives when the CSF was diluted with saline or sorbent. There were no false posi-

tives with the CSF-MHA-TP or CSF-VDRL tests in normal individuals in this study. Other studies revealed that false reactivity did not occur in undiluted CSF using the FTA-ABS test [114,142,286,287]. Similar results were obtained with the TPHA, which is considered reactive in CSF if agglutination occurs at dilutions of 1:10 or higher. However, the CSF-FTA-ABS and CSF-TPHA tests were frequently reactive in previously infected but adequately treated individuals without CNS involvement, in whom serum still remains reactive. IgG antibodies easily pass an intact blood/brain barrier and can therefore be detected in the CSF using sensitive tests. A nonreactive CSF-FTA-ABS and/or CSF-TPHA test usually excludes neurosyphilis [114,142,167,286,287]. The 19S IgM-FTA-ABS test cannot be performed with CSF. The CSF-IgM-SPHA test is considered reactive at titers of 1:1 and higher; positive results were observed in 23 of 24 patients with untreated neurosyphilis, and in none of 69 controls (unpublished studies, A.F.H.L.).

New parameters have been developed in order to provide specific serologic indicators of neurosyphilis. The blood–brain barrier function has been defined by the *albumin quotient,* which relates the CSF albumin to the serum albumin. The *TPHA index* relates the CSF-TPHA titer to the albumin quotient, and the *TPA index* relates the CSF-TPHA-IgG titer to the total amount of CSF-IgG and the serum TPHA-IgG titer to the total amount of serum IgG [142,286]. Initial evaluation of these parameters has shown a considerable margin of error, and the ultimate usefulness of these indices in the diagnosis of neurosyphilis remains to be determined [114,142,286,287].

Diagnosis of activity of neurosyphilis. The activity of neurosyphilis may be assessed using the empirical observations outlined by Dattner and Thomas 30 years ago [57]:

1. Syphilis infection may be very active within the central nervous system and still be asymptomatic; signs and symptoms are not reliable criteria of activity.

2. A positive spinal fluid nontreponemal test alone is not proof of active neurosyphilis. Increased cell counts and total protein determinations are more reliable indicators of activity.

3. In an arrested case of neurosyphilis, cell counts should become normal within 3 to 4 months after treatment, while quantitative nontreponemal tests and protein values show a gradual and steady trend to normal.

4. Following specific therapy with penicillin for active neurosyphilis, the spinal fluid may show a trend toward normal, only to relapse later. Relapses, however, rarely occur more than 1 year following therapy. If the cell count is not normal and no improvement occurs in total protein and quantitative nontreponemal tests 6 months after treatment, further treatment is imperative regardless of the clinical status of the patient.

The above approach outlined by Dattner and Thomas is still useful in modern syphilis therapy. More detailed and analytic studies have led to the development of additional parameters [114,142,286,287]. To the above points, then, the following may be added:

5. A reactive CSF-IgM-SPHA test indicates active infection.

6. A CSF-TPHA index above 100 is strongly suggestive

of active neurosyphilis, provided the albumin quotient does not exceed 20.

7. A nonreactive CSF-FTA-ABS and/or CSF-TPHA usually excludes neurosyphilis.

It is useful to carefully evaluate all available CSF and serologic findings before making the diagnosis of neurosyphilis.

Therapy for syphilis (see Table 201-5)

Introduction. The natural history of untreated early syphilis is provided by studies initiated by Boeck of Oslo, Norway, in 1891. Investigations were continued in 1929 by Bruusgaard, completed by Gjestland in meticulous follow-up of 953 of Boeck's original patients [115], and reviewed by Clark and Danbolt in 1964 [59,60]. Gjestland's studies revealed the following: clinical secondary relapse occurred in the absence of treatment among 23.6 percent, one-fourth of this subgroup having multiple episodes and most occurring within 1 to 2 years; late benign syphilis occurred in 16 percent, observed as early as the first year or as late as the forty-sixth year (average occurring by the fifteenth year) after healing of early syphilis; cardiovascular syphilis occurred in 9.6 percent; and neurosyphilis occurred in 6.5 percent. Among 694 patients known dead on follow-up, syphilis was the primary cause of death in 10.8 percent of the group (15.1 percent for males, 8.3 percent for females), while between 60 and 70 percent of these patients went through life with a minimum of inconvenience and without ever having had treatment for their syphilis.

Boeck was not at all convinced that the toxic therapy available in the late nineteenth century benefited patients in any way. Even today, all therapy must be judged against the natural course of disease. With this information as background, the now widely debated study of untreated late latent syphilis in black males in Macon County, Alabama (Tuskegee), was begun in 1932 [288,289]. At the time, there was a valid question as to whether asymptomatic patients with late latent syphilis were better left untreated rather than subjected to the modalities then available which included mercury, bismuth, iodides, fever therapy, and organic arsenic compounds. The efficacy of these agents was then unproved, side effects not insignificant, and duration of therapy prolonged for months or even years [57,290]. Although syphilitics showed an excess mortality compared to nonsyphilitics to the extent of 140 percent, when treated and untreated syphilitics were compared, the syphilitics classified as "cured through treatment" had a mortality rate 10 to 20 percent higher than those untreated or inadequately treated [291,292]. In addition, the course of cardiovascular disease did not appear to be affected by treatment with arsphenamine [293]. The often quoted figure of 85 percent favorable outcome in treated latency in a Johns Hopkins study, as compared to 35 percent in untreated latency in Bruusgaard's study, represents an extrapolation of data from 40 patients followed for 10 years by Moore et al [292]; it is the main body of evidence cited to support the contention that the Tuskegee study should never have been initiated. However, these figures were too meager to form the basis of public health policy even in 1932. Since a high prevalence of syphilis existed in Macon County at the time—35 percent of the population had evidence of infection—and since arsenic (like mercury)

seemed to do more harm than good for late disease in the modalities used, a central question remained—whether or not to treat asymptomatic late latent disease.

In an attempt to bring order to the prevailing uncertainty in the treatment of syphilis, the clinicians of the Clinical Cooperative Group pooled the experience from their respective clinics: 399 black males with late latent syphilis and 201 nonsyphilitic controls were followed for more than 20 years (during which time almost half of the study subjects received therapy for syphilis). A 30-year follow-up of infected individuals revealed (1) a life expectancy reduced by 17 percent compared with controls, (2) the appearance of late syphilis in 12 percent (64 percent of whom manifested cardiovascular involvement), (3) an estimated 50 percent chance of demonstrating syphilitic cardiovascular involvement at autopsy in those with disease of more than 10 years' duration, and (4) the primary cause of death as syphilitic involvement of the cardiovascular and central nervous systems in 30.4 percent of those coming to autopsy [294,295].

Although criticism of the Tuskegee study is valid—the study should have been discontinued when the potential hazards of disease outweighed the potential dangers of penicillin therapy—even today, we know no more of the effectiveness or ineffectiveness of penicillin in late latent disease than we did in the late 1940s when penicillin became common therapy for syphilis.

The use of mercury, iodides, bismuth, organic arsenicals, and fever in the prepenicillin era comprise a fascinating historical chapter in syphilis therapy, and the interested reader is referred to several reviews [52,57,290]. The organic arsenicals were the most useful drugs among the lot and showed reasonable effectiveness with or without added bismuth for early syphilis during World War II prior to penicillin; however, the long duration of therapy as well as significant morbidity and mortality relegate the arsenicals, as well as the other therapies mentioned, to the annals of history.

Penicillin. Penicillin was first used in the treatment of experimental spirochetosis in 1943 [296] and in the treatment of human syphilis shortly thereafter [297]. It has become the mainstay of drug treatment and the standard on which other modes of therapy are based. There has been no indication that *T. pallidum* has acquired resistance to the drug although organisms have been found to persist in human and experimental animal tissues after adequate therapy, and the inability to culture the organism in vitro until recently has made an accurate assessment of resistance impossible.

Penicillin acts during growth and division of *T. pallidum* by interfering with cell wall synthesis. The cross-linked chains of *N*-acetylglucosamine and *N*-acetylmuramic acid form a matrix in the outer cell wall to contain the inner protoplast, just as the leather coat of a football contains the rubber bladder. The cross-linked chains are breached by the hydrolytic action of a lysozyme manufactured by the organism, thus forming gaps or holes. The gaps are continually being repaired by means of mureine precursors that form within the protoplast and pass to the outer wall where they are incorporated into the cell wall via several enzymes, including carboxypeptidases and transpeptidase, in particular. These enzymes help in the cross-linkings between adjacent re-forming chains. Penicillin has an affinity for these enzymes, particularly transpeptidase, and by preventing their effective performance allows the unbridled lysozyme to continue to cause breaks in the cell wall more rapidly than they can be repaired. Osmotic pressure within the protoplast will then cause a bulge of the inner membrane through the holes of the outer wall, resulting in destruction of the organism [3].

Penicillin does not irreversibly interfere with transpeptidase production; the organism can resume biosynthesis of the enzyme within 20 min and recover from the damage if the penicillin concentration dips below the "effective" level. Since *T. pallidum* divides at a calculated interval of 33 h in early lesions, penicillin levels must be sustained at sufficient levels to be bactericidal. The organism must be in an actively dividing state for penicillin to be effective—if damage to the cell wall is incomplete, insensitive spheroblasts or atypical forms may result. There is no evidence, however, that cell wall-defective viable variants play a role in the resistance of *T. pallidum* to penicillin [298]. Spirochetes in late syphilis may perhaps reproduce more slowly and be less susceptible to short courses of penicillin.

Experimental evidence has demonstrated that concentrations of penicillin must be in the range of 0.0025 units per milliliter in order to kill 50 percent of *T. pallidum* within 16 h. More than 10 times this concentration—0.03 units per milliliter—is recommended for treatment, with a minimum duration at such a level for about 7 to 10 days for early syphilis and longer for late syphilis, presumably providing a two- to threefold margin of safety in treatment in adults [298,299]. Such a level can be attained for early syphilis by a single intramuscular injection of 2.4 million units of benzathine penicillin or via the daily intramuscular injection of 600,000 units of aqueous procaine penicillin for 8 days.

In experimental animals exposed to high concentrations of penicillin, immobilization of *T. pallidum* is essentially complete in 12 h. In human chancres, lesions become darkfield negative in 9 h after treatment. However, increasing the concentration of penicillin in contact with spirochetes beyond a certain level (from 0.1 μg/mL to 5 μg/mL) will not increase the rate at which spirochetes are killed. In rabbit studies of experimental orchitis with *T. pallidum*, it has been found that as the total duration of penicillinemia increases up to 8 days, even at the expense of lower average serum levels produced by injections further apart, the total amount of penicillin required to eradicate the spirochetes diminishes—higher doses of short-acting penicillins given every 24 h may not cure experimental syphilis, whereas low doses of long-acting penicillin given at less frequent intervals will be effective as long as subinhibitory levels are not reached. For instance, aqueous penicillin G 300,000 units given intramuscularly to humans has a duration of 6 h, and the duration of effective penicillinemia is short. Regimens producing continuous and prolonged penicillinemia, sacrificing high levels, have been most successful in the treatment of early experimental syphilis. If only a small fraction of the penicillin is reaching the spirochete in tissue, then a higher serum concentration must be attained in order to be effective. Three million units of benzathine penicillin as a single intramuscular injection produces serum levels of at least 0.1 μg/mL for about 2 weeks [298].

The amount of penicillin required to prevent development of disease increases with the interval between inoc-

ulation and therapy, as well as the number of organisms in the inoculum in experimental infection; both phenomena relate to the number of spirochetes present at the time of treatment. Approximately 3 percent of men with gonococcal urethritis may have incubating syphilis, and the short-acting procaine penicillin used to treat gonococcal infection is enough to abort the lesions of syphilis since so few organisms are present. A more prolonged, continuous level of penicillin is required for lesions of syphilis, however, since a larger number of spirochetes are present. Experimental latent syphilis requires continuous penicillin therapy of even longer duration. This is possibly a function of the number of spirochetes present or, alternatively, perhaps due to the fact that organisms are multiplying more slowly in late compared to early disease.

Oral penicillin has been condemned as having no place in the treatment of syphilis, but problems of patient compliance are more relevant than theoretical or experimental effectiveness, since oral penicillin has been used to abort incubating syphilis and to cure established orchitis in rabbits. Treponemicidal levels are achieved in cerebral spinal fluid with amoxicillin 6 g daily administered with probenecid 2 g daily for 15 days [300]. Such an oral treatment program could theoretically serve as an alternative to parenteral administration of penicillin for early syphilis, if compliance could be assured. Oral penicillin tablets, as well as many other antibiotics self-prescribed by patients in inadequate dosage may abort incubating syphilis, interfere with dark-field examination by reducing the number and mobility of organisms, or allow subclinical infection. Oral penicillin tablets in effective doses may one day even be beneficial in the prophylaxis of syphilis, but such a use is only theoretical at this time and is not recommended.

Microbial persistence [298,301]. Even after "adequate" penicillin therapy, organisms may persist in tissue. Electron micrographic studies of early syphilitic lesions show spirochetes inside of neutrophils, macrophages, plasma cells, and fibroblasts, both within the cytoplasm and even the nuclei of some cells. Organisms are destroyed in macrophages and neutrophils, but spirochetes remain intact inside of plasma cells, fibroblasts, and even spermatocytes. Penetration of these cells is active on the part of the bacterium and passive on the part of the cell.

Intracellular residence of spirochetes is important for several reasons: (1) it is postulated that the organism is protected from the high tissue concentrations of oxygen; (2) intracellular residence may play a positive or negative role in host resistance to the organism; and (3) intracellular residence may protect spirochetes from destruction by antibiotics—after treatment with penicillin, extracellular spirochetes are destroyed within 3 to 6 h, while intracellular organisms remain intact. Long courses of antibiotics (> 7 days) may penetrate living mammalian cells, while short periods of exposure are excluded from cells. It is not known whether intracellular organisms retain their virulence.

Spirochetes infect the eye in secondary syphilis. Spiral forms are found occasionally in the anterior chamber of the eye in patients with treated and untreated late disease. The anterior chamber may be a protected site since antibiotics penetrate poorly—a function of poor lipid solubility. Penicillin G penetrates poorly in the absence of inflammation, while relatively low doses are required to cure

Table 201-5 Syphilis: Centers for Disease Control recommended treatment schedules, 1982

1. Early syphilis (primary, secondary, latent of less than 1 year's duration) should be treated with:
   a. Recommended regimen: Benzathine penicillin G: 2.4 million units total, intramuscular, at a single session
   b. Penicillin-allergic patients:
      (1) Patients who are allergic to penicillin should be treated with: Tetracycline hydrochloride 500 mg by mouth 4 times a day for 15 days. Tetracycline appears to be effective, but has been evaluated less extensively than penicillin. Patient compliance with this regimen may be difficult, so care should be taken to encourage optimal compliance.
      (2) Penicillin-allergic patients who cannot tolerate tetracycline should have their allergy confirmed. For these patients there are 2 options:
          (a) If compliance and serologic follow-up can be assured, administer erythromycin 500 mg by mouth 4 times a day for 15 days.
          (b) If compliance and serologic follow-up cannot be assured, the patient should be managed in consultation with an expert.
2. Syphilis of more than 1 year's duration, except neurosyphilis (latent syphilis of indeterminate or more than 1 year's duration, cardiovascular, or late benign syphilis), should be treated with:
   a. Recommended regimen: Benzathine penicillin G: 2.4 million units, intramuscular, once a week for 3 successive weeks (7.2 million units total). The optimal treatment schedules for syphilis of greater than 1 year's duration have been less well established than schedules for early syphilis. In general, syphilis of longer duration requires more prolonged therapy. Therapy is recommended for established cardiovascular syphilis. Antibiotics may not reverse the pathology associated with this disease, however.
   b. Penicillin-allergic patients: There are no published clinical data that adequately document the efficacy of drugs other than penicillin for syphilis of more than 1 year's duration. Cerebrospinal fluid examinations should be performed before therapy with these regimens.
      (1) Patients who are allergic to penicillin should be treated with: Tetracycline hydrochloride 500 mg by mouth 4 times a day for 30 days. Patient compliance with this regimen may be difficult so care should be taken to encourage optimal compliance.
      (2) Penicillin-allergic patients who cannot tolerate tetracycline should have their allergy confirmed. For these patients there are 2 options:

   (a) If compliance and serologic follow-up can be assured, administer erythromycin 500 mg by mouth 4 times a day for 30 days.
   (b) If compliance and serologic follow-up cannot be assured, the patient should be hospitalized and managed in consultation with an expert.
   Cerebrospinal fluid examination: Cerebrospinal fluid (CSF) examination should be done for patients with clinical symptoms or signs consistent with neurosyphilis. This examination is also desirable for other patients with syphilis of greater than 1 year's duration to exclude asymptomatic neurosyphilis.

3. Neurosyphilis: Published studies show that a total dose of 6.0 to 9.0 million units of penicillin G over a 3- to 4-week period results in a satisfactory clinical response in approximately 90 percent of patients with neurosyphilis. This information must be considered along with the observation that regimens employing benzathine penicillin or procaine penicillin in doses under 2.4 million units daily do not consistently provide treponemicidal levels of penicillin in CSF, and with the knowledge that several case reports show the failure of such regimens to cure neurosyphilis.
   a. Potentially effective drug regimens, none of which has been adequately studied, include: Aqueous crystalline penicillin G, 12 to 24 million units, intravenous, per day (2 to 4 million units every 4 hours) for 10 days, followed by benzathine penicillin G, 2.4 million units, intramuscular, weekly for 3 doses.
      OR
      Acqueous procaine penicillin G, 2.4 million units, intramuscular, daily plus probenecid 500 mg by mouth 4 times a day, both for 10 days, followed by benzathine penicillin G, 2.4 million units, intramuscular, weekly for 3 doses.
      OR
      Benzathine penicillin G, 2.4 million units, intramuscular, weekly for 3 doses.
   b. Penicillin-allergic patients: Patients with histories of allergy to penicillin should have their allergy confirmed and managed in consultation with an expert.
4. Syphilis in pregnancy (for evaluation of pregnant women, see text):
   a. For patients at all stages of pregnancy who are not allergic to penicillin, penicillin should be used in dosage schedules appropriate for the stage of syphilis as recommended for the treatment of nonpregnant patients.
   b. For patients at all stages of pregnancy who have documented allergy to penicillin:

---

acute syphilitic iritis. On the other hand, cephalothin penetrates very well. Antitreponemicidal antibiotics also penetrate poorly into noninflamed bone and cerebrospinal fluid. Late syphilis may have low levels of inflammation in bone, and penetration by penicillin can be expected to be marginal.

Cerebrospinal fluid levels following administration of benzathine penicillin are unreliable in infants [302] and adults [303,304] and are higher following aqueous or procaine penicillin [305]. In 12 or 13 adult patients receiving lumbar puncture for latent syphilis, penicillin levels were undetectable after each dose of 3.6 million units of benzathine penicillin once per week for 4 weeks [303]. In one

patient with asymptomatic neurosyphilis treated with 1.2 million units of benzathine penicillin intramuscularly 3 times weekly for 3 weeks, and a second patient with asymptomatic neurosyphilis treated with 10 days of tetracycline HCl 2 g per day and then with benzathine penicillin G 4.8 million units intramuscularly, *T. pallidum* was demonstrated when the CSF of each patient was inoculated into rabbits [306,307]. In 5 infants treated with a single intramuscular dose of 50,000 units per kilogram of benzathine penicillin G, peak serum levels of 0.38 to 2.1 μg/mL were observed at 24 h, serum concentrations of 0.07 to 0.09 μg/mL were measurable 12 days later, but penicillin activity was detectable in only 1 of 4 CSF samples at 24

Table 201-5 Syphilis: Centers for Disease Control recommended treatment schedules, 1982 (Continued)

(1) If compliance and serologic follow-up can be assured, administer erythromycin in dosage schedules appropriate for the stage of syphilis as recommended for the treatment of nonpregnant patients. Infants born to mothers treated during pregnancy with erythromycin for early syphilis should be treated with penicillin.

(2) If compliance and serologic follow-up cannot be assured, the patient should be hospitalized and managed in consultation with an expert. Tetracycline is not recommended in pregnant women because of potential adverse effects on the fetus.

c. Follow-up: Pregnant women who have been treated for syphilis should have monthly quantitative nontreponemal serologic tests for the remainder of the current pregnancy. Women who show a 4-fold rise in titer should be treated again. After delivery, follow-up is as outlined for nonpregnant patients.

5. Congenital syphilis (for evaluation of infants with suspected prenatal infection, see text): Infants should be treated at birth if maternal treatment for syphilis was inadequate, unknown, or with drugs other than penicillin, or if adequate follow-up of the infant cannot be assured. Infants with congenital syphilis should have a CSF examination before treatment.

a. Symptomatic infants or asymptomatic infants with abnormal cerebrospinal fluid: Aqueous crystalline penicillin G, 500,000 units/kg, intramuscular or intravenous, daily in 2 divided doses for a minimum of 10 days

OR

Aqueous procaine penicillin, 500,000 units/kg, intramuscular, daily for a minimum of 10 days.

b. Asymptomatic infants with a normal cerebrospinal fluid: Benzathine penicillin G, 50,000 units/kg, intramuscular, in a single dose. Although benzathine penicillin has been previously recommended and widely used, published clinical data on its efficacy in congenital neurosyphilis are lacking. If neurosyphilis cannot be excluded, the aqueous crystalline or procaine penicillin regimen is recommended. Only penicillin regimens are recommended for neonatal congenital syphilis. After the neonatal period, penicillin therapy for congenital syphilis should be with the same dosages used for neonatal congenital syphilis. For larger children, the total dose of penicillin need not exceed the dosage used in adult syphilis of more than 1 year's duration. After the neonatal period, the dosage of tetracycline for congenital syphilis in patients who are allergic to penicillin should be individualized but need

not exceed dosages used in adult syphilis of more than 1 year's duration. Tetracycline should not be given to children less than 8 years of age.

6. Follow-up after treatment and re-treatment:

a. All patients with early syphilis and congenital syphilis should be encouraged to return for repeat quantitative nontreponemal tests at least 3, 6, and 12 months after treatment. For these patients, quantitative nontreponemal tests will decline to nonreactive or to reactive with a low titer within a year following successful treatment with benzathine penicillin G. Titers decline more slowly with serologic tests for patients treated for disease of longer duration.

b. Patients with syphilis of more than 1 year's duration should also have a repeat serologic test 24 months after treatment.

c. Careful follow-up serologic testing is particularly important in patients treated with antibiotics other than penicillin. Examination of CSF should be planned as part of the last follow-up visit after treatment with alternative antibiotics.

d. All patients with neurosyphilis must be carefully followed for periodic serologic testing, clinical evaluation at 6-month intervals, and repeat CSF examinations for at least 3 years.

e. The possibility of reinfection should always be considered when patients with early syphilis need to be treated a second time. A CSF examination should be performed before re-treatment unless reinfection and a diagnosis of early syphilis can be established.

f. Re-treatment should be considered when:
  • Clinical signs or symptoms of syphilis persist or recur
  • There is a 4-fold increase in titer with a nontreponemal test
  • A nontreponemal test showing a high titer initially fails to show 4-fold decrease within a year

g. Patients who require re-treatment should be treated according to schedules recommended for syphilis of more than 1 year's duration. In general, a patient should be re-treated only once, since patients may maintain stable, low titers when nontreponemal tests are used or may have irreversible anatomic damage.

7. Epidemiologic treatment: Persons who have been exposed to infectious syphilis within the preceding 3 months and other persons who, on epidemiologic grounds, are at high risk for early syphilis should be treated as for early syphilis. Every effort should be made to determine whether such persons have syphilis.

Source: Centers for Disease Control [311].

to 48 h after therapy [302]. In an infant with early prenatal syphilis who died at age 22 days and whose mother received benzathine penicillin 2.4 million units 10 days before delivery, a nonmotile treponeme was found in the aqueous humor of the eye and the CSF; aqueous humor and eye tissue from this infant produced testicular lesions in rabbits due to a strain of *T. pallidum* that was penicillin-sensitive [308], suggesting inadequate penetration of penicillin into these protected sites. However, this child was also receiving medications which could have interfered with the action of penicillin, stressing the need to follow patients closely to determine response to therapy and the need for additional treatment.

Persisting treponemes have been found in other sites, particularly lymph nodes, arteries affected by temporal arteritis, bone [309], and perilymph of the middle ear [310]. Despite questions about the methodology of these observations, as well as the discovery of treponemal forms in tissues of patients with no evidence of syphilis, the large body of evidence suggests that spirochetes may persist (despite "adequate" antibiotic therapy) in some patients with treated syphilis, both early and late disease.

Treatment guidelines. The therapy of syphilis is based on empirical observations in humans combined with experimental evidence in animals when data in humans are lacking. The treatment schedules recommended by the Centers for Disease Control (USPHS) were updated in 1982 (previous updates were in 1968 and 1976) by an advisory committee on venereal disease control and are the culmination of available information and clinical experience [167,311–313] (Table 201-5).

The most striking feature of the new recommendations is the division of disease into early syphilis (primary, secondary, latent syphilis of less than 1 year's duration) and syphilis of more than 1 year's duration (latent syphilis of indeterminate or more than 1 year's duration, cardiovascular syphilis, late benign syphilis, or neurosyphilis). Penicillin continues to be the drug of choice for all stages of syphilis, and a history of drug allergy should be thoroughly investigated before choosing an alternative antibiotic.

EARLY SYPHILIS (PRIMARY, SECONDARY, LATENT SYPHILIS OF LESS THAN ONE YEAR'S DURATION) [314–316].

Penicillin. Benzathine penicillin G is the drug of choice for primary and secondary syphilis since it provides effective treatment in a single visit—a total of 2.4 million units by intramuscular injection at a single session. Cumulative re-treatment rates in clinical studies using this or a slightly different regimen range from 0 to 11.4 percent [317,318]; reinfection is not differentiated from relapse, and results are pooled for primary and secondary syphilis in one of the studies [317]. Other treatment results collected from multiple studies show that 97 percent of 1381 persons with seronegative primary syphilis were clinically well and serologically negative 2 to 10 years after therapy, with the 3 percent failures counted as reinfections [299].

Among 1030 persons with primary seroreactive syphilis, 93 to 100 percent became serologically nonreactive (as determined by lipoidal antigen tests) and most failures were considered to be reinfections [299]. Approximately 30 percent of this group remained positive to specific treponemal serologic testing after 9 years. Another study suggests that promptness of treatment leads to seroreversal: if treatment is given within 3 months of primary infection, rapid reversal occurs in most cases. If treatment is given more than 3 months after primary infection, even after 1 year the nontreponemal tests are still reactive in over 50 percent of patients [319]. In another study of seroreactive primary syphilis, 100 percent of 175 patients had resolution of lesions and seroreversal 1 year after intramuscular benzathine penicillin G 2.4 million units was given weekly for 2 weeks for a total of 4.8 million units [320]. In 165 patients with secondary syphilis treated with the same two-dose regimen separated by a week, all achieved seronegativity within 24 months; the duration for seroconversion to negative was directly proportional to the duration of the rash before therapy—76 percent of those whose rash was present for 1 to 4 weeks' duration were seronegative in 9 months in contrast to 16 percent of those whose rash was present for 5 weeks or longer (p < 0.001) [321]. In the same study, it was shown that patients with papular and pustular lesions took longer to convert serology to negative than did patients with macular or "maculopapular" lesions, and that the serologic response after tetracycline treatment was slower than that for benzathine penicillin. Excluded in this study were patients with a history of treated syphilis or patients who became reinfected; such patients with recurrent syphilis are thought to have a slower serologic response to treatment. Another study of

40 patients with secondary syphilis showed seroreversal in all cases within 24 months with a treatment schedule consisting of 6 million units of benzathine penicillin given over a 6- to 10-day period [322].

An alternative to benzathine penicillin is aqueous procaine penicillin G 4.8 million units total: 600,000 units by intramuscular injection daily for 8 days. In a study of 41 cases of primary and secondary syphilis treated with this regimen, cumulative re-treatment rates were 3.8 percent at 1 year and 10.7 percent at 2 years [317]. Other studies have shown similar results using higher total doses. Eighty-five patients were reexamined 28 to 36 years after varying treatment schedules during the period 1943–1950; persistent reactivity to the VDRL was present in none of 23 patients treated for primary syphilis, compared to 10 of 57 patients treated for secondary syphilis. Persistent reactivity to the FTA-ABS test and MHA-TP test was present in 20 of 23 and 9 of 23 patients, respectively, treated for primary syphilis, and in 57 of 57 and 49 of 57 patients, respectively, treated for secondary syphilis [255]. Aqueous penicillin G is probably effective, but the requirement for hospitalization and an every 2- to 4-h dosage schedule make this preparation impractical.

Other β-lactam antibiotics like nafcillin, dicloxacillin, oxacillin, methacillin, carbenicillin, and amoxicillin are very effective against *T. pallidum*. Cross-allergenicity to penicillin and the requirement of an every 3- to 6-h administration for adequate serum concentrations, however, make these drugs impractical for routine use.

Therapy for penicillin-allergic individuals. Tetracycline. The CDC recommends tetracycline hydrochloride 500 mg 4 times a day by mouth for 15 days for patients allergic to penicillin. In a combined study of primary and secondary syphilis in which patients were treated with 3 g per day of tetracycline HCl for 10 days, the cumulative re-treatment rates were 9.2 percent at 1 year, and 12.7 percent at 2 years [317]. Lower total doses were associated with higher re-treatment rates. Favorable results have been reported with a total dose of 34 g of chlortetracycline; reports of oxytetracycline are inconclusive [314]. In 21 patients with primary syphilis treated by Fiumara with 500 mg tetracycline HCl 4 times daily for 12 days, all achieved seronegativity within 12 months [320]. In 39 patients with secondary syphilis receiving tetracycline HCl 500 mg 4 times per day for 12 days (24 g), all patients were reported to be cured clinically and all achieved seronegativity within 24 months [321]. "Reinfections" and patients with recurrent syphilis were excluded from these studies.

Erythromycin. Erythromycin (stearate, ethylsuccinate, or base), 500 mg 4 times a day for 15 days may be used for early syphilis in patients with contraindications to penicillin or tetracycline [167,313]. Previous investigations studying erythromycin for primary and secondary disease have shown cumulative re-treatment rates of 10 to 20 percent at 1 and 2 years, respectively, but total doses were smaller than 30 g. In addition, most studies have used the estolate form of the drug which is now believed to be hepatotoxic in adults in the USPHS doses recommended. Although the base and stearate salts are the forms now recommended since they are not believed to be hepatotoxic, studies showing effectiveness at the recommended doses are lacking. There is some indication that 30 g total is more effective than 20 g total over 10 days for primary and secondary syphilis [314]. Further studies are required using the base and stearate forms of erythromycin for early syphilis. The erythromycin regimen is no longer listed as a recommended equally effective alternative to tetracycline for the treatment of nonpregnant patients allergic to penicillin and intolerant to tetracycline (see Table 201-5).

Cephalosporins. For primary syphilis, reports studying cephaloridine 500 to 1000 mg intramuscularly for 6 to 10 days (5 days out of 7 each week), cephalothin 1 g intramuscularly every 12 h for 20 days, and cephalexin 500 mg by mouth 4 times per day for 15 days showed a cumulative re-treatment rate of less than 10 percent [315]. Twenty-five patients with primary or secondary syphilis were treated with 1 g of cephalothin intramuscularly every 12 h for 20 days (primary syphilis) or 25 days (secondary syphilis), and no recurrences were noted at follow-up 6 months to 2 years later [323]. There are no studies of cephalosporins in treatment of latent disease, and the safety of these drugs in the penicillin-allergic individual has not been established. Cross-sensitivity exists in approximately 30 percent of patients allergic to penicillin, but only 10 to 14 percent will exhibit clinical signs and symptoms of allergy after exposure.

Other. Chloramphenicol has been studied with only small numbers of patients at varying doses and it probably has some benefit in primary syphilis, but its well-known bone marrow toxicity makes it a poor choice. Spectinomycin is ineffective in syphilis, both in humans [324] and animals [325]. Rifampin [326], clindamycin [327], kanamycin, and trimethoprim-sulfamethoxazole combination may even enhance growth of *T. pallidum* in BHK-21 cultured tissue cells in vitro [17]. A weak effect on *T. pallidum* has been demonstrated with streptomycin, polymyxin-B, bacitracin, novobiocin, griseofulvin, and the metronidazole derivatives. These drugs may suppress the development of clinical lesions and extend the period of latency but may not prevent the development of late disease.

Abortive treatment. Although never proved, it is believed that larger doses of medication are required for cure as syphilis progresses. This notion forms the basis of treating syphilis in the earliest stage possible, which is during the incubation period. It is therefore recommended that a history of exposure to syphilis, which may result in the development of syphilis in 5 to 20 percent of untreated cases within 3 months [10], requires treatment similar to early syphilis in order to interrupt transmission and progression of disease (abortive treatment). Patients being treated for gonorrhea with the currently recommended schedule of 4.8 million units of procaine penicillin G intramuscularly will abort incubating syphilis which may occur in as many as 3 percent of patients with gonorrhea [328]. The same treatment would be ineffective for established disease.

Latent syphilis. Latent syphilis is defined as that stage of acquired disease that is without clinical manifestations and without CSF evidence of neurosyphilis, and when the only evidence for disease is a positive blood serologic test. There is no substitute for an examination of the CSF in such cases, since neurosyphilis may remain asymptomatic for as long as 20 years [57,303]. Since the treatment of neurosyphilis is different from that in early latent disease, the common practice of not examining the CSF and then treating with 3 weekly injections of benzathine penicillin

2.4 million units may not provide adequate levels of penicillin in the CSF. The significance of this issue requires further investigation.

Although it is stated that "proper treatment during latency will prevent further progress of the disease in at least 95 to 98 percent of cases" [57], adequate data are unavailable to substantiate this claim. The natural progression of untreated syphilis is slow, and follow-up studies require at least 5 to 10 years in order to evaluate the effects of any treatment. The Tuskegee study of late latent syphilis clearly showed an increased mortality in those left untreated (see above); it is estimated that about 25 percent of untreated or inadequately treated individuals with latent syphilis progress to some symptomatic phase [57]. On the other hand, a review of therapeutic studies for latent syphilis confirms the difficulty of recommending a particular drug regimen for this stage of disease [316].

The recommendations for latent disease of less than 1 year's duration are the same as those for primary and secondary disease. Available therapeutic studies (using aqueous procaine penicillin G 600,000 units daily for 10 days, and benzathine penicillin G in several regimens and combinations) suggest that serologic titers will remain elevated in 11 to 45 percent and that there will be no progression to late disease after 1- to 5-year follow-up in most patients [316]. Treatment studies using other antibiotics are too few to allow for definite conclusions. Any therapy for latent disease, therefore, requires long-term follow-up of the patient.

Follow-up after treatment of early syphilis. If the CSF is negative after 2 years' observation of *untreated* latent syphilis, it is unlikely that it will ever become positive. Inadequate or irregular therapy may extend the 2-year period to 4 or 5 years [57]. Follow-up of the patient with early disease is mandatory in order to assess need for re-treatment, development of late disease, or reinfection. After termination of treatment for "early" syphilis, patients should be examined clinically and serologically at 3, 6, and 12 months after treatment and then at 6-month intervals until the end of 2 years, provided that the serologic response is satisfactory. In England, 1379 patients were followed and underwent spinal fluid examination at least 1 year after penicillin treatment for early syphilis, and all showed normal findings [329]. Of 231 patients treated with penicillin for early syphilis, only 3 had inconsequential spinal fluid abnormalities [147]. The examination of the CSF 1 year after primary and secondary syphilis is probably not necessary. For latent disease of less than 1 year's duration with an initial CSF examination negative, reexamination of the CSF is probably indicated at 3 to 5 years to determine possible progression. If the CSF becomes positive for active disease, treatment for neurosyphilis (described below) should be initiated. The serum FTA-ABS test may remain positive in one-third of patients treated for early seropositive syphilis, and there is no evidence to suggest that further treatment is indicated or that symptomatic syphilis will later develop in such patients.

SYPHILIS OF MORE THAN ONE YEAR'S DURATION, EXCEPT NEUROSYPHILIS (LATENT SYPHILIS OF INDETERMINATE OR MORE THAN ONE YEAR'S DURATION, CARDIOVASCULAR, AND LATE BENIGN SYPHILIS).

General recommendations. The recommendation for syphilis of more than 1 year's duration is benzathine penicillin G, 7.2 million units total: 2.4 million units by intramuscular injection weekly for 3 successive weeks. An alternative is aqueous procaine penicillin G, 9 million units total, 600,000 units by intramuscular injection daily for 15 days. For patients allergic to penicillin, one can use tetracycline HCl, 500 mg 4 times a day by mouth for 30 days. For penicillin-allergic patients in whom tetracycline cannot be used, erythromycin (stearate, ethylsuccinate or base) 500 mg 4 times a day by mouth for 30 days is a recommended alternative. Reported morbidity due to late manifestations of syphilis has decreased 88 percent in the last 30 years and appears to continue its decline, suggesting that treatment of early disease with modern-day antibiotics may prevent the onset of later complications [178].

Latent disease. If treatment of latent syphilis is commenced within 2 years of infection, serologic nonreactivity to nontreponemal tests may be expected eventually, as in early symptomatic syphilis of similar duration [330]. The regression of seroreactivity is slower with increasing duration of infection before treatment begins; if treatment is commenced after 4 years of latency, only 20 to 30 percent of diagnosed patients can be expected to achieve nontreponemal test nonreactivity 5 years after treatment, which is similar to spontaneous seroconversion in the natural disease [60]. The FTA-ABS and TPHA will usually remain positive.

The treatment of late latent syphilis (more than 2 years of syphilis infection) has only minimal documentation in the literature. Of a total of 469 patients followed for up to 12 years after treatment with various preparations of penicillin (predominantly procaine, total doses 5 to 15 million units intramuscularly), spinal fluids continued to be normal and no evidence of cardiovascular disease was reported. Serologic reagin nonreactivity resulted in 12 to 77 percent of the patients. Generally, the outcome was good with no progression for the follow-up periods reported for asymptomatic patients treated with adequate doses of penicillin [299]. The minimum dose and best preparation of penicillin for this stage of disease has not clearly been established. There is no documented basis for treatment recommendations for alternative antibiotics in latent syphilis [316].

Late benign syphilis [331]. The essential lesion of late benign syphilis is the gumma, which can occur anywhere, including the brain or other vital organs—the term *benign* is sometimes misleading. There are no controlled studies of penicillin therapy in any large series of patients with this stage of disease, but there are enough case reports to conclude that penicillin is safe, effective, and probably better than heavy metal therapy. The exact dose of penicillin to use is an open question, but since up to 25 percent of such patients will have cardiovascular or neurosyphilis, it is prudent to administer doses of penicillin that are curative for this stage. There is no documented basis for treatment recommendations for alternative antibiotics in late benign syphilis. Healing of the gumma is usually slow and may take several months, depending on extent of tissue destruction [299]. A gumma of the brain will require surgical therapy [116]. Approximately 93 percent of patients with treated late syphilis retain positive reactivity to the FTA-ABS test [178]. Moreover, in syphilis of more than 2 years' duration, an increasing proportion of patients never become reagin negative even after adequate therapy, but titers should be low or decreasing.

NEUROSYPHILIS. A sense of the overall effectiveness of penicillin in the treatment of neurosyphilis is provided by Rothenberg [332] in a review of a total 8706 reported cases—a favorable clinical outcome is the expectation for most patients treated with various preparations of penicillin and doses varying from 2 to 20 million units, with a maximum follow-up from 2 to 18 years. A minimum effective dose cannot be clearly derived from these studies and the effectiveness of penicillin for the various clinical states cannot be easily assessed [332]. Overall clinical results in combined studies are assessed for categories of illness: cure, improvement, or stabilization of disease occurred in 75 percent of patients with general paresis and taboparesis (48 percent cured); in 72 percent of patients with tabes dorsalis (47 percent cured); in 78 percent of patients with meningovascular disease and meningitis (81 percent cured); in 88 percent of patients with miscellaneous conditions (18 percent cured); and in 91 percent patients with asymptomatic disease.

Permanent damage may occur before treatment, in parenchymatous disease especially, and deterioration may occur despite arrest of active disease [333]. Normal pressure hydrocephalus should be excluded in such cases [133]. The tendency to re-treat is greatest in this situation and, according to Hahn et al, about half of those re-treated for clinical progression subsequently improved [334]. Clinical progression was ascribed to low-dose therapy. Re-treatment with massive doses of penicillin for "progression" has shown marked benefit in other reports as well [139,335]. The minimum dose of penicillin G recommended for neurosyphilis, 9 million units over a 3- to 4-week period, is consistent with the weight of evidence and experience described by Rothenberg [332]. The efficacy of benzathine penicillin G for neurosyphilis is less convincing, since available studies disagree on adequacy of response, the number of patients is small, and follow-up is short. A reasonable approach is to hospitalize patients with symptomatic neurosyphilis—especially if initial therapy has failed—and to treat with 12 to 24 million units of aqueous crystalline penicillin G given intravenously each day (2 to 4 million units every 4 h) for 10 days, followed by intramuscular benzathine penicillin G, 2.4 million units, weekly for 3 doses. In a comparison of penicillin vs. metal chemotherapy in more than 1000 patients, Hahn et al have shown that progression had practically ceased after the third year of observation following penicillin therapy but continued after metal therapy [336]. Although malaria fever therapy, alone or combined with metals or penicillin, is out of favor, there is evidence that penicillin penetrates the blood–brain barrier more readily in patients with artificially induced fever. Corticosteroids may be useful in particular cases of neurosyphilis—those with gastric crises and lightning pains of tabes dorsalis.

Alternatives to penicillin include tetracycline, erythromycin (30 to 60 g total), and chloramphenicol. Currently recommended doses for alternatives are based largely on the experience of workers in the field, since adequate drug trials for the minimum effective doses do not exist.

Special problems in the treatment of neurosyphilis include optic atrophy (alone or in conjunction with tabes dorsalis) and VIIIth nerve deafness, both of which are notoriously resistant to treatment. No case of blindness due to optic atrophy was reversible with penicillin, although lack of progression or improvement occurred in 3 to 60 percent with doses of penicillin ranging from 2.0 to

18 million units. Eighth nerve deafness appears to benefit from the combination of penicillin and prednisone, but adequate controlled studies are not available for substantiation (see above).

The Jarisch-Herxheimer reaction in neurosyphilis may be manifested by the appearance of new symptoms, occasionally devastating, with a frequency of 30 per 1086 patients treated and death in 1 patient [334]. Although it has been suggested that steroids be used to "cover" this event, documentation is lacking (see below).

CARDIOVASCULAR SYPHILIS [337]. The optimal dosage, duration, and preparation of penicillin have never been fully evaluated for cardiovascular syphilis, but current recommendations are comparable to the regimens used by early investigators and are judged to be adequate. The preparations used in older studies were chiefly short-acting penicillins, 4 to 11 million units over 1 to 2 weeks or more.

Several problems make assessment of treatment of cardiovascular syphilis difficult. Uncomplicated syphilitic aortitis is usually asymptomatic, difficult to diagnose, and variable in clinical course, and therefore has resisted conclusive evaluation of the effects of treatment. Advanced symptomatic disease—aortic regurgitation, coronary ostial compromise, clinical aneurysm—was associated with poor prognosis no matter what the treatment. In past studies, most symptomatic patients were treated with other measures as well, and the individual effect of penicillin was difficult to evaluate. In the only controlled study of antisyphilitic therapy for cardiovascular involvement in the prepenicillin era [338], 63 patients were adequately studied and followed after treatment or no treatment: there was no difference in the average duration of disease or mortality in the two groups. In the penicillin era, there is suggestive evidence that penicillin had a beneficial effect in the majority of patients in one series [339], although treatment usually included digitalis, bed rest, and diuretics as well. Subjective improvement, reduction in diastolic murmur, and safety of penicillin were the most impressive findings. Another study with follow-up from 6 months to 5 years and well-defined criteria for cardiovascular involvement, found relatively good results with penicillin treatment—asymptomatic patients remained well, with no change in status of aortic insufficiency and no difference between regimens using less than or more than 6 million units of penicillin. In patients with aortic insufficiency, aneurysm, or both, treated with 6 to 11.2 million units of penicillin and followed 6 to 72 months, 62.6 percent had symptomatic improvement, with progression in 4 percent of asymptomatic and 4.5 percent of symptomatic patients. There was a higher mortality in the symptomatic group (32.8 percent) vs. the mildly symptomatic (12.8 percent) [340].

During the prepenicillin era, a relative aggravation of symptoms in patients with cardiovascular syphilis often followed therapy—"therapeutic shock" or "therapeutic paradox." This phenomenon has been attributed to the toxic spirocheticidal agents used and not simply to the Jarisch-Herxheimer reaction [339]. In the penicillin era, it is believed that therapeutic paradox and shock do not occur to any significant extent [337].

Once the patient has become symptomatic, penicillin may have little efficacy, but because of the low cost and lack of toxicity it is recommended (in hopes of arresting the disease) for all patients with cardiovascular syphilis despite the insufficient number of adequately controlled studies. The use of benzathine penicillin or other antibiotics in cardiovascular syphilis is impossible to evaluate because adequate trials are yet to be performed.

SYPHILIS IN PREGNANCY [341]. *Evaluation.* All pregnant women should have a nontreponemal serologic test for syphilis, such as the VDRL or RPR, at the first prenatal visit. For women suspected of being at high risk for syphilis, a second nontreponemal test should be done during the third trimester, and cord blood should be tested similarly. Seroreactive patients should have a quantitative nontreponemal test and a confirmatory treponemal test. If the FTA-ABS is nonreactive and there is no clinical evidence of syphilis, antibiotic therapy may be withheld. However, a quantitative nontreponemal test and a confirmatory treponemal test should be repeated in 4 weeks.

If there is clinical or serologic evidence of syphilis in the pregnant woman, or if syphilis cannot be excluded with certainty, the patient should be treated. Those patients adequately treated in the past need not be re-treated unless there is clinical or serologic evidence of reinfection or relapse, such as dark-field–positive lesions or a 4-fold titer rise of a quantitative nontreponemal test, since the risk of bearing a syphilitic child in subsequent pregnancies is quite small once the patient has had adequate treatment. If the reaginic serology during a subsequent pregnancy is negative and adequate treatment has been given for documented syphilis in the past, the patient does not require re-treatment. If doubt exists, re-treatment is warranted since the potential benefits outweigh the possible risks. The zeal to treat syphilis during pregnancy must be tempered with the knowledge that false-positive reaginic tests are not uncommon in this situation—all positive reaginic tests must be confirmed by specific tests for antitreponemal antibody, including selective IgM tests, if available (see "Serology of Syphilis").

If the pregnant patient receives the currently recommended doses of penicillin prior to or during the first 4 months of pregnancy, the risk of syphilis in the infant is minimal. If therapy is initiated during the latter half of pregnancy, the risk is 1 to 2 percent for the infant. Risk of relapse in the mother is not known. There are no available data for treatment of late syphilis, congenital syphilis, or latent syphilis in pregnancy.

Penicillin for syphilis during pregnancy. The CDC recommendations at all stages of pregnancy for patients not allergic to penicillin are the same dosage schedules appropriate for stages of syphilis recommended in nonpregnant patients. The only potential serious side effect is the Jarisch-Herxheimer reaction, which may precipitate premature labor ("placental shock") [342]; but this phenomenon of associated spontaneous abortion is debatable, and should not delay treatment of maternal syphilis with anything less than full doses of penicillin.

Penicillin readily permeates the placenta, even as early as the tenth week of gestation and throughout the remainder of pregnancy. Benzathine penicillin, aqueous penicillin G, and procaine penicillin G are freely diffusible and produce high fetal blood levels 60 to 90 min after injection, with a peak concentration 25 to 30 percent (rarely 75 percent) of the maternal serum level.

Despite the introduction of penicillin and the reported decrease in prenatal syphilis in the mid-1940s, this form of syphilis has continued to occur for the following reasons:

(1) the clinician often fails to recognize syphilis when it occurs late in pregnancy—in one-third of cases of prenatal syphilis, the mother was seronegative in early pregnancy and seropositive at delivery; and (2) mothers of syphilitic infants often delay in seeking treatment—in 25 percent of the patients, treatment was started at the time of delivery, and in 75 percent no therapy was received prior to conception, and only a few received therapy before the fifth month [342].

There is an unconfirmed conviction that the fetus may easily be cured by the same doses of penicillin that may not be effective for the mother. Documentation of this concept is lacking. However, peak serum ampicillin levels after oral administration are lower during pregnancy vs. the nonpregnant state. Since there is an increased penicillin level in the amniotic fluid compared to maternal serum, this effect is thought not to be dilutional but more likely related to a "third space" phenomenon. A hormonal effect is also possible. There is also a suggestion that any stage of syphilis in pregnant women is more difficult to cure than in nonpregnant women; using therapy with more than 2.4 million units vs. 2.4 million units of penicillin, there is an apparent trend for a better outcome [341].

The prognosis of infants born to syphilitic mothers treated during pregnancy is encouraging: in 414 pregnant women with early syphilis, treated with varying amounts of penicillin (600,000 to 10 million units), there were only 5.3 percent syphilitic children born (11 out of 392 live births) and a "normal" rate of stillbirths. The failures were observed in women treated late in pregnancy and during relapses of reinfection [343].

Erythromycin for syphilis during pregnancy. In patients allergic to penicillin, erythromycin (stearate, ethylsuccinate, or base) is recommended in doses dependent on the stage of syphilis. Erythromycin, however, may not be the *ideal* drug for the pregnant patient. Its ability to cross the placenta is fair to poor, with various studies reporting fetal levels 6 to 20 percent of maternal blood levels after multiple oral doses of various erythromycin preparations (estolate, stearate, base, and ethylsuccinate) [344,345]. One study detected no drug in cord blood after 2 h if a single dose was less than 800 mg of base [346]. Another study, on the other hand, showed that if therapeutically effective amounts are present in the mother's serum, erythromycin *does* cross the placenta in amounts considered adequate [347]. The base has more antibiotic activity than the other forms on a weight-for-weight basis [348], the preparations are variably susceptible to gastric degradation (the base the most, the estolate the least susceptible), and food in the stomach reduces the absorption of the stearate but not that of the estolate [349]. The minimum 30-g dose recommended may be hepatotoxic to pregnant women if the estolate preparation is used—9.6 percent of 167 women developed an elevated SGOT without other symptoms during a 6-week treatment period in the latter half of pregnancy, and all tests returned to normal after therapy was discontinued. A syndrome characterized by cholestatic jaundice, abdominal pain, and acholic stools may complicate the course of therapy of the estolate form, even one tablet in a sensitized patient [350]. Gastrointestinal side effects (nausea, vomiting, cramps, and diarrhea) may occur at a rate of 2 to 50 percent, occurring more with the stearate and less with the estolate preparation. These side effects are less, and blood levels higher, with enteric-coated prep-

arations of erythromycin. Fetal teratogenicity with erythromycin does not appear to be a hazard [351].

Efficacy of erythromycin in the pregnant patient has not been as well documented as for penicillin. Success rates, stated to be 90 percent in curing early or latent syphilis in the nonpregnant patient, appear to be lower in doses less than 30 g, but adequate data are unavailable for clear assessment. Because the estolate is more toxic and the base is irregularly absorbed (unless an enteric-coated preparation is used), the stearate is the preferred form. Infants born to mothers treated with erythromycin for syphilis during pregnancy should be thoroughly evaluated for active disease, treated with penicillin at recommended doses, and followed carefully [352].

Other antibiotics. Tetracycline is well absorbed into the fetal circulation and may even be more effective for syphilis in pregnancy than erythromycin, although adequate data do not exist. Its reported fatal toxicity—progressive azotemia, fatty liver, pancreatitis, and lactic acidosis probably related to intravenous administration in pregnant patients with abnormal renal function—and dental side effects in children when it is used between the fourth month of pregnancy and age 8 (dental fluorescence and staining in deciduous teeth, but probably no relationship to dental hypoplasia or caries in deciduous or permanent teeth) discourage the use of tetracyclines for syphilitic infections in pregnant women. It should be noted, however, that dental side effects are related to the time of usage—formation of deciduous teeth begins at 4 months in utero and the enamel is completed by 10 months postpartum, while formation of permanent teeth begins at 3 to 4 months postpartum and is complete by 5 to 6 years of age [353]. Therefore, discoloration would affect deciduous teeth but not permanent teeth if tetracycline were used during pregnancy.

Cephalosporins are potentially valuable agents in the treatment of syphilis during pregnancy, since placental transfer and treponemicidal fetal blood levels are easily achieved; the compounds appear to be safe in the pregnant patient, and they have been demonstrated to be effective in anecdotal examples in the literature. Theoretical and actual cross-allergenicity to penicillin exists, however, and until more data are available on toxicity, effectiveness, and cross-allergenicity to penicillin, cephalosporins cannot be recommended as routine alternative therapy.

PRENATAL SYPHILIS. Penicillin is the drug of choice for prenatal syphilis, but most of the major trials were conducted in the early penicillin era and employed aqueous penicillin given in intramuscular doses at 3-h intervals. Long-acting parenteral penicillins are less well documented.

An adequate level of penicillin in the treatment of syphilis requires maintenance of serum levels greater than 0.03 units per milliliter for 7 to 10 days [298,299], and the minimum dose of penicillin required to maintain such a level in an infant is aqueous penicillin 50,000 units per kilogram per 24 h in two divided doses, procaine penicillin 50,000 units per kilogram once per day, or benzathine penicillin 50,000 units per kilogram given as a single injection. The duration and type of therapy, however, is dependent on CNS involvement, since benzathine penicillin does not reliably cross the blood–brain barrier. Treatment recommendations, therefore, divide prenatal syphilis according to the results of examination of cerebrospinal fluid: (1) infants with abnormal cerebrospinal fluid require aqueous crystalline penicillin G 50,000 units per kilogram intramuscularly or intravenously daily in two divided doses or aqueous procaine penicillin G 50,000 units per kilogram intramuscularly daily, each for a minimum of 10 days; (2) infants with normal cerebrospinal fluid require only a single intramuscular injection of benzathine penicillin G, 50,000 units per kilogram. Penicillin therapy for prenatal syphilis after the neonatal period should be administered with the same dosages used for early prenatal syphilis. The total dose of penicillin need not exceed the dosage used in adult syphilis of more than 1 year's duration.

Clinically manifest neurologic involvement occurs in 5 to 20 percent of infants with prenatal syphilis [159], but as many as 72 percent may have abnormalities of the cerebrospinal fluid [354]. A satisfactory response in patients with clinical or CSF evidence of neurologic disease occurs in 47 percent followed for 6 months compared to 94 percent of infants without neurologic involvement after treatment with 100,000 units per kilogram of aqueous penicillin [355]. A better response with the same therapy was achieved in another study, all patients having a satisfactory outcome after follow-up for 4 years [356].

There is only one large treatment study of late prenatal syphilis—109 patients treated with 20,000 to 200,000 units per kilogram of aqueous penicillin—and 80 percent were judged to have a satisfactory response, while in only 3 did the disease relapse or progress, with no differences between the high vs. lower dose groups [357]. Interstitial keratitis, occurring in 5 to 9 percent of late prenatal syphilis may be benefitted by topical corticosteroids. Eighth nerve deafness occurs in 2 to 3 percent of late prenatal syphilis and may respond to systemic corticosteroids. Neither of these conditions is related to active infection, and progression may occur despite adequate penicillin therapy.

There are no adequate data for the treatment of prenatal syphilis with antibiotics other than penicillin. Erythromycin may be effective in an oral dose of 30 to 50 mg/kg per day for 15 days. The toxicity of tetracycline for bone and teeth, the cross-allergenicity with penicillin of cephalosporins, and the bone marrow toxicity of chloramphenicol preclude the use of these agents in infancy and early childhood. For children allergic to penicillin and older than 8 years, tetracycline in an oral dose of 30 to 40 mg/kg per day (not to exceed 2 g per day) for 15 days in early disease and 30 days in late disease may be effective.

Careful long-term follow-up and examination must be arranged for patients with prenatal syphilis, especially those with neurologic involvement or those treated with nonpenicillin drugs. In the asymptomatic infant whose mother received adequate therapy during pregnancy, the risk to the child is minimal, but the infant should be followed at frequent intervals until nontreponemal tests are negative. Infants should be treated at birth if maternal treatment was inadequate, unknown, with drugs other than penicillin, or if adequate follow-up of the infant is not assured. Infected infants are frequently asymptomatic at birth and may be seronegative if the maternal infection occurred late in gestation, so the importance of frequent follow-up and examination in such cases cannot be emphasized too strongly.

Follow-up and re-treatment [311]. All patients with syphilis of less than 1 year's duration or prenatal syphilis require repeat quantitative nontreponemal tests at 3, 6, and 12 months after treatment. Patients with syphilis of more than 1 year's duration should have repeat serologic tests for at least 24 months after treatment. Patients treated with antibiotics other than penicillin require an examination of spinal fluid as part of a last follow-up visit.

All patients with symptomatic neurosyphilis must have careful serologic testing for at least 3 years, with clinical reevaluation at 6-month intervals and repeat cerebrospinal fluid examinations yearly until normal. Routine follow-up of spinal fluid in asymptomatic neurosyphilis is more controversial, since the risk of progression to symptoms after a patient has received "adequate" therapy is slight [336].

If re-treatment of a patient is indicated because of a lack of expected fall in serologic titers, reinfection should be considered. If reinfection cannot be established with certainty, examination of spinal fluid should be performed before re-treatment. Re-treatment should be considered when clinical signs or symptoms of syphilis persist or recur, when there is a 4-fold increase in the titer of a nontreponemal test, or when an initially high-titer nontreponemal test fails to show a 4-fold decrease within a year. Re-treatment should be given with schedules recommended for syphilis of more than 1 year's duration. Only one re-treatment course is indicated, in general, since patients may have stable, low titers of nontreponemal tests or irreversible anatomic damage, especially patients with syphilis of more than 1 year's duration. The prognosis of low-titer serofast syphilis does not appear to be affected by prolonged or repeated doses of penicillin [358]. Patients previously diagnosed with syphilis and treated with metal therapy but not penicillin or another antibiotic adequate for syphilis should have an examination of the CSF and be adequately treated unless advanced age or other medical problems make this approach inadvisable.

Complications of therapy. JARISCH-HERXHEIMER (J-H) REACTION [359,360]. The original description by Jarisch (1895) and Herxheimer and Kraus (1902) focused on the apparent flare of mucocutaneous lesions in early syphilis after initiating treatment with mercury. Systemic symptoms and signs were also noted, however, and included fever, headache, pharyngitis, malaise, myalgias, and leukocytosis with lymphopenia. The reaction has subsequently been described after treatment with arsenic, bismuth, penicillin, and immune serum, as well as other antibiotics. The reaction is no less severe in patients treated with bismuth-arsphenamine drugs than with penicillin. Provided the treponemicidal effects reach a critical level, the J-H reaction appears to be an all or none phenomenon. The reaction may occur with subsequent treatment if initial therapy was inadequate to render lesions treponeme free, with the second reaction having characteristics similar to the first. Prognosis after treatment is unrelated to presence or absence of the reaction both in early and late disease.

The J-H reaction occurs after treatment with a frequency of 55 percent in seronegative and 95 percent in seropositive primary syphilis. In secondary syphilis, the reaction occurs with a frequency similar to seropositive primary disease. The onset of the febrile reaction in early syphilis (no difference between primary and secondary disease) begins within 12 h of therapy; peak temperature occurs 6 to 10 h after therapy, persists 8 to 10 h, and resolves usually within 18 to 24 h. Approximately 88 percent of patients have a peak temperature of 39°C (102.2°F) or less, but fever at times reaches 42°C (107.6°F) or higher. Other manifestations of the J-H reaction occurring with or independent of the febrile reaction are worsening of preexisting skin lesions, lymphadenopathy, or recognition of previously inapparent cutaneous lesions. Focal or cutaneous manifestations have occurred in 11 percent of treated early syphilis, and in almost half of those with the febrile reaction. The J-H reaction in early syphilis is of no consequence except to confirm the presence of syphilitic infection in the treated patient. Patient education about the reaction and simple analgesics for symptoms are the only precautions and treatment required.

The frequency of the J-H reaction decreases in late secondary syphilis and is usually not found in latent syphilis. In neurosyphilis, 53 to 95 percent with paresis, 9 to 23 percent with tabes, and 12 to 36 percent with other types of neurosyphilis have developed fever after treatment with penicillin. Febrile reactions are more likely when pretreatment CSF contains increased numbers of cells, protein, or a reactive serologic test for syphilis. New clinical signs, including convulsions, worsened dementia, psychosis, and meningismus have occurred in about 2 percent of persons with neurosyphilis treated with penicillin. Death during such a reaction is uncommon, occurring once among 1086 paretic patients [334]. Convulsions probably can be managed with anticonvulsants. The occurrence of J-H reactions in cardiovascular syphilis is difficult to document. In prenatal syphilis, about half of those with early and 39 percent of those with late disease develop febrile reactions. The early mortality rate of 6 to 12 percent for early prenatal syphilis is felt to reflect the poor health of such children and not the effect of the J-H reaction. The rate of the J-H reaction is difficult to document for syphilis in pregnancy, and "placental" reactions associated with the febrile response to penicillin are often blamed for premature delivery and threatened or spontaneous abortion. These unfortunate events may be due to the disease itself, other associated risk factors, or the systemic reaction to penicillin. The theoretical possibility of a placental reaction should not delay treatment of the pregnant woman with syphilis infection.

Other reported associations with the J-H reaction include the elevation of liver function tests in a case of secondary syphilis with hepatitis [361] and the development (and subsequent resolution) of the nephrotic syndrome in a patient with early syphilis [362]. The histologic changes in the syphilitic lesions, which subside within 18 h, may be a more sensitive indicator of the J-H reaction, especially in the undetectable forms of the reaction. Acute inflammatory changes in both humans and rabbits occur within 4 to 6 h after the beginning of treatment and consist of dilatation of the small dermal vessels followed by endothelial swelling and migration of leukocytes through the vessel walls into the surrounding edematous tissue. Pooled immune serum given to syphilitic rabbits produced histologic changes of the J-H reaction identical to those associated with arsenical or penicillin therapy [363].

Although the J-H reaction has been variously attributed to the release of endogenous pyrogens by the treponemal endotoxin, direct vasotoxicity due to metal therapy, or cell-mediated phenomena, the exact cause of the reaction is unknown. It seems unlikely that plasma kinins play a major role in the pathogenesis since no changes in concentration could be demonstrated during the treatment of patients with early syphilis [364]. Activation of the complement system probably does not play a role in the J-H reaction [365]. Systemic steroids may modify the febrile reaction, but the intensification of syphilitic skin lesions or the characteristic peripheral blood leukocyte patterns seem not to be affected. The effect of corticosteroids on the CNS or cardiovascular lesions during penicillin treatment are unknown, but a 2-day course may be reasonable in patients in whom a local flare of disease could result in permanent physiologic impairment.

Therapeutic paradox, distinguished from the J-H reaction, is defined as a worsening of disease after antisyphilitic therapy, resulting from excessive scarring produced by too rapid destruction of treponemes [359]. It is almost impossible, however, to separate the effects of syphilitic infection and the effects of therapy on particular organ impairment. The problem is most notable in patients with aortic disease, in whom mechanical impairment will lead to aortic incompetence. Although several cases exist in the literature of worsening of the aortic insufficiency murmur 6 to 18 months after penicillin therapy, the problem does not appear to be common and cannot be distinguished from the basic disease process. The theoretical possibility of therapeutic paradox should not prevent adequate therapy for well-documented cardiovascular syphilis.

PENICILLIN REACTIONS. Patients treated with penicillin must be detained for observation for at least 30 min in order to manage a possible life-threatening anaphylaxis. The time interval between drug administration and onset of symptoms for acute anaphylaxis usually begins within seconds. Epinephrine, oxygen, antihistamines, proper equipment, and personnel trained in cardiopulmonary resuscitation must, therefore, be immediately available to persons administering penicillin. The time interval between drug administration and death in one study of six patients dying of acute anaphylaxis varied from 16 min to 2 h [366]. The characteristics of this reaction are vascular collapse with shock, bronchial obstruction and laryngeal edema with wheezing and hypoxemia, and gastrointestinal disturbances including diarrhea. The cutaneous manifestations are urticaria, localized angioedema, and generalized flushing or pruritus [367].

There are at least 20 different adverse reactions to penicillin, not all of which are allergic, but the allergic reactions are the most serious [368]. In a 1969 national survey in the United States of 27,673 patients treated with penicillin in venereal disease clinics, reactions were reported in 183, or 6.61:1000 patients treated, a rate not differing from surveys in 1954, 1959, and 1964 [369]. Of 36,048 patients interviewed, 6.6 percent gave a history of sensitivity to penicillin. Seventy-eight patients who gave a history of penicillin allergy were given penicillin therapy and 10 experienced a reaction, for a rate of 128.2:1000 treated, markedly higher than the overall rate. Even in the absence of a history of penicillin allergy, a reaction rate was observed in 6.22:1000 patients treated. The most common reactions were urticaria (66 patients), serum sickness (3 patients), and "maculopapular" eruptions (17 patients). Anaphylaxis occurred in 11 patients (0.4:1000 patients treated) and was classified as moderate to severe in half these patients; most had previously received penicillin without incident. During the period of the four surveys (1954–1969), only one death occurred among 94,655 patients treated with penicillin, for a fatality rate of 0.001 percent. This study is in agreement with other studies which show the frequency of penicillin reactions to vary between 0.3 to 1.0 percent and the occurrence of severe anaphylactic reactions to range from 0.001 to 0.04 percent, with a fatality rate of 0.0014 percent [370]. In addition, there is no evidence that the incidence of penicillin reactions in venereal disease clinics is increasing—in fact, there has been a trend of decreasing numbers [369].

Another penicillin-associated reaction, the pseudoanaphylactic reaction, is associated with intramuscular procaine penicillin and has been reported predominantly in the treatment of gonorrhea [371–374]. It occurs at a rate of 13/10,479 or approximately 1 per 1000 treatments (0.1 percent, reports ranging from 0.1 to 0.8 percent), is more common in males, and probably occurs in all races [374] despite previous suggestions of predominance in blacks. The reaction is characterized by auditory or visual disturbances, unusual tastes, fears of imminent death, violent combativeness, neuromuscular twitching, and, occasionally, grand mal seizures. Blood pressure is usually elevated, tachycardia is common, the reaction lasts usually no more than 30 min, and treatment includes simply "staying with the patient" or administration of sedatives or anticonvulsants. The mechanism of this reaction is thought to be related to inadvertent intravenous administration of procaine penicillin during intramuscular injection, with the procaine portion of the medication primarily responsible for the toxic reaction. The appearance of procaine in CSF of dogs is rapid after intravenous compared with intramuscular injection. In addition, plasma procaine esterase activity of patients who had experienced systemic toxic reactions was significantly decreased as compared to that of controls [373]. The signs and symptoms are probably related to cortical stimulation by procaine which may occur in an amount no less than 1024 mg per 2.4 megaunits of aqueous procaine penicillin G. As little as 10 mg of procaine administered intravenously has been associated with sudden death.

Epidemiologic considerations [375]. Distinctions must be made among prophylactic, abortive, and epidemiologic treatment of syphilis. Less than therapeutic amounts of penicillin will prevent syphilis and this is called *prophylactic treatment*. Antibiotics administered after exposure but before signs, symptoms, or laboratory evidence of disease is called *abortive treatment*. Patients without signs or symptoms and with a history of contact with syphilis fall into this category. *Epidemiologic treatment* refers to a situation in which antibiotics are given to a patient with signs or symptoms of syphilis but in whom a specific diagnosis cannot be confirmed. Treatment in such a situation can be justified in a pregnant woman in whom serologic findings and history of adequate posttreatment are equivocal, in a clinically normal child born of a syphilitic mother in whom active infection cannot be confirmed or refuted based on laboratory tests, and in a sexually active individual with characteristic signs and symptoms (but not a definite diagnosis) of syphilis in whom adequate follow-up and sexual abstinence cannot be ensured. The prognosis of the unborn child in a syphilitic mother is adversely affected by the

duration of infection; awaiting confirmatory serial VDRL titers or the development of clinical lesions exposes the neonate to severe sequelae; and allowing infectious syphilis to go untreated in a sexually active adult places the community at risk. Epidemiologic treatment has a place in the management of suspected syphilis, although a confirmed diagnosis is optimal for total patient care and contact tracing.

A person exposed to infectious syphilis (primary or secondary) within the previous 30 to 90 days, has a 10 to 62 percent chance of developing syphilis [328,376–379]. The longer the patient remains asymptomatic, the less likely is the possibility of infection. The probability of developing syphilis 48 days after a single contact with an infected person was 16 percent in one study [378]. These figures are confounded by the social milieu of the individual—infection is more likely in a high-risk group and may not be related to the named contact. This risk may approach 20 percent in selected groups associated with infected persons. The benefits of treatment and risks of suspected incubating syphilis must be weighed for each individual and considered in the context of his or her social setting before epidemiologic treatment is given.

For every patient with diagnosed syphilis, there is another person with apparent or inapparent syphilis infection—every attempt must be made to identify the source. Nurse epidemiologists specifically trained in the art of contact interviewing should be utilized to assist in this delicate and time-consuming task. Multiple interviews and many hours working with a patient are often required for complete information. This task should not be assumed lightly by a busy practicing physician. For primary syphilis, the sexual exposures to be investigated in contact tracing must include the duration of the patient's primary chancre plus the 3-month maximum incubation period. For secondary syphilis, the duration of secondary symptoms plus the 6-month maximum incubation period is required. For early latent syphilis, sexual exposures for the previous 2 years must be included unless a nonreactive serologic test for syphilis during that period can be documented. For late latent syphilis, even though infection can probably not be sexually transmitted 2 years after the infection, contact investigation of the family members is indicated to exclude syphilis in a spouse or children.

The goals of contact interview are case finding and case prevention. Each contact must be located and motivated to seek medical evaluation. If an exposure cannot be documented or confirmed in a patient claiming syphilis contact, then the patient is examined and an STS is checked every month for a maximum of 3 months from the last exposure to the contact. A nonreactive STS at the end of 3 months (the maximum incubation period for primary syphilis) is an indication for discharge from follow-up. If a documented exposure has occurred within the past 3 months, treatment is provided even if examination and STS are negative. If exposure has occurred more than 3 months before an examination, treatment is withheld pending the results of the STS.

Nonvenereal treponematoses

Nonvenereal syphilis, yaws, and pinta have been called the "endemic" treponematoses to distinguish them from venereal syphilis. The use of the term *endemic* as a distinguishing factor is not valid, however, when one considers that venereal syphilis has been an endemic disease in many parts of the world for as long as accurate incidence data have been available. *Nonvenereal treponematoses,* therefore, will be the term used to characterize the diseases discussed in this section.

The nonvenereal treponematoses (nonvenereal syphilis, yaws, and pinta) are transmitted via direct and indirect contact among children in groups living under social, economic, and hygienic deprivation. The clinical course usually progresses from primary to secondary eruptions, and then to late manifestations. Cardiovascular, central nervous system, and prenatal involvement are usually not observed in nonvenereal treponematoses, but rare exceptions have been reported [380].

Although the causative organisms of the nonvenereal treponematoses are morphologically identical, variations in their ability to produce infection in various species of experimental animals and subtle differences in immunologic response of experimental infection provide evidence that there are indeed differences among *Treponema pallidum, T. pertenue,* and *T. carateum.* Incomplete cross-immunity as demonstrated in experimental subjects and superinfection immunity studies in rabbits lend support to the differences [381]. Dissimilarities in clinical expression for venereal syphilis and the nonvenereal treponematoses have been attributed to variations or minor mutations of treponeme species as well as host immunity and environment, but supporting experimental evidence is scanty.

Of the treponematoses affecting humans, nonvenereal syphilis is encountered largely in dry areas, while yaws and pinta are diseases of the tropical belt. Pinta and yaws are spread by direct skin-to-skin contact through exuberant infectious skin lesions that flourish on moist, sweaty skins in tropical climates. Insect vectors, trauma, and absence of clothing are probably important factors in transmission. Nonvenereal syphilis, occurring in the dry desert regions and in areas where the affected populations wear clothing, is transmitted mostly via the mucous membrane route and less by skin-to-skin contact [382].

As a result of mass-treatment campaigns during the past 30 years, the younger generation is no longer protected against venereal syphilis via cross-immunity conferred by infection with the nonvenereal treponematoses. Venereal syphilis is now being observed in urban and rural areas of developing countries where it was not noted 35 years ago [383]. In addition, because of the continued low prevalence rate of nonvenereal treponematoses in developing countries and the persisting local problems of poverty and poor social hygiene, the threat of recrudescence of these diseases is ever present. Although tools of diagnosis and mass treatment with penicillin have made eradication possible, the inability of developing countries to support the necessary public health measures may permit these diseases to continue.

Nonvenereal ("endemic") syphilis (bejel, njovera, dichuchwa, frenjak, sibbens, button scurvy, radesyge) [384,385]

The multitude of local names for this disease demonstrates that a common origin was not recognized until the middle of the twentieth century. The disease still exists in Central and South Africa, the Middle East, Lower Mongolia, and Tibet. Foci of nonvenereal syphilis with a prevalence rate as high as 4 percent were present in Europe in Yugoslavia (Bosnia) even after World War II, but have since been eradicated through WHO–UNICEF-sponsored mass-treatment campaigns more than 30 years ago [382]. Small foci of nonvenereal syphilis were described in big cities of Europe and the United States after World War II and during the 1960s, usually ascribed to crowded conditions. The sources of infection in such outbreaks were usually communicable lesions in venereally infected adults [385]. The causative organism is the same as for venereal syphilis, but socioeconomic pressures affect the mode of transmission and age of infection, and these, in turn, modify the disease state. When the opportunity arises, nonvenereal syphilis can cause the venereal form of disease. Available laboratory evidence supports these notions, that one organism may be responsible for both forms of disease, although strains isolated from nonvenereal syphilis may behave somewhat differently in rabbits and hamsters from treponemes of venereal syphilis [381].

Clinical manifestations. Infection occurs in childhood, when a child comes in contact with other infants or adults with contagious lesions. The mode of transmission is presumed to be infected saliva and the portal of entry the mucous membranes of the mouth, tonsils, or larynx. Primary chancres are rarely seen because the inoculum of infection is usually small and invasion is not confined to a circumscribed area. Occasionally, an infected child may infect a previously uninfected mother, producing a primary "throwback" infection, such as a nipple chancre during nursing.

Fig. 201-25 Nonvenereal syphilis. Mucous patches of lips and tongue.

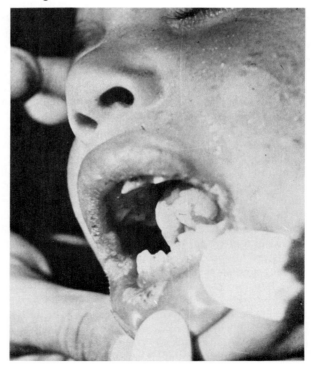

Nonvenereal syphilis usually presents as secondary syphilis. Mucous patches (Fig. 201-25), condylomata lata, and cutaneous lesions similar to those seen with venereal syphilis are common. *T. pallidum* can be demonstrated from condylomata lata and mucous membrane lesions. By the time signs and symptoms are evident, the STS are invariably reactive. Histopathology does not differ from venereal syphilis. Early lesions remain for 6 to 9 months without therapy, healing more slowly than venereal syphilis.

After the secondary lesions heal, there is a prolonged period of latency. In some cases, tertiary lesions appear at a later date. These are gummata that develop in the skin, nasopharynx, and bones—apparently evoked by trauma or reinfection in those individuals sensitized by previous infection. Gummata are most frequent in areas where the prevalence of early disease is highest. Saddle nose deformity, perforation of the palate, or massive destruction of the whole nose and adjacent maxilla including the upper lip (gangosa) (Fig. 201-26) are late complications. The histopathology of late disease is similar to venereal syphilis.

Cardiovascular and neurologic involvement is rare, but has not been well studied. Stigmata of prenatal syphilis are also rare. Since nonvenereal syphilis is a childhood disease, it is usually latent before women become pregnant and the opportunity for prenatal syphilis is remote.

Diagnosis. Diagnosis is provided by dark-field examination and serologic tests for syphilis.

Treatment. Nonvenereal syphilis is very responsive to penicillin and other antibiotics—best managed by mass campaigns, since such cases rarely occur in isolation. Treatment of whole communities can eradicate the disease in a given region. Treatment schedules for nonvenereal syphilis are similar to those described for venereal syphilis, with the stage of disease and size of the patient determining the drug dosage. Penicillin allergy and "contacts" are treated in a manner similar to venereal syphilis with the exception

that close "household" and social contact with an infected person is cause enough for abortive treatment [383].

Yaws [42,386,387]

Yaws, a nonvenereal treponematosis caused by *Treponema pertenue,* is found in hot, humid regions around the equator such as the Caribbean area, Central America, South America, and certain parts of Africa, northern Australia, and the Philippines. In the yaws eradication program in Haiti begun in 1949, the initial prevalence rate was approximately 40 percent in a population of 3.5 million people. After a house-to-house treatment campaign, the prevalence rate of active early and late lesions fell to less than 0.5 percent [383].

Yaws is predominantly a disease of childhood, with about 70 percent of infections occurring before the age of 15. It is transmitted nonvenereally by contact with an infected person. Like nonvenereal syphilis, it is a disease of poverty. Flies have been implicated to be a factor in the transmission of the disease.

Course of the disease. After an incubation period of 2 weeks to 6 months, an initial lesion may appear at the site of inoculation, frequently on the legs below the knees. Secondary lesions appear 3 to 12 weeks after the appearance of the initial lesion. If untreated, healing occurs in 3 to 6 months and the disease becomes latent, but infectious relapses may occur up to 5 years later. Spontaneous cure or permanent latency may follow. Some patients develop tertiary lesions of skin and bones after 5 to 10 years.

Although yaws does not commonly involve the cardiovascular or nervous systems and does not involve the fetus, reports of neuroophthalmologic abnormalities in late yaws confuse the demarcation between yaws and syphilis [380].

The disease is divided into (1) early yaws, which is contagious, and (2) late yaws, which is not.

Clinical manifestations. The primary lesion (mother yaw) is usually single but often multiple. Inoculation occurs at the site of wounds or abrasions, usually from an infected individual or contaminated fomites and flies. The primary lesion usually begins as a nontender papule which bursts open and becomes granulomatous and later ulcerates. Regional nodes are enlarged, firm, and painless. Primary lesions may persist for 2 to 6 months, and heal spontaneously leaving an atrophic and depressed scar with an achromic center.

Secondary lesions in the skin are similar to the primary, but smaller. They are called daughter yaws (Fig. 201-27). In the mucocutaneous areas they resemble condylomata lata and are frequently localized around the orifices (mouth, nose, anus, and vulva). Also, hyperkeratotic lesions can develop on the palms and soles. Osteitis and periostitis may occur in early yaws. Affected bones may be painful and tender, with visible deformity from thickening. These usually are not destructive. The secondary lesions disappear spontaneously within months and the disease becomes early latent.

Late lesions, presenting as gummata of the skin and bones, are localized predominantly on the lower extremities and include nodular or tuberous lesions and gummata

Fig. 201-26 Gangosa may be a late manifestation of venereal and nonvenereal syphilis, as well as yaws.

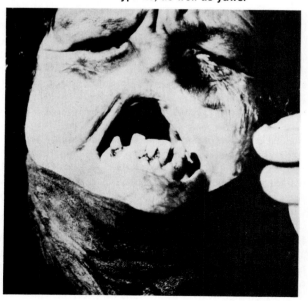

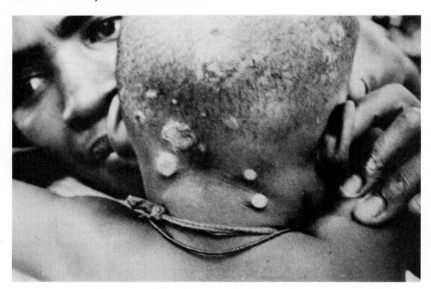

Fig. 201-27 Early secondary lesions of yaws (i.e., "daughter" yaws), showing crusted and ulcerated plaques and papules.

in the skin, and gummatous osteoperiostitis of the bone. Sabre tibia, saddle nose deformity (Fig. 201-28), and gangosa (Fig. 201-26) may occur. Goundou, a rare form of ossifying osteitis, occurring in about 1 percent of patients with yaws, affects the nasal bones and frontal processes of the maxilla, slowly growing over 5 to 20 years and occasionally leading to complete blindness by obstruction.

Histopathology [70]. In the *primary lesion,* there is marked acanthosis and papillomatosis, pronounced epidermal edema, and neutrophils migrating into the epidermis, leading to the formation of epidermal abscesses. The dermis shows infiltration with plasma cells primarily, but also neutrophils, lymphocytes, histiocytes, fibroblasts, and eosinophils. Unlike syphilis, the blood vessels in primary yaws show little or no proliferation of endothelial cells. *Secondary lesions* show histologic changes similar to those in primary lesions, and the epidermal changes resemble those

Fig. 201-28 Late yaws, showing destruction of the nasal septum and vomer and scars of the facial skin of the mother and papulosquamous secondary lesions on the head of the child.

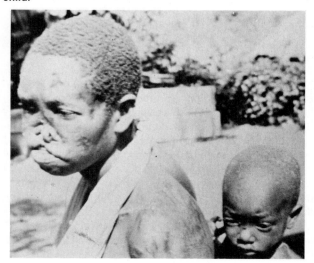

of condylomata lata. Unlike condylomata lata, the inflammatory cell infiltrate has a diffuse rather than a perivascular arrangement. In *late yaws,* ulcerative lesions have a histologic appearance similar to that of late syphilis except that the vascular changes in late yaws are slight or absent. Treponemes can be easily seen between epidermal cells on silver stains of primary and secondary lesions.

Diagnosis. Typical clinical manifestations in an endemic area initially suggest the diagnosis, which is confirmed by demonstrating organisms in primary and secondary lesions using dark-field microscopy of exudates, and using silver stains in routine paraffin sections. Reaginic and treponemal serologic tests for syphilis are positive.

Treatment. Like nonvenereal syphilis, mass treatment with penicillin or other antibiotics is required.

Pinta [42,386,387]

Pinta is a nonvenereal treponematosis caused by *Treponema carateum* and found in Central and South America. Like the other nonvenereal treponematoses, it is a disease of underprivileged people, affecting mostly blacks and native Indians under 20 years of age. Transmission is by direct child-to-child contact and possibly indirectly via insect vectors carrying disease from one child to another. Disease affects only the skin, producing dyschromia and hyperkeratotic eruptions.

Historical aspects. Pinta was well known among Carib and Aztec Indians, under the term *carate,* long before the Spanish Conquest. It was described by Valdéz and Cortéz between 1505 and 1515. The causative microorganism was detected by Grau y Triana and Alfonso Armenteros in Cuba in 1938 and by León y Blanco in Mexico in 1942.

Incidence. The occurrence of pinta is limited to Central and South American regions: Mexico, Venezuela, Colombia, Ecuador, Peru, and Brazil. Less frequently it is found in Guatemala, Honduras, El Salvador, Nicaragua, Haiti, Santo Domingo, Costa Rica, Panama, Bolivia, Cuba, Argentina, Chile, and the Dominican Republic. It is not known for certain outside the Americas [382].

Clinical manifestations. Clinical manifestations are confined to the skin. The primary stage is a patch of desquamating erythema up to 12 mm in diameter, seen on uncovered areas such as the face, arms, and legs. The lesions are usually multiple papules with minimal scaling that enlarge to psoriasiform plaques over a period of months to years. The secondary stage is seen 3 to 5 months later, when further red, scaling patches occur around the primary lesion or become disseminated.

Thereafter, the typical dyschromic areas of hyperpigmentation and depigmentation appear (Figs. 201-29 and A8-33). Beginning as pink or red lesions, they turn brown or yellow, then slate blue or black. Some lesions become white, representing the last stages of the disease. The pigment changes proceed irregularly; in the late stages all varieties of dyschromia, hypochromia, and achromia may be seen in the same patient.

Generalized adenopathy accompanies the last two stages of pinta, but it is difficult to demonstrate treponemes in tissue. Systemic symptoms are absent, and there is no cardiovascular or neurologic involvement.

Histopathology [70]. In early lesions, the epidermis shows slight acanthosis, intra- and extracellular edema, permeation of lymphoid cells into the epidermis, and hydropic degeneration and the loss of melanin in the basal cells. Many melanophages are seen in the upper dermis, which indicates a severe disturbance of pigmentation. Ultrastructural investigations have revealed that the treponeme causes irreversible damage to melanocytes. Dense infiltrates consisting of plasma cells, lymphoid cells, and occasionally histiocytes and neutrophils are found in the upper dermis around enlarged blood and lymph vessels. Treponemes are usually found in large numbers in the epidermis.

Hyperpigmented areas of late pinta are characterized by atrophy of the epidermis, lack of melanin in basal cells, and accumulations of melanophages with slight lymphocytic infiltrates in the dermis. Ample treponemes are still found in the epidermis.

Hypochromic and achromic spots or patches of late pinta show degenerative changes, atrophy of the dermis as well

as the appendages, basophilic degeneration of the elastic fibers, and accumulations of elastotic masses as in actinic elastosis. Melanin is completely absent, even in the dermis. Inflammation is not present, and treponemes cannot be found. Electron microscopic examination reveals the absence of basal epidermal melanocytes, but Langerhans cells are present and some of them contain a few melanosomes enclosed within lysosomes.

Immunity. Immunity from reinfection and superinfection exists during the late stages. Experiments by Medina and Padilha-Goncalves revealed the absence of a cross-immunity among pinta, syphilis, and yaws in their early stages but indicated a variable degree of cross-immunity at late stages, most marked in pinta, and less in syphilis. The investigations of Medina showed that "pintosos" were resistant to inoculation of *T. pallidum* during the late stage of the disease, but patients at any stage of syphilis or yaws could easily be infected with pinta [42]. Antibodies to lipoidal antigens can be found in the serum 2 to 3 months after the onset of the disease, and treponemal tests are also reactive. The cerebrospinal fluid has been found to be nonreactive to tests using lipoidal antigens and to treponemal tests at any stage of pinta.

Diagnosis. Diagnosis of the disease is made by demonstrating *T. carateum* from early skin lesions and a reactive STS.

Treatment. Treatment is similar to that for yaws and non-venereal syphilis.

References

1. Hackett CJ: Diagnostic criteria of syphilis, yaws, treponarid (treponematoses) and some other diseases in dry bones, in *Sitzungsberichte der Heidelberger Akademie der Wissenschaften, Mathematisch—naturwissen schaftliche Klasse.* Berlin/Heidelberg/New York, Springer, 1976, p 1
2. Turner TB: The future direction of research into syphilis, in *Sexually Transmitted Diseases,* edited by RD Catterall, CS Nichol. London, Academic Press, 1976, p 221
3. Willcox PR: Changing patterns of treponemal disease. *Br J Vener Dis* 50:169, 1974
4. Knox JM: The change in clinical manifestations (of syphilis), in *Sexually Transmitted Diseases,* edited by RD Catterall, CS Nichol. London, Academic Press, 1976, p 207
5. Harris JRW: Epidemiologic and social aspects (of syphilis), in *Recent Advances in Sexually Transmitted Diseases,* edited by RS Morton, JRW Harris. Edinburgh, Churchill Livingstone, 1975, p 91
6. Centers for Disease Control: Reported morbidity and mortality in the United States: annual summary 1981. *MMWR* 30:82, 1982
7. Department of Health and Social Security Annual Report: Sexually transmitted diseases. *Br J Vener Dis* 59:206, 1983
8. Judson FN: Sexually transmitted disease in gay men. *Sex Transm Dis* 4:76, 1977
9. Centers for Disease Control: Reported morbidity and mortality in the United States, 1976: annual summary of morbidity and mortality. *MMWR* 25:2, 1977
10. Centers for Disease Control: Syphilis trends in the United States. *MMWR* 35:441, 1981
11. Curtis AC, Philpott OS: Prenatal syphilis. *Med Clin North Am* 48:707, 1964
12. Smibert RM: The spirochetes, in *Bergey's Manual of Deter-*

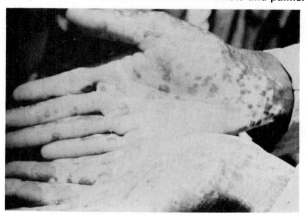

Fig. 201-29 Late phase of pinta. Depigmentation and hyperpigmentation in healed lesions of the wrists and palms.

minative Microbiology, 8th ed, edited by RE Buchanan, NE Gibbons. Baltimore, Williams & Wilkins, 1974, p 167

13. *Syphilis, a Synopsis.* US Dept of HEW, Public Health Service, Publ No 1660. Washington, DC, US Government Printing Office, 1968

14. Willcox RR, Guthe T: *Treponema pallidum. Bull WHO* **35(suppl):**1, 1966

15. Zeigler JA et al: Demonstration of extracellular material at the surface of pathogenic *T. pallidum* cells. *Br J Vener Dis* **52:**1, 1976

16. Horvath I et al: Effects of oxygen and nitrogen on the character of *T. pallidum* in subcutaneous chambers in mice. *Br J Vener Dis* **51:**301, 1976

17. Jones RH et al: Growth and subculture of pathogenic *T. pallidum* (Nichols strain) in BHK-21 cultured tissue cells. *Br J Vener Dis* **52:**18, 1976

18. Rathlev T: Investigations on *in vitro* survival and virulence of *T. pallidum* under aerobiosis. *Br J Vener Dis* **51:**296, 1976

19. Fitzgerald TJ et al: Interaction of *Treponema pallidum* with cultured mammalian cells: effects of oxygen, reducing agents, serum supplements, and different cell types. *Infect Immun* **15:**444, 1977

20. Fieldsteel AH et al: Prolonged survival of virulent *Treponema pallidum* (Nichols strain) in cell-free and tissue culture systems. *Infect Immun* **18:**173, 1977

21. Cover WH et al: The microaerophilic nature of *Treponema pallidum:* enhanced survival and incorporation of tritiated adenine under microaerobic conditions in the presence or absence of reducing compounds. *Sex Transm Dis* **9:**1, 1982

22. Musher DM et al: The immunology of syphilis. *Int J Dermatol* **15:**566, 1976

23. Wright DJM, Grimble AS: Why is the infectious stage of syphilis prolonged? *Br J Vener Dis* **50:**45, 1974

24. Wilkinson AE: Immunity in syphilis, in *Recent Advances in Sexually Transmitted Diseases,* edited by RS Morton, JRW Harris. Edinburgh, Churchill Livingstone, 1975, p 155

25. Magnuson HJ et al: Inoculation syphilis in human volunteers. *Medicine (Baltimore)* **35:**33, 1956

26. Dunlop EMC: Persistence of treponemes after treatment. *Br Med J* **2:**577, 1972

27. Ovcinnikov NM et al: Long-term results of penicillin treatment of early and late forms of syphilis in rabbits. *Br J Vener Dis* **49:**413, 1973

28. Sell S et al: T-cell hyperplasia of lymphoid tissues of rabbits infected with *Treponema pallidum:* evidence for a vigorous immune response. *Sex Transm Dis* **7:**74, 1980

29. Izzat NN et al: Resistance and serological changes in rabbits immunized with virulent *Treponema pallidum* sonicate. *Acta Derm Venereol (Stockh)* **51:**157, 1971

30. Turner TB et al: Effects of passive immunization on experimental syphilis in the rabbit. *Johns Hopkins Med J* **133:**241, 1973

31. Perine PL et al: Immunity to syphilis. I. Passive transfer in rabbits with hyperimmune serum. *Infect Immun* **8:**787, 1973

32. Sepetjian M et al: Attempt to protect rabbits against experimental syphilis by passive immunization. *Br J Vener Dis* **49:**335, 1973

33. Festenstein HC et al: Runting syndrome in neonatal rabbits infected with *Treponema pallidum. Clin Exp Immunol* **2:**311, 1967

34. Miller JN: Immunity in experimental syphilis. VI. Successful vaccination in rabbits with *Treponema pallidum,* Nichols strain, attenuated by gamma irradiation. *J Immunol* **110:**1206, 1973

35. Jensen JR, From E: Alterations in T lymphocytes and T-lymphocyte subpopulations in patients with syphilis. *Br J Vener Dis* **58:**18, 1982

36. Bos JD et al: T-lymphoid cells in primary syphilis. Quantitative studies. *Br J Vener Dis* **56:**74, 1980

37. Jensen JR et al: Fluctuations in natural killer cell activity in early syphilis. *Br J Vener Dis* **59:**30, 1983

38. Jensen JR et al: Depression of natural killer cell activity by syphilitic serum and immune complexes. *Br J Vener Dis* **58:**298, 1982

39. Folds JD et al: Lymphocyte transformation and the effect of circulating immune complexes in humans with syphilis. *Sex Transm Dis* **9:**109, 1982

40. Bos JD: Immune system responses towards *Treponema pallidum* infection. *Antonie Van Leeuwenhoek* **48:**485, 1982

41. Baughn RE et al: Immune complexes in experimental syphilis: a methodologic evaluation. *Sex Transm Dis* **9:**170, 1982

42. Kerdel-Vegas F: Yaws, pinta, in *Textbook of Dermatology,* 3d ed, edited by A Rook et al. Oxford, Blackwell, 1979, p 736

43. Smith JL et al: Neuroophthalmological study of late yaws and pinta. II. The Caracas project. *Br J Vener Dis* **47:**226, 1971

44. Hollander DH: Treponematosis from pinta to venereal syphilis revisited: hypothesis for temperature determination of disease patterns. *Sex Transm Dis* **8:**34, 1981

45. Pavia CS et al: Cell-mediated immunity during syphilis. A review. *Br J Vener Dis* **54:**144, 1978

46. Brause BD, Roberts RB: Attachment of virulent *Treponema pallidum* to human mononuclear phagocytes. *Br J Vener Dis* **54:**218, 1978

47. Logan LC: Rabbit globulin and antiglobulin factors associated with *Treponema pallidum* growth in rabbits. *Br J Vener Dis* **50:**421, 1974

48. Kaplan BS et al: The glomerulopathy of congenital syphilis—an immune deposit disease. *J Pediatr* **81:**1154, 1972

49. Wiggelinkhuizen J et al: Congenital syphilis and glomerulonephritis with evidence for immune pathogenesis. *Arch Dis Child* **48:**375, 1973

50. Wicher KJ et al: An attempt to produce immune complexes in experimental syphilis. *Br J Vener Dis* **50:**319, 1974

51. Praiser H: Infectious syphilis. *Med Clin North Am* **48:**625, 1964

52. Sutton RL: Syphilis, in *Diseases of the Skin,* 11th ed. St Louis, CV Mosby, 1956, p 382

53. Olansky S, Norins LC: Syphilis and other treponematoses, in *Dermatology in General Medicine,* edited by TB Fitzpatrick et al. New York, McGraw-Hill, 1971, p 1955

54. Rudolph AH, Olansky S: Syphilis, in *Clinical Dermatology,* edited by J Demis et al. Hagerstown, MD, Harper & Row, 1976, p 6

55. Lomholt G: Syphilis, in *Textbook of Dermatology,* 2d ed, edited by A Rook et al. London, Blackwell, 1972, p 634

56. Nichals L: Syphilis, in *Dermatology,* edited by SL Moschella et al. Philadelphia, WB Saunders, 1975, p 709

57. Thomas EW: *Syphilis: Its Course and Management.* New York, Macmillan, 1949, p 1

58. Risseeum-Appel IM, Kothe F: Transfusion syphilis: a case report. *Sex Transm Dis* **10:**200, 1983

59. Clark EG, Danbolt N: The Oslo study of the natural history of untreated syphilis: an epidemiologic investigation based on a re-study of Boeck-Bruusgaard material. *J Chronic Dis* **2:**311, 1955

60. Clark EG, Danbolt N: The Oslo study of the natural course of untreated syphilis. *Med Clin North Am* **48:**613, 1964

61. Notowicz A, Menke HE: Atypical primary syphilitic lesions on the penis. *Dermatologica* **147:**328, 1973

62. Drusin LM et al: Infectious syphilis mimicking neoplastic disease. *Arch Intern Med* **137:**156, 1977

63. Starzyci Z: Primary syphilis of the fingers. *Br J Vener Dis* **59:**169, 1983

64. Chang TW et al: Herpetic chancre. *JAMA* **224:**129, 1973

65. Chapel TA et al: How reliable is the morphological diagnosis of penile ulcerations? *Sex Transm Dis* **4:**150, 1977

66. Leibovitz A: An outbreak of pyogenic penile ulcers associated with a microaerophilic streptococcus resembling *Hemophilus ducreyi*. *Am J Syphilol* **38**:203, 1954

67. Dogliotti M: The incidence of syphilis in the Bantu: survey of 587 cases from Baragwanatu Hospital. *S Afr Med J* **45**:8, 1971

68. Lejman K, Bogdaszewaska-Czabanowska J: Syphilitic chancre complicated by fusospirochaetal infection from the same partner. *Br J Vener Dis* **45**:313, 1969

69. Kellogg DS: The detection of *Treponema pallidum* by a rapid direct fluorescent antibody darkfield (DFATP) procedure. *Health Lab Sci* **7**:34, 1970

70. Lever WF, Schaumburg-Lever G: *Histopathology of the Skin*, 6th ed. Philadelphia, JB Lippincott, 1983, p 320

71. Soltani K et al: Demonstration by labeled treponemal antigen of specific antibodies in the tissue infiltrates of secondary syphilis. *J Invest Dermatol* **69**:439, 1977

72. Allyn B: Pruritus in syphilis. *Arch Dermatol* **113**:1295, 1977

73. Chapel TA: The signs and symptoms of secondary syphilis. *Sex Transm Dis* **7**:161, 1980

74. Cole GW et al: Secondary syphilis presenting as a pruritic dermatosis. *Arch Dermatol* **113**:489, 1977

75. Willcox JR: An atypical case of secondary syphilis. *Br J Vener Dis* **57**:30, 1981

76. Lochner JC, Pomeranz JR: Lichenoid secondary syphilis. *Arch Dermatol* **109**:81, 1974

77. Lejman K, Starzycki Z: Keratopustular variety of framboesiform syphilis: a case report. *Br J Vener Dis* **53**:195, 1977

78. Beck MH et al: Secondary syphilis with framboesiform facial lesions. *Br J Vener Dis* **57**:103, 1981

79. Sarojini PA et al: Concentric rings simulating tinea imbricata in secondary syphilis. *Br J Vener Dis* **56**:302, 1980

80. Kennedy CTC, Sanderson KV: Corymbose secondary syphilis. *Arch Dermatol* **116**:111, 1980

81. Lejman K, Starzycki Z: Early varioliform syphilis. *Br J Vener Dis* **57**:25, 1981

82. Mikhail GR, Chapel TA: Follicular papulopustular syphilid. *Arch Dermatol* **100**:471, 1969

83. Petrozzi JW et al: Malignant syphilis—severe variant of secondary syphilis. *Arch Dermatol* **109**:387, 1974

84. Miller RL: Pustular secondary syphilis. *Br J Vener Dis* **50**:459, 1974

85. Sehgal VN, Rege VL: Malignant syphilis and hepatitis. *Br J Vener Dis* **50**:237, 1974

86. French CH: Malignant syphilis. *J R Army Med Corp* **4**:477, 1905

87. Baum EW et al: Secondary syphilis: still the great imitator. *JAMA* **249**:3069, 1983

88. Graham WR, Duvic M: Nodular secondary syphilis. *Arch Dermatol* **118**:205, 1982

89. Matsuda-John SS et al: Nodular late syphilis. *J Am Acad Dermatol* **9**:269, 1983

90. Burkhart CC, Smith MR: Secondary syphilis mimicking mycosis fungoides. *J Am Acad Dermatol* **3**:92, 1980

91. Fiumara NJ, Cahn T: Leukoderma of secondary syphilis: two case reports. *Sex Transm Dis* **9**:140, 1982

92. Pattman RS: Reversible penile leukoderma in a man with secondary syphilis: a case report. *Sex Transm Dis* **9**:96, 1982

93. Pandhi RK et al: Leukoderma in early syphilis. *Br J Vener Dis* **53**:19, 1977

94. Frithz A et al: Leukoderma syphiliticum: ultrastructural observations on melanocyte function. *Acta Derm Venereol (Stockh)* **62**:521, 1982

95. Kingsbury DH et al: Syphilitic paronychia: an unusual complaint. *Arch Dermatol* **105**:458, 1972

96. Shiv SP: Unusual location of syphilitic alopecia. *Sex Transm Dis* **9**:41, 1982

97. Hartsock RJ et al: Luetic lymphadenitis—a clinical and histologic study of 20 cases. *Am J Clin Pathol* **53**:304, 1970

98. Wright DJM: Alcoholic lymphalgia in early syphilis. *Postgrad Med J* **45**:191, 1969

99. Kopf RS: Case records of the Massachusetts General Hospital. *N Engl J Med* **309**:35, 1983

100. Gamble CN, Reardan JB: Immunopathogenesis of syphilitic glomerulonephritis. *N Engl J Med* **292**:449, 1975

101. Feher J et al: Early syphilitic hepatitis. *Lancet* **2**:896, 1975

102. Terry SI et al: Prevalence of liver abnormality in early syphilis. *Br J Vener Dis* **60**:83, 1984

103. Harris JRW: Clinical aspects (of syphilis), in *Recent Advances in Sexually Transmitted Diseases*, edited by RS Morton, JRW Harris. Edinburgh, Churchill Livingstone, 1976, p 97

104. Hira SK, Hira RS: Parotitis with secondary syphilis. *Br J Vener Dis* **60**:121, 1984

105. Waugh MA: Bony symptoms in secondary syphilis. *Br J Vener Dis* **52**:204, 1976

106. Thompson RG, Preston RH: Lesions of the skull in secondary syphilis. *Am J Syphilol* **36**:332, 1952

107. Shore RN et al: Osteolytic lesions in secondary syphilis. *Arch Intern Med* **137**:1465, 1977

108. Tight AR, Warner JF: Skeletal involvement in secondary syphilis detected by bone scanning. *JAMA* **235**:2324, 1976

109. Dismukes WE et al: Destructive bone disease in early syphilis. *JAMA* **236**:2646, 1976

110. Gerster EC et al: Secondary syphilis revealed by rheumatic complaints. *J Rheumatol* **4**:197, 1977

111. Durston JHJ, Jefferiss FJG: Syphilitic myositis. *Br J Vener Dis* **51**:141, 1975

112. MacFaul PA, Catterall RD: Acute choroido-retinitis in secondary syphilis: presence of spiral organisms in the aqueous humor. *Br J Vener Dis* **47**:159, 1971

113. Smith JL: Acute blindness in early syphilis. *Arch Ophthalmol* **90**:256, 1973

114. Stöckli HR: Neurosyphilis heute. *Dermatologica* **165**:232, 1982

115. Gjestland T: The Oslo study of untreated syphilis. *Acta Derm Venereol [Suppl] (Stockh)* **35**:1, 1955

116. Merritt HH: Syphilis, in *A Textbook in Neurology,* 4th ed. Philadelphia, Lea & Febiger, 1967, p 110

117. Trenholme GM et al: Syphilitic meningitis with papilledema. *South Med J* **70**:1013, 1977

118. Vercoe GS: The effect of early syphilis on the inner ear and auditory nerves. *J Laryngol Otol* **90**:853, 1976

119. Biro L et al: Secondary syphilis with unusual clinical and laboratory findings. *JAMA* **206**:889, 1969

120. Ince WE, Mahabir BS: Wenckebach phenomenon occurring in secondary syphilis. *Br J Vener Dis* **50**:97, 1974

121. Abell E et al: Secondary syphilis: a clinicopathological review. *Br J Dermatol* **93**:53, 1975

122. Castigliano SG: Syphilis and oral cancer. *Ann Otol Rhinol Laryngol* **64**:608, 1955

123. Kampmeier RH: The late manifestations of syphilis: skeletal, visceral, and cardiovascular. *Med Clin North Am* **48**:667, 1964

124. Handsfield HH et al: Demonstration of *Treponema pallidum* in a cutaneous gumma by indirect immunofluorescence. *Arch Dermatol* **119**:677, 1983

125. Bonugli FS: Involvement of the aortic valve and ascending aorta in congenital syphilis: a review. *Br J Vener Dis* **37**:257, 1961

126. White RJ: Aortic incompetence associated with congenital syphilis. *Br J Vener Dis* **41**:149, 1965

127. Holt S: Syphilitic ostial occlusion. *Br Heart J* **39**:469, 1977

128. Frater RWM, Jordan A: Syphilitic coronary ostial sclerosis. *Ann Thorac Surg* **6**:463, 1968

129. Grabau W et al: Syphilitic aortic regurgitation—an appraisal of surgical treatment. *Br J Vener Dis* **52**:366, 1976

130. Montgomery BM: The natural history of syphilitic heart disease. *Ann Intern Med* **37**:689, 1952

131. Rosahn PD: *Autopsy Studies on Syphilis: A Monograph.* 6th printing. US Dept of HEW, Public Health Service, Publ No. 433, Washington, DC, US Government Printing Office, 1955

132. Luxon L: Neurosyphilis. *Int J Dermatol* **19**:310, 1980

133. Mosbaek A, Sørensen PS: The incidence and clinical presentation of neurosyphilis in Greater Copenhagen 1974 through 1978. *Acta Neurol Scand* **63**:237, 1981

134. Perdrup A et al: The profile of neurosyphilis in Denmark. *Acta Derm Venereol [Suppl] (Stockh)* **96**:1, 1981

135. Hagedorn HJ: Syphilisantikörper im Liquor cerebrospinalis und ihre diagnostische Bedeutung. *Dtsch Med Wochenschr* **105**:155, 1980

136. Ritter G, Prange H: Serologische Kriterien für die Diagnostik und Therapie der Neurosyphilis. *Med Welt* **32**:1250, 1981

137. Mapelli G et al: Neurosyphilis today. *Eur Neurol* **20**:334, 1981

138. Joffe R et al: Changing clinical picture of neurosyphilis: report of seven unusual cases. *Br Med J* **1**:211, 1968

139. Hooshmand H et al: Neurosyphilis: a study of 241 patients. *JAMA* **219**:726, 1972

140. Harner RE et al: The FTA-ABS test in late syphilis: a serologic study in 1,985 cases. *JAMA* **203**:545, 1968

141. Deacon WE et al: Fluorescent treponemal antibody absorption (FTA-ABS) test for syphilis. *JAMA* **198**:624, 1966

142. McGeeney T et al: Utility of the FTA-ABS test of cerebrospinal fluid in the diagnosis of neurosyphilis. *Sex Transm Dis* **6**:195, 1979

143. Luger A et al: Diagnosis of neurosyphilis by examination of the cerebrospinal fluid. *Br J Vener Dis* **57**:232, 1981

144. Mohr JA et al: Neurosyphilis and penicillin levels in cerebrospinal fluid. *JAMA* **236**:2208, 1976

145. Dijkstra JWE: Asymptomatic neurosyphilis. *Int J Dermatol* **22**:581, 1983

146. Löwhagen G-B et al: Central nervous system involvement in early syphilis. *Acta Derm Venereol (Stockh)* **63**:530, 1983

147. Fernando WL: Cerebrospinal fluid findings after treatment of early syphilis with penicillin: a further series of 80 patients. *Br J Vener Dis* **44**:134, 1968

148. Dippel AL: Relationship of congenital syphilis to abortion and miscarriage, and the mechanism of intrauterine protection. *Am J Obstet Gynecol* **47**:369, 1944

149. Benirschke K: Syphilis, the placenta and the fetus. *Am J Dis Child* **128**:142, 1974

150. Harter CA, Benirschke K: Fetal syphilis in the first trimester. *Am J Obstet Gynecol* **124**:705, 1976

151. Silverstein AM: Ontogeny of the immune response: the development of immunologic responses by the fetus has interesting pathobiologic implications. *Science* **144**:1423, 1964

152. Strag-Pederson B: Economic evaluation of maternal screening to prevent congenital syphilis. *Sex Transm Dis* **10**:167, 1983

153. Rutherford HW: Two cases of third generation syphilis. *Br J Vener Dis* **41**:142, 1965

154. Fiumara NJ: Acquired syphilis in three patients with congenital syphilis. *N Engl J Med* **290**:1119, 1974

155. Tan KC: The re-emergence of early congenital syphilis. *Acta Pediatr Scand* **62**:601, 1973

156. Long WA et al: Congenital syphilitic pneumonia. *Clin Res* **31**:904A, 1983

157. Yuceoglu AM et al: The glomerulopathy of congenital syphilis, a curable immune-deposit disease. *JAMA* **229**:1085, 1974

158. Kashula RO et al: Nephrotic syndrome of congenital syphilis: biopsy studies on four cases. *Arch Pathol* **97**:289, 1974

159. Fiumara NJ, Lessell S: Manifestations of late congenital syphilis—an analysis of 271 patients. *Arch Dermatol* **102**:78, 1970

160. Herman SP: Congenital syphilis—a review. *West Virginia Medical Journal* **70**:290, 1974

161. Hahn RD et al: Treatment of neural deafness with prednisone. *J Chronic Dis* **15**:395, 1962

162. Kerr AG et al: Congenital syphilitic deafness. *J Laryngol Otol* **87**:1, 1973

163. Gray MS, Philip T: Syphilitic arthritis. *Ann Rheum Dis* **22**:19, 1963

164. Parrish DJ, Mitchell JR: Syphilitic paroxysmal cold hemoglobinuria. *J Clin Pathol* **13**:237, 1960

165. Reimer CB et al: The specificity of fetal IgM: antibody or autoantibody. *Ann NY Acad Sci* **254**:77, 1975

166. Kaufman RE et al: Questionnaire survey of reported early congenital syphilis: problems in diagnosis, prevention, and treatment. *Sex Transm Dis* **4**:135, 1977

167. Treponemal Infections. Report of a WHO Scientific Group. *WHO Tech Rep Ser* 674, 1982

168. Müller F, Sinzig G: Spezifität und Sensibilität immunologischer Diagnostik der konnatalen Syphilis mit dem 19S-IgM-FTA-ABS Test. *Z Hautkr* **57**:983, 1982

169. Müller F, Lindenschmidt EG: Demonstration of specific 19S (IgM)-antibodies in untreated and treated syphilis. *Br J Vener Dis* **58**:12, 1982

170. Müller F: Serological tests to identify antibodies in treponematoses. A review. World Health Organization 80.358, Geneva, 1980

171. Schmidt BL: The 19S-IgM-FTA-ABS test in the serum diagnosis of syphilis. World Health Organization 79.362, Geneva, 1979

172. Luger A: Diagnosis of syphilis. *Bull WHO* **59**:647, 1982

173. Rufli T: Lues Serologie—gestern, heute, morgen. *Dermatologica* **165**:221, 1982

174. Rudolph AH: Serologic diagnosis of syphilis: an update. *South Med J* **69**:1196, 1976

175. Wilkerson AE: Syphilis serology, in *Recent Advances in Sexually Transmitted Diseases,* edited by RS Morton, JRW Harris. Edinburgh, Churchill Livingstone, 1975, p 126

176. Jaffe HW: The laboratory diagnosis of syphilis—new concepts. *Ann Intern Med* **83**:846, 1975

177. Olansky S: Serodiagnosis of syphilis. *Med Clin North Am* **56**:1145, 1972

178. Sparling PF: Diagnosis and treatment of syphilis. *N Engl J Med* **284**:642, 1971

179. Catterall RD: Immunität im Verlauf der Syphilis. *Hautarzt* **29**:119, 1979

180. Donaich D: Autoantibodies in syphilis and chronic biological false positive reactions, in *Sexually Transmitted Diseases,* edited by RD Catterall, CS Nichol. New York, Academic Press, 1976, p 210

181. Shannon R et al: Immunological responses in late syphilis. *Br J Vener Dis* **56**:372, 1980

182. Brun R: Essai d'une nouvelle méthode sérologique pour la détection de la syphilis active. *Dermatologica* **165**:254, 1982

183. Müller F: Modellversuche zur Wirkung von IgM-und IgG-Antikörpern auf die Reacktionen des *Treponema pallidum* Hämagglutinations—(TPHA) Testes. *Hautarzt* **27**:26, 1976

184. Luger A: Serology of syphilis by the application of immunological methods, in *Proceedings of the XVIth Congressus internationalis Dermatologiae, Tokyo, 1983.* Tokyo, Univ of Tokyo Press, in press

185. Gschnait F et al: Cerebrospinal fluid immunoglobulins in neurosyphilis. *Br J Vener Dis* **57**:238, 1981

186. Tuffanelli DL: Normal individuals with chronic false-positive (BFP) tests for syphilis, in *Sexually Transmitted Diseases,* edited by L Nichols. Springfield, IL, Charles C Thomas, 1973, p 95

187. McGrew BE, Lantz MA: Quantitative automated reagin test for syphilis. *Am J Med Tech* **36**:1, 1970

188. Wuepper KD et al: Serologic tests for syphilis and the false positive reactor. *Arch Dermatol* **94**:152, 1966

189. Spangler AS et al: Syphilis with a negative blood test reaction. *JAMA* **189**:87, 1964

190. Garner MF, Grantham NM: The VDRL test: significance of "rough" results. *Br J Vener Dis* **44**:131, 1968

191. Wright DJM et al: New antibody in early syphilis. *Lancet* **1**:740, 1970

192. Dorwart BB, Myers AR: Comparison of rapid plasma reagin card test and Venereal Disease Research Laboratory test in the detection of biologic false positive reactions in systemic lupus erythematosus. *Br J Vener Dis* **50**:435, 1974

193. Fiumara NJ: Biologic false-positive reactions for syphilis: Massachusetts, 1954–1961. *N Engl J Med* **268**:402, 1963

194. Luger A et al: Screening for syphilis with the AMHA-TP test. *Eur J Sex Transm Dis* **1**:25, 1982

195. Tuffanelli DL et al: Fluorescent treponemal-antibody absorption tests: studies of false-positive reactions to tests for syphilis. *N Engl J Med* **276**:258, 1967

196. Grossman LJ, Peery TM: Biologically false-positive serological tests for syphilis due to small-pox vaccination. *Am J Clin Pathol* **51**:375, 1969

197. Salo OP et al: Tests for syphilis in young males: an analysis of a seven-year series from a central military hospital. *Milit Med* **132**:258, 1967

198. Quaife RA, Gostling JVT: False positive Wassermann reaction associated with evidence of enterovirus infection. *J Clin Pathol* **24**:120, 1971

199. Moore JE, Mohr CF: Biologically false positive serologic tests for syphilis: type, incidence and cause. *JAMA* **150**:467, 1952

200. Cabrera HA, Carlson J: Biologic false positive reactions and infectious mononucleosis. *Am J Clin Pathol* **50**:643, 1968

201. Hoagland RJ: False positive serology in mononucleosis. *JAMA* **185**:783, 1963

202. Brede HD et al: Detection of biologic false positive syphilis serum reactions. *S Afr Lab Clin Med [Suppl]*, June 12, 1974, p 1191

203. Hare MJ: Serological tests for treponemal disease in pregnancy. *J Obstet Gynecol Br Commw* **80**:515, 1973

204. Salo OP et al: False positive serological tests for syphilis in pregnancy. *Acta Derm Venereol (Stockh)* **49**:332, 1969

205. Moore MB, Knox JM: Sensitivity and specificity in syphilis serology: clinical implications. *South Med J* **58**:963, 1965

206. Kaufman RE et al: Biologic false positive serologic tests for syphilis among drug addicts. *Br J Vener Dis* **50**:350, 1974

207. Cherubin C, Millian SJ: Serologic investigations in narcotic addict. I. Syphilis, lymphogranuloma venereum, herpes simplex and Q fever. *Ann Intern Med* **69**:739, 1968

208. Tuffanelli DL: Narcotic addiction with false-positive reaction for syphilis, immunologic studies. *Acta Derm Venereol (Stockh)* **48**:542, 1968

209. Boak RA et al: Biologic false-positive reactions for syphilis among narcotic addicts. *JAMA* **175**:326, 1961

210. Cushman P, Sherman C: Biologic false-positive reactions in serologic tests for syphilis in narcotic addiction. *Am J Clin Pathol* **61**:347, 1974

211. Willcox RR: Recent advances in venereology. I. Syphilis. *Br J Clin Pract* **27**:115, 1973

212. British Cooperative Clinical Group: Acute and chronic biologic false positive reactors to serologic tests for syphilis. *Br J Vener Dis* **50**:428, 1974

213. Scotti AT et al: Syphilis and biologic false positive reactors among leprosy patients. *Arch Dermatol* **101**:328, 1970

214. Achimastos A et al: Occurrence of biologic false positive reactions with RPR (circle) card test in leprosy patients. *Public Health Rep* **85**:66, 1970

215. Carr RD et al: The biologic false positive phenomenon in elderly men. *Arch Dermatol* **93**:393, 1965

216. Litwin SD, Singer JM: Studies of the incidence and significance of anti-gamma globulin factors in aging. *Arthritis Rheum* **8**:538, 1965

217. Tuffanelli DL: Aging and false positive reactions for syphilis. *Br J Vener Dis* **42**:40, 1966

218. Raskin MA, Eisdorfer C: Screening for syphilis in an aged psychiatrically impaired population. *West J Med* **125**:361, 1976

219. Harvey AM, Shulman LE: Connective tissue disease and the chronic biologic false positive test for syphilis (BFP reaction). *Med Clin North Am* **50**:1271, 1966

220. Shulman LE, Harvey AM: Hashimoto's thyroiditis in false-positive reactors to tests for syphilis. *Am J Med* **36**:174, 1964

221. Catterall RD: Systemic disease and the biologic false positive reaction. *Br J Vener Dis* **48**:1, 1972

222. Mustakallio KK et al: Cryoglobulins and rheumatoid factor in sera from chronic false positive seroreactors for syphilis. *Acta Derm Venereol (Stockh)* **47**:249, 1967

223. Russell Jones R et al: Essential mixed cryoglobulinaemia with false positive tests for syphilis. *Br J Vener Dis* **59**:33, 1983

224. Wuepper KD, Tuffanelli DL: False positive reaction to VDRL test with prozone phenomena, association with lymphosarcoma. *JAMA* **195**:868, 1966

225. Drusin L et al: Waldenström's macroglobulinemia in a patient with a chronic biologic false-positive serologic test for syphilis. *Am J Med* **56**:429, 1974

226. Tuffanelli DL: False positive reactions for syphilis: serological abnormalities in relatives of chronic reactors. *Arch Dermatol* **98**:606, 1968

227. Aho K: Studies of syphilitic antibodies. II. Substances responsible for biologic false positive sero-reactions. *Br J Vener Dis* **44**:49, 1968

228. Tringali GR et al: Effect of 2-mercaptoethanol treatment on anticardiolipin reactivity in sera from syphilitics and false positive reactors. *Br J Vener Dis* **45**:202, 1969

229. Nelson RA, Mayer MM: Immobilization of *Treponema pallidum in vitro* by antibody produced in syphilitic infection. *J Exp Med* **89**:369, 1949

230. Christiansen S: Statistical aspects of the treponemal counts in the TPI test. *Acta Pathol Microbiol Scand [B]* **86**:267, 1978

231. Rein MF et al: Failure of the *Treponema pallidum* immobilization test to provide additional diagnostic information about contemporary problem sera. *Sex Transm Dis* **7**:101, 1980

232. Goldman JN, Lanz MA: FTA-ABS and VDRL slide test reactivity in a population of nuns. *JAMA* **217**:53, 1971

233. Luger A et al: Specificity of the *Treponema pallidum* haemagglutination test. *Br J Vener Dis* **57**:178, 1981

234. Tourville D et al: Evaluation of semi-automated fluoro-kit for FTA-ABS testing. *J Invest Dermatol* **61**:355, 1973

235. Coffey EM et al: Further evaluation of the automated fluorescent treponemal antibody test for syphilis. *Appl Microbiol* **21**:820, 1971

236. Burns RE: Spontaneous reversion of FTA-ABS test reactions. *JAMA* **234**:617, 1975

237. Wright JT et al: False positive FTA-ABS results in patients with genital herpes. *Br J Vener Dis* **51**:329, 1975

238. Dans PE et al: The FTA-ABS test: a diagnostic help or hindrance? *South Med J* **70**:312, 1977

239. Drew FJ, Sarandria JL: False positive FTA-ABS in pregnancy. *J Am Vener Dis Assoc* **1**:165, 1975

240. Buchanan CS, Haserick JR: FTA-ABS test in pregnancy: a probable false-positive reaction. *Arch Dermatol* **102**:322, 1970

241. Pien FD et al: Problems with the beaded fluorescence pattern in the FTA-ABS test. *J Am Vener Dis Assoc* **3**:172, 1976

242. McKenna CH et al: The fluorescent treponemal antibody absorbed (FTA-ABS) test beading phenomenon in connective tissue diseases. *Mayo Clin Proc* **48**:545, 1973

243. Maskey DM et al: Specificity of the FTA-ABS test for syphilis: an evaluation. *JAMA* **207**:1683, 1969

244. Shore RN, Faricelli JA: Borderline and reactive FTA-ABS results in lupus erythematosus. *Arch Dermatol* **113**:37, 1977

245. Strobel PL, Kraus SJ: An electron microscopic study of the FTA-ABS "beading" phenomenon with lupus erythematosus sera, using ferritin-conjugated anti-human IgG. *J Immunol* **108**:1152, 1972

246. Deacon WE et al: Fluorescent treponemal antibody absorption (FTA-ABS) test for syphilis. *JAMA* **198**:624, 1966

247. Sepetjian M et al: New fluorescent antibody test for the serological diagnosis of syphilis. *Br J Vener Dis* **50**:331, 1974

248. Rudolph AH: The microhemagglutination assay for *Treponema pallidum* antibodies (MHA-TP), a new treponemal test for syphilis: where does it fit? *J Am Vener Dis Assoc* **3**:3, 1976

249. Rathlev T: Hemagglutination tests utilizing antigens from pathogenic and apathogenic *Treponema pallidum*. Geneva, WHO document, WHO/RES/77.65, 1965

250. Luger A, Spendlingwimmer I: Appraisal of the *Treponema pallidum* hemagglutination test. *Br J Vener Dis* **49**:181, 1973

251. Luger A, Spendlingwimmer I: Der *Treponema pallidum* Haemagglutinations test. *Wien Klin Wochenschr* **84**:657, 1973

252. Luger A, Spendlingwimmer I: Der Automatisierte Mikrohämagglutinations test mit *Treponema pallidum* Antigen. *Hautarzt* **25**:238, 1974

253. Ķobayashi S et al: Microcapsule agglutination test for *Treponema pallidum* antibodies: a new serodiagnostic test for syphilis. *Br J Vener Dis* **59**:1, 1983

254. Cox PM et al: Automated, quantitative microhemagglutination assay for *Treponema pallidum* antibodies. *Appl Microbiol* **18**:485, 1969

255. Kampmeier RH et al: A survey of 251 patients with acute syphilis treated in the collaborative penicillin study of 1943–1950. *Sex Transm Dis* **8**:266, 1981

256. Morrison-Plummer J et al: Enzyme-linked immunosorbent assay for the detection of serum antibody to outer membrane proteins of *T. pallidum*. *Br J Vener Dis* **59**:75, 1983

257. Pope V et al: Evaluation of the microenzyme-linked immunosorbent assay with *T. pallidum* antigen. *J Clin Microbiol* **15**:630, 1982

258. Larsen SA et al: Specificity, sensitivity, and reproducibility among the fluorescent treponemal antibody absorption, the microhaemagglutination assay for *Treponema pallidum* antibodies, and the haemagglutination treponemal test for syphilis. *J Clin Microbiol* **14**:441, 1981

259. Lindenschmidt EG, Müller A: A treponema-specific soluble antigen for an IgM- and IgG-TP-ABS-ELISA and its application for the serodiagnosis of syphilis. WHO/VDT/RES 81.369, 1981

260. Hunter FF et al: Sodium-desoycholate-extracted treponemal antigen in an enzyme-linked immunosorbent assay for syphilis. *J Clin Microbiol* **16**:483, 1982

261. Pedersen NS et al: Serodiagnosis of syphilis by an enzyme-linked immunosorbent assay for IgG antibodies against the Reiter treponeme flagellum. *Scand J Immunol* **15**:341, 1982

262. Scotti AT, Logan L: A specific IgM antibody test in neonatal congenital syphilis. *J Pediatr* **73**:242, 1968

263. Allansmith M et al: The development of immunoglobulin levels in man. *J Pediatr* **72**:276, 1968

264. Kaufman RE et al: The FTA-ABS (IgM) test for neonatal congenital syphilis: a critical review. *J Am Vener Dis Assoc* **1**:79, 1974

265. Rosen EU, Richardson NJ: A reappraisal of the value of the IgM fluorescent treponemal antibody absorption test in the diagnosis of congenital syphilis. *J Pediatr* **87**:38, 1975

266. Schmidt BL: Der Einsatz der Hochdruckflüssigkeitschromatographie in der Syphilisserologie. *Wien Med Wochenschr* **132**:547, 1982

267. Luger A: Serology of syphilis by the application of immunological methods, in *Proceedings of the XVIth Congressus internationalis Dermatologiae, Tokyo, 1983*. Tokyo, Univ of Tokyo Press, in press

268. Lindenschmidt E-G et al: Microenzyme-linked immunosorbent assay for the detection of specific IgM antibodies in human syphilis. *Br J Vener Dis* **59**:151, 1983

269. Schmidt BL: Solid phase haemabsorption: a method for rapid detection of *Treponema pallidum*-specific IgM. *Sex Transm Dis* **7**:53, 1980

270. Heise H, Doese D: Aktuelle Syphilisdiagnostik in der DDR. *Dermatol Monatsschr* **168**:501, 1982

271. Luger A et al: Die SPHA-Technik (Solid-Phase-Hämabsorption in der Syphilisserologie, einjährige Erfahrung im Routine betrieb). *Hautarzt* **33**:138, 1982

272. Heise H et al: Erste methodische Erfahrungen mit dem Solid Phase-Hämabsorption (SPHA)-Test in der DDR zum Nachweis einer Syphilis. *Dtsch Gesundheitsw* **37**:857, 1982

273. Luger A: Recent developments in the serological diagnosis of syphilis. WHO/VDT/RES 77.354, Geneva, 1977

274. Harner RE et al: The FTA-ABS test in late syphilis: a serologic study of 1,985 cases. *JAMA* **203**:545, 1968

275. Wilkinson AE, Rodin P: IgM-FTA test in syphilis in adults—its relation to clinical findings. *Br J Vener Dis* **52**:219, 1976

276. Rudolph AH: Examination of the cerebrospinal fluid in syphilis. *Cutis* **17**:749, 1976

277. Dattner B et al: Criteria for the management of neurosyphilis. *Am J Med* **10**:463, 1951

278. Delaney P: False positive serology in CSF associated with a spinal cord tumor. *Neurology (Minneap)* **26**:591, 1976

279. Madiedo G et al: False-positive VDRL and FTA in cerebrospinal fluid. *JAMA* **244**:688, 1980

280. McLean AJ, Munger IC: False positive Wassermanns in cerebrospinal fluid. *West J Surg* **46**:455, 1938

281. Gabay EL et al: Computerized tomographic findings in meningovascular syphilis: a case report. *Sex Transm Dis* **10**:39, 1983

282. Burke AW: Syphilis in a Jamaican psychiatric hospital: a review of 52 cases including 17 of neurosyphilis. *Br J Vener Dis* **48**:249, 1972

283. Escobar MR et al: Fluorescent antibody test for syphilis using cerebrospinal fluid: clinical correlation in 15 cases. *Am J Clin Pathol* **53**:886, 1970

284. Mahoney JDH et al: Evaluation of the CSF-FTA-ABS test in latent and tertiary syphilis. *Acta Derm Venereol (Stockh)* **52**:71, 1972

285. Jaffe HW et al: Tests for treponemal antibody in CSF. *Arch Intern Med* **138**:252, 1978

286. Schmidt BL, Luger A: Diagnosis of neurosyphilis by CSF-examination. WHO 80.360, Geneva, 1980

287. Müller F, Moskophides M: Estimation of the local production of antibodies to *Treponema pallidum* in the central nervous system of patients with neurosyphilis. *Br J Vener Dis* **59**:80, 1983

288. Schuman SH et al: Untreated syphilis in the male Negro. *J Chronic Dis* **2**:543, 1955

289. Kampmeier RH: Final report on the "Tuskegee syphilis study." *South Med J* **67**:1349, 1974

290. Kampmeier RH: Syphilis therapy: an historical perspective. *J Am Vener Dis Assoc* **3**:99, 1976

291. Moore JE: Unsolved clinical problems of syphilology. *Am J Syphilol* **23**:701, 1939

292. Moore JE et al: The treatment of latent syphilis. II. The clinical outcome of treatment. *Vener Dis Inform* **13**:371, 1932

293. Moore JE et al: The treatment of latent syphilis. III. Clinical progression and relapse, Wassermann fastness, and death. *Vener Dis Inform* **13**:389, 1932

294. Rockwell DH et al: The Tuskegee study of untreated syphilis—the 30th year of observation. *Arch Intern Med* **114**:792, 1964

295. Peters JJ et al: Untreated syphilis in the Negro male—pathologic findings in syphilitic and nonsyphilitic patients. *J Chronic Dis* **1**:127, 1955

296. Lourie EM, Collier HOJ: The therapeutic action of penicillin on *Spirochaeta recurrentis* and *Spirillum minus* in mice. *Ann Trop Med Parasitol* **37**:200, 1943

297. Mahoney EM: Penicillin treatment of early syphilis. A preliminary report. *Vener Dis Inform* **24**:355, 1943

298. Rein MF: Biopharmacology of syphilotherapy. *J Am Vener Dis* **3**:109, 1976

299. Idsøe O et al: Penicillin in the treatment of syphilis. *Bull WHO* **Suppl 1**:1, 1972

300. Faber WR et al: Treponemicidal levels of amoxicillin in cerebrospinal fluid after oral administration. *Sex Transm Dis* **10**:148, 1983

301. Harris JRW: Experimental syphilis, in *Recent Advances in Sexually Transmitted Diseases,* edited by RS Morton, JRW Harris. Edinburgh, Churchill Livingstone, 1975, p 148

302. Kaplan JM, McCracken GH: Clinical pharmacology of benzathine penicillin G in neonates with regard to its recommended use in congenital syphilis. *J Pediatr* **82**:1069, 1973

303. Mohr JA et al: Neurosyphilis and penicillin levels in cerebrospinal fluid. *JAMA* **236**:2208, 1976

304. Polnikorn N et al: Penicillin concentrations in cerebrospinal fluid after different treatment regimens for syphilis. *Br J Vener Dis* **56**:363, 1980

305. McCracken GH: Penicillin treatment for congenital syphilis, a critical reappraisal. *JAMA* **228**:855, 1974

306. Tramont EC: Persistence of *Treponema pallidum* following penicillin G therapy. Report of 2 cases. *JAMA* **236**:2206, 1976

307. Tramont EC: Persistence of *Treponema pallidum* following penicillin G therapy (letter). *JAMA* **237**:2719, 1977

308. Hardy JB et al: Failure of penicillin in a newborn with congenital syphilis. *JAMA* **212**:1345, 1970

309. Dunlop EMC: Persistence of treponemes after treatment. *Br Med J* **2**:577, 1972

310. Weit RJ, Milko DA: Isolation of spirochetes in perilymph despite prior anti-syphilitic treatment. *Arch Otolaryngol* **101**:104, 1975

311. Centers for Disease Control: Sexually transmitted diseases: treatment guidelines 1982. *MMWR* **31 (suppl 1)**:50s, 1982

312. Centers for Disease Control: Sexually transmitted diseases: treatment guidelines, 1982. *Rev Infect Dis* **4**:729, 1982

313. Brown ST: Update on recommendations for the treatment of syphilis. *Rev Infect Dis* **4 (suppl)**:837, 1982

314. Elliot WE: Treatment of primary syphilis. *J Am Vener Dis Assoc* **3**:128, 1976

315. Brown ST: Treatment of secondary syphilis. *J Am Vener Dis Assoc* **3**:136, 1976

316. Jaffee HW: Treatment of latent syphilis. *J Am Vener Dis Assoc* **3**:143, 1976

317. Schroeter AL et al: Treatment of early syphilis and reactivity of serological tests. *JAMA* **221**:471, 1972

318. Smith CA et al: Benzathine penicillin G in the treatment of syphilis. *Bull WHO* **15**:1087, 1956

319. Lassus A et al: The post-treatment disappearance of reactivity to treponemal and lipoidal tests in early syphilis. *Acta Derm Venereol (Stockh)* **50**:148, 1970

320. Fiumara NJ: Treatment of seropositive primary syphilis: an evaluation of 196 patients. *Sex Transm Dis* **4**:92, 1977

321. Fiumara NJ: Treatment of secondary syphilis: an evaluation of 204 patients. *Sex Transm Dis* **4**:96, 1977

322. Durst RD et al: Dose related seroreversal in syphilis. *Arch Dermatol* **108**:663, 1973

323. Nicolis G, Loucopoulos A: Cephalothin in the treatment of syphilis. *Br J Vener Dis* **50**:270, 1974

324. Lucus JB, Price EV: Cooperative evaluation of treatment for early syphilis. *Br J Vener Dis* **43**:244, 1967

325. Petzoldt D: Effect of spectinomycin on *T. pallidum* in incubating experimental syphilis. *Br J Vener Dis* **51**:305, 1975

326. Huigen E, Stolz E: Action of rifampin on *Treponema pallidum. Br J Vener Dis* **50**:465, 1974

327. Brause BD et al: Relative efficacy of clindamycin, erythromycin and penicillin in treatment of *Treponema pallidum* in skin syphilomas of rabbits. *J Infect Dis* **134**:93, 1976

328. Schroeter A et al: Therapy for incubating syphilis—effectiveness of gonorrhea therapy. *JAMA* **218**:711, 1971

329. Jefferiss FJG: Tests of cure in treated early and latent syphilis. *Br J Vener Dis* **39**:139, 1963

330. Nichols L, Beerman H: Late syphilis: a review of some of the recent literature. *Am J Med Sci* **254**:549, 1967

331. St John RK: Treatment of late benign syphilis: review of literature. *J Am Vener Dis Assoc* **3**:146, 1976

332. Rothenberg R: Treatment of neurosyphilis. *J Am Vener Dis Assoc* **3**:153, 1976

333. Wilner E, Brody JA: Prognosis of general paresis after treatment. *Lancet* **2**:1370, 1968

334. Hahn RD et al: Penicillin treatment of general paresis (dementia paralytica). *Arch Neurol Psychol* **81**:557, 1959

335. Yoder FW: Penicillin treatment of neurosyphilis. Are recommended doses sufficient? *JAMA* **232**:270, 1975

336. Hahn RD et al: Penicillin treatment of asymptomatic central nervous system syphilis: probability of progression to symptomatic neurosyphilis. *Arch Dermatol* **74**:355, 1956

337. St John RK: Treatment of cardiovascular syphilis. *J Am Vener Dis Assoc* **3**:148, 1976

338. Barnett CW, Small AA: The effect of treatment on the prognosis of cardiovascular syphilis. *Am J Syph Gonor Vener Dis* **34**:301, 1950

339. Edeiken J et al: Further observations on penicillin-treated cardiovascular syphilis. *Circ Res* **6**:267, 1952

340. Eisenberg H, Bradfonbrener M: Observations on penicillin treated cardiovascular syphilis. I. Uncomplicated aortitis. II. Complicated aortitis. *Am J Syph Gonor Vener Dis* **37**:439, 1953

341. Thompson SE: Treatment of syphilis in pregnancy. *J Am Vener Dis Assoc* **3**:159, 1976

342. Ingraham NR, Beerman H: The present status of penicillin in the treatment of syphilis in pregnancy and infantile congenital syphilis. *Am J Med Sci* **219**:433, 1950

343. Cole HN et al: Penicillin in the treatment of syphilis in pregnancy. *J Vener Dis Inform* **30**:95, 1949

344. Philipson A et al: Transplacental passage of erythromycin and clindamycin. *N Engl J Med* **288**:1219, 1973

345. Kiefer L et al: The placental transfer of erythromycin. *Am J Obstet Gynecol* **69**:174, 1955

346. Eisenberg GM et al: Bacterial susceptibilities to antibiotics. *Antibiot Chemother* **3**:1026, 1953

347. Heilman FR: Observations on erythromycin. *Proc Staff Meet Mayo Clin* **27**:285, 1952

348. Wick WE, Mallett GE: New analysis for the therapeutic efficacy of propionyl erythromycin and erythromycin base, in *Antimicrobial Agents and Chemotherapy: Proceedings of the Eighth Interscience Conference on Antimicrobial Agents and Chemotherapy, October 1968,* edited by GL Hobby. Bethesda, American Society for Microbiology, 1968, p 410

349. Bell SM: A comparison of absorption after oral administration of erythromycin estolate and erythromycin stearate. *Med J Aust* **2**:1280, 1971

350. Braun P: Hepatotoxicity of erythromycin (editorial). *J Infect Dis* **119**:300, 1969

351. Gladtke E: Effect on the child of drugs taken during late pregnancy. *German Med* **3**:135, 1973

352. Hashisaki P et al: Erythromycin failure in the treatment of syphilis in a pregnant woman. *Sex Transm Dis* **10**:36, 1983

353. Moffitt JM et al: Prediction of tetracycline-induced tooth discoloration. *J Am Dent Assoc* **88**:547, 1974

354. Platou RV et al: Early congenital syphilis: treatment of 252 patients with penicillin. *JAMA* **133**:10, 1947

355. Platou RV: Treatment of congenital syphilis with penicillin. *Adv Pediatr* **4**:39, 1949

356. Ingraham NR: The value of penicillin alone in the prevention and treatment of congenital syphilis. *Acta Derm Venereol (Stockh)* **31(suppl 24):**60, 1951

357. Platou RV, Kometani JT: Penicillin therapy of late congenital syphilis. *Pediatrics* **1:**601, 1948

358. Collart P et al: Significance of spiral organisms found, after treatment, in late human and experimental syphilis. *Br J Vener Dis* **40:**81, 1964

359. Brown ST: Adverse reactions in syphilis therapy. *J Am Vener Dis Assoc* **3:**172, 1976

360. Aronson IK, Soltani K: The enigma of the pathogenesis of the Jarisch-Herxheimer reaction. *Br J Vener Dis* **52:**313, 1976

361. Young E et al: The Jarisch-Herxheimer reaction in syphilitic hepatitis. *Am J Gastroenterol* **61:**476, 1974

362. Scott V, Clark EG: Syphilitic nephrosis as a manifestation of a renal Herxheimer reaction following penicillin therapy for early syphilis. *Am J Syphilol* **30:**463, 1946

363. Sheldon WH et al: The production of Herxheimer reactions by injection of immune serum in rabbits with experimental syphilis. *Am J Syphilol* **35:**405, 1951

364. Zacharias H, Nielsen E: Plasma kinins and the Jarisch-Herxheimer reaction. *Acta Derm Venereol (Stockh)* **54:**401, 1974

365. Aronson IK et al: Jarisch-Herxheimer reaction in complement-depleted rabbits. *Br J Vener Dis* **57:**226, 1981

366. James LP, Austen KF: Fatal systemic anaphylaxis in man. *N Engl J Med* **270:**597, 1964

367. Austen KF: Systemic anaphylaxis in the human being. *N Engl J Med* **291:**661, 1974

368. Fellner MJ: Penicillin allergy 1976: a review of reactions, detection, and current management. *Int J Dermatol* **15:**497, 1976

369. Rudolph AH, Price EV: Penicillin reactions among patients in venereal disease clinics. *JAMA* **223:**499, 1973

370. Odsøe O et al: Nature and extent of penicillin side-reactions with particular reference to fatalities from anaphylactic shock. *Bull WHO* **38:**159, 1968

371. Galpin JE et al: "Pseudoanaphylactic" reactions from inadvertent infusions of procaine penicillin G. *Ann Intern Med* **81:**358, 1974

372. Kraus SJ, Green RL: Pseudoanaphylactic reactions with procaine penicillin. *Cutis* **17:**765, 1976

373. Downham TF et al: Systemic toxic reactions to procaine penicillin G. *Sex Transm Dis* **5:**4, 1978

374. Menke HE, Pepplinkhuizen L: Reactions to aqueous procaine penicillin G. *Arch Dermatol* **108:**856, 1973

375. Hart G: Epidemiologic treatment of syphilis. *J Am Vener Dis Assoc* **3:**177, 1976

376. Moore MB et al: Epidemiologic treatment of contacts to infectious syphilis. *Public Health Rep* **78:**966, 1963

377. Idsøe O et al: A decade of reorientation in the treatment of venereal syphilis. *Bull WHO* **10:**507, 1954

378. Alexander LJ et al: Active treatment of syphilis. *Am J Syph Gonor Vener Dis* **33:**429, 1949

379. Schober PC et al: How infectious is syphilis? *Br J Vener Dis* **59:**217, 1983

380. Harris JRW: Non-venereal treponematoses, in *Recent Advances in Sexually Transmitted Diseases,* edited by RS Morton, JRW Harris. Edinburgh, Churchill Livingstone, 1975, p 124

381. Hardy PH: Pathogenic treponemes, in *The Biology of Parasitic Spirochetes,* edited by RC Johnson. New York, Academic Press, 1976, p 107

382. Willcox RR: The epidemiology of the spirochetoses—a worldwide view, in *The Biology of Parasitic Spirochetes,* edited by RC Johnson. New York, Academic Press, 1976, p 133

383. Cutler JC: Endemic syphilis, yaws and pinta, in *The Biology of Parasitic Spirochetes,* edited by RC Johnson. New York, Academic Press, 1976, p 365

384. Olansky S, Norins LC: Syphilis and other treponematoses, in *Dermatology in General Medicine,* edited by TB Fitzpatrick et al. New York, McGraw-Hill, 1971, p 124

385. Luger A: Non-venereally transmitted "endemic" syphilis in Vienna. *Br J Vener Dis* **48:**356, 1972

386. Kerdel-Vegas F: Yaws, in *Clinical Tropical Dermatology,* edited by O Canizares. Oxford/London/Edinburgh/Melbourne, Blackwell, 1975, p 79

387. Marquez F: Pinta, endemic syphilis, in *Clinical Tropical Dermatology,* edited by O Canizares. Oxford/London/Edinburgh/Melbourne, Blackwell, 1975, p 86

CHAPTER 202

CHANCROID

Andrew H. Rudolph

Definition

Chancroid is an acute, localized autoinoculable genitoinfectious disease caused by the gram-negative bacillus *Haemophilus ducreyi*. It is characterized clinically by necrotic ulcerations which occur at the site of inoculation. These are often accompanied by suppurative regional lymph nodes.

Historical aspects

Chancroid was and still is often confused with other sexually transmitted diseases. In 1852, Bassereau distinguished it from syphilis. The causative bacillus was described by Ducrey in 1889, but even then it was not accepted as the etiologic agent until early in the twentieth century when Koch's postulates had been repeatedly satisfied by producing the disease in humans from pure cultures of the organism.

Etiology

H. ducreyi is a short (0.5 by 1.5 to 2.0 μm), non-spore-bearing, non-acid-fast, gram-negative bacillus with rounded ends (Fig. 202-1) [1]. It is often considered a streptobacillus because of its tendency to develop chain formations, especially in culture. However, the exact taxonomy of *H. ducreyi* is unclear.

Incubation period

The incubation period of chancroid is generally accepted as being 3 to 5 days. It may, however, be as long as 2 weeks. Women may have a longer incubation period than men, their range being 7 to 18 days as compared with 1 to 14 days in men.

Epidemiology

Except for accidental infections of health care professionals, the disease is usually sexually transmitted. Chancroid is reported to occur more frequently in men than in women (male:female ratio, 10:1) [2], but this may be because internal lesions in women often go undetected and therefore unreported. Some evidence suggests that there are asymptomatic carriers of *H. ducreyi*, most commonly women prostitutes, who, while not showing evidence of clinical disease, are named repeatedly by clinically infected male contacts. Cervical cultures of these women may yield *H. ducreyi*. Additionally, a carrier state of *H. ducreyi* may remain after lesions have healed.

Incidence

Chancroid occurs endemically in most parts of the world. It is most common in underdeveloped countries, especially in tropical and subtropical areas, and is more prevalent among poor, urban, and seaport populations. Approximately 700 to 800 cases of chancroid are reported annually

in the United States; however, incomplete bacterial confirmation and lack of reporting make any figures of the actual incidence purely speculative. Although an uncommon disease in the United States, periodic outbreaks and mini-epidemics are often reported [3,4]. In some areas of the United States, a rise in reported cases has recently been documented and the disease may be becoming more common [5].

Clinical signs and symptoms

The disease begins as a macule or papule which becomes a vesicopustule that rapidly breaks down leaving a small, soft, nonindurated, sharply circumscribed, saucer-shaped ulceration. The edges of the ulcer are often ragged, undermined, and surrounded by an erythematous halo. The ulcer is usually covered by a necrotic, yellowish gray exudate and its base is composed of granulation tissue that bleeds easily on manipulation. In contrast to syphilis, the ulcers of chancroid are usually tender and often painful. Individual lesions may vary in diameter from 1 mm to 2 cm and are usually 2 to 5 in number. Adjacent lesions may coalesce to form large ulcerations.

In order of frequency, the lesions occur in the following sites: the preputial orifice, internal surface of prepuce, the frenulum and the glans (Fig. 202-2), the shaft of the penis (Fig. 202-3), the anal orifice in the male; the labia, clitoris, fourchette, vestibule, anus, and cervix in the female. Multiple lesions may develop rapidly by autoinoculation. Au-

Fig. 202-2 Chancroid. Sharply circumscribed ulcer on the glans. (*Courtesy of Dr. A. Eichmann, Zurich, Switzerland.*)

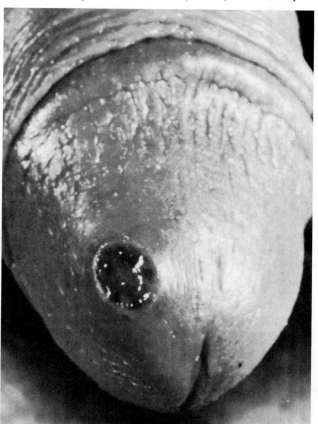

Fig. 202-1 Smear from blood of animal infected with *H. ducreyi*.

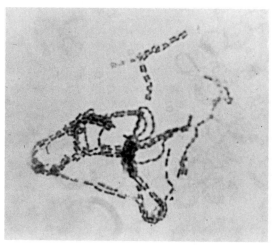

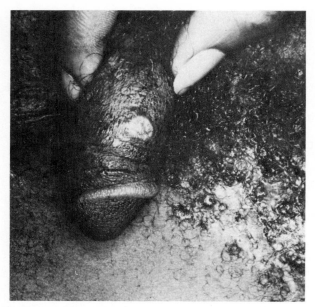

Fig. 202-3   Chancroid. Sharply circumscribed ulcer on the shaft of the penis. (Courtesy of Dr. Louis Fragola.)

toinoculation can also result in lesions located anywhere in the genital area, pubis, abdomen, and thigh. Extragenital lesions have been noted within the mouth or on the umbilicus, lips, breasts, and conjunctivae.

Systemic symptoms rarely occur, and, if present, usually consist of low-grade fever and mild malaise. Chancroid in women may be asymptomatic or be associated with minimal findings such as vaginitis.

Clinical variants

The most common types of chancroid encountered are those described above, i.e., the single ulcerative lesion or multiple ulcerations resulting from autoinoculation. However, a number of variants have been reported [6]:

1. Giant chancroid in which a single lesion extends peripherally and shows extensive ulceration. This form of chancroid may also follow rupture of an inguinal abscess.
2. Lesions that become confluent, spreading by extension and autoinoculation from an original lesion to give rise to a large serpiginous ulcer (ulcus molle serpiginosum). The groin or thigh may be involved. The ulcerations show little tendency to heal and may persist for months or years.
3. Phagadenic chancroid (ulcus molle gangrenosum), a variant felt to occur secondary to a superimposed fusospirochetosis. This form of chancroid may lead to rapid, profound destruction of tissue, but fortunately is rarely encountered.
4. Transient chancroid (chancre mou volant), which consists of a small ulcer that resolves spontaneously without scarring in 4 to 6 days. This may be followed 10 to 20 days later by an acute regional lymphadenitis which may subsequently suppurate. This type is rare and may be confused with lymphogranuloma venereum.
5. Follicular chancroid may be confused with a bacterial folliculitis and consists of small ulcers in a follicular distribution.

6. Papular chancroid (ulcus molle elevatum), which consists of small papules which become ulcerated and may resemble condylomata lata of secondary syphilis.

Bubo (Fig. 202-4)

Inguinal adenitis occurs in one-third to one-half of the cases of chancroid and appears within a few days to 2 weeks (average 1 week) after onset of the primary lesion. The adenitis, when present, may be unilateral or bilateral. Swollen, fixed, matted, erythematous tender nodes are noted first. These may subside without suppuration in over one-half of the cases. Nodes that do not suppurate become soft and fluctuant and, in contrast to the multilocular sinus tracts produced in lymphogranuloma venereum, unilocular suppuration occurs in chancroid. Healing may occur in a few weeks or a large chancroidal ulcer may develop around the opening of the inguinal abscess.

Complications

Suppuration of the inguinal lymph nodes is the most common complication and spontaneous rupture of the bubo may occur with resultant scarring and deformity. However, this is rare if early treatment is initiated. Balanitis, phimosis, and paraphimosis can occur and urethral fistules have been reported. In the phagadenic type of chancroid, superinfection may lead to rapid, marked destruction of the tissues of the penis. Mixed infections with other venereal diseases are also a possible complication. The patient should therefore be followed carefully by repeated clinical and laboratory examinations to exclude this possibility. In this regard, a small percentage of so-called typical chancroids are actually coexistent infections of chancroid and syphilis. In its initial stage, the mixed lesions have all the characteristics of chancroid, but after 15 to 20 days the characteristics of a syphilitic chancre become manifest, particularly if the patient was treated with sulfonamides. The possibility must also be kept in mind of

Fig. 202-4   Bubo in chancroid. (Courtesy of Dr. Louis Fragola.)

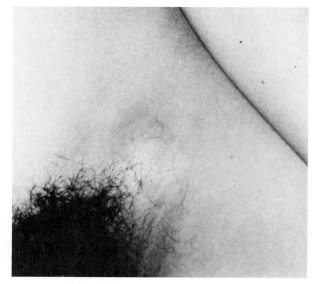

chancroid existing concurrently with lymphogranuloma venereum, granuloma inguinale, or herpes.

Clinical course

The disease is self-limited and systemic spread does not occur. Pain is the most frequent complaint and usually compels the patient to seek early medical care. Infection does not confer immunity and reinfections are possible.

Diagnosis

The diagnosis of chancroid is commonly made on clinical grounds and by excluding other sexually transmitted diseases. However, if possible, the diagnosis should be confirmed by one or more of the following procedures.

Smears

A smear from the base of the ulcer can be examined for *H. ducreyi*. The bacilli (1 to 2 μm by 0.5 μm) are usually found in small clusters or parallel chains of two or three organisms streaming along strands of mucus. This pattern has been described as a "school-of-fish" or "railroad track" appearance. *H. ducreyi* may also be found intracellularly in leukocytes. To obtain a specimen, the lesion should first be thoroughly cleaned with physiologic saline and carefully dried. Serous exudate from the undermined edge of the ulcer is collected on an applicator which is then carefully rolled onto a glass side in one direction only, so that the morphologic appearance of *H. ducreyi* is preserved. Moving the swab back and forth or smearing the exudate disrupts the school-of-fish pattern. The preparation is then stained with Gram's, Unna-Pappenheim, Wright's, Giemsa's, or pyronin methyl green stain. With the Unna-Pappenheim stain, *H. ducreyi* demonstrates a bipolar staining suggesting a "closed safety pin." Observance of organisms in a school-of-fish pattern demonstrating bipolar staining allows a fairly reliable diagnosis of chancroid. Reportedly, *H. ducreyi* can be demonstrated in approximately 50 percent of cases. However, the results from smears are often disappointing and difficult to interpret because of the presence of other organisms which may secondarily contaminate the ulcers and which have a morphologic appearance similar to that of *H. ducreyi*. Material obtained from aspiration of a bubo (Fig. 202-5) can also be similarly examined, and, because of the lack of contamination, may yield more conclusive results. In aspirates from a bubo the organism does not form any definite pattern. To prevent fistula formation, the bubo should be aspirated through normal skin.

Culture

H. ducreyi is traditionally described as a fastidious organism. Careful collection and isolation techniques are required to grow the organism in vitro. Growth is enhanced by high humidity and incubation at a temperature of 33° to 35°C; a 5% CO_2 atmosphere may also be beneficial [6]. Nutritional requirements may vary in different strains, and for optimal recovery several types of plating media should be used. In the past, the use of liquid clotted-blood media (i.e., clotted rabbit or human blood) has been the method

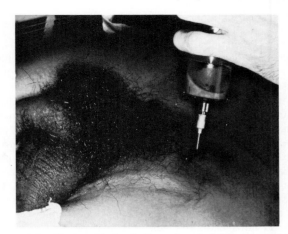

Fig. 202-5　Chancroid. Aspiration of material from a bubo.

most commonly recommended for the initial isolation of *H. ducreyi* [7]. In this regard, Borchardt and Hoke reported culturing *H. ducreyi* in 10 mL of their patients' blood which had been inactivated by warming for 30 min at 56°C in a water bath [8]. Margolis and Hood used 5 to 10 mL of their patient's blood that was inoculated with serum exudate from an ulcer and incubated at 35° C for 48 h in a 5% CO_2-enriched atmosphere [9]. A presumptive diagnosis of chancroid was then made by the identification of gram-negative bacilli from this isolation media. However, other organisms can have an appearance similar to *H. ducreyi* and for its definitive identification, growth on solid media is required. Recently, Kraus et al [10], Hammond et al [11], and Sottnek et al [12] have used a selective solid media containing vancomycin to isolate the organism. The vancomycin inhibits the growth of contaminant bacteria which are often found in chancroidal lesions but does not inhibit the growth of *H. ducreyi* which is resistant to vancomycin. An even more simple medium was used by Carpenter et al [13], who were able to isolate the organism by direct inoculation onto a solid medium consisting of a chocolate agar plate containing 1% IsoVitaleX. The growth of *H. ducreyi* on a solid medium not only facilitates a more definite diagnosis of chancroid but also allows determination of the antibiotic sensitivity of the isolate. This is important because of the changing patterns of resistance to antibiotics that *H. ducreyi* has exhibited.

Biopsy

Biopsy may be a diagnostic aid, but in most cases is not practical. However, typical histologic findings, when present, are sufficiently distinct to permit a presumptive diagnosis of chancroid in many instances. The classical lesion of chancroid is characterized by three vertically arranged zones. Proceeding from the floor of the ulcer inward, these include: (1) a superficial necrotic zone consisting of polymorphonuclear leukocytes, erythrocytes, fibrin, and necrotic tissue; (2) a zone of new blood vessel formation showing marked endothelial proliferation; the endothelial proliferation often leads to occlusion of the vessel lumen, resulting in thrombosis and subsequent necrosis; and (3) a deep zone consisting of a dense infiltrate of lymphocytes and plasma cells. *H. ducreyi* is only rarely demonstrated in tissue sections.

Miscellaneous tests

The Ito-Reenstierna skin test is now of historical importance only. The antigen, made from a suspension of killed *H. ducreyi,* gave a high incidence of nonspecific reactions and is no longer commercially available.

Autoinoculation in which the material from lesions was inoculated into scarified areas of skin of the forearm or thigh with the intent of developing typical chancroidal ulcers which were then smeared for *H. ducreyi* is seldom used as a diagnostic test today. Both false-positive and false-negative reactions were experienced with this technique, and other pathogens could simulate the clinical lesions and the findings on smear.

Complement fixation tests are no longer employed as they are nonspecific and yield both false-positive and false-negative reactions.

An indirect fluorescent antibody technique has been developed for the identification of *H. ducreyi* in culture [14]. However, this technique has not yet been applied to examination of smears from clinical lesions.

Differential diagnosis

Unfortunately, exclusion remains a common method of diagnosing chancroid. Despite the inability to identify or isolate *H. ducreyi,* a presumptive diagnosis of chancroid may be made if: (1) the signs and symptoms are typical, and (2) other venereal diseases are eliminated. Genital herpes simplex, syphilis, lymphogranuloma venereum, granuloma inguinale, infected human bites, and secondarily infected traumatic abrasions must be considered in the differential diagnosis [15]. Even when the diagnosis of chancroid is made, the possibility of mixed infections must be considered. To eliminate the possibility of herpes simplex, appropriately stained materials scraped from the ulcer base should be negative for multinucleated viral giant cells and culture for herpes simplex virus should be negative.

Because of the frequent association of chancroid with syphilis (10 to 15 percent of cases), the possibility of syphilis must be eliminated and at least one, but preferably three, dark-field examinations on three consecutive days should be negative and repeated serologic tests for syphilis should be nonreactive. Serologic tests for syphilis should be obtained initially and then monthly for three successive months. Lymphogranuloma venereum should be eliminated by a negative lymphogranuloma venereum complement-fixation test (titer less than 1:16) and by a failure to demonstrate a significant rise in the titer on repeated testing. "Crush" preparations of tissue stained for Donovan bodies of granuloma inguinale should be negative.

Treatment

The antibiotic susceptibility patterns of *H. ducreyi* have changed, making obsolete the treatments previously recommended. In the past the sulfonamides and tetracyclines, either alone or in combination therapy, were recommended for the treatment of chancroid. However, numerous studies have documented the resistance of *H. ducreyi* to the sulfonamides and to tetracycline [16–19]. Thus, these drugs are no longer recommended [20]. Similarly, doxycycline and minocin, which have proved effective in small numbers of patients, must be suspect [18]. Ideally, the antibiotic sensitivity of the isolate should be obtained prior to initiating antibiotic therapy.

Currently, erythromycin 500 mg orally 4 times a day for 10 days is recommended by the Centers for Disease Control as the treatment of choice for chancroid [21]. An alternative regimen is 800 mg sulfamethoxazole and 160 mg trimethoprim orally 2 times a day for 10 days [21]. Erythromycin has not been studied as much as the sulfamethoxazole/trimethoprim combination, but recent studies have shown it to be very effective in the treatment of chancroid [10,13]. If erythromycin is used, this author feels it should be given on a schedule which would also be effective in treating any possible coexisting syphilis, i.e., erythromycin 500 mg orally 4 times a day for 15 days. Since gastrointestinal side effects are common in patients taking this amount of erythromycin, it must be emphasized that patients complete the full course of therapy. *H. ducreyi* has been shown to be susceptible to the sulfamethoxazole/trimethoprim combination in vitro and also in numerous clinical studies [17,20,22]. An advantage of the sulfamethoxazole/trimethoprim combination is that it is not treponemicidal; therefore, it will not mask primary syphilis [22]. Because of the possibility of a mixed infection with syphilis, a therapeutic trial using sulfamethoxazole/trimethoprim is possible without precluding a diagnosis of syphilis by dark-field or serologic examination. In those patients with chancroid whose isolates are resistant to the above antibiotics, intramuscular streptomycin, intramuscular kanamycin, or intravenous cephalothin have been used successfully [20,23]. Neither penicillin nor ampicillin is effective in treating chancroid.

Local hygiene is important and the involved area should be kept as clean as possible. Saline soaks or compresses may help in this regard. Once the diagnosis of syphilis is eliminated, cleansing with hydrogen peroxide or povidone-iodine may be helpful. Suppurative nodes should not be incised but, if necessary, may be aspirated to prevent spontaneous rupture and sinus tract formation. A large syringe and an 18-gauge or larger needle should be used and the fluctuant buboes entered laterally through normal skin (Fig. 202-5). In patients with phimosis, a circumcision may be necessary, but, if possible, this procedure should be withheld until all active lesions have healed. Regular follow-up evaluation of patients should be encouraged until the lesions are completely healed.

Patients should be advised to abstain from sexual activity until all clinical lesions have cleared. Sexual contacts of the patient should be sought, examined, and if necessary, treated. Epidemiologic treatment of contacts has been recommended and many feel that these individuals should be treated even if clinical disease cannot be demonstrated, since asymptomatic carriage of *H. ducreyi* is possible.

References

1. Marsch WC et al: Ultrastructural detection of *Haemophilus ducreyi* in biopsies of chancroid. *Arch Dermatol Res* **263:**153, 1978
2. Alergant CD: Chancroid. *Practitioner* **209:**624, 1972

3. Lykke-Olesen L et al: Epidemic of chancroid in Greenland. *Lancet* 1:654, 1979

4. Nayyar KC et al: Rising incidence of chancroid in Rotterdam: epidemiological, clinical, diagnostic, and therapeutic aspects. *Br J Vener Dis* **55**:439, 1979

5. Felman YM, Nikitas JA: Chancroid. *Cutis* **26**:464, 1980

6. Gaisin A, Heaton CL: Chancroid: alias the soft chancre. *Int J Dermatol* **13**:188, 1975

7. Deacon WE et al: VDRL chancroid studies. I. A simple procedure for the isolation and identification of *Haemophilus ducreyi*. *J Invest Dermatol* **26**:399, 1956

8. Borchardt KA, Hoke AW: Simplified laboratory technique for diagnosis of chancroid. *Arch Dermatol* **102**:188, 1970

9. Margolis RJ, Hood AF: Chancroid: diagnosis and treatment. *J Am Acad Dermatol* **6**:493, 1982

10. Kraus SJ et al: Pseudogranuloma inguinale caused by *Haemophilus ducreyi*. *Arch Dermatol* **118**:494, 1982

11. Hammond GW et al: Comparison of specimen collection and laboratory techniques for isolation of *Haemophilus ducreyi*. *J Clin Microbiol* **7**:39, 1978

12. Sottnek FO et al: Isolation and identification of *Haemophilus ducreyi* in a clinical study. *J Clin Microbiol* **12**:170, 1980

13. Carpenter JL et al: Treatment of chancroid with erythromycin. *Sex Transm Dis* **8**:192, 1982

14. Denys GA et al: An indirect fluorescent antibody technique for *Haemophilus decreyi*. *Health Lab Sci* **15**:128, 1978

15. Chapel T et al: The microbiological flora of penile ulcerations. *J Infect Dis* **137**:50, 1978

16. Albritton WL et al: Plasmid-mediated sulfonamide resistance in *Haemophilus ducreyi*. *Antimicrob Agents Chemother* **21**:159, 1982

17. Fitzpatrick JE et al: Treatment of chancroid: comparison of sulfamethoxazole-trimethoprim with recommended therapies. *JAMA* **246**:1804, 1981

18. Hammond GW et al: The treatment of chancroid: comparison of one week of sulfisoxazole with single dose doxycycline. *J Antimicrob Chemother* **5**:261, 1979

19. Handsfield HH et al: Molecular epidemiology of *Haemophilus ducreyi* infections. *Ann Intern Med* **95**:315, 1981

20. Fitzpatrick JE, Aeling SL: Chancroid: a review with emphasis on recent changes in incidence and treatment. *J Assoc Milit Dermatol* **8**:31, 1982

21. Centers for Disease Control: Chancroid—California. *MMWR* **31**:173, 1982

22. Rajan VS, Pang R: Treatment of chancroid with Bactrim. *Ann Acad Med Singapore* **8**:63, 1979

23. Hadley AT: Chancroid. *Am Fam Physician* **20**:83, 1979

CHAPTER 203

LYMPHOGRANULOMA VENEREUM

Richard B. Rothenberg

Definition

Lymphogranuloma venereum (LGV) is a sexually transmitted disease of chlamydial etiology with protean clinical manifestations involving the lymphatic system. Though infrequently diagnosed in the United States, its importance lies in the differential diagnosis of syndromes involving lymphadenopathy, genital lesions, proctocolitis, or rectal stricture.

History

The disease has a colorful nosologic history including such designations as tropical or climatic bubo; third, fourth, fifth, or sixth venereal disease; Nicholas-Favre disease—but the current name is now universally accepted. The first major clinical description appeared in 1913 and inclusion bodies in material from lesions were demonstrated 10 years later. In 1930, the disease was produced experimentally by intracerebral inoculation of monkeys with pus from a bubo of LGV [1]. Rake et al [2] grew the organism, then thought to be a filterable virus, in the yolk sac of embryonated eggs in 1940. Development of a number of techniques in the past 20 years, including the use of 5-iodo-2-deoxyuridine-treated McCoy cells for tissue culture [3] and the microimmunofluorescence test [4], has greatly enhanced the study of the chlamydial diseases.

Epidemiology

The resurgence of interest in the laboratory aspects of LGV has not had a parallel in clinical diagnosis. Though probably worldwide in occurrence, reporting is sporadic. In the United States, the reported incidence is continuing to decline (Table 203-1). The chief foci of activity are the District of Columbia and southeastern United States, affecting blacks of low socioeconomic status predominantly. Age-specific attack rates are highest in the 20- to 40-year-old group. LGV organisms have been isolated from cervices of asymptomatic female contacts, who may serve as an important reservoir of infection [5].

Etiology

The disease is caused by *Chlamydia trachomatis* (LGV types I, II, and III) [6]. In the past, differentiation of trachoma inclusion conjunctivitis (TRIC) and LGV organisms rested on (1) clinical source, and (2) increased mouse toxicity of the latter. Since the development of the microimmunofluorescence test, these agents and their sub-

Table 203-1. Reported cases of LGV in the United States, 1970–1976

Year	Cases
1970	621
1971	699
1972	763
1973	410
1974	397
1975	353
1976	365

groups are much more accurately distinguished, permitting more meaningful epidemiologic investigation of the syndromes with which they are associated. The term *Chlamydia* replaces the older term *Bedsonia* for these organisms, whose method of reproduction, structure, metabolism, and DNA and RNA content make them similar to *Rickettsia* [7]. Understanding of the microbiology of chlamydial organisms has burgeoned in recent years, but considerably more attention has devolved on other chlamydial syndromes (pelvic inflammatory diseases, urethral syndrome, pneumonia, etc.) [8].

Clinical manifestations

LGV is contracted by direct contact with infectious secretions, almost exclusively through sexual activity. The portal of entry and the initial symptoms are determined by the nature of the sex act, and though usually genital, it may be rectal or pharyngeal. The incubation period varies from 3 to 30 days if primary lesions occur, but it may be longer if adenopathy is the only manifestation [9]. The period of infectiousness and transmission rates are not clearly defined.

Acute and chronic manifestations characterize both the genital (or inguinal) and rectal syndromes. The primary lesion is a 5- to 8-mm, soft, erythematous, painless erosion

(Fig. 203-1), that heals spontaneously in a few days. Occasionally, a button-like papule may appear which is also transient. Such lesions are reported by a fourth to a third of patients. Secondary inguinal adenopathy begins 1 to 2 weeks after the primary lesion as discrete, movable, tender nodes which later coalesce to form a firm, fist-sized, elongated, immovable mass. These may occur above and below Poupart's ligament, giving rise to the "groove" sign (Fig. 203-2). Nodes are bilateral in one-third of cases [9]. Rupture of fluctuant nodes may lead to chronic sinus formation. Initially, the overlying skin is often slightly reddened and edematous but it later may become thickened and develop a characteristic purplish hue. Generalized systemic symptoms such as fever, chills, and malaise may be prominent. Meningoencephalitis, hepatosplenomegaly, arthralgia, stiff neck, and headache may also occur [5]. In untreated cases, the lymphadenopathy usually subsides spontaneously in 8 to 12 weeks [9]. Late complications of the male inguinal syndrome are rare. Elephantiasis of the penis and scrotum characterized by infiltrative, ulcerative, and fistular lesions occur in approximately 4 percent of cases [9]. Recent reports of LGV mimicking cervical lymphoma in a homosexual male practicing fellatio [11] and a heterosexual male engaging in cunnilingus [12] emphasize the need for a detailed history. The physician must be alert, as well, to the potential for local community outbreaks [13].

The acute rectal syndrome occurs more frequently in women than men. In the latter, direct inoculation of the anal canal is believed to be the mode of entry, whereas the internal lymphatic drainage of the proximal two-thirds of the vagina has been invoked as the source for women. In

Fig. 203-2 Lymphogranuloma venereum. Firm, immovable mass above Poupart's ligament giving rise to the so-called groove sign. (Courtesy of Dr. Louis Fragola.)

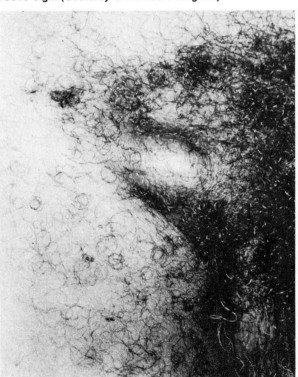

Fig. 203-1 Lymphogranuloma venereum. Soft, painless erosion on the frenulum. (Courtesy of Dr. Louis Fragola.)

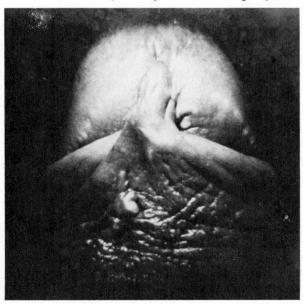

both sexes, acute manifestations include rectal pain, tenesmus, and mucosanguineous rectal discharge, with typical findings of proctocolitis on sigmoidoscopy. It is important to distinguish LGV from other forms of inflammatory bowel disease, particularly in homosexual men [14]. The major late manifestation is rectal stricture. In women, late scarring, fistulas, ulceration, and elephantiasis of the perineum, called esthiomene, may require radical surgical intervention [15].

A variety of dermatologic conditions has been reported in association with acute manifestations, including erythema nodosum, erythema multiforme, scarlatiniform exanthem, and urticaria [1]. In addition, photosensitivity has been reported in as many as 35 percent of patients, occasionally associated with conjunctivitis, joint involvement, and erythema nodosum [1]. Sonck [16] observed a photosensitivity reaction in 140 cases of 400 studied with LGV. This was manifest 1 to 2 months after onset of bubo formation and occurred in 60 percent of the chronic and about 20 percent of subacute cases. Punctiform, red papules appeared on the skin 30 min to 3 h after exposure to sunlight. Accompanying this reaction was conjunctivitis in 19 percent, joint involvement in 33 percent, and erythema nodosum in 16 percent of those with the photosensitivity reaction. The possible allergic or autoimmune nature of these phenomena is supported by the frequent appearance of biologic false-positive tests for syphilis (estimated at 20 percent of cases), the high incidence of cryoprecipitins and rheumatoid factor, and the high serum levels of IgA and IgG in both acute and chronic syndromes [17].

Pathology

Pathologic material is usually nonspecific. Primary ulcers are characterized by an exudate of fibrin, polymorphonuclear leukocytes, and cellular debris [18]. Skin test sites or rectal lesions may contain epithelioid nodules, plasma cells, and occasional giant cells, but these changes are not diagnostic. Stellate triangular abscesses may be observed in lymph node biopsies and are characteristic, but not pathognomonic, of LGV [19].

Diagnosis

The three major methods of diagnosis are: (1) isolation and identification of the organism, (2) the Frei test, (3) chlamydial group complement-fixation test. Culture for *Chlamydia* is now more commonly available in the United States. Typing of organisms is less readily available but may be important in distinguishing non-LGV strains that may cause a similar clinical picture [20]. The Frei test, an intradermal inoculation of killed LGV organisms, was in the past the mainstay of diagnosis. More recently its sensitivity and specificity have been seriously questioned [21] and the test is now of historic interest only, as the antigen is no longer commercially available.

The diagnosis is made on the basis of clinical findings and the complement-fixation test. Although theoretically positive in any chlamydial infection, less than 3 percent of the general population has a titer as high as 1:16 [21]. However, Schachter and Dawson reported that 40 to 50 percent of women with uncomplicated TRIC-agent cervical infection had titers of 1:16 to 1:32; similar titers in men

with TRIC-associated urethritis occurred in 15 to 20 percent [22]. The complement-fixation test generally becomes positive 4 weeks after infection, and is usually positive when buboes are present. A fourfold titer change is, of course, the best diagnostic guide, and a follow-up specimen should be obtained whenever possible. In established cases, however, titers may not change with adequate therapy.

Differential diagnosis

In view of the nonspecific nature of signs and symptoms, acute LGV should be considered in the differential diagnosis of syphilis, herpes progenitalis, granuloma inguinale, and chancroid as well as bacterial, fungal, and tuberculous skin infection. Adenopathy may require consideration of benign and malignant lymphoproliferative disorders (e.g., infectious mononucleosis, Hodgkin's disease), particularly in the presence of oral and cervical infection. Late manifestations must be distinguished from neoplastic skin disease, filariasis, rectal cancer, inflammatory bowel disease, and hidradenitis suppurativa.

Treatment

Antibiotics are effective in the acute illness, but may have little or no effect on late lymphatic pathology. Standard regimens include sulfisoxazole 1 g 4 times daily for 3 weeks, or tetracycline 500 mg 4 times daily for 3 weeks. Other tetracycline derivatives such as minocycline have also been demonstrated to be effective. Buboes should be aspirated, rather than incised and drained, to avoid formation of fistulous tracts. With treatment, prognosis for avoidance of late complications is excellent.

References

1. Koteen H: Lymphogranuloma venereum. *Medicine (Baltimore)* **24**:2, 1945
2. Rake G et al: Agent of lymphogranuloma venereum in the yolk sac of the developing chick embryo. *Proc Soc Biol Med* **43**:332, 1940
3. Wentworth BB, Alexander ER: Isolation of *Chlamydia trachomatis* by use of 5-iodo-2-deoxyuridine-treated cells. *Appl Microbiol* **27**:912, 1974
4. Wang SP: A microimmunofluorescence method. Study of antibody response to TRIC organisms, in *Trachoma and Related Disorders Caused by Chlamydia Agents*, edited by RL Nichols. Amsterdam, Excerpta Medica, 1971, p 273
5. Becker LE: Lymphogranuloma venereum. *Int J Dermatol* **15**:26, 1976
6. Schachter J: Chlamydial infection. *N Engl J Med* **298**:428, 490, 540, 1978
7. Moulder JW: The relationship of the psittacosis group (*Chlamydia*) to bacteria and viruses. *Annu Rev Microbiol* **20**:107, 1966
8. Terho P: *Chlamydia trachomatis* and clinical genital infections: a general review. *Infection* **10 (suppl 1)**:S5, 1982
9. Conizares O: *Modern Diagnosis and Treatment of the Minor Venereal Diseases*. Springfield, IL, Charles C Thomas, 1954, p 62
10. Hopsu-Havu VK, Sonck CE: Infiltrative, ulcerative, and fistular lesions of the penis due to lymphogranuloma venereum. *Br J Vener Dis* **49**:193, 1973

11. Thorsteinsson SB et al: Lymphogranuloma venereum. A cause of cervical lymphadenopathy. *JAMA* **235**:1882, 1976

12. Andrada MT et al: Oral lymphogranuloma venereum and cervical lymphadenopathy: case report. *Milit Med* **139**:99, 1974

13. McLelland BA, Anderson PC: Lymphogranuloma venereum. Outbreak in a university community. *JAMA* **235**:56, 1976

14. Geller SA et al: Rectal biopsy in early lymphogranuloma venereum proctitis. *Am J Gastroenterol* **74**:433, 1980

15. Hirschberg SM, Horton CE: Radical perineal resection for far-advanced lymphogranuloma venereum. *Plast Reconstr Surg* **51**:217, 1973

16. Sonck CE: On the occurrence of solar dermatitis in lymphogranuloma inguinale. *Acta Derm Venereol (Stockh)* **20**:529, 1939

17. Sonck CE et al: Autoimmune serum factors in active and inactive lymphogranuloma venereum. *Br J Vener Dis* **49**:67, 1973

18. Smith EB, Custer RP: The histopathology of lymphogranuloma venereum. *J Urol* **63**:546, 1950

19. Robbins SL (ed): *Pathology.* Philadelphia, WB Saunders, 1967, p 366

20. Schachter J: Confirmatory serodiagnosis of lymphogranuloma venereum proctitis may yield false-positive results due to other chlamydial infections of the rectum. *Sex Transm Dis* **8**:26, 1981

21. Schachter J et al: Lymphogranuloma venereum. I. Comparison of the Frei test, complement-fixation test and isolation of the agent. *J Infect Dis* **120**:372, 1969

22. Schachter J, Dawson C: Lymphogranuloma venereum. *JAMA* **236**:915, 1976

CHAPTER 204

GRANULOMA INGUINALE

Richard B. Rothenberg

Definition

Granuloma inguinale is an indolent, progressive, ulcerative and granulomatous skin disease caused by *Calymmatobacterium granulomatis*. It is probably spread by both venereal and nonvenereal contact [1]. The disease exhibits no tendency to go into spontaneous remission and in later stages may be severely debilitating.

History

The first description is credited to McLoed in 1882, who termed the illness *serpiginous ulcer*. At least a dozen other names have been employed, but, aside from granuloma inguinale, only the term *donovanosis* persists. Donovan, in 1905, first described the bipolar-staining, intracellular inclusions in macrophages from lesion exudate (termed *Donovan bodies*). These were first grown in embryonated eggs in 1943 and finally in artificial media in 1959.

Epidemiology

The disease has been recognized worldwide, but its major incidence appears to be limited to endemic foci in tropical and subtropical environments. Fewer than 100 cases per year are reported in the United States. Certain marked racial and ethnic predilections have been noted: higher incidence in blacks than whites in the United States; in natives other than Europeans in Papua, New Guinea; in Hindus than Mohammedans in India. There is no evidence for specific racial susceptibility. Socioeconomic status and living conditions may be a major risk factor.

The venereal nature of transmission has been debated for many years, and is supported by (1) the genital site of early lesions, (2) the prominence of perirectal disease in male homosexuals, and (3) the predominant occurrence of infection in the sexually active age group [2]. The possibility of nonvenereal transmission is suggested by (1) the occurrence of disease in sexually inactive children, (2) the infrequency of infection in partners exposed repeatedly to open lesions, (3) the infrequency of infection in sexually active people (e.g., prostitutes) in endemic areas [1,3].

Etiology and pathogenesis

The causative agent (formerly termed *Donovania granulomatis*) is a gram-negative rod with some antigenic properties in common with the *Klebsiella* group. It has been demonstrated in fecal flora [4], and there is electron microscopic evidence that it may share bacteriophage with Enterobacteriaceae [5,6]; however, studies using light microscopy in plastic-embedded material with polychromatic staining demonstrate bacteria within vacuoles of cells, and thereby fail to corroborate the presence of bacteriophage-like entities [7]. These data support the hypothesis that disease transmission may occur through fecal contamination in environments with lower levels of hygiene, and may also explain the occurrence in males practicing rectal intercourse.

Antibody against the organism may be detected by complement-fixation test. Circulating antibody which does not affect the relentless course of untreated disease has raised the possibility that a defect in cell-mediated immunity may predispose to clinical illness as is the case in other diseases caused by intracellular organisms (leprosy, tuberculosis) [8].

Clinical manifestations

The primary lesion may be a buttonlike papule, a subcutaneous nodule, or an ulcer. The incubation period is poorly defined and may range from 2 weeks to 3 months. Experimental human inoculation has produced lesions after a latency of 21 days [2]. Papules or nodules are quickly denuded and ulcerate within several days. The subcutaneous nodule, if large enough, may be mistaken for a lymph node, giving rise to the term *pseudobubo*. True adenopathy is rare. The penis, scrotum, and glans are the most common sites of primary lesions in males, and, in females, the labia minora, mons veneris, and fourchette. Typically, the disease then spreads, either by direct extension or autoinoculation, to the inguinal and perineal skin.

Four major clinical varieties are described [9]: (1) the *nodular* variety (Fig. 204-1) is characterized by soft, red nodules which eventually ulcerate and present a bright-red granulating surface; (2) the *ulcerovegetative* variety (most common) (Fig. 204-2) develops from the nodular type and consists of large, spreading, exuberant ulcers (Fig. 204-3); (3) the *hypertropic* form (relatively rare) exhibits a proliferative reaction and formation of large vegetating masses; (4) the *cicatricial* type produces spreading scar tissue formation which is a direct consequence of disease spread per se, rather than healing. Superinfection with fusospirochetal organisms may give rise to necrotic lesions with massive tissue destruction, similar to the situation in so-called phagedenic chancroid. The disease may rarely progress to destroy genital and inguinal tissue, as in the case of mutilating granuloma inguinale described by Fritz et al [10]. Elephantiasis of the penis, scrotum, or vulva may follow involvement with granuloma inguinale.

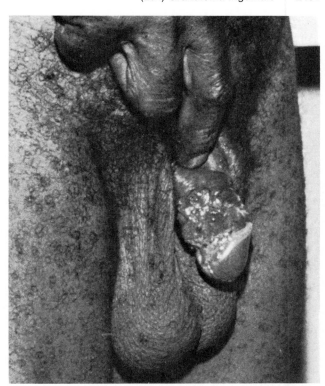

Fig. 204-2 Granuloma inguinale: large ulcerovegetative type. (Courtesy of Dr. Gavin Hart, Adelaide, Australia.)

Fig. 204-3 Granuloma inguinale: exuberant ulcer. (Courtesy of Dr. A. Eichmann, Zurich, Switzerland.)

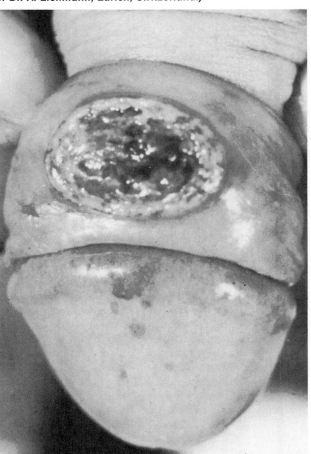

Fig. 204-1 Granuloma inguinale: early nodular variety with central ulceration. (Courtesy of Dr. Gavin Hart, Adelaide, Australia.)

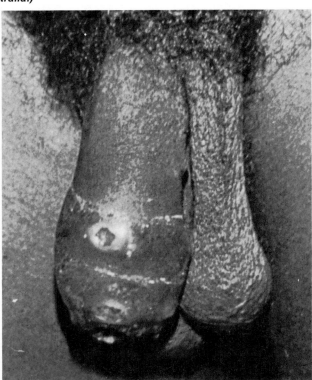

Extragenital lesions are reported in 6 percent of cases, with occasional systemic involvement, notably in gastrointestinal tract and bone [11] including the bony orbit and orbital skin [12]. Chronic ulcerating oral mucosa lesions may occur with or without associated genital lesions [13,14]. The disease shows no tendency toward spontaneous healing, though lesions may be stable for long periods of time. There is believed to be an increased incidence of squamous cell carcinoma of the genital skin in granuloma inguinale [15].

Pathology

Histologically, the skin exhibits a massive cellular reaction, predominantly polymorphonuclear, with occasional plasma cells and rare lymphocytes [6]. The marginal epithelium demonstrates acanthosis, elongation of rete pegs, and pseudoepitheliomatous hyperplasia [2]. These latter changes are highly suggestive of early malignancy and squamous cell carcinoma. Hypertropic and cicatricial forms demonstrate the appropriate increase in fibrous tissue. Typically, large mononuclear cells containing numerous cytoplasmic inclusions (the Donovan bodies) are scattered throughout the lesions. These are considered to be diagnostic of granuloma inguinale [2].

Diagnosis

The diagnosis of granuloma inguinale is usually made by history, clinical appearance, and a crush or touch preparation stained with Wright's or Giemsa's stain from a punch biopsy specimen. Superficial curettings are usually inadequate because of bacterial contamination. Donovan bodies are seen as deeply staining, bipolar, safety pin–shaped rods in the cytoplasm of macrophages (Fig. 204-4). Diagnosis may require multiple specimens since clinical varieties differ in the quantity of organisms present. The complement-fixation test is not currently in general use for routine diagnosis.

In its typical form, granuloma inguinale is easily differentiated from other ulcerative and granulomatous skin diseases, but atypical forms may be difficult to distinguish from syphilis, chancroid, lymphogranuloma venereum, tuberculosis of skin, cutaneous amebiasis, and filariasis, Squamous cell carcinoma with metastases may be closely mimicked by granuloma inguinale and its associated osteolytic bone lesions.

Treatment

Numerous drugs have been found useful in granuloma inguinale, including streptomycin, chloramphenicol, tetracycline, ampicillin, and gentamycin, but controlled trials are not available. Tetracycline, 500 mg 4 times a day for 3 to 4 weeks, appeared to be a good initial choice, but resistance to this therapy, alone or in combination with sulfisoxazole, was observed in U.S. military personnel in Vietnam. Ampicillin was successful in all but 2 of 31 cases of granuloma inguinale acquired in Vietnam, with complete healing of the local lesions which occurred primarily on the penis or in the groin. In the same series, lincomycin

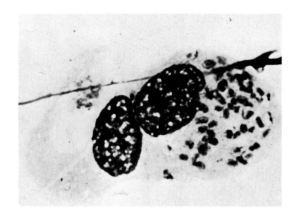

Fig. 204-4 Granuloma inguinale: tissue smear showing Donovan bodies, which are gram-negative and readily stained with Giemsa's stain.

was successfully used in penicillin-allergic individuals [16]. Response may be monitored by clinical appearance and serial biopsies examined for persistent presence of Donovan bodies. In early cases prognosis for complete healing is good. In late cases, irreparable tissue destruction may have supervened and radical surgery may be required.

References

1. Goldberg J: Studies on granuloma inguinale. VII. Some considerations of the disease. *Br J Vener Dis* **40:**140, 1964
2. Rajam RV, Rangiah PN: Donovanosis (granuloma inguinale, granuloma venereum). *WHO Monogr Ser,* no. 24, 1954
3. Kuberski T: Granuloma inguinale (donovanosis). *Sex Transm Dis* **7:**29, 1980
4. Goldberg J: Studies on granuloma inguinale. V. Isolation of bacterium resembling *Donovania granulomatis* from the faeces of a patient with granuloma inguinale. *Br J Vener Dis* **38:**99, 1959
5. Kuberski T et al: Ultrastructure of *Calymmatobacterium granulomatis* in lesions of granuloma inguinale. *J Infect Dis* **142:**744, 1980
6. Davis CM: Granuloma inguinale: a clinical, histological, and ultrastructural study. *JAMA* **211:**632, 1970
7. Dodson RF et al: Donovanosis: a morphologic study. *J Invest Dermatol* **62:**611, 1974
8. Maddock I et al: Donovanosis in Papua New Guinea. *Br J Vener Dis* **52:**190, 1976
9. D'Aunoy R, Von Haam E: Granuloma inguinale. *Am J Trop Med* **17:**747, 1967
10. Fritz GS et al: Mutilating granuloma inguinale. *Arch Dermatol* **111:**1464, 1975
11. Kirkpatrick DJ: Donovanosis (granuloma inguinale): a rare cause of osteolytic bone lesions. *Clin Radiol* **21:**101, 1970
12. Endicott JN et al: Granuloma inguinale of the orbit with bony involvement. *Arch Otolaryngol* **96:**457, 1972
13. Rao M et al: Oral lesions of granuloma inguinale. *J Oral Surg* **34:**1112, 1976
14. Garg BR et al: Donovanosis (granuloma inguinale) of the oral cavity. *Br J Vener Dis* **51:**136, 1975
15. Stewart DB: Ulcerative and hypertrophic lesions of the vulva. *Proc R Soc Med* **61:**363, 1968
16. Breschi LC et al: Granuloma inguinale in Vietnam: successful therapy with ampicillin and lincomycin. *J Am Vener Dis Assoc* **1:**118, 1975

CHAPTER 205

GONORRHEA

David S. Feingold

Definition

Gonorrhea is a bacterial infection caused by *Neisseria gonorrhoeae,* a gram-negative diplococcus whose only natural reservoir is humans. The infection is almost always contracted during sexual activity.

The usual presentation in males is acute urethritis and in females cervicitis, which may be asymptomatic. Other parts of the genitourinary apparatus, the rectum, pharynx, and eye may be infected. Occasionally bacteremia occurs which is regularly associated with arthralgias and skin lesions; metastatic infection in joints or other foci may ensue. Although good treatment is available, the disease remains an important public health problem causing a large percentage of female sterility and considerable morbidity in both sexes.

Historical aspects

The name gonorrhea is attributed to Galen who thought the urethritis represented abnormal flow of semen, hence the combination of *gonos,* "seed," and *rhoea,* "flow." The slang name for gonorrhea, clap, likely derives from a French word for brothel, *clapoir.*

Early confusion among the venereal diseases was augmented by the unfortunate experiment of John Hunter in 1767. He inoculated himself with a presumed gonococcal urethral exudate, only to develop syphilis. With isolation of the causative organism of gonorrhea by Neisser in 1879, positive identification of the disease became possible.

Treatment for gonorrhea has progressed from sandalwood oil to urethral irrigations with potassium permanganate to sulfonamides in the 1930s. Resistance to sulfonamides developed rapidly but, fortunately, in the 1940s the exquisite sensitivity of gonococcal strains to penicillin was discovered. The emerging problem of penicillin resistance of the organism will be discussed later in this chapter.

Epidemiology

The decade between 1965 and 1975 witnessed a threefold increase in the incidence of gonorrhea in the United States. Well over 1 million cases of gonorrhea are reported each year; it is estimated that less than one-third of the new cases are reported. Why has there been such an explosive increase in gonorrhea, a disease for which effective therapy is readily available? Many factors may be responsible: sexual promiscuity, changes in birth control methods, population mobility, paucity of symptoms in many infected patients, high transmissibility of the disease, minimal resistance conferred by previous infection, and frequent delay of patients in seeking care.

Understanding the epidemiology of gonorrhea is central to instituting rational measures to control the disease. The disease is spread almost exclusively by sexual activity, although newborns may be infected by exposure during parturition. Although all age groups are susceptible, infection is more prevalent in the 15- to 35-year age group. The disease is concentrated in high-density population centers, possibly with a core group of active transmitters. However, individual mobility results in the occurrence of gonorrhea everywhere. In 1976, almost 9 million specimens were taken from women as part of the Centers for Disease Control–sponsored gonorrhea testing programs. Positive specimens comprised 4.4 percent. The numbers in different populations ranged from 1.6 percent among family planning groups to 18.7 percent in venereal disease clinics [1].

The Herculean efforts of the U.S. Public Health Service to control the disease are proving effective; the incidence of gonorrhea peaked in the mid-1970s. Recently the incidence has decreased slightly, reflecting fewer reported new cases in males. Sweden witnessed a remarkable decrease in gonorrhea in the 1970s, paralleling the publicity for and widespread use of condoms. However, in other countries of Western Europe, a decrease has also been seen without any special efforts at control.

Etiologic agent and pathogenesis

N. gonorrhoeae are gram-negative diplococci with distinctive morphology; the cocci are flattened and the long axes of the bean-shaped organisms are parallel. Gonococci tolerate oxygen but usually require 2 to 10 percent of CO_2 in the growth atmosphere. The organisms have narrow temperature (35° to 37°C) and pH (7.2 to 7.6) optima for growth. Although fragile, they have relatively simple growth requirements. Defined media are now available on which the organisms will grow readily. Different strains have somewhat different growth requirements. Careful study of these requirements has led to a system of typing gonococcal isolates, auxotyping [2]. Auxotyping was an important advance, since the ability to tell one *N. gonorrhoeae* isolate from another makes epidemiologic studies feasible. Several other efforts to type gonococci are in the developmental stage. These include sensitivity to bacteriocins, the presence of specific lipopolysaccharide antigens, the presence of specific pili or outer membrane proteins, and the use of monoclonal antibodies [3].

Kellogg and coworkers recognized four colony types of *N. gonorrhoeae* [4]. Only types 1 and 2 were pathogenic for humans. These types were also found to possess surface hairlike structures termed pili. The nature of pili as virulence factors has not been clarified; pili may foster adherence of gonococci to mucosal surfaces or resistance to phagocytosis. Other virulence factors are being identified. These may include capsular production in vivo, resistance to the immune bactericidal action of serum, and the ability of gonococci to survive in the presence of various competing commensal organisms. Griffiss and Artenstein [5] point out that all Neisseria are organisms adapted to moist mucous membranes. Of them, the meningococcus and the gonococcus are the ones capable of escaping from host restraints, proliferating rapidly, and even invading the bloodstream. The reason why certain organisms occupy particular ecologic niches and the factors conferring virulence are only beginning to be understood.

Clinical manifestations

Signs, symptoms, complications, and the natural history of gonorrhea differ dramatically between males and females. However, careful studies have exposed the myth that males with gonorrhea are symptomatic and females asymptomatic.

Males

After a single exposure to an infected contact, about 25 percent of males will develop gonorrhea. It has been estimated that 85 percent of men with gonococcal urethritis develop an acute process with discomfort, dysuria, and purulent discharge usually ensuing from 2 to 10 days after exposure. Fifteen percent of urethritis in the male is minimally symptomatic or asymptomatic. Since these patients may not receive treatment they tend to accumulate in the population. The resultant point prevalence of minimally symptomatic or asymptomatic male gonorrhea may be as high as 40 percent [6]. Clearly these men are capable of spreading disease. Untreated symptomatic urethritis subsides over several days to weeks but occasionally local complications such as epididymitis, seminal vesiculitis, and prostatitis occur. Anorectal [7] and pharyngeal [8] gonococcal colonization are not common. The incidence of positive cultures correlates with the practices of passive rectal intercourse and fellatio, respectively. Since symptoms of proctitis and pharyngitis correlate poorly with positive cultures, colonization of these areas rather than overt infection is likely to be what occurs.

Females

When an uninfected woman is exposed to an infected man, gonorrhea ensues over half the time. Once infected, the specific symptoms and signs of acute salpingitis may occur (20 to 40 percent) or the less specific symptoms of dysuria, increased discharge, or abnormal bleeding (20 to 30 percent) may be seen within a few days to a few weeks. Thirty to 60 percent of infected women will be minimally affected or asymptomatic yet remain long-term carriers capable of transferring the infection [9,10]. As described for men, these cases will accumulate since symptomatic gonorrhea is treated preferentially. Since none of the symptoms or signs is diagnostic of gonorrhea, cultures of endocervix, urethra, rectum, and pharynx should be carried out if the disease is suspected or the patient is reported as a contact of gonorrhea.

Pelvic inflammatory disease (PID) is the most important complication of gonococcal infection. PID is the result of ascending infection from the endocervix, causing endo-

metritis and/or salpingitis and/or pelvic peritonitis. Clinical findings can vary from crampy abdominal pain with minimal tenderness in mild cases to fever, severe abdominal pain, and exquisite tenderness with adnexal masses in florid cases. Prompt diagnosis and aggressive treatment are mandatory since infertility, ectopic pregnancy, and chronic pelvic pain are frequent complications. Several organisms other than *N. gonorrhoeae* may cause PID. The etiologic diagnosis, which will be discussed subsequently, may be difficult.

Disseminated gonococcal infections (DGI)

Spread of *N. gonorrhoeae* to the bloodstream has been estimated to occur in 1 to 3 percent of patients with gonorrhea [11], with the majority of cases in females. Although endocarditis, pericarditis, and meningitis have been reported, they are rare complications. Arthritis and skin lesions, on the other hand, are regularly associated with DGI (Fig. A3-18). The syndrome is so characteristic that a presumptive diagnosis can usually be made on clinical grounds alone; the syndrome has been labeled the arthritis-dermatitis syndrome. The onset of gonococcal bacteremia usually occurs with menstruation or pregnancy in females. In males, DGI is most often seen in association with asymptomatic infection. Fever, chills, polyarthralgias, arthritis, and tenosynovitis are common. In the early stages of the disease, skin manifestations occur that are quite characteristic. The skin lesions typically are few in number (often less than a dozen) and concentrated on the extremities, often around the joints. The lesions may be petechial or papular; however, they usually evolve into vesicles or pustules on an erythematous base which may become hemorrhagic. Sometimes they present as hemorrhagic bullae. Prompt diagnosis and therapy are mandatory since delay may result in frank pyogenic arthritis with potential for joint destruction.

Recently, it has been recognized that organisms causing DGI often differ from those causing urethritis. Most strains of gonococci are susceptible to the complement-mediated bactericidal action of normal serum; the strains causing DGI are resistant [11]. This important observation may explain why some gonococci are capable of causing bacteremia while others are restricted to mucous membranes. In support of the necessity for serum resistance in strains causing DGI are the reports that patients deficient in the late complement components are peculiarly susceptible to recurrent neisserial sepsis [12].

The pathogenesis of the arthritis-dermatitis syndrome is unclear. Bacteremia regularly occurs early in the course of DGI but it has been suggested that most signs and symptoms of DGI are manifestations of immune-complex formation.

Miscellaneous clinical manifestations

Rarely, an ulcer or abscess (Fig. 205-1) may appear on the raphe of the penis. Gonococcal perihepatitis is a complication of gonococcal peritonitis with hepatic capsular fibrosis and adhesions (Fitz-Hugh-Curtis syndrome) [13]. Adhesions such as those between the hepatic capsule and the anterior abdominal wall can cause discomfort which may be persistent and difficult to diagnose.

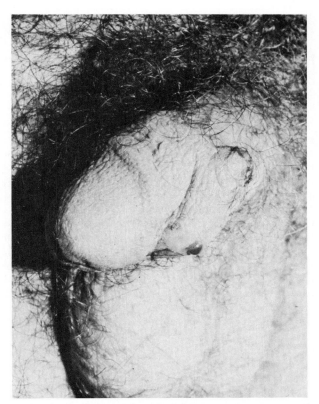

Fig. 205-1   Gonorrhea abscess affecting the median raphe of the penis. (Courtesy of Dr. A. R. Rhodes.)

Gonococcal ophthalmia neonatorum is neonatal purulent conjunctivitis contracted by the newborn in passage through an infected birth canal. Recent reappearance in greater numbers is probably a reflection of the higher incidence of gonorrhea combined with a more casual enforcement or execution of silver nitrate prophylaxis of newborns [14].

Cornified squamous epithelium is quite resistant to infection with *N. gonorrhoeae*, hence vulvovaginitis is infrequent in adult women. However, in children, the vulva and vagina are lined with columnar epithelium; acute vulvovaginitis is the usual manifestation of genital gonococcal infection in the prepubescent female.

Pathology

The picture of active gonococcal infection is usually that of an acute or subacute inflammatory response with polymorphonuclear leukocytes predominating. The histopathology of the vesiculopustular lesions of DGI consists of infiltrates of neutrophils admixed with some mononuclear cells and red blood cells. Fibrinoid necrosis of vessel walls may be seen. The bullae are subepidermal in location [15]. Bacteria are rarely seen or grown in the skin lesions; however, organisms may at times be identified in the lesions using fluorescent antibody techniques [16].

Diagnosis

Definitive diagnosis of gonorrhea depends upon identification of the organisms by Gram's stain and/or culture. A positive Gram's stain consists of characteristic gram-neg-

ative diplococci in the cytoplasm of neutrophils. A positive Gram's stain from the male urethra is considered diagnostic. Gram's stain of endocervical discharge is not usually done since even a positive smear is not considered diagnostic; culture confirmation is required. In women, endocervical cultures give a higher yield of positives than vaginal cultures. In males without exudate, swabs for culture should be inserted several centimeters into the urethra. In women with gonorrhea, not only endocervical cultures, but rectal, urethral, and pharyngeal cultures should be obtained. In DGI, blood, skin lesions, and joint effusions should be cultured. Skin lesions are regularly negative; joint fluid is usually negative until acute purulent arthritis occurs. Blood cultures are positive only early in the disease. Thus, the diagnosis of DGI frequently must be made on clinical grounds only. This rarely presents a problem since frequently the clinical picture, especially the skin lesions and the tenosynovitis, is quite characteristic.

When culturing an area in which a mixed bacterial flora is unusual, e.g., synovial fluid or male urethra, chocolate agar may be used for isolation. When culturing an area which has an exuberant flora such as the throat, rectum, or endocervix, one should use selective media containing antimicrobials which inhibit organisms other than *Neisseria*. Modified Thayer-Martin is the medium usually employed. Transgrow is a similar medium but it also contains CO_2 and is a good transport medium for gonococci.

In addition to *N. gonorrhoeae* several other organisms cause PID including *Chlamydia trachomatis,* endogenous anaerobic and aerobic bacteria, and genital mycoplasmas. It is clearly advantageous for proper therapy to know the causative organism. Endocervical cultures are the only practical way to distinguish between gonococcal and nongonococcal PID; patients in whom gonococci are grown from the cervix are assumed to have gonococcal PID [17].

Several serologic tests for gonorrhea are in the developmental stage. As yet, none shows the requisite sensitivity or specificity. Possibly the greatest value of these tests, if perfected, will be in confirming the etiology of PID and establishing the diagnosis of DGI. No one advocates that they replace culture techniques for the diagnosis of routine gonorrhea, but a possible role for serologic tests for screening or case finding has not been ruled out [18].

Differential diagnosis

The differential diagnosis of genitourinary gonococcal disease in the female includes the following:

1. *Trichomonas vaginalis* infection. This usually presents as a profuse, frothy, foul, vaginal exudate, at times with urethritis. A positive saline preparation for the protozoa is diagnostic.
2. *Candida albicans* infection. Often this presents as a pruritic infection with a creamy or curdy exudate, and diagnosis depends on identification of the organism by smear and/or culture.
3. *Gardnerella vaginalis* and/or anaerobic bacterial vaginitis. There is still dispute about the relative role of these organisms in bacterial vaginitis. However, the syndrome is well defined with malodorous, gray, acidic discharge that shows ''clue'' cells on smear and yields a ''fishy'' amine odor on alkalinization with potassium

hydroxide. All patients with vaginal discharges should be cultured for gonococci. Even though inflammatory vaginitis is rarely seen with gonorrhea alone, mixed infections do occur rather commonly.

In men, urethrits can also be caused by multiple organisms. *T. vaginalis* and *C. albicans* can infect the male and be asymptomatic or cause urethritis or balanitis. Some urethritis has been attributed to *Herpesvirus hominis*. However, even more common than gonorrhea as a cause of urethritis in many populations is so-called nongonococcal or nonspecific or postgonococcal urethritis. This condition is so common and has been the subject of such intensive study recently that it will be discussed separately in the following section.

Nongonococcal urethritis (NGU)

NGU may be the most common sexually transmitted human disease. It is characterized by dysuria, often by urethral discharge or urinary frequency, and by the absence of *N. gonorrhoeae*. In contrast to classic gonococcal urethritis, NGU usually has a longer incubation period, a less acute onset, and scanty urethral discharge; at times, no discharge is evident, only urethral discomfort or tenderness. Occasionally, coinfection with *N. gonorrhoeae* occurs and urethritis remains following effective penicillin therapy for gonorrhea; this has been labeled postgonococcal urethritis.

Until the mid-1970s, causative agents of NGU were not identified; however, it was clear that symptoms usually yielded to therapy with tetracyclines. Now there is good evidence that at least two organisms are responsible for NGU [19]. *Chlamydia trachomatis* has been demonstrated convincingly to cause more than 50 percent of the cases of NGU. Evidence is mounting that *Ureaplasma urealyticus* is responsible for many of the remaining cases of tetracycline-responsive NGU.

The spectrum of disease caused by *C. trachomatis* has expanded steadily since its role in NGU was defined. *C. trachomatis* causes epididymitis, prostatitis, cervicitis, and PID; asymptomatic urethritis, inclusion conjunctivitis, and interstitial pneumonia of the newborn also result from infection with this chlamydia.

Tetracyclines, 2 g per day for 10 days, are effective therapy for most cases of NGU.

Treatment and control

Ideal therapy for gonococcal urethritis would have the following attributes in addition to curing the urethritis. It should be given as a single dose; it should abort coincubating syphilis; it should cure coexisting chlamydial infections. No single drug regimen achieves these ideals. The staff and consultant of the Centers for Disease Control offered their most recent guidelines for treatment of gonorrhea in 1982 [20]. Three regimens for uncomplicated gonococcal urethritis were suggested with no preference offered.

1. Aqueous procaine penicillin G: 4.8 million units injected intramuscularly at two sites, with 1.0 g of probenecid by mouth. An important disadvantage of this regimen is that it is ineffective against chlamydial infections.

2. Tetracycline HCl: 500 mg, by mouth, 4 times a day for 7 days. The disadvantage of this regimen is that it requires compliance with multiple doses.

3. Amoxicillin/ampicillin: Amoxicillin, 3.0 g, or ampicillin, 3.5 g, either with 1.0 g probenecid by mouth. This also is ineffective against chlamydial infections.

Control of gonorrhea was complicated immeasurably by the appearance in the United States in 1975 of penicillinase-producing strains of *N. gonorrhoeae* (PPNG) which resisted any penicillin regimen. Penicillinase synthesis in these organisms depends on the presence of plasmids, extrachromosomal packets of DNA which can be transferred among organisms. Predictions that these organisms would quickly become dominant have not been fulfilled. However, the number of isolates has been increasing yearly. In the first 9 months of 1982, 3424 cases were reported, an increase of 77 percent over the same period in 1981 [21]. In spite of this dramatic increase in PPNG isolates, they comprise only about 0.5 percent of the total gonococcal isolates. It is estimated that if the prevalence of PPNG in any area increases to 5 percent of gonococcal infections, penicillins will cease to be drugs of choice [22]. This has already occurred in the Far East where PPNG comprise over 50 percent of the isolates. Since PPNG are also relatively resistant to tetracyclines the same would apply to these drugs.

In light of the PPNG problem it is now recommended that all patients be recultured within 1 week of therapy to assure that cure has been achieved. If organisms are grown or if the patient is still symptomatic, the patient should be treated with 2 g of spectinomycin intramuscularly in a single injection. The organisms from these patients should be treated for β-lactanase (penicillinase) production and, if positive, an aggressive search for the patient's contacts is mandatory. Cefoxitin (2 g intramuscularly) plus 1 g probenecid and cephotaxime (1 g intramuscularly) are also effective against PPNG.

Control of the gonorrhea epidemic probably depends more on other factors than the details of therapy of acute disease. It is essential to educate the public about venereal disease, including signs and symptoms, methods of prevention and resources available. Medical personnel must also be made aware of the most effective case-finding techniques, including screening of at-risk populations and aggressive search for contacts of patients with gonorrhea.

Possible control of gonorrhea by immunization is being examined. Some success at immunizing chimpanzees has been achieved [23]. Several problems remain, however, including that of serologic specificity among strains, and effective immunization against gonorrhea seems not to be imminent.

References

1. Centers for Disease Control: Results of testing for gonorrhea—United States 12-month period ending December 31, 1976. *MMWR* **26:**217, 1977
2. Carifo K, Catlin BW: *Neisseria gonorrhoeae* auxotyping: differentiation of clinical isolates based on growth responses on chemically defined media. *Appl Microbiol* **26:**223, 1973
3. Tam MR et al: Serological classification of *Neisseria gonorrhoeae* with monoclonal antibodies. *Infect Immun* **36:**1042, 1982
4. Kellogg DS et al: *Neisseria gonorrhoeae*. II. Colonial varia-

tion and pathogenicity during 35 months *in vitro. J Bacteriol* **96:**596, 1968

5. Griffiss JM, Artenstein MS: The ecology of the genus *Neisseria. Mt Sinai J (NY)* **43:**746, 1976

6. Handsfield HH et al: Asymptomatic gonorrhea in men—diagnosis, natural course, prevalence and significance. *N Engl J Med* **290:**117, 1974

7. Klein EJ et al: Anorectal gonococcal infection. *Ann Intern Med* **86:**340, 1977

8. Wiesner PJ et al: Clinical spectrum of pharyngeal gonococcal infection. *N Engl J Med* **288:**181, 1973

9. McCormack WM et al: Clinical spectrum of gonococcal infection in women. *Lancet* **1:**1182, 1977

10. Wiesner PJ, Thompson SE III: Gonococcal diseases. *Disease-a-Month* **XXVI:**2, 1980

11. Schoolnik GK et al: Gonococci causing disseminated gonococcal infection are resistant to the bactericidal action of normal human sera. *J Clin Invest* **58:**1163, 1976

12. Petersen BH et al: Human deficiency of the eighth component of complement. *J Clin Invest* **57:**283, 1976

13. Reichert JA, Valle RF: Fitz-Hugh-Curtis syndrome. *JAMA* **236:**266, 1976

14. Snowe RJ, Wilfert CM: Epidemic reappearance of gonococcal ophthalmia neonatorum. *Pediatrics* **51:**110, 1973

15. Lever WF, Schaumburg-Lever G: *Histopathology of the Skin.* Philadelphia, Lippincott, 1975

16. Tronca E et al: Demonstration of *Neisseria gonorrhoeae* with fluorescent antibody in patients with disseminated infection. *J Infect Dis* **129:**583, 1974

17. Eschenback DA et al: Polymicrobial etiology of acute pelvic inflammatory disease. *N Engl J Med* **293:**166, 1975

18. Dans PE et al: Gonococcal serology: how soon, how useful and how much. *J Infect Dis* **135:**330, 1977

19. Bowie WR et al: Etiology of nongonococcal urethritis. *J Clin Invest* **59:**735, 1977

20. Guidelines for therapy of sexually transmitted diseases. *MMWR* **31:**335, 1982

21. Penicillinase-producing *Neisseria gonorrhoeae. MMWR* **32:**181, 1983

22. McCormack WM: Penicillinase-producing *Neisseria gonorrhoeae*—a retrospective. *N Engl J Med* **307:**438, 1982

23. Arko RJ et al: Immunity in infection with *Neisseria gonorrhoeae:* duration and serologic response in chimpanzee. *J Infect Dis* **133:**441, 1976

Section 30

Animal bites, infestations, and insect bites and stings

CHAPTER 206

BITES OF ANIMAL, ARTHROPOD, AND MARINE LIFE

Ann Sullivan Baker

More than 500,000 animal bites are reported yearly in the United States; dog bites constitute the largest group. The human victim is usually a 7- to 9-year-old boy, often teasing or playing with the dog. The biting dog is usually 6 to 12 months old, is often female, and is usually a working dog, such as a boxer, collie, German shepherd, Great Dane, or Saint Bernard, or a sporting dog, such as a pointer, setter, or retriever. Hounds, for some reason, are relatively safe.

The evaluation and treatment of all bite wounds should include a careful history of the incident, the type of animal, the site of the bite, and the geographic setting. Hand wounds and puncture wounds most often become infected. Most bites should be cultured and a Gram-stained smear prepared; the wound should then be washed, well irrigated, and left open. Selection of an antibiotic depends on the bite history and Gram's stain results. Most patients with deep cat bites, deep cat scratches, and sutured wounds should be treated with penicillin or tetracycline because of the increased incidence of *Pasteurella multocida* infection. Tetanus immune status should be evaluated and rabies immunization considered.

Human bites and monkey bites deserve special mention, since 30 percent become infected with aerobic or anaerobic mouth organisms. Anaerobic infection may spread through the metacarpal-phalangeal space and cause severe damage. The same procedure as for other animal bites should be followed, that is, culture and Gram's stain, thorough washing, and wide dissection. Wounds should be left open if possible, especially hand wounds. Patients with human bites should be treated with penicillin for 7 to 10 days. Clenched fist injuries should be evaluated by a hand surgeon.

Specific bacterial infections

Pasteurella multocida

A common organism infecting bite wounds is *P. multocida*. Disease due to this organism is now diagnosed more frequently; thus, its presence in the nasopharynx in 50 percent of dogs and 75 percent of cats is of public health importance.

Most infections in humans fall into one of three clinical patterns:

1. The most common pattern is that of *local infection with adenitis* after a dog or cat bite or scratch. In patients with a cat bite, this then may progress to tenosynovitis or osteomyelitis due to inoculation of the organism into the periosteum by the long, sharp tooth of the animal. Canine teeth are more blunt and less likely to penetrate the periosteum.

2. *Chronic pulmonary infection*, in which *P. multocida* may occur as the primary pathogen or in association with other organisms. Bacteria may enter through the respiratory tract by inhalation of barn dust or infectious droplets sprayed by the sneeze of an animal. In such cases, the bacteria probably colonize the respiratory tract and lie dormant in the patient with chronic lung disease. Acute infection occurs only after trauma to the bronchial tree. Bronchiectasis, emphysema, peritonsillar abscess, and sinusitis have all been described with this organism.

3. *Systemic infection with bacteremia or meningitis* may occur.

P. multocida is a small, gram-negative, ovoid bacillus that grows well on blood agar, but does not grow on gram-negative media, such as MacConkey agar. Because of its superficial resemblance to *Hemophilus influenzae* and *Neisseria* organisms, respiratory tract and central nervous system infection with *P. multocida* initially may be misdiagnosed. Failure of growth on routine gram-negative media is an important clue.

Treatment of the patient with presumptive *P. multocida* infection (that is, any patient with a deep cat bite or scratch or a deep dog bite) should consist of careful washing and an attempt to leave the wound open. The antibiotic of choice is penicillin, for 7 to 10 days orally, with careful follow-up of the wound. Ampicillin and tetracycline are alternatives; oral cephalosporins are not as useful.

Plague (see Chap. 178)

Tularemia (see Chap. 178)

Rat-bite fever (see Chap. 178)

Cat-scratch disease (see Chap. 195)

Viral infections

Rabies (also see Chap. 172)

The most notorious viral disease caused by an animal bite is rabies. The epidemiology has changed in the past few years. Now, nonimmune dogs account for only 16 percent of cases, whereas sylvatic animals, such as skunks, raccoons, red and gray foxes, bats, and domestic dogs represent the greatest potential danger; rodents, such as squirrels and hamsters, are probably inconsequential as sources of rabies.

Live virus is introduced into nerve tissue at the time of the bite. The virus persists 96 h at the site, and then spreads to the central nervous system. It replicates in gray matter, and then spreads along autonomic nerves to the salivary glands, adrenal glands, and heart. The incubation period varies with the site of the bite from 10 days to as long as one year.

Clinical features include a prodromal period of 1 to 4 days, followed by high fever, headache, and malaise. Paresthesia at the site of inoculation occurs in 80 percent of patients. The next sequence of events is familiar: agitation, hyperesthesia, dysphagia, paralysis, and death.

Diagnosis. The fluorescent antibody method for the viral antigen is the most rapid and sensitive means of making the diagnosis. Brain biopsy of the animal is also useful.

Treatment. Preexposure prophylaxis is important for spelunkers, veterinarians, and virologists. Human diploid vaccine should be given. The neutralizing antibody titer should be followed to assure immunity in high-risk or exposed persons.

Postexposure prophylaxis includes answers to the following questions:

What is the status of animal rabies in the locale where the exposure took place?
Was the attack provoked or unprovoked?
Of what species was the animal?
What was the state of health of the animal?

Most animals transmit rabies virus in saliva only a few days before becoming ill themselves (dog and skunk, five days; fox, three days; cat, one day; bats, however, may harbor the virus for many months).

BITES BY HOUSEHOLD PETS. If the dog or cat is healthy and available for observation for 10 days, do not treat the patient unless the animal develops rabies. At the first sign of rabies in the animal, treat the patient with rabies immune globulin (RIG) and human diploid cell vaccine (HDCV). The symptomatic animal should be killed and tested as soon as possible.

If the pet is rabid, or suspected to be rabid, or if it is a pet from outside of the United States (especially Latin America, Africa, and most of Asia), treat with RIG and HDCV.

BITES BY WILD ANIMALS. All skunks, bats, foxes, coyotes, raccoons, bobcats, and other carnivores should be regarded as rabid unless laboratory tests prove negative. Treat with RIG and HDCV.

BITES BY OTHER ANIMALS. Consider other animals (livestock, rodents, lagomorphs, e.g., rabbits, hares) individually. Local and state public health officials should be consulted on the need for prophylaxis. Bites by the following almost never call for antirabies prophylaxis: squirrels, hamsters, guinea pigs, gerbils, chipmunks, rats, mice and other rodents, rabbits and hares.

SPECIFICS OF TREATMENT. The most important step is to cleanse the wound immediately and with a brush and soap to remove as much virus as possible. Rinse well, then perform a second scrub with green soap or alcohol, which is rabicidal.

Rabies Prophylaxis Information

Local or state laboratory

Centers for Disease Control . . . . 404-329-3534 (any hour)
  1600 Clifton Road
  Atlanta, Georgia 30333

Merieux Institute, Inc. . . . . 1-800-327-2842 (any hour)
  (Florida, Alaska, and Hawaii <u>only</u>. Call collect.)   305-593-9577

If vaccine treatment is indicated, both rabies immune globulin and human diploid cell rabies vaccine should be given as soon as possible, regardless of the interval after exposure.

The administration of RIG is the more urgent procedure. If HDCV is not immediately available, start RIG and give HDCV as soon as it is obtained. Human rabies immunoglobulin should be given to the patient immediately: 50 percent around the site of the bite and 50 percent in the thigh or the arm. The dosage is 20 IU/kg. This passive immunization will result in the early appearance of antibody, but will also inhibit the development of the active antibody from the human diploid vaccine; thus, the reason for prolonged dosage of the vaccines.

Active immunization is accomplished with the new human diploid cell vaccine (HDCV) made by Merieux Institute, Inc. in Miami, Florida (telephone 1-800-327-2842). Human diploid cell rabies vaccine is given intramuscularly for a total of five doses. The doses are given on days 0, 3, 7, 14, and 28. Serum for rabies antibody testing should be collected two weeks after the fifth dose. If there is no antibody response, an additional booster should be given.

MANAGEMENT OF THE PATIENT WITH CLINICAL RABIES. When the rare patient is admitted with the clinical diagnosis of rabies, several steps should be immediately taken.

First, the diagnosis must be made rapidly by fluorescent antibody staining of various tissues, as well as mouse inoculation of the animal's brain tissue. Elevated antibody titers in the absence of immunization are clear evidence of infection. The first signs of clinical rabies are usually nonspecific, such as malaise, anorexia, fatigue, headache, and fever. The acute neurologic illness that follows is most commonly characterized by intermittent episodes of hyperactivity. In some cases, however, a progressive paralysis is most common. The usual period of onset of symptoms to onset of coma is 10 days.

The basic clinical management consists of anticipating and preventing all treatable complications of the rabies infection. Pulmonary hypoxia should be prevented by tracheostomy at the first sign of respiratory difficulty, monitoring of actual PO_2, and use of supplemental oxygen.

Anticonvulsant therapy should also be instituted. Extreme increases in intracranial pressure may be prevented by insertion of a CSF reservoir connected to the lateral ventricle, allowing withdrawal of the intraventricular fluid and measurement of intracranial pressure.

Cardiac arrythmias may be anticipated with careful monitoring.

Unfortunately there are no specific antiviral treatments for rabies at the present time.

Risk of exposure for hospital staff includes contamination of open wounds or mucous membranes with saliva or other potentially infectious material such as neurologic tissue, spinal fluid, or urine. Blood, serum, and stool are not considered infectious.

Rabies has been regarded as uniformly fatal. There have now been several cases that have survived with prolonged cardiorespiratory support. An aggressive approach in the patient with known rabies infection is certainly worthwhile.

Lymphocytic choriomeningitis

Lymphocytic choriomeningitis (LCM) virus is an infectious agent common to the house mouse but rarely transmitted to humans. More recently, outbreaks of LCM virus infection in the United States have been traced to pet hamsters.

Hamsters, like mice, may excrete LCM virus for several months and may become lifelong carriers.

When humans are infected, there may be three major manifestations: a grippe-like illness, meningitis, or encephalitis. The CSF formula usually reveals an increased mononuclear leukocyte count, and hypoglycorrhachia. Symptomatic therapy is all that is available.

Simian herpes B virus

Simian herpes B virus is found in Old World monkeys, especially rhesus and cynomolgus species. Infection is usually caused by a bite, and less commonly after inhalation of monkey saliva or contact with infected monkey cell cultures. A vesicular lesion develops at the wound site, with progressive lymphangitis and fever. Confusion, reduced tendon reflexes in lower extremities, and respiratory paralysis may follow.

Diagnosis depends on viral isolation or intranuclear inclusion bodies in lymph nodes or on a brain biopsy from patient or animal, or on a rise in neutralizing antibody titer to simian herpes B virus. Treatment is supportive.

Orf (contagious ecthyma) (see Chap. 193)

Arthropods

Ticks

Rickettsial infections. ROCKY MOUNTAIN SPOTTED FEVER (see Chap. 183)

Fig. 206-1 Babesiosis. Intracellular parasite *Babesia microti* within the red blood cells.

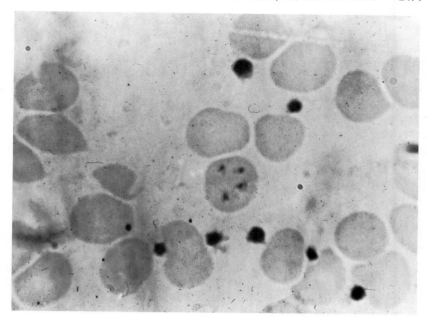

Parasitic infections. BABESIOSIS. Babesiosis, a disease caused by the intracellular red blood cell parasite *Babesia microti* (Fig. 206-1), is also transmitted by ticks. The parasite is carried by the larvae of the deer tick, *Ixodes dammini* (Fig. 206-2). The larvae overwinter and the disease is spread by the nymph from May through July. The nymphs are tiny (1 mm in size), and usually not recognized. Eastern Long Island, Martha's Vineyard, and Nantucket are the major endemic areas.

Fig. 206-2 Deer tick, *Ixodes dammini* (adult female), the major vector of human babesiosis.

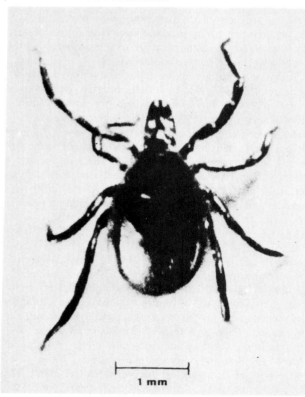

1 mm

There is an increased risk in patients with T-lymphocyte depression or after splenectomy, but several cases have occurred in normal hosts. The clinical syndrome of babesiosis includes fever, drenching sweats, myalgia, and hemolytic anemia. Diagnosis is made by observation of the intracellular red blood cell parasite on a Giemsa-stained smear. The tetrads may be confused with the findings in falciparum malaria, but *Babesia*-infected red blood cells do not have pigment granules. Antibody titers are also helpful in making the diagnosis.

Treatment is symptomatic in the patient with mild infection. In splenectomized patients, exchange transfusions have been helpful. The combination of oral clindamycin 600 mg three times a day and quinine 650 mg three times a day has also been successful.

Spirochetal infections. LYME DISEASE (see Chap. 88)

Toxins. TICK PARALYSIS. Tick paralysis may be caused by 43 different species of ticks, but most human cases in the United States are attributed to *Dermacenter* species.

The paralysis is thought to be caused by a toxin secreted in the saliva of the tick that affects central as well as peripheral nerves. Typically, the tick is attached from 4 to 7 days before the onset of symptoms.

Tick paralysis presents as an ascending flaccid paralysis, acute ataxia, or a combination of the two.

The diagnosis depends on a careful search of the scalp and body for the attached tick.

Treatment consists of removing the tick; improvement is seen in a few hours.

Other tick-related infections. (See also "Tularemia" in Chap. 178.)

Spiders, scorpions, and hymenoptera

Spiders (see Chap. 208)

Scorpion stings (see also Chap. 208). The scorpion is an arthropod of 1 to 8 cm in length. It has an exoskeleton, a

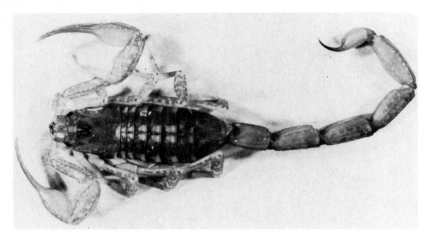

Fig. 206-3 Scorpion. Note the pinching claws, tail, and stinger.

pair of pinching claws, and a tail with a poison gland and stinger (Fig. 206-3). There are about 650 species of scorpions, approximately 40 of which are found in the United States; most are not venomous. The venomous scorpions belong to the family Buthidae. Particularly dangerous species include *Centruroides sculpturatus* and *Centruroides gertschi*, which are found in the southwestern United States.

The clinical symptoms of a scorpion sting are painful burning and/or localized numbness at the site of the sting. Systemic manifestations such as tachycardia, high blood pressure, and respiratory impairment occur rarely.

Therapy includes immersion of the limb in cold water

Fig. 206-4   (1) *Bombus sonorus*, bumblebee. (2) *Apis melifera*, honeybee. (3) *Vespula maculata*, white-faced hornet. (4) *Vespula maculifrons*, yellow jacket. (*From Lichtenstein LM: Anaphylactic reactions to insect stings: a new approach. Hospital Practice 10(3), 1975. Drawing by Nancy Lou Gahan. Reprinted with permission.*)

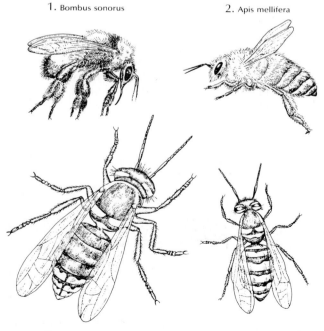

1. Bombus sonorus

2. Apis mellifera

3. Vespula maculata

4. Vespula maculifrons

and a tourniquet about the limb, as well as treatment of symptoms. Antivenom is available by calling Arizona Poison Control Center 602-626-6016.

Hymenoptera stings. Twice as many persons die in the United States from Hymenoptera stings as from snake bites. The order Hymenoptera includes bees, wasps, hornets, and fire ants.

Four prominent members of the order Hymenoptera should be recognized: the bumblebee; the honeybee, with a barbed stinger, fuzzy body, and brown, blunt abdomen; the white-faced hornet; and the yellow jacket, that has a black shiny thorax with long antennae (Fig. 206-4). Hymenoptera venoms contain histamines and other vasoactive substances which are hemolytic and neurotoxic, in addition to being effective hypersensitizing agents.

The clinical syndrome after a sting includes sharp pain, a local wheal, erythema, and intense itching and edema. In the one percent of the population who are hypersensitive, a single sting may produce serious anaphylaxis with urticaria, nausea, abdominal pain, dyspnea, edema of the face and glottis, hypertension, and death.

Treatment requires removal of the venom sac and washing of the area, followed by local supportive care such as cool compresses. The allergic patient may need 0.3 to 0.5 mL of epinephrine (1:1000) injected subcutaneously.

The major factor in the consideration of insect stings is prevention. Desensitization with venom rather than with whole-body extract is now possible. The hypersensitive patient should have available an insect sting kit, such as that made by Hollister-Stier, containing medihaler epinephrine and chlorpheniramine maleate (chlor-Trimeton).

Snake bites

The two major poisonous snakes in the Americas are the pit viper and the coral snake. The coral snake belongs to the family Elapidae. All other poisonous snakes in this hemisphere belong to the family Viperidae. The subfamily of pit vipers includes the rattlesnake, water moccasin, and copperhead. There are about 7000 poisonous snake bites reported in the United States annually; the largest number occur in the Southwestern and Gulf states.

Two poisonous snakes are native to New England. The northern copperhead, also called the highland moccasin,

Snake Bite Information	
Arizona Poison Control Center. 602-626-6016	
Wyeth Laboratory (antivenom). . . . . .215-688-4400 (days)	
	Local Wyeth number (nights)

is pink or reddish brown, and is marked with large barrels of chestnut brown resembling dumbbells or hourglasses (Fig. 206-5). The bite is painful but rarely fatal. The timber rattler is dark brown with chevrons of black and brown (Fig. 206-6).

The degree of toxicity of a snake bite depends on the potency of the venom, the amount injected, the size and condition of the snake, and the size of the person bitten. There are instant clinical manifestations of the pit viper bite. Pain occurs at the site of the bite, as well as a wheal with local edema, numbness, and within moments, ecchymosis and painful lymphadenopathy (Fig. 206-7). Nausea, vomiting, sweating, fever, drowsiness, and slurred speech may then develop. Bleeding of the gums and hematemesis are common hemorrhagic manifestations.

For proper treatment, it is extremely important to establish that the bite is from a poisonous snake. The patient should have distinct fang punctures and immediate local pain, followed by edema and discoloration within 30 min. It is helpful to inspect the snake, since those that are poisonous may be differentiated from those that are not by the presence of fangs and the shape of the pupils (Fig. 206-8).

The limb should be immobilized and a ligature applied proximal to the wound. The ligature should be released for 90 s every 15 min. The physician should make two longitudinal incisions through the fang marks and apply suction intermittently for the first hour. An attempt should be made to neutralize the venom with immune serum. Emergency information and specific immune serum can be obtained

Fig. 206-5 Northern copperhead.

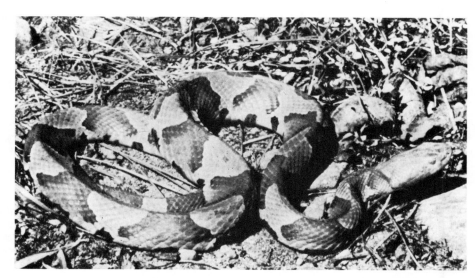

Fig. 206-6 Timber rattler.

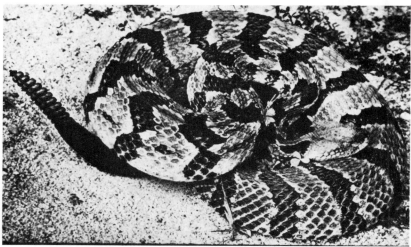

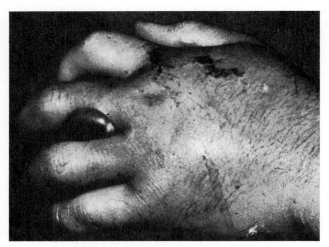

Fig. 206-7 Copperhead snake bite.

from the Oklahoma City Poison Control Center (1-405-271-5454, 24 hours a day). A photograph of snakes common to a specific geographic area is important for all hospital emergency wards.

Polyvalent pit viper antivenin should be used for all severe American snake bites except that of the coral snake. If possible, it should be administered within 1 h of the bite, and the patient should first undergo skin testing for hypersensitivity to horse serum.

The dosage of antivenin for a moderate rattlesnake bite requires 4 to 7 vials (10 cc), severe cases may require 15 to 20 vials; water mocassin bite requires 1 to 4 vials; for copperhead bites, antivenin is usually only necessary for a child or elderly patient. The vials should be diluted in 500 mL of normal saline given intravenously over 30 min. Antitetanus therapy and antibiotic prophylaxis with penicillin 2 g/day or tetracycline 2 g/day should be initiated for severe bites.

Supportive treatment is important, that is, hospitaliza-tion, careful evaluation of baseline hematocrit, platelet count, and prothrombin time.

The wound should be cleansed and covered. Surgical debridement of superficial necrosis should be performed between the third and tenth days.

Marine bites and diseases

Erysipeloid (see Chap. 178)

Seal bite

Normally, a seal bite is on the finger of a trainer or a seal hunter, thus the term *seal finger* or *Spaek finger* (Fig. 206-9). The etiologic agent is unclear; studies are now under way in an attempt to isolate the organism.

The incubation period is 4 to 8 days, followed by throbbing pain, erythema at the site, and swelling of the joint proximal to the bite. Untreated, Spaek finger progresses to cellulitis, tenosynovitis, and arthritis. The treatment before antibiotics were available was amputation of the affected finger to relieve the severe pain and deformity. Tetracycline, 500 mg orally four times a day for 10 days, is now the antibiotic of choice. It is also helpful to immobilize and elevate the finger, as well as soak it several times a day.

Jellyfish sting

Venom is discharged from nematocysts in the tentacles of the larger jellyfish. Stings are characterized by instant burning pain where the tentacles contact the skin, followed by the development of a red, elevated, linear lesion. In more severe cases, the victim experiences nausea, vomiting, abdominal and generalized muscular cramps, and difficulty in breathing. Stings of the sea wasps *Chironex fleckeri* and Chiropsalmus are extremely severe.

On-site resuscitation takes first priority. Pour ocean

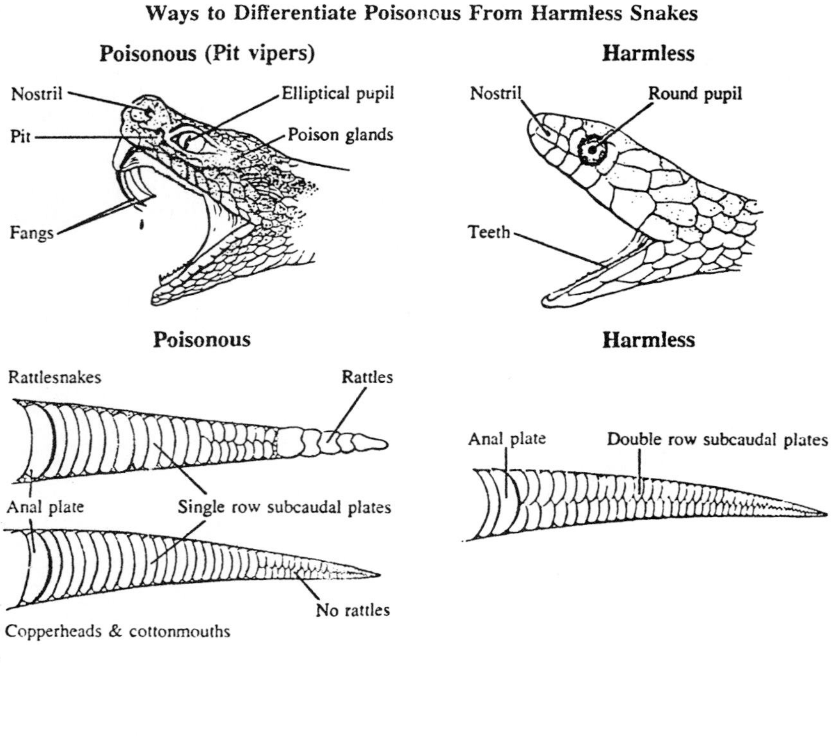

Ways to Differentiate Poisonous From Harmless Snakes

Poisonous (Pit vipers)

Nostril — Elliptical pupil
Pit — Poison glands
Fangs

Harmless

Nostril — Round pupil
Teeth

Poisonous

Rattlesnakes — Rattles
Anal plate — Single row subcaudal plates

Copperheads & cottonmouths — No rattles

Harmless

Anal plate — Double row subcaudal plates

Fig. 206-8 Identification of poisonous and nonpoisonous snakes. *(From Wingert WA, Wainschel W: A quick handbook on snake bites. Resident & Staff Physician, p 56, 1977. Reprinted with permission.)*

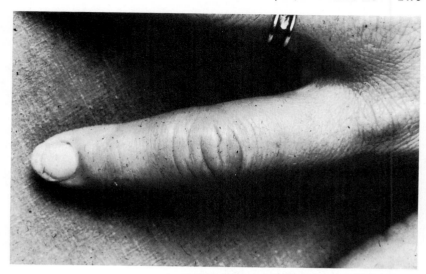

Fig. 206-9 Seal finger. Note edema of the index finger which has erased the skin markings.

water over the wound; do not rub with sand as this will fire the nematocysts that have *not* discharged. Attempt to remove tentacles with gloves. Alcohol or acetic acid (or vinegar) then will inactivate the penetrating nematocysts. Do not use hot water on coelenterate stings; this may cause firing of the nematocysts.

Stingray

Three groups of spiny fish found on the North American coast contain poison: the stingray, scorpion, and cat fish; certain sea urchins; and one shell fish, *Conus californicus*.

Stingrays abound off the coast of southern California, the south Atlantic States, and the Gulf Coast. The body is flattened and pectoral fins are broadened laterally so that they present a flat disk. The tail is long and equipped with barbs. The barb penetrates a foot, releases venom, and lacerates tissue when it is pulled coming out. The pain is sharp and immediate. The jagged wound bleeds and may contain a torn integumentary sheath; the leg becomes edematous.

If a large amount of venom is inoculated, systemic symptoms may also occur.

Treatment includes immediate and thorough irrigation of the wound with salt water to remove venom and act as a vasoconstrictor. Then immerse the wound in hot water for at least $\frac{1}{2}$ to 1 h; the heat will neutralize the toxin. Finally, any remaining pieces of sheath should be searched for. Tetanus toxoid and antibiotics may also be necessary.

Sea urchin

Some varieties may leave a whorl or broken spine that later causes a granulomatous reaction. Remove gross evidence of foreign material with tweezers. Obtain radiographs of the area if irritation persists.

Coral cuts

Coral cuts may produce chronic ulcers if not treated; fragments of calcareous material and animal protein may be left behind. First aid should include thorough cleansing

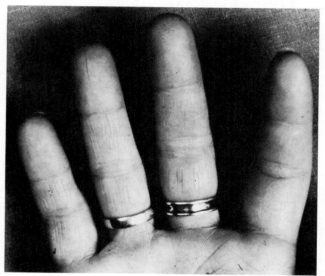

with a soft brush and soapy water, then alcohol rinse, then peroxide to remove bacteria and fine material.

Bibliography

Animal Bites (general references)

Berzon DR et al: Animal bites in a large city—a report on Baltimore, Maryland. *Am J Public Health* **62:**422, 1972

Hubbert WT et al: *Diseases Transmitted from Animal to Man.* Springfield, IL, Charles C Thomas, 1975

Kahrs RF et al: Diseases transmitted from pets to man: an evolving concern for veterinarians. *Cornell Veterinarian* **68:**442, 1978

Steele JH: A bookshelf on veterinary public health. *Am J Public Health* **63:**291, 1973

Strassburg MA et al: Animal bites: patterns of treatment. *Ann Emerg Med* **10:**193, 1981

Babesiosis

Jacoby GA et al: Treatment of transfusion-transmitted babesiosis by exchange transfusion. *N Engl J Med* **303:**1098, 1980

Ruebush TK, Spielman A: Human babesiosis in the United States. *Ann Intern Med* **88:**263, 1978

Wittner M et al: Successful chemotherapy of transfusion babesiosis. *Ann Intern Med* **96:**601, 1982

Cat-scratch disease (see also Chap. 195)

Wear DJ et al: Cat scratch disease: a bacterial infection. *Science* 221:1403, 1983

Coelenterata

Drury JK et al: Jelly fish sting with serious hand complications. *Injury* 12:66, 1980

Hartwick R et al: Disarming the box-jelly fish: nemocyst inhibition in *Chironex fleckeri. Med J Australia* 1:15, 1980

Dog bites

Callaham M: Prophylactic antibiotics in common dog bite wounds: a controlled study. *Ann Emerg Med* 9:410, 1980

Klein D: Friendly dog syndrome. *NY State J Med* 66:2306, 1966

Parris HM et al: Epidemiology of dog bites. *Public Health Rep* 74:891, 1959

Human bites

Mann RJ et al: Human bites of the hand: twenty years of experience. *J Hand Surg* 2:77, 1977

Peeples E et al: Wounds of the hand contaminated by human or animal saliva. *J Trauma* 20:383, 1980

Hymenoptera stings

Emergency treatment of insect sting allergy. *JAMA* 240:27, 1978

Golden DB et al: Regimens of Hymenoptera venom immunotherapy. *Ann Intern Med* 92:620, 1980

Hunt KJ et al: Diagnosis of allergy to stinging insects by skin testing with Hymenoptera venoms. *Ann Intern Med* 85:56, 1976

Lichtenstein LM et al: A case for venom treatment in anaphylactic sensitivity to Hymenoptera sting. *N Engl J Med* 290:1223, 1974

Lymphocytic choriomeningitis

Biggar RJ et al: Lymphocytic choriomeningitis outbreak associated with pet hamsters. *JAMA* 232:494, 1975

Hirsch MS et al: Lymphocytic choriomeningitis virus infection traced to a pet hamster. *N Engl J Med* 291:610, 1974

Marine diseases (general references)

Halstead BW: *Poisonous and Venomous Marine Animals of the World,* vols 1 and 2. Washington, DC, Government Printing Office, 1965, 1967

Pasteurella multocida

Gump GW, Holden RA: Endocarditis caused by a new species of *Pasteurella. Ann Intern Med* 76:275, 1972

Hubbert WT et al: *Pasteurella multocida* infection due to animal bite. *Am J Public Health* 60:1103, 1970

Jarvis WR et al: *Pasteurella multocida* osteomyelitis following dog bites. *Am J Dis Child* 135:625, 1981

Lucas GL, Bartlett DH: *Pasteurella multocida* infection in the hand. *Plast Reconstr Surg* 67:49, 1981

Swartz MN, Kunz LF: *Pasteurella multocida* infection in man. *N Engl J Med* 261:889, 1959

Tindall JP, Harrison CM: *Pasteurella multocida* infections following animal injuries, especially cat bites. *Arch Dermatol* 105:412, 1972

Weber DJ et al: "Pasteurella multocida" infections: report of 34 cases and review of the literature. *Medicine (Baltimore)* 63:133, 1984

Rabies

Anderson LJ et al: Post exposure trial of human diploid cell strain. *J Infect Dis* 142:133, 1980

Corey L, Hattwick MA: Treatment of persons exposed to rabies. *JAMA* 232:272, 1975

Hough SA et al: Human to human transmission of rabies virus by a corneal transplant. *N Engl J Med* 300:603, 1979

Meyer HW: Rabies vaccine. *J Infect Dis* 2:287, 1980

Plotkin SA: Rabies vaccination in the 1980's. *Hosp Pract* 15:65, 1980

Porras C et al: Recovery from rabies in man. *Ann Intern Med* 85:44, 1976

Rabies prevention: recommendation of Immunization Practices Advisory Committee (ACIP). *MMWR* 29(23):265, 1980

Scorpion stings

Horen WP: Insect and scorpion stings. *JAMA* 221:894, 1972

Hunt GR: Bites and stings of uncommon arthropods. *Postgrad Med* 70:107, 1981

Rimsza ME et al: Scorpion envenomization. *Pediatrics* 66:299, 1980

Stahnke HL: Arizona's lethal scorpion. *Arizona Med* 39:490, 1972

Seal bites

Beck B, Smith TG: Seal finger: an unsolved medical problem in Canada. *Technical Report of the Fisheries Research Board of Canada,* No 625. Arctic Biological Station, Fisheries and Marine Service. (Quebec, Ste Anne de Bellevue), 1976

Hilenbrand FKM: Whale finger and seal finger. *Lancet* 2:680, 1953

Markham RB, Polk F: Seal finger. *J Infect Dis* 1:567, 1979

Simian herpes B virus

Davidson WF, Hummeier R: B virus infection in man. *Ann NY Acad Sci* 85:970, 1968

Hull RN: The simian herpes viruses, in *The Herpes Viruses,* edited by AS Kaplan. New York, Academic Press, 1973, p 390

Snake bites

Garlin SR et al: Role of surgical decompression in treatment of rattlesnake bites. *Surg Forum* 30:502, 1979

Glass TG: Early debridement in pit viper bites. *JAMA* 235:2513, 1976

Goldstine EJC: Bacteriology of rattlesnake venom and implications for therapy. *J Infect Dis* 140:818, 1979

Grace TG et al: The management of upper extremity pit viper wounds. *J Hand Surg* 2:168, 1980

Parrish HM et al: Poisonous snake bites in New England. *N Engl J Med* 263:788, 1960

Russell F: Jaws that bite. *Emerg Med* 25:40, 1978

Russell F et al: Snake venom poisoning in the United States. *JAMA* 233:341, 1975

Sutherland SK, Coulter AR: Early management of bites by the eastern diamondback rattlesnake (*Crotalus adamanteus*): studies in monkeys (*Macaca fascicularis*). *Am J Trop Med Hyg* 30:497, 1981

Tick paralysis

Gothe R et al: The mechanisms of pathogenicity in the tick paralysis. *J Med Entomol* 16:357, 1979

Tick paralysis. *MMWR* 30(18): 217, 1981

CHAPTER 207

PROTOZOAN AND HELMINTH INFECTIONS

Fuad S. Farah

Introduction

Parasitic diseases have attracted more medical and public health attention than hitherto, in both the endemic areas and the technologically advanced countries. The World Health Organization has taken the lead in the effort to bring researchers and technologists to the endemic areas. The WHO program is aimed at comprehensive research of six tropical diseases and at training local personnel in the endemic areas who will ultimately carry on and continue the various programs concerned with the endemic problems.

Although endemic, many of the parasitic diseases are being seen in nonendemic areas with greater frequency. The ease and speed of travel has decreased the importance of geographic limitations. It is, therefore, increasingly important for physicians to familiarize themselves with diseases that are not so common in their own environments.

The parasites which cause diseases with cutaneous manifestations belong for the most part to the protozoa and the helminth worms, including the Nematoda (roundworms), Trematoda (flukes), and Cestoidea (tapeworms) of the phylum Platyhelminthes.

Protozoan infections

The protozoa are single-cell organisms capable of performing all necessary functions of life. Those of dermatologic interest include members of superclass Sarcodasica, family Endamoebidae, represented by *E. histolytica,* which infests the human intestine and may occasionally invade the skin. Among the Flagellata (superclass Mastigophorasica) there are two groups of major medical interest, those that inhabit the gastrointestinal and genitourinary tracts and are transmitted from person to person, e.g., *Giardia* and *Trichomonas,* and those that live in the bloodstream and tissue and require an invertebrate vector, e.g., *Leishmania* and *Trypanosoma.*

Helminth infections

The nematodes are roundworms, some of which are completely parasitic while others live freely in water or soil. *Ancylostoma, Necator,* and *Strongyloides* are free-living parasites whose ova hatch in the soil. *Strongyloides stercoralis* is capable of completing its life cycle either in soil or by the larvae infecting animals (ingested by cats or dogs) or humans through the skin, producing ground itch. The larvae reach the bronchi and lung through the bloodstream and are swallowed to reach the intestine and there develop into adults. This type of life cycle also applies to *Ancylostoma duodenale* and *Necator americanus.* Larvae of other species that do not infect the human intestines may penetrate the human skin and produce irritation (creeping eruption).

Ascaris, which does not affect the skin directly although it may be responsible for urticaria in endemic areas, has a similar life cycle to *Strongyloides.* The ova hatch in the human intestine and the larvae migrate to the lung via the bloodstream. They then reach the buccal cavity and are swallowed, eventually reaching the intestine and maturing into adults. The female lays its eggs, which are excreted and await ingestion by the host for continuation of the life cycle. This differs from *Enterobius vermicularis,* another parasite infecting humans, in which the female migrates to the anal region to lay her eggs and the larvae do not migrate in the body.

The adult *Dracunculus* (guinea worm) lives in the connective tissue of humans and other vertebrates, usually just under the skin through which the female discharges large numbers of larval forms when in contact with water. These infect *Cyclops* (water fleas) which upon ingestion by the host repeat the cycle.

Trichinella spiralis is an intestinal parasite of humans and other mammals. Young larvae bore through host tissues to reach the blood vessels through which they disseminate throughout the body. The majority of the larvae encyst in striated muscles. Ingestion of the cysts into the muscle by another host will continue the life cycle.

Wuchereria bancrofti lives in lymphatics, whereas *Onchocera volvulus* and *Loa loa* live in connective tissue; infection of the host is by blood-sucking (*Anopheles*) and tissue-feeding insects, respectively.

The trematodes (flukes) parasitize various cavities of the body (intestines, ducts associated with the gastrointestinal tract, the bladder, or lungs). The discharged eggs require water and a mollusk for further development. The egg is ingested by the snail (or hatches into a free-swimming larva, the miracidium, and finds its way to the snail). In the snail it develops into a spherocyst, divides asexually, and produces many larvae (rediae) which develop into cercariae. These cercariae enter the host either by ingestion (*Fasciola hepatica*) or penetrate the skin of fish (*Clonorchis sinensis*), the latter being ingested by humans. In *Schistosoma,* the cercariae enter the host through the skin. Cercariae of species not infective to humans may enter the skin of humans and produce cutaneous symptoms known as "swimmer's itch" or cercarial dermatitis.

The cestodes parasitize an intermediate host. *Tinea solium* infects humans in the tapeworm stage and pigs in the bladder worm. *Echinococcus* infects the dog in the tapeworm stage and humans in the hydatid cyst form. Cysticercosis may affect the human skin, and may occur in *T. solium* infections. Diphyllobothridae may parasitize humans and affect the skin, causing the condition known as sparganosis.

Protozoan infections

Amebiasis

Amebae are unicellular spherical organisms composed of an ectoplasm and an endoplasm. In the trophozoite stage, amebae reproduce by binary fission. When conditions become unfavorable, the amebae encyst, becoming capable of survival for prolonged periods and of transfer to other hosts. The cysts excyst in the colon, divide, and form new trophozoites. Nonpathogenic forms of amebae may be differentiated from the pathogenic forms morphologically.

In the intestine, *Entamoeba histolytica* usually lives harmlessly in the human bowel (asymptomatic amebiasis). Occasionally, it becomes pathogenic for reasons not presently known, resulting in invasive amebiasis. Colonization occurs by repeated, rapid, binary division. Invasion is accomplished by lytic digestion of the intestinal epithelium. Invasion is not accompanied by a host inflammatory response. However, amebic lesions, especially extraintestinal ones, are prone to secondary infection. Overall, case fatality in amebic dysentery is around 2 percent but is much higher in infants and children (27 percent).

Cutaneous amebiasis occurs less frequently than intestinal amebiasis but it most commonly affects those with active amebiasis, except for a group with cutaneous infection of the genitalia. The skin is involved by direct extension from the involved colon, an amebic hepatic abscess, following surgical intervention in colonic or hepatic amebiasis, or, less commonly, through direct inoculation by contact with infectious material. Common sites of involvement are the anus and the buttocks, penis, or face. Penile amebiasis may appear as the only lesion, acquired by heterosexual or homosexual intercourse with persons who suffer from amebic dysentery. Lesions of the vulva are common in severely ill children with amebic dysentery.

Characteristically, the skin lesions spread quickly. The course is faster in younger patients. Early diagnosis is important; however, the skin lesion itself is not diagnostic and consists of an invading ulcer or an ulcerated granuloma (ameboma). The ulcer (Fig. 207-1) has raised, thickened borders and often undermined edges with an erythematous surrounding zone. It is often covered by a purulent exudate and necrotic slough. It is very painful and is usually associated with regional lymphadenopathy.

Fig. 207-1 Amebiasis of the skin involving the vulva and lower part of the abdomen. (By permission, Biagi FF, Martuscelli QA: Dermatol Trop 2:129, 1963.)

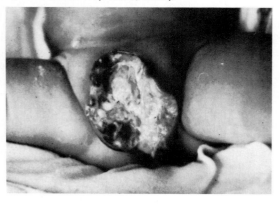

Other skin conditions associated with amebiasis include urticaria and pruritus, which are said to improve with treatment of the amebiasis.

Cutaneous amebiasis should be distinguished from epithelioma, other granulomas, and syphilis. Finding trophozoites at the base of the ulcer on biopsy or in the fresh material from the edge of the ulcer confirms the diagnosis. Repeated stool examinations should be made also, despite a negative history of dysentery. Gel diffusion and latex agglutination tests may be helpful.

The prognosis is good if the diagnosis is made early and treatment initiated immediately. It is, however, serious or fatal in untreated and neglected cases.

The treatment of the skin lesions is with emetine given intramuscularly or subcutaneously in a dose of 1 mg/kg for 10 days. The dose should not exceed 60 mg daily. Local irrigation and cleaning of the ulcer may be helpful. Treatment of the underlying colonic (or hepatic) disease, even if asymptomatic, should be carried out with tetracyclines, diodoquin (diiodohydroxyquinoline), and chloroquine. Metronidazole 750 mg 3 times daily for 5 to 10 days is recommended for intestinal and extraintestinal amebiasis and can be used in combination with other drugs.

Flagellate protozoa of the blood and tissues

Flagellate protozoa that inhabit the human bloodstream and tissues are *Trypanosoma (T. rhodesiense, T. gambiense, T. cruzi,* and *T. rougeti)* and *Leishmania (L. tropica, L. braziliensis,* and *L. donovani).* These organisms require two hosts, a human and an insect or another mammal. *Leishmania, T. gambiense,* and *T. rhodesiense* multiply as flagellates in the midgut of the insect and migrate anteriorly to the proboscis. *T. cruzi* moves posteriorly in the vector's gut and is evacuated with the feces.

Trypanosomiasis

Protozoa of the genus *Trypanosoma* are widely distributed around the equator (15°N-S) in Africa (African trypanosomiasis) and between latitude 42°N in the United States and 43°S in Argentina (American trypanosomiasis).

The *Trypanosoma* are flagellated protozoa. The flagellum arises near the posterior kinetoplast and emerges anteriorly. It has an undulating membrane. It circulates in the bloodstream as a trypomastigote, usually about 15 to 30 μm. When taken up by the vector, it lodges in the midgut, multiplies by binary fission, migrates to the salivary gland, and becomes infective in 2 weeks *(T. rhodesiense)* or 3 weeks *(T. gambiense).*

T. cruzi, the cause of American trypanosomiasis (or Chagas' disease) invades the reticuloendothelial system, myocardium, endocrine glands, and glial cells. Here, the parasite is in the amastigote (leishmanial) form, 1 to 5 μm, and characterized by a larger nucleus. It transforms to the trypomastigote form when outside the cell, is ingested by the vector, passed through the vector's liquid feces while the vector is feeding, and is introduced into the skin wound. In this respect, it differs from African trypanosomiasis and from leishmaniasis.

African trypanosomiasis. Humans are the natural hosts of *T. gambiense* transmitted by tsetse flies of the genus *Glos-*

sina palpalis. *T. rhodesiense* (morphologically similar to *T. gambiense*) is transmitted by *G. morsitans* and primarily infects wild animals, antelopes most notably. *T. rhodesiense* is primarily a zoonosis but infections in humans are fulminant and acute. Age, sex, and occupation do not influence the incidence of infection, except through the degree of exposure to the tsetse fly. *T. gambiense* is more prominent in Central and West Africa and *T. rhodesiense* is more common in East Africa.

Following the infected bite of the fly, dissemination occurs through lymphatics with spread to the central nervous system in *T. gambiense* infections. Often there are no cutaneous lesions, but at times the bite is followed by the formation of a red nodule, 1 to 3 cm in diameter, surrounded by a waxy, white halo (trypanosome chancre) seen mostly in Europeans, not in Africans. It is accompanied by lymphangitis and lymphadenopathy, but not suppuration, and it subsides within a few days. By the second week, fever and constitutional symptoms develop, followed by a generalized pruritic exanthem similar in appearance to erythema multiforme. Lymph node enlargement is prominent, particularly of the posterior cervical chain (Winterbottom's sign). Cardiac involvement may occur. Debility and variable central nervous system (CNS) symptoms appear, including lethargy, irresponsibility, headaches, seizures, ataxia, and paresis; death almost invariably follows.

Edema of the eylids is transient and painful, and the hands and feet are also involved. Large erythematous, often annular, eruptions appear on the trunk. Erythema nodosum sometimes occurs. Intravascular disseminated coagulation occurs in a few patients but cold hemagglutinins are regularly found. Low serum complement levels occur. Pruritus may be prominent.

Diagnosis may be difficult if not suspected in nonendemic areas (as travellers returning home). Immunologic tests may help, including immunofluorescent antibody tests, ELISA, and indirect hemagglutination tests. Finding the parasite in the blood smear should be attempted and is diagnostic.

Treatment should be initiated at the earliest possible time. Suramin (B.P.) or pentamidine isothionate is usually sufficient if given early, in patients without CNS involvement. Suramin is given as 200 mg intravenously as a test dose, and 1 g weekly for 5 weeks therafter. The dose of pentamidine isothionate is 4 mg/kg intramuscularly or intravenously every 1 to 2 days for 10 doses. In more advanced cases, arsenicals, melarsoprol (Mel B), or trimelarsan (Melarsonyl, Mel W) may be used. All these drugs must be used with caution because of their serious side effects.

American trypanosomiasis. Also known as Chagas' disease, American trypanosomiasis is a parasitic disease caused by *Trypansoma cruzi* which is transmitted by blood-sucking insects of the family Triatomidae (order Hemiptera—kissing bugs). The insect vectors are widely distributed in the Western hemisphere, including Texas and the southwestern United States through Central and South America. However, no definite cases have occurred in the United States in spite of the presence of the vector, and the area of distribution of the disease is more limited (42°N–43°S) than the range of the insect distribution. *T. cruzi* exists in many animal reservoirs such as dogs, cats, monkeys, pigs, and rodents like the squirrels.

T. cruzi resembles the trypanosomes responsible for African trypanosomiasis. In the blood, the organism is 15 to 20 mm long, of variable width, with an undulating membrane, and an anteriorly placed flagellum. In tissue cells it assumes the leishmanial form. It is an obligatory intracellular parasite and multiplies only within the cells.

In the tissue, *T. cruzi* invades the cells of the reticuloendothelial system, transforms to Leishman-Donovan forms, and incites an immediate reaction with edema and cellular infiltration manifested as subcutaneous swelling. The infection spreads 4 to 5 days later through lymphatics, and the draining lymph nodes become enlarged, edematous, and infiltrated with lymphocytes and plasma cells. There is hepatosplenomegaly. At a later stage, the parasite escapes to the bloodstream, becomes flagellated, and again penetrates a cell and repeats the cycle. Various tissues and organs are involved, particularly the spleen and liver. In the myocardium, the resultant scarring leads to serious effects. In the brain, localization of parasites leads to neurologic symptoms. The cycles of parasitism are thought to be associated with variations in the trypanosomal antigens. There may be immune hemolysis based on antigen–antibody reactions.

Clinically, the lesions appear at the site of inoculation, within 5 days in the majority of patients. The portal of entry is the conjunctiva (in 80 percent of the cases) evidenced by edema, inflammation of the lacrimal glands known as the "eye sign," "Romana's sign," or "oculoglandular complex" (Fig. 207-2). If the inoculation is in the skin, then a "cutaneous adenopathy complex" or chagoma develops, which is characterized by a tumorlike lesion on the chest, back, or legs. In children, it is often followed by myocarditis or encephalitis and may end fatally. Hepatosplenomegaly, edema, and various forms of cutaneous exanthems appear, some resembling erythema multiforme. Recurrence of the skin lesions is frequent. Subacute or chronic forms of the disease are almost always associated

Fig. 207-2   Romana's sign in Chagas' disease.

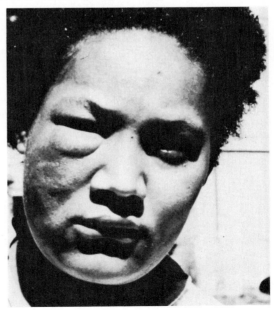

with myocarditis and some possibly with gastrointestinal manifestations such as megacolon or megaesophagus. Chronic heart failure is frequent in advanced cases.

The pathogenesis of the disease is not clarified. It may be related to toxins released by the parasite, or to the deposition of immune complexes with complement (low C3 and C4 have been demonstrated in some patients). It has also been shown that the immune response, both antibody-mediated immunity (ABMI) and cell-mediated immunity (CMI), are suppressed in these infections, possibly through generation of specific suppressor cells.

The diagnosis is suspected by the history and physical findings, especially in individuals living in endemic areas, and is established in early cases by demonstration of the parasite in the blood by smear or culture and in lymph node biopsy material. In subacute and chronic cases, demonstration of antibody by complement fixation, hemagglutination, or immunofluorescence tests is useful.

The treatment is not satisfactory. Arsenical preparations have been used for the treatment of blood trypanosomes. Suramin and trimelarsan as well as pentamidines have been used. Amphotericin B is still under investigation. In the acute stage 8-aminoquinolines may be useful. There is no treatment for the tissue form.

Preventive measures aimed at control of the insects might help. A vaccine preparation is under investigation.

Leishmaniasis

Infections with the *Leishmania* organisms in humans form a wide spectrum of clinical disease. On one side, there is the systemic infection involving the reticuloendothelial system and, on the other side, there are the cutaneous infections localized to the skin without systemic involvement. In the middle of the spectrum there are the mucocutaneous infections characterized by cutaneous lesions and metastatic mucous membrane infection. Three different *Leishmania* species have been designated for the three major clinical diseases, although they are routinely indistinguishable from each other. However, some differences among them might exist in the antigenic composition of the various species as well as those noted by electron

microscopic studies, and by the studies of the parasite DNA density and enzyme electrophoresis. *L. donovani* causes kala-azar, *L. braziliensis* causes the mucocutaneous form, and *L. tropica* causes cutaneous leishmaniasis. However, each of these organisms has variants that are clinically significant (Table 207-1).

The parasite was first discovered in 1885 by Cunningham in India from a case of kala-azar. In 1903, Wright demonstrated the organism in a case of oriental sore. In the same year, Donovan demonstrated the round forms in kala-azar, and Leishman recognized similar forms in trypanosomal infections. Since that time a large volume of literature has been accumulated about leishmaniasis and many excellent reviews on the clinical aspects, the taxonomy, and the biology of *Leishmania* are available.

There are two forms in which the parasite exists. In the tissue, the Leishman-Donovan (LD) bodies, also known as amastigotes, are found intracellularly as small, spherical, oval, uniform bodies 2 to 6 µg long and 1 to 2 µm wide. They have an external membrane, the periblast, and a nearly spherical nucleus with a pointlike kinetoplast from which a thin element emerges and is the root of the flagellum. The flagellar, leptomonad forms or promastigotes are found in cultures in artificial media and in the insect vector. The leptomonad is about 15 to 25 µm long, 1.5 to 3.5 µm wide, with a 15- to 28-µm flagellum. The flagellum is composed of eight fine filaments surrounding a thicker central one, and is responsible for motility. The parasite grows in artificial media containing defibrinated rabbit or human blood or hemoglobin. The organism also can be grown in tissue culture media.

The parasite exists in wild vertebrates, mostly rodents. Different species appear in various regions where the parasite has adapted itself to the mammalian fauna of the endemic area. However, rats, mice, gerbils, and dogs are the common reservoirs.

Mosquitoes of the genus *Phlebotomus* are the principal vectors responsible for the continued cycle of infected animal to mosquito to healthy animal (or human). The phlebotomus must obtain the organism from the reservoir in the leishmanial form. There is a definite association between foci of leishmaniasis and the sand fly population.

Table 207-1   Classification of leishmaniasis

Species	Disease	Most common location
L.d. donovani	Visceral, dermal leishmanoid	India
L.d. infantum	Visceral, dermal leishmanoid	Middle East, Mediterranean, USSR
L.d. sinesis	Visceral, dermal leishmanoid	China
L.d. nilotica	Visceral, mucocutaneous	Africa, especially Sudan and Ethiopia
L.t. major	Cutaneous	Middle East, Mediterranean, China, India
L.t. minor	Cutaneous	Middle East, Mediterranean
L.t. ethiopica	Cutaneous, diffuse cutaneous leishmaniasis (DCL)	Ethiopia
L.m. mexicana	Cutaneous, DCL	Mexico, Central America
L.m. amazonesis	Cutaneous, DCL	Brazil, South America
L.m. pifanoi	DCL, ?cutaneous	Brazil, Central America
L.b. braziliensis	Cutaneous, ?mucocutaneous	Brazil, Central America
L.b. panamensis	Cutaneous, ?mucocutaneous	Central America

The highest incidence appears in fall or early winter and seems to follow the population peak of the phlebotomus by about 3 to 6 months. This pattern has been consistently observed in Iraq and Sudan and is consistent with a 3- to 6-month incubation period. The parasites, ingested by the sand fly feeding on a lesion or from the blood of an animal, are lodged in the intestine of the insect where they become flagellated, multiply, and migrate to the oropharynx in great numbers. Subsequent bites of human skin release the parasite through the insect's proboscis. The parasite enters the macrophages, adopts the leishmanial form, and the cycle is repeated.

In humans, the parasites are found at sites of active lesions: in the skin, mucous membranes, and in the reticuloendothelial system as in kala-azar. They have not been demonstrated in nasal secretions, urine, or other tissues. Human-to-human transmission is not a likely occurrence since the organisms are found deep in lesions. However, in animals, *Leishmania* have been detected in normal skin and in the bloodstream as well as in lesions.

Natural immunity to leishmaniasis seems to exist in endemic areas and appears to play a role in the occurrence and extent of epidemic outbreaks. Epidemics have been observed following the influx of susceptible individuals into an endemic area. This is particularly true in cutaneous leishmaniasis. The inhabitants of endemic areas who are aware that infection protects against repeated inoculations have developed the practice of intentionally infecting the children by scarification and transfer of organisms from active lesions onto nonexposed areas of the skin. On occasion, however, patients with cutaneous leishmaniasis have been reinfected or superinfected. The ability to reinfect only some patients may depend on the use of an antigenically different strain or it may be associated with a defect in the host defense (cell-mediated immune response or an unusual susceptibility of macrophages to parasitization). The same mechanisms might explain the development of diffuse cutaneous leishmaniasis, chronic leishmaniasis, and recidiva lesions in cutaneous leishmaniasis, and may explain the generalization in kala-azar.

Studies of the role of the immune response in the infection and its clinical evolution have been conducted in strains of mice (susceptible to *L. tropica*) and guinea pigs (susceptible to *L. entrietti*). Antibodies were elicited against the infecting parasites, but the level or class of antibody developed did not correlate with the stage or extent of the disease. Passive antibody did not protect against infection. Depression of antibody formation with cyclophosphamide leads to delayed healing and more prolonged infection. Antileishmania antibody causes agglutination of the parasite and disturbs its growth in culture.

Cell-mediated immunity seems to influence the course of the infection also. Suppression of cell-mediated immunity by thymectomy, x-irradiation, antilymphocyte serum, or other means leads to a more prolonged course and nonhealing persistent ulcers. However, sensitized lymphocytes failed to protect animals (and humans in the few cases where they were transferred) against infection.

In the human, infection exists and lesions persist despite a measurable immune response (both antibody-mediated and cell-mediated). The immune response is not able to eradicate the existing infection immediately, but it does, in the majority of cases, prevent reinfection or superinfec-

tion, an observation made also in experimental infections of the guinea pig.

The macrophage appears to play a central role in leishmanial infections. It is a natural habitat of the parasite in which the organism grows and multiplies (Fig. 207-3), perhaps protected by its intracellular status from the effects of the immune response. However, the macrophage processes soluble antigens from the intracellular parasite and, by presenting these on its surface membranes, it may aid in the stimulation of B and T cells involved in the development of the immune response. Obviously, more studies of macrophage function in these diseases are required to elucidate the role it plays, particularly in the areas of chemotaxis.

There exists a definite adaptation of the organism to the host (animal or human) in which it lives. Studies on macrophages obtained from various susceptible species show that the organisms parasitize more efficiently and multiply more in the macrophages of susceptible animals, even if the macrophages come from immunized animals or are otherwise activated, and these do not kill the parasites.

In addition, the parasite may be responsible for depressing cell-mediated immunity locally and generally in the presence of heavy parasite loads, as in diffuse cutaneous leishmaniasis and in kala-azar. The suppression of lymphocyte activity seems to be species-specific, following the same pattern of relationship as between the parasite and the macrophage. The same pattern is noted in the demonstration of macrophage membrane receptors to the *Leishmania* organisms (unpublished data).

Systemic leishmaniasis (kala-azar). Visceral or systemic leishmaniasis, known as kala-azar, is a disease of the reticuloendothelial system caused by *L. donovani*. It is char-

Fig. 207-3 Disseminated anergic cutaneous leishmaniasis. Section of a nodule showing abundant leishmanial forms.

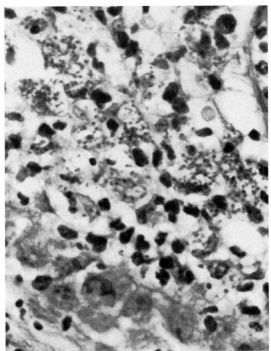

acterized by a prolonged course of fever, emaciation, hepatosplenomegaly, lymph node enlargement, leukopenia, anemia, edema, and, if not successfully treated, by death within 1 to 2 years.

Kala-azar is found throughout large areas of the world. It is prevalent in India, China, Indochina, the Mediterranean Coast, and in some parts of Western Africa. It is found in limited areas in Sudan, Ethiopia, and Kenya, and occurs sporadically in Latin America. The vectors, which are favored by heat and humidity and in some locations dryness, along with the availability of animal reservoirs, determine the incidence of the disease and its epidemic outbreaks.

L. donovani infection is relatively nonspecific among vertebrates. The dog is susceptible to infection by *L. donovani* and other *Leishmania* species and may be an important reservoir in some regions (Italy and the Middle East).

L. donovani parasitizes the reticuloendothelial cells generally and multiplies within the cells, causing them to rupture. The parasites infect other cells and the cycle is repeated. Organisms infect all body tissues, being spread by infected macrophages in the bloodstream. The tissue involvement is most severe in those organs rich in reticuloendothelial cells such as liver, spleen, bone marrow, lymph nodes, lungs, and the skin. There is proliferation of the macrophages in involved tissues. In many of these, typical leishmanial forms (LD bodies) are seen.

The incubation period varies from 1 to 6 months. Fever is usually the initial manifestation. It is above 40°C during the initial period of the illness, irregular, and either continuous or intermittent. It may become less prominent as the disease progresses. Associated symptoms are weakness, fatigue, loss of appetite, emaciation, and, frequently, edema. The hair becomes dry and tends to fall out. The skin becomes pigmented, usually on the face, the malar eminences, temples, and around the mouth (hence the name kala-azar, meaning black death). The spleen is invariably enlarged and is often associated with hepatomegaly and generalized lymphadenopathy.

The diagnosis of kala-azar should be suspected in patients with fever, emaciation, edema, and pigmentation who show splenomegaly, especially those residing in, or who have been in, an endemic area. The diagnosis is confirmed by demonstrating the organisms in smears and cultures of bone marrow puncture materials or, less often, in material obtained by splenic punctures or from lymph node biopsies. There is accompanying severe anemia with marked leukopenia and relative lymphocytosis. The plasma globulin levels are elevated and the formol-gel reaction is positive.

Clinically the condition must be differentiated from Hodgkin's disease, histoplasmosis, tuberculosis, and subacute septicemia.

POST KALA-AZAR DERMAL LEISHMANIASIS. One to two years or more following successful treatment, erythematous papules or patches appear on the face of 6 to 10 percent of patients. Later the lesions involve the rest of the body. Initially hyperpigmented, they may become hypopigmented. The picture is similar to that of lepromatous leprosy or that of diffuse cutaneous leishmaniasis. Parasites are abundant and skin tests with leishmanin may or may not be positive.

TREATMENT. The chemotherapeutic agents used are the trivalent (tartar emetic, Fuadin) or pentavalent antimonial compounds (stibosan, stibamine, or glucantime). Diamadines (stibamine and 2-hydroxy stilbamidine) have also been used. The treatment, when successful, results in reduction in the parasite load, return of the positive leishmanin test, and general improvement of the patient.

Mucocutaneous leishmaniasis (American leishmaniasis). Mucocutaneous leishmaniasis or American leishmaniasis is caused by *L. braziliensis* (and subspecies) and is characterized by a prolonged course and deformities due to the granulomatous lesions of the skin and, in the later stages, of the upper respiratory mucosa.

It is possible that the disease existed in the Americas before the continents were discovered. In 1906 Seidelin demonstrated *Leishmania* in the lesions and in 1909 Lindenberg identified them as the same organisms that produced oriental sore.

Mucocutaneous leishmaniasis is found in Latin America from Mexico to Argentina. Brazil and Peru have the highest incidence. The incidence, as it is with the other forms of leishmaniasis, is related to the population of *Phlebotomus* (*Lutzomyia* in the New World) and is highest during the rainy season. There is no sex or race predilection, but the disease is more frequent in men, particularly in forest workers, because of their increased exposure to the sand fly vector.

The incubation period is variable between 2 to 3 weeks up to 2 months or more. The lesions appear at the site of the insect bite and are consequently localized to the exposed parts of the body. The initial lesion is a small, erythematous, hard, elevated lesion appearing at the site of the insect bite and gradually increasing in size. It frequently ulcerates and is covered by a crust. At this time, lymph nodes are enlarged. Occasionally, there is no ulceration.

The ulcerated skin lesion continues to progress and enlarge (3 to 12 cm in size) with a characteristic raised border (Fig. 207-4). There may be one or several lesions. Secondary bacterial infection is common and a granulating ulcer base bleeds easily. The nonulcerating lesion also enlarges, becomes nodular or verrucose, and may resemble other chronic skin lesions. The lymphatic form may resemble sporotrichosis.

Involvement of the mucous membrane is the most common complication of *L. braziliensis* infection and occurs a few years later (3 to 10 years). Its incidence varies in the different regions and complicates up to one-third of the cases. The mucosal lesions are produced by spread through lymphatics or the bloodstream, and usually start in the nasal mucosa, which becomes inflamed, edematous, and ulcerative. The initial symptoms are referable to the nose, with coryza and variable epistaxis. Commonly, the cartilaginous septum is perforated. Later the lobules of the nose ulcerate, exposing underlying structures with destruction of the nasal fossa, mucosa, and cartilage. The bone is not usually involved, although osteolysis, osteosclerosis, and periostitis may occasionally develop. Anteriorly, the lips are involved, and posteriorly the pharynx, tonsillar area, floor of the mouth, and tongue may be affected. The process may continue into the larynx (with voice changes), trachea, and even the bronchi. The entire mucosa is thickened, granulomatous, bleeds easily, and is malodorous.

Breathing, feeding, and swallowing become painful, with

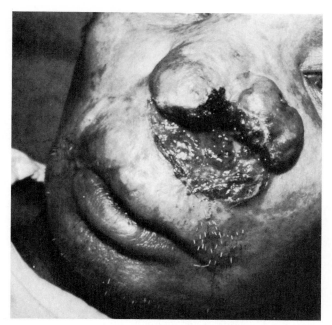

Fig. 207-4 Mucocutaneous leishmaniasis, seen in Hondu- ras. (Courtesy of Dr. Eric Kraus.)

much suffering. Malnutrition develops and contributes to the mortality, which results from acute respiratory involvement.

Occasionally distant cutaneous lesions appear. Some of these contain organisms while others may not (tuberculoid type). The "inhabited" lesions probably spread by lymphatics (regional) or bloodstream (disseminated) and may ultimately ulcerate.

Convit described massive involvement of the skin with papules, nodules, and plaques which contain abundant parasites. These patients are leishmanin-negative and histologically the lesions resemble lepromatous leprosy with macrophages full of parasites (leproid type). *Leishmania tropica* in the same form has been described in Ethiopia.

The cutaneous lesions tend to heal spontaneously except for lesions of the ear (Chiclero's ulcer), which become chronic. However, the mucous membrane complications which occur later in some patients are chronic and progressive, are more difficult to treat, and have a tendency to relapse.

The early lesions show variable proliferation of histiocytes and a corresponding inflammatory infiltrate. Granulomatous reactions (tuberculoid) are seen in some parts of the lesion. The late mucous membrane lesions show similar reactions but tuberculoid granulomas are rare. The epidermis may show pseudoepitheliomatous hyperplasia. Organisms are few and may be difficult to find in mucous membrane lesions. They are abundant in the anergic, disseminated form.

The diagnosis of the disease is established by the identification of the organism in smears, by cultures, or in tissue sections. The leishmanin skin test gives a delayed-hypersensitivity reaction in 97 percent of the cases who have or have had the disease.

Mucocutaneous leishmaniasis must be differentiated from pyoderma, sporotrichosis, syphilis, yaws, chromoblastomycosis, squamous cell carcinoma, and leprosy. When mucous membranes are affected, South American

blastomycosis, rhinoscleroma, and histoplasmosis must be considered.

The two modalities of treatment are antimonials as previously described for kala-azar, and amphotericin B. The effectiveness of the latter was discovered in 1959, but it must be administered under strict medical observation in hospitals. Fifty milligrams in 500 mL of 5% dextrose in water is slowly given by drip over 3 to 4 h. A total of 200 to 1800 mg may be used.

Cutaneous leishmaniasis. ORIENTAL SORE (Fig. A6-10). Oriental sore is a specific granuloma of the skin caused by *L. tropica*. It does not involve the other tissues of the body and, in the majority of patients, healing is associated with permanent immunity. Wright, in 1903, demonstrated the parasite in a patient diagnosed as having leprosy.

The disease is common in tropical and subtropical areas. It is found in China, Syria, Lebanon, Iraq, Israel, Jordan, Saudi Arabia, Egypt, Iran, Pakistan, India, and the Soviet Union. It is found around the Mediterranean coast both in Europe and Africa, where it is also found in Nigeria, Chad, Sudan, and Ethiopia. It is possible to consider the cases in South America that are purely cutaneous (i.e., without mucous membrane lesions) as cutaneous leishmaniasis.

L. tropica, the causative agent of cutaneous leishmaniasis, is not routinely distinguished from *L. braziliensis* or *L. donovani*, although this differentiation is now possible using sophisticated technology as mentioned earlier. The sand fly is the main vector, and *Phlebotomus papatasi* and *Phlebotomus sergenti* are commonly found in the Middle East. There have been reports of epidemics in Syria, Iraq, Iran, and Afghanistan that followed the influx of susceptible populations into the endemic areas. The animal reservoir is the gerbil, although the dog is also incriminated.

There is no sex or racial predilection and children are more affected than others. The incubation period varies from a few weeks to several months. In experimental leishmaniasis the incubation period varies inversely with the size of the inoculum, being shorter when the inoculum is large. Individual susceptibility also plays a role in the determination of the incubation period.

The clinical manifestations of cutaneous leishmaniasis are best considered under the following classifications:

1. Localized cutaneous leishmaniasis
   a. Acute
   b. Chronic
   c. Recidiva
2. Generalized cutaneous leishmaniasis
   a. Diffuse cutaneous leishmaniasis
   b. Leishmanid

ACUTE CUTANEOUS LEISHMANIASIS. The lesions appear on the exposed parts of the body accessible to the phlebotomus. The initial lesion is a 3- to 4-mm papule that resembles a mosquito bite (Fig. 207-5). It is pinkish in color and disappears on pressure. The papule persists and after several weeks begins to enlarge, becomes firm, and attaches to the underlying structures. It feels boggy and develops a smooth and glistening surface. It continues to enlarge and soon develops a dark, livid color. There is no pain, but there may be severe pruritus. At this time, the center may ulcerate and become covered with a brown-gray crust. The crust is adherent and, if removed, shows evidence of follicular plugs on its undersurface and a shallow ulcer with a spongy surface.

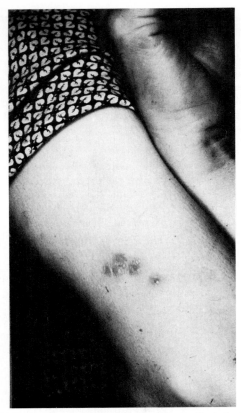

Fig. 207-5   Acute cutaneous leishmaniasis. Early lesions resembling insect bites. Multiple lesions are due to multiple bites. [From Simons RDG, Monshar J (eds): Essays on Tropical Dermatology. Amsterdam, Excerpta Medica, 1969.]

Healing begins at the center of the ulcer beneath the scab and progresses. A characteristic, permanent, depressed, stellate, disfiguring scar (Fig. 207-6) results. The size of the lesion is variable and is larger when the lesions are fewer. The duration is usually about a year, but there are cases that heal faster and others that become chronic, lasting many years.

Fig. 207-6   Scar of healed leishmaniasis on the cheek. The lesion on the ear represents acute leishmaniasis (reinfection). (From Arch Dermatol 103:467, 1971.)

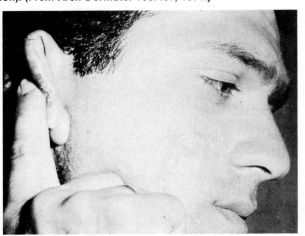

The two types, wet and dry, may coexist in natural infections as they do in experimental infections. Ulceration, however, depends most importantly on external factors such as trauma and not solely on the strain of the infecting parasites.

Usually, cutaneous leishmaniasis appears as a single lesion, although multiple lesions occur occasionally and are the result of multiple infected sand fly bites. Patients with over 200 lesions have been seen. In experimental inoculations in humans, one inoculation produced one lesion.

Superinfection might occur with the development of new lesions distant from the original sore that is still active. It results from a new inoculation and the new lesion usually assumes the morphology and the stage of the existing sores (isophasic response). In other cases the superinfection sore follows the course and evolution of the original lesion but possibly in a shorter period.

Histopathologic studies reveal variable changes in the epidermis. There is hyperkeratosis, some parakeratosis, and follicular plugging. There may be atrophy or acanthosis with occasional intraepidermal abscesses. The basal cell layer may be degenerated. In the dermis there is a heavy infiltrate of histiocytes and mononuclear cells. Eosinophils, neutrophils, and plasma cells are rare and intracellular bodies are abundant.

CHRONIC CUTANEOUS LEISHMANIASIS. In the elderly, the disease may take a more chronic form and lasts for several years in contrast to children, in whom healing occurs within one year. The face is most commonly affected and the lesions may be symmetrical. They may be single or multiple and are plaques of varying sizes, erythematous, boggy, scaly, with follicular prominence (Fig. 207-7). There is no regional lymphadenopathy, discharge, or draining sinuses. Ordinarily the granulomas do not ulcerate and follow a chronic indolent course. The underlying structures and mucosae are not affected.

The diagnosis of this group is difficult, especially because organisms are sparse. This chronic granuloma must be differentiated from lupus vulgaris, leprosy, syphilis,

Fig. 207-7   Chronic cutaneous leishmaniasis. This lesion is of about 15 years' duration. [From Simons RDG, Monshar J (eds): Essays on Tropical Dermatology. Amsterdam, Excerpta Medica, 1969.]

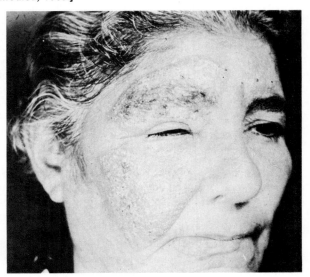

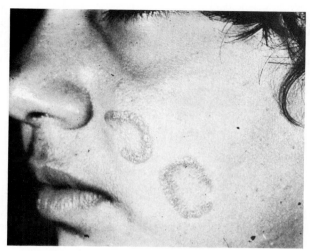

Fig. 207-8 Leishmania recidiva. The active lesions surround the scar in the center. [From Simons RDG, Monshar J (eds): Essays on Tropical Dermatology. Amsterdam, Excerpta Medica, 1969.]

North American blastomycosis, and other deep fungal infections. The prominent histologic feature is the presence of tubercles in the upper and lower dermis composed of epithelial giant cells of Langhans' type. In addition, there are mild to moderate histiocytic and mononuclear infiltrates. Necrosis and LD bodies are scarce.

LEISHMANIA RECIDIVA. This form of leishmaniasis is of special interest. New lesions appear in or around existing scars of healed lesions (Fig. 207-8). The fresh lesions are erythematous, boggy papules that resemble early lesions of acute leishmaniasis, but LD bodies are hard to find. It is possible to assume that intracellular organisms have not been eliminated and have become reactivated, perhaps as a result of changes in the local immunity.

Reinfection occurs when a patient with healed leishmaniasis develops new lesions following fresh inoculation at sites not related to the original infection. The condition is extremely rare and presumably develops when there is a disturbance of immunity acquired as a result of the original infection. It may also result from the inoculation of the patient with a new strain.

The histologic changes of leishmania recidiva combine features of both the acute and the chronic forms. The epidermal changes are variable and the dermis displays a moderate diffuse infiltrate as well as tubercular structure. LD bodies are rarely seen.

DISSEMINATED CUTANEOUS LEISHMANIASIS. A condition seen in South and Central America, Sudan, Ethiopia, and India, disseminated cutaneous leishmaniasis is characterized by the development of disseminated lesions rich in organisms (Fig. 207-9). They are similar to the lesions of lepromatous leprosy and, as in this form of leprosy, the patients show a negative delayed-hypersensitivity response. It is interesting to note that disseminated lesions have been induced in a patient with lepromatous leprosy inoculated experimentally with *L. tropica*.

LEISHMANID. Leishmanid classically represents a generalized eruption in patients with acute leishmaniasis. The leishmanids appear at different sites from the primary focus, do not contain organisms, and are associated with strongly positive leishmanin skin tests. The condition is extremely rare. The eruption is asymptomatic and disappears spontaneously in 2 to 3 months.

DIAGNOSIS. The diagnosis of cutaneous leishmaniasis is made from both clinical and histopathologic features. Definitive diagnosis, however, rests on the isolation and identification of the organism. The leishmanin skin test is positive in about 80 percent of the patients with long-standing or healed leishmaniasis. It is negative in patients with heavy parasite loads, as in diffuse cutaneous leishmaniasis.

TREATMENT. The therapeutic modalities used to date, which include chemotherapy, antibiotics, physical agents, and surgery, leave a lot to be desired. Pentavalent antimonials such as glucantime (methyl glucamine antimoniate) and antimalarials (chloroquine, quinacrine) are the agents most commonly used. The antimonials are effective in patients with multiple lesions and should be administered with care. Toxicity includes headaches, fainting, muscle and joint pain, EKG changes, and seizures. Anti-

Fig. 207-9 Diffuse cutaneous leishmaniasis. Multiple lesions of various forms that are rich in organisms. (Courtesy of Dr. A. D. M. Brycesson, Hospital for Tropical Diseases, London.)

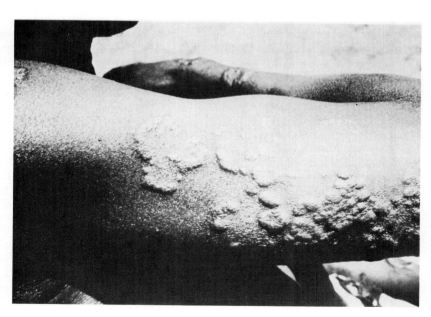

monials should be avoided in patients with myocarditis, hepatitis, or nephritis. The repository antimalarial, cycloguanil pamoate (Camolar), has been recently introduced in the treatment of acute leishmaniasis. Intralesional antimalarials have been used with good results. Antibiotics were advocated at one time but their effect is limited to the control of secondary bacterial infection. Amphotericin B has been used and found effective in the mucocutaneous form.

Surgical and physical methods of treatment include excision (especially of small lesions), electrosurgery, and cryotherapy. All these modalities are destructive and lead to scarring. Surgery has a limited value applicable to single early lesions. It is not, however, a recommended modality for routine treatment. Electrosurgery has application in the treatment of papules of leishmania recidiva. Cryotherapy is useful in acute, chronic, and recidiva cases; although it is destructive, its proper application leads to effective control of the disease process and leaves cosmetically acceptable scars.

In chronic leishmaniasis, systemic treatment with glucantime and cryosurgery are advocated.

The availability of the macrophage cultures that could be infected with leishmania provides an opportunity for the study of the effects of drugs on the intracellular parasite. Many agents have been tried, and some show promise, such as imidazole.

Helminth infections

Helminth is the Greek word for "worm," and in the more restricted sense it refers to parasitic worms. Two large phyla are mostly implicated, the Platyhelminthes (flatworms) and Nematoda (true roundworms). The two classes of Platyhelminthes, the Trematoda (flukes) and Cestoda (tapeworms), are exclusively parasitic throughout their life cycle. Many of the species of Nematoda are free-living and some are parasitic during part or all of their lives.

Platyhelminthes (faltworms)

Schistosomiasis. Also known as bilharziasis in honor of Theodor Bilharz, who in 1851 discovered the causative agent (*Schistosoma haematobium*) in Cairo, Egypt, the disease had been known there much earlier (around 1100 B.C.). The worms live typically in pairs in the portal venous system or in the vesical venules of the caval system but they can be dislodged and carried via the bloodstream to distant sites. The worms may live for up to 30 years or more in the human host.

The life cycle is complex and involves freshwater snails, in which cercariae develop and are released. The free-swimming cercariae penetrate intact skin and reach the bloodstream. The larva matures in the portal veins and lays its eggs mostly in the pelvic veins. *Schistosoma mansoni*, common in Africa and in Central and South America, and *S. japonicum* in the Far East, localize around the rectum and colon and pass their eggs in the feces. *S. haematobium*, common in Africa, India, and the Middle East, especially in the Nile delta of Egypt, localize around the bladder and pass their eggs in the urine. On contact with water the eggs develop into miracidia, which seek the snail and therein develop into free-swimming cercariae.

The cercariae penetrate the human skin and the cycle continues.

The ova may work their way into the tissues where they produce a granulomatous inflammation with a tuberculoid formation and with eosinophils, histiocytes, and occasional giant cells surrounding the ovum, probably dependent on immune mechanisms. These lesions can occur at distant "ectopic" sites.

There are several cutaneous lesions associated with schistosomiasis:

SCHISTOSOMAL DERMATITIS. The cercariae may cause a pruritic papular eruption indistinguishable from cercarial dermatitis due to nonhuman schistosomes.

URTICARIAL REACTIONS. Urticarial reactions appear some 4 to 8 weeks after the cercariae of *S. japonicum* (other human schistosomes less frequently) penetrate the skin. The urticaria is mostly on the trunk and is associated with fever, malaise, abdominal pain, diarrhea, arthralgia, and hepatosplenomegaly. It is referred to as urticarial fever or Katayama disease.

PARAGENITAL GRANULOMAS. These occur frequently in endemic areas of *S. haematobium* infections in the Middle East. Granulomatous lesions involve the vaginal area, perineum, and buttocks and are associated with extensive and communicating fistulas and sinuses (Fig. 207-10).

ECTOPIC CUTANEOUS SCHISTOSOMIASIS. Ova or dislodged flukes in pairs may become deposited in the skin as well as in other areas such as the lung, conjunctiva, or central nervous system. The trunk is most often involved with a granulomatous reaction that is flesh colored, firm, and papular, varying in size but usually 2 to 3 mm. Plaques result from coalescence of the lesions, which desquamate and may ulcerate and ultimately become deeply pigmented. Skin or rectal biopsy reveals the presence of ova.

Treatment is that of the systemic bilharziasis with stibophen, and other trivalent antimonials like Astiban and the recently introduced, promising Ambilhar (niriazole).

Cercarial dermatitis (swimmer's itch). Swimmer's itch describes a pruritic papular eruption caused by the inflammatory reaction incited by the entry of cercariae into the skin. The human blood flukes (schistosomes) described earlier produce an indistinguishable condition from the dermatitis produced by nonpathogenic avian or mammalian flukes. Both freshwater and marine forms are responsible. However, like the pathogenic forms, they require a snail intermediate host, and the endemicity is determined by the availability of the snail.

Collector's itch due to *Trichobilharzia ocellata* and *T. physellae* is common in swamps and in the presence of vegetation. Swimmer's itch is likely due to *T. stagnicolae*, which lives in shallow waters. The condition is found in temperate and tropical regions.

Clinically, itching is manifest at the time of exposure. The cercariae penetrate the skin by means of their spines and by the effects of proteolytic enzymes. The itching results from the acute inflammatory, urticarial (edema and erythema) reaction. This urticarial reaction subsides and is replaced by a papular and pruritic lesion similar to the delayed-hypersensitivity reaction. The eruption is on the exposed parts and spares the areas covered by clothing. It begins to regress after three days and subsides by one to two weeks, although scratching may lead to ulceration.

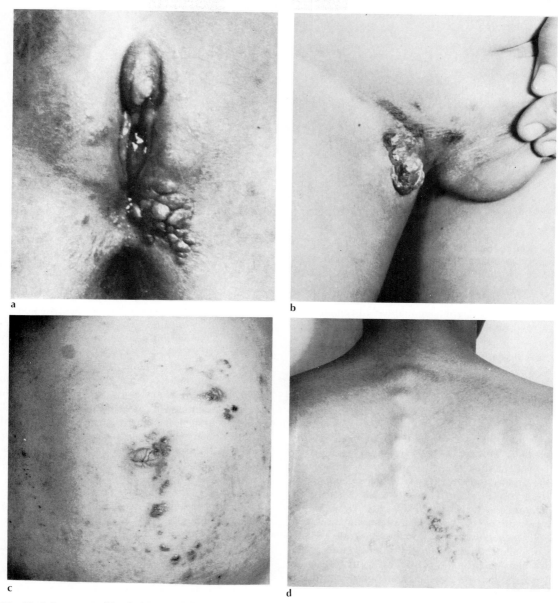

Fig. 207-10   Nodules caused by _S. haematobium._ (a) Vulvar. (b) Inguinal. (c) Periumbilical. (d) Scapular. _[Courtesy of Dr. A. M. El-Mofty; parts (a) and (d) by permission, El-Mofty AM, Cahill KM: Dermatol Trop 3:157, 1964.]_

Treatment is symptomatic with antipruritic preparations to relieve the discomfort. The cercariae do not live in the human skin and the lesions subside spontaneously.

CESTODES. These are tapeworms made up of a scolex (head), neck, and a chain of segments, the proglottids. The scolex attaches to the intestinal mucosa and feeds by means of sucking cups or hooklets. The number of proglottids varies and is characteristic of the species. Cestodes may inhabit the intestines (_Diphelobothrium latum, Taenai saginata, T. salina, Hymenolepis nana_) or the tissues, as with _Echinococcus granulosus_ and _E. sparganosis._

Sparganosis. This condition has a worldwide distribution, but occurs mostly in the Orient and is caused by the procercoid larva (sparganum) of _Spirometra mansonoides_ and _Spirometra mansoni._ The various species do not have characteristics to allow their differentiation. Speciation must depend on the study of the tapeworm in its definitive host (dogs or cats).

Infection occurs after ingestion of the procercoids found in copepod cyclops in drinking water or from ingestion of raw or lightly cooked muscles of the second intermediate host (snakes, birds, pigs, frogs, or other mammals). Application of raw flesh in the form of poultices to open lesions or to the eye or vagina may serve as a source of infection.

The larva penetrates the intestine and develops into spargana in the subcutaneous tissue or muscle. The areas affected are edematous and may be painful. The worm may migrate from one area to the other, and may last indefinitely (Fig. 207-11).

Treatment is by surgical removal and drainage whenever

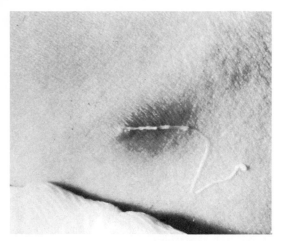

Fig. 207-11 Sparganosis. The worm has been withdrawn from the superficial lesion *(By permission, Miller JA, Abadie SH: J Trop Med Hyg 13:46, 1964.)*

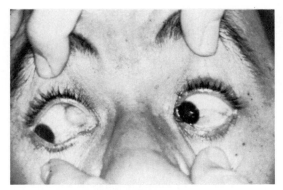

Fig. 207-12 Nodule due to *Cysticercus* under the conjunctiva. *(Courtesy of Dr. Jack Esslinger.)*

feasible. Arsenicals (neoarsphenamine) have been advised and are said to produce a good response.

Echinococcosis (hydatid disease). Two tapeworms, one of dogs (*Echinococcus granulosus*) and one of wild animals (*E. multilocularis*) parasitize humans in the larval stage. Sheep are common intermediate hosts with humans; cattle and pigs are less frequently affected. Humans generally ingest the larvae in contaminated food or water. The larvae penetrate the intestinal wall and are disseminated by the bloodstream to various parts of the body, especially liver, lung, and bone. The life cycle is completed when the predator eats the organs containing hydatid cysts. The skin is occasionally involved with the development of soft, flocculent, subcutaneous cysts of various sizes. They are not painful. Eventually cysts calcify or are resorbed after several years. *E. granulosus* most commonly produces unilocular cysts while *E. multilocularis* produces large, irregular cavities causing prominent tissue destruction, as in the liver. Urticaria may be a common and prominent complication of echinococcosis due to sensitization by the products of the cyst fluid absorbed systemically.

Cysticercosis. *Taenia solium*, the pork tapeworm, produces human intestinal infestation after ingestion of inadequately cooked pork containing *T. solium* cysticerci. The adult worm attaches to the intestinal wall and grows to a length of about 7 m. However, ingested eggs or eggs transferred to the mouth by poor sanitary habits are likely to develop into the larval stage in numerous organs, mostly subcutaneous tissue, with the production of cysticercosis (due to *Cysticercus celulosae*). The growing cyst excites a nonspecific inflammation with ultimate fibrosis and calcification (Fig. 207-12).

The diagnosis is established by x-ray findings, complement fixation, indirect hemagglutination, determination of specific IgE levels, and skin tests. Biopsy is confirmative. The most common form of treatment is surgical. Immunotherapeutic manipulations are being tested. Mebendazole has been recently tried and deserves serious consideration in the treatment of this condition separately and in association with surgery. It probably acts by preventing growth rather than by killing the parasites.

CESTODES. The intestinal cestodes (*T. saginata, T. solium, D. latum* and *H. nana*) are not associated with specific dermatologic symptoms other than cuticarie in some cases. *T. solium* may occur also in tissues where a human serves as an intermediate host. The diagnosis is established by the findings of proglottids or ova in the stools. They all respond to Nicolsamide (2 g as a single dose). Quinarine is also effective and is preferred in *T. solium* infections.

The intestinal worm is asymptomatic and is discovered by finding eggs in the stools (not easily differentiated from *T. saginata*) or by the appearance of gravid proglottids which have characteristic features differing from *T. saginata*. The cysts in the skin are rubbery, round, painless, and

Table 207-2 Parasites that produce cutaneous manifestations

Order	Parasite	Manifestation
Strongyloidea	*Necator americanus*	Uncinarial dermatitis
	Ancylostoma duodenale	(ground itch)
	Ancylostoma capillaria	Larva migrans
Rhabdiasoidea	*Strongyloides sterocalis*	Larva currans
		Strongyloidiasis/
		ground itch
Oxyuroidea	*Enterobius vermicularis*	Oxyuriasis
Spiruroidyea	*Gnathostoma spinigerum*	Gnathostomiasis
Trichuroidea	*Trichinella spiralis*	Trichinosis
Dracunculoidea	*Dracunculus medinensis*	Dracunculosis
Filarioidea	*Onchocerca volvulus*	Onchocerciasis
	Loa loa	Loiasis
	Wuchereria bancrofti	Filariasis
	Burgia malayi	

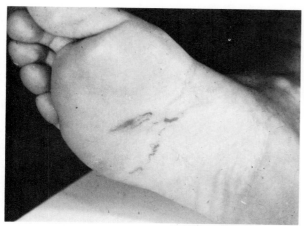

Fig. 207-13 Creeping eruption on the foot. *(Courtesy of Dr. A. Kurban, Division of Dermatology, American University of Beirut, Beirut.)*

may remain unchanged for many years. Immunologic methods such as the precipitin ring test and indirect hemagglutination are more reliable diagnostic tests than skin tests. Histology confirms the diagnosis of cysticercosis cellulosae cutis.

Nicolsamide is the drug of choice for the treatment of the adult worm. Quinacrine hydrochloride may be of value. Removal of all possible cysticerci should be attempted.

Nematodes (roundworms)

Nematodes are elongated, nonsegmented cylindrical animals. Their life cycle depends on the eggs, four larval stages, and the adult stage. Each larval stage ends with development of a new cuticle, the older one being molted. Parasites that produce cutaneous manifestations are listed in Table 207-2.

Larva migrans (creeping eruption). Larva migrans is a characteristic cutaneous eruption caused by larvae of various nematode parasites for which humans are an abnormal final host. When the larvae migrate in and involve viscera, it is called visceral larva migrans in contrast to the cutaneous

larva migrans. The following are examples: *Ancylostoma braziliensis*, in central and southeast United States, and *A. canium*, *Uncinaria stenocephala* (hookworm of dogs), and *Bunostomum phlebotomum* (hookworm of cattle) are the more common species responsible, although transient creeping eruption results from larvae of human hookworm, *A. duodenale* and *Necator americanus*.

The ova of these hookworms are deposited in the soil and hatch into infective larvae which then penetrate human skin. Sandy, warm, shady areas are favorable and children, gardeners, farmers, and sea bathers are more likely to be exposed to the infection.

The various larvae produce a similar reaction in the skin which begins within a few hours as a nonspecific pruritic dermatitis at the site of penetration. The skin areas involved are those in contact with soil, usually the feet (Figs. 207-13 and A6-25) and buttocks (Fig. 207-14). Shortly thereafter the larvae begin to migrate in the skin, or they may remain stationary for a few weeks or months. Migration is manifested by a wandering, thin, linear, raised tunnel-like lesion 2 to 3 mm wide containing serous fluid; the old lesions become dry and crusted. Many larvae may be active at one time, producing bizarre patterns. Migration may stop after a few weeks or months. The larvae move a few millimeters to a few centimeters per day, usually limited to a small area. They rarely travel far. The fast migration is referred to as larva currens (*Strongyloides stercoralis*).

The disease should be self-limited since humans are "dead-end" hosts, but the natural duration of the disease is variable—25 to 81 percent of the larvae disappear in 4 weeks.

Larva migrans may be associated with eosinophilia (10 to 35 percent) and Loeffler's syndrome. Visceral larva migrans due to dog or cat ascarides (*Toxocara canis*) or to other nematode larvae (*Ancylostoma luumbridordis*) may lead to patchy, erythematous urticaria or papular eruptions accompanied by systemic illness, granulomas of liver with hepatomegaly, pneumonitis, eosinophilia, and hyperglobulinemia.

Larva currens is a special form of cutaneous larva migrans caused by *Strongyloides stercoralis*. An intense papular eruption develops at the site of injection, accompa-

Fig. 207-14 Cutaneous larva migrans.

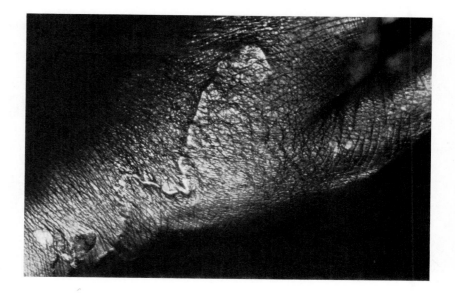

nied often by urticaria, papulovesicular, edematous, or nonspecific eruption. Ordinarily, the eruption is associated with intestinal strongyloidiasis and begins in the skin around the anus and may involve the buttocks, thighs, back, and shoulders. The skin of the abdomen is also affected but the genitalia are spared. The pruritis is intense, and the lesions spread at 5 to 10 cm per h. The larvae leave the skin, enter the blood and later settle in the intestinal mucosa, and the rash fades.

Treatment of larva migrans rests mainly with thiabendazole, given in doses of 25 to 50 mg/kg for 2 to 4 days, rarely longer. Pruritus subsides by the first day and the rest of the lesions disappear in 1 to 2 weeks. Topical thiabendazole is also effective, especially in the early cases. Freezing the involved area of the skin with dry ice or ethyl chloride may be effective if sloughing of the epidermis and the parasite is achieved. The freezing must include the advancing burrow where the parasite might be expected to be.

Intestinal nematodes infecting humans through larvae

Trichinosis. Infection with *Trichinella spiralis* is acquired following the ingestion of inadequately cooked, infected meat (pork, wild pig, bear, or polar bear). The larvae are liberated upon digestion and penetrate the intestinal mucosa where they migrate to the adult stage in about 1 week. In 2 to 3 weeks, the female larva deposits mobile embryos in the tissue. These enter the general circulation and are distributed to all parts of the body. In striated muscles, the embryos develop into larvae which incite an inflammatory reaction leading to encystment of the larvae in fibrous cysts. The larvae may remain infective for several years, but many become calcified during the first year. Passage of embryos through other tissues of the body leads to local, intense inflammation but encystment occurs only in striated muscle (Fig. 207-15). Many animals may be infected with *T. spiralis* but the pig remains the major source of the infection.

Clinical manifestations begin with the stage of muscle invasion (about 1 week following infection) and last for several days to several weeks. An acute illness develops with fever, generalized muscle pain and tenderness, difficulty in respiration and in using tongue muscles, sweating, periorbital edema, and conjunctivitis. The skin is pruritic, and urticaria, macular, papular, or petechial eruptions may occur. Splinter hemorrhages may be seen (Fig. 207-16) and the parasite can be readily demonstrated in biopsy specimens of the nail bed. The severity of the disease depends on the parasite load, and can be fatal in severe infections. Moderate infection improves by the fifth or sixth week, when desquamation may be seen.

The condition is associated with eosinophilia (between 10 and 90 percent). Immunologic evidence of the presence of the infection develops by the third week. Skin tests are not very reliable.

Thiabendazole 50 mg/kg per day given for 7 days has been found useful against the worms in the intestine and against the larval stages. Treatment is effective in early stages, but older infections do not respond. Corticosteroids may be useful in controlling the symptoms because of their anti-inflammatory effects. Prevention of the infection is important and is achieved by the proper cooking of meat.

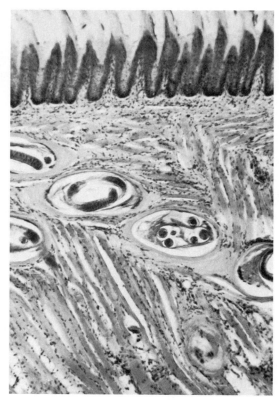

Fig. 207-15 Section of rat tongue showing encysted larvae of *Trichinella*.

Pork cooked at outdoor barbecues is often cooked adequately on the outside, while the center may be insufficiently heated to kill the parasite.

Tissue nematodes

Dracunculosis. Guinea or Medina worm is a chronic infestation of humans caused by *Dracuncula medinensis*. It is common in the Middle East (Arabia, Iran, Pakistan), New Guinea, and Indonesia—areas characterized by dryness and scarcity of water.

D. medinensis is a large nematode, 1 to 2 mm wide and

Fig. 207-16 Splinter hemorrhages in a patient with trichinosis. (Courtesy of Dr. John H. Vaughan.)

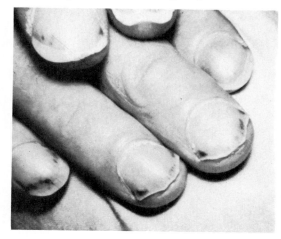

Fig. 207-17 Dracunculosis. Severe, intense inflammatory reaction precedes the rupture of the skin and prolapse of the worm. *(Courtesy of Dr. G. H. Sahba, University of Tehran, Tehran.)*

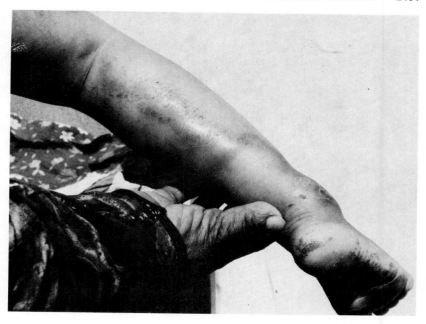

50 to 120 cm long, the male being much shorter, measuring only 4 to 8 and rarely 12 cm. When the female is gravid it travels to the skin of the lower extremities (in 82 percent of cases) and elsewhere in the remainder. It penetrates the skin and discharges large numbers of larvae upon contact with water. Larvae are ingested by copepods (water fleas) of the genus *Cyclops*, where they mature into the infective stage. Humans are infected by drinking water containing infected copepods. The larvae are liberated in the human gastrointestinal tract, and usually migrate to the loose retroperitoneal tissue, where they develop into the adult worms in about 8 months.

There are no clinical signs of the infection until the female worm approaches the skin. Before the skin is broken, severe systemic symptoms develop, including urticaria, erythematous rashes, malaise, and fever. There follows an intense inflammatory reaction around the anterior end of the worm, probably induced by products of the worm or its metabolism (Figs. 207-17 and A6-24). The symptoms subside with the rupture of the skin upon contact with water, when the uterus prolapses, and the larvae are discharged (Fig. 207-18).

It is possible to have more than one worm in the same individual. After several weeks, when the process of larval discharge is completed, the worm dies and may calcify without development of further symptoms. Secondary bacterial infection, chronic pruritus, arthritis, synovitis, ankylosis, and contractures might develop later.

Diethylcarbamazine (Banocide, Hetrazan) is effective in the early stages only. Thiabendazole has been reportedly effective in killing the worm and reducing the inflammation. Extraction of the worm gradually and gently is effective.

Filariasis. Nematodes of the superfamily Filaroides cause a worldwide disease occurring mostly in tropical or subtropical regions between latitude 45°N and 25°S, with the greatest concentration of cases in Africa, Asia, the Pacific, and the northeastern part of South America. *Wuchereria*

bancrofti and *Brugia malayi* produce the diseases of interest to the dermatologist; however, the clinical picture of the two infections is similar.

The adult filaria live in the lymphatics of the extremities and external genitalia. The adults mate in the lymphatics proximal to the lymph nodes. About a year after the infection, the fertilized females discharge the microfilariae in the peripheral blood, in a cyclical manner, and mostly at night (12 P.M. to 2 A.M.). The microfilariae are ingested by anthropophilic mosquitoes (*Culex, Aedes, Mansonia,* and *Anopheles*) when feeding on infected human blood. They metamorphose and mature in the vector's intestine and in 10 days are available for transmission again into the human. Humans are the only known hosts for this parasite.

After an incubation period of about one year or longer,

Fig. 207-18 Dracunculosis. Worm is seen protruding from the skin ulcer. *(Courtesy of Dr. G. H. Sahba, University of Tehran, Tehran.)*

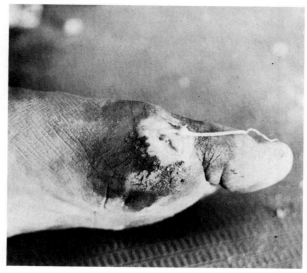

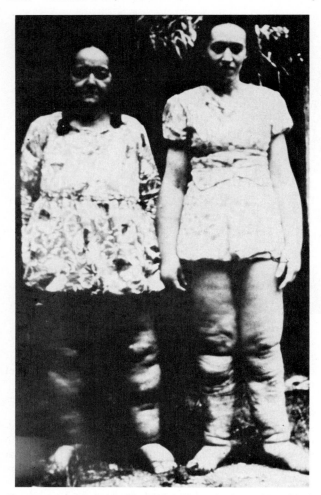

Fig. 207-19 Filariasis. Elephantiasis of the legs. The skin is thickened and hard. (Courtesy of Dr. A. Kurban, Division of Dermatology, American University of Beirut, Beirut.)

clinical manifestations develop. There are episodes of lymphadenitis and lymphangitis, and at times fever. There are recurrent episodes (often monthly), but they may not appear until later in the infection. However, as the infection progresses, the episodes become less severe and the intervals between them more prolonged. Ultimately, after many years, fibrosis and obstruction of the lymphatics develop, leading to elephantiasis of the affected parts, the external genitalia, and the legs (Fig. 207-19). The skin becomes thickened, hard, coarse, and dry. Often it cracks, becomes secondarily infected, and chronic ulcers may develop. Occasionally, urticaria or erythema nodosum may develop.

In endemic areas, it is possible to make an early diagnosis based on the clinical picture, even before the microfilariae appear in the blood. Biopsy of enlarged nodes as well as a positive intradermal test are useful. In the acute symptomatic phase, it is possible to find the parasite on a thick peripheral blood smear taken at night.

Diethylcarbamazine (Banocide), 4 to 6 mg/kg for 10 days to 2 weeks, is the agent of choice for the treatment of microfilariae carriers. Microfilariae are very susceptible to this drug, but adult worms are more resistant. If microfilariae reappear in the blood, retreatment is indicated. The drug is well tolerated but anorexia, nausea, vomiting, headaches, drowsiness, and acute allergic reactions may occur.

Surgical intervention may be successful in reducing the elephantiasis.

Loiasis. *Loa loa* is transmitted to humans by a blood-sucking fly (genus *Chrysops*) which feeds on infected humans. However, monkeys may suffer a similar disease and may act as a reservoir. The larvae enter the skin at the puncture of the proboscis but the adult worm will not appear under the skin or in the conjunctiva before a year. Microfilariae in the blood may, however, appear by the fifth month.

The adult worm characteristically wanders around the viscera of the body. When in the subcutaneous tissue, they cause rapidly developing, distinctive swelling—Calabar swellings—at the sites of migration, which can be painful and last for a few days. They are variable in size and may reach about 5 cm in diameter. They never suppurate.

The eye may be involved when the worm traverses the conjunctiva, where it can even be visible, producing unilateral palpebral swelling and edema. There may also be involvement of the peripheral nerves as well as cerebral involvement. The worm may live 4 to 7 years and it calcifies when it dies.

The diagnosis is made by the clinical picture and the demonstration of the microfilariae in a day-blood sample. A skin test and complement-fixation test are positive in the majority of cases.

Treatment is with diethylcarbamazine given as for filariasis. It has also been used prophylactically in a dose of 200 mg on 3 consecutive days once each month.

Onchocerciasis. *Onchocerca volvulus*, commonly found in tropical Africa, Arabia, Central America, and northern South America, infects about 19 million individuals. The female measures 30 to 70 cm and the male 2 to 5 cm. The disease is spread by the black fly vector (genus *Simulidae*) and the geographic distribution of the disease parallels the distribution of the vector. The microfilariae do not appear in the blood, but reside in the connective tissue and lymphatics of the skin, and in some instances in the eye. The flies become infected by feeding on tissue fluids containing microfilariae, and these develop to the infective stage in the thoracic muscles of the fly in one week. The larvae then migrate to the mouth parts and enter the human skin during subsequent feeding of the fly.

The mature worms and microfilariae are found in the granulomatous dermal nodules situated mostly on the exposed parts—mostly the scalp in Central America and the trunk and extremities in Africa—the differences are probably related to the biting habits of the vectors. The nodules, 3 to 35 mm in diameter, consist of fibrous tissue around the parasite, and of perivascular inflammation, at times with giant cells. Calcification may occur. In the eye, they cause keratitis, iritis, and choroiditis, which may lead to blindness.

The clinical picture is dominated by findings limited to the skin and eyes. The most characteristic lesion is the painless, mobile subcutaneous nodule around the adult worm. There may be one or many nodules present. Pruritus is an early symptom, usually accompanied by an exanthem involving the legs which can extend to other parts of the body. The rash disappears, pruritus continues and chronic lichenification (Fig. A6-23) and multiple scars develop. Pigmentation is prominent. Skin gradually loses elasticity, becomes dry, scaly, and atrophic. Depigmentation also accompanies the skin changes and is particularly common over the bony prominences, especially in African patients. Depigmentation is of variable extent and can be so extensive that the skin with normal pigmentation appears as islands within the depigmented areas.

The diagnosis of onchocerciasis is confirmed by finding the adult worm in the skin. Small superficial snips are taken from the suspected lesion and teased in physiologic saline on a slide. The microfilariae readily migrate from the skin and are seen swimming freely in the saline. Alternatively, nodules may be excised and examined. The filarial skin test and complement-fixation test are positive in the majority of patients. Relative eosinophilia may be found. In the eye lesions, microfilariae are seen moving actively in the anterior chamber.

The treatment is aimed at killing the adult worm and the microfilariae. Diethylcarbamazine (Banocide) kills microfilariae and suramin kills the adult worm. Diethylcarbamazine must be given slowly in increasing dosages to gradually reduce the load of killed parasites and to reduce side effects such as urticaria and exacerbation of the lesions, especially in the eye, and arthralgias. Initially 0.5 to 1.0 mg/kg per day is given for 3 days, and 4 mg/kg for the next 4 days. Then 3 mg and 4 mg/kg are given in the second and third week, respectively. Occasionally, antihistamines might be useful in reducing the severity of the reactions to treatment. Sharp pain following the first dose has been interpreted as a diagnostic test (Mazzotti's test).

Suramin (B.P.) kills the adult worm, and is associated with similar side reactions as is diethylcarbamazine. In addition, toxic reactions (kidney) of the drug itself must be watched for. It is given intravenously as a 10% solution, 1 g weekly for 5 to 6 weeks. For children 20 mg/kg is given weekly.

Trimelarsan (Mel W, Melarsonyl) may be useful against the adult worm.

Intestinal nematodes infecting humans through eggs

Enterobiasis due to pinworms. Infection with *Enterobius (Oxyuris) vermicularis* (pinworms) is the most common helminth infection of humans. It is of worldwide distribution, affecting children (30 percent) more than adults (16 percent), and whites more than blacks. It is more common in the cool and temperate zones than in the tropics.

The pinworm lives in the cecum and in the surrounding areas of the intestine. It is commonly found in the appendix but is probably not related to diseases of that organ. The male, seldom seen, is 2 to 5 mm long; the spindle-shaped female is 8 to 13 mm long. It is the gravid female that migrates to the anal area to deposit its eggs on the perianal and perineal skin, and is at times visible on the skin or in the stools. The eggs containing the larvae become infective about 6 h after oviposition, and may survive for a few days thereafter on fomites, bedclothes, or in dust. A cool, moist environment prolongs survival. The eggs are transferred directly (and with fingers) or indirectly (as an inhalation of airborne eggs) to the mouth and are swallowed; the larvae, released into the duodenum, migrate to the cecum, mature in 2 to 4 weeks, mate, and repeat the cycle. Autoreinfection of an affected individual is common and retroinfection is possible.

Humans are the only known hosts for *E. vermicularis*, and, in most, infection is asymptomatic. When symptomatic, pruritus in the perianal and perineal areas is most common. The pruritus is caused by the movement of the worm and possibly by its products. Itching is most common at night and may lead to disturbance or loss of sleep, irritability, and even anorexia. Occasionally, the worm migrates to the vagina, producing a vulvovaginitis, and rarely it may migrate to the uterus, fallopian tubes, or the peritoneum. These ectopic worms incite a granulomatous reaction which envelops them.

The diagnosis should be suspected in patients with pruritus and/or perineal itching and confirmed by finding the worm on perianal skin or in stools, or the eggs on a cellophane-tape preparation from the perianal skin. The cellophane preparations are best made upon waking and before washing. Eggs are demonstrated in 50 percent if one preparation is studied, and in 90 percent when three consecutive preparations are examined. Routine stool examinations are not generally helpful.

The treatment of enterobiasis is effective in eradicating the infection. Piperazine, pyrantel pamoate, thiabendazole, or mebendazole are effective. However, the treatment of an individual case may fail unless all the family members are treated to eradicate the source of infection. Some recommend repeating the treatment in 2 to 3 weeks. Personal hygiene is helpful in preventing autoinfections.

Bibliography

Botero DL: Epidemiology and public health importance of intestinal infections in Latin America. *Prog Drug Res* **19**:28, 1975

Burke JA: Roundworm infections of the gastrointestinal tract—current concepts. *J Ky Med Assoc* **74**:279, 1976

Faust EC et al: *Animal Agents and Vectors of Human Disease.* Philadelphia, Lea & Febiger, 1975

Amebiasis

AbdusSattar AB: An unusual case of cutaneous amebic ulcer. *J Trop Med Hyg* **82**:201, 1979

Adams EB, MacLeod IN: Invasive amebiasis. I. Amebic dysentery and its complications. *Medicine (Baltimore)* **56**:315, 1977

Biagi F, Martuschelli QA: Cutaneous amebiasis in Mexico. *Dermatol Trop* **2**:129, 1963

Faust EC: The multiple facets of *Entamoeba histolytica* infections. *Int Rev Trop Med* **1**:43, 1961

Fujita WH et al: Cutaneous amebiasis. *Arch Dermatol* **117**:309, 1981

Ganor S: *Entamoeba histolytica*: a possible cause of pruritus. *Int J Dermatol* **20**:26, 1981

Sunarwan E: A case of cutaneous amoebiasis. *Dermatologica* **151**:253, 1975

World Health Organization: Amebiasis. Report of WHO Expert Committee. *WHO Tech Rep Ser* **421**:1, 1969

Trypanosomiasis

Apted FIC: Sleeping sickness in Tanganyika—past, present and future. *Trans R Soc Trop Med Hyg* **56**:15, 1962

Apted FIC: Trypanosomiasis. *Trop Dis Bull* **61**:457, 1964

Chattas A et al: Chagas' disease in children (American trypanosomiasis). *Ann Pediatr* **201**:37, 1963

Davey DG: Human and animal trypanosomiasis in Africa. *Am J Trop Med Hyg* **7**:546, 1958

Greenwood BM, Whittle HC: Complement activation in patients with Gambian sleeping sickness. *Clin Exp Immunol* **24**:133, 1976

Jones IG et al: Electrocardiographic changes in African trypanosomiasis caused by *Trypanosoma brucei rhodensiense. Trans R Soc Trop Med Hyg* **69**:388, 1975

Iayawardena AN, Wakswan BH: Suppressor cells in experimental trypanosomiasis. *Nature* **265**:539, 1977

Kellersberger ER: African sleeping sickness. Review of 9000 cases from central Africa. *Am J Trop Med* **13**:211, 1933

Kierszenbaum F, Budzko DB: Immunization against experimental Chagas' disease by using culture forms of *Trypanosoma cruzi* killed with a solution of sodium perchlorate. *Infect Immun* **12**:461, 1975

Lambert PH, Whittle HC: The pathogenesis of sleeping sickness. *Trans R Soc Trop Med Hyg* **74**:716, 1980

Toledo-Banos HA et al: In vitro cellular immunity in Chagas disease. *Clin Exp Immunol* **38**:376, 1979

World Health Organization: African trypanosomiasis. *WHO Tech Rep Ser* **635**:1, 1979

World Health Organization: Comparative studies of American and African trypanosomiasis. *WHO Tech Rep Ser* **411**:1, 1969

Leishmaniasis

Adler SI: Immunology of leishmaniasis. *Isr J Med Sci* **1**:9, 1965

Berlin C: Leishmaniasis recidiva cutis: leishmanoid. *Arch Dermatol Syphilol* **41**:874, 1940

Berman JD: Activity of imidazole against *Leishmania tropica* in human macrophage culture. *Am J Trop Med* **30**:566, 1981

Brycesson ADM: Diffuse cutaneous leishmaniasis in Ethiopia. I. The clinical and histological features of the disease. *Trans R Soc Trop Med Hyg* **63**:708, 1969

Chance ML: The identification of leishmania. *Parasitology* **17**:55, 1979

Farah FS, Malak JA: Cutaneous leishmaniasis. *Arch Dermatol* **103**:467, 1971

Farah FS et al: The role of the macrophage in cutaneous leishmaniasis. *Immunology* **29**:755, 1975

Farah FS et al: The effect of *L. tropica* on stimulation of lymphocytes with phytohemagglutinin. *Immunology* **30**:629, 1976

Hommel M: The genus leishmania—biology of the parasites and clinical aspects. *Bull Inst Pasteur* **76**:J-102, 1978

Kurban AK et al: Histopathology of cutaneous leishmaniasis. *Arch Dermatol* **93**:396, 1966

Williams P, Coehho M de V: Taxonomy and transmission of leishmania. *Adv Parasitol* **16**:1, 1979

Zuckerman A: Parasitological review: current status of the immunology of blood and tissue parasites. I. Leishmania. *Exp Parasitol* **38**:370, 1975

Schistosomiasis

Abdul-Aziz AH: Cutaneous bilharzial granulomas—a histologic study. *Cutis* **18**:516, 1976

Boros DL: Schistosomiasis mansoni: a granulomatous disease of cell mediated immune etiology. *Ann NY Acad Sci* **278**:36, 1976

El-Mofty AM: Extragenital forms of cutaneous bilharziasis. *Br J Dermatol* **68**:252, 1956

El-Zawakry M: Schistosomal granuloma of the skin. *Br J Dermatol* **77**:344, 1965

Faust EC et al: *Animal Agents and Vectors in Human Disease.* Philadelphia, Lea & Febiger, 1978, p 159

Kagan IG: Recent advances in the diagnosis of schistosomiasis. *Egypt J Bilharz* **3**:121, 1976

Wood MG et al: Schistosomiasis. Paraplegia and ectopic lesions as admission symptoms. *Arch Dermatol* **112**:690, 1976

Cercarial dermatitis

Cart WW: Studies on schistosome dermatitis: status of knowledge after more than twenty years. *Am J Hyg* **52**:251, 1950

Hoeffler DF: "Swimmer's itch" (cercarial dermatitis). *Cutis* **19**:461, 1977

Sparganosis

Mueller JF et al: Human sparganosis in the United States. *J Parasitol* **49**:294, 1963

Swartzwelde JC et al: Sparganosis in southern United States. *Am J Trop Med* **13**:43, 1964

Taylor RL: Sparganosis in the United States. Report of a case. *Am J Clin Pathol* **66**:560, 1976

Echinococcus—hydatid cyst

Baraka A et al: Anaphylactic reaction during hydatid surgery—an immunologic hazard. *Middle East J Anesthesiol* **5**:505, 1980

Dressaint JP et al: Quantitative determination of specific IgE antibodies to *Echinococcus granulosa* and IgE levels in sera from patients with hydatid disease. *Immunology* **29**:813, 1975

Kannereo WS, Miller KL: Echinococcus granulosa—permeability of hydatid cyst to mebendazole in man. *Int J Parasitol* **11**:183, 1981

Kassis A, Tanner CE: Novel approach to the treatment of hydatid disease. *Nature* **262**:588, 1976

Kein P et al: Chemotherapy of *Echinococcus* with mebendazole. Clinical observation in seven patients. *Trop Med Parasitol* **30**:65, 1979

Majdaudzic J et al: Echinococcosis multiloculare. *Med Welt* **32**:1060, 1981

Schantz PM et al: Chemotherapy for larval echinococcosis in animals and humans. Report of workshop 2. *Parasitenka* **67**:5, 1982

Schwabe CW: *Veterinary Medicine and Human Health.* Baltimore, Williams & Wilkins, 1969

Cysticerosis

Mahajan RC et al: Comparative evaluation of indirect hemagglutination and complement fixation tests in serodiagnosis of cysticerosis. *Indian J Med Res* **63**:121, 1975

Larva migrans (creeping eruption)

Beaver PC: Larva migrans. A review. *Exp Parasitol* **5**:587, 1956

Katz R et al: The natural course of creeping eruption and treatment with thiabendazole. *Arch Dermatol* **91**:420, 1965

Stone OJ, Mullins JF: Thiabendazole effectiveness in creeping eruptions. *Arch Dermatol* **91**:427, 1965

Trichinosis

Barriga OO: Reactivity and specificity of *Trichinella spiralis* fractions in cutaneous and serological tests. *J Clin Microbiol* **6**:274, 1977

Gould SE: *Trichinosis in Man and Animals.* Springfield, IL, Charles C Thomas, 1970

Stone OJ et al: Thiabendazole. A probable cure for trichinosis. *JAMA* **187**:536, 1964

Dracunculosis

Faust EC et al: *Animal Agents and Vectors in Human Disease.* Philadelphia, Lea & Febiger, 1975

Muller R: *Dracunculus* and dracunculiusis. *Adv Parasitol* **9**:73, 1971

Loiasis

Duke BOL: Studies on chemotherapy of loiasis. II. Observations on diethylcarbamazine (Banocide) as prophylactic in man. *Ann Trop Med Hyg* **57**:82, 1983

Sacks HN et al: Loiasis—report of a case and review of literature. *Arch Intern Med* **136**:914, 1976

Onchocerosis–onchocerciasis

Rodger FC: A review of recent advances in scientific knowledge of symptomatology, pathology and pathogenesis of onchocereal infections. *Bull WHO* **27**:429, 1962
World Health Organization: Expert Committee on Onchocerciasis. Second report. *WHO Tech Rep Ser* **335**:1, 1966

Enterobiasis

Beaver PC: The detection and identification of some common nematode parasites in man. *Am J Clin Pathol* **22**:481, 1952
Burke JA: Roundworm infections of the gastrointestinal tract. Current concepts. *J Ky Med Assoc* **74**:279, 1976
Tudor RB: Ridding children of common worm infections. *Postgrad Med* **58**:115, 1975

CHAPTER 208

ARTHROPOD BITES AND STINGS

Riley S. Rees and Lloyd E. King, Jr.

Bites and stings due to arthropods cause many patients to consult physicians for relief from these vexatious creatures. Occasionally, death is induced by envenomation, particularly in infants [1]. The clinician primarily diagnoses and treats skin lesions produced by only five of the nine classes of arthropods: Arachnida, Chilopoda, Diplopoda, Cymothoidea, and Insecta [2]. All arthropods are invertebrates with a chitinous exoskeleton, bilateral symmetry, true segmentation, and jointed true appendages that vary from few to many (Fig. 208-1 and Table 208-1).

Arachnida

The Arachnida class includes three orders of medical interest: Acari (ticks and mites), Araneae (spiders), and Scorpiones (scorpions). Although all adults in this class possess four pairs of legs, the cephalothorax may vary but it is typically fused.

Acari

The mites in the order Acari of most interest to the clinician are the follicle mites, food mites, fowl mites, grain mites, harvest mites, murine mites, and scabies. All mites may produce pruritus and/or allergic reactions without any major venom or toxin being detected. Although it is not possible to group all mites that cause human diseases into convenient categories, most of the more common mites can be grouped into three suborders:

Trombidiiformes: Harvest/chigger mites, family Trombiculidae; grain mites, family Pyemotidae; follicle mites, family Demodicidae.
Mesostigmata: Bird/rodent mites, family Dermanyssidae; straw mites, family Hemoganasidae.
Sarcoptiformes: Scabies, family Sarcoptidae; food mites, family Acaridae, family Glycyphagidae; mange, family Psoroptidae.

Follicle mites. *Demodex* mites can be detected in sebaceous glands and hair follicles by skin biopsy of symptomatic and asymptomatic humans and other animal species [3]. Whether the presence of *Demodex* reflects asymptomatic parasitosis or is the etiologic agent in rosacea and other dermatoses is not well documented. Symptoms produced by democidosis, if any, are more likely due to immunologic rather than toxicologic reactions.

Food mites. Several species of mites that infest foodstuffs have been described: grain mite, Acarus; cheese mite, Glycyphagus; grocery mite, Tyrophagus and Tyroglyphus. Exposure to mite-infested foods results in papular urticaria or vesicopapular eruptions due to mites penetrating the epidermis. An occupational history and skin scrapings are frequently required to separate these food mite-induced problems from scabies and other causes of papular urticaria.

Fowl mites. Office workers, homemakers, and bird fanciers are all affected by mites that infest birds, especially pigeons that have nests or roosts near air conditioner intake ducts. *Dermanyssus gallinae* and *D. avium* are the most common fowl ectoparasites identified in the United States. These mites only temporarily infest humans. *Ornithonyssus sylviarum* is an uncommon fowl mite of the northern temperate region that induces human skin lesions.

Grain mites. The best studied grain mite of medical importance is the straw itch mite, *Pyemotes ventricosus* [4], which was identified as the causative agent of one type of Schamberg's disease [5]. *P. ventricosus* is primarily a parasite of insects and the larvae which feed on grain, such as the Angoumois grain moth (*Sitotroga cerealella*) and the wheat joint worm (*Harmolita tritici*). The distribution of *P. ventricosus* is worldwide and it has been identified in over half of the United States. *P. ventricosus* infests both animals and humans, occasionally producing unusual epidemics after an exposure to infested hay, grains, grasses, or straw. It does not burrow into the skin, although affected patients often have systemic symptoms such as fever, diarrhea, anorexia, and malaise. Clinically, the lesions vary from bright red macules to varicelliform eruptions. Treat-

Fig. 208-1 Pictorial key to groups of human ectoparasites. *(C. J. Stojanovich and H. G. Scott. U.S. Department of Health, Education, and Welfare, Public Health Service.)*

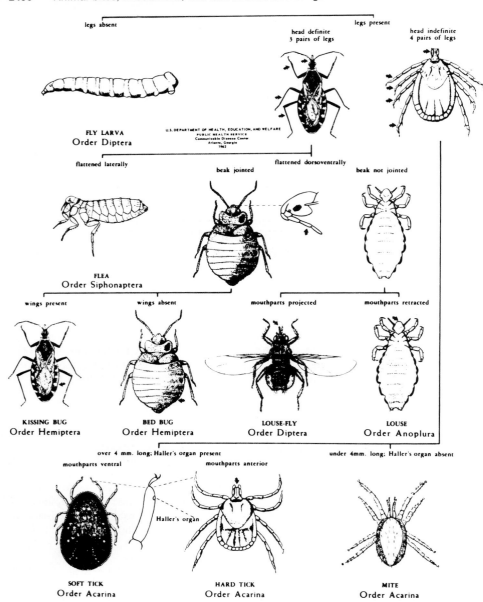

ment with scabicides are considered to be effective for these ectoparasites. However, identification of *P. ventricosus* in various infested grain products is often not made because of the low index of suspicion.

Harvest mites. Perhaps the best known cause of "bites" due to mites in the United States is the chigger, mower, or harvest mite (*Trombicula splendens* and *T. alfreddugesi*). In other parts of the world, *Trombicula* species are the vectors for rickettsia, tsutsugamushi fever, and scrub typhus by *T. deliensis* and *T. akamushi*. Contact with the chigger mite usually occurs during the summer and fall when outdoor activities are maximal. Frequently, the only sign of exposure is intense pruritus on the ankles, legs, or belt line since the bright red mite ("red bugs") may have been scratched off. In nonsensitized individuals, usually only 1- to 2-mm pruritic macules are seen, which require minimal treatment. In sensitized or allergic individuals, the reaction to the chigger infestation may be papular urticaria, vesiculation, or a granulomatous reaction with fever and

lymphadenopathy. Clinically, the distribution of the lesions may be confused with other dermatoses since the type of exposure and the clothing worn greatly affect where the mites attach. Ideally, the mites can be identified by visual inspection.

Murine mites. Two species of murine mites are of medical importance throughout the world: *Ornithonyssus bacoti*, tropical rat mite, and *Allodermanyssus sanguineus*, house-mouse mite, a vector of rickettsialpox. *O. bacoti* has been noted to range widely to obtain its blood meal if the host rats die or leave the infested nest. Persons working in areas rats commonly inhabit (groceries, granaries, restaurants, storehouses) may be affected without ever finding the mite, as it drops off after each feeding. The lesions produced and the treatments used are typical of other arthropod lesions, especially scabies.

Scabies. The mite *Sarcoptes scabiei*, var. *hominis*, is the mite in the order Acari that is of most interest to physicians

Table 208-1   Arthropods that infest, bite, or sting humans

I. Arachnida—mites, ticks, spiders, scorpions (4 pairs of legs)
   A. Acari
      1. Mites—follicle, food, fowl, grain, harvest, murine, scabies
      2. Ticks
   B. Araneae—spiders
   C. Scorpiones
II. Chilopoda and Diplopoda—centipedes, millipedes
III. Insecta (3 pairs of legs)
   A. Anoplura—lice
   B. Coleoptera—beetles
   C. Diptera—flies, mosquitoes
   D. Hemiptera—bedbugs, kissing bugs
   E. Hymenoptera—ants, bees, wasps
   F. Lepidoptera—butterflies, moths
   G. Siphonaptera—fleas

because of its origin in antiquity and prevalence in modern times (for reviews see [6,7]). Therapy for scabies runs the gamut from time-honored sulfur and tar to the newer lindane and crotamiton. Each therapeutic modality has its own limitations which vary from cosmetically unappealing (sulfur) to potential neurotoxicity (lindane). Resistance has been reported to both lindane and crotamiton but these findings have been questioned [6,8]. Most problems encountered with scabies are not therapeutic but diagnostic, as the clinical suspicions wax and wane with fluctuation in scabies prevalence within given populations.

Both the human variant and animal scabies, including sarcoptic mange, can produce human skin lesions. Papules and vesicles are the most common lesions, but the burrow is the characteristic and diagnostic feature of the human variant of scabies. These burrows are either S-shaped or straight lines and have a small vesicle overlying the site of the female mite. Experienced observers can detect and even remove the female mite, which appears as a small dark or gray speck below the vesicle. Excoriations and/or secondary infections may make identification of burrows very difficult. A helpful technique to detect burrows is to put on water-washable ink or topical tetracycline which fluoresces under a Wood's lamp, wash off the excess, and look for the burrows, which retain the ink or tetracycline. In animal scabies, the diagnosis is more difficult because characteristic burrows are seldom found as the mites do not persist on human skin for any length of time. Other clinical variants of human scabies are also well described [6]. In Norwegian scabies, literally thousands of mites instead of the usual 3 to 50 female mites may be found.

Ticks. During their seasonal infestation, ticks are abundant throughout the United States and are vectors for geographic diseases as well as causative agents for local reactions from their bites. Tick activity is maximum in the spring and summer when larval and nymph forms are most abundant, while infestation is rare during the winter months when adult ticks hibernate. Ticks are separated from other mites by the presence of a barbed hypostome which they use for feeding, and are divided into the Argasidae (soft tick) and Ixodidae (hard tick) families [2] (Fig. 208-1). The Ixodidae group, as carriers, has been implicated in the transmission of Rocky Mountain spotted fever [2], Colorado tick fever [9], tularemia [2], and Lyme disease [10,11]. Toxins from tick salivary fluid have been

thought to cause tick-bite paralysis and tick-bite pyrexia [2].

A history of exposure to ticks will aid in the diagnosis, since a tick bite may not show the classic indurated lesion or an erythematous halo. These intensely pruritic lesions may resolve spontaneously or a residual persistent papule may form at the bite site which may require intralesional corticosteroid injections for relief. Tick-bite granulomas may mimic dermatofibromas, histiocytomas, foreign-body granulomas, or lesions of lymphocytoma cutis [12–14]. In contrast to the often obscure clinical diagnosis, histologic findings are quite characteristic. In acute lesions, bloody crusts with disintegrated epidermis overlie an acute dermal inflammatory infiltrate with eosinophils and extravasation of erythrocytes. More chronic lesions may have only perivascular cellular infiltrates, while the oldest lesions may have simply an atrophic epidermis with an underlying dense, fibrous mass.

Lyme disease is an epidemic, immune-mediated inflammatory illness produced by a *Treponema*-like spirochete carried by the ticks *Ixodes dammini* and *I. pacificus* [11–15]. Case reports have been reported from northeastern, midwestern, and western United States. In a representative case, joint, cardiac, or neurologic involvement is preceded by erythema chronicum migrans, which begins as a small papule, frequently at the bite site, and then spreads centripetally with an area of central clearing. In the early stages, myalgias, malaise, fatigue, headache, gastrointestinal upset, and sore throat accompany the rash. The treatment of choice for Lyme disease is tetracycline 250 mg 4 times a day for 10 days; tetracycline has replaced penicillin because it has been shown to prevent major complications of the disease (see also Chap. 88).

In tick-infested areas, the obvious best measure is to avoid tick bites. Ticks may be carefully removed before they are embedded if detected by carefully inspecting exposed body sites and clothing. Once the tick's hypostome is secured to the skin, the tick must be forced to remove it by occluding the spiricles (breathing tubes) with a noxious agent such as gasoline, chloroform, or petrolatum (Vasoline). Burning the tick with a match or other hot object has also been reported to be effective. If the hypostome is retained in the skin when the tick is extracted, then it should be removed with a biopsy punch or a surgical blade. Foreign-body reactions and persistent papules are produced if there are retained tick parts in the wound [2,13].

Araneae

Spiders belong to the class Arachnida and are separated from insects by the absence of antennae, two separate body parts, and five paired appendages. Spiders are carnivorous and either capture their prey in webs or attack them and inject venom through their chelicera (mandibles). In the United States, the genera *Loxosceles* and *Latrodectus* are the only species whose venom produces significant toxic effects in humans although wolf spiders, tarantulas, jumping spiders, orb weavers, and crab spiders may also produce cutaneous lesions [2].

Loxosceles. There are 13 different species of *Loxosceles* in the United States and five of them, *L. reclusa*, *L. deserta*, *L. arizonica*, *L. laeta*, and *L. refuscens*, have been asso-

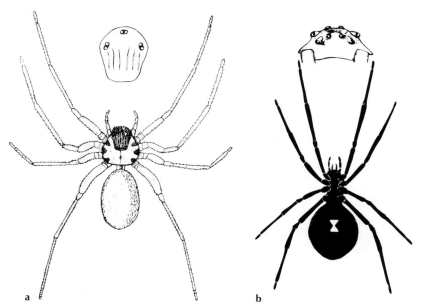

Fig. 208-2 (a) Brown recluse spider. Characteristically there are six eyes in three pairs and fiddle-shaped markings on the cephalothorax. (b) Black widow spider, with eight eyes; it is shiny black, usually with a red hourglass marking on the underside of its abdomen. *U.S. Department of Health, Education, and Welfare, Public Health Service.)*

ciated with cutaneous loxoscelism [2,16]. The brown recluse spider, *L. reclusa,* typifies the species, and is widely distributed throughout the Southeast and the Midwest (Figs. 208-2 and 208-3). Often called the violin or fiddleback spider because of the violin-shaped figure on its dorsal cephalothorax, it varies in size from 0.2 to 2.5 cm in diameter, depending on diet and habitat. Since the brown recluse spider hibernates in the winter, most bites occur between March and October when humans accidentally disturb their habitat (closets, outbuildings, woodpiles). Despite its usual timid nature, this spider is inherently more dangerous than other spiders because it has adapted its habitat to live in close association with humans.

Often initially painless, the bite wound starts with a central papule and produces an irregular erythematous reaction in 6 to 12 h which precedes blister formation and/or skin necrosis [17]. The resultant necrotic skin ulcer heals slowly (Fig. 208-4) and may require skin grafts or flaps to reconstruct the defect. Histologic examination of such bites demonstrates acute vasculitis, platelet thrombi, and leukocyte infiltrates. The lesions are usually not associated with pain or pruritus but may be difficult to diagnose clinically unless the patient saw the spider. Often these bites are confused with Hymenoptera stings, tick bites, allergic reactions, or skin abscesses. Case reports, often unconfirmed, of hemolysis, disseminated intravascular coagulopathy, convulsions, renal failure, or death have been recorded.

The venom of the brown recluse spider contains at least nine protein fractions identifiable by sodium dodecyl sulfate polyacrylamide electrophoresis [18]. One major fraction is a 32,000-dalton protein with sphingomyelinase D activity. This venom fraction aggregates platelets, generates leukocyte chemoattractants, and liberates thromboxane B_2 in vitro while producing typical skin necrosis when injected into rabbits.

The treatment of brown recluse spider bites remains controversial. We have successfully used, both experimentally and clinically, the leukocyte inhibitor dapsone [19]. Ice and elevation are useful in reducing erythema and swelling, while antihistamines will improve accompanying pruritus. Corticosteroids should be reserved for patients with significant systemic symptoms, while antibiotics seem to reduce the incidence of abscess formation and secondary infection in large lesions. Excising the bite site acutely should be avoided since the inflammatory reaction produced by the venom will inhibit wound healing and produce an inferior clinical result [17].

Latrodectus. The black widow spider, sometimes called the "hourglass" or "shoe button" spider, is infamous throughout the continental United States. Notorious for biting people in outdoor privies, the black widow may spin its small web in the grass, over hollow stumps, under woodpiles, or in front of rodent burrows [2,20]. The North American black widows, *Latrodectus mactans, L. variolus,* and *L. hesperus,* have a characteristic red hourglass or double triangle on the ventral surface of the abdomen. The red-legged widow, *L. bishopi,* is found only in southern Florida, while the brown widow, *L. geometricus,* is more cosmotropical in distribution and found rarely in the United States [20].

The venom of the black widow spider is a neurotoxin and alters the structure and function of cholinergic, noradrenergic, and aminergic nerve terminals without producing any significant local reaction. The primary component of the venom has been termed α-*Latrotoxin* and is a 130,000-dalton protein which acts as a calcium ionophore, resulting in release of massive amounts of acetylcholine from nerve terminals [21].

Clinically, generalized pain occurs 1 to 8 h following envenomation with no cutaneous lesions. The characteristic crampy abdominal pain may be associated with pain in the flanks, thighs, or chest, and confusion with acute appendicitis, renal colic, or acute myocardial infarction may occur. Diaphoresis, pallor, nausea, and vomiting accompany most bites. The severity of bites depends on the degree of envenomation and age of the patient. The original reports which suggested a mortality of 5 percent were not well documented and the true incidence is probably much lower.

The treatment is predicated on an accurate diagnosis

Fig. 208-3 (a) Brown recluse spider, fiddle on back. (b) Low-power view of brown recluse spider.

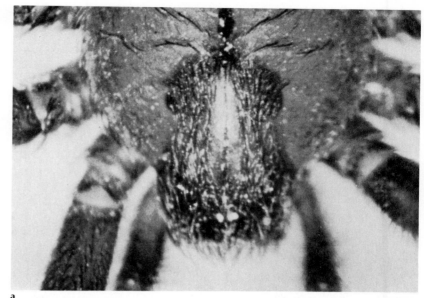

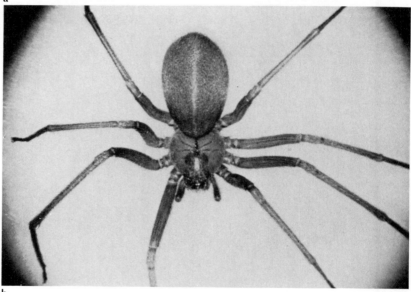

and positive identification of the spider. Traditional therapy with calcium gluconate (10%) and muscle relaxants has proved effective in most patients. Relief of pain with morphine sulfate may reduce the severity of symptoms and muscle spasms [22]. Since antivenom is prepared in horses, it should be used for severe envenomations only in patients not allergic to horse serum.

Scorpions

Scorpions are of medical and sociologic interest primarily in tropical and/or desert areas such as parts of the southwestern United States, Mexico, India, and the Middle East. In the United States, the scorpions commonly encountered are *Centruroides sculpturatus* and its *C. gertschi* variant [2]. Recent studies have identified the characteristics of the toxic components contained in the venoms of several species of scorpions. The three-dimensional structure and amino acid sequence of these proteins have been determined and there is substantial sequence homology [23]. In general, scorpion toxins contain a group or family of small, basic, disulfide-linked proteins (60 to 70 amino acids) responsible for the neurotoxicity [24]. The Old World scorpion toxins (α-toxins) act by binding only to a single class of membrane receptors in electrically excitable cells to affect the sodium inactivation mechanisms involved in depolarizing the sodium channels in excitable membranes. The New World toxins, especially the *Centruorides* toxins (β-toxins), affect the sodium activation process of excitable membranes. In several animal species and humans, crude or pure scorpion venom induces complex cardiac arrhythmias probably due to the release of catecholamines and acetylcholine from postganglionic fibers [25]. These neurotoxic effects of scorpion venom may cause several clinical syndromes which are logical but not always predictable. For example, acute pancreatitis is a common complication of the stings of the Brazilian scorpions (*Tityus* species). In animals, these clinical effects on pancreatic secretion, gastric secretion, excessive salivation, and vomiting were experimentally reproducible by purified scorpion toxin (*Tityus* toxin) [26]. Although a scorpion venom-induced defibrination syndrome is uncommon

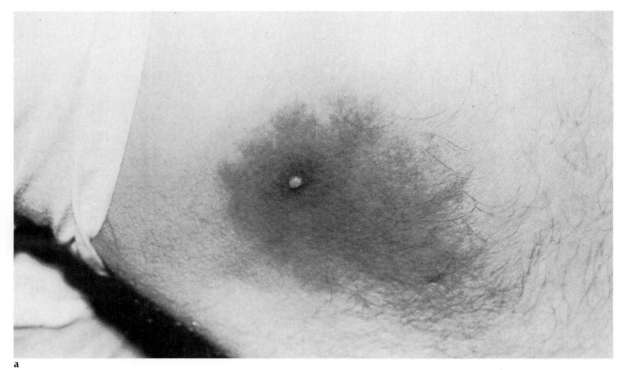

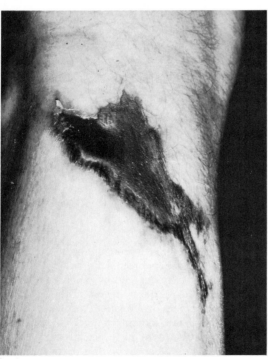

Fig. 208-4 Pustular appearance of necrotic brown recluse spider bite (a and b). *[(b) Courtesy of Dr. C. J. Dillaha, Section of Dermatology, University of Arkansas Medical Center.]*

due to *C. sculpturatus* sting, an adenosine diphosphate-dependent aggregation of dog platelets by *C. sculpturatus* venom has been demonstrated [27]. Whether the venom's effect on platelets or other venom proteins induce the ulcerative skin reactions is not clear. However, the effects of the scorpion venom on neurotransmitter release may be clinically blocked by using alpha-adrenergic agents and chlorpromazine [27]. Complex arrhythmias occurring in the very young and the elderly have to be carefully observed. More serious systemic complications have been

reported in India, Iran, Egypt, and Israel, where the *Buthus* species is common. The *Buthus* venom characteristically produces more severe myotoxic and neurotoxic effects.

Chilopoda and Diplopoda

Centipedes and millipedes superficially resemble each other, having one pair of legs and two pairs of legs per segment, respectively. Millipedes are vegetarians, do not

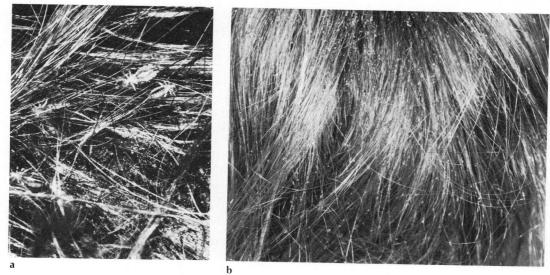

Fig. 208-5 (a) **Full-grown lice in the scalp. (b) Nits in the scalp.**

bite or envenomate, but may produce skin irritation due to an unknown substance secreted from pores on the sides of the body. In contrast, centipedes are nocturnal carnivores which may produce painful bites that become secondarily infected and ulcerated. The *Scolopendra* species found in Hawaii and western United States produces painful skin lesions in the unwary who disturb its habitat.

Insecta

Anoplura

Blood-sucking lice of the order Anoplura have long been successful obligate ectoparasites of humans. Although only two species of Anoplura, *Phthirus pubis* and *Pediculus humanus,* are host-specific parasites of humans, there are three clinical forms of infestation: head, body, and pubic area [2,6]. *P. humanus* var. *capitus,* the head louse (Fig. 208-5) is distinct clinically from *P. humanus* var. *corporis* but morphologically they are very similar (Fig. 208-6). Since interbreeding can occur, it has been speculated that the body louse evolved from the head louse after humans began to wear clothes [6,28,29].

Pediculosis capitis. No age or economic strata are immune to *P. capitis.* The incidence of infestation varies from 5 to 30 percent in certain populations, with crowded conditions and longer hair being associated factors. The adult *P. capitis* is frequently not observed; fewer than 10 lice are detected in over half of the cases. In analogy to Norwegian scabies, more than 1000 head lice on a patient have been observed. *P. capitis* may be transmitted by shared hats, caps, brushes, combs, and even pillows. *P. capitis* is frequently diagnosed by barbers and beauticians who readily observe the nits when the hair is wet (Fig. 208-5). Medically, secondary infections of the scalp or neck with chronic pruritus lead the examiner to inspect the hair shafts closely with a hand lens or Wood's lamp for attached nits (ova). Nonspecific findings such as occipital lymphadenopathy, cervical adenopathy, or mild systemic symptoms make some cases of pediculosis capitis difficult to diagnose.

Treatment may require systemic antibiotics in addition to topical pediculocidal agents such as lindane (gamma benzene hexachloride), DDT, malathion, pyrethrins, copper oleate-tetrahydronaphthalene, or trimethoprim/sulfamethoxazole [6,30,31]. In infants, young children, and

Fig. 208-6 Lice commonly found on humans. (a) Body louse or head louse, *Pediculus humanus.* **(b) Crab louse,** *Phthirius pubis. (U. S. Department of Health, Education, and Welfare, Public Health Service.)*

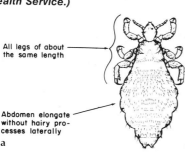

All legs of about the same length

Abdomen elongate without hairy processes laterally

a

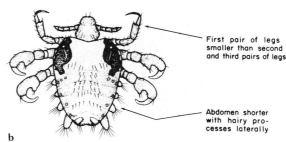

First pair of legs smaller than second and third pairs of legs

Abdomen shorter with hairy processes laterally

b

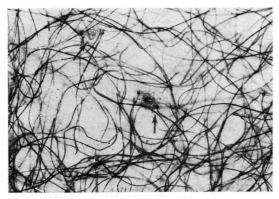

Fig. 208-7   Pediculosis pubis. Arrows point to lice.

pregnant women, potential neurotoxicity of lindane commonly leads to alternative methods of therapy. Shampoos usually are the most convenient pediculocidal vehicle to use in children. Removal of the dead ova or "nits" may be psychologically important as some patients believe that the infestation has not been treated successfully if they remain. In general, if the ova are 1.0 to 1.5 cm from the scalp after otherwise adequate treatment, no active infestation is present.

Pediculosis corporis. Unlike *P. capitis,* the body louse, *P. corporis,* has become relatively more rare in many affluent populations. The eggs of *P. corporis* are found predominantly on clothing and occasionally on body hairs. Since relatively few lice are found on the body, the lice and eggs should be searched for in the seams of clothing. Clinically, only in chronic cases may extreme pruritus with excoriations, urticaria, and pigmentary changes be seen. Small red macules are seen in early cases, with initial lesions often best seen on the back or under the arms. Treatment for the nonsensitized person consists of changes in hygiene (if appropriate) and clothes, and use of the ectoparasiticidal agents noted above. Dry heat is equally effective in killing the lice and their ova in clothing.

Phthiriasis pubis. The crab louse, *Phthirius pubis,* is usually transmitted by sexual contact but may be transferred by articles of clothing or by infested hairs (Fig. 208-7). The lice may be found on hairs all over the body, from the

Fig. 208-8   Pediculosis involving the eyelashes. The black dots are nits of *Phthirius pubis.*

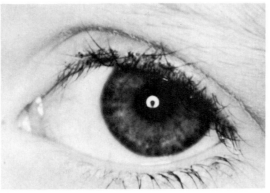

pubis to the edge of the scalp, on eyebrows, eyelashes (Fig. 208-8), thighs, abdomen, and in the axillae. Severe pruritus or secondary infection may be the only sign of infestation. Small blue-gray macules occasionally are seen and are useful diagnostic signs. Careful search with a hand lens for the yellowish adult lice or their ova is the best diagnostic method.

Treatment of phthiriasis pubis is the same as for pediculosis capitis with special attention paid to clothing and bedding infestation. Reinfestation after successful initial therapy is commonly due to reexposure to untreated sexual partners. Allergic and systemic reactions can develop in some patients. All specimens brought by patients should be carefully examined for organisms since delusions of parasitosis and parasitophobia are not uncommon.

Coleoptera

Since there are over 250,000 species of beetles in the Coleoptera order, the largest order in the animal kingdom, it is not surprising that several species are of medical interest [2]. In this section only the beetles whose bodies contain blister-inducing irritants will be discussed. Five families of Coleoptera produce or contain chemicals that induce blistering or vesiculation upon contact with human skin: Meloidea, Staphylinidae, Paussidae, Coccinellidae, and Edemeridae. Only in the family Meloidae is the chemical (cantharidin) which induces blisters well characterized as to its chemical and pathologic effects. Cantharidin is contained in the body of Meloidae beetles, the most famous being *Lytta vesicatoria,* "Spanish fly." Although toxic when given internally, cantharidin is often used topically to cause blisters and to remove verrucae. Several other beetle species, which do not contain cantharidin, may be the cause of blisters in various geographic areas. Rove beetles (*Paedurus* species) are commonly noted in South America. Rarely, the common carpet beetle (*Anthrenus scrophulariae*) may produce a blistering dermatitis via irritant and/or allergic mechanisms. The characteristic clinical features of the "blister beetles" are "kissing" or touching lesions which may produce infection and ulceration.

Diptera

The order Diptera is composed of the two-winged or true flies, and collectively its members are responsible for the transmission of more diseases worldwide than any other arthropod order [2]. At last count, more than 100,000 species in 140 families have been described. The mosquitoes of the family Culicida are vectors for Eastern, Western, and St. Louis encephalitis in the United States, as well as malaria, yellow fever, dengue fever, and filariasis throughout the world. In the continental United States, females of the genus *Aedes* are the most common cause of mosquito bites. The cutaneous reaction is produced when the female mosquito's serrated jaws disrupt the skin and she inserts her blood tube. Irritating salivary secretions are injected to anticoagulate the blood and are responsible for the edema, pruritus, and papular lesions. Mosquito bites may have an urticarial, eczematoid, or granulomatous appearance, depending upon the sensitivity of the victim. Mosquitoes prefer blacks to whites, the young to the old, warm to cool skin, scented to unscented victims. They also are attracted to bright colors and elevated carbon dioxide concentrations in the air, which make summer picnics or gatherings a favorite mosquito haunt [32].

The black flies of the family Simulidae are also bloodsuckers. These stout-bodied insects are found in tremendous swarms near fast-moving water in the late spring and early summer. Because this black fly injects an anesthetic into the wound, the initial bite is painless. However, the bite subsequently becomes extremely painful with itching, erythema, and edema, which may lead to nummular eczema, vesicles, or hard pruritic papules. Histologically, these dermal lesions contain persistent, perivascular accumulations of eosinophilic leukocytes. A systemic reaction termed "black fly fever" producing headache, fever, nausea, and generalized lymphadenitis has been reported [2].

The biting midges, which are also called "punkies," "no seeums," or "sand flies," are another type of bloodsucking arthropod [33]. Most active in the morning and late afternoon, the female midges are vicious biters and require a blood meal to oviposit. The midge bites produce immediate pain with immediate erythema at the bite site, 2- to 3-mm papulovesicles, followed by indurated nodules up to 1.0 cm which persist for many months. These lesions contain focal necrosis of the papillary dermis with lymphocyte, eosinophil, and histiocyte infiltrates in the reticular dermis. Eosinophilic granulomas surrounding necrotic collagen may be found in the subcutaneous tissue of chronic lesions. Unlike black flies and mosquitoes, which pupate in the water, these organisms spend their larval and pupal stages in the ground and metamorphose into adult forms at irregular intervals. Their life cycle makes mass control of this arthropod impossible.

The large family Tabandae are ferocious bloodsucking flies and include horseflies, deerflies, clegs, breeze flies, greenheads, and mango flies. As vectors, these flies are known to transmit anthrax and tularemia in the United States as well as animal trypanosomiasis worldwide [2]. Because they are large flies (6 to 25 mm) with bladelike mouth parts, the bite is quite painful and may bleed vigorously. The cutaneous welt that is produced may be accompanied by urticaria, dizziness, weakness, wheezes, or angioedema. They are a particular problem to campers and hikers in the early spring and summer when the larval forms become adults.

The treatment of Diptera bites requires meticulous attention to wound care by cleansing with soap or other antiseptics to avoid secondary infection. Local application of steroid ointment and systemic treatment with antihistamines will reduce itching and redness. Although systemic allergic reactions are rare, they should be treated aggressively with epinephrine, fluids, corticosteroids, and support care.

Hemiptera

Most of the Hemiptera order feed on plants. Only the Cimicidae and Reduviidae families commonly feed on animals, including humans.

Cimicidae (bedbugs, cimicosis). Several genera have members which are commonly grouped as "bedbugs": *Cimex,*

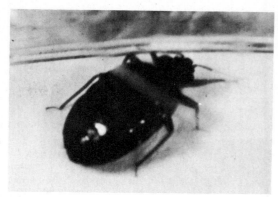

Fig. 208-9 Bedbug.

Leptocimex, Oeciacus, Hematasiphon. The species most common in each geographic area varies—temperate climates, *C. lectularius* (Fig. 208-9); tropical climates, *C. hemopterus*; Africa and South America, *L. bonati.* Bites by the bloodsucking bedbugs are usually not noticed immediately unless large numbers of bugs are present. Bedbugs are nocturnal feeders and can travel great distances to reach a suitable host. They may come from unusual locations: bird's nests, poultry houses, bus upholstery, old houses, and furniture. If only a few linear purpuric macules are present (Fig. 208-10), the diagnosis may not be clinically obvious; however, allergy reaction in sensitized individuals can develop as in other arthropod infestations, bites, or stings.

Reduviidae (kissing bugs, assassin bugs, cone-nosed bugs). Since several species of Reduviidae transmit *Trypanosoma cruzi*, this family is of medical importance. Unlike Cimicidae, Reduviidae produce extremely painful bites. Most species are encountered in the Americas with a few in Africa, Asia, and Europe. Clinically, the lesions described from Reduviidae are similar to those from other arthropods and depend upon the species, type of exposure, and individual sensitivity. The cause of the pain due to the bite of Reduviidae is not clear.

Hymenoptera

The general family of Hymenoptera includes bees (*Apidea*), wasps and hornets (*Vespidea*), and ants (*Formicoi-*

Fig. 209-10 Excoriated bedbug bites.

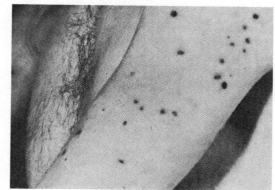

dea) [2]. These insects are notorious for their painful sting which may be associated with an anaphylactic reaction and/or death.

Stings by the female bee, hornet, or wasp from the modified oviposter (stinger apparatus) produce immediate burning and pain followed by an intense, local, erythematous reaction with swelling and urticaria. In the honeybee, the oviposter and paired venom sacs remain impaled in the victim and must be carefully removed to avoid continued envenomation. Severe systemic reactions occur in 0.4 to 0.8 percent of patients and are divided into three categories: angioedema or generalized urticaria; respiratory insufficiency from laryngeal edema or bronchospasm; and shock [34]. Case reports of acute myocardial infarction [35], myasthenia gravis [36], and hemolytic anemia [37] have been reported. Occasionally, major local reactions may persist at the bite site, presumably mediated by cellular immune mechanisms [38].

Venom from the honeybee is a highly complex mixture of pharmacologically active agents. Phospholipase A, which comprises 12 percent of honeybee venom, is responsible for the liberation of acute inflammatory mediators through the nonspecific membrane damage of its breakdown product, lysolecithin. Other venom constituents include hyaluronidase, histamine, norepinephrine, dopamine, melitttin, apamine, mast cell degranulation peptide, and minimine [39].

The acute treatment of Hymenoptera stings is based on the severity of patient response. Cutaneous reactions may be managed by application of ice with local injection of lidocaine for pain relief. Hypotension and respiratory failure must obviously be treated vigorously [34]. Systemic reactions require administration of subcutaneous epinephrine, while corticosteroids and antihistamines may be helpful for urticaria or edema. If a patient experiences an anaphylactic reaction and has a positive skin test, desensitization should be strongly considered. Injection of honeybee whole body extracts has proved clinically unsatisfactory, but lyophilized venom extract injections produced blocking IgG antibodies which afforded protection [40].

Fire ants of the group *Solenopsis* and the harvester ants of the group *Pogonomyrmex* are aggressive and produce local skin necrosis and systemic reactions when they sting [41,42]. Imported fire ant venom contains a nonproteinaceous, hemolytic factor identified as a dialkylpiperidine derivative, Solenopsin D [39,43], which induces the lytic release of histamine and other vasoactive amines from mast cells. Clinically, the bite site starts as an intense local inflammatory reaction which becomes a sterile pustule [39] (Fig. 208-11). In contrast, harvester ant venom is proteinaceous, and contains histamine, kinins, hyaluronidase, hemolysins, phospholipase, smooth muscle stimulants, and other poorly defined proteins [39].

The imported fire ants found only in the southeastern United States are particularly vicious since they attack in groups. By securing its jaw in the victim's skin, the fire ant is able to pivot, thereby leaving a ring of pustules. Since there is no specific therapy for ant stings, therapy is symptomatic. Systemic reactions occur frequently and may require corticosteroids or antihistamines. Desensitization may be helpful to protect allergic patients [34].

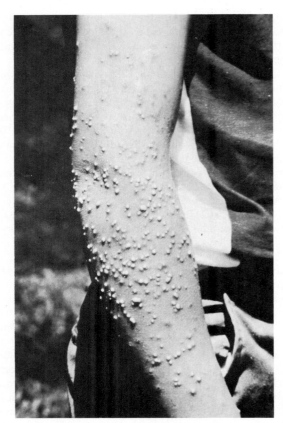

Fig. 208-11 Each wheal is a bite from a fire ant. When disturbed, the imported fire ant will attack anything within its reach. *(Clin Symp 20:75, 1968. U. S. Department of Agriculture, Plant Pest Control Division.)*

Lepidoptera

The medical importance of the Lepidoptera order is due solely to the irritant and allergenic properties of the hairs from caterpillars and moths [44–49]. At least one caterpillar species (gypsy moth, *Lymantria dispar*) may cause irritation due to histamine contained in the lancet hairs, but allergic potential of the same caterpillar hairs was also demonstrated [47]. Exposure to the stinging hairs would be expected in "outdoors" people such as lumbermen, farmers, and even campers. However, wind-borne hairs in areas of heavy infestations have caused an epidemic in New England and even a shipboard epidemic [46,47]. Whether most "urticating" caterpillar dermatoses are due to histamine and/or allergic reactions is not clear at this time [48,49]. The caterpillars and moths most commonly assumed to be a cause of these problems in the United States and Latin America are the following:

Caterpillars. Brown-tailed moth (*Euproctis chrysorrhea*); io moth (*Automeris io*); puss or flannel moth (*Megalopyge oporcularis*); saddleback moth (*Sibine stimulae*).
Moths. Lymantriidae family, tussock moths; brown-tailed moth (*E. chrysorrhea*); gypsy moth (*Lymantria dispar*); Douglas fir tussock moth (*Hemorocampa pseudotsugata* McDonnough); silk or peacock moth (Saturnidae family); silk moth (*Hylesia* species); io moth (*Automeris io*).

As more is known of the true allergenic nature of the reactions to the Lepidoptera, as well as species specificity, some puzzling dermatoses and related mucous membrane reactions may be clarified.

Siphonaptera

The order Siphonaptera contains only two flea families of medical interest: Pulicidae (human, cat, dog, and bird fleas) and Sarcopsyllidae or Tungidae (sand flea, causing tungiasis).

The Pulicidae family is of interest because certain species transmit plague and typhus. All species will bite humans since host specificity is relatively low, i.e., severe attacks may occur where domestic cats (*Ctenocephalides felis*), dogs (*Ct. canus*), and birds (*Ceratophyllus gallinae, C. columbae*) have recently resided. Survival of adult fleas for months in the absence of host animals makes flea-borne epidemics difficult to detect and eradicate. Usually the bite of the human flea (*Pulex irritans*) causes minimal irritation in a nonsensitized person and produces typically linear or clustered urticarial papules (Fig. 208-12). In allergic individuals, lesions are much more severe, with blisters and even erythema multiforme developing.

In the Sarcopsyllidae family, only *Tunga penetrans* is well known to produce problems. The female sand flea burrows into the dermis of the animal host. A painful necrotic abscess forms around the site of the female sand flea and her eggs. Secondary infection and scarring are the usual major complications although tetanus can develop in these wounds. Treatment consists of systemic antibiotics after sterile removal of early lesions, or killing the adult female with a suitable agent such as chloroform. Late lesions resolve by spontaneous ulceration.

Prevention

The biochemical bases of arthropod behavior are just now beginning to be understood [50,51]. Insect repellents such as diethyltoluamide have been the preferred preventive agents for persons bothered by fleas, flies, mites, mosquitoes, and ticks. Passive measures such as screens, nets, and clothing, especially if treated with repellents, are most effective. A number of synthetic arthropod attractants have been discovered [51]. Since pheromones have been identified for Coleoptera (beetles), Diptera (flies), Hymenoptera, and Orthoptora (cockroaches), new forms of prevention and protection from arthropod bites and stings should become available. As no preventive measures other than killing the adult or larval forms of bees, spiders, or wasps are currently very effective, future developments are eagerly anticipated.

References

1. Parrish HM: Analysis of 460 fatalities from venomous animals in the United States. *Am J Med Sci* **245**:129, 1963
2. Harwood RF, James MT (eds): *Entomology in Human and Animal Health,* 7th ed. New York, Macmillan, 1979
3. Ayres S Jr, Ayres S III: Demodectic eruptions (democidosis) in the human. *Arch Dermatol* **83**:816, 1961
4. Betz TG et al: Occupational dermatitis associated with straw itch mites (*Pyemotes ventricosus*). *JAMA* **247**:2821, 1982
5. Goldberger J, Schamberg JF: Epidemic of an urticaroid dermatitis due to a small mite (*Pediculoides ventricosus*) in the straw of mattresses. *Public Health Rep* **24**:973, 1909
6. Orkin M et al (eds): *Scabies and Pediculosis.* Philadelphia, JB Lippincott, 1977
7. Burkhart CG: Scabies: an epidemiologic reassessment. *Ann Intern Med* **98**:498, 1983
8. Rasmussen JE: The problem of lindane. *J Am Acad Dermatol* **5**:507, 1981
9. Goodpasture HC et al: Colorado tick fever: clinical epidemiologic and laboratory aspects of 228 cases in Colorado in 1973–1974. *Ann Intern Med* **88**:303, 1978
10. Burgdorfer W, Keirans JE: Ticks and Lyme disease in the United States. *Ann Intern Med* **99**:121, 1983
11. Steere AC et al: The early clinical manifestations of Lyme disease. *Ann Intern Med* **99**:76, 1983
12. Patterson JW et al: Localized tick bite reaction. *Cutis* **24**:168, 1979
13. Yesuddian P, Thambiah AS: Persistent papules after tick bites. *Dermatologica* **147**:214, 1973
14. Winer LH, Strakosch EA: Tick bites—*Dermacentor variabilis* (SAY). *J Invest Dermatol* **4**:249, 1941
15. Steere AC et al: Treatment of the early manifestations of Lyme disease. *Ann Intern Med* **99**:22, 1983
16. Gertsch WJ: The spider genus *Loxosceles* in North America, Central America and the West Indies. *American Museum Novitates* **1907**:1, 1958
17. Rees RS et al: The management of the brown recluse spider bite. *Plast Reconstr Surg* **68**:768, 1981
18. Rees RS et al: The pathogenesis of systemic *Loxosceles. J Surg Res* **35**:1, 1983
19. King LE Jr, Rees RS: Dapsone treatment of a brown recluse bite. *JAMA* **250**:645, 1983
20. Kaston BJ: *How to Know the Spiders,* 2d ed. Dubuque, IA, William C Brown, 1972
21. Howard BD et al: Effects and mechanisms of polypeptide neurotoxins that act presynaptically. *Annu Rev Pharmacol Toxicol* **20**:307, 1980
22. Key G: A comparison of calcium gluconate and methocarbamol (Robaxin) in the treatment of latrodectism (black widow spider envenomation). *Am J Trop Med Hyg* **30**:273, 1981
23. Catterall WA: Neurotoxins that act on voltage-sensitive so-

Fig. 208-12   Flea bites occurring in a characteristic grouping of three, sometimes referred to as "breakfast, lunch, and dinner."

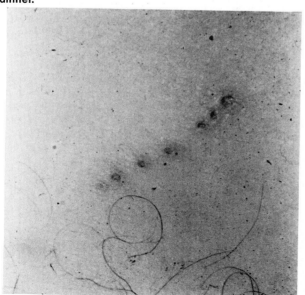

dium channels in excitable membranes. *Annu Rev Pharmacol Toxicol* **20:**15, 1980

24. Fontecilla-Camps JC et al: The three-dimensional structure of scorpion neurotoxins. *Toxicon* **20:**1, 1982
25. Almeida AP et al: Effects of purified scorpion toxin (Tityus toxin) on the isolated guinea pig heart. *Toxicon* **20:**855, 1982
26. Novaes G et al: Effect of purified scorpion toxin (Tityus toxin) on the pancreatic secretion of the rat. *Toxicon* **20:**847, 1982
27. Longenecker GL, Longenecker HE Jr: *Centruroides sculpturates* venom and platelet reactivity: possible role in scorpion venom-induced defibrination syndrome. *Toxicon* **19:**153, 1981
28. Zinssen RH: *Rats, Lice and History.* Boston, Little, Brown, 1935
29. Buxton PA: *The Louse,* 2d ed. London, Arnold, 1947
30. Orkin M et al: Treatment of today's scabies and pediculosis. *JAMA* **236:**1136, 1976
31. Taplin D et al: Malathion for treatment of *Pediculus humanus* var. *capitis* infestation. *JAMA* **247:**3103, 1982
32. Frazier C: Insect reactions related to sports. *Cutis* **19:**439, 1977
33. Steffen C: Clinical and histopathological correlation of midge bites. *Arch Dermatol* **117:**785, 1981
34. Yunginger J: Advances in the diagnosis and treatment of stinging insect allergy. *Pediatrics* **67:**325, 1981
35. Levine H: Acute myocardial infarction following wasp sting. *Am Heart J* **91:**365, 1976
36. Brumlik J: Myasthenia gravis associated with wasp sting. *JAMA* **235:**2120, 1976
37. Monzon C, Miles J: Hemolytic anemia following a wasp sting. *J Pediatr* **96:**1039, 1980
38. Case RL et al: Role of cell-mediated immunity in Hymenoptera allergy. *J Allergy Clin Immunol* **68:**399, 1981
39. Cavagnol RM: The pharmacological effects of Hymenoptera venoms. *Annu Rev Pharmacol Toxicol* **17:**479, 1977
40. Busse WW et al: Immunotherapy in bee sting anaphylaxis: use of honeybee venom. *JAMA* **231:**1154, 1975
41. Clemmer D, Serfling RE: The imported fire ant: dimension of the urban problem. *South Med J* **68:**1133, 1975
42. Pinnas JL et al: Harvester ant sensitivity: in vitro and in vivo studies using whole body extracts and venom. *J Allergy Immunol* **59:**10, 1977
43. Lind NK: Mechanism of action of fire ant (*Solenopsis*) venoms: lytic release of histamine from mast cells. *Toxicon* **20:**831, 1982
44. Hoover AW, Nelson E: Skin symptoms attributed to tussock moth infestation. *Cutis* **13:**597, 1974
45. Berman BA, Ross RN: Gypsy moth caterpillar dermatitis. *Cutis* **31:**251, 1983
46. Shama SK et al: Gypsy-moth-caterpillar dermatitis. *N Engl J Med* **306:**1300, 1982
47. Beaucher WN, Farnham JE: Gypsy-moth-caterpillar dermatitis. *N Engl J Med* **306:**1301, 1982
48. DeJong MCJM et al: A comparative study of the spicule venom of *Euproctis* caterpillars. *Toxicon* **20:**477, 1982
49. Bleumink E et al: Protease activities in the spicule venom of *Euproctis* caterpillars. *Toxicon* **20:**607, 1982
50. Wright RH: Why mosquito repellents repel. *Sci Am* **233:**104, 1975
51. Plimmer JR et al: Insect attractants. *Annu Rev Pharmacol Toxicol* **22:**297, 1982

Section 31

Skin manifestations of immunosuppression

CHAPTER 209

CUTANEOUS MANIFESTATIONS OF IMMUNODEFICIENCY DISORDERS

Arthur J. Ammann

In discussing dermatologic manifestations of immunodeficiency disorders, several approaches may be utilized. Here specific immunodeficiency diseases will be discussed and the dermatologic manifestations that are found detailed. This approach best illustrates the pathogenesis and possible etiology of specific dermatologic manifestations.

The immune system consists of four major components which defend against a constant assault by microbial agents. Each component—T-cell immunity, B-cell immunity, phagocytosis, and complement—provides a unique means of protection, but at the same time the individual components are integrated to provide synergistic immunity. Many of these systems are essential for both systemic and local immunity, and deficiencies of a single component may result in abnormalities of internal organs as well as of the skin and mucous membranes.

Numerous advances have been made in our understanding of basic immunologic mechanisms. As will be pointed out subsequently, for certain immunodeficiency diseases, these advances have reduced confusion in diagnosis and led to more specific therapy. The dermatologist plays an important role in the recognition of immunodeficiency disorders, as the initial manifestation of immunodeficiency disease may be confined to the skin and/or mucous membranes. A contemporary illustration of this fact is the association of Kaposi's sarcoma and acquired immunodeficiency syndrome, an observation which was first made by a dermatologist [1].

B-cell immunity

Historically, B-cell immunodeficiency was the first immunodeficiency disease to be described and occurred in a boy who was diagnosed as agammaglobulinemic [2]. This remained the major immunodeficiency disorder until techniques became available for diagnosing abnormalities of the T-cell system (previously referred to as cell-mediated immunity), the phagocytic system, and complement immunity.

B-cell immunity is derived from two types of mononuclear cells, one which circulates in the peripheral blood and has the appearance of a lymphocyte, and the other which resides in tissue and has the appearance of a plasma cell [3]. B lymphocytes in the peripheral blood make up only 10 to 15 percent of the total lymphocytes, which accounts for the observation that the total lymphocyte count is usually not significantly reduced in individuals who lack circulating B lymphocytes [4]. B lymphocytes have receptors on their surface which resemble or are identical to immunoglobulin molecules and have the capability of recognizing and binding to specific antigens [5]. These immunoglobulin molecules can be identified as belonging to specific classes of immunoglobulin such as IgG, IgM, IgA, IgD, and IgE. Usually, only a single immunoglobulin class is found on the surface of B cells and the relative proportion of the individual classes is similar to that of the serum levels of immunoglobulin; e.g., there is a greater number of IgG-B cells than IgE-B cells. In regard to the latter immunoglobulin, IgE is also found on the surface of mast cells and basophils and accounts for the ability of antigen–antibody reactions involving this class of immunoglobulin to trigger the release of histamine and other vasoactive amines. During ontogeny, IgM or IgD may be found in conjunction with another immunoglobulin class on the surface of B cells [6].

B cells may transform into plasma cells in the tissue. Circulating B lymphocytes have the capability of combining with antigen and, when transformed into plasma cells, produce specific antibody which subsequently circulates throughout the body. The distribution of plasma cells may vary depending on the location of lymphoid tissue. In lymph nodes and spleen, IgG- and IgM-producing plasma cells are abundant, whereas in the lamina propria of the intestinal tract, IgA-producing plasma cells dominate [7].

Each immunoglobulin class has distinct functions. IgG and IgM have the ability to fix complement. IgG diffuses throughout the body and into the interstitial spaces. IgM antibody forms rapidly following infection, whereas IgG antibody is produced more slowly but is sustained at a higher level for longer periods of time. Certain subclasses of IgG cross the placenta well, whereas IgM, IgA, and IgE do not. Although IgA is present in the systemic circulation, its primary function is in the secretions where two molecules of IgA combine with a unique protein termed *secretory component* [8]. Large amounts of secretory IgA are present in saliva, intestinal secretions, and colostrum.

The control of antibody synthesis is much more complex than originally anticipated. Once antibody is produced following exposure to a specific antigen, individual antibody molecules develop unique immunochemical characteristics which are referred to as idiotypes [9]. Idiotypes are recognized as "foreign" by the individual's own immune system and result in the production of anti-idiotypic antibody (sometimes called anti-antibody). The function of anti-idiotypic antibody is to regulate the amount of specific antibody produced.

The B-cell system works in concert with phagocytic and complement immunity. Antibody plus antigen is capable of activating the complement cascade which amplifies the effect of both systems. Phagocytic cells have receptors on their surface for the heavy chain of immunoglobulin molecules, which permits the identification and subsequent ingestion of microbial agents. A deficiency of immunity in the B-cell system usually results in symptoms of recurrent bacterial infection and inadequate protection against viral reinfection. Certain B-cell deficiencies may also result in manifestations of autoimmunity.

The best means of diagnosing an abnormality of the B-cell system is to quantitate specific immunoglobulin levels [10]. The total protein/albumin ratio, although capable of detecting hypogammaglobulinemia, will not detect deficiencies of individual immunoglobulin classes such as IgA deficiency. Patients who have elevated levels of immunoglobulins may also have abnormalities in the B-cell system which are secondary to T-cell abnormalities [11]. Hypergammaglobulinemia should be considered as evidence of immunologic dysregulation and should be investigated with the same degree of detail as hypogammaglobulinemia. Certain patients with elevated levels of immunoglobulin may be unable to produce specific antibody following immunization. It is important to emphasize at this point, however, that patients suspected of having immunodeficiency should never be immunized with live or attenuated viral vaccines to determine whether or not they are capable of producing an antibody response.

B-cell immunodeficiency

Hypogammaglobulinemia

Two major types of hypogammaglobulinemia occur: X-linked or congenital hypogammaglobulinemia, and common variable or acquired hypogammaglobulinemia [12–14]. Clinical manifestations are similar in both groups except for age of onset. In congenital hypogammaglobulinemia, recurrent, severe bacterial infection usually begins sometime after six months of age following the loss of maternally derived IgG in the infant. Initial symptoms consist of pneumonia, meningitis, and recurrent otitis media. Chronic infectious manifestations usually involve the lungs, sinuses, gastrointestinal tract, and skin. Occasionally patients may present with what appears to be an autoimmune disease such as juvenile rheumatoid arthritis.

In a male patient it may be difficult to differentiate congenital hypogammaglobulinemia with late onset of symptomatology from that of acquired hypogammaglobulinemia. In the former disorder circulating B cells are absent, although this may be occasionally observed in patients with acquired hypogammaglobulinemia [15,16]. Infectious manifestations of hypogammaglobulinemia may have a more subtle onset in adult patients, who may present with chronic sinusitis, persistent cough following an acute infection, and recurrent or chronic diarrhea usually of unknown etiology but occasionally associated with protozoal infection. As in children with congenital hypogammaglobulinemia, the initial presentation in acquired hypogammaglobulinemia may be that of an autoimmune disorder. The onset of symptoms in acquired hypogammaglobulinemia may be as late as 70 years of age.

Dermatologic manifestations of hypogammaglobulinemia are frequent. Patients may develop recurrent pustules, although more often the skin is found to have eczematoid lesions which are chronically infected with common skin bacteria. Detailed histologic examination of skin lesions in patients with hypogammaglobulinemia has not been performed as the lesions usually respond to local and/or systemic therapy. Chronic infection of the skin or oral mucous membrane with fungi is unusual in patients with hypogammaglobulinemia as they have intact T-cell immunity. The chronic diarrhea which is frequently observed may be a result of protozoal infection or alteration of the normal microbial flora of the intestinal tract. Acute or chronic conjunctivitis is frequently present and may be due to a variety of organisms.

A diagnosis of hypogammaglobulinemia can be established if the level of IgG is less than 250 mg/dL. IgM and IgA are usually less than 30 mg/dL, although an occasional patient may have a normal or elevated IgM value. In infants it is important to compare IgG values to those of age-matched controls, as IgG levels may be low between 6 and 18 months of age.

Treatment of hypogammaglobulinemia is best accomplished utilizing gamma globulin. Gamma globulin is made from pooled plasma obtained from over 1000 individual donors and offers passive protection against a variety of infectious agents. Intravenous gamma globulin is slowly replacing intramuscular gamma globulin as higher serum levels of immunoglobulin can be achieved following intravenous use and the discomfort of intramuscular injections can be avoided [17]. Gamma globulin preparations contain primarily IgG and only trace amounts of other immunoglobulins. In most patients, the infectious manifestations of hypogammaglobulinemia are well controlled with 100 mg/kg of gamma globulin given intravenously on a monthly basis. Occasionally, larger doses are required (up to 400 mg/kg) or the infusions may be required on an every 2- to 3-week basis. Both systemic and dermatologic manifestations of the disease respond readily; however, on occasion, systemic antibiotic therapy may be required. Local antibiotic treatment of chronic conjunctivitis may be necessary.

Selective IgA deficiency

Selective IgA deficiency is the most common immunodeficiency disorder recognized [18,19]. In the general population, it has an incidence of between 1 in 400 and 1 in 600. In studies of allergic populations, patients are found more frequently (about 1 in 200) [20]. Originally, selective IgA deficiency was described in healthy adults and was somewhat of a laboratory curiosity [21,22]. As larger numbers of cases accumulated, it became apparent that many patients had a variety of associated diseases. These fell into several broad categories, including gastrointestinal tract disease, recurrent or chronic sinopulmonary infection, autoimmune disease, allergy, and malignancy. Initially, it was difficult to determine why a broad range of diseases was associated with selective IgA deficiency. However, detailed studies of the function of IgA, in particular secretory IgA, indicated that this system had an important role in local immunity and in restricting the access of microbial agents and antigens to the systemic circulation. Thus, if microbial agents were not effectively excluded by the pulmonary and gastrointestinal tract mucosa, patients might present with a variety of diseases, the manifestations of which might vary with the type of infectious exposure as well as the duration of exposure.

Clinical symptoms may begin at any age, although they are most frequently present sometime after 1 to 2 years of age. Recurrent upper respiratory tract infections, diarrhea, sinusitis, arthritis, or otitis media may be a presenting complaint. Patients who develop autoimmune disease or malignancy usually present during adult life. Severe systemic infection, such as is observed in hypogammaglobulinemia or severe T-cell immunodeficiency disorders, is usually not found in patients with selective IgA deficiency.

A diagnosis of selective IgA deficiency is best accomplished utilizing quantitative immunoglobulins. The level of IgA in the serum should be less than 5 mg/dL. A protein electrophoresis cannot be used to detect selective IgA deficiency. In most instances, patients with selective IgA deficiency have intact T-cell immunity. However, there are subsets of patients who may have additional immunologic abnormalities which account for more severe clinical symptomatology. Abnormalities of interferon production, T-cell function, and immunoglobulin G subclass production have been described [23,24]. Because it is important to determine how extensive the immunologic abnormalities are in patients diagnosed with immunodeficiency, it is recommended that T-cell studies be performed in patients with selective IgA deficiency. This is particularly important in young patients where selective IgA deficiency may be the initial laboratory abnormality; for example, in a young child who has not yet developed all of the features of the ataxia-telangiectasia syndrome. As some forms of selective IgA deficiency are inherited, quantitative immunoglobulin levels should be obtained on all family members.

There are probably several etiologies of selective IgA deficiency. In some families, selective IgA deficiency occurs as an autosomal dominant, while in others it may be an autosomal recessive or occur sporadically. The incidence of selective IgA deficiency is over 1 out of 5 in patients who are treated with diphenylhydantoin. In some instances the IgA deficiency remains, even after withdrawal of the drug.

Dermatologic manifestations of selective IgA deficiency are rare. An association between vitiligo and selective IgA deficiency has been reported. Patients who present with dermatologic manifestations of autoimmune disease, such as Raynaud's syndrome, vasculitis, or a systemic lupus erythematosus rash, should have quantitative immunoglobulins performed to determine whether the patient has selective IgA deficiency. Although the presence of IgA deficiency does not appear to influence the course of the underlying disease, it is important to recognize this additional abnormality in relation to other symptoms which may be present such as sinopulmonary infection and gastrointestinal tract disease.

There is no specific treatment for selective IgA deficiency. It is essential that these patients not be treated with gamma globulin, as there are insufficient amounts of IgA in gamma globulin to correct the abnormality. In addition, patients are capable of making antibodies to proteins, including IgA, and may therefore recognize foreign antigens in gamma globulin and develop allergic reactions. Caution must also be exercised when patients receive blood transfusions. A common cause of transfusion reactions is the presence of antibody to IgA in patients with unrecognized selective IgA deficiency [24]. Patients should receive packed, washed red cells to avoid this type of reaction. The frequent use of antibiotics has decreased the occurrence of recurrent and chronic sinopulmonary infection. Diseases associated with selective IgA deficiency, such as systemic lupus erythematosus or rheumatoid arthritis, are treated in a manner identical to that of the disease when IgA deficiency is not present.

T-cell immunodeficiency disorders

The T-cell system is composed of distinct subpopulations of lymphocytes, each having unique function and producing a large number of lymphokines which have effects on subpopulations of T cells, B cells, and other mononuclear cells such as natural killer cells. The original concept of an independent T- and B-cell system is no longer accepted and, in fact, normal T-cell immunity is a requirement for normal B-cell immunity.

Precursors of T cells are initially derived from the bone marrow and are subsequently modified within the thymus, where maturation and specific function are acquired. The various stages of maturation are identified using monoclonal antibodies against surface antigens [25]. Monoclonal antibodies are also useful in identifying subpopulations of T cells which have specific functions. The monoclonal antibody OKT4 (Leu 3) identifies T cells which have a helper and inducer function, while the OKT8 (Leu 2) monoclonal antibody recognizes a population of T cells with suppressor and cytotoxic function. Activated T cells have a surface receptor termed Ia which functions in conjunction with a T-cell receptor for antigen [25,26]. The ability of T cells to recognize specific antigen is comparable in degree to that of B cells but is mediated by these two unique receptors rather than the immunoglobulin-like molecule present on the surface of B cells.

T cells have the ability to produce a variety of lymphokines. Interleukin 2, produced by both helper and cytotoxic T cells, is capable of enhancing the response of T cells to antigen, mitogen, and alloantigen and increasing both antibody response and natural killer cell activity [27]. Certain interferons are also produced by T cells and are capable of mediating a wide variety of immunologic reactions [28].

In order for a normal immune response to occur, there must be interaction between cells of the immune system. Antigen processing by monocytes is the first step in an immunologic reaction. Subsequently, monocytes release monokines, specifically interleukin 1, which enhance the immunologic reaction of activated T cells [27]. The interaction between monocytes and T cells is dependent on the presence of Ia, shared histocompatibility antigens, and a specific T-cell receptor. Subsequent activation of B cells is dependent on the presence of Ia and specific antigen recognition through the immunoglobulin receptor. As a generalization, patients with severe T-cell immunodeficiency always have an impairment of B-cell immunity, even if immunoglobulins are present at normal levels.

A deficiency of T-cell immunity results in susceptibility to infection with fungi, protozoa, and viruses. Certain complications such as graft-versus-host reaction may also occur. Patients with selective T-cell deficiency may have limited clinical symptoms, such as recurrent *Candida* infection, or may have broad-based immunodeficiency with susceptibility to all microbial agents.

Chronic mucocutaneous candidiasis

Patients with chronic mucocutaneous candidiasis (CMC) have an increased susceptibility to skin and mucous mem-

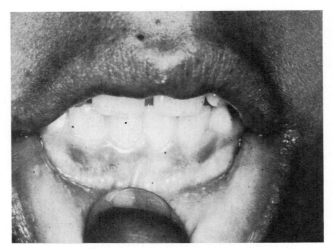

Fig. 209-1   Child with chronic mucocutaneous candidiasis and Addison's disease. Generalized pigmentation of the skin and gums is present. Angular cheilosis secondary to *Candida* infection is also seen.

brane infection with *Candida* [28–30]. They rarely have systemic infection with *Candida* and usually do not have susceptibility to other fungal agents. The onset of the disorder may occur as early as several months of age or as late as adult life. CMC is also associated with idiopathic endocrinopathy. Patients with this form of the disease may initially present with endocrine dysfunction and develop evidence of *Candida* infection only after years of difficulty with a specific endocrinopathy. Alternatively, chronic *Candida* infection may be the initial manifestation in a patient who will subsequently develop endocrine deficiency. This sequence is essential to recognize, as the mortality in CMC is usually associated with the development of an unrecognized endocrine disorder such as Addison's disease, rather than a result of *Candida* infection. The increased skin pigmentation characteristic of Addison's disease may be the first clinical feature recognized (Fig. 209-1). The most common endocrinopathy is that of hypoparathyroidism followed by Addison's disease, pernicious anemia, diabetes, gonadal dysfunction, and growth hormone abnormalities.

The initial manifestations of *Candida* infection may be confined to small areas of the oral mucosa or skin. As the disease persists, however, more diffuse involvement occurs and the *Candida* infection results in severely disfiguring skin lesions or debilitating mucosal involvement. Skin infection may have a "stocking-glove" distribution Fig. 209-2). Occasionally, the only manifestation of *Candida* infection is isolated infection of the nails (Fig. 209-3).

The etiology of CMC is unknown. The association of autoantibodies directed against endocrine organs has led to the suggestion that the disease has an autoimmune basis, with the thymus gland representing another endocrine organ [31]. Patients with CMC have characteristic laboratory abnormalities, the most important of which is an absent delayed-hypersensitivity skin test to *Candida* antigen. This is the single most useful test for diagnosis and is easily performed. The delayed-hypersensitivity skin test must be read carefully, as many patients have antibody to *Candida* antigen that will result in an Arthus reaction, which is usually observed 6 to 24 h following injection of antigen. If a strong Arthus reaction occurs, the "carryover" of this

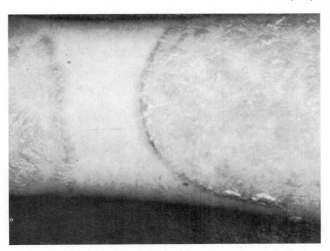

Fig. 209-2   Severe granulomatous form of *Candida* infection involving the skin with demonstration of involved and uninvolved areas. Note clearly demarcated borders.

reaction into the 24- to 48-h delayed-hypersensitivity reaction period may be misinterpreted as a positive delayed-hypersensitivity skin test. Some patients with CMC have an inability to produce migration inhibition factor following stimulation of peripheral blood mononuclear cells. More profound defects in T-cell immunity have also been reported, including an abnormal lymphocyte response to mitogen. Other patients may have defects in monocyte function which result in susceptibility to infection with bacterial agents. Patients who have *Candida* infection of the mucous membrane or skin should have a complete evaluation of their immunologic status as *Candida* infection is a common manifestation of severe immunodeficiency disorders.

A variety of antifungal drugs is available for the treatment of *Candida* infection. Mycostatin, which is frequently used, is usually ineffective. Clotrimazole appears to be more effective but resistance is sometimes rapidly encoun-

Fig. 209-3   Isolated nail involvement in a patient with chronic nail candidiasis. *Candida* infection may precede the appearance of the endocrinopathy.

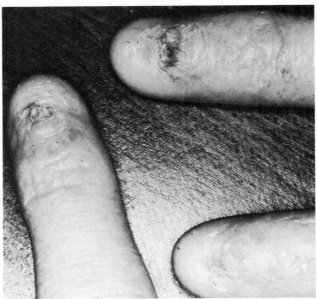

tered. Miconazole appears to be the most effective antifungal agent that can be used topically. Ketoconazole may be an effective agent for systemic treatment, but caution should be observed as ketoconazole may result in liver disease and patients with CMC are predisposed to developing hepatitis. Patients who have severe *Candida* infection of the skin or mucous membranes may require treatment with intravenous amphotericin-B. The systemic toxicity of this antifungal agent is a major limitation in its repeated use, but it is the single most effective agent. Some studies indicate that patients may respond more readily to a combination of amphotericin-B and transfer factor [32]. The role of transfer factor in the treatment of T-cell immunodeficiency disorders remains controversial.

Biotin-responsive multiple carboxylase enzyme deficiency

Several disorders have been described in association with biotin deficiency. A particularly interesting group of patients is one that has abnormalities in carbohydrate and branched chain amino acid catabolism and is responsive to the oral administration of biotin. These disorders include deficiencies of the enzyme propionyl-CoA carboxylase (PCC), which is required for the catabolism of isoleucine and valine; deficiency of α-methylcrotonyl-CoA carboxylase (MCC), which is required for the catabolism of leucine; and combined deficiencies of PCC, MCC, and pyruvate carboxylase (PC) [33]. Multiple carboxylase deficiencies are probably the result of an abnormality in the metabolism of biotin, which is a necessary cofactor for all of the carboxylases [34].

Biotin-responsive multiple carboxylase deficiencies are inherited in an autosomal-recessive manner and have two distinctive clinical presentations. The more severe form has an onset in the newborn period. The immunodeficiency is usually associated with severe and overwhelming bacterial infections. The second form has a delayed onset and occurs sometime after the first year of life. It is associated with clinical evidence of mucocutaneous candidiasis, a desquamative dermatitis, keratoconjunctivitis, and alopecia (Fig. 209-4). These patients are at risk for developing pneumonia, bacteremia, septicemia, overwhelming viral infections, and recurrent otitis media. Patients usually develop a progressive ataxia which is associated with progressive neurologic deterioration. Without supplemental biotin, both forms of the disease are fatal. The clinical features of biotin-responsive multiple carboxylase deficiencies are similar to those of biotin deficiency associated with nutritional biotin deprivation [35]. Biotin deficiency may occur in individuals who ingest large amounts of uncooked egg white, which contains large amounts of avidin, capable of binding to biotin. Biotin deficiency has also been described in patients receiving hyperalimentation, where biotin has been omitted from the vitamin supplementation of the hyperalimentation fluids.

Immunologic studies in patients with biotin-responsive multiple carboxylase deficiencies are normal if the studies are performed in culture media containing biotin, whereas pronounced T-cell defects can be demonstrated in biotin-depleted culture media. Other laboratory abnormalities include organic aciduria, ketonuria, lactic acidosis, hypoglycemia, hyperammonemia, hyperphosphatemia, and hyperglycinemia.

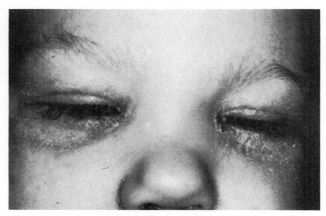

Fig. 209-4 Desquamative dermatitis in a patient with biotin-dependent multiple carboxylase deficiency. Involvement of the skin surrounding the eyes is typical.

Patients with all forms of biotin deficiency and patients with biotin-responsive multiple carboxylase deficiencies can be effectively treated with oral biotin. Treatment is capable of reversing immunologic, dermatologic, metabolic, and neurologic abnormalities [36].

Severe combined immunodeficiency disease

Several forms of severe combined immunodeficiency disease (SCID) exist, indicating that there are several etiologies of this disorder. Approximately one-third of patients with SCID have an absence of the enzyme adenosine deaminase (ADA) [37]. Two inherited patterns of SCID, unassociated with ADA deficiency, have been observed: autosomal recessive and X-linked [38].

The phenotype of severe combined immunodeficiency disease, regardless of the etiology, is similar. Patients present early in infancy with severe bacterial, viral, or fungal infection. They usually exhibit failure to thrive, recurrent otitis media, pneumonia, and chronic diarrhea. Occasionally, the onset of symptoms may be delayed to beyond 1 year of age. Without treatment, the disease is usually fatal by 2 years of age. Diagnosis is readily established utilizing assays of T- and B-cell immunity. If the infant is over 6 months of age, maternal immunoglobulin is not present and hypogammaglobulinemia can be detected. Lymphopenia is commonly present. Specific evaluation of T-cell immunity reveals a deficiency in both number and function. The response of T cells to mitogens such as phytohemagglutinin (PHA), concanavalin A, antigen, or alloantigen is either markedly diminished or absent. Patients who are diagnosed as SCID, based on immunologic studies, should also have biochemical studies to determine the activity of adenosine deaminase, as the presence of this enzyme deficiency will permit specific genetic counseling and intrauterine diagnosis [39].

Dermatologic manifestations in SCID may result either from infection or from complications of the disease such as graft-versus-host reaction. *Candida* infection of the mucous membranes is one of the earliest manifestations of the disease. Initially, fungal infection of the skin may be thought to be a simple *Candida* diaper dermatitis. However, the chronicity of infection and its resistance to local antifungal therapy should suggest that an underlying im-

munodeficiency disorder is present. Graft-versus-host disease may be observed in SCID. This complication is associated with a variety of dermatologic manifestations and will be discussed subsequently.

The treatment of choice for SCID is the transplantation of a histocompatible bone marrow from a sibling donor. Recently, lectin-separated bone marrow or monoclonal-treated bone marrow has been utilized to transplant non-histocompatible bone marrow [40,41]. As soon as a diagnosis of SCID is established, supportive therapy should be instituted. Intravenous gamma globulin in a dose of 100 to 400 mg/kg will reduce the susceptibility to both viral and bacterial infections. Broad-spectrum antibiotic treatment may be necessary for established infections. Trimethoprim-sulfamethoxazole given prophylactically is necessary to prevent *Pneumocystis carinii* infection. Aggressive diagnostic measures may be necessary in patients to establish the etiology of infection, in particular, an open lung biopsy for the diagnosis of *Pneumocystis carinii* pneumonia.

Immunodeficiency with thrombocytopenia and eczema (Wiskott-Aldrich syndrome)

The Wiskott-Aldrich syndrome (WAS) is inherited in an X-linked manner. The etiology of this disease is unknown. Patients usually present in early infancy with either bleeding or recurrent infection. Bleeding is a result of thrombocytopenia, which may be present at birth and varies in severity [42]. Although platelet counts are always low, if they fall in a range above 60,000/μL, bleeding problems may be minimal and may result in a delay in diagnosis. Initially, patients have repeated infections due to *Streptococcus pneumoniae* or *Hemophilus influenzae*. As the disease progresses, recurrent viral infections are also present. In later life there is an increased susceptibility to malignancy [43].

The primary dermatologic manifestation of WAS is that of eczema, which cannot be distinguished from that found in atopic patients. Secondary infection of the eczema is frequently present. Petechial lesions secondary to thrombocytopenia may be present at any time but are more frequent following viral infections (Fig. 209-5).

A diagnosis of WAS can be established more readily by hematologic evaluation than by immunologic evaluation. Characteristically, platelet counts are less than 100,000/μL and the platelet size is small. In almost all other disorders associated with thrombocytopenia, the platelet size is larger than normal. Immunologic studies demonstrate a normal IgG level, a reduced IgM level, and increased IgA and IgE levels, although there are some exceptions to this pattern. Isohemagglutinins are usually absent as is the antibody response following immunization with pneumococcal polysaccharide antigens [44,45]. T-cell immunity, which may be normal initially, becomes abnormal with time and includes a reduction in both T-cell number and function.

Specific treatment of WAS is not available. Histocompatible bone marrow transplantation has been successful in a number of cases [46]. Supportive therapy includes intravenous gamma globulin for the prevention of bacterial and viral infection, and broad-spectrum antibiotic treatment as necessary. The eczema in WAS does not respond readily to treatment. Systemic corticosteroid ther-

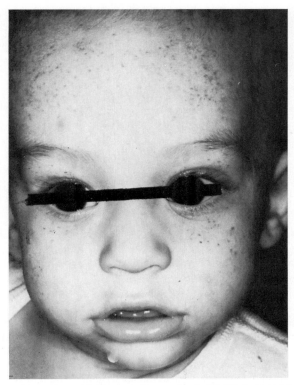

Fig. 209-5   Petechial lesions in a patient with Wiskott-Aldrich syndrome. Petechial purpura and ecchymoses may only appear following an acute viral illness in spite of the thrombocytopenia which is present at birth.

apy should not be utilized as it may increase the susceptibility to infection. A chronic keratitis, secondary to viral infection, is frequently observed in older WAS patients and is resistant to treatment.

Immunodeficiency with ataxia-telangiectasia

Ataxia-telangiectasia (AT), is inherited in an autosomal recessive manner and is associated with distinctive clinical and immunologic features [47,48]. When present simultaneously, the finding of ataxia, telangiectasia, and recurrent sinopulmonary infection establishes a diagnosis. As in other immunodeficiency disorders, however, the onset of individual symptoms may be variable, making a diagnosis difficult during the first several years of life. Initially, the ataxia may be thought to be a result of a post-viral disorder. Its persistence should arouse suspicion. Subsequently, patients may develop telangiectases involving the skin and bulbar conjunctiva. Recurrent sinopulmonary infection may follow. The clinical presentation may vary, however, and any one of the major manifestations may appear first or be delayed until 6 to 8 years of age. Patients are also susceptible to malignancy, with lymphosarcoma as the most common type, and others such as Burkitt's lymphoma less frequent [49]. Studies of cultured cells from patients indicate abnormalities of DNA repair mechanisms with increased susceptibility of cells to damaging effects of cytotoxic agents [50]. It is of interest that patients who develop malignancy and are subsequently treated, have an exquisite sensitivity to radiation therapy or systemic treatment with cytotoxic agents.

A diagnosis of AT can be readily established on a clinical basis when all of the major manifestations of the disease are present. Prior to that time, determination of serum alpha-fetoprotein, which is elevated in almost all patients, may be the most useful laboratory study [51]. Immunologic abnormalities are not consistently present during the early phase of the disease. The most common immunologic abnormality detected is IgA deficiency (approximately 40 percent of the cases). Decreased T-cell numbers, abnormal T-cell function, and impairment of B-cell immunity are also observed. AT is a progressive disorder, in relation to both clinical symptomatology and immunologic studies. Older patients become incapacitated from ataxia, develop mental retardation, and succumb to severe sinopulmonary tract infection or malignancy. The increased susceptibility to infection is associated with deteriorating immunologic function.

There are several dermatologic abnormalities that occur in AT. The telangiectases involve the bulbar conjunctiva, the skin over the bridge of the nose, ears, and antecubital fossa. Telangiectasia becomes more severe with time. Additional dermatologic manifestations consist of cutaneous atrophy simulating scleroderma and becoming more prominent with disease progression, areas of hypo- and hyperpigmentation, atopic dermatitis, nummular eczema, café au lait macules, and cutaneous malignancies [52,53].

There is no effective prevention or correction of the abnormalities found in AT. Bone marrow transplantation has not been successfully performed, although it is theoretically possible. Supportive therapy consists of intravenous gamma globulin and broad-spectrum antibiotics when indicated.

Immunodeficiency with short-limbed dwarfism

There are three major forms of immunodeficiency with short-limbed dwarfism (SLD). Type I is associated with combined immunodeficiency, Type II with T-cell immunodeficiency and Type III with B-cell immunodeficiency. Patients who have SLD with combined immunodeficiency present with a clinical picture similar to that of severe combined immunodeficiency disease [54]. They have susceptibility to viral, bacterial, fungal, and protozoal infection and usually succumb to overwhelming infection in the first year of life. Patients with SLD and T-cell immunodeficiency are susceptible to recurrent sinopulmonary tract infection, progressive vaccinia, and fatal varicella [55]. They may develop a malabsorption-like syndrome. Patients with B-cell immunodeficiency and SLD have recurrent pyogenic infections such as otitis media, meningitis, and pneumonia.

Characteristically, patients with SLD have short, pudgy hands and extremities. Unlike achondroplasia, the head is of normal size. During infancy, redundant skin folds are seen around the neck and large joints and the patients may be misdiagnosed as having Turner's syndrome (Fig. 209-6). The hair is characterized as light in color, reduced in diameter, and sparse (Fig. 209-7). Examination of the hair under a microscope reveals an absence of the central pigment core (Fig. 209-8). Patients with SLD and combined immunodeficiency disease are also susceptible to graft-versus-host disease and may have associated dermatologic abnormalities when this complication is present. Progres-

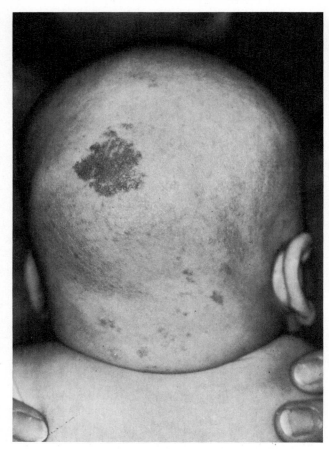

Fig. 209-6   Patient with short-limbed dwarfism during neonatal period. Note redundant skin folds of the neck. Similar skin folds may be seen over the large joints of the arms and legs. These folds disappear as the child grows older.

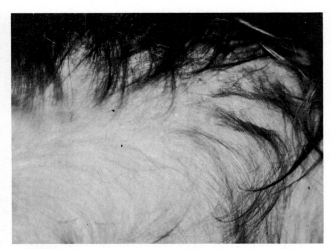

Fig. 209-7   Thin and sparse hair, usually of light color, in a patient with short-limbed dwarfism, cartilage-hair hypoplasia, and T-cell immunodeficiency.

sive vaccinia, a complication of smallpox immunization, is rarely observed (Fig. 209-9).

Immunologic abnormalities vary with the degree of immunodeficiency. In SLD with B-cell immunodeficiency, only abnormalities of B-cell immunity are found, including hypogammaglobulinemia and the inability to form antibody following immunization. Patients with combined immunodeficiency have defects in both T- and B-cell immunity and are phenotypically similar to patients with severe combined immunodeficiency. Patients with SLD and T-cell immunodeficiency have a more selective T-cell abnormality. The response of lymphocytes to mitogens is usually normal.

Treatment of patients with SLD and immunodeficiency is identical to that of the associated immunodeficiency disorder when SLD is not present. It is important to recognize that some patients with SLD are entirely normal immunologically.

Graft-versus-host disease

Graft-versus-host disease (GVHD) was first studied in animals as early as 1916, when chick embryos were utilized to assay splenic enlargement as a consequence of GVHD [56]. GVHD in a human was first recognized following transplantation of allogeneic bone marrow for the treatment of leukemia [57]. Because GVHD is a protean disorder, and usually appears several weeks following administration of viable leukocytes, it frequently masquerades as other seemingly well-established disease entities. GVHD has been misdiagnosed as an allergic reaction to drugs, acute viral infection, acrodermatitis enteropathica, and histiocytosis X [58–60].

Viable leukocytes capable of dividing and attacking the host in an unopposed manner are responsible for GVHD. However, before GVHD can occur, several requirements must be met. First, there must be histocompatibility differences between the graft (donor) and the host (recipient). Second, the recipient must be unable to reject the foreign cells which produce the graft-versus-host reaction (the host must be immunodeficient). Third, the donor cells must be immunocompetent and have the ability to recognize and react against host cells. The specific antigens which evoke GVHD are related to the major histocompatibility complex and are termed *human leukocyte antigens* (HLA). Several loci are known, including HLA-A, HLA-B, HLA-D, and HLA-DR. The HLA-D locus determines whether graft cells will react against the histocompatibility antigens HLA-A, B, D or DR. In a host who has significant T-cell immunodeficiency, there is an absence of an ability to recognize and react against transfused leukocytes. The donor cells are therefore free to proliferate in an unopposed manner and will cause extensive damage to the host as they recognize histocompatibility differences. Untreated, GVHD is fatal.

The administration of a number of blood products has been associated with GVHD and include packed red cells, frozen cells, platelets, fresh plasma, and leukocyte-poor red cells [58,61]. GVHD may also occur following attempts at immunologic reconstitution using fetal thymus, fetal liver, or bone marrow transplantation [62,63]. Maternal–fetal GVHD is probably a result of infusion of small amounts of maternal leukocytes prior to, or during, delivery of an infant with immunodeficiency.

GVHD may first be observed as early as 5 to 7 days following infusion of viable lymphocytes but on occasion may be delayed as long as 30 days. The clinical and labo-

Fig. 209-8 Hair from a patient with short-limbed dwarfism and cartilage-hair hypoplasia (A) compared with a normal (B). The hair is thin and lacks the central pigmented core.

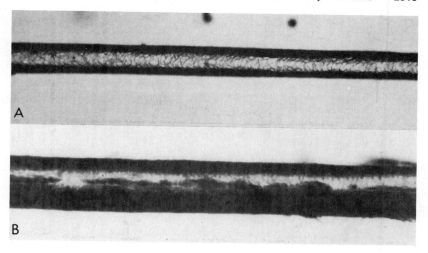

ratory diagnosis of GVHD is not dependent on a single clinical or laboratory feature and may therefore cause confusion. Most of the clinical features are explained on the basis of cell destruction, which is caused by the graft cells reacting against host cells. Although only red blood cells lack histocompatibility antigens, graft cells are capable of producing antibody which may be directed against other host antigens, e.g., hemolytic anemia.

Three distinct clinical forms of GVHD exist: acute, hyperacute, and chronic. The hyperacute form of GVHD usually begins as a macular and papular rash and rapidly progresses to a form resembling toxic epidermal necrolysis [63]. Toxic epidermal necrolysis is not associated with staphylococcal infection or prior drug therapy but is associated with a significant degree of histocompatibility mismatch between donor and recipient and/or infusion of large numbers of immunocompetent cells. The disease is associated with other clinical features of GVHD but is always rapidly fatal.

Acute GVHD, which initially presents with a macular and papular rash, is frequently mistaken for a viral or allergic disorder (Fig. 209-10). At first the rash will blanch with pressure and may be transient in appearance. As the GVHD progresses the macular and papular rash becomes

confluent and, if persistent, scaling dermatitis is observed. A lichen planus-like reaction may be present. Jaundice, difficulty in breathing, diarrhea, hepatosplenomegaly, cardiac irregularities, central nervous system irritability, and pulmonary infiltrates may occur sometime during GVHD. An increased susceptibility to infection is almost always present and can further exacerbate the underlying susceptibility to infection in a patient with primary immunodeficiency disease.

Chronic GVHD may be observed following blood transfusions, attempts at histocompatible bone marrow transplantation, or maternal–fetal transfusion. The clinical and laboratory features may vary from slight abnormalities of the skin, such as intermittent desquamation, to severe chronic desquamation and a sclerodermatous-like picture. Alopecia, vertical ridging of the nails, and loss of eyebrows and eyelashes may be observed (Figs. 209-11 to 209-13). Lymphadenopathy, hepatosplenomegaly, chronic diarrhea, and failure to thrive are seen in both pediatric and adult patients.

Chronic GVHD has been confused with a variety of

Fig. 209-10 Early graft-versus-host disease following an unirradiated blood transfusion in a patient with undiagnosed severe combined immunodeficiency. The initial macular and papular rash may be confused with a viral eruption or drug reaction.

Fig. 209-9 Progressive vaccinia following smallpox immunization in a patient with short-limbed dwarfism. This fatal lesion is rarely seen since routine smallpox immunization has been abandoned.

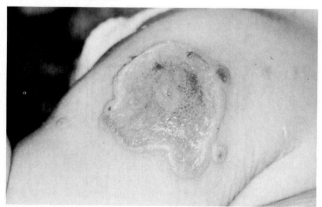

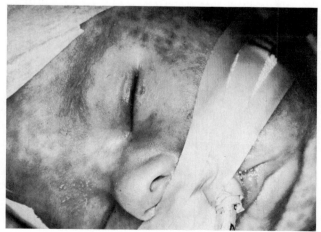

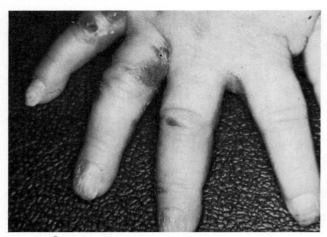

Fig. 209-11 Chronic graft-versus-host disease interfering with normal nail growth. This usually results in vertical ridging of the nails. Also note secondary infection of the skin.

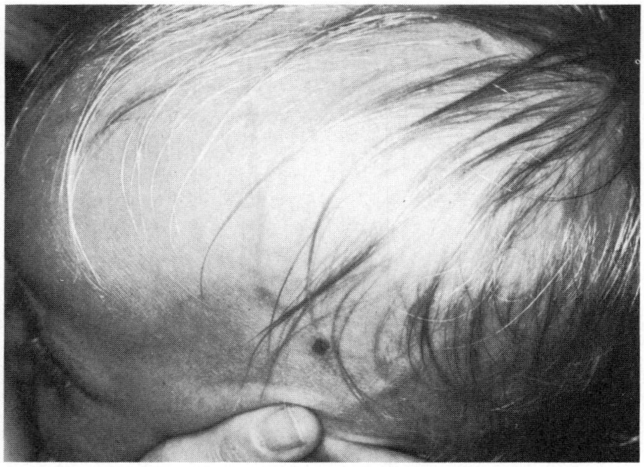

Fig. 209-12 Chronic graft-versus-host disease resulting in loss of hair from the scalp. Eyebrows and eyelashes may also be lost.

clinical disorders. Because of the presence of lymphadenopathy, hepatosplenomegaly, and skin rash (frequently associated with a histiocytic infiltration) an erroneous diagnosis of Letterer-Siwe disease may be made. Patients with Letterer-Siwe disease have normal T- and B-cell immunity, in contrast to patients with GVHD, who have severely depressed T-cell immunity. Acrodermatitis enteropathica has also been confused with chronic GVHD [64]. Since patients with chronic GVHD usually have diarrhea and malabsorption, secondary zinc deficiency is a frequent complication. Although the administration of zinc may provide transient improvement in GVHD, the severe immunodeficiency remains.

Laboratory studies of patients with GVHD are variable. Eosinophilia usually appears at the same time as skin rash. Lymphopenia, chronic anemia, hemolytic anemia, hypogammaglobulinemia, T-cell deficiency, elevated liver enzymes, abnormal urine sediment, and abnormal chest x-rays may be present individually or simultaneously.

Biopsy of skin lesions of patients with GVHD is most useful in the chronic phase. During the early phase, the histologic appearance is often nonspecific. The histologic features of chronic GVHD are felt to be diagnostic and include liquefaction or hydropic degeneration of the epidermal basal layer with focal discrete coagulation necrosis [64]. Intercellular edema is evident. In the dermis there is perivascular lymphoid infiltration of the upper dermis or submucosa. Edema of the dermal papillae is found. More specific abnormalities include (1) prominent coagulation necrosis of cells of the basal and malpighian layers and melanocytes, (2) single groups of acantholytic necrotic epithelial cells, (3) focal liquefaction degeneration of basal epithelial cells, (4) extensive intracellular edema, and (5) occasional interepithelial bullae. Dermal findings include diffuse or focal subepithelial infiltrates with lymphocytes, macrophages, and eosinophils. In the upper dermis there are "mummified" cells. Free or phagocytized melanin pigment may be seen in the epidermis.

There is no curative treatment for GVHD other than eradication of the GVHD by intensive immunosuppression and transplantation with histocompatible bone marrow. When GVHD occurs after a histocompatible bone marrow

transplant, it is usually mild and does not require specific treatment. Severe or chronic forms have been treated with immunosuppression, but caution must be used as immunosuppression without immunologic reconstitution provides only temporary improvement in clinical and laboratory features, while producing additional immunodeficiency. A variety of immunosuppressive agents has been utilized, including high-dose steroids, cyclophosphamide, antithymocyte globulin, methotrexate, and cyclosporin A [65–67].

Because GVHD is difficult to treat once it is established, it is essential to prevent the disease. If a patient is receiving immunologically competent cells for purposes of immunologic reconstitution, careful histocompatibility typing must be performed. If histoincompatible bone marrow transplantation is utilized, newer procedures using lectin-separated cells or monoclonal-treated bone marrow are required. When patients who are known to have immunodeficiency, either as a primary cause or secondary to immunosuppression, receive blood products, blood should be irradiated with 3000 R. This dose of radiation will destroy viable lymphocytes without interfering with red cell

Fig. 209-13 Chronic graft-versus-host disease interfering with growth of the toenails. Secondary fungal infection may also be present.

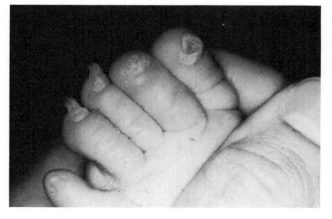

or platelet function. Patients who should receive irradiated blood products include those with primary immunodeficiency disease, acquired immunodeficiency disease, infants receiving intrauterine transfusions, premature infants, patients on large doses of immunosuppressant agent, and patients with severe lymphopenia secondary to malignancy, immunosuppression, or viral infection.

Acquired immunodeficiency syndrome (AIDS)

AIDS was recognized in early 1979 and by 1984 there were over 3000 new cases reported to the Centers for Disease Control [68,69]. AIDS has been defined as "T-cell immunodeficiency in a previously healthy adult in association with opportunistic infection or Kaposi's sarcoma." It is now apparent that this initial description was too restrictive and that many AIDS-related disorders exist, e.g., additional forms of malignancy and the lymphadenopathy syndrome [70,71]. The major clinical forms of AIDS include opportunistic infection, Kaposi's sarcoma, other malignancies, and a lymphadenopathy syndrome. It is important to emphasize that these categories are not mutually inclusive or exclusive.

The etiologic agent in AIDS has not been identified with certainty, although a retrovirus is the prime candidate. Recently, a retrovirus termed HTLV-III (human T-cell leukemia virus), a retrovirus termed LAV (lymphadenopathy-associated virus), and a retrovirus termed ARV (AIDS-related retrovirus) have been isolated from the peripheral blood and tissue of patients, and antibodies to these retroviruses have been identified in the serum of patients with AIDS and associated risk factors [72–74]. It is probable that all three retroviruses are identical. Retrovirus is considered to be the most likely cause of AIDS, since the virus is known to infect T cells and is highly associated with AIDS and related disorders. However, it is not clear whether an AIDS retrovirus by itself is capable of producing the severe immunodeficiency that is seen in AIDS.

Epidemiologic studies have defined specific risk factors associated with AIDS, including homosexuality, intravenous drug abuse, hemophilia with administration of factor VIII concentrate, multiple blood transfusions in a susceptible host, and individuals of Haitian origin [75–79]. In the homosexual group, individuals with multiple sexual partners and those who are passive partners in rectal intercourse appear to be at greatest risk. Blood transfusion-related AIDS is associated with multiple transfusions and the identification of donors with AIDS or risk factors associated with AIDS.

AIDS has not been confined to the adult population. Over 120 infants have been described who have clinical, laboratory, and epidemiologic features similar to those of AIDS in adults [80]. Most patients with pediatric AIDS are born to mothers who are intravenous drug abusers. This suggests vertical transmission of an infectious agent. Infants with AIDS have also been described who have developed immunodeficiency following multiple blood transfusions where a donor with AIDS or a specific AIDS risk factor has been identified. Other pediatric patients have been born to mothers of Haitian origin.

Patients with AIDS have a history of multiple opportunistic infections or Kaposi's sarcoma [81–85]. However, clinical symptoms may vary among groups who have dif-

fering risk factors. A history of hepatitis is frequently obtained in patients who are intravenous drug abusers and/or homosexual partners. Chronic diarrhea may be due to a variety of organisms including *Giardia, Entamoeba histolytica,* or *Cryptosporidium.* Homosexual patients have a high incidence of syphilis, gonorrhea, and enteritis secondary to organisms associated with chronic diarrhea. Viral agents are a frequent cause of both acute and chronic infection and include herpes simplex, herpes zoster, cytomegalovirus, adenovirus, and Epstein-Barr virus. Central nervous system manifestations may be present and are usually secondary to encephalitis or meningitis as a consequence of viral infection, cryptococcosis, or disseminated toxoplasmosis. Leukodystrophy has been reported. Acute or chronic dyspnea may be a result of several infectious agents, but *Pneumocystis carinii* is the most common organism identified. Patients with the lymphadenopathy syndrome develop fluctuating lymphadenopathy, splenomegaly, fevers, weight loss, and chronic diarrhea. Lymph node biopsies may show malignant cells, but the usual histologic pattern is that of reactive hyperplasia.

Dermatologic manifestations of AIDS are secondary to the severe T-cell immunodeficiency and, in most instances, can be related to the presence of opportunistic infection. Chronic candidal infection of the mucous membranes may be present and can result in erosive esophagitis. Infection with herpes simplex and herpes zoster results in characteristic skin manifestations which are of a severe and chronic nature. Viral infections may be present on mucous membranes, periorally or perianally. The typical lesions of Kaposi's sarcoma may be observed on the extremities (Fig. 209-14), but may appear anywhere on the skin (Fig. 209-15) or mucous membranes. The lesions are dark blue (Fig. 209-16) or purple-brown plaques or nodules. Biopsy of these lesions demonstrates characteristic histologic features including atypical spindle cells, capillary-like spaces, and erythrocytes (see Chap. 96). Patients may also have squamous cell carcinoma of the oral cavity and cloacogenic carcinoma of the rectum. Patients with *Pneumocystis carinii* pneumonia who are treated with trimethoprim-sulfamethoxazole have a high incidence of systemic reactions

Fig. 209-14 Lesions of AIDS: tiny purplish-brown plaques appearing on the dorsum of the left foot.

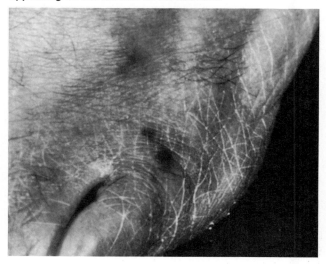

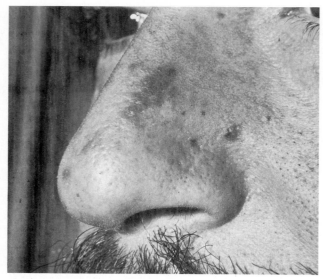

Fig. 209-15 Lesions of AIDS: purple-brown plaques on the nose.

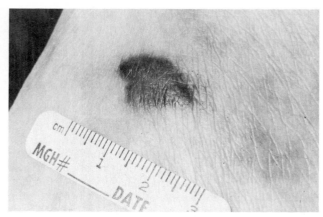

Fig. 209-16 Lesions of AIDS: dark blue plaque which may simulate nodular melanoma or blue nevus.

to the drug (over 40 percent in some series) [86]. The reaction is associated with fever, a diffuse macular and papular skin eruption, thrombocytopenia, leukopenia, and anemia.

A diagnosis of AIDS is established utilizing epidemiologic, clinical, and laboratory observations. A documentation of immunodeficiency is essential to confirming a diagnosis of AIDS. Lymphopenia is marked (<600/μL) and is associated with a reduction in the percentage of total T cells (<30 percent; normal, >60 percent). The helper/suppressor T-cell ratio is usually <0.5 (normal, >1.5). Functional studies of T-cell immunity are abnormal, including stimulation of peripheral lymphocytes with mitogen and antigen. Patients have reduced to absent delayed-hypersensitivity skin test responses. Immunoglobulin levels are usually elevated, but most patients fail to form adequate antibody following immunization [87–89]. Natural killer cell activity and lymphocyte cytotoxicity against virally infected cells is reduced [90]. Complement levels are normal or increased and most patients have circulating immune complexes. Lymphokine production is reduced.

The most severe immunologic abnormalities are observed in patients with AIDS. Patients with lymphadenopathy syndrome or individuals with risk factors associated with AIDS have less significant abnormalities. It is important to emphasize that a reduced helper/suppressor cell ratio, or evidence of immunodeficiency, without additional clinical and epidemiologic evidence of AIDS, does not establish a diagnosis. Many common viral infections and most immunosuppressive drugs will result in similar transient immunologic abnormalities in otherwise healthy individuals [91–94].

Currently, there is no treatment for combating the immunodeficiency of AIDS. Aggressive diagnostic measures are recommended in an attempt to identify microbial agents which can be treated with specific therapy. Mycobacterial infection usually requires treatment with multiple agents but is generally ineffective. *Pneumocystis carinii* infection does not respond readily to treatment with pentamidine or trimethoprim-sulfamethoxazole. Antiviral agents such as acylovir may be successful in the treatment of herpes zos-

ter and herpes simplex. Amphotericin B is usually required for the treatment of local and systemic *Candida* infection. No specific treatment is available for cytomegalovirus, Epstein-Barr virus, *Cryptosporidium*, or retrovirus. Treatment of malignancy in patients with AIDS has not been successful. Immunosuppressive therapy results in additional immunodeficiency and susceptibility to infection. Attempts at immunologic reconstitution have not been successful, although some encouraging results have been obtained in early experimental studies.

Phagocytic abnormalities

A number of specific phagocytic disorders have been defined. They may be divided into those diseases which have an intrinsic or extrinsic abnormality. Extrinsic defects include deficiencies of substances which are necessary for normal opsonization and ingestion of microbial agents. The most widely recognized extrinsic deficiencies are a result of deficiency of antibody or complement factors. Patients with hypogammaglobulinemia are unable to opsonize and phagocytize microbial agents. This defect can be corrected by the passive administration of gamma globulin. Patients with complement deficiencies are unable to activate the complement pathway, a necessary step in amplifying the effect of antibody and phagocytosis. Extrinsic abnormalities may also include the presence of autoantibody directed against neutrophils. These antibodies may be found in such autoimmune diseases as systemic lupus erythematosus or may occur spontaneously, unassociated with a defined autoimmune disease. Passive transfer of antibody directed against neutrophils may occur during the newborn period and result in significant neutropenia with susceptibility to infection.

Intrinsic defects, which result in abnormal phagocytosis, include several enzymatic abnormalities such as the inability to generate hydrogen peroxide and superoxide as found in chronic granulomatous disease or a complete absence of leukocyte glucose 6-phosphate dehydrogenase or myeloperoxidase deficiency [95–98]. Several phagocytic disorders do not have clearly defined biochemical abnormalities. These include the Chédiak-Higashi syndrome and the hyperimmunoglobulin E-recurrent infection syndrome [99,100].

All phagocytic disorders have, as a characteristic, sus-

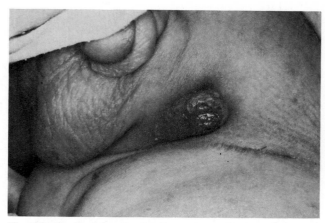

Fig. 209-17 Draining inguinal lymph node in a young infant with chronic granulomatous disease. The early appearance of this lesion and repeated isolation of *Staphylococcus epidermidis* resulted in an early diagnosis.

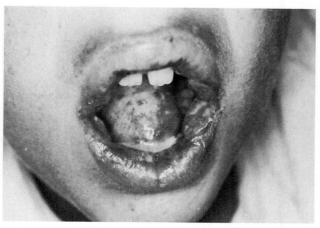

Fig. 209-18 Recurrent aphthous ulcers in a patient with chronic granulomatous disease.

ceptibility to infection with bacterial organisms. In some patients the infections remain confined to the skin, but in most instances systemic infection with abscess formation is found. Acute and chronic infection may occur within the first several months of life, as in chronic granulomatous disease, or symptoms may be delayed until adult life, as in myeloperoxidase deficiency. Specific diagnostic tests are available which assist in differentiating among the various phagocytic disorders as well as complement deficiency states [100].

Chronic granulomatous disease

Chronic granulomatous disease is inherited as an X-linked or autosomal disorder with onset of symptoms in the first two years of life. The most frequent clinical abnormalities consist of lymphadenopathy, hepatosplenomegaly, chronic draining lymph nodes (Fig. 209-17), pneumonia, chronic rhinitis, osteomyelitis, and chronic diarrhea. A major clue to diagnosis is the isolation of a normally nonpathogenic or unusual organism. Organisms that have been isolated from patients with chronic granulomatous disease include *S. aureus, S. epidermidis, S. marcescens, Pseudomonas, Candida,* and *Aspergillus.*

A number of dermatologic manifestations are associated with chronic granulomatous disease. Patients frequently have an ulcerative stomatitis; the etiology is unknown, but it is similar in appearance to aphthous ulceration (Fig. 209-18). Chronic conjunctivitis may also be present. Chronic or acute infection of the skin in the form of multiple small abscesses may be found. Culture of these abscesses reveals normally nonpathogenic or unusual organisms and may provide an important clue to early diagnosis. Female carriers of chronic granulomatous disease have a high incidence of discoid or systemic lupus erythematosus. The carrier state, although not predisposing to infection, apparently does predispose to autoimmune disease. In contrast to carriers, only a few patients with chronic granulomatous disease have developed systemic lupus erythematosus.

A diagnosis of chronic granulomatous disease is best established utilizing either the nitroblue tetrazolium dye test or quantitative intracellular killing of an organism iso-

lated from the patient. The reduction of nitroblue tetrazolium dye is dependent on the generation of hydrogen peroxide and superoxide and does not occur in its absence. Patients with chronic granulomatous disease are unable to kill certain bacteria normally in vitro [101]. Both of the above tests may also be used to diagnose the carrier state. More recently, the nitroblue tetrazolium dye test and quantitative intracellular killing assays have been replaced with measurements of chemiluminescence (the amount of light generated by a phagocytizing cell).

Chronic granulomatous disease was originally termed fatal granulomatous disease because of the poor response to treatment. Recently, however, aggressive diagnostic measures, coupled with immediate treatment, have improved the survival of patients significantly. Drainage of an abscess, open lung biopsy, liver biopsy, and aspiration of the site of infection in osteomyelitis are all procedures that are indicated in patients with chronic granulomatous disease when a specific site of infection is identified. The prompt institution of broad-spectrum antibiotic therapy is necessary until a specific organism is isolated and appropriate bacterial sensitivities are known.

Chédiak-Higashi syndrome

The Chédiak-Higashi syndrome is a multisystem autosomal recessive disorder with symptoms of recurrent bacterial infections, hepatosplenomegaly, central nervous system abnormalities, and an increased incidence of malignancies [102]. A diagnosis of this disorder is easily established by examination of the peripheral blood and observation of giant cytoplasmic granular inclusions in leukocytes and platelets. These abnormalities are observed on routine peripheral blood smears. Immunologic abnormalities include abnormal neutrophil chemotaxis, delayed intracellular killing of certain bacteria, and depressed natural killer cell activity.

A single dermatologic manifestation, partial albinism, is present in these patients. This may be an initial clue to the diagnosis of this syndrome as patients initially appear normal, but subsequently progress and develop recurrent infection, central nervous system deterioration and, eventually, malignancy.

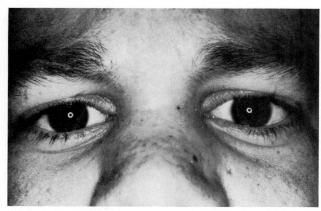

Fig. 209-19 Thickened skin, coarse facial features, and small "cold" abscesses in a patient with the hyperimmunoglobulin IgE-recurrent infection syndrome.

Hyperimmunoglobulin E-recurrent infection syndrome

In 1966, a disorder termed *Job's syndrome* was described [103]. The patients were fair-skinned, red-headed girls with recurrent "cold" staphylococcal abscesses of the lymph nodes, subcutaneous tissue, and skin. As additional cases were reported, it was apparent that systemic infection occurred involving the lungs, abdominal cavity, or liver. Subsequently, similar clinical features were described in a disorder termed the *hyperimmunoglobulin E-recurrent infection syndrome* [101,104]. It is currently felt that Job's syndrome and the hyperimmunoglobulin E-recurrent infection syndrome are identical.

Clinical features include eczematoid skin lesions, coarse facial features (Fig. 209-19), chronic nasal discharge, otitis media, and a history of repeated surgical procedures. A characteristic feature of the disease is the presence of large abscesses with large amounts of purulent material but paucity of local inflammatory reactions. Fever and leukocytosis may be present with the development of infected, swollen lymph nodes. In early studies *Staphylococcus aureus* was the primary organism cultured from lesions. Recently, however, additional organisms have been identified including *Streptococcus pneumoniae,* Group A streptococci, *Hemophilus influenzae,* and *Candida* [102]. Prolonged antibiotic therapy is necessary to control the recurrent and/or chronic infections that result from these organisms.

As more investigators agreed on the diagnostic criteria for the hyperimmunoglobulin E-recurrent infection syndrome, additional clinical and laboratory features were described. Both males and females may be affected. Immunoglobulin E levels are usually >1000 IU. Abnormal neutrophil chemotaxis is present and neutrophils from patients produce a serum factor which is capable of inhibiting the neutrophil chemotaxis of normal individuals [104]. Patients may have decreased percentages and function of suppressor T cells and elevated levels of IgE antibody against staphylococcal antigens [105].

Although early recognition of this disorder and an aggressive approach to antibiotic therapy have resulted in clinical improvement, patients continue to have a high degree of morbidity and a guarded prognosis. Antibiotic therapy should be directed toward specific agents isolated from the patient. There is no specific therapy available to reverse the immunologic abnormalities that have been described.

Complement abnormalities and immunodeficiency

Of the nine major complement components, a deficiency of each has been described. Specific diseases are associated with deficiencies of C1 to C8 [106]. C9 deficiency has not been associated with a disease state.

Complement is a necessary component for amplification of B-cell immunity, as well as phagocytosis. Activation of early complement components is a result of antibody–antigen reaction. The alternative complement pathway may be activated by a number of factors other than antibody. The best diagnostic test to determine whether complement deficiency exists is a measurement of total hemolytic complement levels. In this assay, antibody directed against red cells is utilized in conjunction with a fresh serum sample from a patient. The amount of hemolysis that the serum sample supports is a measurement of complement activity in the sample. If a component of complement is absent, abnormal hemolytic complement activity will be observed. The hemolytic complement assay is used to screen for a deficiency of any of the major components in the complement pathway, although this method does not define the specific complement component that may be deficient.

Deficiencies in or absence of early complement components, C1q, C1r, C1s, and C4, are usually associated with autoimmune diseases such as systemic lupus erythematosus, dermatomyositis, and anaphylactoid purpura. The dermatologic lesions in these diseases are identical to those of the disease unassociated with congenital complement deficiency. It is postulated that the role of complement is to prolong the clearance of immune complexes and, in the absence of complement, immune complexes are immediately deposited into tissue—hence, the susceptibility to autoimmune disease in congenital complement deficiency. Deficiencies of the later complement components C3 and C5 to C8 are associated with susceptibility to infection rather than autoimmune disease, although there are some exceptions. Deficiency of C3 results in susceptibility to generalized bacterial infection, while deficiency of C5 to C8 may predispose to infection with such organisms as *Streptococcus pneumoniae, H. influenzae* or *Neiserria.* A complement deficiency should be suspected in any patient who has recurrent infection with these organisms. A form of C3 deficiency has been reported to be associated with partial lypodystrophy.

There is no specific treatment for complement deficiency. Prophylactic antibiotics should be utilized in those patients who have susceptibility to specific bacterial organisms. Fresh-frozen plasma may provide a source of complement but it also provides a substrate which can be consumed and underlying autoimmune disease may worsen.

References

1. Centers for Disease Control: Kaposi's sarcoma and *Pneumocystis* pneumonia among homosexual men—New York City and California. *MMWR* **30:**305, 1981

2. Bruton OC: Agammaglobulinemia. *Pediatrics* **9**:722, 1952

3. Paul WE: Lymphocyte biology, in *Clinical Immunology,* edited by CW Parker. Philadelphia, WB Saunders, 1980, p 19

4. Cooper MD, Lawton AR: Circulating B cells in patients with immunodeficiency. *Am J Pathol* **69**:513, 1972

5. Warner NL: Membrane immunoglobulins and antigen receptors on B and T lymphocytes. *Adv Immunol* **19**:67, 1974

6. Vitetta ES, Uhr JW: IgD and B cell differentiation. *Immunol Rev* **37**:50, 1977

7. McWilliams M et al: Mesenteric lymph node B lymphoblasts which home to the small intestine are precommitted to IgA synthesis. *J Exp Med* **145**:866, 1977

8. Tomasi TB, Binenstock J: Secretory immunoglobulins. *Adv Immunol* **9**:1, 1968

9. Eichmann K: Expression and function of idiotypes on lymphocytes. *Adv Immunol* **26**:195, 1978

10. Stiehm ER: Immunoglobulins and antibodies, in *Immunologic Disorders in Infants and Children,* edited by ER Stiehm, V Fulginiti. Philadelphia, WB Saunders, 1973, p 42

11. Ammann AJ, Hong R: Cellular immunodeficiency, in *Immunologic Disorders in Infants and Children,* edited by ER Stiehm, V Fulginiti. Philadelphia, WB Saunders, 1973, p 236

12. Ammann AJ: Immunodeficiency diseases, in *Basic and Clinical Immunology,* edited by DP Stites et al. Palo Alto, Lange, 1985, p 384

13. Douglas SD et al: Clinical, serologic and leukocyte function studies on patients with idiopathic "acquired" agammaglobulinemia and their families. *Am J Med* **48**:48, 1970

14. Rosen FS, Janeway CA: The gamma globulins. III. The antibody deficiency syndromes. *N Engl J Med* **275**:709, 1966

15. Dickler HB et al: Lymphocytes in patients with variable immunodeficiency and panhypogammaglobulinemia. *J Clin Invest* **53**:834, 1974

16. Dosch H-M et al: Functional differentiation of B lymphocytes in congenital agammaglobulinemia. I. Generation of hemolytic plaque-forming cells. *J Immunol* **119**:1959, 1977

17. Ammann AJ et al: Use of intravenous γ-globulin in antibody immunodeficiency: results of a multicenter controlled trial. *Clin Immunol Immunopathol* **22**:60, 1982

18. Hansen LA: Aspects of the absence of the IgA system, in *Immunologic Diseases in Man,* edited by D Bergsma, RA Good. Baltimore, Williams & Wilkins, 1968, p 292

19. Ammann AJ, Hong R: Selective IgA deficiency and autoimmunity. *Clin Exp Immunol* **7**:833, 1970

20. Bachmann R: Studies on the serum γ-A-globulin level. III. The frequency of a γ-A-globulinemia. *Scand J Clin Lab Invest* **17**:316, 1965

21. Rockey JH et al: Beta-2A aglobulinemia in two healthy men. *J Lab Clin Med* **63**:205, 1964

22. Goldberg LS et al: Selective absence of IgA: a family study. *J Lab Clin Med* **72**:204, 1968

23. Cowan MJ et al: Cellular immune defect in selective IgA deficiency using a microculture method for PHA stimulation and limiting dilution. *Clin Immunol Immunopathol* **17**:595, 1980

24. Hong R, Ammann AJ: Selective absence of IgA. *Am J Pathol* **69**:491, 1972

25. Reinherz EL et al: Separation of functional subsets of human T cells by a monoclonal antibody. *Proc Natl Acad Sci USA* **76**:4061, 1979

26. Germain RN et al: Role of I-region gene products in T cell activation. I. Stimulation of T lymphocyte proliferative responses by subcellular membrane preparations containing Ia alloantigens. *J Immunol* **128**:506, 1982

27. Wagner H et al: The in vivo effects of interleukin 2 (TCGF). *Immunobiology* **161**:139, 1982

28. Gordon J, Minks MA: The interferon renaissance: molecular aspects of induction and action. *Microbiol Rev* **45**:244, 1981

29. Hermans PE et al: Chronic mucocutaneous candidiasis as a surface expression of deep seated abnormalities: report of a syndrome of superficial candidiasis, absence of delayed hypersensitivity and aminoaciduria. *Am J Med* **47**:503, 1969

30. Kirkpatrick CH et al: Chronic mucocutaneous candidiasis: model-building in cellular immunity. *Ann Intern Med* **74**:955, 1971

31. Blizzard RM, Gibbs JH: Candidiasis: studies pertaining to its association with endocrinopathies and pernicious anemia. *Pediatrics* **42**:231, 1968

32. Kirkpatrick CH et al: Effect of transfer factor on lymphocyte function in anergic patients. *J Clin Invest* **51**:733, 1971

33. Wolf B et al: Multiple carboxylase deficiency: clinical and biochemical improvement following neonatal biotin treatment. *Pediatrics* **68**:113, 1981

34. Thoene J et al: Biotin-responsive carboxylase deficiency associated with subnormal plasma and urinary biotin. *N Engl J Med* **304**:817, 1981

35. Sweetman L et al: Clinical and metabolic abnormalities in a boy with dietary deficiency of biotin. *Pediatrics* **68**:553, 1981

36. Cowan MJ et al: Multiple biotin-dependent carboxylase deficiencies associated with defects in T-cell and B-cell immunity. *Lancet* **2**:115, 1979

37. Hirschhorn R: Defects of purine metabolism in immunodeficiency diseases. *Prog Clin Immunol* **3**:67, 1977

38. Gitlin D, Craig JM: The thymus and other lymphoid tissues in congenital agammaglobulinemia. I. Thymic alymphoplasia and lymphocytic hypoplasia and their relation to infection. *Pediatrics* **32**:517, 1963

39. Cowan MJ, Ammann AJ: Immunodeficiency syndromes associated with inherited metabolic disorders. *Clin Haematol* **10**:139, 1981

40. Hale G et al: Removal of T cells from bone marrow for transplantation: a monoclonal antilymphocyte antibody that fixes human complement. *Blood* **62**:873, 1983

41. Reisner Y et al: Allogeneic bone marrow transplantation using stem cells fractionated by lectins: VI. In vitro analysis of human and monkey bone marrow cells fractionated by sheep red blood cells and soybean agglutinin. *Lancet* **2**:1320, 1980

42. Aldrich RA et al: Pedigree demonstrating a sex-linked recessive condition characterized by draining ears, eczematoid dermatitis and bloody diarrhea. *Pediatrics* **13**:133, 1954

43. Waldman TA et al: Immunodeficiency disease and malignancy. *Ann Intern Med* **77**:605, 1972

44. Krivit W, Good RA: Aldrich's syndrome (thrombocytopenia, eczema and infection in infants). *Am J Dis Child* **97**:137, 1959

45. Cooper MD et al: Wiskott-Aldrich syndrome: immunologic deficiency disease involving the afferent limb of immunity. *Am J Med* **44**:499, 1968

46. Bach FH et al: Bone-marrow transplantation in a patient with the Wiskott-Aldrich syndrome. *Lancet* **2**:1364, 1968

47. Boder E, Sedgwick RP: Ataxia-telangiectasia: a review of 101 cases, in *Cerebellum, Posture and Cerebral Palsy,* edited by G Walsh. London, The National Spastics Society and Heinemann Medical Books, Ltd, 1963, p 110

48. Ammann AJ et al: Immunoglobulin E deficiency in ataxia-telangiectasia. *N Engl J Med* **281**:469, 1969

49. Peterson RDA et al: Ataxia-telangiectasia: its association with defective thymus, immunological deficiency disease and malignancy. *Lancet* **1**:1189, 1964

50. Barfknecht TR, Little JB: Hypersensitivity of ataxia telangiectasia skin fibroblasts to DNA alkylating agents. *Mutat Res* **94**:369, 1982

51. Waldman TA, McIntire KR: Serum alpha fetoprotein levels in patients with ataxia-telangiectasia. *Lancet* **2**:1112, 1972

52. Epstein WL et al: Dermatologic aspects of ataxia telangiectasia. *Cutis* **4**:1324, 1968

53. Reed WB et al: Cutaneous manifestations of ataxia-telangiectasia. *JAMA* **195**:746, 1966

54. McKusick VA et al: Dwarfism in the Amish. II. Cartilage-hair hypoplasia. *Bull Johns Hopkins Hosp* **116**:285, 1964

55. Lux SE et al: Chronic neutropenia and abnormal cellular

immunity in cartilage-hair hypoplasia. *N Engl J Med* **282**:234, 1970

56. Murphy JB: The effect of adult chicken organ graft on the chick embryo. *J Exp Med* **24**:1, 1916

57. Mathe G et al: Nouveaux essais de greffe de moelle osseuse homologue après irradiation totale chez des enfants atteints de leucémie aiguë en remission. Le problème du syndrome secondaire chez l'homme. *Rev Hematol* **15**:115, 1960

58. Parkman R et al: Graft-versus-host disease after intrauterine and exchange transfusions for hemolytic disease of the newborn. *N Engl J Med* **290**:359, 1974

59. Copenhagen Study Group of Immunodeficiencies: Circumvention of early graft versus host disease in hemiallogeneic bone marrow transplantation in a case of severe combined immunodeficiency. *Scand J Immunol* **2**:551, 1973

60. Lerner KG et al: Histopathology of graft-vs-host reaction (GvHR) in human recipients of marrow from HL-A-matched sibling donors. *Transplant Proc* **6**:367, 1974

61. Wara DW et al: Graft vs host disease: pathogenesis, recognition, prevention and treatment. *Curr Probl Pediatr* **8**:1, 1978

62. Hathaway WE et al: Aplastic anemia, histiocytosis and erythrodermia in immunologically deficient children. Probable human runt disease. *N Engl J Med* **273**:953, 1965

63. Peck GL et al: Toxic epidermal necrolysis in a patient with graft-vs-host reaction. *Arch Dermatol* **105**:561, 1972

64. Slavin RE, Santos GW: The graft versus host reaction in man after bone marrow transplantation: pathology, pathogenesis, clinical features and implication. *Clin Immunol Immunopathol* **1**:472, 1973

65. Thomas ED et al: Bone-marrow transplantation (first of two parts). *N Engl J Med* **292**:832, 1975

66. Thomas ED et al: Bone-marrow transplantation (second of two parts). *N Engl J Med* **292**:895, 1975

67. Storb R et al: Treatment of established human graft-versus-host disease by antithymocyte globulin. *Blood* **44**:57, 1974

68. Gottlieb MS et al: The acquired immune deficiency syndrome. *Ann Intern Med* **99**:208, 1983

69. Friedman-Kien AE: Epidemic Kaposi's sarcoma: a manifestation of the acquired immune deficiency syndrome. *J Dermatol Surg Oncol* **9**:637, 1983

70. Fauci AS et al: Acquired immunodeficiency syndrome: epidemiologic, clinical, immunologic, and therapeutic considerations. *Ann Intern Med* **100**:92, 1984

71. Cochran AJ et al: Tumor infiltrates in acquired immunodeficiency syndrome patients with Kaposi's sarcoma. *Lancet* **1**:416, 1983

72. Gallo RC, Wong-Staal F: Origin of human T cell leukaemia-lymphoma virus. *Lancet* **2**:962, 1983

73. Gallo RC et al: Isolation of human T cell leukemia virus in acquired immune deficiency syndrome (AIDS). *Science* **220**:865, 1983

74. Kalyanaraman VS et al: Antibodies to the core protein of lymphadenopathy-associated virus (LAV) in patients with AIDS. *Science* **225**:321, 1984

75. Weintrub PS et al: Immunologic abnormalities in patients with hemophilia A. *J Pediatr* **103**:692, 1983

76. Deresinski SC et al: AIDS transmission via transfusion therapy. *Lancet* **1**:102, 1984

77. Rubinstein A: Acquired immunodeficiency syndrome in infants. *Am J Dis Child* **137**:825, 1983

78. Jaffe HW et al: Acquired immune deficiency syndrome in the United States: the first 1,000 cases. *J Infect Dis* **148**:339, 1983

79. Jaffe HW et al: National case-control study of Kaposi's. *Ann Intern Med* **99**:145, 1983

80. Ammann AJ: Is there an acquired immune deficiency syndrome in infants and children? *J Pediatr* **72**:430, 1983

81. Anderson KP et al: Central nervous system toxoplasmosis in homosexual men. *Am J Med* **75**:877, 1983

82. Giron JA et al: Mycobacterial culture in acquired immunodeficiency syndrome. *Ann Intern Med* **98**:1028, 1983

83. Hawley DA et al: Cytomegalovirus encephalitis in acquired immunodeficiency syndrome. *Am J Clin Pathol* **80**:874, 1983

84. Honig C, Soave R: Cryptosporidium in acquired immunodeficiency syndrome. *Lab Invest* **48**:36A, 1983

85. Kochen MM et al: Pentamidine or co-trimoxazole for *Pneumocystis carinii* pneumonia. *Lancet* **2**:1300, 1983

86. Jaffe HS et al: Complications of co-trimoxazole in treatment of AIDS-associated *Pneumocystis carinii* pneumonia in homosexual men. *Lancet* **2**:1109, 1983

87. Ammann AJ et al: B-cell immunodeficiency in acquired immune deficiency syndrome. *JAMA* **251**:1447, 1984

88. Lane HC et al: Abnormalities of B cell activation and immunoregulation in patients with the acquired immunodeficiency syndrome. *N Engl J Med* **309**:453, 1983

89. Lane HC et al: Abnormalities of peripheral blood B cell function in the acquired immune deficiency syndrome. *Clin Res* **31**:492A, 1984

90. Rook AH et al: Interleukin-2 enhances the depressed natural killer and cytomegalovirus-specific cytotoxic activities of lymphocytes from patients with the acquired immune deficiency syndrome. *J Clin Invest* **72**:398, 1983

91. Hoffman SL et al: Reduction of suppressor T lymphocytes in the tropical splenomegaly syndrome. *N Engl J Med* **310**:337, 1984

92. Moxley JH, Roeder PC: Abnormal T-lymphocyte subpopulations in healthy subjects after tetanus booster immunization (letter). *N Engl J Med* **310**:198, 1984

93. Van Wauwe J, Goossens J: Monoclonal anti-human T-lymphocyte antibodies: enumeration and characterization of T-cell subsets. *Immunology* **42**:157, 1981

94. Nowinski RC et al: Monoclonal antibodies for diagnosis of infectious diseases in humans. *Science* **219**:637, 1983

95. Holmes B et al: Studies of the metabolic activity of leukocytes from patients with a genetic abnormality of phagocytic function. *J Clin Invest* **46**:1422, 1967

96. Baehner RL et al: Comparative study of the metabolic and bacteriocidal characteristics of severely glucose-6-phosphate dehydrogenase deficient polymorphonuclear leukocytes and leukocytes from children with chronic granulomatous disease. *J Reticuloendothel Soc* **12**:150, 1972

97. Lehrer RI, Cline MJ: Leukocyte myeloperoxidase deficiency and disseminated candidiasis: the role of myeloperoxidase in resistance to Candida infection. *J Clin Invest* **48**:1478, 1969

98. Boxer LA et al: Correction of leukocyte function in Chédiak-Higashi syndrome by ascorbate. *N Engl J Med* **295**:1041, 1970

99. Oliver JM: Impaired microtubule function correctable by cyclic GMP and cholinergic agonists in the Chédiak-Higashi syndrome. *Am J Pathol* **85**:395, 1976

100. Cline MJ, Territo MC: Phagocytosis, in *Clinical Immunology,* edited by CW Parker. Philadelphia, WB Saunders, 1980, p 298

101. Hill HR: The syndrome of hyperimmunoglobulinemia E and recurrent infections. *Am J Dis Child* **136**:767, 1982

102. Donabedian H, Gallin JL: Mononuclear cells from patients with the hyperimmunoglobulin E-recurrent infection syndrome produce an inhibitor of leukocyte chemotaxis. *J Clin Invest* **69**:1155, 1982

103. Davis SD et al: Job's syndrome: recurrent, "cold," staphylococcal abscesses. *Lancet* **1**:1013, 1966

104. Donabedian H, Gallin JL: The hyperimmunoglobulin E recurrent-infection (Job's) syndrome. *Medicine (Baltimore)* **62**:195, 1983

105. Geha RS et al: Deficiency of suppressor T cells in the hyperimmunoglobulin E syndrome. *J Clin Invest* **68**:783, 1981

106. Cooper NR: The complement system, in *Basic and Clinical Immunology,* edited by DP Stites, JD Stobo. Palo Alto, Lange, 1985, p 119

PART SIX

THERAPEUTICS

Section 32

Topical modalities

CHAPTER 210

PHARMACOKINETICS AND TOPICAL APPLICATIONS OF DRUGS

Wolfgang Schalla and Hans Schaefer

In this chapter we will emphasize some practical aspects of pharmacokinetics after topical application. For more detailed information the reader is referred to review articles and specialized books [1–13].

A pharmacologic effect upon an organism (or part of it) is caused by two simultaneous actions:

1. Effects of the drug upon the body, i.e., causing respective changes in the body (pharmacodynamics)
2. Effects of the body upon the drug, i.e., inducing changes to the drug on the body surface and in the body (pharmacokinetics)

Therapeutic regimen should be based on the data from either of these analytical approaches, but only the latter is within the scope of this chapter.

Topical versus systemic therapy of skin diseases

In dermatology, one has a choice of treating by systemic (oral, intravenous, intramuscular, subcutaneous) or local (topical or epicutaneous, and intradermal) administration. The difference between topical and systemic therapy is illustrated in Fig. 210-1, using a simple pharmacokinetic model. After topical application, the drug first enters the skin as the target organ, then becomes distributed (diluted) in the whole body, and is finally eliminated. After systemic administration, the drug is at first diluted by distribution in the whole body, i.e., only a portion of the drug will reach the target organ and act on the skin. The elimination in the latter instance is not a subsequent event following drug action in the skin; rather it takes place concomitantly, as does metabolization of the drug by the liver. In consequence, for the same drug level in the skin, the load on the whole body is much higher with a given drug after systemic administration. In other words, *drugs that are too toxic for systemic therapy can still be used for topical treatment,* particularly if they are applied to the restricted

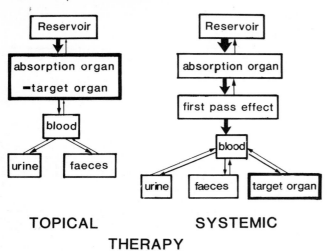

TOPICAL

SYSTEMIC

THERAPY

Fig. 210-1 Comparison of topical and systemic administration using simple pharmacokinetic models.

Table 210-1 Factors in dermatologic therapy that favor the topical and oral route

	Topical	Oral
Target site within the body	+*	+
Target site in the skin	+	
Target in deep skin layers	(+)	+
Small skin areas involved	+	
Large skin areas involved	+	+
High first-pass effect in liver	+	(+)
Hydrophilic drug		+
Lipophilic drug	+	+
Drugs with higher allergic potency		+

*Note: Only in the case of desired transdermal delivery; not for the common topical therapy in dermatology.

surface areas and if some other rules of pharmacokinetics for topical treatment are taken into account. Another conclusion is that the term *bioavailability* has to be redefined for topical therapy: bioavailability characterizes, by pharmacokinetic data, the rate and the extent to which one or more active ingredients from a preparation become available to the therapy target(s) and to the body. It is separated into *topical* bioavailability (at the target sites) and *systemic* bioavailability. The latter is usually measured in serum or in elimination compartments; reference must be made to the target of the former (intestinal lumen, lens of the eye, epidermis, and so on).

Looking at the concentration profile of a drug in the skin indicates that the concentration declines from the skin surface to the subcutis after topical application, whereas the opposite is true for systemic administration (Fig. 210-2). This relation favors the use of topical application if the pathologic process being treated resides in the epidermis or papillar dermis. For processes in the lower part of the dermis or subcutis one has to consider whether the drug concentrations necessary will be obtained by topical application (concentration gradient), and, even if so, whether the percutaneous absorption and thereby the drug load for the whole body does not exceed that obtained by systemic administration for the same effect in these deeper skin layers.

Table 210-1 summarizes the aspects determining the route of choice. Factors that influence the pharmacokinetics of a drug after topical application include the skin, the drug, and the treatment regimen (Table 210-2).

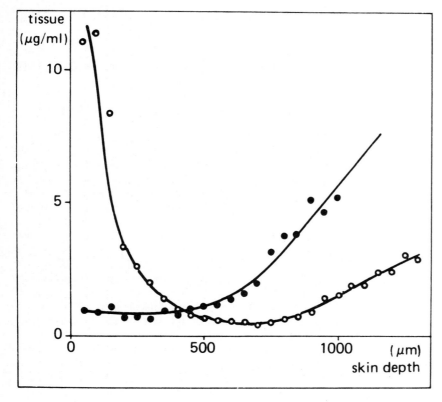

Fig. 210-2 Cyproterone acetate distribution in the skin of the rat after oral (●) and topical (o) administration of equal doses over 7 days. Oral dose: 7 × 0.4 mg/200 g rat. Topical dose: 7 × 0.4 mg/16 cm² skin. (From Träuber [14].)

Table 210-2   Factors influencing the pharmacokinetics of a drug after topical application

Pharmaceutical and pharmacologic factors:
   Chemical structure
   Concentration in the vehicle
   Quantity applied to a given surface area
   Liberation from the vehicle
   Interactions between vehicle or other drugs with that drug
    and the skin
   Binding
   Drug metabolism
Horny layer structure:
   Regional variations
   Hydration/occlusion
   Environmental factors (e.g., ultraviolet [UV] hyperkeratosis,
    solvents, bacterias)
   Age
   Modification by the vehicle
   Modification by other drugs (e.g., keratolytics)
   Disease (hyper-, para-, and orthokeratotic disorders)
Other skin factors:
   Surface area treated
   Density of hair follicles
   Density of sweat glands
   Skin blood flow (resorption, skin temperature)
   pH (e.g., intertriginous areas)
Treatment schedules:
   Frequency of application (if twice daily or less)
   Rhythm of application (regular vs. discontinuous, e.g., ap-
    plication for 4 days followed by a pause of 3 days (see
    [14a])
   Continuous vs. short contact therapy (see [15–18])

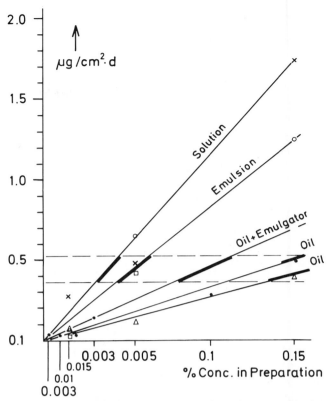

Fig. 210-3   Concentration of tritium-labeled 8-methoxypsoralen in the skin after 100-min penetration. Mean values for the total skin thickness, *d*, calculated from serial sections parallel to the skin surface. (From Schaefer et al [12].)

Properties of the skin for permeation

No evidence will indicate an active transport of drugs in the skin, i.e., the permeation of topically applied drugs can be characterized by passive diffusion processes.

If interest is focused on the risk of systemic toxicity with topical application, the skin can be regarded as a uniform membrane, and some constants that describe the diffusion of substances through the skin can be measured. In a simplified form, the steady-state flux through the whole skin (or epidermis or horny layer sheets) is often described by the following formula (for more details, see [13]):

$$J = \frac{K \cdot D \cdot \Delta C}{\delta} = Kp \cdot \Delta C$$

where

      J = flow of the diffusing drug, mol · cm^{-2} · s^{-1}
  K = partition coefficient between the membrane (horny layer)
        and the vehicle
     D = diffusion coefficient, cm^2 · s^{-1}
ΔC = concentration gradient between the two sides of the mem-
        brane, mol · cm^{-3}
     δ = thickness of the membrane, cm
  Kp = permeability coefficient, cm · s^{-1}

If, on the other hand, emphasis is on the optimization of treatment modalities for skin disorders, on skin pharmacology, or on skin toxicology, then the skin itself is the target and can no longer be regarded as a uniform membrane. Direct measurements of the time course of drug concentrations in the various skin compartments then pertain.

The film on the skin surface built up by sebum and sweat (0.04 to 0.24 mg/cm^2) does not seem of major importance for skin permeability after topical application. If more than 2 to 3 mg of a formulation is applied per square centimeter, the flux into the skin usually cannot be increased to a greater extent unless the vehicle exerts an occlusive effect. The vehicle, the physicochemical properties, and the concentration of the drug therein, on the other hand, influence to a great extent the permeation of the drug (Fig. 210-3) by influencing the flux directly or via the stratum corneum structure and the partitioning between vehicle and stratum corneum.

The stratum corneum is the most important barrier in which every single layer of horny cells diminishes the penetration to the same extent. A linear relation exists (using a log scale) for the amount found in successive strippings (Fig. 210-4). It was previously assumed that the drugs penetrate the stratum corneum transcellularly, i.e., they would have to pass multiple lipophilic (interstitial space and cell membranes) and hydrophilic (intracellular components) structures within the stratum corneum. Recently, it was shown that for lipophilic topical drugs the intercellular route could also be an important penetration pathway [19]. Thereby, lamellar bodies seem to play a major role in the formation of the permeability barrier. For hydrophilic substances, the stratum granulosum also inhibits the permeation. These barriers make the stratum corneum (and the granulosum) act as a reservoir from which

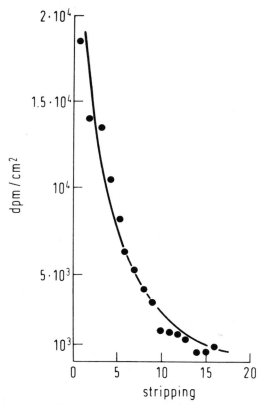 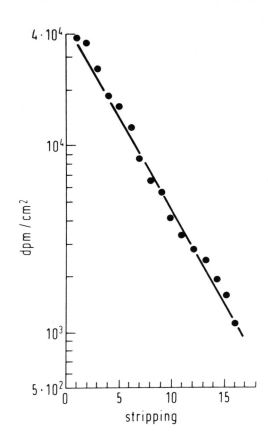

Fig. 210-4 Distribution of radioactivity in the horny layer (4-chlortestosterone acetate. Left: linear plot; right: log plot. (From Schaefer et al [12].)

the drug progressively penetrates into the viable skin layers over a longer time period (Fig. 210-5).

The viable epidermis and dermis add some resistance to free diffusion. But the importance of the barrier function of the viable layers of the skin for lipophilic drugs is not yet clear because no clear difference in skin permeability has been demonstrated between incomplete or complete removal of the stratum corneum and removal of the entire epidermis. Such measures cause an increase of the flux into the skin by a factor of 5 to 10 and more [20].

Besides specific binding to special skin structures, an accumulation of the lipophilic substances in the hair follicle/sebaceous gland unit and sometimes also in the subcutaneous fat is observed. But it is believed that the follicular pathway is not a major route of penetration because of the relatively small surface area involved compared to the interfollicular epidermis. However, for drugs that have a low flux the transfollicular route may play a role at the early stage of the penetration process.

The sweat glands are of no major importance for skin permeability of topical drugs, although they can excrete drugs which thereby can reach the skin surface and the horny layer [21].

According to the laws of diffusion a concentration gradient from the skin surface to the subcutis pertains which, under in vitro conditions, decreases with time. In vivo, however, most of the drug reaching the dermis is resorbed by blood (and lymph) vessels. Therefore, the gradient is constant after a certain time, and equilibrium is never obtained (Fig. 210-6).

Practical aspects of skin permeation

Regional and individual variations

Feldmann and Maibach [22] observed striking variations of skin permeability in respect to various regions of the body. Taking the percutaneous absorption of hydrocortisone on the forearm as 1, that on the soles was diminished by a factor of 7, whereas scrotal skin was 40 times as permeable as that of the forearm. For other drugs these ratios probably would be somewhat different according to their lipophilicity and hydrophilicity. The same authors also were able to demonstrate important individual variations in the same body region [23].

Age

Pharmacodynamic data, in particular from systemic intoxication and systemic side effects after topical application, can only be interpreted with restrictions. The skin surface to body weight ratio in infants is about 3 times that of adults. In newborn infants, the metabolization and elimination processes are not yet fully developed, thereby interfering with the behavior of the percutaneously absorbed drug. Thus the pharmacologic response to the same drug concentration can vary.

Summarizing the very few pharmacokinetic data that bypass these problems, the skin permeability seems to be increased in preterm infants. In mature newborns or slightly older infants the permeability barrier for hydro-

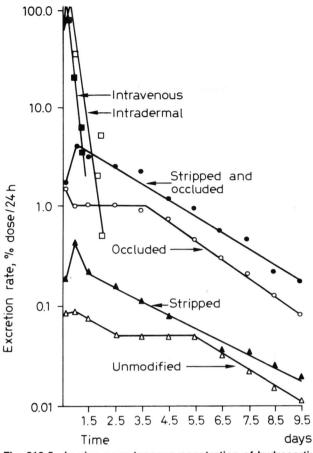

Fig. 210-5   In vivo percutaneous penetration of hydrocorti-sone as determined from urinary excretion. The vertical axis is the excretion rate in percentage of dose per 24 h; the horizontal axis is time in days after a single application of 4 μg/cm² on the forearm. *(From Maibach [6].)*

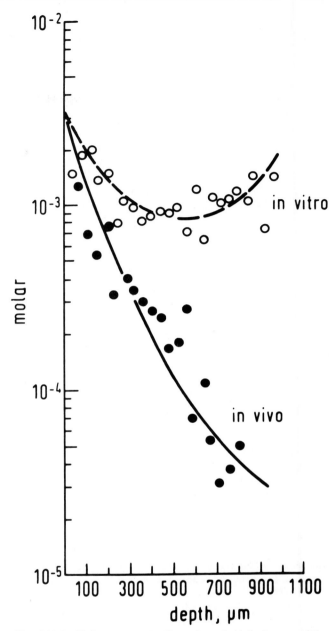

Fig. 210-6   Molar concentration of cortisol in human skin depending on the distance from the skin surface (1% [¹⁴C]-cortisol in polyethylene glycol; penetration period = 1000 min). *(From Schaefer et al [12].)*

philic compounds becomes probably as efficient as in adults, whereas that for lipophilic substances appears to be impaired even in children ([20,24] and unpublished results). No solid data related to changes in skin perme-ability in the elderly are available.

Application frequency and placebo

Nearly all epicutaneously applied drugs will enter the skin with a constant flux for many hours (see Fig. 210-5). In consequence, neither the flux of a drug [20,25] nor its therapeutic efficacy [26–29] can be increased by frequent epicutaneous application. *For most drugs the maximal flux is reached with once- or twice-daily applications of the preparation containing them.*

Additional applications of the vehicle alone make sense because it is applied directly onto the diseased areas, thereby adding a beneficial effect to the treatment on its own (although sometimes also aggravating a dermatosis). In other words, *placebos do not exist in topical therapy.* Therefore a treatment schedule using the application of the active drug (a corticoid) in the morning and the vehicle alone at night was found as effective as applying the active drug twice a day.

Effect of the dermatosis

Because the stratum corneum is the most important barrier against diffusion, disorders of keratinization influence per-meation. Such disorders change the number of horny cells, as well as the thickness and the composition of the stratum corneum. In untreated psoriatic plaques, the water loss is often doubled or tripled (unpublished data) and the perme-ability of lipophilic drugs is increased up to five to tenfold (Fig. 210-7). Recently, such an increase in percutaneous absorption through psoriatic lesions could not be found by using the urinary elimination of hydrocortisone after its

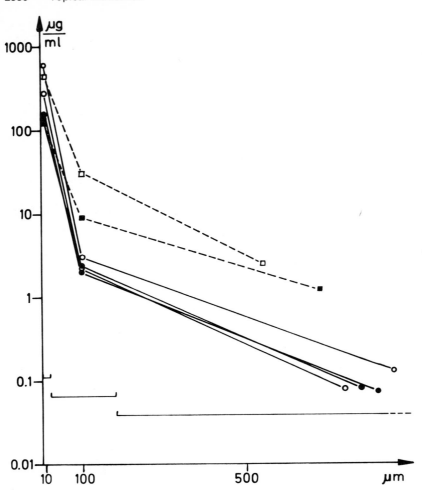

Fig. 210-7 Mean values of desoxymethasone concentrations in the different skin layers in the psoriatic lesion (- - -) and in the uninvolved skin (——); in vivo applications of 0.05% (closed symbols) and 0.25% (open symbols) desoxymethasone preparation. The thicknesses of the horny layer, epidermis, and dermis are indicated in the lower part of the graph. *(From Schalla et al [30].)*

topical application [31]. This could indicate that despite higher skin concentrations the resorption by skin blood vessels is unchanged in psoriatic lesions, i.e., the distribution or binding could be modified in involved skin. In eczema, the skin permeability can also be increased.

An efficient treatment will turn the keratinization slowly back to normal (although powerful corticosteroids can cause a reduction in the number of overlying horny cells). The restoration of the barrier function will diminish the flux of a given topically applied drug, thus decreasing the therapeutic efficacy. It explains why it is useful to increase the drug concentration in a given formulation in the course of treatment, as is recommended, for example, in most anthralin regimens for psoriasis.

Short-contact therapy

Such differences in skin permeability between involved and uninvolved skin (i.e., drug enters diseased areas more rapidly) lead to the process of short-contact therapy [15–17]. Removal of the drug excess from the skin surface after 15 to 60 min diminishes permeation, particularly in the uninvolved skin, within the following hours compared to continuous application for the same total period, whereas there is no or only a minor reduction in the involved areas (Fig. 210-8). This treatment regimen based on pharmacokinetic considerations is confirmed in clinical studies [16,18].

Properties of drugs for permeation

According to the target site, after topical application the drug acts (1) on the skin surface or within the stratum corneum, (2) in the viable part of the skin, or (3) in the rest of the body.

In the first case (sunscreens, ion exchangers, keratolytics, many disinfectants, and so on), these chemicals should not pass the stratum corneum in an active form because the desired actions are located more superficially. Drugs of group (2) should permeate the stratum corneum and reach the targets in the skin. Ideally the flux from the reservoir within the stratum corneum would give optimal concentration at the target structure, but the drug would be metabolized to inactive substances before reaching the general circulation. Thereby, the risk of systemic side effects would be greatly reduced. Drugs which should act after percutaneous absorption and distribution in the whole body (group [3]) are at present of only hypothetical interest in dermatology but recently have been used for extracutaneous disorders.

The permeability of a given drug depends upon its physicochemical properties and its binding capacity to skin structures. For the former the lipophilicity influences the liberation from the vehicle, the diffusion pathway (extracellular or transcellular), and the resistance against penetration. Highly lipophilic drugs which also have some hydrophilic character permeate best, whereas purely hy-

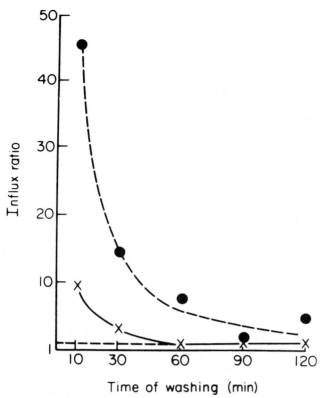

Fig. 210-8 The ratio of the noninfluenced influx into the skin to that influenced by washing off the excess drug (ordinate) vs. the time at which the drug excess was washed off (abscissa) is shown. The total penetration period was always 1000 min. Removal of this drug excess within the first hour after application diminishes further penetration much more strongly when the barrier function of the horny layer is intact (- - -) than when this function is disturbed (———). Tritium-labeled anthralin (0.1%) in petrolatum; in vitro. *(From Schalla et al [17].)*

drophilic or lipophlic substances enter the skin poorly. Therefore, it was believed that skin permeability could be increased by reducing the hydrophilicity of drugs by masking polar groups. Such a product would then liberate the active drug within the skin by splitting off that part which masks the polar group. Such mechanisms could be demonstrated for some esterified pro-drugs such as hydrocortisone acetate, fluocortinbutylester, and recently for 5-fluorouracilesters (see Chap. 28). For the majority of compounds, however, such esters are not fully hydrolyzed; rather they are new derivatives that have intrinsic pharmacologic action.

A recent study of the permeability of nails [32] has suggested that highly polar substances can be easily delivered through hydrated human nail plates, but that there probably also exists a parallel lipid pathway. The permeability of the nail therefore seems quite different from that of the stratum corneum.

Conclusion

The pharmacokinetic and skin permeability data available at present have been analyzed in an experimental environment and are more applicable to pharmaceutical and basic pharmacologic purposes than to clinical pharmacology,

i.e., they do not yet directly allow dose adjustments to individual dermatoses and patients. Nevertheless, there are some recent pharmacokinetic models that are steps in this direction [33–35].

The following general rules pertain for the pharmacokinetics of topically applied drugs:

1. The percutaneous absorption is exclusively a diffusion process. It is usually very slow because the permeation through the stratum corneum, not the elimination, is the rate-limiting step. If the horny layer is lacking, the viable skin layers are the next most important barrier.
2. A concentration gradient is maintained with the highest concentration of a drug in the horny layer and the lowest in the subcutaneous side of the dermis (Figs. 210-2, 210-6, and 210-7).
3. Factors such as metabolism, binding to proteins, and accumulation in subcutaneous fat may play a role, but they generally have little influence on the total percutaneous absorption rates.
4. The factors influencing the pharmacokinetics after topical application (Table 210-1) vary considerably inter- and intraindividually under clinical conditions.
5. In parakeratotic skin disorders, the barrier is disturbed in involved areas; therefore the skin concentration is increased compared to uninvolved skin (Fig. 210-7). In the course of the healing process the skin permeability will return to normal, thereby diminishing the actual concentration of the drug in the skin.

References

1. Ainsworth M: Methods for measuring percutaneous absorption. *J Soc Cosmet Chem* **11**:69, 1960
2. Brandau R, Lippold BH (eds): *Dermal and Transdermal Absorption*. Stuttgart, Wissenschaftliche Verlagsgesellscheft, 1982
3. Drill VA, Lazar P (eds): *Cutaneous Toxicity*. New York/San Francisco/London, Academic Press, 1977
4. Katz M, Poulsen BJ: Absorption of drugs through the skin, in *Handbook of Experimental Pharmacology*, vol 28/1, edited by O Eichler et al. Berlin/Heidelberg/New York, Springer, 1971, p 103
5. Katz M: Design of topical drug products: pharmaceutics, in *Drug Design*, vol 4, edited by EJ Ariëns. New York/London, Academic Press, 1973, p 93
6. Maibach HI: In vivo percutaneous penetration of corticoids in man and unresolved problems in their efficacy. *Dermatologica* **152(suppl 1)**:11, 1976
7. Marzulli FN, Maibach HI (eds): *Dermatotoxicology*, 2d ed. Washington/New York/London, Hemisphere, 1983
8. Malkinson FD, Rothman S: Percutaneous absorption, in *Handbuch Haut- und Geschlechtskrankheiten*, vol I/3, edited by A Marchionini, HW Spier, Berlin/Göttingen/Heidelberg, Springer, 1963, p 90
9. Mauvais-Jarvis P et al (eds): *Percutaneous Absorption of Steroids*. London/New York/Toronto/Sydney/San Francisco, Academic Press, 1980
10. Montagna W et al (eds): *Pharmacology and the Skin*, vol XII of *Advances in Biology of Skin*. New York, Appleton-Century-Crofts, 1972
11. Polano MK et al (eds): Advances in topical corticosteroid therapy. *Dermatologica* **152(suppl 1)**:1, 1976
12. Schaefer H et al: *Skin Permeability*. Berlin/Heidelberg/New York, Springer, 1982
13. Scheuplein RJ: The skin as a barrier (p 1669), Skin permeation (p 1693), Site variations in diffusion and permeability (p 1731),

in *The Physiology and Pathophysiology of the Skin,* vol 5, edited by A Jarret. London/New York/San Francisco, Academic Press, 1978

14. Träuber U: Metabolism of drugs on and in the skin, in *Dermal and Transdermal Absorption,* edited by R Brandau, BH Lippold. Stuttgart, Wissenschaftliche Verlagsgesellscheft, 1982, p 133

14a. Schmitz H, Flinzer E: Zur Frage einer periodisierten Anwendung topischer Corticosteroide—Praktikabilität und Wirksamkeit. *Drug Res* **32(I)**:430, 1982

15. Schalla W et al: Penetration studies in short-term therapy with dithranol. *Arch Dermatol Res* **267**:203, 1980

16. Schaefer H et al: Limited application period for dithranol in psoriasis. *Br J Dermatol* **102**:571, 1980

17. Schalla W et al: Skin permeability of anthralin. *Br J Dermatol* **105(suppl 20)**:104, 1981

18. Runne U, Kunze J: Short duration ("minutes") therapy with dithranol for psoriasis: a new out-patient regimen. *Br J Dermatol* **106**:135, 1982

19. Elias PM: Membranes, lipids and the epidermal permeability barrier, in *The Epidermis in Disease,* edited by R Marks, E Christophers. Lancaster, MTP Press, 1981, p 1

20. Schalla W: Penetration von essentiellen Fettsäuren und Triglyzeriden in die menschliche Haut beim Säugling und Erwachsenen—in vitro und in vivo Daten und ihre klinische Bedeutung. M.D. Thesis, Freie Universität, Berlin, 1978

21. Harris R et al: The role of eccrine sweat in delivery of ketoconazole to human stratum corneum (abstr). *J Invest Dermatol* **80**:314, 1983

22. Feldmann R, Maibach H: Regional variations in percutaneous penetration of ^{14}C-cortisol in man. *J Invest Dermatol* **48**:181, 1967

23. Feldmann R, Maibach H: Percutaneous penetration of steroids in man. *J Invest Dermatol* **52**:89, 1969

24. Schalla W et al: Influx of essential fatty acids (EFA) and triglycerides into the skin in relation to the age of human beings. *J Invest Dermatol* **72**:287, 1979

25. Wester RC et al: Frequency of application on percutaneous absorption of hydrocortisone. *Arch Dermatol* **113**:620, 1977

26. Eaglstein WH et al: Topical corticosteroid therapy: efficacy of frequent application. *Arch Dermatol* **110**:955, 1974

27. Fredriksson T et al: Treatment of psoriasis and atopic dermatitis with halcinonide cream applied once and three times daily. *Br J Dermatol* **101**:575, 1980

28. Hauss H, Proppe A: Kortikoidsparende Behandlungsweisen in der Dermatologie. *Therapiewoche* **27**:5340, 1977

29. Sudilovsky A et al: A comparison of single and multiple applications of halcinonide cream. *Int J Dermatol* **20**:609, 1981

30. Schalla W et al: Beeinflussungsgrössen der Penetration von Steroidexterna. *Aktuelle Dermatol* **6(suppl 1)**:3, 1980

31. Wester R et al: In vivo percutaneous absorption of hydrocortisone in psoriatic patients and normal volunteers. *J Am Acad Dermatol* **8**:645, 1983

32. Walters KA et al: Physicochemical characterization of the human nail: permeation pattern for water and the homologous alcohols and differences with respect to the stratum corneum. *J Pharm Pharmacol* **35**:28, 1983

33. Guy RH et al: A pharmacokinetic model for percutaneous absorption. *Int J Pharmacol* **11**:119, 1982

34. Guy RH et al: Percutaneous absorption: multidose pharmacokinetics. *International Journal of Pharmaceutics* **17**:23, 1983

35. Shrewsbury RP et al: Percutaneous absorption of hydroxyurea through psoriatic lesions. *Curr Ther Res* **28**:1002, 1980

CHAPTER 211

THE PHARMACOLOGY OF TOPICAL THERAPY

Kenneth A. Arndt and Paula V. Mendenhall

One of the most rewarding aspects of the practice of dermatology is the ability to improve or eliminate most of the diverse cutaneous conditions that cause patients to consult their physicians. Just as the skin is uniquely available for inspection and for diagnostic procedures, it is easily accessible for the delivery of a myriad of effective chemical (pharmaceutical preparations) and physical (ultraviolet, laser, and ionizing radiation, cryosurgery, electrosurgery, cold steel surgery) therapeutic modalities. Furthermore, the outcome of most therapeutic interventions is positive, i.e., the patient's disease gets objectively better. Those learning about dermatology find that they not only can diagnose previously obscure "rashes" with relative ease, but also that it is possible to successfully treat the great majority of cases in a field formerly reputed to be plagued by chronic and incurable ills. As in the practice of other medical specialities it is not necessary to have an exact etiologic diagnosis in order to be able to offer appropriate therapy. If the physician is adept at classifying disease by reaction patterns, e.g., eczematous, benign hyperplastic, acneform, etc., then useful treatment can be administered even if the specific cause of the eruption is not known.

In order to deliver successful dermatologic therapy it is necessary to (1) be able to accurately assess the type of eruption, (2) understand the principles of use of topical agents, (3) know the differences between dermatologic bases and what they can do, (4) be acquainted with the structure and presumed mode of action of the many pharmaceutically active compounds available for topical use, and (5) be skilled in the delivery of the physical modes of therapy. Types of topical preparations, the composition of pharmaceutical drug preparations, and the appropriate administration of topical medications will be discussed in this chapter. More detailed disease-related discussion and structural formulas of therapeutic agents are available in some monographs [1–3].

Types of preparations and when to use

The commonly used topical agents are available as liquids (for wet dressings, soaks, and baths; as lotions, solutions, tinctures, and aerosols) or as solids (powders, creams, gels, ointments, fixed dressings, and pastes). The liquid preparations are most useful for acute exudative problems and also are easiest to apply to hairy areas. Creams and ointments are more lubricating.

Liquid preparations

Wet dressings consist of cloths or pads soaked in solutions. They soothe, cool, and dry through evaporation of water and are indicated in the therapy of acute inflammatory states manifested by oozing, weeping, and accumulation of superficial crusts, and in treating bullous disease, erosions, and ulcers. Application of these dressings leads to vasoconstriction and hence alleviates the erythema and warmth associated with inflammation. When dressings are changed, the skin is cleansed of exudates and crusts. If dressings are left to dry in place, accumulated debris is more efficiently, though more painfully, removed ("wet-to-dry" dressings). The most important ingredient of solutions used for wet dressings is water. Although many additives may be used, the cleansing and drying effects of the aqueous base are paramount.

Agents used for wet dressing solutions are generally either astringents or antimicrobial agents. The astringents decrease exudation through the precipitation of protein. The most commonly used additive is aluminium acetate (Burow's solution; Blu-Boro; Domeboro); a 5% concentration is diluted 1:20 to 1:40 in water, and the resultant solution is easy to use, and does not stain. Potassium permanganate was formerly used extensively in the treatment of fungal infections and was felt to act as a germicide through its oxidizing action. It is more difficult to use; it stains skin, nails, and clothing; and undissolved crystals can cause chemical burns. Antimicrobial agents used for compresses include 0.1% to 0.5% silver nitrate, 1.0% acetic acid (especially for wounds infected with *Pseudomonas aeruginosa*), and solutions of povidone-iodine and of neosporin and polymyxin.

Open wet dressing solutions should be liberally applied on multiple layers of an absorbent but nonirritating dressing (old bed linen, handkerchiefs, Kerlix, gauze fluffs) to the affected area for 10 to 30 min 3 to 4 times a day. The cloth is immersed in the solution, and gently squeezed to remove excess water. Optimally, the dressings should be changed every 10 to 20 min. Overenthusiastic use of open wet compresses can lead to excessive drying and cooling; the latter is particularly a consideration in children. In general, no more than one-third of the total body surface should be treated at any time.

Closed wet dressings result when an impermeable cover such as plastic wrap is placed over a compress. This technique prevents evaporation, retains heat and causes maceration, and may be useful in the treatment of cellulitis or abscesses but is used much less often for dermatologic eruptions.

Baths and soaks, in which parts or all of the body are immersed, are used in treating more widespread, less exudative conditions. Baths may both cleanse the skin of scales or adherent debris and be used to deliver medication to affected skin. Less drying and cooling take place as exposure to air and hence evaporation are decreased, yet baths and soaks are soothing, subdue itching and other cutaneous discomfort, and tend to decrease vasodilatation. Prolonged immersion may result in maceration; therefore, the duration of bathing should be limited to 30 min. The agents used for wet dressings can also be utilized for baths. Often, however, either colloid additives such as colloidal oatmeal (Aveeno) or, less often, starch are used for their soothing and antipruritic effects, or bath oils are added to prevent drying of the skin. The latter are oil emulsions that are dispersed throughout the bath and coat the skin surface as the patient leaves the tub, thereby presumably decreasing evaporative water loss and thus acting as an emollient.

Some *lotions* consist of suspensions of a powder in water. If suspending agents are not present it is necessary to shake before application (shake lotions, such as calamine lotion). As the aqueous phase evaporates, there is drying and cooling and a therapeutic film of powder is left on the skin. In other lotions or *solutions,* the active ingredients are dissolved and they are consequently clear and used as vehicles for medications such as corticosteroids, antibiotics, and antineoplastic agents. All types of lotions are particularly well suited for use in hairy and intertriginous regions, and in acute exudative dermatoses. *Aerosols* and *sprays* are sophisticated (and often expensive) vehicles for delivering lotions or solutions to the skin. The medication is suspended in a propellant, which allows application without touching the skin. There are relatively few general indications for their use except when the amount of inflammation, tenderness, blistering, and oozing makes direct application difficult or painful, as may occur in acute contact dermatitis such as poison oak or poison ivy. The cooling sensation of the spray may itself be antipruritic.

Solid preparations

Powders promote drying. They are often used in body fold areas to increase evaporation, reduce accumulation of moisture and maceration, and to decrease friction between skin surfaces. Powders may contain active medications or may be inert. There is a tendency to presume all powders are the same, but their physiochemical properties vary greatly. Talc, a common ingredient of baby and other dusting powders, is hydrous magnesium silicate, which is totally nonabsorbent. Starch or cellulose, conversely, are quite absorbent but will form potentially abrasive conglomerates unless assiduously washed off before reapplying. Other powders used include zinc oxide or stearate, magnesium stearate, and bentonite. Starch-containing powders should not be used in intertriginous eruptions when infection, particularly with *Candida albicans,* is present since the glycogen can be easily metabolized by these microorganisms, leading to exacerbation of the infection. Powders containing antibacterial antibiotics (neomycin, polymyxin B, bacitracin) are good for erosions and ulcers and antifungal or antimonilial antibiotics (tolnaftate, nystatin) are commonly used in intertriginous areas.

Creams are emulsions of oil-in-water (O/W). In a cream the oil droplets (such as oils, fats, and waxes) represent the discontinuous phase and are dispersed in water, the continuous phase. These formulations also contain emulsifying agents and preservatives. Occasionally the preservatives can act as allergens and produce an allergic contact dermatitis. Creams are easily washable, will be completely absorbed into the skin (''vanishing'' creams), will take up more water, but are not themselves soluble. *Gels* are transparent, colorless semisolid colloidal dispersions prepared in a solid or semisolid state that liquefy on contact with the warm skin, drying as a greaseless, nonocclusive film. Aqueous, acetone, alcohol, or propylene glycol gels of organic polymers are primarily used. As with lotions, creams and gels are preferable when water-washable, nongreasy, cosmetically more elegant vehicles are needed.

Ointments may be classified into three types: water-soluble, emulsifiable, and water-repellent. *Water-soluble ointments* consist of polyethylene glycol preparations (Carbowax). These are completely water-soluble inert oils and may act as lubricants or water-soluble bases. *Emulsifiable ointments* are further divided into two varieties. *Water-in-oil (W/O) absorbent ointments* have water droplets (the discontinuous phase) dispersed in oil (the continuous phase), are difficult to wash off, and are insoluble in water, but will take up water in significant amounts. *Absorbent ointments* such as hydrophilic petrolatum USP and Aquaphor contain oils and emulsifying agents but no water. They are difficult to wash off and are insoluble in water but also will absorb water to become W/O emulsions. *Water-repellent ointments* consist of inert oils, are insoluble in water, are difficult to wash off, do not dry out, and change little with time. Petrolatum, a purified semisolid mixture of hydrocarbons obtained from petroleum, is the most commonly used base for ointments. White petrolatum, a decolorized preparation, is more esthetically appealing and is most often used. Liquid petrolatum (mineral oil) is also a mixture of purified hydrocarbons obtained from petroleum. Ointments spread easily to form a protective film over the skin and act as lubricants for dry skin and vehicles for active medications. Petrolatum is the optimal hydrophobic base, that is, it can act as a protective barrier to prevent the drying effect of aqueous compounds on the skin. If skin is hydrated by soaking in water before the application of petrolatum, the petrolatum seals in the water and becomes one of the most effective lubricants available. Ointment vehicles generally provide better penetration of incorporated medications than do creams or lotion vehicles because of their occlusive nature.

Pastes are made by incorporating a fine powder into an ointment. Powders usually constitute 20 to 50 percent of the paste. Pastes, relatively little used in today's therapeutics, are more absorptive (i.e., drying), less greasy, and often better tolerated than ointments. They are useful for treatment of ulcers, subacute and chronic dermatoses, and for psoriasis when, for example, anthralin is incorporated into zinc oxide paste.

Fixed dressings include tapes and plasters. In medicated tapes, the active ingredient (e.g., corticosteroid) is incorporated into the tape's adhesive. There are also several types of nonmedicated adhesive tapes that may aid wound healing when applied to lesions such as leg ulcers. Plasters may contain keratolytics such as salicylic acid. They are thick and spongy and protect skin from pressure and rubbing as well as acting as a drug vehicle.

Topical drug preparations and administration

Pharmaceutical drug preparations are used both systemically and topically to treat dermatologic conditions. For many drugs, topical administration is the preferred route as systemic administration may have serious drawbacks. Since most drugs used by oral administration to treat dermatologic conditions do not concentrate in the skin, medications often have to be administered at high levels in order to get effective therapeutic levels of drugs to epidermis and dermis. Such large doses not uncommonly cause untoward systemic side effects. Also, some drugs that are effective in treating dermatologic diseases are simply too toxic for systemic administration at any dose. Topical therapy, on the other hand, has many advantages. Drugs can actually be applied directly to the diseased site. The amount of drug applied can be sufficient for a therapeutic response in the skin and yet small enough not to cause other effects after entering the systemic circulation. Further, some drugs due to their physical characteristics can only be applied topically and some preparations are used topically simply for their surface effects on the outermost layers of the skin.

Percutaneous absorption

Because of the importance of topical therapy in dermatologic conditions it is worthwhile discussing some of the myriad of factors involved in designing a pharmaceutical for topical use. In order for any drug to be effective topically, it must be formulated at the proper concentration and in the proper vehicle. Formulation design, therefore, must take into account the characteristics of percutaneous absorption, including the principles of diffusion both in the drug product itself and from the drug product through the skin. In addition, factors affecting percutaneous absorption, including interactions among the skin, drug, and vehicle should be considered. Percutaneous absorption is now generally recognized as a process that is dependent on the principles of diffusion, and the stratum corneum is considered to be the rate-limiting step in this process. This can be demonstrated by removing the stratum corneum by successive strippings with cellophane tape, thus removing the barrier to penetration of most drugs, and by the fact that diseased or defective stratum corneum is also much more permeable.

There have been many studies and much speculation on how drugs diffuse through the stratum corneum. The possible routes of penetration include the skin appendages (pilosebaceous follicles or sweat glands) and the continuous stratum corneum (intercellular or intracellular). In a review of available information, Barry [4] concludes that routes through the appendages (shunt routes) cannot contribute appreciably to steady-state diffusion although they may contribute in the very early stages or may be important for ions and large polar molecules (e.g., anti-inflammatory topical steroids). He also concludes that permeation is not via the intercellular route but across the bulk of the stratum corneum (intracellular). The intracellular keratin is composed of polar and nonpolar regions where drugs pass through according to their chemical properties.

Diffusion is a passive process for the stratum corneum

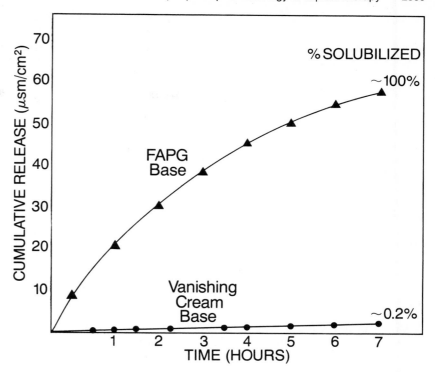

Fig. 211-1 This figure shows the effect of solubility of drug vehicle on its release into skin: the more fluocinonide in the solution, the greater the release of this corticosteroid from the vehicle.

is a nonliving tissue and there is not active transport across this membrane. Passive diffusion may be regarded as a process where a solute moves from a region of high activity or concentration down a gradient to a region of lower activity or concentration. In the percutaneous absorption of drugs, the solute at high concentration is the drug in its vehicle, while the area of lower activity is the skin itself. The rate of diffusion can be determined using Fick's law where flux or movement across the stratum corneum is shown to be *directly* proportional to (a) the partition coefficient of the drug between its vehicle and the stratum corneum, (b) the diffusion constant of the drug across the stratum corneum, (c) the difference in concentration of the drug across the stratum corneum, and *inversely* proportional to the thickness of the stratum corneum. A detailed description of Fick's law for molecules in general appears in Chap. 28. The partition coefficient is a factor that can be manipulated to some degree by dosage design and can therefore influence percutaneous absorption. We will discuss it here in more detail.

The *partition coefficient* is a term that defines the distribution of a solute between two different phases. In percutaneous absorption, the drug in solution is the solute while the two phases are the drug vehicle and the stratum corneum. If a drug is loosely held by its vehicle, it will have a large partition coefficient and will partition readily into the stratum corneum. A drug that is tightly held will have a small partition coefficient and tend to remain in its vehicle rather than partition into the skin. For any drug, the partition coefficient is dependent on the composition of each phase. The composition of the stratum corneum and the solubility of the drug in the stratum corneum cannot be controlled by the formulation scientist; however, the composition of the drug vehicle phase and the solubility of the drug in this phase can be designed to affect percutaneous absorption [5].

One of the more important factors in dosage design to optimize percutaneous absorption is the solubilization of the drug in its vehicle. If a drug is not completely in solution, release of the drug from the vehicle may be decreased due to slow diffusion through the vehicle. On the other hand, if a drug is completely in solution and a large excess of drug solvent is present in the vehicle, then the drug will have a tendency to remain there and not readily partition into the stratum corneum. Thus, to optimize partition of drugs into the skin, the formulation chemist should design a vehicle with the optimum amount of the proper solvent system: sufficient to completely solubilize the drug but not so much as to hold the drug in the vehicle. This solvent system will be different for each drug and also for different concentrations of the same drug [6] (Fig. 211-1).

Interactions

There are many complex factors that can affect the percutaneous absorption of drugs. These can be divided into biologic factors and physiochemical factors. The biologic factors are generally well known. These include general biologic variability, varying penetration rates according to regional skin site, changes in peripheral circulation, and skin metabolism [7]. The physiochemical factors that can affect percutaneous absorption may not be as well known to clinicians. These factors have been well organized by Katz and Poulsen [8] and we will here look at the following categories: drug–skin interactions, vehicle–skin interactions, and drug–vehicle interactions.

Drug–skin interactions. One type of drug–skin interaction involves skin hydration. Hydration of the stratum corneum increases its permeability. It is possible that, in addition to other ways of hydrating the stratum corneum, some drugs themselves may increase hydration by exerting an osmotic effect if they are soluble enough to reach high concentrations in the tissue. Drugs or chemicals that have been shown to increase hydration in the stratum corneum include a complex mixture of materials called the *natural moisturizing factor* (NMF) of skin, urea, and steroids such as prenenolone and estrogens [9].

A second type of drug–skin interaction that may affect percutaneous absorption involves the binding of chemicals to the skin. If drugs bind strongly, it may be necessary to administer loading doses to bind available sites before therapeutic activity can occur. Also, binding of a chemical by the skin may affect or be affected by the application of a second chemical. Complex interactions may occur and these have not yet been studied in detail. One type of interaction that has been looked at is the binding effect of topical corticosteroids. It is known that potent fluorinated steroids form depots or reservoirs in the stratum corneum. Although it is possible to elicit vasoconstrictive responses for several days after application of these steroids, whether or not these reservoirs have therapeutic significance is not clear.

Vehicle–skin interactions. When pharmaceutical vehicles are applied to the skin they may affect permeability by alteration of the skin's physical state. This alteration may occur as a result of effects on the hydration of the stratum corneum or on skin temperature, by solvent effects on the stratum corneum, or by combinations of these processes [10]. Different vehicles, depending on their composition, may have either positive or negative effects on stratum corneum hydration. Petrolatum-type ointments may increase hydration due to occlusive effects. Emulsions may increase the hydration of the stratum corneum to some degree either through occlusive effects or by adding water to the tissue, depending on the type of emulsion (O/W or W/O) and the ratio of water phase to oil phase. Water-in-oil emulsions will generally be more occlusive than oil-in-water emulsions. Glycol lotions or gels are humectants and may absorb water from the skin.

Temperature can also have an effect on drug permeability because the stratum corneum itself is a poor heat insulator and, under normal conditions, usually reflects the temperature of the environment. A rise in skin temperature can increase drug diffusion, as the diffusion constant is directly proportional to temperature. Although the use of occlusive dressings will cause a small increase in temperature, any increase in drug permeability due to this change is small compared to that caused by increased hydration of the stratum corneum. In real life, therefore, the effect of temperature on drug permeability is probably of minor importance.

The effectiveness of specific solvents in vehicles to increase percutaneous absorption can be significant. Detailed lists of ideal properties of these penetration enhancers have been developed which state that the ideal penetration enhancer should be pharmacologically inert, nontoxic, nonirritating, and nonallergenic [11,12]. It should be an excellent solvent for drugs and be compatible with a wide range of ingredients used in vehicles. The ideal material would also be cosmetically elegant and be easily incorporated into all types of vehicles, and its action should be reversible. While it is unlikely that the ideal solvent will be discovered, there are several chemicals available that do

meet some of the criteria. Dimethyl sulfoxide (DMSO) is perhaps the best known and most widely studied penetration enhancer. While DMSO is an excellent solvent and penetration enhancer for molecules of low molecular weight, it does not increase penetration of macromolecules. Also, the exact mechanism of action of penetration enhancement by DMSO has not been elicited. The possibility of putative toxic effects has prevented its use in drug products in the United States although drugs containing DMSO are available in some European countries. Dimethylacetamide (DMAC) and dimethylformamide (DMF) are two other organic solvents with properties similar to DMSO but they have not been as extensively studied. Other compounds that have been reported to enhance penetration include alkyl sulfoxides, phosphine oxides, sugar esters, 2-pyrrolidone, azocycloalkan-2-ones, tetrahydrofurfuryl alcohol, and various surfactants [13]. Propylene glycol and ethanol have also been reported to be penetration enhancers. These chemicals may increase penetration, however, by acting as cosolvents to increase the amount of dissolved drug in the vehicle without having specific effects on the barrier properties of the stratum corneum itself unless used at very high concentrations.

Drug–vehicle interactions. There are certain cases in which the stratum corneum is not the rate-determining step in percutaneous absorption. It may be defective or even absent due to injury or disease, or there may exist times when for various reasons diffusion of a drug within the drug product itself may be very slow. In both of these cases, the release rate of the drug from the vehicle into the skin may be the limiting step in absorption [14]. It should be recognized, however, that as the skin begins to heal with time, the barrier capacity of the stratum corneum may be reestablished. As this occurs, absorption of the same drug product may be determined by the newly formed barrier.

There are many factors that may affect drug diffusion through the vehicle. Topical drug products are heterogeneous systems which contain many ingredients, some of which may interact, complex, or bind chemically to the drug in such a manner as to affect diffusion of the drug out of the vehicle and into the skin. Such products are generally multiphase systems and drugs may partition into the various phases and affect the amount of drug available for absorption, because it is the external phase of a product that has the greatest amount of skin contact. The drug which has partitioned into the internal phase or phases may be less available for release into the skin. In addition, many drugs exist as polymorphs, which are different crystalline forms of the drugs, each having different physiochemical properties. The use of one particular polymorph in a product or the conversion with time of one polymorph to another may affect the drug's solubility and availability [15].

Transdermal delivery systems

Transdermal devices are systems that are used to deliver drugs to the systemic circulation via the skin. Although not used to treat skin disorders, transdermal devices do use the skin as the portal of entry of drugs into the body for systemic effects. In this case, it is the device itself, not the stratum corneum, that controls the rate at which the drug diffuses through the skin. In the Transdermal Therapeutic System device, a drug reservoir is separated from the skin by a polymeric membrane. This microporous membrane controls the rate at which drug is delivered to the skin and thus controls rate of absorption. A loading or priming dose may be contained in the contact adhesive which affixes the device to the skin.

The advantages of this type of drug delivery system include eliminating the variabilities of gastrointestinal absorption and the "first pass effect" of the liver on drug metabolism, and providing constant controlled administration of a drug with a steady rate of entrance into the systemic circulation. Not every drug can be given by this method. In order to be effective in a transdermal device, the drug must be potent enough so that small doses are effective, the drug cannot irritate or sensitize the skin, and it must possess the correct physiochemical properties to partition into the stratum corneum and reach the systemic circulation [16]. Scopolamine for motion sickness is one drug that is effectively administered using a transdermal device. Drugs may also be applied topically for systemic effect without the use of specific devices as, for instance, the use of topical nitroglycerin creams for the treatment of angina.

Vehicle ingredients

There are literally thousands of raw materials or supposedly inert ingredients that can be used in formulating topical vehicles. As a general rule, however, those ingredients used in topical drug products tend to be less exotic than some of the newer raw materials used in some cosmetic products.

In order to review ingredients used in topical preparations, it is convenient to divide them into general classes and look at the most common members of each class. It should be recognized that many ingredients may serve more than one function in a particular vehicle. The general classes we will look at are emulsifying agents, stabilizers, solvents, thickening agents, emollients, and humectants (Table 211-1) [17].

Emulsifying agents

Emulsions, which are dispersions of two or more immiscible liquid phases (usually an aqueous phase and an oil phase), are thermodynamically unstable. In time, they will separate into their phases due to flocculation or coalescence of the dispersed droplets. Emulsifying agents, added to these systems to improve stability, are surface-active agents (surfactants) which decrease surface tension. By adsorption they form a film around each droplet of dispersed material, imparting an adequate electric potential to these droplets so that mutual repulsion will occur [18]. There is no one ideal emulsifying agent available because the properties of the phases will vary. Also, there is no ideal amount of emulsifier to use; the pharmaceutical scientist uses the minimum amount of the best emulsifying agent for a particular system necessary to impart maximum stability.

Emulsifying agents may be divided into synthetic and naturally occurring types. In practice, synthetic agents are the most widely used in pharmaceutical preparations. Synthetic emulsifying agents may be further divided into anionic, cationic, and nonionic surfactants. Soaps and sodium lauryl sulfate are common examples of anionic surfactants. Alkali soaps are stable only at a high pH (>10) as, at lower pHs, the fatty acid precipitates out of solution. Sodium lauryl sulfate is widely used in topical products as a detergent, wetting agent, and emulsifying agent. Unlike soaps, sodium lauryl sulfate is compatible with dilute acids and calcium and magnesium ions. As an emulsifying agent, sodium lauryl sulfate is usually combined with auxiliary agents. Sodium lauryl ether sulfate (sodium laureth sulfate) is an ethoxylated agent often used in place of sodium lauryl sulfate as it is less irritating to skin.

Cationic emulsifying agents are weak emulsifiers and are generally used in combination with other auxiliary agents. Quaternary ammonium compounds are examples of cationic agents. They form emulsions with pHs of 4 to 6. Cationic agents are incompatible with anionic surfactants.

By far the most widely used emulsifying agents are the nonionics and the most commonly used of these are combinations of polysorbates and sorbitan esters. Polysorbates are water-soluble polyoxyethylene sorbitan esters. There are many polysorbates available containing varying amounts of oxyethylene groups and different fatty acid esters. In general, the polysorbates form oil-in-water emulsions which are stable and little affected by high concentrations of electrolytes or by pH changes. There are also many sorbitan esters available. These fatty acid esters of sorbitol and its anhydrides are oil-soluble, water-dispersible surfactants. They form water-in-oil emulsions which have the same stability characteristics as the polysorbate emulsions. Because of their differing solubilities in oil and water and their tendency to form different types of emulsions (O/W vs. W/O), the polysorbates and sorbitans are commonly used together to form stable fine-textured emulsions.

In addition to true emulsifying agents, there are also many chemicals that are used as auxiliary emulsifying agents or emulsion stabilizers. Cetyl alcohol is used to build viscosity into emulsions and improve emulsion texture. Glyceryl monostearate is a poor water-and-oil emulsifying agent used by itself, but helps stabilize emulsions when used as an auxiliary agent. Lanolin has some emulsifying action due to its cholesterol and aliphatic alcohol content. Lanolin alcohol imparts a high gloss and creamy texture to emulsions and may help stabilize emulsions by absorption of water. Polyethylene glycols are strongly hydrophilic and useful as emulsion stabilizers. Stearyl alcohol has some surfactant properties, increases the ability of emulsions to retain large quantities of water, and thus increases emulsion stability. It also builds viscosity into emulsions and produces firmer emulsions than cetyl alcohol.

Stabilizers

Included in this category is a wide variety of chemicals that are added to pharmaceutical preparations to increase or help preserve their stability both initially and over time. Agents may be used to increase the stability of the drug itself or the stability of the vehicle. Preservatives, antiox-

Table 211-1 Vehicle ingredients—examples of commonly used agents

Emulsifying agents	Solvents
Cholesterol	Alcohol
Disodium monooleamidosulfosuccinate	Diisopropyl adipate
Emulsifying wax, NF	Glycerin
Polyoxyl 40 stearate	1,2,6-Hexanetriol
Polysorbates	Isopropyl myristate
Sodium laureth sulfate	Propylene carbonate
Sodium lauryl sulfate	Propylene glycol
Sorbitan esters	Water
Stearic acid	
	Thickening agents
Auxiliary emulsifying agents/emulsion	Beeswax
stabilizers	Carbomer
Carbomer	Petrolatum
Cetearyl alcohol	Polyethylene
Cetyl alcohol	Xanthan gum
Glyceryl monostearate	
Lanolin and lanolin derivates	Emollients
Polyethylene glycols	Caprylic/capric triglycerides
Stearyl alcohol	Cetyl alcohol
	Glycerin
Stabilizers (including preservatives,	Isopropyl myristate
antioxidants, and chelating agents)	Isopropyl palmitate
Benzyl alcohol	Lanolin and lanolin derivates
Butylated hydroxyanisole (BHA)	Mineral oil
Butylated hydroxytoluene (BHT)	Petrolatum
Chlorocresol	Squalane
Citric acid	Stearic acid
Edetate disodium	Stearyl alcohol
Glycerin	
Parabens	Humectants
Propyl gallate	Glycerin
Propylene glycol	Propylene glycol
Sodium bisulfite	Sorbitol solution
Sorbic acid/potassium sorbate	

idants, and chelating agents are all examples. of chemical stabilizers.

Preservatives are agents that are used to prevent or inhibit microbial growth. Preservatives should be used at a level that will inhibit microbial growth throughout the life of the product including the period of patient use. This is particularly important in topical products, because every patient use is a possible source of contamination, especially if the product is dispensed in a jar. Products dispensed in tubes are less prone to contamination by bacteria present on the patient's skin or in the air. The parabens are probably the preservatives most widely used in pharmaceutical preparations. Parabens are esters of *p*-hydroxybenzoic acid. There are several esters that are used including the methyl, ethyl, propyl, and butyl esters. As preservatives, the parabens are active against molds, fungi, and yeasts, but less effective against bacteria. They are commonly used as mixtures because of their varying activities and solubilities and may be the cause of an allergic contact reaction to vehicle contents. The activity of parabens is reduced in the presence of nonionic surfactants such as the polysorbates. Other preservatives commonly used include benzyl alcohol and sorbic acid or potassium sorbate. Propylene glycol and glycerin exhibit antimicrobial activity when they are used in high concentrations (>20%).

Antioxidants are agents that inhibit oxidation and are used in products where either the active ingredient or the vehicle may deteriorate through oxidative processes. Butylated hydroxyanisole (BHA) and butylated hydroxytoluene (BHT) are used to retard oxidative degradation in oils and fats. Propyl gallate prevents rancidity in oils and fats and also inhibits the development of peroxides in ethers and similar substances. *Chelating agents,* such as citric acid and edetate disodium (disodium EDTA), are used to form complexes with heavy metals. They are sometimes used as synergists with antioxidants, for heavy metals may accelerate oxidative reactions.

Solvents

Solvents are used to increase the solubility of the active drug in the vehicle or to solubilize other necessary ingredients in the product. Water, alcohol, glycerin, and propylene glycol are commonly used solvents.

Thickening agents

Thickening agents include those materials that are used to thicken or increase the viscosity of products or to suspend ingredients in the vehicle. They may act as emulsion stabilizers or as ointment bases. Beeswax is used to increase viscosity in ointments and enables the incorporation of water to produce water-in-oil emulsions. Carbomers are synthetic, high-molecular-weight polymers. When dispersed in water as the free acid, they form thin cloudy products. Upon neutralization with alkali hydroxides or amines, carbomers will form clear gels of varying viscosities. Carbomers are also used as suspending agents. Petrolatum may be used by itself as an ointment vehicle or in emulsions to increase viscosity and emolliency. Although petrolatum is compatible with most drugs available in ointments, it may not release certain drugs readily. Polyethylene is a polymer of ethylene monomers. It is resistant to oxidation and is used as a stiffening agent to replace natural waxes.

Emollients

Emollients are agents that make the skin soft and pliable by increasing hydration of the stratum corneum. They are all occlusive to some degree. The greater the occlusiveness, the greater the decrease in water loss and resulting increased hydration of the stratum corneum. Petrolatum is probably the most occlusive and, therefore, the best emollient available. Its inherent greasy feel, however, precludes wide use by itself. Petrolatum is often mixed with more cosmetically acceptable materials to produce an acceptable feeling for skin. However, because the product has been made more acceptable by decreasing occlusiveness, it also functions less efficiently as an emollient. Compromises are made by the formulation chemist to produce products that are acceptable to the patient and yet retain emollient action. As a result, there are many emollient agents used in topical products. Cetyl alcohol and stearyl alcohol are mixtures of solid aliphatic alcohols. They are used as emollients as they lubricate without being greasy and impart a smooth feeling to the skin. Isopropyl myristate and isopropyl palmitate are light mobile liquids which act as emollients without leaving a heavy, greasy feel on the skin.

Humectants

Humectants are agents which are added to vehicles on the premise that they are hygroscopic and will draw moisture into the skin. Under dry atmospheric conditions, however, humectants will act in a manner opposite to that desired and actually withdraw water from the skin. Glycerin, propylene glycol, and sorbitol solutions are examples of humectants used in topical products.

Application of topical medications

Amount

It is important to prescribe adequate amounts of medication for the patient. Estimate the total amount of material needed either until the patient is scheduled to return or until the eruption clears, and dispense the medication in one large tube, jar, or bottle; this will ensure a higher degree of patient compliance and a greater chance of successful therapy, and offer the possibility of cost savings to the patient. If the medication is expensive, as with corticosteroids, patients should be told the approximate cost of both generic and trade products. This information is available in the yearly editions of the American Druggist *Blue Book* [19], the *Drug Topics Red Book* [20], or in the *Manual of Dermatologic Therapeutics* [1]. One gram of cream will cover an area approximately 10 by 10 cm; an ointment will spread up to 10 percent further. The approximate amount needed for the single application of a cream or ointment to the face or hands is 2 g; to one arm or the anterior or posterior trunk, 3 g; to one leg, 4 g; and to the entire body, 30 g.

Frequency

The absorption, distribution, and excretion characteristics of parenterally administered medications are known in enough detail that it is usually possible to instruct the patient regarding the exact amount and frequency of use. The same type of dose/response pharmacokinetic information is much more difficult to obtain for topically applied agents; however, some interesting data concerning application frequency are now available. One study found that six treatments a day of topically applied corticosteroid were no more effective than three applications a day in a study on 12 patients with corticosteroid-responsive dermatoses [21]. An investigation into the percutaneous absorption of radioactive labeled hydrocortisone on the shaved forearm of the rhesus monkey demonstrated no substantial difference in total absorption when a given amount was applied as a single dose or when one-third of the same amount was applied 3 times daily [22]. However, when the larger amount was applied as a single dose, absorption was substantially increased over the smaller amount (one-third) applied either once or 3 times. The clinical relevance of the results for humans needs further study, but the absorption characteristics of monkey and human skin are known to be similar. One recent investigation revealed that one daily application of fluocinonide ointment was as effective as 4-times-daily application in 52 patients with stable psoriasis [23], while another demonstrated that once-daily application of betamethasone dipropionate or diflorasone diacetate ointment to 139 patients with psoriasis showed statistically significant improvement compared to subjects using vehicle alone [24]. It may be that a single large daily application of medication, at least of corticosteroids, could be the most efficient means of delivering medication to the skin. Acute tolerance (tachyphylaxis) to the vasoconstrictive and antimitotic effects of topically applied glucocorticoids may occur within 1 week of repeated application. After a 4-day rest period, responsiveness to the corticosteroid effects returns to the original level [25].

Absorption characteristics

There is marked regional variation in the amount of medication absorbed from different body areas. Approximately 1 percent of a hydrocortisone solution will penetrate normal skin on the forearm. Compared to the forearms, hydrocortisone is absorbed only one-seventh as well through the plantar foot arch, but 6 times more through forehead skin and 42 times more through scrotal skin [26]. Inflamed eczematous skin has increased percutaneous penetration, and with conditions such as exfoliative psoriasis there seems to be little barrier to absorption at all.

When medications such as corticosteroids are applied to the skin under an airtight occlusive plastic dressing, their efficacy and absorption are increased 10 to 100 times. Occlusion with a plastic dressing increases the skin surface area, increases hydration and temperature, and also appears to induce a reservoir of corticosteroid in the stratum corneum that lasts for several days after application. The increased absorption of medications applied under plastic occlusive dressings may also lead more rapidly to the appearance of undesirable side effects such as local atrophy and suppression of the HPA axis when corticosteroids are used. Also, greatly enhanced irritant or toxic side effects occur with occlusive dressings when other agents are used, e.g., tar. Occlusive therapy also can promote infection, folliculitis, and miliaria, and result in an interference in heat exchange.

Simple hydration of skin prior to application of topical corticosteroids may increase penetration up to fivefold. The optimal technique for applying topical medications, therefore, is first to hydrate skin by immersion in water for about 5 min and then immediately apply the cream or ointment. If occlusion techniques are to be employed, the plastic dressing or body suit should be put on directly thereafter.

References

1. Arndt KA: *Manual of Dermatologic Therapeutics. With Essentials of Diagnosis,* 3d ed. Boston, Little, Brown, 1983
2. Landow RK: *Handbook of Dermatologic Treatment.* Greenbrae, CA, Jones Medical Publications, 1983, p 219
3. Madden SW (ed): *Current Dermatologic Therapy,* 3d ed. Philadelphia, WB Saunders, 1982
4. Barry B: *Dermatological Formulations—Percutaneous Absorption.* New York, Dekker, 1983, p 96
5. Poulsen B: *In Drug Design,* vol IV, edited by E Ariens. New York, Academic Press, 1973, p 168
6. Flynn G: *In Modern Pharmaceutics,* edited by G Banker, C Rhodes. New York, Dekker, 1979, p 317
7. Barry B: *Dermatological Formulations—Percutaneous Absorption.* New York, Dekker, 1983, p 129
8. Katz M, Poulsen B: In *Handbook of Experimental Pharmacology,* vol 28, part I, edited by B Brodie, J Gillette. New York, Springer-Verlag, 1971, p 117
9. Barry B: *Dermatological Formulations—Percutaneous Absorption.* New York, Dekker, 1983, p 145
10. Katz M, Poulsen B: In *Handbook of Experimental Pharmacology,* vol 28, part I, edited by B Brodie, J Gillette. New York, Springer-Verlag, 1971, p 121
11. Katz M, Poulsen B: In *Handbook of Experimental Pharmacology,* vol 28, part I, edited by B Brodie, J Gillette. New York, Springer-Verlag, 1971, p 125
12. Barry B: *Dermatological Formulations—Percutaneous Absorption.* New York, Dekker, 1983, p 160
13. Barry B: *Dermatological Formulations—Percutaneous Absorption.* New York, Dekker, 1983, p 163
14. Poulsen B: In *Drug Design,* vol IV, edited by E Ariens. New York, Academic Press, 1973, p 185
15. Haleblian J, McCrone W: Pharmaceutical applications of polymorphism. *J Pharm Sci* 58:911, 1969
16. Barry B: *Dermatological Formulations—Percutaneous Absorption.* New York, Dekker, 1983, p 181
17. *The Base Book.* Palo Alto, CA, Syntex Laboratories, 1982
18. Higuchi W et al: In *Remington's Pharmaceutical Sciences,* edited by A Osol. Easton, PA, Mack Publishing, 1980, p 310
19. *1983 Blue Book.* New York, American Druggist, 1983
20. *Drug Topics Red Book.* Oradell, NJ, Topics, 1983
21. Eaglstein WH et al: Topical corticosteroid therapy: efficacy of frequent application. *Arch Dermatol* 110:955, 1974
22. Wester RC et al: Frequency of application on percutaneous absorption of hydrocortisone. *Arch Dermatol* 113:620, 1977
23. Senter RP: Topical fluocinonide and tachyphylaxis. *Arch Dermatol* 119:363, 1983
24. Lane AT et al: Once-daily treatment of psoriasis with topical glucocorticosteroid ointments. *J Am Acad Dermatol* 8:523, 1983
25. deVivier A: Acute tolerance to effects of topical glucocorticoids. *Br J Dermatol* 94 (suppl 12):25, 1976
26. Feldman RJ, Maibach HI: Regional variation in percutaneous penetration of ^{14}C cortisol in man. *J Invest Dermatol* 48:181, 1967

CHAPTER 212

TOPICAL CORTICOSTEROIDS

Christopher F. H. Vickers

Topical corticosteroids are the most widely used preparations in dermatology; the multiplicity of different corticosteroids on the market is matched only by the many different bases, steroid antimicrobial combinations, and in addition, the combination with agents aimed at increasing penetration such as urea. Many manufacturers have produced ranges of concentrations, and there are also variations especially designed for certain body sites, e.g., the scalp.

The introduction of topical hydrocortisone in the early 1950s represented a great advance on previously available therapy, but it was the first of the halogenated steroids, triamcinolone acetonide, introduced in 1954 [1], that began the revolution which culminated in the appearance of the very potent agents now available to dermatologists. The large number of available topical corticosteroids, combinations, and dilutions means that each dermatologist has a group of steroids he or she regularly uses as first-line therapy, resorting to others only in difficult situations.

Grading of the potency of topical corticosteroids has in general been based on a combination of comparative clinical trials [2,3] and the assay of McKenzie and Stoughton

[4]. It is a fact of the 1980s that, owing to adverse publicity, many dermatologists and primary care physicians have become opposed to the use of the high-potency topical corticosteroids [5], thus depriving their patients of essential therapy. Careful monitoring of the amount of topical corticosteroids being applied is essential, and guidelines for different age groups are available.

The mechanism of action of corticosteroids is as follows: penetration of the stratum corneum is followed by passage across the cell membrane, binding to specific cytoplasmic receptors, translocation of the complex to the nucleus, and interaction with high-affinity binding sites via the process of mRNA transcription which results in the formation of new proteins [6–8]. When topical corticosteroids are applied to the skin, the initial changes are vasoconstriction followed by reduction of inflammatory change, and finally reduction in mitotic rate and thus epidermopoiesis [9,10]. Vasoconstriction from corticosteroids is not well understood but may be due to alteration of cátecholamine and histamine effects on peripheral blood vessels. The reduction of inflammation and mitotic rate occurs by a mechanism similar to that seen with systemic corticosteroids [11].

Of recent years, much care has been taken by pharmaceutical companies to increase the delivery of the steroid to the skin by techniques such as micronization of the steroid powder, and to increase the percutaneous absorption of the applied corticosteroid by careful control of the base (e.g., addition of propylene glycol) [12,13] and by the addition of hydrating agents, such as urea, which are known to increase the penetration of topically applied agents. The most recent tendency has been the attempt to develop topical corticosteroids with an increased topical/systemic potency ratio.

Side effects of topical corticosteroids

These can be divided into (1) systemic, first recognized with 9α-fludrocortisone by Fitzpatrick et al [14] in 1955 and occurring more frequently with the halogenated corticosteroids and also when topical corticosteroids are applied under plastic occlusion, and (2) local, which are more frequent in these same situations, and possibly in the very young or the very old patient. Local side effects are certainly more common on the face and in the flexures where percutaneous absorption is known to be greater [15,16].

Systemic side effects

The overenthusiastic use of high-potency topical corticosteroids, especially under plastic occlusion, can give rise to systemic side effects. Edema due to sodium retention was first described with the application of 9α-fludrocortisone [14] and has been regularly reported with all the halogenated topical corticosteroids; hyperglycemia and glycosuria, hypertension, Cushing's syndrome [17] with striae, buffalo hump, moon face, and hirsuties have all been seen. Hypokalemia and the induction of peptic ulceration by topical corticosteroids have also been reported. Certainly the plasma cortisol levels can be depressed as a result of the suppression of the pituitary-adrenal axis [18,19]. The delayed healing of wounds in the presence of topical corticosteroid therapy may be a local rather than a systemic effect. Whether osteoporosis and growth retardation in children can be ascribed to topical corticosteroid therapy is subject to considerable disagreement. Most researchers would accept the fact that growth retardation is unlikely from topical corticosteroid application.

Local side effects

These are easily recognized but occasionally cause diagnostic problems. Side effects are more common on facial and flexural skin after occlusion with plastic and in advanced age. They are best divided into three groups.

Skin damage. Classically, the epidermis becomes atrophic; the dermal collagen shows changes identical with those seen in the aging process (solar elastosis). The skin becomes translucent, yellowish due to the visibility of the dermal collagen, and telangiectasia appears, again an effect of altered light transmission through epidermis and collagen and not an increase in the numbers of cutaneous blood vessels [20]. ''Shear purpura'' is also commonly seen and results from the epidermal atrophy with flattening of the dermal-epidermal interface [21]. Striae may be found, especially in the flexures [16], though many of the reported cases have been in teen-age children where such striae may be physiologic in origin. The measurement of these steroid side effects now constitutes one of the elegant assessments of topical corticosteroids. In one technique, a topical corticosteroid is applied to the skin in a special chamber and measurement of telangiectasia and atrophy is made after a period of several days [22].

Infections and infestations. Especially after plastic occlusion therapy but also after application of topical corticosteroids to the flexures, candidiasis is not uncommon and can be severe if not quickly recognized. Many dermatologists favor the use of topical corticosteroid anticandidal combinations in such cases. Bacterial infections may also complicate therapy in the same situation and often follow poral occlusion during occlusive therapy.

The inappropriate application of topical corticosteroids to dermatophyte infections may mask the clinical signs and make the diagnosis very difficult (tinea incognito) [23]. A mild condition may also be made much more severe; a low-grade impetigo may rapidly spread and again make diagnosis difficult if a topical corticosteroid is applied. If topical corticosteroids are applied in the early stages of scabies, the diagnosis may similarly be masked; this is especially likely to occur in an infant, where the itching baby is presumed to have infantile eczema [24]. Examination of the axillae and the soles would almost certainly avoid this pitfall. The application of topical corticosteroids to patients with rosacea may initially suppress the reaction, but there is usually rapid breakthrough of the disease or, if the therapy is discontinued, a very severe flare-up [25]. Most authors believe that the perioral dermatitis syndrome is caused by the application of high-potency topical corticosteroids to facial skin in a patient with rosacea or in the early stages of the disease [26].

Other effects on the skin. Depigmentary changes have been reported following the use of corticosteroids, notably with a steroid-impregnated adhesive tape [27].

Gluteal granulomata in the diaper area have been thought

Table 212-1 Classification of topical corticosteroids

	Strength available	Trade name	
		British	**American**
Very potent			
Clobetasol	0.05%	Dermovate	
Halcinonide	0.01%	Halciderm	Halog
Beclomethazone diproprionate	0.5%	Propaderm Forte	
Diflucortalone valerate	0.3%	Nerisone Forte	
Fluocinolone acetonide	0.2%	Synalar Forte	
Potent			
Beclomethazone diproprionate	0.025%	Propaderm	
Betamethazone 17-valerate	0.1%	Betnovate	Valisone
Diflucortalone valerate	0.1%	Nerisome	
Fluocinolone acetonide	0.025%	Synalar	Synalar
Fluocinonide	0.05%	Metosyn	Topsyn, Lidex
Moderately potent			
Desonide	0.5%	Tridesilon	Tridesilon
Triamcinolone acetonide	0.1%	Many names	Kenalog
Flurandrenolide	0.05%	Haelan X	Cordran
Hydrocortisone butyrate	0.1%	Locoid	
Fluprednylidene	0.1%	Decoderm	
Mildly potent			
Clobetazone butyrate	0.05%	Eumovate	
Fluocortolone hexonate	0.1% }	Ultradil	
Fluocortolone pivalate	0.1% }		
Fluocortolone	0.25% }	Ultralanum	
Fluocortolone hexonate	0.25% }		
Flurandrenalide	0.0125%	Haelan	Cordran
Weak			
Hydrocortisone	0.1–2.5%	Many commercial preparations	
Methylprednisolone	0.025%	Medrone	

to follow the use of high-potency topical corticosteroids in this area [28], but such granulomata frequently occur in the Jacquet type of diaper erythema, and it is doubtful that this is a true side effect of topical corticosteroids.

The conversion of classical psoriasis to acute pustular psoriasis by the sudden withdrawal of topical corticosteroids is well documented [29], and probably comparable to the exacerbations seen in rosacea [25].

The application of topical corticosteroids in combination with antibacterials has been advocated by some authors in the therapy of gravitational ulceration but this may result in a chronic nonhealing ulcer. Vasoconstriction easily visible around the ulcer may account for the nonhealing because of reduction of skin blood flow at the ulcer edge. Similarly, nonhealing of minor injuries has been noted in patients applying topical corticosteroids to the surrounding skin.

Classification of topical corticosteroids (Table 212-1)

In 1983 there were 93 different topical corticosteroids on the market in the United Kingdom. Nearly all the basic corticosteroids are available in ointment, cream, and lotion bases, several in special alcoholic lotions for application to hair-bearing areas and a few in aerosol sprays. One adhesive tape impregnated with flurandrenolide in a concentration of 4 μg/cm² can be very valuable in the management of chronic discoid lupus erythematosus and keloid scarring. Corticosteroid suppositories and special steroid

ointment applicators for the rectum are designed for the management of pruritus ani. Triamcinolone acetonide 0.1% in Orobase is very useful when corticosteroids are applied to ulcerative lesions in the buccal mucosa, while pellets of hydrocortisone succinate are also beneficial in recurrent aphthous ulceration. Recently many physicians have used inhalation steroids (as used in bronchial asthma) with a special oral adaptor in the management of painful ulceration of the mouth in Behçet's syndrome, pemphigus, and other conditions [30].

Topical corticosteroids in combination with other agents

Antimicrobials

There are many corticosteroid antimicrobial combinations; the most frequently added substances are nystatin, neomycin, iodochlorhydroxyquin, and clioquinol. The full list is shown in Table 212-2. Whether such combinations should ever be used is still a subject of considerable disagreement [31]. Allergic sensitivity to the antimicrobial may be masked by the action of the topical corticosteroid and thus the underlying condition may be aggravated and unrecognized. More important than this is the question of whether infection is controlled in the presence of the corticosteroid. Many believe that if the underlying disease is complicated by secondary infection, then topical antimicrobials should be applied first, followed by a return to

Table 212-2   Antimicrobials that are combined with corticosteroids

Antibacterial	Antifungal
Neomycin	Nystatin
Tetracycline	Miconazole
Gentamycin	
Sodium fusidate	
Framycetin	
Polymixin	
Bacitracin	
Chlorhexidine	
Clioquinol	

corticosteroid. There are, however, many clinical situations where the combinations are of value, such as the child with infantile eczema, where the possibility of secondary infection is very real in the "crawling-toddling" age, or in seborrheic eczema, with its well-established tendency to secondary bacterial and candidal infections. Combinations of low-potency corticosteroids with anticandidal agents make good sense in diaper-area conditions, where candidiasis is such a frequent complication. The addition of miconazole may lead to a false sense of security in the differentiation of a foot eczema from tinea pedis. However, the combination may be useful in certain situations. Double or even triple combinations of corticosteroid, antibacterial, and anticandidal agents may at first seem like "blunderbuss" polypharmacy but, again, may have a place in secondarily infected flexural lesions such as seborrheic eczema or diaper rashes. Indeed one, Timodine, from the United Kingdom, is of proven value in the intertrigo resulting from urinary incontinence in the very young and the very old. This is one of only two topical corticosteroid preparations in a water-resistant silicone base.

Other additives

Urea 10% has been added to some topical corticosteroids following experimental evidence that this increases the percutaneous absorption of hydrocortisone in the in vitro situation. Whether the effectiveness of the corticosteroid is greatly enhanced is arguable but the combinations are helpful for patients with very dry (xerotic) skin; they probably act by increasing hydration of the stratum corneum [32]. Stinging is an occasional problem with urea-containing materials. Allantoin and coal tar have been combined with the corticosteroids in several preparations and these may be beneficial in atopic eczema and psoriasis, especially as the usual steroid is hydrocortisone. The addition of the antipruritic crotamiton is of help in some extreme pruritic dermatoses but allergic sensitivity is not unknown. Finally, chymotrypsin and heparin have been added to some preparations; their value is as yet unknown. The addition of salicylic acid to topical corticosteroids has a rational basis but has not in general been held to be successful [33].

The choice of bases

New developments during the last few years have brought forward many new bases, some with more cosmetic acceptability and others claiming to treat associated dryness, but most attempting to deliver the corticosteroid more effectively by the addition of substances such as propylene glycol (claimed to increase the effectiveness of hydrocortisone by a factor of 10) [34]. Other bases have been introduced both to increase penetration of the corticosteroid and to avoid the use of lanolin and parabens, both potential sensitizers. Several new gel bases appear to have all these advantages—cosmetic acceptability, better drug delivery, and the avoidance of potential allergens in the base [33,35].

With the bewildering array of bases available, choice is very much a personal matter. The old adage of lotions and creams for weeping lesions and ointments for dry lesions still applies, but many dermatologists ask their patients which they would like—a good route to better patient compliance. There is no doubt, however, that it is wise not to use ointment bases in flexures or hair-bearing areas where lotions or creams are preferable; specially formulated gels and alcoholic solutions are best for these areas. Likewise, in children with atopic eczema and associated ichthyosis, the use of ointment bases is preferred. In many situations, the dermatologist or primary care physician may wish to apply a more dilute form of topical corticosteroid and there are a number of these on the market; they are made up in sterile pharmaceutical conditions using the selected base best designed for delivery of the particular corticosteroid. Dilution of commercially available topical corticosteroid preparations in hospital or local pharmacies has certain financial advantages but several major drawbacks [36]. The main problem is one of sterility; cases of contamination with *Pseudomonas* organisms have occurred with disastrous results. The second problem concerns the diluent base which must be compatible with or identical to the original base. The pH of the base is also vital, as changes may lead to degeneration of the steroid molecule if it is significantly altered. In some instances, the carefully micronized corticosteroid aggregates with resulting loss of activity. Some steroids are dissolved in propylene glycol before being incorporated into the base; again, this solution may be "broken" in the dilution process. Creams that are basically water-in-oil or oil-in-water emulsions are also easily "broken" by addition of incorrect material.

Other problems with topical corticosteroids

Allergic reactions

Most allergic hypersensitive reactions to topical corticosteroids arise from added antimicrobials such as neomycin, preservatives such as parabens, or the lanolin used in the base [37–40]. Very occasional reactions to corticosteroids themselves have been reported [41–43]. In view of the vast amounts of topical corticosteroids used each year all over the world, these cases are exceptionally rare, though some authors have pointed out that they may be missed, as sensitivity to one corticosteroid only may occur, and failure to respond may merely lead to a change in topical preparation.

Tachyphylaxis

Many patients report that the topical corticosteroid they are using is losing its effectiveness and most dermatologists would agree that a change of corticosteroid is often beneficial. It was often believed that the effect was in the patient's imagination rather than in the skin, until 1975 when DuVivier and Stoughton reported experimental tachyphylaxis [44]. These authors showed a decreasing vasoconstrictor response to topical corticosteroids if applications were repeated at 48-h intervals. There was a linear relation with increasing intervals of application. The explanation is not clear; it may be a more rapid dispersal of the corticosteroid after repeated local application, or it may even be similar to the phenomenon of enzyme induction occurring after the oral administration of certain drugs.

General principles

Once the diagnosis of corticosteroid-responsive dermatosis has been made, a suitable local application must be chosen. The question of the base is dealt with elsewhere. In general it is wiser to start with a moderate- or low-potency corticosteroid [45] if the disease is not severe or not very active, in which case it is rational to use the weakest corticosteroid and then review the situation in a few days. The next move depends on the diagnosis. With acute contact dermatitis due to a removable antigen, no further therapy is required if the skin has been cleared. A more chronic disease such as atopic eczema, when there has been an acute exacerbation treated with a very potent topical corticosteroid, should be "titrated" slowly down, first to a corticosteroid in the next group down and then the next group and so on until the lowest-potency steroid group is reached that will maintain a reasonable level of skin activity. The patient should be instructed to apply the corticosteroid two or three times daily using a very thin coat. If the skin is very dry it is advisable to prescribe an emollient that may be applied more generously after the corticosteroid. In the special situation of pompholytic eczema of the palms and soles, soaking in warm saline for 10 min before application of the corticosteroid will enhance penetration and thus the clinical efficiency. Some dermatologists recommend soaking in a bath for 10 to 15 min before each application of the corticosteroid. Soap should be avoided and emollients used as soap substitutes with either of these techniques.

The use of plastic occlusion over an application of topical corticosteroid is probably less common nowadays with the more potent topical corticosteroids available. The technique is based on the resultant increase of percutaneous absorption [46,47]. Complications are frequent, the most common being secondary infection by staphylococci and *Candida albicans*. For this reason, corticosteroid antimicrobial mixtures are usually prescribed. Any area of the body can be occluded, and at the present time the most popular devices are bathing caps for covering corticosteroid on the scalp in psoriasis and gloves or plastic bags for hands and feet. It is important that all air is excluded from the surface and that tubular bandages are applied over the plastic. The dressings are normally left in place overnight and the patient showers or bathes using a soap substitute the following morning. Finally, corticosteroid-impregnated gauze bandages are valuable in the control of itching dermatoses, especially in children.

Intralesional corticosteroid therapy

The use of intralesional injections of hydrocortisone and triamcinolone has been widespread in the treatment of many diseases [48]. Generally favorable results have been reported, especially in chronic discoid lupus erythematosus, hypertrophic lichen planus, resistant local patches of psoriasis, lichen simplex, and granuloma annulare. Use of intralesional injections of hydrocortisone in keloid scarring, acne cysts, and sarcoidosis is also widely accepted [49]. In alopecia areata, tufts of regrowth may occur and give the patient a psychological boost. Variable reports of results in necrobiosis lipoidica have indicated that ulceration may become a problem, and in sarcoidosis the effects are quite unpredictable though the technique is always worth a trial. There is considerable controversy over the effect of periungual injection of corticosteroid in psoriasis of the nails, some claiming an 80 percent cure rate [50] but only if onycholysis is absent. Nowadays, triamcinolone acetonide is usually the drug of choice and most dermatologists use the needleless pressure jet injector which is much less painful and delivers approximately 0.1 ml per injection. Care must be taken not to exceed a total dose of 60 to 70 mg as adrenal suppression will result above this dose [51].

References

1. Vickers CFH, Tighe SM: Topical triamcinolone in eczema. *Br J Dermatol* **72**:352, 1960
2. Wilson L: The clinical assessment of topical corticosteroid activity. *Br J Dermatol* **94 (suppl 12)**:33, 1976
3. Anjo DM et al: Methods for predicting percutaneous absorption in man, in *Percutaneous Absorption of Steroids*, edited by P Mauvais Jarvais, CFH Vickers. London, Academic Press, 1980, p 185
4. McKenzie AW, Stoughton RB: Method for comparing percutaneous absorption of steroids. *Arch Dermatol* **86**:608, 1962
5. Scott M et al: Effect on plasma cortisol level and urinary cortisol excretion, in healthy volunteers, after application of three different topical steroid ointments under occlusion. *Acta Derm Venereol (Stockh)* **61**:543, 1981
6. Gorski J, Gannon F: Current models of hormone action. *Annu Rev Physiol* **38**:437, 1976
7. Marks R, Williams K: The action of topical corticosteroids on the epidermal cell cycle, in *Mechanisms of Topical Corticosteroid Activity*, edited by LC Wilson, R Marks. London, Churchill Livingstone, 1976, p 39
8. Altura BM, Altura BT: Effects of local anaesthetics, antihistamines and glucocorticosteroids on peripheral blood flow and vascular smooth muscle. *Anaesthesiology* **41**:197, 1974
9. Allison F et al: Studies on the pathogenesis of acute inflammation. *J Exp Med* **102**:669, 1955
10. MacGregor RR: Granulocyte adherence changes induced by hemodialysis, endotoxin, epinephrine and glucocorticoids. *Ann Intern Med* **86**:35, 1977
11. Hammarström S et al: Glucocorticoid in inflammatory proliferative skin disease reduces arachidonic and hydroxlyeicosatetraenoic acid. *Science* **197**:994, 1977
12. Malone T et al: Development and evaluation of ointment and cream vehicles for a new topical steroid, fluclorolone acetonide. *Br J Dermatol* **90**:187, 1974
13. Barry BW, Woodford R: Comparative bioavailability of proprietary topical corticosteroid preparations. Vasoconstrictor assays on 30 creams and gels. *Br J Dermatol* **91**:323, 1974
14. Fitzpatrick TB et al: Sodium retention and edema from percutaneous absorption of fludrocortisone acetate. *JAMA* **158**:1149, 1955
15. Cronin EA, Stoughton RB: Percutaneous absorption, regional variations and the effect of hydration and epidermal stripping. *Br J Dermatol* **74**:265, 1962

16. Sneddon IB: Atrophy of the skin. *Br J Dermatol* **94 (suppl 12)**:121, 1971

17. Himathongkam T et al: Florid Cushing's syndrome and hirsutism induced by desoximetasone. *JAMA* **239**:430, 1978

18. Scoggins RB, Kliman B: Percutaneous absorption of corticosteroids. *N Engl J Med* **273**:831, 1965

19. Munro DD: The effect of percutaneously absorbed steroids on hypothalamic-pituitary-adrenal function after intensive use in in-patients. *Br J Dermatol* **94 (suppl 12)**:67, 1976

20. Kirby JD, Munro DD: Steroid induced atrophy in an animal and human model. *Br J Dermatol* **94 (suppl 12)**:111, 1976

21. Scarborough J, Shuster S: Corticosteroid purpura. *Lancet* **1**:93, 1960

22. Frosch PJ et al: The Duhrung chamber test for assaying corticosteroid atrophy in humans, in *Percutaneous Absorption of Steroids*, edited by P Mauvais Jarvais, CFH Vickers. London, Academic Press, 1980

23. Ive FA, Marks R: Tinea incognito. *Br Med J* **111**:149, 1968

24. MacMillan AL: Unusual features of scabies associated with topical fluorinated steroids. *Br J Dermatol* **87**:496, 1972

25. Sneddon IB: Adverse effect of topical fluorinated corticosteroids in rosacea. *Br Med J* **1**:671, 1969

26. Sneddon IB: A trial of hydrocortisone butyrate in the treatment of rosacea and perioral dermatitis. *Br J Dermatol* **89**:505, 1973

27. Kestel JL Jr: Hypopigmentation following the use of Cordran tape. *Arch Dermatol* **103**:460, 1971

28. Tappenheimer J, Pfleger L: Gluteal granulomata. *Hautarzt* **22**:383, 1971

29. Baker H: Corticosteroids and pustular psoriasis. *Br J Dermatol* **94 (suppl 12)**:83, 1976·

30. Tyldesley WR, Harding SM: Betamethazone 17 valerate aerosol in the treatment of oral lichen planus. *Br J Dermatol* **96**:659, 1977

31. Leyden JJ, Kligman AM: The case for steroid antibiotic combinations. *Br J Dermatol* **96**:179, 1977

32. Feldman RJ, Maibach HI: Percutaneous penetration of hydrocortisone with urea. *Arch Dermatol* **109**:58, 1974

33. Sarkany I, Gaylarde PM: Effects of bases and accelerants on the anti-inflammatory activity of topical corticosteroids. *Dermatologica* **152 (suppl 1)**:81, 1976

34. Almeyda J, Burt BW: Double blind controlled study of treatment of atopic eczema with a preparation of hydrocortisone in a new drug delivery system versus betamethasone 17 valerate. *Br J Dermatol* **91**:579, 1974

35. Polano MK, Ponec M: Bioavailability and effects of various vehicles on percutaneous absorption, in *Percutaneous Absorption of Steroids*, edited by P Mauvais Jarvais, CFH Vickers. London, Academic Press, 1980

36. Mooney AF: Dilution of topical cortico-steroid formulations. *Br J Dermatol* **90**:109, 1974

37. Epstein S: Parabens sensitivity—subtle trouble. *Ann Allergy* **26**:185, 1968

38. Provost TT, Jilson OF: Ethylene diamine contact dermatitis. *Arch Dermatol* **96**:231, 1967

39. Shore RN, Shelley WB: Contact dermatitis from stearyl alcohol and propylene glycol in fluocinolide cream. *Arch Dermatol* **109**:397, 1974

40. Coskey RJ: Contact dermatitis due to clindamycin. *Arch Dermatol* **114**:115, 1978

41. Church RE: Sensitivity to hydrocortisone acetate ointment. *Br J Dermatol* **72**:341, 1960

42. Alan MD, Alan SD: Allergic contact dermatitis due to corticosteroids. *Ann Allergy* **30**:181, 1972

43. Comaish S: A case of hypersensitivity to corticosteroids. *Br J Dermatol* **81**:919, 1969

44. DuVivier A, Stoughton RB: Acute tolerance to effects of topical glucocorticosteroids. *Br J Dermatol* **94 (suppl 12)**:32, 1976

45. Vickers CFH et al: The use of topical steroids of differing potency in the management of the atopic child. *Br J Dermatol* **94 (suppl 12)**:129, 1976

46. Fritsch WC, Stoughton RB: The effect of temperature and humidity on percutaneous absorption. *J Invest Dermatol* **41**:307, 1963

47. Vickers CFH, Fritsch WC: A hazard of plastic film therapy. *Arch Dermatol* **87**:633, 1963

48. Verbov JL: The place of intralesional steroid therapy in dermatology. *Br J Dermatol* **94 (suppl 12)**:51, 1976

49. Scoggins RB: Decrease of urinary corticosteroids following local application of fluocinalone acetonide under an occlusive dressing. *J Invest Dermatol* **39**:473, 1962

50. Bleeker JJ: Intradermal triamcinolone acetonide treatment of psoriatic nail dystrophy with Port-o-Jet. *Br J Dermatol* **92**:479, 1975

51. McGugan AD, Shuster S: A hazard of intralesional steroid therapy. *J Invest Dermatol* **40**:271, 1963

CHAPTER 213

NONCORTICOSTEROID AGENTS

Christopher F. H. Vickers

Despite the long-time usage of many noncorticosteroid agents in dermatology, the mode of action of many of these classical remedies remains an enigma. In this chapter an attempt will be made to discuss most of the major agents and their mode of action, where known; such a discussion cannot be comprehensive, since dermatologists have a vast pharmacopeia.

Metals (Table 213-1)

Aluminum acetate as a 3% solution has long been used for its astringent effect [1] and is favored by some as a treatment for hyperhidrosis [2]. Its chloride and chlorhydrate form the basis for most of the OTC pharmaceutical antiperspirants which have been produced as lotions, aerosols,

Table 213-1 Various topical therapeutic agents in dermatology

Metals:
  Aluminum:
    Acetate
    Chloride
    Chlorhydrate
    Oxide
  Calcium hydroxide
  Lead acetate
  Magnesium:
    Oxide
    Sulfate
  Mercury:
    Ammoniated
    Biniodide
    Perchloride
  Potassium permanganate
  Selenium disulfide
  Silver:
    Nitrate
    Sulfadiazine
  Titanium dioxide
  Zinc oxide
Antipruritic, anti-inflammatory, antimicrobial, and keratolytic
    agents:
  Benzalkalonium
  Benzoic acid
  Benzoyl peroxide
  Benzyl benzoate
  Bufexamac
  Camphor
  Chlorhexidine
  Dyes:
    Gentian violet
    Brilliant green
  Ethyl lactate
  Formaldehyde
  Gamma benzene hexachloride
  Glutaraldehyde
  Hydrogen peroxide
  Hydroxy (alpha) acids
  Ichthammol
  Lactic acid
  Malic acid
  Menthol
  Monosulfram
  Phenol
  Resorcinol
  Salicyclic acid
  Sodium chloride
  Sulfur
  Tar
  Urea
  Undecylinic acid
  Vitamin A acid
Antipsoriatics:
  Allantoin
  Chrysarobin
  Dithranol
  Pyrogallic acid

and roll-ons. Aluminum oxide, like magnesium oxide, titanium dioxide, and zinc oxide, is used as an inert filler as well as in the preparation of certain sunscreens and shake lotions.

Lead acetate was often prescribed for its astringent and antipruritic effects. It is certainly a safe and soothing preparation and is a common dermatologic preparation in developing countries.

Magnesium sulfate 25% in a paste in glycerol is a very old remedy for the treatment of boils and carbuncles. It is relied on for its osmotic effects in loosening crusts and is of value in such conditions as acute paronychia, digital arterial occlusions in scleroderma, and similar problems.

Mercury salts, once extensively used in the treatment of psoriasis, impetigo, and other infections, have fallen into disrepute due to the nephrotoxic effects [3–5] following percutaneous absorption. Sensitization is also fairly frequent [6,7] and the only remaining salts in at all common use are the perchloride and biniodide added to many preparations for their astringent and antibacterial action.

Potassium permanganate is probably the most widely used astringent for its antibacterial effect on weeping and infected dermatoses. It is applied either in the form of wet dressings or as an addition to the bath.

Selenium disulfide is a beneficial agent in the control of dandruff though its use should be limited to fairly short periods, as brittleness of the hair may occur, possibly due to breakage of disulfide cross-bonds [8]. It is also commonly used as a twice-daily application, for seven days, in the treatment of tinea versicolor.

Silver nitrate 0.5% in aqueous solution is an extremely valuable lotion for the wet dressing of infected eczemas, gravitational ulcers, and indeed any weeping and/or infected skin lesions [9]. Its cosmetic disadvantages (staining the skin black) are outweighed by the rapid resolution of weeping and the control of superficial infection, often by resistant organisms. Forty percent silver nitrate in alcohol is helpful in the management of severe folliculitis.

Silver sulfadiazine, a recently introduced preparation, is valuable in the management of gravitational ulceration and burns. It has a good antistaphylococcal effect both prophylactically and therapeutically [10]. Sensitization is extremely rare, which is interesting in view of the frequent hypersensitivity to locally applied sulfonamide creams.

Various anti-inflammatory and antimicrobial agents
(Table 213-1)

Benzalkalonium as an antiseptic agent is also used as a 25% solution in the treatment of plantar warts.

Benzoic acid is one of the classic agents of dermatology, used in Whitfield's ointment, predominantly for the treatment of fungal infections. It also has a place in the management of hyperkeratotic conditions and, in smaller concentrations, in many preparations designed to loosen slough.

Benzoyl peroxide probably owes most of its action to the fact that it is a powerful oxidizer. It was originally a treatment for acne, but a recent development has been the use of higher concentrations (20% to 50%) in chronic gravitational ulceration and to clean slough in pressure and trophic ulcers. Its value as a comedolytic in acne [11,12] is well established and it is also effective as an antimicrobial against *Propionibacterium acnes.* Whether its action in reducing fatty acid content in sebum is secondary to its antimicrobial effect or primary is undecided [13]. Many preparations are available, but care needs to be exercised in the early stage of treatment as it is an irritant. Bleaching of skin and hair has also been reported [14,15]. Despite this, benzoyl peroxide preparations are the mainstay of topical therapy in acne vulgaris.

Benzyl benzoate, best known as a scabicide, also appears in low concentrations in several preparations for the management of diaper area eruptions.

Bufexamac (n-butoxyphenylacethydroxine acid) is the only nonsteroidal anti-inflammatory cream currently on the market. Its initial promise has not been borne out; irritation and sensitization are unacceptably high and its anti-inflammatory effect is low. One interesting fact is that it appears to act as a sunscreen in the UVA range.

Camphor has two uses: first, as an addition to shake lotions for its cooling and antipruritic effect, notably in urticaria and lichen planus; second, and for a similar reason, it is added to many chilblain preparations.

Menthol is used interchangeably with camphor and indeed the two are often combined in one preparation. The method of action of both drugs is probably due to an induced feeling of cold which competitively inhibits itching.

Chlorhexidine is chiefly an antimicrobial and is contained in some antidandruff shampoos.

Two dyes, *gentian violet* and *brilliant green* in aqueous solution, retain their place in dermatology for their astringent and antimicrobial (especially anticandidal) action. One new gel preparation for gravitational ulceration contains 1% brilliant green.

Formaldehyde solution 3% to 7% and gluteraldehyde 5% to 10% are beneficial in the treatment of warts, especially in children, as are lactic acid 2% to 10% and salicylic acid 5% to 10%.

Gamma benzene hexachloride, helpful as a scabicide, also has a place in the management of infestations and papular urticaria.

Hydrogen peroxide, 5 to 20 volumes, has been in wide use for many years as a cleansing agent to remove purulent debris; it has a distinct antibacterial effect and the effervescent quality helps loosen crusts and debris. Recently a 1.5% cream has become available which shows great promise in the management of gravitational ulceration and infected wounds.

Alpha hydroxy acids have interested dermatologists for their keratolytic effects for many years. Lactic, malic, and pyruvic acids in convenient bases have been shown to have a beneficial effect on ichthyosis and hyperkeratotic eczema [16]. Many proprietary preparations contain these solutions as well as salicylic acid, which is probably the most effective keratolytic in 5% to 40% concentrations in yellow or white soft paraffin.

Ichthammol is one of the time-honored traditional therapies in dermatology. It originates from shale oil which undergoes chemical degradation with ammonia and sulfuric acid to form a sulfur-rich substance. Only certain bases, usually containing glycerin, are suitable for formulations containing ichthammol. It is believed to have anti-inflammatory and vasoactive properties and has been a standard agent in the management of eczema (especially seborrheic) and rosacea and is used in a glycerol solution in the management of acute otitis externa where its soothing properties are legendary. There is little formal evidence of pharmacologic activity but its continued use is testimony to its

safety [17], patient acceptance, and the symptomatic relief it gives.

Lactic acid and *malic acid,* already mentioned for their keratolytic effect, have been employed in combinations in solutions in propylene glycol for the removal of slough from ulcers and wounds.

Monosulfuran is an effective antiparasitic agent that is used in the management of scabies and papular urticaria. It is the only such agent available in the form of a soap.

Resorcinol is mentioned only to be dismissed. Sensitization, irritation, and absorption leading to methemoglobinemia have caused it to be abandoned in the management of acne vulgaris. There are also many more effective agents available at present. It is still a constituent of Castellani's paint (magenta paint).

Salicylic acid is the oldest keratolytic known and can be used in concentrations of 0.5% to 60% in almost any base, although some emulsions are "cracked" by the addition of too high a concentration. Its widespread and prolonged use has been reported to give rise to salicylism, especially in children. Sensitization is unknown and irritation uncommon if care is taken to introduce low concentrations at first. It enhances percutaneous absorption of other agents in the same base and has been added to some topical corticosteroid preparations for this purpose. Its action on hyperplastic keratin is probably twofold: to decrease keratinocyte adhesion [18], and to increase water binding, thus hydrating the keratin [19]. Some reports have suggested a direct anti-inflammatory effect, though only equivalent to 0.1% hydrocortisone [20,21].

Sodium chloride has probably an even older place in dermatology than salicylic acid. The use of saline soaks to remove dressings, sloughs, crusts, and debris dates back to early medical history. Normal saline soaks still have the same part to play and are often of great value prior to the administration of topical corticosteroids to hand and foot eczema, although it is probably the hydration of the keratin that leads to enhanced penetration of the corticosteroid.

Sodium chloride 10% to 40% in a greasy base has been recommended in the management of hyperkeratotic and ichthyotic conditions and in the treatment of inoperable cutaneous carcinomas to reduce crust, slough, and unpleasant odors. It probably acts by attracting water to the keratin.

Salabrasion is a technique for removing either accidental or deliberate tattoos. Rough sodium chloride crystals are rubbed vigorously into the skin which has been previously infiltrated with local anesthetic. Occlusive dressings are applied and a vigorous inflammatory response is followed in favorable cases by the transepidermal elimination of the tattoo pigment. As an alternative to dermabrasion it offers certain attractions [22].

Sulfur, another time-honored remedy, is still extensively used in seborrheic conditions, in scabies (as a 10% ointment), and by some in acne; however, many experiments have now shown its comedogenicity [23]. Some authors doubt whether sulfur has any other than a placebo effect. In seborrheic conditions it is often combined with many other agents so that it is difficult to be certain whether any specific response can be said to result. Sensitization is rare and it is likely to continue in use. Sodium thiosulfate 20% solution is one choice in the management of widespread tinea versicolor, but, like selenium disulfide, it has tended to be displaced by the newer imidazole antifungals. In developing countries where cost is a consideration, it continues as one of the most effective remedies.

Tar. Most dermatologists when prescribing tar are thinking of crude coal tar but two other types need to be mentioned briefly. One, shale tar (ichthammol), has already been discussed above. Wood tars, of which only oil of cade has any widespread use outside Scandinavia, are obtained by distilling wood under controlled conditions. Oil of cade has a strong and distinctive odor. It can be added to arachis oil or simple bases as an application to the scalp in seborrheic eczema and psoriasis. Other wood tars are used in Scandinavia in similar fashion to oil of cade.

Coal tar is the product of distillation of coal during the production of gas. Very few such distilleries now exist in the Western world since the discovery of natural gas deposits. The thick black viscous fluid is a combination of at least 10,000 different chemicals and only about 4 to 5 percent of them have been identified [24], though these constitute the large majority by weight of the crude material.

One problem that exists in analyzing the active ingredients is that all coal tars are different depending on the source of the coal and the type and temperature of the distillation. The method by which crude coal tar exerts its influence is still not well understood.

Many confusing reports have appeared concerning different fractions of tars. Phenolic constituents have been suggested as lysosomal-release agents which stimulate mitosis—hardly the desired effect in psoriasis. Other extracts appear to produce acanthosis [25]. The coal tars and their actions remain one of the most intriguing and stimulating conundrums in dermatologic therapy. Many efforts have been made to produce cosmetically acceptable preparations and most have failed. Patient compliance is always difficult but therapeutic results in chronic eczema, especially atopic dermatitis, are gratifying. Tars are usually prescribed in ointment or paste bases and there are tar-impregnated bandages available that are very valuable in the management of childhood atopic eczema.

That tar is carcinogenic in animal experiments is beyond doubt [26]. Workers in the tar and pitch industry develop carcinomata, but there are very few reports of carcinomata resulting from the therapeutic use of crude coal tar to which hundreds of thousands of patients have been exposed in all parts of the world [27]. The few reports that exist suggest that carcinomata develop when tar is applied to the flexures.

Tar undoubtedly is phototoxic and tar undoubtedly induces phototoxic reactions in a number of patients who have used it for long periods [28], such as in the Goeckerman regime or in atopic eczema in childhood, photosensitivity appearing sometimes many years after discontinuation of therapy. This phototoxic reaction is the rationale for adding UV radiation to the Goeckerman regime, but recent studies have cast doubt on its value (see Chap. 131).

Urea is proteolytic at high concentrations (ca. 40%) and it has been used in aqueous solution in the management of black hairy tongue [29] and to remove nails affected by fungal infections or psoriasis. In the latter situation, the nail is isolated by occlusive collodion and 40% urea in a lanolin base is applied as an ointment. The whole is occluded for several days (P. D. Samman, personal communication). Urea has also been added to some topical cor-

ticosteroid preparations. Five to ten percent urea in various bases is commonly recommended in the management of ichthyosis but many patients experience burning.

Vitamin A acid (tretinoin). Vitamin A has long been known to profoundly affect the process of keratinization [30] but topical application of vitamin A, usually in a lotion, was without significant effect. In 1962 the application of topical vitamin A acid was first reported and has since found widespread use in acne in the form of a gel or solution at 0.025% to 0.5% [31–33]. Initially there may be redness and soreness of the skin but the comedones then start to extrude [34,35] and do not usually re-form if therapy is continued. It is one of the most successful local therapies in the modern antiacne armamentarium.

Ichthyosis vulgaris and lamellar ichthyosis have both benefited considerably from local use of vitamin A acid 0.1% in simple base [36].

Simplistically, it might be expected that as one of the actions of vitamin A acid is to induce a granular layer, it might benefit psoriasis, but this has not been shown in most published work [37]. Darier's disease occasionally responds dramatically but these results again are very variable [32]. Lichen planus, plane warts, and solar keratoses have also been treated with variable success. The benign, common keratosis pilaris often improves considerably although initial irritation is common [38,39].

The profound effect of vitamin A analogues on (1) keratinization, (2) epidermopoiesis, with the capability of restoring near-normal keratinization when that process is disorganized, (3) DNA synthesis, (4) lysosomal stabilization, and (5) prostaglandin synthesis has led to the uncovering of more potent derivatives, such as isotretinoin and 13-*cis*-retinoic acid.

Antipsoriatics (Table 213-1)

Allantoin (5-ureidohydantoin) derived from comfrey root has been synthesized and is used in various bases.

Chrysarobin is a derivative of the plant *Andira arobata* and a mixture of anthranols. It is still occasionally prescribed for patients who burn easily with dithranol, its synthetic analogue.

Dithranol, a mainstay of topical therapy in psoriasis, is a synthetic derivative of chrysarobin and it is used widely in many different bases, paints, pastes, and wax sticks. There are also special pomades for the scalp. It stains normal skin dark brown or black and for this reason as well as its irritation of normal skin it is usual to apply it in a base that remains where it is placed and does not spread over the surface of the skin. Dithranol in white soft paraffin is used, however, in the newly described short-contact therapy. Salicylic acid is added to many preparations to prevent oxidative processes leading to the production of an inactive anthrone.

The mode of action of dithranol is incompletely understood but it certainly inhibits glycolytic enzymes [40] and this may result from lipoid peroxidation [41].

Curiously, the inhibition of enzyme activity appears to be preceded by an acanthotic effect similar to that which is observed with tar [42]. DNA uptake is inhibited [43]. Glucose 6-phosphate dehydrogenase activity in human skin is also strongly inhibited by dithranol and less so by more cosmetically acceptable derivatives such as triacetoxyanthracene [44].

The mechanism of the staining has been extensively investigated but no full explanation has yet been offered. Attempts to prepare a dithranol derivative that does not stain skin have been so far unsuccessful.

Dithranol clearly acts by inhibiting mitosis though there is a contributing epidermopoietic stimulating effect.

Pyrogallic acid (1,2,3-trihydroxybenzene) has been utilized for many years in the treatment of psoriasis of the scalp, especially where scales are very thick. Patient compliance is apt to be rather low as the material tends to be very dark in color, the result of oxidative reduction.

Oils

Oils of many kinds are mainstays of dermatology mainly as bath additives (mineral oil). Coconut oil is the basis of some useful remedies for scalp psoriasis, especially in the presence of tar allergy and dithranol irritation. Sunflower seed oil has been shown to correct the results of essential fatty acid deficiency. Its clinical use in ichthyosis and atopic eczema has been disappointing.

Agents of doubtful usage

Finally, mention must be made of several agents that probably should no longer be used. *Topical anesthetics* are almost without exception (the sole safe agent being lignocaine [Brit] or lidocaine [USA]) sensitizers and should be avoided entirely. *Topical antihistamine* may have a transient antipruritic effect but sensitization is very common. *Boric acid,* once a common dermatologic preparation, has now been outlawed in view of the problems of neurotoxicity in children treated for diaper area eruptions with agents containing boric acid. Likewise, *hexachlorophene,* a very effective antimicrobial, has come under a cloud for the same reason. It is still used and as far as is known, is safe for adults.

References

1. Martindale W: *The Extra Pharmacopoeia.* London, Pharmaceutical Press, 1982, p 216
2. Shelley WB, Hurley HJ: Aluminum chloride in the treatment of hyperhidrosis. *Arch Dermatol* **111:**1004, 1975
3. Turk JL, Baker H: Nephrotic syndrome due to ammoniated mercury. *Br J Dermatol* **80:**623, 1968
4. Barr RD et al: Nephrotic syndrome in adult Africans in Nairobi. *Br Med J* **2:**131, 1972
5. Ross AT: Mercuric polyneuropathy with albumino-cytologic disassociation and eosinophilia. *JAMA* **188:**830, 1964
6. Epstein E: Allergy to dermatologic agents. *JAMA* **198:**517, 1966
7. Kligman AM: The identification of contact allergen by human assay. *J Invest Dermatol* **47:**393, 1966
8. Grover AW: Diffuse hair loss associated with selenium sulphide shampoo. *JAMA* **160:**1397, 1956
9. Cason JS, Lowbury EJL: Mortality and infection in extensively burned patients treated with silver nitrate compresses. *Lancet* **1:**651, 1968
10. Lowbury EJL et al: Topical chemoprophylaxis with silver sulphadiazine and silver nitrate chlorhexidine cream. Emergence of sulphadiazine resistant gram negative bacteria. *Br Med J* **1:**493, 1976
11. Vasarinsch P: Benzoyl peroxide versus sulphur lotion. *Arch Dermatol* **98:**183, 1968
12. Kirton V, Wilkinson D: Benzoyl peroxide in acne. *Practitioner* **204:**683, 1979
13. Fulton JE, Pablo G: Topical antibacterial therapy for acne. *Arch Dermatol* **110:**83, 1974
14. Bleiberg J et al: Bleaching of hair after use of topical benzoyl peroxide acne lotion. *Arch Dermatol* **108:**583, 1973
15. Bushkell LL: Bleaching by benzoyl peroxide. *Arch Dermatol* **110:**465, 1974
16. Swanbeck G: A new treatment of ichthyosis and other hyperkeratotic conditions. *Acta Derm Venereol (Stockh)* **48:**123, 1968
17. *Drug and Therapeutics Bulletin* **12:**102, 1974
18. Baden HP: A keratolytic gel containing salicylic acid in propylene glycol. *J Invest Dermatol* **61:**330, 1974
19. Huber C, Christophers E: Keratolytic effects of salicylic acid. *Arch Dermatol Res* **257:**293, 1977
20. Davies M, Marks R: Studies on the effect of salicylic acid on normal skin. *Br J Dermatol* **95:**187, 1976
21. Weirich EG et al: Dermatopharmacology of salicylic acid. *Dermatologica* **152:**87, 1976
22. Manchester GH: Tattoo removal: a new simple technique. *Calif Med* **118:**10, 1973
23. Mills OH, Kligman AM: Is sulphur helpful or harmful in acne? *Br J Dermatol* **86:**620, 1972
24. Frank HG: Coal tar constituents. *Indust Eng Chem* **55:**38, 1963
25. Wrench R, Britten AZ: Evaluation of coal tar fractions for use in psoriasiform diseases using the mouse tail test. *Br J Dermatol* **92:**569, 1975
26. Berenblum I: Liquor picis carbonis—carcinogenic agent. *Br Med J* **2:**601, 1948
27. Rook AJ et al: Squamous epithelioma possibly induced by therapeutic application of tar. *Br J Cancer* **10:**12, 1956
28. Kaidby KH, Kligman AM: Clinical and histological study of coal tar photosensitivity in humans. *Arch Dermatol* **112:**592, 1977
29. Pegum J: Urea in the treatment of black hairy tongue. *Br J Dermatol* **84:**602, 1971
30. Kligman AM et al: Acne therapy with tretinoin in combination with antibiotics. *Acta Derm Venereol (Stockh)* **55 (suppl 74):**111, 1975
31. Valles-Jones JC: Retinoic acid in the treatment of acne. *Practitioner* **213:**387, 1974
32. Günther S: Vitamin A acid in Darier's disease. *Acta Derm Venereol (Stockh)* **55 (suppl 74):**145, 1975
33. Stutgen C: The local handling of keratin by vitamin A ointments. *Dermatologica* **124:**65, 1962
34. Kligman AM et al: Topical vitamin A acid in acne vulgaris. *Arch Dermatol* **99:**469, 1969
35. Mills OH et al: Acne vulgaris. *Arch Dermatol* **106:**200, 1972
36. Peck GL: Treatment of lamellar ichthyosis and other keratinising disorders with oral synthetic retinoids. *Lancet* **2:**1172, 1977
37. Günther S: The therapeutic value of retinoic acid in chronic discoid, acute guttate and erythrodermic psoriasis: clinical observations in 25 patients. *Br J Dermatol* **89:**55, 1973
38. Goette DK: Keratosis pilaris clearing with topical vitamin A acid. *Acta Derm Vernereol (Stockh)* **55 (suppl 74):**146, 1975
39. Günther S: Use of topical retinoic acid. *Acta Derm Venereol (Stockh)* **55 (suppl 74):** 159, 1975
40. Rassner G: Enzymaktivitätshemmung in vitro durch Dithranol. *Arch Dermatol Forsch* **243:**47, 1972
41. Diezel W et al: Experiments concerning the mode of action of dithranol, increased lipid peroxidation and enzyme inhibition. *Dermatologica* **150:**154, 1975
42. Cox AJ, Watson W: Histological variations in lesions of psoriasis. *Arch Dermatol* **106:**503, 1972
43. Liden S, Michaelson G: Dithranol in psoriasis. *Br J Dermatol* **91:**447, 1974
44. Raab WP: Dithranol (Anthrolin) versus triacetoxyanthracene. *Br J Dermatol* **95:**193, 1976

CHAPTER 214

ANTIBACTERIAL AGENTS

David S. Feingold

Antibacterial agents can be divided into natural products, usually called antibiotics, and synthetic chemicals, which comprise most of the so-called antiseptics. Traditionally, topical antibiotics are used to prevent and treat skin and wound infections; antiseptics are used to decrease bacterial numbers on the skin or "degerm" the skin. This is an artificial distinction. We will use here the inclusive term topical antibacterial or antimicrobial agents.

Because rigorous clinical proof of efficacy is lacking for most topical antibacterial agents for most indications, conclusions expressed herein will be the opinion of the author based on theory, available data, and personal experience. Topical antifungal compounds will be discussed in Chap. 215. Disinfectants, antimicrobial compounds used on inanimate objects, will not be discussed.

The rationale for trying topical antibacterial agents is compelling. Compounds may be applied directly to the wound or infection. Hence, with a small amount of antibacterial preparation, very high local drug concentrations can be achieved. This broadens the spectrum of antibacterials and permits the use of compounds that might be too toxic if larger amounts or systemic medication were required. Finally the treatment of a wide range of pathogens and even mixed infections is theoretically possible since mixtures of antibacterials can be used; mixtures may also result in synergistic effects and may delay the selection of resistant organisms.

In Table 214-1 some of the uses of topical antibacterial agents are listed. In the following paragraphs these uses will be discussed and evaluated.

Degerming the skin

Topical antibacterials are effective at decreasing the number of bacteria on the skin [1]. Thus they are used to kill and prevent growth of pathogens on the skin when these may present problems. The ideal skin degerming agent has the following properties: broad antimicrobial spectrum; rapidly bactericidal; persistent activity on the skin; not

Table 214-1 Some uses for topical antibacterials

Degerming the skin:
  Hand cleaning
  Preparation of operative sites
  Prevention of recurrent skin infections
  Protection of susceptible hosts, e.g.,
    Immunosuppressed patients
    Newborns in nursery
Prophylaxis of clean wounds (first aid)
Treatment of burns
Treatment of skin infections
Treatment of acute dermatitis
Treatment of acne

irritating or allergenic or toxic; not absorbed into the circulation; active in presence of body fluids such as blood; cosmetically acceptable. No compound fulfills all of these criteria. For particular uses certain properties are more important. For repeated hand washings, as performed by surgeons and nurses, nonirritancy and persistance on the skin are essential criteria. For preparation of operative sites, rapid bactericidal effect is important. For skin degerming in impaired hosts, broad antimicrobial spectrum is essential. In newborns, a particularly nontoxic preparation is required.

Prophylaxis of clean wounds

When a wound results in a break in the continuity of the epidermis, an antibacterial agent is applied to prevent infection from developing. The wound may be accidental (abrasions, cuts, bites) or intentional (surgical wounds or IVs). For centuries, patients, their mothers, and their professional health advisors have employed favorite unctions for such wounds. In no case has any formulation been proved to help. Possibly no preparation ever will be rigorously proven effective for this purpose since so few clean wounds become infected that the number that must be studied to achieve significance, for even a very effective compound, is extremely large.

Although the efficacy of first-aid preparations is questionable, it seems clear they will continue to be used by us all. Thus the most important principle may be that the preparations do no harm. They should not be irritating or toxic. They should not be sensitizing. They should not apply selection pressure for the accumulation of bacterial strains with resistance to therapeutically important antimicrobial agents. The use of topical antimicrobials in superficial wounds makes sense. The right agents should be able to prevent contamination by pathogens of limited areas for a few days until the integrity of the epidermis is reestablished. The longer the epidermal barrier remains defective, the more likely infection is to occur. For example, chronic ulcers regularly become infected.

Treatment of burns

Infection kills burn patients who survive the initial acute fluid and electrolyte problems. Prevention of infection is extremely difficult since burn sites are favorable for bacterial overgrowth, the epidermal barrier is often defective for extended periods, and the patients are in hospital where multiple resistant organisms abound. Treatment tactics should be to debride the burn frequently and to establish the epidermis or a surrogate as fast as possible with skin grafts or the placement of skin substitutes. The use of topical antimicrobials to retard bacterial overgrowth in burn patients is well established but difficult to achieve. With large burned surfaces, systemic absorption of the antimicrobial must be minimal or the agent nontoxic. Another consideration in burn patients is that pain on application and removal of some compounds is often extreme. The antibacterial used in these patients must also remain effective in the presence of serum and necrotic debris.

Treatment of skin infections

Should topical antibacterials be used to treat impetigo? There are no adequate data to support use of topicals for impetigo. Systemic antibiotics do help, and they should be used to treat moderate to extensive impetigo. For limited impetigo one may opt not to use systemic antibiotics. In this instance one can argue for topicals, but with the goal of preventing spread of the infection to uninvolved skin. If the process spreads or does not begin to heal within a few days, then systemic antimicrobials are indicated.

Topical antibacterials have no role in the treatment of erysipelas, cellulitis, or furuncles. Erythrasma probably does respond to topicals.

Treatment of acute dermatitis

The numbers of *Staphylococcus aureus* are often very high on the skin involved with an acute dermatitis such as atopic dermatitis. Leyden and Kligman have argued persuasively that the high density of organisms results in the generation of "toxic" products which contribute further to the inflammation [2]. Since topical antibacterials can dramatically lower bacterial counts, the use of topical antibacterials as well as topical glucocorticoids is a logical treatment for acute dermatitis.

Treatment of acne

Topical antibacterials are helpful in the treatment of inflammatory acne [3]. The rationale and details of usage in acne are discussed in Chap. 67.

Major topical antibacterial compounds in use

Dozens if not hundreds of topical antibacterials are available. Some of those that are commonly used are listed in Table 214-2. Many are available in a variety of concentrations, vehicles, and mixtures. Some properties, advantages, and disadvantages will be discussed in the order listed in the table.

Alcohols are rapidly bactericidal but the action is transient and they are irritating, especially with repeated use or when applied to damaged skin. They should be restricted to preparation of operative or venipuncture sites.

Aluminum salts may have strong, broad-spectrum antibacterial as well as antifungal actions. Aluminum chloride hexahydrate (20%) as in Drysol is particularly effective and its drying properties make it ideal for treating macerated, mixed infections in intertriginous areas such as digit web spaces [4]. Six percent aluminum chloride hexahydrate (Xerac AC) may be effective against folliculitis, especially of the buttocks and thighs [5]. Aluminum diacetate (Burow's solution) in the recommended use concentrations is not an effective antibacterial.

Bacitracin, a polypeptide product of *Bacillus subtilis,* has a narrow action spectrum limited to gram-positive organisms. It is generally an effective bactericidal agent against the pathogens *S. aureus* and *Streptococcus pyogenes.* Unfortunately it is not stable in water-miscible formulation and thus is not a good choice when the occlusive properties of an ointment are undesirable. Hypersensitivity is rare. Bacitracin is often formulated in combination with neomycin and/or polymyxin B. Bacitracin ointment twice daily to the anterior nares may be helpful for nasal carriers of *S. aureus.* It is also frequently used on clean, small wounds to prevent infection.

Chlorhexadine is the most ideal agent for skin cleaning and surgical scrubs. It shares with hexachlorophene a remarkable persistence on the skin when used regularly. It is rapidly bactericidal, has a broad spectrum, shows little irritancy or allergy, remains active in body fluids, and is minimally absorbed. Logically, chlorhexidine is now widely used in hospitals and the community when it is important to decrease bacterial numbers on the skin. Chlorhexidine is available in a sudsing base and an isopropyl alcohol solution. Chlorhexidine as a first-aid cream would be an excellent addition to our formulary but this type of preparation is not available in the United States.

Clindamycin and *erythromycin* are antibiotics that effectively inhibit growth of most gram-positive bacteria. They are approved for topical treatment of inflammatory acne and available as 1% to 2% solutions in ethanol and propylene glycol. Clindamycin phosphate is not absorbed from the skin so antibiotic-associated colitis is not a risk.

Gentamicin cream is a controversial agent that has been

Table 214-2   Commonly used topical antibacterial agents

Agents	Some recommended uses
Alcohols	Preparation of surgical sites
Aluminum salts	Treatment of mixed, intertriginous infections
Bacitracin	Decrease *S. aureus* in nares; first-aid uses
Chlorhexidine	Skin degerming uses of all types
Clindamycin	Treatment of acne
Erythromycin	Treatment of acne
Gentamicin	Should not be used
Hexachlorophene	Limitation of *S. aureus* epidemics in nurseries
Iodophors	Skin degerming and first-aid uses
Neomycin	Decrease in bacterial numbers in acute dermatitis
Polymyxin B	Prevention of *Pseudomonas* infections
Silver sulfadiazine	Burns and first-aid uses

used most often for prophylaxis of burned skin; it has a broad gram-negative spectrum. The emergence of resistant strains and the occurrence of allergic sensitization have been associated with topical use of gentamicin. Since gentamicin and related aminoglycoside antibiotics are such important agents for systemic therapy of infections, topical gentamicin should not be used.

Hexachlorophene has lost favor as a skin degerming agent because it does not have a very effective gram-negative spectrum, and absorption with subsequent toxicity, especially in newborns, has been a concern. Use on small areas of the skin (e.g., the umbilicus of newborns) aimed at limiting spread of virulent *S. aureus* is acceptable.

Iodophors are organic complexes with iodine that slowly liberate iodine on reduction. They have a broad range of microbicidal activity. The disadvantages of the iodophors are that activity does not persist on the skin and they may be inactivated by body fluids. Iodophors, available in many vehicles, are widely used for preoperative skin preparation, hand scrubbing, and for treatment and prevention of skin infections.

Neomycin is the most widely used topical antibiotic in various combinations with other antibiotics and glucocorticoids. It is an aminoglycoside like gentamicin; it shares the broad gram-negative spectrum and the spotty gram-positive one. Most *S. aureus* are sensitive to neomycin. *S. pyogenes* is relatively resistant but at the high concentrations achieved on the skin these organisms also are probably killed by topical neomycin preparations. Allergic contact dermatitis does occur with neomycin. In North America there is a very high incidence of positive patch tests [6]. Sensitivity is most likely to occur with chronic usage on inflamed skin. The allergy may be manifest as a mild dermatitis and thus confused with the lesion being treated. The possibility of cross-sensitization to important systemic aminoglycosides is a worry although proof that this occurs is not available. Neomycin in its various combinations is used more than its properties can justify. The extensive use of neomycin in Mycolog cream (also containing nystatin and triamcinolone) cannot be condoned.

Polymyxin B, a cyclic polypeptide product of *B. polymyxin,* has an effective activity spectrum limited to gram-negative bacilli. Although some gram-negatives, notably *Proteus* and *Serratia* species, are resistant, *Pseudomonas aeruginosa* and other major hospital pathogens are sensitive. It is hard to justify the use of polymyxin B topically for *Pseudomonas,* however, since its activity is promptly neutralized by divalent cations at the concentrations found in body fluids.

Silver sulfadiazine is made by substituting one molecule of silver for the ionizable hydrogen atom in sulfadiazine. It has been used widely for prevention and treatment of wound sepsis in patients with second- and third-degree burns. It is a good agent for this purpose by dint of a broad microbicidal spectrum and the absence of the staining and electrolyte problems caused by silver nitrate. Its antimicrobial effect is not reversed by *p*-aminobenzoic acid or other metabolites that may be found in wounds or body fluids. It is rarely painful to apply or remove as is mafenide (Sulfamylon). Care must be taken since sulfadiazine blood levels are found when silver sulfadiazine is applied to large areas. This agent has many of the properties one would design into a first-aid cream and it deserves more extensive use.

Summary

Topical antibacterial compounds effectively reduce the colony counts of bacteria on the skin. Thus they may interrupt the spread of pathogenic bacteria, prevent infection of damaged skin or, less likely, help treat skin infections. Unfortunately, data supporting these contentions are meager. Since topical antibacterials will continue to be used we should foster use of those that do least harm and have the most potential to be effective. Chlorhexidine, silver sulfadiazine, and iodophors are agents that merit wide usage for many of the indications listed. Efficiency of the other agents is limited to narrow indications or not indicated.

References

1. Leyden JJ et al: Updated *in vivo* methods for evaluating topical antimicrobial agents on human skin. *J Invest Dermatol* **72**:165, 1979
2. Leyden JJ, Kligman AM: The case for steroid-antibiotic combinations. *Br J Dermatol* **96**:179, 1977
3. Melski JW, Arndt KA: Topical therapy for acne. *New Engl J Med* **302**:503, 1980
4. Leyden JJ, Kligman AM: Aluminum chloride in the treatment of symptomatic athlete's foot. *Arch Dermatol* **111**:1004, 1975
5. Shelley WB, Hurley HJ: Anhydrous formulation of aluminum chloride for chronic folliculitis. *JAMA* **244**:1956, 1980
6. Prystowsky SD et al: Allergic contact hypersensitivity to nickel, neomycin, ethylenediamine and benzocaine: relationships between age, sex, history of exposure, and reactivity to standard patch tests in a general population. *Arch Dermatol* **115**:959, 1979

ANTIFUNGAL AGENTS

Ernesto Gonzalez

Historical background

The specialty of mycology has the distinction of having laid the foundation of the field of infectious diseases with the discoveries of the thrush fungus by Langenbeck and the cause of favus by Schoenlein, both in 1839 [1]. Although great advances were made earlier in the identification and classification of fungi, the therapeutic approach to the superficial mycoses was limited to a few topical agents with a variable, albeit venerable, history of success. Most of the older topical preparations with low antifungal activity depended in large measure on their keratolytic effect to eradicate the fungus from its habitat in the stratum corneum. An important limiting factor among these preparations was their irritant effect, which limited their application to noninflammatory and nonocclusive areas.

With the introduction of griseofulvin in 1959 [2], the first oral antifungal agent for superficial mycoses, a new era in the treatment of these infections was begun. Although its impact was limited to dermatophyte infections, it had wide application to these conditions. It was effective against acute and chronic infections, with or without inflammation, and could eradicate dermatophytes from glabrous skin as well as from hair, where topical treatment was not beneficial.

The breakthrough to topical antifungal therapy, however, occurred in 1972 with the introduction of the first broad-spectrum agent, haloprogin [3]. Soon to follow, the imidazole group of topical and oral antimycotics revolutionized the therapeutic approach to superficial fungal infections by offering medications that were equally effective on all cutaneous mycoses without the irritant drawbacks of the older remedies. More importantly, it is now obvious that this extensive group of chemicals has been barely tapped, even though several of them are already on the market, and promise a future of more effective and safe topical, and probably oral, antifungal agents. Table 215-1 lists the most common topical antifungal agents available.

General principles of topical antifungal therapy

The topical treatment of fungal infections is confined to those that are classified as superficial, collectively called dermatomycoses. The three most important groups included in this division of mycology are tinea versicolor, candidiasis, and dermatophytosis. They probably constitute the most prevalent of all infectious diseases. According to a national health survey published in 1978 [5], for example, approximately 10 percent of the population in the United States was infected with these groups of fungi. In Europe, these fungal infections account for 4 to 8 percent of new outpatient referrals to dermatology clinics, while in certain parts of the tropics, where humidity and heat prevail, it is estimated that these infections account for 15 to 20 percent of new cases [6]. Therefore, the magnitude of this public health problem becomes apparent.

Some superficial fungal infections are not responsive to topical therapy and in those cases systemic treatment with or without topical treatment is indicated. Several factors influence the selection of topical antifungal agents over systemic therapy. The species of fungus, especially in the case of dermatophyte infections, establishes an important host–parasite relationship which can affect the response to therapy. Infections with *Trichophyton rubrum,* for example, are more chronic and recalcitrant to therapy, probably due to the inability of the host to mount an adequate inflammatory response to stimulate immunologic surveillance. In these cases, prolonged topical therapy and, sometimes, systemic therapy might be required to reduce the incidence of recurrences. Species that stimulate an inflammatory response by the host, e.g., *T. mentagrophytes,* on the other hand, will be more responsive to therapy.

The anatomic location of the infection, especially in the case of dermatophytes, is also a very important consideration in the choice of topical vs. systemic antifungal therapy. Characteristically, fungal infections involving the scalp, body, palms, and face are notoriously resistant to topical therapy alone and almost invariably will require a systemic approach. It should be borne in mind that dermatophyte infections are classified by anatomic areas since one species can produce different infections depending on the anatomic location and, conversely, many species can produce similar morphologic changes in the same anatomic area.

The severity and extent of infection constitute another factor in the selection of therapy. In tinea versicolor, for example, the amount of skin surface involved will determine the use of a cream vs. a lotion. Systemic therapy will be the treatment of choice in severe and extensive cases of dermatophyte and candidal infections.

Other factors that have a bearing on therapy are age, sex, habitus, occupation, and general health, with emphasis on the two most important environmental variables that optimize fungal growth—heat and humidity.

For the diagnosis and treatment of fungal infections of the skin, the character of host response to the different species and the anatomic site are the two most important considerations.

Dermatophyte infections

Topical agents

The newer broad-spectrum antifungal agents such as imidazoles and haloprogin have replaced some of the traditional remedies such as benzoic acid compound ointment

Table 215-1   Topical antifungal agents

	Available formulations	OTC	Relative cost* ($)	Comments	Irritation
Dermatophytosis					
Benzoic acid compound ointment (Whitfield's ointment)	Ointment	Yes	.83		Yes
Undecylenic acid	Ointment, powder	Yes	2.51 (.9 oz)		Mild
Tolnaftate	Cream, powder aerosol, solution	Yes	3.05		Rare
Candidiasis					
Polyenes:					
Nystatin	Ointment, powder	Yes	6.83		No
Amphotericin B	Lotion, ointment	No	8.70		No
Tinea versicolor					
Sodium thiosulfate	Lotion	Yes	5.75 (6 oz)		Mild
Selenium sulfide 2.5%	Shampoo, lotion	No	4.28 (6 oz)	Adjunctive for tinea capitis [4]	Mild
Dermatophytosis, candidiasis, and tinea versicolor					
Imidazoles:					
Miconazole	Cream, lotion	Yes	4.36		No
Clotrimazole	Cream, solution	No	4.26		No
Econazole	Cream	No	4.05		No
Haloprogin	Cream, solution	No	4.91		No
Ciclopirox olamine	Cream	No	4.25		No

* Cost to pharmacist for 15 g of cream unless otherwise noted.

(Whitfield's ointment), undecylenic acid ointment, and even tolnaftate. This is due in part to the fact that the broad-spectrum antifungals are effective for the three types of superficial mycoses and it is therefore not necessary to establish a diagnosis of the specific group before instituting therapy.

The new agents are not irritating and are cosmetically more acceptable than the traditional remedies. Interestingly, however, controlled studies show that some of the established medications, such as undecylenic acid, Whitfield's ointment, and more recently, tolnaftate, fared very well when compared to the newer broad-spectrum antifungal agents [7–9]. Even when these new broad-spectrum antifungal agents are cross-matched there is no evidence that one is more effective than another [10,11]. The consensus seems to indicate, however, that miconazole or clotrimazole are preferable to haloprogin [12].

In addition to clotrimazole and miconazole, marketed in England in 1973 and 1974 as the first imidazoles [13], a new imidazole, econazole has recently become available in the United States. It appears to be equal in effectiveness and safety to the previous imidazole preparations [14,15].

The mode of action of the imidazoles, like that of the polyene antibiotics, appears to involve alterations to the structure and thus the properties of the fungal cell membrane by inhibition of ergosterol synthesis which is essential for the integrity of the membrane, and the accumulation of lanosterol, a sterol intermediate that cannot support the growth of yeast in the absence of ergosterol [16,17]. This activity on the cell membrane by the imidazoles is less dependent on the sterol content than the similar effect by polyene antibiotics (e.g., amphotericin B). A more acute, lethal effect, independent of ergosterol synthesis, has been described in a laboratory model which indicates that the

imidazoles may have fungistatic and fungicidal effects depending on the concentration [17].

Ciclopirox olamine, which is chemically unrelated to the imidazoles or any other antifungal agent now used in the United States, is a hydroxypyridone with an in vitro activity against a wide variety of fungi, yeasts, and bacteria brought about by interfering with their metabolism [18]. Except for the possible effect on dermatophyte infection of the nails, its effectiveness and safety seem comparable to the imidazoles.

It is not within the scope of this chapter to discuss the individual merits of all of these studies, but it is apparent that, until controlled studies are carried out, definite conclusions as to the relative effectiveness of these medications cannot be made. Such studies will have to take into consideration percutaneous penetration of the vehicle, environmental factors, anatomic site, the species of fungus, host–parasite relationship, as well as adequate parameters to assess cure, reinfection, and relapse rates with more realistic treatment and follow-up courses. It would be simplistic, however, to conclude that the proliferation of these new topical antifungal agents has streamlined the therapeutic approach to fungal infections of the skin. Although it is a fact that an assortment of safe, effective, and cosmetically acceptable products are now available, it is also true that the newer medications are much more expensive, and it is therefore incumbent upon the physician to provide cost-effective treatment.

The dilemma for the practitioner, however, is not so much what type of topical agent to use, but when and where and for how long. It is now evident that systemic therapy is required to eradicate certain infections on glabrous skin as well as all dermatophyte infections of the hair and nails. Although no controlled data are available,

Table 215-2 Dermatophyte fungal infections

Type	Recommended therapy			Remarks
	Topical*	Oral	Maintenance†	
Tinea pedis:				
Webspace	3–4 weeks	No	Yes, topical	
Vesicular	Adjunctive	Yes	No	Topical therapy can be irritating
Diffuse-scaly	Adjunctive	Yes	Yes, topical	Keratolytics might be helpful‡
Tinea cruris	3–4 weeks	Extensive cases only	Yes, topical	Topical therapy might irritate scrotal skin
Tinea corporis:				
Acute, inflammatory	2–3 weeks	Extensive cases only	No	
Extensive chronic, scaly	No	Yes	Yes, oral	
Tinea manum	No	Yes	No	Adjunctive topical therapy can be used (keratolytic)‡
Tinea facei	No	Yes	No	
Tinea capitis	No	Yes	No	Selenium sulfide might reduce infectivity [4]
Tinea barbae	No	Yes	No	
Onychomycosis	No	Yes	±	Ciclopirox under occlusion might be effective
Majocchi's granuloma	No	Yes	No	

* Miconazole, clotrimazole, econazole, haloprogin, ciclopirox.
† Whitfield's ointment, undecylenic acid, tolnaftate.
‡ Whitfield's ointment, undecylenic ointment.

empirical observations suggest that the duration of therapy is variable and dependent not only on the species of the fungus and anatomic area but on other factors as well. The aim of this chapter, therefore, is to provide guidelines for the use of topical medications and for the duration of treatment.

Relapse or reinfection still remains the most important problem in the therapy of dermatophyte infection. The cause of this phenomenon has not been elucidated but it is probably dependent on the host–parasite relationship, since the emergence of resistant strains of dermatophytes during treatment with the imidazoles or other topical antifungal agents has never been reported [19].

Treatment based on site of infection

In general, it can be stated that topical therapy alone will eradicate lesions from glabrous skin, except in widespread and chronic infections, particularly those caused by *T. rubrum,* as well as the more severe types of granulomatous lesions produced by *T. verrucosum* and other fungi of animal origin, which require systemic therapy [19]. Systemic treatment, as mentioned previously, is essential for infections of nails and hair. Chronic, indolent dermatophyte infections tend to be extensive and more difficult to eradicate because of the host immune response to the pathogen [20]. Conversely, intense inflammatory dermatophyte infections are limited to small areas of the skin and can either remit spontaneously or respond to antifungal agents.

Ideally, the duration of topical antifungal therapy should continue until no clinical evidence of acute or chronic changes is evident, and should be confirmed by negative direct examination and/or culture. When laboratory facilities are not available, the treatment should continue for one to two weeks after all clinical evidence of infection has disappeared. In indolent, chronic infection of the feet and recurrent infection of the groin, maintenance therapy

with less expensive medications, e.g., undecylenic acid or tolnaftate, is recommended. Table 215-2 provides guidelines for duration of therapy according to the anatomic area. For oral therapy, refer to Chap. 181. As a rule, however, griseofulvin or ketoconazole should be used four to six weeks for infections of glabrous skin, six to eight weeks in tinea capitis [21], and longer than six months for onychomycosis. Recently, the adjunctive use of selenium sulfide shampoo or lotion 2.5% twice a week has been recommended to reduce the infectivity in children with tinea capitis produced by *T. tonsurans* [4].

Pityriasis (tinea) versicolor

This infection is produced by a normal inhabitant of the skin, *Pityrosporum orbiculare,* when it changes from its saprophytic yeast form to its pathogenic mycelial form [22]. The predisposing factors for the metamorphosis of this organism are not well understood but seem to include endogenous and exogenous factors. Production of lymphokines [23], genetic factors, nutrition, and hyperhidrosis are considered important endogenous factors [24]. Heat and humidity as well as the use of lipid-containing topical preparations seem to enhance the growth of the pathogenic phase of this fungus. Although it is considered to be the most superficial of the dermatomycoses, *P. orbiculare* is found not only in the stratum corneum but also intracellularly, in the viable epidermal cell layers, and it seems to induce an inflammatory infiltrate in the dermis [25]. The interplay of all these factors may explain the chronicity of this disease and its high incidence of relapse.

Treatment

The treatment of tinea versicolor should be topical and, until a safe oral antifungal agent is developed, the use of oral antifungal agents (e.g., ketoconazole) is not recommended. Although most of the old remedies with keratolytic activity and the newer broad-spectrum agents can be used, the present standard treatment is selenium sulfide 2.5% shampoo or lotion or zinc pyrithone shampoo. With the aid of a Wood's lamp, the areas of hypopigmentation and/or fluorescence should be identified for the patient so that all affected areas can be treated. Otherwise the medication should be applied to the glabrous skin surface, avoiding the face and intertriginous areas, including forearms and thighs. Two methods of application have been described: weekly overnight application for two weeks [26] or 30- to 45-min daily application for two weeks. The author prefers the second method because irritation is reduced. Relapse rates are about 50 percent after one year [26] and, therefore, re-treatment at periodic intervals is recommended. The use of imidazole creams is advised for the face and intertriginous areas to prevent irritation.

Candidiasis (see Chap. 181)

Candida albicans is a member of the normal flora of the alimentary tract in humans and, although not a regular member of the cutaneous microflora, it can be carried in the skin of healthy adults in tropical climates where heat and humidity induce maceration of intertriginous regions. Under certain conditions where the host characteristics are altered, *C. albicans* undergoes a metamorphosis similar to *P. orbiculare,* changing from the saprophytic yeast form to a pathogenic mycelial state. Predisposing factors for this opportunistic fungus to become a pathogen include: local events that can alter the cutaneous barrier, e.g., occlusion, topical medication; alteration of gastrointestinal flora, e.g., oral antibiotics; and systemic factors that can alter the host–parasite relationship, e.g., cancer, pregnancy, immunosuppressants. The management of superficial candidiasis, therefore, consists of specific anticandidal chemotherapy as well as the control of predisposing factors. As with dermatophytosis, superficial candidiasis presents as a spectrum of clinical entities that require individualized treatment according to anatomic location and host–parasite interaction.

Topical therapy specific for candidiasis includes four groups of medications: the polyene antibiotics which include nystatin and amphotericin B, the imidazole group (clotrimazole, miconazole, and econazole), haloprogin, and more recently, ciclopirox olamine. The polyene group has a narrow spectrum of activity and both medications seem to be equally effective against *C. albicans.* The other three groups are broad-spectrum antifungal agents that are effective against all superficial mycoses as well as bacteria. Since not infrequently gram-negative bacteria act as co-pathogens in superficial candidiasis, the broad-spectrum agents are preferred to the polyenes. Controlled studies, however, have not shown any advantage of haloprogin and the imidazoles over nystatin in the treatment of candidiasis [7,8,27]. It also appears that there is no significant difference in effectiveness among the different imidazoles [10]. As with the dermatophytes, there is no evidence of natural resistance to any of these drugs by *C. albicans.*

Drying agents such as gentian violet, Castellani's paint, and aluminum chloride 20% to 30% have limited application because of their irritant effect, discoloration of the skin, and low efficiency in eradicating *C. albicans.* The same drawbacks apply to the quinolines such as iodochlorhydroxyquin except that the irritant effect is minimal.

Treatment based on site of infection

The naturally occluded areas of the perineum, interdigital spaces of the toes and third space of the hands, the axillae, and inframammary regions are most prone to develop candidiasis. The basic prerequisite for yeast overgrowth, namely humidity and maceration, should be controlled by drying out these surfaces with adequate ventilation or the use of a non-starch-containing, absorbent powder. The application of one of the polyene or imidazole group of medications in a cream formulation twice a day for two to three weeks is usually adequate. Talcum or a medicated powder can be used prophylactically after a bath or shower to prevent recurrences, especially during hot and humid weather. Hygiene is important, especially in cases of perineal infections, and the patients should be instructed to avoid seeding the perineal region with feces to avoid *C. albicans* colonization. If relapses are frequent, a course of oral treatment with polyenes (nystatin) or an imidazole (ketoconazole) might be advisable to reduce overgrowth of *C. albicans* in the gut.

Chronic paronychia as a manifestation of candidiasis is normally treated with topical medications, in contrast to onychomycosis where topical therapy is ineffective. It is a therapeutic challenge because of the inability of the patient to avoid exposure to humidity and trauma, the major predisposing factors, and because of the relative inaccessibility of the nail fold to receive an adequate concentration of the antifungal medication. The use of thymol 4% to 5% in chloroform or alcohol or the immersion of the affected finger in alcohol for several minutes are helpful measures to reduce the moisture content of the affected area. Liquid preparations of polyene or imidazole will enhance penetration of the antifungal agent by capillary diffusion into the nail fold. This medication, preceded by the drying agent, should be applied several times a day for at least two months. Compliance, therefore, is poor and relapses frequent. The use of oral imidazole (ketoconazole) should be limited to severe cases with multiple nail involvements because of possible side effects.

Chronic mucocutaneous candidiasis presents another therapeutic challenge since immunologic unresponsiveness on the part of the host is almost invariable. Topical therapy is usually ineffective and this syndrome is probably the best indication for the use of ketoconazole orally. Oral treatment with polyene (nystatin) and less frequently, ketoconazole, is also indicated for oral candidiasis.

Future of topical antifungal agents

The discovery of the imidazoles as a broad-spectrum, effective, and relatively safe group of antifungal agents has inaugurated a new and exciting field in medical mycology. Their therapeutic impact, with the diversity of topical and oral derivatives, has not yet been fully researched but promises to be rewarding in the future. Recently, a new imidazole, terconazole, was reported to be superior to clotrimazole in controlled laboratory conditions [28]. The ideal antifungal agent that could eradicate cutaneous and systemic fungal infections by both topical and oral routes with no major side effects may not be an unreachable goal. Unbiased, controlled evaluations of these new products should be encouraged to avoid unnecessary and costly proliferation of new chemicals that add to the confusion of the practitioner and the patient.

References

1. Baum GL: Antifungal therapy, 1978. *Postgrad Med J* **55:**587, 1979
2. Blank H et al: Treatment of dermatomycoses with orally administered griseofulvin. *Arch Dermatol* **79:**259, 1959
3. Herman HW: Clinical efficacy studies of haloprogin, a new topical antimicrobial agent. *Arch Dermatol* **106:**839, 1972
4. Allen HB et al: Selenium sulfide: adjunctive therapy for tinea capitis. *Pediatrics* **69:**81, 1982
5. National Health Survey: *Skin conditions and Related Need for Medical Care Among Persons 1–74 Years. United States 1971–1974.* DHEW Publication No (PHS) 79–1660. Hyattsville, MD, United States Department of Health, Education and Welfare (Public Health Service), National Center for Health Statistics, November 1978
6. Hay RJ: Treatment of superficial fungal infections. *Clin Exp Dermatol* **6:**509, 1981
7. Clayton YM, Connor BL: Comparison of clotrimazole cream, Whitfield's ointment and nystatin ointment for topical treatment of ringworm infections, pityriasis versicolor, erythrasma and candidiasis. *Br J Dermatol* **89:**297, 1973
8. Comaish JS: Double-blind comparison of clotrimazole with Whitfield's and nystatin ointments. *Postgrad Med J* **50(suppl):**73, 1974
9. Keczkes K et al: Topical treatment of dermatophytoses and candidoses. *Practitioner* **214:**412, 1975
10. Clayton IM, Knight AG: A clinical double-blind trial of topical miconazole and clotrimazole against superficial fungal infections and erythrasma. *Clin Exp Dermatol* **1:**225, 1976
11. Clayton IM et al: A clinical double-blind trial of topical hal-

oprogin and miconazole against superficial fungal infections. *Clin Exp Dermatol* **4:**65, 1979
12. *Med Lett Drugs Ther* **18(24),** Nov 19, 1976
13. Milne JLR: The antifungal imidazoles: clotrimazole and miconazole. *Scott Med J* **23:**149, 1978
14. Fredricksson T: Treatment of dermatomycoses with topical econazole and clotrimazole. *Curr Ther Res* **25:**590, 1979
15. MacKie RM: Topical econazole in cutaneous fungal infections. *Practitioner* **224:**1311, 1980
16. Holt JR: Topical pharmacology of imidazole antifungals. *J Cutan Pathol* **3:**45, 1976
17. Sud IJ, Feingold DS: Mechanisms of action of the antimycotic imidazoles. *J Invest Dermatol* **76:**438, 1981
18. *Med Lett Drugs Ther* **25(647),** Oct 28, 1983
19. Clayton IM: Dermatophyte infections. *Postgrad Med J* **55:**605, 1979
20. Jones HE: Therapy of superficial fungal infection. *Med Clin North Am* **66:**873, 1982
21. Krowchuk DP et al: Current status of the identification and management of tinea capitis. *Pediatrics* **69:**81, 1983
22. Feagerman J, Fredricksson T: Tinea versicolor: some new aspects on etiology, pathogenesis, and treatment. *Int J Dermatol* **21:**8, 1982
23. Sohnle PG, Collins-Lech C: Cell mediated immunity to *Pityrosporum orbiculare* in tinea versicolor. *J Clin Invest* **62:**45, 1978
24. Burke RC: Tinea versicolor: susceptibility factors and experimental infections in human beings. *J Invest Dermatol* **36:**389, 1961
25. Montes LF: Systemic abnormalities and intracellular site of infections of the stratum corneum. *JAMA* **213:**1469, 1970
26. Roberts SOB: Treatment of superficial and cutaneous mycoses, in *Antifungal Chemotherapy,* edited by DCE Speller. New York, John Wiley & Sons, 1980, p 259
27. Carter VH, Olansky S: Haloprogin and nystatin therapy for cutaneous candidiasis. Comparison of the efficacy of haloprogin and nystatin therapy. *Arch Dermatol* **110:**81, 1974
28. Van Cutsem J et al: Terconazole—a new broad spectrum antifungal. *Chemotherapy* **29:**322, 1983

CHAPTER 216

DERMATOLOGIC SURGERY: MICROSCOPICALLY CONTROLLED SURGICAL EXCISION (THE MOHS TECHNIQUE)

Jessica Fewkes and Frederic E. Mohs

Microscopically controlled surgery in the treatment of nonmelanoma skin cancer

Definition

Mohs micrographic surgery is the official nomenclature recently adopted by the American College of Chemosurgery for the surgical technique developed by Mohs to treat certain cutaneous tumors. The technique consists of the excision of successive layers of the involved tissue with frozen section examination of the entire undersurface of each layer for precise histographic control. These factors are responsible for its unique ability to follow any contiguously spreading lesion to tumor-free margins regardless of shape, size, depth, or invasion of bone or cartilage. Many synonyms for the technique survive such as chemosurgery: fixed tissue technique, chemosurgery: fresh tissue technique, microscopically controlled surgery, microcontrolled surgery, Mohs microscopic surgery, Mohs histographic surgery, Mohs technique, Mohs surgery, and the acronym MOHS (microscopically oriented histographic surgery) [1]. The official name will be used exclusively in this chapter.

Historical aspects

While a medical student, Mohs was experimenting with the injection of irritants into normal and cancerous tissues of rats to compare the leukocytic reaction in the two tissues. One of the chemicals was a 20% solution of zinc chloride which inadvertently was of a strength sufficient to produce necrosis rather than just irritation. When the tissue was removed, Mohs noted the excellent preservation of the microscopic features of the specimen; thus evolved the idea of applying the chemical to a cancerous growth which fixes it in situ and then removing the cancer for immediate microscopic examination. This resulted in the publication of Mohs' fixed tissue technique for tumor extirpation [2–4]. In 1953, a modification, the fresh tissue technique, was inaugurated by Mohs mainly for cancers on the eyelid margins, where swelling and discomfort from the action of the zinc chloride was a particular disadvantage; also described was its use for small cancers in other sites [3]. Beginning in 1958 the fresh tissue technique for the treatment of eyelid cancer was described in numerous presentations and articles [5–9]. A significant impetus to the more widespread use of the fresh tissue technique was a paper on its use in 75 cases of skin cancer presented by Dr. Theodore Tromovitch at the 1970 meeting of the American College of Chemosurgery. In subsequent years, the fresh tissue technique came to be used for almost all cutaneous carcinomas regardless of size or location, and the statistics showed the same high, long-term cure rates as the fixed tissue technique [10,11]. These favorable results were not surprising since the same complete microscopic control of excision was achieved by both techniques. Most Mohs surgeons today use the fresh tissue technique exclusively, but Mohs and some of his trainees [12] still find the fixed tissue technique advantageous in certain complicated, far-advanced cancers following bony structures, for penile cancers invading the erectile tissues, and for melanomas. The technique of Mohs surgery has proved itself to be a tremendous advantage in the removal of many skin lesions. It provides the highest cure rates for recurrent tumors and it conserves the maximum amount of normal tissue as it creates a tumor-free defect [13]. There are now over 100 members of the American College of Chemosurgery and a chemosurgeon in most major teaching hospitals. The technique is well recognized as a major modality used for the treatment of selected skin cancers.

Methods

Fixed tissue technique. The original Mohs technique involved the application of a 40% zinc chloride paste [2–4,14,15]. The lesion is first prepared with a keratolytic agent, dichloracetic acid; this penetrates any stratum corneum overlying it that may act as a barrier to the paste. Then the chemical fixative is applied to the lesion and to a narrow rim of clinically normal skin. The thickness of the application and the length of time it remains on the skin surface will determine the depth of penetration of the zinc chloride. These variables are used to adjust the tech-

nique to the different areas of the skin and the different types of neoplasms on which it is used. An occlusive dressing is then placed. When the appropriate amount of time has elapsed, the tissue is excised. The histographic technique of examining the fixed tissue as described below is then performed. If the tumor is found in an area, the fixative is reapplied just to that spot, and the whole procedure is repeated until a tumor-free plane is reached.

The advantage of the zinc chloride is its ability to fix the tissue in situ causing relatively little pain and bleeding at the time of removal. Since the tissue is fixed at the time of removal, no implantation of tumor cells can occur during excision. Its disadvantages include the discomfort, which may require analgesia, resulting from the inflammation and swelling in the area due to the necrosis of the tissue. The time the fixative is permitted to act may range from 10 min to 48 h depending on the depth of penetration desired and convenience of scheduling. With small lesions, two or three fixation–excision sequences can be completed in one day as an outpatient procedure, but some extensive lesions may require several days and occasionally require hospitalization [4].

After a tumor-free plane has been reached, the final layer of fixed tissue is allowed to separate naturally, and most defects are allowed to heal by granulation and epithelialization. This obviates frequent follow-up visits and further surgery. It has also provided a wealth of information regarding wound healing. In many cases, and certainly for many elderly, who comprise the majority of these patients, spontaneous granulation provides an excellent alternative to surgical repair. For large tumors, aggressive reconstruction is often delayed for 12 months following removal of the tumor to facilitate surveillance and treatments to the area. Granulation does not interfere with this yet covers the defect [15–17].

Fresh tissue technique (Fig. 216-1). The fresh tissue technique was originally used mainly for lesions on the eyelid margins where the zinc chloride fixative was poorly tolerated. In the early 1970s, the technique was adapted to all other areas and became the method that most Mohs surgeons use today [18].

The area is first anesthetized by local infiltration or field block with injectable lidocaine. The tumor is then debulked using a sharp curette or scalpel. This removes excess tissue and gives a truer definition of the margins of the lesion. Then a saucer-shaped excision of the cancer-containing tissue is performed including in it a narrow rim of clinically normal-appearing skin. This is accomplished by angling the scalpel at 45° to cut the sides of the piece of tissue and a single flat plane for the bottom. These are critical features of this step.

A unique feature of Mohs surgery is its histographic control. At the time of tissue removal, several steps are taken to ensure proper orientation of the excised piece in relation to the surface from which it was removed. Before the piece of tissue is completely taken off, landmarks are made on the excised tissue and on the surrounding skin at corresponding points using a scalpel or a dye. A map is drawn to show the tissue and the landmarks and their location in relation to the area of the body from which it was taken.

The tissue is then cut into manageable-sized pieces.

Fig. 216-1 Schematic representation of the technique of Mohs surgery. (Courtesy of Neil A. Swanson, M.D.)

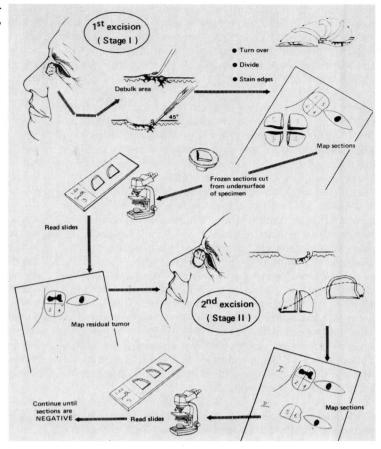

Each piece is individually marked with dye to designate right and left, superior and inferior. Each is flattened and frozen; horizontally cut sections are prepared and stained; and then each is examined under the microscope. Because of the 45° angle of the site and the flat bottom of the piece of tissue that is removed from the patient, when the tissue is flattened in the cryostat, all of its undersurface (that which was in closest contact with the patient) is accessible to examination. No areas are "sampled," that is, having only a portion examined. The entire undersurface and sides of the excised piece are carefully examined under the microscope. If tumor is found in a portion of the tissue, and the tumor does not have skip areas, it is assumed that the tumor has been transected during its removal, and *at that site,* there must be more tumor. If no more tumor is found in the piece of tissue, then all has been excised. Because of the histographic control, any tumor cells that are identified on a slide can be precisely located on the map and, therefore, also on the patient. The next step, then, is to excise only those areas in which tumor has been found and not disturb the rest of the defect. The entire procedure as outlined above is then repeated until no tumor is found on any slide. The main advantage of this technique is its complete removal of a tumor while preserving the maximum amount of surrounding normal tissue. This may be critical if the tumor is periorbital, on a digit, on the penis, or on the nasal tip.

The technique is usually performed on an outpatient basis as it requires only local anesthesia and usually can be accomplished, with the fresh tissue technique, in one day. This obviates hospitalization and general anesthesia, and allows the patient to come from long distances and go home the same day. Since such excellent cure rates have been found with this technique, it is also possible to immediately repair defects created by removal of a neoplasm by Mohs micrographic surgery [19]. Thus extirpation of a tumor and its repair may be done in one day, saving the patient multiple trips to the hospital. Because the wounds made by this technique using either fixed or fresh tissue are clean, they are often left to heal by secondary intention. For many patients this may be preferable because there is no need for further surgery or trips to the hospital for removal of sutures. For large lesions or extremely aggressive tumors, granulation tissue will not cover or bury recurrences, allowing early detection. Scar revision is always possible at a later date should the resultant scar be unacceptable to the patient. However, in certain anatomic locations, such as the lips, the eyelids, and the nasal rim, immediate repair is often preferable to prevent distortion [19].

Indications for use

Mohs micrographic surgery is now accepted as the treatment of choice for many cutaneous carcinomas. There are approximately 400,000 nonmelanoma skin cancers occurring each year in the United States [20]. Eighty percent are on the head and neck area [21]. They are mostly basal cell carcinomas and squamous cell carcinomas. Conventional modalities, excisional surgery, cryosurgery, electrodesiccation and curettage, and radiation therapy can cure skin cancers in 80 to 92 percent of cases [14,22,23]. That leaves approximately 40 to 80 thousand tumors per year requiring additional therapy. If the tumor falls into one of the following categories, then Mohs is the procedure of choice.

Recurrent tumors. Mohs micrographic surgery found its first major application in the extirpation of recurrent tumors. Recurrent tumors have had unacceptable cure rates, approximately 50 percent, when treated with conventional modalities [24]. Mohs micrographic surgery has shown a 97 percent cure rate for these tumors [4,14,18,25]. The reason lies in its ability to visually trace all silent tumor extensions which may be encased in scar tissue, invisible to clinical examination. Basal cell carcinoma extends in the direction of least resistance and invades between or into plates of cartilage or embryonic fusion planes, travels along perineural or perivascular sheaths [26], skims along periosteum and perichondrium or over the tarsal plate to conjunctival mucosa, but may also invade these structures [27,28]. This technique can follow the neoplasm into all areas, sacrificing only involved tissue and preserving the vital structures next to but not invaded by it. It may give a very discouraged patient the first substantial tumor-free period in years. This encourages patients to keep follow-up appointments, which may make a critical difference in early detection of recurrences.

Critical locations. Since 80 percent of skin tumors occur on the head and neck region [21], there is a high probability that they will be located in or adjacent to an important structure such as the eye [29], nose, or vermilion border of the lip. In these areas, conservation of the maximum amount of normal tissue is important to minimize distortion and dysfunction of the area involved and ensure good cosmetic results [30]. Thus, Mohs micrographic surgery may be the therapy of choice for a primary as well as a recurrent lesion in these areas. With the low probability of recurrence when utilizing this technique, such locations can be repaired immediately after surgery. For eyelids and lips where wound contraction during healing can cause distortion, it is a very important aspect in the selection of treatment modality. For lesions overlying the facial nerve, stepwise conservative removal and examination of tissue may prevent injury to this vital structure, sacrificing neural tissue only when it is already involved by the tumor. The locations that have the highest recurrence rates as noted below are the locations where growth patterns of the neoplasm render it inaccessible except to excision with the Mohs technique [15].

Areas of high recurrence. Specific areas of the face have been noted to have high recurrence rates of basal cell and squamous cell carcinomas. These include the postauricular sulcus, inner canthi, scalp [31,32], the ear [33], the junction of the nasal ala and the nasal labial fold, the nose, and the forehead [22,23]. Part of the reason is that these areas present difficulties for conventional treatment modalities. Areas with cartilaginous support allow perichondrial extensions of tumor which are very hard to pick up and eradicate with techniques other than Mohs micrographic surgery. The areas at the junction of the nasal ala and the

nasal labial fold and the postauricular sulcus and periauricular skin allow intercalation of tumor between embryonic fusion planes and very deep penetration of what appear to be small papular lesions [34,35]. The forehead has a high incidence of morpheaform tumors which often extend far beyond their clinical borders, and basal or squamous cell carcinomas which extend along the supraorbital nerve sheath gaining access to the brain via the foramen. They may also travel in the fascial planes on the temples [36]. These tumors can be devastating, but if found early and traced with this technique, it is possible to greatly reduce morbidity and mortality. Treatment of recurrent tumors by Mohs micrographic surgery has resulted in excellent cure rates of 97 percent.

Aggressive tumors. There are many tumors that fall into this category either by their locations in the mid face [37], over embryonic fusion planes (especially the postauricular sulcus or tragus [33]), at the nasal labial fold junction with the nasal ala; or by rapid growth; or by their duration [34]. Tumors that occur in young people who have no stigmata of syndromes involving increased incidence of skin carcinomas may also be very aggressive and need to be treated accordingly. Squamous cell carcinomas occurring on or around the auricle have a high rate of recurrence and metastasis. Their initial treatment with this technique and ascertainment of extension into the parotid or lymph glands may be critical for the patient's survival. Patients with the basal cell nevus syndrome may have many tumors over their lifetime and conservation of the maximum amount of tissue is very important [38].

Histology of neoplasm. As more cancers are treated by Mohs micrographic surgery, the correlation of the histology and growth patterns of a tumor is evident to the chemosurgeon at the time of surgery. Different histologic types and different areas are being identified as behaving more aggressively than a nonmetastasizing, slow-growing, non-invasive basal cell carcinoma. A particularly aggressive type is the metatypical basal cell carcinoma, which has a higher than usual degree of recurrence and invasion and perhaps also metastasis [39,40]. This requires an equally aggressive method for its removal.

Morpheaform or sclerosing basal cell carcinoma has a higher recurrence rate than other basal cell carcinomas [27]. It may send long silent extensions into areas beyond the clinically apparent margins [28]. Microcystic adnexal carcinoma may cause minimal epidermal changes, but invades deeply into bone and cartilage and may travel along nerves [41]. Sebaceous carcinomas have been reported to have skip areas, have a high recurrence rate, and the most aggressive are located on eyelids. Squamous cell carcinomas can be very aggressive tumors on the head. Knowing these characteristics, the Mohs surgeon is able to apply his/her skills and technique to provide the best management of these neoplasms.

Large tumors. With very large tumors, when they occur on the head and neck, the Mohs technique provides very important maximum conservation of surrounding tissues. These tumors are very difficult to eradicate. It has been shown that even utilizing the Mohs technique, tumors over 2 cm in size have a lower cure rate than those that are under 2 cm in diameter [4,25,32]. Thus, it is critical to manage early and with the appropriate modality tumors that are rapidly growing or close to 2 cm at the time of detection. Repair following removal of large tumors by Mohs micrographic surgery is usually delayed in order to avoid complicated reconstructive surgery that covers a possible recurrence and prevents early detection [17]. Follow-up for these, and for any patient with a cutaneous neoplasm, is essential to his/her care and may prevent many difficult tumors from ever occurring.

Poorly defined borders. If there is doubt as to the clinical size of a tumor, and it falls into any of the locations noted above, then it should be treated with Mohs micrographic surgery. Large tumors and morpheaform basal cell carcinomas, tumors in scars, and tumors on the nose are usually responsible for the majority of lesions in this category. They may send silent, filamentous extensions beyond the clinically visible or palpable borders of the lesion, and thus require sacrifice of large amounts of normal skin or risk inadequate treatment.

Other carcinomas. There are many lesions that are now being treated with Mohs micrographic surgery other than those already mentioned. Usually they have one or more characteristics of the tumors noted above. This is true of such lesions as dermatofibrosarcoma protuberans [42], microcystic adnexal carcinoma [41], verrucous carcinoma [4,43], sebaceous carcinoma [44], Bowen's disease [45], Merkel cell carcinoma [46], and extramammary Paget's disease [47]. As more is learned about the behavior of other cutaneous tumors, the unique features of Mohs micrographic surgery may also make it applicable to their treatment.

Conclusions

The Mohs surgeon combines knowledge of the behavior of a tumor and its particular location with skills in excision, histographic control, and microscopic examination utilizing the Mohs micrographic surgery to remove cutaneous neoplasms. These factors interweave to give the highest cure rates for large or recurrent tumors. They also provide maximum conservation of uninvolved tissue and allow immediate repair of defects following tumor removal when appropriate. These two factors may be critical for many areas on the head and neck where most of these tumors occur.

These factors also make this procedure cost-effective for the patient. High cure rates will reduce recurrences. They will encourage patients to keep follow-up appointments, and any recurrences can be detected early and treated when small. Most lesions are treated on an outpatient basis.

With the proven efficacy of the Mohs technique, many Mohs surgeons have developed a strong interdisciplinary relationship with surgeons in fields such as ophthalmology, otolaryngology, and plastic surgery to treat many complicated head and neck tumors [48]. The tissue-conserving advantage of this technique has allowed removal of periorbital tumors, oral mucosal tumors, and other lesions, and has resulted in saving the patient an exenteration, a mandibulectomy, the removal of an ear or a digit.

Microscopically controlled surgery in the treatment of primary melanoma of the skin

In common with cutaneous carcinomas, melanomas often send out slender strands of malignant cells for a considerable distance beyond the clinically visible and palpable borders of the tumors. However, in contrast with carcinomas, melanomas also relatively frequently invade the walls of lymphatic vessels and spread by embolism to form satellites in the peritumoral lymphatics. In an attempt to encompass the ''silent'' contiguous outgrowths and also the noncontiguous satellites, the conventional management long has been wide and deep excision, usually followed by placement of a graft but sometimes by advancement of a flap or by primary closure. Such surgical treatment usually was successful in eradicating the local disease when the lesion was in anatomical areas where such radical management was not too disfiguring or disruptive of important functions. However, in areas such as the face where there is strong motivation to spare maximal amounts of normal tissue, there is a greater likelihood of transecting silent outgrowths or of cutting into clinically invisible satellites. The results could be that the highly malignant melanoma cells could be disseminated in the wound during undermining to close the defect or concealed for a considerable time by covering with a graft or flap. By the time the recurrence of the melanoma would become evident the primary lesion would be more difficult to eradicate, and metastasis might have occurred. Microscopically controlled surgery provides a means by which the danger of these complications can be significantly reduced because the microscopic guidance assures complete removal of the unpredictable outgrowths from the main tumor mass, and because any clinically invisible satellites remain localized and can be removed readily as soon as they become visible.

Advantages of chemosurgery

Advantages of microscopically controlled surgery in the treatment of cutaneous melanomas may be listed as follows:

1. *Reliability,* as reported in previous publications [4,49,50], is evidenced by an overall five-year cure rate of 50 percent, and in the Stage 1 cases of 65 percent. When it is considered that 69 percent of the series were of the most dangerous nodular type of melanoma and that 64 percent of them had invaded to the subcutaneous tissues (Level V) these cure rates are impressive. Moreover, microscopically controlled surgery yielded a higher five-year rate of cure than did conventional surgery for each of the four Clark's levels of invasion as follows: Level II, 100 cf 90 percent; Level III, 92 cf 57 percent; Level IV, 64.3 cf 40.7 percent; and Level V, 32.7 cf 18.8 percent. Also in the series of 103 cases there were only three recurrences of the primary melanoma and two of these had long-term cures after retreatment with the same method. The reasons for the exceptionally high degree of reliability are several. First, the microscopic control ensures eradication of the unpredictable outgrowths as well as the main mass of the primary melanoma. Second, the removal of an extra margin of tissue after reaching a microscopically

melanoma-free level increases the likelihood of eradicating invisible satellites in the peritumoral lymphatics. Third, if a clinically invisible satellite is transected, the neoplasm remains localized and on the surface where it can be detected early and removed; it is not seeded in the wound as it could be with conventional surgery during undermining to permit primary closure or during covering of the wound with a graft or flap. Fourth, chemical fixation in situ has no tendency to increase metastasis from malignant tumors as has been shown by animal experiments [2] and by many years of clinical experience [4,51]. This is in contrast with electrosurgical procedures in which the heat produces tissue steam that can propel clumps of melanoma cells through the lymphatics or blood vessels [52]. Also the in situ fixation avoids the danger of dislodging melanoma cells dangling in the lumens of invading vessels by the ''milking'' action that might occur with any but the most gentle handling of the tissues during surgical excision.

2. *Conservation* of maximal amounts of normal tissues is a particular advantage in treating facial melanomas, especially those near important structures such as the eye or the facial nerve. Since the microscopic control ensures eradication of silent contiguous outgrowths, the only reason for removing an extra margin is to remove possible satellites. This margin can be quite flexible because if clinically invisible satellites were missed, or even if they were transected, they remain localized and can be safely removed as they become grossly visible [53]. Since satellites and in-transit metastases are the result of embolic spread rather than continuous permeation through lymphatic vessels, there is no need to remove all of the tissue between the satellite and the site of the primary melanoma.

A viable option besides wide excision and grafting for the treatment of cutaneous melanoma is microscopically controlled surgery using the fixed tissue technique for all except eyelid and conjunctival melanomas for which the fresh tissue technique followed by chemical cauterization is used to avoid damaging the eye.

References

1. Shelley WB: Microscopically oriented histographic surgery. *Arch Dermatol* 114:1097, 1978
2. Mohs FE, Guyer MF: Pre-excisional fixation of tissues in the treatment of cancer in rats. *Cancer Res* 1:49, 1941
3. Mohs FE: *Chemosurgery in Cancer, Gangrene and Infections.* Springfield, IL, Charles C Thomas, 1956
4. Mohs FE: *Chemosurgery: Microscopically Controlled Surgery for Skin Cancer.* Springfield, IL, Charles C Thomas, 1978
5. Mohs FE: Chemosurgery for microscopically controlled excision of external cancer. *Arch Belg Dermatol Syphiligr* 14:1, 1958
6. Mohs FE: The chemosurgical method for the microscopically controlled excision of external cancer with reference to cancer of the eyelids. (Course 483, Instruction section.) *Trans Am Acad Ophthalmol Otolaryngol* 62:355, 1958
7. Mohs FE: Chemosurgical excision of cancer of the skin with microscopic control. *Vopr Onkol* 7:24, 1961 (in Russian)
8. Mohs FE: Microscopically guided excision of cancer of the skin by means of chemosurgery. *J Arkansas Med Soc* 65:203, 1968
9. Mohs FE: Chemosurgery for microscopically controlled excision of skin cancer, in *Proceedings of the 6th National Cancer Conference (Denver).* Philadelphia, JB Lippincott, 1970, p 517
10. Tromovitch TA, Stegman SJ: Microscopically controlled excision of skin tumors. *Arch Dermatol* 110:231, 1974
11. Mohs FE: Chemosurgery for skin cancer: fixed tissue and fresh tissue techniques. *Arch Dermatol* 112:211, 1976
12. Braun M: The case for Mohs surgery for the fixed-tissue technique. *J Dermatol Surg Oncol* 7:634, 1981
13. Cottell WI, Proper S: Mohs surgery, fresh-tissue technique: our technique with a review. *J Dermatol Surg Oncol* 8:576, 1982
14. Mohs FE: Chemosurgery for the microscopically controlled excision of skin cancer. *J Surg Oncol* 3:257, 1971
15. Pollack SV: Mohs chemosurgery for skin cancer. *Prog Dermatol* 14:1, 1980
16. Swanson NA: Mohs surgery. *Arch Dermatol* 119:261, 1983
17. Bumstead RM et al: Delayed skin grafting in facial reconstruction, when to use and how to do. *Arch Otolaryngol* 109:178, 1983
18. Tromovitch TA, Stegman SJ: Microscopic-controlled excision of cutaneous tumors: chemosurgery, fresh-tissue technique. *Cancer* 41:653, 1978
19. Robins P et al: Immediate repair of wounds following operations by Mohs fresh-tissue technique. *J Dermatol Surg Oncol* 5:329, 1979
20. Silverberg E: Cancer statistics, 1984. *CA* 37:7, 1984
21. Robins P: Mohs surgery in the treatment of basal cell and squamous cell carcinomas of the skin, in *Cancer of the Skin,* edited by R Andrade et al. Philadelphia, WB Saunders, 1976, p 1537
22. Dubin N, Kopf AW: Multivariate risk score for recurrence of cutaneous basal cell carcinomas. *Arch Dermatol* 119:373, 1983
23. Kopf A: Computer analysis of 3531 basal-cell carcinomas of the skin. *J Dermatol (Tokyo)* 6:267, 1979
24. Menn H et al: The recurrent basal epithelioma. *Arch Dermatol* 103:628, 1971
25. Robins P: Chemosurgery: my fifteen years of experience. *J Dermatol Surg Oncol* 7:779, 1981
26. Mark GJ: Basal cell carcinoma with intraneural invasion. *Cancer* 40:2181, 1977
27. Mohs FE, Lathrop TG: Modes of spread of cancer of skin. *Arch Dermatol* 66:427, 1952
28. Robinson JK et al: Invasion of cartilage by basal cell carcinoma. *J Am Acad Dermatol* 2:499, 1980
29. Callahan A et al: Cancer excision from eyelids and ocular adnexa: the Mohs fresh tissue technique and reconstruction. *Cancer* 32:322, 1982
30. Ceilley RI, Anderson RL: Microscopically controlled excision of malignant neoplasms on and around eyelids followed by immediate surgical reconstruction. *J Dermatol Surg Oncol* 4:55, 1978
31. Mohs FE, Zitelli JA: Microscopically controlled surgery in the treatment of carcinoma of the scalp. *Arch Dermatol* 117:764, 1981
32. Burg G et al: Histographic survey: accuracy of visual assessment of the margins of basal-cell epithelioma. *J Dermatol Surg* 1:21, 1975
33. Bumstead RM, Ceilley RI: Auricular malignant neoplasms. Identification of high-risk lesions and selection of method of reconstruction. *Arch Otolaryngol* 108:225, 1982
34. Levine H: Cutaneous carcinoma of the head and neck: management of massive and previously uncontrolled lesions. *Laryngoscope* 93:87, 1983
35. Panje WR, Ceilley RI: The influence of embryology of the midface on spread of epithelial malignancies. *Laryngoscope* 89:1914, 1979
36. Carruthers IA et al: Basal cell carcinomas of the temple. *J Dermatol Surg* 9:759, 1983
37. Mora RG, Robins P: Basal-cell carcinomas in the center of

the face: special diagnostic, prognostic, and therapeutic considerations. *J Dermatol Surg Oncol* **4:**315, 1978

38. Mohs FE et al: Microscopically controlled surgery for carcinomas in patients with nevoid basal cell carcinoma syndrome. *Arch Dermatol* **116:**777, 1980

39. Farmer ER, Helwig EB: Metastatic basal cell carcinoma: a clinicopathologic study of seventeen cases. *Cancer* **46:**748, 1980

40. Borel PM: Cutaneous basosquamous carcinoma. *Arch Pathol* **95:**293, 1973

41. Goldstein DJ et al: Microcystic adnexal carcinoma: a distinct clinicopathologic entity. *Cancer* **50:**566, 1982

42. Peters CW et al: Chemosurgical reports: dermatofibrosarcoma protuberans of the face. *J Dermatol Surg Oncol* **8:**823, 1982

43. Mora RG: Microscopically controlled surgery (Mohs chemosurgery) for treatment of verrucous squamous cell carcinoma of the foot (epithelioma cuniculatum). *J Am Acad Dermatol* **8:**354, 1983

44. Harvey JT, Anderson RL: The management of Mebomian gland carcinoma. *Ophthalmic Surg* **13:**56, 1982

45. Mikhail GR: Brown's disease and squamous cell carcinoma of the nail bed. *Arch Dermatol* **110:**267, 1970

46. Pollack SV, Goslen JB: Small-cell neuroepithelial tumor of skin: a Merkel-cell neoplasm? *J Dermatol Surg Oncol* **8:**116, 1982

47. Mohs FE, Blanchard L: Microscopically controlled surgery for extramammary Paget's disease. *Arch Dermatol* **115:**706, 1979

48. Swanson NA et al: Mohs surgery: techniques, indications, and applications in head and neck surgery. *Head Neck Surg* **6:**683, 1983

49. Mohs FE: Chemosurgery for melanoma. *Arch Dermatol* **113:**285, 1977

50. Mohs FE et al: Chemosurgery for familial malignant melanoma. *J Dermatol Surg Oncol* **5:**127, 1979

51. Mohs FE: Chemosurgery: microscopically controlled surgery for skin cancer—past, present and future. *J Dermatol Surg Oncol* **4:**41, 1978

52. Amadon PD: Electrocoagulation of melanoma and its dangers. *Surg Gynecol Obstet* **56:**943, 1933

53. Mohs FE: The width and depth of the spread of malignant melanoma as observed by a chemosurgeon. *Am J Dermatopathol* **6** (**suppl 1**):123, 1984

Section 33

Systemic therapy

CHAPTER 217

SYSTEMIC CORTICOSTEROIDS

Richard F. Spark

Systemic corticosteroid therapy, introduced in 1949 as treatment for rheumatoid arthritis, was shortly thereafter proposed as treatment for a variety of dermatologic disorders. Since then, corticosteroid treatment has been reported to be effective in a spectrum of illnesses as diverse as pemphigus vulgaris, systemic lupus erythematosus (SLE), acute allergic dermatitis, cystic acne, and hirsutism.

Three different biologic actions of systemic corticosteroids account for their effectiveness in a majority of dermatologic disorders.

1. Inhibition of inflammatory response
2. Immunosuppression
3. Suppression of the hypothalamic-pituitary-adrenal (H-P-A) axis

It is not possible to selectively segregate any one of the desirable actions of the systemic corticosteroids from the other two. A physician who uses steroids for their anti-inflammatory potential must recognize that as long as these drugs are used, and in many cases after they have been discontinued, immune responses and the ability of the H-P-A axis to respond to stress will be impaired.

Other actions of corticosteroids have no known benefit in dermatologic disorders, but must be reckoned with as part of the undesirable pharmacologic baggage that attends the use of systemic corticosteriod treatment. Included are steroid-induced abnormalities in carbohydrate, protein, and fat metabolism and fluid balance, including glucose intolerance, negative nitrogen balance, proximal myopathy, cushingoid habitus, and lipolysis.

Metabolism

Carbohydrate metabolism

Steroids are derivatives of the physiologic glucocorticoid hormones, hydrocortisone and cortisone. In therapeutic doses, these compounds block the action of insulin at the insulin receptor, and invariably create some degree of insulin resistance. In normal persons, mild glucose intolerance ensues. In diabetic patients, such therapy will provoke significant hyperglycemia, worsen diabetic control, and rarely induce diabetic ketoacidosis.

Protein metabolism

Steroids are catabolic hormones and in pharmacologic doses cause a negative nitrogen balance and a selective myopathy of the proximal muscles of the shoulder and pelvic girdle.

Fat metabolism

Redistribution of body fat with increased deposition of lipid in the central body core creating truncal obesity, buffalo hump, and moon facies, characteristic of cushingoid habitus, has been recognized as an adverse consequence of steroid treatment since Sulzberger's original paper in 1951. Corticosteroids also have a lipolytic effect on peripheral fat stores, thinning out subcutaneous fat and thereby revealing underlying vascular channels which are unusually friable, and without the cushion of surrounding fat are vulnerable to minimal trauma. This accounts for the multiple peripheral ecchymoses commonly seen in patients on chronic corticosteroid therapy.

Fluid status

Sodium and water retention, edema, and hypertension occur with corticosteroids such as cortisone and hydrocortisone. Minor modifications in the structure of the steroid molecule (see below) have minimized or eliminated this deleterious mineralocorticoid effect of systemic corticosteroids.

Therapeutic uses

Despite the seemingly endless catalogue of side effects, systemic corticosteroid therapy has been successfully incorporated as an integral element in the dermatologic pharmacopeia. Multiple treatment schedules and high-dose, moderate-dose, single-dose, and alternate-day corticosteroid administration have been proposed as effective therapeutic regimens. To maximize clinical benefit and minimize side effects, it is useful to have an appreciation of the etiology and natural history of the specific clinical disorder to be treated, a familiarity with basic steroid pharmacology, and an understanding of the normal physiology of the H-P-A axis.

Etiology and natural history

For acute self-limited dermatoses, such as poison ivy dermatitis, where a specific allergen can be identified, a few days of a moderately high dose of corticosteroids followed by a short rapid tapering course will be more than adequate. This schedule will not suffice in pemphigus vulgaris, where very high doses of corticosteroids, 200 to 300 mg per day prednisone equivalent as initial therapy, have proved to be most effective. In those conditions such as SLE, where the etiology is obscure, a more prolonged continuous therapeutic schedule is required. Alternate-day

steroid therapy seems to be most effective in those clinical disorders associated with the production of an abnormal immunoglobulin. Alternate-day steroid schedule will disrupt synthesis of the immunoglobulin if administered on a schedule of every other or, in the rare case, every third day, and provide therapeutic benefit. In cystic acne or hirsutism, where adrenal androgen excess is demonstrable, a single low dose of corticosteroid will suffice, administered at bedtime when the H-P-A axis is most vulnerable to suppression. In other disorders, reliance on clinical experience and empiric observation has helped define specific schedules of corticosteroid treatment.

Pharmacology

The steroids with their "chicken wire structure" are unnecessarily forbidding and intimidating. In reality, all corticosteroids have the same basic structure, three hexanes and a single pentane ring. By convention, these rings are designated A, B, C, and D, and individual sites of the molecule are numbered in sequence. A few sites are critical for corticosteroid bioactivity. Modifications at these loci can materially alter and enhance the potency of individual steroids.

A basic steroid "skeleton" with sites critical for bioactivity is illustrated in Fig. 217-1a. This structure of hydrocortisone (cortisol), the adrenal corticosteroid, is represented in Fig. 217-1b. Sites critical for continued bioactivity include the ketone at the 3 position of ring A and the dihydroxyketone moiety at the 17-21 position in ring D. Reduction of the ketone to a hydroxyl results in the formation of dihydrocortisol, an inert corticosteroid. Insertion of a double bond at the 1-2 position in the A ring serves to protect this molecule from too rapid metabolic degradation and enhances biologic activity. This new compound is prednisolone (Fig. 217-2), which on a milligram per milligram basis is four times more potent than the native hydrocortisone. Further protection from metabolic degradation and a fivefold enhanced potency is achieved with the addition of a methyl group at position 6, forming methyl prednisolone.

Hydrocortisone, and to a lesser degree prednisolone, has intrinsic mineralocorticoid activity and will cause some sodium retention and potassium iron excretion. Enhanced mineralocorticoid activity results when a halogen atom, most commonly fluorine (F), is added to the native hydrocortisone at position 9. This compound, 9-alpha fluorohydrocortisone (Fig. 217-3a), has 150 times the sodium-retaining capacity of cortisol, and, as such, is beneficial in conditions of mineralocorticoid deficiency, such as primary adrenal insufficiency, but is not useful in dermatologic disorders.

Paradoxically, this strikingly enhanced mineralocorticoid activity is completely abolished when another methyl group is added at position 16. This substitution protects the 17-21 dihydroxyketone moiety of ring D from too rapid degradation. This new molecule is basically prednisolone with a fluorine at position 9, and the methyl at 16. This is dexamethasone (Fig. 217-3b) which is 25 times more potent than hydrocortisone.

Treatment of dermatologic conditions often requires a potent anti-inflammatory agent that is devoid of mineralocorticoid activity. Relative anti-inflammatory and miner-

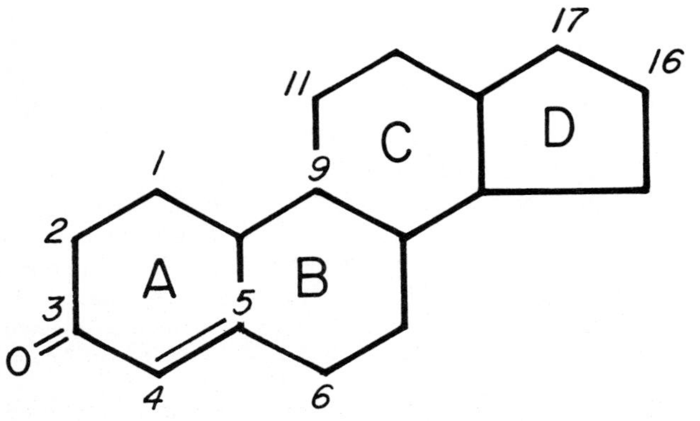

Fig. 217-1 (a) A basic steroid skeleton with sites critical for continued bioactivity, indicated by number. (b) The structure of hydrocortisone (cortisol).

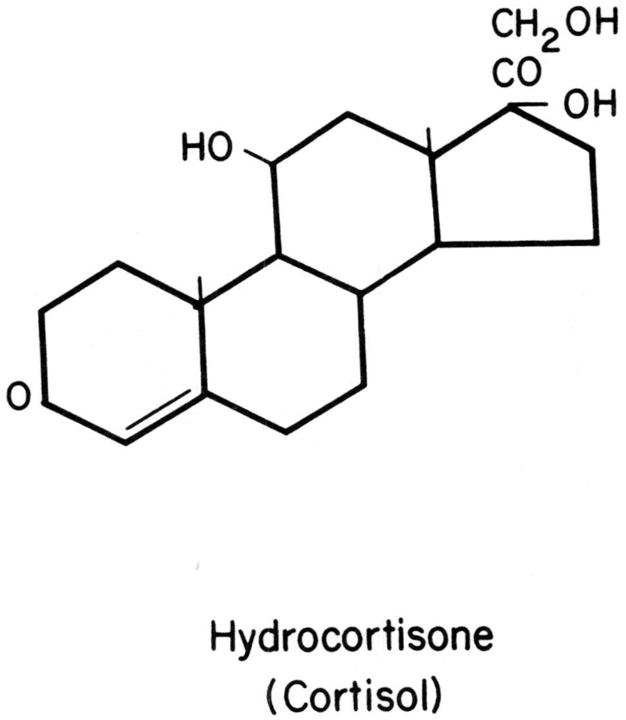

alocorticoid acitivity of the compounds listed above, as well as prednisone (like prednisolone but with a ketone at the 11 position) is given in Table 217-1.

Metabolic disposition of the corticosteroids was initially defined by studies of plasma half-life of specific molecules, but results of these kinetic studies have proved to be misleading for they do not account for binding of the individual steroid molecule to target tissue. Thus, dexamethasone has a plasma half-life of only 240 min, but may bind to the hypothalamus and pituitary for up to 36 h, making this synthetic steroid unacceptable for use in alternate-day steroid therapy. Conversely, prednisone and prednisolone, whose binding to the hypothalamus and pituitary is less prolonged, may be useful in alternate-day steroid therapy.

Therapeutic schedules

The basic premise attending the use of alternate-day steroid therapy is the concept that such a schedule would maintain the desired therapeutic effect and avoid suppressing the H-P-A axis.

The hypothalamic-pituitary-adrenal axis (Fig. 217-4)

Hypothalamic corticotropin-releasing factor, a 41 amino acid peptide, traverses the hypothalamic-hypophyseal portal system to stimulate the pituitary corticotroph to release adrenocorticotrophin (ACTH), a 39 amino acid peptide. Pituitary ACTH released into the circulation binds to specific receptors on the adrenal cortex, stimulating cyclic AMP production and cortisol secretion.

Cortisol secretion has an intrinsic diurnal rhythm linked to a normal sleep–wake schedule. Serum ACTH and cortisol levels are highest on awakening in the morning, may fall to undetectable levels at midnight, remain low during sleep, and then, between 3 and 4 A.M., ACTH secretion spontaneously increases and stimulates cortisol production so that, on arising the following morning, serum ACTH and cortisol levels are once again elevated.

Superimposed on the intrinsic diurnal rhythm is a critical emergency reserve system that allows the H-P-A axis to increase both ACTH and cortisol secretion in response to stress at any time of the day.

In the absence of stress, the H-P-A axis secretes no more than 20 mg of cortisol daily. Any daily amount of

corticosteroid greater than 20 mg a day of hydrocortisone or its equivalent will suppress the H-P-A axis. All oral steroid preparations are "pegged to the 20 mg hydrocortisone standard." A single tablet of prednisone 5 mg, 6-methylprednisolone (Medrol) 4 mg, and dexamethasone 0.75 mg is equivalent to 20 mg hydrocortisone. Systemic steroid therapy, when prescribed in doses to achieve circulating levels of steroid in excess of 20 mg cortisol or its equivalent, will always suppress the H-P-A axis.

No problems occur if this therapy is given for short periods of time, up to a month. Endogenous H-P-A function will be restored within 48 h after exogenous steroid therapy has been stopped.

However, when systemic corticosteroids are continued for periods greater than one month, H-P-A function is more profoundly suppressed and recovery may not be evident for periods of up to one year after all steroid therapy has been discontinued. During this interval, the patient is in a state of chronic pituitary-adrenal insufficiency, and will not be able to increase ACTH and cortisol secretion in reponse to stress. As a consequence, profound hypotension and shock may attend an otherwise trivial stress, such as minor infection or minimal trauma. In such hypotensive episodes, a prior history of systemic corticosteroid therapy suggests the presence of underlying occult pituitary-adrenal insufficiency. Once recognized, appropriate "stress" doses of hydrocortisone can be administered, and along with appropriate fluids and antibiotics will reverse what is in essence an iatrogenic "acute pituitary-adrenal crisis." These crises only develop when, by virtue of either dose or duration of therapy, systemic corticosteroids have produced such profound suppression of the H-P-A axis that the anticipated stress-induced augmentation of cortisol secretion cannot be accomplished. Certainly, this degree of H-P-A inhibition would be expected in those individuals treated

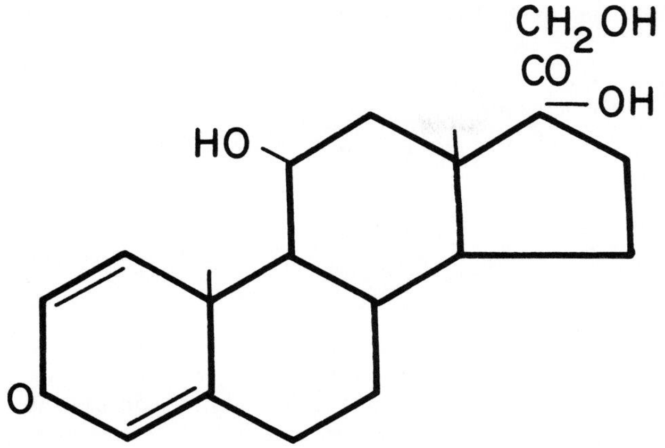

Prednisolone

a

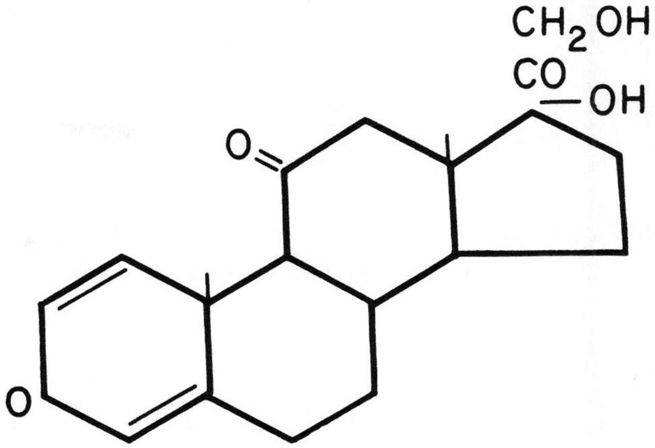

Fig. 217-2   (a) The structure of prednisolone, similar to hydrocortisone, but fortified by the insertion of a double bond at the 1-2 position. (b) The structure of prednisone, similar

Prednisone

b

to prednisolone, but with a ketone instead of a hydroxyl at the 11 position.

with high-dose, long-term steroid therapy. Recent studies have indicated that an impaired cortisol response to hypoglycemic stress is present in individuals who have been treated with doses of steroids as low as 5 mg of prednisone daily for several months.

Evaluation of pituitary-adrenal reserve

There are times when it is important to know whether an individual currently or previously treated with systemic corticosteroids has sufficient H-P-A reserve to respond to

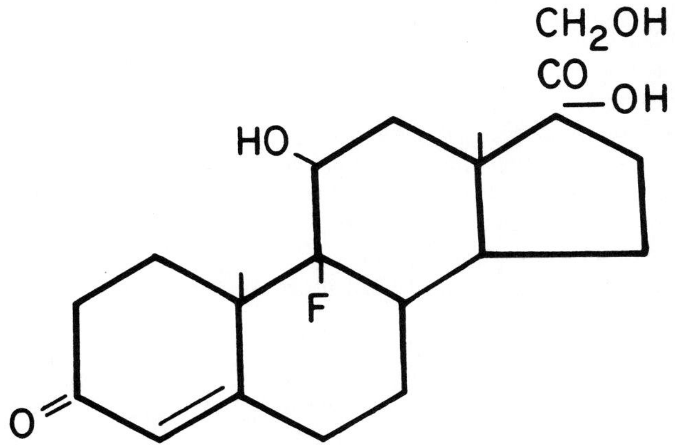

Fig. 217-3   (a) 9α-Fluorohydrocortisone (Florinef), a potent mineralocorticoid. The structure is identical to hydrocortisone, but with the insertion of a fluorine atom at position 9. (b) The structure of dexamethasone, prednisolone, with a fluorine at position 9 and a methyl group at position 16, and completely devoid of mineralocorticoid activity.

9α-Fluorocortisol
(Florinef)

a

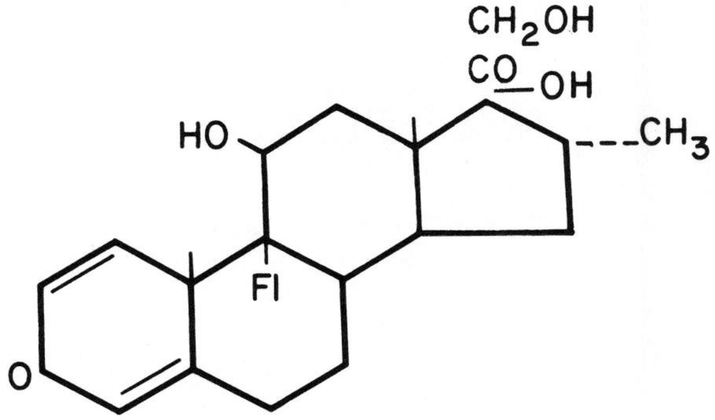

16α-Methyl-9α-fluoroprednisolone
(Dexamethasone)

b

Table 217-1   Anti-inflammatory and sodium-retaining potencies of systemic corticosteroids

Compound	Single tablet dose (mg)	Anti-inflammatory	Mineralo-corticoid
Hydrocortisone	20	1	1
Cortisone	25	0.8	0.8
Prednisone	5	4	0.8
6α-Methylprednisolone	4	5	0.5
Dexamethasone	0.75	25	0

the stress of surgery, infection, trauma, etc. When systemic corticosteroid therapy suppresses the hypothalamus, serum ACTH levels fall, and the adrenal is unstimulated and will eventually atrophy. When this occurs, the adrenal is unresponsive to *exogenous* ACTH. Baseline cortisol levels will be low and will not increase after stimulation with beta 1-24 ACTH 250 μg intramuscularly. However, this occurs only after long-term chronic steroid therapy.

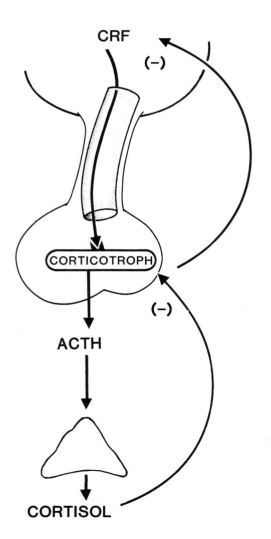

Fig. 217-4   The hypothalamic-pituitary-adrenal axis. CRF, corticotropin-releasing factor; ACTH, adrenocorticotrophin.

REGULATION OF CORTISOL SECRETION

The hypothalamus and pituitary are the first sites suppressed by chronic steroid therapy and are the first sites that must be activated to respond to the stress of surgery, infection, or trauma. It is important to know not only that the adrenal can respond to exogenous ACTH, but that the individual is capable of producing sufficient *endogenous* ACTH to facilitate the normal response to stress.

Two tests currently in use, the insulin tolerance test and the metyrapone test, have been useful to evaluate endogenous ACTH reserve. The insulin tolerance test relies on insulin-induced hypoglycemia as a stress to provoke increased pituitary ACTH secretion, while metyrapone induces a pharmacologic blockade of cortisol biosynthesis and defines the ability of the hypothalamus and pituitary to respond to a subnormal cortisol level. Both tests are most safely accomplished in hospital and can only be done on a prospective basis to determine, for example, whether a patient scheduled for surgery has sufficient pituitary-adrenal reserve to respond adequately to the surgical stress.

In clinical practice, one rarely has the luxury of sufficient time to perform such tests prospectively. More commonly, the need to determine the status of pituitary-adrenal reserve is urgent, for patients with acute pituitary-adrenal insufficiency will present in extremis. A single plasma cortisol level, if "normal," implies pituitary-adrenal insufficiency, for with a degree of stress sufficient to cause hypotension, plasma cortisol levels should be elevated greater than 30 μg/dL. However, this may be considered supportive evidence, for pituitary-adrenal insufficiency must be presumed and treated if there is a history of chronic systemic corticosteroid therapy.

Alternate-day steroid (ADS) therapy

ADS therapy has been enthusiastically championed by those who presume that with this schedule, beneficial effects of systemic corticosteroid therapy will be maximized and deleterious side effects minimized. While clinical experience has established the value of ADS therapy in some conditions, this treatment schedule is of no therapeutic benefit in other disorders.

Conditions that are most likely to respond to ADS therapy are those conditions where immunosuppression is desirable. Corticosteroids may interrupt a step in the chain of immunoglobulin synthesis, an effect which may be sustained for up to 36 or 48 h. Conversely, in those conditions where an acute inflammatory process is active, corticosteroids are effective while being administered, but the inflammatory process recurs promptly after corticosteroid levels decline.

ADS therapy was originally designed to protect the H-P-A axis from suppression, the rationale being that on the day that steroids were not administered, the H-P-A axis would function normally. Within limits, this appears to be a valid concept. However, the hypothalamus and pituitary are not impervious to the effects of corticosteroids when they are administered in very high doses. Thus, from a pragmatic standpoint, ADS therapy will protect the H-P-A axis when administered in doses of prednisone equivalent to 40 mg every other day. At doses higher than this, even when corticosteroids are administered on an alternate-day schedule, suppression of the H-P-A axis is likely to occur.

Nocturnal single-dose corticosteroid therapy

There are certain clinical conditions in which suppression of the H-P-A axis is desirable. In addition to cortisol, the adrenal makes a variety of other steroid compounds, including a group classified as androgens. The most prominent adrenal androgen is a compound called dehydroepiandrosterone sulfate (DHEA-S). This adrenal androgen appears to be important physiologically only at the time of puberty, when secretion increases and allows for the development of axillary and pubic hair in young men and women. Postpuberty plasma levels of DHEA-S vary between 150 to 400 mg, decline with aging, and, other than the development of public and axillary hair, have no known physiologic significance. Although DHEA-S is an androgen, it is a weak androgen which can exert an androgen effect only when secreted in large amounts. ACTH controls DHEA-S secretion. Secretion of DHEA-S is elevated in certain forms of congenital adrenal hyperplasia and specific types of hirsutism and chronic cystic acne. Since DHEA-S secretion is controlled by ACTH, suppression of ACTH will, in turn, suppress DHEA-S secretion. This can be achieved with relatively small doses of corticosteroids, 5 to 7.5 mg prednisone, administered at midnight at a time when the H-P-A axis is most vulnerable to suppression. Such therapy will lower DHEA-S levels to or below the normal range and be of clinical benefit in selected cases of hirsutism or cystic acne. Nocturnal single-dose corticosteroid therapy, by design, suppresses the H-P-A axis and suppresses not only DHEA-S secretion, but also cortisol secretion. The consequences of this were discussed above.

Nocturnal single-dose corticosteroid therapy in the doses described above is generally not associated with other complications of chronic corticosteroid use.

This therapy is of no benefit to those patients with hirsutism or cystic acne in whom there is no demonstrable elevation in secretion of adrenal androgen hormones.

In addition to the problems that may attend the use of corticosteroid therapy, there are other problems that may persist after corticosteroid therapy has been discontinued. Suppression of the H-P-A axis and its consequences have been discussed in detail above. There are, in addition, two troublesome problems that may occur after corticosteroid therapy has been discontinued. These include (1) a flare of the primary disease for which corticosteroids were first administered, and (2) the corticosteroid withdrawal syndrome.

From the earliest days of corticosteroid use, once it had been established that a patient's illness responded to pharmacologic corticosteroid doses, it was equally apparent that in many cases, these patients became dependent on the corticosteroids as long as the underlying factors responsible for the disease remained active. Corticosteroid responsiveness might suggest some degree of corticosteroid dependence. Gradual reduction of steroid dose and careful clinical observation of the patient will be required in such instances. The only treatment for a flare of a corticosteroid-responsive disease is reinstitution of corticosteroid therapy. If, because of corticosteroid-induced side effects reintroduction of corticosteroids is not possible, then other therapeutic options must be considered.

The corticosteroid withdrawal syndrome

The corticosteroid withdrawal syndrome has been recognized and documented since the early 1950s. It is independent of the flare of the primary disease noted above and may exist independent of, or coexist with, the clinical deterioration of the patient. In the steroid withdrawal syndrome, the patient complains bitterly of weakness, fatigue, anorexia, and has a low-grade fever rarely exceeding 39°C (101°F). When this occurs, the appearance of a peculiar desquamation of the fingertips may lead to the diagnosis. The syndrome may occur in patients who have been given a course of corticosteroids for as short a time as three weeks. Abrupt cessation of corticosteroids appears to be critical for the development of the steroid withdrawal syndrome. Corticosteroids inhibit the conversion of beta carotene to vitamin A and since the syndrome has some of the characteristics of mild vitamin A intoxication, it was postulated that the corticosteroid-induced block conversion of beta carotene to vitamin A resulted in an initial excess of the beta carotene. Abrupt discontinuation of steroids allowed for the rapid conversion of the excessive beta carotene to an excessive amount of circulating vitamin A. Whatever the etiology, recognition of this syndrome is crucial for prompt reinstitution of corticosteroids followed by gradual tapering which will result in an amelioration and eventual resolution of the steroid withdrawal syndrome. ADS therapy may be most helpful in this condition.

Corticosteroid-induced osteonecrosis

Osteonecrosis (ON) deserves special attention. The pathogenesis of this complication of systemic corticosteroid therapy is unknown. ON may occur in any bone, but most commonly it is the femur that is affected. Treatment for ON of the femur is total hip replacement. Patients at risk for developing ON are those with SLE and others who have been treated with high *initial* but *not total* corticosteroid doses. However, since ON may also develop in hypoadrenal patients receiving *physiologic* replacement doses of corticosteroids, other factors, including individual idiosyncratic response, must be considered.

ON may occur in as many as 6 percent of corticosteroid-treated patients, a statistic of enormous medicolegal significance.

In summary, systemic corticosteroids are firmly entrenched as an effective form of dermatologic therapy. Still, because of the problems that may attend the use of this medication, today's physicians are justifiably wary of initiating systemic corticosteroids. Ultimately, as with any other medication, a decision on the benefit/risk ratio must be considered. For systemic corticosteroids, benefits can be maximized and risks can be minimized. When this is done, systemic corticosteroids prove to be an invaluable addition to the dermatologic therapeutic armamentarium.

Bibliography

Abeles M et al: Aseptic necrosis of bone in systemic lupus erythematosus. *Arch Intern Med* **138**:750, 1978

Amatruda TT et al: Certain endocrine and metabolic factors of the steroid withdrawal syndrome. *J Clin Endocrinol Metab* **25**:1207, 1965

Boyd RE et al: Acute effects of steroids on immune complex profile of patients with systemic lupus erythematosus. Correlation of profile with development of target organ involvement. *Arthritis Rheum* **26**:637, 1983

Cupps TR et al: Multiple mechanisms of B cell immunoregulation in man after administration of in vivo corticosteroids. *J Immunol* **132**:170, 1984

Fauci AS et al: Glucocorticoid therapy, mechanisms of action and clinical considerations. *Ann Intern Med* **84**:304, 1976

Fujieda K et al: Pituitary-adrenal function in women treated with low doses of prednisone. *Am J Obstet Gynecol* **137**:962, 1980

Graber AL et al: Natural history of pituitary-adrenal recovery following long-term suppression with corticosteroids. *J Clin Endocrinol Metab* **25**:11, 1965

Harris ED Jr et al: Low dose prednisone therapy in rheumatoid arthritis: a double blind study. *J Rheumatol* **10**:713, 1983

Lever WF, Schaumburg-Lever G: Treatment of pemphigus vulgaris. Results obtained in 84 patients between 1961 and 1982. *Arch Dermatol* **120**:44, 1984

MacGregor RR et al: Alternate-day prednisone therapy, evaluation of delayed hypersensitivity responses, control of disease and steroid side effects. *N Engl J Med* **280**:1427, 1969

Marynick SP et al: Androgen excess in cystic acne. *N Engl J Med* **308**:991, 1983

Spiegel RJ et al: Adrenal suppression after short-term corticosteroid therapy. *Lancet* **1**:630, 1979

Williams PL, Corbett M: Avascular necrosis of bone complicating corticosteroid replacement. *Ann Rheum Dis* **42**:276, 1983

CHAPTER 218

DAPSONE

Stephen I. Katz

Historical aspects

In 1940, Costello first described the dramatic success of sulfapyridine in treating a patient with dermatitis herpetiformis, a disease he believed represented a form of bacterial allergy [1]. Swartz and Lever later reported the regular response of all their patients with dermatitis herpetiformis to sulfapyridine therapy [2]. In the early 1950s, a group of drugs chemically related to sulfapyridine, the sulfones (dapsone and related compounds), were first used in treating patients with this disease [3,4]. Since dapsone is the most widely used drug among these compounds for the treatment of dermatitis herpetiformis, some other neutrophilic dermatoses, and leprosy, there has been an enormous amount of research into its metabolism, mechanisms of action, and toxicity.

Pharmacology

The chemical structure of dapsone (4,4'-diaminodiphenylsulfone, DDS) is shown in Fig. 218-1. The only difference between dapsone and sulfoxone, a water-soluble sulfone, is that the latter is substituted on the amino groups by a $-CH_2OSONa$ radical. Sulfoxone is no longer available in the United States. This and other derivatives of dapsone are thought to be metabolized to the parent dapsone structure. Sulfapyridine resembles dapsone in that it has an aminophenyl group attached to a sulfone (SO_2); however, on the other side of the sulfone, there is a pyridine group

(Fig. 218-1). Although other sulfonamides have an aminophenyl group attached to a sulfone, they have different groups on the other side of the sulfone, and none is as effective as sulfapyridine in the treatment of inflammatory diseases.

After oral administration approximately 80 to 85 percent of dapsone is absorbed, with peak levels being reached at 4 to 6 h after a single dose. Sulfoxone, however, is only 50 percent absorbed. In patients taking 50 to 300 mg/day of dapsone, the peak levels of dapsone and its major metabolite reach 0.5 to 7 mg/L and 0.2 to 5 mg/L, respectively [5]. The half-life of dapsone in the circulation is anywhere from 2 to 4 days. Its retention in the body, however, is prolonged, perhaps because of its enterohepatic recirculation, since high concentrations have been detected in the bile. Dapsone and its metabolites are excreted by way of the kidneys.

Dapsone is metabolized in the liver. The two major metabolic pathways involve (1) acetylation and (2) N-hydroxylation (Fig. 218-2). As with isoniazid and certain hydrazides and sulfonamides, dapsone and its derivatives are acetylated polymorphically, i.e., some patients rapidly acetylate dapsone to monoacetyldapsone (MADDS), the major metabolite, while in others this occurs slowly. However, in humans MADDS is rapidly deacetylated. Thus, there is an equilibrium that is rapidly reached and sustained between MADDS and dapsone. The half-life in the body seems to be unrelated to the rate of acetylation. From a clinical standpoint, it seems that in the control of symp-

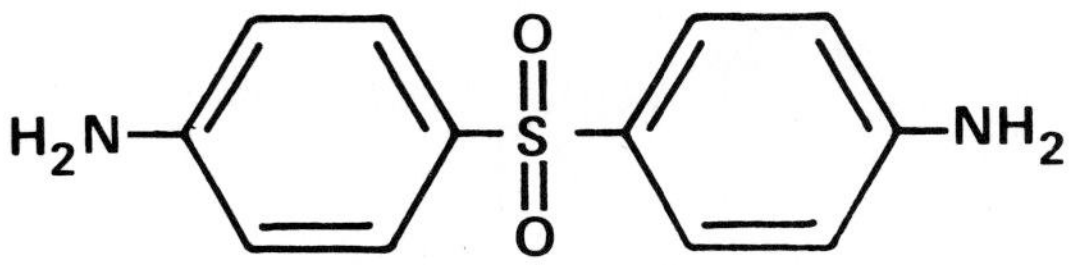

Fig. 218-1 Chemical structure of dapsone, sulfoxone, and sulfapyridine.

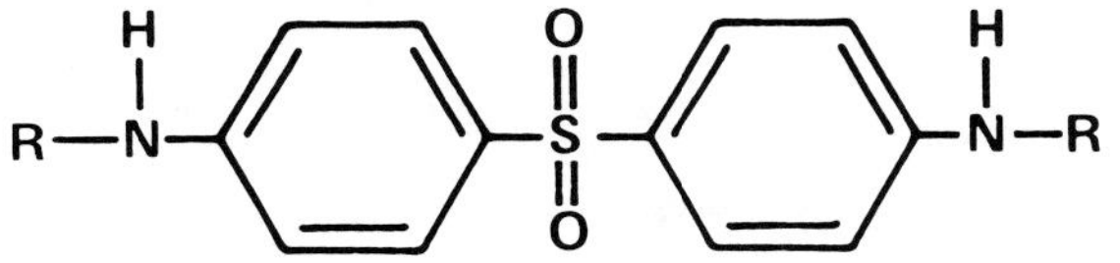

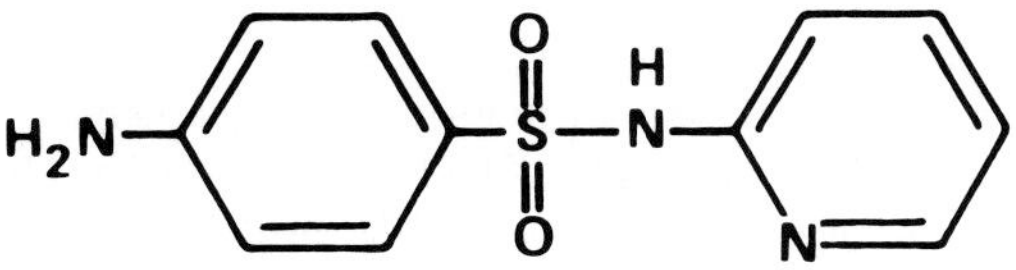

toms of dermatitis herpetiformis and even in its efficacy as an antileprosy drug, the dapsone dosage requirement is unrelated to acetylator phenotype [5,6].

The other major metabolic pathway involves hydroxylation of one of the amino groups to form the aminohydroxylaminodiphenylsulfone. This compound is responsible for the methemoglobinemia, hemolysis, and Heinz body formations which occur regularly when dapsone is administered [7]. Thus, these effects represent pharmacologic side effects that must be anticipated.

Drugs that interfere with the effect of dapsone include probenecid and rifampin. Probenecid has been reported to block the renal excretion of dapsone; however, serum dapsone levels are not significantly affected [8]. When given concurrently with dapsone, rifampin increases the rate of dapsone clearance, the most likely cause of which is the induction of microsomal enzymes.

Indications

Since its introduction into clinical medicine, dapsone has had therapeutic trials in a multitude of diseases. Its use in leprosy and malaria chemoprophylaxis is beyond the scope of this chapter. Long lists of inflammatory diseases that have responded to dapsone therapy have been generated [9]. Some of the individual reports are difficult to assess critically. Two diseases that invariably respond to dapsone therapy are dermatitis herpetiformis and erythema elevatum diutinum [10]. The dramatic dependence of patients on dapsone is best exemplified by the prompt exacerbations that follow withdrawal of the drug.

Other diseases in which dapsone therapy has been reportedly effective in some patients are rheumatoid arthritis, acne conglobata, actinomycetoma, pyoderma gangrenosum, bullous pemphigoid, scarring pemphigoid, relapsing polychondritis, the bullous eruption of systemic lupus erythematosus (SLE), granuloma faciale, subcorneal pustular dermatosis, and certain forms of leukocytoclastic vasculitis. The preferred dosage of dapsone in each of these diseases is listed in the relevant chapters. As a unifying feature, these diseases have the presence of granulocytes (neutrophils or eosinophils) as the preponderant infiltrating cell. In most diseases, the neutrophils appear early in the pathologic process. The response to dapsone therapy is not as rapid, regular, or predictable in any of these diseases as it is in dermatitis herpetiformis or erythema elevatum diutinum. McConkey et al [11] have provided controlled data that show dapsone therapy to be modestly effective in the treatment of some patients with rheumatoid arthritis. High dosages (up to 400 mg/day) are usually required in the treatment of otherwise unresponsive patients with cystic acne. With the advent of the new synthetic retinoids, however, a trial of dapsone therapy may no longer be necessary. A small group of patients with bullous pemphigoid has responded fairly dramatically to dapsone therapy [12]. A group of patients with scarring pemphigoid has reportedly benefited from dapsone therapy as well [13].

Patients with SLE occasionally have subepidermal vesicular lesions that closely simulate dermatitis herpetiformis, histologically [14]. These patients do not have an "admixture" of dermatitis herpetiformis and SLE, although the eruption is extraordinarily responsive to dapsone therapy [15]. A potentially exciting report, which was too brief and could not be evaluated, has also recently suggested the efficacy of dapsone therapy in discoid LE [16]. Some patients with subcorneal pustular dermatosis respond to and become dependent on dapsone, while others are unresponsive. This may reflect the heterogeneity of this disease, of which the nosologic features have been a source of considerable debate [17].

Although there are several reports which suggest that dapsone therapy is remarkably effective in the treatment of relapsing polychondritis, this author's experience with dapsone therapy in several patients with this condition has been uniformly unsuccessful. Occasionally, there are patients with chronic leukocytoclastic vasculitis in addition to those with erythema elevatum diutinum in whom dapsone therapy provides the prompt cessation of lesions. Since there is no uniformly successful therapy for these patients, many of whom do not seem to have associated internal problems, a short trial of dapsone therapy is warranted. In general, when a pathologic lesion is characterized by a neutrophilic infiltrate and is unassociated with an infectious agent, a trial of dapsone therapy should be considered.

In this regard there are occasional patients who have a subepidermal blistering disease which is not readily classifiable by clinical, histologic, immunofluorescence and immunoelectron microscopic findings. These patients have small, vesicular lesions that are pruritic and widespread, and some have scarring lesions. All have linear IgG deposits at the dermal-epidermal junction; in some patients,

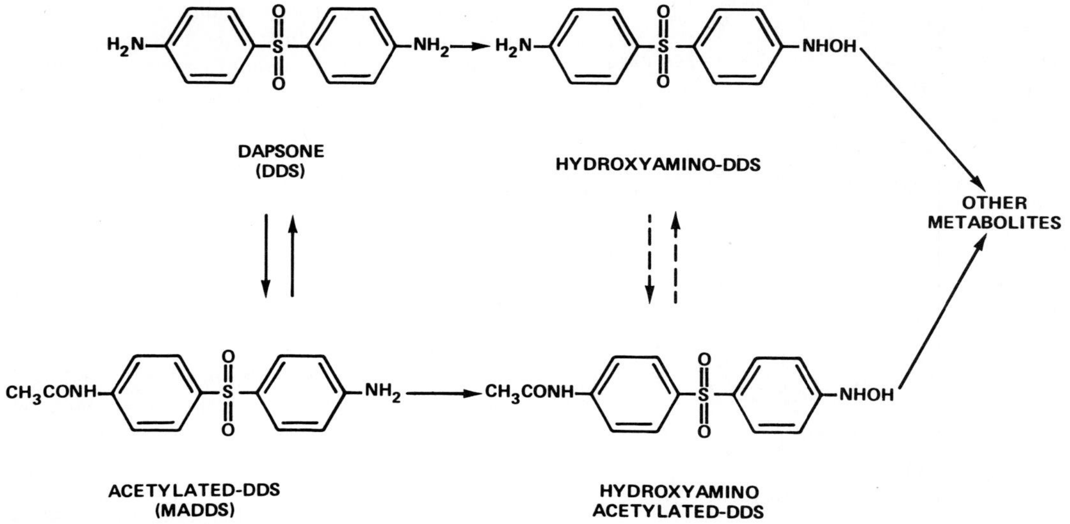

Fig. 218-2 Dapsone metabolism in humans.

the IgG deposits are within the lamina lucida (as in pemphigoid), and, in others, the deposits are below the lamina densa. The uniform findings are the subepidermal blisters, the linear IgG deposits by immunofluorescence microscopy, and the presence of neutrophils in an almost single file in the dermis just below the dermal-epidermal junction. There are also occasional collections of neutrophils at the dermal-epidermal junction. Some of these patients have responded dramatically to dapsone therapy, with a portion requiring long-term treatment, while others have a disease that is shorter lived. The conditions of some of these patients might be classified as vesicular pemphigoid, and some as acquired epidermolysis bullosa, although the conditions of other patients fall outside of this realm.

Adverse effects

Dapsone therapy produces hemolysis and methemoglobinemia. The metabolite responsible for both these pharmacologic effects of sulfones has been identified as aminohydroxylaminodiphenylsulfone. It can be anticipated that patients taking more than 50 mg/day of dapsone will have some degree of hemolysis that will be reflected in a lowered hemoglobin level. At 150 mg/day, dapsone may produce a decrease of as much as 2 g of hemoglobin [18]. Patients with glucose-6-dehydrogenase deficiency have a greater decrease in the hemoglobin level. Most patients tolerate this fall in the level of hemoglobin well, but the conditions of older patients or those with cardiopulmonary problems should be closely monitored or they should be given sulfapyridine. An increase in the reticulocyte count will accompany the fall in the hemoglobin level. Several months after treatment has begun, the hemoglobin level may rise to almost pretreatment levels but will usually remain 1 g below the original level.

Methemoglobinemia will also regularly occur in patients treated with sulfones but not as often as in patients treated with sulfapyridine. Methemoglobinemia is not a major problem in most patients. Even in patients taking 200 mg/day of dapsone, the level usually does not exceed 12 percent of the total hemoglobin level and is often less than 5 percent. The methemoglobin level is more pronounced at the onset of treatment and, as with hemolysis, it is somewhat dose dependent. The cyanosis (which may seem more gray than blue) that results from methemoglobinemia may be seen in anyone with a methemoglobin level greater than 3 percent but may not be apparent in some patients with a level as high as 12 percent. Symptoms of methemoglobinemia include weakness, tachycardia, nausea, headache, and abdominal pains, but should not be attributed to methemoglobinemia until levels of 20 percent or greater are present. Some of these symptoms may be seen in patients taking dapsone in the absence of methemoglobinemia.

Other than these pharmacologic side effects, adverse effects of dapsone may be idiosyncratic or allergic in nature [9,19,20] (Table 218-1). Peripheral neuropathies are one such example and usually occur at high-dose levels. Loss of motor function is the most common type of neuropathy and it is reversible on withdrawal of dapsone. Recent studies have suggested that dapsone may rarely induce a pronounced hypoalbuminemia [21]. Other less well-known side effects include the induction of acute psychosis [22,23] and a potentially fatal mononucleosis-like syndrome that occurs during induction of dapsone therapy in patients with leprosy [24]. Although agranulocytosis has been reported, it is an extremely rare complication and occurs during the first 3 to 4 months of therapy. Generally, when adverse reactions occur as a result of therapy with dapsone, dapsone derivatives or even sulfapyridine cause the same types of problems.

Recent information from two independent carcinogenicity studies suggests that dapsone is a "weak carcinogen" in rats [25,26]. However, similar evidence does not exist in humans.

A frequently asked question is whether dapsone is safe if given during pregnancy. In one study of leprosy patients there were two infants born with congenital malformations out of 56 live births [27]. However, there are no controlled studies in animals or people which address this point.

Monitoring of dapsone therapy

Before the institution of therapy with the sulfones or sulfapyridine, a complete blood cell (CBC) count should be obtained. In addition, Asians, blacks, and persons of Mediterranean descent should be tested for glucose-6-phosphate dehydrogenase deficiency, because sulfones can cause profound hemolysis in persons lacking this enzyme. After therapy is begun, leukocyte count with differential and hemoglobin levels should be obtained weekly or twice a month during the first 3 months. Thereafter, CBC counts should be obtained every 3 to 4 months. Liver and renal function tests should also be obtained before institution of therapy and periodically thereafter. Once the disease being treated is under control, the dosage of dapsone should be reduced to be sure that the patient is using the minimum amount of drug required. Although in some diseases, such as dermatitis herpetiformis, the patients may alter the drug dosage according to the severity of the disease, they should be reminded not to increase the dosage by large amounts very abruptly. As the blue-gray color of methemoglobinemia may be attributed to other causes by emergency room physicians, patients should be advised to carry a medication card in their wallets.

Mechanisms of action

The mechanisms of action of dapsone in leprosy and inflammatory diseases have been the subject of considerable study. Dapsone and its derivatives are potent oxidants with a notable influence on glutathione. Their bacteriostatic effect is by way of interference with the folate biosynthetic pathway of bacteria. Less well-known activities of dapsone relate to its inhibition of choline incorporation into the lecithin of the cell membranes, thereby decreasing phospholipid synthesis [28]. Also, dapsone administered in the diet decreases visceral lesions and mortality in chickens infected with Marek's disease (herpes virus), which induces a lymphocytic malignant neoplasm in chickens.*

There have been numerous studies that have attempted to identify the mechanism by which dapsone exerts its anti-inflammatory effects. Considerable evidence suggests that it is not related to its antibacterial effect. Various investigators have shown that dapsone inhibits lysosomal enzyme activity [29,30] and interferes with the myeloperoxidase-H_2O_2-halide-mediated cytotoxic system in polymorphonuclear leukocytes [31,32]. Although these findings may account for the effect of the drug on neutrophils or on their lysosomal enzymes at the site of injury, they probably do not account for the lack of flux of neutrophils into the dermis in treated patients. There are few data to support suggestions that dapsone interferes with complement activation and deposition [33]. Some in vivo studies have shown that dapsone inhibits adjuvant-induced arthritis and carrageenin-induced inflammation in rats at doses of 100 to 200 mg/kg [34].

Several studies have suggested that dapsone and its derivatives do not exert an effect on the response of neutrophils to chemotactic stimuli. However, two studies have suggested that dapsone inhibits neutrophils from responding to some chemotactic stimuli [35,36]. More extensive studies using various chemotactic stimuli in varied concentrations are required to evaluate more fully the possibility that dapsone may interfere with a specific chemotactic factor or with the response of neutrophils to such a factor.

Table 218-1   Adverse reactions to sulfones*

Pharmacologic effects
  Hemolysis
  Methemoglobinemia
Headache
Gastric irritation
Nausea
Anorexia
Fatigue
Hepatitis, infectious mononucleosis-like with adenopathy
Cholestatic jaundice
Morbiliform eruptions
Erythema nodosum
Erythema multiforme
Exfoliative dermatitis
Toxic epidermal necrolysis
Psychosis
Leukopenia
Agranulocytosis
Peripheral neuropathy (primarily motor)

*Modified from Lang [9], Alexander [19], and Katz et al [20].

References

1. Costello MJ: Dermatitis herpetiformis treated with sulphapyridine. *Arch Dermatol Syphilol* **41**:134, 1940
2. Swartz JH, Lever WF: Dermatitis herpetiformis: immunology and therapeutic considerations. *Arch Dermatol Syphilol* **47**:680, 1943
3. Cornbleet R: Sulfoxone (Diasone) sodium for dermatitis herpetiformis. *Arch Dermatol Syphilol* **64**:684, 1951
4. Kruizinga EE, Hamminga H: Treatment of dermatitis herpetiformis with diaminodiphenylsulphone (DDS). *Dermatologia* **106**:386, 1953
5. Ellard GA et al: Dapsone acetylation in dermatitis herpetiformis. *Br J Dermatol* **90**:441, 1974
6. Ellard GA et al: Dapsone acetylation and the treatment of leprosy. *Nature* **239**:159, 1972
7. Hjelm M, deVerdier CH: Biochemical effects of aromatic amines: I. Methaemoglobinaemia, haemolysis and Heinz-body formation induced by 4,4'-diaminodiphenylsulphone. *Biochem Pharmacol* **14**:1119, 1965
8. Goodwin CS, Sparell G: Inhibition of dapsone excretion by probenecid. *Lancet* **2**:884, 1969
9. Lang P: Sulfones and sulfonamides in dermatology today. *J Am Acad Dermatol* **1**:479, 1979
10. Katz SI et al: Erythema elevatum diutinum: skin and systemic manifestations, immunologic studies, and successful treatment with dapsone. *Medicine (Baltimore)* **56**:443, 1977
11. McConkey B et al: Dapsone in rheumatoid arthritis. *J Rheumatol Rehab* **15**:230, 1976
12. Person JR, Rogers RS III: Bullous pemphigoid responding to sulfapyridine and the sulfones. *Arch Dermatol* **113**:610, 1977
13. Rogers RS et al: Treatment of cicatricial (benign mucous membrane) pemphigoid with dapsone. *J Am Acad Dermatol* **6**:215, 1982
14. Penneys NS, Wiley HE III: Herpetiformis blisters in systemic lupus erythematosus. *Arch Dermatol* **115**:1427, 1979
15. Hall RP et al: Bullous eruption of systemic lupus erythema-

---

* Shen TY et al: Read before the American Chemical Society Abstracts Meeting. September 12–16, 1971.

tosus: dramatic response to dapsone therapy. *Ann Intern Med,* in press

16. Coburn PR, Shuster S: Dapsone and discoid lupus erythematosus. *Br J Dermatol* **106:**105, 1982

17. Chimenti S, Ackerman AB: Is subcorneal pustular dermatitis of Sneddon and Wilkinson an entity sui generis? *Am J Dermatopathol* **3:**363, 1981

18. Cream JJ, Scott GL: Anaemia in dermatitis herpetiformis: the role of dapsone-induced haemolysis and malabsorption. *Br J Dermatol* **82:**333, 1970

19. Alexander JO: Dermatitis herpetiformis, in *Major Problems in Dermatology,* edited by A Rook. Philadelphia, WB Saunders, 1975, p 291

20. Katz SI et al: Dermatitis herpetiformis: the skin and the gut. *Ann Intern Med* **93:**857, 1980

21. Kingham JGC et al: Dapsone and severe hypoalbuminaemia. *Lancet* **2:**662, 1979

22. Sahu DM: Dapsone-induced psychosis: a case report. *Indian J Dermatol* **17:**47, 1972

23. Fine JD et al: Psychiatric reaction to dapsone and sulfapyridine. *J Am Acad Dermatol* **9:**274, 1983

24. Frey AM et al: Fatal reaction to dapsone during treatment of leprosy. *Ann Intern Med* **94:**777, 1981

25. *Bioassay of Dapsone for Possible Carcinogenicity,* US Dept of Health, Education, and Welfare publication 77–820. National Cancer Institute Carcinogenesis Technical Reports Series, 1977

26. Griciute L, Tomatis L: Carcinogenicity of dapsone in mice and rats. *Int J Cancer* **25:**123, 1980

27. Maurus JM: Hansen's disease in pregnancy. *Obstet Gynecol* **52:**22, 1978

28. Shigeura HT et al: Metabolic studies on dapsone and sulfone derivatives in chick macrophages. *Biochem Pharmacol* **24:**687, 1975

29. Barranco VP: Inhibition of lysosomal enzymes by dapsone. *Arch Dermatol* **110:**563, 1974

30. Mier PD, Van Den Hurk JJMA: Inhibition of lysosomal enzymes by dapsone. *Br J Dermatol* **93:**471, 1975

31. Stendahl O et al: The inhibition of polymorphonuclear leukocyte cytotoxicity by dapsone: a possible mechanism in the treatment of dermatitis herpetiformis. *J Clin Invest* **62:**214, 1978

32. Kazmierowski JA et al: Dermatitis herpetiformis: effects of sulfones and sulfonamides on neutrophil myeloperoxidase-mediated iodinations and cytotoxicity. *J Clin Immunol,* in press

33. Katz SI et al: Effect of sulfones on complement deposition in dermatitis herpetiformis and on complement-mediated guinea pig reactions. *J Invest Dermatol* **67:**688, 1976

34. Williams K et al: Anti-inflammatory actions of dapsone and its related biochemistry. *J Pharm Pharmacol* **28:**555, 1976

35. Anderson R et al: In vitro and in vivo effects of dapsone on neutrophil and lymphocyte functions in normal individuals and patients with lepromatous leprosy. *Antimicrob Agents Chemother* **19:**495, 1981

36. Harvath L et al: Selective inhibition of neutrophil chemotaxis by sulfones. *Clin Res* **31:**571A, 1983

CHAPTER 219

AMINOQUINOLINES

Gunnar Swanbeck

The aminoquinolines are derived from quinine, a compound extracted from the bark of the cinchona tree native to South America. They have been used mainly as antimalarials. Even in dermatologic literature these compounds are generally described under the heading of antimalarials. The antimalarials that are of dermatologic interest may all be regarded as aminoquinolines: chloroquine, hydroxychloroquine, amodiaquin, and quinacrine (see Fig. 219-1). The latter compound is of course more correctly classified as an acridine derivative. These four compounds are all 4-aminoquinolines. In the following discussion the word aminoquinolines designates the four compounds mentioned above.

Mode of action

The aminoquinolines have several relatively well-defined effects on biochemical and cellular systems, the significance of which is not fully understood. Some of the more important will be mentioned here.

Interactions with nucleic acids

Aminoquinolines bind to DNA. They also affect DNA and RNA polymerase activity and inhibit DNA replication and transcription to RNA [1–3]. This may be a process that is directly related to the DNA binding and may be noteworthy for the antimalarial properties of these compounds and also for their inhibition of the lupus erythematosus-cell phenomenon and antinuclear antibody reactions [4,5]. This is one possible explanation for the clinical effect of the aminoquinolines on lupus erythematosus.

Immunologic effects

The aminoquinolines may suppress lymphocyte transformation in vitro [6]. They may also interfere with complement-dependent antigen–antibody reactions [7]. No effect on the development of primary or secondary antibody response has been found [7,8].

Anti-inflammatory activity

Chloroquine has been shown to be a lysosomal stabilizer but it also inhibits hydrolytic enzymes [9]. It has also been demonstrated that chloroquine interferes with prostaglandin synthesis [10]. Another important property may be its influence on the neutrophil, macrophage, and eosinophil chemotaxis [11,12].

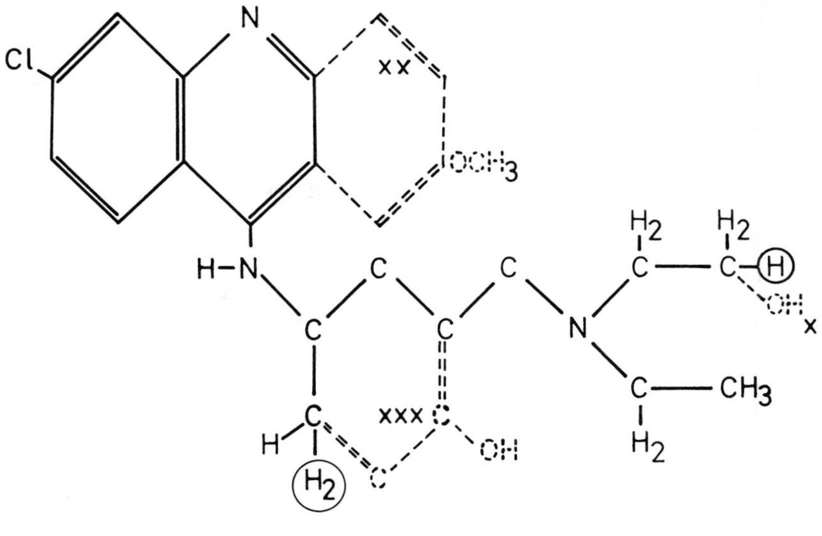

Fig. 219-1 The aminoquinolines used in dermatology are all 4-aminoquinolines and may be regarded as derivatives of chloroquine, which is illustrated by the solid line. The other compounds are indicated by dotted lines: x = hydroxychloroquine, xx = quinacrine, xxx = amodiaquine. The two hydrogens within circles are substituted in the respective derivatives.

Photodermatologic properties

There has been much work and speculation concerning the possible sunscreening effect of systemically administered chloroquine. Chloroquine absorbs in the UVA region of the spectrum and is bound in epidermis in a relatively high concentration; however, there is no effect on the minimal erythema dose [13]. The clinical action on lupus erythematosus and polymorphous light eruption may very well be explained by the effect of chloroquine on immunologic reactions.

Pharmacokinetics and distribution

The aminoquinolines are all water-soluble and are readily absorbed in the gastrointestinal tract. The plasma concentration reaches a peak within about 8 h, but plasma is not cleared of the aminoquinoline within 24 h [14]. Giving daily doses, the plasma concentration increases to an equilibrium value after some weeks, but remains relatively low, while the concentration in some organs may become many thousand times higher than in the plasma. The liver, spleen, lungs, and adrenal glands store chloroquine in large amounts [15]. Melanin-containing cells have a particular affinity for chloroquine [16]. The high uptake of chloroquine in the liver may be of importance for the use of this drug in porphyria cutanea tarda, and the melanin affinity may be the basis for the ocular side effects.

The equivalent doses of three of the aminoquinolines are: chloroquine 250 mg, hydroxychloroquine 400 mg, and quinacrine 100 mg.

Side effects

Only side effects that are specific for the aminoquinolines will be discussed here. The acute symptoms resulting from very large doses of chloroquine are weakness, dyspnea, hypotension, tremor, coma, convulsions, and cardiopulmonary arrest [15]. A lethal dose of chloroquine for an adult is 3 to 6 g.

All the aminoquinolines may induce leukopenia within the first few months of treatment. Aplastic anemia has been reported with use of quinacrine but it is a very rare side effect.

The aminoquinolines are to be regarded as teratogenic. Chloroquine is capable of crossing the placenta, and congenital defects such as deafness, mental retardation, and convulsions have been described in newborn children of women who have taken chloroquine during pregnancy [17].

Toxic psychosis, headache, and irritability have been reported as consequences of the use of both chloroquine and quinacrine [18]. These are, however, usually reversible and disappear when the medication is discontinued.

Among the cutaneous side effects of aminoquinolines, the exacerbation of psoriasis is well known and may lead to a generalized exfoliation. There are conflicting reports in the literature on the actual risk of using aminoquinolines in psoriasis. It is curious that antimalarials are quite widely used by rheumatologists for the treatment of psoriatic arthritis and they do not believe that these drugs have caused flare-ups of preexisting psoriasis.

Discoloration of the skin may occur as a long-term cutaneous side effect [15,19]. A moderate dose of quinacrine rather regularly gives a yellow discoloration after a few months.

All the aminoquinolines may cause a bluish black pigmentation of the pretibia, palate, face, and nail beds. These effects on the skin are reversible over time.

Ocular side effects are the greatest problem of the aminoquinolines, especially after long administration. Both chloroquine and hydroxychloroquine may give deposits in the cornea that are reversible and may produce only slight symptoms in the form of halos around bright objects [20].

Irreversible retinopathy is probably the most limiting factor for use of the aminoquinolines. Most of the cases described involve chloroquine and hydroxychloroquine. This does not mean that the other aminoquinolines are safe in this respect. The retinopathy is certainly dose-related. There are two common views about this problem. One is that the accumulated dose of chloroquine should not exceed 200 g. The other is that the daily dose of chloroquine "should not exceed 2 mg per pound of body weight" 4.4 mg/kg) [21,22]. Some ophthalmologists claim that for an adult a daily dose of about 250 mg of chloroquine will be safe if there is a yearly interruption of therapy for about 2 months. The patient should also be seen by an ophthalmologist at regular intervals. An interruption of the medication is, however, no guarantee against progression of the ocular problems. Systemic lupus erythematosus may itself produce ocular changes similar to those seen with amino-quinolines. However, ocular changes have also been observed in rheumatoid arthritis patients who are taking chloroquine [23].

Indications for use

Malaria and rheumatoid arthritis are two of the chief indicators for aminoquinolines. They will not be discussed here as they are outside the field of dermatology. With regard to skin diseases, there are positive reports on the use of aminoquinolines for more than a dozen different conditions. Some of these findings have withstood the test of time; in other cases a single report on a rare disease has not been verified in spite of a long lapse of time since the original report was published.

Diseases where the risk/benefit ratio seems to be favorable are lupus erythematosus, polymorphous light eruption, and porphyria cutanea tarda, and these diseases will be dealt with in more detail. Other diseases where positive results with the use of aminoquinolines have been reported are sarcoidosis, DNA-autosensitivity reaction, solar urticaria, scleroderma, lymphocytic infiltration of the skin, disseminated granuloma annulare, cutaneous cryptococcosis, cutaneous leishmaniasis, epidermolysis bullosa, acrodermatitis chronica atrophicans, and lichen sclerosus et atrophicus [24].

Lupus erythematosus

As early as the nineteenth century lupus erythematosus was treated with quinine, the forerunner of the aminoquinolines. However, it was not until the 1950s that chloroquine and its derivatives came into more general use for this disease. The first report was by Page in 1951 [25] but several more were to follow.

Generally the full effect of the aminoquinolines is obtained within a month. Cutaneous symptoms respond better than do systemic involvements [26]. The seriously ill patient with fever, renal damage, and hematologic abnormalities does not benefit from these compounds.

Today the aminoquinolines are mainly used in combination with steroids in lupus erythematosus. The clinical effect of steroids and aminoquinolines seems to be additive. However, their side effects are different and a more favorable risk/benefit ratio is obtained by the combined use of the two types of drugs.

Although there are no convincing double-blind studies with aminoquinolines in lupus erythematosus, the clinical evidence for their efficacy is overwhelming. Also the large number of studies that show a high recurrence rate after discontinuation of the treatment strongly support the clinical evidence [27,28].

Polymorphous light eruption

This disease is confined to the sun-exposed areas of the skin, and the histology of the lesions indicates that there are immunologic factors involved in the pathogenesis. There are several reports indicating that chloroquine is effective in this disease [13,29]. In those parts of the world where there is a season with little sun radiation it is pos-

sible for the patient to discontinue aminoquinolines for some months and thereby decrease the risk of long-term side effects. In polymorphous light eruption, aminoquinoline medication is often combined with the use of topical suncreening agents.

Porphyria cutanaea tarda

Chloroquine has been found to be a beneficial drug in the treatment of porphyria cutanea tarda. Its effect in this disease is most probably dependent on mechanisms other than those in lupus erythematosus and polymorphous light eruption. It is tempting to believe that the high affinity of chloroquine for liver tissue is of primary importance.

Following a daily dose of 250 mg of chloroquine to a patient with porphyria cutanea tarda, the following will be observed on the third to fourth day of medication: headache, nausea, fever, elevated transaminases, massive excretion of uroporphyrins in the urine [30]. If the medication is stopped after a week of daily doses of 250 mg, the patient will continue to excrete porphyrins in the urine for two months. By the end of the third month the patient usually has normal excretion of porphyrins, no other symptoms of disease, and remains symptomless for two years or more.

The problem with this type of treatment is the acute reaction and the possible risk for the liver. Two regimens have been proposed to circumvent this problem. One is to give a small dose, 125 mg of chloroquine, twice a week over a long period of time [31]. The other is to use phlebotomies three times, before 250 mg chloroquine is given daily to the patient for 7 days [32]. Both methods seem to work satisfactorily.

Several theories have been proposed for the mode of action of chloroquine in porphyria cutanea tarda. It seems reasonable to assume, however, that uroporphyrins and chloroquine compete for the same binding sites in the liver tissue and that chloroquine is able to displace porphyrins from the tissue.

References

1. Kurnick NB, Radcliffe IE: Reaction between DNA and quinacrine and other anti-malarials. *J Lab Clin Med* **60:**669, 1962
2. Cohen SN, Yielding KL: Stabilization of the structure of native DNA by chloroquine and observations on the nature of the chloroquine-DNA complex. *Arthritis Rheum* **6:**767, 1963
3. Cohen SN, Yielding KL: Further studies on the mechanism of action of chloroquine: inhibition of DNA and RNA polymerase reactions. *Arthritis Rheum* **7:**302, 1964
4. Dubois EL: Effect of quinacrine (Atabrine) upon lupus erythematosus phenomenon. *Arch Dermatol Syphilol* **71:**570, 1955
5. Bencze G, Johnson GD: Inhibition of antinuclear factor reaction by chloroquine. *Immunology* **9:**201, 1965
6. Harvitz D, Hirschorn K: Suppression of in vitro lymphocyte responses by chloroquine. *N Engl J Med* **273:**23, 1965
7. Neblett TR et al: Chloroquine: its mechanism of action upon immune phenomena. *Arch Dermatol* **92:**720, 1965
8. Kalmanson GM, Guze LB: Studies of the effects of hydroxychloroquine on immune responses. *J Lab Clin Med* **65:**484, 1965
9. Weissman G: Labilization and stabilization of lysosomes. *Fed Proc* **23:**1038, 1964

10. Greaves MW, McDonald-Gibson WJ: Anti-inflammatory agents and prostaglandin biosynthesis. *Br Med J* **3**:527, 1972

11. Ward PA: The chemosuppression of chemotaxis. *J Exp Med* **124**:209, 1966

12. Ganderer CA, Gleich CJ: Inhibition of eosinophilotaxis by chloroquine and corticosteroids. *Proc Soc Exp Biol Med* **157**:129, 1978

13. Cahn MM et al: Polymorphous light eruption—the effect of chloroquine phosphate in modifying reactions to ultraviolet light. *J Invest Dermatol* **26**:201, 1956

14. Rubin M, Zvaifler N: The metabolism of chloroquine. *Clin Res* **10**:22, 1962

15. Dubois EL: Anti-malarials in the management of discoid and systemic lupus erythematosus. *Semin Arthritis Rheum* **8**:33, 1978

16. Zvaifler NJ et al: Chloroquine deposition in ocular tissues. *Arthritis Rheum* **5**:667, 1962

17. Lewis R et al: Malaria associated with pregnancy. *Obstet Gynecol* **42**:696, 1973

18. Sapp OL: Toxic psychosis due to quinacrine and chloroquine. *JAMA* **187**:373, 1964

19. Tuffanelli DL et al: Pigmentation associated with anti-malarial therapy. Its possible relationship to the ocular lesions. *Arch Dermatol* **88**:419, 1963

20. Hobbs RF, Calnan CD: Visual disturbances with anti-malarial drugs with particular reference to chloroquine keratopathy. *Arch Dermatol* **80**:557, 1959

21. Bernstein HN: Chloroquine ocular toxicity. *Surv Ophthalmol* **12**:415, 1967

22. MacKenzie AH: An appraisal of chloroquine. *Arthritis Rheum* **13**:280, 1970

23. Scherbel AL et al: Ocular lesions in rheumatoid arthritis and related disorders with particular reference to retinopathy: study of 741 patients treated with and without chloroquine. *N Engl J Med* **273**:360, 1965

24. Isacson D et al: Antimalarials in dermatology. *Int J Dermatol* **21**:379, 1982

25. Page F: Treatment of lupus erythematosus with mepacrine. *Lancet* **2**:755, 1951

26. Dubois EL: Quinacrine (Atabrine) in treatment of systemic and discoid lupus erythematosus. *Arch Intern Med* **94**:131, 1954

27. Christiansen JV, Nielsen JP: Treatment of lupus erythematosus with mepacrine. Results and relapses during a long observation. *Br J Dermatol* **68**:73, 1956

28. Merwin C, Winkelmann R: Dermatologic clinics 2. Antimalarial drugs in therapy of lupus erythematosus. *Proc Mayo Clin* **37**:253, 1962

29. Christiansen JV, Brodthagen H: The treatment of polymorphic light eruptions with chloroquine. *Br J Dermatol* **68**:204, 1956

30. Cripps DJ, Curtis AC: Toxic effect of chloroquine on porphyria hepatica. *Arch Dermatol* **86**:575, 1962

31. Kordac V et al: Chloroquine in the treatment of PCT. *N Engl J Med* **296**:949, 1977

32. Swanbeck G, Wennersten G: Treatment of porphyria cutanea tarda with chloroquine and phlebotomy. *Br J Dermatol* **97**:77, 1977

CHAPTER 220

CYTOTOXIC AGENTS IN DERMATOLOGY

Michael M. Wick

The modern era of chemotherapy with cytotoxic agents began with the introduction of the antimetabolite, amethoprin, by Farber in 1948 [1]. Since that time, a large number of synthetic and natural substances have been identified whose primary role is to exert their effects through the inhibition of intracellular processes, often leading to cell death. Agents such as methotrexate, 5-fluorouracil, azathioprine, hydroxyurea, and cytoxan have achieved important roles in the treatment of human disease. Although the basis of selectivity of these agents in the treatment of disease is often obscure, certain correlates of activity have been developed [1–3].

Dermatologic conditions offer a unique opportunity to circumvent the intrinsic lack of selectivity of these agents by offering the possibility, through topical application, of avoiding effects upon the usual target organs—the rapidly proliferating bone marrow and the gastrointestinal mucosa. Generally, the therapeutic effects of these drugs in dermatology are the consequence of direct antiproliferative effects mediated through the immune system.

The life cycle of the mammalian cell can be classified according to events that occur in an orderly fashion through growth and division. These temporal markers provide a convenient framework within which to classify the various cytotoxic agents according to that portion of the cell cycle during which they exert their biologic effects [4].

The length of the cell cycle, the generation time, is the time required for a cell to develop from the midpoint of mitosis to the midpoint of a subsequent mitosis in the daughter cell. The events occurring between these two time points may be divided into several discrete segments. The G_1 phase is a presynthetic period in which the cells conduct those metabolic activities that are necessary for DNA synthesis. Following a G_1 period, the cells duplicate their DNA during the S period of the cell cycle. Following the cessation of DNA synthetic activity, a second gap, the G_2 period, occurs. Following the G_2 period is the mitotic (M) phase. Alternatively, a cell may enter a G_0 phase, which is found in either G_1 or G_2, where there is very little metabolic activity. The viability and clonogenic potential of the cell, however, remain intact, and cells may return from this resting state and undergo active cell division. Weinstein and McCullough [5], Gelfant [6], and Voorhees et al [7] extended these observations directly to cell cycle events and related biochemical changes in normal human and abnormal human skin. It is within this setting that we can classify the chemotherapeutic agents used in dermatology.

Drugs

Antimetabolites

Antimetabolites are generally inhibitors of specific enzymes involved in cellular replication. The majority of clinically useful agents interfere with enzymes required for DNA synthesis and therefore are generally most effective against relatively rapidly dividing cells during the S phase.

Methotrexate

Methotrexate (MTX) is the most frequently used chemotherapeutic agent in dermatology [8]. An analog of folic acid, it inhibits the enzyme dihydrofolate reductase. Reduced folate is required for the synthesis of thymidine and purines, and following the depletion in intracellular pool of these substances, DNA synthesis is inhibited [9,10]. The binding of this inhibitor to the enzyme is extremely tight, with virtually complete inhibition of DNA synthesis occurring in normal bone marrow when drug concentrations in the extracellular fluid exceed levels of 10^{-8} M. Methotrexate, therefore, tends to act during the S phase of the cell cycle.

The cytotoxicity of MTX is largely influenced by pharmacokinetic factors, the major one being the duration of exposure and the drug concentration reached. The minimum cytotoxic concentration present in the plasma is approximately 10^{-8} M, although cytotoxicity is also proportional to the duration of exposure [11]. The effects of MTX can be aborted by the administration of a rescue agent, leucovorin (5-formotetrahydrofolate), which can be interconverted to the other reduced folates and bypass the block in folate reduction caused by MTX [12]. Interestingly, the administration of leucovorin does not interfere with the antipsoriatic effect of MTX and the adjunctive immunologic effect in pemphigus and may be useful in limiting other toxicities of methotrexate as well [13].

Methotrexate may be administered intramuscularly, intravenously, or orally, with essentially 100 percent of the oral dose absorbed. However, small alterations in renal function can have profound effects on the duration of the plasma levels, leading to toxicity. A second important aspect of MTX pharmacokinetics is the variability of excretion from patient to patient. This is especially true in the presence of significant third spaces; for example, malignant effusions. Effusions apparently concentrate the drug and can act as a reservoir for later drug release, especially in the presence of diminished renal function [14]. Third, because MTX is bound to plasma protein, concomitant administration of a drug such as aspirin, which may displace it, can also have a profound enhancing effect [15]. In conventional regimens, peak plasma concentrations of about 10^{-6} to 10^{-5} M are achieved.

5-Fluorouracil

5-Fluorouracil (5-FU) is probably the second most commonly used cancer chemotherapeutic agent in dermatol-

ogy. The mechanism of action of 5-FU inhibition involves at least two pathways. The first is through the formation of 5-fluoro-2′-deoxyuridine 5′-monophosphate, a tight-binding inhibitor of thymidylate synthetase capable of inhibiting the synthesis of thymidine [16]. More recent evidence supports the concept that 5-FU may have an alternative mechanism of action that is preferential in tumor cells. Specifically, 5-FU may be incorporated into RNA, thereby rendering the RNA molecule defective [17]. Because RNA synthesis generally occurs throughout the cell cycle, whereas DNA synthesis is restricted to the S phase, this alternative mechanism may be of relevance to dermatology. This is true because the growth rate of the lesions for which 5-FU is used is generally not much larger than that of surrounding skin. Therefore, an alternative mechanism must be invoked in order to explain the relative selectivity observed with this agent.

Hydroxyurea

Hydroxyurea is a simple compound that exerts a marked cytotoxic effect both in vitro and in vivo. The major biochemical action is the causation of an immediate inhibition of DNA synthesis [18]. Biochemical evidence supports the inhibition of the enzyme ribonucleotide disphosphate reductase as the principal site of action. This enzyme is critically important for converting ribonucleotides to deoxyribonucleotides and is most active during the S phase of the cell cycle. The rate of DNA synthesis in mammalian cells is controlled by the supply of deoxyribonucleotides, which in turn is controlled by production through the enzyme ribonucleotide diphosphate reductase. Therefore, a small inhibition of this enzyme results in a marked decrease in the rate of DNA synthesis.

Azathioprine

Azathioprine is a purine analog derived from 6-mercaptopurine by the addition of an imidazole ring onto sulfur. This compound is largely converted to 6-mercaptopurine, an active metabolite, in the body. Its major effect occurs in the inhibition of purine synthesis, resulting in inhibition of both RNA and DNA synthesis [19]. It appears to be most effective during the S phase of the cell cycle. Azathioprine has gained widespread use because it appears to have a good therapeutic index and is frequently chosen for immunosuppression. The drug is well absorbed orally, with a recommended initial daily dose of 2 to 3 mg/kg followed by a maintenance dose of 1 to 2 mg/kg [20]. Because allopurinol inhibits the metabolic degradation of azathioprine to 6-mercaptopurine, a downward adjustment (25 percent) is seriously recommended when allopurinol is given concomitantly.

Alkylating agents

A variety of alkylating agents have undergone extensive use in dermatology. These include cyclophosphamide, chlorambucil, nitrogen mustard, and 1,3-bis(2-chloroethyl)-1-nitrosourea. The alkylating agents differ from the antimetabolites, principally because the former rely on the physical alteration of the DNA molecule for their effect. These DNA–drug interactions include alkylation, cross-linking, and carbamoylation. Cyclophosphamide differs from the others in that it requires prior hepatic activation by microsomal enzyme systems for activity [21]. Because these enzymes are shared by other drugs, marked drug interactions can occur; for example, high-dose steroids or barbiturates can markedly increase its toxicity. In addition to DNA damage, these drugs also interfere with the synthesis of RNA. The net effect of these actions is that alkylating agents, unlike the antimetabolites, tend to be active against slowly growing cells throughout all stages of the cell cycle. Unfortunately, they are also among the most potent in terms of mutagenicity, teratogenicity, and carcinogenicity [22]. The therapeutic index and risk/benefit ratios of the alkylating agents are among the most marginal of those used in dermatology.

Although bleomycin, a polypeptide antibiotic, is not, strictly speaking, an alkylating agent, it shares many properties with the alkylating agents. It appears to exert its antitumor activity through the breaking of double-stranded DNA [23]. This action appears to be more selective than that observed with the alkylating agents, and unique areas of DNA are susceptible with the formation of free-thymine bases. Although bleomycin is more active against proliferating cells, it does appear to be toxic to cells in the S phase.

Clinical applications

Methotrexate

Methotrexate has demonstrated a beneficial effect in a variety of benign and malignant dermatologic disorders. Its effects can be classified as either antimitotic (for example, as in the treatment of benign proliferative keratinizing disorders such as psoriasis, pityriasis rubra pilaris, severe cases of epidermolytic ichthyosis, or mycosis fungoides) or immunosuppressive, as in the treatment of the pemphigus–pemphigoid group. A large body of experience has indicated that it is generally a safe drug when given carefully and does not appear to be mutagenic, as it acts primarily by metabolic inhibition [24]. The major use of MTX in dermatology has been in the treatment of psoriasis. Its utility has been established in multiple, noncontrolled and controlled trials [25–27]. In general, MTX is capable of inducing remissions in 80 to 90 percent of patients treated and of maintaining these remissions for long periods with continued therapy. A large variety of schedules have been utilized with weekly administration as a single or divided dose, ranging from 25 to 50 mg/m^2 and 2.5 to 7.5 mg every 12 h for three doses, respectively. In general, the daily schedules have fallen into disfavor, as they appear to be related to a higher incidence of hepatic toxicity.

The major long-term concern in the use of MTX in dermatology has been the development of chronic hepatic toxicity. Recently, Nyfors reported his long experience with the effects and side effects of MTX [28]. In a 10-year prospective therapeutic trial of 248 patients, major risks of hepatic toxicity appeared to be related to total cumulative dose of MTX, with total cumulative doses of 2000 to 4000 mg correlating with a high percentage of patients in whom fibrosis/cirrhosis developed. Other risk factors appeared to be age, obesity, and, possibly, intercurrent alcohol consumption during MTX therapy. Because liver function tests can be normal in the presence of hepatic toxicity, a repeat liver biopsy was strongly urged in patients having total doses of more than 2000 mg. The second major concern in the use of MTX has been the possibility of carcinogenesis, teratogenicity, and pulmonary toxicity. There is no clinical or experimental evidence suggesting that MTX has a carcinogenic effect. Bailin et al [29], in a study of more than 200 patients followed for seven years, were unable to show an increased rate of malignancy. Although MTX is teratogenic in pregnant females [30], there is no evidence that MTX taken by males or nonpregnant females has any effect on fertility or offspring. Methotrexate does occasionally cause oligospermia, which is reversible. Pulmonary toxicity is related to a hypersensitivity syndrome that rapidly reverses on discontinuance of MTX and treatment with systemic steroids.

Although stomatitis is the most frequently reported side effect of MTX therapy, other cutaneous side effects have been observed, including alopecia, photoreactions, acneform lesions, macular and papular exanthems, ulcerations, erythema, hyperpigmentation, and exfoliated dermatitis limited to the hands and feet [31,32]. These side effects appear to be related to the dose and schedule of administration, in addition to being idiosyncratic. Side effects, unless severe, do not warrant either a decrease in dosage or a change in treatment schedule, in view of the severity of the underlying disease for which MTX is generally used.

In addition to its use in psoriasis, MTX has also been used in such diseases as dermatomyositis and polymyositis [33], Wegener's granulomatosis [34], Reiter's disease [35], mycosis fungoides [36], pityriasis lichenoides and lymphomatoid papulosis [37], pustular psoriasis [38], congenital ichthyosiform erythroderma [39], and pityriasis rubra pilaris [40]. MTX is also useful in the treatment of pemphigus vulgaris [41]. Like azathioprine, MTX tends to reduce the dose of prednisone required to moderate and maintain remissions.

5-Fluorouracil

5-Fluorouracil (5-FU) is an excellent example of the potentially unique application of cancer chemotherapeutic agents in dermatology. The major use of 5-FU is via topical application, which permits its use with a minimum of adverse side effects. Topical 5-FU has received extensive use for the treatment of superficial basal and squamous cell carcinomas [42] and actinic keratoses [43,44]. It is available in 1% and 5% strengths, although the original enthusiasm for this agent in the treatment of basal and squamous cell carcinomas has been blunted somewhat by apparent high recurrence rates [45]. The treatment of actinic keratoses is complicated by a marked irritant reaction [46], as well as the potential for subsequent permanent scarring, alopecia, and hypo- and hyperpigmentation. 5-FU has also been used in the treatment of porokeratosis [47], keratoacanthomas (intralesional) [48], facial warts [49], and, inadvisably, lentigo maligna [50] with varying success. 5-FU has the added advantage of uncovering not only clinically undetectable keratoses, but malignant epitheliomas as well.

Stomatitis and alopecia are the most common side effects of systemic treatment. Systemic 5-FU therapy has also been associated with nail changes, hyperpigmentation of skin and nails, and phototoxicity. Patients receiving 5-FU at a dose of 15 mg/kg once weekly note severe xeroderma, especially involving the palms and soles, often progressing to fissuring. The specific toxic effects following topical administration may include irritation, scarring, alopecia, and hyper- and hypopigmentation.

Hydroxyurea

The principal use of hydroxyurea in dermatology has been for the treatment of psoriasis vulgaris. This use is based on observations of a large number of adverse cutaneous reactions in patients with chronic lymphocytic leukemia undergoing maintenance therapy with hydroxyurea. In 7 of 28 patients, partial alopecia, increased pigmentation, skin atrophy, nail changes, and erythema were noted [51]. Subsequent controlled and uncontrolled studies have indicated response rates of 50 to 60 percent [52]. The drug has also been evaluated in pustular psoriasis without impressive results.

Although hydroxyurea is not a first choice for the systemic treatment of psoriasis, it remains a possible alternative for those patients with underlying liver disease who are unable to tolerate MTX. The usual maintenance doses are 1 to 2 g per day in divided doses.

Cutaneous side effects in patients treated with hydroxyurea occur in 25 to 35 percent of cases. A variety of cutaneous reactions have been described, including allergic cutaneous vasculitis, macular and papular eruptions, alopecia, stomatitis, and xeroderma. Interestingly, fixed drug eruptions and nail changes, as well as increased erythema in previously irradiated sites, have also been described [31].

Azathioprine

Azathioprine has been the most popular immunosuppressive agent used in dermatology, and marked immunosuppression can occur at doses that do not cause significant leukopenia. The precise mechanism of action of this agent in the immunologically mediated dermatologic diseases of the pemphigus–pemphigoid group is not known, although it appears to have an effect on the humoral arm of the immune system. The first report of the effectiveness of azathioprine in treating pemphigus vulgaris was in 1969 [53]. Subsequent studies have confirmed its activity in this disease [41]. The principal role of azathioprine is in reducing the steroid dose required for the induction and maintenance of remission. In pemphigus erythematosus and pemphigus foliaceus it is rarely capable of maintaining a remission without prednisone. Bullous pemphigoid is more responsive to azathioprine alone or in combination with systemic steroids and in essentially all patients showing control of blister formation. Azathioprine, although not effective in psoriasis, does show some activity in pityriasis rubra pilaris [54].

Cyclophosphamide

Cyclophosphamide is an alkylating agent that has a marked effect on the primary and secondary humoral immune response in humans. It has received significant use in the treatment of pemphigus [55] and has proved effective when other immunosuppressants have failed. Like azathioprine, it exerts a steroid-sparing effect when used in combination

with steroids for the treatment of pemphigus and pemphigoid [56,57]. A dramatic reduction in the mortality of pemphigus vulgaris has been reported, although in a retrospective analysis. It is equally effective in the treatment of Wegener's granulomatosis where cyclophosphamide alone may maintain long-term remissions [58]. Case reports exist for the use of cyclophosphamide in the treatment of Behçet's syndrome and necrotizing vasculitis [59] and lichen myxedematosus [60].

Merchlorethamine is an alkylating agent that can be conveniently formulated for topical therapy of a variety of dermatologic disorders, including early phases of mycosis fungoides [61]. Using daily applications, most patients will undergo a significant clinical improvement and remission of their disease. The treatment, however, is complicated by the subsequent development of allergic contact dermatitis, which usually necessitates the cessation of therapy [62]. Attempts to induce tolerance to merchlorethamine in sensitized patients have met with varying success. Topical merchlorethamine has also been used as a treatment for hyperhydrosis [63], acrodermatitis [64], and psoriasis [65]. Two patients with histiocytosis of skin were reported to have responded to topical nitrogen mustard [66]. Topical nitrosourea (BCNU, CCNU) has also been shown to be effective in the control of early cutaneous mycosis fungoides [67]. The nitrosoureas are especially valuable in those patients who have become sensitized to merchlorethamine, as cross-sensitization is not observed. It is significant that the more lipid-soluble nitrosoureas readily penetrate skin, causing significant plasma levels and leading to myelosuppression.

Conclusion

Cytotoxic agents have found an important role in the treatment of multiple dermatologic disorders. However, since they appear to control rather than cure various dermatoses, the new issues of chronic as opposed to acute toxicities have emerged. Concern has focused particularly upon the potential for carcinogenesis. As these agents have become more effective in the treatment of human malignancies and the achievement of disease-free intervals, increases in the development of second malignancies, especially of the lymphoreticular system [68–71], have been observed. The agents of most concern as carcinogens are the alkylating agents, since they are capable of inducing permanent alterations in cellular genetic material. It is with this group in particular that caution in use must be advised until the relevance of these observations to dermatology is assessed.

References

1. Farber S et al: Temporary remissions in acute leukemia in children produced by the folic acid antagonist, 4-aminopterolglutamic acid (aminopterin). *N Engl J Med* **238**:787, 1948
2. Wick MM et al: Cancer chemotherapy in dermatology, in *Dermatology Update 1982,* edited by SL Moschella. New York, Elsevier, 1982, p 339
3. Capizzi RL: Introduction: the place of pharmacology in cancer medicine, in The Pharmacologic Basis of Cancer Chemotherapy. *Semin Oncol* **IV(2)**:131, 1977
4. Hill TB, Baserga R: The cell cycle and its significance for cancer treatment. *Cancer Treat Rev* **2**:159, 1975

5. Weinstein GD, McCullough JC: Cytokinetics and chemotherapy of psoriasis. *J Invest Dermatol* **67**:26, 1976
6. Gelfant S: A new concept of tissue and tumor cell proliferation. *Cancer Res* **37**:3845, 1977
7. Voorhees JJ et al: Cyclic AMP, cylic GMP, and glucocorticoids as potential metabolic regulators of epidermal proliferation and differentiation. *J Invest Dermatol* **65**:179, 1975
8. Bergstresser PR et al: Systemic chemotherapy for psoriasis. A national survey. *Arch Dermatol* **112**:977, 1976
9. Goldman ID: The mechanism of action of methotrexate. I. Interaction with a low-affinity intracellular site required for maximum inhibition of deoxyribonucleic acid synthesis in L-cell mouse fibroblast. *Mol Pharmacol* **10**:257, 1974
10. Goldman ID: Analysis of the cytotoxic determinants for methotrexate. A role for "free" extracellular drug. *Cancer Treat Rep* **6**:51, 1975
11. Pinedo HM, Chabner BA: The role of drug concentration, duration of exposure, and endogenous metabolites in determining MTX cytotoxicity. *Cancer Treat Rep* **61**:709, 1977
12. Nixon PF, Bertino JR: Effective absorption and utilization of oral formyltetrahydrofolate in man. *N Engl J Med* **286**:175, 1972
13. Hanno R et al: Methotrexate in psoriasis. *J Am Acad Dermatol* **2**:171, 1980
14. Wan SH et al: Effect of route of administration and effusions on methotrexate pharmacokinetics. *Cancer Res* **34**:3487, 1974
15. Taylor JR, Halprin KM: Effect of sodium salicylate on methotrexate-serum albumin binding. *Arch Dermatol* **113**:588, 1977
16. Santi DV et al: Mechanism of interaction of thymidylate synthetase with 5-fluorodeoxyuridylate. *Biochemistry* **13**:471, 1974
17. Carrico CK, Glazer RI: Effect of 5-fluorouracil on the synthesis and translation of polyadenylic acid-containing RNA from regenerating rat liver. *Cancer Res* **39**:3694, 1979
18. Timson J: Hydroxyurea. *Mutat Res* **32**:115, 1975
19. Rosman M, Bertino JR: Azathioprine. *Ann Intern Med* **79**:694, 1973
20. Moschella SL: The present status of chemotherapy in dermatology. *Med Clin North Am* **56**:725, 1972
21. Cox PJ et al (eds): Symposium on the Metabolism and Mechanism of Action of Cyclophosphamide. *Cancer Treat Rep* **60**:299, 1976
22. Sieber SM, Adamson RH: Toxicity of antineoplastic agents in man. Chromosomal aberrations, antifertility effects, congenital malformations, and carcinogenic potential, in *Advances in Cancer Research,* edited by G Klein et al. New York, Academic Press, 1975, p 57
23. Ishida R, Takahashi T: Increased DNA chain breakage by combined action of bleomycin and superoxide radical. *Biochem Biophys Res Commun* **66**:1432, 1975
24. Newberger AE et al: Biologic and biochemical actions of methotrexate in psoriasis. *J Invest Dermatol* **70**:183, 1976
25. Roenigk HH Jr et al: Methotrexate therapy for psoriasis. *Arch Dermatol* **108**:35, 1973
26. Weinstein GD: Methotrexate. *Ann Intern Med* **86**:199, 1977
27. Weinstein GD, Frost P: Methotrexate for psoriasis. *Arch Dermatol* **103**:33, 1971
28. Nyfors A: *Methotrexate Therapy for Psoriasis: Effect and Side Effects with Particular Reference to Hepatic Changes. A Survey.* Aarhus, Denmark, Laegeforeningens Forlag, 1980
29. Bailin PL et al: Is methotrexate therapy for psoriasis carcinogenic? A modified retrospective–prospective analysis. *JAMA* **232**:359, 1975
30. Carless RG: Methotrexate in young females with psoriasis. *N Engl J Med* **285**:296, 1971
31. Adrian RM et al: Mucocutaneous reactions to antineoplastic agents. *CA* **30**:143, 1980
32. Levine N, Greenwald ES: Mucocutaneous side effects of cancer chemotherapy. *Cancer Treat Rep* **5**:67, 1978
33. Giannini M, Callen JP: Treatment of dermatomyositis with methotrexate and prednisone. *Arch Dermatol* **115**:1251, 1979
34. Capizzi RL, Bertino JR: Methotrexate therapy of Wegener's granulomatosis. *Ann Intern Med* **74**:74, 1971
35. Jetton RL, Duncan WC: Treatment of Reiter's syndrome with methotrexate. *Ann Intern Med* **70**:349, 1969
36. Groth O et al: Tumor stage of mycosis fungoides treated with bleomycin and methotrexate: report from the Scandinavian Mycosis Fungoides Study Group. *Acta Derm Venereol (Stockh)* **59**:59, 1979
37. Lynch PJ, Saied NK: Methotrexate treatment of pityriasis lichenoides and lymphomatoid papulosis. *Cutis* **23**:634, 1979
38. Hoffman TE, Watson W: Methotrexate toxicity in the treatment of generalized pustular psoriasis. *Cutus* **21**:68, 1978
39. Herskowitz LJ et al: Acute pancreatitis associated with long-term azathioprine therapy in patients with systemic lupus erythematosus. *Arch Dermatol* **115**:179, 1979
40. Knowles WR, Chernosky ME: Pityriasis rubra pilaris prolonged treatment with methotrexate. *Arch Dermatol* **102**:603, 1970
41. Lever WF, Schaumburg-Lever G: Immunosuppressants and prednisone in pemphigus vulgaris. *Arch Dermatol* **113**:1236, 1977
42. Reymann F: Treatment of basal cell carcinoma of the skin with 5-fluorouracil ointment, a 10-year follow-up study. *Dermatologica* **158**:368, 1979
43. Breza T et al: Non-inflammatory destruction of actinic keratoses by fluorouracil. *Arch Dermatol* **112**:1258, 1976
44. Epstein E: Treatment of lip keratoses (actinic chelitis) with topical 5-fluorouracil. *Arch Dermatol* **113**:906, 1977
45. Mohs FE et al: Tendency of fluorouracil to conceal deep foci of invasive basal cell carcinoma. *Arch Dermatol* **114**:1021, 1978
46. Kaplan LA et al: Hypertrophic scarring as a complication of fluorouracil Rx. *Arch Dermatol* **115**:1452, 1979
47. Dupre A, Cristol B: Mibelli's porokeratosis of the lips. *Arch Dermatol* **114**:1841, 1978
48. Odom RB, Goette DK: Treatment of keratoacanthomas with intralesional fluorouracil. *Arch Dermatol* **114**:1779, 1978
49. Lockshin NA: Flat facial warts treated with 5-fluorouracil. *Arch Dermatol* **115**:929, 1979
50. Gromet MA: Treatment of lentigo maligna with 5-FU. *Arch Dermatol* **113**:1128, 1977
51. Kennedy BJ et al: Skin changes secondary to hydroxyurea therapy. *Arch Dermatol* **111**:183, 1975
52. Moschella SL, Greenwald MA: Psoriasis with hydroxyurea. An 18-month study of 60 patients. *Arch Dermatol* **107**:363, 1973
53. Krakewski A: Pemphigus vulgaris. *Arch Dermatol* **110**:117, 1969
54. Ahmed AR et al: Bullous pemphigoid. Clinical and immunologic follow-up after successful therapy. *Arch Dermatol* **113**:1043, 1977
55. Sabbour MS, Osman LM: Comparison of chlorambucil, azathioprine, or cyclophosphamide combined with corticosteroids in the treatment of lupus nephritis. *Br J Dermatol* **100**:113, 1975
56. Brody JH, Pirozzi DJ: Benign mucous membrane pemphigoid response to treatment with cytoxan. *Arch Dermatol* **113**:1598, 1977
57. Fellner MJ et al: Successful use of cyclophosphamide and prednisone for initial treatment of pemphigus vulgaris. *Arch Dermatol* **114**:889, 1978
58. Novack SN, Pearson CM: Cyclophosphamide therapy in Wegener's granulomatosis. *N Engl J Med* **284**:938, 1971
59. Fauci AS et al: Cyclophosphamide therapy of severe systemic necrotizing vasculitis. *N Engl J Med* **301**:235, 1979
60. Jessen RT et al: Lichen myxedematosus treatment with cyclophosphamide. *Int J Dermatol* **17**:833, 1978

61. Vonderheid EC et al: A 10-year experience with topical merchlorethamine for mycosis fungoides: comparison with patients treated by total skin electron beam radiation therapy. *Cancer Treat Rep* **63**:681, 1979

62. Molin L et al: Mycosis fungoides plaque stage treated with topical nitrogen mustard with and without attempts to tolerate induction: report from the Scandinavian Mycosis Fungoides Study Group. *Acta Derm Venereol (Stockh)* **59**:64, 1979

63. Cullen SI: Topical methenamine therapy for hyperhidrosis. *Arch Dermatol* **111**:1158, 1975

64. Notowicz A et al: Treatment of Hallopeau's acrodermatitis with topical merchlorethamine. *Arch Dermatol* **114**:129, 1978

65. Handcer RM, Medansky RS: Treatment of psoriasis with topical nitrogen mustard. *Int J Dermatol* **18**:758, 1979

66. Zachariae H: Histiocytosis X in two infants treated with topical nitrogen mustard. *Br J Dermatol* **100**:433, 1979

67. Zackheim HS, Epstein EH Jr: Treatment of mycosis fungoides with topical nitrosourea compounds. *Arch Dermatol* **111**:1564, 1975

68. Canellos GP et al: Second malignancies complicating Hodgkin's disease in remission. *Lancet* **1**:947, 1975

69. Coleman CN et al: Hematologic neoplasia in patients treated for Hodgkin's disease. *N Engl J Med* **297**:1249, 1977

70. Penn I: Chemical immunosuppression and human cancer. *Cancer* **34**:1474, 1974

71. Reimer RR et al: Acute leukemia after alkylating-agent therapy of ovarian cancer. *N Engl J Med* **297**:177, 1977

CHAPTER 221

RETINOIDS

Gary L. Peck and John J. DiGiovanna

Vitamin A is a necessary dietary nutrient which is important in growth, vision, reproduction, and the maintenance and differentiation of epithelial tissue for all vertebrates. Except for its role in vision, the exact molecular mechanisms regulating these funtions are unknown. Today, the term *vitamin A* is used to characterize the biologic activity of this group of compounds rather than a particular compound. In mammals vitamin A activity is fulfilled by three major compounds: retinol, retinal, and retinoic acid; and perhaps by a number of their metabolites. The term *retinoid* refers to the entire group of compounds which includes retinol, with its naturally occurring and synthetic derivatives.

Historical perspective

Awareness of therapies containing vitamin A activity can be traced back to the ancient Egyptians (ca 1500 B.C.) as evidenced by writings describing the benefits of liver as a treatment of night blindness [1]. In 1909, a fat-soluble extract from egg yolk was found to be necessary for life [2,3]. McCollum and Davis later used the term *fat-soluble factor A* for a dietary component that was important for the normal growth of animals [4–6]. The active factor ''A'' was associated with yellow vegetables as well as with animal fats and fish oils [7] and was subsequently named vitamin A [8].

In 1931, vitamin A (retinol) was purified from halibut liver oil and its structural formula was determined [9,10]. In 1935, another vitamin A derivative, later identified to be retinal, was demonstrated by Wald and later by others to be important in the visual cycle [11–14]. In 1946, vitamin A acid (retinoic acid) was synthesized and shown to promote growth [15].

Vitamin A was first used clinically during World War I in the treatment of xerophthalmia and in the prevention of night blindness. The significance of retinoids to dermatology dates back to 1925, when epithelial changes were identified in vitamin A-deficient animals and low levels of vitamin A were thereby related to dyskeratotic skin conditions [16,17]. Systemic vitamin A was then used clinically in the treatment of disorders involving abnormal keratinization such as Darier's disease and pityriasis rubra pilaris, in which follicular keratoses resembled the lesions of vitamin A deficiency [18,19]. Once the beneficial effects of vitamin A were observed in these disorders, its use spread to the treatment of other diseases of the epidermis and epidermal appendages. Vitamin A deficiency provides a conceptual link in understanding how retinoids may be effective as therapy for a wide range of dermatologic disorders, since it is characterized by squamous metaplasia of a variety of epithelia with increased cell proliferation and hyperkeratosis. Vitamin A was initially related to cancer in 1926 when rats fed a vitamin A-deficient diet were found to develop carcinomas of the stomach [20].

All-*trans*-retinoic acid (tretinoin), a naturally occurring metabolite of retinol, has been used clinically in the treatment of pityriasis rubra pilaris, various ichthyoses, psoriasis, acne, and actinic keratoses [21–25]. This compound is currently accepted as standard topical therapy for acne vulgaris. Experience with the systemic use of tretinoin has been limited by prominent side effects [26].

In an effort to develop compounds that might possess a better therapeutic index than retinol or retinoic acid in the prophylaxis and treatment of cancer, a group of synthetic derivatives of retinoic acid were synthesized and developed beginning in 1968 [27]. Many chemical variations, both of the cyclic and carboxylic end groups and also the side chain of the retinoic acid molecule are possible [28]. More than 1500 analogues have been synthesized and are being tested in various in vivo and in vitro models [29,30]. Only a few of them have so far been used in clinical trials.

Table 221-1   Oral synthetic retinoids

Generic name	Chemical name	Trade name	Principal indications	Other indications
Isotretinoin	13-*cis*-Retinoic acid	Accutane (USA) Roaccutane (Europe)	Cystic acne	Darier's disease Pityriasis rubra pilaris
Etretinate	Trimethylmethoxyphenyl analog of retinoic acid ethyl ester	Tegison (USA) Tigason (other than USA)	Psoriasis	Lamellar ichthyosis, etc.

At the time of this writing, two synthetic retinoids of appreciably different action spectra, pharmacokinetics, and side effects (Table 221-1) are commercially available: 13-*cis*-retinoic acid (isotretinoin) and the trimethylmethoxyphenyl analog of retinoic acid ethyl ester (etretinate). 13-*cis*-Retinoic acid is a naturally occurring metabolite of vitamin A found in tissues in small quantities [31]; however, its usefulness in dermatology evolved before this was known [32]. With the dramatic response of severe cystic acne, psoriasis, and many of the disorders of keratinization, and the wide spectrum of benign and malignant conditions noted to be partially responsive, the retinoids have ushered in a new era in the therapy of skin disease.

Retinoid structures and functions

The structures and functions of the major naturally occurring retinoids are outlined in Fig. 221-1. The structures of natural and synthetic retinoids are presented in Fig. 221-2. Vitamin A is necessary for growth, differentiation, the maintenance of epithelial tissues and reproduction. Retinol can be reversibly oxidized to retinal, the aldehyde derivative which is important in vision. Retinoic acid is an important oxidative metabolite of retinol which can substitute for some vitamin A functions. In vitamin A-deficient animals, retinoic acid can replace retinol in supporting growth promotion, and in the maintenance and differentiation of epithelial tissues. Retinoic acid, however, cannot substitute for retinol in maintaining reproductive function nor for retinal in the visual cycle.

Retinoid uptake: dietary intake, serum transport, and delivery to target cells

The pathway traveled by the naturally occurring retinoids from dietary precursors through absorption, serum transport, storage, and delivery to target cells is shown in Fig. 221-3. Retinoids are derived from retinyl esters contained in dietary animal sources (fats, fish liver oils) and from carotenoids in yellow and green leafy vegetables. Ingested retinyl esters are hydrolyzed in the intestine leaving free retinol to be absorbed into the mucosal cells. Alternatively, a range of carotenoids can act as retinoid precursors, the most common and efficient precursor being all-*trans*-β-carotene. β-carotene is not absorbed directly [34]. In the gut, carotenoids undergo oxidative cleavage of the central double bond by the action of β-carotene-15,15'-dioxygenase to yield retinal. In the intestinal mucosa, the retinal is reduced by retinaldehyde reductase to retinol, the alcohol form [35,36].

In the intestinal cell, the free retinol is then esterified (mainly as retinyl palmitate), complexed with long-chain fatty acids into chylomicrons, and transported through the lymph and then into the blood to the liver [37,38]. In the liver, retinol is stored in the ester form in a small number

Fig. 221-1   Structures and functions of the major naturally occurring retinoids. (Adapted with permission from Pawson et al [33]. Copyright 1982, American Chemical Society.)

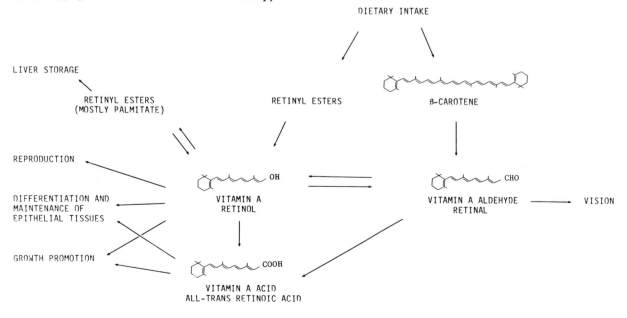

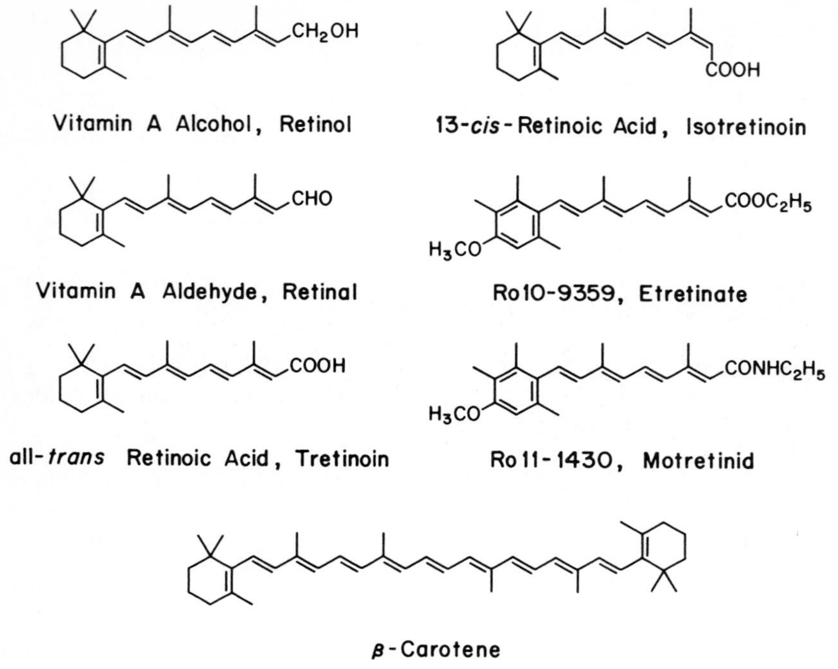

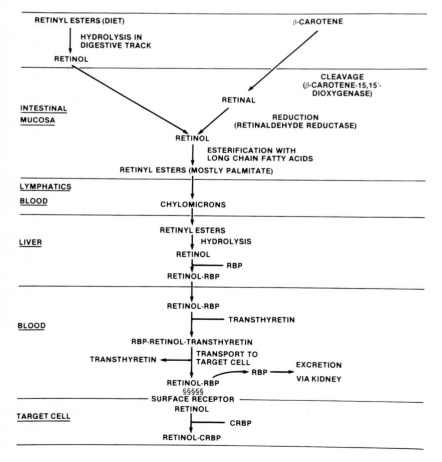

Fig. 221-2 Structures of natural and synthetic retinoids.

Vitamin A Alcohol, Retinol

13-*cis*-Retinoic Acid, Isotretinoin

Vitamin A Aldehyde, Retinal

Ro10-9359, Etretinate

all-*trans* Retinoic Acid, Tretinoin

Ro11-1430, Motretinid

β-Carotene

of fat-storing, stellate cells called *vitamin A storage* or *Ito cells* [39]. Upon demand the ester is hydrolyzed to the free alcohol and complexed with its transport protein, the serum retinol binding protein (RBP) [40], which is synthe-

sized in the liver [41]. Free retinol is not released from the liver alone, but only in a 1:1 ratio with RBP.

Upon release from the liver, the RBP–retinol complex binds to prealbumin, a serum protein which has recently

Fig. 221-3 Retinoid uptake, storage, serum transport, and delivery to target tissues. (Adapted with permission from Pawson et al [33]. Copyright 1982, American Chemical Society.)

RETINYL ESTERS (DIET)   β-CAROTENE

HYDROLYSIS IN DIGESTIVE TRACK

RETINOL

CLEAVAGE (β-CAROTENE-15,15'-DIOXYGENASE)

RETINAL

REDUCTION (RETINALDEHYDE REDUCTASE)

INTESTINAL MUCOSA

RETINOL

ESTERIFICATION WITH LONG CHAIN FATTY ACIDS

RETINYL ESTERS (MOSTLY PALMITATE)

LYMPHATICS

BLOOD

CHYLOMICRONS

RETINYL ESTERS

LIVER   HYDROLYSIS

RETINOL

RBP

RETINOL-RBP

RETINOL-RBP

TRANSTHYRETIN

BLOOD

RBP-RETINOL-TRANSTHYRETIN

TRANSPORT TO TARGET CELL

TRANSTHYRETIN

RBP   EXCRETION VIA KIDNEY

RETINOL-RBP
§§§§
SURFACE RECEPTOR

TARGET CELL   RETINOL

CRBP

RETINOL-CRBP

been termed *transthyretin* (TTR) to signify its role as a transport protein for both thyroxin and the RBP–retinol complex. Thyroxin is bound to TTR at a site that is independent from the RBP–retinol binding site. In the blood, retinol circulates as a complex of RBP–retinol–TTR.

On the molecular level, retinol arrives at a target cell bound to the serum RBP transport protein. The RBP–retinol complex binds to specific membrane receptors of target cells. These membrane receptors interact with the RBP–retinol complex but not to either free retinol or RBP. Retinol is then translocated into the cell. A specific cytosol binding protein for retinol is present within target cells; it is called the cellular retinol binding protein (CRBP). This intracellular binding protein is distinct from the serum transport protein (RBP) and binds specifically and saturably to retinol. Its exact function is unknown.

All-*trans*-retinoic acid is not a normal dietary constituent. When administered, this compound is not absorbed via the lymphatics in association with lipoproteins like retinol, but is absorbed directly into the portal blood [42,43]. In addition, it does not bind to RBP but circulates in the serum bound to albumin [43]. Retinoic acid also has a specific intracellular binding protein, the cellular retinoic acid binding protein (CRABP).

Vitamin A is transported in the serum as all-*trans*-retinol and that is the form which is presented to target cells. But once inside a cell, retinol must often be converted to other metabolites before it is physiologically active. For example, retinol must be converted to retinal before it can react with opsin and function in the visual process.

Retinoid metabolism

While the active tissue metabolites and the mechanisms of vitamin A degradation and removal from epithelial tissues are not known, a number of retinoid metabolites have been identified. A small amount of retinoic acid is formed from retinol in tissues and this is quickly converted to other metabolites [44]. 13-*cis*-Retinoic acid has potent biologic effects but even further metabolic products of 13-*cis*-retinoic acid have been identified [45].

Retinol and a hydroxylated derivative of retinoic acid have been found to be phosphorylated and then glycosylated, primarily with mannose [46–48]. Retinyl phosphate and retinyl-P-sugar derivatives act as carriers of monosaccharides and may function as intermediates in cellular glycosylation reactions. The specific role of each of these retinoid metabolites has not been elucidated. Identification of further retinoid metabolites and clarification of the biologic activity of each compound will be necessary to further clarify the exact mechanisms accounting for the varied retinoid effects.

Mechanisms of retinoid action

Retinoids have a variety of biologic effects. These actions include: (1) the regulation of differentiation in epithelial and other cells, (2) inhibition of tumor promotion during experimental carcinogenesis, (3) effects on tumor growth, (4) effects on the immune system and inflammation, and (5) alterations in cellular cohesiveness and interaction. These effects can be understood at a cellular level by retinoid action on three parameters: proliferative capacity,

differentiation state, and cell surface composition [33]. On a molecular level, several retinoid actions have been identified which may be responsible for modulation of these parameters. These include retinoid influences on RNA synthesis [49–52], protein synthesis [53], posttranslational glycosylation of protein [47,54–56], prostaglandin synthesis [57,58], labilization of membranes, and effects on specific enzymes such as ornithine decarboxylase and collagenase.

Retinoid effects on proliferative capacity

Vitamin A deficiency is known to be associated with inhibition of proliferation in many systems [59–61]. While the lack of vitamin A can suppress growth, the treatment of cultured cells with excess retinoid can also cause growth inhibition, the lengthening of generation time, and a reduction of saturation density.

Retinoid effects on differentiation state

Retinoids are involved in regulating cellular differentiation. During retinoid deficiency, the normal growth and differentiation of a variety of tissues and organs (including bronchi, trachea, stomach, intestine, uterus, kidney, bladder, testis, prostate, pancreatic ducts, and skin) also do not occur [16,62]. In tissues that are normally a mucous epithelium, physiologic doses of retinoids promote differentiation in the direction of mucus secretion, while inhibiting keratinization. The bladder, lung, and trachea are dependent on retinoid for maintenance of their columnar epithelia. Vitamin A deficiency in these tissues results in the development of a stratified squamous epithelium. Furthermore, vitamin A in excess can inhibit keratinization in a broad variety of stratified squamous epithelia and induces mucous metaplasia in chick skin and hamster cheek pouch [63]. When chick embryo epidermis is maintained in organ culture under the influence of large amounts of retinoid, the epidermal cells become columnar mucus-secreting cells [64].

Retinoids are involved in the relationship between differentiation and malignant transformation. For example, without retinoids the tracheal and bronchial epithelia undergo squamous metaplasia, a premalignant condition [16,65,66]. In animal studies, vitamin A deficiency yields an enhanced susceptibility to chemical carcinogenesis of the respiratory system, bladder, and colon [67–70]. Conversely, naturally occurring retinoids have been shown to protect animals against the development of carcinomas of the stomach, vagina, cervix, bronchi, trachea, and lung, and against skin papillomas and carcinomas. Furthermore, some malignant cell lines can also be induced to differentiate under retinoid influence. Several teratocarcinoma cell lines have been induced to differentiate on exposure to retinoic acid [71]. The F9 cell line, for instance, differentiates into endoderm and produces plasminogen activator, collagen-like proteins, and alkaline phosphatase [72]. When the retinoic acid-treated F9 cell line is subsequently exposed to dibutyryl cyclic adenosine monophosphate, these cells differentiate into neural-like cells [73]. The embryonal carcinoma cell membranes are in a relatively higher fluid state than their differentiated derivatives and the biologically active retinoids increase the membrane viscosity of these cells while inducing their differentiation

[74]. The observed effects of retinoids on differentiation, however, are not completely consistent. Retinoids can inhibit the differentiation of mesodermal tissues in chondrogenesis, osteogenesis, and in the conversion of fibroblasts to adipocytes [75–78]. Similarly, while retinoids have been shown to stimulate the differentiation of human melanoma [79] and promyelocytic leukemia cells [80,81], differentiation is suppressed in another human [82] and a hamster [83] melanoma line, and in a murine leukemia line [84].

Cell surface alterations

Under the influence of retinoids, cell surface alterations can occur which often result in increased adhesiveness of the treated cells [85–87]. Retinoids can alter membrane microviscosity [88] and may interact directly with membranes [89]. Another direct effect on cell membranes is the production of gap junctions that allow cell-to-cell coupling and facilitate intercellular communication [90,91].

On a molecular level, cells exposed to retinoids develop alterations in surface protein profiles [83,87,92], increased protein glycosylation [47,56,93], modulation of glycosaminoglycan synthesis [85,94], and quantititive changes in surface protein receptors [89].

Effects on transformation, tumor promotion, tumor growth, and ornithine decarboxylase

One characteristic feature of vitamin A deficiency is a squamous metaplasia of a variety of epithelia [95]. Retinoids suppress malignant transformation, in vitro, caused by chemical carcinogens, ionizing radiation, growth factors, or viruses [69,95–100]. Using experimental models of carcinogenesis, retinoids interfere with tumor development in several tissues, including urinary bladder, breast, and skin.

Tumor promotors are agents that enhance carcinogenesis when administered after initiation by a carcinogen. While the initiation step is irreversible, the effect of the promoter is reversible. Retinoids can interfere with the promotion phase of carcinogenesis. After dimethylbenzanthracene (DMBA) initiation of mouse skin carcinogenesis, for example, retinoids administered during the croton-oil promotion phase can inhibit the development of skin papillomas [101]. Retinoids have a prophylactic effect against DMBA-induced heratoacanthomas in the rabbit ear; animals fed etretinate after topical application of DMBA failed to develop keratoacanthomas [102]. In other animal model systems, retinoids inhibit tumor formation in a variety of organs (Table 221-2). In addition to the skin, chemopreventive effects of retinoids against cancer have been documented in the breast [105], urinary bladder [103], lung [109], prostate [117], and cervix and forestomach [96]. In female Sprague-Dawley rats, breast tumors induced by N-methylnitrosurea and 7,12-dimethylbenzanthracene were inhibited with retinyl acetate and retinyl methyl ether [105,106]. The incidence of tumors in animals continuously fed retinoid was approximately one-third of controls, but in animals whose diets were changed from retinoid to placebo the tumor incidence approached controls. This indicates that a continuous exposure to retinoid is required to sustain the chemoprotective effect.

Some retinoids manifest tissue specificity. 4-Hydroxyphenyl retinamide is effective in preventing breast cancer in the rat. The tissue levels of this retinoid are markedly elevated in the breast but not in the liver [107]. This retinoid has a strong antiproliferative effect on normal mammary epithelium. Eventually it may be possible to develop retinoid molecules that can be targeted for specific organs.

Retinoids are effective chemopreventative agents in bladder cancer [103]. 13-cis-Retinoic acid is effective in the inhibition of transitional cell papillomas and carcinomas and squamous cell carcinomas induced by N-methylnitrosourea or N-butyl-N-(4-hydroxybutyl)nitrosamine [104]. In these chemoprevention studies, animals were not treated with retinoids until they had received full exposure to the carcinogens, thereby excluding the possibility that the retinoids were inhibiting the initiation phase of carcinogenesis. Accordingly, retinoids are considered to be "antipromoting" agents in these experimental carcinogenesis systems, as discussed above. Tumor promoters, such as phorbol esters, the active agents in croton oil, increase ornithine decarboxylase (ODC) activity early during experimental carcinogenesis in skin [118,119]. ODC is the rate-limiting enzyme in the synthesis of polyamines, which are involved in cell proliferation and differentiation [120]. Retinoids interfere with the ability of phorbol esters to induce ODC [120–123]. When many retinoids were tested, the degree of ODC inhibition was found to correlate with the ability of the retinoid to inhibit the development of skin papillomas [123]. Retinoids that do not interefere with tumor promotion do not block ODC activity [124]. When retinoids inhibit proliferation of other cell types, they also appear to suppress the increase in ODC activity [76,125,126].

Ornithine decarboxylase induction during the G_1 phase of the cell cycle may be a requirement for cell cycle progression, and, therefore, the antiproliferative effects of retinoids may be related to their ability to block the cell cycle in the G_1 phase and thereby inhibit ODC induction [127]. In support of this concept, retinoic acid treatment of melanoma cell lines and synchronized spinner cultures of HeLa cells has been shown to increase the proportion of cells in the G_1 phase of the cell cycle [128,129].

Retinoids have been extensively studied as antipromo-

Table 221-2 Retinoids and cancer: laboratory studies

	Reference
Inhibit proliferation of malignant cell lines	[95]
Inhibit chemical carcinogenesis in vivo:	
Bladder	[103, 104]
Breast	[105–107]
Skin	[108]
Lung	[109]
Cervix	[96]
Forestomach	[96]
Inhibition of tumor promotion and induction of ornithine decarboxylase by phorbol esters	[110, 111]
Might interefere with tumor initiation:	[112]
Inhibit carcinogen-induced aryl-hydrocarbon hydroxylase	
Inhibit binding of carcinogen to DNA	
Suppress malignant transformation in vivo:	
Chemical carcinogenesis	[113]
Ionizing radiation	[114]
Sarcoma growth factor	[115]

Reprinted from Peck [116].

ters. However, retinyl acetate has been shown to inhibit the rate of proliferation of mouse epidermal cells in culture, reduce the activity of aryl hydrocarbon hydroxylase induced by benz[a]anthracene, and markedly decrease the binding of 7,12-dimethylbenz[a]anthracene to DNA, suggesting a possible interference in the initiation phase of carcinogenesis [112].

While retinoids are most potent as prophylactic agents before tumor development has occurred, they can interfere with the proliferation of many but not all malignant cell lines in vitro [130]. The growth of some types of malignant cells can be unaffected or actually stimulated [124].

Retinoids have a wide variety of effects on in vitro malignant transformation. Retinoids reverse the anchorage-independent growth of transformed mouse fibroblasts [131] and suppress malignant transformation caused by chemical carcinogens [113], ionizing radiation [114], and transforming peptides from virally transformed cells [115]. The trimethylmethoxyphenyl analogue of N-ethylretinamide (Ro 11-1430) inhibits transformation of mouse embryo fibroblasts exposed to ^{60}Co gamma rays [114].

Retinoids may suppress malignant transformation induced by the sarcoma growth factor (SGF), suggesting that retinoids are more than antipromoting agents since this factor directly affects cell transformation [115]. SGF is a polypeptide produced by murine sarcoma virus-transformed cells. SGF stimulates cell growth, causes proliferation in soft agar, and leads to abnormal growth patterns in cell culture. The factor induces cell growth of rat fibroblasts in soft agar; the disordered growth pattern of these cells in culture is inhibited by retinoids [115]. Retinylidene dimedone was found to be the most efficient inhibitor of these changes although retinyl acetate, retinoic acid, and retinyl methyl ether are also effective.

Retinoids also interfere with viral-induced transformation. Etretinate was found to be effective in the treatment of lesions of epidermodysplasia verruciformis induced by the oncogenic human papilloma virus, types 5 and 3 [132–134].

Retinoid effects on the immune system

Retinoids are generally thought to stimulate humoral and cellular immunity, but inhibitory effects have also been observed. They can act as adjuvants in this process, enhancing antibody production in response to a variety of antigens and they can have diverse effects on cell-mediated immunity. Part of the antitumor effects of retinoids may be due to these immune effects [135–138].

Antilymphocyte serum has been found to oppose the vitamin A-induced growth inhibition of the S91 melanoma in mice [135] and a vitamin A-accelerated rejection of skin homografts [138]. When mice were inoculated with Lewis lung tumor cells, treatment with BCG and vitamin A was found to markedly decrease the incidence of primary tumors and lung metastases [139].

Low doses of retinoic acid in vitro stimulate cell-mediated cytotoxicity against tumors, while, in contrast, high doses abolish it [140]. Retinoic acid is a specific adjuvant for the induction of cytotoxic (killer) T lymphocytes and is not a general T-cell mitogen or adjuvant. Etretinate and Ro 13-6298, a benzoic acid derivative of retinoic acid, have been shown to stimulate two in vitro tests of tumor immunity: (1) an increased capacity of treated spleen cells to lyse antibody-coated chick erythrocytes, and (2) a strong activation of peritoneal macrophages making them highly cytostatic for P815 mastocytoma cells [141]. However, Ro 13-6298 also induced nonspecific suppressor cells.

Arginase released by activated macrophages is thought to be responsible for the differential killing of tumor cells. Retinoic acid and retinol in nontoxic concentrations completely inhibit the expression of Fc receptors and enhance the production of arginase [142]. It is possible that the retinoid effects on macrophages may occur through inhibition of prostaglandins since prostaglandins E_1 and E_2 inhibit the tumoricidal activity of macrophages [143].

Retinoids may also affect mitogen-stimulated lymphocyte proliferation. Vitamin A enhances the lymphocyte proliferation stimulated by extracts of *Candida albicans* and *Trichophyton mentagrophytes* [144], while retinoic acid does not enhance the proliferative response of mixed lymphocyte cultures to phytohemagglutinin (PHA) [140]. In contrast, the trimethylmethoxyphenyl derivative of retinoic acid (Ro 10-1670), the main metabolite of etretinate, inhibits the response of human peripheral blood lymphocytes to mitogenic stimuli [145]. Ro 10-1670 treatment of lymphocytes and lectins inhibits the usual increase in DNA synthesis seen with lectin (concanavalin A, pokeweed mitogen, and PHA) treatment of lymphocytes.

Lymphocytes from patients with Darier's disease have abnormally high lectin responsiveness [146]. Treatment of these lymphocytes with etretinate decreases the excessive response. Etretinate also has a blocking effect on immunoglobulin secretion by both normal and psoriatic B cells [147,148].

Since retinoids can directly inhibit the proliferation of transformed cells in vitro, in the absence of immunoregulatory cells, these immune effects are probably not the sole mechanism of retinoid antitumor activity. Nevertheless, the immunostimulatory effects of retinoids have led to their use as adjuvant therapy for cancer patients [95]. Further studies are needed to define more precisely the influence that retinoids might exert on immunoregulatory cells in vivo and to clarify the extent to which these effects mediate the antitumor activity of the retinoids.

Intracellular binding proteins

Some retinoid actions may be mediated through intracellular receptor proteins similar to the mechanism of action of several hormones. Many hormones are known to bind to specific intracellular receptor proteins which are identified in vivo by their ability to bind radiolabeled ligand (hormone). In a unified concept of steroid hormone action, the intracellular receptor protein has been postulated to bind to a hormone as it enters the cytoplasm and translocate it to the nucleus. In the nucleus, another receptor protein could further facilitate hormone action.

A similar receptor mechanism has been proposed for retinoid action. In 1973, a specific, soluble cellular retinol binding protein (CRBP) was identified in several tissues of the rat [149]. A distinct cellular retinoic acid binding protein (CRABP) was found in chick embryo skin [150]. This discovery highlighted the physiologic significance of retinoic acid in vivo and its potential importance as a separate entity from retinol.

Both CRBP and CRABP have been isolated and partially characterized [151–154], have molecular weights of approximately 14,000 to 15,000, and appear to have a single specific retinoid binding site [155,156], i.e., CRBP is specific for retinol while CRABP is specific for retinoic acid [156,157]. These two proteins are immunologically different but have a related amino acid sequence [158]. They have been identified in many tissues in a variety of species [159,160]. The binding of [³H]retinol to CRBP can be competitively inhibited by an excess of nonradiolabeled all-*trans*-retinol, α-retinol, and 3-dehydroretinol (vitamin A₂), but not by retinal nor retinoic acid [160,161], indicating the requirement for an alcohol function at carbon 15. 13-*cis*-Retinoic acid and etretinate bind to CRABP and are potent competitors of [³H]retinoic acid binding [162–164]. The binding of these retinoids to CRABP may indicate one mechanism by which they exert their clinical effects.

One possible role for these binding proteins is in the translocation of retinoid from the cytosol into the nucleus, where effects on DNA, RNA, or protein synthesis may be initiated. Wiggert et al [165], using Y-79 retinoblastoma cells provided evidence to suggest translocation of the retinoic acid-CRABP complex into the nucleus. In contrast, the complex of retinol bound to CRBP apparently did not enter the nucleus.

The levels of both CRBP and CRABP have been found to vary among different tissues [166], during development [167], and between normal and malignant tissues [168]. CRABP is not as widely distributed as CRBP among different tissues. While both have been found in rat brain, eye, skin, ovary, testis, and uterus [151,167], only CRBP was detected in small intestine, kidney, liver, lung, and spleen [151], and neither was detected in heart, skeletal muscle, or serum [151].

CRBP has been identified in rat and human skin, and CRABP in chick embryo, human and rat skin, and dermal fibroblast cultures. When adult human skin was analyzed to determine the relative contribution of epidermis and dermis to the binding found in skin, the binding from both CRBP and CRABP was confined predominantly to the epidermis, with no detectable binding in the dermis [169]. 13-*cis*-Retinoic acid does compete with all-*trans*-retinoic acid for binding epidermal and sebaceous follicle CRABP obtained from human facial skin, but with less affinity [170].

These binding proteins also vary with development. For example, in the rat, CRBP is present in most fetal and adult tissues, but in the adult, CRABP is found only in the brain, eye, and skin [155]. The presence of CRABP in developing tissues and its disappearance in adult tissues implicate retinoic acid and CRABP in the promotion of differentiation. This concept is supported by the fact that retinoic acid is generally more effective than retinol in promoting differentiation [95] and that a correlation exists between the ability of some retinoids to promote differentiation and to compete for binding to CRABP [95,163,171].

In some malignant tumors, the total amount of binding to these proteins is altered compared to the normal counterpart. Breast tumors [159,160,172–174] often show more binding to CRABP compared to normal breast tissue [168,172]. The amount of CRBP binding has also been found to vary between normal and malignant tissues [174]. While these binding proteins may be intimately involved in the mechanism of natural and synthetic retinoid action, their exact molecular role is still unclear.

Membrane effects

Labilization of membranes

Some retinoid effects may be due to direct action on cell membranes. In the blood, the binding of retinol to the transport protein, RBP, minimizes this effect. Free retinol can have a detergent-like effect, altering membrane microviscosity, possibly through insertion directly into the membrane [88,89]. One result of this detergent-like effect is the labilization of lysosomal membranes [175,176], which may result in lysosomal enzyme release and subsequent retinoid toxicity [177,178]. Membrane labilization seems to be dose-dependent, occurring only at high doses; retinoids at lower doses may stabilize membranes [179,180]. In Darier's disease treated with isotretinoin, there is no evidence of lysosomal enzyme release from the epidermis [181].

Gap junctions

Gap junctions are communication links between cells which allow for passage of electrical signals, ions, and molecules [182]. These channels are probably important in the control of tissue organization and growth. During the development of malignancy, the number of gap junctions decreases [183–185]. In response to retinoids gap junctions proliferate rapidly in neoplastic and embryonic keratinizing epithelia. The rapidity of the response suggests that retinoids act on these structures through a direct effect [91,186].

Elias et al [90] have found that topical retinoic treatment of basal cell carcinomas in humans induced a twofold increase in gap junction density with a 35 percent decrease in desmosome density when analyzed by the freeze-fracture technique. In contrast, neither gap junction nor desmosome density in basal cell carcinomas was altered by oral 13-*cis*-retinoic acid. This suggests that the antineoplastic effects of retinoids may occur through different mechanisms depending on the route of administration and the particular compound employed.

Glycoconjugate biosynthesis

During vitamin A deficiency there is a decrease in the biosynthesis of carbohydrate containing macromolecules in epithelial tissues [187,188]. In vitamin A-deficient animals the synthesis of specific glycoproteins can be stimulated by the addition of vitamin A [47,187,189]. Retinoids are known to be involved in the transfer of monosaccharides, an important step in the formation of membrane glycoproteins. Retinol and a hydroxylated derivative of retinoic acid can be phosphorylated and then glycosylated, primarily with mannose [47,48,56]. These glycosyl retinyl phosphates can serve as intermediates in glycosylation, acting as sugar carriers that donate monosaccharides to membrane proteins. Changes in cell surface glycoproteins have been related to changes in cell morphology and adhesiveness [190–192]. In addition, retinoids can modify glycolipid biosynthesis but the mechanism is not known [193].

Glycosaminoglycan (GAG) synthesis is also affected by retinoids, but in a manner that varies with the tissue studied. Retinoic acid treatment of a human intestinal epithelial line was found to lead to an increase in the amount of

Table 221-3   Retinoid-responsive diseases

Acne:
  Cystic acne*
  Papular acne‡
  Acne rosacea*
  Gram-negative folliculitis*
  Hidradenitis suppurativa†
  Steroid acne‡
  Oil acne‡
Disorders of keratinization:
  The ichthyoses:*
    Ichthyosis vulgaris
    Lamellar ichthyosis
    Nonbullous congenital ichthyosiform erythroderma
    Epidermolytic hyperkeratosis
    X-linked ichthyosis
    Keratoderma palmaris et plantaris
    Mal de Meleda‡
    Papillon-Lefèvre syndrome‡
  Darier's disease*
  Pityriasis rubra pilaris*
  Erythrokeratodermia variabilis*
  Kyrle's disease‡
  Pachyonychia congenita‡
Skin cancer and precancer chemotherapy and
    chemoprophylaxis:
  Basal cell carcinoma†
  Squamous cell carcinoma†
  Actinic keratoses*
  Keratoacanthoma*
  Leukoplakia†
  Bowen's disease†
  Mycosis fungoides†
  Cutaneous metastases of malignant melanoma†
Psoriasis:
  Psoriasis vulgaris*
  Pustular psoriasis of von Zumbusch*
  Pustular psoriasis of palms and soles*
  Erythrodermic psoriasis*
  Psoriatic arthritis†
Miscellaneous diseases:‡
  Verrucous epidermal nevi
  Subcorneal pustular dermatosis
  Impetigo herpetiformis
  Reiter's syndrome
  Warts
  Epidermodysplasia verruciformis
  Discoid lupus erythematosus
  Lichen planus
  Acanthosis nigricans
  Cutaneous sarcoidosis [216]
  Scleromyxedema [217]

* Very effective
† Somewhat effective
‡ Reported

heparan sulfate, a decrease in chondroitin 4-sulfate, dermatan sulfate, and chondroitin 6-sulfate released into the medium, with a concomitant inhibition of cell growth [194]. Vitamin A acetate treatment of dermal cell cultures revealed that sulfate incorporation into heparin, heparan sulfate, or both was increased, whereas incorporation into chondroitin 4-sulfate was decreased, and chondroitin 6-sulfate was unchanged [195]. In a transplantable rat chondrosarcoma, etretinate and two similar aromatic retinoids induced a 95 percent inhibition of GAG biosynthesis but had no effect on normal cartilage [196]. In pig and human epidermis, retinoic acid stimulated glucosamine incorpo-

ration into extracellular, surface-associated (trypsin released) GAG but had no effect on glycoproteins that are integral components of plasma membranes [197].

The increased cellular adhesiveness observed with retinoid treatment may be due to alterations in cell surface glycoproteins and glycosaminoglycans. Transformed mouse fibroblasts are poorly adherent to each other and to the culture dish. Under the influence of retinol or retinoic acid their morphologic appearance becomes more normal and the cells firmly adhere to the dish [191].

Since these glycoconjugates are involved in cellular recognition and adhesion, this may be one manner in which retinoids affect differentiation [198].

Retinoid effects on proteases and prostaglandins

Increased secretion of plasminogen activator has been found after retinoid treatment of a variety of cell lines of mesenchymal origin including embryonal carcinoma cells, chick embryo muscle cells, chick fibroblasts, human synovial cells, and others [92,199–208]. Plasminogen activator is a protease that cleaves plasminogen to plasmin—the enzyme that catalyzes fibrinolysis. Plasminogen activator may be important in tissue remodeling.

Collagenase is another protease whose production is affected by retinoids. In contrast to plasminogen activator, collagenase is usually suppressed by retinoids [209–213].

Retinoids have also been shown to be inhibitors of prostaglandin production in rheumatoid synovial cells [210]. N-(4-hydroxyphenyl)retinamide inhibits prostaglandin synthesis and also inhibits breast carcinogenesis [214,215].

Clinical studies

Synthetic retinoids have profound effects on many skin diseases. Either used alone or in combination with other agents, the retinoids have been successful in clinical trials over the past decade in the treatment of cystic acne, psoriasis, a variety of disorders of keratinization, multiple basal cell carcinomas, cutaneous T-cell lymphoma, and other skin diseases (Table 221-3). A decade of clinical and laboratory investigation into the therapeutic spectrum and the mechanisms of action of natural and synthetic retinoids preceded the clinical accomplishments in dermatologic disease observed with synthetic retinoids. For example, the chemoprevention of experimental carcinogenesis with isotretinoin provided a theoretical rationale for its use in patients with multiple basal cell carcinomas.

Cystic acne (see also Chap. 67)

With the historical use of oral vitamin A and topical tretinoin (all-*trans*-retinoic acid) in the treatment of acne, and with the observation that patients with disorders of keratinization treated with oral isotretinoin developed drying and chapping of their facial skin similar to that observed with topical tretinoin, it appeared reasonable to treat acne patients with oral isotretinoin. In the initial trial, 14 previously treatment-resistant cystic acne patients responded dramatically to isotretinoin, at an average maximum dosage of 2.0 mg/kg per day, and had an 85 percent mean reduction in lesion counts at the end of the 4-month treatment period [218]. Thirteen went on to completely clear after discontinuation of therapy, indicating that therapy

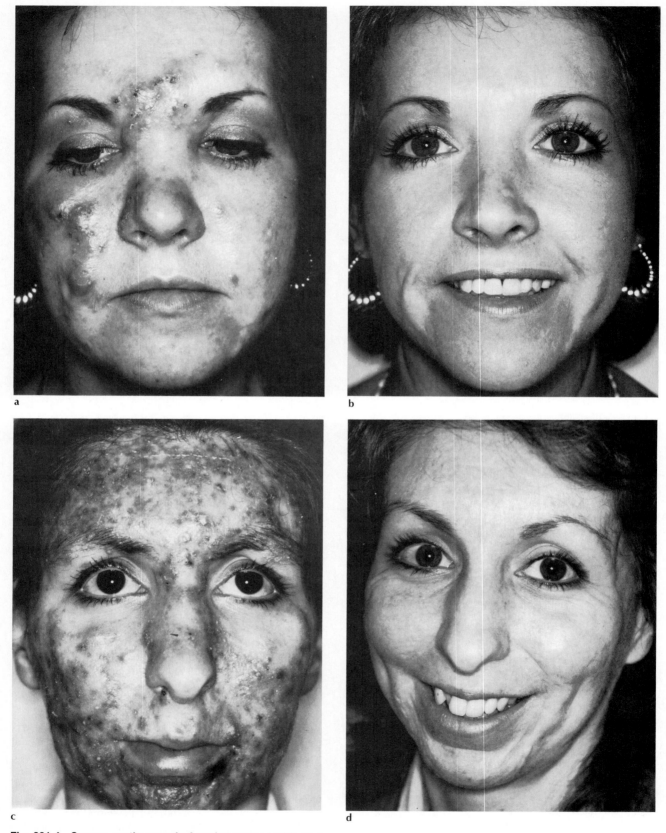

Fig. 221-4   Severe cystic acne in females treated with oral isotretinoin. (a, c, e, and g) Before treatment. (b, d, f, and h) After treatment.

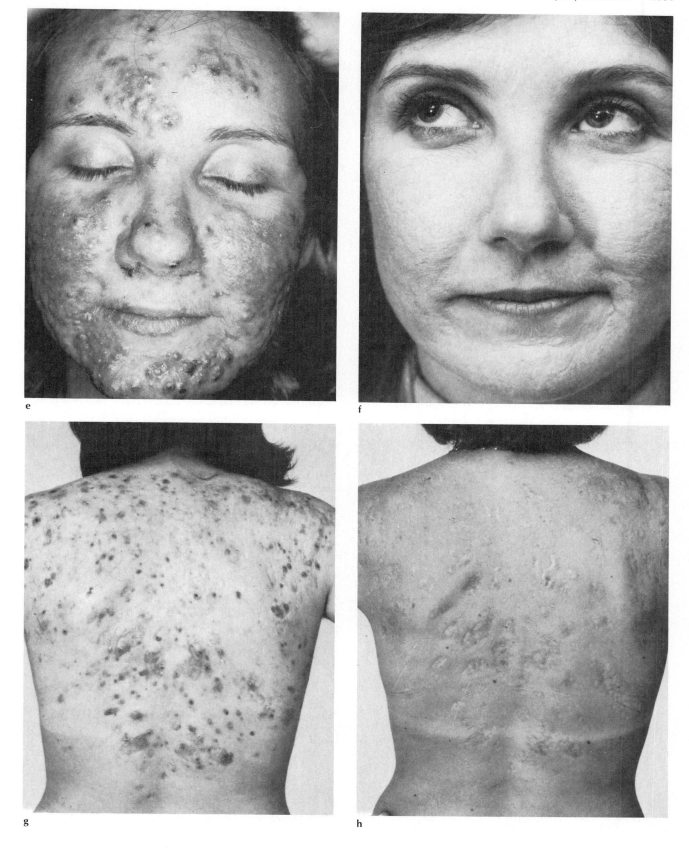

e

f

g

h

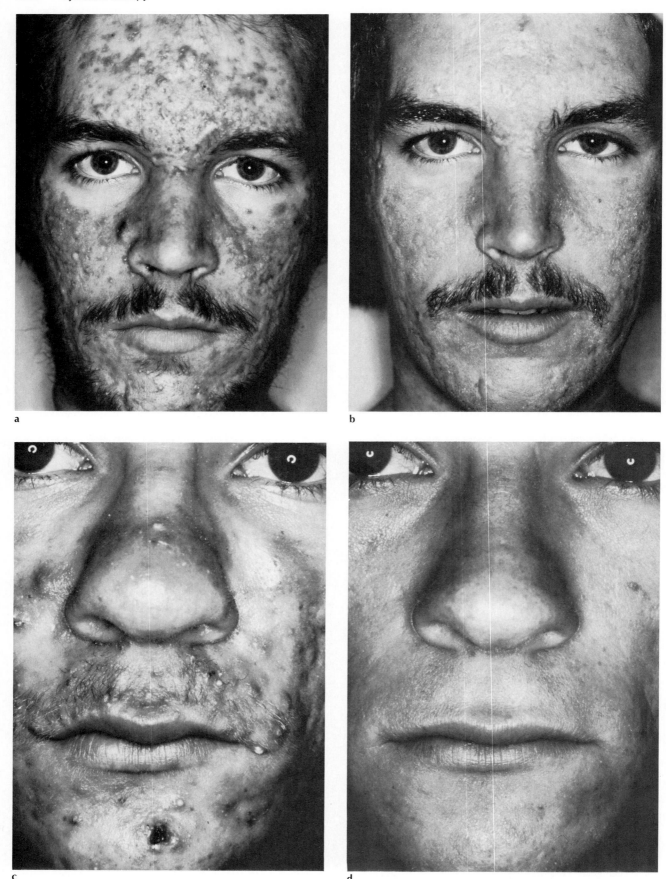

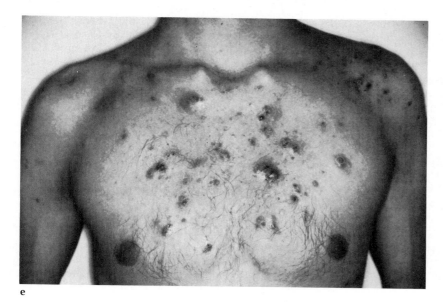

e

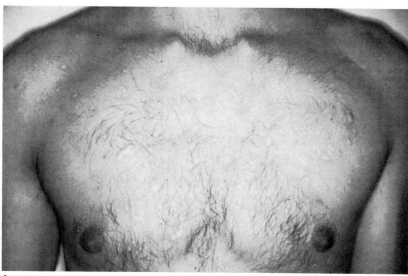

f

Fig. 221-5 Severe cystic acne in males treated with oral isotretinoin. (a, c, and e) Before treatment. (b, d, and f) After treatment.

need not be maintained until total improvement is observed. This continued healing was followed by prolonged remissions in all cases, currently lasting seven years.

In a subsequent clinical trial involving 32 patients, the therapeutic effects of isotretinoin were demonstrated clearly not to be a placebo response [219]. Doses as low as 0.5 mg/kg per day were found to be effective. Facial acne was observed to respond more rapidly and at a lower dosage than truncal acne. Continued healing after discontinuation of therapy was particularly evident in this trial. Of the 18 patients in the study who cleared completely with one 4-month course of therapy, only one cleared during the treatment period. Complete clearing in the other patients occurred at a mean time of 6 months after therapy (Figs. 221-4 and 221-5).

Cystic acne is unique among retinoid-responsive diseases in that most cases of even the greatest severity can be successfully treated with only one 4- or 5-month course at doses of 0.5 to 2.0 mg/kg per day. Only about one-third of acne patients require a second course and only a few require a third to completely clear. Because of the contin-

ued healing seen after discontinuing therapy, 2-month treatment-free evaluation periods are useful in determining which patients require additional therapy. Generally, patients with severe cystic acne located predominantly on the trunk require higher doses, up to 2.0 mg/kg per day, and longer treatment periods than do patients with facial acne.

Although isotretinoin has proved to be the most effective therapy for cystic acne, there is typically a lag period before the onset of the therapeutic effect. The usual time for a 50 percent decrease in the number of acne nodules and cysts on the face is at 8 weeks of therapy and on the trunk is at 12 weeks. Of those patients who clear completely, two-thirds remain totally free of cysts. The remaining one-third of patients have an occasional cyst or two at follow-up examinations. Only 10 percent of acne patients have had mild relapses sufficient to require further therapy with isotretinoin. Tendency to relapse is dose-dependent, i.e., patients treated with 0.1 mg/kg per day have a much greater tendency to relapse than those treated with 1.0 to 2.0 mg/kg per day [220–224]. When mild relapses do occur, a trial of conventional acne therapy should be given. If this fails, then a second course of isotretinoin is indicated.

Current dosage recommendations are that 1.0 mg/kg per day of isotretinoin be used for 4 or 5 months as an initial course of therapy. Although doses as low as 0.05 mg/kg per day have been used, a higher relapse rate with only a moderate reduction in incidence of side effects has been observed with these doses. This argues against the usefulness of low doses in cystic acne.

An alternative initial dosage schedule was designed after observing the continuing therapeutic effects regularly seen after the discontinuation of therapy with isotretinoin. Comparable therapeutic results could be achieved if high initial doses (1 to 2 mg/kg per day) were given for only 2 weeks followed by a low maintenance dose (0.25 to 0.5 mg/kg per day) for the remainder of a 16-week treatment period. The higher doses (2.0 and maintenance at 0.5 mg/kg per day) were used for patients with predominantly truncal acne and the lower doses (1.0 and maintenance at 0.25 mg/kg per day) for facial acne patients. This high-initial, low-maintenance dose schedule was superior to both a 2-week high-dosage schedule followed by placebo and to a constant low-dosage schedule. Specifically, the constant low-dosage schedule (0.5 mg/kg per day) led to an initial 20 percent increase in the lesion count at 2 weeks and, at the end of the 16-week treatment period, only a 50 percent reduction in lesions. In contrast, the high-low dosage schedule led to no mean increase in lesions at 2 weeks and a 75 percent reduction at 16 weeks.

Dosage recommendations for patients who require a second course of therapy may require higher doses, such as 1.5 to 2.0 mg/kg per day, for an additional 4- to 6-month course of therapy. This is particularly true for persistent acne of the nuchal region, the low back, buttocks, and thighs. Doses higher than 2.0 mg/kg per day are generally not necessary.

Occasionally an increased number of acne cysts was seen during the first 2 weeks of isotretinoin therapy in the initial clinical trials prior to the marketing of this agent [225]. This may have been due either to isotretinoin paradoxically and temporarily increasing the number of lesions, similar perhaps to the effect seen during initial therapy with topical tretinoin, or it could have been due to the abrupt discontinuation of previously used, partially effective therapy, such as oral antibiotics, 4 weeks prior to patients entering into experimental protocols with isotretinoin. Higher initial doses of isotretinoin (2.0 mg/kg per day) may minimize this initial flare. One other uncommon reaction in treating cystic acne with isotretinoin is the evolution of acne cysts, particularly on the trunk, into crusted pyogenic granuloma-like lesions [226–230]. These lesions rarely may occur in severe acne untreated with isotretinoin, but are probably more commonly observed during isotretinoin therapy; they readily respond to debridement of the crusts and either intralesional injection or topical application or a short course of systemic administration of corticosteroids.

In addition to cystic acne, isotretinoin therapy is effective in acne vulgaris, gram-negative folliculitis [231], acne fulminans, acne conglobata, hidradenitis suppurativa, dissecting folliculitis of the scalp, and acne rosacea [231]. However, the treatment of hidradenitis may require pro-

longed therapy with 2 mg/kg per day and the response may be partial. The rapid therapeutic response of gram-negative folliculitis to low-dose isotretinoin is not considered to be a direct antibacterial effect but rather a secondary effect of alterations in the microenvironment. Additionally, colonization of the anterior nares with *Staphylococcus aureus* has been noted during isotretinoin therapy. The use of an antibiotic ointment to the nares has been suggested for the prevention of subsequent staphylococcal folliculitis and furunculosis.

Inhibition of sebum production with alterations in skin surface lipid film chemistry may represent a key mechanism of action of isotretinoin leading to clinical improvement in acne [232]. At peak levels of sebum suppression, the relative percentage of the skin surface lipid film comprising wax esters and squalene, which are derived from the sebaceous glands, is reduced, and the percentage of cholesterol and cholesterol esters is increased. Isotretinoin is the most effective known inhibitor of sebum production, being superior to estrogen and x-irradiation. Inhibition of quantitative sebum production (or sebum excretion rate) is almost maximal by the fourth week of treatment with isotretinoin and thus usually occurs prior to clinical improvement. Inhibition is dose-dependent and doses of 0.5 to 1.0 mg/kg per day lead to an 80 to 90 percent inhibition after 12 to 16 weeks of therapy [233]. After treatment is stopped quantitative sebum production returns toward pretreatment levels, but long-term follow-up from 20 to 99 weeks posttreatment shows an overall persistent 38 percent (range, 0 to 80 percent) inhibition [234]. Patients who received two courses, for a total of 10 months, of therapy with isotretinoin showed a persistent 60 percent decrease in quantitative sebum production when measured one year or more after treatment [235]. These data suggest that prolonged remission in some patients may be related at least in part to continued partial sebaceous gland inhibition. The histologic changes parallel and reflect the inhibition of sebum production and reveal that the sebaceous glands virtually disappear during treatment with isotretinoin and gradually recover after discontinuation of therapy [236].

The inhibition of the wax ester secretion rate by isotretinoin was studied specifically using a bentonite clay technique [237,238]. The mean rates of wax ester secretion were greatly elevated in untreated acne patients, but were suppressed below the normal range (as measured in patients without acne) during therapy. However, the posttreatment secretion rates again rose above the normal range at all dose levels (0.1 to 1.0 mg/kg per day), indicating that other factors must contribute to the continued healing of acne and to the prolonged remissions observed after discontinuing therapy.

In addition to inhibition of sebum production, anti-inflammatory antibacterial, inhibitory effects on microbial enzyme activity and desquamative effects on poral occlusion should be considered as possible mechanisms by which isotretinoin is effective in the treatment of acne [239–243]. Isotretinoin reduces the number of *Propionibacterium acnes* on the skin surface, probably reflecting decreased follicular colonization of *P. acnes* secondary to the decrease in sebaceous secretion.

Isotretinoin does not appear to be acting as an antiandrogen since no change has been noted in serum testosterone levels or gonadotropins, nor have there been any signs of feminization in males during therapy. Furthermore, the androgen-sensitive parts of the hamster flank organ, aside from the sebaceous component, do not involute during treatment with isotretinoin [244].

Psoriasis

Unlike acne in which a single 4- or 5-month course of therapy with isotretinoin can lead to prolonged remissions in most cases, the treatment of psoriasis with retinoids usually requires long-term administration because of the relapses that eventually occur if therapy is discontinued (Fig. 221-6). The prolonged administration of retinoids thus places psoriasis patients at greater potential risk of developing chronic retinoid toxicity than acne patients. The major emphasis of the treatment of psoriasis with synthetic retinoids has focused on etretinate at a dosage of 0.5 to 1.0 mg/kg per day [245–248]. Etretinate is of particular value in the treatment of pustular psoriasis and erythrodermic psoriasis, both of which are characteristically treat-

ment-resistant, often requiring therapy with chemotherapeutic agents such as methotrexate. Etretinate has been used both alone and in combination with other active agents such as anthralin, ultraviolet radiation (UVB, 280 to 320 nm), photochemotherapy (PUVA), methotrexate, and topical and systemic corticosteroids [249–254]. Several small uncontrolled studies have indicated that most patients with psoriatic arthritis improve when treated with etretinate [255–258]. The etretinate-induced improvement allowed patients to decrease or discontinue their use of nonsteroidal anti-inflammatory agents.

Etretinate markedly augmented the response of psoriasis patients to photochemotherapy using oral methoxsalen and long-wave ultraviolet radiation (UVA, 320 to 400 nm) or PUVA [249–251] (see Chap. 132). The regimen combining a retinoid with photochemotherapy has been termed *RePUVA*. In many studies of RePUVA, etretinate has been given for 1 to 4 weeks followed by the addition of PUVA. The combined treatment considerably decreased the total amount of UVA required for clearing and accelerated the response of psoriasis to PUVA. Moreover, it was effective

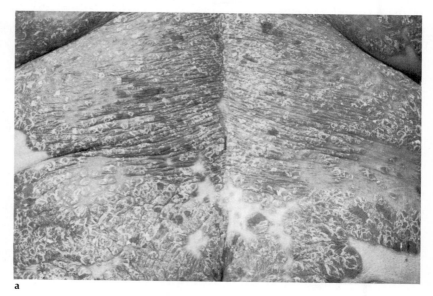

a

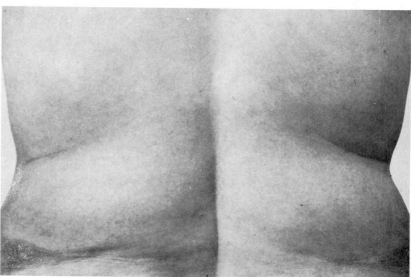

b

Fig. 221-6 Generalized chronic plaque type psoriasis before (a) and after (b) treatment with etretinate.

in patients who had been PUVA failures previously. Re-PUVA produced longer remissions than did PUVA. Fewer side effects from etretinate were seen during the RePUVA than with etretinate used alone because of the lower doses employed.

RePUVA using isotretinoin at a dose of 1 mg/kg per day was compared prospectively to RePUVA with etretinate [259]. The retinoids were given alone for 5 days prior to adding PUVA and were discontinued once psoriasis had cleared completely, at which time the patients were placed on PUVA maintenance. No significant difference between the two treatment regimens was observed in regard to duration of treatment required for clearing, number of UVA exposures required, and cumulative UVA dose, even though etretinate is superior to isotretinoin when used alone in the treatment of psoriasis vulgaris. Recently, iso-tretinoin was demonstrated to be effective in a small series of patients with pustular psoriasis [260].

Once psoriasis has cleared or markedly improved with etretinate, the subsequent posttreatment clinical course is variable. Some patients have prolonged remissions without maintenance therapy. In other patients the therapeutic ef-fect can often be maintained with conventional topical therapy and ultraviolet radiation with or without low-dose etretinate, 25 mg/day. However, relapses may occur even if etretinate therapy is maintained. Therefore, chronic maintenance therapy with etretinate may best be reserved for patients with pustular psoriasis, erythrodermic pso-riasis, and for those patients with severe psoriasis vulgaris who have proved to be otherwise treatment-resistant and who regularly demonstrate relapse on withdrawal of etre-tinate. In one report chronic maintenance therapy of pso-riasis with etretinate for six years failed to induce chronic toxicity [261].

Initial dosage recommendations for the treatment of pso-riasis with etretinate have been that therapy of erythro-dermic psoriasis may begin at 25 to 35 mg/day and increase to 50 to 60 mg/day within 2 to 4 weeks [262]. Pustular

Fig. 221-7   Epidermolytic hyperkeratosis before (a) and after (b) treatment with etretinate.

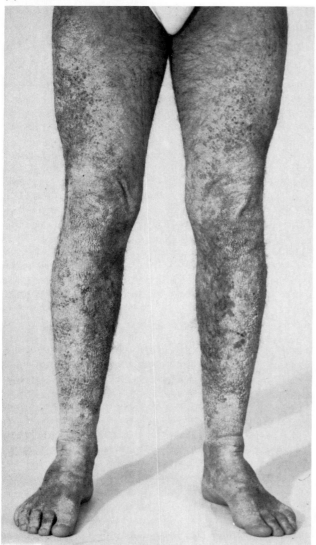

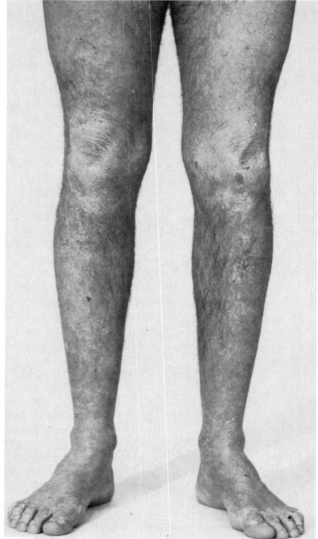

a

b

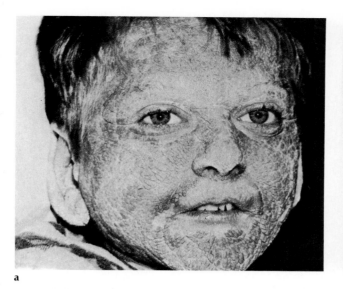
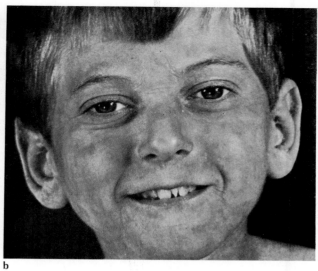

a   b

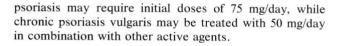

Fig. 221-8 A 13-year-old boy with erythrokeratodermia figurata variabilis before (a) and after (b) treatment with etretinate.

psoriasis may require initial doses of 75 mg/day, while chronic psoriasis vulgaris may be treated with 50 mg/day in combination with other active agents.

Cutaneous disorders of keratinization

The demonstration of isotretinoin's effectiveness in previously recalcitrant cases of disorders of keratinization, such as Darier's disease and pityriasis rubra pilaris, stimulated interest in the use of synthetic retinoids in these diseases [263,264]. Since 1976, numerous reports have indicated that these and other disorders of keratinization respond both to isotretinoin and etretinate [265]. In contrast to results in acne, for which isotretinoin is more effective than etretinate, etretinate and isotretinoin gave comparable responses in Darier's disease, lamellar ichthyosis, nonbullous congenital ichthyosiform erythroderma, and pityriasis rubra pilaris [266–268]. Etretinate was superior to isotretinoin in the treatment of psoriasis, epidermolytic hyperkeratosis (Fig. 221-7), keratoderma palmaris et plantaris, X-linked ichthyosis, ichthyosis vulgaris, erythrokeratodermia variabilis (Fig. 221-8), and lichen planus.

Patients with the dry, brown hyperkeratotic type of Darier's disease respond better (Fig. 221-9) and may have more prolonged remissions than those with the red, inflamed, infected variety of Darier's disease who also have marked intertriginous involvement. The latter patients are much more difficult to treat and relapse very quickly after therapy is discontinued. Although there was no initial worsening of disease, as occasionally occurs with psoriasis, in one report isomorphic reactions did occur in one-third of patients with Darier's disease treated with etretinate [267].

In a report of 45 patients with pityriasis rubra pilaris of varying duration prior to therapy with intermittent courses of isotretinoin, long-term remissions were noted after discontinuation of treatment [268] (Fig. 221-10). Although most cases of adult-onset pityriasis rubra pilaris sponta-

neously clear within three years, this finding could indicate either that isotretinoin therapy induced or accelerated a spontaneous remission or was merely coincidental with it. In patients who did not have a complete remission after a course of therapy, new areas of involvement did not occur and the return of disease did not reach the pretreatment degree of severity, as had been observed in Darier's disease after stopping treatment with isotretinoin. Intermittent courses of therapy with prolonged treatment-free intervals may be effectively used in patients such as these. However, not all patients with pityriasis rubra pilaris respond in this manner. For instance, two patients with chronic pityriasis rubra pilaris, characterized by childhood onset, myriads of follicular papules, and a duration longer than 10 years, responded very dramatically to treatment initially with isotretinoin and subsequently with etretinate and relapsed dramatically and completely after each 4- to 6-month course of therapy over a more than 8-year period of retinoid therapy [266].

Patients with lamellar ichthyosis treated with retinoids had a reduction in scale, increased heat tolerance and ability to sweat, and improved ectropion. Clearing in these patients is usually not complete and may be greater in the summer than in the winter, when their disease is typically more severe.

Since disorders of keratinization, unlike acne, may require long-term therapy with retinoids, it must be emphasized that the safety of chronic administration of retinoids has not been determined beyond eight years. Of particular concern is bone toxicity in children with regard to premature closure of epiphyses [269] and fractures [270] and changes in the axial skeleton resembling diffuse idiopathic skeletal hyperostosis in both children and adults [271–273].

Unusual responses to therapy have been observed [274]. During etretinate therapy of patients with keratoderma palmaris et plantaris (epidermolytic type), epidermolytic hyperkeratosis, and pachyonychia congenita, palmoplantar blistering was enhanced. Patients with Hailey-Hailey dis-

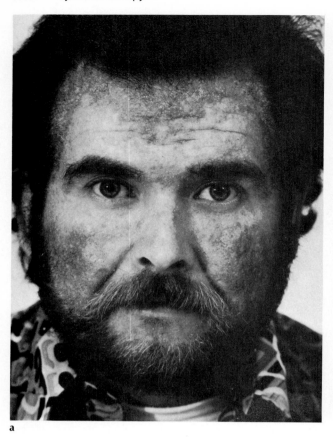 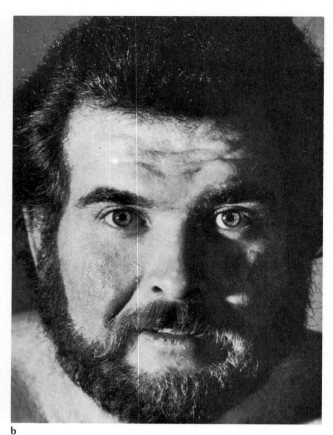

a   b

Fig. 221-9 Darier's disease before (a) and after (b) treatment with isotretinoin

ease and atopic dermatitis have worsened with both retinoids.

Cancer

The synthetic retinoids, isotretinoin and etretinate, have been used in the treatment and prevention of cutaneous malignancy in patients with chronic actinic dermatitis (basal cell carcinoma, actinic keratosis) [275], nevoid basal cell carcinoma syndrome [264,276,277], xeroderma pigmentosum (basal cell carcinoma, keratoacanthoma, actinic keratosis) [278], multiple keratoacanthomas (Ferguson-Smith) [279,280], porokeratosis of Mibelli with malignant degeneration (squamous cell carcinoma, Bowen's disease) [281], epidermodysplasia verruciformis [132–134], oral leukoplakia [282], cutaneous metastases of malignant melanoma [283,284], and cutaneous T-cell lymphoma (mycosis fungoides and Sézary's syndrome) [285–290]. As a general statement, synthetic retinoids usually do not cure cutaneous tumors but do produce variable degrees of partial regression when given at high dosage. Induction of inflammation by high-dose isotretinoin is not a necessary prerequisite for the regression of basal cell carcinoma, since both inflamed and noninflamed tumors will undergo regression [264,276,277]. However as the goal is changed from chemotherapy to chemoprevention, it appears that synthetic retinoids at low dosage are of value in preventing the formation of new skin tumors as long as therapy is

maintained [277]. Discontinuation of therapy is often followed by relapse.

Several reports have described the beneficial responses of synthetic retinoids either alone or in combination with other chemotherapeutic agents and with PUVA in the treatment of cutaneous T-cell lymphoma [285–290]. When synthetic retinoids were used alone, tumors and plaques underwent marked partial regression clinically. Relapse occurred in most patients after withdrawal of therapy, indicating that treatment with synthetic retinoids is not curative. Complete remissions were described in a report in which etretinate was added to a combination chemotherapy program of bleomycin, cyclophosphamide, prednisone, and transfer factor [290]. The synthetic retinoids may be active in cutaneous T-cell lymphoma by virtue of direct effects on the function of subsets of T lymphocytes.

Acute toxicities

The acute toxicities observed to date with the synthetic retinoids, isotretinoin and etretinate, are well tolerated, not life threatening, are dose-dependent in incidence and severity, treatable with bland therapies, and reversible on discontinuation of treatment. The acute toxicities of the synthetic retinoids mimic many of the findings of vitamin A intoxication, but are less severe than those seen with vitamin A and involve primarily the skin and mucous membranes.

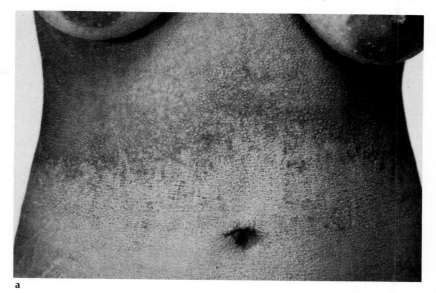

a

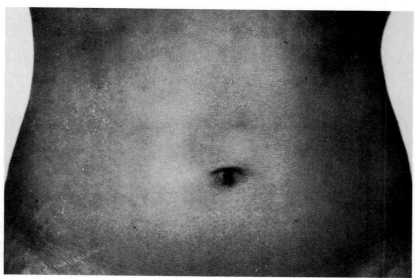

Fig. 221-10 Chronic pityriasis rubra pilaris before (a) and after (b) treatment with isotretinoin.

b

The major symptoms of synthetic retinoid acute toxicity are those of mucocutaneous drying and chapping: cheilitis, facial dermatitis, conjunctivitis [291], xerosis with itching, dryness of the nasal mucosa with minor nosebleeds, dry mouth with thirst, excessive palmoplantar desquamation, stratum corneum fragility (increased peeling with minor trauma), and hair loss. Rarely, corneal opacities have been observed during treatment with isotretinoin [292] (Table 221-4). These epithelial changes have disappeared after discontinuation of therapy.

In addition to these mucocutaneous toxicities, systemic toxicities have been observed, and include: (1) transient, minor elevations in liver function tests that return to pretreatment levels without discontinuation of therapy in most cases [293]; (2) hyperlipidemia with elevations primarily in the very-low-density lipoproteins and triglycerides, and occasionally in low-density lipoproteins and cholesterol [294,295]; (3) other laboratory abnormalities such as increased platelet count, hypercalcemia, hyperuricemia with gout in two cases, and elevated creatine phosphokinase in association with muscle pain after exercise [296,297]; (4) arthralgias; (5) photosensitivity [298]; and (6) teratogenicity [299,300], as both etretinate and isotretinoin have led to birth defects in humans. Unusual systemic toxicities include: (1) pseudotumor cerebri with headache, papilledema, and visual changes; (2) premature epiphyseal closure [269]; (3) mental depression [301]; and (4) leukopenia. It is not clear whether urticaria, erythema nodosum, inflammatory bowel disease, and idiopathic seizures observed in a few patients treated with isotretinoin are drug related.

Because the acute toxicities of the two synthetic retinoids, isotretinoin and etretinate, overlap but are not identical, it appears likely that each new synthetic retinoid will have a unique spectrum of clinical toxicity as well as efficacy. Under certain circumstances the differences in relative toxicity could influence retinoid selection in diseases in which the therapeutic effects are comparable.

As with vitamin A toxicity, the synthetic retinoids can alter tests of liver function. The tests most commonly elevated are the transaminases (AST, ALT), but occasionally other tests (alkaline phosphatase, lactic dehydroge-

Table 221-4 Retinoid toxicity

Acute:
  Mucocutaneous:
    Cheilitis
    Facial dermatitis
    Xerosis with pruritus
    Conjunctivitis
    Dry nasal mucosa
    Minor nosebleeds
    Stratum corneum fragility
    Palmoplantar peeling
    Hair loss
    Dry mouth with thirst
    Paronychia
    Stickiness of skin*
    Chills*
    Inflamed urethral meatus*
    Nail plate abnormalities*
    Corneal opacities†
    Pyogenic granuloma-like lesions in acne†
  Systemic:
    Headache*
    Arthralgias*
    Myalgias*
    Teratogenicity (head, ear, and heart abnormalities)
    Spontaneous abortion
    Pseudotumor cerebri†
    Mental depression†
    Inflammatory bowel disease†
  Laboratory:
    Hyperlipidemia:
      Increased triglycerides, VLDL
      Increased cholesterol, LDL*
      Decreased HDL*
      Eruptive xanthoma†
      Acute hemorrhagic pancreatitis†
    Elevated liver function tests:
      AST, ALT, alkaline phosphatase, LDH, bilirubin
    Elevated platelet counts*
    Leukopenia
    Hyperuricemia with gout†
    Hypercalcemia†
    Elevated CPK and myalgias after exercise†
Chronic:
  Mucocutaneous - none
  Systemic:
    Vertebral abnormalities resembling diffuse idiopathic
      skeletal hyperostosis:
      Osteophyte and bony bridge formation
      Anterior spinal ligament calcification
    Premature epiphyseal closure†
  Laboratory - none

* Uncommon
† Rare

nase, bilirubin) can also be abnormal. Elevations of transaminase occur in approximately 15 percent of patients, return to normal within two to four weeks, and remain normal even with continued therapy with the retinoids. However, one case of an acute hepatotoxic reaction to etretinate has occurred associated with fever and eosinophilia, possibly indicating a hypersensitivity reaction [302]. Continuous therapy with etretinate for up to six years did not lead to chronic liver toxicity (as measured by liver function tests but not by liver biopsies) even in patients with preexisting liver disease [261].

Vitamin A toxicity includes pain and tenderness in bones and joints. Arthralgias have been seen in only a minority of patients treated with synthetic retinoids, and the arthralgias disappear after discontinuation of therapy. In contrast to these retinoid-induced arthralgias, treatment of psoriatic arthritis with etretinate has led to objective improvement.

Another acute toxicity common to both vitamin A and the synthetic retinoids has been hypertriglyceridemia. The observed elevations of plasma triglycerides and VLDL levels have been dose-dependent and reversible on discontinuation of therapy [294,295]. Dosages of isotretinoin above 1 mg/kg per day are needed to elevate triglyceride levels markedly beyond the normal range. For example, one patient who may have had a preexisting hyperlipoproteinemia developed eruptive xanthomas while being treated with isotretinoin at a dose of 2.5 mg/kg per day [303]. Another patient developed acute hemorrhagic pancreatitis after the plasma triglycerides exceeded 1400 mg/dL [226]. This has led to a recommendation to discontinue therapy if triglyceride levels reach 800 mg/dL. In one report of 20 men with cystic acne of the trunk who were treated with isotretinoin at a maximum dosage of 2 mg/kg per day, the maximum increases from baseline levels were for triglycerides, 67 percent; VLDL, 56 percent; LDL, 22 percent; and cholesterol, 16 percent. The maximum decrease in high-density lipoproteins was 10 percent [294]. Hypertriglyceridemia has also been observed with etretinate, particularly in patients with one of the following predisposing factors: obesity, high alcohol intake, diabetes, and pretreatment hypertriglyceridemia [304]. Certainly, if patients with pretreatment elevations in the level of plasma triglycerides are to be treated with retinoids, their condition must be monitored very closely. The long-term importance of this observation and the effect of dietary management of plasma triglyceride levels during therapy with retinoids remains to be determined.

Conjunctivitis, which may interfere with a patient's ability to wear contact lenses during therapy, may be a result of a decrease in the outer lipid layer of the tear film with subsequent evaporation of the aqueous phase [305]. Furthermore, *Staphylococcus aureus* has been cultured from eyelids of patients with isotretinoin-induced blepharoconjunctivitis [291]. If artificial tears and topical ophthalmologic antibiotic therapy fail to relieve the conjunctivitis, then ophthalmologic consultation should be sought.

Of 16 women who took isotretinoin during pregnancy, nine had spontaneous abortions and seven had children with birth defects. The birth defects included hydrocephalus, deformed external ears, and cardiac abnormalities [296,299,300].

Ten cases of pseudotumor cerebri have developed during treatment with isotretinoin. If patients receiving isotretinoin develop persistent headache with visual changes, the drug should be discontinued promptly and the patient should be examined for papilledema with retinal hemorrhages. In five cases the patients were also being treated with tetracycline or minocycline, drugs that are known to rarely produce increased intracranial hypertension. This finding would suggest caution in combining these therapies.

Hair loss is an additional toxicologic finding that occurs both with hypervitaminosis A and also with synthetic retinoid therapy, particularly with etretinate. The hair loss usually occurs 3 to 8 weeks after beginning etretinate ingestion and after a minimum total dose of 2 g. It ceases 6 to 8 weeks after discontinuation of therapy. In the majority of cases the hair loss is a telogen effluvium; occasionally, dystrophic anagen roots are found [306].

Although retinoids at high doses may inhibit spermatogenesis in animals, semen analyses from patients receiving oral retinoids have revealed no abnormalities. In fact, a return toward normal of abnormally low pretreatment sperm counts in isotretinoin-treated acne patients has been noted [307].

Chronic toxicity

The most common findings observed in animals and humans during chronic hypervitaminosis A intoxication have been bony changes. Demineralization, thinning of the long bones, cortical hyperostosis, periostitis, and permature closure of the epiphyses have been documented [308–314]. There are several indications that the synthetic retinoids may be capable of inducing chronic bone toxicities similar to chronic hypervitaminosis A. Etretinate accelerated ossification of the epiphyseal line in rats given 3 mg/kg per day [315]. Radiographic evidence of partial closure of the proximal epiphysis of the right tibia, demineralization, and altered bone remodeling occurred in a 10-year-old boy treated with high doses (3.5 mg/kg per day) of oral isotretinoin over $4\frac{1}{2}$ years for epidermolytic hyperkeratosis [269].

Children with epidermolytic hyperkeratosis, lamellar ichthyosis, psoriasis, and other disorders of keratinization have been safely and successfully treated with etretinate for over three years. One child treated with etretinate, however, developed two traumatic fractures during therapy [270]. Radiologically this patient's long bones were abnormally slender, but pretreatment x-rays had not been performed. It is known that in rats high-dose vitamin A and high-dose etretinate (3 mg/kg per day) may induce fractures and modeling defects of the long bones with enhanced bone resorption. The administration of etretinate did not interfere with the overall growth and development of these children as monitored by sequential height and weight measurements.

Hypervitaminosis A in adult cats causes confluent exostosis formation of the cervical spine [316,317]. Similarly, in 50 patients, 37 receiving etretinate and 13 receiving isotretinoin for periods greater than two years, 9 had osteophytes present at two or three vertebral levels with anterior spinal ligament calcification, but without disc space narrowing [272]. Lack of disc space narrowing eliminates degenerative joint disease as a cause of these changes. Nine patients had bone bridging, that is, the osteophytes connected two vertebrae. Patients treated with isotretinoin for longer than two years at a minimum dose of 1.5 mg/kg per day were considered to be at significant risk for developing vertebral osteophyte, anterior spinal ligament calcification, and bony bridging, similar to the findings of idiopathic skeletal hyperostosis and hypervitaminosis A in the adult. Furthermore, in a prospective study, vertebral osteophytes were observed to form within 12 months after the initiation of therapy with isotretinoin at 2.0 mg/kg per day [226,273].

Factors in the decision to use retinoids

As with other medications a risk/benefit ratio is often useful in determining whether or not to treat a patient with synthetic retinoids. Pertinent criteria in determining a risk/benefit ratio would include:

1. Responsiveness of the disorder to retinoids. The complete and often prolonged benefit of isotretinoin in the treatment of severe cystic acne is optimal in contrast to the minimal improvement and characteristic relapse after withdrawal of therapy seen in some of the disorders of keratinization.

2. Dose of retinoid required. Some diseases such as nonbullous congenital ichthyosiform erythroderma and cystic acne limited to the face respond well to lower doses of isotretinoin, whereas other diseases such as inflammatory Darier's disease may require higher doses. Particularly in regard to psoriasis treated with etretinate, the use of lower doses in combination with other treatments such as PUVA (RePUVA) may eliminate some toxicities that require a minimum or threshold dose.

3. Availability of alternative treatments. In psoriasis, acne, and certain disorders of keratinization, such as lamellar ichthyosis, alternative therapies are available. However, synthetic retinoids may represent the only effective treatment in other diseases, such as severe cases of Darier's disease and epidermolytic hyperkeratosis.

4. Chronicity of retinoid therapy. Some diseases, such as inflammatory Darier's disease and epidermolytic hyperkeratosis, may relapse rapidly on withdrawal of synthetic retinoids. Other diseases, such as cystic acne, psoriasis, and hyperkeratotic Darier's disease, may have prolonged partial or complete remissions that permit retinoid-free intervals. Patients with diseases that require continuous retinoid administration may be at increased risk for developing chronic toxicity.

5. Severity of the disease. One is more inclined to initiate retinoid therapy in patients with severe diseases. This is especially true when educational, psychological, or physical development may be compromised. For example, early retinoid treatment of lamellar ichthyosis may prevent the development of ectropion.

6. Age of the patient. Children with disorders of keratinization requiring chronic, moderate-to-high-dose retinoid therapy are at highest risk to develop bony toxicity. Not only would they be at risk of premature epiphyseal closure but because of the anticipated greater lifetime exposure to drug they would also be at higher risk of eventually developing the vertebral changes resembling diffuse idiopathic skeletal hyperostosis.

7. Sex of the patient. Retinoid teratogenicity entails special risks for the female patient of childbearing age. While isotretinoin is rapidly cleared from the body within days, etretinate can be detected in the serum for months or even years after discontinuation of therapy. Thus it is not known when it is safe to conceive after discontinuation of etretinate. Current guidelines suggest at least 12 to 18 months.

8. Presence of other disorders which may be aggravated by retinoid usage. Renal or hepatic compromise, preexisting hyperlipidemia, or a family history of hyperlipidemia or premature atherosclerotic cardiovascular disease should be considered in the therapeutic assessment.

9. Concomitant use of other drugs with similar toxicities. Estrogens and corticosteroids may elevate serum lipids. Tetracycline may rarely produce benign intracranial hypertension. In addition to retinoids, many drugs are hepatotoxic, e.g., methotrexate.

Conclusions

The synthetic retinoids, isotretinoin and etretinate, represent a new class of drugs that are highly effective in the treatment of a broad spectrum of dermatologic disease. Although there is overlap in therapeutic efficacy between isotretinoin and etretinate, each agent has unique clinical indications. For instance, isotretinoin is the drug of choice for severe cystic acne at dose levels of 0.5 to 2.0 mg/kg per day. The development of optimum dosage schedules for acne of varying severity and for facial and truncal locations is continuing. The use of etretinate either alone or in combination with presently available therapies for psoriasis has been very effective, especially for the typically treatment-resistant pustular and erythrodermic varieties. Maintenance therapy with etretinate is necessary for many psoriatic patients. This raises questions about the long-term safety and the duration of teratogenic potential of this retinoid, especially since etretinate is stored in fat and blood levels of etretinate have been detected for prolonged periods after discontinuation of therapy [318,319]. So far, no serious chronic toxicity has been observed in patients who have received etretinate for more than six years [261].

Synthetic retinoids must now also be considered the most effective treatment for Darier's disease and certain other disorders of keratinization. The degree of clinical response and duration of posttreatment remission varies with the different disorders treated.

The use of synthetic retinoids in cancer prevention and therapy for both cutaneous and internal tumors is potentially the most significant clinical use of these drugs, requiring further investigation and clarification. Based on the results of preliminary studies, it appears that chronic maintenance therapy is needed for successful chemoprevention of cancer with retinoids.

Acute side effects have been predominantly limited to the skin and mucous membranes and were reversible after discontinuation of treatment. Systemic toxicities include hypertriglyceridemia, elevations in liver function tests, arthralgias, pseudotumor cerebri, and teratogenicity. The only chronic toxicity known to date is radiographic changes in the vertebral column after long-term, high-dose isotretinoin. These changes include calcification of the anterior spinal ligament and osteophyte and bony bridge formation, similar to the findings of diffuse idiopathic skeletal hyperostosis.

Based on the experience obtained with isotetrinoin and etretinate, the future of the retinoids appears most promising, particularly with the expanding spectrum of retinoid-responsive diseases and with the continuing development of new synthetic compounds, such as the arotinoids [320], that may improve still further their efficacy or tolerability.

References

1. Mandel HG, Cohn VH: Fat-soluble vitamins, in *The Pharmacological Basis of Therapeutics*, 6th ed, edited by AG Gilman et al. New York, Macmillan, 1980, p 1583

2. Stepp W: Versuche uber Futterung mit lipoidfreier Nahrung. *Biochem Z* **22**:452, 1909

3. Stepp W: Experimentelle Untersuchungen über die Bedeutung der Lipoide für die Ernährung. *Z Biol* **57**:135, 1911

4. McCollum EV, Davis M: The necessity of certain lipids in the diet during growth. *J Biol Chem* **15**:167, 1913

5. McCollum EV, Davis M: The nature of the dietary deficiencies of rice. *J Biol Chem* **23**:181, 1915

6. McCollum EV, Kennedy C: The dietary factors operating in the production of polyneuritis. *J Biol Chem* **24**:491, 1916

7. Steenbock H: White corn *vs* yellow corn and a (probable) relationship between the fat soluble vitamins and yellow plant pigments. *Science* **50**:352, 1919

8. Drummond JC: The nomenclature of the so-called accessory food factors (vitamins). *Biochem J* **14**:660, 1920

9. Karrer P et al: Zur kenntnis des Vitamins-A aus Frischtränen II. *Helv Chir Acta* **14**:1431, 1931

10. Euler HV, Karrer P: The study of vitamin A concentrates. *Helv Chir Acta* **14**:1040, 1931

11. Wald GJ: Vitamin A in eye tissues. *J Gen Physiol* **18**:905, 1935

12. Wald GJ: Carotenoids and the visual cycle. *J Gen Physiol* **19**:351, 1935

13. Morton RA: Chemical aspects of the visual process. *Nature* **153**:69, 1944

14. Morton RA, Goodwin TW: Preparation of retinene in vitro. *Nature* **153**:405, 1944

15. Arens JF, van Dorp DA: A new method for the synthesis of α,β-unsaturated aldehydes. *Recl Trav Chim Pays-Bas* **67**:973, 1948

16. Wolbach SB, Howe PR: Tissue changes following deprivation of fat-soluble A vitamin. *J Exp Med* **42**:753, 1925

17. Mori SJ: Primary changes in eyes of rats which result from deficiency of fat-soluble A in diet. *JAMA* **79**:197, 1922

18. Peck SM et al: Keratosis follicularis (Darier's disease). *Arch Dermatol Syphilol* **43**:223, 1941

19. Porter AD: Vitamin A in some congenital anomalies of the skin. *Br J Dermatol* **63**:123, 1951

20. Fujimaki Y: Formation of carcinoma in albino rats fed on deficient diets. *J Cancer Res* **10**:469, 1926

21. Stuttgen G: Zur Lokalbehandlung von Keratosen mit Vitamin-A-Saure. *Dermatologica* **124**:65, 1962

22. Beer P: Studies of the effects of vitamin A acid. *Dermatologica* **124**:192, 1962

23. Frost P, Weinstein GD: Topical administration of vitamin A acid for ichthyosiform dermatoses and psoriasis. *JAMA* **207**:1863, 1969

24. Kligman AM et al: Topical vitamin A acid in acne vulgaris. *Arch Dermatol* **99**:469, 1969

25. Bollag W, Ott R: Therapy of actinic keratoses and basal cell carcinomas with local application of vitamin A acid. *Cancer Chemother Rep* **55**:59, 1971

26. Stuttgen G: Oral vitamin A acid therapy. *Acta Derm Venereol (Stockh)* **55** (**suppl 74**):174, 1975

27. Bollag W: Belgian patent 752,924, July 3, 1970

28. Pawson BA: A historical introduction to the chemistry of vitamin A and its analogs (retinoids), in *Modulation of Cellular Interaction by Vitamin A and Derivatives (Retinoids)*, edited by LM DeLuca, SS Shapiro. New York, The New York Academy of Sciences, 1981, p 1

29. Bollag W, Matter A: From vitamin A to retinoids in experimental and clinical oncology: achievements, failures, and outlook, in *Modulation of Cellular Interaction by Vitamin A and Derivatives (Retinoids)*, edited by LM DeLuca, SS Shapiro. New York, The New York Academy of Sciences, 1981, pp 9

30. Sporn MB et al: Relationship between structure and activity of retinoids. *Nature* **263**:110, 1976

31. Frolik CA: In vitro and in vivo metabolism of all-*trans*- and 13-*cis*-retinoic acid in the hamster, in *Modulation of Cellular*

Interaction by Vitamin A and Derivatives (Retinoids), edited by LM DeLuca, SS Shapiro. New York, The New York Academy of Sciences, 1981, p 37

32. Bollag W: Belgian patent 762,344, August 2, 1971
33. Pawson BA et al: Retinoids at the threshold: their biological significance and therapeutic potential. *J Med Chem* **25(11)**:1269, 1982
34. Huang H, Goodman D: Vitamin A and carotenoids. I. Intestinal adsorption and metabolism of ^{14}C-labeled vitamin A alcohol and β-carotene in the rat. *J Biol Chem* **240**:2839, 1965
35. Goodman DS: Vitamin A and retinoids: recent advances. *Fed Proc* **38**:2501, 1979
36. Goodman DS, Olson JA: The conversion of all-*trans* beta carotene into retinal, in *Methods in Enzymology,* vol 15, edited by RB Clayton. New York, Academic Press, 1969, p 462
37. Goodman DS et al: The intestinal absorption and metabolism of vitamin A and beta carotene in man. *J Clin Invest* **45**:1615, 1966
38. Goodman DS et al: Tissue distribution and metabolism of newly absorbed vitamin A in the rat. *J Lipid Res* **6**:390, 1965
39. Hirosawa K, Yamada K: The localization of the vitamin A in the mouse liver as revealed by electron microscope radioautography. *J Electron Microsc (Tokyo)* **22**:337, 1973
40. Kanai M et al: Retinol-binding protein: the transport protein for vitamin A in human plasma. *J Clin Invest* **47**:2025, 1968
41. Muto Y et al: Regulation of retinol binding protein metabolism by vitamin A status in the rat. *J Biol Chem* **247**:2542, 1972
42. Fidge NH et al: Pathways of absorption of retinal and retinoic acid in the rat. *J Lipid Res* **9**:103, 1968
43. Smith JE et al: The plasma transport and metabolism of retinoic acid in the rat. *Biochem J* **132**:821, 1973
44. Zile M et al: Characterization of retinol β-glucuronide as a minor metabolite of retinoic acid in bile. *Proc Natl Acad Sci USA* **77**:3230, 1980
45. Napoli J et al: Identification of 5,8-oxyretinoic acid isolated from small intestine of vitamin A-deficient rats dosed with retinoic acid. *Proc Natl Acad Sci USA* **75**:2603, 1978
46. Peterson P et al: Formation and properties of retinylphosphate galactose. *J Biol Chem* **251**:4986, 1976
47. DeLuca LM: The direct involvement of vitamin A in glycol transfer reactions of mammalian membranes. *Vitam Horm* **35**:1, 1977
48. Bhat PV, DeLuca LM: The biosynthesis of a mannolipid containing a metabolite of retinoic acid by 3T12 mouse fibroblasts. *Ann NY Acad Sci* **359**:135, 1981
49. Zachman RD: The stimulation of RNA synthesis in vivo and in vitro by retinol in the intestine of vitamin A deficient rats. *Life Sci* **6**:2207, 1967
50. Johnson BC et al: Vitamin A and nuclear RNA synthesis. *Am J Clin Nutr* **22**:1048, 1969
51. Sporn MB et al: Retinyl acetate: effect on cellular content of RNA in epidermis in cell culture in chemically defined medium. *Science* **182**:722, 1973
52. Tsai CH, Chytil F: Effect of vitamin A deficiency on RNA synthesis in isolated cat liver nuclei. *Life Sci* **23**:1446, 1978
53. Smith KB: Early effects of vitamin A on protein synthesis in the epidermis of embryonic chick skin cultured in serum-containing medium. *Dev Biol* **30**:241, 1973
54. DeLuca LM et al: Biosynthetic studies of mannolipids and mannoproteins of normal and vitamin A-depleted hamster livers. *Biochim Biophys Acta* **409**:342, 1975
55. Hassell HR et al: Stimulation of mannose incorporation into specific glycolipids and glycopeptides of rat liver by high doses of retinyl palmitate. *J Biol Chem* **253**:1627, 1978
56. Wolf G et al: Recent evidence for the participation of vitamin A in glycoprotein synthesis. *Fed Proc* **38**:2540, 1979
57. Ziboh VA et al: Effects of retinoic acid on prostaglandin biosynthesis in guinea-pig skin. *J Invest Dermatol* **65**:370, 1975
58. Aso K et al: The role of prostaglandin E, cyclic AMP, and cyclic GMP in the proliferation of guinea-pig ear skin stimulated by topical application of vitamin A acid. *J Invest Dermatol* **6**:231, 1976
59. Friedenwald J et al: Mitotic activity and wound healing in the corneal epithelium of vitamin A deficient rats. *J Nutr* **29**:299, 1945
60. Zile M et al: Effect of vitamin A deficiency on intestinal cell proliferation in the rat. *J Nutr* **107**:552, 1977
61. Zile M et al: On the physiological basis of vitamin A-stimulated growth. *J Nutr* **109**:1787, 1979
62. Moore T: Effects of vitamin A deficiency in animals: pharmacology and toxicology of vitamin A, in *The Vitamins,* 2nd ed, vol 1, edited by WH Sebrell, RS Harris. New York, Academic Press, 1967, pp 245, 280
63. Peck GL et al: Effects of retinoic acid on embryonic chick skin. *J Invest Dermatol* **69**:463, 1977
64. Fell H: The effect of excess vitamin A on cultures of embryonic chicken skin explanted at different stages of differentiation. *Proc R Soc Lond [Biol]* **146**:242, 1957
65. Wong Y, Buck R: An electron microscopic study of metaplasia of the rat tracheal epithelium in vitamin A deficiency. *Lab Invest* **24**:55, 1971
66. Harris CC et al: Histogenesis of squamous metaplasia in the hamster tracheal epithelium caused by vitamin A deficiency or benzo-(a)pyrene-ferric oxide. *J Natl Cancer Inst* **48**:743, 1972
67. Nettesheim P et al: Effect of vitamin A on lung tumor induction in rats. *Proc Am Assoc Cancer Res* **16**:54, 1975
68. Cohen SM et al: Effect of hyper- and avitaminosis A on urinary bladder carcinogenicity of N-[4-(5-nitro-2-furyl)-2-thiazolyl]-formamide (FANFT). *Fed Proc* **33**:602, 1974
69. Newberne PM, Rogers AE: Rat colon carcinomas associated with aflatoxin and marginal vitamin A. *J Natl Cancer Inst* **50**:439, 1973
70. Rogers AE et al: Induction by dimethylhydrazine of intestinal carcinoma in normal rats and rats fed high or low levels of vitamin A. *Cancer Res* **33**:1003, 1973
71. Sherman MI et al: Studies on the mechanism of induction of embryonal carcinoma cell differentiation by retinoic acid. *Ann NY Acad Sci* **359**:91, 1981
72. Strickland S, Mahdavi V: The induction of differentiation in teratocarcinoma stem cells by retinoic acid. *Cell* **15**:393, 1978
73. Kuff EL, Fewell JW: Induction of neural-like cells and acetylcholinesterase activity in cultures of F9 teratocarcinoma treated with retinoic acid and dibutyryl cyclic adenosine monophosphate. *Dev Biol* **77**:103, 1980
74. Jetten AM et al: Specific and nonspecific alterations in membrane microviscosity induced by retinoids in embryonal carcinoma and fibroblast cells. *Ann NY Acad Sci* **359**:91, 1981
75. Lewis CA et al: Inhibition of limb chondrogenesis in vitro by vitamin A: alterations in cell surface characteristics. *Dev Biol* **64**:31, 1978
76. Takigawa M et al: Polyamine and differentiation: induction of ornithine decarboxylase by parathyroid hormone is a good marker of differentiated chondrocytes. *Proc Natl Acad Sci USA* **77**:1481, 1980
77. DiSimone DP, Reddi AH: The influence of vitamin A (retinoic acid) on matrix induced endochondral bone differentiation. *J Cell Biol* **91**:147a, 1981
78. Murray T, Russell TR: Inhibition of adipose conversion in 3T3-L2 cells by retinoic acid. *J Supramol Struct* **14**:255, 1980
79. Lotan R, Lotan D: Stimulation of melanogenesis in a human melanoma cell line by retinoids. *Cancer Res* **40**:3345, 1980
80. Breitman TR et al: Induction of differentiation of the human promyelocytic leukemia cell line (HL-60) by retinoic acid. *Proc Natl Acad Sci USA* **77**:2936, 1980
81. Honma Y et al: Induction of differentiation of cultured hu-

man promyelocytic leukemia cells by retinoids. *Biochem Biophys Res Commun* **95**:507, 1980

82. Hoal EG et al: Inhibition of pigmentation by retinoic acid in a human melanoma cell line. *Fed Proc* **41**:683, 1982

83. Avdalovic N et al: The effect of retinoic acid on the morphology and cell surface properties of a non-adhesive variant of hamster melanoma cells. *Proc Am Assoc Cancer Res* **22**:121, 1981

84. Takenaga K et al: Production of differentiation-inhibiting factor in cultured mouse myeloid leukemia cells treated with retinoic acid. *Cancer Res* **41**:1948, 1981

85. Jetten AM et al: Characterization of the action of retinoids on mouse fibroblast cell lines. *Exp Cell Res* **119**:289, 1979

86. Christophers E: Growth stimulation of cultured postembryonic epidermal cells by vitamin A acid. *J Invest Dermatol* **63**:450, 1974

87. Hassell JR et al: Enhanced cellular fibronectin accumulation in chondrocytes treated with vitamin A. *Cell* **17**:821, 1979

88. Jetten AM et al: Enhancement in 'apparent' membrane microviscosity during differentiation of embryonal carcinoma cells induced by retinoids. *Exp Cell Res* **138**:494, 1982

89. Jetten AM: Modulation of cell growth by retinoids and their possible mechanisms of action. *Fed Proc* **43**:134, 1984

90. Elias PM et al: Influence of topical and systemic retinoids on basal cell carcinoma membranes. *Cancer* **48**:932, 1981

91. Prutkin L: Mucous metaplasia and gap junctions in the vitamin A acid-treated skin tumor, keratoacanthoma. *Cancer Res* **35**:364, 1975

92. Lotan R et al: Retinoic acid-induced modifications in the growth and cell surface components of a human carcinoma (HeLa) cell line. *Exp Cell Res* **130**:401, 1980

93. Sasak W et al: Effect of retinoic acid on cell-surface glycopeptides of cultured spontaneously-transformed mouse fibroblast (Balb/c 3T12-3 cells). *Cancer Res* **40**:1944, 1980

94. Shapiro SS, Poon JP: Retinoic acid-induced alterations of growth and morphology in an established epithelial line. *Exp Cell Res* **119**:349, 1979

95. Lotan R: Effects of vitamin A and its analogs (retinoids) on normal and neoplastic cells. *Biochim Biophys Acta* **605**:33, 1908

96. Chu EW, Malmgren RA: An inhibitory effect of vitamin A on the induction of tumors of forestomach and cervix in the Syrian hamster by carcinogenic polycyclic hydrocarbons. *Cancer Res* **25**:884, 1965

97. Davies RE: Effects of vitamin A on 7,12-dimethylbenz(a)anthracene-induced papillomas in rhino mouse skin. *Cancer Res* **27**:237, 1967

98. Genta VM et al: Vitamin A deficiency enhances binding of benzo(a)pyrene to tracheal epithelial DNA. *Nature* **247**:48, 1974

99. Cohen SM et al: Effect of avitaminosis A and hypervitaminosis A on urinary bladder carcinogenicity of N-(4-(5-nitro-2-furyl)-2-thiazolyl) formamide. *Cancer Res* **36**:2334, 1976

100. Narisewa T et al: Effect of vitamin A deficiency of rat colon carcinogenesis by N-methyl-N'-nitro-N-nitrosoguanidine. *Cancer Res* **36**:1379, 1976

101. Bollag W: Therapy of chemically induced skin tumors of mice with vitamin A palmitate and vitamin A acid. *Experientia* **27**:90, 1971

102. Mahrle G, Berger H: Protective effect of aromatic retinoic acid analog on skin tumor. *J Invest Dermatol* **70**:235, 1978

103. Sporn MB et al: 13-*cis*-Retinoic acid: inhibition of bladder carcinogenesis in the rat. *Science* **195**:487, 1977

104. Becci PJ et al: Inhibitory effect of 13-*cis*-retinoic acid on urinary bladder carcinogenesis induced in C57BL/6 mice by N-butyl-N-(4-hydroxybutyl)-nitrosamine. *Cancer Res* **38**:4463, 1978

105. Thompson HG et al: Continual requirements of retinoid for maintenance of mammary cancer inhibition. *Proc Am Assoc Cancer Res* **19**:74, 1978

106. Grubbs CJ et al: Inhibition of mammary cancer by retinyl methyl ether. *Cancer Res* **37**:599, 1977

107. Moon RC et al: N-(4-Hydroxyphenyl)-retinamide, a new retinoid for prevention of breast cancer in the rat. *Cancer Res* **39**:1339, 1979

108. Mayer H et al: Retinoids: a new class of compounds with prophylactic and therapeutic activities in oncology and dermatology. *Experientia* **34**:1105, 1978

109. Saffiotti U et al: Experimental cancer of the lung. Inhibition by vitamin A of the induction of tracheobronchial squamous metaplasia and squamous cell tumors. *Cancer* **20**:857, 1967

110. Verma AK et al: Inhibition of mouse skin carcinogenesis by a retinoid, steroid, and protease inhibitor. *Proc Am Assoc Cancer Res* **21**:93, 1980

111. Weeks CE et al: Inhibition of phorbol ester-induced tumor promotion in mice by vitamin A analog and antiinflammatory steroid. *JNCI* **63**:401, 1979

112. Yuspa SH et al: Retinyl acetate modulation of cell growth kinetics and carcinogen-cellular interaction in mouse epidermal cell cultures. *Chem Biol Interact* **16**:251, 1977

113. Merriman RL, Bertram JS: Reversible inhibition by retinoids of 3-methylcholanthrene-induced neoplastic transformation in C3H/10T 1/2 CL8 cells. *Cancer Res* **39**:1661, 1979

114. Harisiadis L et al: A vitamin A analogue inhibits radiation-induced oncogenic transformation. *Nature* **274**:486, 1978

115. Todaro GJ et al: Retinoids block phenotypic cell transformation produced by sarcoma growth factor. *Nature* **276**:272, 1978

116. Peck GL: Retinoids in clinical dermatology, in *Progress in Diseases in the Skin*, vol 1, edited by R Fleischmajer. New York, Grune & Stratton, 1981, p 227

117. Lasnitzki I: Reversal of methylcholanthrene-induced changes in mouse prostates in vitro by retinoic acid and its analogues. *Br J Cancer* **34**:239, 1976

118. O'Brien TG: The induction of ornithine decarboxylase as an early, possibly obligatory, event in mouse skin carcinogenesis. *Cancer Res* **36**:2644, 1976

119. O'Brien TG et al: Induction of the polyamine-biosynthetic enzymes in mouse epidermis and their specificity for tumor promotion. *Cancer Res* **35**:2426, 1975

120. Russell DH, Durie GM: *Polyamines as Biochemical Markers of Normal and Malignant Growth*. New York, Raven Press, 1978

121. Verma AK, Boutwell RK: Vitamin A acid (retinoic acid), a potent inhibitor of 12-O-tetradecanoyl-phorbol-13-acetate-induced ornithine decarboxylase activity in mouse epidermis. *Cancer Res* **37**:2196, 1977

122. Verma AK et al: Inhibition of 12-O-tetradecanoyl-phorbol-13-acetate-induced ornithine decarboxylase activity in mouse epidermis by vitamin A analogs (retinoids). *Cancer Res* **38**:793, 1978

123. Verma AK et al: Correlation of the inhibition by retinoids of tumor promoter-induced mouse epidermal ornithine decarboxylase activity and of skin tumor promotion. *Cancer Res* **39**:419, 1979

124. Boutwell RK, Verma AK: The influence of retinoids on polyamine and DNA synthesis in mouse epidermis. *Ann NY Acad Sci* **359**:275, 1981

125. Kensler TW et al: Effects of retinoic acid and juvenile hormone on the induction of ornithine decarboxylase activity by 12-O-tetradecanoyl-phorbol-13-acetate. *Cancer Res* **38**:2896, 1978

126. Chapman SK: Antitumor effects of vitamin A and inhibitors of ornithine decarboxylase in cultured neuroblastoma and glioma cells. *Life Sci* **26**:1359, 1980

127. Russell DH, Haddox MK: Antiproliferative effects of retinoids related to the cell cycle-specific inhibition of ornithine decarboxylase. *Ann NY Acad Sci* **359**:281, 1981

128. Lotan R et al: Characterization of retinoic acid-induced alterations in the proliferation and differentiation of a murine and a human melanoma cell line in culture. *Ann NY Acad Sci* **359**:389, 1981

129. Dion LD, Gifford GE: Vitamin A-induced modulation of the transformed cell phenotype in vitro. *Ann NY Acad Sci* **359**:389, 1981

130. Yuspa SH, Harris CC: Altered differentiation of mouse epidermal cells treated with retinyl acetate in vitro. *Exp Cell Res* **86**:95, 1974

131. Dion LD et al: Retinoic acid and the restoration of anchorage dependent growth to transformed mammalian cells. *Exp Cell Res* **117**:15, 1978

132. Lutzner M, Blanchet-Bardon C: Oral retinoid treatment of human papillomavirus type 5-induced epidermodysplasia verruciformis. *N Engl J Med* **302**:1091, 1980

133. Jablonska S et al: Ro 10-9359 in epidermodysplasia verruciformis: preliminary report, in *Retinoids: Advances in Basic Research and Therapy,* edited by CE Orfanos et al. New York, Springer-Verlag, 1981, p 401

134. Edelson Y et al: Treatment of epidermodysplasia verruciformis or multiple verrucae planae by oral aromatic retinoid (Ro 10-9359-Tigason), in *Retinoids: Advances in Basic Research and Therapy,* edited by CE Orfanos et al. New York, Springer-Verlag, 1981, p 446

135. Felix EL et al: Inhibition of the growth and development of a transplantable murine melanoma by vitamin A. *Science* **189**:886, 1975

136. Dennert G: Retinoids and the immune system: immunostimulation by vitamin A, in *The Retinoids,* vol 2, edited by MB Sporn et al. New York, Academic Press, 1984, p 373

137. Patek PQ et al: Antitumor potential of retinoic acid; stimulation of immune mediated effectors. *Int J Cancer* **24**:624, 1979

138. Medawar PB, Hunt R: Anti-cancer action of retinoids. *Immunology* **42**:349, 1981

139. Kurata T, Micksche M: Immunoprophylaxis in Lewis lung tumor with vitamin A + BCG. *IRCS Journal of Medical Science* **5**:277, 1977

140. Dennert G, Lotan R: Effects of retinoic acid on the immune system: stimulation of T killer cell induction. *Eur J Immunol* **8**:23, 1978

141. Hercend T et al: In vivo immunostimulating properties of two retinoids: Ro 10-9359 and Ro 13-6298, in *Retinoids: Advances in Basic Research and Therapy,* edited by CE Orfanos et al. New York, Springer-Verlag, 1981, p 21

142. Rhodes J, Oliver S: Retinoids as regulators of macrophage function. *Immunology* **40**:467, 1980

143. Schultz RM et al: Regulation of macrophage tumoricidal function: A role for prostaglandins of the E series. *Science* **202**:320, 1978

144. Levis WR, Emden RG: Enhancing effect of vitamin A on in vitro antigen stimulated lymphocyte proliferation. *Proc Am Assoc Cancer Res* **17**:446, 1976

145. Bauer R, Orfanos CE: Influence of retinoid on human blood cells in vitro. TMMP-retinoid inhibits the mitogenic properties of lectins and modulates the lymphocytic response, in *Retinoids: Advances in Basic Research and Therapy,* edited by CE Orfanos et al. New York, Springer-Verlag, 1981, p 153

146. Soppi AM et al: Effect of systemic Ro 10-9359 treatment of immunological parameters in Darier's disease, in *Retinoids: Advances in Basic Research and Therapy,* edited by CE Orfanos et al. New York, Springer-Verlag, 1981, p 321

147. Bialasiewicz AA et al: Suppression of pokeweed mitogen-activated human peripheral blood lymphocytes by Ro 10-9359: evaluation of plaque forming cells (PFC) (poster exhibit), in *Symposium on Retinoids: Advances in Basic Research and Therapy,* Berlin, October 13–15, 1980

148. Bialasiewicz AA et al: Immunological features of psoriasis: effects of Ro 10-9359, concanavalin A (con A), pokeweed mitogen (PWM), and methotrexate (MTX) on cultivated lymphocytes, in *Retinoids: Advances in Basic Research and Therapy,* edited by CE Orfanos et al. New York, Springer-Verlag, 1981, p 335

149. Bashor M et al: In vitro binding of retinol to rat-tissue components. *Proc Natl Acad Sci USA* **70**:3483, 1973

150. Sani B, Hill D: Retinoic acid: a binding protein in chick embryo metatarsal skin. *Biochem Biophys Res Commun* **61**:1267, 1974

151. Ong D, Chytil F: Retinoic acid-binding protein in rat tissue. Partial purification and comparison to rat tissue retinol-binding protein. *J Biol Chem* **250**:6113, 1975

152. Ong D, Chytil F: Cellular retinoic acid-binding protein from rat testes. Purification and characterization. *J Biol Chem* **253**:4551, 1978

153. Ong D, Chytil F: Cellular retinol-binding protein from rat liver. Purification and characterization. *J Biol Chem* **253**:828, 1978

154. Ross A et al: The binding protein for retinol from rat testes cytosol. *J Biol Chem* **253**:6591, 1978

155. Chytil F, Ong DE: Cellular retinol and retinoic acid-binding proteins in vitamin A action. *Fed Proc* **38**:2510, 1979

156. Ong DE, Chytil F: Specificity of cellular retinol-binding protein for compounds with vitamin A activity. *Nature* **255**:74, 1975

157. Cogan U et al: Binding affinities of retinol and related compounds to retinol-binding proteins. *Eur J Biochem* **65**:71, 1976

158. Eriksson U et al: The NH_2-terminal amino acid sequence of cellular retinoic-acid binding protein from rat testis. *FEBS Lett* **135**:70, 1981

159. Chytil F, Ong DE: Cellular-binding protein for compounds with vitamin A activity, in *Receptors and Hormone Action,* edited by BW O'Malley, L Birmbaumer. New York, Academic Press, 1978, p 573

160. Chytil F, Ong DE: Cellular vitamin A binding proteins, in *Vitamins and Hormones,* vol 36, edited by PL Munson et al. New York, Academic Press, 1978, p 1

161. Saari JC et al: Cellular retinol- and retinoic acid-binding proteins of bovine retina. *J Biol Chem* **253**:6432, 1978

162. Sani BP et al: Determination of binding affinities of retinoids to retinoic acid-binding protein and serum albumin. *Biochem J* **171**:711, 1978

163. Jetten AM, Jetten MER: Possible role of retinoic acid binding protein in retinoid stimulation of embryonal carcinoma cell differentiation. *Nature* **278**:180, 1979

164. Chytil F, Ong DE: Mediation of retinoic acid-induced growth and anti-tumor activity. *Nature* **260**:49, 1976

165. Wiggert B et al: Differential binding to soluble nuclear receptors and effects on cell viability of retinol and retinoic acid in cultured retinoblastoma cells. *Biochem Biophys Res Commun* **79**:218, 1977

166. Bashor M, Chytil F: Cellular retinol-binding protein. *Biochim Biophys Acta* **411**:87, 1975

167. Ong D, Chytil F: Changes in levels of cellular retinol- and retinoic acid-binding proteins of liver and lung during perinatal development of rat. *Proc Natl Acad Sci USA* **73**:3976, 1976

168. Ong D et al: Retinoic acid binding protein: occurrence in human tumors. *Science* **190**:60, 1975

169. DiGiovanna JJ et al: Quantitative and qualitative analysis of cytosol retinoid binding proteins in human skin. *J Invest Dermatol* **80**:356, 1983

170. Puhvel SM, Sakamoto M: Cellular retinoic acid-binding proteins in human epidermis and sebaceous follicles. *J Invest Dermatol* **82**:79, 1984

171. Trown PW et al: Relationship between binding affinities to cellular retinoic acid binding protein and in vivo and in vitro properties for 18 retinoids. *Cancer Res* **40**:212, 1980

172. Sani BP, Corbett TH: Retinoic acid-binding protein in normal tissues and experimental tumors. *Cancer Res* **37**:209, 1977

173. Sani BP, Titus BC: Retinoic acid-binding protein in experimental tumors and in tissues with metastatic tumor foci. *Cancer Res* **37**:4031, 1977

174. Ong DE et al: Cellular binding proteins for vitamin A in colorectal adenocarcinoma of rat. *Cancer Res* **38**:4422, 1978

175. Fell HG, Dingle JT: Studies on the mode of action of excess of vitamin A: VI. Lysosomal protease and the degradation of cartilage matrix. *Biochem J* **87**:403, 1963

176. Wang CC et al: Destabilization of mouse liver lysosomes by vitamin A compounds and analogues. *Biochem Pharmacol* **25**:471, 1976

177. Lazarus GS et al: Lysosomes and the skin. *J Invest Dermatol* **65**:259, 1975

178. Sporn MB, Newton DL: Chemoprevention of cancer with retinoids. *Fed Proc* **38**:2528, 1979

179. Dingle JT: Vacuoles, vesicles, and lysosomes. *Br Med Bull* **24**:141, 1968

180. Roels OA et al: Vitamin A and membranes. *J Clin Nutr* **22**:1020, 1969

181. Farb RM et al: The effect of 13-*cis*-retinoic acid on epidermal lysosomal hydrolase activity in Darier's disease and pityriasis rubra pilaris. *J Invest Dermatol* **75**:133, 1980

182. McNutt NS: Freeze-fracture techniques and applications to the structural analysis of the mammalian plasma membrane, in *Cell Surface Reviews*, vol 4, edited by G Poste, GL Nicolson. Amsterdam, North-Holland, 1977, p 75

183. McNutt NS, Weinstein RS: Carcinoma of the cervix: deficiency of nexus intercellular junctions. *Science* **165**:597, 1969

184. Sheridan JD: Low-resistance junctions between cancer cells in various solid tumors. *J Cell Biol* **45**:91, 1970

185. Weinstein RS et al: The structure and function of intercellular junctions in cancer. *Adv Cancer Res* **23**:23, 1976

186. Elias PM, Friend DS: Vitamin A-induced mucous metaplasia. An in vitro system for modulating tight and gap junction differentiation. *J Cell Biol* **68**:173, 1976

187. DeLuca LM: Vitamin A, in *Handbook of Lipid Research*, vol 2, edited by LM DeLuca. New York, Plenum Publishing, 1978, p 1

188. DeLuca LM: Epithelial membranes and vitamin A, in *Mammalian Cell Membranes*, edited by GA Jamieson, DM Robinson. Boston, Butterworth, 1977, p 231

189. Wolf G: Retinal-linked sugars in glycoprotein synthesis. *Nutr Rev* **35**:97, 1977

190. DeLuca LM et al: Recent developments in studies on biological functions of vitamin A in normal and transformed tissues, in *Pure and Applied Chemistry*, vol 51. New York, Pergamon Press, 1979, p 581

191. Adamo S et al: Retinoid-induced adhesion in cultured transformed mouse fibroblast. *JNCI* **62**:1473, 1979

192. Sasak W et al: Role of retinoids in the induction of adhesion and mannosylation of glycoconjugates of cultured spontaneously-transformed mouse fibroblasts (Balb/c 3T12-3 cells). *J Cell Biol* **79**:CS206, 1978

193. Patt LM et al: Retinol induces density-dependent growth inhibition and changes in glycolipids and LETS. *Nature* **273**:379, 1978

194. Poon JP, Shapiro SS: Retinoic acid mediated inhibition of growth in transformed epithelial cells. *Fed Proc* **37**:1392, 1978

195. Poon JP et al: Effect of vitamin A acetate on glycosaminoglycan biosynthesis in epidermal and dermal cells in vitro. *Fed Proc* **36**:748, 1977

196. Shapiro SS et al: Effect of aromatic retinoids on rat chondrosarcoma glycosaminoglycan biosynthesis. *Cancer Res* **36**:3702, 1976

197. King IA, Tabiowo A: Long-term effects of all-*trans*-retinoic acid on epidermal glycosaminoglycan, glycoprotein, and protein synthesis in vitro, in *Retinoids: Advances in Basic Research and Therapy*, edited by CE Orfanos et al. New York, Springer-Verlag, 1981, p 473

198. Shapiro SS, Mott DJ: Modulation of glycosaminoglycan biosynthesis by retinoids, in *Modulation of Cellular Interactions by Vitamin A and Derivatives (Retinoids)*, edited by LM De Luca, SS Shapiro. New York, The New York Academy of Sciences, 1981, p 306

199. Sherman MI et al: Differentiation of early mouse embryonic and teratocarcinoma cells in vitro: plasminogen activator production. *Cancer Res* **36**:4208, 1976

200. Linney E, Levinson BB: Teratocarcinoma differentiation: plasminogen activator activity associated with embryoid body formation. *Cell* **10**:297, 1977

201. Miskin R et al: Plasminogen activator in chick embryo muscle cells: induction of enzyme by RSV, PMA and retinoic acid. *Cell* **15**:1301, 1978

202. Wilson EL, Reich E: Plasminogen activator in chick fibroblasts. Induction of synthesis by retinoic acid: synergism with viral transformation and phorbol ester. *Cell* **15**:385, 1978

203. Jetten AM et al: Stimulation of several murine embryonal carcinoma cell lines by retinoids. *Exp Cell Res* **124**:381, 1979

204. Strickland S, Sawey MJ: Studies on the effect of retinoids on the differentiation of teratocarcinoma cells in vitro and in vivo. *Dev Biol* **78**:76, 1980

205. Wilson EL, Dowdle EB: Effects of retinoids on normal and neoplastic human cells cultured in vitro. *Cancer Res* **40**:4817, 1980

206. Schroder EW et al: Effects of retinoic acid on plasminogen activator and mitogenic responses of cultured mouse cells. *Cancer Res* **40**:3089, 1980

207. Paravicini U: Pharmacokinetics and metabolism of oral aromatic retinoids, in *Retinoids: Advances in Basic Research and Therapy*, edited by CE Orfanos et al. New York, Springer-Verlag, 1981, p 13

208. Hamilton JA: Stimulation of the plasminogen activator activity of human synovial cells by retinoids. *Fed Proc* **40**:779, 1981

209. Schindler J et al: Isolation and characterization of mouse mutant embryonal carcinoma cells which fail to differentiate in response to retinoic acid. *Proc Natl Acad Sci USA* **78**:1077, 1981

210. Brinckerhoff CE et al: Inhibition by retinoic acid of collagenase production in rheumatoid synovial cells. *N Engl J Med* **303**:432, 1980

211. Brinckerhoff CE, Harris ED Jr: Modulation by retinoic acid and corticosteroids of collagenase production by rabbit synovial fibroblasts treated with phorbol myristate acetate or poly(ethylene glycol). *Biochim Biophys Acta* **677**:424, 1981

212. Bolmer SD, Wolf G: Suppression of ornithine decarboxylase, fibronectin, and collagenase by retinoic acid of phorbol ester-promoted mouse skin in vivo. *Fed Proc* **40**:1814, 1981

213. Bauer EF et al: Inhibition of collagen degradative enzymes by retinoic acid in vitro. *J Am Acad Dermatol* **6**:603, 1982

214. Levine L: N-(4-hydroxyphenyl)-retinamide: a synthetic analog of vitamin A that is a potent inhibitor of prostaglandin synthesis. *Prostaglandins Med* **4**:285, 1980

215. Moon RC et al: N-(4-hydroxyphenyl)-retinamide, a new retinoid for prevention of breast cancer in the rat. *Cancer Res* **39**:1339, 1979

216. Waldinger TP et al: Treatment of cutaneous sarcoidosis with isotretinoin. *Arch Dermatol* **119**:1003, 1983

217. Brenner S, Yust I: Treatment of scleromyxedema with etretinate. *J Am Acad Dermatol* **10**:295, 1984

218. Peck GL et al: Prolonged remissions of cystic and conglobate acne with 13-*cis*-retinoic acid. *N Engl J Med* **300**:329, 1979

219. Peck GL et al: Isotretinoin versus placebo in the treatment of cystic acne. *J Am Acad Dermatol* **6**:735, 1982

220. Jones DH et al: A dose-response study of 13-*cis*-retinoic acid in acne vulgaris. *Br J Dermatol* **108**:333, 1983

221. Strauss JS et al: Isotretinoin therapy for acne: results of a

multicenter dose-response study. *J Am Acad Dermatol* **10**:490, 1984

222. Gollnick H et al: Oral treatment of conglobate acne with isotretinoin. Cooperative multicenter study group from 19 departments of dermatology (abstr). *J Invest Dermatol* **80**:376, 1983

223. Jones GH et al: 13-*cis*-Retinoic acid in acne (a double-blind study of dose response), in *Retinoids: Advances in Basic Research and Therapy,* edited by CE Orfanos et al. New York, Springer-Verlag, 1981, p 255

224. Plewig G et al: Effects of two retinoids in animal experiments and after clinical application in acne patients: 13-*cis*-retinoic acid Ro 4-3780 and aromatic retinoid Ro 10-9359, in *Retinoids: Advances in Basic Research and Therapy,* edited by CE Orfanos et al. New York, Springer-Verlag, 1981, p 219

225. Katz R et al: Flare of cystic acne from oral isotretinoin. *J Am Acad Dermatol* **8**:132, 1983

226. Shalita AR et al: Isotretinoin treatment of acne and related disorders: an update. *J Am Acad Dermatol* **9**:629, 1983

227. Exner JG et al: Pyogenic granuloma-like acne lesions during isotretinoin therapy. *Arch Dermatol* **119**:808, 1983

228. Valentic JP et al: Inflammatory neovascular nodules associated with oral isotretinoin treatment of severe acne. *Arch Dermatol* **119**:871, 1983

229. Campbell JP et al: Retinoid therapy is associated with excess granulation tissue responses. *J Am Acad Dermatol* **9**:708, 1983

230. Holland DB et al: Inflammatory responses in acne patients treated with 13-*cis*-retinoic acid (isotretinoin). *Br J Dermatol* **110**:343, 1984

231. Plewig G et al: Action of isotretinoin in acne rosacea and gram-negative folliculitis. *J Am Acad Dermatol* **6**:766, 1982

232. Farrell LN et al: The treatment of severe cystic acne with 13-*cis*-retinoic acid. *J Am Acad Dermatol* **3**:602, 1980

233. Goldstein JA et al: Comparative effect of isotretinoin and etretinate on acne and sebaceous gland function. *J Am Acad Dermatol* **6**:760, 1982

234. Strauss JS et al: The effect of marked inhibition of sebum production with 13-*cis*-retinoic acid on skin surface lipid composition. *J Invest Dermatol* **74**:66, 1980

235. Gross EG et al: Long-term inhibition of quantitative sebum production with isotretinoin (abstr). *J Invest Dermatol* **80**:357, 1983

236. Landthaler M et al: Effects of 13-*cis*-retinoic acid on sebaceous glands in humans, in *Retinoids: Advances in Basic Research and Therapy,* edited by CE Orfanos et al. New York, Springer-Verlag, 1981, p 259

237. Stewart ME et al: Effect of 13-*cis*-retinoic acid at three dose levels on sustainable rates of sebum secretion and on acne. *J Am Acad Dermatol* **8**:532, 1983

238. Stewart ME et al: Suppression of sebum secretion with 13-*cis*-retinoic acid: effect on individual skin surface lipids and implications for their anatomic origin. *J Invest Dermatol* **82**:74, 1984

239. Camisa C et al: The effects of retinoids on neutrophil functions in vitro. *J Am Acad Dermatol* **6**:620, 1982

240. Norris DA et al: 13-*cis*-Retinoic acid has major anti-inflammatory activity in vivo. *Clin Res* **31**:593A, 1983

241. King K et al: A double-blind study of the effects of 13-*cis*-retinoic acid on acne, sebum excretion rate and microbial population. *Br J Dermatol* **107**:583, 1982

242. Leyden JJ, McGinley KJ: Effect of 13-*cis*-retinoic acid on sebum production and *Propionibacterium acnes* in severe nodulocystic acne. *Arch Dermatol Res* **272**:331, 1982

243. Jones H et al: Effect of 13-*cis*-retinoic acid on pilosebaceous duct obstruction. *Br J Dermatol* **107** (suppl 22):35, 1982

244. Gomez EC: Differential effect of 13-*cis*-retinoic acid and an aromatic retinoid (Ro 10-9359) on the sebaceous glands of the hamster flank organ. *J Invest Dermatol* **76**:68, 1981

245. Ward A et al: Etretinate: a review of its pharmacological properties and therapeutic efficacy in psoriasis and other skin disorders. *Drugs* **26**:9, 1983

246. Ehmann CW, Voorhees JJ: International studies of the efficacy of etretinate in the treatment of psoriasis. *J Am Acad Dermatol* **6**:692, 1982

247. Mahrle G et al: Oral treatment of keratinizing disorders of skin and mucous membranes with etretinate. *Arch Dermatol* **118**:97, 1982

248. Goerz G, Orfanos CE: Systemic treatment of psoriasis with a new aromatic retinoid. *Dermatologica* [Suppl 1] **157**:38, 1978

249. Fritsch PO et al: Augmentation of oral methoxsalen-photochemotherapy with an oral retinoic acid derivative. *J Invest Dermatol* **70**:178, 1978

250. Grupper C, Berretti B: Treatment of psoriasis by oral PUVA-therapy combined with aromatic retinoid (Re-PUVA), in *Retinoids: Advances in Basic Research and Therapy,* edited by CE Orfanos et al. New York, Springer-Verlag, 1981, p 341

251. Lauharanta J et al: Aromatic retinoid (Ro 10-9359), Re-PUVA, and PUVA in the treatment of psoriasis, in *Retinoids: Advances in Basic Research and Therapy,* edited by CE Orfanos et al. New York, Springer-Verlag, 1981, p 201

252. Orfanos CE et al: Oral retinoid and UVB radiation: a new alternative treatment for psoriasis on an outpatient basis. *Acta Derm Venereol (Stockh)* **59**:241, 1979

253. Van der Rhee HJ, Polano MK: Treatment of psoriasis vulgaris with a low-dosage Ro 10-9359 orally combined with corticosteroids topically, in *Retinoids: Advances in Basic Research and Therapy,* edited by CE Orfanos et al. New York, Springer-Verlag, 1981, p 193

254. Orfanos CE, Runne U: Systemic use of a new retinoid with and without local dithranol treatment in generalized psoriasis. *Br J Dermatol* **95**:101, 1976

255. Brackertz D, Muller W: Die Beeinflussung der arthropathia Psoriatica und der chronischen Polyarthritis durch ein oral wirksames aromatisches Retinoid. *Verh Dtsch Ges Inn Med* **85**:1343, 1979

256. Rosenthal M: Retinoid in der Behandlung von Psoriasis-arthritis. *Schweiz Med Wochenschr* **109**:1912, 1979

257. Stollenwerk R et al: Clinical observations on oral retinoid therapy of psoriatic arthropathy (Ro 10-9359) in *Retinoids: Advances in Basic Research and Therapy,* edited by CE Orfanos et al. New York, Springer-Verlag, 1981, p 205

258. Thivolet J et al: L'Association retinoide aromatique PUVA-therapie dans le traitement des psoriasis arthropathiques. *Ann Dermatol Venereol* **106**:1037, 1979

259. Hönigsmann H, Wolff K: Isotretinoin-PUVA for psoriasis, *Lancet* **1**:236, 1983

260. Sofen HL et al: Treatment of generalized pustular psoriasis with isotretinoin. *Lancet* **1**:40, 1984

261. Ott F: Long-term biological tolerance of Ro 10-9359, in *Retinoids: Advances in Basic Research and Therapy,* edited by CE Orfanos et al. New York, Springer-Verlag, 1981, p. 355

262. Orfanos CE et al: Neue Aspekte und Entwicklungen der antipsoriatischen Retinoid therapie. *Hautarzt* **32**:275, 1981

263. Peck GL, Yoder FW: Treatment of lamellar ichthyosis and other keratinising dermatoses with an oral synthetic retinoid. *Lancet* **2**:1172, 1976

264. Peck GL et al: Treatment of Darier's disease, lamellar ichthyosis, pityriasis rubra pilaris, cystic acne, and basal cell carcinoma with oral 13-*cis*-retinoic acid. *Dermatologica* [Suppl 1] **157**:11, 1978

265. Ward A et al: Isotretinoin: a review of its pharmacological properties and therapeutic efficacy in acne and other skin disorders. *Drugs* **28**:6, 1984

266. Peck G et al: Comparative analysis of two retinoids in the treatment of disorders of keratinization, in *Retinoids: Advances in Basic Research and Therapy,* edited by CE Orfanos et al. New York, Springer-Verlag, 1981, p 279

267. Lowhagen GB et al: Effects of etretinate (Ro 10-9359) on Darier's disease. *Dermatologica* **165:**123, 1982

268. Goldsmith LA et al: Pityriasis rubra pilaris response to 13-cis-retinoic acid (isotretinoin). *J Am Acad Dermatol* **6:**710, 1982

269. Milstone LM et al: Premature epiphyseal closure in a child receiving oral 13-cis-retinoic acid. *J Am Acad Dermatol* **7:**663, 1982

270. Tamayo L, Ruiz-Maldonado R: Long-term follow-up of 30 children under oral retinoid Ro 10-9359, in *Retinoids: Advances in Basic Research and Therapy,* edited by CE Orfanos et al. New York, Springer-Verlag, 1981, p 287

271. Pittsley RA, Yoder FW: Retinoid hyperostosis. *N Engl J Med* **308:**1012, 1983

272. Gerber LH et al: Vertebral abnormalities associated with synthetic retinoid use. *J Am Acad Dermatol* **10:**817, 1984

273. Ellis CN et al: Isotretinoin therapy is associated with early skeletal radiographic changes. *J Am Acad Dermatol* **10:**1024, 1984

274. Fritsch PO: Oral retinoids in dermatology. *Int J Dermatol* **20:**314, 1981

275. Moriarty M et al: Etretinate in the treatment of actinic keratosis. *Lancet* **1:**364, 1982

276. Peck GL et al: Treatment of basal cell carcinomas with 13-cis-retinoic acid. *Proc Am Assoc Cancer Res* **20:**56, 1979

277. Peck GL et al: Chemoprevention of basal cell carcinoma with isotretinoin. *J Am Acad Dermatol* **6:**815, 1982

278. Braun-Falco O et al: Tumor prophylaxe bei Xeroderma pigmentosum mit aromatischen Retinoid (Ro 10-9359), *Hautarzt* **33:**445, 1982

279. Haydey RP et al: Treatment of keratoacanthomas with oral 13-cis-retinoic acid. *N Engl J Med* **303:**560, 1980

280. Berretti B et al: Aromatic retinoid in the treatment of multiple superficial basal cell carcinoma, arsenic keratosis and keratoacanthoma, in *Retinoids: Advances in Basic Research and Therapy,* edited by CE Orfanos et al. New York, Springer-Verlag, 1981, p 397

281. Schnitzler L, Verret JL: Retinoid and skin cancer prevention, in *Retinoids: Advances in Basic Research and Therapy,* edited by CE Orfanos. New York, Springer-Verlag, 1981, p 385

282. Koch HF: Effect of retinoids on precancerous lesions of oral mucosa, in *Retinoids: Advances in Basic Research and Therapy,* edited by CE Orfanos et al. New York, Springer-Verlag, 1981, p 307

283. Levine N, Meyskens FL: Topical vitamin A acid therapy for cutaneous metastatic melanoma. *Lancet* **2:**224, 1980

284. Cassidy J et al: Phase II trial of 13-cis-retinoic acid in metastatic breast cancer and other malignancies. *Proc Am Soc Clin Oncol* **22:**441, 1981

285. Souteyrand P et al: Treatment of parapsoriasis en plaques and mycosis fungoides with an oral aromatic retinoid (Ro 10-9359), in *Retinoids: Advances in Basic Research and Therapy,* edited by CE Orfanos et al. New York, Springer-Verlag, 1981, p 313

286. Warrell RP Jr et al: Isotretinoin in cutaneous T-cell lymphoma. *Lancet* **2:**629, 1983

287. Kessler JF et al: Treatment of cutaneous T-cell lymphoma (mycosis fungoides) with 13-cis-retinoic acid. *Lancet* **1:**1345, 1983

288. Claudy AL et al: Treatment of cutaneous lymphoma with etretinate. *Br J Dermatol* **109:**49, 1983

289. Ippolito F, Giacalone B: Sur un cas de mycosis fongoide avec manifestations tumorales traite avec Ro 10-9359 (Tigason). *Ann Dermatol Venereol* **109:**65, 1982

290. Zachariae H et al: Oral retinoid in combination with bleomycin, cyclophosphamide, prednisone and transfer factor in mycosis fungoides. *Acta Derm Venereol (Stockh)* **62:**162, 1982

291. Blackman HF et al: Blepharoconjunctivitis: a side effect of 13-cis-retinoic acid therapy for dermatologic diseases. *Ophthalmology* **86:**753, 1979

292. Weiss J et al: Bilateral corneal opacities. Occurrence in a patient treated with oral isotretinoin. *Arch Dermatol* **117:**182, 1981

293. Glazer SD et al: Ultrastructural survey and tissue analysis of human livers after a 6-month course of etretinate. *J Am Acad Dermatol* **10:**632, 1984

294. Zech LA et al: Changes in plasma cholesterol and triglyceride levels after treatment with oral isotretinoin: a prospective study. *Arch Dermatol* **119:**987, 1983

295. Bershad S et al: Changes in plasma lipids and lipoproteins during isotretinoin therapy for acne. *N Engl J Med* **313:**981, 1985

296. Editorial: Adverse effects with isotretinoin. *J Am Acad Dermatol* **10:**519, 1984

297. McBurney EI, Rosen DA: Elevated creatine phosphokinase with isotretinoin. *J Am Acad Dermatol* **10:**528, 1984

298. McCormack LS, Turner MLC: Photosensitivity and isotretinoin therapy. *J Am Acad Dermatol* **9:**273, 1983

299. Lammer EJ et al: Retinoic acid embryopathy. *N Engl J Med* **313:**837, 1985

300. Stern RS et al: Isotretinoin and pregnancy. *J Am Acad Dermatol* **10:**851, 1984

301. Hazen PG et al: Depression—a side effect of 13-cis-retinoic acid therapy. *J Am Acad Dermatol* **9:**278, 1983

302. Weiss VC et al: Hepatotoxic reactions in a patient treated with etretinate. *Arch Dermatol* **120:**104, 1984

303. Dicken CH, Connolly SM: Eruptive xanthomas associated with isotretinoin (13-cis-retinoic acid). *Arch Dermatol* **116:**951, 1980

304. Gollnick H: Elevated levels of triglycerides in patients with skin disease treated with oral aromatic retinoid. The significance of risk factors, in *Retinoids: Advances in Basic Research and Therapy,* edited by CE Orfanos et al. New York, Springer-Verlag, 1981, p 503

305. Ensink BW, Van Voorst Vader PC: Ophthalmological side effects of 13-cis-retinoid therapy. *Br J Dermatol* **108:**627, 1983

306. Orfanos CE: Oral retinoids—present status. *Br J Dermatol* **103:**473, 1980

307. Schill WB et al: Aromatic retinoid and 13-cis-retinoic acid: spermatological investigations, in *Retinoids: Advances in Basic Research and Therapy,* edited by CE Orfanos et al. New York, Springer-Verlag, 1981, p 389

308. Caffey J: Chronic poisoning due to excess of vitamin A. *Am J Roentgenol* **65:**12, 1951

309. Frame B et al: Hypercalcemia and skeletal effects in chronic hypervitaminosis A. *Ann Intern Med* **80:**44, 1974

310. Bartolozzi G, Bernini G: Chronic hypervitaminosis A. *Helv Paediatr Acta* **25:**301, 1970

311. Di Benedetto RJ: Chronic hypervitaminosis A in an adult. *JAMA* **201:**700, 1967

312. Hellriegel KP, Reuter H: Side effects of vitamins, in *Meyler's Side Effects of Drugs,* vol 8, edited by MNG Dukes. Amsterdam, Excerpta Medica, 1975, p 799

313. Pease CN: Focal retardation and arrestment of growth of bones due to vitamin A intoxication. *JAMA* **182:**980, 1962

314. Ruby LK, Mohinder AM: Skeletal deformities following chronic hypervitaminosis A. *J Bone Joint Surg* **56A:**1283, 1974

315. Teelmann K: Experimental toxicology of the aromatic retinoid Ro 10-9359 (etretinate), in *Retinoids: Advances in Basic Research and Therapy,* edited by CE Orfanos et al. New York, Springer-Verlag, 1981, p 41

316. Seawright AA et al: Hypervitaminosis A and hyperostosis of the cat. *Nature* **206:**1171, 1965

317. Seawright AA et al: Hypervitaminosis A and deforming cervical spondylosis of the cat. *J Comp Pathol* **77:**29, 1967

318. Rollman O, Vahlquist A: Retinoid concentration in skin,

serum, and adipose tissue of patients treated with etretinate. *Br J Dermatol* **109**:439, 1983

319. DiGiovanna JJ et al: Etretinate: persistent serum levels of a potent teratogen. *J Invest Dermatol* **82**:434, 1984

320. Orfanos CE et al: Current developments of oral retinoid therapy with three generations of drugs. *Curr Probl Dermatol* **13**:33, 1985

CHAPTER 222

ANTIVIRAL AGENTS

Donna Felsenstein and Martin S. Hirsch

For the past two centuries, live and inactivated vaccines have been our major weapons against viral infections. Judicious prophylactic use of vaccines has helped control a multitude of pathogenic viruses, many with diverse dermatologic manifestations, including smallpox, measles, and rubella.

Over the past decade, efforts have shifted from vaccines toward the chemoprophylaxis and chemotherapy of viral infections. A greater understanding of the mechanisms involved in virus replication has resulted in the ability to target metabolic functions unique to certain viruses and produce selective inhibition of viral replication. In no area of medical virology is this more evident than in the approach to the herpesvirus group. Recognition of viral enzymes such as herpes simplex virus thymidine kinase and DNA polymerase have permitted successful pharmacologic attacks. As a result, prevention and treatment of certain forms of herpes infections are now possible.

Advances in herpes chemotherapy are occurring rapidly, and a chapter on antiviral therapy runs the risk of being soon outdated. Nevertheless, an understanding of the present status of antiherpes agents has become essential to the proper practice of dermatology. Two agents, vidarabine and acyclovir, are now licensed in the United States for the systemic treatment of herpesvirus group infections and several other drugs are on the horizon. Topical antiherpes preparations for ophthalmologic and dermatologic use are also available.

Herpesviruses are not the only agents against which antivirals have been developed. Amantidine hydrochloride is licensed for the prophylaxis and early therapy of influenza A virus infections. Methisazone has demonstrated prophylactic effects against smallpox, and aerosolized ribavirin shows promise against respiratory syncitial virus infection of children. These agents will not be covered in this chapter because of their limited current relevance to the practice of dermatology, and because they have been extensively reviewed elsewhere [1–7]. We will concentrate, rather, on the available nucleoside derivatives for herpes therapy, particularly vidarabine and acyclovir.

Vidarabine

Vidarabine (9-β-D-arabinofuranosyladenine, adenine arabinoside, Ara-A, Vira-A), a purine nucleoside analogue, was the first antiviral agent to be approved for intravenous use in life-threatening disorders. It has some activity against all members of the human herpesvirus group, as well as against some poxviruses, retroviruses, and rhabdoviruses.

Vidarabine is rapidly deaminated in vivo by adenosine deaminase. Its metabolite, arabinosyl hypoxanthine, has significantly less antiviral activity than the parent compound. Once within cells, vidarabine is phosphorylated to the mono-, di-, and triphosphate forms. It is the latter form that acts as a relatively selective competitive inhibitor of viral DNA polymerase. Vidarabine may also become incorporated into the viral DNA molecule, resulting in early chain termination. Following intravenous administration, vidarabine is widely distributed throughout the body, including the cerebrospinal fluid [8]. Its half-life in the circulation is 3 to 4 h. Excretion is primarily by the renal route, and dose adjustment is necessary in patients with renal failure [9].

Varicella-zoster in the immunosuppressed

Immunosuppressed patients, particularly those with lymphoproliferative neoplasms, are at increased risk from complications of both primary varicella and herpes zoster. Placebo-controlled trials have shown that immunosuppressed patients with primary varicella infection have decreased duration of fever, decreased time to cessation of new vesicle formation, and a lower incidence of visceral complications when treated with vidarabine within 72 h of onset of disease [10].

Initial controlled trials of vidarabine in immunosuppressed patients with herpes zoster also demonstrated acceleration of virus clearance from vesicles, and decreased time to cessation of new vesicle formation and to total pustulation, when treatment was begun within the first six days [11]. Vidarabine was later shown to accelerate cutaneous healing, lower rates of cutaneous dissemination (from 24 to 8 percent) and of visceral complications (from 19 to 5 percent), and shorten duration of postherpetic neuralgia when compared with placebo in this patient population. Treatment within 72 h of onset was essential for beneficial effects. Patients with lymphoproliferative disorders and patients older than 38 years of age are more likely to develop complications, and benefit most from treatment with vidarabine [12].

Herpes simplex infections

Topical vidarabine 3% ointment was approved in the United States for use in the treatment of acute and recurrent herpetic keratoconjunctivitis in 1977. It is one of three agents licensed for this purpose, the others being idoxuridine (IDU) (Stoxil, Herplex) and trifluorothymidine (Viroptic). All are useful in the treatment of dendritic and geographic herpes simplex ulcers, although higher efficacy rates of approximately 90 percent have been seen with vidarabine and trifluorothymidine [13–16]. Vidarabine and trifluorothymidine interfere less with corneal healing than IDU and are especially useful in patients allergic to IDU or in whom IDU-resistant strains have developed [14,16–18]. Vidarabine penetrates the corneal epithelium poorly, and is therefore not beneficial in the treatment of stromal ulcers or herpetic uveitis. Vidarabine should be administered as the 3% ointment 5 times a day at 3-h intervals until healing, and at reduced dosage for an additional 7 days. Side effects may include superficial punctate keratitis, lacrimal punctal occlusion, follicular conjunctivitis, and contact dermatitis [15]. In contrast to its effects on ocular herpes infections, topical use of 3% adenine arabinoside cream has been demonstrated to have no influence on the course of either primary or recurrent herpes simplex genital infection [19].

Intravenous vidarabine is beneficial in the treatment of neonatal herpes simplex virus (HSV) infections. Placebo-controlled trials have shown that vidarabine lowers mortality in newborns with central nervous system (CNS) involvement and disseminated disease (from 74 to 38 percent), and in those with localized CNS involvement (from 50 to 10 percent). Morbidity was decreased from 90 to 50 percent in localized CNS disease, and from 89 to 71 percent in disseminated disease with localized CNS disease [20]. When only skin involvement is evident, initiation of therapy in the newborn is also appropriate, to prevent visceral dissemination and CNS involvement.

In adults with herpes simplex encephalitis, vidarabine reduces mortality from approximately 70 to 40 percent and decreases significant morbidity by 45 percent [21,22]. Treatment started early in the course of illness, following appropriate diagnostic procedures, is most effective if begun prior to the development of significant CNS depression, and in patients under 30 years of age [22]. However, prospective, randomized studies comparing vidarabine and acyclovir in the treatment of herpes simplex encephalitis have shown acyclovir to be more effective in reducing mortality, making it the drug of choice [23, NIAD—Antiviral Collaborative Study, 23a].

Dosage and toxicity

The recommended dose for varicella-zoster infections in immunosuppressed patients is 10 mg/kg per day for 5 days. For herpes encephalitis, vidarabine should be given at a dose of 15 mg/kg per day for 10 days. Newborns tolerate higher doses, and 30 mg/kg per day for 10 days is appropriate in the treatment of neonatal HSV infection. The drug is poorly soluble and should be given at a concentration of approximately 0.5 mg/ml as a 12-h continuous infusion. A final in-line membrane filter is recommended. As previously mentioned, reduced doses are needed in patients with impaired renal function. The metabolism of vidarabine is inhibited by allopurinol, and reduced doses are recommended in patients receiving this agent [3].

Toxicity of vidarabine is minimal at recommended doses. Adverse effects include nausea, vomiting, diarrhea, anorexia, paresthesias, tremors, erythematous rash, elevated serum glutamic oxalacetic transaminase levels and serum alanine aminotransferase levels [3,11,12,21–24]. When higher doses of the drug (20 mg/kg per day) are used in adults or when renal dysfunction is present, bone marrow toxicity with anemia, thrombocytopenia, leukopenia, and megaloblastic changes in the erythroid series can be seen, as can significant neurologic abnormalities [24–26]. Toxicity is usually reversible with discontinuation of the drug. Mutagenicity, teratogenicity, and carcinogenicity have been demonstrated in experimental situations, emphasizing the need for judicious use of this agent, particularly in infants and pregnant females.

Acyclovir

Acyclovir (acycloguanosine, 9-(2-hydroxyethoxymethyl)-guanine, Zovirax) is an acyclic purine nucleoside analogue which has shown great promise in the treatment of herpesvirus infections. Topical, intravenous, and oral preparations have recently been licensed in the United States.

Acyclovir is selectively phosphorylated by herpes simplex or varicella-zoster virus-coded thymidine kinases to a monophosphate derivative [27]. The monophosphate form is subsequently converted to acycloguanosine triphosphate (acyclo-GTP) by cellular enzymes. Acyclo-GTP inhibits herpesvirus DNA polymerase 10 to 30 times more effectively than it inhibits cellular DNA polymerase [27,28]. It may also function by acting as a substitute for viral DNA polymerase, causing early chain termination of viral DNA, thus interfering with DNA synthesis by another mechanism [29]. The preferential uptake and conversion of acyclovir to an active form by herpesvirus-infected cells accounts for its low toxicity in normal host cells.

Clinical isolates of HSV-1 and HSV-2 are exquisitely sensitive to acyclovir. Although strains of varicella-zoster (VZV) are somewhat less sensitive than HSV strains (mean 50% inhibitory dose for HSV-1 0.15 μM, HSV-2 1.6 μM, VZV 3.8 μM), clinical isolates of VZV are inhibited by serum levels obtainable with intravenous acyclovir [30,31]. Despite the absence of a virus-specified thymidine kinase, inhibition of Epstein-Barr virus (EBV) occurs through the interaction of acyclo-GTP with the sensitive EBV DNA polymerase [32]. Acyclovir has little effect on the replication of cytomegalovirus [30], and appears to have little clinical applicability to its treatment.

Acyclovir is widely distributed throughout the body with good penetration into the cerebrospinal fluid. Following intravenous administration, the serum half-life is 2 to 4 h. Peak plasma levels following an intravenous dose of 5 mg/kg are 30 to 40 μM [33], whereas following oral administration of 200 mg, peak levels of 1.4 to 4.0 μM are achieved [34]. The kidney is its primary source of excretion, and dose adjustments need to be made in patients with renal insufficiency [33]. Hemodialysis removes approximately 60 percent of an administered dose [35].

Varicella-zoster

Varicella-zoster infection in the immunosuppressed patient is responsive to the use of intravenous acyclovir. In one controlled study, acyclovir decreased the incidence of varicella pneumonitis in immunocompromised children [36]. Its use in the treatment of herpes zoster in immunocompromised patients has also been well documented. Intravenous acyclovir halts progression of localized cutaneous zoster, as well as the development or further progression of disseminated cutaneous or visceral zoster. It accelerates healing of lesions and cessation of viral shedding. The best results are seen when acyclovir is initiated within 72 h of onset of the exanthem, although beneficial effects may occasionally be seen when therapy is begun after three days. The effect on postherpetic neuralgia in these patients remains to be established [37]. Intravenous acyclovir also facilitates healing of herpes zoster in nonimmunocompromised patients, although dissemination is generally less likely to occur in this group [38,39]. Acyclovir has been most helpful in the reduction of acute pain, particularly in patients over the age of 66, or if treatment is initiated within 72 h of onset of pain [39]. Thus far, it has not proved to be efficacious in the immunocompetent host in preventing the occurrence of postherpetic neuralgia [38,39]. This needs to be evaluated further by the use of longer treatment protocols (greater than five days of therapy). As it is not feasible to hospitalize all patients with herpes zoster for intravenous acyclovir, further studies are needed to evaluate the efficacy of an oral outpatient regimen. These studies are in progress.

Herpes simplex

Perhaps acyclovir's most widespread use will occur in the prophylaxis and treatment of mucocutaneous herpes simplex virus infections. Since these infections account for considerable morbidity among the immunosuppressed, prophylaxis with antiviral agents may be of particular value in high-risk patients, including those in the early posttransplant or cancer chemotherapy periods. HSV-seropositive patients can be protected against the development of lesions, as well as asymptomatic viral shedding, when prophylaxis with intravenous acyclovir is begun early during immunosuppressive therapy. Latent infection is not eliminated, however, and recurrences develop if treatment is not continued during the time the patient remains maximally immunocompromised [40,41]. Acyclovir does not worsen the hematologic abnormalities in these patients, nor does it inhibit hematopoietic recovery after chemotherapy [40]. Prophylactic oral acyclovir appears to have the same efficacy as the intravenous preparation [42].

All three acyclovir preparations (intravenous, oral, topical) have been successful in the treatment of established mucocutaneous infections in the immunosuppressed population. Intravenous acyclovir decreases the time to cessation of viral shedding, time to crusting and healing of lesions, and duration of pain [43–45]. The drug has no effect on latency, and reactivation may occur when it is discontinued. Anecdotal reports suggest that symptomatic recurrences can be suppressed on an outpatient basis with oral acyclovir [46]. This needs to be confirmed by controlled trials. Topical acyclovir (5% ointment in a polyethylene glycol base) has been shown to be effective in de-creasing viral shedding, duration of pain, and time to healing in immunosuppressed patients [47,48]. Accelerated resolution of pain and time to healing may be most significant in patients with lesions >50 mm^2 [48].

Topical, intravenous, and oral preparations of acyclovir have been licensed in the United States for treatment of primary herpes genitalis. In primary genital herpes infection, topical acyclovir can significantly reduce the local signs and symptoms of infection by 3 to 4 days. Use of the drug results in decreased viral shedding, decreased time to crusting and healing of lesions, and decreased duration of pain or itching. It has no effect on systemic symptoms, frequency of recurrence, or time to recurrence [49,50]. The beneficial effects of this therapy are less evident in the treatment of recurrent infections. Although a decrease in duration of viral shedding and time to healing of only 1 to 2 days is seen in men with recurrent HSV genitalis treated with acyclovir, even this minimal benefit is not evident in females with recurrent infection [49,50]. Topical acyclovir thus has little role in the treatment of recurrent HSV genitalis. Of note, topical application has been associated with transient burning. This appears to be due to the polyethylene glycol base, since patients treated with placebo complained of symptoms as commonly as did patients in the acyclovir group [49]. The drug is not approved for intravaginal use, since the polyethylene glycol base may cause vaginal erythema [51].

Intravenous acyclovir is more effective than topical therapy in the resolution of both local and systemic signs and symptoms of primary genital herpes infection. When intravenous treatment is initiated within six days of the appearance of vesicles, duration of viral shedding from genital lesions, as well as from cervix, urethra, and pharynx is shortened by 85 to 90 percent (8 to 11 days). Duration of local and systemic symptoms such as formation of new vesicles, pain, itching, and dysuria, is decreased by 50 to 60 percent (3 to 4 days). Rate of healing is accelerated, and there is a lower rate of complications such as extragenital lesions and urinary retention [52,53]. Rate of recurrence is not affected. Cost of hospitalization for intravenous treatment can be significant, so that use of oral acyclovir may prove to be more realistic. In primary genital herpes, oral acyclovir can shorten the clinical course by approximately one week and can reduce the severity of the disease (decreased viral shedding, decreased new vesicle formation in men and women, and decreased duration of pain). Latency is not affected, and, therefore, time to recurrence is not altered, as is the case with other acyclovir preparations [54]. Less of a beneficial effect is observed in recurrent disease [55]. Studies are being conducted to evaluate the benefit of prophylactic oral acyclovir in patients with recurrent genital infections. Initial trials confirm a decreased incidence of recurrence in patients treated with oral acyclovir when compared with placebo [56,57]. With discontinuation of the prophylactic drug, recurrences develop. Theoretically, long-term use of oral acyclovir may be of benefit in patients with frequent and severe recurrent episodes of genital herpes. The benefit of this therapy must be weighed against the possible emergence of resistance (to be discussed) and the theoretical possibility of long-term effects on host DNA.

Unlike genital infection, recurrent perioral infection (herpes labialis) in the healthy host is not effectively treated by acyclovir when used as a 5% or 10% ointment

[58]. Further studies are being conducted to evaluate efficacy when a cream base is used. No studies have been published on the usefulness of parenteral or oral acyclovir on recurrent or primary orolabial herpes in healthy subjects.

Acyclovir appears to be safe for the treatment of neonates [59], and trials comparing vidarabine and acyclovir in the treatment of herpes neonatorum are under way. At present, vidarabine remains the drug of choice for treatment of herpes simplex infection of the newborn. As mentioned, acyclovir has now been shown to be the drug of choice for treatment of herpes simplex encephalitis [23, NIAD—Antiviral Collaborative Study, 23a].

Other viruses

Human papilloma (wart) viruses, like herpesviruses, are DNA viruses, and might therefore be sensitive to acyclovir. Since wart viruses cannot be grown in tissue culture, tests of chemotherapeutic sensitivity to this antiviral agent are virtually impossible, and clinical trials will need to be done. Good results were reported in one patient with the application of topical acyclovir (2.5% ointment) in the treatment of extensive, recurrent plantar warts [60], but anecdotal case reports are no substitute for controlled trials. Acyclovir is also undergoing clinical trials in the prophylaxis and treatment of Epstein-Barr virus infections.

Dosage and toxicity

The intravenous acyclovir dose for adults with mucocutaneous herpes simplex virus infections is 15 mg/kg per day (750 mg/m^2 per day) in three divided doses. Treatment of primary HSV genital infection and progressive mucocutaneous disease should be continued for 5 to 7 days. A higher dose of 30 mg/kg per day for 10 days is necessary in the treatment of herpes simplex encephalitis. Intravenous dosage for varicella in immunosuppressed patients has been recommended at 15 mg/kg per day for 7 days, and for herpes zoster, 1500 mg/m^2 per day for 7 days. As mentioned, the drug is primarily excreted by the kidney, and dosage adjustments need to be made in patients with renal failure [33]. Currently recommended regimens for oral acyclovir include the following: 200 mg five times daily for 10 days for the initial attacks of genital herpes or for treatment of mucocutaneous herpes infections in the immunocompromised host, and 200 mg three to five times daily for no longer than 4 to 6 months for suppression of frequently recurrent genital herpes or mucocutaneous lesions in the immunocompromised host. The topical preparation should be used as a 5% ointment and administered five times daily for 5 to 7 days.

Side effects of topical preparations have already been mentioned. The most common side effect of intravenous acyclovir is phlebitis, particularly if minor extravasation occurs, due to the preparation's alkalinity (pH 10 to 11) [44,53]. Transient crystalluria with impairment of renal function occurs, particularly if the drug is given as a rapid intravenous bolus [61]. Neurologic toxicity, consisting of tremor, disorientation, lethargy, and paresthesias, has been reported in cancer patients receiving intrathecal methotrexate. It occurred several days after initiation of acyclovir and did not resolve until 4 to 15 days after its discontinuation [62]. Rash is a rare side effect [44]. No teratogenicity, carcinogenicity, or mutagenicity has been reported. Nausea is the most common side effect of oral acyclovir.

Acyclovir-resistant strains of herpes simplex have been isolated in the laboratory, as well as from at least a dozen patients [43,63–65]. Resistant mutant strains have lacked the thymidine kinase necessary for selective acyclovir incorporation [66,67]. These thymidine kinase-deficient mutants may be less virulent than wild-type strains [65], but conclusions regarding pathogenicity are premature. Resistance in vitro may also result from mutations altering thymidine kinase substrate specificity [67] or DNA polymerase susceptibility [66]. Whether these resistant viruses will become clinical problems remains to be determined.

Idoxuridine (5-iodo-2′deoxyuridine, IDU, IUDR, Stoxil, Herplex, idoxene)

IDU is an iodinated pyrimidine used exclusively in the treatment of herpes simplex keratitis. Its mechanism of action has been reviewed in detail elsewhere [68]. The primary site of action has not been clearly defined, although incorporation into viral DNA may play a role. In vitro, it is effective against DNA viruses such as vaccinia, polyoma, varicella-zoster, cytomegalovirus, and hepatitis B [6,68], but its principal clinical efficacy has been demonstrated against herpes simplex virus. It is available as a 0.1% ophthalmic solution in distilled water, which is administered as one drop in the conjunctival sac hourly during the day, and every 2 h during the night. A 0.5% ophthalmic ointment in a petrolatum base is also available, and is administered five times a day (every 4 h), while awake. Both preparations should be continued for 3 to 5 days after healing is completed.

Allergic reactions have been reported with IDU [13], as has the development of resistant strains. Vidarabine and trifluorothymidine have proved to be effective in such cases [16–18]. In view of the development of IDU resistance, and because they interfere less with corneal healing, vidarabine and trifluorothymidine may be of greater value than IDU in the treatment of herpetic keratoconjunctivitis [16,17]. IDU should be used with caution in pregnant females due to possible teratogenic effects [5].

Trifluorothymidine (trifluoridine, Viroptic, F3T)

Trifluorothymidine is a thymidine analogue with potent antiherpes activity. It functions by reversibly inhibiting thymidilate synthetase, resulting in inhibition of DNA synthesis. Direct incorporation into DNA can occur, with the production of defective viral progeny. A short serum half-life and significant systemic toxicity prohibit its use as a systemic antiviral agent [16].

Topical trifluorothymidine was approved for use in the United States in 1980, for the treatment of ocular herpes. It is more successful in producing healing of dendritic or geographic ulcers when compared to idoxuridine, although rate of healing is equivalent [16,69]. Efficacy appears to be as good as that seen with vidarabine [70]. Trifluorothymidine is available as a 1% ophthalmic solution, and is administered as one drop in the infected eye every 2 h while awake, for a maximum number of nine times per day.

Prolonged therapy, greater than three weeks, is not advised [5]. Adverse reactions to topical therapy include conjunctivitis, punctate keratitis, and a subjective sensation of irritation [16].

Bromovinyldeoxyuridine

Bromovinyldeoxyuridine [E-5-(2-bromovinyl)-2′-deoxyuridine, BVDU] is a nucleoside analogue under investigation as an antiherpetic agent. The mechanism of action is similar to that of acyclovir [71]. Briefly, upon entry into an infected cell, a virus-specified thymidine kinase phosphorylates the drug to the 5′-monophosphate form. After conversion to the triphosphate by cellular enzymes, the converted form of the drug competes more effectively with dTTP for viral DNA polymerases than with cellular DNA polymerases [72]. This may account for its diminished toxicity in host cells [73].

In vitro studies have demonstrated its efficacy in the inhibition of HSV-1 and HSV-2, although HSV-2 is far less sensitive [73]. Animal studies comparing BVDU, IDU, trifluorothymidine, and Ara-A have shown BVDU to be equally beneficial in the treatment of superficial keratitis and superior in the treatment of stromal keratitis and iritis [74–77]. BVDU can be administered orally, with achievement of significant serum inhibitory levels for HSV-1 and VZV [77,78]. Clinical trials are under way in HSV-1 and VZV infections.

Phosphonoacetic acid and phosphonoformate

Phosphonoacetic acid (PAA) and its analogue phosphonoformate (PFA) have been shown to have antiviral properties against HSV-1 and HSV-2 [79]. Both compounds preferentially inhibit HSV DNA polymerase, as opposed to mammalian cellular DNA polymerase, but this preference is dependent on enzyme concentration [80].

PAA and PFA appear comparable in the treatment of cutaneous herpes simplex infection in animal studies [79,81]. Dermal toxicity, however, appears greater with the former agent [81]. Due to increased dermal toxicity by PAA, as well as retention of this compound in bone [5], greater interest has focused on the less toxic analogue, PFA. Topical application of PFA as a 3% ointment has been evaluated in one study in the treatment of herpes labialis. PFA shortened the papular and vesicular stages of the disease, but did not significantly affect time to healing [82]. Further clinical evaluation of this agent is warranted.

Interferons

Interferons differ significantly from the chemotherapeutic agents previously discussed. They are proteins with both antiviral and antineoplastic activities. Only their antiviral properties will be dealt with in this chapter.

As antiviral agents, interferons function in two ways. First, they induce an antiviral state by binding to receptors on the cell surface of an infected cell, stimulating the production of several cellular enzymes with antiviral activity [83,84]. In many viral systems, these enzymes inhibit the translation of viral messenger RNA into viral protein. Inhibition of transcription, assembly, and release of certain viruses has also been described. Second, interferons function through regulatory effects on the immune system. This has been reviewed elsewhere [85] and will not be pursued here. Because of their indirect inhibitory effect on viral replication, interferons are effective against a wide range of DNA and RNA viruses.

Interferons are classified into three major types. (1) Interferon-alpha (IFN-α)—produced by lymphocytes, largely in response to viral infection; (2) interferon-beta (IFN-β)—produced by fibroblasts in response to viral or nonviral stimulation; (3) interferon-gamma (IFN-γ)—produced by sensitized T or B cells in response to antigens or mitogens [86]. All three major types can now be produced by genetic recombination techniques in bacteria, and are undergoing extensive clinical trials.

IFN-α is usually administered by intramuscular injection. The serum half-life is 4 to 6 h when given by this route [87]. IFN-β should be given intravenously, since much higher serum levels can be obtained by this route [88]. Pharmacologic studies with IFN-γ are under way, but little information has been gathered to date. Interferons do not readily penetrate into the cerebrospinal fluid [87,89,90].

IFN-α, at doses of 3.5×10^5 U/kg per day for 48 h, followed by 1.75×10^5 U/kg per day for 72 h, is effective in the treatment of primary varicella in immunocompromised children, if initiated within 72 h of appearance of the exanthem. A decrease in the number of days to cessation of new lesion formation, as well as a decrease in the incidence of life-threatening dissemination, has been demonstrated [91]. Similar beneficial effects are seen in patients with underlying malignancies and localized herpes zoster infections when treated with 5.1×10^5 U/kg per day for 2 days, followed by 2.55×10^5 U/kg per day for a total of 8 days. A lower incidence of visceral complications, decreased progression of lesions in the primary dermatome, and decreased cutaneous dissemination are observed, as well as diminished incidence and duration of postherpetic neuralgia [92]. Shorter courses of therapy (i.e., 48 h) seem to be of little benefit [93].

IFN-α has been effective as a prophylactic agent in patients with a history of herpes labialis who are at high risk for reactivation following trigeminal ganglion surgery [94]. Latent infection is not eliminated, and rate of recurrence is unaffected [95]. In renal transplant patients, prophylactic IFN-α has little effect on the incidence of herpes simplex infections or viral shedding [96].

Unlike other antiviral agents, IFN-α, when combined with debridement, may prove to be effective in the prevention of recurrences of herpetic keratitis [97,98]. Further controlled studies in ophthalmic herpes are needed.

Controlled trials have shown that the morbidity of cytomegalovirus infections in renal transplant patients can be decreased with the use of IFN-α [96,99]. This agent may also reduce EBV reactivation in the transplant population [100].

Toxicity of interferons includes fever, local pain, anorexia, fatigue, malaise, alopecia [101], lymphocytopenia, granulocytopenia, and thrombocytopenia. Hematologic toxicity is dose dependent and reversible [87,89]. Neurologic toxicity has been reported with the use of high-dose therapy [102]. At present, interferon is used for investigational purposes only. With the increased availability of interferon preparations, multiple clinical trials in different settings are under way.

Table 222-1   Indications and guidelines for the use of varicella-zoster immune globulin (VZIG) for the prophylaxis of chickenpox (varicella)

1. One of the following underlying illnesses or conditions:
   a. Leukemia or lymphoma
   b. Congenital or acquired immunodeficiency
   c. Under immunosuppressive treatment
   d. Newborn of mother who had onset of chickenpox less than 5 days before delivery or within 48 h after delivery
2. One of the following types of exposure to chickenpox or zoster patients:
   a. Household contact
   b. Playmate contact (more than 1 h play indoors)
   c. Hospital contact (in same 2- to 4-bed room or adjacent beds in a large ward)
   d. Newborn contact (newborn of mother who had onset of chickenpox less than 5 days before delivery or within 48 h after delivery)
3. Negative or unknown prior history of chickenpox
4. Age of less than 15 years, with administration to older patients on an individual basis
5. Time elapsed after exposure is such that VZIG can be administered within 96 h

Adapted from [118].

Other antiviral therapies

Prior to the use of present antiviral agents, several other forms of therapy had been tried for many years without success. Although topical 2-deoxy-D-glucose was reported to decrease the severity and frequency of primary and recurrent genital herpes infections, results of the study were questioned [103]. Efficacy of this drug in the treatment of HSV infections has not been substantiated in animal experiments [104]. L-Lysine, levamisole, photodynamic activation, and use of topical ether and chloroform are all of no proven clinical value in the treatment of herpetic infections [105–112].

One approach to viral prophylaxis is the use of varicella-zoster immune globulin (VZIG). It is prepared from the plasma of healthy blood donors identified as having high titers of varicella-zoster antibodies. Although VZIG is of considerable value in the prophylaxis of exposed seronegative high-risk patients [113–117], it is not of benefit in the therapy of ongoing infection. Use of VZIG should be restricted to those patients meeting the five criteria listed in Table 222-1 [118].

References

1. Hirsch MS, Swartz MN: Antiviral Agents I. *N Engl J Med* **302**:903, 1980
2. National Institutes of Health Conference: Amantadine: Does it have a role in the prevention and treatment of influenza? A National Institutes of Health Consensus Development Conference. *Ann Intern Med* **92**:256, 1980
3. Hermans PE, Cockerill FR III: A Symposium on Antimicrobial Agents. IV. Antiviral Agents. *Mayo Clin Proc* **58**:217, 1983
4. Liu C: Antiviral drugs. *Med Clin North Am* **66**:235, 1982
5. Galasso GJ: An assessment of antiviral drugs for the management of infectious diseases in humans. *Antiviral Res* **1**:73, 1981
6. Galasso GJ et al (eds). *Antiviral Agents and Viral Diseases of Man*. New York, Raven Press, 1979
7. Hall CB et al: Aerosolized ribavarin treatment of infants with respiratory syncytial viral infection. *N Engl J Med* **308**:1443, 1983
8. Whitley R et al: Vidarabine: a preliminary review of its pharmacological properties and therapeutic use. *Drugs* **20**:267, 1980
9. Aronoff GR et al: Hypoxanthine arabinoside pharmacokinetics after adenine arabinoside administration to a patient with renal failure. *Antimicrob Agents Chemother* **18**:212, 1980
10. Whitley R et al: Vidarabine therapy of varicella in immunosuppressed patients. *J Pediatr* **101**:125, 1982
11. Whitley RJ et al: Adenine arabinoside therapy of herpes zoster in the immunosuppressed. NIAID Collaborative Antiviral Study. *N Engl J Med* **294**:1193, 1976
12. Whitley RJ et al: Early vidarabine therapy to control the complications of herpes zoster in immunosuppressed patients. *N Engl J Med* **307**:971, 1982
13. Pavan-Langston D, Dohlman CH: A double-blind clinical study of adenine arabinoside therapy of viral keratoconjunctivitis. *Am J Ophthalmol* **74**:81, 1972
14. Pavan-Langston D: Clinical evaluation of adenine arabinoside and idoxuridine in the treatment of ocular herpes simplex. *Am J Ophthalmol* **80**:495, 1975
15. Pavan-Langston D et al: Acyclovir and vidarabine in the treatment of ulcerative herpes simplex keratitis. *Am J Ophthalmol* **92**:829, 1981
16. Pavan-Langston D, Foster CS: Trifluorothymidine and idoxuridine therapy of ocular herpes. *Am J Ophthalmol* **84**:818, 1977
17. Hyndiuk RA et al: Adenine arabinoside in idoxuridine unresponsive and intolerant herpetic keratitis. *Am J Ophthalmol* **79**:655, 1975
18. Nesburn AB et al: Adenine arabinoside effect on experimental idoxuridine-resistant herpes simplex infection. *Invest Ophthalmol* **13**:302, 1974
19. Adams HG et al: Genital herpetic infection in men and women: clinical course and effect of topical application of adenine arabinoside. *J Infect Dis* **133** (suppl A):151, 1976
20. Whitley RJ et al: Vidarabine therapy of neonatal herpes simplex virus infection. *Pediatrics* **66**:495, 1980
21. Whitley RJ et al: Adenine arabinoside therapy of biopsy-proved herpes simplex encephalitis. *N Engl J Med* **297**:289, 1977
22. Whitley RJ et al: Herpes simplex encephalitis. Vidarabine therapy and diagnostic problems. *N Engl J Med* **304**:313, 1981
23. Skoldenberg B et al: Acyclovir versus vidarabine in herpes simplex encephalitis. Randomized multicenter study in consecutive Swedish patients. *Lancet* **2**:707, 1984
23a. Whitley RJ et al: Herpes simplex encephalitis: adenine arabinoside verus acyclovir therapy. *N Engl J Med*, in press
24. Ross AH et al: Toxicity of adenine arabinoside in humans. *J Infect Dis* **133** (suppl A):192, 1976
25. Gottlieb JA, Bodey GP Sr: Possible bone-marrow depression by Ara-A therapy for disseminated herpes zoster (letter). *N Engl J Med* **290**:914, 1974
26. Lauter CB et al: Microbiologic assays and neurological toxicity during use of adenine arabinoside in humans. *J Infect Dis* **134**:75, 1976
27. Elion GB et al: Selectivity of action of an antiherpetic agent, 9-(2-hydroxyethoxymethyl) guanine. *Proc Natl Acad Sci USA* **74**:5716, 1977
28. Allaudeen HS et al: Mode of action of acyclovir triphosphate on herpesviral and cellular DNA polymerases. *Antiviral Res* **2**:123, 1982
29. McGuirt PV, Furman PA: Acyclovir inhibition of viral DNA

chain elongation in herpes simplex virus-infected cells. *Am J Med* **73(1A):**67, 1982

30. Crumpacker CS et al: Growth inhibition by acycloguanosine of herpes viruses isolated from human infections. *Antimicrob Agents Chemother* **15:**642, 1979

31. McLaren C et al: Spectrum of sensitivity to acyclovir of herpes simplex virus clinical isolates. *Am J Med* **73(1A):**376, 1982

32. Pagano JS, Datta AK: Perspectives on interactions of acyclovir with Epstein-Barr and other herpes viruses. *Am J Med* **73(1A):**18, 1982

33. Whitley RJ et al: Pharmacokinetics of acyclovir in humans following intravenous administration. A model for the development of parenteral antivirals. *Am J Med* **73(1A):**165, 1982

34. Van Dyke RB et al: Pharmacokinetics of orally administered acyclovir in patients with herpes progenitalis. *Am J Med* **73(1A):**172, 1982

35. Laskin O et al: Acyclovir kinetics in end-stage renal failure. *Clin Pharmacol Ther* **31:**594, 1982

36. Prober CG et al: Acyclovir therapy of chickenpox in immunosuppressed children—a collaborative study. *J Pediatr* **101:**622, 1982

37. Balfour HH Jr et al: Acyclovir halts progression of herpes zoster in immunocompromised patients. *N Engl J Med* **38:**1448, 1983

38. Bean B et al: Acyclovir therapy for acute herpes zoster. *Lancet* **2:**118, 1982

39. Esmann V et al: Therapy of acute herpes zoster with acyclovir in the nonimmunocompromised host. *Am J Med* **73(1A):**320, 1982

40. Saral R et al: Acyclovir prophylaxis of herpes-simplex virus infections: a randomized, double-blind controlled trial in bone-marrow transplant recipients. *N Engl J Med* **305:**63, 1981

41. Saral R et al: Acyclovir prophylaxis against herpes simplex virus infections in patients with leukemia: a randomized, double-blind, placebo controlled study. *Ann Intern Med* **99:**773, 1983

42. Wade JC et al: Oral acyclovir prophylaxis of herpes simplex virus infections after marrow transplant. 22nd Interscience Conference on Antimicrobial Agents and Chemotherapy. American Society for Microbiology. Miami Beach, Florida, Oct 4–6, 1982

43. Wade JC et al: Intravenous acyclovir to treat mucocutaneous herpes simplex virus infection after marrow transplantation. *Ann Intern Med* **96:**265, 1982

44. Meyers JD et al: Multicenter collaborative trial of intravenous acyclovir for treatment of mucocutaneous herpes simplex virus infection in the immunocompromised host. *Am J Med* **73(1A):**229, 1982

45. Mitchell CD et al: Acyclovir therapy for mucocutaneous herpes simplex infections in immunocompromised patients. *Lancet* **1:**1389, 1981

46. Straus SE et al: Acyclovir for chronic mucocutaneous herpes simplex virus infection in immunosuppressed patients. *Ann Intern Med* **96:**270, 1982

47. Whitley R et al: Mucocutaneous herpes simplex virus infections in immunocompromised patients, a model for evaluation of topical antiviral agents. *Am J Med* **73(1A):**236, 1982

48. Whitley R et al: Infections caused by herpes simplex virus in the immunocompromised host: natural history and topical acyclovir therapy. *J Infect Dis* **150:**323, 1984

49. Corey L et al: Double-blind controlled trials of topical acyclovir in genital herpes simplex virus infections. *Am J Med* **73(1A):**326, 1982

50. Corey L et al: A trial of topical acyclovir in genital herpes simplex virus infections. *N Engl J Med* **306:**1313, 1982

51. Corey L, Holmes KK: Genital herpes simplex virus infec-

52. Mindel A et al: Intravenous acyclovir treatment for primary genital herpes. *Lancet* **1:**697, 1982

53. Corey L et al: Intravenous acyclovir for the treatment of primary genital herpes. *Ann Intern Med* **98:**914, 1983

54. Bryson YJ et al: Treatment of first episodes of genital herpes simplex virus infection with oral acyclovir. *N Engl J Med* **308:**916, 1983

55. Nilsen AE et al: Efficacy of oral acyclovir in the treatment of initial and recurrent genital herpes. *Lancet* **2:**571, 1982

56. Straus SE et al: Suppression of frequently recurring genital herpes: a placebo-controlled double-blind trial of oral acyclovir. *N Engl J Med* **310:**1545, 1984

57. Douglas JM et al: A double-blind study of oral acyclovir for suppression of recurrences of genital herpes simplex virus infection. *N Engl J Med* **310:**1551, 1984

58. Spruance SL et al: Treatment of herpes simplex labialis with topical acyclovir in polyethylene glycol. *J Infect Dis* **146:**85, 1982

59. Yeager AS: Use of acyclovir in premature and term infants. *Am J Med* **73(1A):**205, 1982

60. Bauer DJ: Treatment of plantar warts with ACV. *Am J Med* **73(1A):**313, 1982

61. Brigden D et al: Renal function after acyclovir intravenous injection. *Am J Med* **73(1A):**182, 1982

62. Wade JC, Meyers JD: Neurologic symptoms associated with parenteral acyclovir treatment after marrow transplantation. *Ann Intern Med* **98:**921, 1983

63. Burns WH et al: Isolation and characterization of resistant herpes simplex virus after acyclovir therapy. *Lancet* **1:**421, 1982

64. Crumpacker CS et al: Resistance to antiviral drugs of herpes simplex virus isolated from a patient treated with acyclovir. *N Engl J Med* **306:**343, 1982

65. Sibrack CD et al: Pathogenicity of acyclovir resistant herpes simplex virus type 1 from an immunodeficient child. *J Infect Dis* **146:**673, 1982

66. Schnipper LE, Crumpacker CS: Resistance of herpes simplex virus to acycloguanosine: role of viral thymidine kinase and DNA polymerase loci. *Proc Natl Acad Sci USA* **77:**2270, 1980

67. Darby G et al: Altered substrate specificity of herpes simplex virus thymidine kinase confers acyclovir-resistance. *Nature* **289:**81, 1981

68. Prusoff WH: Antiviral iodinated pyrimidine deoxyribonucleosides: 5-iodo-2'-deoxyuridine; 5-iodo-2'-deoxycytidine; 5-iodo-5'-amino-2',5'-dideoxyuridine. *Pharmacol Ther* **7:**1, 1979

69. Wellings PC et al: Clinical evaluation of trifluorothymidine in the treatment of herpes simplex corneal ulcers. *Am J Ophthalmol* **73:**932, 1972

70. Costar DJ et al: Clinical evaluation of adenine arabinoside and trifluorothymidine in the treatment of corneal ulcers caused by herpes simplex virus. *J Infect Dis* **133 (suppl A):**173, 1976

71. Sim IS et al: E-5-(2-Bromovinyl)-2'-deoxyuridine (BVDU), pharmacology and clinical experience, in *Herpesvirus: Clinical, Pharmacological and Basic Aspects,* edited by H Shiota et al. Amsterdam, Excerpta Medica, 1981, p 157

72. Allaudeen HS et al: On the mechanism of selective inhibition of herpesvirus replication by (E)-5-(2-bromovinyl)-2'-deoxyuridine. *Proc Natl Acad Sci USA* **78:**2698, 1981

73. DeClercq EJ et al: Comparative efficacy of antiherpes drugs against different strains of herpes simplex virus. *J Infect Dis* **141:**563, 1980

74. Maudgal PC et al: (E)-5-(2-Bromovinyl)-2'-deoxyuridine in the treatment of experimental herpes simplex keratitis. *Antimicrob Agents Chemother* **17:**8, 1980

75. Hettinger ME et al: Ac₂IDU, BVDU and thymine arabinoside therapy in experimental herpes keratitis. *Arch Ophthalmol* **99:**1618, 1981

76. Maudgal PC et al: Experimental stromal herpes simplex keratitis. Influence of treatment with topical bromovinyldeoxyuridine and trifluridine. *Arch Ophthalmol* **100:**653, 1982

77. Maudgal PC et al: Oral and topical treatment of experimental herpes simplex iritis with bromovinyldeoxyuridine. *Arch Ophthalmol* **100:**1337, 1982

78. DeClercq E et al: Oral therapy with (E)-5-(2-bromovinyl)-2'-deoxyuridine for severe herpes zoster infections. *Br Med J* **281:**1178, 1980

79. Kern ER et al: A comparison of phosphonoacetic acid and phosphonoformic acid activity in genital herpes simplex virus type 1 and type 2 infections in mice. *Antiviral Res* **1:**225, 1981

80. Helgstrand E et al: Trisodium phosphonoformate, a new antiviral compound. *Science* **201:**819, 1978

81. Alenius S et al: Therapeutic effect of trisodium phosphonoformate on cutaneous herpesvirus infection in guinea pigs. *Antimicrob Agents Chemother* **14:**408, 1978

82. Wallin J et al: Therapeutic efficacy of trisodium phosphonoformate in treatment of recurrent herpes labialis, in *The Human Herpes Viruses—An Interdisciplinary Perspective,* edited by AJ Nahmias et al. New York, Elsevier, 1981, p 680

83. Friedman RM: Antiviral activity of interferon. *Bacteriol Rev* **41:**543, 1977

84. Dianzani F, Baron S: Activation by interferon of the events leading to the antiviral state. *Tex Rep Biol Med* **35:**297, 1977

85. Stiehm ER et al: Interferon: immunobiology and clinical significance. UCLA Conference. *Ann Intern Med* **96:**80, 1982

86. National Institute of Allergy and Infectious Diseases and the World Health Organization: Interferon nomenclature. *Nature* **286:**110, 1980

87. Pollard RB, Merigan TC: Experience with clinical application of interferon and interferon inducers. *Pharmacol Ther* **2A:**783, 1978

88. Hanley DF et al: Pharmacology of interferons I. Pharmacologic distinctions between human leukocyte and fibroblast interferons. *Int J Immunol Pharmacol* **1:**219, 1979

89. Merigan TC: Pharmacokinetics and side effects of interferon in man. *Tex Rep Biol Med* **35:**541, 1977

90. Emodi G et al: Circulating interferon in man after administration of exogenous human leukocyte interferon. *J Natl Cancer Inst* **54:**1045, 1975

91. Arvin AM et al: Human leukocyte interferon for the treatment of varicella in children with cancer. *N Engl J Med* **306:**761, 1982

92. Merigan TC et al: Human leukocyte interferon for the treatment of herpes zoster in patients with cancer. *N Engl J Med* **298:**981, 1978

93. Merigan TC et al: Short course human leukocyte interferon in the treatment of herpes zoster in patients with cancer. *Antimicrob Agents Chemother* **19:**193, 1981

94. Pazin GJ et al: Prevention of reactivated herpes simplex infection by human leukocyte interferon after operation on the trigeminal root. *N Engl J Med* **301:**225, 1979

95. Haverkos HW et al: Follow-up of interferon treatment of herpes simplex (letter). *N Engl J Med* **303:**399, 1980

96. Cheeseman SH et al: Controlled clinical trials of prophylactic human-leukocyte interferon in renal transplantation: effects on cytomegalovirus and herpes simplex virus infections. *N Engl J Med* **300:**1345, 1979

97. Sundmacher R et al: Successful treatment of dendritic keratitis with human leukocyte interferon. A controlled clinical study. *Albrecht Von Graefes Arch Klin Exp Ophthalmol* **201:**39, 1976

98. Dunnick JK, Galasso GJ: Clinical trials with exogenous interferon: summary of a meeting. *J Infect Dis* **139:**109, 1979

99. Hirsch MS et al: Effects of interferon-alpha on cytomegalovirus reactivation syndromes in renal-transplant recipients. *N Engl J Med* **308:**1489, 1983

100. Cheeseman SH et al: Epstein-Barr virus infection in renal transplant recipients. Effects of antithymocyte globulin and interferon. *Ann Intern Med* **93:**39, 1980

101. Ingimarsson S et al: Side effects of long term treatment with human leukocyte interferon. *J Infect Dis* **140:**560, 1979

102. Smedley H et al: Neurological effects of recombinant human interferon. *Br Med J* **286:**262, 1983

103. Blough HA, Giuntoli RL: Successful treatment of human genital herpes infections with 2-deoxy-D-glucose. *JAMA* **241:**2798, 1979

104. Kern ER et al: Failure of 2-deoxy-D-glucose in the treatment of experimental cutaneous and genital infections due to herpes simplex virus. *J Infect Dis* **146:**159, 1982

105. Milman N et al: Failure of lysine treatment in recurrent herpes simplex labialis (letter). *Lancet* **2:**942, 1978

106. Milman N et al: Lysine prophylaxis in recurrent herpes simplex labialis: a double-blind controlled crossover study. *Acta Derm Venereol (Stockh)* **60:**85, 1980

107. Russell AS et al: A double-blind controlled trial of levamisole in the treatment of recurrent herpes labialis. *J Infect Dis* **137:**597, 1978

108. Roome AP et al: Neutral red with photoinactivation in the treatment of herpes genitalis. *Br J Vener Dis* **51:**130, 1975

109. Myers MG et al: Photodynamic inactivation in recurrent infections with herpes simplex virus. *J Infect Dis* **133 (suppl A):**145, 1976

110. Myers MG et al: Failure of neutral-red photodynamic inactivation in recurrent herpes simplex virus infections. *N Engl J Med* **293:**945, 1975

111. Corey L et al: Ineffectiveness of topical ether for the treatment of genital herpes simplex virus infection. *N Engl J Med* **299:**237, 1978

112. Taylor CA et al: Topical treatment of herpes labialis with chloroform. *Arch Dermatol* **113:**1550, 1977

113. Brunell PA et al: Prevention of varicella by zoster immune globulin. *N Engl J Med* **280:**1191, 1969

114. Brunell PA et al: Prevention of varicella in high risk children: a collaborative study. *Pediatrics* **50:**718, 1972

115. Gershon AA et al: Zoster immune globulin. A further assessment. *N Engl J Med* **290:**243, 1974

116. Orenstein WA et al: Prophylaxis of varicella in high-risk children: dose-response effect of zoster immune globulin. *J Pediatr* **98:**368, 1981

117. Zaia JA et al: Evaluation of varicella-zoster immune globulin: protection of immunosuppressed children after household exposure to varicella. *J Infect Dis* **147:**737, 1983

118. Centers for Disease Control: Varicella-zoster immune globulin—United States. *MMWR* **30(2):**15, 21, 1981

PART SEVEN

PEDIATRIC DERMATOLOGY

Section 34

Pediatric dermatology

CHAPTER 223

PEDIATRIC (NEONATAL) DERMATOLOGY

William L. Weston

Pediatric dermatology overlaps considerably with adult dermatology and therefore the discussions in this chapter are limited to those conditions which are characteristically seen in newborns. For those individuals interested in the scope of pediatric dermatology, the following "cross-reference–index" is provided for convenience in locating discussions throughout the book.

Premature and normal newborn skin biology

The newborn period constitutes the first 30 days following birth. Evaluation of newborn skin requires a thorough knowledge of the structure and function of skin of the developing embryo and fetus (see also Chap. 9).

Embryonic cells formed after fertilization contain the entire genetic code required for production of each component of skin [1]. These embryonic cells divide to form a single-layer ectoderm and a single-layered mesoderm which are the precursors to the primordial epidermis and dermis.

The epidermis

The single-layered ectoderm produces a second single layer of cells designated the *periderm* [1–4]. This appears in the eighth gestational week. The periderm consists of flattened polygonal cells modified by surface microvilli. A complex polysaccharide coat covers the microvilli surface. Periderm cells divide independently of the underlying epidermis and remain on the skin surface until the underlying epidermis completely keratinizes [1–4]. The periderm sloughs into the amniotic fluid and becomes one component of the vernix caseosa. The function of the periderm is uncertain. It is believed that the periderm may participate in the transport of fluids, electrolytes, and sugars into the developing embryo, or that it may provide a barrier function for the skin surface while keratinization is incomplete [1–4].

Cross-reference to chapters in which pediatric dermatologic entities are discussed (Continued)

Maturation and keratinization of epidermal cells is completed by approximately 28 weeks [1–3]. The primordial ectoderm cell has some characteristics of germinative adult keratinocytes (basal cells) by 8 weeks with recognizable keratin filaments and desmosomes present. The cytoplasm of primordial ectodermal cells is filled with glycogen. Active proliferation of the keratinocytes occurs until week 12 with formation of several cell layers which move outward from the basal cell layer and interpose themselves between the basal cell layer and the periderm. By the 12th week, immunoreactive cell surface antigens are acquired by the keratinocytes including the pemphigus and pemphigoid antigens as well as the ABO blood group antigens [5]. Interaction with maternally transferred antibody is possible at the 12th week. The Langerhans cells, the antigen-presenting cell of the epidermis and thus an immunologic outpost for antigens applied to the skin surface, are first detectable by 12 weeks [1–4]. Their functional capacity in the developing skin is unknown.

Nails keratinize first at 16 weeks, but the remainder of the epidermis does not completely keratinize until 26 to 28 weeks. After the nail, the scalp keratinizes, followed by keratinization of the remainder of the skin in a caudad progression [1–4]. Establishment of an epidermal barrier equal to that of adult skin is accomplished by 37 weeks [6–12]. Preterm infants less than 32 weeks have an abnormal epidermal barrier with increased percutaneous absorption and exaggerated transepidermal water loss [7,8,10–12]. Between 32 and 37 weeks, the epidermal barrier may be more permeable than adult or normal newborn skin [7,8,10–12].

Preterm babies have excess vernix caseosa on their skin surface at delivery, particularly those from 35 to 38 weeks gestation. The vernix becomes scantier and limited to the flexural areas after 38 weeks and is absent in postmature infants [13–15]. Vernix appears as a greasy or cheesy substance which may be admixed with meconium, giving a green stain, or with maternal blood. Vernix is composed of periderm cells, sebum, and desquamated stratum corneum cells [13].

Pigmentation of the epidermis may begin by 16 weeks when melanocytes containing melanosomes and the enzymes necessary for the synthesis of melanin are noted in the epidermis [2–4]. Melanocytes migrate from the neural crest through the primordial dermis to the epidermis. By 20 weeks the epidermis has its full complement of melanocytes [2–4]. However, even in the term or postterm babies, melanization is not complete. Newborns have much lighter skin color than they will later acquire in infancy and childhood [13,14].

Epidermal appendages

The epidermal appendages begin as downward buds from the basal keratinocyte layer as crowded clusters of basal cells called *pregerm*. For pilosebaceous structure, pregerm first appears on areas corresponding to the eyebrows, upper lip, and chin [2–4]. They later appear on the scalp. By 16 weeks, the downward projection of these clusters of basal cells is complete, and by 20 weeks club-shaped follicles with follicular channels are formed. Hair follicles grow at an oblique angle to the skin surface such that hair will emerge from the skin surface in a caudal direction [2–4]. Most hair follicles on newborn infants' bodies point downward. Hair formation begins on the scalp and proceeds in a cephalocaudad direction. Sebaceous glands form in much the same fashion as hair, and are first observed on hairy areas of skin, buccal mucosa, lips, esophagus, and vagina [2–4]. Sebaceous glands may be observed on the lip and buccal mucosa on newborns as 1- to 3-mm discrete yellow macules [2–4]. By 16 weeks, hydroxysteroid dehydrogenase enzymes are established in the sebaceous germ, and sebaceous tissues exhibit very high enzyme activity prior to birth [2–4]. Steroid hormone conversion by these enzymes is efficient and the 30- to 36-week fetus has larger sebaceous glands than a term infant. However, neonatal acne is usually not observed until 2 to 4 weeks after birth. Apocrine glands appear after sebaceous glands are completely differentiated. They begin in the areola, axilla, scalp, umbilicus, and the perineum at 28 weeks, and are not differentiated until 34 to 36 weeks. Scalp hair which is thin in caliber, soft and fine, and designated *lanugo hair,* covers the scalp and brow of the preterm infant. Excessive facial hair may be observed in certain preterm infants [13,14]. At delivery, scalp hairs are synchronous in their growth phase, with 80 percent of hairs in a resting or telogen state. Following birth, shedding of the majority of the scalp hairs occurs during the first three months of postnatal life.

Eccrine sweat glands first appear at 26 weeks as germ buds and the sweat ducts may be patent and sweating functional as early as 30 to 32 weeks [3,4,16]. Harpin and Rutter showed that babies over 36 weeks of age were able to sweat on their birth day, whereas preterm infants under 36 weeks required up to 13 days following birth to initiate sweating [16]. Sweating was observed first on the forehead, and although sweating was present early, it was not complete and the ability of term or preterm babies to sweat sufficiently to have functional thermal regulation was considered doubtful [16]. Not all sweat ducts are patent at birth, and sweat duct obstruction giving rise to miliaria crystallina or miliaria rubra is commonly observed in term infants [13,14].

The development of the fetal nail, the skin ridges, and the volar pads is linked in the developing digit. These structures form simultaneously at 8 weeks just after the digits separate [2–4]. The proximal and distal nail folds and volar pads are formed by 12 weeks. The distal nail fold is the first epithelial structure to keratinize and forms a complete nail plate by 17 weeks. Dermal ridges are completed by 16 weeks and sweating of the digits is possible after 32 weeks. The requirement for early formation of the nail is unclear [3–5]. Nails at birth are thin and concave, particularly the great toenails and the index fingernails. Nails may remain thin for 18 months following birth.

The dermis

The primordial dermis begins as a cellular mesenchyme which is watery and without fibrous structure between cells [3,6,17]. By 6 weeks the first evidence of collagen appears as a fine network without distinct fibers [17]. As epidermal appendages project deeply into the dermis at 16 weeks of age, collagen fibers appear and the dermis organizes into two distinct regions: the papillary dermis with fine collagen fibrils and the reticular dermis with thick collagen bundles. By 20 weeks, fetal dermis is similar to adult dermis but thicker and contains fibronectin and collagen types I, III, and V [3,6,17]. Elastic fibers are recognized in the 22-week dermis, but the adult form of mature elastic fibers does not appear until two years following birth [3,6,17].

The orderly arrangement of cutaneous blood vessels with a superficial and deep dermal plexus is recognizable after 17 weeks [3,14]. Vasomotor control of cutaneous vessels is uncoordinated in preterm babies, with mottling of the skin prominent, and is related to low skin temperature or metabolic acidosis [14,15,18,19]. Within a few hours after birth, the skin of a newborn turns intensely red and remains red for a few hours thereafter. Thermal regulation of heat loss by the skin vessels is poor [18,19]. The harlequin color change is a phenomenon observed in infants of low birth weight. When an infant is placed on its side, a pale upper half of the body is observed, with a sharp line of demarcation of the red lower half of the body. Such episodes have no importance.

The development of cutaneous innervation has not been rigorously studied. Specialized sensory nerve endings such as Merkel corpuscles are present in the fingertips and the palms at birth [3,6,14]. These are thought to be important in two-point discrimination. Innervation of the arrector pili muscles, sweat glands, and the vessels is complete at birth, but functional responses of the corresponding innervating organ are not at adult levels.

The fat

Fat initially forms with discrete areas of fat within the dermis at 16 to 18 weeks, then demarcation of the distinct fat layer, which coincides with the completed development of hair follicles [3,6,14]. The subcutaneous fat pad is thin and poorly developed in preterm infants. The lack of subcutaneous tissue will also contribute to difficulties in thermal regulation.

Thermoregulation and cold injury

The preterm and low-birth-weight infant is susceptible to hypothermia and often requires rigorous control of the environment by heated delivery areas and by incubators [18,19]. Heat loss occurs in the newborn by evaporation of amniotic fluid from the skin surface of the newly delivered baby and by radiation of heat from the dilated superficial dermal blood vessels observed as red skin occurring hours after birth. Lack of subcutaneous tissue contributes with loss of insulation [18,19]. Neonates do not shiver in response to cold stress, but may increase muscular activity in an attempt to generate heat, or assume a flexed or fetal position to minimize heat loss by diminishing the skin surface area [18,19]. The critical temperature for newborns is 32° to 34°C, below which severe neonatal cold injury can occur.

Neonatal cold injury is manifested by redness of the face, hands, and feet, by cold pale skin elsewhere, by edema of the hands and feet, and by general lethargy of the infant. Warming the baby by 0.5° to 1°C per hour and applying energy by intravenous glucose will support the baby's recovery. Fat necrosis is a frequent result of cold injury, with warm, red, indurated plaques appearing within a few hours to a few days after injury [14]. Sclerema neonatorum manifests by diffuse hardening of the skin with

Table 223-1 Symptoms and signs of bacterial sepsis in the newborn

Symptom	Sign
Lethargy	Pustules
Poor feeding	Jaundice
Irritability	Petechiae
Diarrhea	Pallor
	Cyanosis
	Omphalitis
	Conjunctivitis
	Enlarged liver or spleen
	Hypothermia

coldness and pallor [14]. It is associated with debilitated infants and preterm infants with cold exposure. Respiratory distress and infections may ensue, resulting in death (see below and Chap. 99).

Transient skin conditions in the newborn

Pustules

Pustules are yellow, discrete, 1- to 8-mm raised lesions which frequently display a red base. The appearance of pustules in the newborn should bring to mind immediately the possibility of bacterial sepsis [20–23]. Pustules in association with other signs and symptoms of sepsis in the newborn (Table 223-1) or of prolonged rupture of maternal membranes should make one suspect bacterial sepsis. Bacterial culture of the pustules and other body fluids such as blood, urine, and CSF should be performed. There is no rapid, completely reliable method of determining whether or not a baby has bacterial sepsis, and one should always maintain a high index of suspicion.

The incidence of bacterial sepsis is estimated to be 1/1000 term births and 1/200 preterm births, and makes bacterial sepsis an uncommon cause of pustules in the newborn [20], but the high mortality rate of unrecognized bacterial sepsis makes it imperative for the clinician to consider this possibility [20–26].

Other causes of pustules in the newborn may be considered after bacterial sepsis is eliminated as a possibility. They are listed in Table 223-2. Erythema toxicum may occasionally be pustular, particularly if skin involvement is extensive [27–29]. Transient neonatal pustular melanosis mimics erythema toxicum and is predominantly observed in black infants [30]. It is characterized by pustules that evolve to hyperpigmented macules in 3 to 10 days. Herpes simplex skin infection may be pustular but is usually ve-

Table 223-2 Differential diagnosis of pustules in the newborn

Bacterial sepsis
Erythema toxicum
Transient neonatal pustular melanosis
Herpes simplex virus
Acne neonatorum
Candidiasis
Infantile acropustulosis
Nevus comedonicus
Pustular psoriasis

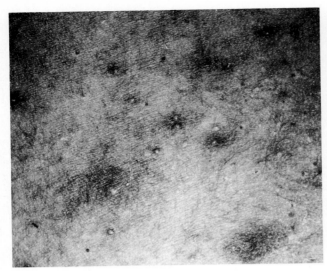

Fig. 223-1 Erythema toxicum.

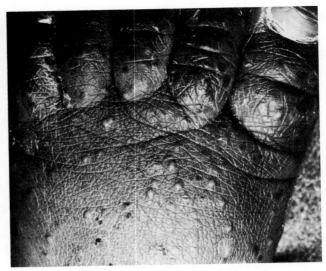

Fig. 223-2 Transient neonatal pustular melanosis.

sicular [31–33]. Acne neonatorum usually is not present in the first 14 days of life, and evolution to the pustular stage requires several more days. Acne is limited to the face, chest, and perineum of newborns [34]. Candidiasis in the diaper area or other intertriginous areas may be pustular, and satellite pustules are frequently observed at a distance from the margins of confluent areas of candidiasis [35]. Candidiasis acquired in utero may also be pustular, with discrete pustules located within a diffusely eczematous skin [36]. Infantile acropustulosis may begin at birth or within the newborn period, and present with discrete pustules limited to the distal extremities with prominent involvement of the palms and soles [37,38]. Nevus comedonicus is a birthmark consisting of patulous follicular openings [39]. Pustule formation or abscesses rarely occur. Psoriasis rarely appears in the newborn period but may be extensive and pustular [40,41].

Erythema toxicum

Erythema toxicum usually first appears at 24 to 48 hours of age with blotchy red macules 2 to 3 cm in diameter that have a tiny central vesicle [27,28] (Fig. 223-1). Erythema toxicum will develop in up to 50 percent of term infants, but is rare in preterm infants [28]. Erythema toxicum skin lesions are often present at birth but rarely begin after the fifth postnatal day. Smear of the central vesicle or pustule contents reveals a predominance of eosinophils. If skin lesions are numerous, a peripheral blood eosinophilia of up to 20 percent may be observed [27]. Skin lesions fade and disappear by 5 to 7 days of age.

Transient neonatal pustular melanosis (Fig. 223-2)

This condition closely mimics erythema toxicum, with a similar natural history, age of onset, and distribution of skin lesions [30]. The presence of neutrophils within the central vesicle rather than eosinophils is used to differentiate this condition from erythema toxicum. Further, since this condition occurs predominantly in black infants, post-inflammatory hyperpigmentation is an expected result in

the areas of evolving skin lesions [30]. The hyperpigmentation may last several months. No treatment is necessary.

Miliaria [42]

Obstruction of sweat ducts is frequently observed in infants in the first 30 days of life. Immaturity of the sweat ducts in premature infants leads to distal obstruction with hundreds of 1- to 3-mm vesicles on an inflammatory base, observed on the neck, cheeks, and trunk. Lesions are developed by heating the cutaneous surface enough to induce sweating. Miliaria with multiple, tiny vesicles without erythema is designated *miliaria crystallina*. Miliaria crystallina is seen primarily in premature infants, and lesions may resolve spontaneously in 24 to 72 h. Full-term and older infants will develop sweat duct obstruction deeper within the midepidermis, with rupture of the duct and an inflammatory response. This produces a clinical picture with red papules or vesicles with a red base which are distributed predominantly on the upper chest and neck, but may be extensive. Drying heat lamps or phototherapy used for hyperbilirubinemia in the nursery may also result in miliaria [15]. Relief of overheating results in spontaneous resolution of the eruption. If continued sweating occurs, repeated daily episodes of miliaria may occur in an overlapping fashion.

Milia

Milia are multiple, 1- to 2-mm, white papules observed on the face and forehead of infants and in the oral cavity where they are designated as *Epstein's pearls* [43]. Up to 40 percent of term infants have milia on the skin and 64 percent have milia on the palate. The superficial cysts rupture and empty their keratinous contents onto the epithelial surface. No treatment is necessary.

Acne neonatorum (see also Chap. 67)

Neonatal acne is rarely present at birth but appears as multiple, discrete papules at 2 to 4 weeks of age [34,44].

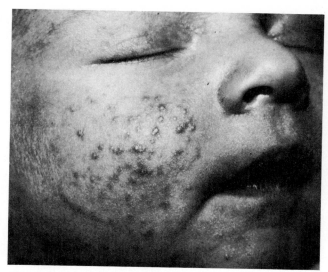

Fig. 223-3 Acne neonatorum.

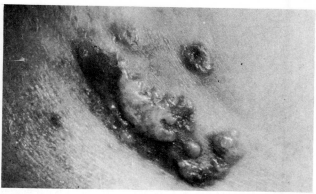

Fig. 223-4 Herpes simplex. Grouped vesicles and vesico-pustules on the extremity of a newborn infant. Herpes simplex virus 2 was cultured.

Involvement of the face, chest, back, and groin are the usual areas for cutaneous lesions (Fig. 223-3). Papules evolve into pustules after a few weeks. The sebaceous glands are hyperplastic and hydroxysteroid dehydrogenase activity is high in the month prior to birth and at birth [8]. There is some evidence that newborns with acne experience transient increases in circulating androgens [44]. Neonatal acne may persist up to 8 months of age [34,44]. There is some suggestion that infants with extensive neonatal acne may experience severe acne as an adolescent. Treatment of neonatal acne is usually not recommended since spontaneous resolution is the expected outcome.

Sebaceous gland hyperplasia

Yellow, 1-mm macules or papules are seen at pilosebaceous openings over the nose and cheeks of newborns [45]. Sebaceous gland hyperplasia is responsible for this observation. These yellow lesions resolve by 4 to 6 weeks of age and no treatment is recommended.

Mottling

Dusky erythema in a lacy pattern appears over the extremities and trunk of newborns when exposed to lowering of skin temperature [46,47]. The erythema is especially prominent in preterm infants. Rewarming of the skin surface will result in resolution of the mottling. It is felt to be the result of poor autonomic nervous system control of cutaneous blood vessels and inappropriate shunting of blood from superficial to deep plexuses in certain skin segments. Persistent mottling may be a sign of congenital hypothyroidism. Mottling is expected to disappear by 6 months of age.

Herpes simplex virus infection (see also Chap. 190)

Grouped vesicles on an erythematous base should bring to mind neonatal herpes simplex virus (HSV) infection [32,33,48–50] (Fig. 223-4). Any area of skin may be involved, but vesicles on the scalp or buttocks are particu-

larly common. Skin sites used for monitoring electrodes may produce sufficient skin trauma to induce HSV skin lesions [32,33,48]. Vesicles may be present at birth but onset after birth is more likely, with the mean age of onset 6 days of age [32,33,48,50]. Some infants with neonatal HSV will not have skin lesions, but 70 percent will. Mucous membrane involvement is common. Eighty percent of neonatal infections are HSV type 2, with 20 percent HSV type 1 [32,33,48,50]. Prior to the availability of antiviral agents, mortality was high (70 percent).

A Tzanck smear of a vesicle base will demonstrate multinucleated giant cells and balloon cells. Fluorescein-tagged anti-HSV-specific antibody may be used to examine vesicle smears or snap-frozen biopsy sections of skin to make a rapid diagnosis. Viral culture of HSV requires 12 to 120 h to grow, and on all infected or suspected neonates, cultures of skin lesions, urine, nasopharynx, eyes, and CSF are indicated [48–50]. The infant's eyes should be evaluated for corneal involvement. Serum antibodies for HSV are of little assistance in making the diagnosis in the acute stages of the disease. Electron microscopy of blister fluid may identify HSV infections, but is available only in a few large medical centers [48–50]; where available, electron microscopy provides HSV detection by the negative staining method in less than half an hour. Rapid diagnosis is essential, and a high index of suspicion must be maintained because 70 percent of mothers are symptomatic and 70 percent of HSV-infected infants who present with skin vesicles as the first sign will later develop CNS disease or disseminated HSV [48–50]. Both adenosine arabinoside and acyclovir have been demonstrated to be efficacious when administered intravenously [33,51].

HSV-infected infants have an increased incidence of premature births, may have signs that mimic bacterial sepsis, and may develop psychomotor retardation even if obvious signs of dissemination of HSV are not evident during the neonatal period [33,50].

Varicella (see also Chap. 191)

Congenital varicella is quite rare but may mimic HSV infections of the newborn [52–54]. Lesions appear as crops of macules and papules which evolve into vesicles and then crust. Age of onset is within the first 10 days, with a mortality of 20 percent reported [52,53]. Scarring of skin lesions, hypotrophic muscles, and eye changes may result [54]. Tzanck smear and skin biopsy demonstrate the same changes as with HSV, and maternal history of varicella/zoster exposure or cutaneous lesions compatible with varicella are most useful in making a diagnosis. Immediate administration of zoster-immune globulin to the infant is recommended if maternal infection was present from five days before delivery to two days after delivery [52,53].

Impetigo (see also Chap. 176)

Bacterial impetigo may be observed in the newborn period. Flaccid, well-demarcated bullae may be seen, which evolve with moist crusts [55,56]. Any area of skin may be involved but the scalp and face are common sites. *Staphylococcus aureus* is the predominant organism, including those strains capable of producing the staphylococcal scalded-skin syndrome. Therefore, prompt recognition and treatment is necessary. Bacterial culture of skin lesions in the nasopharynx will yield the organism within 24 h [57]. Smear of vesicle contents and Gram's stain will demonstrate the bacteria. Group A and Group B streptococci as well as *Escherichia coli* may also occasionally cause impetigo in the newborn period. Appropriate antibiotics should be administered promptly in order to prevent sepsis and diminish spread of the bacteria to other patients and hospital personnel [56].

Staphylococcal scalded-skin syndrome (Ritter's disease) (see also Chap. 55)

Infants 2 to 30 days of age may develop an abrupt onset of generalized erythema, followed in 24 h by bullae, with subsequent exfoliation of large sheets of skin within 48 h. The skin injury is an intraepidermal cleavage through the granular layer due to a circulating exotoxin produced by *Staphylococcus aureus*. Small amounts of staphylococci, less than 10^8 organisms, may be all that is required to produce enough exotoxin to exfoliate a human [57,58]. Culture of the nasopharynx is the most likely to yield the organism, with skin lesions positive in only 30 percent [58]. *S. aureus* of phage group 2 is the organism most responsible. Isolation of the affected newborn is essential to prevent nursery epidemics [57]. Antistaphylococcal antibiotics should be administered systemically and fluid and electrolyte replacement provided much like that for burns.

Breast abscess

Swelling, erythema, and fluctuance in one breast of a newborn infant signifies the possibility of a breast abscess [59]. *Staphylococcus aureus* and gram-negative organisms are the most likely pathogens. Onset is usually 5 to 20 days after birth. Fever may accompany the infection, but most infants are otherwise asymptomatic. Needle aspiration of the infection may be necessary to obtain a positive bacterial culture [59]. Systemic antibiotic therapy is necessary.

Omphalitis

Redness and induration of the umbilical region is due to bacterial infection through the cut surface of the umbilical cord [25]. Prophylactic bacteriostatic agents applied to the cord have reduced the likelihood of this condition in most nurseries. It is predominantly due to *Staphylococcus aureus* and if untreated may progress to bacterial sepsis [25]. Administration of systemic antistaphylococcal antibiotics is the treatment of choice.

Sucking blisters

At birth, a solitary, oval bulla or erosion, 5 to 20 mm in diameter, is noted over the dorsum of the fingers, the thumb, or the radial aspect of the forearm. It is said to occur as frequently as 1 in 240 deliveries [60]. The newly born infant may aggressively suck on the involved area giving a clue to the diagnosis. The characteristic location helps make the diagnosis with forms of epidermolysis bullosa which may present with only a solitary bulla or erosion at birth, and may mimic sucking blisters. No therapy is necessary.

Caput succedaneum and cephalohematoma

Edema of the scalp or hemorrhage of the scalp, which occurs on the occipital areas as a deep swelling with or without purpura, may be noted. This swelling is observed in vertex deliveries, particularly those with prolonged labor, and resolves spontaneously in 7 to 10 days [61,62]. If purpura is extensive in cephalohematoma, it can serve as a source of hyperbilirubinemia. Secondary bacterial infection of cephalohematomas may rarely occur, resulting in cellulitis [61,62]. Sepsis or osteomyelitis of the underlying scalp bones has also been described [61]. *Staphylococcus aureus* and gram-negative bacteria may be responsible.

Petechiae and purpura

Petechiae and purpura may be a presenting feature of congenital infection, particularly when the newborn is small for gestational age and has hepatosplenomegaly. An acronym used for these congenital infections is the *torch syndrome* (Table 223-3) [63]. Petechiae and purpura are the most common cutaneous symptoms for this group of congenital infections and may be an important clue for diagnosis. Newborns with congenital infection may also demonstrate microcephaly, microphthalmia, congenital heart defects, cataracts, and psychomotor retardation [64–67].

Serologic tests for toxoplasmosis, syphilis, rubella, cytomegalovirus, and herpes simplex should be performed on infants, and viral cultures performed when necessary.

Table 223-3 Features of the "TORCH" syndrome

Petechiae and purpura
Jaundice
Chorioretinitis
Anemia and thrombocytopenia
Hepatosplenomegaly
Small for gestational age

T = Toxoplasmosis
O = Other (congenital syphilis and viruses)
R = Rubella
C = Cytomegalovirus
H = Herpes simplex virus

Effective therapy is available for congenital syphilis (penicillin), herpes simplex (adenosine arabinoside, acyclovir), and possibly toxoplasmosis (sulfadiazine and pyrimethamine) [33,51,64–67]. The success of therapy is highest if few signs and symptoms of congenital infection are present at birth.

Other causes of petechiae and purpura in the newborn include trauma, with facial and scalp petechiae common in difficult vertex deliveries. Neonatal thrombocytopenia due to maternal autoantibodies, as in idiopathic thrombocytopenic purpura or systemic lupus erythematosus, may also produce neonatal petechiae a few hours after birth. Hypoprothrombinemia may result in purpura in the newborn older than 2 or 3 days, due to vitamin K deficiency. Prophylactic administration of vitamin K at birth will prevent this eventuality. Neonatal petechiae and purpura are unusual in the hemophilia states, but bleeding from circumcision sites may be the first manifestation of hemophilia in the newborn period. Neonatal purpura secondary to platelet dysfunction may be observed in the Wiskott-Aldrich syndrome although eczematous lesions do not appear until after the newborn period.

Subcutaneous fat necrosis (see also Chap. 99)

Sharply circumscribed, firm nodules with an overlying dusky bluish hue are found over the buttocks, cheeks, or proximal extremities of infants 1 to 7 days of age [14,68]. These areas of fat necrosis are usually solitary and develop slowly. Increased susceptibility of the newborn fat to cold injury is felt to be the cause. The warm, red, indurated plaques appear within a few hours to a few days after injury [14]. After first appearance, the plaques may assume a violaceous color and remain firm and immobile. Lesions evolve over several weeks, healing with a depression in the skin surface, calcifying to form a firm nodule with occasional drainage onto the skin surface, or healing without change in the overlying skin.

Sclerema neonatorum (see also Chap. 99)

A diffuse hardening and immobilization of skin with coldness and pallor occurs in sick infants due to cold injury. Often the entire trunk is involved [14,69]. Undernourished infants, preterm infants, and infants with hypoglycemia or metabolic acidosis are particularly susceptible. Respiratory distress and infections may ensue, resulting in death. The appearance of sclerema formerly was considered a poor prognostic sign, but with improved neonatal care some infants have recovered [14,69].

Birthmarks

Congenital malformations are most often observed in skin [70,71]. The two most frequently recognized are flat hemangiomas of faint red color (salmon patch) and Mongolian spots [70,71]. Salmon patches are observed with high frequency in both white infants (703/1000 births) [70] and black infants (592/1000 births) [70]. Mongolian spots are more frequently observed in Orientals (910/1000 births) [72] and black infants (880/1000 births) [70], but are less common in white infants (48/1000 births) [70]. Mongolian spots

and the salmon patch are observed at least 100 times more than any other skin birthmarks [70,71].

Vascular birthmarks (see also Chap. 95)

Flat hemangiomas. Flat hemangiomas are divided into those that are light red or pink in color, the frequently observed salmon patch, and those that are red or red-purple in color, the port-wine stain [70,71,73–76]. The *salmon patch* appears as a light red macule at the nape of the neck, the upper eyelids, and the glabella. A salmon patch is present over the back of the neck in up to 50 percent of all infants [70,71]. All salmon patches tend to fade with time as normal skin pigment increases, but remnants will persist well into adult life. Generally, the eyelid lesions may fade by 3 to 6 months of age, and the glabella lesions by 5 to 6 years of age. Lesions of the nape of the neck never fade completely.

Port-wine stains appear as deep red or red-purple macules over the face or extremities [73–75]. They are almost always unilateral. Occasionally they are extensive and cover large areas of skin and are bilateral. Port-wine stains over the face or an extremity may be associated with soft tissue and bony hypertrophy [73–75].

A port-wine stain over the face may be a clue to the Sturge-Weber syndrome, particularly if the skin served by the ophthalmic branch of the trigeminal nerve is involved with the flat hemangioma. The Sturge-Weber syndrome is characterized by seizures, mental retardation, glaucoma, and hemiplegia [73–75]. The glaucoma may appear at birth, and may be unrecognized [73]. Calcification of the hemangioma of the brain in the Sturge-Weber syndrome may be detected by skull x-rays. Most babies with port-wine stain over one portion of the face, however, do not have the Sturge-Weber syndrome and do not have involvement of the skin served by the ophthalmic branch of the trigeminal nerve.

When port-wine stains are found over an extremity and are associated with soft tissue bony hypertrophy of the affected extremity, the condition is called the Klippel-Trénaunay-Weber syndrome [76]. Elongation of an extremity can cause orthopedic deformity. Arteriovenous fistulas are present in 25 percent of such patients. Absence of the deep venous channels in the affected limb may be observed in most affected infants [76].

Treatment of salmon patches is unnecessary. Treatment of port-wine stains is quite difficult. Although laser therapy has been successful in some instances, its long-term results are still uncertain. Covering the flat hemangioma with makeup may be satisfactory in certain infants. X-irradiation, tattooing, and skin grafting have poor cosmetic results, often worse than the port-wine stain.

Raised hemangiomas. Raised hemangiomas are usually not observed at birth, but a circumscribed area of blanched skin with a few telangiectases may be present, representing a precursor lesion of a developing hemangioma [77]. By 2 to 4 weeks of age, this precursor lesion begins to become raised with the appearance of red nodules on the surface and at deeper palpable portions. The lesion grows out of proportion to the baby for the first 8 months of life, stretching and distorting the skin above it (Fig. 223-5a). Raised hemangiomas begin to show signs of involution at age 15

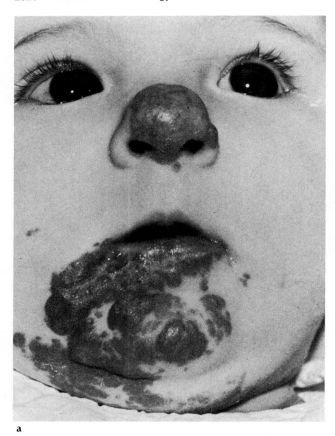

a

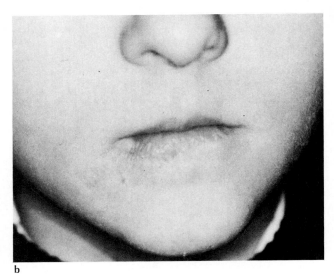

b

Fig. 223-5 (a) Raised hemangioma on the face of a girl 3 weeks of age. (b) The same girl at age 6 years showing spontaneous regression of hemangioma with minimal scarring. *(Courtesy of K. Wolff, M.D.)*

months, when pale areas appear within the red nodule. At 16 months of age the first sign of flattening appears. The raised lesion regresses to skin level by 5 years of age in 50 percent of the patients, and by puberty in most all patients (Fig. 223-5b). Most often, only redundant, loose skin that was stretched during the rapid growth phase remains [78]. In large, raised hemangiomas, ulceration of the epithelial surface often occurs and secondary bacterial suprainfection may result (Fig. 223-6).

There are several major complications of raised hemangiomas including (1) platelet trapping, (2) airway obstruction, (3) visual obstruction, and (4) cardiac decompensation [79–81]. Platelet trapping in the so-called Kasabach-Merritt syndrome occurs within the sluggish circulation of the raised hemangioma. It is observed primarily in the patient with a single hemangioma and develops within the first 6 months of life [79] (Fig. 223-6). Platelet trapping produces easy bruising and petechiae in the areas of the body not involved with hemangioma and may progress to frank hemorrhage due to consumption coagulopathy. Platelet trapping within the hemangioma itself may result in a firm, hard, deep-purple nodule. [79].

Obstruction of the airway results in respiratory stridor and usually is due to subglottic hemangiomas. Infants with hemangiomas of the airway usually have multiple hemangiomas involving the skin of the head and neck [80,81].

Visual obstruction by the eyelid enlarged by a hemangioma may result in decreased vision in that eye because of lack of use of the eye for vision by the infant [80,81]. Rarely, large raised hemangiomas may pool sufficient blood to produce high output cardiac failure.

The indications for treatment of hemangiomas are obstruction of a vital orifice such as the airway or excretory channel, visual obstruction, platelet trapping syndrome, and cardiac decompensation [80,81]. The treatment of choice is prednisone at doses from 1 to 4 mg/kg per day. Alternate-day therapy may be sufficient in certain instances. Treatment for at least 4 to 8 weeks is often necessary [80,81]. Treatment initiated during the growing phase of the hemangioma, from 1 month of age to 8 months of age, produces the best results [80,81].

Diffuse neonatal hemangiomatosis is a rare syndrome consisting of multiple, small, raised cutaneous hemangiomas plus hemangiomas observed in the liver, lungs, gastrointestinal tract, and the central nervous system. These raised hemangiomas may be present at birth and more may develop with time [82]. Such infants may succumb to serious hemorrhage, but spontaneous involution of the lesions has been reported. At the present time, there is no method by which one can predict the outcome of such infants.

The *blue rubber bleb nevus syndrome* is a rare disorder consisting of multiple cavernous hemangiomas of the skin and bowel. The lesions are blue in color and measure from 3 to 4 cm in diameter. They may be painful and associated with excessive sweating.

Depressed hemangiomas (congenital phlebectasia). In congenital phlebectasia a mottled pattern of blue or dusky red erythema is seen from birth [83]. Often, a single extremity is involved, but the lesions may occur bilaterally on the extremities, or involvement of the trunk may be observed [83]. Skin overlying the dusky areas may be depressed. A gradual increase in size of the lesions is expected over the first few years of life, with progressive involvement of more skin surface. Most of the lesions fade by adult life. Rigorous natural history studies of congenital phlebectasia are not available.

Lymphatic birthmarks

Lymphangiomas may be circumscribed skin papules or deep cavernous nodules [84,85]. Circumscribed lymphangiomas appear as a solitary group 2- to 4-mm, gelatinous, skin-colored papules limited to a skin area less than 10 cm. They are often connected to underlying venous channels, and hemorrhage in one or more of the gelatinous papules may occur producing sudden darkening. The lesions are usually present at birth but may be overlooked until later in infancy or childhood [84,85]. Cavernous lymphangiomas are rubbery, skin-colored nodules that may result in grotesque enlargement of soft tissues. They are solitary and may involve the face, trunk, and extremities. They are particularly common over the parotid area where they are called cystic hygromas. They may have a rapid growth similar to that of a raised hemangioma [84,85]. There is no satisfactory treatment for lymphangiomas at present, and the precise incidence of these lesions is not known, but they are considered to be quite rare.

Pigment cell birthmarks (see also Chaps. 79 and 80)

Hyperpigmented lesions observed at birth. Infants' skin color is always light at birth and it becomes darker later in life [13,14]. Hyperpigmentation of the scrotum and the linea alba is common in dark-skinned infants. The most commonly observed pigmentary abnormality in infancy is the Mongolian spot.

Localized hyperpigmentation. LOCALIZED FLAT HYPERPIGMENTATION. The *Mongolian spot* is a blue-black macule found over the lumbosacral area and up to 90 percent of Oriental, black, and American Indian babies are affected [70,71,77,85]. They are occasionally noted over the shoulders and back and may extend over the buttocks and extremities. Pathology of Mongolian spots consists of spindle-shaped pigment cells located deep within the dermis. Mongolian spots fade somewhat with time and the difference in the pigmentation from the normal skin pigment becomes less obvious as the newborn's pigment increases in color. Some traces of Mongolian spots may persist into adult life.

Café au lait spots are light brown, oval macules which may appear more dark brown on black skin; they may be found anywhere on the body. Café au lait macules at birth are far less prevalent (19/1000 live births) than Mongolian spots (255/1000 live births) [70,86].

The chance for two or more café au lait macules to be present at birth occurs only in 2 to 6/1000 live births. Black infants are far more likely (120/1000 live births) than white infants (3/1000 live births) to have a café au lait macule at birth. These lesions persist through childhood and may increase in number with age. The presence of six or more café au lait macules, greater than 1.5 cm in their greatest diameter, is considered by most authorities a major clue to multiple neurofibromatosis [86]. Although it has recently been suggested that the melanocytes of café au lait macules and neurofibromatosis contain giant pigment granules, this is not often the case in newborns or infants, and the absence of giant pigment granules does not rule out the possibility of multiple neurofibromatosis.

Junctional nevocellular nevi present at birth are quite

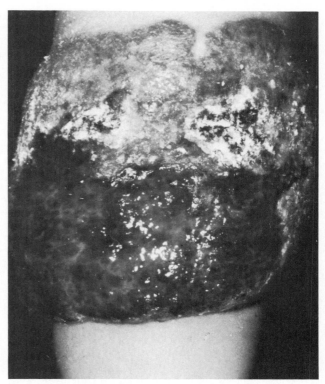

Fig. 223-6 Giant, partially ulcerated hemangioma in a 1-month-old infant. This child later developed the Kasabach-Merritt syndrome. (Courtesy of K. Wolff, M.D.)

uncommon, occurring in approximately 11/1000 live births [70,71,86]. They appear as dark brown or black macules and represent clones of melanocytes at the junction of the epidermis and dermis. With aging they may become raised and papular and contain intradermal melanocytes as well, creating a compound nevus. Often the surface of the lesion at birth is irregular and roughened.

LOCALIZED RAISED PIGMENT CELL LESIONS (RAISED NEVOCELLULAR NEVI). Skin-colored to tan, to brown, solitary papules with smooth surfaces represent intradermal nevi [70,71,86]. Most such nevi are small, measuring less than 1 to 1.5 cm in their greatest diameter, and their occurrence is of cosmetic interest only. There is a controversy over the cancer potential regarding large congenital melanocytic nevi [86–90]. Various authorities define large melanocytic nevi (Fig. 223-7) by different criteria. Kopf et al use greater than 20 cm in its greatest diameter as a definition for large congenital melanocytic nevi [88], while others consider those greater than 10 cm [86], in identifying those with cancer potential. The estimate of cancer potential ranges from 6 percent [87] to 12 percent [88]. The incidence is at least 20 times greater than in infants without these lesions. There is a slightly increased frequency of large congenital pigmented lesions in blacks and in those infants born to mothers with acute illnesses [90]. There is no correlation of large pigmented nevi with sex, twinning, parental consanguinity, parental age, birth order, radiation exposure, or drug intake [90]. If malignant melanoma occurs, it is likely to occur within the first 6 years of age, and it has been uniformly fatal [86–88,91].

Most authorities recommend removal of large nevocel-

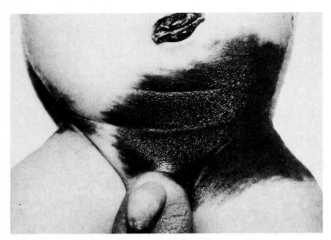

Fig. 223-7 Large congenital melanocytic nevus.

lular pigmented nevi within the first year of life as prophylaxis against melanoma [86–91]. Since congenital pigmented nevi often involve the subcutaneous fat and the periappendage projections into the subcutaneous fat area, removal of the subcutaneous tissue should be included in any procedure [88]. A controversy exists as to whether those less than 20 cm in their greatest diameter or small lesions should be removed [86–89]. Most authorities would recommend that these be removed if you take into account the potential for cosmetic improvement. Whether such smaller lesions have any malignant potential is uncertain [88,89].

Hypopigmentation. CIRCUMSCRIBED HYPOPIGMENTATION. Localized areas of hypopigmented skin are uncommon in infants [70]. A hypopigmented area of the skin is found in approximately 8/1000 live births [70], and a hypopigmented tuft of hair is found in 3/1000 live births [70].

Piebaldism. Piebaldism is a disorder where there is an absence of melanocytes within segments of skin [92,93]. Most commonly the disorder is transmitted in an autosomal dominant pattern [92,93]. The white patches of skin are completely devoid of pigment cells, but may be difficult to detect at birth because of the light skin color at birth. The use of a Wood's lamp to examine the infant may accentuate the difference in color [92,93]. In several kinships, the piebald trait has been linked to cerebellar ataxia, neurosensory hearing loss, or retardation [92,93]. A hypopigmented tuft of hair, usually in the frontal region, is a feature of the *Waardenburg syndrome* [93]. This autosomal dominant syndrome exhibits white forelock, white patches on the skin, heterochromia of the irides, and deafness. The deafness may affect one or both ears. Most authorities view Waardenburg's syndrome as a variant of the piebald syndrome.

White spots of *tuberous sclerosis* appear as hypopigmented macules in the shape of a leaf [94]. The macules may be rounded on one end and pointed on the other, and range from 5 to 50 mm in diameter. In the newborn period, they may be the only sign of tuberous sclerosis, and in families in which this condition occurs, involvement of a newborn infant may be suspected first by the presence of these lesions [94]. A Wood's lamp examination is neces-

sary to detect these lesions, and not all macules are leaf-shaped. They may be found anywhere on the skin, but are most predominant on the posterior trunk and the extremities [95].

Hypomelanosis of Ito. Newborns with hypomelanosis of Ito have bizarre hypopigmented swirls that follow Blaschko's lines [94–97]. The hypopigmentation may be zosteriform in distribution or may be quite extensive and unilateral or bilateral. In all these patients, hypopigmentation is secondary to a decreased number of melanosomes within the pigment cells and within keratinocytes [94]. The inheritance of hypomelanosis of Ito is not known.

DIFFUSE HYPOPIGMENTATION. *Chédiak-Higashi syndrome.* Newborns with this syndrome have white skin like albinos, blond hair, and blue eyes [94]. Melanosomes in the skin and hair of persons with Chédiak-Higashi syndrome are dispersed in an irregular fashion and have large abnormal melanosomes. Such patients also have abnormal lysosomes within their circulating white cells and have an inability to kill bacteria, although clinical infection does not usually occur in the newborn period [94].

Albinism. At least four varieties of albinism have been described in humans, all of them inherited in an autosomal recessive pattern [94,98,99]. Newborns with this disorder have fine white hair, pink skin, severe nystagmus, photophobia, and nevi which are not pigmented. The disease is due to complete lack of functional tyrosinase, the enzyme necessary in the production of melanin.

One subtype of albinism has tyrosinase enzyme present. These infants are born with fair complexions and gray eyes, and have poor visual acuity and nystagmus. Although tyrosinase is present, melanin formation is slow. With increasing age, they may tan [94]. The third type of albino, the yellow mutant [94,99], has yellowish hair at birth that becomes more reddish as the child becomes older. They have similar visual problems as other albinos.

The fourth form of albinism, the *Hermansky-Pudlak syndrome,* is albinism associated with a platelet dysfunction which results in a clinical bleeding disorder [94,99]. The tyrosinase enzyme is also present in Hermansky-Pudlak syndrome.

Phenylketonuria. Patients with phenylketonuria lack the enzymes needed to utilize phenylalanine, an amino acid which binds tightly to the receptor sites of tyrosinase such that the enzyme cannot oxidize it to melanin. Newborns with phenylketonuria have blond hair, blue eyes, and fair skin. Because of the severe mental retardation, prompt recognition of this syndrome is necessary, and initiation of a phenylalanine-free diet required [94]. Blood tests for the presence of phenylalanine are routinely performed in many institutions as a screening procedure for phenylketonuria.

Epidermal cell birthmarks

Birthmarks of epidermal cells are quite uncommon when contrasted with pigment cells and vascular structures. They occur in up to 3/1000 live births [70,86,89].

Epidermal nevus. Epidermal nevi have a warty surface and often are linear or curvilinear in appearance and are noted on the head or neck [70,86,89,100]. Most are present at birth but may become more prominent and evident later on during the neonatal period. At birth, the lesions are barely palpable and may not be warty or irregular on the surface.

Most lesions are 2 to 5 cm in length, but occasionally they appear as long unilateral streaks involving an entire extremity or one side of the trunk, where they may be designated nevus unius lateris [100]. The lesions may be so extensive as to involve most of the body. The term *ichthyosis hystrix* has been applied to such extensive nevi. Epidermal nevi may become erythematous and itchy with episodes of redness and inflammation and may be designated *inflammatory linear verrucous epidermal nevus* (IL-VEN) [100,101]. In up to 60 percent of infants with epidermal nevi, associated skeletal defects, seizure disorders, and mental retardation, flat hemangiomas have been found. Patients with the most extensive skin involvement are those most likely to have an associated skeletal or central nervous system deformity [100].

Epidermal nevi show thickening of the epidermis and hyperkeratosis. In some cases, a peculiar vacuolization of the granular layer appears with separation of the cells of that layer, resulting in a microscopic blister cavity. Overgrowth of sebaceous glands and aprocrine glands may be found underlying the epidermal proliferations [100]. Surgical excision for small lesions is the best treatment. Extensive lesions may be treated with keratolytics with varying degrees of success [100,101].

Nevus sebaceous. The sebaceous nevus of Jadassohn appears at birth as a slightly raised, oval or linear area with yellow or orange color [102,103]. These nevi are common on the scalp and are characteristically devoid of hair, producing a congenital circumscribed hair loss, and may be seen on the face. They have a curvilinear or oval configuration, similar to that of epidermal nevi. Sebaceous nevi may be contiguous to an epidermal nevus and may be considered part of the epidermal nevus syndrome [100–102]. Sebaceous nevi occur in up to 3/1000 live births and are the most common of all epidermal nevi.

Development of basal cell carcinoma, squamous cell carcinoma, or sebaceous carcinoma within the nevus sebaceous has been reported following puberty. The chance for such development is estimated at 15 to 20 percent [102,103]. Surgical excision just before puberty is recommended because of the risk of skin cancer following puberty.

Nevus comedonicus. In nevus comedonicus, linear or oval groups of widely dilated, follicular openings plugged with keratin are present at birth on the face and scalp [39]. The precise incidence is not known but they are observed far less commonly than nevus sebaceous or epidermal nevi [70,86,89]. Individual lesions may become inflamed and pustular and may mimic acne. Bilateral and widespread involvement of skin may occur rarely. In small lesions simple surgical excision is the treatment of choice. Larger, extensive lesions may be controlled with the application of keratolytics [39].

Connective tissue nevi

The term *connective tissue nevi* refers to skin lesions consisting predominantly of the elements of extracellular collagen tissue and products of fibroblasts, i.e., collagen, elastin, and proteoglycans. All connective tissue nevi are quite rare although the precise incidence is not known.

Collagenoma. Collagenoma may be isolated or appear in a zosteriform pattern [104]. They appear as localized areas of thickened skin with multiple skin-colored papules and plaques. Stretching and overlying skin will give a yellowish discoloration to the area. Biopsy shows thickened, abundant collagen bundles with or without associated increases in elastic tissue. Biopsy must include normal adjacent skin for comparison in order to detect the involvement of lesional skin [104].

Shagreen patch. A shagreen patch is a connective tissue nevus with increased collagen; it may be red or skin-colored, depending on the number of increased blood vessels within the lesion [104]. Shagreen patches are irregularly thickened tumors or plaques and can appear anywhere on the skin. A shagreen patch may be present at birth but it is more likely for it to become detectable after birth. It is observed in tuberous sclerosis.

Elastoma. Increases in elastic and in proteoglycans have been found in isolated elastomas which are present at birth [104]. Elastomas may be solitary or they may be multiple in the *Buschke-Ollendorff syndrome*. This autosomal dominant syndrome appears as symmetrically distributed skin-colored papules or nodules with a predilection for the lower trunk or extremities [104]. Lesions may assume a peau d'orange appearance and develop a lacy pattern over the trunk. Lesions may be present at birth or they may appear later in life. X-rays of the ends of the long bones, the pelvis, and the hands reveal sclerotic densities which are asymptomatic, although they may occasionally be mistaken for metastatic bone lesions [104].

Common congenital malformations that involve skin

Congenital malformations involving skin are frequently observed in newborns [70,105–107]. Even if one discounts Mongolian spots or the salmon patch, congenital malformations occur in up to 7 percent of live births [105,106]. The common congenital malformations are listed in Table 223-4.

Ear anomalies

Minor abnormalities in the formation of the ear constitute the most common malformations other than Mongolian spots or salmon patches [105,106]. Loss of the fold of the skin in the superior part of the helix is the most common, whereas low-set ears that angle away from the eye, periauricular skin tags, auricular or preauricular pits, or sinuses and small ears are less common [105–107]. The latter four ear anomalies may be a clue to deafness.

Digital anomalies

A simian crease (a single crease on one or both upper palms) occurs in 2 percent of all live births (Table 223-4). It is one feature of Down's syndrome but may also be observed in a variety of other syndromes, including trisomy-13, Cornelia de Lange syndrome, Seckel's syn-

Table 223-4 Common congenital malformations

	Prevalence, cases/1000 births
1. Mongolian spots in blacks and Orientals	916
2. Capillary hemangiomas	702
3. Lack of usual fold of helix	35.2
4. Simian crease	20.4
5. Clinodactyly	9.9
6. Hydrocele	8.8
7. Hypospadias	6.0
8. Pigmented nevi	4.9
9. Epicanthal folds	4.2
10. Meningocele, encephalocele, anecephaly	4.0
	2.5
11. Ears slant away from eye	2.3
12. Preauricular skin tags	1.6
13. Partial syndactyly 2nd to 3rd toes	1.4
14. Small ears	1.2
15. Auricular sinus	1.0
16. Club foot	0.8
17. Cleft lip and palate	0.5
18. Cleft palate	0.03
19. Aplasia cutis congenita	

drome, and the cri-du-chat syndrome [107]. Clinodactyly with curvature of a digit is often observed in the 5th finger, or overlapping of the 2nd toe with the 3rd toe [107]. Partial or complete fusion (syndactyly of the 2nd or 3rd toes) and club foot also occur with relative frequency [105,106].

Genital anomalies

Hydrocele of one testis or hypospadias are the most common genital anomalies observed [105–107]. They may be clues to other urinary tract anomalies and investigations of the urinary tract may be indicated. They also may be associated with undescended testes and may be clues to chromosome abnormality [107].

Epicanthal folds

Epicanthal folds on the inner aspect of the eye are frequently observed [105–107]. This malformation is present in chromosomal abnormalities such as the Down's syndrome, Turner's syndrome, and Klinefelter's syndrome [107].

Neural tube defects

Primary defects in neural tube closures such as meningomyelocele, encephalocele, and anencephaly are relatively frequent [105–107]. In some instances, a tuft of hair that is longer and more pigmented than the adjacent hair overlies the affected area and may be a diagnostic clue to an underlying defect in the newborn [105–107].

Abnormalities of the lip and mouth

Pits in the lips have been described in up to 2 percent of normal newborns [43] and cleft lip and palate or cleft lip alone are slightly less common [105–107]. The finding of lip pits or cleft lip or cleft palate may be a part of the first-arch syndrome which includes a small jaw and ocular hypertelorism. This encompasses the Pierre Robin syndrome, the oral-facial-digital syndrome, and the Treacher Collins syndrome [107].

Scalp defects

Aplasia cutis congenita occurs in 1/3000 births as an oval, sharply marginated, depressed area on the scalp [105–108]. Lesions are hairless and may appear as an ulcer with a red base, or as a depression covered by a finely wrinkled epithelial membrane [108]. It is usually located on the posterior scalp, but may be noted on the trunk (Fig. 223-8) or on the extremities and may be quite extensive in these locations. On the scalp it is thought that vascular thrombi might be responsible for this defect [108]. Saggital sinus hemorrhage has been noted later in infancy [109]. It is seen as an autosomal dominant trait or may be associated with dystrophic forms of epidermolysis bullosa [108]. Simple excision or hair transplant into the scalp area may be performed to correct the cosmetic defect [110].

Major chromosomal abnormalities (see also Chap. 138)

Chromosomal abnormalities occur in 1/2000 live births, in 5 to 10 percent of perinatal deaths, and in up to 50 percent of spontaneous abortions [105]. Discussed briefly are the major recognizable chromosomal abnormalities with cutaneous features.

Trisomy 21 (Down's syndrome). Trisomy 21 is seen in 1/800 live births [105–107]. There is an increased number in infants born to mothers over 40 years of age [111]. Cutaneous features are the most useful in the recognition of this syndrome: prominent epicanthal folds, eyes slanting upward, small ears, simian palmar creases, excessive skin over the back of the neck, and clinodactyly of the 5th finger [107]. These features plus hypotonia and evidence of congenital heart disease are the main characteristics. Chromosomal analysis will confirm the diagnosis [107]. Mental retardation may be severe and growth failure associated with congenital heart disease make the prognosis poor.

Trisomy 18, trisomy 13-15. Trisomy 18 is observed in 1/3000 births, and trisomy 13-15 in 1/5000 births [105–107]. In both instances, increased parental age has been associated [107]. Such babies are small for gestational age, have low-set ears, simian creases, congenital heart disease, and severe mental retardation [107]. The presence of cleft lip and palate makes trisomy 13-15 more likely, while rocker-bottom feet and a flexion contracture of the fingers makes trisomy 18 more likely to be diagnosed. Chromosomal analysis, however, is required to make a precise diagnosis [107].

Turner's syndrome. The most common sex chromosome anomaly is Turner's syndrome in which only one X chromosome is present (XO) [107]. The newborns exhibit webbing of the neck and marked edema of the hands and feet. The neck is quite short [107]. Coarctation of the aorta may

Fig. 223-8 Congenital absence of skin in a newborn. The abdomen is covered by a shiny, translucent membrane. (Courtesy of K. Wolff, M.D.)

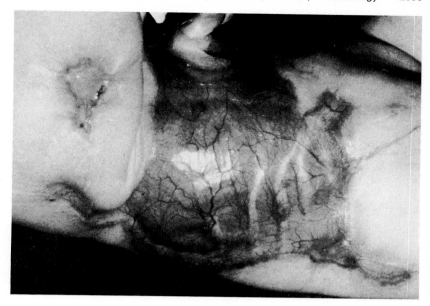

be present. Chromosomal analysis will confirm the diagnosis.

Klinefelter's syndrome. Extra sex chromosomes are characteristic of Klinefelter's syndrome (XXY, XXXY, XXXXY). Low birth weight, undescended testes, and a small penis lead to suspicion of this syndrome [107]. Hypotonia and a variety of other anomalies may also be observed. Chromosomal analysis is diagnostic. Mental deficiency is usually severe in this syndrome [107].

Chronic skin conditions as manifest in the newborn period

This section will be restricted to those chronic skin conditions as they appear and develop within the first 30 days of life. The reader should consult the appropriate section of this text for detailed descriptions of these conditions at other ages (see also "Cross-Reference Index" at the beginning of this chapter).

The red scaly newborn

Physiologic scaling and redness. The scaly and often red newborn may be an enigma to the inexperienced observer. For example, a postmature baby may exhibit desquamation that is marked over the hands, feet, and lower trunk, and if observed during the first day of life when newborn skin is quite red, an erroneous diagnosis of ichthyosis may be made [13–15,19]. Similarly, preterm infants born at 32 weeks of gestational age or earlier will have a red, glistening skin which may be confused with ichthyosis [13–15,19]. Such changes are transient and resolve within the newborn period.

Collodion baby. Newborns with an encasement of shiny, tight, inelastic scale are designated as having a collodion membrane. The membrane is composed of greatly thickened stratum corneum which has been saturated with water. As the water content evaporates in extrauterine life, large fissures appear in the membrane, and the membrane

is shed, revealing red skin underneath (Fig. 223-9). The presence of a collodion membrane does not allow one to predict that the affected baby will develop ichthyosis since spontaneous healing may occur without subsequent development of an ichthyotic state [112,113]. Skin biopsy of the collodion membrane is usually not diagnostic. Most collodion babies do have a form of ichthyosis, with most developing features of lamellar ichthyosis, although bullous ichthyosis (congenital bullous ichthyosiform erythroderma) and X-linked ichthyosis have presented as collodion babies [112–118].

Harlequin fetus. Although harlequin fetus has been considered a more severe form of lamellar ichthyosis, it is now thought to represent a distinct, rare, autosomal recessive disease [112,113,115,118]. Harlequin fetus is incompatible with extrauterine life, and presents as a dead fetus with massive dense platelike scales which produce severe deformities of the skeletal tissues and soft tissues restricting respiration. This phenotype may be produced by defects in both lipid and protein metabolism [115].

Lamellar ichthyosis (congenital nonbullous ichthyosiform erythroderma). This is an autosomal recessive disorder in which most infants are born as collodion babies [112–114]. After shedding of the collodion membrane, the skin becomes red and large platelike white scales appear over the first week of life. Ectropion and eclabion are prominent in the newborn period and the skin remains red throughout the entire newborn period [113,116,118]. Skin biopsy after the collodion membrane is shed will demonstrate hyperkeratosis, but is otherwise not diagnostic.

Bullous ichthyosis (congenital bullous ichthyosiform erythroderma, epidermolytic hyperkeratosis). This rare autosomal dominant condition presents with scattered blisters and scaling in the newborn [116,118] (Fig. 223-10). Rarely they may present with a collodion membrane. Recurrent crops of blisters develop during the first 30 days of life, and *Staphylococcus aureus* infection of the blister cavities is usually observed. Treatment with antistaphylococcal

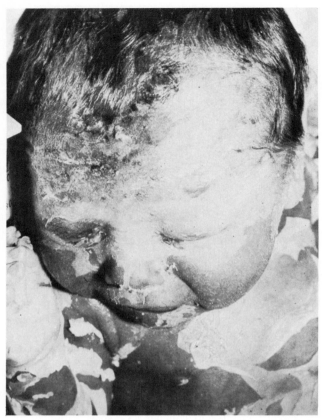

Fig. 223-9 Collodion baby. Lamellar ichthyosis eventuated.

systemic antibodies is mandatory. The skin remains red throughout the newborn period with scales increasing in thickness, encasing the scalp hair, and assuming a greasy brown appearance. Skin biopsy will reveal enlargement of the granular cell layer with bizarre vacuolization of the epidermal granular cells.

X-linked ichthyosis. X-linked ichthyosis is an uncommon recessive disorder in which the newborn may be relatively unaffected [112,116–118]. Scaling is usually mild during the

first 30 days of life, and the skin is of a normal color. The hyperpigmented scale characteristic of this disorder does not appear until later in childhood. This condition has been linked to steroid sulfatase deficiency [117]. Mothers of affected babies have low urinary estrogen levels, and often fail to spontaneously initiate labor [117]. Examination of the mother may reveal comma-shaped corneal opacities, but the newborn will not have these lesions. Measurement of steroid sulfatase levels in red cells, white cells, or in skin, confirms the diagnosis. Skin biopsy is usually not very helpful [112,113,118].

Ichthyosis vulgaris. This autosomal dominant disorder is the most common of all ichthyoses, occurring in 1/200 live births, but does not present any diagnostic features in the immediate newborn period [112,113,118]. Skin in ichthyosis vulgaris remains normal throughout the newborn period [118].

Dermatitis

Atopic dermatitis, seborrheic dermatitis. Atopic dermatitis is said to have its onset after the newborn period, with the most frequently observed age of onset at 2 to 3 months [119–125]. If a dermatitis begins within the newborn period, it is often designated seborrheic dermatitis [119]. It is clear that infants who later develop typical atopic dermatitis have the onset of their skin eruption within the newborn period. Yates and coworkers, in a prospective study with two-year follow-up, recognized that there was significant overlap between seborrheic and atopic dermatitis, both in distribution of the lesions with involvement of the scalp, diaper area, and flexural areas in both diseases, and in the history of pruritus, feeding patterns, food intolerance, and family members with atopic disease [119]. In 60 percent of the cases they could not make a diagnosis with certainty. Physiologic overproduction of sebum occurs in the newborn period, giving any dermatitis a greasy feel to the skin surface, which adds to the confusion in making a precise diagnosis. Dermatitis within the first month of life is so confusing it may be best diagnosed as simply dermatitis. Seventy percent of the cases eventuate into seborrheic dermatitis and approximately 25 percent are atopic der-

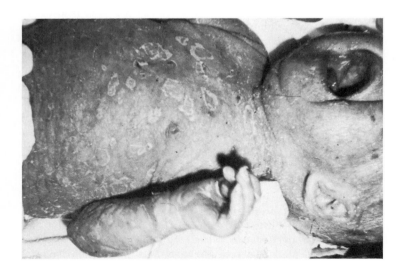

Fig. 223-10 Bullous ichthyosis (bullous congenital ichthyosiform erythroderma). Newborn with scaling and multiple bullae over the trunk, face, and arms.

Table 223-5   Differential diagnosis of eczematous disorders in the newborn

Diaper dermatitis
Atopic dermatitis
Seborrheic dermatitis
Contact dermatitis
Acrodermatitis enteropathica
Leiner's disease
Severe combined immunodeficiency
Histiocytosis X
Scabies
Candidiasis
Multiple carboxylase deficiency

matitis. Treatment with a low-potency glucocorticosteroid topical preparation for 7 to 14 days may be sufficient to control the eruption. Involvement of the diaper area in both seborrheic and atopic dermatitis is frequent although other skin areas are almost always involved [119–125]. It has frequently been observed that babies with either atopic or seborrheic dermatitis may begin with a dermatitis in the diaper area and if secondary candidiasis occurs the dermatitis will flare in other areas of skin. Occasionally, both atopic dermatitis and seborrheic dermatitis will progress to involvement of most of the newborn's cutaneous surface. The differential diagnoses of eczematous changes in the newborn are listed in Table 223-5. The eczematous eruptions associated with Wiskott-Aldrich syndrome, ataxia-telangiectasia, and hypogammaglobulinemia are usually not observed in the first 30 days of life [126].

Diaper dermatitis. Dermatitis involving the skin covered by a diaper is usually considered a primary irritant contact dermatitis resulting from prolonged contact with urine and feces [125]. Diaper dermatitis present for longer than 72 h should be considered superinfected with *Candida albicans* and treated with topically applied antiyeast agents. Any of the disorders listed in Table 223-5 may begin in the diaper area for several days and then involve other skin areas [125]. Increasing the frequency of diaper changes and keeping the skin dry are strategies crucial to the successful therapy of diaper dermatitis.

Scabies. During the newborn period, eczematous eruptions may appear that progress to generalized dermatitis. Infants with scabies may have thousands of lesions and involvement of the head and neck, which evolves into a generalized dermatitis that will mimic seborrheic or atopic dermatitis. Individual burrows may be obscured [127,128]. Scabies mites can be recovered from burrows or papules primarily on the hands and feet (Fig. 223-11). Treatment of scabies within the first 30 days of life remains problematical because of concerns regarding the toxicity of the most effective scabicide, gamma benzene hexachloride [128,129]. It is unclear whether other forms of therapy are less toxic and they may be less efficacious; usually, however, treatment with dimethyldiphenylene disulfide will cure the condition. Cautious therapy with 1% gamma benzene hexachloride still remains the treatment of choice, leaving the preparation on the skin for 4 h. Careful supervision of therapy is recommended.

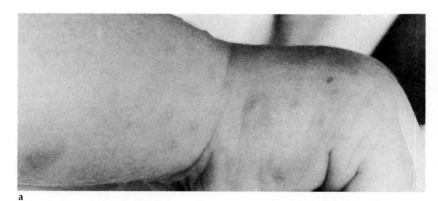

a

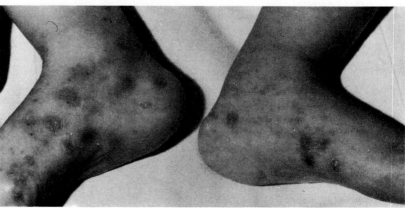

b

Fig. 223-11   Scabies in a baby. Burrows are often not seen; instead, papulovesicles and crusted lesions are found characteristically on the lateral dorsum of the hand (a) and the insteps (b). *(Courtesy of K. Wolff, M.D.)*

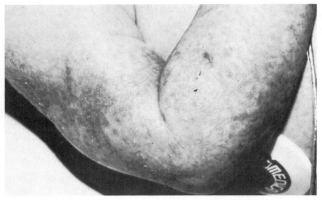

Fig. 223-12 Multiple carboxylase deficiency. Eczematous lesions over the arm in an infant responsive to biotin.

Severe combined immunodeficiency, Leiner's disease, and multiple carboxylase deficiency. This group of disorders will mimic each other in clinical features. The onset of the eczematous skin eruption is late in the newborn period, and is often associated with diarrhea, respiratory infections, and failure to thrive [126,130–132]. Diagnosis is confirmed by analysis of the number and function of T lymphocytes in the case of severe combined immunodeficiency [126,130], by analysis of opsonin function of C5 and failure to generate C5a chemotactic factors in Leiner's disease [126], and by carboxylase analysis of lymphocytes or cultured skin fibroblasts in multiple carboxylase deficiency [130,131]. Each of these conditions is quite rare but each may be improved with therapy. Severe combined immunodeficiency may respond to thymic transplants or bone marrow transplants, Leiner's disease to fresh plasma infusions [126], and multiple carboxylase deficiency to administration of biotin [130,131]. In each of these disorders a generalized dermatitis which may mimic seborrheic dermatitis has been described (Fig. 223-12).

Histiocytosis X. A generalized dermatitis or a dermatitis that mimics seborrheic dermatitis may appear in the newborn affected with histiocytosis X [133,134]. The skin eruption may be present at birth [125]. A very characteristic feature of this eruption is the appearance of purpuric papules or petechiae within the dermatitis, especially occurring on the head and neck, axillae, and groin [133,134] (Fig. 223-13). Chronic draining ears may accompany the skin lesions and enlargement of the liver and spleen may be present. Diagnosis may be made by skin biopsy and bone x-rays. Response to chemotherapy protocols may be expected.

Candidiasis. Congenital candidiasis may present with generalized eczematous skin [36]. Direct microscopic examination of scales dissolved in 10% potassium hydroxide will demonstrate yeast forms and a fungal culture of skin scrapings will confirm the diagnosis [36]. Response to topical anti-*Candida* agents is prompt.

Acrodermatitis enteropathica. Eczematous eruptions about the eyes, mouth, groin, and distal extremities may be the presenting sign of acrodermatitis enteropathica (Fig. 223-14). The skin disease may precede the diarrhea and be the presenting symptom at about the fourth week following birth [132,135]. Secondary infection of the skin lesions with *Candida albicans* is frequent. The newborn will exhibit

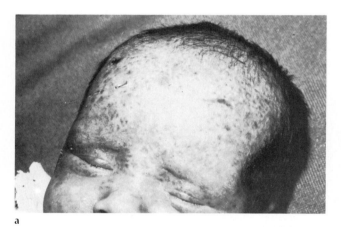

a

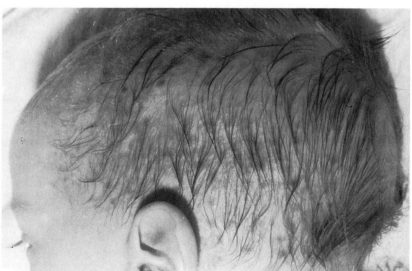

b

Fig. 223-13 Histiocytosis X. (a) Eczematous and pruritic papules and petechiae over the head and face of a newborn infant. (b) More discrete lesions on the scalp of an infant one month of age. *(b, Courtesy of K. Wolff, M.D.)*

Fig. 223-14 Acrodermatitis enteropathica. Erosive dermatitis over the ears, cheeks, and fingers of an infant with documented zinc deficiency.

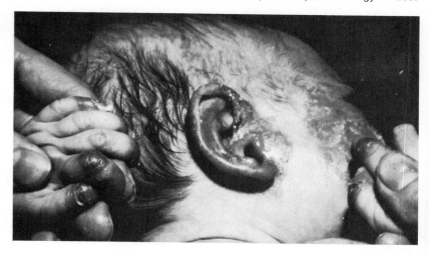

apathy and poor feeding as an early sign. This condition is a recessively inherited disorder of zinc deficiency, and oral zinc therapy results in improvement of apathy within 24 h and improvement of the skin lesions within 7 to 10 days [135].

Blistering diseases

Epidermolysis bullosa (see also Chap. 64). Diagnosis in the immediate newborn period may be difficult, particularly in the instance of epidermolysis bullosa letalis in which the baby may have few or no blisters in the first 30 days of life, only to develop severe blisters in the second or third month [136]. Also, in the generalized form of epidermolysis bullosa simplex, many blisters may be present at birth but few after the first month of life. In all forms of epidermolysis bullosa, the evolution of lesions during the first month of life may confuse the clinician. Extreme care must be taken in obtaining and interpreting skin biopsies from newborns to distinguish among these mechanobullous diseases. Shave or ellipse biopsies of the edge of a blister that is less

than 12 h old is preferred. Both light and electron microscopy should be performed. Immunofluorescence mapping of antigenic sites at the basement membrane zone provides a rapid diagnosis [137].

Incontinentia pigmenti. Incontinentia pigmenti is an X-linked dominant disorder which often presents with linear blisters on the extremities at birth or within the first three days of life [138] (Fig. 223-15). It is common for new blisters to appear during the entire newborn period. The pigmentary changes and verrucous lesions are not observed in the newborn period. Occasionally the mother will have curvilinear hyperpigmented areas remaining. Strabismus and other ocular findings may not be detectable in the newborn period.

Diffuse cutaneous mastocytosis. Newborns with diffuse cutaneous mastocytosis usually have normal-appearing skin at birth. Within the first 30 days of life, vesicles appear on the skin which do not have a red base [139–141]. Dermographism may be prominent. Vesicles may appear any-

Fig. 223-15 Incontinentia pigmenti. Linear papules and vesicles with an inflammatory base over the extremity of a newborn.

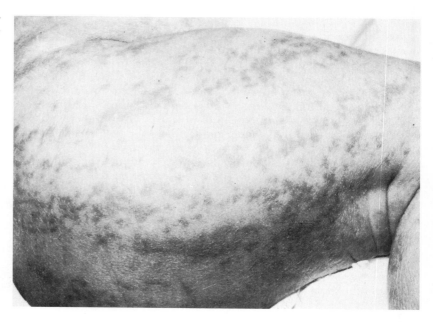

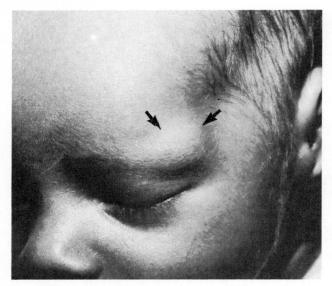

Fig. 223-16 Epithelial cyst (arrows) in the characteristic lateral eyebrow location in a newborn infant.

where on the skin including the scalp and evolve to become more numerous with new crops appearing daily. Itching and irritability may be prominent. Rarely, massive blistering may occur in a single episode such that giant bullae are formed on the trunk with diffuse redness of the skin, and large sheets of skin are desquamated [139–141]. After a refractory period, this massive blistering process may be repeated in 7 to 14 days. The staphylococcal scalded-skin syndrome is often misdiagnosed.

Hepatosplenomegaly may be present and an evaluation for systemic involvement is recommended. X-rays of long bones and a bone marrow examination are useful. Epidermal thickening designated "Morrocan leather skin" is not observed in the newborn period, and usually not until 3 to 6 months of age. Skin biopsy will demonstrate a bandlike collection of mast cells in the mid to upper dermis [139–141]. Three major mediators released by mast cells account for the various symptoms and signs observed in bullous mastocytosis [142–145]. Histamine appears to be responsible for the dermographism, the blister formation within skin lesions, wheezing, and diarrhea [142,145]. Prostaglandin D_2 is responsible for cutaneous flushing episodes, hypotension, and syncopal attacks [144]. It perhaps is also involved in sudden death observed in these infants. Heparin is responsible for the cutaneous bleeding observed [139].

Treatment of urticaria, blistering, and diarrhea may be effective with H_1 blockers such as hydroxyzine or chlorpheniramine [142,145]. Oral sodium dichromoglycate or similar agents may also help with diarrhea, but other symptoms are usually not influenced by these drugs [142,143,145]. The addition of H_2 blocking agents may or may not be useful. Syncopal attacks, flushing episodes, and hypotension may respond to H_1 blocking agents, plus the use of aspirin in doses up to 40 mg/kg per day [145]. The use of aspirin in these infants should be with extreme caution since massive degranulation of mast cells has been reported with aspirin therapy. Severe hypotension and pro-

longed syncopy has responded to intravenous or subcutaneous epinephrine [145].

Common skin nodules which may be present at birth or which appear within the newborn period

In the newborn period, the two most commonly observed skin nodules are epithelial cysts which account for 60 percent of such nodules, and pilomatrixomas which account for 15 percent of skin nodules [146,147].

Epithelial cysts. In the newborn, epithelial cysts are found predominantly at the lateral border of the eyebrow (Fig. 223-16) or under the scalp [147]. They are sometimes found on the bridge of the nose, and rarely on the trunk or extremities. Whether or not the cysts contain follicular or other adnexal structures (dermoid cysts) does not vary their location [147]. Slow growth of the cyst may be anticipated and surgical removal may be desired for cosmetic improvement.

Pilomatrixomas. Pilomatrixoma (calcifying epithelioma of Malherbe) is believed to be a hamartoma of hair follicle origin. Pilomatrixomas occur as discrete firm nodules located on the eyebrow, eyelid, neck, upper back, or upper arm of newborns [146]. Simple excision is the treatment of choice.

Neurofibromas. Neurofibromas may be present at birth as a soft nodule usually greater than 3 cm in diameter, and are common on the palm or sole but may appear anywhere on the skin [148]. In multiple neurofibromatosis, café au lait macules may accompany the neurofibroma, but few café au lait macules may be present at birth, and six or more café au lait macules are rarely observed in the newborn period in patients with multiple neurofibromatosis [148]. In the newborn approximately one-third of babies who have a cutaneous neurofibroma will have multiple neurofibromatosis. Elective excision can be performed.

Lipomas. Soft nodules on the trunk or proximal extremities may be present at birth and represent lipomas [146]. Usually, they are well demarcated on palpation and are clearly within the subcutaneous tissue with a freely mobile skin overlying the nodule. Diagnosis is by biopsy.

Juvenile xanthogranulomas. Orange to yellow-brown intradermal soft nodules appear on the skin of infants. They may be present at birth and more may appear during the newborn period [149]. Juvenile xanthogranulomas often number 5 to 10 and they will involute spontaneously within a year or two. The skin predominantly is involved but xanthogranulomas may be noted in the ocular iris where they mimic retinoblastoma [149]. Lesions have been described in the lung, liver, spleen, pericardium, and testes. Biopsy of the skin nodule reveals Touton giant cells and granulomatous inflammation in the middermis.

Urticaria pigmentosa (papular mastocytosis). At birth, one or two macular, red or red-brown lesions of urticaria pigmentosa may be present, usually on the trunk [140,142]. More lesions appear during the newborn period and hundreds of lesions may appear during the first eight months of life. Some of the macular lesions present at birth become more nodular and darker with increasing age. Individual lesions develop blisters by stroking of the skin surface in the newborn period, which occurs in addition to developing urticaria within the macule and a prominent erythematous flare [140,141]. The erythematous flare may be subject to misinterpretation because dermographism is so prevalent in newborns. Skin biopsy will reveal excessive mast cells within the dermis [140]. Systemic mastocytosis occurs in up to 10 percent of the newborns with urticaria pigmentosa [140].

References

1. Holbrook KA: Human epidermal embryogenesis. *Int J Dermatol* **18**:329, 1979
2. Breathnach AS, Wolff K: Structure and development of skin, in *Dermatology in General Medicine,* 2d ed, edited by TB Fitzpatrick et al. New York, McGraw-Hill, 1979, p 41
3. Holbrook KA, Smith LT: Ultrastructural aspects of human skin during the embryonic, fetal, premature, neonatal and adult periods of life. *Birth Defects* **17**:9, 1981
4. Holbrook KA, Odland GF: Regional development of the human epidermis in the first trimester embryo and the second trimester fetus. *J Invest Dermatol* **80**:161, 1980
5. Muller HK et al: Ontogeny of pemphigus and bullous pemphigoid antigens in human skin. *Br J Dermatol* **88**:443, 1973
6. Holbrook KA: A histological comparison of infant and adult skin, in *Neonatal Skin: Structure and Function,* edited by HI Maibach, EK Boisits. New York, Marcel Dekker, 1982, p 3
7. Harpin VA, Rutter N: Barrier properties of the newborn infants skin. *J Pediatr* **102**:419, 1983
8. West DP et al: Pharmacology and toxicology of infant skin. *J Invest Dermatol* **76**:147, 1981
9. Fairley JA, Rasmussen JE: Comparison of stratum corneum thickness in children and adults. *J Am Acad Dermatol* **8**:652, 1983
10. Nachman RL, Esterly NB: Increased skin permeability in preterm infants. *J Pediatr* **97**:628, 1971
11. Rutter N, Hull D: Water loss from the skin of term and preterm babies. *Arch Dis Child* **54**:858, 1979
12. Cunico RL et al: Skin barrier properties in the newborn. *Biol Neonate* **32**:177, 1977
13. Schaffer AJ, Avery ME: *Diseases of the Newborn,* 4th ed. Philadelphia, WB Saunders, 1977, p 65
14. Esterly NB, Solomon LM: The skin, in *Neonatal-Perinatal Medicine,* edited by AA Fanaroff, RJ Martin. St Louis, CV Mosby, 1983, p 939
15. Philip AGS: *Neonatology,* 2d ed. Garden City, NY, Medical Examination Publishing Co, 1980, pp 16, 45, 68
16. Harpin VA, Rutter N: Sweating in preterm babies. *J Pediatr* **100**:614, 1982
17. Smith LT, Holbrook KA: Development of dermal connective tissue in human embryonic and fetal skin. *Scan Electron Microsc* **4**:1745, 1982
18. Smales ORC, Kime R: Thermoregulation in babies immediately after birth. *Arch Dis Child* **53**:58, 1978
19. Smith CA, Nelson NM: *The Physiology of the Newborn Infant,* 4th ed. Springfield, IL, Charles C Thomas, 1976
20. Philip AGS, Hewitt JR: Early diagnosis of neonatal sepsis. *Pediatrics* **65**:1036, 1980
21. Jeffrey H et al: Early neonatal bacteremia: comparison of group B streptococcal, other gram positive and gram negative infections. *Arch Dis Child* **52**:683, 1977
22. Philip AGS: *Neonatology,* 2d ed. Garden City, NY, Medical Examination Publishing Co, 1980, p 193
23. Wilson HD, Eichenwald JF: Sepsis neonatorum. *Pediatr Clin North Am* **21**:571, 1974
24. Naeye RL, Peters E: Causes and consequences of premature rupture of fetal membranes. *Lancet* **1**:192, 1980
25. McKenna H, Johnson D: Bacteria in neonatal omphalitis. *Pathology* **9**:111, 1977
26. Remington JS, Klein JO: *Infectious Diseases of the Fetus and Newborn Infant.* Philadelphia, WB Saunders, 1976, p 71
27. Levy HL, Cothram F: Erythema toxicum neonatorum present at birth. *Am J Dis Child* **103**:617, 1962
28. Carr JA et al: Relationship between toxic erythema and infant maturity. *Am J Dis Child* **112**:129, 1966
29. Freeman RG et al: Histopathology of erythema toxicum neonatorum. *Arch Dermatol* **82**:586, 1960
30. Ramamurthy RS, Esterly NB: Transient neonatal pustular melanosis. *J Pediatr* **88**:831, 1976
31. Hanshaw JB, Dudgeon JA: *Viral Diseases of the Fetus and Newborn.* Philadelphia, WB Saunders, 1978
32. Light IJ: Post-natal acquisition of herpes simplex virus by the newborn infant: review of the literature. *Pediatrics* **63**:480, 1979
33. Whitley RJ et al: The natural history of herpes simplex virus infection of mother and newborn. *Pediatrics* **66**:489, 1980
34. Tromovitch TA et al: Acne in infancy. *Am J Dis Child* **106**:230, 1963
35. Weston WL et al: Diaper dermatitis: current concepts. *Pediatrics* **66**:532, 1980
36. Kamm LA, Giacola GP: Congenital cutaneous candidiasis. *Am J Dis Child* **129**:1215, 1975
37. Jarratt M, Ramsdell W: Infantile acropustulosis. *Arch Dermatol* **115**:834, 1979
38. Kahn G, Rywlin AM: Acropustulosis of infancy. *Arch Dermatol* **115**:831, 1979
39. Cantu JM et al: Familial comedones. *Arch Dermatol* **114**:1807, 1978
40. Farber EM, Jacobs AH: Infantile psoriasis. *Am J Dis Child* **131**:1266, 1977
41. Nyfors A: Psoriasis in children. *Acta Derm Venereol [Suppl] (Stockh)* **95**:47, 1981
42. Sulzberger MB, Harris DR: Miliaria and anhidrosis. III. Multiple small patches and the effects of different periods of occlusion. *Arch Dermatol* **105**:845, 1972
43. Jorgenson RJ et al: Intraoral findings and anomalies in neonates. *Pediatrics* **69**:577, 1982
44. Duke EMC: Infantile acne associated with transient increases in plasma concentrations of luteinising hormone, follicle-stimulating hormone and testosterone. *Br Med J* **282**:1275, 1981
45. Gordon J: Miliary sebaceous cysts and blisters in the healthy newborn. *Arch Dis Child* **24**:286, 1949
46. South DA, Jacobs AH: Cutis marmorata telangiectatica congenita. *J Pediatr* **93**:944, 1978
47. Fitzsimmons JS, Starks M: Cutis marmorata telangiectatica congenita or congenital generalized phlebectasia. *Arch Dis Child* **45**:724, 1970
48. Nahmias AJ et al: Perinatal risk associated with maternal genital herpes simplex infection. *Am J Obstet Gynecol* **110**:825, 1974
49. Kibrick S: Herpes simplex infection at term: what to do with mother, newborn and nursery personnel. *JAMA* **243**:147, 1980
50. Nahmias AJ et al: Infection of the newborn with herpes virus hominis. *Adv Pediatr* **17**:185, 1970
51. Whitley RJ et al: Vidarabine therapy of neonatal herpes simplex virus infection. *Pediatrics* **66**:495, 1980

52. Meyers JD: Congenital varicella in term infants: risk reconsidered. *J Infect Dis* **129**:215, 1974

53. Brice JEH: Congenital varicella resulting from infection during the second trimester of pregnancy. *Arch Dis Child* **51**:474, 1976

54. Webster MH, Smith CS: Congenital abnormalities and maternal herpes zoster. *Br Med J* **2**:1193, 1977

55. Davies PA: Bacterial infection in the fetus and newborn. *Arch Dis Child* **46**:1, 1971

56. Belgaumker TK: Impetigo neonatorum congenita due to group B betahemolytic streptococcus infection. *J Pediatr* **86**:982, 1975

57. Curran FP, Al-Salihi FL: Neonatal staphylococcal scalded skin syndrome: massive outbreak due to an unusual phage type. *Pediatrics* **66**:285, 1980

58. Rasmussen JE: Toxic epidermal necrolysis. *Arch Dermatol* **111**:1135, 1975

59. Rudoy RC, Nelson, JD: Breast abscess during the neonatal period. A review. *Am J Dis Child* **129**:1031, 1975

60. Murphy WF, Langley AL: Common bullous lesions—presumably self-inflicted—occurring *in utero* in the newborn infant. *Pediatrics* **32**:1099, 1963

61. Ellis SS et al: Osteomyelitis complicating neonatal cephalohematoma. *Am J Dis Child* **127**:100, 1974

62. Lee Y-H, Berg RB: Cephalohematoma infected with bacteroides. *Am J Dis Child* **121**:77, 1971

63. Nahmias AJ: The TORCH complex. *Hospital Practice* **9**:65, 1974

64. Desmonts G, Couvreur J: Congenital toxoplasmosis: a prospective study of 378 pregnancies. *N Engl J Med* **290**:1110, 1974

65. Fiumara NJ: Syphilis in newborn children. *Clin Obstet Gynecol* **18**:183, 1975

66. Dudgeon JA: Congenital rubella. *J Pediatr* **87**:1078, 1975

67. Stagno S et al: Auditory and visual defects resulting from symptomatic and subclinical congenital cytomegaloviral and toxoplasma infections. *Pediatrics* **59**:669, 1977

68. Marks MB: Subcutaneous adipose derangements of the newborn. *Am J Dis Child* **104**:122, 1962

69. Anagnostakis A et al: Neonatal cold injury: evidence of defective thermogenesis due to impaired norepinephrine release. *Pediatrics* **53**:24, 1974

70. Alper JC, Holmes LB: The incidence and significance of birthmarks in a cohort of 4,641 newborns. *Pediatr Dermatol* **1**:58, 1983

71. Jacobs AH, Walton RG: The incidence of birthmarks in the neonate. *Pediatrics* **58**:218, 1976

72. Lau JTK, Ching RML: Mongolian spots in Chinese children. *Am J Dis Child* **136**:863, 1982

73. Alexander GL, Norman RM: *The Sturge-Weber Syndrome.* Bristol, England, J Wright, 1960

74. Barsky SH et al: The nature and evolution of port-wine stains: a computer-assisted study. *J Invest Dermatol* **74**:154, 1980

75. O'Connell A, Crick RP: Facial naevus and unsuspected visual loss from glaucoma. *Br Med J* **2**:1750, 1978

76. Lindenauer SM: The Klippel-Trénaunay syndrome. *Ann Surg* **162**:303, 1965

77. Hidano A, Nakajima S: Earliest features of the strawberry mark in the newborn. *Br J Dermatol* **87**:138, 1972

78. Simpson JR, Lond MB: Natural history of cavernous hemangiomata. *Lancet* **2**:1057, 1959

79. Shim WKT: Hemangiomas of infancy complicated by thrombocytopenia. *Am J Surg* **116**:896, 1968

80. Esterly NB: Kasabach-Merritt syndrome in infants. *J Am Acad Dermatol* **8**:504, 1983

81. Edgerton MT: The treatment of hemangiomas with special reference to the role of steroid therapy. *Ann Surg* **183**:517, 1976

82. Wishnick MM: Multinodular hemangiomatosis with partial biliary obstruction. *J Pediatr* **92**:960, 1978

83. Lynch PJ, Zelickson AS: Congenital phlebectasia. *Arch Dermatol* **95**:98, 1967

84. Flanagan BP, Helwig EB: Cutaneous lymphangioma. *Arch Dermatol* **113**:24, 1977

85. Peachey RDG: Lymphangioma of skin: a review of 65 cases. *Br J Dermatol* **83**:519, 1970

86. Alper J et al: Birthmarks with serious medical significance: nevocellular nevi, sebaceous nevi, and multiple café-au-lait spots. *Pediatrics* **95**:696, 1979

87. Rhodes AR: Pigmented birthmarks and precursor melanocytic lesions of cutaneous melanoma identifiable in childhood. *Pediatr Clin North Am* **30**:435, 1983

88. Kopf AW et al: Congenital nevocytic nevi and malignant melanomas. *J Am Acad Dermatol* **1**:123, 1979

89. Jacobs AH: Birthmarks II. Melanocytic and epidermal nevi. *Pediatrics in Review* **1**:47, 1979

90. Castilla EE et al: Epidemiology of congenital pigmented naevi. II. Risk factors. *Br J Dermatol* **104**:307, 1981

91. Trozak DJ et al: Metastatic malignant melanoma in prepubertal children. *Pediatrics* **55**:191, 1975

92. Telfer MA et al: Dominant piebald trait (white forelock and leukoderma) with neurological impairment. *Am J Hum Genet* **23**:383, 1971

93. Bard LA: Heterogeneity in Waardenburg's syndrome. *Arch Ophthalmol* **96**:1193, 1979

94. Nordlund JJ: Genetic basis of pigmentation and the disorders of pigmentation, in *Pathology of Malignant Melanoma*, edited by AB Ackerman. New York, Masson, 1981, p 23

95. McWilliam RC, Stephenson JBP: Depigmented hair. The earliest sign of tuberous sclerosis. *Arch Dis Child* **53**:961, 1978

96. Nordlund JJ et al: Hypomelanosis of Ito. *Acta Derm Venereol (Stockh)* **57**:261, 1977

97. Jackson R: The lines of Blaschko: a review and reconsideration. *Br J Dermatol* **95**:349, 1976

98. O'Donnell FE et al: X-linked ocular albinism. *Arch Ophthalmol* **94**:1883, 1976

99. Jay B et al: Human albinism. *Birth Defects* **12**:415, 1976

100. Solomon LM et al: The epidermal nevus syndrome. *Arch Dermatol* **97**:273, 1968

101. Hurwitz S: Epidermal nevi and tumors of epidermal origin. *Pediatr Clin North Am* **30**:483, 1983

102. Jones EQ, Heyl T: Nevus sebaceus. A report of 140 cases with special regard to the development of secondary malignant tumors. *Br J Dermatol* **82**:99, 1970

103. Domingo J, Helwig EB: Malignant neoplasms associated with nevus sebaceus of Jadassohn. *J Am Acad Dermatol* **1**:545, 1979

104. Uitto J et al: Connective tissue nevi of the skin. *J Am Acad Dermatol* **3**:441, 1980

105. Holmes LB: Congenital malformations. *N Engl J Med* **295**:204, 1976

106. Marden DM et al: Congenital anomalies in the newborn infant, including minor variations. *J Pediatr* **64**:357, 1964

107. Smith DW: *Recognizable Patterns of Human Malformation.* Philadelphia, WB Saunders, 1970

108. Levin DL et al: Congenital absence of skin. *J Am Acad Dermatol* **2**:203, 1980

109. Schneider BM et al: Aplasia cutis congenita complicated by sagittal sinus hemorrhage. *Pediatrics* **66**:948, 1980

110. McCray MK, Roenigk HH: Scalp reduction for correction of cutis aplasia congenita. *J Dermatol Surg Oncol* **7**:655, 1981

111. Holmes LB: Genetic counseling for the older age pregnant

woman: new data and questions. *N Engl J Med* **298:**1419, 1978

112. Reed WB et al: Lamellar ichthyosis of the newborn. A distinct clinical entity: its comparison to the other ichthyosiform dermatoses. *Arch Dermatol* **105:**394, 1972

113. Williams ML: The ichthyoses—pathogenesis and prenatal diagnosis: a review of recent advances. *Pediatr Dermatol* **1:**1, 1983

114. Frenk E: A spontaneously healing collodion baby. A light and electron microscopic study. *Acta Derm Venereol (Stockh)* **61:**168, 1981

115. Baden HP et al: Keratinization in the harlequin fetus. *Arch Dermatol* **118:**14, 1982

116. Goldsmith LA: The ichthyoses. *Prog Med Genet* **1:**185, 1976

117. Shapiro LJ et al: X-linked ichthyosis due to steroid sulphatase deficiency. *Lancet* **2:**70, 1978

118. Rand RE, Baden HP: The ichthyoses—a review. *J Am Acad Dermatol* **8:**285, 1983

119. Yates VM et al: Early diagnosis of infantile seborrheic dermatitis and atopic dermatitis. Clinical features. *Br J Dermatol* **108:**633, 1983

120. Vickers CFH: The natural history of atopic eczema. *Acta Derm Venereol [Suppl] (Stockh)* **92:**113, 1980

121. Moller H: Clinical aspects of atopic dermatitis in childhood. *Acta Derm Venereol [Suppl] (Stockh)* **95:**25, 1981

122. Rajka G: *Atopic Dermatitis.* Philadelphia, WB Saunders, 1975

123. Marsh DG et al: The epidemiology and genetics of atopic allergy. *N Engl J Med* **305:**1551, 1981

124. Yates VM et al: Early diagnosis of infantile seborrheic dermatitis and atopic dermatitis. Total and specific IgE levels. *Br J Dermatol* **108:**639, 1983

125. Weston WL et al: Diaper dermatitis: current concepts. *Pediatrics* **66:**532, 1983

126. Weston WL: Cutaneous manifestations of defective host defenses. *Pediatr Clin North Am* **24:**395, 1977

127. Honig PJ: Bites and parasites. *Pediatr Clin North Am* **30:**563, 1983

128. Hurwitz S: Scabies in babies. *Am J Dis Child* **126:**226, 1973

129. Rasmussen JE: The problem of lindane. *J Am Acad Dermatol* **5:**507, 1981

130. Cowan MJ et al: Multiple biotin-dependent carboxylase deficiencies associated with defects in T & B cell immunity. *Lancet* **2:**115, 1979

131. Burri B et al: Mutant holocarboxylase synthetase: evidence for the enzyme defect in early infantile biotin-responsive multiple carboxylase deficiency. *J Clin Invest* **68:**1491, 1981

132. Arlette JP: Zinc and the skin. *Pediatr Clin North Am* **30:**583, 1983

133. Cohen DM et al: Letterer-Siwe disease in a newborn. *Arch Pathol* **81:**347, 1966

134. Smith PJ et al: Improved prognosis in disseminated histiocytosis. *Med Pediatr Oncol* **2:**371, 1976

135. Neldner KH et al: Acrodermatitis enteropathica. *Int J Dermatol* **17:**380, 1978

136. Eady RAJ, Tidman MJ: Diagnosing epidermolysis bullosa. *Br J Dermatol* **108:**621, 1983

137. Hintner H et al: Immunofluorescence mapping of antigenic determinants within the dermal-epidermal junction in mechanobullous diseases. *J Invest Dermatol* **76:**113, 1981

138. Carney RG Jr: Incontinentia pigmenti. *Arch Dermatol* **112:**535, 1976

139. Campbell EW Jr et al: Heparin activity in systemic mastocytosis. *Ann Intern Med* **90:**940, 1979

140. Demis DJ: The mastocytosis syndrome: clinical and biological studies. *Ann Intern Med* **59:**194, 1963

141. Orkin M et al: Bullous mastocytosis. *Arch Dermatol* **101:**547, 1970

142. James MD: The treatment of urticaria pigmentosa. *Clin Exp Dermatol* **7:**311, 1982

143. Czarnetzki BM: A double-blind cross-over study of the effect of ketotifen in urticaria pigmentosa. *Dermatologica* **166:**44, 1983

144. Roberts LJ 2nd et al: Increased production of prostaglandin D_2 in patients with systemic mastocytosis. *N Engl J Med* **303:**1400, 1980

145. Roberts LJ 2nd et al: Shock syndrome associated with mastocytosis. Pharmacologic reversal of the acute episode and therapeutic prevention of recurrent attack. *Adv Shock Res* **8:**145, 1982

146. Knight PJ, Reiner CB: Superficial lumps in children: what, when, and why? *Pediatrics* **72:**147, 1983

147. Pollard ZF et al: Dermoid cysts in children. *Pediatrics* **57:**379, 1976

148. Riccardi VM: Pathophysiology of neurofibromatosis. *J Am Acad Dermatol* **3:**157, 1980

149. Webster SB et al: Juvenile xanthogranuloma with extracutaneous lesions. *Arch Dermatol* **93:**71, 1966

INDEX

INDEX

Page references in **boldface** indicate illustrations or tables.